KUMAR
&
CLARK

CLINICAL MEDICINE

SIXTH EDITION

EDITED BY

PROFESSOR PARVEEN KUMAR

CBE BSc MD FRCP FRCP (Edin)

Professor of Clinical Medical Education, Barts and the London,
Queen Mary's School of Medicine and Dentistry, University of London, and
Honorary Consultant Physician and Gastroenterologist, Barts and The London
NHS Trust and Homerton Hospital NHS Foundation Trust, London, UK

DR MICHAEL CLARK

MD FRCP

Honorary Senior Lecturer, Barts and the London, Queen Mary's School of
Medicine and Dentistry, University of London, UK

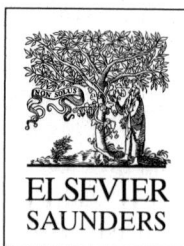

ELSEVIER
SAUNDERS

EDINBURGH   LONDON   NEW YORK   OXFORD
PHILADELPHIA   ST LOUIS   SYDNEY   TORONTO 2005

CLINICAL MEDICINE

SIXTH EDITION

ELSEVIER
SAUNDERS

First edition 1987
Second edition 1990
Third edition 1994
Fourth edition 1998
Fifth edition 2002
Sixth edition 2005

ISBN 0702027634
International Student Edition ISBN 0702027642

British Library Cataloguing in Publication Data
A catalogue record for this book is available from the British Library

Library of Congress Cataloging in Publication Data
A catalog record for this book is available from the Library of Congress

Note
Medical knowledge is constantly changing. Standard safety precautions must be followed, but as new research and clinical experience broaden our knowledge, changes in treatment and drug therapy may become necessary or appropriate. Readers are advised to check the most current product information provided by the manufacuturer of each drug to be administered to verify the recommended dose, the method and duration of administration, and contraindications. It is the responsibility of the practitioner, relying on experience and knowledge of the patient, to determine dosages and the best treatment for each individual patient. Neither the Publisher nor the editors assumes any liability for any injury and/or damage to persons or property arising from this publication.   *The Publisher*

Working together to grow
libraries in developing countries

www.elsevier.com | www.bookaid.org | www.sabre.org

ELSEVIER   BOOK AID International   Sabre Foundation

your source for books,
journals and multimedia
in the health sciences
www.elsevierhealth.com

Commissioning Editor: Ellen Green
Development Editor: Clive Hewat
Project Manager: Frances Affleck
Design Direction: George Ajayi
Illustrations: Richard Morris; Ethan Danielson

The
publisher's
policy is to use
**paper manufactured
from sustainable forests**

Printed in Spain

Contents

ONLINE CONTENTS
STUDENTCONSULT

The sixth edition of Kumar & Clark: *Clinical Medicine* has an online version which can be accessed via www.studentconsult.com. The online version consists of the full text and illustrations for the sixth edition as well as other additional features, some of which are unique to Kumar & Clark. To access the online version, readers should follow the instructions on the inside front cover. The list below provides a guide to some of the online features, and you can also find them listed online in the 'extras' folder.

Online Appendix *edited by Professor Janaka de Silva*

This appendix, which will be updated regularly, provides supplementary information on diseases and problems that are more prevalent in certain parts of the world. The need for this material – which enlarges on what can be found in the print version – became plain to the Editors from their travels to various parts of the world. We are grateful to members of the Kumar & Clark International Advisory Panel and other colleagues for their contributions to this unique resource.

- **Dengue** *Dr R Sood*
- **Diarrhoeas including amoebiasis** *Dr S A Azer*
- **Fluorosis** *Professor S Hough*
- **Helminth infections and filariasis** *Professor N de Silva*

- **IgA nephropathy** *Professor K N Lai*
- **Leprosy** *Dr S A Kamath*
- **Leptospirosis** *Professor M Ellis*
- **Malaria** *Dr S A Kamath*
- **Poisoning** *Professor J de Silva, Dr A K Kundu*
- **Pyogenic meningitis** *Dr S Shafqat*
- **Rheumatic fever** *Dr K N Viswanathan*
- **Severe acute respiratory syndrome (SARS)** *Professor K N Lai*
- **Tuberculosis** *Professor S K Sharma*
- **Vitamin B$_{12}$ and folic acid deficiency** *Professor V J Louw*

Interactive Surface Anatomy *from Drake et al: Gray's Anatomy for Students*

This programme relates anatomy to the skills of clinical examination. Over 40 interactive animations take the student through the seven body regions, demonstrating major anatomical features, surface landmarks and other palpable structures. By working through each module students see their role when performing a general physical examination, listening for heart sounds, examining movements of the eye, and many others. We are grateful to the authors of *Gray's Anatomy for Students* for the opportunity to provide Kumar & Clark readers with the benefits of this unique interactive learning tool and to introduce them to this outstanding new anatomy textbook.

BACK
- How to identify specific vertebral spinous processes
- Visualizing the inferior ends of the spinal cord and subarachnoid space

THORAX
- How to count ribs
- Surface anatomy of the breast in women
- Visualizing structures at the T4/5 vertebral level
- Visualizing structures in the superior mediastinum
- Visualizing the margins of the heart
- Where to listen for heart sounds

- How to visualize the pleural cavities and lungs
- Where to listen to right lung sounds
- Where to listen to left lung sounds

PELVIS AND PERINEUM
- Identification of structures in the urogenital triangle of women
- Identification of structures in the urogenital triangle of men

ABDOMEN
- How to find the superficial inguinal ring
- How to determine lumbar vertebral levels

- Visualizing structures at the LI vertebral level
- Visualizing the position of major blood vessels
- Using abdominal quadrants to locate major viscera
- Defining surface regions to which pain from the gut is referred
- Where to find the kidneys and spleen

LOWER LIMB
- Avoiding the sciatic nerve
- Finding the femoral artery in the femoral triangle
- Identifying structures around the knee
- Visualizing the contents of the popliteal fossa
- Finding the tarsal tunnel
- Identifying tendons around the ankle and in the foot
- Finding the dorsalis pedis artery
- Identifying major superficial veins
- Where to take peripheral arterial pulses in the lower limb

UPPER LIMB
- Visualising the axilla, its contents and related structures
- Locating the brachial artery in the arm

- Locating the triceps brachii tendon and the position of the radial nerve
- Identifying the cubital fossa and its contents
- Identifying tendons and locating major vessels and nerves in the distal forearm
- Identifying the position of the flexor retinaculum and the recurrent branch of the median nerve
- Visualizing the positions of the superficial and deep palmar arches
- Where to take peripheral arterial pulses in the upper limb

HEAD AND NECK
- Visualizing structures at the CIII/CIV and CVI vertebral levels
- How to outline the anterior and posterior triangles of the neck
- How to locate the cricothyroid ligament (membrane)
- How to find the thyroid gland
- Where to take peripheral arterial pulses in the head and neck
- Testing eye movements – demonstration illustrating the muscle involved in each activity.

Animations of practical procedures

This feature brings to life a selection of key practical procedures in a way not usually possible outside the clinic or skills laboratory. Once again, the existence of the online version has made it possible to provide this unique feature, which builds on the descriptions given in the 'practical boxes' in Kumar & Clark. This list gives a selection of currently available and forthcoming animations.

- Bladder catheterisation
- Intercostal drainage
- Internal jugular vein cannulation
- Joint aspiration
- Lumbar puncture
- Radial artery cannulation
- Simple aspiration
- Taking the blood pressure

Heart and lung sounds *by Dr Salvatore Mangione*

This feature provides readers with the opportunity to improve their clinical skills by listening to 10 pulmonary and 12 cardiac sounds. The sounds can be heard on their own or accompanied by an instructive narrative. This workshop has been prepared by Dr Salvatore Mangione, and we are grateful for the opportunity to make it available to readers of Kumar & Clark.

- PULMONARY AUSCULTATION:
  Bronchial breath sounds
  Crackles
  Wheezes
  Vesicular breath sounds
  Rhonchi
  Pleural friction rub
  Bronchial breath sounds and late-inspiratory crackles

  Late-inspiratory squeak
  Amphoric breath sounds
  Whispered pectoriloquy

- CARDIAC AUSCULTATION:
  Opening snap
  Aortic regurgitation and systolic flow murmur
  Pericardial friction rub
  S3 gallop

  Mid-systolic click
  Patent ductus arteriosus
  Early-systolic ejection sound
  Aortic stenosis
  S4 gallop
  Mitral regurgitation
  Aortic regurgitation
  Mitral stenosis and opening snap

Ask the author

This popular feature from the fifth edition of Kumar & Clark is being carried on into the sixth edition. It gives readers the opportunity to submit questions to the editors and to read the answers online. Readers can view the most recent questions, or can access the complete list of questions and answers that have been logged on the site.

Cecil Textbook of Medicine Online

A year's free access to the online version of the 22nd edition of *Cecil Textbook of Medicine* is available as a special extra feature on the Kumar & Clark website. This feature will provide readers with a powerful extra resource of additional information, and will give them the opportunity to become acquainted with this outstanding medical reference work, consulted by students, practitioners and researchers all over the world.

Contributors

Jane Anderson PhD FRCP

Consultant Physician
Centre for the Study of Sexual Health & HIV
Homerton University Hospital NHS Foundation Trust
London, UK
Sexually transmitted diseases

John Anderson MD MA MB BS FRCP

Consultant Physician
Homerton University Hospital NHS Foundation Trust,
and Barts and the London NHS Trust, London, UK
Diabetes mellitus and lipids

Carol Black DBE PRCP FMedSci

President
Royal College of Physicians, London, UK
Connective tissue disorders, vasculitis

Nicholas H Bunce MB BS MD

Consultant Cardiologist
St George's Healthcare NHS Trust
London, UK
Cardiovascular disease

Andrew K Burroughs MB ChB (Hons) FRCP

Consultant Physician and Hepatologist
The Royal Free Hospital Hampstead NHS Trust, London;
Professor of Hepatology, Royal Free and University
College Medical School, London, UK
Liver disease

A John Camm MD FRCP

Chairman of the Division of Cardiac and Vascular Sciences
St George's University of London, UK
Cardiovascular disease

Anthony W Clare MD FRCP FRCPI FRCPsych MPhil

Associate Professor of Psychiatry, Dublin University;
Consultant Psychiatrist, St Patrick's Hospital, Dublin,
Ireland
Psychological medicine

Michael L Clark MD FRCP

Honorary Senior Lecturer
Barts and the London, Queen Mary's School of Medicine
and Dentistry, University of London, UK
Editor; Gastrointestinal disease; Environmental medicine

Charles R A Clarke MA FRCP MB BCh

Consultant Neurologist
National Hospital for Neurology and Neurosurgery, and
Whipps Cross University Hospital NHS Trust, London,
UK
Neurological disease; Environmental medicine

Brian T Colvin MA MB BChir FRCP FRCPath

Senior Lecturer in Haematology & Director of the
Haemophilia Centre
The Royal London Hospital, Queen Mary's School of
Medicine and Dentistry,
University of London, Barts and the London NHS Trust,
London, UK
Bleeding disorders, thrombosis

Juliet Compston BSc MB BS MD FRCPath FRCP
FMedSci

Professor of Bone Medicine and Honorary Consultant
Physician
University of Cambridge School of Clinical Medicine
Cambridge, UK
Bone disease

Christopher P Denton PhD FRCP

Senior Lecturer & Consultant Rheumatologist
Royal Free Hampstead NHS Trust, London, UK
Rheumatology

Len Doyal BA MSc

Professor of Medical Ethics
Barts and the London, Queen Mary's School of Medicine
and Dentistry, University of London, UK;
Honorary Consultant, Barts and the London NHS Trust,
London, UK
Ethics

Marinos Elia MD BSc (Hons) FRCP

Professor of Clinical Nutrition and Metabolism
Institute of Human Nutrition
University of Southampton, UK;
Honorary Consultant Physician
Southampton University Hospitals NHS Trust, UK
Nutrition

Roger G Finch MB BS FRCP FRCPath FRCP (Edin)
FFPM

Professor of Infectious Diseases
University of Nottingham, UK;
Consultant, Nottingham City Hospital NHS Trust
Nottingham, UK
Infectious diseases and tropical medicine

Anthony J Frew MA MD FRCP

Professor of Allergy and Respiratory Medicine
School of Medicine, University of Southampton, UK
Respiratory disease

Edwin A M Gale MB FRCP

Professor of Diabetic Medicine
University of Bristol, UK
Diabetes mellitus and other disorders of metabolism

Christopher J Gallagher MB ChB PhD FRCP

Consultant, Medical Oncology
Barts and the London NHS Trust, London, UK
Malignant disease

Alasdair M Geddes CBE MB ChB FRCP (Lond & Edin)
FRCPath FFPH FMedSci

Emeritus Professor of Infectious Diseases
The University of Birmingham, UK
Biological warfare

Meredydd Harries BSc MB BS FRCS MSc

Consultant ENT Surgeon
Brighton and Sussex University Hospitals NHS Trust
and Worthing and Southlands Hospitals NHS Trust, UK
Disorders of the ear, nose and throat

Charles J Hinds FRCA FRCP

Professor of Intensive Care Medicine
Barts and the London, Queen Mary's School of Medicine
and Dentistry, London, UK;
Consultant, Department of Anaesthesia and Intensive
Care, William Harvey Research Institute, London, UK
Intensive care medicine

Stephen T Holgate MD DSc FRCP FRCPath FMedSci
FIBiol

Medical Research Council Clinical Professor of
Immunopharmacology
School of Medicine, University of Southampton, UK
Respiratory disease

Trevor A Howlett MD FRCP

Consultant Physician and Endocrinologist
University Hospitals of Leicester NHS Trust, Leicester
Royal Infirmary, UK
Endocrine disease

Ray K Iles BSc MSc PhD CBiol MIBiol

Professor of Biomedical Science and Director of Research
and Postgraduate Studies, Institute of Social and Health
Research, Middlesex University, London, UK
Cell and molecular biology, and genetic disorders

Donald J Jeffries MB BS FRCP FRCPath

Professor of Virology
Barts and the London, Queen Mary's School of Medicine
and Dentistry, University of London, UK;
Head of Medical Microbiology, Barts and the London
NHS Trust, London, UK
Virology

Parveen J Kumar CBE BSc MD FRCP FRCP (Edin)

Professor of Clinical Medical Education, Barts and the
London, Queen Mary's School of Medicine and
Dentistry, University of London, UK; Honorary
Consultant Physician and Gastroenterologist, Barts and
The London NHS Foundation Trust and Homerton
Hospital NHS Trust, London, UK; Academic Vice-
President, Royal College of Physicians, London (2003-
2005); Chairman, Medicines Commission UK (2001-2005)
Editor

Andrew Lister MD FRCP FRCPath FRCR FMedSci

Director, Cancer Research UK Medical Oncology Unit;
Professor of Medical Oncology
Barts and the London, Queen Mary's School of Medicine
and Dentistry, London, UK
Malignant disease

Christopher N Mallinson FRCP

Emeritus Consultant Physician and Gastroenterologist
University Hospital Lewisham, London, UK
Communication

Peter Moss MD FRCP DTMH

Consultant in Infectious Diseases & Associate Medical
Director
Hull and East Yorkshire Hospitals NHS Trust, UK
Infectious diseases and tropical medicine

Michael F Murphy MD FRCPath FRCP

Professor of Blood Transfusion Medicine
University of Oxford; Consultant Haematologist and
Clinical Director - Patients, National Blood Service and
Oxford Radcliffe Hospitals NHS Trust, Oxford, UK
Haematological disease

Donncha O'Grádaigh MB PhD MRCPI

Consultant Rheumatologist
Waterford Regional Hospital, Ireland
Bone Disease

David G Paige MA MB BS FRCP

Consultant Dermatologist and Lead Clinician
Barts and the London NHS Trust, London, UK
Skin disease

Jacqueline Parkin PhD MB BS FRCP

Honorary Consultant
Barts and the London NHS Trust, London, UK
Clinical immunology

Anthony J Pinching D Phil FRCP

Associate Dean for Cornwall and Professor of Clinical
Immunology
Peninsula Medical School, Truro, UK
Clinical immunology

Sir Michael Rawlins MD FMedSc FRCP

Professor of Clinical Pharmacology
University of Newcastle-upon-Tyne;
Chairman
National Institute for Health and Clinical Excellence,
London, UK
Drug therapy

Michael Shipley MA MD FRCP

Consultant Rheumatologist and Clinical Director
University College London Hospitals, London, UK
Rheumatology

David B Silk MD FRCP

Professor of Clinical Nutrition
Department of Surgical Oncology and Technology
Imperial College London, St Mary's Hospital NHS Trust,
London, UK
Gastrointestinal disease

Allister Vale MD FRCP FRCPE FRCPG FFOM FAACT

Consultant Clinical Pharmacologist and Director
National Poisons Information Service (Birmingham
Centre) and West Midlands Poisons Unit, City Hospital,
Birmingham, UK
Poisoning

Francis Vaz FRCS (ORL-HNS) BSc (Hons)

Specialist Registrar in Otolaryngology South Thames
Guy's and St Thomas' Hospitals, London, UK
Disorders of the ear, nose and throat

Seema Verma MD FRCOphth

Consultant Ophthalmic Surgeon
Moorfields Eye Hospital NHS Foundation Trust
London, UK
Disorders of the eye

James Wainscoat FRCP FRCPath

Consultant Haematologist
The Oxford Radcliffe Hospital NHS Trust, The John
Radcliffe, Oxford, UK
Haematological disease

David Watson BSc (Hons) MB BS FRCA

Consultant and Senior Lecturer in Intensive Care Medicine
William Harvey Research Institute, Barts and the
London NHS Trust, Queen Mary's School of Medicine
and Dentistry, London, UK
Intensive care medicine

David Westaby MA FRCP

Consultant Physician and Gastroenterologist
Chelsea and Westminster Healthcare NHS Trust
London, UK
Biliary and pancreatic disease

Peter D White OBE MD FRCP FRCPsych

Professor of Psychological Medicine
Bart's and the London NHS Trust, Queen Mary's School
of Medicine and Dentistry, London, UK
Psychological medicine

Muhammad M Yaqoob MD FRCP

Professor of Nephrology
Department of Renal Medicine and Transplantation
Barts and the London, Queen Mary's School of Medicine
and Dentistry, London, UK
*Water, electrolytes and acid-base balance; Renal
disease*

International Advisory Panel

AUSTRALIA

Dr S A Azer
Senior Lecturer in Medical Education
Faculty of Medicine, Dentistry and Health Sciences
University of Melbourne
Victoria

Associate Professor P Katelaris
Senior Consultant Gastroenterologist
Gastroenterology Department
Concord Hospital
University of Sydney

Professor N Thomson
Professor and Head
Department of Medicine and
Central and Eastern Clinical School
Monash University Medical School
The Alfred Hospital, Melbourne
Victoria

BANGLADESH

Professor M Tahir
Professor and Chairman, Department of Medicine
and Pro-Vice-Chancellor
Department of Medicine
Bangabandhu Sheikh Mujib Medical University Hospital
Dhaka

Professor (Dr) MA Azhar
Department of Medicine
Sir Salimullah Medical College
Dhaka

CHINA

Professor K N Lai
Chair, Professor and Head
Department of Medicine
University of Hong Kong

Professor Wang De-bing
Department of Medicine
Peking University Health Science Center
Beijing

EGYPT

Professor R Barsoum
Professor and Former Chairman
Department of Internal Medicine, Cairo University

INDIA

Professor G Abraham
Professor
Department of Medicine
Sri Ramachandra Medical College and Research Institute
Chennai

Professor D Bandyopadhyay
Professor and Head
Department of Dermatology, STD and Leprosy
R G Karr Medical College
Kolkata

Professor A Deshpande
Professor of Medicine and Head
Department of Internal Medicine
Grant Medical College and Sir JJ Group of Govt. Hospitals
Mumbai

Dr R Dewan
Professor
Department of Medicine
Maulana Azad Medical College
New Delhi

Dr N Gill
Professor of Medicine
KJ Somaiya Medical College
Mumbai

Dr R Gupta
Assistant Professor
Department of Medicine
All India Institute of Medical Sciences
New Delhi

Dr S A Kamath
Professor
Department of Medicine
Topiwala National Medical College
Mumbai

Dr D R Karnad
Professor of Medicine
Department of Medicine
Seth GS Medical College and King Edward Memorial
Hospital
Mumbai

Dr M R Khandakar
Professor and Head
Department of Medicine
National Medical College
Kolkata

Professor (Dr) B D Mankad
Professor and Head
Department of Medicine
BJ Medical College
Ahmedabad

Dr D Mathai
Professor and Head
Department of General Medicine Unit-1 and Infectious
Diseases
Christian Medical College
Vellore

Dr V K Rajamani
Professor
Institute of Internal Medicine
Madras Medical College and Research Institute
Chennai

Dr S.M. Rajendran
Professor and Head
Department of Medicine and Diabetology
Stanley Medical College
Chennai

Professor S K Sharma
Chief
Division of Pulmonary and Critical Care Medicine
Chair, Department of Medicine
All India Institute of Medical Sciences
New Delhi

Dr S K Sharma
Professor and Head
Department of Medicine
Lady Harding Medical College
New Delhi

Professor Shivakumar
Professor
Department of Medicine
Stanley Medical College & Hospital
Chennai

Dr R Sood
Professor
Department of Medicine
All India Institute of Medical Sciences
New Delhi

Dr K N Viswanathan
Professor of Medicine and Consultant
in Internal and Tropical Medicine
Department of Medicine
Sri Ramachandra Medical College
and Research Institute
Chennai

JORDAN

Professor K Ajlouni
Professor and Head
National Center for Diabetes, Endocrinology
and Genetics
Jordan University Hospital
Amman

Dr A Saadeh
Professor of Medicine and Head of
Department of Internal Medicine and Cardiology
Jordan University of Science and Technology
Irbid

KUWAIT

Professor N A Abdella
Professor of Medicine
Head of Diabetes Unit and General Medical Unit
Department of Medicine
Kuwait University

OMAN

Dr N Woodhouse
Professor of Medicine and Head of Endocrine Unit
Department of Medicine
Sultan Qaboos University
Muscat

PAKISTAN

Professor T Ahmed
Principal and Professor of Medicine
Dow Medical College & Civil Hospital
Karachi

Professor (Dr) M A Chaudhry
Principal, Professor and Head of Department
Department of Medicine
Fatima Jinnah Medical College
Sir Ganga Ram Hospital
Lahore

Dr S S Hamid
Professor and Consultant Gastroenterologist
Department of Medicine
The Aga Khan University
Karachi

Dr M Hasan
Principal, Professor and Head
Department of Medicine
King Edward Medical College/Mayo Hospital
Lahore

Dr M A Khan
Karim Jiwa Professor
Department of Medicine
Aga Khan University and Hospital
Karachi

Professor M H Khan
Professor of Medicine and Vice Chancellor DUHS
Department of Medicine
Dow University of Health Sciences
Karachi

Dr S Shafqat
Associate Professor
Department of Neurology
Aga Khan University Medical College
Karachi

SAUDI ARABIA

Professor M M Al-Nozha
Professor and President
Taibah University
King Fahad Hospital
Madinah Munawwarah

SOUTH AFRICA

Professor S Hough
Professor and Chairman
Department of Internal Medicine
University of Stellenbosch, the Tygerberg Academic
Hospital
Cape Town

Professor V J Louw
Professor and Head, Clinical Haematology
Department of Internal Medicine
Free State University/Universitas Academic Health
Complex
Bloemfontein

Professor A P MacPhail
Professor and Head
Department of Internal Medicine
University of the Witwatersrand
Johannesburg

Professor J L Seggie
Professor and Head
Division of General Internal Medicine
Department of Medicine
University of Cape Town and Groote Schuur Hospital
Cape Town

SRI LANKA

Professor N R de Silva
Coordinator Medical Education and Professor of
Parasitology
Faculty of Medicine
University of Kelaniya
Ragama

Professor H J de Silva
Professor of Medicine
Department of Medicine
University of Kelaniya
Ragama

Professor R Sheriff
Professor of Medicine and Head of Department
Department of Medicine
Colombo Medical College

SUDAN

Professor S S Fedail
Professor
Department of Medicine
University of Khartoum

UNITED ARAB EMIRATES

Professor S G Carruthers
Professor of Internal Medicine and Dean
United Arab Emirates University
Faculty of Medicine and Health Sciences
Al Ain

Professor M Ellis
Professor of Medicine
Consultant in Infectious Diseases and Tropical Medicine
Department of Medicine
Faculty of Medical and Health Sciences
Al Ain

Dr J M Muscat-Baron
Professor of Medicine, Clinical Dean
Department of Medicine
Dubai Medical College

Preface to the Sixth Edition

Clinical Medicine has now been in print for approximately 20 years. With each successive edition, we have been gratified by the book's growing success, and keenly aware of our responsibility to keep the contents up to date so that it can continue to make a significant contribution to medical education.

The previous edition of *Clinical Medicine* took the book into the electronic era with a full-text website. This innovation was very well received and introduced the book to an even larger global readership. It also led directly to the creation by the publishers of *Student Consult*, a community of medical textbooks available in print and electronic formats. We are pleased that *Clinical Medicine* should have pioneered this significant development.

As part of our preparation for this sixth edition, we have been privileged to travel to many parts of the world, including Asia and the Middle and Far East. It gave us the opportunity to speak directly to our readers and to hear their views on how the book could be improved. These visits led to the creation for this edition of the International Advisory Panel (see page xii). We would like to thank these colleagues for their support and advice. Our travels made us aware of the importance of providing supplementary information on diseases and problems that are more prevalent in certain parts of the world. We have therefore introduced a new online appendix to the book, which provides detailed advice and a local emphasis that cannot be covered in the printed text. It includes topics such as SARS, viral haemorrhagic (dengue) fever, TB, malaria, snake bite, pesticide and plant poisoning, fluorosis and leprosy. Because this appendix is online, we will be able to enlarge and extend it during the life of this edition. We would like to thank our colleagues who have contributed to the online appendix, in particular, the overall editor Professor Janaka de Silva. We would welcome suggestions from readers for additional topics.

One of the challenges of editing a book such as *Clinical Medicine* is to decide what changes should be made for each new edition. For the last edition, we included a new chapter on ethics and communication, a change that was very well received. For this edition, we have added a new chapter on The Special Senses – eyes, and ENT – in response to readers' suggestions and to our appreciation of the frequency with which these conditions are encountered in general practice medicine. As always,

each chapter in the book has been thoroughly revised and updated by our expert contributors. In particular, the chapters on drug therapy, nutrition, renal, pancreatic-biliary disease, and cardiology have been very extensively re-written. The chapter on oncology has been re-titled Malignant Disease to reflect its change in scope and emphasis.

The book's reputation as a colourful and attractive textbook has always contributed to its popularity. For this edition every line drawing has been redone in a new and much more modern style, which we hope will be appreciated by the younger (as well as the older!) generation of readers. We have also 'animated' a selection of common practical procedures, e.g. lumbar puncture, to aid clinical skills. There is also an interactive surface anatomy programme to help readers with the skills of clinical examination. The opportunity to *hear* heart and lung sounds online is also an exciting innovation. These are all available on the book's electronic website.

In our capacity as editors of *Clinical Medicine*, and in our clinical practice, we are constantly brought into contact with the wider needs of medical students, junior doctors and general physicians. We are also aware that this book is widely used by other health care professionals. This has led to the development of other books, now known as the 'Kumar and Clark Family', which we hope will supplement and extend the useful-ness of *Clinical Medicine*. For an easier-to-carry version, *Pocket Essentials of Clinical Medicine* by A. Ballinger and S. Patchett is already popular in both print and electronic (PDA) versions. We have also recently updated our own *Acute Clinical Medicine*, which is also available in two formats – print and electronic. In preparing for exams, students and junior doctors should find Smith et al: *Pass Finals – a companion to Kumar and Clark* and Baliga: *Self-assessment in Clinical Medicine* particularly useful.

As always, we would like to acknowledge the debt we owe to our families – both our own and those of our authors – for their patience and quiet support during the inevitable periods when 'book work' intruded on family life.

PJK
MLC

Acknowledgements

As always, we would like to thank many of our colleagues who have helped in the preparation of this edition. Many have given us useful advice, helped us to collect photographs and indeed read the manuscripts to make sure that the contents are up-to-date. These include Alison McLean, Susannah Leaver, Peter Fairclough and Paul Kelly.

Some of our authors have left after many years of commitment and loyalty to the book. We would like to thank Dr Paul Drury, Dr Larry Baker, Professor Nigel Benjamin, and Dr Stephen Kelsey. We welcome our new authors who have contributed much to this edition.

Our ward rounds and outpatient reviews are a continuing source of evidence-based education and we are grateful to our specialist registrars, senior house officers, house officers and our own medical students who continue to stimulate us by asking penetrating questions.

We are extremely grateful for the skill and support of our publishers. Ellen Green has now taken us through the last three editions. Clive Hewat has meticulously co-ordinated the whole project with unfailing good humour and patience. The production team, Frances Affleck, Project Manager, and George Ajayi, Designer, have produced a high quality edition of the book. We are also grateful for the meticulous work of the copy editor, Sue Beasley, who has been associated with the book for the last 2 editions, and for the contribution of Caroline Cockrell, Departmental Assistant, for her help in arranging endless couriers and parcels, and most particularly for her careful management of the 'Ask the Author' questions and answers included in the book's website. We would also like to express our thanks to the many people behind the scenes who have contributed in so many ways to the book's preparation.

We are particularly grateful to Ms Jillian Linton who did most of the preparation and co-ordination of the numerous chapters.

Special acknowledgements

Chapter 1 Ethics and communication
Professor Len Doyal would like to thank Sharon Burton of the General Medical Council.

Chapter 6 Gastrointestinal disease
Professor David Silk would like to thank Dr Iain Beveridge for his contribution to the colon polyps and cancer section of the chapter. The editors would like to thank Professor Cliona O'Farrelly.

Chapter 9 Malignant disease
Dr Christopher J Gallagher would like to thank Professor A Rohatiner (St Bartholomew's Hospital Dept of Medical Oncology).

Chapter 13 Cardiovascular disease
Professor AJ Camm would like to thank Dr Aodhan Breathnach and Dr Derek Macallan (Dept of Infectious Diseases, PHLS Collaborating Centre & Dept of Medical Microbiology, St George's Hospital) for their work on the infective endocarditis section of the chapter; Dr Nab Al-Saady (Senior Registrar, Cardiological Sciences, St George's Hospital Medical School) for general assistance with the chapter and Dr Jonathon Goldman for his assistance with the echocardiology section of the chapter.

Crown copyright material is reproduced with the permission of the controller of Her Majesty's Stationery Office.

Important note

Every effort has been made to check the drug dosages given in this book. However, as it is possible that dosage schedules have been revised, the reader is strongly urged to consult the drug companies' literature before administering any of the drugs listed. Drugs mentioned in this book are given their generic Recommended International Non-Proprietary Names in accordance with Directive, 97/27/EEC.

Ethics and communication

ETHICS

WHY STUDY ETHICS AND LAW APPLIED TO MEDICINE?

Professional concern about ethics and law

Many clinical choices created by advances in medical technology are essentially ethical rather than scientific. Doctors may be expert in understanding and applying clinical science, yet this expertise does not in itself answer many ethical questions about the circumstances in which such science should and should not be applied. For example, they may know a great deal technically about advanced life-support systems or the termination of pregnancy. Their knowledge, however, will not tell them whether or not it is ethical to withdraw ventilatory support from a severely brain-damaged patient who will not otherwise die or to perform a termination on a 13-year-old girl who does not want her parents to know that she is pregnant. Answers to these questions derive from moral beliefs and arguments.

Patients are increasingly aware of what they believe to be their human rights and expect doctors to respect them.

- Rights are claims for specific types of goods or services that individuals are believed to be entitled to make on others (e.g. free speech, access to primary and secondary education, access to an acceptable standard of medical care).
- In the UK, if patients believe their rights have been ignored by doctors, they may formally complain to the General Medical Council (GMC) or seek legal redress.
- As it pertains to medicine, the law establishes boundaries for what government and the courts – through statute and common law – have deemed to be acceptable professional practice. The GMC – the UK

regulatory body – sets boundaries for acceptable standards of conduct and care through its guidance documents and decisions in cases heard by its Professional Conduct and Performance Committees.
- Whether or not legal actions or formal complaints against doctors are successful, they contribute toward bringing the medical profession into disrepute.

The three duties of clinical care

The rights of patients may be summarized by three corresponding duties of care which apply to all patients for whom doctors have clinical responsibility.

1. **Protect life and health**. Clinicians should practise medicine to a high standard, taking care not to cause unnecessary harm or suffering. Patients should only be given treatments which they need. Treatments should not be prescribed, for example, just because patients request them.
2. **Respect autonomy**. Humans have autonomy – the ability to reason, plan and make choices about the future. Respect for these attributes goes hand in hand with respect for human dignity. Doctors should respect the autonomy, and thus the dignity, of their patients. This respect for the autonomy of patients leads to two further rights – informed consent and confidentiality. Competent adult patients should be able to choose to accept proposed treatments and to control personal information which they divulge concerning such treatments. Denying patients such choice and control robs them of their human dignity.
3. **Protect life and health and respect autonomy with fairness and justice**. In the conduct of public and professional life, it is generally thought that people

have the right to expect to be treated equally. Medicine is no exception and doctors have a duty to practise accordingly. The access to, and quality of, clinical care should be based only on the dictates of need rather than arbitrary prejudice or favouritism.

Why should doctors take the duties of care seriously?

Professional regulation

Within the UK, the practice of medicine is regulated by the General Medical Council (GMC). It is responsible for the registration of doctors, setting and monitoring the quality of their education and disciplining for unprofessional conduct. Doctors have no professional choice but to conform to the standards laid down by the GMC, which are based on the three duties of care (Box 1.1). These same duties are confirmed by other professional bodies like the Royal College of Physicians, the Royal College of Surgeons, the British Medical Association and the Medical Research Council.

National practices differ but all countries have similar regulatory bodies.

The law

The three duties of care are also enshrined in statute and common law, which also regulate medical practice. Doctors may be sued in civil law for financial compensation for any harm that they may cause while failing in their professional duties. If it can be shown that this failure is intentional, or reckless causing extreme harm or death, doctors may face prosecution in the criminal courts and, if found guilty, imprisonment.

 Box 1.1 General Medical Council (UK), Good Medical Practice: 2–4

The importance of protecting life and health:

- 'an adequate assessment of the patient's condition … (and) … if necessary, an appropriate examination'
- 'providing or arranging investigations or treatments where necessary'
- 'competence when making diagnoses and when giving or arranging treatment'

The importance of respect for autonomy:

- 'listen to patients and respect their views and beliefs'
- 'giving patients the information they ask for or need about their condition, its treatment and prognosis'
- 'respecting patients' privacy and dignity'

The importance of fairness and justice:

- '… (not allowing) … views about a patient's lifestyle, culture, beliefs, race, colour, gender, sexuality, disability, age or social or economic status, to prejudice … treatments'
- '… (not refusing or delaying) treatment because you believe that patients' actions have contributed to their condition, or because you may be putting yourself at risk'

Similar statements are made by a variety of professional bodies in many countries.

 Box 1.2 European Convention on Human Rights

Substantive rights which apply to evaluating good medical practice

Right to life (Article 2)
Prohibition of torture, inhuman or degrading treatment or punishment (Article 3)
Prohibition of slavery and forced labour (Article 4)
Right to liberty and security (Article 5)
Right to a fair trial (Article 6)
No punishment without law (Article 7)
Right to respect for private and family life (Article 8)
Freedom of thought, conscience and religion (Article 9)
Freedom of expression (Article 10)
Right to marry (Article 12)
Prohibition of discrimination (Article 14)

UK law includes the Human Rights Act 1998. This law incorporates the European Convention on Human Rights, making it legally binding in the UK (Box 1.2). The provisions of the Act impose duties on doctors to ensure that their clinical practice is not in violation of these rights – the same duties that all other doctors in Europe must observe. The Act also thus helps to ensure that what constitutes legal practice in the UK is judged by broader, trans-national moral standards.

Rational self-interest

The most rational way for doctors to ensure that their own medical treatment (as well as the treatment of those for whom they have deep personal feelings) meets high standards of care is to support, through the usual professional and legal channels, the right of all patients to the same high standards of care.

The clinical importance of trust

Patients will not trust doctors whom they suspect may ignore their human rights. Without trust, patients will not cooperate in their diagnosis and treatment, undermining the prospect for clinical success. Lack of trust also engenders a defensive and impersonal approach to medicine by both clinicians and patients, potentially spoiling the quality of patient care and professional life.

The doctor/patient relationship

Doctors are expected to treat patients, and their carers where appropriate, as active partners in the healing process.

FURTHER READING

British Medical Association (2000) *The Impact of the Human Rights Act 1998 on Medical Decision* Making. London: BMA.

General Medical Council (2001) *Good Medical Practice.* London: GMC.

Royal College of Surgeons (1997) *The Surgeon's Duty of Care.* London: RCS.

THE NATURE OF MEDICAL MISTAKES

Doctors have a duty to protect the life and health of patients to an acceptable professional standard. What does this mean in practice and what are the penalties for not doing so?

Clinical negligence

If clinicians are suspected not to have provided an acceptable standard of clinical care, they may be sued for negligence – a breach of their professional duty. To win a legal action and financial damages for negligence, patients/claimants must provide convincing evidence to a judge that:

■ they were harmed
■ the harm was caused by the accused doctor
■ the action which caused the harm was a breach of professional duty.

However, in practice, demonstrating that these three things have occurred may be more difficult. For example, the alleged harm may have occurred against the background of a complex medical condition or course of treatment, making it difficult to establish the actual cause.

When has a breach of professional duty occurred?

In the UK, whether or not a doctor has acted inconsistently with the duty to protect life and health to an acceptable standard, is ordinarily decided in civil cases by a judge on the basis of testimony from expert witnesses.

■ Such experts are selected to represent a responsible body of professional opinion. The testimony of these experienced clinicians will be used to help the court determine a professional standard which doctors working in their specializations should meet in clinical practice of the kind under dispute. Both the patient/claimant and defendant/doctor will try to produce experts to support their case.
■ There will be clinical conduct so unreasonable that its negligence speaks for itself (e.g. a dramatic and harmful mistake about drug dosage).
■ If expert witnesses are found for the doctor/defendant who will state that under similar circumstances, they would have clinically responded in the same way as the doctor then the patient/claimant will probably lose. Provided that their testimony is logically consistent and compatible with other widely accepted professional beliefs about good clinical practice, it is likely that the doctor's actions will be found to be reasonable. This will be so irrespective of how representative the clinical opinions given in court are of other doctors practising in the same field. Experts can differ about what is and is not clinically acceptable.
■ Because only a minority opinion is required for doctors to defend claims of negligence against them, the professional standard employed in deciding such claims can make it difficult for patients/claimants to win damages.

Inexperience is irrelevant

Lack of experience is not taken into account in legal determinations of negligence or the GMC's formal hearings. All doctors are expected to work to a professional standard of expertise based on similar clinical work of experienced clinicians. This does not mean that doctors have to be experts in everything. In the face of doubts about their ability or training to provide treatment to a reasonable standard, doctors should seek appropriate supervision and refuse to proceed otherwise.

Mistakes are not necessarily to be feared

Poor professional practice – for example, clinical care which is overly defensive – can result from unfounded fears of patients' readiness to make formal complaints or take legal action.

■ All doctors make clinical mistakes in their professional careers. Yet it should be clear that a clinical error is not necessarily a negligent error. Responsible and experienced clinicians may testify that the erroneous action was and is unavoidable in that type of clinical practice. Under similar circumstances, they too sometimes make – or might make – the same error.
■ Just because doctors can make professionally defensible mistakes does not mean that they should in any way relax their professional standards.
■ Professional bodies within medicine, and the defence associations which insure doctors against negligence, recommend that doctors should be honest and apologetic about their mistakes, remembering that to do so is not necessarily an admission of negligence. As a result of such honesty and humility, there is mounting evidence that patients will feel that they have been respected and are less likely to take legal action or to make formal complaints.

For all of these reasons, there is less to fear legally from patients than doctors sometimes believe. The law offers wide protection for clinicians provided that they do their best to act reasonably and responsibly in protecting the lives and health of their patients.

FURTHER READING
Mason JK, McCall Smith RA (2002) *Law and Medical Ethics*. London: Butterworths.
Montgomery J (2003) *Health Care Law*. Oxford: Oxford University Press.

RESPECT FOR AUTONOMY

Legally valid consent

Obtaining the consent of patients to treatment is just as fundamentally a part of good medical care as is proper clinical diagnosis and good therapeutic management. Doctors seeking consent for a particular procedure must be competent in the knowledge of how the procedure is performed and its problems.

For agreement to treatment to be legally acceptable it must meet three conditions:

- Consent must be informed to an adequate standard.
- Patients must be competent to consent to treatment.
- Patients must not be coerced into accepting treatment against their wishes.

Patients need to weigh up the pros and cons of proposed treatments with other objective interests in their personal lives. They cannot do so without the basic ability to reason about information concerning what is wrong with them, what their doctors propose to do about it, and with what potential benefits and risks. If patients are coerced into making choices about treatment, the ethical and legal right to exercise control over their personal life is ignored. In these circumstances, such choices become more those of clinicians who unduly pressure patients rather than of patients themselves.

Battery

It is an unlawful battery intentionally to touch a competent person without their consent.

- For competent adult patients to be touched lawfully, they must be given information in broad terms about the proposed treatment – what it is and why it is being suggested. Thus a clinician will commit a battery if such a patient is given an injection without permission, irrespective of the need for it.
- Treatment can be given legally to adult patients without consent if they are temporarily or permanently incompetent to provide it and the treatment is *necessary* to save their life, or to prevent them from incurring serious and permanent injury. Otherwise, consent must be obtained, however inconvenient this may be for the patient or clinician.

Negligence: information about risks

Clinicians may also be in breach of their professional duty to obtain adequate consent through not providing a reasonable amount of information about the *risks* of proposed treatment. Here the legal claim of a patient/claimant would be for negligence.

The reasonable doctor standard of disclosure:
- Success will depend on the court being convinced that the patient/claimant had been harmed by the treatment and would not have agreed to it if they had been given more information about its risks.
- The patient/claimant must also show the amount of information provided about risks was unreasonable. If the clinician/defendant can find expert witnesses deemed to constitute a reasonable body of medical opinion who will say that they too (at that point in time) would have provided no more information about risks, the patient/plaintiff will probably lose, just as we saw in the case of litigation for clinical negligence.
- This 'professional standard' of disclosure of information about risks is open to dispute.

The reasonable patient standard of disclosure. Patients may disagree with clinicians about how much information they require to protect their personal interests. Indeed, in deciding what information to disclose to patients about risks, clinicians may know little about how they perceive their interests. Since it is the health and lives of patients that are potentially at risk, the moral focus of such disclosure should be on what is acceptable to them rather than the medical profession.

- It is increasingly argued that clinicians obtaining consent to treatment should ask what sort of information about risks a 'reasonable person' in the position of the patient would want before agreeing to treatment. To do otherwise constitutes an unacceptable threat to the moral rights and dignity of patients and entails a potential loss of trust in the medical profession.
- Practically, clinicians should interpret this standard of disclosure of the reasonable person as meaning that they should ask what sort of imformation someone in the position of the patient needs, in order to make an informed choice. When in doubt, clinicians should also ask what sort of information they would want for themselves, their families and friends. They should also remember that the graver the risk, the more important it is to disclose information about it, even when the chance of it occurring is small.

Express vs implied consent

Consent to treatment may be obtained in two ways:

- Express consent may be verbal or written, usually through the patient signing a consent form. Here consent is given explicitly in relation to specific information about the proposed treatment. Consent to surgical treatment is usually express and written. Consent to lesser forms of physical intervention (e.g. venepuncture) is ordinarily express and verbal. Clinicians should always remember that a signed consent form is not legal or professional proof that proper express consent has been obtained. Informed consent should be viewed as an educational process. Signed consent forms are symbols of the completion rather than the success of this process.
- Consent may also be implied by the fact that the patient accepts treatment without question, protest or any other physical sign that might be associated with rejection. Implied consent is ordinarily given against the background of an express consent to a specific treatment which has already been obtained. For example, once patients have given their express consent for being connected to a drip, there is no need for them to given further consent whenever its contents are replenished.
- Patients have not given their implied consent to a specific treatment simply because they have presented themselves for care in a hospital. They must be given appropriate information about the proposed care and provide express consent to it.

Medical students or their supervisors should always obtain the explicit consent of patients to provide case histories or to be examined for purely educational purposes. Students should always make it clear to patients that they are not qualified doctors.

Confidentiality

If clinicians violate the confidentiality of their patients, they risk causing harm rather than protecting patients from it. Through violating the right of patients to control information which they divulge as part of their medical care, such clinicians disrespect autonomy, undermine trust and call the medical profession into disrepute. These rights are protected by common and statute law. Doctors who breach the confidentiality of patients face severe professional and legal sanctions.

Respecting confidentiality in practice

Patients should be informed of the ways in which information about them will need to be shared with other clinicians and healthcare workers involved in their treatment. On the basis of this information, unless patients state the contrary, they give their implied consent for this information to be shared. Where patients object to particular information being shared, their wish should be respected unless this interferes with the successful execution of their treatment. Information should be sought from patients as early as possible about who, if anyone, they wish to be given information about their condition and treatment. A note should be made of their wishes in the clinical record. Clinicians or healthcare workers not involved in the care of a patient have no right of access to related information without the patient's consent, simply because such information is considered useful for other purposes. In almost all clinical circumstances, therefore, the confidentiality of patients must be respected.

When confidentiality must or may be breached

The principle of confidentiality in medicine is not absolute. Sometimes, the law dictates that clinicians must reveal private information about patients to others in contexts that they may or do object to. At other times, they have the discretion to do so, in accordance with good professional practice. Both circumstances highlight the difficult ethical tension which can be posed between the rights of individual patients and the interests of the public. The right to privacy does not entail the right to harm others in exercising it.

Therefore, clinicians must breach confidentiality when (among others):

- patients have infectious diseases which must be notified, through informing the relevant local authority officer
- police request information about patients who have been involved in a traffic accident
- patients are suspected of engaging in terrorist activity in the UK
- they are presented with a court order by a judge or asked to do so by a judge in judicial proceedings.

Clinicians have the discretion to breach confidentiality when they become aware of, for example:

- past or potential criminal and violent behaviour that has resulted, or is likely to result, in serious harm to the patient or others, such as child abuse – note that in these circumstances, the ordinary expectation would be in favour of discretion
- refusal of patients to comply with their own legal obligations to provide information about their medical condition to the relevant authority (e.g. to the Driver and Vehicle Licensing Agency); again, it would usually be expected for this discretion to be exercised
- infectious patients who pose a threat to specific individuals through undisclosed risks
- infectious patients who pose a potential threat to unknown members of the public through undisclosed risks.

In all these circumstances, patients should be informed of any intent to breach their confidentiality, unless doing so may place the clinician or others at risk of serious harm. Clinicians should always remember that they are professionally accountable for discretionary breaches and may be asked to justify in court, or by the GMC in the UK, their decision either to disclose or not to disclose.

Respect for autonomy in the treatment of vulnerable patients

We have seen that for consent to treatment to be valid, patients must be competent to give it.

What is competence?

Competence should be understood as task-oriented. People may be competent to do some things but incompetent to do others. This means that they should not be judged to be either competent or incompetent in absolute terms. Legally, if patients are competent they must be able to:

- understand information about their condition and treatment
- remember this information
- deliberate about the therapeutic choices posed by the information
- believe that the information applies to them and is not, for example, being made up for other reasons.

Competence to consent to treatment may be compromised by many things – age, mental illness, congenital disease, accident and injury (among others).

Children

In the UK, the legal age of presumed competence to consent to treatment is 16. Below this age, those with parental responsibility are the legal proxies of their children and usually consent to treatment on their behalf. Yet:

- The age of 16 is somewhat arbitrary and many children below this age clearly possess the abilities associated with competence. For example, they may be mature enough to understand and reason about information given to them about their condition and treatment.

- Clinicians should ordinarily respect the dignity of such children through asking them if they agree to the proposed treatment, even when the consent of parents is also obtained.
- If such children wish to have clinical consultations and clinically indicated care without the knowledge of their parents then this – along with their confidentiality – should be respected.
- Young children may be incompetent to make important decisions about their medical care, although they may have developed some degree of autonomy in this regard. They should be consulted about their care and due consideration given to their wishes.
- In England, unlike Scotland, young people do not acquire the right to refuse medical treatment thought to be in their best interest until the age of 18. In practice, the legal ability to force treatment on mature children against their wishes should only be contemplated in circumstances where life is at risk or there is a risk of serious and permanent injury. Doing otherwise is not in the best interests of young people because of the potentially dangerous alienation that it may create toward doctors and medicine.

Those with parental responsibility have questionable legal authority to direct clinicians to administer or withdraw treatments deemed necessary to protect children from death or serious harm. The court should be consulted about such disagreements, unless an emergency dictates otherwise.

Psychiatric illness

The vast majority of patients being treated for psychiatric illness are competent to consent and to refuse treatment. There is no difference between their rights and those of other competent patients. Because of the danger of stigma associated with mental illness, great care should be taken to protect their confidentiality. If patients with severe psychiatric illness are incompetent to understand the nature and consequences of their illness, they will be unable to provide valid consent to treatment. Here, the ethical duty of care shifts from respect for autonomy of such patients to protecting them.

The 1983 Mental Health Act (England and Wales). Mental illness may so compromise the autonomy of patients that they become a danger to themselves and/or to others. Provided that their illness is treatable, such patients may be detained under the 1983 Mental Health Act for further examination and treatment. Because of the terrible risks and ethical significance of denying someone their ordinary civil liberties, the conditions of detainment under the Act are highly specific: the longer the period of detainment, the more safeguards there are to ensure the clinical need for it (see Table 22.29, p. 1314).

Psychiatric treatment without consent. Under certain circumstances, detained patients may be given psychiatric treatment without their consent. However, attempts should be made to obtain consent, if possible. Unless their mental illness has made them incompetent to do so, such patients must still give their consent to proposed treatments for physical disorders. Again, incompetence in one respect does not entail incompetence in all respects. However, if patients are unable competently to consent because of the severity of their psychiatric condition – and treatment is required to save their life or to prevent serious and permanent disability – they can be given necessary care without it. If treatment can wait, without seriously compromising their interests, then patients should be asked to consent to it when they become competent to do so.

Other forms of incompetence to provide consent to treatment

Patients may also be incompetent because of congenital, developmental or accidental brain damage. With children, those with parental responsibility consent to treatment on their behalf. With adults, there is no provision in English law for adults to act as legal proxies for other adults, although this is not so in other legal jurisdictions (e.g. Scotland). The moral argument for this being so is that some people might not be motivated by protecting the best interests of their family members. Therefore, relatives should not have the final say over treatment decisions. However, relatives should be asked their views about the wishes or concerns of the patient and consulted about medically relevant information which might be used to optimize the success of the patient's care. They should not be given the impression as a result of such consultation that it is they who are determining treatment decisions. Within the jurisdiction of English law, doctors and no one else must decide what is and is not in the best clinical interests of patients. All forms of treatment can be administered to permanently incompetent adults on this basis. Of course, the moral coherence of these arguments depends on the assumption that clinicians are best placed to protect the interest of vulnerable patients and this, in turn, rests on consistently high standards of clinical care and reflection about ethics and law.

FURTHER READING

British Medical Association (1999) *Confidentiality and the Disclosure of Health Information.* London: BMA.

British Medical Association (2001) *Consent, Rights, and Choices in Healthcare for Children and Young People.* London: BMJ Press.

Doyal L, Tobias J (eds) (2001) *Informed Consent in Medical Research.* London: BMJ Books.

General Medical Council (1998) *Seeking Patient's Consent: The Ethical Considerations.* London: GMC.

General Medical Council (2001) *Confidentiality: Protecting and Providing Information.* London: GMC.

ETHICAL AND LEGAL BOUNDARIES OF THE DUTY TO PROTECT LIFE AND HEALTH

Generally speaking, clinicians are professionally obligated to intervene to save the lives of patients for whom they have clinical responsibility. However, there are a range of circumstances where the duty of care to provide life-sustaining treatment is superseded by other ethical and legal responsibilities.

Competent refusal

The right of competent refusal supersedes the ordinary duty clinicians have to try to save the lives of such patients, along with any preferences others might have that they should be forced to accept treatment (Box 1.3). Patients may refuse life-sustaining treatment explicitly when it is offered or they may formulate an 'advance directive' which stipulates the circumstances under which they refuse it, should they become incompetent to do so in the future. Competent refusals of life-sustaining treatment (e.g. refusal of blood transfusion by Jehovah's Witnesses) must be made on the basis of clear information about the consequences of refusal. Equally, decisions not to attempt to sustain life medically should also only be made with the consent of competent patients (e.g. a decision not to provide cardiopulmonary resuscitation). Such patients may have arrangements which they need to make that their clinicians will know nothing about and it would be ethically wrong to pre-empt this.

The best interests of the incompetent

There will be some situations where the provision of life-sustaining treatment will not be regarded as being in the best interests of permanently incompetent patients, even though not providing it will lead to their death occurring before it otherwise would. This is when prolongation of patients' lives will be of no benefit to them, against the background of their dire clinical circumstances. For example, it is acceptable not to use medical means to prolong the lives of patients when:

- it is believed on good evidence that further treatment will not save life
- patients are already imminently and irreversibly close to death
- patients are so permanently or irreversibly brain damaged that they are incapable of any future self-directed activity or intentional social interaction.

One ethical justification for the latter two provisions is that such patients have no further need for medical treatment because they have no further objective interest in continuing to live. Because of their clinical condition, they can no longer do or achieve anything in life. However, because of potential differences in moral and religious belief, decisions not to provide or continue life-sustaining treatment should always be made with as much consensus as possible among the clinical team responsible for the patient's care and people close to the patient who are consulted about their care. Where there is unsolvable conflict, especially in relation to children and their parents, the court should be consulted. In emergencies, judges are always available in the appropriate court, usually the Family Law Division.

Clinicians may decide not to prolong the lives of imminently dying and/or extremely brain-damaged patients for the legally acceptable reason that they are acting in the best interests of their patients to attempt to minimize their suffering rather than intending to kill them. To do the latter would be murder. Clearly, when contemplating not providing or withdrawing life-sustaining treatments, doctors should do their best to act within the law. However, it should also not be forgotten that much debate continues about whether or not there is a much closer ethical link between clinical decisions not to save life and decisions actively to end it. The law concerning such matters may change at some point in the future.

The duty as a doctor to be fair and just

The principle of equality of persons should dominate the way in which the duties of care are discharged in clinical practice. Clinicians may show technical mastery of treatment options and great ability and sensitivity in obtaining informed consent to treatment and maintaining confidentiality. However, if in the process of doing so, they actively discriminate against individual or groups of patients, they are still acting unprofessionally and should be penalized accordingly. For example, discrimination on the basis of race, age, social worth, class, intelligence or occupation should not be tolerated (Box 1.4).

Scarce resources

As a matter of right in the UK, the National Health Service (NHS) provides *equal* access to appropriate medical care on the basis of need alone. This right is mitigated by scarce resources and the courts have made it clear that they will not force health authorities or trusts to provide treatments which are beyond their means. However, the courts also demand that decisions about such means must be made on reasonable grounds and that patients have a clear right to expect this. Thus on both ethical and legal grounds, prejudice or favouritism is not acceptable in the allocation of scarce resources. If

---

 Box 1.3 Competent refusal

Prima facie every adult has the right and capacity to decide whether or not he will accept medical treatment, even if a refusal may risk permanent injury to his health or even lead to premature death. Furthermore, it matters not whether the reasons for the refusal were rational or irrational, unknown or even non-existent. This is so notwithstanding the very strong public interest in preserving the life and health of all citizens.

Re T (adult: refusal of medical treatment) [1992]

Box 1.4 The duty as a doctor to be fair and just

Injustice can occur in medicine through treating patients unequally according to (among others):

- race
- age
- fitness
- social worth
- class
- intelligence
- physical attractiveness
- profession
- parenthood.

rationing healthcare is inevitable in the NHS, as many believe to be the case, then ways must be found to do so which are fair and just. In practice this means that scarce resources should be allocated to patients on the basis of the similarity and extremity of their need (e.g. triage) and the time at which they presented themselves for treatment (e.g. the randomness imposed by the 'lottery of nature'). To the degree that this procedure of allocation is followed, all patients will be said to have had an equal opportunity to be treated on the basis of equal need. It is respect by clinicians and healthcare teams for these principles of equality – equal need and equal chance – that guarantees fairness and justice in the delivery of healthcare. In the UK, the National Institute for Clinical Excellence (NICE) is a body set up to evaluate treatments on a clinical and cost-effective basis, and to ensure equal access to care across the country. In circumstances of scarcity, waste and inefficiency are clearly matters of great ethical concern.

More specifically, any well-run A&E department within the United Kingdom will follow precisely these moral principles in the way in which decisions are made about who to treat first and with what. The treatments on offer will be those that have been shown to deliver optimal results for minimal expense. Patients who are in the most need – as determined by the triage nurse – will be seen first. Everyone else will receive treatment in relation to the assessment of the urgency of their need and when they initially register for treatment. In this way a waiting list will be constructed for each clinical session. So long as no one attempts to jump the queue, patients traditionally respect these rules – sometimes to a point of waiting for long periods to be seen without complaint. Waiting lists in other clinical settings should be similarly constructed, although here other variables will come into play (e.g. the accuracy with which general practitioners communicate the urgency of need to hospital consultants). What is unacceptable in any aspect of the allocation of scarce healthcare resources is for prejudice or favouritism – treating equals unequally – to influence their construction.

Lifestyle
Patients should not be denied potentially beneficial treatments on the grounds that their lifestyles have been more unhealthy than others with whom they compete for the same treatments. Decisions to do so are almost always prejudicial. For example, why single out smokers or the obese for blame as opposed to those who engage in dangerous sports? Patients are not equal in their abilities to lead healthy lives and to make correct healthcare choices for themselves. Some are better educated and informed, more emotionally confident and more supported by their social environment. To ignore this, to regard all patients as equal competitors and to reward the already better off is unjust and unfair. In this situation it is incorrect to treat unequals equally.

FURTHER READING
British Medical Association (2001) *Withholding and Withdrawing Life-prolonging Medical Treatment.* London: BMJ Press.
Butler J (1999) *The Ethics of Health Care Rationing.* London: Cassell.
Harris J (1984) *The Value of Life.* London: Routledge.
Samanta A, Samanta J (2003) Legal standard of care: a shift from the traditional Bolam test. *Clinical Medicine* **3**: 443–446.

GENERAL READING
Beauchamp T, Childress J (2001) *Principles of Biomedical Ethics.* New York: Oxford University Press.
British Medical Association (2004) *Medical Ethics Today: The BMA's Handbook of Ethics and Law.* London: BMJ Books.
Parker M, Dickenson D (2001) *Medical Ethics Workbook.* Cambridge: Cambridge University Press.
Tallis R (2004) *Hippocratic Oaths: Medicine and Its Discontents.* London: Atlantic Books.

COMMUNICATION

COMMUNICATION IN HEALTHCARE

During the last 50 years, the subject of communication in healthcare has become a serious study. At the beginning of the 21st century it is now established in the curriculum of every training institute for healthcare professionals at every level. Evidence is that healthcare fails without a conscious informed effort of communication which is the personal and professional responsibility of everyone concerned with the care of the sick: healthcare professionals including nurses, doctors, therapists and pharmacists as well as ancillary staff and managers. It is a major issue in the strategies of all health organizations representing providers, consumers, managers or governmental departments.

Healthcare is seldom a simple matter of 'find it and fix it', in spite of the unquestionable advances of biomedical science. Rather it is a complicated interaction of at least four elements: physical care – surgical or medical; cognitive care to provide clear information for patients to help themselves and to adhere to advice; behavioural care whereby patients can modify their habits and lives; psychological care, either of coincident primary psychological factors or those secondary to physical illness.

It is the aim and mission of the modern healthcare professional to provide care that is evidence-based, unconditionally patient centred and shared in a collaborative partnership. Effective communication is an absolute necessity at every stage in each and every clinical interview. It cannot be delegated.

Communication, good or bad, affects in opposite ways every one of the four aspects of care above and it has an immense potential for influencing the use of healthcare resources and finances on a grand scale.

Health outcomes

Effect of communication on biomedical care and its outcome

The best biomedical outcome obviously depends upon accurate diagnosis and appropriate treatment. Communication styles that are 'patient centred' provide a more complete clinical picture upon which diagnosis and treatment can be based and lead to improvement in health outcomes (Box 1.5). Patients describe several consistent failures of communication (Box 1.6) which lead to an incomplete history and a poor professional relationship.

Adherence to treatment

Health outcomes also depend on the extent to which patients adhere to their clinical advice. Patients do not do so for many reasons. The correctable factors are all matters of communication: letting patients know why their treatment is being given and what benefits they stand to gain, what the pros and cons may be, what options exist, and doing so in a way which builds trust and collaboration (Box 1.7). The annual economic cost of non-adherence to advice runs into many millions of pounds in the UK.

Social outcomes

Patient satisfaction is the result of their:

- knowing that they are getting the best appropriate biomedical healthcare

> **Box 1.5 Communication improves health outcomes**
>
> **Outcome improved with better communication**
>
> Symptom resolution
> Psychological distress reduced
> Health and functional status improved
> Blood pressure control improved
> Pain control improved
> Patient anxiety reduced
>
> From Stewart M (1995). Effective physician–patient communication and health outcomes: a review. *Canadian Medical Association Journal* **152**: 1423–1433.

> **Box 1.6 Failures of communication**
>
> Patients reported the following problems in interviews:
>
> - 54% of their complaints were not elicited
> - 45% of their concerns were not elicited
> - 50% of psychological problems were not elicited
> - In 50% of visits, patients and doctors disagreed on main presenting problem
> - In 50% of cases, their history was blocked by interruption within 24 seconds.
>
> Simpson M et al. (1991) The Toronto Consensus Statement. *British Medical Journal* **303**: 1385–1387.

> **Box 1.7 Factors in communication which improve patients' adherence to clinical advice**
>
> - Clinician understands the patient
> - Clinician's tone of voice
> - Clinician elicits all the patient's health concerns
> - Patient is comfortable asking questions
> - Patient perceives that sufficient time is spent with the clinician
>
> Stewart M et al. (1999) Evidence on patient communication. *Cancer Prevention and Control* **3(i)**: 25–30.

- knowing that they are being treated as individuals and not items on a conveyor belt
- being treated in a humane manner.

These are all strongly related to good communication.

Satisfaction also affects psychological well-being and adherence to treatment, both of which have a knock-on effect on physical health outcomes.

Discord between patients and clinicians

Modern healthcare is carried out in a climate of consumerism and critical participation. With this has come an increasing number of complaints and lawsuits from what is nevertheless a small proportion of patients. The majority of complaints are not based on failures of biomedical practice but on poor communication (Box 1.8). In contrast, Box 1.9 shows the qualities that patients describe in interviews with primary care physicians who have never been sued.

Complaints and lawsuits, however, represent the tip of an iceberg. There is widespread failure of even the most basic communication in hospital and general practice, at least in the UK. Box 1.8 shows the results of a very large study of what patients experience rather than their opinion of it. A very large proportion of patients were not provided with even basic civility let alone simple information about their future care.

The monetary costs of these failures of communication is enormous.

Clinician satisfaction

While staffing shortages and inadequate resources and facilities for biomedical care are commonly cited as causes of discontent amongst clinicians of all kinds, it is the quality of their relationships with their patients

> **Box 1.8 Factors leading to poor relationships with clinicians**
>
> Factors cited by 75% of complaining patients as the cause of their complaint against their clinician:
>
> - Feeling deserted
> - Feeling devalued
> - Information poorly delivered
> - Lack of understanding.
>
> Stewart M et al. (2000) The impact of patient-centred care on outcomes. *Journal of Family Practice* **49**: 796–804.

Box 1.9 Qualities leading to good relationships

Primary care physicians (who have never been sued):

- orientated patients to the process of the visit, e.g. introductory comments: 'We are going to do this first and then go on to that'
- used facilitative comments
- asked patients their opinion
- used active listening
- used humour and laughter
- conducted slightly longer visits (18 versus 15 minutes).

Stewart M et al. (2000) The impact of patient-centred care on outcomes. *Journal of Family Practice* **49**: 796–804.

and colleagues which is the most reliable global indicator of clinician satisfaction and happiness. Healthcare professionals have a very high incidence of occupational morbidity, a major source of which is seen to be due to difficulties with personal relationships including clinician–patient relationships. The health of clinicians as well as their patients is closely connected with the development of skill, knowledge and above all attitude to communication.

The cost of loss of work, early retirement, healthcare for clinicians and poor performance is a further heavy burden on any health service.

POOR COMMUNICATION BETWEEN DOCTORS AND PATIENTS

Difficulties clinicians have in communicating with patients

Lack of knowledge

Clinicians usually concentrate on the biomedical model of clinical medicine rather than the psychosocial model, as they are often ignorant of the qualitative research on the latter. This can lead to major diagnostic and therapeutic errors, for example:

- numerous illnesses have physical symptoms without an organic basis
- physical illnesses are prolonged by psychological factors (p. 1280)
- 20% of medical patients have psychiatric disease (p. 1280).

Many clinicians 'know' that patients never remember what they are told so think it is a waste of time giving them more than reassurance. The evidence is that patients' memory for even complicated matters is good if they are informed skilfully, as outlined on page 13.

Attitude

Clinicians who take an authoritarian role and have a negative attitude to shared care and multiprofessional teamwork tend to reveal themselves in their questioning styles and are unlikely to be self-critical of their com-

munication skills even when they are shown the evidence of their poor performance.

Lack of skill

- *Time.* It takes coaching and practice to acquire the skill to integrate good communication into every interview and to make patients feel that they have had enough time devoted to them. Clinicians often see communication as desirable but too time-consuming. However, time skimped at a critical moment deprives the patient and involves someone else in more time later.
- *Uncomfortable topics and patients.* Lack of skill also leaves clinicians uneasy in certain difficult interviews, and Box 1.10 shows the different strategies patients notice clinicians use to avoid uncomfortable topics or 'difficult patients'. These strategies are largely the result of clinicians' fears and inadequate training. It is necessary for clinicians to find their own ways of managing patients who are widely found to be difficult.

Failure of empathy

One of the things which distinguishes the healthcare professions from others is that patients expect humanity from their doctors as well as competence. Clinicians provide this by demonstrating empathy (p. 12). This may require an effort from doctors who have never been ill themselves. It takes commitment as well as skill to demonstrate empathy to a large number of similar patients in a morning.

Personal failures

Like anyone else, clinicians can be unhappy, short-tempered, rushed and interrupted, ignorant on some subjects, or charmless. But this is not the patients' problem and it is a professional obligation not to allow doctors' problems to affect a patient's experience or care.

 Box 1.10 Strategies which patients find their doctors use to distance themselves from their patients

Strategy	Example
Selective attention to cues	Chooses biomedical topics, avoids others
Normalizing	'Everyone feels that. Forget it.'
Premature reassurance	'I am sure everything will be OK.'
False reassurance	'Everything is OK.'
Switching the topic	'A headache? Tell me about your feet.'
Passing the buck	'Nurse will tell you all about that.'
Jollying along	'Worse things happen at sea.'
Physical avoidance	Waving but not stopping

Maguire P (2000) *Communication Skills for Doctors*. London: Arnold.

Difficulties for patients in communicating with doctors

Inferiority

Patients commonly feel themselves to be in the weaker position in a medical interview. This may be exacerbated by their own problems or by their clinicians. The aim of shared care is to overcome this inequality.

Anxiety and its consequences

Most patients are anxious to some extent and often try to hide it. Anxiety can make patients seem to regress in behaviour, mental power and memory. Free-floating anxiety may cause ideas which are worse than reality and contribute to complex misconceptions.

Misconceptions

Anxiety and medical ignorance commonly create misconceptions in patients' minds about their illnesses which in turn profoundly affect their symptoms and the ability to recover. Such misconceptions need detecting and uprooting, without which correct information will not register. Simple reassurance will not supplant a misconception.

Conflicting information

Apart from friends, family and the media, patients get varied information from many different healthcare professionals. Clinicians seldom record what they tell patients. Conflicting information can lie long undetected whilst it contributes to misconceptions.

Forgetfulness

Patients, like most of us who are provided with numerous new and alarming facts, tend to forget all but a few, unless care is taken to aid their memory. This is compounded if they are told information in words they do not understand. However, if information is given carefully, 70–80% of the facts will be remembered by a patient after 6 weeks, or even indefinitely. An exception is evident in well-informed surgical patients who often forget most of what they were told within weeks of their operation.

Disinclination to disclose their concerns

Patients may not disclose all their concerns if they feel nothing can be done, or they are wasting the doctors' time, or fear being thought neurotic with non-physical problems. They are less likely to be forthcoming if their first questions are blocked or answered incomprehensibly, if they fear their effective treatment may be withdrawn, if they are distracted or distressed, or if they do not like or trust their doctor.

Impaired faculties of communication

Patients with impaired hearing or speech or vision or mental function or whose clinician does not speak their language all experience substandard healthcare as a direct result of their inability to communicate.

One in five medical patients have psychiatric illnesses, diagnosed or otherwise, which may affect their ability or inclination to communicate.

FURTHER READING

Lewin B (1995) The place of psychological therapies in coronary artery disease. In: *Psychiatric Aspects of Physical Disorder.* London: Royal College of Physicians/Royal College of Psychiatrists.

Maguire P (2000) *Communication Skills for Doctors.* London: Arnold.

Pendleton, D et al. (2003) *The New Consultation.* Oxford: Oxford University Press.

Simpson M et al. (1991) The Toronto Consensus Statement. *British Medical Journal* **303**: 1385–1387.

Stewart M et al. (2000) The impact of patient-centred care on outcomes. *Journal of Family Practice* **49**: 796–804.

THE MEDICAL INTERVIEW

Clinicians conduct about 200 000 interviews during their careers. Such interviews often provide more critical information than do clinical tests and they also form the basis of the relationship which leads to collaborative partnership with their patients.

There is no single prescription for a medical interview because each patient is different, but well-researched guiding principles and well-coached skills will allow clinicians to use their time to the greatest benefit of their patients.

The overriding principle is to find out not only the medical facts in detail, but what patients have experienced and what impact this experience has had upon them. This information is essential to expand the diagnosis and recommend appropriate action and also to gain the confidence, the trust and the compliance of the patient.

The example below is in the context of a first medical interview in a consulting room. Obviously this is different from a follow-up interview, or an emergency.

It is helpful to regard the interview in three phases (Box 1.11).

Opening

The start of the interview will be helped by well-organized arrangements for appointments, reception and punctuality. If possible, the clinician should come out of the room to greet each patient. Otherwise it is polite to rise, look at the patient, establish eye contact and shake hands if appropriate. Greet them and find out the way the patient prefers to be addressed. The patient sits beside the clinician, not on the far side of a desk. The clinician sits in a posture which conveys attention and friendliness.

 Box 1.11 **The three phases of an interview**

Opening		Engage
Exploring and focusing	During which the clinician will	Empathize
Closing		Educate
		Enlist

Clinicians should introduce themselves indicating a name badge and their status and responsibility to the patient. On no account should the patient be undressed before the first meeting.

First impressions are critical. The patients' non-verbal cues indicate their emotional state, and the main influences on the emotional tone of the interview are the clinicians' own non-verbal messages, facial expression, body language and unspoken attitudes.

Start by discovering what the patient expects from the interview and indicate how long it will last.

Exploring and focusing

Taking a full history

The components of a complete history are shown in Table 1.1. A clear factual account of the biomedical details is, of course, essential, but is not enough. The order of taking a history is not prescribed, for example many experienced clinicians begin with the social history: 'To start with, can you tell me something about yourself?'

Listening skills and questioning styles

Questioning style determines whether the clinician or the patient talks more. Clinicians will obtain more information by starting with open questions, letting the patients speak more than they do, then guiding the history by using closed questions for further detail, rather than asking closed questions of their own (Box 1.12). The aim is to obtain all the patients' concerns, remembering that they usually have at least three (range 1–12). Only then can the agenda be prioritized, balancing the patients' concerns with the clinician's main points of interest.

It is a failure on the part of the clinician if a serious point is raised only as the patient has a hand on the door knob, preparing to leave.

Facilitating the patient

If the clinician sits in complete silence, the patient will flounder and lose confidence. The patient will be helped by some eye contact, a grunt even or a smile to show that the clinician is listening attentively. Reflecting questions (see Box 1.12) guide the history, allowing the clinician to take up unexpected points as they arise or expand topics, without interrupting the patient. As the history unfolds, detail can be brought into focus by using screening and closed questions.

Table 1.1 Components of a medical interview

The nature of the key problems
Clarification of these problems
Date and time of onset
Development over time
Precipitating factors
Help given to-date
Impact of the problem on patient's life
Availability of support
Patient's ideas and fears
Patient's attitude to similar problems in others
Screening question

 Box 1.12 Questioning style

Question	Example
Open question	'What has brought you to see me today?'
Open screening question	'Is there anything else you want to tell me?'
Open directive question	'How did the treatment for your headache go?'
Reflecting question	'Could you tell me a bit more about that?'
Closed question	'What date exactly did the headache start?'
Rhetorical leading question	'The headache has got better on my treatment hasn't it?'

Leading questions may be helpful but they should not end in the rhetorical 'isn't it?', 'wouldn't it?' challenge which makes the questions difficult for the patient to discuss even when they are completely wrong.

Ideas and fears and their validation

While the clinician may be mainly interested in the biomedical explanation, patients seek help because of their own interpretation of their condition. They need to know that their ideas have been heard and acknowledged and are henceforth incorporated in their clinician's interpretation of their complaints. Otherwise the patient may tend to believe that the clinician has not got things right, which increases the risk of the patient not adhering to the recommendations that follow. So hearing these ideas and then acknowledging them, i.e. *validating* them, is an essential step in engaging a patient's trust, and beginning to 'treat the whole patient'.

If clinicians habitually summarize their biomedical and psychosocial notes at each interview, such misunderstandings can be avoided and their interview is immediately well founded.

Empathizing

Empathy has been described as 'imagination for others'. An empathic response is one which demonstrates a genuine interest in patients' experiences. This is a key skill in building the patient–clinician relationship and is highly therapeutic. Like other communication skills, it can be taught and learnt but it cannot be counterfeited by a repertoire of routine mannerisms.

Techniques which demonstrate empathy are:

- seeing, hearing and accepting patients as they are – illustrated in Box 1.13
- reflecting what the patients are feeling as they talk and what the patient sees as important and what the patient may be thinking
- using the patient's own words and ideas
- letting the patient correct any misunderstanding that arises
- using appropriate self-disclosure without capping the patient's story.

Box 1.13 Demonstrating empathy by showing the patient that their experiences are recognized and accepted

Demonstration	Questioning style
The patient experiences being seen	'That last point made you look worried. Is there something more serious about that point you would like to tell me?'
The patient experiences being heard	'I notice that you have talked about the death of your mother but could I ask you to tell me something about how your brother died?'
The patient experiences being accepted	'I can tell you that most people in your circumstances get angry at some point, even with the people who have helped them.'
The clinician shows self-disclosure	'I'm a bit like you. Whenever I get heartburn I think it's a heart attack.'

Giving information – educating the patient

When information is given skilfully, patients are able to understand what is said, to remember it and to find it helpful. Patients are more likely to adhere to clinical advice if they get comprehensible information, if it makes sense of their problems and if they can get easy access to more if they need it. The whole point of giving information is to allow patients to understand their problem and use their information to help themselves. This aspect of patient partnership is a keystone of modern medical practice.

One study of junior doctors showed that they gave information poorly because they lacked both clear objectives and a systematic technique of giving information.

There is a large amount of research to show that:

- Information must be related not only to the biomedical facts, but to the patients' ideas about their condition.
- While most patients are voracious for information, this is not invariably the case, particularly when the information is sensitive or threatening. The pacing of information is discussed further in 'Breaking bad news' on page 14.
- Most patients will understand and recall 70–80% of even the most unfamiliar, complex or alarming information if it is provided along the following guidelines:
  - (a) Use a logical sequence to explain the cause and effect of the condition in the context of the patient's symptoms. (Be proactive about explaining causes; patients always want to know.)
  - (b) Talk about one thing at a time and check that the patient understands before you move on to the next.

Box 1.14 Possible aids to giving information

Method	Example
Write it down	As you go – make a copy for your records
Use a diagram	
Send the patient a copy of your report	With a patient's paragraph as a routine
Make an audio tape	Desk-top recorder £20; tapes 50p each
Use prepared information	Leaflets, audio or video
Provide address of support organization	BACUP for cancer patients NHS Direct for help of all kinds. Tel: 0845 4647
Provide a website reference	Patient UK: http://www.patient.co.uk

  - (c) Use simple language; translate any unavoidable medical terms and write them down.
  - (d) Make your information and instructions direct, detailed and concrete.
  - (e) At the outset show patients that you will write down the key words, use a simple diagram, and can offer them other aids to memory as shown in Box 1.14. Otherwise patients may be alarmed to find that they are forgetting half of what you say, perhaps distracted by some of the earlier information. Write out the risks of operations for patients, which tend to be rapidly forgotten after operations, however well understood before.
  - (f) For the numerous patients who need more information than you can provide in the time, give them prepared information, or a source of it.
  - (g) Do not be exasperated when patients refer to the Internet; have a useful website reference ready and written out (see Box 1.14).

Negotiating the next steps – enlisting the patient's collaboration

To achieve optimum adherence, the clinician's suggestions about diagnosis or treatment must be negotiated with the patient. This requires an explanation of the benefits and disadvantages and the risks of these suggestions and any alternatives, all with the aim of enlisting patients to take an active part in their own care.

Patients adhere best to suggestions about investigation and treatment when they are thus enlisted as partners as a result of:

- a frank exchange of information
- a negotiation of options
- involving the patient in decisions.

Summarizing

Misunderstanding can be greatly reduced if clinicians make a brief summary first of the patient's agenda and then their own. This may include matters which have to be postponed to a further interview, and certainly should include the arrangements for any such interview or the commitment to informing other healthcare professionals involved with the patient. It is good, but still rare, practice to make a note together of what the patient has been told and what has been understood.

Closing
Any human contact ends with an appropriate farewell, not forgetting some words of encouragement.

FURTHER READING
Bedell SE et al. (2001) The doctor's letter of condolence. *New England Journal of Medicine* **344**: 1162–1163.
Keller V (1994) A new model for physician–patient communication. *Patient Education and Counselling* **23**: 131–140.
Maguire, P et al. (2003) Managing the difficult consultation. *Clinical Medicine* **3**: 532–537.
Silverman J et al. (1998) *Skills for Communicating with Patients*. London: Radcliffe Press.

INTERVIEWS IN WHICH DIFFICULTIES IN COMMUNICATION CAN BE EXPECTED

Some interviews are bound to be difficult for patients or clinicians or both. Usually this is because they have a high emotional content – frightening, painful or embarrassing – and there is no straightforward medical solution. So clinicians have to rely on their personal qualities to an extent which their training may not have prepared them for and can rely less, if at all, on biomedical knowledge.

The three commonest subjects requested on communication courses for doctors reflect problems commonly reported by patients:

- breaking bad news
- complaints and lawsuits
- cultural differences.

These are discussed below.

Other popular topics are: hostility and anger, 'difficult' patients and colleagues, taking a sexual history, and eliciting a psychiatric history, which is discussed in detail on page 1274.

These are all interviews in which, patients find, many clinicians exhibit the distancing strategies listed in Box 1.10. Every clinician has a professional responsibility to recognize interviews they find difficult. Otherwise they will make difficult matters even worse than they need be for their patients and themselves.

The basic principles of the medical interviews described above hold good for all of the above examples but certain details become more prominent.

Breaking bad news

Bad news is any information which is likely to alter drastically a patient's view of the future. It is one of the most potent causes of distress and psychological morbidity and of complaints and lawsuits.

Those interviews may be difficult because:

- bad news commonly means that biomedical measures are of little or no help; so the clinician's familiar basis of experience and authority is discounted

- the patient can be expected to be upset, behave unpredictably and require emotional support which may be beyond what the clinician can give
- the clinician is upset as well
- the patient may blame the clinician, and indeed there may be an element of medical mishap to complicate matters
- the clinician may have had little experience in such interviews (being ushered out during training) or have had bad previous experiences and no help subsequently.

Breaking bad news is a professional skill which is acquired by practice under supervision. It should give a clinician confidence and satisfaction rather than alarm, although it can never be painless.

The way that bad news is broken has a major psychological and physical effect upon patients. For example, the main predictive factor for patients developing full-blown psychiatric disorders on learning of the diagnosis of cancer depends upon the way their bad news is broken. Likewise the memories and well-being of the relatives now and later depends on the way that the subject is introduced; for example, the rehabilitation of patients after acute coronary events depends, damage for damage, on the way in which the news is broken and patients' ideas about it are educated.

Relatives may ask that bad news is withheld from the patient. The information belongs to the patient not to relatives; moreover the evidence is clear that patients:

- usually know more than anyone has guessed
- may imagine things to be worse than they are
- welcome clear information even about the worst news
- welcome the liberty to speak as they wish about their illness and their future rather than join in a charade of deception decided by others
- differ in how much they can take at a time.

The interview
The basic clinical interview described above requires particular attention to certain points:

Opening
- The patient is seen as soon as possible once the current information has been gathered.
- If possible, the patient should have someone with them.
- The interview should take place with everyone introduced, sitting in a quiet place.
- Clinicians must indicate their status and the extent of their responsibility toward the patient and the amount of time available.

Exploring and focusing
- The clinician should find out if anything new has happened since the last encounter.
- What does the patient know and how does the patient react to it? In detail.
- The clinician should then introduce a warning that the news is bad: 'I'm afraid it looks more serious than we hoped.' Then the details.

- At this point the clinician should pause and allow the patient to think, and only continue when the patient gives some lead to follow. This pause may be a long one while thoughts go round in the patient's head, and is often accompanied by shutdown which makes patients unable to hear anything further until these thoughts settle down and allow them to re-emerge.

Only then should the clinician:

- Discover how much the patient is likely to be able to take in at this point – methods for finding this out are shown in Table 1.2.
- Give the information without fudging, in small chunks and make sure that the patient understands each one before moving on.
- Be prepared for the patient to have disorderly emotional responses of some kind and acknowledge them early on as being what you expect and understand and wait for them to settle before continuing. The clinician must learn to judge which patients wish to be touched and which do not. You can always reach out and touch their chair.
- Watch out for shutdown; when it occurs, just wait. When the patient emerges it is best to deal with what they then say, and only after that take up the running.
- Keep pausing to allow the patient to think.
- Stop the interview if necessary and arrange to resume later.

Focusing on planning and support

- The clinician can emphasize that some things are fixable and others are not. A broad time frame can be given for the fixable aspects of care.

Table 1.2 Two ways to find out how much a patient in an oncology clinic wants to know

Buckman (Canada)	An open screening question: 'If this condition turns out to be something serious are you the type of person who likes to know exactly what is going on?'
Sanson-Fisher (Australia)	Explicit categorization by direct questions in succession: 'If you would like to know, I will tell you … 1. What the diagnosis is' 2. What the treatment will be' 3. What sort of symptoms you will have' 4. What examinations and tests will be necessary' 5. What can be done for any physical discomfort or pain you may have' 6. What the outcome might be.'

Buckman R (1994) *How to Break Bad News*. London: Papermac. Reynolds PM, Sanson-Fisher RW et al. (1981) Cancer and Communication. *British Medical Journal* 282: 1449–1451.

- No time frame is ever accurate for the unfixable, but the clinician must be prepared for the question: 'How long have I got?' and avoid the trap of providing a figure which is bound to be inaccurate. Rather stress the importance of ensuring that the quality of life is made as good as possible from day to day.
- The patient must be provided with some positive information and hope tempered with realism.

Closing

The clinician must be sure that:

- the patient has understood what has been discussed so far and that crucial information has been written down for the patient
- the patient knows how to contact the appropriate team member and thus has a safety net in place
- the next interview date – preferably soon – has been agreed, for what purpose and with whom
- other members of the family have been invited to meet the clinicians as the patient wishes
- written material and further sources of information are readily available
- everyone is bid goodbye, starting with the patient.

After the bad news is broken

Patients who are facing the loss of life, limb or liberty can be expected to have many questions that are difficult to answer and to exhibit their own pattern of the disorderly emotions summarized in Table 1.3. The way questions are answered and emotions are empathically treated has a major long-term effect on patients and clinicians alike.

Patients want to know if they are going to die and if so when? Will they be able to stay at home? Will they be in pain? Must they eat if they don't want to? Patients facing the end of life have different priorities from the clinicians, and need clear information about their pain and symptom control, the extent to which they can influence this and how long active treatment will continue. Settling family matters and completing unfinished business come high on their agenda, and must be reconciled with attempts at palliation or treatment, particularly if these are of uncertain benefit. It is the clinician's responsibility to mediate between the patient, other medical staff and the patients' relatives.

Even if there is no medical solution, the clinician has a valuable role at this stage as an empathic experienced professional who can help the patient in many ways.

Table 1.3 Emotional responses to the fact or threat of loss: some or all of these can be expected but in no particular pattern

Despair
Denial
Anger
Bargaining
Depression
Acceptance

Kubler Ross E (1970) *On Death and Dying*. New York: Macmillan

DEALING WITH ADVERSITY

Complaints and lawsuits

The enormous increase in complaints and medicolegal lawsuits is one indication of the importance of communication in healthcare in these consumerist times.

Unfortunately adversity is as unavoidable in healthcare as it is in life. However, hardworking clinicians doing their best do not always respond appropriately to adverse criticism of any kind. They tend not to deal effectively with grumbles and complaints at the appropriate time, which is as soon as they are made, but use avoiding strategies as for other forms of difficulty (see Box 1.10).

In a national commission on patients' complaints, the two main recommendations were that all healthcare professionals should have training in communication and should be aware of their responsibility for dealing promptly with complaints made by patients in their care and not dump them automatically on managers or complaints officers – especially when patients have suffered the results of a mistake or a mishap.

Complaints

The majority of complaints come from the exasperation of patients who:

- have not been able to get clear information
- feel that they are owed an apology
- are concerned that other patients will go through what they have.

Many complaints are resolved satisfactorily once these points are satisfied, and the sooner the better. In these consumerist times, clinicians should not take criticism as a personal affront but respond professionally by providing the information that patients need, not just by a defence or a medical account but in answer to the patient's specific questions. A personal apology, as medical defence organizations emphasize, is not an expression of guilt; it is a common courtesy. Nor should it be wrapped up so cautiously as to become a worthless token.

Clinicians should work in a professional culture which regards complaints as a valuable source of feedback which deserve to be noted, collected systematically and acted upon if need be. The constructive use of complaints is built into the concept of patient involvement in achieving quality in healthcare.

When clinicians learn of a complaint they should:

- be objective, not resentful or defensive – remember that there is a duty of care to the patient in this as every way
- remember that the complainant is still a patient
- allow all the facts to speak through a clear account, verbal or written
- explain the reasons and circumstances behind the facts
- express regret
- explain how things will improve
- leave the medical records strictly unaltered.

Lawsuits

Lawsuits, the extreme form of complaint, are commonly rooted in poor communication arising from:

- delay in providing information to complainants
- misinformation which comes from unclear language and medical jargon
- different words being used by the large number of different healthcare professionals that many patients see
- no clear explanation being given to patients as situations change or when they are discharged
- misunderstanding of the medical records
- failure to provide adequate information during consent procedures.

The difficulty of unravelling these issues is usually complicated by the absence of any record of what the patient was told.

The communication styles that distinguish clinicians who have never been sued (shown in Box 1.9) can help to prevent these frustrations.

A lawsuit is the ultimately wasteful and damaging way of resolving these failures of communication. As in complaints procedures, many patients abandon a lawsuit when they get a clear exposition of the facts which they can see explains their circumstances; something which could usually have been provided long before and should not have arisen in the first place.

Reports

Certain points should be borne in mind when writing in response to a complaint or a court.

The report is for the use of the tribunal (the judge) and not just for representatives of one side. It should be the same regardless of whether the clinician is instructed by the plaintive or the defence.

Writing a legal report is complex and requires the clear separation of the recorded facts from the evidence-based opinions of the experts. It must be comprehensible to the lay members (nearly all) of the tribunal. The clinician who takes on the work of expert witness would be well advised to seek training in the preparation of reports, court procedure and cross-examination. Training is best provided by the firms of solicitors which specialize in this work. Without preparation, the clinician risks failing the court and having an unforgettably bruising experience.

PATIENTS WITH IMPAIRED FACULTIES FOR COMMUNICATION

All healthcare professionals need to exert particular patience and ingenuity, and acquire some special knowledge, when communicating with certain patients with impaired faculties for communication.

Patients with limited understanding or speech. With certain patients, for example with organic brain disease or severe mental disease, clinicians require energy and

Table 1.4 Dos and don'ts of communicating with people who are deaf or hard of hearing (from RAD – Royal Association in Aid of Deaf People)

Smile and use eye contact
If you are stuck write it down
Speak normally, don't mouth slowly
Put your face in a good light
Stay still and don't put things in your mouth
Trim moustaches and beards, avoid sunglasses, big
  earrings or background activity
Never say 'forget it'

imagination to make the best of the limited lines of communication. Open questions are often impossible for them; open directive questions have to be adjusted to the ability of each patient together with every non-verbal gesture, mime or murmur that can help. Just as much ingenuity may be called upon to confirm the meaning of the responses. Third parties involved in the care of the patient can help. Much can be learnt by watching a specialized speech therapist at work.

Patients with impaired hearing. Patients with severely impaired hearing may be accompanied by a signer in one of the two sign languages. Deaf patients who do not use signing are helped by several factors shown in Table 1.4, many of which would not occur to the uninformed.

It is a help for deaf patients to have access to a Minicom – a telephone adapted for the deaf.

Patients whose doctors do not share their cultural background. Patients who do not have the language of their host country or their doctor suffer poor healthcare relative to their socio-economic status, sometimes shamefully so. When such patients depend upon a third party in the form of an interpreter, clinicians must remember to talk to the patient, and not to the interpreter or other third party, to avoid marginalizing the patient and missing what non-verbal communication occurs. Clinicians should also be aware of certain taboos concerning shaking hands, eye contact or topics that cannot be discussed, for example with unmarried women. It is difficult to produce prepared written material for every ethnic group, particularly when these change rapidly. However, members of the patient's community may be able to find appropriate material on the Internet or acquire it otherwise. Another source of help would be a fellow healthcare professional from the same cultural background.

The role of third parties. It has been suggested that all patients are in need of a third party 'advocate' to help them through the foreign language and culture of healthcare. 'I speak perfect English, but I don't speak Biology.'

Patients in all of the above groups often depend on third parties either for their care or as interpreters, as do very many other patients, particularly at the extremes of life.

With the best of intentions third parties may take over the patients in their care, reading their minds and taking

responsibility for them. Whether the patient is with a carer, a relative, another doctor or an interpreter, the clinician should if possible speak to the patient and not to the third party, and make a distinction between what is a straight translation and what the third party is contributing. However, third parties also deserve respect; paediatricians have often been found to communicate more considerately with children than with parents, and the army of carers who look after the disabled are often disregarded by the professionals and family members who may know their charges much less well.

FURTHER READING
Littlewood R, Lipsedge M (1997) *Aliens and Alienists*, 3rd edn. London: Routledge.
Silverman J et al. (1998) *Skills for Communicating with Patients*. London: Radcliffe Press.

IMPROVING COMMUNICATION

In the UK, improving communication is a stated objective in the policy statement of every national, governmental, professional and academic body concerned with healthcare, particularly in respect of increasing the extent to which patients take part in their own healthcare and its management and reducing the wastage of resources from complaints and non-adherence to treatment.

Most UK institutions which offer undergraduate, postgraduate and continuing education diplomas to healthcare professionals now teach and examine the communication skills of the candidates.

The challenge to the professional bodies and to healthcare management equally is:

- to provide facilities, time, resources and trained personnel to develop and support good communication practice in every healthcare professional
- at the same time to motivate healthcare professionals in communication
- to provide patients with accurate accessible information
- to organize systematic regular feedback from patients and the community and respond to the evidence therefrom.

This requires consistent and persistent strategic initiative, money, an effective programme for change management, and the capacity to provide the individual coaching that is needed to change the performance of individuals. In this sort of strategy it is the peer pressure of senior and influential professionals which has the greatest influence.

Improving communication in individuals

There are certain basic factors which contribute to improving communication skills:

- Having clear objectives about the work, the nature of communication and medical interviews and how the basic interview can be adapted to all others.

- Teaching in small groups of learners who get to know each other, all of whom go through the same process. This allows each member to reveal difficulties and weaknesses and to discuss and improve them comfortably.
- Experiential methods are needed; learning by doing it, not by reading the manual.
- Role-play is one cornerstone of learning communication skill – role-play with experienced actors as simulated patients rather than amateur role-players selected from the group.
- Discussion of each simulated consultation is carried out along pre-decided rules of feedback, designed to explore what has happened; working from the strengths of the learner towards weaknesses; among friendly, discreet and equally vulnerable colleagues. Learning from feedback can be enhanced by using a video-recording of the process.
- A few hours' work can only raise awareness. A new skill needs to be practised at least three times and often more before it will stick. Improvement in performance requires coaching until the skill is established, and like any other human activity communication skills need to be exercised regularly.

Teaching the teachers

Widespread improvement in communication will require a lot more teachers and well-motivated learners. All teachers should be taught to teach and supported adequately.

Research

One reason that many clinicians do not know the results of research on communication is that the qualitative and meta-analytic methods used are unfamiliar and are dispersed in non-clinical literature.

Qualitative research seeks to ask broad questions concerning social phenomena in a natural rather than an experimental setting – questions about the meaning, the experience, the views and values of healthcare issues to all participants.

The methods used – observation, in-depth interviews, focus groups and detailed case studies – are complementary rather than antithetical to quantitative research. They are designed to answer the questions that quantitative research cannot reach. For example, while quantitative research demonstrates the dangers of smoking, qualitative research examines what makes people stop or continue doing it.

Research into the effect of communication on health is complicated because in the same patient at the same time, good or bad communication influences every one of the four categories of healthcare issues above. Separating the effects of these variables under research conditions requires meticulous techniques of qualitative care, achieved in certain studies hitherto, but only with great difficulty.

Many questions on communication issues remain to be answered:

- What are the most effective methods of practice and teaching?
- How can clinicians become more self-aware and why do they resist learning communication skills?
- How can clinicians get fast personal feedback?
- To what extent does improved communication influence outcome?
- How can cost–benefit calculations be made in communication practice and how can these best be explained to hard-pressed managers?

FURTHER READING

Crowe, R et al. (1999) The role of expectancies in the placebo effect and their use in the delivery of healthcare: a systematic review. *Health Technology Assessment* **3**(3): 1–96.

Di Blasi, Z (2001) Influence of context effects on health outcomes: a systemic review. *Lancet* **357**: 757–762.

Fallowfield L, Jenkins V (2004) Communicating sad, bad and difficult news in medicine. *Lancet* **363**:312.

Pope C et al. (1995) Reaching the parts other methods cannot reach: an introduction to qualitative methods in health and health services research. *British Medical Journal* **31**: 42–51.

GENERAL READING

Audit Commission of the UK (1993) *What Seems to be the Matter? Communication Between Hospital and Patients*. London: HMSO.

Department of Health (2000) *The NHS Plan: A Plan for Investment. A Plan for Reform*. London: The Stationery Office.

Di Blasi Z et al. (2001) Influence of context effects on health outcomes: a systematic review. *Lancet* **357**: 757–762.

Royal College of Physicians of London (1997) *Improving Communications Between Doctors and Patients*. London: Royal College of Physicians of London.

SIGNIFICANT WEBSITES

http://www.wma.net/e/policy.html
World Medical Association policy
http://www.bma.org.uk/ethics
British Medical Association ethics site
http://www.nih.gov/sigs/bioethics/UK
National Institute of Health website: bioethics pages
http://www.clinical-skills-net.org.uk
UK Clinical Skills Network
http://www.nivel.nl/each
European Association for Communication in Healthcare
http://www.ethics-network.org.uk
UK Clinical Ethics Network
http://www.gmc-uk.org/
General Medical Councul

Infectious diseases, tropical medicine and sexually transmitted diseases

2

INFECTION AND INFECTIOUS DISEASE

Infection remains the main cause of morbidity and mortality in man, particularly in underdeveloped areas where it is associated with poverty and overcrowding. In the developed world increasing prosperity, universal immunization and antibiotics have reduced the prevalence of infectious disease. However, antibiotic-resistant strains of microorganisms and diseases such as human immunodeficiency virus (HIV) infection, variant Creutzfeldt–Jakob disease (vCJD), and severe acute respiratory syndrome (SARS) have emerged. There is increased global mobility, both enforced (as a result of war, civil unrest, and natural disaster), and voluntary (for tourism and economic benefit). This has aided the spread of infectious disease and allowed previously localized pathogens such as SARS and West Nile virus to establish themselves world-wide. An increase in the movement of livestock and animals has enabled the spread of zoonotic diseases like monkeypox, while changes in farming and food-processing methods have contributed to an increase in the incidence of food and water-borne diseases. Deteriorating social conditions in the inner city areas of our major conurbations have facilitated the resurgence of tuberculosis and other infections. Prisons and refugee camps, where large numbers of people are forced to live in close proximity, often under poor conditions, are providing a breeding ground for devastating epidemics of infectious disease. There are new concerns about the deliberate release of infectious agents such as smallpox or anthrax by terrorist groups or national governments.

In the developing world successes such as the eradication of smallpox have been balanced or outweighed by the new plagues. Infectious diseases cause nearly 25% of all human deaths (Table 2.1). Two billion people – one-third of the world's population – are infected with tuberculosis, 500 million people catch malaria every year, and 200 million are infected with schistosomiasis. Infections are often multiple, and there is synergy both between different infections, and between infection and other factors such as malnutrition. Many of the infectious diseases affecting developing countries are preventable or treatable, but continue to thrive owing to lack of money and political will.

The climate also has consequences on diseases. The El Nino Southern Oscillation (ENSO) is a climatic event originating in the Pacific Ocean that affects the weather world-wide, causing droughts and floods. ENSO affects, for example, the cholera risk and malaria epidemics.

Table 2.1 World-wide mortality from infectious diseases

Disease	Estimated deaths (in 2002/2003)
HIV/AIDS	5 million
Acute lower respiratory infection	3.8 million
Tuberculosis	2.5 million
Diarrhoeal disease	1.8 million
Malaria	1.2 million
Measles	760 000
Tetanus	292 000
Whooping cough	301 000
Meningitis	175 000
Leishmaniasis	51 000
Trypanosomiasis	48 000

Infectious agents

The causative agents of infectious diseases can be divided into four groups.

Prions are the most recently recognized and the simplest infectious agents, consisting of a single protein molecule. They contain no nucleic acid and therefore no genetic information: their ability to propagate within a host relies on inducing the conversion of endogenous prion protein PrPc into a protease resistant isoform PrPres.

Viruses contain both protein and nucleic acid, and so carry the genetic information for their own reproduction. However, they lack the apparatus to replicate autonomously, relying instead on 'hijacking' the cellular machinery of the host. They are small (usually less than 200 nanometres in diameter) and each virus possesses only one species of nucleic acid (either RNA or DNA).

Bacteria are usually, though not always, larger than viruses. Unlike the latter they have both DNA and RNA, with the genome encoded by DNA. They are enclosed by a cell membrane, and even bacteria which have adopted an intracellular existence remain enclosed within their own cell wall. Bacteria are capable of fully autonomous reproduction, and the majority are not dependent on host cells.

Eukaryotes are the most sophisticated infectious organisms, displaying subcellular compartmentalization. Different cellular functions are restricted to specific organelles, e.g. photosynthesis takes place in the chloroplasts, DNA transcription in the nucleus and respiration in the mitochondria. Eukaryotic pathogens include unicellular protozoa, fungi (which can be unicellular or filamentous), and multicellular parasitic worms.

Other higher classes, notably the insects and the arachnids, also contain species which can parasitize man and cause disease: these are discussed in more detail on page 117.

Host–organism interactions

Each of us is colonized with huge numbers of microorganisms (10^{14} bacteria, plus viruses, fungi, protozoa, and worms) with which we coexist. The relationship with some of these organisms is symbiotic, in which both partners benefit, while others are commensals, living on the host without causing harm. Infection and illness may be due to these normally harmless commensals and symbiotes evading the body's defences and penetrating into abnormal sites. Alternatively, disease may be caused by exposure to exogenous pathogenic organisms which are not part of our normal flora.

The symptoms and signs of infection are a result of the interaction between host and pathogen. In some cases, such as the early stages of influenza, symptoms are almost entirely due to killing of host cells by the invading organism. Usually, however, the harmful effects of infection are due to a combination of direct microbial pathogenicity, and the body's response to infection. In meningococcal septicaemia, for example, much of the tissue damage is caused by cytokines released in an attempt to fight the bacteria. In a few instances, such as chronic South American trypanosomiasis (Chagas' disease), morbidity is almost entirely immunological, with the parasite itself having little effect once the inflammatory process has been triggered. The molecular mechanisms underlying host–pathogen interactions are discussed in more detail on page 199.

Sources of infection

The endogenous skin and bowel commensals can cause disease in the host, either because they have been transferred to an inappropriate site (e.g. bowel coliforms causing urinary tract infection), or because host immunity has been attenuated (e.g. candidiasis in an immunocompromised host). Many infections are acquired from other people, who may be symptomatic themselves or be asymptomatic carriers. Some bacteria, like the meningococcus, are common transient commensals, but cause invasive disease in a small minority of those colonized. Infection with other organisms, such as the hepatitis B virus, can be followed in some cases by an asymptomatic but potentially infectious carrier state.

Zoonoses are infections that can be transmitted from wild or domestic animals to man. Infection can be acquired in a number of ways: direct contact with the animal, ingestion of meat or animal products, contact with animal urine or faeces, aerosol inhalation, via an arthropod vector, or by inoculation of saliva in a bite wound. Many zoonoses can also be transmitted from person to person. Some zoonoses are listed in Table 2.2.

Most microorganisms do not have a vertebrate or arthropod host but are free-living in the environment. The vast majority of these environmental organisms are non-pathogenic, but a few can cause human disease (Table 2.3). Person-to-person transmission of these infections is rare. Some parasites may have a stage of their life cycle which is environmental (for example the free-living

Table 2.2 Zoonotic infections

Disease	Pathogen	Animal reservoir	Mode of transmission
Prions			
vCJD	Prion protein	Cattle	Ingestion (CNS tissue)
Viral			
Lassa fever	Arenavirus	Multimammate rat	Direct contact
Japanese encephalitis	Flavivirus	Pigs	Mosquito bite
Rabies	Rhabdovirus	Dog and other mammals	Saliva, faeces (bats)
Yellow fever	Flavivirus	Primates	Mosquito bite
Monkey pox	Orthopox virus	Rodents, small mammals	Uncertain
SARS	Coronavirus	Civet cats and small mammals	Droplet
Bacterial			
Gastroenteritis	*Escherichia coli* 0157	Cattle, chickens	Ingestion (meat)
	Salmonella enteritidis and others	Chickens, cattle	Ingestion (meat, eggs)
	Campylobacter jejuni	Various, e.g. chicken	Ingestion (meat, milk, water)
Leptospirosis	*Leptospira interrogans*	Rodents	Ingestion (urine)
Brucellosis	*Brucella abortus*	Cattle	Contact; ingestion of
	Brucella melitensis	Sheep, goats	milk/cheese
Anthrax	*Bacillus anthracis*	Cattle, sheep	Contact; ingestion
Lyme disease	*Borrelia burgdorferi*	Deer	Tick bite
Cat scratch fever	*Bartonella henselae*	Cats	Flea bite
Plague	*Yersinia pestis*	Rodents	Flea bite
Typhus	Various *Rickettsia* spp.	Various	Arthropod bite
Psittacosis (ornithosis)	*Chlamydia psittaci*	Psittacine and other birds	Aerosol
Others			
Toxoplasmosis	*Toxoplasma gondii*	Cats and other mammals	Ingestion (meat, faeces)
Cryptosporidiosis	*Cryptosporidium parvum*	Cattle	Ingestion (faeces)
Hydatid disease	*Echinococcus granulosus*	Dogs	Ingestion (faeces)
Trichinosis	*Trichinella spiralis*	Pigs, beans	Ingestion (meat)
Toxocariasis	*Toxocara canis*	Dogs	Ingestion
Cutaneous larva migrans	*Ancylostoma caninum*	Dogs	Penetration of skin by larvae
Leishmaniasis	*Leishmania* spp.	Dogs	Ingestion

vCJD, variant Creutzfeldt–Jakob disease; SARS, severe acute respiratory syndrome

larval stage of *Strongyloides stercoralis* and the hookworms) even though the adult worm requires a vertebrate host. Other pathogens can survive for periods in water or soil and may be transmitted from host to host via this route (see below): these should not be confused with true environmental organisms.

Routes of transmission

Endogenous infection
The body's own endogenous flora can cause infection if the organism gains access to an inappropriate area of the body. This can happen by simple mechanical transfer, for example colonic bacteria entering the female urinary tract. The non-specific host defences may be breached, for example by cutting or scratching the skin and allowing surface commensals to gain access to deeper tissues; this is frequently the aetiology of cellulitis. There may be more serious defects in host immunity owing to disease or chemotherapy, allowing normally harmless skin and bowel flora to produce invasive disease.

Airborne spread
Many respiratory tract pathogens are spread from person to person by aerosol or droplet transmission.

Secretions containing the infectious agent are coughed, sneezed, or breathed out, and are then inhaled by a new victim. Some enteric viral infections may also be spread by aerosols of faeces or vomit. Environmental pathogens such as *Legionella pneumophila*, and zoonoses such as psittacosis, are also acquired by aerosol inhalation, while rabies virus may be inhaled in the dust from bat droppings.

Faeco-oral spread
Transmission of organisms by the faeco-oral route can occur by direct transfer (usually in small children), by contamination of clothing or household items (usually in institutions or conditions of poor hygiene), or most commonly via contaminated food or water. Human and animal faecal pathogens can get into the food supply at any stage. Raw sewage is used as fertilizer in many parts of the world, contaminating growing vegetables and fruit. Poor personal hygiene can result in contamination during production, packaging, preparation or serving of foodstuffs. In the western world, the centralization of food supply and increased processing of food has allowed the potential for relatively minor episodes of contamination to cause widely disseminated outbreaks of food-borne infection.

Table 2.3 Environmental organisms which can cause human infection

Organism	Disease (most common presentations)
Bacteria	
Burkholderia pseudomallei	Melioidosis
Burkholderia cepacia	Lung infection in cystic fibrosis
Pseudomonas spp.	Various
Legionella pneumophila	Legionnaires' disease (pneumonia)
Bacillus cereus	Gastroenteritis
Listeria monocytogenes	Various
Clostridium tetani	Tetanus
Clostridium perfringens	Gangrene, septicaemia
Mycobacteria other than tuberculosis (MOTT)	Pulmonary infections
Fungi	
Candida sp.	Local and disseminated infection
Cryptococcus neoformans	Meningitis, pulmonary infection
Histoplasma capsulatum	Pulmonary infection
Coccidioides immitis	Pulmonary infection
Mucor spp.	Mucormycosis (rhinocerebral, cutaneous)
Sporothrix schenkii	Lymphocutaneous sporotrichosis
Blastomyces dermatitidis	Pulmonary infection
Aspergillus fumigatus	Pulmonary infections

Table 2.4 Infections transmitted by arthropod vectors

Disease	Infective organism	Vector
Dengue	Flavivirus	Mosquito
Yellow fever		
West Nile fever		
Scrub typhus	*Orientiae tsutsugamushi*	Mite
Rickettsial spotted fevers	*Rickettsia* sp.	Hard tick
Tick-borne relapsing fever	*Borrelia duttoni*	Soft tick
Louse-borne relapsing fever	*Borrelia recurrentis*	Body louse
Carrión's disease	*Bartonella bacilliformis*	Sandfly
Lyme disease	*Borrelia burgdorferi*	Hard tick
Plague	*Yersinia pestis*	Flea
Malaria	*Plasmodium* sp.	Mosquito
Lymphatic filariasis	*Wuchereria bancrofti*	Mosquito
	Brugia malayi	Mosquito
Onchocerciasis	*Onchocerca volvulus*	Blackfly
Leishmaniasis	*Leishmania* sp.	Sandfly
African trypanosomiasis	*Trypanosoma brucei*	Tsetse fly
South American trypanosomiasis	*Trypanosoma cruzi*	Reduviid bug

Water-borne faeco-oral spread is usually the result of inadequate access to clean water and safe sewage disposal, and is common throughout the developing world. Global coverage for access to clean drinking water is 83% of the world population but global sanitation coverage is currently 58%.

Vector-borne disease

Many tropical infections, including malaria, are spread from person to person or from animal to person by an arthropod vector. Vector-borne diseases are also found in temperate climates, but are relatively uncommon. In most cases part of the parasite life cycle takes place within the body of the arthropod, and each parasite species requires a specific vector. Simple mechanical transfer of infective organisms from one host to another can occur, but is rare. Some vector-borne diseases are shown in Table 2.4.

Direct person-to-person spread

Organisms can be passed on directly in a number of ways. Sexually transmitted infections are dealt with on page 117. Skin infections such as ringworm, and ectoparasites such as scabies and head lice, can be spread by simple skin-to-skin contact. Other organisms are passed on by blood- (or occasionally other body fluid) to-blood transmission. In some cases such as HIV and hepatitis B virus this is the only route: in others such as malaria and Chagas' disease it is an unusual alternative to the normal arthropod vector. Blood-to-blood transmission can occur during sexual contact, from mother to infant peripartum, between intravenous drug users sharing any part of their injecting equipment, when infected medical equipment is reused, if contaminated blood or blood products are transfused, or in any sporting or accidental contact when blood is spilled.

Direct inoculation

Infection can occur when pathogenic organisms breach the normal mechanical defences by direct inoculation. Some of the circumstances in which this can occur are covered under endogenous infection and blood-to-blood transmission above. Some environmental organisms may be inoculated by accident: this is a common mode of transmission of tetanus and certain fungal infections. Rabies virus may be inoculated by the bite of an infected animal.

Consumption of infected material

Although many food-related zoonotic infections are due to contamination of food with animal faeces (and are thus, strictly speaking, faeco-oral), several diseases are transmitted directly in animal products. These include some strains of salmonella (eggs, chicken meat), brucellosis (unpasteurized milk), and the prion diseases kuru and vCJD (neural tissue).

Prevention and control

Methods of preventing infection depend upon the source and route of transmission, as described above.

- *Eradication of reservoir.* In a few diseases, for which man is the only natural reservoir of infection, it may be possible to eliminate disease by an intensive programme of case finding, treatment and immunization. This has been achieved in the case of smallpox. If there is an animal or environmental reservoir complete eradication is unlikely, but local control methods may decrease the risk of human infection (for example killing of rodents to control plague, leptospirosis, and other diseases).

■ *For arthropod-vector-borne infections:*
  – destroying vector species (which may be practical in certain circumstances)
  – taking measures to avoid being bitten (e.g. insect repellent sprays, bed nets).
■ *For food-borne infections.* Improvements in food handling and preparation result in less contamination during processing, transport or preparation. Organisms intrinsically present in food can be killed by appropriate preparation and cooking. Improved surveillance and regulation of the food industry, as well as better health education for the public is necessary.
■ *For faeco-oral infections.* Thirty per cent of the world's population do not have access to adequate safe drinking water, and over half do not have adequate sanitation. Improvements in water supply could dramatically decrease the prevalence of faeco-oral infections.
■ *For blood-borne infections.* Prevention of blood transfer, e.g. in blood transfusions and contaminated medical equipment. Donated blood is routinely tested for infection in most developed countries.
■ *For infections spread by airborne and direct contact.* Some airborne-transmitted respiratory infections, and some infections spread by direct contact, can be controlled by isolating patients. This is often difficult, but isolation is useful in patients with severe immunodeficiency to protect them from infection.
■ *Immunization* (p. 42).

Cases of some infectious diseases should be notified to the public health authorities so that they are aware of cases and outbreaks. Diseases that are notifiable in England and Wales are listed in Table 2.5.

FURTHER READING
Kovats, RS et al. (2003) El Nino and health. *Lancet* **362**: 1481–1489.
Health Protection Agency website:
  http://www.hpa.org.uk
[Various authors] (2000) Articles on all aspects of zoonoses. *Revue Scientifique et Technique* **19**(1): 33–317.
World Health Report 2003. Online. Available:
  http://www.who.int/whr/2003/en.

PRINCIPLES AND BASIC MECHANISMS

Man constantly interacts with the world of microorganisms from birth to death. The majority cause no harm and some play a role in the normal functioning of the mouth, vagina and lower intestinal tract. However, many microorganisms have the potential to produce

Table 2.5   Notifiable diseases in England & Wales under the Public Health (Infectious Diseases) Regulations 1988

Acute encephalitis
Acute poliomyelitis
Anthrax
Cholera
Diphtheria
Dysentery (amoebic or bacillary)
Food poisoning
Leprosy
Leptospirosis
Malaria
Measles
Meningitis
Meningococcal septicaemia (without meningitis)
Mumps
Ophthalmia neonatorum
Paratyphoid fever
Plague
Rabies
Relapsing fever
Rubella
Scarlet fever
Smallpox
Tetanus
Tuberculosis
Typhoid fever
Typhus
Viral haemorrhagic fever
Viral hepatitis
Whooping cough
Yellow fever

disease. This may result from inoculation of damaged tissues, tissue invasion, a variety of virulence factors or toxin production.

Specificity

Microorganisms are often highly specific with respect to the organ or tissue they infect. For example, a number of viruses are hepatotropic, such as those responsible for hepatitis A, B, C and E and yellow fever. This predilection for specific sites in the body relates partly to the immediate environment in which the organism finds itself; for example, anaerobic organisms colonize the anaerobic colon, whereas aerobic organisms are generally found in the mouth, pharynx and proximal intestinal tract. Other organisms that show selectivity include:

■ *Streptococcus pneumoniae* (respiratory tract)
■ *Escherichia coli* (urinary and alimentary tract).

Even within a species of bacterium such as *E. coli*, there are clear differences between strains with regard to their ability to cause gastrointestinal disease (p. 69), which in turn differ from uropathogenic *E. coli* responsible for urinary tract infection.

Within an organ a pathogen may show selectivity for a particular cell type. In the intestine, for example, rotavirus predominantly invades and destroys intestinal epithelial cells on the upper portion of the villus, whereas reovirus selectively enters the body through the specialized epithelial cells, known as M cells, that cover the Peyer's patches (see p. 287).

Pathogenesis

Figure 2.1 summarizes some of the steps that occur during the pathogenesis of infection. In addition, pathogens have developed a variety of mechanisms to evade host defences. For example, some pathogens produce toxins directed at phagocytes – *Staphylococcus aureus* (α-toxin), *Strep. pyogenes* (streptolysin) and *Clostridium perfringens* (γ-toxin), while others such as *Salmonella* spp. and *Listeria monocytogenes* can survive within macrophages. Several pathogens possess a capsule that protects against complement activation (*Strep.*

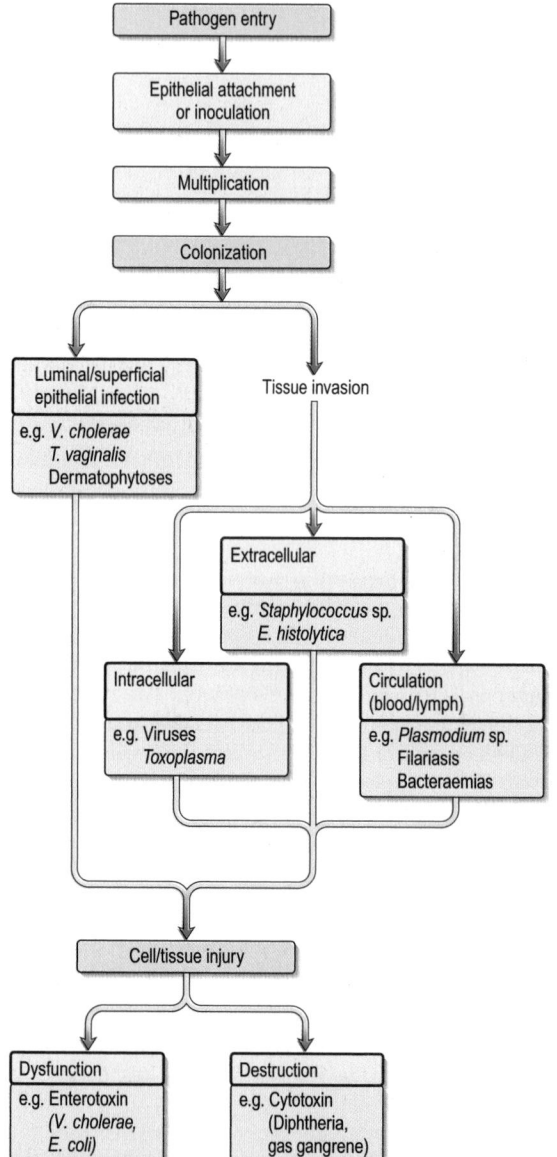

Fig. 2.1 **The pathogenesis of infection.**

pneumoniae). Antigenic variation is an additional mechanism for evading host defences that is recognized in viruses (antigenic shift and drift in influenza), bacteria (flagella of salmonella and gonococcal pili), and protozoa (surface glycoprotein changes in *Trypanosoma*).

Epithelial attachment

Many bacteria attach to the epithelial substratum by specific organelles called pili (or fimbriae) that contain a surface lectin(s) – a protein or glycoprotein that recognizes specific sugar residues on the host cell. This family of molecules is known as adhesins (see p. 198). Following attachment, some bacteria, such as coagulase-negative staphylococci (*Staph. epidermidis*), produce an extracellular slime layer and recruit additional bacteria, which cluster together to form a biofilm. These biofilms can be difficult to eradicate, and are a frequent cause of medical device-associated infections which affect prosthetic joints and heart valves as well as indwelling catheters. Some viruses (e.g. HIV) and protozoa (e.g. *Plasmodium* spp., *Entamoeba histolytica*) attach to specific target-cell receptors. Other parasites such as hookworm have specific attachment organs (buccal plates) that firmly grip the intestinal epithelium.

Colonization

Following epithelial attachment, pathogens may either remain on the surface epithelium or within the lumen of the organ they have colonized. Tissue invasion may follow.

Invasion may result in:

■ an intracellular location for the pathogen (e.g. viruses, *Toxoplasma gondii*, *Mycobacterium* spp., *Plasmodium* spp.)
■ an extracellular location for the pathogen (e.g. pneumococci, *E. coli* and *Entamoeba histolytica*)
■ invasion directly into the blood or lymph circulation (e.g. schistosome schistosomula and trypanosomes).

Once the pathogen is firmly established in its target tissue, a series of events follows that usually culminates in damage to the host.

Tissue dysfunction or damage

Microorganisms produce disease by a number of well-defined mechanisms:

Exotoxins and endotoxins

■ *Exotoxins* have many diverse activities including inhibition of protein synthesis (diphtheria toxin), neurotoxicity (*Clostridium tetani* and *C. botulinum*) and enterotoxicity, which results in intestinal secretion of water and electrolytes (*E. coli*, *Vibrio cholerae*).
■ *Endotoxin* is a lipopolysaccharide (LPS) in the cell wall of Gram-negative bacteria. It is responsible for many of the features of septic shock (see p. 967), namely hypotension, fever, intravascular coagulation and, at high doses, death. The effects of endotoxin are mediated predominantly by release of tumour necrosis factor.

Staph. aureus presents an excellent example of the repertoire of microbial virulence. The clinical expression of disease varies according to site, invasion and toxin production and is summarized in Table 2.6. Furthermore, host susceptibility to infection may be linked to genetic or acquired defects in host immunity that may complicate intercurrent infection, injury, ageing and metabolic disturbances (Table 2.7).

Host response to infection

Natural defences

The natural host defences to infection are those of an intact surface epithelium with local production of secretions, antimicrobial enzymes (e.g. lysozyme in the eye) and in the stomach, gastric acidity. The mucociliary escalator of the large airways is unique to the lung,

Table 2.6 Clinical conditions produced by *Staphylococcus aureus*

Due to invasion	Bones and joints
Skin	Osteomyelitis, arthritis
Furuncles	
Cellulitis	**Miscellaneous**
Impetigo	Parotitis
Carbuncles	Pyomyositis
	Septicaemia
Lungs	Enterocolitis
Pneumonia	
Lung abscesses	**Due to toxin**
	Staphylococcal food
Heart	poisoning
Endocarditis	Scalded skin syndrome
Pericarditis	Bullous impetigo
	Staphylococcal scarlet fever
Central nervous system	Toxic shock syndrome
Meningitis	
Brain abscesses	

Table 2.7 Examples of host factors that increase susceptibility to staphylococcal infections (predominantly *S. aureus*)

Injury to skin or mucous membranes	Abnormal leucocyte function
Abrasions	Job's syndrome
Trauma (accidental or surgical)	Chediak–Higashi syndrome
	Steroid therapy
Burns	Drug-induced leucopenia
Insect bites	
	Postviral infections
Metabolic abnormalities	Influenza
Diabetes mellitus	
Uraemia	**Miscellaneous conditions**
	Excess alcohol consumption
Foreign bodies*	Malnutrition
Intravenous and other indwelling catheters	Malignancies
	Old age
Cardiac and orthopaedic prosthesis	
Tracheostomies	

* Often *Staphylococcus epidermidis*

Immunological defences

Antibody and cell-mediated immune mechanisms play a vital role in combating infection. All organisms can initiate secondary immunological mechanisms, such as complement activation, immune complex formation and antibody-mediated cytolysis of cells. The immunological response to infection is described in Chapter 4.

Metabolic and immunological consequences of infection

Fever

Body temperature is controlled by the thermoregulatory centre in the anterior hypothalamus in the floor of the third ventricle. Gram-negative bacteria contain lipo-polysaccharide (LPS) and peptidoglycan, which is also a component of Gram-positive bacterial cell walls. Toll-like receptors (TLR, p. 202) on monocytes and dendritic cells recognize these lipopolysaccharides and generate signals leading to formation of inflammatory cytokines, e.g. IL-1, -6, -12, TNF-α and many others. These cytokines act on the thermoregulatory centre by increasing prostaglandin (PGE$_2$) synthesis. The antipyretic effect of salicylates is brought about, at least in part, through its inhibitory effects on prostaglandin synthase.

Fever production has a positive effect on the course of infection. However, for every 1°C rise in temperature, there is a 13% increase in resting metabolic rate and oxygen consumption. Fever therefore leads to increased energy requirements at a time when anorexia leads to decreased food intake. The normal compensatory mechanisms in starvation (e.g. mobilization of fat stores) are inhibited in acute infections. This leads to an increase in skeletal muscle breakdown, releasing amino acids, which, via gluconeogenesis, are used to provide energy.

Tumour necrosis factor (TNF)

TNF-α is released from a variety of phagocytic cells (macrophages/monocytes) and TNF-β from non-phagocytic cells (lymphocytes, natural killer cells) in response to infections (bacterial endotoxin) and inflammatory stimuli. TNF itself then stimulates the release of a cascade of other mediators involved in inflammation and tissue remodelling, such as interleukins (IL-1 and IL-6), prostaglandins, leukotrienes and corticotropin. TNF is therefore responsible for many of the effects of an infection.

The biological behaviour of the pathogen and the consequent host response are responsible for the clinical expression of disease that often allows clinical recognition. The incubation period following exposure can be helpful (e.g. chickenpox 14–21 days). The site and distribution of a rash may be diagnostic (e.g. shingles) while symptoms of cough, sputum and pleuritic pain point to lobar pneumonia. Fever and meningismus characterize classical meningitis. Infection may remain localized or become disseminated and give rise to the sepsis syndrome and disturbances of protein metabolism

FURTHER READING
Bassler BL (2002) Small talk: cell-to-cell communication in bacteria. *Cell* **109**: 421–424.
Ghannoum M, O'Toole GA (2004) *Microbial Biofilm.* Washington DC: ASM Press.
Opal SM, DePalo V (2000) Anti-inflammatory cytokines. *Chest* **117**: 1162–1172.
Opal SM, Huber CE (2002) The toll-like receptors and their role in septic shock. *Critical Care* **6**: 125–136.
Vallance BA, Finlay BB (2000) Exploitation of host cells by enteropathogenic *Escherichia coli. Proceedings of the National Academy of Sciences of the United States of America* **97**(16): 8799–8806.

and acid–base balance (Ch. 15). Many infections are self-limiting, and immune and non-immune host defence mechanisms will eventually clear the pathogens. This is generally followed by tissue repair, which may result in complete resolution or leave residual damage.

APPROACH TO THE PATIENT WITH A SUSPECTED INFECTION

Infectious diseases can affect any organ or system, and can cause a wide variety of symptoms and signs. Fever is often regarded as the cardinal feature of infection, but not all febrile illnesses are infections, and not all infectious diseases present with a fever. History-taking and examination should aim to identify the site(s) of infection, and also the likely causative organism(s).

History

A detailed history is taken with specific questions about epidemiological risk factors for infection. These are based on the sources of infection and routes of transmission discussed above.

- Travel history: some diseases are more prevalent in certain geographical locations, and many infections common in the tropics are seen rarely if at all in the UK.
- Food and water history: systemic as well as gastro-enteric infections can be caught via this route.
- Occupational history.
- Animal contact: domestic, farm and wild animals can all be responsible for zoonotic infection.
- Sexual activity: as well as the traditional sexually trans-mitted diseases, HIV, hepatitis B and very occasionally hepatitis C can all be transmitted sexually. Some enteric infections are more common among male homosexuals.
- Intravenous drug use: as well as blood-borne viruses, drug injectors are susceptible to a variety of bacterial and fungal infections due to inoculation. Tattooing, body piercing and receipt of blood products (especially outside the UK) are also risk factors for blood-borne viruses.
- Leisure activities: certain pastimes may predispose to water-borne infections or zoonoses.

Clinical examination

A thorough examination covering all systems is required. Skin rashes and lymphadenopathy are common features of infectious diseases, and the ears, eyes, mouth and throat should also be inspected. Infections commonly associated with a rash are listed in Box 2.1. Rectal, vaginal and penile examination is required in sexually transmitted infections.

The fever pattern may occasionally be helpful, e.g. the tertian fever of falciparum malaria, but too much weight should not be placed on the pattern or degree.

Investigations

In some infections such as chickenpox the clinical presentation is so distinctive that no investigations are normally necessary to confirm the diagnosis. Other cases require investigation.

 Box 2.1 Infections commonly associated with a rash

Macular/maculopapular
Measles
Rubella
Enteroviruses
Human herpesvirus 6
Epstein–Barr virus
Cytomegalovirus
Parvovirus
Human immunodeficiency virus (HIV)
Dengue
Typhoid
Secondary syphilis
Rickettsia – spotted fevers

Vesicular
Chickenpox (herpes zoster virus)
Shingles (herpes zoster virus)
Herpes simplex virus
Hand, foot and mouth disease (Coxsackie virus)
Herpangina (Coxsackie virus)

Petechial/haemorrhagic
Meningococcal septicaemia
Any septicaemia with disseminated intravascular coagulation (DIC)
Tick typhus
Viruses (Table 2.23)

Erythematous
Scarlet fever
Lyme disease (erythema chronicum migrans)
Toxic shock syndrome

Urticarial
Toxocariasis
Strongyloidiasis
Schistosomiasis
Cutaneous larva migrans

Others
Tick typhus (eschar)
Primary syphilis (chancre)
Anthrax (ulcerating papule)

General investigations (to assess health and identify organ(s) involved)

These will vary depending on circumstances:

- **Blood tests**. Routine blood count, ESR and C-reactive protein, biochemical profile, urea and electrolytes are performed in the majority of cases (Box 2.2).
- **Imaging**. X-ray, ultrasound, echocardiography, CT and MR scanning are used to identify and localize infections. Biopsy or aspiration of tissue for microbiological examination may also be facilitated by ultrasound or CT guidance.
- **Radionuclide scanning** after injection of indium- or technetium-labelled white cells (previously harvested from the patient) may occasionally help to localize infection. It is most effective when the peripheral white cell count is raised, and is of particular value in localizing occult abscesses.

Microbiological investigations (to identify causative organism)

Diagnostic services range from simple microscopy to molecular probes. It is often helpful to discuss the clinical problem with a microbiologist to ensure that appropriate tests are performed, and that specimens are collected and transported correctly.

Microscopy and culture

Specimens to be sent for microscopy and culture (Box 2.3).

Box 2.2 General investigations for a patient with suspected infection

Investigation	Possible cause
Full blood count	
Neutrophilia	Bacterial infection
Neutropenia	Viral infection
	Brucellosis
	Typhoid
	Typhus
	Overwhelming sepsis
Lymphocytosis	Viral infection
Lymphopenia	HIV infection (not specific)
Atypical lymphocytes	Infectious mononucleosis
Eosinophilia	Invasive parasitic infection
Thrombocytopenia	Overwhelming sepsis
	Malaria
ESR or C-reactive protein	All
Urea and electrolytes	Potentially deranged in severe illness from any cause
Liver enzymes	
Minor elevation of transferases	Non-specific feature of many infections
	Mild viral hepatitis
Grossly deranged transferases, elevated bilirubin	Viral hepatitis (usually A, B or E)
Coagulation	May be deranged in hepatitis, and in overwhelming infection of any type

Box 2.3 Specimens and indications for microscopy and culture

Specimen	Investigation	Indication
Blood	Giemsa stain for malaria	Any symptomatic traveller returning from a malarious area
	Stains for other parasites	Specific tropical infections
	Culture	All suspected bacterial infections
Urine	Microscopy and culture	All suspected bacterial infections
	Tuberculosis (TB) culture	Suspected TB
		Unexplained leucocytes in urine
Faeces	Microscopy ± iodine stain	Suspected protozoal diarrhoea
	Culture	All unexplained diarrhoea
	Electron microscopy/viral culture (not usually necessary to do both)	Suspected viral diarrhoea in children
		Viral meningitis
	Clostridium difficile toxin	Diarrhoea following hospital stay or antibiotic treatment
Throat swabs	Culture	Suspected bacterial tonsillitis and pharyngitis
	Viral culture	Viral meningitis
		Viral respiratory infections where urgent diagnosis is considered necessary
Sputum	Microscopy and culture	Unusual chest infections; pneumonia
	Auramine stain/TB culture	Suspected TB
	Other special stains/cultures	Immunocompromised patients
		Suspected fungal infections
Cerebrospinal fluid	Microscopy and culture	Suspected meningitis
	Auramine stain/TB culture	Suspected TB, meningitis
	Other special stains/cultures	Immunocompromised patients
		Suspected fungal infections
	Polymerase chain reaction	Suspected encephalitis or viral or bacterial meningitis
Rash aspirate:		
Petechial	Microscopy and culture	Meningococcal disease
Vesicular	Viral culture	Herpes simplex/zoster

■ *Blood and urine* should routinely be sent for bacterial culture regardless of whether fever is present at the time.

■ *Cerebrospinal fluid, sputum and biopsy* specimens are sent if clinically indicated.

■ *Special culture techniques* are required for fungi, mycobacteria, and some other bacteria such as *Brucella* spp., and the laboratory must be informed if these are suspected.

■ *Faeces* should not routinely be sent for viral investigations: viral gastroenteritis is rare except in infants and the institutionalized elderly, and is self-limiting. Protozoa should be considered as a cause of diarrhoea in returning travellers, immunocompromised patients, toddlers, homosexual men, farm workers, and in any cases of prolonged unexplained diarrhoea. Detection of a specific clostridial toxin is a more reliable test for diarrhoea caused by *Clostridium difficile* than culture of the organism itself. Stool culture is a costly routine test and is often requested indiscriminately.

Immunodiagnostic tests

These can be divided into two types:

■ tests that detect viral or bacterial antigen, using a polyvalent antiserum or a monoclonal antibody
■ tests that detect serological response to infection.

These investigations are valuable in the identification of organisms that are difficult to culture, especially viruses and fungi, and can also be helpful when antibiotics have been administered before samples were obtained. However, care is needed in the interpretation of serological tests. Elevated antibody titres on a single occasion (especially of IgG) are rarely diagnostic, and in some infections it may be difficult to distinguish between old and acute infection. Paired serological tests a few weeks apart, or specific assays for IgM (indicating an acute infection) are more helpful.

Nucleic acid detection

Specific genes from many pathogenic microorganisms have been cloned and sequenced. Nucleic acid probes can be designed to detect these sequences, identifying pathogen-specific nucleic acid in body fluids or tissue. The utility of this approach has been greatly enhanced by the development of amplification techniques such as the polymerase chain reaction (PCR), which increases the amount of target DNA/RNA in the sample to be tested. However PCR assays for many organisms are still in the process of development.

Treatment

Many infections, particularly those caused by viruses, are self-limiting and require no treatment. The mainstay of treatment for most infectious diseases is antimicrobial chemotherapy. The choice of antibiotic should be governed by:

■ the clinical state of the patient
■ the likely cause of the infection.

Serious infections may require supportive therapy in addition to antibiotics. It is always preferable to have a definite microbial diagnosis before starting treatment, so that an antibiotic with the most appropriate spectrum of activity and site of action can be used. However, some patients are too unwell to wait for results (which in the case of culture may take days). In diseases such as meningitis or septicaemia delay in treatment may be fatal and therapy must be started on an empirical basis. Appropriate samples for culture should be taken before the first dose of antibiotic, and an antibiotic regimen chosen on the basis of the most likely causative organisms. Usually patients are less unwell, and specific therapy can be deferred pending results. Antibiotic therapy is discussed in more detail on page 30.

Special circumstances

Overseas travellers. A detailed travel itinerary, including any flight stopovers should be taken from anyone who is unwell after arriving in this country from abroad. Previous travel should also be covered as some infections may be chronic or recurrent. It is necessary to find out not just which countries were visited but also the type of environment: a stay in a remote jungle village carries different health risks from a holiday in an air-conditioned coastal holiday resort. Food and water consumption, bathing and swimming habits, animal and insect contact, and contact with human illness all need to be recorded. Enquiry should be made about sexual contacts, drug use and medical treatment (especially parenteral) while abroad. In some parts of the world over 90% of professional sex workers are HIV positive, and hepatitis B and C are very common in parts of Africa and Asia. In addition to the investigations described in the previous section, special tests may be needed depending on the epidemiological risks and clinical signs, and malaria films are mandatory in anyone who is unwell after being in a malarious area. Some of the more common causes of a febrile illness in returning travellers to the UK are listed in Table 2.8.

Table 2.8 Causes of febrile illness in travellers returning to the UK	
Tropical countries	**Specific geographical areas**
Malaria	**(see text)**
Schistosomiasis	Histoplasmosis
Dengue	Brucellosis
Tick typhus	
	World-wide
Economically less-	Pneumonia
developed countries	URTI
Typhoid	UTI
Tuberculosis	Traveller's diarrhoea
Dysentery	Viral infection
Hepatitis A	
Amoebiasis	
URTI, upper respiratory tract infection; UTI, urinary tract infection	

Immunocompromised patients. Advances in medical treatment over the past three decades have led to a huge increase in the number of patients living with immuno-deficiency states. Cancer chemotherapy, the use of immunosuppressive drugs and the world-wide AIDS epidemic have all contributed to this. The presentation may be very atypical in the immunocompromised patient with few, if any, localizing signs or symptoms. Infection can be due to organisms which are not usually pathogenic, including environmental bacteria and fungi. The normal physiological responses to infection (e.g. fever, neutro-philia) may be diminished or absent. The onset of symptoms may be sudden, and the course of the illness fulminant. A high index of suspicion for infections in people who are known to be immunosuppressed is required. These patients should usually be given early and aggressive antibiotic therapy without waiting for the results of investigations. Samples for culture should be sent before starting treatment, but therapy should not be delayed if this proves difficult. The choice of antibiotics should be guided by the likely causative organisms: these are shown in Box 2.4.

Highly transmissible infections. Relatively few patients with infectious disease present a serious risk to healthcare workers (HCW) and other contacts. However, the appearance of diseases like severe acute respiratory syndrome (SARS), the occasional importation of zoonoses like Lassa fever, and concerns about the bioterrorist use of agents such as smallpox mean that there is still the potential for unexpected outbreaks of life-threatening disease. During the world-wide SARS outbreak in 2003, scrupulous infection control procedures reduced spread of infection. However, in the 'inter-epidemic' period it is difficult to maintain the same level of 'alert'. HCWs should remain vigilant because the early symptoms of many of these diseases are non-specific.

Pyrexia of unknown origin

History, clinical examination and simple investigation will reveal the cause of a fever in most patients. In a small number, however, no diagnosis is apparent despite continuing symptoms. The term pyrexia (or fever) of unknown origin (PUO) is sometimes used to describe this problem. Various definitions have been suggested for PUO: a useful one is 'a fever persisting for > 2 weeks, with no clear diagnosis despite intelligent and intensive investigation'. Patients who are known to have HIV or other immunosuppressing conditions are normally excluded from the definition of PUO, as the investigation and management of these patients is different.

Successful diagnosis of the cause of PUO depends on a knowledge of the likely and possible aetiologies. These have been documented in a number of studies, and are summarized in Box 2.5.

ⓘ Box 2.4 Common causes of infection in immunocompromised patients

Deficiency	Causes	Organisms
Neutropenia	Chemotherapy Myeloablative therapy Immunosuppressant drugs	*Escherichia coli* *Klebsiella pneumoniae* *Staphylococcus aureus* *Staph. epidermidis* *Aspergillus* spp. *Candida* spp.
Cellular immune defects	HIV infection Lymphoma Myeloablative therapy Congenital syndromes	Respiratory syncytial virus Cytomegalovirus Epstein–Barr virus Herpes simplex and zoster *Salmonella* spp. *Mycobacterium* spp. (esp. *M. avium-intracellulare*) *Cryptococcus neoformans* *Candida* spp. *Cryptosporidium parvum* *Pneumocystis carinii* *Toxoplasma gondii*
Humoral immune deficiencies	Congenital syndromes Chronic lymphocytic leukaemia Corticosteroids	*Haemophilus influenzae* *Streptococcus pneumoniae* Enteroviruses
Terminal complement deficiencies (C5–C9)	Congenital syndromes	*Neisseria meningitidis* *N. gonorrhoeae*
Splenectomy	Surgery Trauma	*Strep. pneumoniae* *N. meningitidis* *H. influenzae* Malaria

Box 2.5 Causes of pyrexia of unknown origin

Infection (20–40%)
Pyogenic abscess
Tuberculosis
Infective endocarditis
Toxoplasmosis
Epstein–Barr virus (EBV) infection
Cytomegalovirus (CMV) infection
Primary HIV infection
Brucellosis
Lyme disease

Malignant disease (10–30%)
Lymphoma
Leukaemia
Renal cell carcinoma
Hepatocellular carcinoma

Collagen vascular disease (15–20%)
Adult Still's disease
Rheumatoid arthritis
Systemic lupus erythematosus
Wegener's granulomatosis
Giant cell arteritis

Miscellaneous (10–25%)
Drug fevers
Thyrotoxicosis
Inflammatory bowel disease
Sarcoidosis
Granulomatous hepatitis
Factitious fever
Familial Mediterranean fever

Undiagnosed (5–25%)

and temporal artery biopsy should be considered in the elderly (p. 583). Bronchoscopy can be used to obtain samples for microbiological and histological examination if sputum specimens are not adequate. Serological tests have greatly improved the diagnosis of infectious causes of PUO, but should be used with caution. The more tests that are done, the greater is the danger of a false positive or misleading result, and serological tests should only be ordered and interpreted in the context of the clinical findings and epidemiology.

Treatment of a patient with a persistent fever is aimed at the underlying cause, and if possible only symptomatic treatment should be used until a diagnosis is made. Blind antibiotic therapy may make diagnosis of an occult infection more difficult, and empirical steroid therapy may mask an inflammatory response without treating the underlying cause. In a few patients no cause for the fever is found despite many months of investigation and follow-up. In most of these the symptoms do eventually settle spontaneously, and if no definite cause has been identified after 2 years the long-term prognosis is good.

FURTHER READING
Ellis C (2004) The returned traveller. *Clinical Medicine* **4**: 506–509.
Mourad O, Palda A, Detsky A (2003) A comprehensive evidence-based approach to fever of unknown origin. *Archives of Internal Medicine* **163**: 545–551.
Vanderschuerren S, Knochaert D, Adrianssens T et al. (2003) Prolonged febrile illness to fever of unknown origin. *Archives of Internal Medicine* **163**: 1033–1041.

A detailed history and examination is essential, taking into account the possible causes, and the examination should be repeated on a regular basis in case new signs appear. Investigation findings to date should be reviewed, obvious omissions amended and abnormalities followed up. Confirm that the patient does have objective evidence of a raised temperature: this may require admission to hospital if the patient is not already under observation. Some people have an exaggerated circadian temperature variation (usually peaking in the evening), which is not pathological.

The range of tests available is discussed above. Obviously investigation is guided by particular abnormalities on examination or initial test results, but in some cases 'blind' investigation is necessary. Some investigations, especially cultures, should be repeated regularly, and serial monitoring of inflammatory markers such as C-reactive protein allows assessment of progress.

Improvements in imaging techniques have diminished the need for invasive investigations in PUO, and scanning has now superseded the blind diagnostic laparotomy. Ultrasound, echocardiography, CT, MRI, and labelled white cell scanning can all help in establishing a diagnosis if used appropriately: the temptation to scan all patients with PUO from head to toe as a first measure should be avoided. Biopsy of liver and bone marrow may be useful even in the absence of obvious abnormalities,

ANTIMICROBIAL CHEMOTHERAPY

Principles of use

Antibiotics are among the safest of drugs, especially those used to treat community infections. They have had a major impact on the life-threatening infections and reduce the morbidity associated with surgery and many common infectious diseases. This in turn is, in part, responsible for the overprescribing of these agents which has led to concerns with regard to the increasing incidence of antibiotic resistance.

Most antibiotic prescribing, especially in the community, is empirical. Even in hospital practice, microbiological documentation of the nature of an infection and the susceptibility of the pathogen is generally not available for a day or two. Initial choice of therapy relies on a clinical diagnosis and, in turn, a presumptive microbiological diagnosis. Such 'blind therapy' is directed at the most likely pathogen(s) responsible for a particular syndrome such as meningitis, urinary tract infection or pneumonia. Initial therapy in the severely ill patient is often broad spectrum in order to cover the range of possible pathogens but should be narrowed down once microbiological information becomes available.

Bactericidal versus bacteriostatic

In the majority of infections there is no firm evidence that bactericidal drugs (penicillins, cephalosporins, aminoglycosides) are more effective than bacteriostatic drugs, but it is generally considered necessary to use the former in the treatment of bacterial endocarditis and in patients in whom host defence mechanisms are compromised, particularly in those with neutropenia.

Combinations of drugs are occasionally required for reasons other than providing broad-spectrum cover. Tuberculosis is initially treated with three or four agents to avoid resistance emerging. Synergistic inhibition is achieved by using penicillin and gentamicin in enterococcal endocarditis or gentamicin and ceftazidime in life-threatening pseudomonas infection.

Pharmacokinetic factors

To be successful, sufficient antibiotic must penetrate to the site of the infection. Knowledge of the standard pharmacokinetic considerations of absorption, distribution, metabolism and excretion for the various drugs is required. Difficult sites include the brain, eye and prostate, while loculated abscesses are inaccessible to most agents.

Many mild-to-moderate infections can be treated effectively with oral antibiotics provided that the patient is compliant. Parenteral administration is indicated in the severely ill patient to ensure rapid high blood and tissue concentrations of drug. Some antibiotics can only be administered parenterally, such as the aminoglycosides and extended-spectrum cephalosporins. Parenteral therapy is also required in those unable to swallow or where gastrointestinal absorption is unreliable.

Dose and duration of therapy

This will vary according to the nature, severity and response to therapy.

Prolonged treatment (up to 6 weeks) is necessary for some varieties of infective endocarditis, while pulmonary tuberculosis is treated for at least 6 months. In treating many common infections, improvement occurs within 2–3 days; once the patient is afebrile or the leucocytosis has settled, oral administration should be considered for those commenced on parenteral therapy. Treatment for 5–7 days is adequate for most infections. Shorter-course therapy (3 days or less) is appropriate for those with symptomatic uncomplicated bacteriuria (cystitis). Minimizing the duration of therapy lowers the risks of adverse reactions and superinfection with *Candida* spp. or *Clostridium difficile*, as well as the cost of therapy.

Drugs which are concentrated intracellularly, such as erythromycin, quinolones and tetracyclines are used in treating mycoplasma, brucella and legionella infections.

Renal and hepatic insufficiency

Many drugs require dose reduction in renal failure to avoid toxic accumulation. This applies to the β-lactams and especially the aminoglycosides and vancomycin. Tetracyclines, other than doxycycline and minocycline, should be avoided. In those with hepatic insufficiency, caution or dose reduction is required for agents such as isoniazid, ketoconazole, clindamycin, interferon and rifampicin.

Therapeutic drug monitoring

To ensure therapeutic yet non-toxic drug concentrations, serum concentrations of drugs such as the aminoglycosides and vancomycin are monitored, especially in those with impaired or changing renal function. Peak (1 hour post-dose) and trough (pre-dose) serum samples are assayed. However, with the increasing use of once-daily aminoglycoside dosage regimens, random but timed serum assays are being adopted.

Antibiotic chemoprophylaxis

The value of antibiotic chemoprophylaxis has been questioned as there are few controlled trials to prove efficacy (p. 832). However, there are still a number of indications for which the prophylactic use of antibiotics is still advised (Table 2.9). These include surgical procedures where the risk of infection is high (colon surgery) or the consequences of infection are serious (endocarditis, post-splenectomy sepsis). The choice of agent(s) is determined by the likely infectious risk and the established efficacy and safety of the regimen.

Table 2.9 Antibiotic chemoprophylaxis		
Clinical problem	**Aim**	**Drug regimen***
Infective endocarditis (IE)	To prevent infection in: **High risk**, e.g: Previous IE Prosthetic heart valves Mitral valve prolapse with MR or thickened valve leaflets Complex congenital heart disease	**Dental, oral, respiratory tract or oesophageal procedures** Amoxicillin, 3 g oral 1 hour pre-procedure or 2 g IV < 30 min pre-procedure Note: with previous IE add gentamicin 1.5 mg/kg IV < 30 min pre-procedure If allergic to penicillin use clindamicin
	Moderate risks, e.g. Acquired valvular heart disease Non-cyanotic congenital heart defects Structural cardiac abnormalities	**Genitourinary or gastrointestinal procedures** Amoxicillin and gentamicin If allergic to penicillin use vancomicin and gentamicin
Splenectomy/spleen malfunction	To prevent serious pneumococcal sepsis	Phenoxymethylpenicillin 500 mg 12-hourly *Cont'd*

Table 2.9 (Cont'd) Antibiotic chemoprophylaxis

Clinical problem	Aim	Drug regimen*
Rheumatic fever	To prevent recurrence and further cardiac damage	Phenoxymethylpenicillin 250 g × 2 daily or sulfadiazine 1g if allergic to penicillin
Meningitis: Due to meningococci	To prevent infection in close contacts	Adults: rifampicin 600 mg twice-daily for 2 days (Children < 1 year: 5 mg/kg; > 1 year: 10 mg/kg) Alternatives (single dose) ciprofloxacin 500 mg (p.o.) or ceftriaxone 250 mg (i.m)
Due to *H. influenzae* type b	To reduce nasopharyngeal carriage and prevent infection in close contacts	Adults: rifampicin 600 mg daily for 4 days (Children: < 3 months 10 mg/kg; > 3 months 20 mg/kg)
Tuberculosis	To prevent infection in exposed (close contacts) tuberculin-negative individuals, infants of infected mothers and immunosuppressed patients	Oral isoniazid 300 mg daily for 6 months (Children: 5–10 mg/kg daily)

* Unless stated, doses are those recommended in adults
Note: new guidelines for IE laid down by AGREE (Appraisal of Guidelines for Research and Evaluation), http://www.agreecollabration.org/

Mechanisms of action and resistance to antimicrobial agents

Antibiotics act at different sites of the bacterium (Table 2.10).

Resistance to an antibiotic can be the result of:

- impaired or altered permeability of the bacterial cell envelope, e.g. penicillins in Gram-negative bacteria
- active expulsion from the cell by membrane efflux systems
- alteration of the target site (e.g. single point mutations in *E. coli* or a penicillin-binding protein in *Strep. pneumoniae* leading to acquired resistance – see below)
- specific enzymes which inactivate the drug before or after cell entry
- development of a novel metabolic bypass pathway.

Table 2.10 Site of action of antibiotics

Site of action	Antibiotic
Cell wall	Penicillin, cephalosporins, vancomycin, monobactams
Inhibits protein synthesis	Macrolides, aminoglycosides, tetracyline, oxazolidinones
Inhibits RNA synthesis	Rifampicin
Inhibits DNA synthesis	Quinolones and metronidazole
Folic acid antagonists	Sulphonamides and trimethoprim

The development or acquisition of resistance to an antibiotic by bacteria invariably involves either a mutation at a single point in a gene or transfer of genetic material from another organism (Fig. 2.2).

Fig. 2.2 **Some mechanisms for the development of resistance to antimicrobial drugs.** These involve either a single point mutation or transfer of genetic material from another organism (transformation, transduction or R factor transfer).

Larger fragments of DNA may be introduced into a bacterium either by transfer of 'naked' DNA or via a bacteriophage (a virus) DNA vector. Both the former (transformation) and the latter (transduction) are dependent on integration of this new DNA into the recipient chromosomal DNA. This requires a high degree of homology between the donor and recipient chromosomal DNA.

Finally, antibiotic resistance can be transferred from one bacterium to another by conjugation, when extra-chromosomal DNA (a plasmid) containing the resistance factor (R factor) is passed from one cell into another during direct contact. Transfer of such R factor plasmids can occur between unrelated bacterial strains and involve large amounts of DNA and often codes for multiple antibiotic resistance.

Transformation is probably the least clinically relevant mechanism, whereas transduction and R factor transfer are usually responsible for the sudden emergence of multiple antibiotic resistance in a single bacterium. Increasing resistance to many antibiotics has developed (Table 2.11).

FURTHER READING

Finch RG, Williams RJ (eds) (1999) Antibiotic resistance. Baillière's Clinical Infectious Diseases. London: Baillière Tindall.

Hughes WT, Armstrong D, Bodey GP et al. (2002) Guidelines for the use of antimicrobial agents in neutropenic patients with cancer. *Clinical Infectious Diseases* **34**: 730–751.

Murray BE (2000) Vancomycin-resistant enterococcal infections. *New England Journal of Medicine* **342**: 710–721.

Ramsdale DR, Turner-Stokes L (2004) Prophylaxis and treatment of infective endocarditis in adults. *Clinical Medicine* **4**: 545–55.

Stalam M, Kaye D (2000) Antibiotic agents in the elderly. *Infectious Disease Clinics of North America* **14**: 357–369.

Steinke D, Davey P (2001) Association between antibiotic resistance and community prescribing: a critical review of bias and confounding in published studies. *Clinical Infectious Diseases* **33** (Suppl 3): S193–S205.

ANTIBACTERIAL DRUGS

β-Lactams (penicillins, cephalosporins and monobactams)

Penicillins (Table 2.12)

Structure. The β-lactams share a common ring structure (Fig. 2.3). Changes to the side-chain of benzylpenicillin (penicillin G) render the phenoxymethyl derivative (penicillin V) acid resistant and allow it to be orally absorbed. The presence of an amino group in the phenyl radical of benzylpenicillin increases its antimicrobial spectrum to include many Gram-negative and Gram-positive organisms. More extensive modification of

Table 2.11 Some bacteria that have developed resistance to common antibiotics

Pathogen	Previously fully sensitive to
Streptococcus pneumoniae	Penicillin, erythromycin, cefotaxime
Strep. pyogenes	Erythromycin, tetracycline
Staphylococcus aureus	Penicillin, methicillin, ciprofloxacin
Neisseria gonorrhoeae	Penicillin, ciprofloxacin
Haemophilus influenzae	Amoxicillin, chloramphenicol
Enterobacteria	Amoxicillin, trimethoprim, ciprofloxacin, gentamicin
Salmonella spp.	Amoxicillin, sulphonamides, ciprofloxacin
Shigella spp.	Amoxicillin, trimethoprim, tetracycline
Pseudomonas aeruginosa	Gentamicin

Table 2.12 Classification of penicillins

Benzylpenicillin and its long-acting parenteral relatives	Extended-spectrum penicillins
Benzylpenicillin	Ampicillin, pivampicillin,* talampicillin*
Benethamine penicillin*	Amoxicillin
Benzathine penicillin*	Co-amoxiclav, pivmecillinam
Clemizole penicillin*	Co-fluampicil
Procaine benzylpenicillin (procaine penicillin)	
	Penicillins active against *Pseudomonas*
Oral alternatives to benzylpenicillin	Azlocillin,* mezlocillin,* piperacillin, ticarcillin
Azidocillin*	
Phenoxymethylpenicillin (penicillin V)	
β-Lactamase-stable penicillins	
Flucloxacillin	
Oxacillin*	
Methicillin*	
Nafcillin*	

* Not available in the UK

Fig. 2.3 The structure of penicillins.

the side-chain (e.g. as in flucloxacillin) renders the drug insensitive to bacterial penicillinase. This is useful in treating infections caused by penicillinase (β-lactamase)-producing staphylococci.

Mechanisms of action. β-lactams block bacterial cell wall mucopeptide formation by binding to and inactivating specific penicillin-binding proteins (PBPs), which are peptidases involved in the final stages of cell wall assembly and division. Methicillin-resistant *Staph. aureus* (MRSA) (see p. 63) produce a low-affinity PBP which retains its peptidase activity even in the presence of high concentrations of methicillin.

Indications for use. Benzylpenicillin can only be given parenterally and is often the drug of choice for serious infections, notably infective endocarditis, meningococcal, streptococcal, clostridial infections (tetanus, gas gangrene), actinomycosis, anthrax, and spirochaetal infections (syphilis, yaws).

Phenoxymethylpenicillin (penicillin V) is an oral preparation that is used chiefly to treat streptococcal pharyngitis and as prophylaxis against rheumatic fever.

Flucloxacillin is used in infections caused by penicillinase-producing staphylococci.

Ampicillin is susceptible to penicillinase, but its antimicrobial activity includes streptococci, pneumococci and enterococci as well as Gram-negative organisms such as *Salmonella* spp., *Shigella* spp., *E. coli*, *H. influenzae* and *Proteus* spp. Drug resistance has, however, eroded its efficacy against these Gram-negatives. It is widely used in the treatment of respiratory tract infections. Amoxicillin has similar activity to ampicillin, but is better absorbed when given by mouth.

The extended-spectrum penicillin, ticarcillin is active against pseudomonas infections, as is the acylureido-penicillin piperacillin in combination with sulbactam.

Clavulanic acid is a powerful inhibitor of many bacterial β-lactamases and when given in combination with an otherwise effective agent such as amoxicillin (co-amoxiclav) or ticarcillin can broaden the spectrum of activity of the drug. Sulbactam acts similarly and is available combined with ampicillin, while tazobactam in combination with piperacillin is effective in appendicitis, peritonitis, pelvic inflammatory disease, and complicated skin infections. The penicillin β-lactamase combinations are also active against β-lactamase-producing staphylococci.

Pivmecillinam has significant activity against Gram-negative bacteria including *E. coli*, *Klebsiella*, *Enterobacter* and salmonellae but no activity against pseudomonas.

Interactions. Penicillins inactivate aminoglycosides when mixed in the same solution.

Toxicity. Generally, the penicillins are very safe. Hypersensitivity (skin rash (common), urticaria, anaphylaxis), encephalopathy and tubulointerstitial nephritis can occur. Ampicillin also produces a hypersensitivity rash in

Fig. 2.4 **The structure of a cephalosporin.**

approximately 90% of patients with infectious mononucleosis who receive this drug. Co-amoxiclav causes a cholestatic jaundice six times more frequently than amoxicillin.

Cephalosporins and cephamycins (Fig. 2.4)

The cephalosporins have an advantage over the penicillins in that they are resistant to staphylococcal penicillinases (but are still inactive against methicillin-resistant staphylococci) and have a broader range of activity that includes both Gram-negative and Gram-positive organisms, but excludes enterococci and anaerobic bacteria. Ceftazidime and cefpirome are active against *Pseudomonas aeruginosa*. Cefoxitin is a cephamycin.

Indications for use (Table 2.13). These potent broad-spectrum antibiotics are useful for the treatment of serious systemic infections, particularly when the precise nature of the infection is unknown. They are commonly used for serious sepsis in postoperative and immuno-compromised patients, particularly during cytotoxic chemotherapy of leukaemia and other malignancies. They are used in pneumonia, meningitis, peritonitis and urinary tract infections.

Interactions. There are relatively few interactions.

Toxicity. The toxicity is similar to that of the penicillins but is less common. Some 10% of patients are allergic to both groups of drugs. The early cephalosporins caused proximal tubule damage, although the newer derivatives have fewer nephrotoxic effects.

Monobactams

Aztreonam is currently the only member of this class available. It is a synthetic β-lactam and, unlike the penicillins and cephalosporins, has no ring other than the β-lactam, hence its description as a monobactam.

Its mechanism of action is by inhibition of bacterial cell wall synthesis. It is resistant to most β-lactamases and does not induce β-lactamase production.

Indications for use. Aztreonam's spectrum of activity is limited to aerobic Gram-negative bacilli. With the exception of urinary tract infections, aztreonam should be used in combination with metronidazole (for anaerobes) and an agent active against Gram-positive cocci (a

Table 2.13 Some examples of cephalosporins

	Activity	Use
First generation Cefalexin (oral) Cefradine (oral) Cefadroxil (oral)	Gram-positive cocci and Gram-negative organisms Penicillin allergy	Urinary tract infections

Second generation
Cefuroxime
Cefamandole
	Extended spectrum
	More effective than first generation against
	  E. coli, Klebsiella spp. and *Proteus mirabilis*,
	  but less effective against Gram-positive
	  organisms
		Prophylaxis and treatment of Gram-negative
		  infections and mixed aerobic–anaerobic infections

Cefoxitin Cefaclor (oral) Cefuroxime (oral) Cefprozil (oral)	Includes *Bacteroides fragilis*	Peritonitis

Third generation
Cefotaxime
Ceftazidime
	Broad-spectrum
	More potent against aerobic Gram-negative
	  bacteria than first or second generation
		Especially severe infection with Enterobacteriaceae,
		  Pseudomonas aeruginosa (ceftazidime, cefpirome)
		  and *Neisseria gonorrhoeae, N. meningitidis,* Lyme
		  disease (ceftriaxone)

Cefpirome Ceftriaxone Cefpodoxime (oral) Cefixime (oral)		Urinary tract infections and infections with neutropenia Once daily. Septicaemia, pneumonia, meningitis
Fourth generation Cefepime*	Aerobic Gram-negative bacteria including *P. aeruginosa*	Febrile, neutropenic patients

* Unavailable in the UK

penicillin or erythromycin). It is a useful alternative to aminoglycosides in combination therapy, largely for the treatment of intra-abdominal sepsis.

Toxicity.   As for the β-lactam antibiotics.

Carbapenems

The carbapenems are semisynthetic β-lactams and include imipenem, meropenem and ertapenem. They are currently the most broad spectrum of antibiotics, being active against the majority of Gram-positive and Gram-negative as well as anaerobic bacterial pathogens. Ertapenem, unlike the others, is not active against *Pseudomonas* or *Acinetobacter* spp. They differ in their dosage and frequency of administration. Imipenem is partially inactivated in the kidney by enzymatic inactivation and is therefore administered in combination with cilastatin.

Indications for use.   They are used for serious nosocomial infections when multiple-resistant Gram-negative bacilli or mixed aerobe and anaerobe infections are suspected.

Toxicity.   This is similar to that of β-lactam antibiotics. Nausea, vomiting and diarrhoea occur in less than 5% of cases. Imipenem may cause seizures and should not be used to treat meningitis; meropenem is safe for this indication.

Aminoglycosides

Structure.   These antibiotics are polycationic compounds of amino sugars (Fig. 2.5).

Mechanism of action.   Aminoglycosides interrupt bacterial protein synthesis by inhibiting ribosomal function (messenger and transfer RNA).

Indications for use.   Streptomycin is bactericidal and is rarely used except for the treatment of tuberculosis. Occasional indications include endocarditis (with penicillin/ampicillin). Neomycin is used only for the topical treatment of eye and skin infections. Even though it is poorly absorbed, prolonged oral administration can produce ototoxicity.

Gentamicin and tobramycin are given parenterally. They are highly effective against many Gram-negative organisms including *Pseudomonas* spp. They are

Fig. 2.5   **The structure of an aminoglycoside.**

synergistic with a penicillin against *Enterococcus* spp. Netilmicin and amikacin have a similar spectrum but are more resistant to the aminoglycoside-inactivating enzymes (phosphorylating, adenylating or acetylating) produced by some bacteria. Their use should be restricted to gentamicin-resistant organisms.

Interactions Enhanced nephrotoxicity occurs with other nephrotoxic drugs, ototoxicity with some diuretics, and neuromuscular blockade with curariform drugs.

Toxicity. This is dose-related. Aminoglycosides are nephrotoxic and ototoxic (vestibular and auditory), particularly in the elderly. Therapeutic drug monitoring is necessary in ensuring therapeutic and non-toxic drug concentrations.

Tetracyclines

Structure. These are bacteriostatic drugs possessing a four-ring hydronaphthacene nucleus (Fig. 2.6). Included among the tetracyclines are tetracycline, oxytetracycline, demeclocycline, lymecycline, doxycycline and minocycline.

Mechanism of action. Tetracyclines inhibit bacterial protein synthesis by interrupting ribosomal function (transfer RNA).

Indications for use. Tetracyclines are active against Gram-positive and Gram-negative bacteria but their use is now limited, partly owing to increasing bacterial resistance. A tetracycline is used for the treatment of acne and rosacea. Tetracyclines are also active against *V. cholerae*, *Rickettsia* spp., *Mycoplasma* spp., *Coxiella burnetii*, *Chlamydia* spp. and *Brucella* spp. Resistance is now common with *Strep. pneumoniae*.

Interactions. The efficacy of tetracyclines is reduced by antacids and oral iron-replacement therapy.

Toxicity. Tetracyclines are generally safe drugs, but they may enhance established or incipient renal failure, although doxycycline is safer than others in this group.

Tetracycline

Fig. 2.6 **The structure of a tetracycline.** Substitution of CH_3, OH or H at positions A to D produces variants of tetracycline.

They cause brown discoloration of growing teeth, and thus these drugs are not given to children or pregnant women. Photosensitivity can occur.

Macrolides

Erythromycin

Structure. Erythromycin consists of a lactone ring with unusual sugar side-chains.

Mechanism of action. Erythromycin inhibits protein synthesis by interrupting ribosomal function.

Indications for use. Erythromycin has a similar (but not identical) antibacterial spectrum to penicillin and is useful in individuals with penicillin allergy. It can be given orally or parenterally. It is the preferred agent in the treatment of pneumonias caused by *Legionella* spp. and *Mycoplasma* spp. It is also effective in the treatment of infections due to *Bordetella pertussis* (whooping cough), *Campylobacter* spp., *Chlamydia* spp. and *Coxiella* spp.

Other macrolides

These include clarithromycin, azithromycin and telithromycin. They have a broad spectrum of activity that includes selective Gram-negative organisms, mycobacteria and *Toxoplasma gondii*. Compared with erythromycin, they have superior pharmacokinetic properties with enhanced tissue and intracellular penetration and longer half-life that allows once or twice daily dosage. Clarithromycin is widely recommended as a component of triple therapy regimens (usually with a proton pump inhibitor and amoxicillin) for the eradication of *Helicobacter pylori*. Azithromycin is used for trachoma (see p. 84).

Interactions. Erythromycin and other macrolides interact with theophyllines, carbamazepine, digoxin and ciclosporin, occasionally necessitating dose adjustment of these agents.

Toxicity. Diarrhoea, vomiting and abdominal pain are the main side-effects of erythromycin (less with clarithromycin and azithromycin) and are, in part, a consequence of the intestinal prokinetic properties of the macrolides. Macrolides may also rarely produce cholestatic jaundice after prolonged treatment. QT_c prolongation is a recognized cardiac effect of the macrolides. This may have serious consequences if the syndrome of 'torsades de pointes' is induced.

Chloramphenicol

Structure. Chloramphenicol is the only naturally occurring antibiotic containing nitrobenzene (Fig. 2.7). This structure probably accounts for its toxicity in humans and for its activity against bacteria.

Fig. 2.7 **The structure of chloramphenicol.**

Mechanism of action. Chloramphenicol competes with messenger RNA for ribosomal binding. It also inhibits peptidyl transferase.

Indications for use. Chloramphenicol is rarely used in developed countries. In developing countries it has been invaluable in the treatment of severe infections caused by *Salmonella typhi* and *S. paratyphi* (enteric fevers) and *H. influenzae* (meningitis and acute epiglottitis) which are still prevalent in countries where Hib vaccination has not been introduced. It is also active against *Yersinia pestis* (plague) and is used topically for the treatment of purulent conjunctivitis. Drug resistance is currently eroding the efficacy of chloramphenicol.

Interactions. Chloramphenicol enhances the activity of anticoagulants, phenytoin and oral hypoglycaemic agents.

Toxicity. Severe irreversible bone marrow suppression is rare but nevertheless now restricts the usage of this drug to only the severely ill patient. Chloramphenicol should not be given to premature infants or neonates because of their inability to conjugate and excrete this drug; high blood levels lead to circulatory collapse and the often fatal 'grey baby syndrome'.

Fusidic acid

Structure. Fusidic acid has a structure resembling that of bile salts (see p. 350).

Mechanism of action. It is a potent inhibitor of bacterial protein synthesis. Its entry into cells is facilitated by the detergent properties inherent in its structure.

Indications for use. Fusidic acid is mainly used for penicillinase-producing *Staph. aureus* infections such as osteomyelitis (it is well concentrated in bone) or endo-carditis, and for other staphylococcal infections accompanied by septicaemia. The drug is well absorbed orally but is relatively expensive and should be used in combination with another staphylococcal agent to prevent resistance emerging.

Resistance. Resistance may occur rapidly and is the reason why fusidic acid is given in combination with another antibiotic.

Toxicity. Fusidic acid may occasionally be hepatotoxic but is generally a safe drug and if necessary can be given during pregnancy.

Sulphonamides and trimethoprim

Structure. The sulphonamides are all derivatives of the prototype sulphanilamide. Trimethoprim is a 2,4-diaminopyrimidine.

Mechanism of action. Sulphonamides block thymidine and purine synthesis by inhibiting microbial folic acid synthesis. Trimethoprim prevents the reduction of dihydrofolate to tetrahydrofolate (see Fig. 8.12).

Indications for use. Sulfamethoxazole is mainly used in combination with trimethoprim (as co-trimoxazole). Its use is now largely restricted to the treatment and prevention of *Pneumocystis carinii* infection and listeriosis in developed countries, although it is still in widespread use in developing countries. It may also be used for toxoplasmosis and nocardiosis and as a second-line agent in acute exacerbations of chronic bronchitis and in urinary tract infections. Trimethoprim alone is often used for urinary tract infections and acute-on-chronic bronchitis, as the side-effects of co-trimoxazole are most commonly due to the sulphonamide component. Sulfapyridine in combination with 5-aminosalicylic acid (i.e. sulfasalazine) is used in inflammatory bowel disease.

Resistance. Resistance to sulphonamides is often plasmid-mediated and results from the production of sulphonamide-resistant dihydropteroate synthetase from altered bacterial cell permeability to these agents.

Interactions. Sulphonamides potentiate oral anti-coagulants and hypoglycaemic agents.

Toxicity. Sulphonamides cause a variety of skin eruptions, including toxic epidermal necrolysis, the Stevens–Johnson syndrome, thrombocytopenia, folate deficiency and megaloblastic anaemia with prolonged usage. It can provoke haemolysis in individuals with glucose-6-phosphate dehydrogenase deficiency and therefore should not be used in such people. Co-trimoxazole should also be avoided in the elderly if possible, as deaths have been recorded, probably owing to the sulphonamide component.

Quinolones

The quinolone antibiotics, such as ciprofloxacin, norfloxacin, ofloxacin and levofloxacin, are useful oral broad-spectrum antibiotics, related structurally to nalidixic acid. The latter achieves only low serum

Fig. 2.8   The structure of a quinolone (ciprofloxacin).

Fig. 2.9   The structure of linezolid, an oxazolidinone.

concentrations after oral administration and its use is limited to the urinary tract where it is concentrated. Newer quinolones, including moxifloxacin, gemifloxacin and gatifloxacin, have greater activity against Gram-positive pathogens. The structure is shown in Figure 2.8.

Mechanism of action.   The quinolone group of bactericidal drugs inhibit bacterial DNA synthesis by inhibiting topoisomerase IV and DNA gyrase, the enzyme responsible for maintaining the superhelical twists in DNA.

Indications for use.   The extended-spectrum quinolones such as ciprofloxacin have activity against Gram-negative, including *Pseudomonas aeruginosa*, and some Gram-positive bacteria (e.g. anthrax, p. 82). They are useful in Gram-negative septicaemia, skin and bone infections, urinary and respiratory tract infections, meningococcal carriage, in some sexually transmitted diseases such as gonorrhoea and non-specific urethritis due to *Chlamydia trachomatis*, and in severe cases of travellers' diarrhoea (see p. 70). The newer oral quinolones provide an alternative to β-lactams in the treatment of community-acquired lower respiratory tract infections.

Resistance.   In many countries 10–20% of *E. coli* are resistant.

Interactions.   Ciprofloxacin can induce toxic concentrations of theophylline.

Toxicity.   Gastrointestinal disturbances, photosensitive rashes and occasional neurotoxicity can occur. Avoid in childhood and pregnancy. Tendon damage including rupture has been reported.

Oxazolidinones

Structure.   The oxazolidinones are a novel class of antibacterial agents of which linezolid (Fig. 2.9) is the first to become available.

Mechanism of action.   The oxazolidinones inhibit protein synthesis by binding to the bacterial 23S ribosomal RNA of the 59S sub-unit, thereby preventing

the formation of a functional 70S complex essential to bacterial translation.

Indications for use.   Linezolid is active against a variety of Gram-positive pathogens including vancomycin-resistant *Enterococcus faecium* (unfortunately resistant organisms have already been reported), methicillin-resistant *Staph. aureus* and penicillin-resistant *Strep. pneumoniae*. It is also active against group A and group B streptococci. Clinical experience has demonstrated efficacy in a variety of hospitalized patients with severe to life-threatening infections, such as bacteraemia, hospital-acquired pneumonia and skin and soft tissue infections. It can be given both intravenously and by mouth.

Interactions.   Linezolid interacts reversibly as a non-selective inhibitor of monoamine oxidase, and has the potential for interacting with serotoninergic and adrenergic agents.

Toxicity.   Side-effects include gastrointestinal disturbances, headache, rash, hypertension and reversible thrombocytopenia. Safety has not yet been shown in pregnancy.

Nitroimidazoles

Structure.   These agents are active against anaerobic bacteria and some pathogenic protozoa. The most widely used drug is metronidazole (Fig. 2.10). Others include tinidazole and nimorazole.

Mechanism of action.   After reduction of their nitro group to a nitrosohydroxyl amino group by microbial enzymes, nitroimidazoles cause strand breaks in microbial DNA.

Fig. 2.10   The structure of metronidazole, a nitroimidazole.

Indications for use. Metronidazole plays a major role in the treatment of anaerobic bacterial infections, particularly those due to *Bacteroides* spp. It is also used prophylactically in colonic surgery. It may be given orally, by suppository (well absorbed and cheap) or intravenously (very expensive). It is also the treatment of choice for amoebiasis, giardiasis and infection with *Trichomonas vaginalis.*

Interactions. Nitroimidazoles can produce a disulfiram-like reaction with ethanol and enhance the anticoagulant effect of warfarin.

Toxicity. Nitroimidazoles are tumorigenic in animals and mutagenic for bacteria, although carcinogenicity has not been described in humans. They cause a metallic taste, and polyneuropathy with prolonged use. They should be avoided in pregnancy.

Glycopeptides

The glycopeptides are antibiotics active against Gram-positive bacteria and act by inhibiting cell wall synthesis.

Vancomycin

Vancomycin is given intravenously for methicillin-resistant *Staph. aureus* and other multiresistant Gram-positive organisms. It is also used for treatment and prophylaxis against Gram-positive infections in penicillin-allergic patients. It is used for *Strep. pneumoniae* meningitis when caused by penicillin-resistant strains. By mouth it is an alternative to metronidazole for *Clostridium difficile*-associated colitis. Vancomycin-resistant enterococci (VRE) are now seen, as well as vancomycin-resistant *Staphylococcus* (p. 63).

Toxicity. Vancomycin can cause ototoxicity and nephrotoxicity and thus serum levels should be monitored. Care must be taken to avoid extravasation at the injection site as this causes necrosis and thrombophlebitis. Too rapid infusion can produce symptomatic release of histamine (red man syndrome).

Teicoplanin

This glycopeptide antibiotic is less nephrotoxic than vancomycin. It has more favourable pharmacokinetic properties, allowing once-daily dosage.

Other antibiotics

Clindamycin is not widely used because of its toxic side-effect, antibiotic-associated colitis (pseudomembranous colitis). It is active against Gram-positive cocci including some penicillin-resistant staphylococci. It is also active against anaerobes, especially bacteroides. It is well concentrated in bone and used for osteomyelitis.

Quinupristin and dalfopristin. A combination of these streptogramin antibiotics is used for Gram-positive bacteria which have failed to respond to other antibacterials.

Table 2.14	Antifungal agents
Polyenes	**Allylamines**
Amphotericin, nystatin	Terbinafine
Echinocandins	**Other antifungals**
Caspofungin	Amorolfine (topical only)
	5-Flucytosine
Azoles	Griseofulvin
Miconazole, ketoconazole, fluconazole, itraconazole, voriconazole	
Topical clotrimazole, sulconazole, tolnaftate, econazole, tioconazole	

ANTITUBERCULOSIS DRUGS

These are described on page 932. Rifampicin is also used in other infections apart from tuberculosis.

ANTIFUNGAL DRUGS (Table 2.14)

Polyenes

Polyenes react with the sterols in fungal membranes, increasing permeability and thus damaging the organism. The most potent is amphotericin, which is used intravenously in severe systemic fungal infections. Nephrotoxicity is a major problem and dosage levels must take background renal function into account. Liposomal amphotericin is less toxic but very expensive. Nystatin is not absorbed through mucous membranes and is therefore useful for the treatment of oral and enteric candidiasis and for vaginal infection. It can only be given orally or as pessaries.

Azoles

Imidazoles such as ketoconazole, miconazole and clotrimazole are broad-spectrum antifungal drugs. They are predominantly fungistatic and act by inhibiting fungal sterol synthesis, resulting in damage to the cell wall. Ketoconazole is active orally but can produce liver damage. It is effective in candidiasis and deep mycoses including histoplasmosis and blastomycosis but not in aspergillosis and cryptococcosis.

Clotrimazole and miconazole are used topically for the treatment of ringworm and cutaneous and genital candidiasis. Econazole and tioconazole are used for the topical treatment of cutaneous and vaginal candidiasis and dermatophyte infections.

Triazoles. These include fluconazole, voriconazole and itraconazole. Fluconazole is noted for its ability to enter CSF and is used for candidiasis and for the treatment of central nervous system (CNS) infection with *Cryptococcus neoformans.* Itraconazole fails to penetrate CSF. It is the agent of choice for non-life-threatening blastomycosis and histoplasmosis. It is also moderately effective in invasive aspergillosis. Toxicity is mild. The problem associated with poor absorption of the capsules in the absence of food has been overcome with the liquid formulation. Voriconazole has broad-spectrum activity that includes *Candida*, *Cryptococcus* and *Aspergillus* spp. and other filamentous fungi. It is available for oral and intravenous use. Adverse effects include rash, visual disturbance and abnormalities of liver enzymes. It is indicated for invasive aspergillosis and severe candida infections unresponsive to amphoteracin and fluconazole respectively.

Allylamines

Terbinafine has antifungal and anti-inflammatory activity orally and is useful for the treatment of superficial mycoses such as dermatophyte infections, onychomycosis and cutaneous candidiasis. A topical formulation is also available to treat fungal skin infections.

Echinocandins

This is a new class of antifungals which act by inhibiting the cell wall polysaccharide, glucan. Caspofungin is active against *Candida* spp. and *Aspergillus* spp. and is indicated for serious aspergillosis unresponsive to other drugs. It is administered intravenously.

Other antifungals

Flucytosine. The fluorinated pyridine derivative, flucytosine, is used in combination with amphotericin B for systemic fungal infection. Side-effects are uncommon, although it may cause bone marrow suppression. It is active when given orally or parenterally.

Griseofulvin. Griseofulvin, a naturally occurring antifungal, is widely used for the treatment of more extensive superficial mycoses and onychomycosis.

Amorolfine. Amorolfine is available for the topical treatment of fungal skin and nail infections.

ANTIVIRAL DRUGS

Drugs for HIV infection are discussed on page 144.

Nucleoside analogues

Aciclovir. Aciclovir (Fig. 2.11) is an acyclic nucleoside analogue which acts as a chain terminator of herpesvirus DNA synthesis. This drug is converted to aciclovir monophosphate by a virus-encoded thymidine kinase produced by alpha herpesviruses, herpes simplex types 1 and 2 and varicella zoster virus (Table 2.15). Conversion to the triphosphate is then achieved by cellular enzymes. Aciclovir triphosphate competes with deoxyguanine triphosphate and the drug is incorporated into the growing chains of herpesvirus DNA. This highly specific mode of activity, targeted only to virus-infected cells, means that aciclovir has very low toxicity. Intravenous,

Aciclovir

Fig. 2.11 The structure of aciclovir.

Table 2.15 Antiviral agents (for drugs against HIV see Table 2.53)

Drug	Use
Nucleoside analogues	
Aciclovir	Topical – HSV infection
	Oral and intravenous – VZV and HSV
Famciclovir	Oral – VZV and HSV
Valaciclovir	Oral – VZV and HSV
Ganciclovir	Intravenous and oral – CMV
Valganciclovir	Oral – CMV
Adefovir	Oral – HBV infection
Cidofovir	Intravenous – CMV
Pyrophosphate analogues	
Foscarnet	Intravenous – CMV
Adamantanes	
Amantadine	Oral – influenza A
Neuraminidase inhibitors	
Zanamivir	Topical (inhalation) – influenza A and B
Oseltamivir	Oral – influenza A and B
Ribavirin	Topical (inhalation) – RSV
	Oral – Lassa fever, hepatitis C
Palivizumab	Prevention of RSV
Alpha-interferon (INF-α)	HBV, HCV, some malignancies (e.g. renal cell carcinoma)
(Pegylated INF-α)	(Given once weekly)

oral and topical preparations are available for the treatment of herpes simplex and varicella zoster virus infections (Table 2.15).

A pro-drug of aciclovir, valaciclovir, has been developed. Coupling of the amino acid valine to the acyclic side-chain of aciclovir allows better intestinal absorption. The valine is removed by enzymic action and aciclovir is released into the circulation. A similar pro-drug of a related nucleoside analogue (penciclovir) is the antiherpes drug, famciclovir. The mode of action and efficacy of famciclovir are similar to those of aciclovir.

Ganciclovir. This guanine analogue is structurally similar to aciclovir, with extension of the acyclic side-chain by a carboxymethyl group. It is active against herpes simplex viruses and varicella zoster virus by the same mechanism as aciclovir. In addition, phosphorylation by a protein kinase encoded by the UL97 region of cytomegalovirus renders it potently active against this virus. Thus ganciclovir is currently the first-line treatment for cytomegalovirus disease. Intravenous and oral preparations are available as is an oral pro-drug, valganciclovir. Unlike aciclovir, ganciclovir has a significant toxicity profile including neutropenia, thrombocytopenia and the likelihood of sterilization by inhibiting spermatogenesis. For this reason, it is reserved for the treatment or prevention of life- or sight-threatening cytomegalovirus infection.

Cidofovir. This is a phosphonate derivative of an acyclic nucleoside which is a DNA polymerase chain inhibitor. It is administered intravenously for the treatment of severe cytomegalovirus (CMV) infections in patients with AIDS. It is given with probenecid, and as it is nephrotoxic, particular attention should be given to hydration and to monitoring renal function.

Adefovir dipivoxil is used in the treatment of chronic hepatitis B (see p. 372).

Pyrophosphate analogues

Foscarnet (sodium phosphonoformate) is a simple pyrophosphate analogue which inhibits viral DNA polymerases. It is active against herpesviruses and its main roles are as a second-line treatment for severe cytomegalovirus disease and for the treatment of aciclovir-resistant herpes simplex infection. It is given intravenously and the potential for severe side-effects, particularly renal damage, limits its use.

Amantadine. Amantadine is a synthetic symmetrical amine which is active prophylactically and therapeutically against influenza A virus (it is inactive against influenza B virus). Its prophylactic efficacy is similar to that of influenza vaccine and it is occasionally used to prevent the spread of influenza A in institutions such as nursing homes. Although CNS side-effects such as insomnia, dizziness and headache may occur (it is also used as a treatment for Parkinson's disease), these are not usually produced by the lower doses currently recommended.

Neuraminidase inhibitors

Two drugs that inhibit the action of the neuraminidase of influenza A and B have been introduced. Zanamavir is administered by inhalation and oseltamivir is an oral preparation. Both have been shown to be effective in reducing the duration of illness in influenza.

Ribavirin

This synthetic purine nucleoside derivative which interferes with 5'-capping of messenger RNA, is active against several RNA viruses. It is administered by a small-particle aerosol generator (SPAG) to infants with acute respiratory syncytial virus (RSV) infection. In a clinical trial in Sierra Leone it was shown to reduce the mortality of Lassa fever virus infection. Individuals with hepatitis C virus infection, treated with alpha-interferon–ribavirin combinations, have lower relapse rates than those receiving interferon alone.

Palivizumab

This monoclonal antibody is specifically indicated to prevent seasonal respiratory syncytial virus (RSV) infection in infants at high risk of this infection. It is administered by intramuscular injection.

Interferons (see also p. 202)

These are naturally occurring proteins produced by virus-infected cells, macrophages and lymphocytes. Interferons are stimulated by a number of factors, including viral nucleic acid, and render uninfected cells resistant to infection with the same – or in some circumstances different – viruses. They have been synthesized commercially by either culture of lymphoblastoid cells or by recombinant DNA technology and are licensed for therapeutic use.

The potency of INF-α has been enhanced by coupling the protein with polyethylene glycol. The resulting PEG interferon given once weekly has been shown to improve the response to treatment of hepatitis B and C.

FURTHER READING

[Anon] (2004) Caspofungin and voriconazole for fungal infections. *Drugs and Therapeutics Bulletin* **1**: 5–8.

Finch RG, Greenwood D, Norrby R, Whitley R (2003) *Antibiotic and Chemotherapy*, 8th edn. Edinburgh: Churchill Livingstone.

Herbrecht R, Denning DW, Patterson TF et al. (2002) for the Invasive Fungal Infections Group of the European Organisation for Research and Treatment of Cancer and the Global Aspergillus Study Group. Voriconazole versus amphotericin B for primary therapy of invasive aspergillosis. *New England Journal of Medicine* **347**(6): 408–415.

Jacoby GA, Munoz-Price LS (2004) The new β-Lactamases. *New England Journal of Medicine* **352**: 380–391.

Stevens DL, Herr D, Lampiris H et al. (2002) Linezolid versus vancomycin for the treatment of methicillin-resistant *Staphylococcus aureus* infections. *Clinical Infectious Diseases* **341**: 1481–1490.

Walsh TJ (2002) Echinocandins – an advance in the primary treatment of invasive candidiasis. *New England Journal of Medicine* **347**(25): 2070–2072.

IMMUNIZATION AGAINST INFECTIOUS DISEASES

Although effective antimicrobial chemotherapy is available for many diseases, the ultimate aim of any infectious disease control programme is to prevent infection occurring. This is achieved either by:

- eliminating the source or mode of transmission of an infection (p. 22)
- reducing host susceptibility to environmental pathogens.

Immunization, immunoprophylaxis and immunotherapy

Immunization has changed the course and natural history of many infectious diseases. Passive immunization by administering preformed antibody, either in the form of immune serum or purified normal immunoglobulin, provides short-term immunity and has been effective in both the prevention (immunoprophylaxis) and treatment (immunotherapy) of a number of bacterial and viral diseases (Table 2.16). The active immunization schedule currently recommended is summarized in Box 2.6. Long-lasting immunity is achieved only by active immunization with a live attenuated or an inactivated organism (Table 2.17). Active immunization may also be performed with microbial toxin (either native or modified) – that is, a toxoid. Immunization should be kept up to date with booster doses throughout life. Travellers to developing countries, especially if visiting rural areas, should in addition enquire about further specific immunizations.

In 1974 the World Health Organization introduced the Expanded Programme on Immunization (EPI). Twenty years later more than 80% of the world's children had been immunized against tuberculosis, diphtheria, tetanus, pertussis, polio and measles. It is hoped that poliomyelitis will shortly be eradicated world-wide, which will match the past success of global smallpox eradication. Introduction of conjugate vaccines against *Haemophilus influenzae* type b (Hib) has proved highly effective in controlling invasive *H. influenzae* infection, notably meningitis (see p. 898).

FURTHER READING

Ada G (2001) Vaccines and vaccination. *New England Journal of Medicine* **345**: 1042–1053.

Beverley P (ed.) (2002) Vaccination. *British Medical Bulletin* **62**.

High KP (2001) Nutritional strategies to boost immunity and prevent infection in elderly individuals. *Clinical Infectious Diseases* **33**: 1892–1900.

Jackson LA, Neuzil KM, Yu O et al. for the Vaccine Safety Datalink (2003) Effectiveness of pneumococcal polysaccharide vaccine in older adults. *New England Journal of Medicine* **348**(18): 1747–1755.

John TJ (2000) The final stages of the global eradication of polio. *New England Journal of Medicine* **343**: 806–807.

Public Health Laboratory Service (2002) Immunoglobulin handbook. London: PHLS. Online. Available: http://www.hpa.org.uk/infections/topics_az/immunoglobulin/immunoglobulinHandbook.pdf.

Salisbury DM, Begg NT (eds) (1996) *Immunization Against Infectious Diseases*. London: HMSO.

Protection for travellers to developing/tropical countries

There has been a huge increase in the number of people travelling to developing countries, mainly for recreation and leisure. The risk of infection depends on the area to be visited, the type of activity and the underlying health

Box 2.6 Recommended immunization schedules: (i) in the UK; (ii) WHO model schedule for developing countries

Time of immunization	Vaccine
(i) UK*	
2 months	DPT, Hib, OPV, MenC, BCG[†]
3 months	DPT, Hib, OPV, MenC
4 months	DaPT, Hib, OPV, MenC
12–15 months	MMR
3–5 years	DTaP, OPV, MMR
10–14 years	BCG[‡]
15–18 years	Td, OPV
(ii) Developing countries[§]	
Birth (or first contact)	OPV, BCG
6 weeks	DPT, OPV, HBV
10 weeks	DPT, OPV, HBV
14 weeks	DPT, OPV, HBV
9 months	Measles, YF[¶]

DPT, adsorbed diphtheria, whole cell pertussis, tetanus triple vaccine; Hib, *Haemophilus influenzae* b vaccine; OPV, oral polio vaccine; MenC, meningococcus group C conjugate vaccine; aP, acellular pertussis; MMR, measles, mumps, rubella triple vaccine; BCG, bacille Calmette–Guérin (tuberculosis vaccine); d, adsorbed low-dose diphtheria; HBV, hepatitis B vaccine; YF, yellow fever vaccine

* Changing from OPV to inactivated polio vaccine; ? HBV vaccine to be added to schedule
[†] Children at high risk of contact with tuberculosis
[‡] Tuberculin-negative children at low risk of contact with tuberculosis
[§] Model scheme, adapted locally depending on need and availability of vaccines
[¶] In endemic areas

of the traveller. Advice should therefore always be based on an individual assessment.

Protection for travellers can be divided into three categories:

- Personal protection, e.g.
  - insect repellent
  - bed netting
  - avoidance of animals
  - care with food and drink
- Chemoprophylaxis, e.g. antimalarials
- Immunization, e.g.
  - yellow fever
  - hepatitis A and B
  - typhoid.

Because situations and risks can change rapidly, websites (which can be regularly updated) are often the best source of advice on travel health.

FURTHER READING

CDC travel health site: http://www.cdc.gov/travel

Dupont H, Steffen R (2000) *Textbook of Travel Medicine and Health*. Hamilton, Ontario: Decker.

WHO Travel Health Site: http://www.who.int/ith

Table 2.16 Examples of passive immunization available

Infection	Antibody	Indication	Efficacy
Bacterial			
Tetanus	Human tetanus immune globulin	Prevention and treatment	+
Diphtheria	Horse serum	Prevention and treatment	+
Botulism	Horse serum	Treatment	+
Viral			
Hepatitis A / Measles	Human normal immune globulin	Prevention (rarely required since vaccine introduced)	+
Hepatitis B	Human hepatitis B immune globulin	Prevention	+
Varicella zoster	Human varicella zoster immune globulin	Prevention	+
Rabies	Human rabies immune globulin	Prevention	+

Table 2.17 Preparations available for active immunization

Live attenuated vaccines
Oral polio (Sabin)
Measles
Mumps
Rubella
Yellow fever
BCG
Typhoid

Inactivated conjugate vaccines
Hepatitis A
Pertussis
Typhoid – whole cell and Vi antigen
Polio
Influenza
Cholera
Meningococci (groups A and C)
Meningococcus group C
Rabies
Pneumococcal
Haemophilus influenzae type b

Toxoids
Diphtheria
Tetanus

Recombinant vaccines
Hepatitis B

BCG, bacille Calmette–Guérin

VIRAL INFECTIONS: AN INTRODUCTION

Viruses are much smaller than other infectious agents (see Tables 2.18 and 2.20) and contain either DNA or RNA, not both as in bacteria and other microorganisms. Since they are metabolically inert, they must live intra-cellularly, using the host cell for synthesis of viral proteins and nucleic acid. Viruses have a central nucleic acid core surrounded by a protein coat that is antigenically unique for a particular virus. The protein coat (capsid) imparts a helical or icosahedral structure to the virus. Some viruses also possess an envelope consisting of lipid and protein.

Hepatitis viruses are discussed on page 362.

DNA VIRUSES

Details of the structure, size and classification of human DNA viruses are shown in Table 2.18.

ADENOVIRUSES

Adenovirus infection commonly presents as an acute pharyngitis, and extension of infection to the larynx and trachea in infants may lead to croup. By school age the majority of children show serological evidence of previous infection. Certain subtypes produce an acute conjunctivitis associated with pharyngitis. In adults, adenovirus causes acute follicular conjunctivitis and rarely pneumonia that is clinically similar to that produced by *Mycoplasma pneumoniae* (see p. 924). Adenoviruses have also been implicated as a cause of gastroenteritis (see p. 52) without respiratory disease and may be responsible for acute mesenteric lymphadenitis in children and young adults. Mesenteric adenitis due to adenoviruses may lead to intussusception in infants.

HERPESVIRUSES

Members of the herpesviruses are important causes of a wide range of human diseases. Details are summarized in Table 2.19. The hallmark of all herpesvirus infections is the ability of the viruses to establish latent (or silent) infections that then persist for the life of the individual.

Herpes simplex virus (HSV) infection
(Fig. 2.12)

Two types of HSV have been identified: HSV-1 is the major cause of herpetic stomatitis, herpes labialis ('cold sore'), keratoconjunctivitis and encephalitis, whereas

Table 2.18   Human DNA viruses

Structure		Approximate size	Family	Viruses
Symmetry	**Envelope**			
Icosahedral	–	80 nm	Adenovirus	Adenoviruses
Icosahedral	+	100 nm (160 nm with envelope)	Herpesvirus	Herpes simplex virus (HSV) types 1 and 2
				Varicella zoster virus
				Cytomegalovirus
				Epstein–Barr virus (EBV)
				Human herpesvirus type 6 (HHV-6)
				Human herpesvirus type 7 (HHV-7)
				Human herpesvirus type 8 (HHV-8)
Icosahedral	+	42 nm	Hepadnavirus	Hepatitis B virus (HBV)
Icosahedral	–	50 nm	Papovavirus	Human papillomavirus
				Polyomavirus
Icosahedral	–	23 nm	Parvovirus	Parvovirus B19
Complex	+	300 nm × 200 nm	Poxvirus	Variola virus
				Vaccinia virus
				Monkeypox
				Cowpox
				Orf
				Molluscum contagiosum

Table 2.19   Major diseases caused by human herpesviruses

Subfamily	Virus	Children	Adults	Immunocompromised
α-Herpesvirus	Herpes simplex type 1	Stomatitis*	Cold sores	Dissemination
			Keratitis	
			Erythema multiforme	
	Herpes simplex type 2		Primary genital herpes*	Dissemination
			Recurrent genital herpes	
	Varicella zoster virus	Chickenpox*	Shingles	Dissemination
β-Herpesvirus	Cytomegalovirus	Congenital*		Pneumonitis
				Retinitis
				Gastrointestinal
	Human herpesvirus type 6	Roseola infantum*		Pneumonitis
	Human herpesvirus type 7	Roseola infantum*		
γ-Herpesvirus	Epstein–Barr virus		Infectious mononucleosis*	Lymphoma
			Burkitt's lymphoma	
			Nasopharyngeal carcinoma	
	Human herpesvirus type 8		Kaposi's sarcoma	Kaposi's sarcoma

* Signifies primary infection

Fig. 2.12   Electronmicrograph of herpes simplex virus.

HSV-2 causes genital herpes and may also be responsible for systemic infection in the immunocompromised host. These divisions, however, are not rigid, for HSV-1 can give rise to genital herpes and HSV-2 can cause pharyngitis.

The portal of entry of HSV-1 infection is usually via the mouth or occasionally the skin. The primary infection may go unnoticed or may produce a severe inflammatory reaction with vesicle formation leading to painful ulcers (gingivostomatitis; see Fig. 2.13). The virus then remains latent, most commonly in the trigeminal ganglia, but may be reactivated by stress, trauma, febrile illnesses and ultraviolet radiation, producing the recurrent form of the disease known as herpes labialis ('cold sore'). Approximately 70% of the population are infected with HSV-1 and recurrent infections occur in one-third of individuals.

Fig. 2.13 **Primary herpes simplex type 1** (gingivostomatitis).

Reactivation often produces localized paraesthesiae in the lip before the appearance of a cold sore.

Complications of HSV-1 infection include transfer to the eye (dendritic ulceration, keratitis), acute encephalitis (p. 1167), skin infections such as herpetic whitlow, and erythema multiforme (see p. 1342).

In genital herpes the primary infection is usually more severe and recurrences are common. The virus remains latent in the sacral ganglia and during recurrence can produce a radiculomyelopathy, with pain in the groin, buttocks and upper thighs. Primary anorectal herpes infection is common in male homosexuals (see p. 125).

Immunocompromised patients such as those receiving intensive cancer chemotherapy or those with the acquired immunodeficiency syndrome (AIDS) may develop disseminated HSV infection involving many of the viscera. In severe cases death may result from hepatitis and encephalitis.

Neonates may develop primary HSV infection following vaginal delivery in the presence of active genital HSV infection in the mother. The disease in the baby varies from localized skin lesions to widespread visceral disease often with encephalitis. Caesarean section should therefore be considered if active genital HSV infection is present during labour.

Humoral antibody develops following primary infection, but mononuclear cell responses are probably more important in preventing dissemination of disease.

The clinical picture, diagnosis and treatment are described on page 132.

Varicella zoster virus (VZV) infection

VZV produces two distinct diseases, varicella (chickenpox) and herpes zoster (shingles). The primary infection is chickenpox. It usually occurs in childhood, the virus entering through the mucosa of the upper respiratory tract. It should be noted that in some countries (e.g. the Indian subcontinent) a different epidemiological pattern exists with most infections occurring in adulthood. Chickenpox rarely occurs twice in the same individual.

Infectious virus is spread from fresh skin lesions by direct contact or airborne transmission and the period of infectivity in chickenpox extends from 2 days before the appearance of the rash until the skin lesions are all at the crusting stage. Following recovery from chickenpox the virus then remains latent in dorsal root and cranial nerve ganglia.

Clinical features of chickenpox

Fourteen to twenty-one days after exposure to VZV, a brief prodromal illness of fever, headache and malaise heralds the eruption of chickenpox, characterized by the rapid progression of macules to papules to vesicles to pustules in a matter of hours (Fig. 2.14). In young children the prodromal illness may be very mild or absent. The illness tends to be more severe in older children and can be debilitating in adults. The lesions occur on the face, scalp and trunk, and to a lesser extent on the extremities. It is characteristic to see skin lesions at all stages of development on the same area of skin. Fever subsides as soon as new lesions cease to appear. Eventually the pustules crust and heal without scarring.

Important complications of chickenpox include pneumonia, which generally begins 1–6 days after the skin eruption, and bacterial superinfection of skin lesions. Pneumonia is more common in adults than in children and cigarette smokers are at particular risk. Pulmonary symptoms are usually more striking than the physical findings, although a chest radiograph usually shows diffuse changes throughout both lung fields. CNS involvement occurs in about 1 per 1000 cases and most commonly presents as an acute truncal cerebellar ataxia. The immunocompromised are susceptible to disseminated infection with multiorgan involvement.

Clinical features of shingles

Shingles (see p. 1321) occurs at all ages but is most common in the elderly, producing skin lesions similar to chickenpox, although classically they are unilateral and restricted to a sensory nerve (dermatomal) distribution (Fig. 2.15). Shingles never occurs as a primary infection but results from reactivation of latent VZV from dorsal

Fig. 2.14 **Chickenpox in an adult.** Generalized VZV.

Fig. 2.15 **Shingles – VZV affecting a dermatome.**
Reproduced with kind permission of Imperial College School
of Medicine.

root and/or cranial nerve ganglia. The onset of the rash of
shingles is usually preceded by severe dermatomal pain,
indicating the involvement of sensory nerves in its
pathogenesis. Virus is disseminated from freshly formed
vesicles and may cause chickenpox in susceptible
contacts.

Diagnosis

The diseases are usually recognized clinically but can be
confirmed by electronmicroscopy, immunofluorescence
or culture of vesicular fluid and by serology.

Prophylaxis and treatment

Chickenpox usually requires no treatment in healthy
children and infection results in lifelong immunity.
However, the disease may be fatal in the immunocompromised, who can be offered protection, after exposure to the virus, with zoster immune immunoglobulin
(ZIG).

Anyone with chickenpox who is over the age of
16 years should be considered for antiviral therapy with
aciclovir, or a similar drug, if they present within 72 hours
of onset. Women in pregnancy are prone to severe
chickenpox and, in addition, there is a risk of intrauterine
infection with structural damage to the fetus (mainly in
the mid trimester – risk rate 2%). For these reasons
prophylactic ZIG is recommended for women in pregnancy exposed to varicella zoster virus and, if chickenpox
develops, aciclovir treatment should be given. (NB:
aciclovir has not been licensed for use in pregnant
women.) If a woman has chickenpox at term, her baby
should be protected by ZIG if delivery occurs within
5 days of the onset of the mother's illness. An effective
varicella vaccine is used in many parts of the USA; it is
available on a named-patient basis in the UK.

Shingles is also treated with aciclovir and the duration
of lesion formation and time to healing can be reduced by
early treatment. Aciclovir, valaciclovir and famciclovir
have all been shown to reduce the burden of zoster-
associated pain when treatment is given in the acute
phase. Shingles involving the ophthalmic division of the

trigeminal nerve has an associated incidence of acute and
chronic ophthalmic complications of 50%. Early treatment with aciclovir reduces this to 20% or less. As for
chickenpox, all immunocompromised individuals should
be given aciclovir at the onset of shingles.

Cytomegalovirus (CMV) infection

Infection with CMV is found world-wide and has its most
profound effects as an opportunistic infection in the
immunocompromised, particularly in recipients of bone-
marrow and solid organ transplants and in patients with
AIDS. Over 50% of the adult population have serological
evidence of latent infection with the virus, although
infection is generally symptomless. As with all herpesviruses, the virus persists for life, usually as a latent
infection in which the naked DNA is situated extra-
chromosomally in the nuclei of the cells in the
endothelium of the arterial wall and in T lymphocytes.

Clinical features

In healthy adults CMV infection is usually asymptomatic
but may cause an illness similar to infectious mononucleosis, with fever, occasionally lymphocytosis with
atypical lymphocytes, and hepatitis with or without
jaundice. The Paul–Bunnell test for heterophile antibody
is negative. Infection may be spread by kissing, sexual
intercourse or blood transfusion, and transplacentally to
the fetus. Disseminated fatal infection with widespread
visceral involvement occurs in the immunocompromised
(see p. 138) and may cause encephalitis, retinitis,
pneumonitis and diffuse involvement of the gastrointestinal tract.

Intrauterine infection usually occurs in primary
infection acquired during pregnancy and may have
serious consequences in the fetus; CNS involvement may
cause microcephaly and motor disorders. Jaundice and
hepatosplenomegaly are common, and thrombocytopenia and haemolytic anaemia also occur. Evidence
of CNS involvement may be provided by demonstration
of periventricular calcification on X-ray.

Diagnosis

Serological tests can identify latent (IgG) or primary
(IgM) infection. The virus can also be identified in tissues
by the presence of characteristic intranuclear 'owl's eye'
inclusions (Fig. 2.16) on histological staining and by direct
immunofluorescence. Culture in human embryo fibroblasts is usually slow but diagnosis can be accelerated by
immunofluorescent detection of antigen in the cultures.
The polymerase chain reaction, which can be quantitative, provides a sensitive way of detecting CMV in
blood and other body fluids.

Treatment

In the immunocompetent, infection is usually self-
limiting and no specific treatment is required. In the
immunosuppressed, ganciclovir (5 mg/kg daily for
14–21 days) reduces retinitis and gastrointestinal damage
and can eliminate CMV from blood, urine and respiratory

Fig. 2.16 Typical 'owl-eye' inclusion-bearing cell infected with cytomegalovirus.

secretions. It is less effective against pneumonitis. In patients who are continually immunocompromised, particularly those with AIDS, maintenance therapy may be necessary. Drug resistance has been reported in AIDS patients and transplant recipients. Bone marrow toxicity is common. No antiviral drugs are currently available for routine treatment of CMV in neonates and the toxicity of ganciclovir prohibits its use in most cases. Two other drugs, foscarnet and cidofovir, are available for the treatment of CMV infection but both are nephrotoxic and their use should be restricted to those with severe disease.

Epstein–Barr virus (EBV) infection

This virus causes an acute febrile illness known as infectious mononucleosis (glandular fever), which occurs world-wide in adolescents and young adults. EBV is probably transmitted in saliva and by aerosol.

Clinical features

The predominant symptoms are fever, headache, malaise and sore throat. Palatal petechiae and a transient macular rash are common, the latter occurring in 90% of patients who have received ampicillin (inappropriately) for the sore throat. Cervical lymphadenopathy, particularly of the posterior cervical nodes, and splenomegaly are characteristic. Mild hepatitis is common, but other complications such as myocarditis, meningitis, encephalitis, mesenteric adenitis and splenic rupture are rare.

Although some young adults remain debilitated and depressed for some months after infection, the evidence for reactivation of latent virus in healthy individuals is controversial, although this is thought to occur in immunocompromised patients. Following primary infection, EBV remains latent in resting memory B lymphocytes. It has been shown in vitro that of nearly 100 viral genes expressed during replication, approximately only 10 are expressed in the latently infected B cells. Severe, often fatal infectious mononucleosis may result from a rare X-linked immunoproliferative syndrome affecting young boys. Those who survive have an increased risk of hypogammaglobulinaemia and/or lymphoma.

EBV is the cause of oral hairy leucoplakia in AIDS patients and is the major aetiological agent responsible for Burkitt's lymphoma, nasopharyngeal carcinoma, post-transplant lymphoma, and the immunoblastic lymphoma of AIDS patients and Hodgkin's lymphoma. Different levels of expression of EBV latency genes occur in the various clinical conditions caused by the virus.

Diagnosis

EBV infection should be strongly suspected if atypical mononuclear cells (glandular fever cells) are found in the peripheral blood. It can be confirmed during the second week of infection by a positive Paul–Bunnell reaction, which detects heterophile antibodies (IgM) that agglutinate sheep erythrocytes. False-positives can occur in other conditions such as viral hepatitis, Hodgkin's lymphoma and acute leukaemia. The Monospot test is a sensitive and easily performed screening test for heterophile antibodies. Specific EBV IgM antibodies indicate recent infection by the virus. Clinically similar illnesses are produced by CMV and toxoplasmosis but these can be distinguished serologically.

Treatment

The majority of cases require no specific treatment and recovery is rapid. Corticosteroid therapy is advised when there is neurological involvement (e.g. encephalitis, meningitis, Guillain–Barré syndrome) or when there is marked thrombocytopenia or haemolysis.

Human herpesvirus type 6 (HHV-6)

This human herpesvirus infects CD4+ T lymphocytes, occurs world-wide, and exists as a latent infection in over 85% of the adult population. It is spread by contact with oral secretions. The virus causes roseola infantum (exanthem subitum) which presents as a high fever followed by generalized macular rash in infants. HHV-6 is a common cause of febrile convulsions, and aseptic meningitis or encephalitis may occur as rare complications. Reactivation in the immunocompromised may lead to severe pneumonia.

Treatment

Supportive management only is recommended for the common infantile disease. Ganciclovir can be used in the immunocompromised.

Human herpesvirus type 7 (HHV-7)

This virus is similar to HHV-6 in being a T lymphotropic herpesvirus. It is also present as a latent infection in over 85% of the adult population and it is known to infect CD4+ helper T cells by using the CD4 antigen (the main receptor employed by HIV). The full spectrum of disease due to HHV-7 has not yet been fully characterized, but, like HHV-6, it is known to cause roseola infantum in infants.

Human herpesvirus type 8 (Kaposi's sarcoma-associated herpesvirus)

This human herpesvirus is strongly associated with the aetiology of classical and AIDS-related Kaposi's sarcoma. Antibody prevalence is high in those with tumours but relatively low in the general population of most industrialized countries. High rates of infection (> 50% population) have been described in central and southern Africa and this matches the geographic distribution of Kaposi's sarcoma before the era of AIDS. HHV-8 can be sexually transmitted among homosexual men, through heterosexual sex and through exposure to blood from needle sharing. It is thought that salivary transmission may be the predominant route in Africa. HHV-8 RNA transcripts have been detected in Kaposi's sarcoma cells and in circulating mononuclear cells from patients with the tumour. This virus may also have a pathogenetic role in primary pulmonary hypertension.

PAPOVAVIRUSES

These viruses tend to produce chronic infections, often with evidence of latency. They are capable of inducing neoplasia in some animal species and were among the first viruses to be implicated in tumorigenesis. Human papillomaviruses, of which there are at least 70 types, are responsible for the common wart and have been implicated in the aetiology of carcinoma of the cervix (mainly types 16 and 18) and oral cancer (type 16). The human BK virus, a polyomavirus, is generally found in immunocompromised individuals and may be detected in the urine of 15–40% of renal transplant patients, in patients receiving cytotoxic chemotherapy, and in those with immunodeficiency states. A related virus, JC, is the cause of progressive multifocal leucoencephalopathy (PML) which presents as dementia in the immuno-compromised and is due to progressive cerebral destruction resulting from accumulation of the virus in brain tissue.

For genital warts see page 126.

HUMAN PARVOVIRUS B19

Human parvovirus B19 produces erythema infectiosum (fifth disease), a common infection in schoolchildren. The rash is typically on the face (the 'slapped-cheek' appearance). The patient is well and the rash can recur over weeks or months. Asymptomatic infection occurs in 20% of children. Moderately severe self-limiting arthro-pathy (see p. 573) is common if infection occurs in adulthood. Aplastic crisis may occur in patients with chronic haemolysis (e.g. sickle cell disease). Chronic infection with anaemia occurs in immunocompromised subjects. Hydrops fetalis (3% risk) and spontaneous abortion (9% risk) may result from infection during the first and second trimesters of pregnancy.

POXVIRUSES

Smallpox (variola)

This disease was eradicated in 1977 following an aggressive vaccination policy and careful detection of new cases coordinated by the World Health Organization. Its possible use in bioterrorism has resulted in the reintroduction of smallpox vaccination in some countries (p. 1031).

Monkeypox

This is a rare zoonosis that occurs in small villages in the tropical rainforests in several countries of western and central Africa. Its clinical effects, including a generalized vesicular rash, are indistinguishable from smallpox, but person-to-person transmission is unusual. Serological surveys indicate that several species of squirrel are likely to represent the animal reservoir.

Cowpox

Cowpox produces large vesicles which are classically on the hands in those in contact with infected cows. The lesions are associated with regional lymphadenitis and fever. Cowpox virus has been found in a range of species including domestic and wild cats, and the reservoir is thought to exist in a range of rodents.

Vaccinia virus

This is a laboratory virus and does not occur in nature in either humans or animals. Its origins are uncertain but it has been invaluable in its use as the vaccine to prevent smallpox. Vaccination is now not recommended except for laboratory personnel handling certain poxviruses for experimental purposes or in contingency planning to manage a deliberate release of smallpox virus. It is being assessed experimentally as a possible carrier for new vaccines.

Orf

This poxvirus causes contagious pustular dermatitis in sheep and hand lesions in humans (see p. 1322).

Molluscum contagiosum

This is discussed on page 1322.

FURTHER READING
Cohen JI (2000) Epstein–Barr infection. *New England Journal of Medicine* **343**: 1778–1787.
Frey SE, Belshe RB (2004) Poxvirus zoonoses. *New England Journal of Medicine* **350**: 324–327.
Gnann JW, Whitley RJ (2002) Herpes zoster. *New England Journal of Medicine* **347**: 340–346.
Prober C (2005) Sixth disease and the ubiquity of human herpes viruses. *New England Journal of Medicine* **352**: 753–755.
Whitley R, Roizman B (2001) Herpes simplex infections. *Lancet* **357**: 1513–1518.
Young NS, Brown KE (2004) Parvovirus B19. *New England Journal of Medicine* **350**: 586–598.

RNA VIRUSES (Table 2.20)

PICORNAVIRUSES

Poliovirus infection (poliomyelitis)

Poliomyelitis occurs when a susceptible individual is infected with poliovirus type 1, 2 or 3. These viruses have a propensity for the nervous system, especially the anterior horn cells of the spinal cord and cranial nerve motor neurones. Poliomyelitis is found world-wide but its incidence has decreased dramatically following improvements in sanitation, hygiene and the widespread use of polio vaccines. Spread is usually via the faeco-oral route, as the virus is excreted in the faeces.

Clinical features

The incubation period is 7–14 days. Although polio is essentially a disease of childhood, no age is exempt. The clinical manifestations vary considerably.

Inapparent infection

Inapparent infection is common and occurs in 95% of infected individuals.

Abortive poliomyelitis

Abortive poliomyelitis occurs in approximately 4–5% of cases and is characterized by the presence of fever, sore throat and myalgia. The illness is self-limiting and of short duration.

Non-paralytic poliomyelitis

Non-paralytic poliomyelitis has features of abortive poliomyelitis as well as signs of meningeal irritation, but recovery is complete.

Paralytic poliomyelitis

Paralytic poliomyelitis occurs in approximately 0.1% of infected children (1.3% of adults). Several factors predispose to the development of paralysis:

- male sex
- exercise early in the illness
- trauma, surgery or intramuscular injection, which localize the paralysis
- recent tonsillectomy (bulbar poliomyelitis).

This form of the disease is characterized initially by features simulating abortive poliomyelitis. Symptoms subside for 4–5 days, only to recur in greater severity with

Table 2.20 Human RNA viruses

Symmetry	Envelope	Approximate size	Family	Viruses
Icosahedral	–	30 nm	Picornavirus	Poliovirus Coxsackievirus Echovirus Enterovirus 68–72 Rhinovirus
Icosahedral	–	80 nm	Reovirus	Reovirus Rotavirus
Icosahedral	+	50–80 nm	Togavirus	Rubella virus Alphaviruses Flaviviruses
Spherical	+	80–100 nm	Bunyavirus	Congo–Crimean haemorrhagic fever Hantavirus
Spherical	–	35–40 nm	Calicivirus	Noravirus Hepatitis E
Spherical	–	28–30 nm	Astrovirus	Astrovirus
Helical	+	80–120 nm	Orthomyxovirus	Influenza viruses A, B and C
Helical	+	100–300 nm	Paramyxovirus	Measles virus Mumps virus Respiratory syncytial virus Human metapneumovirus Nipah virus Hendra virus
Helical	+	80–220 nm	Coronavirus	URTI (229E, OC43) SARS
Helical	+	60–175 nm	Rhabdovirus	Lyssavirus – rabies
Helical	+	100 nm	Retrovirus	Human immunodeficiency viruses (HIV 1 and 2) Human T cell lymphotropic virus (HTLV 1 and 2)
Helical	+	100–300 nm	Arenavirus	Lassa virus Lymphocytic choriomeningitis virus
Pleomorphic	+	Filaments or circular forms; 100 × 130–2600 nm	Filovirus	Marburg virus Ebola virus

signs of meningeal irritation and muscle pain, which is most prominent in the neck and lumbar region. These symptoms persist for a few days and are followed by the onset of asymmetric paralysis without sensory involvement. The paralysis is usually confined to the lower limbs in children under 5 years of age and the upper limbs in older children, whereas in adults it manifests as paraplegia or quadriplegia.

Bulbar poliomyelitis

Bulbar poliomyelitis is characterized by the presence of cranial nerve involvement and respiratory muscle paralysis. Soft palate, pharyngeal and laryngeal muscle palsies are common.

Aspiration pneumonia, myocarditis, paralytic ileus and urinary calculi are late complications of poliomyelitis.

Diagnosis

The diagnosis is a clinical one. Distinction from Guillain–Barré syndrome is easily made by the absence of sensory involvement and the asymmetrical nature of the paralysis in poliomyelitis. Laboratory confirmation and distinction between the wild virus and vaccine strains is achieved by virus culture, neutralization and temperature marker tests.

Treatment

Treatment is supportive. Bed rest is essential during the early course of the illness. Respiratory support with intermittent positive-pressure respiration is required if the muscles of respiration are involved. Once the acute phase of the illness has subsided, occupational therapy, physiotherapy and occasionally surgery have important roles in patient rehabilitation.

Prevention and control

Immunization has dramatically decreased the prevalence of this disease world-wide and global eradication of the virus, coordinated by the World Health Organization, is expected within the next 1–2 years. However, there have been recent outbreaks in West Africa where cultural taboos have disrupted the polio vaccination campaign and recently in the Sudan. Trivalent oral poliovaccine (OPV) (active virus) is currently used (see Box 2.6); occasionally, inactivated poliovirus vaccine (IPV) is used intramuscularly for the immunocompromised and their family contacts and for women in pregnancy. Recent studies using inactivated poliovirus vaccine have revealed greater potency than the original Salk IPV. The greater reliability of IPV in hot climates and the scientific and ethical problems of continuing to use OPV in countries free from poliomyelitis, mean that IPV is to be introduced for immunization schedules in the UK in the future.

Coxsackievirus, echovirus and other enterovirus infections

These viruses are spread by the faeco-oral route. They each have a number of different types and are responsible for a broad spectrum of disease involving the skin and mucous membranes, muscles, nerves, the heart (Table 2.21) and, rarely, other organs, such as the liver and pancreas. They are frequently associated with pyrexial illnesses and are the most common cause of aseptic meningitis.

Herpangina

This disease is mainly caused by Coxsackie A viruses and presents with a vesicular eruption on the fauces, palate and uvula. The lesions evolve into ulcers. The illness is usually associated with fever and headache but is short-lived, recovery occurring within a few days.

Hand, foot and mouth disease

This disease is mainly caused by Coxsackievirus A16 or A10. Oral lesions are similar to those seen in herpangina but may be more extensive in the oropharynx. Vesicles and a maculopapular eruption also appear, typically on

Table 2.21 Picornavirus infections (excluding poliovirus and rhinovirus)				
Disease	**Coxsackievirus**		**Echovirus** (types 1–9, 11–7, 29–33)	**Enterovirus** (types 68–71)
	A (types A_1–A_{22}, A_{24})	**B** (types B_1–B_6)		
Cutaneous and oropharyngeal				
Herpangina	+++	+	+	
Hand, foot and mouth	+++	+		+
Erythematous rashes	+	+	+++	
Neurological				
Paralytic	+		±	+
Meningitis	++	++	+++	+
Encephalitis	++	++	±	+
Cardiac				
Myocarditis and pericarditis	+	+++	+	
Muscle				
Myositis (Bornholm disease)	+	+++	+	

+++, often causes; ++, sometimes causes; +, rarely causes; ±, possibly causes the palms of the hands and the soles of the feet, but also on other parts of the body. This infection commonly affects children. Recovery occurs within a week.

Neurological disease

Other enteroviruses in addition to poliovirus can cause a broad range of neurological disease, including meningitis, encephalitis, and a paralytic disease characteristic of poliomyelitis.

Heart and muscle disease

Enteroviruses are cause of acute myocarditis and pericarditis, from which, in general, there is complete recovery. However, these viruses can also cause chronic congestive cardiomyopathy and, rarely, constrictive pericarditis.

Skeletal muscle involvement, particularly of the intercostal muscles, is a feature of *Bornholm disease*, a febrile illness usually due to Coxsackievirus B. The pain may be of such an intensity as to mimic pleurisy or an acute abdomen. The infection affects both children and adults and may be complicated by meningitis or cardiac involvement.

Rhinovirus infection

Rhinoviruses are responsible for the common cold (see p. 895). Chimpanzees and humans are the only species to develop the common cold. ICAM-1 is the cellular receptor (p. 199) for rhinovirus and it is only in these two species that the specific binding domain is present. Peak incidence rates occur in the colder months, especially spring and autumn. There are multiple rhinovirus immunotypes (>100), which makes vaccine control impracticable. In contrast to enteroviruses, which replicate at 37°C, rhinoviruses grow at 33°C (the temperature of the upper respiratory tract), which explains the localized disease characteristic of common colds.

REOVIRUSES

Reovirus infection

Reovirus infection occurs mainly in children, causing mild respiratory symptoms and diarrhoea. A few deaths have been reported following disseminated infection of brain, liver, heart and lungs.

Rotavirus infection

Rotavirus (Latin *rota* = wheel) is so named because of its electronmicroscopic appearance with a characteristic circular outline with radiating spokes (Fig. 2.17). It is responsible world-wide for both sporadic cases and epidemics of diarrhoea, and is currently one of the most important causes of childhood diarrhoea. More than 870 000 children under the age of 5 years are estimated to die annually in resource-deprived countries, compared with 75–150 in the USA. The prevalence is higher during the winter months in non-tropical areas. Asymptomatic

Fig. 2.17 Electronmicrograph of human rotavirus.

infections are common, and bottle-fed babies are more likely to be symptomatic than those that are breast-fed.

Adults may become infected with rotavirus but symptoms are usually mild or absent. The virus may, however, cause outbreaks of diarrhoea in patients on care of the elderly wards.

Clinical features

The illness is characterized by vomiting, fever, diarrhoea, and the metabolic consequences of water and electrolyte loss.

Diagnosis and treatment

The diagnosis can be established by ELISA for the detection of rotavirus antigen in faeces and by electronmicroscopy of faeces. Histology of the jejunal mucosa in children shows shortening of the villi, with crypt hyperplasia and mononuclear cell infiltration of the lamina propria.

Treatment is directed at overcoming the effects of water and electrolyte imbalance with adequate oral rehydration therapy and, when indicated, intravenous fluids (see Box 2.9). Antibiotics should not be prescribed.

Rhesus–human reassortant vaccines have been developed whereby a human rotavirus VP7 is expressed on the surface of a rhesus rotavirus. The tetravalent vaccine contains three reassortants for human rotavirus G-types 1, 2 and 4 plus the rhesus rotavirus (G-type 3). This vaccine (IRRV-TV; rhesus (human) rotavirus – tetravalent vaccine) has been shown to give high levels of protection in children in resource-deprived countries. Although initially licensed by the FDA in the USA, it has been withdrawn owing to an increased incidence of intussusception in the vaccinees.

Other viruses

Other viruses associated with gastroenteritis are shown in Table 2.22. These include members of two major families which can be recognized by their electronmicroscopic appearance. Caliciviruses, which include the noraviruses

Table 2.22 Viruses associated with gastroenteritis

Rotavirus (groups A, B, C, D and E)
Enteric adenovirus (types 40 and 41)
Noravirus (Norwalk-like viruses of calicivirus family)
Astrovirus

(previously known as Norwalk agent, a small round structured virus) and astroviruses, are responsible for winter vomiting. Although gastroenteritis viruses are normally spread by the faeco-oral route, aerosol spread also occurs.

TOGAVIRUSES

This family comprises three genera: the rubiviruses, which include rubella virus; and the alphaviruses and flaviviruses, which each include some of the arthropod-borne viruses.

Rubella

Rubella ('German measles') is caused by a spherical, enveloped RNA virus which is easily killed by heat and ultraviolet light. While the disease can occur sporadically, epidemics are not uncommon. It has a world-wide distribution. Spread of the virus is via droplets; maximum infectivity occurs before and during the time the rash is present.

Clinical features

The incubation period is 14–21 days, averaging 18 days. The clinical features are largely determined by age, with symptoms being mild or absent in children under 5 years.

During the prodrome the patient may develop malaise and fever. Mild conjunctivitis and lymphadenopathy may be present. The distribution of the lymphadenopathy is characteristic and involves particularly the suboccipital, postauricular and posterior cervical groups of lymph nodes. Small petechial lesions on the soft palate (Forchheimer spots) are suggestive but not diagnostic. Splenomegaly may be present.

The eruptive or exanthematous phase usually occurs within the first 7 days of the initial symptoms. The rash first appears on the forehead and then spreads to involve the trunk and the limbs. It is pinkish red, macular and discrete, although some of these lesions may coalesce (Fig. 2.18). It usually fades by the second day and rarely persists beyond the third day after its appearance.

Complications

Complications are rare. They include superadded pulmonary bacterial infection, arthralgia, haemorrhagic manifestations due to thrombocytopenia, encephalitis and the congenital rubella syndrome. Rubella affects the fetuses of up to 80% of all women who contract the infection during the first trimester of pregnancy. The incidence of congenital abnormalities diminishes in the second trimester and no ill-effects result from infection in the third trimester.

Fig. 2.18 Rubella rash.

Congenital rubella syndrome is characterized by the presence of fetal cardiac malformations, especially patent ductus arteriosus and ventricular septal defect, eye lesions (especially cataracts), microcephaly, mental retardation and deafness.

The expanded rubella syndrome consists of the manifestations of the congenital rubella syndrome plus other effects including hepatosplenomegaly, myocarditis, interstitial pneumonia and metaphyseal bone lesions.

Diagnosis and treatment

The diagnosis may be suspected clinically, but laboratory diagnosis is essential to distinguish the illness from other virus infections (e.g. echovirus) and drug rashes. This is achieved by demonstrating a rising antibody titre (measured using the sensitive haemagglutination-inhibiting antibody (HAI) test or ELISA) in two successive blood samples taken 14 days apart or by the detection of rubella-specific IgM. The virus can be cultured from throat swabs (or oral fluid samples), urine and, in the case of intrauterine infection, the products of conception.

Treatment is supportive.

Prevention

Human immunoglobulin can decrease the symptoms of this already mild illness, but does not prevent the teratogenic effects. Several live attenuated rubella vaccines have been used with great success in preventing this illness and these have been successfully combined with the measles and mumps (MMR) vaccine. The side-effects of vaccination have been dramatically decreased by using vaccines prepared in human embryonic fibroblast cultures (RA 27/3 vaccine). Use of the vaccine is contraindicated during pregnancy or if there is a likelihood of pregnancy within 3 months of immunization. Inadvertent use of the vaccine during pregnancy has not, however, revealed a risk of teratogenicity.

Arbovirus (arthropod-borne) infection

Arboviruses are zoonotic viruses, with the possible exception of the O'nyong-nyong fever virus of which humans are the only known vertebrate hosts. They are transmitted through the bites of insects, especially mosquitoes, and ticks. Over 385 viruses are classified as arboviruses. *Culex*, *Aedes* and *Anopheles* mosquitoes account for the transmission of the majority of these viruses.

Although most arbovirus diseases are generally mild, epidemics are frequent and when these occur the mortality is high. In general, the incubation period is less than 10 days. The illness tends to be biphasic and, as in other viral fevers, pyrexia, conjunctival suffusion, a rash, retro-orbital pain, myalgia and arthralgia are common. Lymphadenopathy is seen in dengue. Lifelong immunity to a particular virus is usual. In some of these viral fevers, haemorrhage is a feature (Table 2.23). Increased vascular permeability, capillary fragility and consumptive coagulopathy have been implicated as causes of the haemorrhage. Encephalitis resulting from cerebral invasion may be prominent in some fevers.

Alphaviruses

The 24 viruses of this group are all transmitted by mosquitoes; eight result in human disease. These viruses are globally distributed and tend to acquire their names from the location where they were first isolated (such as Ross River, Eastern Venezuelan, and Western encephalitis viruses) or by the local expression for a major symptom caused by the virus (such as chikungunya, meaning 'doubled up'). Infection is characterized by fever, skin rash, arthralgia, myalgia and sometimes encephalitis.

Table 2.23   Viral infections associated with haemorrhagic manifestations*

Togavirus
Flavivirus
Yellow fever (urban and sylvan)
Dengue haemorrhagic fever
Kysanur Forest disease
Omsk haemorrhagic fever
Rift Valley fever
Alphavirus
Chikungunya

Bunyavirus
Congo–Crimean haemorrhagic fever
Hantavirus infections

Arenavirus
Argentinian haemorrhagic fever
Bolivian haemorrhagic fever
Lassa fever
Epidemic haemorrhagic fever

Filovirus
Marburg
Ebola

---

* Most of these are arboviruses. Some (e.g. hantavirus, Lassa fever) have a rodent vector. The source and transmission route of filoviruses is not known.

Flaviviruses

There are 60 viruses in this group, some of which are transmitted by ticks and others by mosquitoes.

Yellow fever

Yellow fever, caused by a flavivirus, results in an illness of widely varying severity so that the disease is under-reported. It is a disease confined to Africa (90% of cases) and South America between latitudes 15° N and 15° S. For poorly understood reasons, yellow fever has not been reported from Asia, despite the fact that climatic conditions are suitable and the vector, *Aedes aegypti*, is common. The infection is transmitted in the wild by *A. africanus* in Africa and the *Haemagogus* species in South and Central America. Extension of infection to humans (via the mosquito or from monkeys) leads to the occurrence of 'jungle' yellow fever. *A. aegypti*, a domestic mosquito which lives in close relationship to humans, is responsible for human-to-human transmission in urban areas (urban yellow fever). Once infected, a mosquito remains so for its whole life.

Clinical features

The incubation period is 3–6 days. When the infection is mild, the disease is indistinguishable from other viral fevers such as influenza or dengue.

Three phases in the severe (classical) illness are recognized. Initially the patient presents with a high fever of acute onset, usually 39–40°C, which then returns to normal in 4–5 days. During this time, headache is prominent. Retrobulbar pain, myalgia, arthralgia, a flushed face and suffused conjunctivae are common. Epigastric discomfort and vomiting are present when the illness is severe. Relative bradycardia (Faget's sign) is present from the second day of illness. The patient then makes an apparent recovery and feels well for several days. Following this 'phase of calm' the patient again develops increasing fever, deepening jaundice and hepatomegaly. Ecchymosis, bleeding from the gums, haematemesis and melaena may occur. Coma, which is usually a result of uraemia or haemorrhagic shock, occurs for a few hours preceding death. The mortality rate is up to 40% in severe cases. The pathology of the liver shows mid-zone necrosis, and eosinophilic degeneration of hepatocytes (Councilman bodies) (see p. 362).

Diagnosis and treatment

The diagnosis is established by a careful history of travel and vaccination status, and by isolation of the virus (when possible) from blood during the first 3 days of illness. Serodiagnosis is possible, but in endemic areas cross-reactivity with other flaviviruses is a problem.

Treatment is supportive. Bed rest (under mosquito nets), analgesics, and maintenance of fluid and electrolyte balance are important.

Prevention and control

Yellow fever is an internationally notifiable disease. It is easily prevented using the attenuated 17D chick embryo vaccine. Vaccination is not recommended for children under 9 months and immunosuppressed patients unless there are compelling reasons. For the purposes of international certification, immunization is valid for 10 years, but protection lasts much longer than this and probably for life. The WHO Expanded Programme of Immunization includes yellow fever vaccination in endemic areas.

Dengue

This is the commonest arthropod-borne viral infection in humans: over 100 million cases occur every year in the tropics, with over 10 000 deaths from dengue haemorrhagic fever. Dengue is caused by a flavivirus and is found mainly in Asia, South America and Africa, although it has been reported from the USA. Four different antigenic varieties of dengue virus are recognized and all are transmitted by the daytime-biting *A. aegypti* which breed in standing water in refuse dumps in inner cities. *A. albopictus* is a less common transmitter. Humans are infective during the first 3 days of the illness (the viraemic stage). Mosquitoes become infective about 2 weeks after feeding on an infected individual, and remain so for the rest of their lives. The disease is usually endemic. Immunity after the illness is partial.

Clinical features

The incubation period is 5–6 days following the mosquito bite. Asymptomatic or mild infections are common. Two clinical forms are recognized.

Classic dengue fever

Classic dengue fever is characterized by the abrupt onset of fever, malaise, headache, facial flushing, retrobulbar pain which worsens on eye movements, conjunctival suffusion and severe backache, which is a prominent symptom. Lymphadenopathy, petechiae on the soft palate and skin rashes may also occur. The rash is transient and morbilliform. It appears on the limbs and then spreads to involve the trunk. Desquamation occurs subsequently. Cough is uncommon. The fever subsides after 3–4 days, the temperature returns to normal for a couple of days, and then the fever returns, together with the features already mentioned, but milder. This biphasic or 'saddleback' pattern is considered characteristic. Severe fatigue, a feeling of being unwell and depression are common for several weeks after the fever has subsided.

Dengue haemorrhagic fever (DHF)

Dengue haemorrhagic fever is a severe form of dengue fever and is believed to be the result of two or more sequential infections with different dengue serotypes. It is a disease of children and has been described almost exclusively in South East Asia. The disease has a mild start, often with symptoms of an upper respiratory tract infection. This is then followed by the abrupt onset of shock and haemorrhage into the skin and ear, epistaxis, haematemesis and melaena known as the dengue shock syndrome. Serum complement levels are depressed and there is laboratory evidence of a consumptive coagulopathy.

Diagnosis and treatment

Isolation of dengue virus by tissue culture in sera obtained during the first few days of illness is diagnostic. Demonstration of rising antibody titres by neutralization (most specific), haemagglutination inhibition 'ELISA' or complement-fixing antibodies in sequential serum samples is evidence of dengue virus infection. Blood tests show leucopenia and thrombocytopenia.

Treatment is supportive with analgesics and adequate fluid replacement; in DHF, blood transfusion may be necessary.

Prevention

Travellers should be advised to sleep under impregnated nets but this is not very effective as the mosquito bites in daytime. Topical insect repellents should be used. Adult mosquitoes should be destroyed by sprays, and breeding sites should be eradicated.

Rift Valley fever

Rift Valley fever, caused by a flavivirus, is primarily an acute febrile illness of livestock – sheep, goats and camels. It is found in southern and eastern Africa. The vector in East Africa is *Culex pipiens* and in southern Africa, *Aedes caballus*. Following an incubation period of 3–6 days, the patient has an acute febrile illness that is difficult to distinguish clinically from other viral fevers. The temperature pattern is usually biphasic. The initial febrile illness lasts 2–4 days and is followed by a remission and a second febrile episode. Complications are indicative of severe infection and include retinopathy, meningo-encephalitis, haemorrhagic manifestations and hepatic necrosis. Mortality approaches 50% in severe forms of the illness. Treatment is supportive.

Japanese encephalitis

Japanese encephalitis is a mosquito-borne encephalitis caused by a flavivirus. It has been reported most frequently from the rice-growing countries of South East Asia and the Far East. *Culex tritaeniorhynchus* is the most important vector and this feeds mainly on pigs as well as birds such as herons and sparrows. Humans are accidental hosts.

As with other viral infections, the clinical manifestations are variable. The onset is heralded by severe rigors. Fever, headache and malaise last 1–6 days. Weight loss is prominent. In the acute encephalitic stage the fever is high (38–41°C), neck rigidity occurs and neurological signs such as altered consciousness, hemiparesis and convulsions develop. Mental deterioration occurs over a period of 3–4 days and culminates in coma. Mortality varies from 7–40% and is higher in children. Residual neurological defects such as deafness, emotional lability and hemiparesis occur in about 70% of patients who have had CNS involvement. Convalescence is prolonged.

Antibody detection in serum and CSF by IgM capture ELISA is a useful rapid diagnostic test. An inactivated mouse brain vaccine is effective and available. Treatment is supportive.

West Nile virus

In 1999, the West Nile virus was first recognized in the western hemisphere (New York, USA) and it had previously been reported in Africa, Asia and parts of Europe. The outbreak in the USA produced thousands of symptomatic and symptomless infections with 1% resulting in encephalitis. It is spread by mosquitoes and infects birds, humans and horses. It can also be transmitted with blood transfusions, breast-feeding and organ donation.

BUNYAVIRUSES

Bunyaviruses belong to a large family of more than 200 viruses, most of which are arthropod-borne.

Congo–Crimean haemorrhagic fever

This is found mainly in Asia and Africa. The primary hosts are cattle and hares and the vectors are the *Hyalomma* ticks. Following an incubation period of 3–6 days there is an influenza-like illness with fever and haemorrhagic manifestations. The mortality is 10–50%.

Hantaviruses

Hantaviruses are enzootic viruses of wild rodents which are spread by aerosolized excreta and not by insect vectors. The most severe form of this infection is Korean haemorrhagic fever (or haemorrhagic fever with renal syndrome – HFRS). This condition has a mortality of 5–10% and is characterized by fever, shock and haemorrhage followed by an oliguric phase. Milder forms of the disease are associated with related viruses (e.g. Puumala virus) and may present as nephropathia epidemica, an acute fever with renal involvement. It is seen in Scandinavia and in other European countries in people who have been in contact with bank voles. In the USA, a new hantavirus (transmitted by the deer mouse) termed Sin Nombre was identified as the cause of outbreaks of acute respiratory disease in adults, referred to as hantavirus pulmonary syndrome (HPS). Other hantavirus types and rodent vector systems have been associated with this syndrome.

Diagnosis of hantavirus infection is made by an ELISA technique for specific antibodies.

ORTHOMYXOVIRUSES

Influenza

Three types of influenza virus are recognized: A, B and C. The influenza virus is a spherical or filamentous enveloped virus. Haemagglutinin (H), a surface glycopeptide, aids attachment of the virus to the wall of susceptible host cells at specific receptor sites. Cell penetration, probably by pinocytosis, and release of replicated viruses from the cell surface is effected by budding through the cell membrane facilitated by the action of the enzyme neuraminidase (N) which is also present on the viral envelope. ISH subtypes (H1–H15) and nine N subtypes (N1–N9) have been identified for influenza A viruses but only H1, H2, H3 and N1 and N2 have established stable lineages in the human population since 1918.

- Influenza A is generally responsible for pandemics and epidemics.
- Influenza B often causes smaller or localized and milder outbreaks, such as in camps or schools.
- Influenza C rarely produces disease in humans.

Antigenic shift describes the capacity of influenza A to develop new antigenic variants at irregular intervals. This results from genetic recombination of the RNA of the virus (which is arranged in eight segments) with that of an animal orthomyxovirus.

Antigenic drift (minor changes in influenza A and B viruses) results from point mutations leading to amino acid changes in the two surface glycoproteins, haemagglutinin (H) and neuraminidase (N), which induce humoral immunity.

Thus, changes due to antigenic shift or drift render the individual's immune response less able to combat the new variant.

Major shifts in the antigenic make-up of influenza A viruses provide the necessary conditions for major pandemics, whereas minor antigenic drifts give rise to less severe epidemics because immunity in the population is less blunted.

The most serious pandemic of influenza occurred in 1918, and was associated with more than 20 million deaths world-wide. In 1957, a major shift in the antigenic make-up of the virus led to the appearance of influenza A2 type H2-N2, which caused a world-wide pandemic. A further pandemic occurred in 1968 owing to the emergence of Hong Kong influenza type H3-N2, and minor antigenic drifts have caused outbreaks around the world ever since. In 1997, avian H5-N1 strain of influenza A was found in humans and represented a major change in viral surface antigens. Avian flu re-emerged in 2004–5.

Purified haemagglutinin and neuraminidase from recently circulating strains of influenza A and B viruses are incorporated in current vaccines.

Sporadic cases of influenza and outbreaks among groups of people living in a confined environment are frequent. The incidence increases during the winter months. Spread is mainly by droplet infection but fomites and direct contact have also been implicated.

The clinical features, diagnosis, treatment and prophylaxis of influenza are discussed on page 898.

PARAMYXOVIRUSES

These are a heterogeneous group of enveloped viruses of varying size that are responsible for parainfluenza, mumps, measles and other respiratory infections (Fig. 2.19).

Fig. 2.19 **Electronmicrograph of a paramyxovirus (mumps).**

Fig. 2.20 **Measles.** Courtesy of Dr MW McKendrick, Royal Hallamshire Hospital, Sheffield.

Parainfluenza

Parainfluenza is caused by the parainfluenza viruses types I–IV; these have a world-wide distribution and cause acute respiratory disease. Type IV appears to be less virulent than the other types and has been linked only to mild upper respiratory diseases in children and adults.

Parainfluenza is essentially a disease of children and presents with features similar to the common cold. When severe, a brassy cough with inspiratory stridor and features of laryngotracheobronchitis (croup) are present. Fever is usually present for 2–3 days and may be more prolonged if pneumonia develops. The development of croup is due to submucosal oedema and consequent airway obstruction in the subglottic region. This may lead to cyanosis, subcostal and intercostal recession and progressive airway obstruction. Infection in the immunocompromised is usually prolonged and may be severe. Treatment is supportive with oxygen, humidification and sedation when required. The role of steroids is controversial.

Measles (rubeola)

Measles is a highly communicable disease that occurs world-wide. With the introduction of aggressive immunization policies, the incidence of measles has fallen dramatically in the West, but it still remains one of the most common childhood infections in resource-deprived countries, where it is associated with a high morbidity and mortality. It is spread by droplet infection and the period of infectivity is from 4 days before until 2 days after the onset of the rash.

Clinical features

The incubation period is 8–14 days. Two distinct phases of the disease can be recognized.

Typical measles

- *The pre-eruptive and catarrhal stage*. This is the stage of viraemia and viral dissemination. Malaise, fever, rhinorrhoea, cough, conjunctival suffusion and the pathognomonic Koplik's spots are present during this stage. Koplik's spots are small, greyish, irregular lesions surrounded by an erythematous base and are found in greatest numbers on the buccal mucous membrane opposite the second molar tooth. They occur a day or two before the onset of the rash.
- *The eruptive or exanthematous stage*. This is characterized by the presence of a maculopapular rash that initially occurs on the face, chiefly the forehead, and then spreads rapidly to involve the rest of the body (Fig. 2.20). At first the rash is discrete but later it may become confluent and patchy, especially on the face and neck. It fades in about 1 week and leaves behind a brownish discoloration.

Although measles is a relatively mild disease in the healthy child, it carries a high mortality in the malnourished and in those who have other diseases. Complications are common in such individuals and include bacterial pneumonia, bronchitis, otitis media and gastroenteritis. Less commonly, myocarditis, hepatitis and encephalomyelitis may occur. In those who are malnourished or those with defective cell-mediated immunity, the classical maculopapular rash may not develop and widespread desquamation may occur. The virus also causes the rare condition, subacute sclerosing panencephalitis, which may follow measles infection occurring early in life (<18 months of age). Persistence of the virus with reactivation pre-puberty results in accumulation of virus in the brain, progressive mental deterioration and a fatal outcome (see p. 1240).

Maternal measles, unlike rubella, does not cause fetal abnormalities. It is, however, associated with spontaneous abortions and premature delivery.

Atypical measles

In the past, a severe illness called atypical measles occurred in individuals given an inactivated vaccine (now withdrawn). This vaccine conferred incomplete protection and on exposure to the wild measles virus they developed high fever, myalgia, abdominal pain and a variety of skin rashes which could be mistaken for scarlet fever, meningococcal disease or varicella. Pneumonia was invariably present and pulmonary infiltrates persisted for years in some cases.

Diagnosis and treatment

Most cases of measles are diagnosed clinically but, if necessary, immunofluorescence, virus culture and serological tests (complement fixation test (CFT), haemagglutination inhibition tests) are used to confirm the diagnosis.

Treatment is supportive. Antibiotics are indicated only if secondary bacterial infection occurs.

Prevention

A previous attack of measles confers a high degree of immunity and second attacks are uncommon. Normal human immunoglobulin given within 5 days of exposure effectively aborts an attack of measles. It is indicated for previously unimmunized children below 3 years of age, during pregnancy, and in those with debilitating disease.

Active immunization. Children are immunized with the combined mumps–measles–rubella (MMR) vaccine (Box 2.6).

Mumps

Mumps is the result of infection with a paramyxovirus. It is spread by droplet infection, by direct contact or through fomites. Humans are the only known natural hosts. The peak period of infectivity is 2–3 days before the onset of the parotitis and for 3 days afterwards.

Clinical features

The incubation period averages 18 days. Although no age is exempt, it is primarily a disease of school-aged children and young adults; it is uncommon before the age of 2 years. The prodromal symptoms are non-specific and include fever, malaise, headache and anorexia. This is usually followed by severe pain over the parotid glands, with either unilateral or bilateral parotid swelling. The enlarged parotid glands obscure the angle of the mandible and may elevate the ear lobe, which does not occur in cervical lymph node enlargement. Trismus due to pain is common at this stage. Submandibular gland involvement occurs less frequently.

Complications

CNS involvement is the most common extrasalivary-gland manifestation of mumps. Clinical meningitis occurs in 5% of all infected patients, and 30% of patients with CNS involvement have no evidence of parotid gland involvement.

Epididymo-orchitis develops in about one-third of patients who develop mumps after puberty. Bilateral testicular involvement results in sterility in only a small percentage of these patients. Pancreatitis, oophoritis, myocarditis, mastitis, hepatitis and polyarthritis may also occur.

Diagnosis and treatment

The diagnosis of mumps is on the basis of the clinical features. In doubtful cases, serological demonstration of a fourfold rise in antibodies detected by complement fixation or indirect haemagglutination or neutralization tests on acute and convalescent sera is diagnostic. Virus can be isolated in cell culture from saliva, throat swab, urine and CSF and identified by immunofluorescence or haemadsorption.

Treatment is supportive. Attention should be given to adequate nutrition and mouth care. Analgesics should be used to relieve pain.

Prevention

Active immunization. Children are immunized with the MMR vaccine (Box 2.6). Vaccination is contraindicated in immunosuppressed individuals, during pregnancy, or in those with severe febrile illnesses.

Respiratory syncytial virus infection

Respiratory syncytial virus (RSV) is a paramyxovirus that causes many respiratory infections in epidemics each winter. It is a common cause of bronchiolitis in infants, which is complicated by pneumonia in approximately 10% of cases. The infection normally starts with upper respiratory symptoms. After an interval of 1–3 days a cough and low-grade fever may develop. The onset of bronchiolitis is characterized by dyspnoea and hyper-expansion of the chest with subcostal and intercostal recession. The disease may be severe and potentially fatal in babies with underlying cardiac or respiratory disease. RSV infection has been associated with the occurrence of sudden infant death syndrome (SIDS). Immunity is short-lived and, consequently, reinfection can occur throughout life. RSV is occasionally the cause of outbreaks of pneumonia in the elderly and in the immunocompromised.

Transfer of infection between children in hospital commonly occurs unless infected patients are isolated or cohorted. Meticulous attention to handwashing and other infection control measures reduces the risk of transmission by staff members.

Diagnosis and treatment

Immunofluorescence on nasopharyngeal aspirates, virus culture and serology are the usual ways of confirming the diagnosis.

Treatment is generally supportive, but aerosolized ribavirin can be given to severe cases, particularly those with underlying cardiac or respiratory disease see p. 41).

Prevention

No vaccine is available for RSV but high-risk children (including those with bronchopulmonary dysplasia and congenital heart disease) can be protected against severe disease by monthly administration of either a hyper-immune globulin against RSV, or a humanized mono-clonal antibody Palivizumab, during the winter months (see p. 41).

Metapneumovirus

This recently discovered virus causes approximately 20% of lower respiratory tract infections in infants and young children.

Hendra and Nipah viruses

Hendra virus (formerly called equine morbillivirus) and Nipah virus are newly recognized zoonotic viruses that have caused disease in humans who have been in contact with infected animals (horses and pigs respectively). The viruses are named after the locations where they were first isolated, Hendra in Australia and Nipah in Malaysia, and both are classified as paramyxoviruses. Hendra virus has caused severe respiratory distress in horses and humans and Nipah virus caused a major outbreak of viral encephalitis (265 cases and 105 deaths) in Malaysia between September 1998 and April 1999. Treatment of these conditions is largely supportive, although there is some evidence that early treatment with ribavirin may reduce the severity of the diseases.

CORONAVIRUSES

Human coronaviruses were first isolated in the mid 1960s and the majority of isolates (related to the reference strains 229E and OC43) have been associated with common colds. In November 2002, an apparently new viral disease occurred in China (Guangdong province) and this spread rapidly in other parts of the Far East and also in Canada (Toronto and Vancouver).

This disease, known as 'severe acute respiratory syndrome' (SARS-COV) of which bronchopneumonia has been a major feature, is caused by a previously unknown coronavirus. Similarity of this virus to coronaviruses isolated from civet cats, raccoons and ferret badgers indicates the likelihood that SARS is a zoonotic disease.

The epidemic was finally brought under control in the summer of 2003 and by then there had been > 8000 cases with approximately 800 deaths.

RHABDOVIRUSES

Rabies

Rabies is a major problem in some countries, and established infection is invariably fatal. It is a genotype 1, single-stranded RNA virus of the Lyssavirus genus. The rabies virus is bullet-shaped and has spike-like structures arising from its surface containing glycoproteins that cause the host to produce neutralizing, haemagglutination-inhibiting antibodies. The virus has a marked affinity for nervous tissue and the salivary glands. It exists in two major epidemiological settings:

- *Urban rabies* is most frequently transmitted to humans through rabid dogs and, less frequently, cats.
- *Sylvan (wild) rabies* is maintained in the wild by a host of animal reservoirs such as foxes, skunks, jackals, mongooses and bats.

With the exception of Australia, New Zealand and the Antarctic, human rabies has been reported from all continents. Transmission is usually through the bite of an infected animal. However, the percentage of rabid bites leading to clinical disease ranges from 10% (on the legs) to 80% (on the head). Other forms of transmission, if they occur, are rare.

Having entered the human body, the virus replicates in the muscle cells near the entry wound. It penetrates the nerve endings and travels in the axoplasm to the spinal cord and brain. In the CNS the virus again proliferates before spreading to the salivary glands, lungs, kidneys and other organs via the autonomic nerves.

There have been only two recorded cases of survival from clinical rabies.

Clinical features

The incubation period is variable and may range from a few weeks to several years; on average it is 1–3 months. In general, bites on the head, face and neck have a shorter incubation period than those elsewhere. In humans, two distinct clinical varieties of rabies are recognized:

- furious rabies – the classic variety
- dumb rabies – the paralytic variety.

Furious rabies

The only characteristic feature in the prodromal period is the presence of pain and tingling at the site of the initial wound. Fever, malaise and headache are also present. About 10 days later, marked anxiety and agitation or depressive features develop. Hallucinations, bizarre behaviour and paralysis may also occur. Hyper-excitability, the hallmark of this form of rabies, is precipitated by auditory or visual stimuli. Hydrophobia (fear of water) is present in 50% of patients and is due to severe pharyngeal spasms on attempting to eat or drink. Aerophobia (fear of air) is considered pathognomonic of rabies. Examination reveals hyperreflexia, spasticity, and evidence of sympathetic overactivity indicated by pupillary dilatation and diaphoresis.

The patient goes on to develop convulsions, respiratory paralysis and cardiac arrhythmias. Death usually occurs in 10–14 days.

Dumb rabies

Dumb rabies, or paralytic rabies, presents with a symmetrical ascending paralysis resembling the Guillain–Barré syndrome. This variety of rabies commonly occurs after bites from rabid bats.

Diagnosis

The diagnosis of rabies is generally made clinically. Skin-punch biopsies are used to detect antigen with an immunofluorescent antibody test on frozen section. Viral RNA can be isolated using the reverse transcription polymerase chain reaction (RT-PCR). Isolation of viruses from saliva or the presence of antibodies in blood or CSF may establish the diagnosis. The corneal smear test is not recommended as it is unreliable. The classic Negri bodies are detected at post-mortem in 90% of all patients with rabies; these are eosinophilic, cytoplasmic, ovoid bodies, 2–10 nm in diameter, seen in greatest numbers in the neurones of the hippocampus and the cerebellum. The diagnosis should be made pathologically on the biting animal using RT-PCR, immunofluorescence assay (IFA) or tissue culture of the brain.

Treatment

Once the CNS disease is established, therapy is symptomatic as death is virtually inevitable. The patient should be nursed in a quiet, darkened room. Nutritional, respiratory and cardiovascular support may be necessary.

Drugs such as morphine, diazepam and chlorpromazine should be used liberally in patients who are excitable.

Prevention

Pre-exposure prophylaxis. This is given to individuals with a high risk of contracting rabies, such as laboratory workers, animal handlers and veterinarians. Two doses of human diploid cell vaccine (HDCV) 1.0 mL deep subcutaneously or intramuscularly given 4 weeks apart provides effective immunity. A reinforcing dose is given after 12 months and additional reinforcing doses are given every 1–3 years depending on the risk of exposure. Vaccines of nervous-tissue origin are still used in some parts of the world. These, however, are associated with significant side-effects and are best avoided if HDCV is available.

Postexposure prophylaxis. The wound should be cleaned carefully and thoroughly with soap and water and left open. Human rabies immunoglobulin should be given immediately (20 IU/kg); half should be injected around the area of the wound and the other half should be given intramuscularly. Five 1.0 mL doses of HDCV should be given intramuscularly: the first dose is given on day 0 and is followed by injections on days 3, 7, 14 and 28. Reaction to the vaccine is uncommon.

Control of rabies

Domestic animals should be vaccinated if there is any risk of rabies in the country. In the UK, control has been by quarantine of imported animals and no indigenous case of rabies has been reported for many years. The quarantine laws are under revision at the present time. The Pet Travel Scheme (PETS) introduced as a pilot scheme in 2000 enables certain pet animals to enter or re-enter Great Britain without quarantine if they come from qualifying countries via designated routes, are carried by authorized transport companies, and meet the conditions of the scheme. Wild animals in 'at risk' countries must be handled with great care.

RETROVIRUSES

Retroviruses (Table 2.24) are distinguished from other RNA viruses by their ability to replicate through a DNA intermediate using an enzyme, reverse transcriptase.

Table 2.24 Human lymphotropic retroviruses

Subfamily	Virus	Disease
Lentivirus	HIV-1	AIDS
	HIV-2	AIDS
Oncovirus	HTLV-1*	Adult T cell leukaemia/ lymphoma
		Tropical spastic paraparesis
	HTLV-2	Myelopathy

* HTLV, human T cell lymphotropic virus

HIV-1 and the related virus, HIV-2, are further classified as lentiviruses ('slow' viruses) because of their slowly progressive clinical effects.

HIV-1 and HIV-2 are discussed on page 130.

HTLV-1 causes adult T cell leukaemia/lymphoma and tropical spastic paraparesis (see p. 1193).

ARENAVIRUSES

Arenaviruses are pleomorphic, round or oval viruses with diameters ranging from 50–300 nm. The virion surface has club-shaped projections, and the virus itself contains a variable number of characteristic electron-dense granules that represent residual, non-functional host ribosomes. The prototype virus of this group is lymphocytic choriomeningitis virus, which is a natural infection of mice. Arenaviruses are also responsible for Argentinian and Bolivian haemorrhagic fevers and Lassa fever.

Lassa fever

This illness was first documented in the town of Lassa, Nigeria, in 1969 and is confined to sub-Saharan West Africa (Nigeria, Liberia and Sierra Leone). The multi-mammate rat, *Mastomys natalensis*, is known to be the reservoir. Humans are infected by ingesting foods contaminated by rat urine or saliva containing the virus. Person-to-person spread by body fluids also occurs. Only 10–30% of infections are symptomatic.

Clinical features

The incubation period is 7–18 days. The disease is insidious in onset and is characterized by fever, myalgia, severe backache, malaise and headache. A transient maculopapular rash may be present. A sore throat, pharyngitis and lymphadenopathy occur in over 50% of patients. In severe cases epistaxis and gastrointestinal bleeding may occur – hence the classification of Lassa fever as a viral haemorrhagic fever. The fever usually lasts 1–3 weeks and recovery within a month of the onset of illness is usual. However, death occurs in 15–20% of hospitalized patients, usually from irreversible hypovolaemic shock.

Diagnosis

The diagnosis is established by serial serological tests (including the Lassa virus-specific IgM titre) or by culturing the virus from the throat, serum or urine. Molecular diagnosis by means of the reverse transcriptase polymerase chain reaction has become available and this provides a sensitive and reasonably rapid diagnostic test.

Treatment

Treatment is supportive. In addition, clinical benefit and reduction in mortality can be achieved with ribavirin therapy, if given in the first week.

In non-endemic countries, strict isolation procedures should be used, the patient ideally being nursed in a flexible-film isolator. Specialized units for the management of Lassa fever and other haemorrhagic fevers have been established in the UK. As Lassa fever virus and other causes of haemorrhagic fever (Marburg/Ebola and Congo–Crimean haemorrhagic fever viruses) have been transmitted from patients to staff in healthcare situations, great care should be taken in handling specimens and clinical material from these patients.

Lymphocytic choriomeningitis (LCM)

This infection is a zoonosis, the natural reservoir of LCM virus being the house mouse. Infection is characterized by:

- non-nervous-system illness, with fever, malaise, myalgia, headache, arthralgia and vomiting
- aseptic meningitis in addition to the above symptoms.

Occasionally, a more severe form occurs, with encephalitis leading to disturbance of consciousness.

This illness is generally self-limiting and requires no specific treatment.

MARBURG VIRUS DISEASE AND EBOLA VIRUS DISEASE

These severe, haemorrhagic, febrile illnesses are discussed together because their clinical manifestations are similar. The diseases are named after Marburg in Germany and the Ebola river region in the Sudan and Zaire where these viruses first appeared. The natural reservoir for these viruses has not been identified and the precise mode of spread from one individual to another has not been elucidated.

Epidemics have occurred periodically in recent years, mainly in sub-Saharan Africa. The mortality from Marburg and Ebola has ranged from 25% to 90% and recovery is slow in those who survive.

The illness is characterized by the acute onset of severe headache, severe myalgia and high fever, followed by prostration. On about the fifth day of illness a non-pruritic maculopapular rash develops on the face and then spreads to the rest of the body. Diarrhoea is profuse and is associated with abdominal cramps and vomiting. Haematemesis, melaena or haemoptysis may occur between the seventh and sixteenth day. Hepato-splenomegaly and facial oedema are usually present. In Ebola virus disease, chest pain and a dry cough are prominent symptoms.

Treatment is symptomatic. Convalescent human serum appears to decrease the severity of the attack.

POSTVIRAL/CHRONIC FATIGUE SYNDROME
(see also p. 1281)

Viral illnesses have been implicated aetiologically, including those due to EBV, Coxsackie B viruses, echoviruses, CMV and hepatitis A virus. Non-viral causes such as allergy to *Candida* spp. have also been proposed.

The proportion of patients with 'organic' diagnoses remains uncertain. Studies have suggested that two-thirds of patients with a symptom duration of more than 6 months have an underlying psychiatric disorder.

TRANSMISSIBLE SPONGIFORM ENCEPHALOPATHIES (TSE OR PRION DISEASE)

Transmissible spongiform encephalopathies are caused by the accumulation in the nervous system of a protein, termed a 'prion', which is an abnormal isoform Pr Pres of a normal, host protein (Pr Pc).

Although familial forms of prion disease are known to exist, these conditions can be transmissible, particularly if brain tissue enters another host. There is no convincing evidence for the presence of nucleic acid in association with prions; thus these agents cannot be considered orthodox viruses and it is the abnormal prion protein itself that is infectious and can trigger a conversion of the normal protein into the atypical isoform. After infection, a long incubation period is followed by CNS degeneration associated with dementia or ataxia which invariably leads to death. Histology of the brain reveals spongiform change with an accumulation of the abnormal prion protein in the form of amyloid plaques.

The human prion diseases are Creutzfeldt–Jakob disease, including the sporadic, familial, iatrogenic and variant forms of the disease, Gerstmann–Straussler–Scheinker syndrome, fatal familial insomnia, and kuru.

- *Creutzfeldt–Jakob disease* (CJD) usually occurs sporadically world-wide with an annual incidence of one per million of the population. Although, in most cases, the epidemiology remains obscure, transmission to others has occurred as a result of administration of human cadaveric growth hormone or gonadotrophin, from dura mater and corneal grafting, and in neurosurgery from reuse of contaminated instruments and electrodes (iatrogenic CJD).
- *Variant CJD.* In the UK, knowledge that large numbers of cattle with the prion disease, bovine spongiform encephalopathy (BSE) had gone into the human food chain, led to enhanced surveillance for emergence of the disease in humans. The evidence is convincing, based on transmission studies in mice and on glycosylation patterns of prion proteins, that this has occurred and, to date, there have been approximately 150 confirmed and suspected cases of variant CJD

(human BSE) in the UK and 12 in the rest of the world. In contrast to sporadic CJD, which presents with dementia at a mean age of onset of 60 years, variant CJD presents with ataxia, dementia, myoclonus and chorea at a mean age of onset of 29 years (Fig. 2.21).

- *Gerstmann–Straussler–Scheinker syndrome* and *fatal familial insomnia* are rare prion diseases usually occurring in families with a positive history. The pattern of inheritance is as an autosomal dominant with some degree of variable penetrance.
- *Kuru* was described and characterized in the Fore highlanders in NE New Guinea. Transmission was associated with ritualistic cannibalism of deceased relatives. With the cessation of cannibalism by 1960, the disease has gradually diminished and recent cases had all been exposed to the agent before 1960.

The infectious agents of prion disease have remarkable characteristics. In the infected host there is no evidence of inflammatory, cytokine or immune reactions. The agent is highly resistant to decontamination, and infectivity is not reliably destroyed by autoclaving or by treatment with formaldehyde and most other gas or liquid disinfectants. It is very resistant to γ irradiation. Autoclaving at a high temperature (134–137°C for 18 minutes) is used for decontamination of instruments, and hypochlorite (20 000 p.p.m. available chlorine) or 1 molar sodium hydroxide are used for liquid disinfection. Uncertainty about the reliability of any methods for safe decontamination of surgical instruments has necessitated the introduction of guidelines for patient management.

Fig. 2.21 **Creutzfeldt–Jakob disease.** Deaths of confirmed and sporadic cases of CJD (* to 28/2/03) in the UK. Courtesy of Prof JW Ironside, Director National CJD Surveillance Unit, University of Edinburgh.

FURTHER READING
Banatvala JE, Brown DWG (2004) Rubella. *Lancet* **363**: 1127–1136.
Collins ST et al. (2004) Transmissible spongiform encephalopathies. *Lancet* **363**: 51–61.
Hien TT, deJong M, Farrar J (2005) Avian Influenza. *New England Journal of Medicine* 351: 2363–2365.
Nicholson KG et al. (2003) Influenza. *Lancet* **362**: 1733–1745.
Peiris JSM et al. (2003) The severe acute respiratory syndrome. *New England Journal of Medicine* **349**: 2431–2441.
Robertson SE, Hull BP, Tomori O et al. (1995) Yellow fever. A decade of resurgence. *Journal of the American Medical Association* **276**: 1157–1162.
Warrell MJ, Warrell DA (2004) Rabies and other lyssavirus diseases. *Lancet* **363**: 959–969.

BACTERIAL INFECTIONS

Classification of bacteria

Bacteria are unicellular organisms (prokaryotes). A small fraction are of medical importance. Unusual infections may result from exposure under circumstances of altered host defences, notably in the severely immunocompromised patient.

Bacteria have traditionally been classified according to the Gram stain which distinguishes Gram-positive from Gram-negative organisms. Using light microscopy, these can then largely be divided into cocci and bacilli (rods). Some have a spiral appearance (spirochaetes) while others, such as *Clostridium* spp., may contain spores (Table 2.25). The cell wall arrangement of Gram-positive cocci contains a phospholipid bilayer surrounded by peptidoglycan made up of repeating units of *N*-acetylglucosamine and *N*-acetylmuramic acid. In contrast, Gram-negative bacilli possess a second outer lipid bilayer containing protein and lipopolysaccharide (endotoxin). Some pathogens are encapsulated, which is an anti-phagocytic virulence factor.

Bacteria can often be cultured in broth or on solid agar. Those growing in the absence of oxygen are strict anaerobes (e.g. *Bacteroides* spp.), whilst oxygen-dependent bacteria are known as aerobes (e.g. *Pseudomonas* spp.). Many pathogens can tolerate reduced concentrations of oxygen (e.g. *E. coli*). Some organisms are more demanding in their growth requirements and require special laboratory media (e.g. *Mycoplasma* spp. and *Mycobacterium* spp.); others require more prolonged incubation (e.g. *Brucella* spp.).

Genetic classification is defining bacteria in terms of DNA sequence information and has led to the reclassification of several bacteria. DNA fingerprinting is also being increasingly applied to distinguishing similar isolates, which has applications in defining the epidemiology of infection.

Diagnosis and management of bacterial infections

The history and examination usually localizes the infection to a specific organ or body site. A systemic response may accompany such localized disease or, in the

Table 2.25 Classification of bacteria affecting humans

Aerobic bacteria	Cocci	Bacilli
Gram-positive	*Staphylococcus aureus*	*Listeria monocytogenes*
	Staph. epidermidis	*Corynebacterium diphtheriae*
	Streptococcus pneumoniae	*Bacillus anthracis*
	Strep. pyogenes (group A)	*B. cereus*
	Strep. agalactiae (group B)	
	Enterococci	
	Viridans streptococci	
Gram-negative	*Neisseria gonorrhoeae*	*Escherichia coli*
	N. meningitidis	*Klebsiella* spp.
	Moraxella catarrhalis	*Proteus* spp.
	Bordetella pertussis	*Haemophilus influenzae*
		Legionella spp.
		Salmonella spp.
		Shigella spp.
		Campylobacter jejuni
		Helicobacter pylori
		Pseudomonas spp.
		Brucella spp.
		Acinetobacter spp.
		Burkholderia spp.
		Vibrio cholerae
		Yesinia pestis
		Gram-positive
Anaerobes	Peptococci	*Actinomyces* spp.
	Peptostreptococci	*Clostridium perfringens*
		C. difficile
		C. botulinum
		C. tetani
		Gram-negative
		Bacteroides fragilis group
		Fusobacterium spp.
Spirochaetes	*Treponema pallidum*	
	Leptospira spp.	
	Borrelia spp.	
Others	*Mycobacterium* spp.	
	Mycoplasma pneumoniae	
	Ureaplasma spp.	
	Chlamydia spp.	

case of bloodstream infections, be the primary mode of presentation. The microbiological diagnosis is difficult to establish in most community-managed infections, and even in hospital where there is ready access to diagnostic laboratories only a minority of infections are documented. For these reasons, a clinical approach to bacterial diseases has been adopted.

SKIN AND SOFT TISSUE INFECTION

Superficial infections

Infections of the skin and the soft tissues beneath are common. These are usually fungal (see p. 1322) or bacterial. Although a wide range of bacteria have been recovered from skin and soft tissue infections (Table 2.26), the majority are caused by the Gram-positive cocci *Staphylococcus aureus* and *Streptococcus pyogenes*. Staphylococci are part of the normal microflora of the human skin and

Table 2.26 Bacterial causes of superficial skin and soft tissue infection

Specific risk factors	Likely organisms
None	*Staphylococcus aureus*
	Streptococcus pyogenes
Diabetes, peripheral vascular disease	Group B streptococci
Animal bite	*Pasteurella multocida*, *Capnocytophaga canimorsus*
Fresh water exposure	*Aeromonas hydrophila*
Sea water exposure	*Vibrio vulnificans*
Lymphoedema, stasis dermatitis	Groups A, C and G streptococci
Hot tub exposure	*Pseudomonas aeruginosa*
Malignant otitis externa	*Pseudomonas aeruginosa*
Human bite	*Fusobacterium* spp.

Table 2.27 Classification of bacterial skin and superficial soft tissue infections

Infection	Subgroup	Site	Common cause
Pyoderma	Impetigo	Skin	*Streptococcus pyogenes* *Staphylococcus aureus*
	Bullous impetigo	Skin	*Staph. aureus*
	Folliculitis	Skin, hair follicles	*Staph. aureus*
Abscesses	Furuncle (boil)	Subcutaneous tissue	*Staph. aureus*
	Hidradenitis suppurativa (acne inversa)	Multiple apocrine glands (axillae, groins)	*Staph. aureus*, anaerobes (secondary infection)
	Carbuncle	Dense group of furuncles: back of neck, shoulders	*Staph. aureus*
Cellulitis		Skin and subcutaneous tissue	*Staph. aureus* *Strep. pyogenes* Group C and G streptococci
Erysipelas		Skin	*Strep. pyogenes*
Ecthyma		Skin and subcutaneous tissue	*Strep. pyogenes* *Staph. aureus*

nasopharynx; up to 25% of people are carriers of *S. aureus*, which is the species responsible for the majority of staphylococcal infections. Although soft tissue infections are the most common manifestation of *S. aureus* disease, numerous other sites can be affected (Table 2.6).

The classification of soft tissue infections is complex, because imprecise and overlapping terms are in use. The commonly encountered infections (Table 2.27) are described in more detail on page 1318.

The majority of skin and superficial soft tissue infections are due to bacteria on the skin surface penetrating the dermis or the subcutaneous tissues. Infection can take place via hair follicles, insect bites, cuts and abrasions, or skin damaged by superficial fungal infection. Sometimes infection is introduced by an animal bite or a penetrating foreign body: in these cases more unusual organisms may be found. A number of factors predispose to cellulitis and other soft tissue infections (Table 2.28).

Pasteurellosis

Pasteurella multocida is found in the oropharynx of up to 90% of cats and 70% of dogs. It can cause soft tissue infections following animal bites. Although the infection initially resembles other forms of cellulitis, there is a much higher incidence of spread to deeper tissues, resulting in osteomyelitis, tenosynovitis or septic arthritis. The organism is sensitive to penicillin, but as infections following animal bites are often polymicrobial, co-amoxiclav is used.

Table 2.28 Predisposing factors for skin and soft tissue infection

Diabetes mellitus
Chronic lymphoedema
Peripheral vascular disease
Steroid treatment
Malnutrition
Some immunodeficiency states (e.g. Job's syndrome)
Nasal carriage of *Staphylococcus aureus*

Meticillin-resistant *Staphylococcus aureus* (MRSA)

S. aureus are commonly resistant to penicillin, and isolated resistance to other β-lactam antibiotics such as meticillin and flucloxacillin has been recognized since the development of the first semisynthetic penicillins in the early 1960s. However, in the last 25 years, strains of MRSA with resistance to a much wider range of antibiotics have emerged. In some cases only the glycopeptide antibiotics vancomycin and teicoplanin are effective, and a few organisms have been isolated with decreased sensitivity even to these. Vancomycin-insensitive *Staphylococcus aureus* (VISA) develop because the organism produces a thick cell wall by changing the synthesis of cell wall material. Vancomycin resistant *Staphylococcus aureus* (VRSA) acquires resistance by receiving the van A gene from vancomycin-resistant enterococci (see Fig. 2.2). Two classes of antibiotics, the streptogramins (e.g. quinupristin with dalfopristin) and the oxazolidinones (e.g. linezolid) are effective against Gram-positive bacteria, including MRSA. They should usually be reserved for multi-resistant organisms. Control of the use of antibiotics in hospitals and good infection control policies are vital to prevent spread.

MRSA is usually found as a harmless skin commensal, especially in hospitalized patients or nursing home residents. However, it can cause a variety of infections in soft tissues and elsewhere, and can cause death. It is particularly associated with surgical wound infections. Eradication of the organism is difficult, and people who are known to be colonized should be isolated from those at risk of significant infection. Topical treatment with antibiotics is often used, but is of limited efficacy. Hand-washing is more effective.

Cat scratch disease

Cat scratch disease is a zoonosis caused by *Bartonella henselae*. Asymptomatic bacteraemia is relatively common in domestic and especially feral cats, and human infection is probably due to direct inoculation from the claws or via cat flea bites. Regional lymphadenopathy appears

1–2 weeks after infection; the nodes become tender and may suppurate. Histology of the nodes shows granuloma formation, and the illness may be mistaken for myco-bacterial infection or lymphoma. There are usually few systemic symptoms in immunocompetent patients, although more severe disease may be seen in the immunocompromised. In these patients tender cutaneous or subcutaneous nodules are seen (bacillary angiomatosis) which may ulcerate. The lymphadenopathy resolves spontaneously over weeks or months, although surgical drainage of very large suppurating nodes may be necessary. *B. henselae* is sensitive to doxycycline, but the clinical benefit of treatment is unproven.

Toxin-mediated skin disease

A number of skin conditions, although caused by bacteria, are mediated by exotoxins rather than direct local tissue damage.

Staphylococcal scalded skin syndrome

The scalded skin syndrome is caused by a toxin-secreting strain of *S. aureus*. It principally affects children under the age of 5. The toxin, exfoliatin, causes intra-epidermal cleavage at the level of the stratum corneum leading to the formation of large flaccid blisters that shear readily. It is a relatively benign condition, and responds to treatment with flucloxacillin.

Toxic shock syndrome (TSS)

TSS is usually due to toxin-secreting staphylococci, but toxin-secreting streptococci have also been implicated. Although historically associated with vaginal colonization and tampon use in women, this is not always the case. The exotoxin (normally toxic shock syndrome toxin 1, TSST-1) causes abrupt onset of fever and shock, with a diffuse macular rash and desquamation of the palms and soles. Many patients are severely ill and mortality is about 10%. Treatment is mainly supportive, although the organism should be eradicated.

Scarlet fever (see p. 65)

Deep soft tissue infections

Infections of the deeper soft tissues are much less common than superficial infections, and tend to be more serious. Usually they are related to penetrating injuries or to surgery, and the causative organisms relate to the nature of the wound.

Necrotizing fasciitis

Necrotizing fasciitis is a fulminant, rapidly spreading infection associated with widespread tissue destruction and a high mortality. There are two forms. Type 1, caused by a mixture of aerobic and anaerobic bacteria, is usually seen following abdominal surgery or in diabetics. Type 2, caused by group A streptococci, arises spontaneously in previously healthy people. Both types are characterized by severe pain at the site of initial infection, rapidly

followed by tissue necrosis. Infection tracks rapidly along the tissue planes, causing spreading erythema, pain and sometimes crepitus. The only chance of survival is with urgent surgical debridement and aggressive antibiotic therapy. Type 2 necrotizing fasciitis is treated with high doses of benzylpenicillin and clindamycin; type 1 with a broad-spectrum combination.

Gas gangrene

Gas gangrene is caused by deep tissue infection with *Clostridium* spp., especially *C. perfringens*, and follows contaminated penetrating injuries. It is particularly associated with battlefield wounds, but is also seen in intravenous drug users, and following surgery. The initial infection develops in an area of necrotic tissue caused by the original injury; toxins secreted by the bacteria kill surrounding tissue and enable the anaerobic organism to spread rapidly. Toxins are also responsible for the severe systemic features of gas gangrene. Treatment consists of urgent surgical removal of necrotic tissue, and treatment with benzylpenicillin and clindamycin.

FURTHER READING
Bisno AL, Stevens DL (1996) Streptococcal infections in skin and soft tissues. *New England Journal of Medicine* **334**: 240–245.
Huskins WC, Goldmann DA (2005) Controlling meticillin-resistant Staph aureus. *The Lancet* **365**: 273–275.
Seal KV (2001) Necrotizing fasciitis. *Current Opinion in Infectious Disease* **14**: 127–132.

RESPIRATORY TRACT INFECTIONS

Infections of the respiratory tract are divided into infections of the upper and lower respiratory tract, which are separated by the carina. In health, the lower respiratory tract is normally sterile owing to a highly efficient defence system (p. 881). Infections of the upper respiratory tract are particularly common in childhood when they are usually the result of virus infection. The paranasal sinuses and middle ear are contiguous structures and can be involved secondary to viral infections of the nasopharynx. The lower respiratory tract is frequently compromised by smoking, air pollution, aspiration of upper respiratory tract secretions and chronic lung disease, notably chronic bronchitis and chronic obstructive pulmonary disease. Infections of the respiratory tract are defined clinically, sometimes radio-logically, as in the case of pneumonia, and by appropriate microbiological sampling.

Upper respiratory tract infections

- The common cold (acute coryza) (p. 895)
- Sinusitis (p. 1158)
- Rhinitis (p. 895)
- Pharyngitis (p. 898).

Fig. 2.22 Scarlet fever rash, showing desquamation.

Scarlet fever

Scarlet fever occurs when the infectious organism (usually a group A streptococcus) produces erythrogenic toxin in an individual who does not possess neutralizing antitoxin antibodies.

Clinical features

The incubation period of this relatively mild disease, which mainly affects children, is 2–4 days following a streptococcal infection, usually in the pharynx. Regional lymphadenopathy, fever, rigors, headache and vomiting are present. The rash, which blanches on pressure, usually appears on the second day of illness; it initially occurs on the neck but rapidly becomes punctate, erythematous and generalized. It is typically absent from the face, palms and soles, and is prominent in the flexures. The rash usually lasts about 5 days and is followed by extensive desquamation of the skin (Fig. 2.22). The face is flushed, with characteristic circumoral pallor. Early in the disease the tongue has a white coating through which prominent bright red papillae can be seen ('strawberry tongue'). Later the white coating disappears, leaving a raw-looking, bright red colour ('raspberry tongue'). The patient is infective for 10–21 days after the onset of the rash, unless treated with penicillin.

Scarlet fever may be complicated by peritonsillar or retropharyngeal abscesses and otitis media.

Diagnosis

The diagnosis is established by the typical clinical features and culture of a throat swab. Elevated anti-streptolysin O and anti-DNase B levels in convalescent serum are indicative of streptococcal infection.

Treatment

Penicillin is the drug of choice and is given orally as phenoxymethylpenicillin 500 mg four times daily for 10 days. Individuals allergic to penicillin can be treated effectively with erythromycin 250 mg four times daily for 10 days. Treatment is usually effective in preventing rheumatic fever (p. 76) and acute glomerulonephritis (p. 629), which are non-suppurative complications of streptococcal pharyngitis. Unlike acute rheumatic fever, streptococcal nephritis may also complicate streptococcal skin infection.

Prevention

Chemoprophylaxis with penicillin or erythromycin should be given in epidemics.

Diphtheria

Diphtheria caused by *Corynebacterium diphtheriae* occurs world-wide. Its incidence in the West has fallen dramatically following widespread active immunization, but it is epidemic in Russia and Eastern Europe. Transmission is mainly through airborne droplet infection and rarely through fomites.

C. diphtheriae is a Gram-positive bacillus. Only strains which carry the tox+ gene, are capable of toxin production. The toxin has two subunits, A and B. Subunit A is responsible for clinical toxicity. Subunit B serves only to transport the toxin component to specific receptors, present chiefly on the myocardium and in the peripheral nervous system. Humans are the only natural hosts.

Clinical features

Diphtheria was formerly a disease of childhood but is increasingly affecting adults in countries where childhood immunization has been interrupted as in Russia and Eastern Europe. The incubation period is 2–7 days. The manifestations may be regarded as local (due to the membrane) or systemic (due to exotoxin). The presence of a membrane, however, is not essential to the diagnosis. The illness is insidious in onset and is associated with tachycardia but only low-grade fever. If complicated by infection with other bacteria such as *Strep. pyogenes*, fever is high and spiking.

Nasal diphtheria is characterized by the presence of a unilateral, serosanguineous nasal discharge that crusts around the external nares.

Pharyngeal diphtheria is associated with the greatest toxicity and is characterized by marked tonsillar and pharyngeal inflammation and the presence of a membrane. This tough greyish yellow membrane is formed by fibrin, bacteria, epithelial cells, mononuclear cells and polymorphs, and is firmly adherent to the underlying tissue. Regional lymphadenopathy, often tender, is prominent and produces the so-called 'bull-neck'.

Laryngeal diphtheria is usually a result of extension of the membrane from the pharynx. A husky voice, a brassy cough, and later dyspnoea and cyanosis due to respiratory obstruction are common features.

Clinically evident myocarditis occurs, often weeks later, in patients with pharyngeal or laryngeal diphtheria. Acute circulatory failure due to myocarditis may occur in convalescent individuals around the tenth day of illness and is usually fatal. Neurological manifestations occur either early in the disease (palatal and pharyngeal wall paralysis) or several weeks after its onset (cranial nerve palsies, paraesthesiae, polyneuropathy or, rarely, encephalitis).

Cutaneous diphtheria is increasingly being seen in association with burns and in individuals with poor

> ### Box 2.7 Antitoxin administration
>
> - Many antitoxins are heterologous and therefore dangerous
> - Hypersensitivity reactions are common
>
> **Prior to treatment**
> Question patient about:
> (a) allergic conditions (e.g. asthma, hay fever)
> (b) previous antitoxin administration.
>
> Read instructions on antitoxin package carefully. Always give a subcutaneous test dose.

personal hygiene. Typically the ulcer is punched-out with undermined edges and is covered with a greyish white to brownish adherent membrane. Constitutional symptoms are uncommon.

Diagnosis

This must be made on clinical grounds since therapy is usually urgent and bacteriological results of culture studies and toxin production cannot be awaited.

Treatment

The patient should be isolated and bed rest advised. Antitoxin therapy is the only specific treatment. It must be given promptly to prevent further fixation of toxin to tissue receptors, since fixed toxin is not neutralized by antitoxin. Depending on the severity, 20 000–100 000 units of horse-serum antitoxin should be administered intramuscularly after an initial test dose to exclude any allergic reaction. Intravenous therapy may be required in a very severe case. There is a risk of acute anaphylaxis after antitoxin administration and of serum sickness 2–3 weeks later (Box 2.7). However, the risk of death outweighs the problems of anaphylaxis. Antibiotics should be administered concurrently to eliminate the organisms and thereby remove the source of toxin production. Benzylpenicillin 1.2 g four times daily is given for 1 week.

The cardiac and neurological complications need intensive therapy.

Prevention

Diphtheria is prevented by active immunization in childhood (see p. 42). Booster doses should be given to those travelling to endemic areas if more than 10 years has elapsed following their primary course of immunization. All contacts of the patient should have throat swabs sent for culture; those with a positive result should be treated with penicillin or erythromycin and active immunization or a booster dose of toxoid given.

Pertussis (whooping cough)

Pertussis occurs world-wide. Humans are both the natural hosts and reservoirs of infection. The disease is caused by *Bordetella pertussis* which is a Gram-negative coccobacillus. *B. parapertussis* and *B. bronchiseptica* produce milder infections. Pertussis is highly contagious and is spread by droplet infection. In its early stages it is indistinguishable from other types of upper respiratory tract infection.

Epidemic disease occurred in the UK when the safety of the whooping cough vaccine was questioned. Currently, uptake exceeds 95% and the disease is uncommon.

Clinical features

The incubation period is 7–10 days. It is a disease of childhood, with 90% of cases occurring below 5 years of age. However, no age is exempt.

During the catarrhal stage the patient is highly infectious, and cultures from respiratory secretions are positive in over 90% of patients. Malaise, anorexia, mucoid rhinorrhoea and conjunctivitis are present. The paroxysmal stage, so called because of the characteristic paroxysms of coughing, begins about a week later. Paroxysms with the classic inspiratory whoop are seen only in younger individuals in whom the lumen of the respiratory tract is compromised by mucus secretion and mucosal oedema. The whoop results from air being forcefully drawn through the narrowed tract. These paroxysms usually terminate in vomiting. Conjunctival suffusion and petechiae and ulceration of the frenulum of the tongue are usual. Lymphocytosis due to the elaboration of a lymphocyte-promoting factor by *B. pertussis* is characteristic; lymphocytes may account for over 90% of the total white blood cell count. This stage lasts approximately 2 weeks and may be associated with several complications, including pneumonia, atelectasis, rectal prolapse and inguinal hernia. Cerebral anoxia may occur, especially in younger children, resulting in convulsions. Bronchiectasis is a rare sequel.

Diagnosis

The diagnosis is suggested clinically by the characteristic whoop and a history of contact with an infected individual. It is confirmed by isolation of the organism. Cultures of swabs of nasopharyngeal secretions result in a higher positive yield than cultures of 'cough plates'.

Treatment

If the disease is recognized in the catarrhal stage, erythromycin will abort or decrease the severity of the infection. In the paroxysmal stage, antibiotics have little role to play in altering the course of the illness.

Prevention and control

Affected individuals should be isolated to prevent contact with others, e.g. in hostels and boarding schools. Pertussis is an easily preventable disease and effective active immunization is available (Box 2.6). Convulsions and encephalopathy have been reported as rare complications of vaccination but they are probably less frequent than after whooping cough itself. Any exposed susceptible infant should receive prophylactic erythromycin.

Acute epiglottitis (p. 898)

This has been virtually eliminated among children in those countries which have introduced *Haemophilus influenzae* vaccine, as in the UK. Occasionally, infections are being recognized in adults. The clinical features are described on page 898.

Acute laryngotracheobronchitis (p. 898)

Influenza (pp. 55 and 898)

Lower respiratory tract infections

Pneumonia: community-acquired (p. 922); hospital-acquired (p. 929); in immunocompromised persons (p. 926).

Psittacosis (ornithosis)
Although originally thought to be limited to the psittacine birds (parrots, parakeets and macaws), it is known that the disease is widely spread amongst many species of birds, including pigeons, turkeys, ducks and chickens (hence the broader term 'ornithosis'). Human infection is related to exposure to infected birds and is therefore a true zoonosis. The causative organism, *Chlamydia psittaci*, is excreted in avian secretions; it can be isolated for prolonged periods from birds who have apparently recovered from infection. The organism gains entry to the human host by inhalation.

Clinical features and treatment
These are discussed on page 925.

Other respiratory infections (see also p. 925)

Chlamydia pneumoniae causes a relatively mild pneumonia in young adults, clinically resembling infection caused by *Mycoplasma pneumoniae*. Diagnosis can be confirmed by specific IgM serology. Treatment is with erythromycin 500 mg 6-hourly, tetracycline 500 mg every 6–8 hours, or a fluoroquinolone, e.g. ciprofloxacin 500 mg twice daily.

Other chlamydial infections include trachoma (p. 84), lymphogranuloma venereum (p. 122) and other genital infections.

Legionnaires' disease. This is caused by *Legionella pneumophila* and other *Legionella* spp. It is described on page 925.

Lung abscess (p. 929).

Tuberculosis (pp. 86 and 930).

FURTHER READING
Munoz FM, Keitel Wa (2003) Progress in the diagnosis, prevention and treatment of pertussis. *Current Infectious Disease Reports* 5: 213–219.

GASTROINTESTINAL INFECTIONS

Gastroenteritis

The most common form of acute gastrointestinal infection is gastroenteritis, causing diarrhoea with or without vomiting. Children in the developing world can expect, on average, three to six bouts of severe diarrhoea every year. Although oral rehydration programmes have cut the death toll significantly, at least 2.25 million people die every year as a direct result of diarrhoeal disease. In the western world diarrhoea is both less common and less likely to cause death. However, it remains a major cause of morbidity, especially in the elderly. Other groups who are at increased risk of infectious diarrhoea include travellers to developing countries, homosexual men, and infants in day care facilities. Viral gastroenteritis (p. 51) is a common cause of diarrhoea and vomiting in young children but is rarely seen in adults. Protozoal and helminthic gut infections (p. 109) are rare in the West but relatively common in developing countries. The most common cause of significant adult gastroenteritis world-wide is bacterial infection.

Mechanisms
Bacteria can cause diarrhoea in three different ways (Table 2.29). Some species may employ more than one of these methods.

Table 2.29	Pathogenic mechanisms of bacterial gastroenteritis		
Pathogenesis	**Mode of action**	**Clinical presentation**	**Examples**
Mucosal adherence	Effacement of intestinal mucosa	Moderate watery diarrhoea	Enteropathogenic *E. coli* (EPEC)
Mucosal invasion	Penetration and destruction of mucosa	Dysentery	*Shigella* spp. *Campylobacter* spp. Enteroinvasive *E. coli* (EIEC)
Toxin production Enterotoxin	Fluid secretion without mucosal damage	Profuse watery diarrhoea	*Vibrio cholerae* *Salmonella* spp. *Campylobacter* spp. Enterotoxigenic *E. coli* (ETEC) *Bacillus cereus* *Staphylococcus aureus* producing enterotoxin B *Clostridium perfringens* type A
Cytotoxin	Damage to mucosa	Dysentery	*Salmonella* spp. *Campylobacter* spp. Enterohaemorrhagic *E. coli* 0157 (EHEC)

Mucosal adherence

Most bacteria causing diarrhoea must first adhere to specific receptors on the mucosa. A number of different molecular adhesion mechanisms have been elaborated; for example, adhesions at the tip of the pili or fimbriae which protrude from the bacterial surface aid adhesion. For some pathogens this is merely the prelude to invasion or toxin production but others such as enteropathogenic *Escherichia coli* (EPEC) cause attachment-effacement mucosal lesions on EM and produce a secretory diarrhoea directly as a result of adherence. Enteroaggregative *E. coli* (EAggEC) adhere in an aggregative pattern with the bacteria clumping on the cell surface and its toxin causes persistent diarrhoea in developing countries. Diffusely adhering *E. coli* (DAEC) adheres in a uniform manner and may also cause diarrhoea in children and in developing countries.

Mucosal invasion

Invasive pathogens such as *Shigella* spp., enteroinvasive *E. coli* (EIEC) and *Campylobacter* spp. penetrate into the intestinal mucosa. They destroy the epithelial cells and produce the symptoms of dysentery: low-volume bloody diarrhoea, with abdominal pain.

Toxin production

Gastroenteritis can be caused by different types of bacterial toxins:

- *Enterotoxins*, produced by the bacteria adhering to the intestinal epithelium, induce excessive fluid secretion into the bowel lumen, leading to watery diarrhoea, without physically damaging the mucosa, e.g. cholera, enterotoxigenic *E. coli* (ETEC). Some enterotoxins preformed in the food primarily cause vomiting, e.g. *Staph. aureus* and *Bacillus cereus*. A typical example of this is 'fried rice poisoning', in which *B. cereus* toxin is present in cooked rice left standing overnight at room temperature.
- *Cytotoxins* damage the intestinal mucosa and, in some cases, vascular endothelium as well.

Clinical syndromes

Bacterial gastroenteritis can be divided on clinical grounds into two broad syndromes: *watery diarrhoea* (usually due to enterotoxins, or adherence), and *dysentery* (usually due to mucosal invasion and damage) (Box 2.8). With some pathogens such as *Campylobacter jejuni* there may be overlap between the two syndromes.

Salmonella

Gastroenteritis can be caused by many of the numerous serotypes of salmonella (all of which are members of a single species, *S. choleraesuis*), but the most commonly implicated are *S. enteritidis* and *S. typhimurium*. These organisms, which are found all over the world, are commensals in the bowels of livestock (especially poultry) and in the oviducts of chicken. They are usually transmitted to man in contaminated foodstuffs.

> **Box 2.8 Bacterial causes of watery diarrhoea and dysentery**
>
> **Watery diarrhoea**
> *Bacillus cereus* ⎫
> *Staphylococcus aureus* ⎬ plus profuse vomiting
> *Vibrio cholerae*
> Enterotoxigenic *Escherichia coli* (ETEC)
> Enteropathogenic *Escherichia coli* (EPEC)
> *Salmonella* spp.
> *Campylobacter jejuni*
> *Clostridium perfringens*
> *Clostridium difficile*
>
> **Dysentery**
> *Shigella* spp.
> *Salmonella* spp.
> *Campylobacter* spp.
> Enteroinvasive *Escherichia coli* (EIEC)
> Enterohaemorrhagic *Escherichia coli* (EHEC)
> *Yersinia enterocolitica*
> *Vibrio parahaemolyticus*
> *Clostridium difficile*

Salmonellae can affect both the large and small bowel, and induce diarrhoea both by production of enterotoxins and by epithelial invasion. The typical symptoms commence abruptly 12–48 hours after infection and consist of nausea, cramping abdominal pain, diarrhoea, and sometimes fever. The diarrhoea can vary from profuse and watery to a bloody dysentery syndrome. Spontaneous resolution usually occurs in 3–6 days, although the organism may persist in the faeces for several weeks. Bacteraemia occurs in 1–4% of cases and is more common in the elderly and the immunosuppressed. Occasionally bacteraemia is complicated by metastatic infection, especially of atheroma on vascular endothelium, with potentially devastating consequences. In healthy adults salmonella gastroenteritis is usually a relatively minor illness, but young children and the elderly are at risk of significant dehydration.

Specific diagnosis is made by culturing the organism from blood or faeces, but management is usually empirical. Antibiotic therapy (ciprofloxacin 500 mg twice daily) may decrease the duration and severity of symptoms, but is rarely warranted (see Box 2.10).

Campylobacter jejuni

C. jejuni is also a zoonotic infection, existing as a bowel commensal in many species of livestock. It is found world-wide, and is a common cause of childhood gastroenteritis in developing countries. Adults in these countries may be tolerant of the organism, excreting it asymptomatically. In the West it is a common cause of sporadic food-borne outbreaks of diarrhoea, especially in the summer when barbecued beefburgers are a frequent vehicle.

Like salmonella, campylobacter can affect large and small bowel and can cause a wide variety of symptoms. The incubation period is usually 2–4 days, after which there is an abrupt onset of nausea, diarrhoea and abdominal cramps. The diarrhoea is usually profuse and watery, but an invasive haemorrhagic colitis is sometimes seen. Bacteraemia is very rare, and infection is usually self-limiting in 3–5 days. Diagnosis is made from stool cultures. If symptoms are severe, azithromycin 500 mg once daily is the drug of choice (see Box 2.10).

Shigella

Shigellae are enteroinvasive bacteria which cause classical bacillary dysentery. The principal species causing gastroenteritis are *S. dysenteriae*, *S. flexneri* and *S. sonnei*, which are found with varying prevalence in different parts of the world. All cause a similar syndrome, as a result of damage to the intestinal mucosa. Some strains of *S. dysenteriae* also secrete a cytotoxin affecting vascular endothelium. Although shigellae are found world-wide, transmission is strongly associated with poor hygiene. The organism is spread from person to person, and only small numbers need to be ingested to cause illness (< 200, compared to 10^4 for campylobacter and $> 10^5$ for salmonella). Bacillary dysentery is far more prevalent in the developing world, where the main burden falls on children.

Symptoms start 24–48 hours after ingestion and typically consist of frequent small-volume stools containing blood and mucus. Dehydration is not as significant as in the secretory diarrhoeas, but systemic symptoms and intestinal complications are worse. The illness is usually self-limiting in 7–10 days, but in children in developing countries the mortality may be as high as 20%. Antibiotic treatment decreases the severity and duration of diarrhoea, and possibly reduces the risk of further transmission (see Box 2.10). Resistance to antibiotics is widespread: in some areas amoxicillin or co-trimoxazole may still be effective, but in many places nalidixic acid or ciprofloxacin is needed.

Enteroinvasive *Escherichia coli* (EIEC)

This causes an illness indistinguishable from shigellosis. Definitive diagnosis is made by stool culture.

Enterohaemorrhagic *Escherichia coli* (EHEC)

EHEC (usually serotype O157:H7, and also known as verotoxin-producing *E. coli*, or VTEC) is a well recognized cause of gastroenteritis in man. It is a zoonosis usually associated with cattle, and there have been a number of major outbreaks (notably in Scotland and Japan) associated with contaminated food. EHEC secrete a toxin (Shiga-like toxin 1) which affects vascular endothelial cells in the gut and in the kidney. After an incubation period of 12–48 hours it causes diarrhoea (frequently bloody), associated with abdominal pain and nausea. Some days after the onset of symptoms the patient may develop thrombotic thrombocytopenic purpura (p. 471) or haemolytic uraemic syndrome (HUS, p. 636). This is more common in children, and may lead to permanent renal damage or death. Treatment is mainly supportive: there is evidence that antibiotic therapy might precipitate HUS by causing increased toxin release.

Enterotoxigenic *Escherichia coli* (ETEC)

ETEC produce both heat-labile and heat-stable enterotoxins which stimulate secretion of fluid into the intestinal lumen. The result is watery diarrhoea of varying intensity, which usually resolves within a few days. Transmission is normally from person to person via contaminated food. The organism is common in developing countries, and is a major cause of travellers' diarrhoea (see below).

Vibrio

Cholera, due to *Vibrio cholerae* is the prototypic pure enterotoxigenic diarrhoea: it is described on page 84.

Vibrio parahaemolyticus causes acute watery diarrhoea after eating raw fish or shellfish that has been kept for several hours without refrigeration. Explosive diarrhoea, abdominal cramps and vomiting occurs with a fever in 50%. It is self-limiting, lasting up to 10 days.

Yersiniosis

Yersinia enterocolitica infection is a zoonosis of a variety of domestic and wild mammals. Human disease can arise either via contaminated food products, e.g. pork, or from direct animal contact. *Y. enterocolitica* can cause a range of gastroenteric symptoms including watery diarrhoea, dysentery, and mesenteric adenitis. The illness is usually self-limiting, but ciprofloxacin may shorten the duration. *Y. pseudotuberculosis* is a much less common human pathogen: it causes mesenteric adenitis and terminal ileitis.

Staphylococcus aureus

Some strains of *Staph. aureus* can produce a heat-stable toxin (enterotoxin B) which causes massive secretion of fluid into the intestinal lumen. It is a common cause of food-borne gastroenteritis in Europe and the USA, outbreaks usually occurring as a result of poor food hygiene. Because the toxin is preformed in the contaminated food, onset of symptoms is rapid, often within 2–4 hours of consumption. There is violent vomiting, followed within hours by profuse watery diarrhoea. Symptoms have usually subsided within 24 hours.

Bacillus cereus

B. cereus produces two toxins. One produces watery diarrhoea up to 12 hours after ingesting the organism. The other toxin is preformed in food and causes severe vomiting, e.g. 'fried rice poisoning' (p. 72).

Clostridial infections

C. difficile is found as part of the normal bowel flora in 3–5% of the population and even more commonly in hospitalized people. *C. difficile* produces two toxins: toxin A is an enterotoxin and toxin B is cytotoxic and causes bloody diarrhoea. It usually causes illness after other bowel commensals have been eliminated by antibiotic therapy. Almost all antibiotics have been linked with *C. difficile* diarrhoea, which can begin anything from 2 days to a month after taking antibiotics. Elderly hospitalized patients are most frequently affected.

Symptoms can range from mild diarrhoea to haemorrhagic colitis: sometimes the ulcerated colonic mucosa may be covered by a membrane-like material (pseudomembranous colitis). The diagnosis is made by detecting A or B toxins in the stools by ELISA techniques. Treatment is with metronidazole 400 mg three times daily or oral vancomycin 125 mg four times daily; causative antibiotics should be discontinued if possible. The disease is usually more severe in the elderly, and can cause intractable diarrhoea leading to death.

Clostridium perfringens infection is due to inadequately cooked food, usually meat or poultry allowed to cool for a long time during which the spores germinate. The ingested organism produces an enterotoxin causing watery diarrhoea with severe abdominal pain, usually without vomiting.

Travellers' diarrhoea

Travellers' diarrhoea is defined as the passage of three or more unformed stools per day in a resident of an industrialized country travelling in a developing nation. Infection is usually food- or water-borne, and younger travellers are most often affected (probably reflecting behaviour patterns). Reported attack rates vary from country to country, but approach 50% for a 2-week stay in many tropical countries. The disease is usually benign and self-limiting: treatment with quinolone antibiotics may hasten recovery but is not normally necessary. Prophylactic antibiotic therapy may also be effective for short stays, but should not be used routinely. The common causative organisms are listed in Table 2.30.

Management of acute gastroenteritis

In children, untreated diarrhoea has a high mortality due to dehydration, especially in hot climates. Death and serious morbidity are less common in adults but still occur, particularly in developing countries and in the

Table 2.30 Common causes of travellers' diarrhoea (TD)

Organism	Frequency (varies from country to country)
ETEC	30–70%
Shigella spp.	0–15%
Salmonella spp.	0–10%
Campylobacter spp.	0–15%
Viral pathogens	0–10%
Giardia intestinalis	0–3%

ETEC, enterotoxigenic *Escherichia coli*

elderly. The mainstay of treatment for all types of gastroenteritis is oral rehydration solutions (ORS): antibiotics have a subsidiary role in some cases (Fig. 2.23; Boxes 2.9 and 2.10 and p. 85). The use and formulation of ORS are discussed under cholera on p. 85. It should also be remembered that other diseases, notably urinary tract infections and chest infections in the elderly, and malaria at any age, can present with acute diarrhoea.

Food poisoning

Food poisoning is a legally notifiable disease in England and Wales, and is defined as 'any disease of an infective or toxic nature caused by or thought to be caused by the consumption of food and water'. Not all cases of gastroenteritis are food poisoning, as the pathogens are not always food- or water-borne. Common bacterial causes of food poisoning are listed in Table 2.31. Food poisoning may also be caused by a number of non-infectious organic and inorganic toxins (Table 2.32). Illnesses such as botulism (p. 73) are also classified as food poisoning, even though they do not primarily cause gastroenteritis. Listeriosis is described on p. 78.

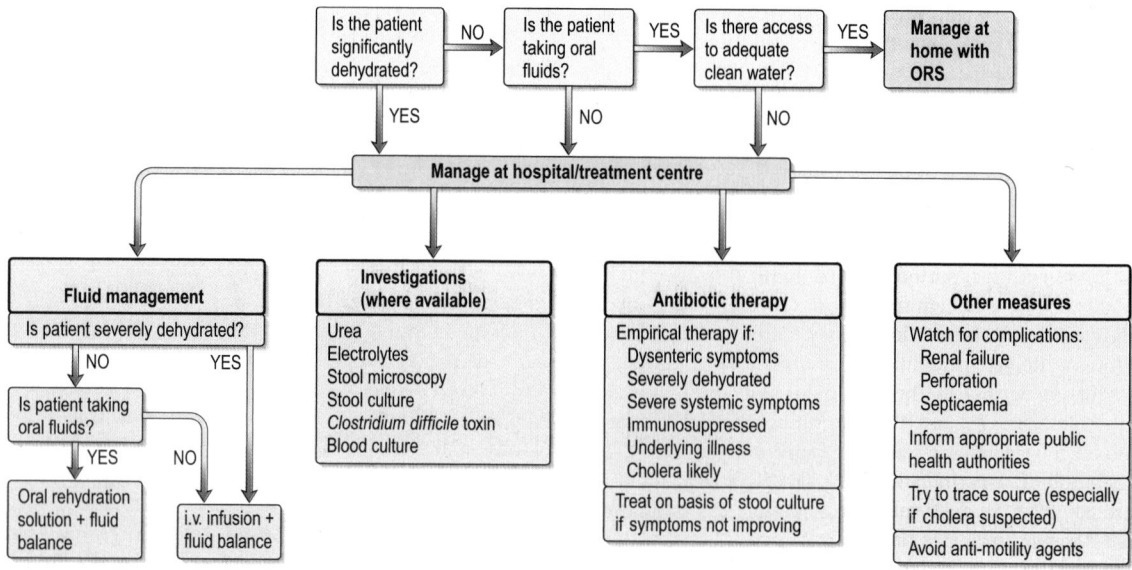

Fig. 2.23 **Gastroenteritis – management plan.** ORS, oral rehydration solution.

Box 2.9 Oral rehydration solutions (ORS) and intravenous solutions in moderate and severe diarrhoea

	Salts (mmol per litre)				Substance added (per litre of water)	
	Na⁺	K⁺	Cl⁻	Glucose		
Oral						
WHO New reduced osmolality formulation	75	20	65	75	NaCl Na citrate KCl Glucose	2.6 g 2.9 g 1.5 g 13.5 g
Cereal-based	85	–	80	–	80 g cooked rice 5 g salt (NaCl)	
Household	85	–	80	111	20 g glucose 5 g salt (NaCl)	
UK/Europe	35–60	20	37	90–200	Pre-prepared solutions	
Intravenous						
Ringer's lactate	131	4	109	0	Pre-prepared	

(Na⁺ column header rendered as Na^+; K⁺ as K^+; Cl⁻ as Cl^-)

Box 2.10 Antibiotics in adult acute bacterial gastroenteritis

Condition	Indications	Drug of choice	Alternatives	Benefits
Dysentery	Most patients	Ciprofloxacin 500 mg twice daily	Nalidixic acid 1 g four times daily Ampicillin 500 mg four times daily Co-trimoxazole 960 mg twice daily	Relieve symptoms Shorten illness Decrease transmission
Cholera	All patients	Ciprofloxacin	Tetracycline 250 mg four times daily Nalidixic acid Co-trimoxazole	Relieve symptoms Shorten illness Decrease transmission
Empirical therapy of watery diarrhoea	Severe symptoms Prolonged illness Elderly patients Immunosuppressed	Ciprofloxacin	Azithromycin 500 mg once daily Co-trimoxazole	Relieve symptoms Shorten illness May decrease complications
Travellers' diarrhoea	Rarely used	Ciprofloxacin	Co-trimoxazole	Relieve symptoms Shorten illness
Treatment of confirmed *Salmonella, Shigella, Campylobacter*	Symptoms not improving (rarely needed)	Ciprofloxacin Azithromycin	Erythromycin Co-trimoxazole	May shorten illness
Clostridium difficile	Most cases (unless symptoms resolved)	Metronidazole 400 mg three times daily	Vancomycin 125 mg four times daily	Relieve symptoms Shorten illness

The increase in reported food poisoning in developed countries is at least in part due to changes in the production and distribution of food. Livestock raised and slaughtered under modern intensive farming conditions is frequently contaminated with salmonella or campylobacter. However, the main problem is not at this stage. Only 0.02–0.1% of the eggs from a flock of chickens infected with *S. enteritidis* will be affected, and then only at a level of less than 20 cells per egg – harmless to most healthy individuals. It is flaws in the processing, storage and distribution of food products which allow massive amplification of the infection, resulting in extensive contamination. The internationalization of food supply encourages widespread and distant transmission of the resulting infections.

Enteric fever (p. 85)

Other gastrointestinal infections

Gastric infection with *Helicobacter pylori* is discussed on page 283, Whipple's disease on page 305, and bacterial peritonitis on page 344.

Table 2.31 Bacterial causes of food poisoning

Organism	Source/vehicles	Incubation period	Symptoms	Diagnosis	Recovery
Staphylococcus aureus	Man – contaminated food and water	2–4 h	Diarrhoea, vomiting and dehydration	Culture organism in vomitus or remaining food	< 24 h
E. coli	Salads, water, ice	24 h	Watery diarrhoea	Stool culture	1–4 days
E. coli O157:H7	Cattle – meat, milk	12–48 h	Watery diarrhoea ± haemorrhagic colitis, HUS	Stool culture	10–12 days
Yersinia enterocolitica	Milk, pork	2–14 h	Abdominal pain, vomiting, diarrhoea	Stool culture	2–30 days
Bacillus cereus	Environment – rice, ice-cream, chicken	1–6 h / 6–14 h	Vomiting / Diarrhoea	Culture organism in faeces and food	Rapid
Clostridium perfringens	Environment – contaminated food	8–22 h	Watery diarrhoea and cramping pain	Culture organism in faeces and food	2–3 days
Listeria monocytogenes	Environment – milk, raw vegetables dairy products, unpasteurized cheese	?	Colic, diarrhoea and vomiting	Stool culture	?
Vibrio parahaemolyticus	Seafood	2–48 h	Diarrhoea, vomiting	Stool, food	2–10 days
Clostridium botulinum	Environment – bottled or canned food	18–24 h	Brief diarrhoea and paralysis due to neuromuscular blockade	Demonstrate toxin in food or faeces	10–14 days
Salmonella spp.	Cattle and poultry – eggs, meat	12–48 h	Abrupt diarrhoea, fever and vomiting	Stool culture	Usually 3–6 days, but may be up to 2 weeks
Campylobacter jejuni	Cattle and poultry – meat, milk	48–96 h	Diarrhoea ± blood, fever, malaise and abdominal pain	Stool culture	3–5 days
Shigella spp.	Man – contaminated food and water	24–48 h	Acute watery, bloody diarrhoea	Stool culture	7–10 days

HUS, haemolytic uraemic syndrome

Table 2.32 Organic toxins causing food poisoning (see p. 1020)

Toxin	Source	Illness
Scombotoxin	Tuna, mackerel	Histamine fish poisoning
Ciguatoxin	Barracuda, snapper	Ciguatera (diarrhoea and paraesthesia)
Dinoflagellate plankton toxin	Shellfish	Neurotoxic shellfish poisoning
Haemagglutinins	Inadequately-prepared dried kidney beans	Diarrhoea and vomiting
Unknown	Buffalo fish	Haff disease (toxic rhabdomyolysis)
Phallotoxins, amatoxins	Mushrooms	Various

FURTHER READING

Bartlett JG (2002) Antibiotic associated diarrhoea. *New England Journal of Medicine* **346**: 334–339.

De Bruyn G, Hahn S, Borwick A (2001) Antibiotic treatment for travellers' diarrhoea. Cochrane database of systematic reviews, Issue 1. Oxford: Update Software.

Musher DM, Musher BL (2004) Contagious acute gastrointestinal infections. *New England Journal of Medicine* **351**: 2417–2427.

INFECTIONS OF THE CARDIOVASCULAR SYSTEM

- Infective endocarditis (p. 828).

INFECTIONS OF THE NERVOUS SYSTEM

The central and peripheral nervous systems can be affected by a variety of microorganisms either directly or via toxins, e.g. viral (p. 1239), protozoal (p. 95) and prion diseases (pp. 60 and 1242).

Bacterial meningitis (see p. 1236)

The most common bacterial disease affecting the central nervous system is acute meningitis, which causes about 175 000 deaths per year, predominantly in the developing world. Epidemic meningitis due to *Neisseria meningitidis* (usually group A) is common in a broad belt across sub-Saharan Africa and is also seen in parts of Asia. In Europe and North America bacterial meningitis is usually sporadic, with B and C strains predominating. A conjugate vaccine for serogroup C meningococcus has resulted in a fall in the number of cases of C meningitis in those countries where it is now part of the childhood immunization schedule, such as the UK.

Streptococcus pneumoniae is the other major cause throughout the world, while tuberculous meningitis (p. 1238) is common in sub-Saharan Africa and parts of Asia.

Haemophilus influenzae b (Hib) was once a common cause of meningitis in children, but since an effective vaccine has been available, serious *H. influenzae* infections have become rare in western countries. Many developing countries have also instituted immunization programmes, but invasive *H. influenzae* infection remains common in some parts of the world.

Other less common causes of meningitis in adults include group B streptococci, *Listeria monocytogenes* (see p. 78), *Staph. aureus*, and Gram-negative bacilli. These organisms are usually associated with an underlying illness or immunocompromising condition, or with a cerebrospinal fluid leak.

Cerebral abscess

This is covered on page 1243.

Toxin-mediated infections

Botulism

Clostridium botulinum is a common environmental organism, and produces spores which can survive heating to 100°C. It causes botulism, an illness caused by contamination of canned or bottled foodstuff, in which the anaerobic organism can multiply and elaborate a neurotoxin. After ingestion the toxin causes profound neuromuscular blockade, leading to autonomic and motor paralysis. The first symptoms, occurring 18–24 hours after ingestion, are nausea and diarrhoea. These are followed by cranial nerve palsies and then progressive symmetrical paralysis, leading to respiratory failure.

The diagnosis is usually clinical, and is confirmed by detection of toxin in faeces or in the contaminated food. Treatment is mainly supportive, with mechanical ventilation if necessary. Antitoxin is available in some countries (including the UK); the risk of anaphylaxis is relatively high, and it should only be used in severe cases. A subcutaneous test dose should be given before intravenous or intramuscular injection. Antibiotics have no proven role. The overall mortality from botulism is high, but patients who survive the acute paralysis can make a full recovery.

Botulism may also follow the contamination of wounds and street heroin injection with *C. botulinum*, and in infants may be related to bowel colonization by the organism.

Tetanus

Tetanus is also due to a toxin-secreting clostridium: *C. tetani*. The organism is found in soil, and illness usually results from a contaminated wound. The injury itself may be trivial and disregarded by the individual. It has also complicated intravenous drug misuse. In developing countries neonatal tetanus follows contamination of the umbilical stump, often after dressing the area with dung.

The organism is not invasive, and clinical manifestations of the disease are due to the potent neurotoxin, tetanospasmin. Tetanospasmin acts on both the α and δ motor systems at synapses, resulting in disinhibition. It also produces neuromuscular blockade and skeletal muscle spasm, and acts on the sympathetic nervous system. The end result is marked flexor muscle spasm and autonomic dysfunction.

Clinical features

The incubation period varies from a few days to several weeks. The most common form of the disease is generalized tetanus. General malaise is rapidly followed by trismus (lockjaw) due to masseter muscle spasm. Spasm of the facial muscles produces the characteristic grinning expression known as risus sardonicus. If the disease is severe, painful reflex spasms develop, usually within 24–72 hours of the initial symptoms. The interval between the first symptom and the first spasm is referred to as the 'onset time'. The spasms may occur spontaneously but are easily precipitated by noise, handling of the patient, or by light. Respiration may be impaired because of laryngeal spasm; oesophageal and urethral spasm lead to dysphagia and urinary retention, respectively, and there is arching of the neck and back muscles (opisthotonus). Autonomic dysfunction produces tachycardia, a labile blood pressure, sweating and cardiac arrhythmias. Patients with tetanus are mentally alert.

Death results from aspiration, hypoxia, respiratory failure, cardiac arrest or exhaustion. Mild cases with rigidity usually recover. Poor prognostic indicators include short incubation period, short onset time, and extremes of age.

Localized tetanus is a milder form of the disease. Pain and stiffness are confined to the site of the wound, with increased tone in the surrounding muscles. Recovery usually occurs.

Cephalic tetanus is uncommon but invariably fatal. It usually occurs when the portal of entry of *C. tetani* is the middle ear. Cranial nerve abnormalities, particularly of the seventh nerve, are usual. Generalized tetanus may or may not develop.

Neonatal tetanus is usually due to infection of the umbilical stump. Failure to thrive, poor sucking, grimacing and irritability are followed by the rapid development of intense rigidity and spasms. Mortality approaches 100%. One aim of the WHO Expanded Programme on Immunization (EPI) is to eliminate this condition by immunizing all women of childbearing age, providing clean delivery facilities and strengthening surveillance in high-risk areas.

Diagnosis

Few diseases resemble tetanus in its fully developed form, and the diagnosis is therefore usually clinical. Rarely, *C. tetani* is isolated from wounds. Phenothiazine overdosage, strychnine poisoning, meningitis and tetany can occasionally mimic tetanus.

Management

Suspected tetanus. Any wound must be cleaned and debrided if necessary, to remove the source of toxin. Human tetanus immunoglobin 250 units should be given along with an intramuscular injection of tetanus toxoid. If the patient is already protected a single booster dose of the toxoid is given; otherwise the full three-dose course of adsorbed vaccine is given (see below).

Established tetanus management is supportive medical and nursing care. Improvement in this area has contributed more than any other single measure to the decrease in the mortality rate from 60% to nearer 20%. Patients are nursed in a quiet, isolated, well-ventilated, darkened room. Benzodiazepines are used to control spasm and sedate the patient; if the airway is compromised intubation and mechanical ventilation may be necessary.

Antibiotics and antitoxin should be administered, even in the absence of an obvious wound. Intravenous metronidazole is the drug of choice, although penicillin is also effective. Human tetanus immunoglobulin (HTIG) 500 IU should be given by intramuscular injection to neutralize any circulating toxin. If HTIG is not available, immune equine tetanus immunoglobulin 10 000 IU should be given intramuscularly: this is probably as effective as HTIG, but there is a high incidence of severe allergic reactions. If the patient recovers, active immunization should be instituted, as immunity following tetanus is incomplete.

Prevention

Tetanus is an eminently preventable disease and all persons should be immunized regardless of age. Those who work in a contaminated environment, such as farmers, are particularly at risk and should have regular booster injections. Active immunization with the alum-adsorbed toxoid should be given. Initially two doses of 0.5 mL of the toxoid are given intramuscularly with an 8-week interval. The third dose is given 6–12 months later as a booster. Subsequent boosters are required at 5-year intervals. Infant immunization schedules in all countries include tetanus (Box 2.6). Protection by passive immunization with either the equine or human anti-tetanus immunoglobulin is short-lived, lasting only about 2 weeks.

FURTHER READING

Begg N, Cartwright KA, Cohen J et al. (1999) Overview of acute and chronic meningitis. *Neurologic Clinics* **17**(4): 691–710.

Gold R (1999) Epidemiology of bacterial meningitis. *Infectious Disease Clinics of North America* **13**(3): 515–525.

BONE AND JOINT INFECTIONS

- Infective arthritis (p. 571)
- Osteomyelitis (p. 573).

URINARY TRACT INFECTIONS

- Complicated versus uncomplicated infections (p. 638)
- Acute pyelonephritis (p. 639)
- Reflux nephropathy (p. 639)
- Perinephric abscess (renal carbuncle) (p. 642)
- Bacterial prostatitis (p. 642)
- Tuberculosis of the urinary tract (p. 642)
- Peritonitis complicating continuous ambulatory peritoneal dialysis (p. 677).

SYSTEMIC/MULTISYSTEM INFECTIONS

Many infections are confined to a particular body organ or system, owing to the metabolic requirements of the organism, the route of infection, or the response of host defences. Other infections can potentially affect several systems or the entire body. Under unusual circumstances such as altered host immunity, infections which are normally circumscribed may become systemic. This section describes those infections which commonly cause multisystem disease in an immunocompetent host.

Bacteraemia and septicaemia

Bacteraemia, the transient presence of organisms in the blood, can occur in healthy people without causing symptoms. It can follow surgery, dental treatment, and even tooth-brushing. Bacteraemia can also occur from the bowel or bladder, especially in the presence of local inflammation. Unless a site of metastatic infection is established (such as the heart valves), most organisms are rapidly cleared from the blood.

Septicaemia. Some invading bacteria such as *Staph. aureus* or *E. coli* are less likely to be dealt with by the immune system and more likely to cause disease. Illness arising from such blood-borne infection is called septicaemia, and may occur in isolation or secondary to a focal infection. Septicaemia usually causes severe systemic symptoms including high fever, rigors, hypotension, myalgia and headache. It can also lead to the establishment of metastatic foci of infection and, in its most severe form, to septic shock.

Patients presenting with symptoms and signs suggesting septicaemia should be examined carefully for

Table 2.33 Causes of septicaemia in a previously healthy adult

Site of origin	Usual pathogen(s)
Skin	*Staphylococcus aureus* and other Gram-positive cocci
Urinary tract	*Escherichia coli* and other aerobic Gram-negative rods
Respiratory tract	*Streptococcus pneumoniae*
Gall bladder or bowel	*Enterococcus faecalis*, *E. coli* and other Gram-negative rods *Bacteroides fragilis*
Pelvic organs	*Neisseria gonorrhoeae*, anaerobes

Table 2.34 Causes of septicaemia in hospitalized patients

Clinical problem	Usual pathogen(s)
Urinary catheter	*Escherichia coli*, *Klebsiella* spp., *Proteus* spp., *Serratia* spp., *Pseudomonas* spp.
Intravenous catheter	*Staphylococcus aureus* and *Staph. epidermidis*, *Klebsiella* spp., *Pseudomonas* spp., *Candida albicans*
Peritoneal catheter	*Staph. epidermidis*
Post-surgery:	
Wound infection	*Staph. aureus*, *E. coli*, anaerobes (depending on site)
Deep infection	Depends on anatomical location
Burns	Gram-positive cocci, *Pseudomonas* spp., *Candida albicans*
Immunocompromised patients	Any of the above

evidence of a source: common sites of infection and organisms leading to septicaemia are listed in Tables 2.33 and 2.34. Because of the potential severity of septicaemia, treatment with antibiotics should usually be started empirically as soon as appropriate cultures have been taken. The choice of agent is governed by the likely pathogen: if there are no clues, a broad-spectrum regimen should be used (e.g. piperacillin plus gentamicin, or cefotaxime, with or without metronidazole). In hospital units with epidemic MRSA infection, it is common practice to add vancomycin or teicoplanin to this empiric regimen. Antibiotic therapy should be reviewed daily as the illness progresses and the results of investigations become available. The general management of septic shock is covered on page 978.

Meningococcal septicaemia

Neisseria meningitidis is found world-wide, in five major serogroups. In sub-Saharan Africa and parts of Asia where group A meningococcus is prevalent it usually causes epidemic disease. Groups Y and W can also cause epidemic infection, while groups B and C (which are the predominant strains in Europe and North America) tend to be sporadic. In England and Wales approximately 2000 cases of meningococcal disease are reported annually.

Man is the only known reservoir for the organism, which is carried asymptomatically in the nasopharynx of 5–20% of the general population. Meningococcal disease occurs when the bacteria invade the nasal mucosa and enter the bloodstream: this only happens in a small percentage of those colonized. Invasion depends on both host and bacterial factors. It is more likely to take place soon after colonization has taken place, and following viral upper respiratory infections.

Clinical features

Invasive meningococcal infection may cause meningitis, septicaemia, or both. Meningitic disease (see p. 1236) usually presents with the classical triad of headache, fever, and neck stiffness. Vomiting, diminished consciousness, and focal neurological signs occur, although some patients, especially in the early stages, only have mild symptoms. Meningococcal septicaemia causes the typical features of septic shock such as fever, myalgia, and hypotension (p. 967), and may be accompanied by a petechial or haemorrhagic rash (Fig. 2.24). In some cases the patient can deteriorate rapidly, with shock, disseminated intravascular coagulation, and multiorgan failure.

Diagnosis

The presence of meningitis and septicaemia with a typical rash is strongly suggestive of meningococcal disease. Gram-negative diplococci may be seen on Gram stain of CSF or of aspirate from petechiae, and meningococci can also be cultured from CSF or blood, or detected by PCR. A rising titre of antibody to meningococcal outer membrane protein (OMP) can also be used in diagnosis.

Management

N. meningitidis is sensitive to benzylpenicillin, chloramphenicol, and third-generation cephalosporins: antibiotic treatment for meningococcal meningitis should be started *immediately* (see emergency box 21.1, page 1238) and continued parenterally for 7 days. Meningococcal septicaemia should be managed in the same way as any

Fig. 2.24 Meningococcal infections, showing a purpuric rash.

other septicaemic illness (p. 973). The mortality from meningococcal septicaemia in developed countries is currently approximately 10%, while that from meningococcal meningitis alone is less than 5% (see below). Mild neurological sequelae (especially vestibular nerve damage) are common, but serious brain damage is relatively unusual.

The meningococcal C conjugate vaccine has led to an overall reduction of meningococcal C disease in the UK but unfortunately an increase in infection of other serotypes may occur. A serogroup B vaccine is not available. A combined A and C vaccine is also available (p. 42).

For close contacts of a case of meningococcal disease, household and 'kissing' contacts should be given prophylaxis with oral rifampicin or ciprofloxacin to eradicate the bacteria from the nasopharynx. In the case of group C disease, contacts should be offered immunization.

Rheumatic fever

Rheumatic fever is an inflammatory disease that occurs in children and young adults (the first attack usually occurs at between 5 and 15 years of age) as a result of infection with group A streptococci. It affects the heart, skin, joints and central nervous system. It is common in the Middle and Far East, eastern Europe and South America. It is rare in the UK, western Europe and North America. This decline in the incidence of rheumatic fever (from 10% of children in the 1920s to 0.01% today) parallels the reduction in all streptococcal infections and is largely due to improved hygiene and the use of antibiotics.

Pharyngeal infection with group A streptococcus is followed by the clinical syndrome of rheumatic fever. This is thought to develop because of an autoimmune reaction triggered by molecular mimicry between the cell wall M proteins of the infecting *Strep. pyogenes* and cardiac myosin and laminin. The condition is not due to direct infection of the heart or to the production of a toxin.

Pathology

All three layers of the heart may be affected. The characteristic lesion of rheumatic carditis is the Aschoff nodule, which is a granulomatous lesion with a central necrotic area occurring in the myocardium, particularly in the subendocardium of the left ventricle. Small, warty vegetations may develop on the endocardium, particularly on the heart valves. This leads to some degree of valvular regurgitation. A serofibrinous effusion characterizes the acute pericarditis that occurs.

The synovial membranes are acutely inflamed during rheumatic fever, and subcutaneous nodules (which are also granulomatous lesions) are seen in the acute stage of the disease.

Clinical features

The disease presents suddenly, with fever, joint pains, malaise and loss of appetite. The clinical features depend on the organs that are involved. Diagnosis relies on the presence of two or more major clinical manifestations or

Table 2.35 Revised Duckett Jones criteria for the diagnosis of rheumatic fever. The diagnosis is made on the basis of two or more major criteria or one major plus two or more minor criteria

Major criteria
Carditis
Polyarthritis
Chorea
Erythema marginatum
Subcutaneous nodules

Minor criteria
Fever
Arthralgia
Previous rheumatic fever
Raised ESR/C-reactive protein
Leucocytosis
Prolonged PR interval on ECG

Plus evidence of antecedent streptococcal infection, e.g. positive throat cultures for group A streptococci, elevated antistreptolysin O titre (> 250 U) or other streptococcal antibodies, or a history of recent scarlet fever

ESR, erythrocyte sedimentation rate

one major manifestation plus two or more minor features. These are known as the Duckett Jones criteria (Table 2.35).

Carditis manifests as:

- new or changed heart murmurs
- development of cardiac enlargement or cardiac failure
- appearance of a pericardial effusion and ECG changes of pericarditis (raised ST segments) or myocarditis (inverted or flattened T waves), first-degree or greater AV block or other cardiac arrhythmias
- transient diastolic mitral (Carey–Coombs) murmur due to mitral valvulitis.

Non-cardiac features include the following:

- There is usually a fever with an apparently excessive tachycardia.
- The arthritis associated with rheumatic fever is classically a fleeting migratory polyarthritis affecting large joints such as the knees, elbows, ankles and wrists. The joints are swollen, red and tender. As the inflammation in one joint recedes, another becomes affected. Once the acute inflammation disappears, the rheumatic process leaves the joints normal.
- Sydenham's chorea (or St Vitus' dance, see p. 1232) is involvement of the central nervous system that develops late after a streptococcal infection. Sufferers are noticeably 'fidgety' and display spasmodic, unintentional choreiform movements. Speech is often affected.
- Skin manifestations include erythema marginatum, a transient pink rash with slightly raised edges, which occurs in 20% of cases. The erythematous areas found mostly on the trunk and limbs coalesce into crescent- or ring-shaped patches. Subcutaneous nodules, which are painless, pea-sized, hard nodules beneath the skin, may also occur, particularly over tendons, joints and bony prominences.

Investigations

- **Throat swabs** are cultured for the group A streptococcus.
- **Serological changes** may indicate a recent streptococcal infection. The antistreptolysin O titre, and sometimes others such as the antistreptokinase titre, are performed.
- **Non-specific indicators of inflammation** such as the ESR and the C-reactive protein levels are usually elevated.
- **Cardiac investigations**, e.g. ECG, echocardiogram.

Treatment

Patients with fever, active arthritis or active carditis should be completely rested in bed. When the clinical syndrome has subsided (e.g. no pyrexia, normal pulse rate, normal ESR, normal white cell count) the patient may be mobilized.

Residual streptococcal infections should be eradicated with oral phenoxymethylpenicillin 500 mg four times daily for 1 week. This therapy should be administered even if nasal or pharyngeal swabs do not culture the streptococci.

High-dose salicylate (preferably acetylsalicylate, i.e. aspirin) therapy is given to the limit of tolerance determined by the development of tinnitus. If carditis is present, systemic corticosteroids are given. Prednisolone 60–120 mg in four divided doses each day is administered until the clinical syndrome is improved and the ESR has fallen to normal. Steroids are then tapered off over 2–4 weeks. However, the efficacy of steroids is unproven.

Recurrences are most common when persistent cardiac damage is present, and are prevented by the continued administration of oral phenoxymethylpenicillin 250 mg twice daily until the age of 20 years or for 5 years after the latest attack (see p. 32). A sulphonamide (e.g. sulfadiazine) may be used if the patient is allergic to penicillin. Any streptococcal infection that does develop should be treated very promptly.

Prognosis

More than 50% of those who suffer acute rheumatic fever with carditis will later (after 10–20 years) develop chronic rheumatic valvular disease, predominantly affecting the mitral and aortic valves (Table 13.35).

Leptospirosis

Leptospirosis is a zoonosis caused by the spirochaete *Leptospira interrogans*. There are over 200 serotypes: the main types affecting humans are *L. i. icterohaemorrhagiae* (rodents), *L. i. canicola* (dogs and pigs), *L. i. hardjo* (cattle), and *L. i. pomona* (pigs and cattle). Leptospires are excreted in the animal urine, and enter the host through a skin abrasion or through intact mucous membranes. Leptospirosis can also be caught by ingestion of contaminated water. The organism can survive for many days in warm fresh water, and for up to 24 hours in sea water.

In England and Wales only about 30 cases of leptospirosis are reported every year (although many mild infections probably go undiagnosed), and it remains largely an occupational disease of farmers, vets, and others who work with animals. In some parts of the world (e.g. Hawaii, where the annual incidence is about 130/100 000) it is associated with a variety of recreational activities which bring people into closer contact with rodents. Outbreaks of leptospirosis have also been associated with flooding.

Clinical features

Weil, in 1886, described a severe illness consisting of jaundice, haemorrhage, and renal impairment caused by *L. i. icterohaemorrhagiae*, but fortunately 90–95% of infections are subclinical or cause only a mild fever. The incubation period of leptospirosis is usually 7–14 days, and the illness typically has two phases. A leptospiraemic phase, which lasts for up to a week, is followed after a couple of days' interval by an immunological phase. The first phase is characterized by severe headache, malaise, fever, anorexia and myalgia. Most patients have conjunctival suffusion. Hepatosplenomegaly, lymphadenopathy and various skin rashes are sometimes seen. The second phase is usually mild. Fifty per cent of patients have meningism, about a third of whom have a CSF lymphocytosis. The majority of patients recover uneventfully at this stage.

In severe disease there may not be a clear distinction between phases. Following the initial symptoms, patients progressively develop hepatic and renal failure, haemolytic anaemia, and circulatory collapse. Cardiac failure and pulmonary haemorrhage may also occur. Even with full supportive care the mortality is around 10%, rising to 15–20% in the elderly.

Diagnosis

The diagnosis is usually a clinical one. Leptospires can be cultured from blood or CSF during the first week of illness, but culture requires special media and may take several weeks. A minority of patients may also excrete the organism in their urine from the second week onwards. Specific IgM antibodies start to appear from the end of the first week and the diagnosis is often made retrospectively with a microscopic agglutinating test (MAT) showing a four-fold rise. There is typically a leucocytosis and in severe infection, thrombocytopenia and an elevated creatine phosphokinase.

Management

Early antibiotic therapy will limit the progress of the disease, but treatment should still be initiated whatever the stage of the infection. Oral doxycycline may be used in mild cases: intravenous penicillin or erythromycin is given in more severe disease. Intensive supportive care is needed for those patients who develop hepatorenal failure.

Brucellosis

Brucellosis (Malta fever, undulant fever) is a zoonosis and has a world-wide distribution, although it has been virtually eliminated from cattle in the UK. The highest incidence is in the Mediterranean countries, the Middle

East and the tropics; there are about 500 000 new cases diagnosed per year.

The organisms usually gain entry into the human body via the mouth; less frequently they may enter via the respiratory tract, genital tract or abraded skin. The bacilli travel in the lymphatics and infect lymph nodes. This is followed by haematogenous spread with ultimate localization in the reticuloendothelial system. Spread is usually by the ingestion of raw milk from infected cattle or goats, although occupational exposure is also common. Person-to-person transmission is rare.

Clinical features

The incubation period of acute brucellosis is 1–3 weeks. The onset is insidious, with malaise, headache, weakness, generalized myalgia and night sweats. The fever pattern is classically undulant, although continuous and intermittent patterns are also seen. Lymphadenopathy, hepato-splenomegaly and spinal tenderness sacro-iliitis (20–30%) may be present; arthritis, osteomyelitis, epididymo-orchitis (up to 40%), meningoencephalitis and endocarditis have all been described.

Untreated brucellosis can give rise to chronic infection, lasting a year or more. This is characterized by easy fatiguability, myalgia, and occasional bouts of fever and depression. Splenomegaly is usually present. Occasionally infection can lead to localized brucellosis. Bones and joints, spleen, endocardium, lungs, urinary tract and nervous system may be involved. Systemic symptoms occur in less than one-third.

Diagnosis

Blood (or bone marrow) cultures are positive during the acute phase of illness in 50% of patients (higher in *B. melitensis*), but prolonged culture is needed. If using automated blood culture systems (BACTEC) incubate longer than the usual 5–7 days. This is less helpful in chronic disease where serological tests are of greater value. The brucella agglutination test, which demonstrates a fourfold or greater rise in titre (> 1 in 160) over a 4-week period, is highly suggestive of brucellosis. However, non-agglutinating IgG and IgA molecules can block the agglutinating reaction (prozone phenomenon) and the test should be carried out to a high dilution to avoid this. An elevated serum IgG level is evidence of current or recent infection; a negative test excludes chronic brucellosis. In localized brucellosis antibody titres are low, and diagnosis is usually established by culturing the organisms from the involved site. PCR for detection of Brucella in blood gives a rapid diagnosis, and along with measurement of IgG or IgM antibodies by ELISA, are highly sensitive and specific.

Management and prevention

Brucellosis is treated with a combination of doxycycline 200 mg daily and rifampicin 600–900 mg daily for 6 weeks, but relapses occur. Alternatively, tetracycline can be combined with streptomycin, which is usually given for only the first 2 weeks of treatment. Prevention and control involve careful attention to hygiene when handling infected animals, vaccination with the eradication of infection in animals, and pasteurization of milk. No vaccine is available for use in humans.

Listeriosis

Listeria monocytogenes is an environmental organism which is widely disseminated in soil and decayed matter. It affects both animals and man: the most common route of human infection is in contaminated foodstuffs. The organism can grow at temperatures as low as 4°C, and the most commonly implicated foods are unpasteurized soft cheeses, raw vegetables and chicken pâtés. Listeriosis is a rare but serious infection affecting mainly neonates, pregnant women, the elderly, and the immunocompromised. *L. monocytogenes* has also been recognized as a cause of self-limiting food-borne gastroenteritis in healthy adults, but the incidence of this is unknown.

In pregnant women listeria causes a flu-like illness, but infection of the fetus can lead to septic abortion, premature labour, and stillbirth. Early treatment of listeria in pregnancy may prevent this, but the overall fetal loss rate is about 50%. Listeria in the elderly and the immuno-compromised usually causes meningoencephalitis, although septicaemia and a variety of other focal infections have been described.

The diagnosis is established by culture of blood, CSF, or other body fluids. The treatment of choice for adult listeriosis is ampicillin plus gentamicin. Co-trimoxazole is also effective, but the organism is resistant to cephalosporins.

Q fever

Q (query) fever is a zoonosis caused by the rickettsia-like organism *Coxiella burnetii*. Infection is widespread in domestic, farm and other animals, birds and arthropods: spread is mainly by ticks. Modes of transmission to humans are by dust, aerosol, and unpasteurized milk from infected cows. The formation of spores means that *C. burnetii* can survive in extreme environmental conditions for long periods. The infective dose is very small, so that minimal animal contact is required. One reported outbreak occurred among inhabitants of a village through which infected sheep had passed.

Clinical features

Symptoms begin insidiously 2–4 weeks after infection. Fever is accompanied by flu-like symptoms with myalgia and headache. The acute illness usually resolves spontaneously but pneumonia or hepatitis may develop. Occasionally infection can become chronic, with endocarditis, myocarditis, uveitis, osteomyelitis or other focal infections.

C. burnetii is an obligate intracellular organism, and does not grow on standard culture media. Diagnosis is made serologically using an immunofluorescent assay. Antibody tests for two different bacterial antigens allow distinction between acute and chronic infection; a nested PCR assay is now available.

Management

Treatment with doxycycline 200 mg daily (or a quinolone as an alternative) reduces the duration of the acute illness, but it is not known whether this correlates with eradication of the organism. For chronic Q fever, including endocarditis, doxycycline is often combined with rifampicin or clindamycin. Even prolonged courses of treatment may not clear the infection.

Lyme disease

Lyme disease is caused by a spirochaete *Borrelia burgdorferi,* which has at least 11 different genomic species. It is a zoonosis of deer and other wild mammals. The syndrome was first recognized and named following an 'outbreak' of arthritis in the town of Lyme, Connecticut, in the mid-1970s. Since then the disease has increased in both incidence and detection: it is now known to be widespread in the USA, Europe, Russia and the Far East. Infection is transmitted from animal to man by ixodid ticks, and is most likely to occur in rural wooded areas in spring and early summer.

Clinical features

The first stage of the illness, which follows 7–10 days after infection, is characterized by the skin lesion, erythema migrans at the site of the tick bite. This is often accompanied by headache, fever, malaise, myalgia, arthralgia and lymphadenopathy. Many people have no further illness after this. A second stage may follow weeks or months later, when some patients develop neurological symptoms (meningoencephalitis, cranial or polyneuropathies), radiculopathies, cardiac problems (conduction disorders, myocarditis) or arthritis. These manifestations, which are often fluctuant and changing, usually resolve spontaneously over months or years. Some patients, however, develop chronic and persistent neurological disease (e.g. paraparesis) or rheumatological disease ('late Lyme disease'). Acrodermatitis chronica atrophicans, usually on the backs of the hands and feet can occur if the disease does not resolve spontaneously.

Diagnosis

The clinical features and epidemiological considerations are usually strongly suggestive. The diagnosis can only rarely be confirmed by isolation of the organisms from blood, skin lesions or CSF. IgM antibodies are detectable in the first month, and IgG antibodies are invariably present late in the disease. Commercial tests (ELISA, immunofluorescence, haemagglutination) are available but false positive results do occur. A genuine positive IgG may be a marker of previous exposure rather than of ongoing infection.

Management

Amoxicillin or doxycycline given early in the course of the disease shortens the duration of the illness in approximately 50% of patients. Late disease should be treated with 2–4 weeks of intravenous benzylpenicillin or ceftriaxone. However, treatment is unsatisfactory, and preventative measures are necessary. In tick-infested areas, repellents and protective clothing should be worn. Prompt removal of any tick is essential as infection is unlikely to take place until the tick has been attached for more than 48 hours. Ticks should be grasped with forceps near to the point of attachment to the skin and then withdrawn by gentle traction. Antibiotic prophylaxis following a tick bite is not usually justified, even in areas where Lyme disease is common. A vaccine was available but has recently been withdrawn.

Tularaemia

Tularaemia is due to infection by *Francisella tularensis*, a Gram-negative organism. It is primarily a zoonosis, acquired mainly from rodents. Infection is normally transmitted by arthropod vectors, including ticks and blood-sucking flies. Humans may be infected by this route or by handling infected animals, when the micro-organisms enter through minor abrasions or mucous membranes. Occasionally infection occurs from contaminated water or from eating uncooked meat. The disease is widely distributed in North America, Northern Europe and Asia. It is relatively rare, occurring mainly in hunters, trappers, and others in close contact with animals.

The incubation period of 2–7 days is followed by a generalized illness. The most common presentation is ulceroglandular tularaemia. A papule occurs at the site of inoculation. This ulcerates and is followed by tender, suppurative lymphadenopathy. Rarely this can be followed by bacteraemia, leading to septicaemia, pneumonia, or meningitis. These forms of the disease carry a high mortality if untreated.

Diagnosis is by culture of the organism or by a rising titre seen on a bacterial agglutination test.

Tularaemia should be treated with streptomycin or gentamicin.

FURTHER READING

Galvin JE, Hemric ME, Ward K, Cunningham MW (2000) Cytotoxic Mab from rheumatic carditis recognizes heart valves and laminin. *Journal of Clinical Investigation* **106**: 217–224.

Hotchkiss R, Karl I (2003) The pathophysiology and treatment of sepsis. *New England Journal of Medicine* **348**: 138–150.

Levett PN (1999) Leptospirosis: re-emerging or re-discovered disease? *Journal of Medical Microbiology* **48**: 417–418.

Parola P, Raoult D (2001) Ticks and tick-borne bacterial diseases in humans. *Clinical Infectious Diseases* **32**: 897–928.

Rosenstein NE et al. (2001) Meningococcal disease. *New England Journal of Medicine* **344**: 1378–1389.

Stanek G, Strle F (2004) Lyme borreliosis. *Lancet* **362**: 1639–1647.

Pappas G et al (2005) Brucellosis. *New England Journal of Medicine* **352**: 2325–2336.

BACTERIAL INFECTIONS SEEN IN DEVELOPING AND TROPICAL COUNTRIES

SKIN, SOFT TISSUE AND EYE DISEASE

Leprosy

Leprosy (Hansen's disease) is caused by the acid-fast bacillus *Mycobacterium leprae*. Unlike other mycobacteria, it does not grow in artificial media or even in tissue culture. Apart from the nine-banded armadillo, man is the only natural host of *M. leprae*, although it can be grown in the footpads of mice.

The WHO campaign to control leprosy has been hugely successful, with more than 13 million people having been cured of the disease. The number of people with active leprosy has fallen from 5.4 million in 1985 to about 600 000, largely as the result of supervised multi-drug treatment regimens. India has 70% of the world cases with Brazil having the next highest. It is also common across Africa and Asia.

The precise mode of transmission of leprosy is still uncertain but it is likely that nasal secretions play a role. Infection is related to poverty and overcrowding. Once an individual has been infected, subsequent progression to clinical disease appears to be dependent on several factors. Males appear to be more susceptible than females, and there is evidence from twin studies of a genetic susceptibility. The main factor, however, is the response of the host's cell-mediated immune system.

Two *polar types* of leprosy are recognized (Ridley–Jopling system) (Fig. 2.25):

- *Tuberculoid leprosy*, a localized disease that occurs in individuals with a high degree of cell-mediated immunity (CMI). The T cell response to the antigen releases interferon which activates macrophages to destroy the bacilli (Th1 response) but with associated destruction of the tissue. The lepromin test (see below) is positive.
- *Lepromatous leprosy*, a generalized disease that occurs in individuals with impaired CMI (Fig. 2.25). Here the tissue macrophages fail to be activated and the bacilli multiply intracellularly. Th2 cytokines are produced (see p. 208). The lepromin test is negative.

The WHO classification of leprosy depends on the number of skin lesions and the number of bacilli detected on the skin smears: paucibacillary leprosy has 5 or fewer skin lesions with no bacilli; multibacillary leprosy has 6 more lesions which may have bacilli.

In practice many patients will fall between these two extremes and some may move along the spectrum as the disease progresses or is treated.

Clinical features

The incubation period varies from 2–6 years, although it may be as short as a few months or as long as 20 years. The onset of leprosy is generally insidious. Acute onset is known to occur, and patients may present with a transient rash, with features of an acute febrile illness, with evidence of nerve involvement, or with any combination of these. The major signs of leprosy are:

- Skin lesions, usually anaesthetic (generally tuberculoid).
- Thickened peripheral nerves, nerves of predilection which are superficial or lie in fibro-osseous tunnels – ulnar (elbow), median (wrist), radial cutaneous (wrist), common peroneal (knee), posterior tibial and sural (ankle), facial (crossing zygomatic arch) and greater auricular (posterior triangle of the neck).

The spectrum of disease can be divided into five clinical groups.

Tuberculoid leprosy (TT)

In tuberculoid leprosy the infection is localized because the patient has unimpaired cell-mediated immunity. The characteristic, usually single, skin lesion is a hypopigmented, anaesthetic patch with thickened, clearly demarcated edges, central healing, and atrophy. The face, gluteal region and extremities are most commonly affected. The nerve leading to the hypopigmented patch, and the regional nerve trunk, are often thickened and tender. Unlike other parts of the body, a tuberculoid patch on the face is not anaesthetic. Nerve involvement leads to marked muscle atrophy. Tuberculoid lesions are known to heal spontaneously. The prognosis is good.

Borderline tuberculoid (BT) leprosy

This resembles TT but skin lesions are usually more numerous, smaller, and may be present as small 'satellite' lesions around larger ones. Peripheral but not cutaneous nerves are thickened, leading to deformity of hands and feet.

Borderline (BB) leprosy

Skin lesions are numerous, varying in size and form (macules, papules, plaques). The annular, rimmed lesion

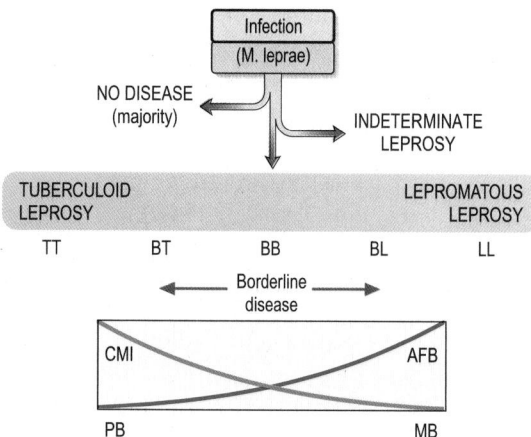

Fig. 2.25 Clinical spectrum of leprosy with the combined Ridley–Jopling and WHO classification. BT, borderline tuberculoid; BB, borderline; BL, borderline lepromatous; CMI, cell-mediated immunity; AFB, acid-fast bacilli; PB, paucibacillary; MB, multibacillary. Modified from Jacobson R (1999) Krahenbuhl JL *Lancet* **353**: 655.

with punched-out, hypopigmented anaesthetic centre is characteristic (Fig. 2.26). There is widespread nerve involvement and limb deformity (Fig. 2.27).

Borderline lepromatous (BL) leprosy

There are a large number of florid asymmetrical skin lesions of variable form, which are strongly positive for acid-fast bacilli. Skin between the lesions is normal and often negative for bacilli.

Lepromatous leprosy (LL)

Although practically every organ can be involved, the changes in the skin are the earliest and most obvious manifestation. Peripheral oedema and rhinitis are the earliest symptoms. The skin lesions predominantly occur on the face, the gluteal region and the upper and lower limbs. They may be macules, papules, nodules or plaques: of these, the macule is the first to appear. Infiltration is most noticeable in the ear lobes. Thinning of the lateral margins of the eyebrows is characteristic. The mucous membranes are frequently involved, resulting in nasal stuffiness, laryngitis and hoarseness of the voice. Nasal septal perforation with collapse of the nasal cartilages produces a saddle-nose deformity. With progression of the disease the typical leonine facies due to infiltration of the skin becomes apparent. Glove and stocking anaesthesia, gynaecomastia, testicular atrophy, ichthyosis and nerve palsies (facial, ulnar, median and radial) develop late in the disease. Neurotrophic atrophy affecting the phalanges leads to the gradual disappearance of fingers. Nerve involvement is less pronounced than in TT.

Lepra reactions

These are immunologically mediated acute reactions that occur in patients with the borderline or lepromatous spectrum of disease, usually during treatment. Two forms are recognized.

Non-lepromatous lepra reaction (type I lepra reaction). This is seen following treatment of patients with borderline disease; it is a type IV delayed hypersensitivity reaction. Both upgrading (or reversal) reactions (i.e. a clinical change towards a more tuberculoid form) and downgrading reactions (i.e. a change towards the lepromatous form) can occur. Neurological deficits such as an ulnar nerve palsy may occur abruptly.

Erythema nodosum leprosum (ENL; type II lepra reaction). This is a humoral antibody response to an antigen–antibody complex (i.e. a type III hypersensitivity reaction). It is seen in 50% of patients with treated LL. ENL is characterized by fever, arthralgia, iridocyclitis, crops of painful, subcutaneous erythematous nodules, and other systemic manifestations. It may last from a few days to several weeks.

Diagnosis

The diagnosis of leprosy is essentially clinical with:

- hypopigmented/reddish patches with loss of sensation
- thickening of peripheral nerves
- acid-fast bacilli (AFB) seen on skin-slit smears/biopsy. Small slits are made in pinched skin and the fluid obtained is smeared on a slide and stained for AFB.

Patients should be examined carefully for skin lesions in adequate natural light. Occasionally nerve biopsies are helpful. Detection of *M. leprae* DNA is possible in all forms of leprosy using the polymerase chain reaction, and can be used to assess the efficacy of treatment.

Management

Multidrug therapy (MDT) is essential because of developing drug resistance (up to 40% of bacilli in some areas are resistant to dapsone). Much shorter courses of treatment are now being used: the current WHO recommended drug regimens for leprosy are shown in Box 2.11 but

Fig. 2.26   Multiple asymmetrical hypopigmented anaesthetic patches. Courtesy of Dr P Matondo, Zambia.

Fig. 2.27   Leprosy – claw hand due to median and ulnar nerve damage.

Box 2.11 Recommended treatment regimens for leprosy in adults (modified WHO guidelines)

Multibacillary leprosy (LL, BL, BB)
Rifampicin 600 mg once-monthly, supervised
Clofazimine 300 mg once-monthly, supervised
Clofazimine 50 mg daily, self-administered
Dapsone 100 mg daily, self-administered
Treatment continued for 12 months

Paucibacillary leprosy (BT, TT)
Rifampicin 600 mg once-monthly, supervised
Dapsone 100 mg daily, self-administered
Treatment continued for 6 months

Single lesion paucibacillary leprosy
Rifampicin 600 mg ⎫
Ofloxacin 400 mg ⎬ as a single dose
Minocycline 100 mg ⎭

LL, lepromatous; BL, borderline lepromatous; BB, borderline;
BT, borderline tuberculoid; TT, tuberculoid

longer therapy may be required in severe cases. Follow up including skin smears is essential.

Patient education is essential. Patients should be taught self-care of their anaesthetic hands and feet to prevent ulcers. If ulcers develop, no weight-bearing should be permitted. Cheap canvas shoes with cushioned insoles are protective.

Leprosy should be treated in specialist centres with adequate physiotherapy and occupational therapy support. Surgery and physiotherapy also play a role in the management of trophic ulcers and deformities of the hands, feet and face.

Treatment of lepra reactions. This is urgent, as irreversible eye and nerve damage can occur. Antileprosy therapy must be continued. Type II lepra reactions (ENL) can be treated with analgesics, chloroquine, clofazimine and antipyretics. Thalidomide was previously used for ENL and is effective. However, because of its teratogenicity, it is no longer recommended by WHO. Prednisolone 40–60 mg daily for 3–6 months is effective in type I reactions.

Prevention

The prevention and control of leprosy depends on rapid treatment of infected patients, particularly those with LL and BL, to decrease the bacterial reservoir.

Anthrax

Anthrax is caused by *Bacillus anthracis*. The spores of these Gram-positive bacilli are extremely hardy and withstand extremes of temperature and humidity. The organism is capable of toxin production and this property correlates most closely with its virulence. The disease occurs world-wide. Epidemics have been reported in The Gambia, in both North and South America and in southern Europe. Transmission is through direct contact with an infected animal; infection is most frequently seen in farmers, butchers, and dealers in wool and animal hides. Spores can also be ingested or inhaled. There have been recent cases in the USA due to the deliberate release of anthrax spores as a bioterrorist weapon (p. 1031).

Clinical features

The incubation period is 1–10 days. Cutaneous anthrax is the most common. The small, erythematous, maculo-papular lesion is initially painless. It may subsequently vesiculate and ulcerate, with formation of a central black eschar. The illness is self-limiting in the majority of patients, but occasionally perivesicular oedema and regional lymphadenopathy may be marked, and toxaemia can occur.

Inhalational anthrax (woolsorter's disease) follows inhalation of spores, and bioterrorism should be suspected. A febrile illness is accompanied by non-productive cough and retrosternal discomfort; pleural effusions are common. Untreated, the mortality is about 90%, and in the recent cases in the USA it was 45% despite treatment.

Gastrointestinal anthrax is due to consumption of undercooked, contaminated meat. It presents as severe gastroenteritis; haematemesis and bloody diarrhoea can occur. Toxaemia, shock and death may follow.

Diagnosis

The diagnosis is established by demonstrating the organism in smears from cutaneous lesions or by culture of blood and other body fluids. Serological confirmation can be made using ELISAs detecting antibodies to both the organism and a toxin.

Management

Ciprofloxacin is considered the best treatment. In mild cutaneous infections, oral therapy for 2 weeks is adequate but therapy for 60 days was used in the recent outbreaks in the USA. In more severe infections high doses of intravenous antibiotics are needed, along with appropriate supportive care. Any suspected case should be reported to the relevant authority.

Control

Any infected animal that dies should be burned and the area in which it was housed disinfected. Where animal husbandry is poor, mass vaccination of animals may prevent widespread contamination, but needs to be repeated annually. A human vaccine is available for those at high risk, and prophylactic antibiotics may be indicated following exposure. Some countries are establishing public health policies to deal with the deliberate release of anthrax spores.

Mycobacterial ulcer (Buruli ulcer)

Buruli ulcer is seen world-wide in rural areas in the tropical rainforests. *Mycobacterium ulcerans*, the causative organism, is found in pools and rivers, and infection is usually due to bathing, swimming or collecting water. A small subcutaneous nodule at the site of infection gradually ulcerates, involving subcutaneous tissue, muscle and fascial planes. The ulcers are usually large with undermined edges and markedly necrotic bases due to mycolactone. Smears taken from necrotic tissue generally reveal numerous acid-fast bacilli. The only effective treatment is wide surgical excision with skin grafts, but this is often unavailable in areas where the disease is prevalent. Antituberculous therapy is ineffective.

Endemic treponematoses (bejel, yaws and pinta)

These diseases are found in various parts of the tropics and subtropics, mainly in impoverished rural areas (Fig. 2.28). The WHO treated over 50 million cases in the 1950s and 1960s, reducing the prevalence of these diseases, but subsequently there has been a resurgence of infection. The latest estimate of global prevalence is 2.5 million cases. Improvements in sanitation and an increase in living standards will be required to eradicate the diseases completely as organisms are transmitted by bodily contact, usually in children.

Clinical features

Yaws

Yaws (caused by *Treponema pertenue*) is the most wide-spread and common of the endemic treponemal diseases. It is spread by direct contact, the organism entering through damaged skin. After an incubation period of

weeks or months a primary inflammatory reaction occurs at the inoculation site, from which organisms can be isolated. Dissemination of the organism leads to multiple papular lesions containing treponemes; these skin lesions usually involve the palms and soles. There may also be bone involvement, particularly affecting the long bones and those of the hand.

Approximately 10% of those infected go on to develop late yaws. Bony gummatous lesions may progress to cause gross destruction and disfigurement, particularly of the skull and facial bones, the interphalangeal joints and the long bones. Plantar hyperkeratosis is characteristic. Like syphilis, there may be a latent period between the early and late phases of the disease, but visceral, neurological and cardiovascular problems do not occur.

Bejel (endemic syphilis)

Bejel is seen in Africa and the Middle East. The causative organism (*Treponema endemicum*) enters through abrasions in the skin or from contaminated drinking vessels. It differs from venereal syphilis in that a primary lesion is not commonly seen. The late stages resemble syphilis, but cardiological and neurological manifestations are rare.

Pinta

Pinta, caused by *Treponema carateum*, is restricted mainly to Central and South America. It is milder than the other trepanomatoses and is confined to the skin. The primary lesion is a pruritic red papule, usually on the hand or foot. It may become scaly but never ulcerates and is generally associated with regional lymphadenopathy. In the later stages similar lesions can continue to occur for up to

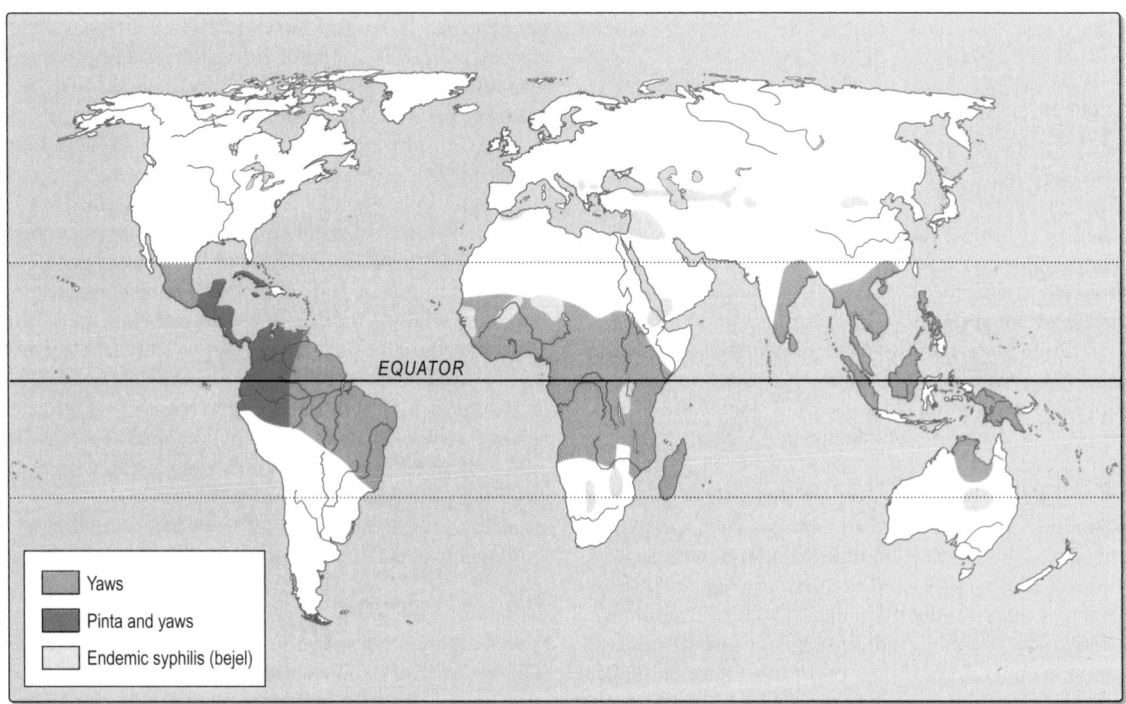

Fig. 2.28 **Bejel, yaws and pinta – geographical distribution.**

1 year, associated with generalized lymphadenopathy. Eventually the lesions heal leaving hyperpigmented or depigmented patches.

Diagnosis and management

In endemic areas the diagnosis is usually clinical. The causative organism can be identified from the exudative lesions under dark-ground microscopy. Serological tests for syphilis are positive but do not differentiate between the conditions.

The treatment is with long-acting penicillin (e.g. intramuscular benzathine penicillin, 1.2 million units) given as a single dose. Doxycycline is used when penicillin is ineffective or contra-indicated.

Trachoma

Trachoma, caused by the intracellular bacterium *Chlamydia trachomatis*, is the most common cause of blindness in the world. It is estimated that there are 150 million current infections, and 6 million people who have been blinded by trachoma. It is a disease of poverty which is found mainly in the tropics and the Middle East: it is entirely preventable. Trachoma commonly occurs in children, and is spread by direct transmission or by flies. Isolated infection is probably self-limiting, and it is repeated infection which leads to chronic eye disease.

Clinical features

Infection is bilateral and begins in the conjunctiva, with marked follicular inflammation and subsequent scarring. Scarring of the upper eyelid causes entropion, leaving the cornea exposed to further damage with the eyelashes rubbing against it (trichiasis). The corneal scarring that eventually occurs leads to blindness.

Trachoma may also occur as an acute ophthalmic infection in the neonate.

Diagnosis and management

The diagnosis is generally established by the typical clinical picture. It can be confirmed by cell culture techniques or species-specific fluorescent monoclonal antibodies, but these are rarely available in endemic areas.

Tetracycline ointment applied locally each day for 6–8 weeks is effective but compliance is poor. Systemic therapy with a single dose of azithromycin 20 mg/kg is the treatment of choice. In endemic areas repeated courses of therapy are necessary. Once infection has been controlled, surgery may be required for eyelid reconstruction and for treatment of corneal opacities.

Prevention

Community health education, improvements in water supply and sanitation (pit latrines) and earlier case reporting could have a substantial impact on disease prevalence. This is reflected in the WHO 'SAFE' approach to trachoma: surgery, antibiotics, facial cleanliness, environmental improvement. A WHO target is global eradication by 2020.

FURTHER READING

Barlett JG et al. (2002) Management of anthrax. *Clinical Infectious Diseases* **35**: 851–858.

Britton WJ, Lockwood DNJ (2004) Leprosy. *Lancet* **363**: 1209–1219.

Mabey D, Solomon A, Foster A (2003) Trachoma. *Lancet* **362**: 223–229.

Swartz MN (2001) Recognition and management of anthrax. *New England Journal of Medicine* **345**: 1621–1626.

GASTROINTESTINAL INFECTIONS

Cholera

Cholera is caused by the curved, flagellated Gram-negative bacillus, *Vibrio cholerae*. The organism is killed by temperatures of 100 °C in a few seconds but can survive in ice for up to 6 weeks. One major pathogenic serogroup possesses a somatic antigen (O1) with two biotypes: classical and El Tor. The El Tor biotype replaced the classical biotype as the major cause of the seventh pandemic which began in the 1960s. Infection with the El Tor biotype generally causes milder symptoms, but can still cause severe and life-threatening disease.

The fertile, humid Gangetic plains of West Bengal have traditionally been regarded as the home of cholera. However, a series of pandemics have spread the disease across the world, usually following trade routes. The seventh pandemic has affected large areas of Asia, North Africa, Kenya and southern Europe. It has spread to South and Central America in recent years, claiming thousands of lives. A new serogroup (O139 Bengal) is now responsible for an increasing number of cases in Bangladesh, India and South East Asia. It has a characteristic pattern of antibiotic resistance (sulfamethoxazole, trimethoprim and streptomycin), and may prove to be the cause of the next pandemic.

Transmission is by the faeco-oral route. Contaminated water plays a major role in the dissemination of cholera, although contaminated foodstuffs and contact carriers may contribute in epidemics. Achlorhydria or hypochlorhydria facilitates passage of the cholera bacilli into the small intestine. Here they proliferate, elaborating an exotoxin which produces massive secretion of isotonic fluid into the intestinal lumen (see p. 332). Cholera toxin also releases serotonin (5-HT) from enterochromaffin cells in the gut, which activates a neural secretory reflex in the enteric nervous system. This may account for at least 50% of cholera toxin's secretory activity. *V. cholerae* also produces other toxins (zona occludens toxin, ZOT, and accessory cholera toxin, ACT) which contribute to its pathogenic effect.

Clinical features

The incubation period varies from a few hours to 6 days. The majority of patients with cholera have a mild illness that cannot be distinguished clinically from diarrhoea due to other infective causes. Classically, however, three phases are recognized in the untreated disease.

The *evacuation phase* is characterized by the abrupt onset of painless, profuse, watery diarrhoea, associated with vomiting in the severe forms. 'Rice water' stools, so called because of mucus flecks floating in the watery stools, are typical of this stage.

If appropriate supportive treatment is not given, the patient passes on to the *collapse phase*. This is characterized by features of circulatory shock (cold clammy skin, tachycardia, hypotension and peripheral cyanosis) and dehydration (sunken eyes, hollow cheeks and a diminished urine output). The patient, though apathetic, is usually lucid. Muscle cramps may be severe. Children may present with convulsions owing to hypoglycaemia. At this stage renal failure and aspiration of vomitus present major problems.

If the patient survives the collapse stage the *recovery phase* starts, with a gradual return to normal clinical and biochemical parameters in 1–3 days.

Diagnosis

This is largely clinical. Examination of freshly passed stools may demonstrate rapidly motile organisms. This is not diagnostic, as *Campylobacter jejuni* may also give a similar appearance. However, demonstration of the rapidly motile vibrios by dark-field illumination and subsequent inhibition of their movement with type-specific antisera is diagnostic. Stool and rectal swabs should be taken for culture.

Management

The mainstay of treatment is rehydration, and with appropriate and effective rehydration therapy mortality has decreased to less than 1%. Oral rehydration is usually adequate, but intravenous therapy is occasionally required.

Oral rehydration solutions (ORS) are based on the observation that glucose (and other carbohydrates) enhances sodium and water absorption in the small intestine, even in the presence of secretory loss due to toxins. Additions such as amylase-resistant starch to glucose-based ORS have been shown to increase the absorption of fluid. Cereal-based electrolyte solutions have been found to be as effective as sugar/salt ORS, and actually reduce stool volume as well as rehydrating. The WHO has recently recommended the use of reduced osmolarity ORS for all types of diarrhoea, although concerns remain about the risk of hyponatraemia. Suitable solutions for rehydration are listed in Box 2.9 (p. 71).

Mildly dehydrated individuals are given ORS 50 mL/kg in the first 4 hours, followed by a maintenance dose of 100 mL/kg daily until the diarrhoea stops. For moderate dehydration, ORS 100 mL/kg is given within the first 4 hours followed by 10–15 mL/kg/hour.

Intravenous rehydration is required only for severely dehydrated individuals with features of collapse. Several litres of intravenous fluid (Ringers Lactate) are usually required to overcome the features of shock. Maintenance of hydration is effectively carried out by oral rehydration solutions.

Antibiotics such as tetracycline 500 mg four times daily for 3 days help to eradicate the infection, decrease stool output, and shorten the duration of the illness. Drug resistance is becoming an increasing problem, and ciprofloxacin is now used more frequently.

Immunization is now recommended by the WHO in potential or actual outbreak situations. Live attenuated and killed vaccine (both oral) are available: neither protect against the 0139 strain. Chemoprophylaxis with tetracycline 500 mg twice-daily for 3 days for adults, or 125 mg daily for children, is effective. The best preventative measures, however, are good hygiene and improved sanitation.

Enteric fever

Over 16 million new cases of enteric fever occur worldwide, mainly in India and Africa, causing 600 000 deaths per year. Enteric fever is an acute systemic illness characterized by fever, headache, and abdominal discomfort. *Typhoid*, the typical form of enteric fever, is caused by *Salmonella typhi*. A similar but generally less severe illness known as paratyphoid is due to infection with *S. paratyphi* A, B, or C. Man is the only natural host for *S. typhi*, which is transmitted in contaminated food or water. The incubation period is 10–14 days.

Clinical features

After ingestion, the bacteria invade the small bowel wall via Peyer's patches, from where they spread to the regional lymph nodes and then to the blood. The onset of illness is insidious and non-specific, with intermittent fever, headache, and abdominal pain. Physical findings in the early stages include abdominal tenderness, hepatosplenomegaly, lymphadenopathy, and a scanty maculopapular rash ('rose spots'). Without treatment (and occasionally even after treatment) serious complications can arise, usually in the third week of illness. These include meningitis, lobar pneumonia, osteomyelitis, intestinal perforation and intestinal haemorrhage. The fourth week of the illness is characterized by gradual improvement, but in developing countries up to 30% of those infected will die, and 10% of untreated survivors will relapse. This compares with a mortality rate of 1–2% in the USA.

After clinical recovery 5–10% of patients will continue to excrete *S. typhi* for several months: these are termed convalescent carriers. Between 1% and 4% will continue to carry the organism for more than a year: this is chronic carriage. The usual site of carriage is the gall bladder, and chronic carriage is associated with the presence of gallstones. However, in parts of the Middle East and Africa where urinary schistosomiasis is prevalent, chronic carriage of *S. typhi* in the urinary bladder is also common.

Diagnosis

The definitive diagnosis of enteric fever requires the culture of *S. typhi* or *S. paratyphi* from the patient. Blood culture is positive in most cases in the first 2 weeks. Culture of intestinal secretions, faeces, and urine is also used, although care must be taken to distinguish acute infection from chronic carriage. Bone marrow culture is more sensitive than blood culture, but is rarely required except in patients who have already received antibiotics. Leucopenia is common but non-specific. Serological tests such as the Widal antigen test are of little practical value and are easily misinterpreted.

Management

Increasing antibiotic resistance is seen in isolates of *S. typhi*, especially in the Indian subcontinent. Chloramphenicol, co-trimoxazole and amoxicillin may all still be effective in some cases, but quinolones (e.g. ciprofloxacin 500 mg twice daily) are now the treatment of choice, although increased resistance to these agents is being seen: in such cases azithromycin may be effective. Infection from the Indian subcontinent, Middle East and South East Asia is often resistant to multiple antibacterial agents. The patient's temperature may remain elevated for several days after starting antibiotics, and this alone is not a sign of treatment failure. Prolonged antibiotic therapy may eliminate the carrier state, but in the presence of gall bladder disease it is rarely effective. Cholecystectomy is not usually justified on clinical or public health grounds.

Prevention

This is mainly through improved sanitation and clean water. Travellers should avoid drinking untreated water, ice in drinks and eating ice creams. Vaccination with injectable inactivated or oral live attenuated vaccines gives partial protection.

SYSTEMIC INFECTIONS

Tuberculosis

Tuberculosis is caused by *Mycobacterium tuberculosis*, and occasionally *M. bovis* or *M. africanum*. These are slow-growing bacteria, and unlike other mycobacteria, are facultative intracellular organisms. The prevalence of tuberculosis increases with poor social conditions, inadequate nutrition, and overcrowding. In developing countries it is most commonly acquired in childhood.

The impact of tuberculosis in the developing world has been magnified in the past 20 years by the emergence of the HIV pandemic (p. 129) (Fig. 2.29).

Widespread misuse of antibiotics, combined with the breakdown of healthcare systems in parts of Africa, Russia and East Europe, has led to the emergence of drug-resistant tuberculosis. The most serious form, known as multidrug-resistant tuberculosis (MDRTB), is caused by bacteria that are resistant to both rifampicin and isoniazid, two drugs which form the mainstay of treatment. MDRTB is very difficult to treat, and has a significant mortality even with the best medical care.

In most people, the initial primary tuberculosis is asymptomatic or causes only a mild illness.

Occasionally the primary infection progresses locally to a more widespread lesion. Haematogenous spread at this stage may give rise to miliary tuberculosis.

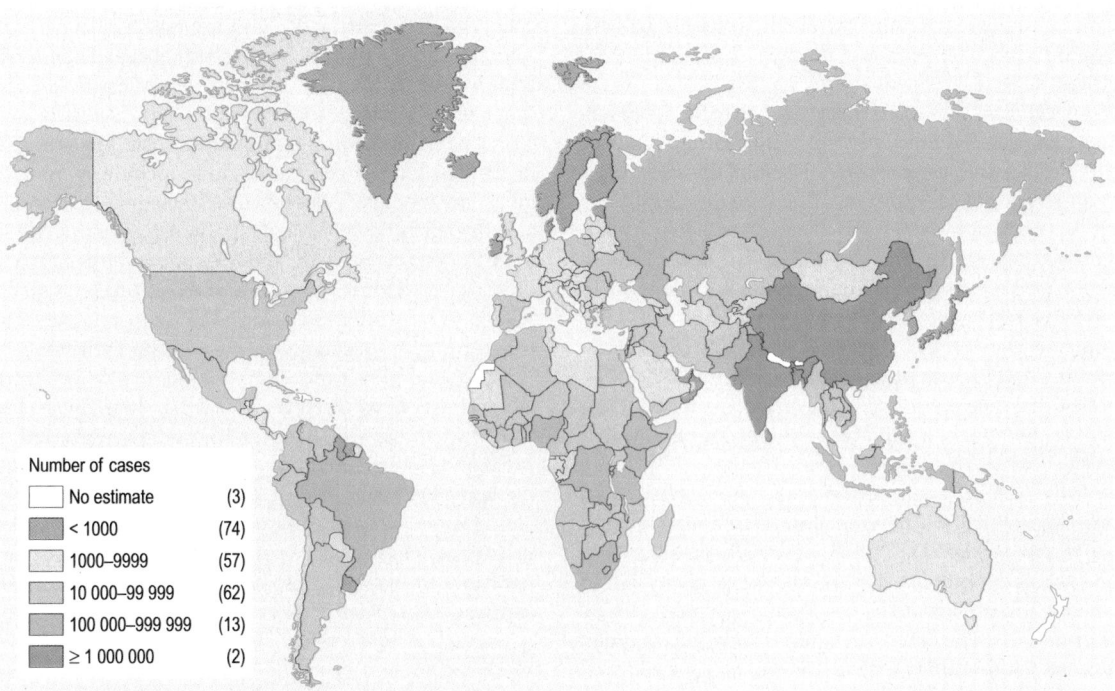

Number of cases

No estimate	(3)
< 1000	(74)
1000–9999	(57)
10 000–99 999	(62)
100 000–999 999	(13)
≥ 1 000 000	(2)

Fig. 2.29 **Tuberculosis – geographical distribution.** From Frieden TR, Sterling TR, Munsiff SS et al. (2003) Tuberculosis. Reprinted with permission from Elsevier (*Lancet* **362**: 888).

Tuberculosis in the adult may be the result of reactivation of old disease (post-primary tuberculosis), primary infection, or more rarely reinfection.

Pulmonary tuberculosis is the most common form; this is described on page 306, along with the chemotherapeutic regimens. Tuberculosis also affects other parts of the body:

- The gastrointestinal tract, mainly the ileocaecal area, but occasionally the peritoneum, producing ascites (see p. 344).
- The genitourinary system. The kidneys are most commonly involved, but tuberculosis can also cause painless, craggy swellings in the epididymis, and salpingitis, tubal abscesses, and infertility in females.
- The central nervous system, causing tuberculous meningitis and tuberculomas (p. 1238).
- The skeletal system, leading to septic arthritis and osteomyelitis.
- The skin, giving rise to lupus vulgaris.
- The eyes, where it can cause choroiditis or iridocyclitis.
- The pericardium, producing constrictive pericarditis (p. 856).
- The adrenal glands, causing destruction and producing Addison's disease.
- Lymph nodes. This is a common mode of presentation, especially in young adults and children. Any group of lymph nodes may be involved, but hilar and para-tracheal lymph nodes are the most common. Initially the nodes are firm and discrete but later they become matted and can suppurate with sinus formation. Scrofula is the term used to describe massive cervical lymph node enlargement with discharging sinuses. Mycobacterial lymph node disease may also be caused by non-tuberculous mycobacteria.

Non-tuberculous mycobacterial infections

The majority of mycobacterial species are environmental organisms, and are rarely pathogenic. Some have been found to cause disease in man, particularly in immuno-compromised patients or those with pre-existing chronic lung disease (Table 2.36).

Plague

Plague is caused by *Yersinia pestis*, a Gram-negative bacillus. Sporadic cases of plague (as well as occasional epidemics) occur world-wide: about 2500 cases per year are reported to the WHO, with a 10% mortality. The majority of cases are seen in sub-Saharan Africa, although the disease is occasionally seen in developed countries in people undertaking outdoor pursuits. The main reservoirs are woodland rodents, which transmit infection to domestic rats (*Rattus rattus*). The usual vector is the rat flea, *Xenopsylla cheopis*. These fleas bite humans when there is a sudden decline in the rat population. Occasionally, spread of the organisms may be through infected faeces being rubbed into skin wounds, or through inhalation of droplets.

Table 2.36 Non-tuberculous mycobacteria causing disease in man

Clinical	Common cause	Rare cause
Chronic lung disease	*Mycobacterium avium-intracellulare* *M. kansasii*	*M. malmoense* *M. xenopi*
Local lymphadenitis	*M. avium-intracellulare* *M. scrofulaceum*	*M. malmoense* *M. fortuitum*
Skin and soft tissue infection		
Fish tank granuloma	*M. marinum*	
Abscesses, ulcers, sinuses	*M. fortuitum* *M. chelonae*	*M. haemophilum*
Bone and joint infection	*M. kansasii* *M. avium-intracellulare*	*M. scrofulaceum*
Disseminated infection (in HIV)	*M. avium-intracellulare*	

Clinical features

Four clinical forms are recognized: bubonic, pneumonic, septicaemic and cutaneous.

Bubonic plague

This is the most common form and occurs in about 90% of infected individuals. The incubation period is about 1 week. The onset of illness is acute, with high fever, chills, headache, myalgia, nausea, vomiting and, when severe, prostration. This is rapidly followed by the development of lymphadenopathy (buboes), most commonly involving the inguinal region. Characteristically these are matted and tender, and suppurate in 1–2 weeks. Petechiae, ecchymoses and bleeding from the gastrointestinal tract, the respiratory tract and the genitourinary tract may occur. Mental confusion follows the development of toxaemia.

Pneumonic plague

This is characterized by the abrupt onset of features of a fulminant pneumonia with bloody sputum, marked respiratory distress, cyanosis and death in almost all affected patients.

Septicaemic plague

This presents as an acute fulminant infection with evidence of shock and disseminated intravascular coagulation (DIC). If left untreated, death usually occurs in 2–5 days. Lymphadenopathy is unusual.

Cutaneous plague

This presents either as a pustule, eschar or papule or an extensive purpura, which can become necrotic and gangrenous.

Diagnosis

A rapid diagnostic test on samples (bubo aspirate, sputum) has been developed. This is an easy to read, hand held immunodermatographic dipstick assay relying on conjugated gold particles to detect *Y. pestis*-specific F1 capsular antigen. It has an extremely high sensitivity and specificity. The diagnosis can also be established by demonstrating the organism in lymph node aspirates, in blood cultures or on examination of sputum.

Management

Treatment is urgent and should be instituted before the results of culture studies are available. The treatment of choice is intramuscular streptomycin 1 g twice daily or gentamicin 2 mg/kg i.v. three times daily for 10 days. Oral tetracycline 500 mg four times daily and chloramphenicol are also effective.

Prevention

Prevention of plague is largely dependent on the control of the flea population. Outhouses, or huts, should be sprayed with insecticides that are effective against the local flea. During epidemics rodents should not be killed until the fleas are under control, as the fleas will leave dead rodents to bite humans. Tetracycline 500 mg four times daily or sulphonamides 2–4 g daily for 7 days are effective chemoprophylactic agents. A partially effective formalin-killed vaccine is available for use by travellers to plague-endemic areas.

Relapsing fevers

These conditions are so named because, after apparent recovery from the initial infection, one or more recurrences may occur after a week or more without fever. They are caused by spirochaetes of the genus *Borrelia*.

Clinical features

Louse-borne relapsing fever (caused by *B. recurrentis*) is spread by body lice, and only humans are affected. Classically it is an epidemic disease of armies and refugees, although it is also endemic in the highlands of Ethiopia, Yemen and Bolivia. Lice are spread from person to person when humans live in close contact in impoverished conditions. Infected lice are crushed by scratching, allowing the spirochaete to penetrate through the skin. Symptoms begin 3–10 days after infection and consist of a high fever of abrupt onset with rigors,

generalized myalgia and headache. A petechial or ecchymotic rash may be seen. The general condition then deteriorates, with delirium, hepatosplenomegaly, jaundice, haemorrhagic problems and circulatory collapse. Although complete recovery may occur at this time, the majority experience one or more relapses of diminishing intensity over the weeks following the initial illness. The severity of the illness varies enormously, and some cases have only mild symptoms. However, in some epidemics mortality has exceeded 50%.

Tick-borne relapsing fever is caused by *B. duttoni* and other *Borrelia* species, spread by soft (argasid) ticks. Rodents are also infected, and humans are incidental hosts, acquiring the spirochaete from the saliva of the infected tick. This disease is mainly found in countries where traditional mud huts are the form of shelter, but is occasionally associated with old houses and camp sites in the USA. The illness is generally similar to the louse-borne disease, although neurological involvement is more common.

Diagnosis and management

Spirochaetes can be demonstrated microscopically in the blood during febrile episodes: organisms are more numerous in louse-borne relapsing fever. Treatment is usually with tetracycline or doxycycline (see p. 36). A severe Jarisch–Herxheimer reaction (p. 124) occurs in many patients, often requiring intensive nursing care and intravenous fluids.

Prevention

Control of infection relies on elimination of the vector. Ticks live for years and remain infected, passing the infection to their progeny. These reservoirs of infection should be controlled by spraying houses with insecticides and by reducing the number of rodents. Patients infested with lice should be deloused by washing with a suitable insecticide. All clothes must be thoroughly disinfected.

Typhus

Typhus is the collective name given to a group of diseases caused by *Rickettsia* species (Table 2.37). Rickettsia (and the closely related Orientiae) are small intracellular bacteria that are spread to humans by arthropod vectors,

Table 2.37 Infections caused by rickettsiae			
Disease	**Organism**	**Reservoir**	**Vector**
Typhus fever group			
Epidemic typhus	*Rickettsia prowazekii*	Man	Human body louse
Endemic (murine) typhus	*R. typhi*	Rodents	Rat flea
Scrub typhus	*Orientia tsutsugamushi*	Trombiculid mite	Trombiculid mite
Spotted fever group			
African tick typhus	*R. africae*	Various mammals	Hard tick
Mediterranean spotted fever	*R. conorii*	Rodents, dog	Hard tick
Rocky Mountain spotted fever	*R. ricketsii*	Rodents	Hard tick
Rickettsial pox	*R. akari*	Rodents	Mite
Flea-borne spotted fever	*R. felis*	Various mammals	Flea

including body lice, fleas, hard ticks, and larval mites. Rickettsiae inhabit the alimentary tract of these arthropods and the disease is spread to the human host by inoculation of their faeces through broken human skin, generally produced by scratching. Rickettsiae multiply intracellularly and can enter most mammalian cells, although the main lesion produced is a vasculitis due to invasion of endothelial cells of small blood vessels. Multisystem involvement is usual.

Clinical features

Typhus fever group

Epidemic typhus

The vector of epidemic typhus is the human body louse, and like louse-borne relapsing fever, epidemics are associated with war and refugees. Outbreaks have occurred in Africa, Central and South America, and Asia.

The incubation period of 1–3 weeks is followed by an abrupt febrile illness associated with profound malaise and generalized myalgia. Headache is severe and there may be conjunctivitis with orbital pain. A measles-like eruption appears around the fifth day, the macules increasing in size and eventually becoming purpuric in character. At the end of the first week, signs of meningo-encephalitis appear and CNS involvement may progress to stupor or coma, sometimes with extrapyramidal involvement. At the height of the illness, splenomegaly, pneumonia, myocarditis, and gangrene at the peripheries may be evident. Oliguric renal failure occurs in fulminating disease, which is usually fatal. Recovery begins in the third week but is generally slow. The disease may recur many years after the initial attack owing to rickettsiae that lie dormant in lymph nodes. The recrudescence is known as Brill–Zinsser disease. The factors that precipitate recurrence are not clearly defined, although other infections may play a role.

Endemic (murine) typhus

This is an infection of rodents that is inadvertently spread to humans by rat fleas. The disease closely resembles epidemic typhus but is much milder and rarely fatal.

Scrub typhus

Found throughout Asia and the Western Pacific, this disease is spread by larval trombiculid mites (chiggers). An eschar (a black, crusted, necrotic papule) can often be found at the site of the bite. The clinical illness is very variable, ranging from a mild illness to fulminant and potentially fatal disease. The more severe cases resemble epidemic typhus. Unlike other types of typhus the organism is passed on to subsequent generations of mites, which consequently act as both reservoir and vector.

Spotted fever group

A variety of *Rickettsia* species, collectively known as the spotted fever group rickettsiae, cause the illnesses known as spotted fevers. In all except for rickettsial pox (which is transmitted by a rodent mite) the vector is a hard tick. Although the causative organism and the name of the

illness vary from place to place the clinical course is common to all. After an incubation period of 4–10 days an eschar may develop at the site of the bite in association with regional lymphadenopathy. There is abrupt onset of fever, myalgia and headache, accompanied by a maculo-papular rash which may become petechial. Neurological, haematological and cardiovascular complications occur as in epidemic typhus, although these are uncommon.

Diagnosis

The diagnosis is generally made on the basis of the history and clinical course of the illness. It can be confirmed serologically by the indirect fluorescent antibody test (the most sensitive and specific), or the latex agglutination test. The Weil–Felix agglutination test, although previously widely used, is not specific or sensitive.

Treatment and prevention

Doxycycline or tetracycline given for 5–7 days is the treatment of choice. Ciprofloxacin is also effective. Doxycycline 200 mg weekly protects against scrub typhus; it is reserved for highly endemic areas. Rifampicin is also used when resistance to tetracycline has occurred. Seriously ill patients need intensive care. Control of typhus is achieved by eradication of the arthropod vectors. Lice and fleas can be eradicated from clothing by insecticides (0.5% malathion or DDT). Control of rodents is necessary in endemic typhus and some of the spotted fevers. Areas of vegetation infested with trombiculid mites can be cleared by chemical spraying from the air. Bites from ticks and mites should be avoided by wearing protective clothing on exposed areas of the body. The likelihood of infection from ticks is related to the duration of feeding, and in high-risk areas the body should be inspected twice a day and any ticks removed (p. 79).

Bartonellosis and ehrlichiosis

Bartonella spp. and *Ehrlichia* spp. are intracellular bacteria closely related to the rickettsiae. A number of human diseases can be caused by these organisms; like rickettsial disease, infection is usually spread from animals via an arthropod vector (Table 2.38).

Carrión's disease

This disease is restricted mainly to the habitat of its main vector, the sandfly, in the river valleys of the Andes mountains at an altitude of 500–3000 m. Two clinical presentations are seen, which may occur alone or consecutively. *Oroya fever* is an acute febrile illness causing myalgia, arthralgia, severe headache, and confusion, followed by a haemolytic anaemia. *Verruga peruana* consists of eruptions of reddish-purple haemangiomatous nodules, resembling bacillary angiomatosis. It may follow 4–6 weeks after Oroya fever, or be the presenting feature of infection. Spontaneous resolution may occur over a period of months or years. Carrión's disease is

Table 2.38 Human infections caused by *Bartonella* spp. and *Ehrlichia* spp.

Disease	Organism	Reservoir	Vector
Bartonella			
Carrión's disease	*Bartonella bacilliformis*	Unknown	Sandfly
Cat scratch disease	*B. henselae*	Cat	Cat flea
Bacillary angiomatosis	*B. henselae*	Cat	Cat flea
Trench fever	*B. quintana*	Human	Body louse
Ehrlichia			
Human ehrlichiosis	*Ehrlichia chafeensis*	Deer	Hard ticks
'Human granulocytic ehrlichia' (HE)	*A. phagocytophilum**	Small mammals and deer	Hard ticks

*Formerly known as *Ehrlichia phagocytophilia*

frequently complicated by superinfection, especially with *Salmonella* spp.

The diagnosis is made by culturing bacilli from blood or peripheral lesions. Serological tests have been developed but are not widely available.

Treatment with chloramphenicol or tetracycline is very effective in acute disease, but less so in verruga peruana.

Cat-scratch disease and bacillary angiomatosis

These are described on page 63.

Trench fever

Trench fever is caused by *Bartonella quintana*, and transmitted by human body lice. It is mainly seen in refugees and the homeless. It is characterized by cyclical fever (typically every 5 days), chills, and headaches, accompanied by myalgia and pretibial pain. The disease is usually self-limiting but it can be treated with erythromycin or doxycycline if symptoms are severe.

Melioidosis

The term melioidosis refers to infections caused by the Gram-negative bacteria *Burkholderia pseudomallei*. This environmental organism, which is found in soil and surface water, is distributed widely in the tropics and subtropics. The majority of clinical cases of melioidosis occur in South East Asia. Infection follows inhalation or direct inoculation. More than half of all patients with melioidosis have predisposing underlying disease: it is particularly common in diabetics.

B. pseudomallei causes a wide spectrum of disease, and the majority of infections are probably subclinical. Illness may be acute or chronic, localized or disseminated, but one form of the disease may progress to another and individual patients may be difficult to categorize. The most serious form is septicaemic melioidosis, which is often complicated by multiple metastatic abscesses: this is frequently fatal. Serological tests are available, but definitive diagnosis depends on isolating the organism from blood or appropriate tissue. *B. pseudomallei* has extensive intrinsic antibiotic resistance. The most effective agent is ceftazidime, which is given intravenously for 2–4 weeks; this should be followed by several months of co-amoxiclav to prevent relapses.

Actinomycosis

Actinomyces spp. are Gram-positive, branching higher bacteria which are normal mouth and intestine commensals; they are particularly associated with poor mouth hygiene. Actinomyces have a world-wide distribution but are a rare cause of disease in the West.

Clinical features

- *Cervicofacial actinomycosis*, the most common form, usually occurs following dental infection or extraction. It is often indolent and slowly progressive, associated with little pain, and results in induration and localized swelling of the lower part of the mandible. Lymphadenopathy is uncommon. Occasionally acute inflammation occurs. Sinuses and tracts develop with discharge of 'sulphur' granules.
- *Thoracic actinomycosis* follows inhalation of organisms, usually into a previously damaged lung. The clinical picture is not distinctive and is often mistaken for malignancy or tuberculosis. Symptoms such as fever, malaise, chest pain and haemoptysis are present. Empyema occurs in 25% of patients and local extension produces chest-wall sinuses with discharge of 'sulphur' granules.
- *Abdominal actinomycosis* most frequently affects the caecum. Characteristically, a hard indurated mass is felt in the right iliac fossa. Later, sinuses develop. The differential diagnosis includes malignancy, tuberculosis, Crohn's disease and amoeboma. The incidence of pelvic actinomycosis appears to be increasing with wider use of intrauterine contraceptive devices.

Occasionally actinomycosis becomes disseminated to involve any site.

Diagnosis and management

Diagnosis is by microscopy and culture of the organism. Treatment often involves surgery as well as antibiotics: penicillin is the drug of choice. Intravenous penicillin 2.4 g 4-hourly is given for 4–6 weeks, followed by oral penicillin for some weeks after clinical resolution. Tetracyclines are also effective.

Nocardia infections

Nocardia spp. are Gram-positive branching bacteria, which are found in soil and decomposing organic matter. *N. asteroides*, and less often *N. brasiliensis*, are the main human pathogens.

Clinical features

Mycetoma is the most common illness. This is a result of local invasion by *Nocardia* spp. and presents as a painless swelling, usually on the sole of the foot (Madura foot). The swelling of the affected part of the body continues inexorably. Nodules gradually appear which eventually rupture and discharge characteristic 'grains', which are colonies of organisms. Systemic symptoms and regional lymphadenopathy are rare. Sinuses may occur several years after the onset of the first symptom. A similar syndrome may be produced by other branching bacteria, and also by species of eumycete fungi such as *Madurella mycetomi* (p. 95).

Pulmonary disease, which follows inhalation of the organism, presents with cough, fever, and haemoptysis: it is usually seen in the immunocompromised. Pleural involvement and empyema occur. In severely immuno-suppressed patients initial pulmonary infection may be followed by disseminated disease.

Diagnosis and management

The diagnosis is often difficult to establish, as *Nocardia* is not easily detected in sputum cultures or on histological section. Severe pulmonary or disseminated infection may require parenteral treatment: effective agents include ceftriaxone and amikacin. Local infection is usually treated with prolonged courses of oral sulphonamides, combined with surgical drainage of pus if necessary.

FURTHER READING
Cole ST et al (eds) (2005) *Tuberculosis and the Tubercle Bacillus*. Washington: ASM Press.
Guerrant R, Carneiro F, Dillingham R (2003) Cholera, diarrhea, and oral rehydration therapy: triumph and indictment. *Clinical Infectious Diseases* **37**: 398–405.
Parry CM et al. (2002) Typhoid fever. *New England Journal of Medicine* **347**: 1770–1782.
Ustianowski A, Lockwood D (2003) Leprosy: current diagnostic and treatment approaches. *Current Opinion in Infectious Disease* **16**: 421–427.
Watt G, Parola P (2003) Scrub typhus and tropical rickettsioses. *Current Opinion in Infectious Disease* **16**: 429–436.

FUNGAL INFECTIONS

Morphologically, fungi can be grouped into three major categories:

- yeasts and yeast-like fungi, which reproduce by budding
- moulds, which grow by branching and longitudinal extension of hyphae

Table 2.39 Common fungal infections

Systemic	Subcutaneous
Histoplasmosis	Sporotrichosis
Cryptococcosis	Subcutaneous zygomycosis
Coccidioidomycosis	Chromoblastomycosis
Blastomycosis	Mycetoma
Zygomycosis (mucormycosis)	**Superficial**
Candidiasis	Dermatophytosis
Aspergillosis	Superficial candidiasis
Pneumocystis carinii (previously classed as a protozoan)	*Malassezia* infections

- dimorphic fungi, which behave as yeasts in the host but as moulds in vitro (e.g. *Histoplasma capsulatum* and *Sporothrix schenckii*).

Despite the fact that fungi are ubiquitous, systemic fungal infections are uncommon, although increasing in selected populations of patients such as the immunocompromised and transplant patients, those managed in high dependency units and in those with severe immunodeficiency, including HIV. Fungal infections are transmitted by inhalation of spores or by contact with the skin. Opportunistic mycoses can cause disease in immunocompromised patients. Fungi do not produce endotoxin, but exotoxin (e.g. aflatoxin) production has been documented in vitro. Fungi may also produce allergic pulmonary disease. Some fungi such as *Candida albicans* are human commensals. Diseases are usually divided into systemic, subcutaneous or superficial (Table 2.39).

SYSTEMIC FUNGAL INFECTIONS

Candidiasis

Candidiasis is the most common fungal infection in humans and is predominantly caused by *Candida albicans* although other species of *Candida* are increasingly recognized. *Candida* are small asexual fungi. Most species that are pathogenic to humans are normal oropharyngeal and gastrointestinal commensals. Candidiasis is found world-wide.

Clinical features

Any organ in the body can be invaded by candida, but vaginal infection and oral thrush are the most common forms. This latter is seen in the very young, in the elderly, following antibiotic therapy and in those who are immunosuppressed. Candidal oesophagitis presents with painful dysphagia. Cutaneous candidiasis typically occurs in intertriginous areas. It is also a cause of paronychia. Balanitis and vaginal infection are also common (see p. 127).

Chronic mucocutaneous candidiasis is a rare manifestation, usually occurring in children, and is associated with a T cell defect. It presents with hyperkeratotic plaque-like lesions on the skin, especially the face, and on the fingernails. It is associated with several endocrinopathies, including hypothyroidism and hypoparathyroidism. Dissemination of candidiasis may lead to haematogenous spread, with meningitis, pulmonary involvement, endocarditis or osteomyelitis.

Diagnosis and treatment

The fungi can be demonstrated in scrapings from infected lesions, tissue secretions or in invasive disease, from blood cultures.

Treatment varies depending on the site and severity of infection. Oral lesions respond to nystatin, oral amphotericin B or fluconazole. For systemic infections, parenteral therapy with fluconazole, itraconazole or amphotericin B is necessary. Polysymptomatic patients often complaining of widespread candidiasis can have a psychiatric disorder (see p. 1283).

Histoplasmosis

Histoplasmosis is caused by *Histoplasma capsulatum*, a non-encapsulated, dimorphic fungus. Spores can survive in moist soil for several years, particularly when it is enriched by bird and bat droppings. Histoplasmosis occurs world-wide but is only commonly seen in Ohio and the Mississippi river valley regions where over 80% of the population have been subclinically exposed. Transmission is mainly by inhalation of the spores, particularly when clearing out attics, barns and bird roosts or exploring caves.

Clinical features

Figure 2.30 summarizes the pathogenesis, main clinical forms and sequelae of histoplasma infection. Primary pulmonary histoplasmosis is usually asymptomatic. The only evidence of infection is conversion of a histoplasmin skin test from negative to positive, and radiological features similar to those seen with the Ghon primary complex of tuberculosis (see p. 930). Calcification in the lungs, spleen and liver occurs in patients from areas of high endemicity. When symptomatic, primary pulmonary histoplasmosis generally presents as a mild influenza-like illness, with fever, chills, myalgia and cough. The systemic symptoms are pronounced in severe disease.

Complications such as atelectasis, secondary bacterial pneumonia, pleural effusions, erythema nodosum and erythema multiforme may also occur.

Chronic pulmonary histoplasmosis is clinically indistinguishable from pulmonary tuberculosis (see p. 931). It is usually seen in white males over the age of 50 years. Radiologically, pulmonary cavities, infiltrates and characteristic fibrous streaking from the periphery towards the hilum are seen.

The presentation of disseminated histoplasmosis resembles disseminated tuberculosis clinically. Fever, lymphadenopathy, hepatosplenomegaly, weight loss, leucopenia and thrombocytopenia are common. Rarely, features of meningitis, hepatitis, hypoadrenalism, endocarditis and peritonitis may dominate the clinical picture.

Diagnosis

Definitive diagnosis is possible only by culturing the fungi or by demonstrating them on histological sections.

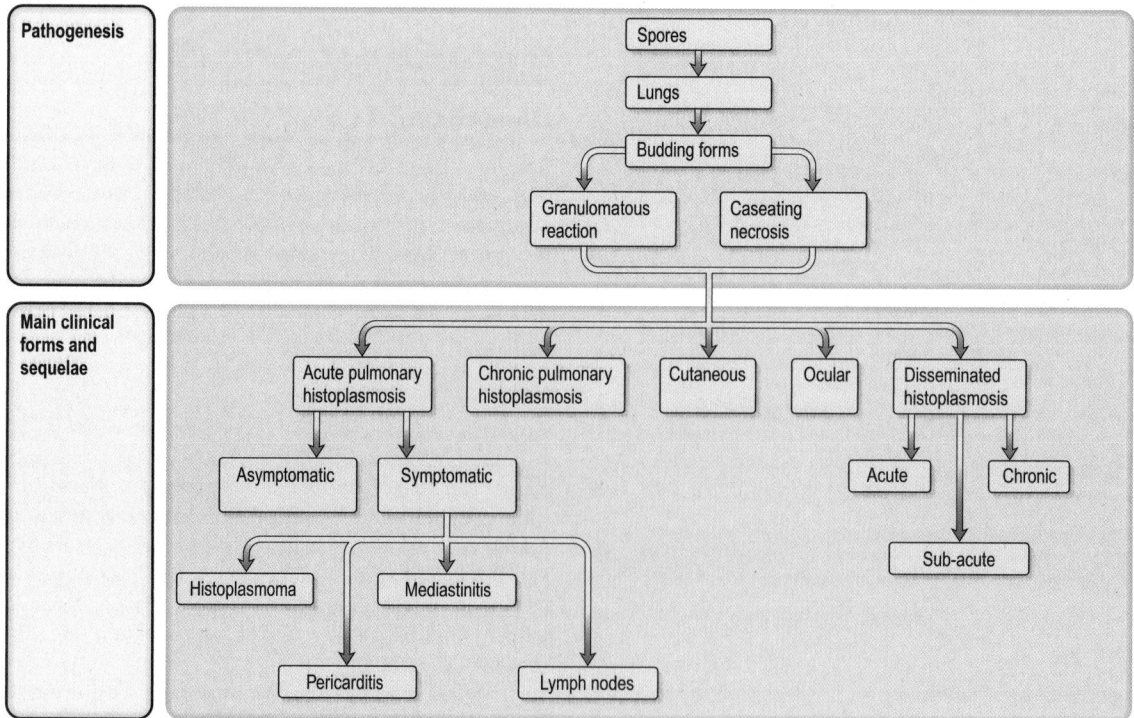

Fig. 2.30 **Histoplasma infection.** Summary of pathogenesis, main clinical forms and sequelae.

The histoplasmin skin test is of limited diagnostic value and can be negative in acute disseminated disease. Antibodies usually develop with 3 weeks of the onset of illness and are best detected by complement-fixation, immunodiffusion or radioimmunoassay.

Definitive diagnosis is possible only by culturing the fungi or by demonstrating them on histological sections. The histoplasmin skin test is of limited diagnostic value and can be negative in acute disseminated disease. Antibodies usually develop within 3 weeks of the onset of illness and are best detected by the complement-fixation, immunodiffusion or the counter-immunoelectrophoretic tests.

Management

Only symptomatic acute pulmonary histoplasmosis, chronic histoplasmosis and acute disseminated histoplasmosis require therapy. Itraconazole or ketoconazole are indicated for moderate disease. Severe infection is treated with intravenous amphotericin B to a total dose of 1.5 g followed by itraconazole. Patients with AIDS usually require treatment with parenteral amphotericin B followed by lifelong maintenance therapy with itraconazole 200 mg twice daily. Surgical excision of histoplasmomas (pulmonary granuloma due to *H. capsulatum*) or chronic cavitatory lung lesions and release of adhesions following mediastinitis are often required.

African histoplasmosis

This is caused by *Histoplasma duboisii*, the spores of which are larger than those of *H. capsulatum*. Skin lesions (e.g. abscesses, nodules, lymph node involvement and lytic bone lesions) are prominent. Pulmonary lesions do not occur. Treatment is similar to that for *H. capsulatum* infection.

Aspergillosis

Aspergillosis is caused by one of several species of dimorphic fungi of the genus *Aspergillus*. Of these, *A. fumigatus* is the most common, although *A. flavus* and *A. niger* are also recognized. These fungi are ubiquitous in the environment and are commonly found on decaying leaves and trees. Humans are infected by inhalation of the spores. Disease manifestation depends on the dose of the spores inhaled as well as the immune response of the host. Three major forms of the disease are recognized:

- Bronchopulmonary allergic aspergillosis (see p. 939) shows symptoms suggestive of bronchial asthma.
- Aspergilloma (see p. 940) is sometimes referred to as a pulmonary mycetoma.
- Invasive aspergillosis, which occurs in immunosuppressed patients and presents as acute pneumonia, meningitis or an intracerebral abscess, lytic bone lesions, and granulomatous lesions in the liver; less commonly endocarditis, paranasal *Aspergillus* granuloma or keratitis may occur. Urgent treatment with intravenous amphotericin B is required.

The diagnosis and treatment are described in more detail on page 939.

Cryptococcosis

Cryptococcosis is caused by the yeast-like fungus, *Cryptococcus neoformans*. It has a world-wide distribution and appears to be spread by birds, especially pigeons, in their droppings. The spores gain entry into the body through the respiratory tract, where they elicit a granulomatous reaction. Pulmonary symptoms are, however, uncommon; meningitis which usually occurs in those with HIV or lymphoma is the usual mode of presentation and often develops subacutely. Less commonly, lung cavitation, hilar lymphadenopathy, pleural effusions and occasionally pulmonary fibrosis occur. Skin and bone involvement is rare.

Diagnosis and treatment

This is established by demonstrating the organisms in appropriately stained tissue sections. A positive latex cryptococcal agglutinin test performed on the CSF is diagnostic of cryptococcosis.

Amphotericin B (0.7 mg/kg daily i.v.) alone or in combination with flucytosine (100–200 mg/kg daily) for 2 weeks followed by fluconazole 400 mg daily has reduced the mortality of this once universally fatal condition. Therapy should be continued for 3 months if meningitis is present. Fluconazole has greater CSF penetration and is used when toxicity is encountered with amphotericin B and flucytosine and as maintenance therapy in immunocompromised patients, especially those with HIV in whom the recommended treatment is followed by lifelong fluconazole 200 mg daily, unless they are responding to HAART.

Coccidioidomycosis

Coccidioidomycosis is caused by the non-budding spherical form (spherule) of *Coccidioides immitis*. This is a soil saprophyte and is found in the southern USA, Central America and parts of South America. Humans are infected by inhalation of the thick-walled barrel-shaped spores called arthrospores. Occasionally epidemics of coccidioidomycosis have been documented following dust storms.

Clinical features

The majority of patients are asymptomatic and the infection is only detected by the conversion of a skin test using coccidioidin (extract from a culture of mycelial growth of *C. immitis*) from negative to positive. Acute pulmonary coccidioidomycosis presents, after an incubation period of about 10 days, with fever, malaise, cough and expectoration. Erythema nodosum, erythema multiforme, phlyctenular conjunctivitis and, less commonly, pleural effusions may occur. Complete recovery is usual.

Pulmonary cavitation with haemoptysis, pulmonary fibrosis, meningitis, lytic bone lesions, hepatosplenomegaly, skin ulcers and abscesses may occur in severe disease.

Diagnosis

Because of the high infectivity of this fungus, and consequent risk to laboratory personnel, serological tests (rather than culture of the organism) are widely used for diagnosis. These include the highly specific latex agglutination and precipitin tests (IgM) which are positive within 2 weeks of infection and decline thereafter.

A positive complement-fixation test (IgG) performed on the CSF is diagnostic of coccidioidomycosis meningitis within 4–6 weeks and may remain positive for many years.

Treatment

Mild pulmonary infections are self-limiting and require no treatment, but progressive and disseminated disease requires urgent therapy. Ketoconazole or itraconazole 400 mg daily for 6 months is the treatment of choice for primary pulmonary disease with more prolonged courses for cavitating or fibronodular disease. Fluconazole in high dose (600–1000 mg daily) is given for meningitis. Amphotericin B is indicated for life-threatening infection. Surgical excision of cavitatory pulmonary lesions or localized bone lesions may be necessary. When occurring in those with HIV, amphotericin B, followed by maintenance itraconazole or fluconazole is indicated.

Blastomycosis

Blastomycosis is a systemic infection caused by the biphasic fungus *Blastomyces dermatitidis*. Although initially believed to be confined to certain parts of North America, it has been reported in Canada, Africa, Israel, Eastern Europe and Saudi Arabia.

Clinical features

Blastomycosis primarily involves the skin, where it presents as non-itchy papular lesions that later develop into ulcers with red verrucous margins. The ulcers are initially confined to the exposed parts of the body but later involve the unexposed parts as well. Atrophy and scarring may occur. Pulmonary involvement presents as a solitary lesion resembling a malignancy or gives rise to radiological features similar to the primary complex of tuberculosis. Systemic symptoms such as fever, malaise, cough and weight loss are usually present. Bone lesions are common and present as painful swellings.

Diagnosis and treatment

The diagnosis is confirmed by demonstrating the organism in histological sections or by culture, although results can be negative in 30–50% of cases. Enzyme immunoassay may be helpful although there is some cross-reactivity of antibodies to blastomyces with histoplasma.

Itraconazole is preferred for treating mild to moderate disease in the immunocompetent for periods up to 6 months. Ketoconazole or fluconazole are useful alter-

natives. In severe or unresponsive disease and in the immunocompromised, amphotericin B is indicated.

Invasive zygomycosis

Invasive zygomycosis (mucormycosis) is rare and is caused by several fungi, including *Mucor* spp., *Rhizopus* spp. and *Absidia* spp. It occurs in severely ill patients. The hallmark of the disease is vascular invasion with marked haemorrhagic necrosis.

Rhinocerebral mucormycosis is the most common form. Nasal stuffiness, facial pain and oedema, and necrotic, black nasal turbinates are characteristic. It is rare and is mainly seen in diabetics with ketoacidosis. Other forms include pulmonary and disseminated infection (immunosuppressed), gastrointestinal infection (in malnutrition), and cutaneous involvement (in burns).

Treatment is with amphotericin B and sometimes judicious debridement. This condition is invariably fatal if left untreated.

FURTHER READING

Chapman SW, Bradsher RW Jr, Campbell GD Jr et al. (2000) Practice guidelines for the management of patients with blastomycosis. *Clinical Infectious Diseases* **30**: 679–683.

Pappas PG, Rex JH, Sobel JD et al. (2004) Guidelines for treatment of candidiasis. *Clinical Infectious Diseases* **38**: 161–189.

Saag MS, Graybill RJ, Larsen RA (2000) Practice guidelines for the management of cryptococcal disease. *Clinical Infectious Diseases* **30**: 710–718.

Singh N (2001) Trends in the epidemiology of opportunistic fungal infections: predisposing factors and the impact of antimicrobial use practices. *Clinical Infectious Diseases* **33**: 1692–1696.

Stevens DA, Kan VL, Judson MA (2000) Practice guidelines for disease caused by *Aspergillus*. *Clinical Infectious Diseases* **30**: 696–709.

Wheat LJ, Sarosi GA, McKinsey DS (2000) Practice guidelines for the management of patients with histoplasmosis. *Clinical Infectious Diseases* **30**: 688–695.

SUBCUTANEOUS INFECTIONS

Sporotrichosis

Sporotrichosis is due to the saprophytic fungus *Sporothrix schenckii*, which is found world-wide. Infection usually follows cutaneous inoculation, at the site of which a reddish, non-tender, maculopapular lesion develops – referred to as 'plaque sporotrichosis'. Pulmonary involvement and disseminated disease rarely occur.

Treatment with saturated potassium iodide (10–12 mL daily orally for adults) is curative in the cutaneous form. Itraconazole 100–200 mg/day for 3–6 months is a useful alternative.

Subcutaneous zygomycosis

Subcutaneous zygomycosis, a disease seen in children in Africa and Indonesia, is caused by several filamentous fungi of the *Basidiobolus* genus. The disease usually remains confined to the subcutaneous tissues and muscle fascia. It presents as a brawny, woody infiltration involving the limbs, neck and trunk. Less commonly, the pharyngeal and orbital regions may be affected.

Treatment is with saturated potassium iodide solution given orally.

Chromoblastomycosis

Chromoblastomycosis (chromomycosis) is caused by fungi of the genera *Phialophora*, *Cladosporium* and *Fonsecaea*. These are found mainly in tropical and subtropical countries. It presents initially as a small papule, usually at the site of a previous injury. This persists for several months before ulcerating. The lesion later becomes warty and encrusted and gradually spreads. Satellite lesions may be present. Itching is frequent. The drug of choice is flucytosine, sometimes in combination with ketoconazole or amphotericin B. Itraconazole may also prove effective. Cryosurgery is used to remove local lesions.

Mycetoma (Madura foot)

Mycetoma may be due to subcutaneous infection with fungi (*Eumycetes* spp.) or bacteria (see p. 91). Infection results in local swelling which may discharge through sinuses. Bone involvement may follow.

Treatment is with ketoconazole or antibacterials according to the aetiological agent.

Pneumocystis carinii infection

Genetic analysis has shown this organism to be homologous with fungi. It exists as a trophozoite which is probably motile and reproduces by binary fission. After invasion the trophozoite wall thickens and forms a cyst. On maturation further division takes place to yield eight merozoites which after cell wall rupture develop into trophozoites. Infection probably occurs in infancy but in otherwise healthy infants it remains undetected. It is usually cleared from the lungs. *P. carinii* disease in adults is associated with immunodeficiency states, particularly AIDS, and is discussed on page 136.

SUPERFICIAL INFECTIONS

Dermatophytosis

Dermatophytoses are chronic fungal infections of keratinous structures such as the skin, hair or nails. *Trichophyton* spp., *Microsporum* spp., *Epidermophyton* spp. and *Candida* spp. can also infect keratinous structures.

Malassezia infection

Malassezia spp. are found on the scalp and greasy skin and are responsible for seborrhoeic dermatitis, pityriasis versicolor (hypo- or hyperpigmented rash on trunk) and *Malassezia* folliculitis (itchy rash on back).

Treatment is with topical antifungals or oral ketoconazole if infection is extensive.

FURTHER READING

Ribes JA, Vanover-Sams CL, Baker DJ (2000). Zygomycetes in human disease. *Clinical Microbiology Reviews* **13**: 236–301.
Richardson MD, Warnock DW (eds) (2003) *Fungal Infection: Diagnosis and Management,* 3rd edition. Oxford: Blackwell Science.
Silveira F, Nucci M (2001). Emergence of black moulds in fungal disease: epidemiology and therapy. *Current Opinion in Infectious Disease* **14**: 679–684.

PROTOZOAL INFECTIONS

Protozoa are unicellular eukaryotic organisms. They are more complex than bacteria, and belong to the animal kingdom. Although many protozoa are free-living in the environment some have become parasites of vertebrates, including man, often developing complex life cycles involving more than one host species. In order to be transmitted to a new host, some protozoa transform into hardy cyst forms which can survive harsh external conditions. Others are transmitted by an arthropod vector, in which a further replication cycle takes place before infection of a new vertebrate host. Major protozoan parasites of man are listed in Table 2.40.

BLOOD AND TISSUE PROTOZOA

Malaria

Human malaria can be caused by four species of the genus *Plasmodium*: *P. falciparum*, *P. vivax*, *P. ovale*, *P. malariae*. Ocassionly other species of malaria usually found in primates can affect man. Malaria probably originated from animal malarias in central Africa, but was spread around the globe by human migration. Public health measures and changes in land use have eradicated malaria in most developed countries, although the potential for malaria transmission still exists in many areas. Five hundred million people are infected every year,

Table 2.40	Major protozoal diseases of man	
Blood	**Tissues**	**Gastrointestinal tract**
Malaria	Leishmaniasis	Giardiasis
Trypanosomiasis	Toxoplasmosis	Amoebiasis
		Cryptosporidiosis

and over one million die yearly. Twenty five thousand international travellers per year are infected.

Epidemiology

Malaria is transmitted by the bite of female anopheline mosquitoes. The parasite undergoes a temperature-dependent cycle of development in the gut of the insect, and its geographical range therefore depends on the presence of the appropriate mosquito species and on adequate temperature. The disease occurs in endemic or epidemic form throughout the tropics and subtropics (Fig. 2.31) except for areas above 2000 m: Australia, the USA, and most of the Mediterranean littoral are also malaria-free. In hyperendemic areas (51–75% rate of para-sitaemia, or palpable spleen in children 2–9 years of age) and holoendemic areas (> 75% rate) where transmission of infection occurs year round, the bulk of the mortality is seen in infants. Those who survive to adulthood acquire significant immunity; low-grade parasitaemia is still present, but causes few symptoms. In mesoendemic areas (11–50%) there is regular seasonal transmission of malaria. Mortality is still mainly seen in infants, but older children and adults may develop chronic ill health due to repeated infections. In hypoendemic areas (0–10%), where infection occurs in occasional epidemics, little immunity is acquired and the whole population is susceptible to severe and fatal disease.

Malaria can also be transmitted in contaminated blood transfusions. It has occasionally been seen in injecting drug users sharing needles and as a hospital-acquired infection related to contaminated equipment. Rare cases are acquired outside the tropics when mosquitoes are transported from endemic areas ('airport malaria'), or when the local mosquito population becomes infected by a returning traveller.

Parasitology

The female mosquito becomes infected after taking a blood meal containing gametocytes, the sexual form of the malarial parasite (Fig. 2.32). The developmental cycle in the mosquito usually takes 7–20 days (depending on temperature), culminating in infective sporozoites migrating to the insect's salivary glands. The sporozoites are inoculated into a new human host, and those which are not destroyed by the immune response are rapidly taken up by the liver. Here they multiply inside hepatocytes as merozoites: this is pre-erythrocytic (or hepatic) sporogeny. After a few days the infected hepatocytes rupture, releasing merozoites into the blood from where they are rapidly taken up by erythrocytes. In the case of *P. vivax* and *P. ovale*, a few parasites remain dormant in the liver as hypnozoites. These may reactivate at any time subsequently, causing relapsing infection.

Inside the red cells the parasites again multiply, changing from merozoite, to trophozoite, to schizont, and finally appearing as 8–24 new merozoites. The erythrocyte ruptures, releasing the merozoites to infect further cells. Each cycle of this process, which is called erythrocytic schizogony, takes about 48 hours in *P. falciparum*, *P. vivax* and *P. ovale*, and about 72 hours in *P. malariae*. *P. vivax* and *P. ovale* mainly attack reticulocytes and young erythrocytes, while *P. malariae* tends to attack older cells; *P. falciparum* will parasitize any stage of erythrocyte.

A few merozoites develop not into trophozoites but into gametocytes. These are not released from the red

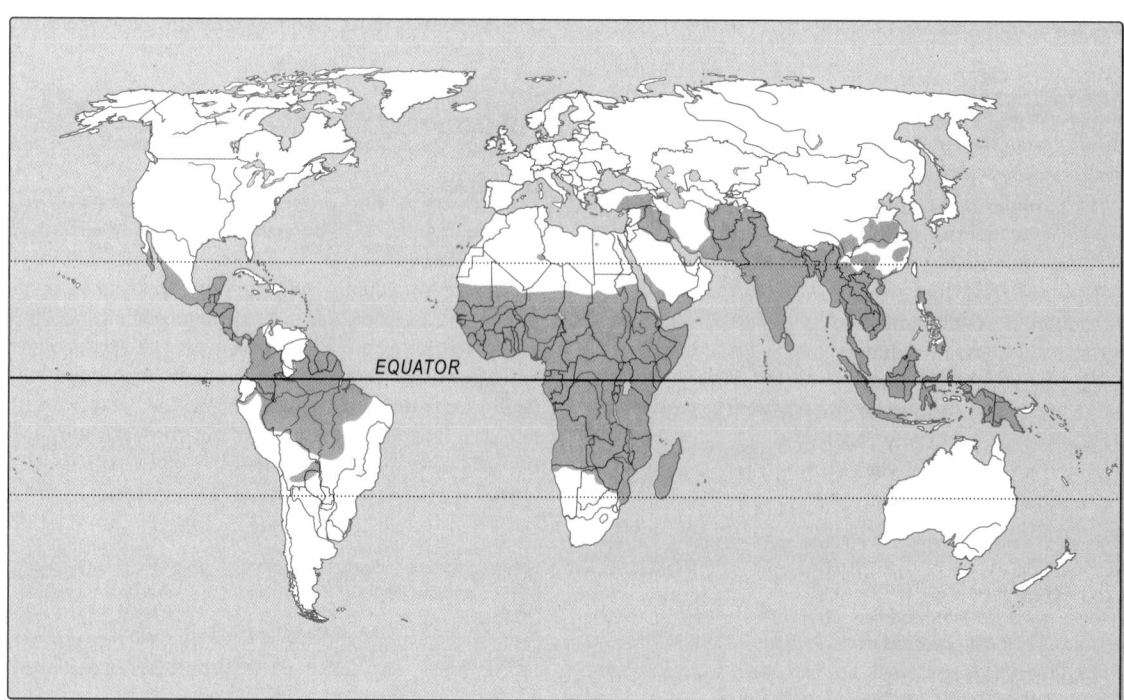

Fig. 2.31 **Malaria – geographical distribution.** From Baird 2005, Copyright: © Massachusetts Medical Society. All rights reserved.

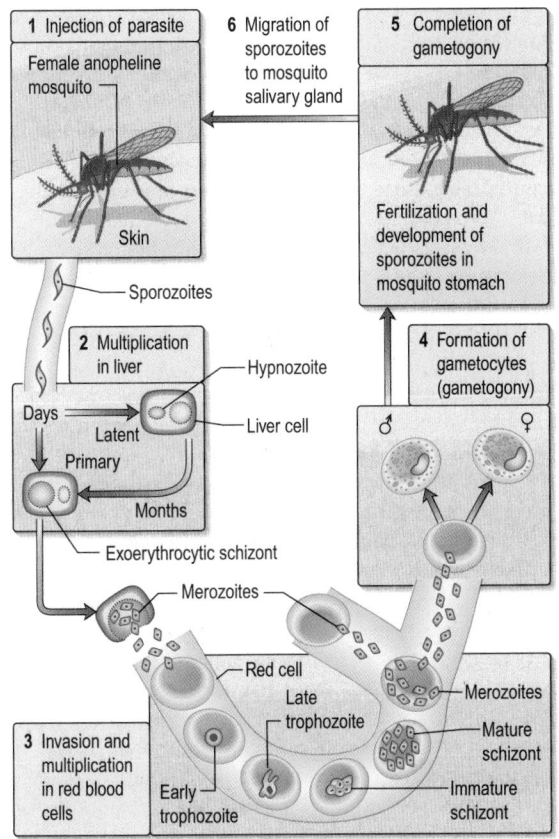

Fig. 2.32 A schematic life cycle of *Plasmodium vivax*.

(Figure labels)
1 Injection of parasite
Female anopheline mosquito
Skin
Sporozoites
2 Multiplication in liver
Hypnozoite
Liver cell
Days
Latent
Primary
Months
Exoerythrocytic schizont
Merozoites
Red cell
Late trophozoite
3 Invasion and multiplication in red blood cells
Early trophozoite
Merozoites
Mature schizont
Immature schizont
6 Migration of sporozoites to mosquito salivary gland
5 Completion of gametogony
Fertilization and development of sporozoites in mosquito stomach
4 Formation of gametocytes (gametogony)
♂ ♀

cells until taken up by a feeding mosquito to complete the life cycle.

Pathogenesis

The pathology of malaria is related to anaemia, cytokine release, and in the case of *P. falciparum*, widespread organ damage due to impaired microcirculation. The anaemia seen in malaria is multifactorial (Table 2.41). In *P. falciparum* malaria, red cells containing schizonts adhere to the lining of capillaries in the brain, kidneys, gut, liver and other organs. As well as causing mechanical obstruction these schizonts rupture, releasing toxins and stimulating further cytokine release.

After repeated infections partial immunity develops, allowing the host to tolerate parasitaemia with minimal ill effects. This immunity is lost if there is no further infection for a couple of years. Certain genetic traits also confer some immunity to malaria. People who lack the

Table 2.41　Causes of anaemia in malaria infection

Haemolysis of infected red cells
Haemolysis of non-infected red cells (blackwater fever)
Dyserythropoiesis
Splenomegaly and sequestration
Folate depletion

Duffy antigen on the red cell membrane (a common finding in West Africa) are not susceptible to infection with *P. vivax*. Certain haemoglobinopathies (including sickle cell trait) also give some protection against the severe effects of malaria: this may account for the persistence of these otherwise harmful mutations in tropical countries. Iron deficiency may also have some protective effect. The spleen appears to play a role in controlling infection, and splenectomized people are at risk of overwhelming malaria. Some individuals appear to have a genetic predisposition for developing cerebral malaria following infection with *P. falciparum*. Pregnant women are especially susceptible to severe disease.

Clinical features

Typical malaria is seen in non-immune individuals. This includes children in any area, adults in hypoendemic areas, and any visitors from a non-malarious region.

The normal incubation period is 10–21 days, but can be longer. The most common symptom is fever, although malaria may present initially with general malaise, headache, vomiting, or diarrhoea. At first the fever may be continual or erratic: the classical tertian or quartan fever only appears after some days. The temperature often reaches 41°C, and is accompanied by rigors and drenching sweats.

P. vivax or P. ovale infection

The illness is relatively mild. Anaemia develops slowly, and there may be tender hepatosplenomegaly. Spontaneous recovery usually occurs within 2–6 weeks, but hypnozoites in the liver can cause relapses for many years after infection. Repeated infections often cause chronic ill health due to anaemia and hyperreactive splenomegaly.

P. malariae infection

This also causes a relatively mild illness, but tends to run a more chronic course. Parasitaemia may persist for years, with or without symptoms. In children, *P. malariae* infection is associated with glomerulonephritis and nephrotic syndrome.

P. falciparum infection

This causes, in many cases, a self-limiting illness similar to the other types of malaria, although the paroxysms of fever are usually less marked. However it may also cause serious complications (Box 2.12), and the vast majority of malaria deaths are due to *P. falciparum*. Patients can deteriorate rapidly, and children in particular progress from reasonable health to coma and death within hours. A high parasitaemia (> 1% of red cells infected) is an indicator of severe disease, although patients with apparently low parasite levels may also develop complications. Cerebral malaria is marked by diminished consciousness, confusion, and convulsions, often progressing to coma and death. Untreated it is universally fatal. *Blackwater fever* is due to widespread intravascular haemolysis, affecting both parasitized and unparasitized red cells, giving rise to dark urine.

Box 2.12 Some features of severe falciparum malaria

CNS
Cerebral malaria (coma convulsion)

Renal
Haemoglobinuria (blackwater fever)
Oliguria
Uraemia (acute tubular necrosis)

Blood
Severe anaemia (haemolysis and dyserythropoiesis)
Disseminated intravascular coagulation (DIC)

Respiratory
Acute respiratory distress syndrome

Metabolic
Hypoglycaemia (particularly in children)
Metabolic acidosis

Gastrointestinal/liver
Diarrhoea
Jaundice
Splenic rupture

Other
Shock – hypotensive
Hyperpyrexia

Hyperreactive malarial splenomegaly (tropical splenomegaly syndrome, TSS)

This is seen in older children and adults in areas where malaria is hyperendemic. It is associated with an exaggerated immune response to repeated malaria infections, and is characterized by anaemia, massive splenomegaly, and elevated IgM levels. Malaria parasites are scanty or absent. TSS usually responds to prolonged treatment with prophylactic antimalarial drugs.

Diagnosis

Malaria should be considered in the differential diagnosis of anyone who presents with a febrile illness in, or having recently left, a malarious area. Falciparum malaria is unlikely to present more than 3 months after exposure, even if the patient has been taking prophylaxis, but vivax malaria may cause symptoms for the first time up to a year after leaving a malarious area.

Diagnosis is usually made by identifying parasites on a Giemsa-stained thick or thin blood film (thick films are more difficult to interpret, and it may be difficult to speciate the parasite, but they have a higher yield). At least three films should be examined before malaria is declared unlikely. An alternative microscopic method is quantitative buffy coat analysis (QBC), in which the centrifuged buffy coat is stained with a fluorochrome which 'lights up' malarial parasites. A number of antigen-detection methods for identifying malarial proteins and enzymes have been developed. Some of these are available in card or dipstick form, and are potentially suitable for use in resource-poor settings. Serological tests are of no diagnostic value.

Parasitaemia is common in endemic areas, and the presence of parasites does not necessarily mean that malaria is the cause of the patient's symptoms. Further investigation, including a lumbar puncture, may be needed to exclude bacterial infection.

Management

The drug of choice for susceptible parasites is chloroquine (Box 2.13). *P. vivax*, *P. ovale* and *P. malariae* are almost always sensitive to this drug, the only exception being some strains of *P. vivax* from Oceania.

There is now widespread chloroquine resistance among *P. falciparum*, and there are few parts of the world where all infections will be susceptible. Despite this, cost

Box 2.13 Drug treatment of uncomplicated malaria in adults

Type of malaria	Drug treatment	
Plasmodium vivax, P. ovale, P. malariae, CQ-sensitive *P. falciparum*	Chloroquine:	600 mg 300 mg 6 hours later 300 mg 24 hours later 300 mg 24 hours later
CQ-resistant, SP-sensitive *P. falciparum*	Fansidar (SP): 3 tablets as single dose	
CQ- and SP-resistant *P. falciparum*	Quinine: 600 mg 3 times daily for 7 days *plus* Tetracycline: 500 mg 4 times daily for 7 days or Fansidar (SP): 3 tablets as single dose	
	Alternative therapies Mefloquine: 20 mg/kg in 2 doses 8 hours apart	
	or Malarone: 4 tablets daily for 3 days or Coartemether: 4 tablets 12-hourly for 3 days or Lapdap (chlorproguanil/dapsone)	

CQ, chloroquine; SP, Fansidar = pyrimethamine/sulfadoxine; Malarone = atovaquone/proguanil; Coartemether = artemether lamufantrine
Chloroquine doses quoted are for base drug
Quinine dose applies to sulphate, hydrochloride or dihydrochloride

and availability mean that chloroquine is still the most commonly used antimalarial.

Treatment should ideally be based on a knowledge of local sensitivity, but this is often not known. In developed countries *P. falciparum* is commonly treated with quinine, usually as quinine sulphate. In mild cases this can be given orally, but in more severe illness it is given by intravenous infusion. Tinnitus and nausea are predictable side-effects of quinine, and do not require dose reduction unless severe. Some resistance to quinine is emerging, and another antimalarial (either Fansidar (pyrimethamine/sulfadoxine) or tetracycline) should be given at the end of the course of quinine.

Other available antimalarial drugs include mefloquine, artemisinin derivatives, and the fixed-dose combination preparations Malarone (atovaquone/proguanil), coartemether (artemether/lamufantrine), and Lapdap (chlorproguanil/dapsone). The way in which these drugs should be distributed and used, particularly in the poorer developing countries, is still a matter for debate. Multidrug combinations are available but costly (e.g. Artemisinin combination therapy ACT). These extend the usefulness of existing drugs and limit the development of resistance to new agents. Trials of these combination therapies are being completed.

Severe malaria, indicated by the presence of any of the complications discussed above, or a parasite count above 1% in a non-immune patient, is a medical emergency. Quinine should be given intravenously as shown in Emergency box 2.1: the loading dose should be omitted if the patient has already received quinine or mefloquine. Intensive care facilities may be needed, including mechanical ventilation and dialysis. Severe anaemia may require transfusion. Careful monitoring of fluid balance is essential: both pulmonary oedema and prerenal failure are common. Hypoglycaemia can be induced both by the infection itself and by quinine treatment. Superadded bacterial infection is common. In very heavy infections (parasitaemia > 10%), there may be a role for exchange transfusion, if the facilities are available.

Following successful treatment of *P. vivax* or *P. ovale* malaria, it is necessary to give a 2- to 3-week course of primaquine (15 mg daily) to eradicate the hepatic hypnozoites and prevent relapse. This drug can precipitate haemolysis in patients with G6PD deficiency (p. 446).

Prevention and control

As with many vector-borne diseases, control of malaria relies on a combination of case treatment, vector eradication, and personal protection from vector bites, e.g. insecticide treated nets. Mosquito eradication is usually achieved either by the use of insecticides, house spraying with DDT, or by manipulation of the habitat (e.g. marsh drainage). After some initial successes, a

---

> **!** **Emergency Box 2.1**
> **Drug treatment of severe *Plasmodium falciparum* malaria in adults**

	Full hospital facilities	No infusion available	No injection available
CQ-sensitive *P. falciparum*	Chloroquine: 10 mg/kg infused over 8 hours, followed by 15 mg/kg over 24 hours	Chloroquine: 2.5 mg/kg every 4 hours by intramuscular injection (to total of 25 mg/kg)	Chloroquine: by nasogastric tube (as in oral regimen) *or*
CQ-resistant *P. falciparum*	Quinine salt: 20 mg/kg infused over 4 hours, followed by 10 mg/kg over 4 hours every 8 hours *or* Artesunate 2.4 mg/kg by intravenous injection, then 1.2 mg/kg	Quinine dihydrochloride given by divided intramuscular injection (regimen as for i.v.)	Artemisinin rectal suppositories (limited availability)

Chloroquine (CQ) doses quoted are for base drug. Quinine doses apply to sulphate, hydrochloride and dihydrochloride.

> **(i)** **Box 2.14** **Malaria prophylaxis for adult travellers**

Area visited	Prophylactic regimen	Alternatives
No chloroquine resistance	Chloroquine 300 mg weekly	Proguanil 200 mg daily
Limited chloroquine resistance	Chloroquine 300 mg weekly *plus* Proguanil 200 mg daily	Doxycycline 100 mg daily *or* Mefloquine 250 mg weekly
Significant chloroquine resistance	Mefloquine 250 mg weekly	Doxycycline 100 mg daily *or* Malarone 1 tablet daily

WHO campaign to eliminate malaria foundered in the mid-1960s. Since then the emergence of both parasite resistance to drugs and mosquito resistance to insecticides has rendered the task more difficult. However, malaria is once again a priority for the WHO, which announced a new 'Roll Back Malaria' campaign in 1998.

Non-immune travellers to malarious areas should take measures to avoid insect bites, such as using insect repellent and sleeping under mosquito nets. Antimalarial prophylaxis should also be taken in most cases, although this is never 100% effective (Box 2.14). The precise choice of prophylactic regimen depends both on the individual traveller and on the specific itinerary; further details can be found in National Formularies or from travel advice centres. Despite considerable efforts, there is still no effective vaccine available for malaria.

Trypanosomiasis

African trypanosomiasis (sleeping sickness)

Sleeping sickness is caused by trypanosomes transmitted to humans by the bite of the tsetse fly (genus *Glossina*). It is endemic in a belt across sub-Saharan Africa, extending to about 14° N and 20° S: this marks the natural range of the tsetse fly. Two subspecies of trypanosome cause human sleeping sickness: *Trypanosoma brucei gambiense* ('Gambian sleeping sickness'), and *T. b. rhodesiense* ('Rhodesian sleeping sickness').

Epidemiology

West African sleeping sickness is found from Uganda in Central Africa, west to Senegal and south as far as Angola. Man is the major reservoir, and infection is transmitted by riverine *Glossina* species (e.g. *G. palpalis*). Sleeping sickness due to *T. b. rhodesiense* occurs in East and Central Africa from Ethiopia to Botswana. It is a zoonosis of both wild and domestic animals. In endemic situations it is maintained in game animals and transmitted by savanna flies such as *G. morsitans*. Epidemics are usually related to cattle, and the vectors are riverine flies.

Recent political upheavals and wars have both disrupted established treatment and control programmes, and led to large population movements. This has resulted in major epidemics of *T. b. gambiense* disease in Angola and the Democratic Republic of Congo, and *T. b. rhodesiense* in Uganda. Although the majority of cases are unreported the prevalence may be as high as 500 000 cases per year, with about 65 000 deaths.

Parasitology

Tsetse flies bite during the day, and unlike most arthropod vectors both males and females take blood meals. An infected insect may deposit metacyclic trypomastigotes (the infective form of the parasite) into the subcutaneous tissue. These cause local inflammation ('trypanosomal chancre') and regional lymphadenopathy. Within 2–3 weeks the organisms invade the bloodstream, subsequently spreading to all parts of the body including the brain.

Clinical features

T. b. gambiense causes a chronic, slowly progressive illness. Episodes of fever and lymphadenopathy occur over months or years, and hepatosplenomegaly may develop. Eventually infection reaches the central nervous system, causing headache, behavioural changes, confusion, and daytime somnolence. As the disease progresses patients may develop tremors, ataxia, convulsions and hemiplegias; eventually coma and death supervene. Histologically there is a lymphocytic meningoencephalitis, with scattered trypanosomes visible in the brain substance.

T. b. rhodesiense sleeping sickness is a much more acute disease. Early systemic features may include myocarditis, hepatitis and serous effusions, and patients can die before the onset of CNS disease. If they survive, cerebral involvement occurs within weeks of infection, and is rapidly progressive.

Diagnosis

Trypanosomes may be seen on Giemsa-stained smears of thick or thin blood films, or of lymph node aspirate. Blood films are usually positive in *T. b. rhodesiense*, but may be negative in *T. b. gambiense*: concentration techniques may increase the yield. The quantitative buffy coat test (QBC, see p. 98) developed for diagnosing malaria is also used to identify trypanosomes. Serological tests are useful for screening for infection: the card agglutination test for trypanosomiasis (CATT) is a robust and easy-to-use field assay. Examination of cerebrospinal fluid is essential in patients with evidence of trypanosomal infection. CNS involvement causes lymphocytosis and elevated protein in the CSF, and parasites may be seen in concentrated specimens.

Management

The treatment of sleeping sickness has remained largely unchanged for more than 40 years, although there have been developments in the management of *T. b. gambiense* infection. In both forms, treatment is usually effective if given before the onset of CNS involvement, but much less so in neurological disease. The drug of choice in early trypanosomiasis is suramin, given intravenously at a dose of 20 mg/kg at 5 to 7-day intervals up to a total dose of 5 g. Severe reactions are relatively common, and a test dose of 100 mg is usually given prior to this regimen. Intramuscular pentamidine is effective against *T. b. gambiense* only: a number of different regimens are in use. A single dose of suramin should be given to patients with parasitaemia prior to lumbar puncture, to avoid inoculation into the CSF.

The only effective drugs which penetrated the CSF in trypanocidal concentrations were the arsenicals, of which the most widely used is melarsoprol. These are given intravenously; a variety of dosing schedules are in use. Melarsoprol is extremely toxic: 2–10% of patients develop an acute encephalopathy, with a 50–75% mortality, and peripheral neuropathy and hepatorenal toxicity are also common. Prednisolone 1 mg/kg/day decreases the treatment-related mortality by 50% in *T. b. gambiense* infection; it has not been fully assessed in *T. b. rhodesiense* disease. Between 3–6% of patients relapse following melarsoprol treatment. In *T. b. gambiense* sleeping sickness, eflornithine (difluoromethylornithine) is effective, clearing parasites from blood and CSF: it has a variable effect on *T. b. rhodesiense* infection. Eflornithine is much less toxic than the arsenical drugs, but cost prevents it from being used as a first-line treatment in most cases.

Control

The morbidity and mortality of sleeping sickness could be considerably reduced by early detection and treatment of cases. Control programmes have been effective in some areas, but many have been discontinued because of lack of funding, or political upheaval. As in many vector-borne diseases, prevention depends largely on elimination, control or avoidance of the vector. Again this requires considerable coordination and money, and has only been implemented in a few places.

South American trypanosomiasis (Chagas' disease)

Chagas' disease is widely distributed in rural areas of South and Central America. It is caused by *Trypanosoma cruzi*, which is transmitted to humans in the faeces of blood-sucking reduviid bugs (also called cone-nose, or assassin bugs). The bugs, which live in mud or thatch buildings, feed on a variety of vertebrate hosts at night, defecating as they do so. Faeces infected with *T. cruzi* trypomastigotes are rubbed in through skin abrasions, mucosa or conjunctiva. The parasites spread in the bloodstream, before entering host cells and multiplying. Cell rupture releases them back into the circulation, where they can be taken up by a feeding bug. Further multiplication takes place in the insect gut, completing the trypanosome life cycle. Human infection can also occur via contaminated blood transfusion, or occasionally by transplacental spread.

Clinical features

Acute infection, which usually occurs in children, often passes unnoticed. A firm reddish papule is sometimes seen at the site of entry, associated with regional lymphadenopathy. In the case of conjunctival infection there is swelling of the eyelid, which may close the eye (Romaña's sign). There may be fever, lymphadenopathy, hepatosplenomegaly, and rarely meningoencephalitis. Acute Chagas' disease is occasionally fatal in infants, but normally there is full recovery within a few weeks or months.

After a latent period of many years, some people go on to develop *chronic Chagas' disease*. The pathogenesis of this is unclear: it is possibly due to an autoimmune response triggered by the initial infection, although recently the demonstration of parasites on PCR has thrown doubt on this mechanism. The heart is commonly affected, with conduction abnormalities, arrhythmias, aneurysm formation and cardiac dilatation. Gastrointestinal involvement leads to progressive dilatation of parts of the gastro-intestinal tract: this commonly results in megaoesophagus (causing dysphagia and aspiration pneumonia) and mega-colon (causing severe constipation).

Diagnosis

Trypanosomes may be seen on a stained blood film during the acute illness. In chronic disease, parasites may be detected by xenodiagnosis: infection-free reduviid bugs are allowed to feed on the patient, and the insect gut subsequently examined for parasites. Serological tests can detect both acute and chronic Chagas' disease.

Management and control

Nifurtimox is the drug of choice for treating Chagas' disease, but it is variably available throughout the world. Benznidazole (5–10 mg/kg/day for 60 days) is also used. The cure rate is about 80% in acute infection. Both are toxic with adverse reactions in up to 50% of patients. The drug treatment of chronic infection is controversial, as most of the tissue damage is thought to be immune-mediated and there is little clinical evidence that parasite elimination influences the outcome. Antiarrhythmic drugs and pacemakers may be needed in cardiac disease, and surgical treatment is sometimes needed for gastro-intestinal complications. In the long term, prevention of Chagas' disease relies on improved housing and living conditions. In the interim, local vector control programmes may be effective and the countries of the 'Southern Cone' of South America have a joint programme to control the disease by spraying houses with insecticide.

Leishmaniasis

This group of diseases is caused by protozoa of the genus *Leishmania*, which are transmitted by the bite of the female phlebotomine sandfly (Table 2.42). Leishmaniasis

Table 2.42 *Leishmania* species causing visceral and cutaneous disease in man

	Species complex	Species
Visceral leishmania	L. donovani	L. donovani L. infantum L. chagasi
Cutaneous leishmania	L. tropica L. major L. aethiopica L. mexicana	L. tropica L. major L. aethiopica L. mexicana L. amazonensis L. garnhami L. pifanoi L. venezuelensis
	L. braziliensis	L. braziliensis L. guyanensis L. panamanensis L. peruviana
Mucocutaneous leishmania		L. braziliensis

is seen in localized areas of Africa, Asia (particularly India and Bangladesh), Europe, the Middle East and South and Central America. Certain parasite species are specific to each geographical area. The clinical picture is dependent on the species of parasite, and on the host's cell-mediated immune response. Asymptomatic infection, in which the parasite is suppressed or eradicated by a strong immune response, is common in endemic areas, as demonstrated by a high incidence of positive leishmanin skin tests. Symptomatic infection may be confined to the skin (sometimes with spread to the mucous membranes), or widely disseminated throughout the body (visceral leishmaniasis). Relapse of previously asymptomatic infection may be seen in patients who become immuno-compromised, especially those with HIV infection.

In some areas leishmania is primarily zoonotic, whereas in others, man is the main reservoir of infection. In the vertebrate host the parasites are found as oval amastigotes (Leishman–Donovan bodies). These multiply inside the macrophages and cells of the reticulo-endothelial system, and are then released into the circulation as the cells rupture. Parasites are taken into the gut of a feeding sandfly (genus *Phlebotomus* in the Old World, genus *Lutzomyia* in the New World), where they develop into the flagellate promastigote form. These migrate to the salivary glands of the insect, where they can be inoculated into a new host.

Visceral leishmaniasis
Clinical features

Visceral leishmaniasis (kala azar) is caused by *L. donovani*, *L. infantum* or *L. chagasi*, and is prevalent in localized areas of Asia, Africa, the Mediterranean littoral and South America. In India, where man is the main host, the disease occurs in epidemics. In most other areas it is endemic, and it is mainly children and visitors to the area who are at risk. The main animal reservoirs in Europe and Asia are dogs and foxes, while in Africa it is carried by various rodents.

The incubation period is usually 1–2 months, but may be several years. The onset of symptoms is insidious, and the patient may feel quite well despite markedly abnormal physical findings. Fever is common, and although usually low-grade, it may be high and inter-mittent. The liver, and especially the spleen, become enlarged; lymphadenopathy is common in African kala azar. The skin becomes rough and pigmented. If the disease is not treated, profound pancytopenia develops, and the patient becomes wasted and immunosuppressed. Death usually occurs within a year, and is normally due to bacterial infection or uncontrolled bleeding.

Diagnosis

Specific diagnosis is made by demonstrating the parasite in stained smears of aspirates of bone marrow, lymph node, spleen or liver. The organism can also be cultured from these specimens. Specific serological tests are positive in 95% of cases. Pancytopenia, hypoalbuminaemia and hypergammaglobulinaemia are common. The

leishmanin skin test is negative, indicating a poor cell-mediated immune response.

Management

The most widely used drugs for visceral leishmaniasis are the pentavalent antimony salts (e.g. sodium stibogluconate, which contains 100 mg of antimony per mL), given intra-venously or intramuscularly at a dose of 20 mg of anti-mony per kg for 21 days. In India, meglumine antimonate is used. Resistance to antimony salts is increasing, and relapses may occur following treatment. The drug of choice where resources permit is intravenous amphotericin B (preferably given in the liposomal form). However, this drug is expensive and not widely available in many areas where the disease is prevalent. Intravenous pentamidine is also effective, and an oral drug, miltefosine, has been shown in India to be highly effective. Intercurrent bacterial infections are common and should be treated with antibiotics. Blood transfusion may occasionally be required.

Successful treatment may be followed in a small proportion of patients by a skin eruption called *post-kala azar dermal leishmaniasis* (PKDL). It starts as a macular maculopapular nodular rash which spreads over the body. It is most often seen in the Sudan and India. Current trials are looking at the use of miltefosine for treating PKDL.

Cutaneous leishmaniasis

Cutaneous leishmaniasis is caused by a number of geographically localized species, which may be zoonotic or anthroponotic. Following a sandfly bite, leishmania amastigotes multiply in dermal macrophages. The local response depends on the species of leishmania, the size of the inoculum, and the host immune response. Single or multiple painless nodules occur on exposed areas within 1 week to 3 months following the bite. These enlarge and ulcerate with a characteristic erythematous raised border. An overlying crust may develop. The lesions heal slowly over months or years, sometimes leaving a disfiguring scar.

L. major and *L. tropica* are found in Russia and Eastern Europe, the Middle East, Central Asia, the Mediterranean littoral, and sub-Saharan Africa. The reservoir for *L. major* is desert rodents, while *L. tropica* has a mainly urban distribution with dogs and humans as reservoirs. *L. aethiopica* is found in the highlands of Ethiopia and Kenya, where the animal reservoir is the hyrax. The skin lesions usually heal spontaneously with scarring: this may take a year or more in the case of *L. tropica*. Leishmaniasis recidivans is a rare chronic relapsing form caused by *L. tropica*.

L. mexicana is found predominantly in Mexico, Guatemala, Brazil, Venezuela and Panama: infection usually runs a benign course with spontaneous healing within 6 months. *L. braziliensis* infections (which are seen throughout tropical South America) also usually heal spontaneously, but may take longer.

L. mexicana amazonensis and *L. aethiopica* may occasion-ally cause diffuse cutaneous leishmaniasis. This is rare, and is characterized by diffuse infiltration of the skin by Leishman–Donovan bodies. Visceral lesions are absent.

Diagnosis and treatment

The diagnosis can often be made clinically in a patient who has been in an endemic area. Giemsa stain on a split-skin smear will demonstrate leishmania parasites in 80% of cases. Biopsy tissue from the edge of the lesion can be examined histologically, and parasites identified by PCR; culture is less often successful. The leishmanin skin test is positive in over 90% of cases, but does not distinguish between active and resolved infection. Serology is unhelpful.

Small lesions usually require no treatment. Large lesions or those in cosmetically sensitive sites can sometimes be treated locally, by curettage, cryotherapy or topical antiparasitic agents. In other cases, systemic treatment (as for visceral leishmaniasis) is required, although treatment is less successful as antimonials are poorly concentrated in the skin; L. aethiopica is not sensitive to antimonials.

Mucocutaneous leishmaniasis

Mucocutaneous leishmaniasis occurs in 3–10% of infections with L. b. braziliensis, and is commonest in Bolivia and Peru. The cutaneous sores are followed months or years later by indurated or ulcerating lesions affecting mucosa or cartilage, typically on the lips or nose ('espundia'). The condition can remain static, or there may be progression over months or years affecting the nasopharynx, uvula, palate and upper airways.

Diagnosis and treatment

Biopsies usually show only very scanty organisms, although parasites can be detected by PCR; serological tests are frequently positive.

Amphotericin B is the treatment of choice if available, although systemic antimonial compounds are widely used; miltefosine may also be effective. Relapses are common following treatment. Patients may die because of secondary bacterial infection, or occasionally laryngeal obstruction.

Prevention

Prevention of leishmaniasis relies on control of vectors and/or reservoirs of infection. Insecticide spraying, control of host animals, and treating infected humans may all be helpful. Personal protection against sandfly bites is also necessary, especially in travellers visiting endemic areas.

Toxoplasmosis

Toxoplasmosis is caused by the intracellular protozoan parasite Toxoplasma gondii. The sexual form of the parasite lives in the gut of the definitive host, the cat, where it produces oocysts. After a period of maturing in the environment, these oocysts become the source of infection for secondary hosts which may ingest them. In the secondary hosts (which include man, cattle, sheep, pigs, rodents, and birds) there is disseminated infection.

Following a successful immune response the infection is controlled, but dormant parasites remain encysted in host tissue for many years. The life cycle is completed when carnivorous felines eat infected animal tissue. Humans are infected either from contaminated cat faeces, or by eating undercooked infected meat; transplacental infection may also occur.

Clinical features

Toxoplasmosis is common: seroprevalence in adults in the UK is about 25%, rising to 90% in some parts of Europe. Most infections are asymptomatic or trivial. Symptomatic patients usually present with lymphadenopathy, mainly in the head and neck. There may be fever, myalgia, and general malaise; occasionally there are more severe manifestations including hepatitis, pneumonia, myocarditis, and choroidoretinitis. Lymphadenopathy and fatigue can sometimes persist for months after the initial infection.

Congenital toxoplasmosis may also be asymptomatic, but can produce serious disease. Clinical manifestations include microcephaly, hydrocephalus, encephalitis, convulsions and mental retardation. Choroidoretinitis is common; occasionally this may be the only feature.

Immunocompromised patients, especially those with HIV infection, are at risk of serious infections with T. gondii. In acquired immunodeficiency states this is usually due to reactivation of latent disease (p. 137).

Diagnosis

Diagnosis is usually made serologically. IgG antibodies detectable by the Sabin–Feldman dye test remain positive for years; acute infection can be confirmed by demonstrating a rising titre of specific IgM.

Management

Acquired toxoplasmosis in an immunocompetent host rarely requires treatment. In those with severe disease (especially eye involvement) sulfadiazine 2–4 g daily and pyrimethamine 25 mg daily are given for 4 weeks, along with folinic acid. The management of pregnant women with toxoplasmosis aims to decrease the risk of fetal complications. Treatment of early infection (before the parasite has crossed the placenta) with spiramycin cuts the rate of fetal infection significantly. If the fetus has already been infected, treatment with sulfadiazine and spiramycin (± pyrimethamine, which is itself teratogenic) appears to decrease the severity of complications. Infected infants should be treated from birth. The treatment of toxoplasmosis in HIV-positive patients is covered on page 137.

Babesiosis

Babesiosis is a tick-borne parasitic disease, diagnosed most commonly in North America and Europe. It is a zoonosis of rodents and cattle, and is occasionally transmitted to humans: infection is more common and more severe in those who are immunocompromised following splenectomy. The causative organisms are the plasmodium-like *Babesia microti* (rodents) and *B. divergens* (cattle).

The incubation period averages 10 days. In patients with normal splenic function, the symptoms are mild and usually comprise fever, nausea, myalgia, chills, vomiting and abdominal pain. Hepatosplenomegaly and haemolytic anaemia may also be present. In splenectomized individuals, systemic symptoms are more pronounced and haemolysis is associated with haemoglobinuria, jaundice and renal failure. Examination of a peripheral blood smear may reveal the characteristic plasmodium-like organisms.

The standard treatment was a combination of quinine 650 mg and clindamycin 600 mg orally three times daily for 7 days but a regimen of atovaquone and azithromycin is as effective, with fewer adverse reactions.

GASTROINTESTINAL PROTOZOA

The major gastrointestinal parasites of man are shown in Table 2.43.

Amoebiasis

Amoebiasis is caused by *Entamoeba histolytica*. The organism formerly known as *E. histolytica* is now known to consist of two distinct species: *E. histolytica*, which is pathogenic, and *E. dispar*, which is non-pathogenic. Cysts of the two species are identical, but can be distinguished by molecular techniques after culture of the trophozoite. *E. histolytica* can be distinguished from all amoebae except *E. dispar*, and from other intestinal protozoa, by microscopic appearance. Amoebiasis occurs world-wide, although much higher incidence rates are found in the tropics and subtropics.

The organism exists both as a motile trophozoite and as a cyst that can survive outside the body. Cysts are transmitted by ingestion of contaminated food or water, or spread directly by person-to-person contact. Trophozoites emerge from the cysts in the small intestine and then pass on to the colon, where they multiply.

Table 2.43 Pathogenic human intestinal protozoa
Amoebae *Entamoeba histolytica*
Flagellates *Giardia intestinalis*
Ciliates *Balantidium coli*
Coccidia *Cryptosporidium parvum* *Isospora belli* *Sarcocystis* spp. *Cyclospora cayetanensis*
Microspora *Enterocytozoon bieneusi* *Encephalitozoon* spp.

Clinical features

It is believed that many individuals can carry the pathogen without obvious evidence of clinical disease (asymptomatic cyst passers). However, this may be due in some cases to the misidentification of non-pathogenic *E. dispar* as *E. histolytica*, and it is not clear how often true *E. histolytica* infection is symptomless. In affected people *E. histolytica* trophozoites invade the colonic epithelium, probably with the aid of their own cytotoxins and proteolytic enzymes. The parasites continue to multiply and finally frank ulceration of the mucosa occurs. If penetration continues, trophozoites may enter the portal vein, via which they reach the liver and cause intrahepatic abscesses. This invasive form of the disease is serious and may even be fatal.

The incubation period of intestinal amoebiasis is highly variable and may be as short as a few days or as long as several months. The usual course is chronic, with mild intermittent diarrhoea and abdominal discomfort. This may progress to bloody diarrhoea with mucus, and is sometimes accompanied by systemic symptoms such as headache, nausea and anorexia. Less commonly, infection may present as acute amoebic dysentery, resembling bacillary dysentery or acute ulcerative colitis.

Complications are unusual, but include toxic dilatation of the colon, chronic infection with stricture formation, severe haemorrhage, amoeboma, and amoebic liver abscess. Amoebomas, which develop most commonly in the caecum or rectosigmoid region, are sometimes mistaken for carcinoma. They may bleed, cause obstruction or intussuscept. Amoebic liver abscesses often develop in the absence of a recent episode of colitis. Tender hepatomegaly, a high swinging fever and profound malaise are characteristic, although early in the course of the disease both symptoms and signs may be minimal. The clinical features are described in more detail on page 392.

Diagnosis

Microscopic examination of fresh stool or colonic exudate obtained at sigmoidoscopy is the simplest way of diagnosing colonic amoebic infection. To confirm the diagnosis motile trophozoites containing red blood cells must be identified: the presence of amoebic cysts alone does not imply disease. Sigmoidoscopy and barium enema examination may show colonic ulceration but are rarely diagnostic.

The amoebic fluorescent antibody test is positive in at least 90% of patients with liver abscess and in 60–70% with active colitis. Seropositivity is low in asymptomatic cyst passers.

Management

Metronidazole 800 mg three times daily for 5 days is given in amoebic colitis; a lower dose (400 mg three times daily for 5 days) is usually adequate in liver abscess. Tinidazole is also effective: dehydroemetine and chloroquine are alternative drugs, but are rarely used. After treatment of the invasive disease, the bowel should be cleared of parasites with a luminal amoebicide such as diloxanide furoate.

Prevention

Amoebiasis is difficult to eradicate because of the substantial human reservoir of infection. The only progress will be through improved standards of hygiene and better access to clean water. Cysts are destroyed by boiling, but chlorine and iodine sterilizing tablets are not always effective.

Giardiasis

Giardia intestinalis is a flagellate (Fig. 2.33) that is found world-wide. It causes small intestinal disease, with diarrhoea and malabsorption. Prevalence is high throughout the tropics, and it is the most common parasitic infection in travellers returning to the UK. In certain parts of Europe, and in some rural areas of North America, large water-borne epidemics have been reported. Person-to-person spread may occur in day nurseries and residential institutions. Like *E. histolytica*, the organism exists both as a trophozoite and a cyst, the latter being the form in which it is transmitted.

The organism sometimes colonizes the small intestine and may remain there without causing detriment to the host. In other cases, severe malabsorption may occur which is thought to be related to morphological damage to the small intestine. The changes in villous architecture are usually mild partial villous atrophy; subtotal villous atrophy is rare. The mechanism by which the parasite causes alteration in mucosal architecture and produces diarrhoea and intestinal malabsorption is unknown: there is evidence that the morphological damage may be immune-mediated. Bacterial overgrowth has also been found in association with giardiasis and may contribute to fat malabsorption.

Clinical features

Many individuals excreting giardia cysts have no symptoms. Others become ill within 1–3 weeks after ingesting cysts: symptoms include diarrhoea, often watery in the early stage of the illness, nausea, anorexia, and abdominal discomfort and bloating. In most people affected, these resolve after a few days, but in some the symptoms persist. Stools may then become paler, with the characteristic features of steatorrhoea. If the illness is prolonged, weight loss ensues, which can be marked. *Chronic giardiasis* frequently seen in developing countries can result in growth retardation in children.

Diagnosis

Both cysts and trophozoites can be found in the stool, but negative stool examination does not exclude the diagnosis since the parasite may be excreted at irregular intervals. The parasite can also be seen in duodenal aspirates (obtained either at endoscopy or with an Enterotest capsule), and in histological sections of jejunal mucosa.

Management

Metronidazole 2 g as a single dose on 3 successive days will cure the majority of infections, although sometimes a second or third course is necessary. Alternative drugs include tinidazole, mepacrine and albendazole. Preventative measures are similar to those outlined above for *E. histolytica*.

Cryptosporidiosis

This organism is found world-wide, cattle being the major natural reservoir. It has also been demonstrated in supplies of drinking water in the UK. The parasite is able to reproduce both sexually and asexually; it is transmitted by oocysts excreted in the faeces.

In healthy individuals cryptosporidiosis is a self-limiting illness. Acute watery diarrhoea is associated with fever and general malaise lasting for 7–10 days. In immunocompromised patients, especially those with HIV, diarrhoea is severe and intractable (see p. 138).

Diagnosis is usually made by faecal microscopy, although the parasite can also be detected in intestinal biopsies. As yet there is no effective antimicrobial treatment for this infection.

Balantidiasis

Balantidium coli is the only ciliate that produces clinically significant infection in humans. It is found throughout the tropics, particularly in Central and South America, Iran, Papua New Guinea and the Philippines. It is usually carried by pigs, and infection is most common in those

Fig. 2.33 *Giardia intestinalis* **on small intestinal mucosa.** Courtesy of Dr A Phillips, Department of Electron Microscopy, Royal Free Hospital, London.

communities that live in close association with swine. Its life cycle is identical to that of *E. histolytica*. *B. coli* causes diarrhoea, and sometimes a dysenteric illness with invasion of the distal ileal and colonic mucosa. Trophozoites rather than cysts are found in the stool. Treatment is with tetracycline or metronidazole.

Blastocystis hominis infection

B. hominis is a strictly anaerobic protozoan pathogen that inhabits the colon. For decades its pathogenicity for humans was questioned, but there is increasing evidence that it may cause diarrhoea. It is sensitive to metronidazole.

Cyclospora cayetanensis infection

Cyclospora cayetanensis, a coccidian protozoal parasite, was originally recognized as a cause of diarrhoea in travellers to Nepal. It has been detected in stool specimens from immunocompetent and immunodeficient people world-wide. Infection is usually self-limiting, but can be treated with co-trimoxazole.

Microsporidiosis

Protozoa of the phylum Microsporea can cause diarrhoea in patients with HIV/AIDS (see p. 138).

FURTHER READING

Baird JK (2005) Effectiveness of anti-malarial drugs. *New England Journal of Medicine* 352: 1565–1577.

Barrett M et al. (2003) Trypanosomiasis. *Lancet* 362: 1469–1478.

Duffy PE, Mutabingwa TK (2004) Drug combinations for malaria – time to ACT? *Lancet* 363: 3–4.

Greenwood BM et al (2005) Malaria. *Lancet* 365: 1487–1498.

Maitland K, Bejon P, Newton-Charles R (2003) Malaria. *Current Opinion in Infectious Disease* 16: 389–395.

Stanley SL (2003) Amoebiasis. *Lancet* 361: 1025–1034.

Sundar S, Jha T, Thakur C et al. (2002) Oral miltefosine for Indian visceral leishmaniasis. *New England Journal of Medicine* 347: 1739–1746.

WHO Tropical Diseases Research page: http://www.who.int/tdr.

HELMINTHIC INFECTIONS

Worm infections are very common in developing countries, causing much disease in both humans and domestic animals. They are frequently imported into industrialized countries. The most common human helminth infections are listed in Table 2.44.

Helminths are the largest internal human parasite. They reproduce sexually, generating millions of eggs or larvae. *Nematodes* and *trematodes* have a mouth and intestinal tract, while *cestodes* absorb nutrients directly through the outer tegument. All worms are motile,

although once the adults are established in their definitive site they rarely migrate further. Adult helminths may be very long-lived: up to 30 years in the case of the schistosomes.

Many helminths have developed complex life cycles, involving more than one host. Both primary and intermediate hosts are often highly specific to a particular species of worm. In some cases of human infection man is the primary host, while in others, humans are a non-specific intermediary or coincidentally infected.

NEMATODES

Human infections can be divided into:

- Tissue-dwelling worms including the filarial worms, and the Guinea worm *Dracunculus medinensis*.
- Human intestinal worms, including the human hookworms, the common roundworm (*Ascaris lumbricoides*) and *Strongyloides stercoralis*, which are the most common helminthic parasites of man. The adult worms live in the human gut, and do not usually invade tissues, but many species have a complex life cycle involving a migratory larval stage.
- Zoonotic nematodes which accidentally infect man and are not able to complete their normal life cycle. They often become 'trapped' in the tissues, causing a potentially severe local inflammatory response.

Tissue-dwelling worms

Filariasis

Several nematodes belonging to the superfamily Filarioidea can infect humans. The adult worms are long and threadlike, ranging from 2 cm to 50 cm in length; females are generally much larger than males. Larval stages are inoculated by various species of biting flies, each specific to a particular parasite. The adult worms which develop from these larvae mate, producing millions of offspring (microfilariae), which migrate in the blood or skin. These are taken up by feeding flies, in which the remainder of the life cycle takes place. Disease, which may be caused by either the adult worms or by microfilariae, is caused by host immune response to the parasite and is characterized by massive eosinophilia. Adult worms are long-lived (10–15 years), and reinfection is common, so that disease tends to be chronic and progressive.

Lymphatic filariasis

Lymphatic filariasis, which may be caused by different species of filarial worm, has a scattered distribution in the tropics and subtropics (Table 2.45). Nearly 1 billion people in developing countries are at risk. *Wuchereria bancrofti* is transmitted to man by a number of mosquito species, mainly *Culex fatigans*. Adult female worms (which are 5–10 cm long) live in the lymphatics, releasing large numbers of microfilariae into the blood. Generally this occurs at night, coinciding with the nocturnal feeding

Table 2.44 Helminths commonly infecting man

	Helminth	Common name/disease caused
Nematodes (roundworms)		
Tissue-dwelling worms	*Wuchereria bancrofti*	Filariasis
	Brugia malayi/timori	Filariasis
	Loa loa	Loiasis
	Onchocerca volvulus	River blindness
	Dracunculus medinensis	Dracunculiasis
	Mansonella perstans	Mansonellosis
Intestinal human nematodes	*Enterobius vermicularis*	Threadworm
	Ascaris lumbricoides	Roundworm
	Trichuris trichiura	Whipworm
	Necator americanus	Hookworm
	Ancylostoma duodenale	Hookworm
	Strongyloides stercoralis	Strongyloidosis
Zoonotic nematodes	*Toxocara canis*	Toxocariasis
	Trichinella spiralis	Trichinellosis
Trematodes (flukes)		
Blood flukes	*Schistosoma* species	Schistosomiasis
Lung flukes	*Paragonimus* species	Paragonimiasis
Intestinal/hepatic flukes	*Fasciolopsis buski*	
	Fasciola hepatica	
	Clonorchis sinensis	
	Opisthorchis felineus	
Cestodes (tapeworms)		
Intestinal adult worms	*Taenia saginata*	Beef tapeworm
	Taenia solium	Pork tapeworm
	Diphyllobothrium latum	Fish tapeworm
	Hymenolepis nana	Dwarf tapeworm
Larval tissue cysts	*Taenia solium*	Cysticercosis
	Echinococcus granulosus	Hydatid disease
	Echinococcus multilocularis	Hydatid disease
	Spirometra mansoni	Sparganosis

Table 2.45 Diseases caused by the filarial worms

Organism	Adult worm	Microfilariae	Major vector	Clinical signs	Distribution
Wuchereria bancrofti	Lymphatics	Blood	*Culex* species	Fever, Lymphangitis, Elephantiasis	Tropics
Brugia timori/malayi	Lymphatics	Blood	*Mansonia* species	Fever, Lymphangitis, Elephantiasis	East and South East Asia, South India, Sri Lanka
Loa loa	Subcutaneous	Blood	*Chrysops* species	'Calabar' swellings, Urticaria	West and Central Africa
Onchocerca	Subcutaneous	Skin, eye	*Simulium* species	Subcutaneous nodules, Eye disease	Africa, South America
Mansonella perstans	Retroperitoneal	Blood	*Culicoides* species	Allergic eosinophilia	Sub-Saharan Africa, South America

pattern of *C. fatigans*. Non-periodic forms of *W. bancrofti*, transmitted by day-biting species of mosquito, are found in the South Pacific. *Brugia malayi* (and the closely related *B. timori*) are very similar to *W. bancrofti*, exhibiting the same nocturnal periodicity. The usual vectors are mosquitoes of the genus *Mansonia*, although other mosquitoes have been implicated.

Clinical features

Following the bite of an infected mosquito, the larvae enter the lymphatics and are carried to regional lymph nodes. Here they grow and mature for 6–18 months.

Adult worms produce allergic lymphangitis. The clinical picture depends on the individual immune response, which in turn may depend on factors such as age at first exposure. In endemic areas many people have asymptomatic infection. Sometimes early infection is marked by bouts of fever accompanied by pain, tenderness and erythema along the course of affected lymphatics. Involvement of the spermatic cord and epididymis are common in Bancroftian filariasis. These acute attacks subside spontaneously in a few days, but usually recur. Recurrent episodes cause intermittent lymphatic obstruction, which in time can become fibrotic and irreversible. Obstructed lymphatics may rupture, causing cellulitis and further fibrosis; there may also be chylous pleural effusions and ascites. Over time there is progressive enlargement, coarsening, and fissuring of the skin, leading to the classical appearances of elephantiasis. The limbs or scrotum may become hugely swollen. Eventually the adult worms will die, but the lymphatic obstruction remains and tissue damage continues. Elephantiasis takes many years to develop, and is only seen in association with recurrent infection in endemic areas.

Occasionally the predominant features of filarial infection are pulmonary. Microfilariae become trapped in the pulmonary capillaries, generating intense local allergic response. The resulting pneumonitis causes cough, fever, weight loss, and shifting radiological changes, associated with a high peripheral eosinophil count. This is known as *tropical pulmonary eosinophilia* (see p. 940).

Diagnosis

The diagnosis of filariasis is usually made on clinical grounds, supported by a high eosinophil count. Serological tests are sensitive, especially in the earlier stages, but can cross-react with other nematodes: they become negative 1–2 years after effective treatment. PCR assays are being developed. Microfilariae start to appear in the peripheral blood about a year after infection, and may be detected on a stained nocturnal blood film. Parasitological diagnosis is difficult in established elephantiasis. The clinical picture is usually diagnostic, but similar lymphatic damage may occasionally be caused by silicates absorbed through the feet from volcanic soil.

Treatment

Diethylcarbamazine (DEC) kills both adult worms and microfilariae. Serious allergic responses may occur as the parasites are killed, and particular care is needed when using DEC in areas endemic for loiasis. Old multi-dose regimens are now being replaced by single-dose treatment often in combination with albendazole. Associated bacterial infections should be treated promptly, and reconstructive surgery may be needed to remove excess tissue. Mass chemotherapy can decrease the prevalence and severity of infection in endemic areas and 80 million people have already been treated under the WHO eradication programme. Early diagnosis and treatment prevent the development of elephantiasis. These approaches must be combined with vector control to achieve permanent results, while individual protection depends on avoidance of mosquito bites.

Loiasis

Loiasis, seen in humid forest areas of West and Central Africa and affects 3–13 million people – in some areas, up to 40% of the population. It is caused by infection with *Loa loa*. This is a small (3–7 cm) filarial worm which is found in the subcutaneous tissues. The microfilariae circulate in the blood during the day, but cause no direct symptoms. The vectors are day-biting flies of the genus *Chrysops*, known as the tabanid fly (horse or deer fly).

Adult worms migrate around the body in subcutaneous tissue planes. Worms do not replicate in humans and may be present for years, frequently without causing symptoms. From time to time localized, tender, hot, soft tissue swellings occur due to hypersensitivity (Calabar swellings) often near to a joint. These are produced in response to the passage of a worm and usually subside over a few days or weeks. There may also be more generalized urticaria and pruritus. Occasionally a worm may be seen crossing the eye under the conjunctiva; they may also enter retro-orbital tissue, causing severe pain. Short-term residents of endemic areas often have more severe manifestations of the disease.

Microfilariae may be seen on stained blood films, although these are often negative. Serological tests are relatively insensitive, and cross-react with other microfilariae. There is usually massive eosinophilia. DEC may cause severe allergic reactions (including fever, urticaria, myalgia, and occasionally encephalitis) associated with parasite killing and is being replaced by newer agents. Ivermectin in single doses of 200–400 µg/kg is effective: it may occasionally cause severe reactions. Albendazole, which causes a more gradual reduction in microfilarial load, may be preferable in heavily-infected patients. Drug reactions are more likely if there is a high microfilarial load, or if there is co-infection with *Onchocerca volvulus*. Mass treatment with either DEC or ivermectin can decrease the transmission of infection, but the mainstay of prevention is vector avoidance and control.

Onchocerciasis

Onchocerciasis (river blindness) affects 18 million people world-wide, mostly in West and Central Africa. It also occurs in the Yemen, and parts of Central and South America. It is the result of infection with *Onchocerca volvulus*. Infection is transmitted by day-biting flies of the genus *Simulium*: principally *S. damnosum* in West Africa, *S. neavei* in East Africa, and *S. metallicum* in America.

Pathogenesis

Infection occurs when larvae are inoculated by the bite of an infected fly. The worms mature in 2–4 months, and can live for more than 15 years. Adult worms, which can reach lengths of 50 cm (although less than 0.5 mm in diameter), live in the subcutaneous tissues. They may form fibrotic nodules, especially over bony prominences and sites of trauma. Huge numbers of microfilariae are distributed in the skin, and may invade the eyes. Live microfilariae cause relatively little harm, but dead parasites may cause severe allergic reactions, with hyaline necrosis and loss of tissue collagen and elastin. In the eye a similar process causes conjunctivitis, sclerosing keratitis, uveitis, and secondary glaucoma. Choroidoretinitis is also occasionally seen.

Clinical features

Symptoms usually start about a year after infection. Initially there is generalized pruritus, with urticaria and fleeting oedema. Subcutaneous nodules (which can be detected by ultrasound) start to appear, and in dark-skinned individuals, hypo- and hyperpigmentation from excoriation and inflammatory changes. Over time more chronic inflammatory changes appear, with roughened, inelastic skin. Superficial lymph nodes become enlarged, and in the groin may hang down in loose folds of skin ('hanging groin'). Eye disease, which is associated with chronic heavy infection, usually first manifests as itching and conjunctival irritation. This gradually progresses to more extensive eye disease and eventually to blindness. Short-term travellers are unlikely to become infected as the black flies are not efficient vectors of the disease.

Diagnosis

In endemic areas the diagnosis can often be made clinically, especially if supported by finding eosinophilia on a blood film. In order to identify parasites, skin snips taken from the iliac crest or shoulder are placed in saline under a cover slip. After 4 hours, microscopy will show microfilariae wriggling free on the slide. If this is negative, DEC can be applied topically under an occlusive dressing: this will provoke an allergic rash in the majority of infected people (modified Mazzotti reaction) but this is not routinely performed as it is unpleasant. Slit-lamp examination of the eyes may reveal the microfilariae. Serological tests are frequently positive in endemic areas, but this does not imply current infection. ELISA and Western blots have been used. Tests may be negative in expatriates with a low worm load.

Management and prevention

Ivermectin, in a single dose of 150 µg/kg, kills microfilariae and prevents their return for 6–12 months. There is little effect on adult worms, so annual (or more frequent) retreatment is needed. In patients co-infected with *Loa loa*, ivermectin may occasionally induce severe allergic reactions, including a toxic encephalopathy.

Since 1974 the WHO Onchocerciasis Control Programme has had a considerable impact on onchocerciasis in West Africa. A combination of vector control measures and, more recently, mass treatment with ivermectin, has led to a decrease in both infection rates and progression to serious disease. Humans are the only host but measures are required over a long period because of the longevity of the worm (10–15 years).

Mansonellosis

Mansonella perstans is a filarial worm transmitted by biting midges of the genus *Culicoides*. Small numbers of microfilariae are found in the blood, and although they do not cause serious disease there may be minor allergic reactions and an eosinophilia.

Dracunculiasis

Infection with the Guinea worm, *Dracunculus medinensis*, occurs when water fleas containing the parasite larvae are swallowed in contaminated drinking water. Ingested larvae mature, penetrate the intestinal wall, and mate, after which the male usually dies. The female worm, which can reach over a metre in length, migrates through connective and subcutaneous tissue for 9–18 months before surfacing, usually on the skin of the leg. An allergic blister forms, and then bursts, exposing the anterior end of the worm. The uterus of the worm ruptures, releasing larvae: the worm is attracted to the surface by cooling, and so the larvae are likely to be deposited in water. They are ingested by the small crustacean water fleas, and the cycle is completed. The disease is found in sub-Saharan Africa, Egypt, the Arabian peninsula, and parts of Central Asia (India is now Guinea worm free). It is usually acquired by people collecting water at water holes.

A persistent skin ulcer may develop at the site of rupture: bacterial infection is common, and tetanus can occur. If the worm is broken there may be a systemic allergic reaction.

The diagnosis is usually clinical.

The traditional treatment, extracting the worm over several days by winding it round a stick, is probably still the most effective. The worm should not be damaged. Antibiotics may be needed to control secondary infection. Anthelminthic drugs are of little value.

Water fleas (and thus infective larvae) can be removed from drinking water by chemical treatment or by simple filtration. Large-scale eradication programmes have been in place for several years and the incidence of infection has fallen dramatically, with only 75 000 cases reported in the year 2000: 75% of these were from the Sudan. Man is the only host of *D. medinensis*, and it should therefore be possible to completely eradicate this parasite.

Human intestinal nematodes

Adult intestinal nematodes (also sometimes referred to as soil-transmitted helminths, or geohelminths) live in the human gut. There are two main types of life cycle, both including a soil-based stage. In some cases infection is spread by ingestion of eggs (which often require a period of maturation in the environment), while in others the eggs hatch in the soil and larvae penetrate directly through the skin of a new host (Fig. 2.34). *Ascaris lumbricoides* deviates from the simplified life cycle shown in that the larvae invade the duodenum and enter the venous system, via which they reach the lungs. They are eventually expectorated and swallowed, entering the intestine where they complete their maturation. Strongyloides is also unusual, in that it is the only nematode that is able to complete its life cycle in humans. Larvae may hatch before leaving the colon, and so are able to reinfect the host by penetrating the intestinal wall and entering the venous system.

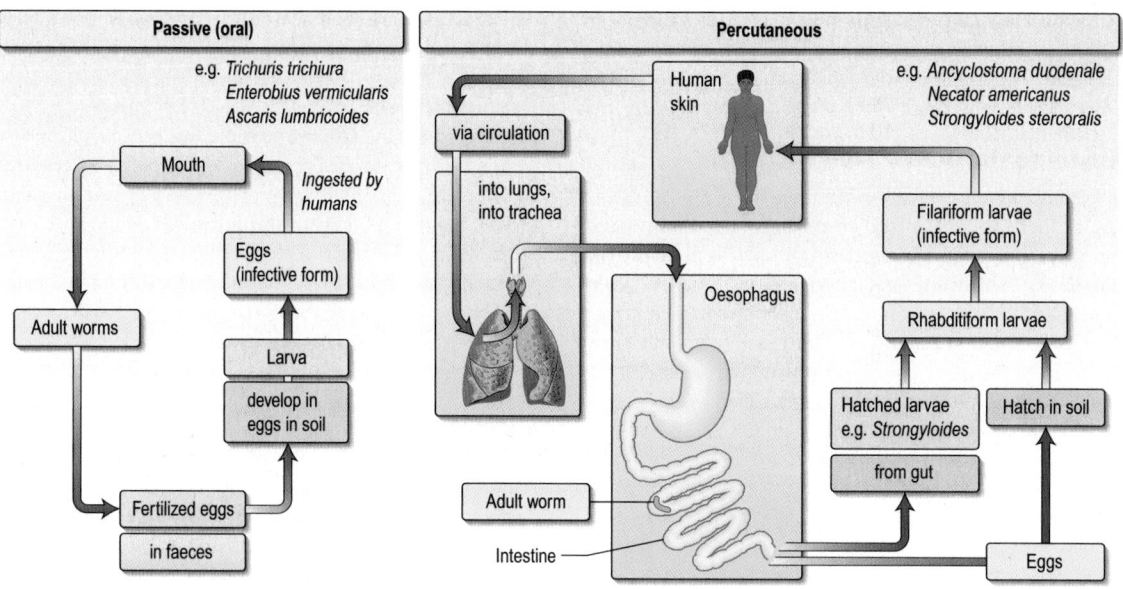

Fig. 2.34 A schematic life cycle of intestinal nematodes.

Ascariasis (roundworm infection)

A. lumbricoides is a pale yellow worm, 20–35 cm in length (Fig. 2.35). It is found world-wide but is particularly common in poor rural communities, where there is heavy faecal contamination of the immediate environment. Larvae migrate through the tissues to the lungs before being expectorated and swallowed; adult worms are found in the small intestine. Ova are deposited in faeces, and require a 2- to 4-month maturation in the soil before they are infective.

Infection is usually asymptomatic, although heavy infections are associated with nausea, vomiting, abdominal discomfort and anorexia. Worms can sometimes obstruct the small intestine, the most common site being at the ileocaecal valve. They may also occasionally invade the appendix, causing acute appendicitis, or the bile duct, resulting in biliary obstruction and suppurative cholangitis. Larvae in the lung may produce pulmonary eosinophilia. Heavy infection in children, especially those who are already malnourished, may have significant effects on nutrition and development. Serious morbidity and mortality are rare in ascariasis, but the huge number of people infected means that on a global basis roundworm infection causes a significant burden of disease, especially in children.

Ascaris eggs can be identified in the stool, and occasionally adult worms emerge from the mouth or the anus. They may also be seen on barium enema studies. Appropriate drug treatments are shown in Box 2.15. Very rarely, surgical or endoscopic intervention may be required for intestinal or biliary obstruction.

Threadworm (*Enterobius vermicularis*)

E. vermicularis is a small (2–12 mm) worm, which is common throughout the world. Larval development takes place mainly in the small intestine, and adult worms are normally found in the colon. The gravid female deposits eggs around the anus causing intense itching, especially at night. Unlike *A. lumbricoides*, the eggs do not require a maturation period in soil, and infection is often directly transmitted from anus to mouth via the hands. Eggs may also be deposited on clothing and bed linen, and are subsequently either ingested or inhaled. Apart from discomfort and local excoriation, infection is usually harmless.

Ova can be collected either using a moistened perianal swab, or by applying adhesive cellophane tape to the perianal skin. They can then be identified by microscopy.

The most commonly used drugs in the UK are mebendazole and piperazine (Box 2.15). However, isolated treatment of an affected person is often ineffective. Other family members (especially small children) may also need to be treated, and the whole family should be given advice about personal hygiene. Two courses of treatment 2 weeks apart may break the cycle of autoinfection.

Whipworm (*Trichuris trichiura*)

Infections with whipworm are common world-wide, especially in poor communities with inadequate sanitation.

Fig. 2.35 *Ascaris lumbricoides*, approximately 20 cm long.

Box 2.15 Drugs used for treating human intestinal nematodes (single dose unless otherwise stated)

		Ascaris	Hookworm	*Enterobius*	*Trichuris*	*Strongyloides*
Piperazine	75 mg/kg	++	+	++	–	–
Pyrantal pamoate	10 mg/kg	++	+	++	–	–
Oxantel pamoate	10 mg/kg	++	+	n/a	++	–
Albendazole	400 mg*	++	++	++	+	+
Mebendazole	500 mg†	++	++	++	+	+
Tiabendazole	25 mg/kg*	n/a	n/a	n/a	n/a	++
Levamisole	5 mg/kg	++	+	n/a	n/a	–
Ivermectin	200 µg/kg‡	n/a	n/a	n/a	n/a	++

++, highly effective; +, moderately effective; –, ineffective; n/a, drug not used for this indication/no data available

* Twice daily for 3 days in strongyloidiasis
† WHO recommended dose for developing countries; in UK commonly given as 100 mg single dose for threadworm, or 100 mg twice daily for 3 days for whipworm
‡ Once daily for 2 days

Adult worms, which are 3–5 cm long, inhabit the terminal ileum and caecum, although in heavy infection they are found throughout the large bowel. The head of the worm is embedded in the intestinal mucosa. Ova are deposited in the faeces, and require a maturation period of 3–4 weeks in the soil before becoming infective.

Infection is usually asymptomatic, but mucosal damage can occasionally be so severe that there is colonic ulceration, dysentery, or rectal prolapse.

Diagnosis is made by finding ova on stool microscopy, or occasionally by seeing adult worms on sigmoidoscopy. Drug treatment is shown in Box 2.15.

Hookworm infection

Hookworm infections, caused by the human hookworms *Ancylostoma duodenale* and *Necator americanus*, are found world-wide. They are relatively rare in developed countries, but very common in areas with poor sanitation and hygiene: overall about 25% of the world's population are affected. Hookworm infection is a major contributing factor to anaemia in the tropics. *A. duodenale* is found mainly in East Asia, North Africa and the Mediterranean, while *N. americanus* is the predominant species in South and Central America, South East Asia and sub-Saharan Africa.

Adult worms (which are about 1 cm long) live in the duodenum and upper jejunum, where they are often found in large numbers. They attach firmly to the mucosa using the buccal plate, feeding on blood. Eggs passed in the faeces develop in warm moist soil, producing infective filariform larvae. These penetrate directly through the skin of a new host, and are carried in the bloodstream to the lungs. Having crossed into the alveoli, the parasites are expectorated and then swallowed, thus arriving at their definitive home.

Clinical features

Local irritation as the larvae penetrate the skin ('ground itch') may be followed by transient pulmonary signs and symptoms, often accompanied by eosinophilia. Light infections, especially in a well-nourished person, are often asymptomatic. Heavier worm loads may be associated with epigastric pain and nausea, resembling peptic ulcer disease. Chronic heavy infection, particularly on a background of malnourishment, may cause iron deficiency anaemia. Blood loss has been estimated at about 0.15 mL/worm/day for *A. duodenale*, and 0.03 mL/worm/day for *N. americanus*; other factors may also be involved in the development of anaemia, which may be accompanied by hypoproteinaemia. Heavy infection in children is associated with delays in physical and mental development.

Diagnosis and treatment

The diagnosis is made by finding eggs on faecal microscopy. In infections heavy enough to cause anaemia these will be present in large numbers. The aim of treatment in endemic areas is reduction of worm burden rather than complete eradication: albendazole or mebendazole, which can both be given as a single dose, are the best drugs (Box 2.15). The WHO is promoting mass treatment programmes for schoolchildren in many parts of the world, together with treatment for schistosomiasis where appropriate.

Strongyloidiasis

Strongyloides stercoralis is a small (2 mm long) worm which lives in the small intestine. It is found in many parts of the tropics and subtropics, and is especially common in Asia. Eggs hatch in the bowel, and larvae are found in the stool. Usually these are non-infective rhabditiform larvae, which require a further period of maturation in the soil before they can infect a new host, but sometimes this maturation can occur in the large bowel. Infective filariform larvae can therefore penetrate directly through the perianal skin, reinfecting the host. In this way autoinfection may continue for years or even decades. Some war veterans who were imprisoned in the Far East during the Second World War have been found to have active strongyloidiasis over 50 years later. After skin penetration the life cycle is similar to that of the hookworm, except that the adult worms may burrow into the intestinal mucosa, causing a local inflammatory response.

Clinical features

Skin penetration by *S. stercoralis* causes a similar local dermatitis to hookworm. In autoinfection this manifests as a migratory linear weal around the buttocks and lower abdomen (cutaneous larva currens). In heavy infections damage to the small intestinal mucosa can cause malabsorption, diarrhoea and even perforation. There is usually a persistent eosinophilia. In patients who are immunosuppressed (e.g. by corticosteroid therapy or intercurrent illness) filariform larvae may penetrate directly through the bowel wall in huge numbers, causing an overwhelming and usually fatal generalized infection (the strongyloidiasis hyperinfestation syndrome). This condition is often complicated by septicaemia due to bowel organisms.

Diagnosis and treatment

Motile larvae may be seen on stool microscopy, especially after a period of incubation. Serological tests are also useful. The best drug for treating strongyloidiasis is ivermectin (200 µg/kg daily for 2 days); albendazole and tiabendazole are also used.

Zoonotic nematodes

A number of nematodes which are principally parasites of animals may also affect man. The most common are described below.

Trichinosis

The normal hosts of *Trichinella spiralis*, the cause of trichinosis, include pigs, bears and warthogs. Man is infected by eating undercooked meat from these animals. Ingested larvae mature in the small intestine, where adults release new larvae which penetrate the bowel wall and migrate through the tissues. Eventually these larvae encyst in striated muscle.

Light infections are usually asymptomatic. Heavier loads of worms produce gastrointestinal symptoms as the adults establish themselves in the small intestine, followed by systemic symptoms as the larvae invade. The latter include fever, oedema, and myalgia. Massive infection may occasionally be fatal, but usually the symptoms subside once the larvae encyst.

The diagnosis can usually be made from the clinical picture, associated eosinophilia, and serological tests. If necessary it can be confirmed by muscle biopsy a few weeks after infection. Albendazole (20 mg/kg for 7 days) given early in the course of the illness will kill the adult worms and decrease the load of larvae reaching the tissues. Analgesia and steroids may be needed for symptomatic relief.

Toxocariasis (visceral larva migrans)

Eggs of the dog roundworm, *Toxocara canis*, are occasionally ingested by humans, especially children. The eggs hatch and the larvae penetrate the small intestinal wall and enter the mesenteric circulation, but are then unable to complete their life cycle in a 'foreign' host. Many are held up in the capillaries of the liver, where they generate a granulomatous response, but some may migrate into other tissues including lungs, striated muscle, heart, brain, and eye. In most cases infection is asymptomatic, and the larvae die without causing serious problems. In heavy infections there may be generalized symptoms (fever and urticaria) and eosinophilia, as well as focal signs related to the migration of the parasites. Pulmonary involvement may cause bronchospasm and chest X-ray changes. Ocular infection may produce a granulomatous swelling mimicking a retinoblastoma, while cardiac or neurological involvement may occasionally be fatal. Rarely, larvae survive in the tissues for many years, causing symptoms long after infection.

Isolation of the larvae is difficult, and the diagnosis is usually made serologically. Albendazole 400 mg daily for a week is the most effective treatment.

Cutaneous larva migrans (CLM)

CLM is caused by the larvae of the non-human hookworms *Ancylostoma braziliense* and *A. caninum*. Like human hookworms, these hatch in warm moist soil, and then penetrate the skin. In man they are unable to complete a normal life cycle, and instead migrate under the skin for days or weeks until they eventually die. The wandering of the larva is accompanied by a clearly-defined, serpiginous, itchy rash ('creeping eruption'), which progresses at the rate of about 1 cm per day. There are usually no systemic symptoms. The diagnosis is purely clinical. Single larvae may be treated with a 10% solution of topical tiabendazole; multiple lesions may require systemic therapy with tiabendazole or albendazole or ivermectin.

FURTHER READING
Bundy DAP, de Silva NR (1998) Can we deworm this wormy world? *British Medical Bulletin* **54**: 421–432.
Hoerauf A, Buttner D, Adjei O, Pearlman E (2003) Onchocerciasis. *British Medical Journal* **326**: 207–210.
Hotez DJ et al. (2004) Hookworm infections. *New England Journal of Medicine* **353**: 799–807.

TREMATODES

Trematodes (flukes) are flat leaf-shaped worms. They have complex life cycles, often involving fresh water snails and intermediate mammalian hosts. Disease is caused by the inflammatory response to eggs or to the adult worms.

Water-borne flukes

Schistosomiasis

Schistosomiasis affects over 200 million people in the tropics and subtropics, most of whom live in sub-Saharan Africa. Chronic infection causes significant morbidity, and after malaria it has the most socio-economic impact of any parasitic disease. Schistosomiasis is largely a disease of the rural poor, but has also been associated with major development projects such as dams and irrigation schemes.

Parasitology and pathogenesis

There are three main species of schistosome which commonly cause disease in man: *Schistosoma mansoni*, *S. haematobium*, and *S. japonicum*. *S. intercalatum* and *S. mekongi* are less important. The geographical distribution is shown in Figure 2.36. Eggs are passed in the urine or faeces of an infected person, and hatch in fresh water to release the miracidia (Fig. 2.37). These ciliated organisms penetrate the tissue of the intermediate host, a species of water snail specific to each species of schistosome. After multiplying in the snail, large numbers of fork-tailed cercariae are released back into the water, where they can survive for 2–3 days. During this time the cercariae can penetrate the skin or mucous membranes of the definitive host, man. Transforming into schistosomulae, they pass through the lungs before reaching the portal vein, where they mature into adult worms (the male is about 20 mm long, and the female a little larger). Worms pair in the portal vein before migrating to their final destination: mesenteric veins in the case of *S. mansoni* and *S. japonicum*, and the vesicular plexus for *S. haematobium*. Here they may remain for many years, producing vast numbers of eggs. The majority of these are released in urine or faeces, but a small number become embedded in the bladder or bowel wall, and a few are carried in the circulation to the liver or other distant sites.

The pathology of schistosome infection varies with species and stage of infection. In the early stages there may be local and systemic allergic reactions to the migrating parasites. As eggs start to be deposited there may be a local inflammatory response in the bowel or bladder, while ectopic eggs may produce granulomatous lesions anywhere in the body. Chronic heavy infection, in

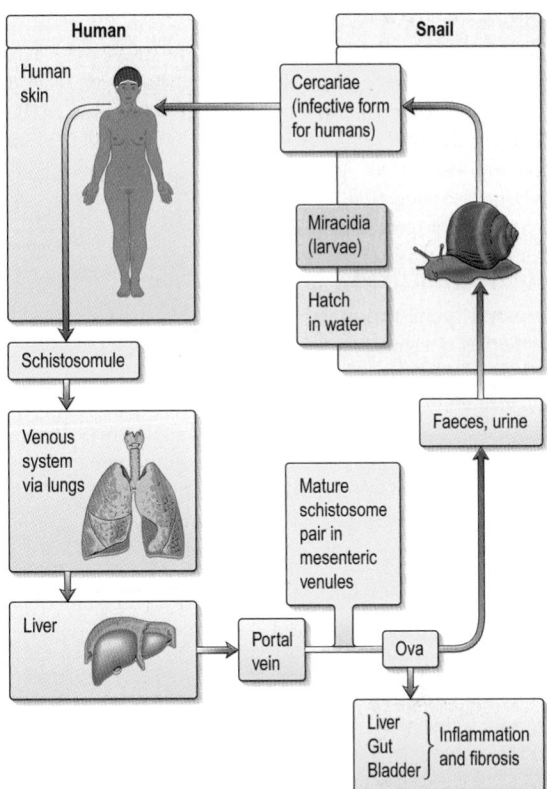

Fig. 2.37 A schematic life cycle of *Schistosoma*.

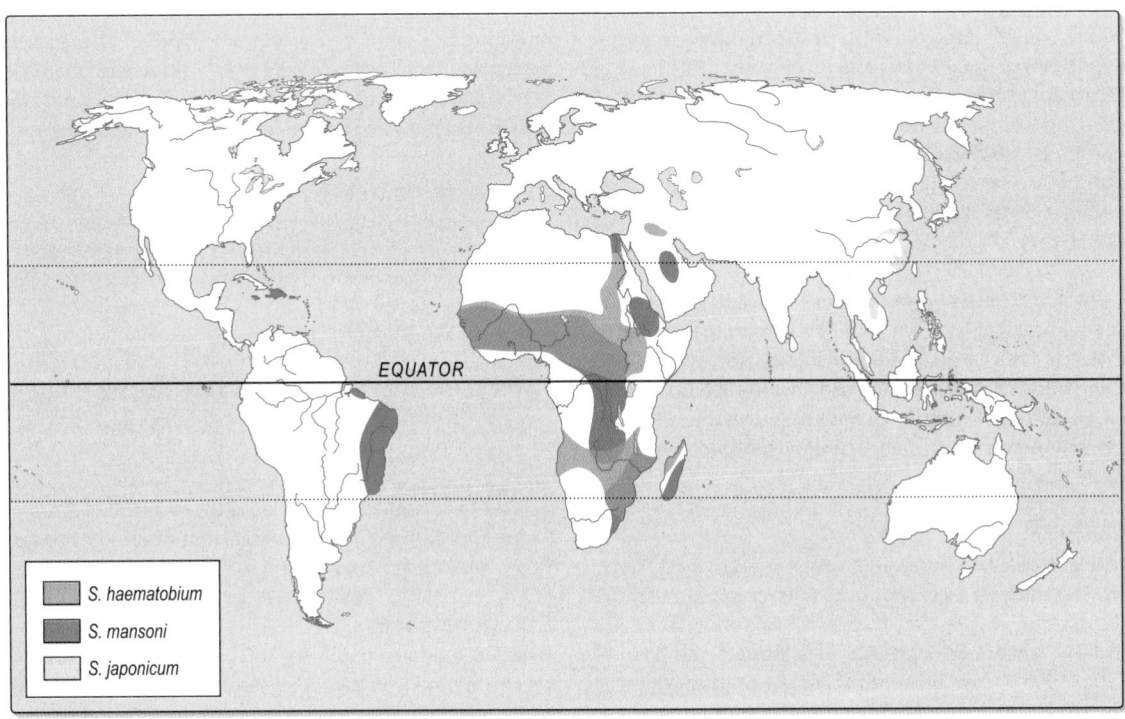

Fig. 2.36 Schistosomiasis – geographical distribution.

which large numbers of eggs accumulate in the tissues, leads to fibrosis, calcification, and in some cases, dysplasia and malignant change. Morbidity and mortality are related to duration of infection and worm load, as well as to the species of parasite. Children in endemic areas tend to have the heaviest worm load, because of both increased exposure to infection, and differences in the immune response between adults and children.

Clinical features

Cercarial penetration of the skin may cause local dermatitis ('swimmer's itch'). After a symptom-free period of 3–4 weeks, systemic allergic features may develop, including fever, rash, myalgia, and pneumonitis (Katayama fever). These allergic phenomena are common in non-immune travellers, but are rarely seen in local populations, who are usually exposed to infection from early childhood onwards. If infection is sufficiently heavy, symptoms from egg deposition may start to appear 2–3 months after infection.

S. haematobium infection (bilharzia). The earliest symptom is usually painless terminal haematuria. As bladder inflammation progresses there is increased urinary frequency and groin pain. Obstructive uropathy develops, leading to hydronephrosis, renal failure, and recurrent urinary infection. There is a strong association between chronic urinary schistosomiasis and squamous cell bladder carcinoma. The genitalia may also be affected, and ectopic eggs may cause pulmonary or neurological disease.

S. mansoni usually affects the large bowel. Early disease produces superficial mucosal changes, accompanied by blood-stained diarrhoea. Later the mucosal damage becomes more marked, with the formation of rectal polyps, deeper ulceration, and eventually fibrosis and stricture formation. Ectopic eggs are carried to the liver, where they cause an intense granulomatous response. Hepatitis is followed by progressive periportal fibrosis, leading to portal hypertension, oesophageal varices and splenomegaly (p. 392). Hepatocellular function is usually well preserved.

S. japonicum, unlike the other species, infects numerous other mammals apart from man. It is similar to *S. mansoni,* but infects both large and small bowel, and produces a greater number of eggs. Disease therefore tends to be more severe, and rapidly progressive. Hepatic involvement is more common, and neurological involvement is seen in about 5% of cases.

Diagnosis

Schistosomiasis is suggested by relevant symptoms following fresh water exposure in an endemic area. In the early allergic stages the diagnosis can only be made clinically. When egg deposition has started, the characteristic eggs (with a terminal spine in the case of *S. haematobium,* and a lateral spine in the other species) can be detected on microscopy. In *S. haematobium* infec-

tion, the best specimen for examination is a filtered mid-day urine sample. Parasites may also be found in semen, and in rectal snip preparations. *S. mansoni* and *S. japonicum* eggs can usually be found in faeces or in a rectal snip. Serological tests are available, and may be useful in the diagnosis of travellers returning from endemic areas, although the test may not become positive for 12 weeks after infection: a parasitological diagnosis should always be made if possible. X-rays, ultrasound examinations, and endoscopy may show abnormalities of the bowel or urinary tract in chronic disease, although these are non-specific. Liver biopsy may show the characteristic periportal fibrosis.

Management

The aim of treatment in endemic areas is to decrease the worm load and therefore minimize the chronic effects of egg deposition. It may not always be possible (or even desirable) to eradicate adult worms completely, and reinfection is common. However, a 90% reduction in egg output has been achieved in mass treatment programmes, and in light infections where there is no risk of re-exposure the drugs are usually curative. The most widely used is praziquantel (40 mg/kg as a single dose), which is effective against all species of schistosome, well-tolerated, and reasonably cheap.

Prevention

Prevention of schistosomiasis is difficult, and relies on a combination of approaches. Mass treatment of the population (especially children) will decrease the egg load in the community. Health education programmes, the provision of latrines, and access to a safe water supply should decrease the contact with infected water. Attempts to eradicate the snail host have generally been unsuccessful, although man-made bodies of water can often be made less 'snail-friendly'. Travellers should be advised to avoid potentially infected water. Oral artemether is safe and shows a prophylactic effect against *S. mansoni.*

FURTHER READING

Magnusson P (2003) Treatment and re-treatment strategies for schistosomiasis control in different settings: a review of 10 years' experiences. *Acta Tropica* **86**: 243–254.

Partners for parasite control: http://who.int/wormcontrol.

Utzinger J et al. (2003) Sustainable schistosomiasis control. *Lancet* **362**: 1932–1934.

Food-borne flukes

Many flukes infect man via ingestion of an intermediate host, often fresh water fish.

Paragonimiasis

Over 20 million people are infected with lung flukes of the genus *Paragonimus*. The adult worms (of which the major species is *P. westermani*) live in the lungs, producing eggs which are expectorated or swallowed and passed in the faeces. Miracidia emerging from the eggs penetrate the first intermediate host, a fresh water snail. Larvae released from the snail seek out the second intermediate host, fresh water crustacea, in which they encyst as metacercariae. Humans and other mammalian hosts become infected after consuming uncooked shellfish. Cercariae penetrate the small intestinal wall, and migrate directly from the peritoneum to the lungs across the diaphragm. Having established themselves in the lung, the adult worms may survive for 20 years.

The common clinical features are fever, cough and mild haemoptysis. In heavy infections the disease may progress, sometimes mimicking pneumonia or pulmonary tuberculosis. Ectopic worms may cause signs in the abdomen or the brain.

The diagnosis is made by detection of ova on sputum or stool microscopy. Serological tests are also available. Radiological appearances are variable and non-specific. Treatment is with praziquantel 25 mg/kg three times daily for 3 days. Prevention involves avoidance of inadequately cooked shellfish.

Liver flukes

The human liver flukes, *Clonorchis sinensis*, *Opisthorchis felineus*, and *O. viverrini*, are almost entirely confined to East and South East Asia, where they infect more than 20 million people. Adults live in the bile ducts, releasing eggs into the faeces. The parasite requires two intermediate hosts, a fresh water snail and a fish, and humans are infected by consumption of raw fish. The cycle is completed when excysted worms migrate from the small intestine into the bile ducts.

Infection is often asymptomatic, but may be associated with cholangitis and biliary carcinoma. The diagnosis is made by identifying eggs on stool microscopy. Treatment is with a single dose of praziquantel (40 mg/kg), and infection can be avoided by cooking fish adequately.

Other fluke infections

Man can also be infected with a variety of animal flukes, notably the liver fluke *Fasciola hepatica*, and the intestinal fluke *Fasciolopsis buski*. Both require a water snail as an intermediate host; cercariae encyst on aquatic vegetation, and then are consumed by animals or man. After ingestion, *F. hepatica* penetrates the intestinal wall before migrating to the liver: during this stage it causes systemic allergic symptoms. After reaching the bile ducts, it causes similar problems to those of the other liver flukes. *F. buski* does not migrate after it excysts, and causes mainly bowel symptoms.

The best treatment for *F. buski* is praziquantel 25 mg/kg, three doses in 24 hours, and for *F. hepatica*, triclabendazole 10 mg/kg as a single dose (which may need repeating).

CESTODES

Cestodes (tapeworms) are ribbon-shaped worms which vary from a few millimetres to several metres in length.

Adult worms live in the human intestine, where they attach to the epithelium using suckers on the anterior portion (scolex). From the scolex arises a series of progressively developing segments, called proglottids. The mature distal segments contain eggs, which may either be released directly into the faeces, or are carried out with an intact detached proglottid. The eggs are consumed by intermediate hosts, after which they hatch into larvae (oncospheres). These penetrate the intestinal wall of the host (pig or cattle) and encyst in the tissues. Man ingests the cysts in undercooked meat or fish, and the cycle is completed when the parasites excyst in the stomach and develop into adult worms in the small intestine. Infections are usually solitary, but several adult tapeworms may coexist. The exceptions to this life cycle are the dwarf tapeworm, *Hymenolepis nana*, which has no intermediate host and is transmitted from person to person by the faeco-oral route and *Taenia solium* which produces cysticercosis (see below).

Taenia saginata

T. saginata, the beef tapeworm, may reach a length of several metres. It is common in all countries where undercooked beef is eaten. The adult worm causes few if any symptoms. Infection is usually discovered when proglottids are found in faeces or on underclothing, often causing considerable anxiety. Ova may also be seen on stool microscopy. Infection can be cleared with a single dose of praziquantel (10 mg/kg). It can be prevented by careful meat inspection, or by thorough cooking of beef.

Taenia solium and cysticercosis

T. solium, the pork tapeworm, is generally smaller than *T. saginata*, although it can still reach 6 metres in length. It is particularly common in South America, South Africa, China, and parts of South East Asia. As with *T. saginata* infection is usually asymptomatic. The ova of the two species are identical, but the proglottids can be distinguished on inspection.

Tapeworms are mainly acquired by eating uncooked pork while cysticercosis follows the ingestion of eggs from contaminated food and water. Faeco-oral auto-infection can occur but is rare. Patients with tapeworms do not usually develop cysticercosis and patients with cysticercosis do not usually harbour tapeworms. Following the ingestion of eggs, the larvae are liberated, penetrate the intestinal wall, and are carried to various parts of the body where they develop into cysticerci (Fig. 2.38). These are cysts, 0.5–1 cm diameter, containing the scolex of a new adult worm. Common sites for cysticerci include subcutaneous tissue, skeletal muscle and brain.

Superficial cysts may be felt under the skin, but usually cause no significant symptoms. Cysts in the brain can cause a variety of problems including epilepsy, personality change, hydrocephalus and focal neurological signs (p. 1241). These may only appear many years after infection.

Muscle cysts tend to calcify, and are often visible on X-rays. Cutaneous cysts can be excised and examined. Brain cysts are less prone to calcification, and are often

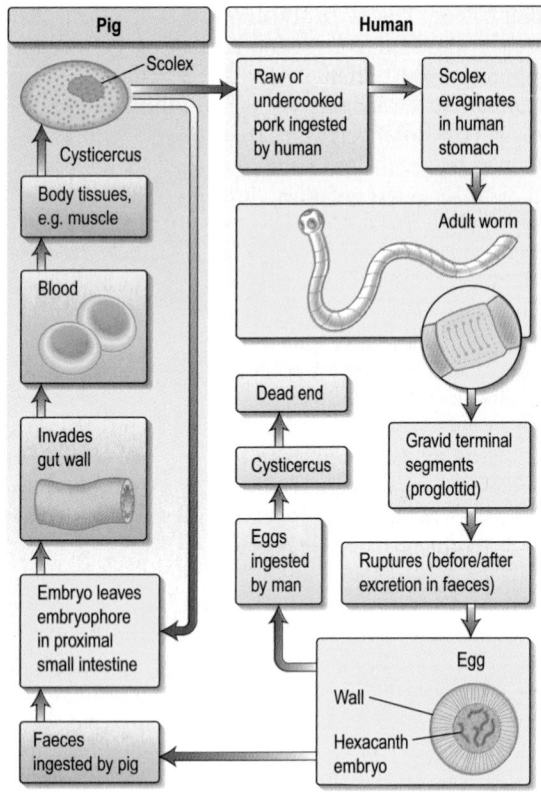

Fig. 2.38 A schematic life cycle of *Taenia solium.*

Fig. 2.39 A schematic life cycle of *Echinococcus granulosus.*

only seen on CT or MRI scan. Serological tests may support the diagnosis.

Treatment is again with praziquantel: niclosamide 1 g repeated after 2 hours is also effective. There is no evidence that drug treatment should be accompanied by a purgative, as was previously believed.

Treatment of cerebral cysticercosis (p. 1241)

The role of anthelminthics in cysticercosis remains controversial. Even in neurocysticercosis there is little evidence of benefit, although symptomatic patients with viable neurocysts should probably be treated. Albendazole 15 mg/kg daily for 8–20 days is the drug of choice; the alternative is praziquantel 50 mg/kg daily (in divided doses) for 15 days.

Successful treatment is accompanied by increased local inflammation, and corticosteroids should be given during and after the course of anthelminthic. Anticonvulsants should be given for epilepsy, and surgery may be indicated if there is hydrocephalus. Prevention of cysticercosis depends on good hygiene, as well as on the eradication of human *T. solium* infection.

Diphyllobothrium latum

Infection with the fish tapeworm, *D. latum*, is common in northern Europe and Japan, owing to the consumption of raw fish. The adult worm reaches a length of several metres, but like the other tapeworms usually causes no symptoms. A megaloblastic anaemia (due to competitive utilization of B_{12} by the parasite) may occur. Diagnosis and treatment are the same as for *Taenia* species.

Hydatid disease

Hydatid disease occurs when humans become an intermediate host of the dog tapeworm, *Echinococcus granulosus* (Fig. 2.39). The adult worm lives in the gut of domestic and wild canines, and the larval stages are usually found in sheep, cattle and camels. Man may become infected either from direct contact with dogs, or from food or water contaminated with dog faeces. After ingestion the parasites excyst, penetrate the small intestine wall, and are carried to the liver and other organs in the bloodstream. A slow-growing, thick-walled cyst is formed, inside which further larval stages of the parasite develop. The life cycle cannot be completed unless the cyst is eaten by a dog. Hydatid disease is prevalent in areas where dogs are used in the control of livestock, especially sheep. It is common in Australia, Argentina, the Middle East, and parts of East Africa; small foci of infection are still found in North Wales and rural Scotland.

Symptoms depend mainly on the site of the cyst. The liver is the most common organ affected (60%), followed by the lung (20%), kidneys (3%), brain (1%) and bone (1%). The symptoms are those of a slowly growing benign tumour. Pressure on the bile ducts may cause jaundice. Rupture into the abdominal cavity, pleural cavity or biliary tree may occur. In the latter situation, intermittent jaundice, abdominal pain and fever associated with eosinophilia result. A cyst rupturing into a bronchus may result in its expectoration and spontaneous cure, but if secondary infection supervenes a chronic pulmonary abscess will form. Focal seizures can occur if cysts are present in the brain. Renal involvement produces lumbar pain and haematuria. Calcification of the cyst occurs in about 40% of cases.

A related parasite of foxes, *E. multilocularis*, causes a similar but more severe infection, alveolar hydatid disease. These cysts are invasive and metastases may occur.

The diagnosis and treatment of hydatid liver disease are described on page 392.

ARTHROPOD ECTOPARASITES

Arthropods, which include the arachnid ticks and mites as well as insects, may be responsible for human disease in several ways.

Local hypersensitivity reactions

Local lesions may be caused by hypersensitivity to allergens in arthropod saliva. This common reaction, known as papular urticaria, is non-specific and is seen in the majority of people in response to the bite of a variety of blood-sucking arthropods including mosquitoes, bugs, ticks, lice, and mites. Occasionally tick bites may cause a more severe systemic allergic response, especially in previously sensitized individuals.

Most of these parasites alight on man only to feed, but some species of lice live in very close proximity to the skin: body lice in clothing, and head and pubic lice on human hairs (p. 1325).

Resident ectoparasite infections

Other ectoparasites are actually resident within the skin, causing more specific local lesions.

Scabies (p. 1325)

Jiggers

Jiggers is due to infection with the jigger flea, *Tunga penetrans*, and is common throughout South America and Africa. The pregnant female flea burrows into the sole of the foot, often between the toes. The egg sac grows to about 0.5 cm in size, before the eggs are discharged onto the ground. The main danger is bacterial infection or tetanus. The flea should be removed with a needle or scalpel, and the area kept clean until it heals.

Myiasis

Myiasis is caused by invasion of human tissue by the larva of certain flies, principally the Tumbu fly, *Cordylobia anthropophaga* (found in sub-Saharan Africa), and the human botfly, *Dermatobia hominis* (Central and South America). The larvae, which hatch from eggs laid on

laundry and linen, burrow into the skin to form boil-like lesions: a central breathing orifice may be visible. Again, the main risk is secondary infection. It is not always easy to extract the larva: covering it with petroleum jelly may bring it up in search of air.

Systemic envenoming

Many arthropods can cause local or systemic illness through envenoming, i.e. injection of venom.

The main role of arthropods in causing human disease is as vectors of parasitic and viral infections. Some of these infections are shown in Table 2.4, and discussed in detail elsewhere.

FURTHER READING
Garcia HH (2003) *Taenia solium* cysticercosis. *Lancet* **362**: 547–556.
Heukelbach J, Feldmeier H (2004) Ectoparasites – the underestimated realm. *Lancet* **363**: 889–891.
McManus DP et al. (2003) Echinococcosis. *Lancet* **362**: 1295–1304.
Moss PJ, Beeching NJ (2003) *Ectoparasites in Infectious Diseases*, 2nd edn. London: Mosby.

SEXUALLY TRANSMITTED INFECTIONS

Sexually transmitted infections (STIs) are among the most common causes of illness in the world and remain epidemic in all societies. The public health, social and economic consequences are extensive, both of the acute infections and their longer-term sequelae. There has been a recent sharp increase in the incidence of STIs in the UK (as in the rest of the world). New presentations at genitourinary medicine (GUM) clinics in the UK rose by 37% from 1 546 812 in 2002 to 2 125 243 in 2003.

Between 1997 and 2002 there has been an increase in both gonorrhoea (97%) and syphilis (716%) infections. There has been a steady rise in the incidence of *Chlamydia trachomatis* with a 103% increase over the same time period. Viral conditions, particularly herpes simplex virus (HSV) and human papillomavirus, have also increased substantially. Increased numbers may also reflect recent public health campaigns promoting STI screening and the use of increasingly sensitive diagnostic tests. Substantial rises in human immunodeficiency virus (HIV) infection in the UK have further heightened awareness of STIs. In 2002 over 49 000 adults were estimated to have HIV, with up to one-third being unaware of their infection. Many people attend GUM clinics to seek information, advice and checks of their sexual health, but have no active STI.

Those most likely to acquire STIs are young people, homo- and bisexual men and black and ethnic minority populations. Changes in incidence reflect high-risk sexual behaviour and inconsistent use of condoms. Increased travel both within and between countries, recreational drug use, alcohol and more frequent partner change are also implicated. Multiple infections frequently coexist, some of which may be asymptomatic and facilitate spread.

Approach to the patient

Patients presenting with possible STIs are frequently anxious, embarrassed and concerned about confidentiality. Staff must be alert to these issues and respond sensitively. The clinical setting must ensure privacy and reinforce confidentiality.

History

The history of the presenting complaint frequently focuses on genital symptoms, the three most common being vaginal discharge (Table 2.46), urethral discharge (Table 2.47), and genital ulceration (Table 2.48). Details should be obtained of any associated fever, pain, itch, malodour, genital swelling, skin rash, joint pains and eye symptoms. All patients should be asked about dysuria, haematuria and loin pain. A full general medical, family and drug history, particularly of any recent antibacterial or antiviral treatment, allergies and use of oral contraceptives, must be obtained. In women, menstrual, contraception and obstetric history should be obtained. Any past or current history of drug misuse should be explored.

A detailed sexual history should be taken and include the number and types of sexual contacts (genital/genital, oral/genital, anal/genital, oral/anal) with dates, partner's sex, whether regular or casual partner, use of condoms and other forms of contraception, previous history of STIs including dates and treatment received, HIV testing and results and hepatitis B vaccination status.

Enquires should be made concerning travel abroad to areas where antibiotic resistance is known or where particular pathogens are endemic.

Examination

General examination must include the mouth, throat, skin and lymph nodes in all patients. Signs of HIV infection are covered on page 144. The inguinal, genital and perianal areas should be examined with a good light source. The groins should be palpated for lymphadenopathy and hernias. The pubic hair must be examined for nits and lice. The external genitalia must be examined for signs of erythema, fissures, ulcers, chancres, pigmented or hypopigmented areas and warts. Signs of trauma may be seen.

In men, the penile skin should be examined and the foreskin retracted to look for balanitis, ulceration, warts or tumours. The urethral meatus is located and the presence of discharge noted. Scrotal contents are palpated and the consistency of the testes and epididymis noted. A rectal examination/proctoscopy should be performed in patients with rectal symptoms, those who practise anoreceptive intercourse and patients with prostatic symptoms. A search for rectal warts is indicated in patients with perianal lesions.

Table 2.46	Causes of vaginal discharge
Infective	**Non-infective**
Candida albicans	Cervical polyps
Trichomonas vaginalis	Neoplasms
Bacterial vaginosis	Retained products (e.g. tampons)
Neisseria gonorrhoeae	Chemical irritation
Chlamydia trachomatis	
Herpes simplex	

Table 2.47	Causes of urethral discharge
Infective	**Non-infective**
Neisseria gonorrhoeae	Physical or chemical trauma
Chlamydia trachomatis	Urethral stricture
Mycoplasma genitilium	Non-specific (aetiology
Ureaplasma urealyticum	unknown)
Trichomonas vaginalis	
Herpes simplex virus	
Human papillomavirus (meatal warts)	
Urinary tract infection (rare)	
Treponema pallidum (meatal chancre)	

Table 2.48	Causes of genital ulceration
Infective	**Non-infective**
Syphilis:	
Primary chancre	Behçet's syndrome
Secondary mucous patches	Toxic epidermal necrolysis
Tertiary gumma	Stevens–Johnson
Chancroid	syndrome
Lymphogranuloma venereum	Carcinoma
Donovanosis	Trauma
Herpes simplex:	
Primary	
Recurrent	
Herpes zoster	

In women, Bartholin's glands must be identified and examined. The cervix should be inspected for ulceration, discharge, bleeding and ectopy and the walls of the vagina for warts. A bimanual pelvic examination is performed to elicit adnexal tenderness or masses, cervical tenderness, and to assess the position, size and mobility of the uterus. Rectal examination and proctoscopy are performed if the patient has symptoms or practises anoreceptive intercourse.

Investigations

Although the history and examination will guide investigation, it must be remembered that multiple infections may coexist, some being asymptomatic. Full screening is indicated in any patient who may have been in contact with an STI.

In men
- Urethral smears for Gram staining
- Urethral swabs for gonococcal culture and *Chlamydia* testing

- Two-glass urine test and urinalysis
- Rectal swabs for Gram staining and culture for *N. gonorrhoeae* and *C. trachomatis*
- Throat swab for culture for *N. gonorrhoeae*
- Blood for syphilis and HIV serology (with counselling).

In women

- Smears from the lateral vaginal wall for Gram staining
- Vaginal swab for culture of *Candida* and *Trichomonas*
- A wet preparation is made from the posterior fornix for *Trichomonas* and for the potassium hydroxide test for bacterial vaginosis
- The pH of vaginal secretions using narrow-range indicator paper
- Endocervical smears and swabs for Gram staining, gonococcal culture and *Chlamydia* tests
- Urethral smears and swabs for Gram staining and gonococcal culture
- Rectal and throat swabs for *N. gonorrhoeae* and *C. trachomatis*, if indicated
- Urinalysis
- Cervical cytology
- Blood for syphilis and HIV serology (with counselling).

Additional investigations when indicated

- Urine sample for nucleic acid amplification tests if available locally
- Blood for hepatitis B and C serology
- Swabs for HSV and *Haemophilus ducreyi* from clinically suspicious lesions into special media
- Smears and swabs from the subpreputial area in men with balanoposthitis (inflammation of glans penis and prepuce) for candidiasis
- Scrapings from lesions suspicious of early syphilis for immediate dark-ground microscopy
- Pregnancy testing
- Cervical cytology
- Stools for *Giardia*, *Shigella* or *Salmonella* from those practising oral/anal sex.

Treatment, prevention and control

The treatment of specific conditions is considered in the appropriate section. Many GUM clinics keep basic stocks of medication and dispense directly to the patient.

Tracing the sexual partners of patients is crucial in controlling spread of STIs. The aims are to prevent the spread of infection within the community and to ensure that people with asymptomatic infection are properly treated. Appropriate antibiotic therapy may be offered to those who have had recent intercourse with someone known to have an active infection (epidemiological treatment). Interviewing people about their sexual partners requires considerable tact and sensitivity, and specialist health advisors are available in GUM clinics.

Prevention starts with education and information. People begin sexual activity at ever-younger ages and education programmes need to include school pupils as well as young adults. Education of health professionals is also crucial. Public health campaigns aimed at informing groups at particular risk are being implemented at a national level. Appropriate and accessible services must be well advertised. Avoiding multiple partners, correct and consistent use of condoms and avoiding sex with people who have symptoms of infection may reduce the risks of acquiring an STI. For those who change their sexual partners frequently, regular check-ups (approximately 3-monthly) are advisable. Once people develop symptoms they should be encouraged to seek medical advice as soon as possible to reduce complications and spread to others.

Sexual assault

The medical and psychological management of people who have been sexually assaulted requires particular sensitivity and should be undertaken by an experienced clinician in ways that reduce the risks of further trauma. Post-traumatic stress disorder is common. Although most frequently reported by women, both women and men may suffer sexual assault. Investigations for and treatment of sexually transmitted infections in people who have been raped can be carried out in GUM departments. Collection of material for use as evidence, however, should be carried out within 7 days of the assault by a physician trained in forensic medicine and must take place before any other medical examinations are performed.

History

In addition to the general medical, gynaecological and contraceptive history, full details of the assault, including the exact sites of penetration, ejaculation by the assailant and condom use should be obtained, together with details of the sexual history both before and after the event.

Examination

Any injuries requiring immediate attention must be dealt with prior to any other examination or investigations. Accurate documentation of any trauma is necessary. Forced oral penetration may result in small palatal haemorrhages. In cases of forced anal penetration, anal examination including proctoscopy should be carried out, noting any trauma.

Investigations

A full STI screen at presentation with a second examination 2 weeks later is recommended. Cultures for *Neisseria gonorrhoeae* and tests for *Chlamydia trachomatis* should be obtained from all sites of actual or attempted penetration. *C. trachomatis* culture is the only test currently accepted as evidence. Gram-stained slides of urethral, cervical and rectal specimens for microscopy for gonococci should be performed. Bacterial vaginosis, yeasts and *Trichomonas vaginalis* (TV) tests should be carried out on vaginal material. Syphilis serology should be requested and a serum saved. Hepatitis B, HIV and hepatitis C testing should be offered. Specimens should be identified as having potential medicolegal implications.

Management

Preventative therapy for gonorrhoea and chlamydia may be advised using a single dose combination of ciprofloxacin 500 mg and azithromycin 1 g. Hep B vaccine should be offered and may be of value up to 3 weeks after the event. HIV prophylaxis may be offered within 72 hours of the assault, based upon a specific risk assessment. Post-coital oral contraception may be given within 72 hours of assault. Psychological care provision and appropriate referral to support agencies should be arranged. Sexual partners should be screened and treated if necessary.

Initial follow-up at 2 weeks should be arranged to review the patient's needs and the prophylaxis regimens that are in place, with further follow-up as needed.

Fig. 2.40 *Neisseria gonorrhoeae* – Gram-negative intracellular diplococci. Courtesy of Dr B Goh.

CLINICAL SYNDROMES

HIV and AIDS

These are discussed in the section starting on page 129.

Gonorrhoea (GC)

Neisseria gonorrhoeae is a Gram-negative intracellular diplococcus (Fig. 2.40), which infects epithelium particularly of the urogenital tract, rectum, pharynx and conjunctivae. Humans are the only host and the organism is spread by intimate physical contact. It is very intolerant to drying and although occasional reports of spread by fomites exist, this route of infection is extremely rare.

Clinical features

Up to 50% of women and 10% of men are asymptomatic. The incubation period is 2–14 days with most symptoms occurring between days 2 and 5. In men the most common syndrome is one of anterior urethritis causing dysuria and/or urethral discharge (Fig. 2.41). Complications include ascending infection involving the epididymis or prostate leading to acute or chronic infection. In homosexual men rectal infection may produce proctitis with pain, discharge and itch.

In women the primary site of infection is usually the endocervical canal. Symptoms include an increased or altered vaginal discharge, pelvic pain due to ascending infection, dysuria, and intermenstrual bleeding. Complications include Bartholin's abscesses and in rare cases a perihepatitis (Fitzhugh–Curtis syndrome) can develop. On a global basis GC is one of the most common causes of female infertility. Rectal infection, due to local spread, occurs in women and is usually asymptomatic, as is pharyngeal infection. Conjunctival infection is seen in neonates born to infected mothers and is one cause of ophthalmia neonatorum.

Disseminated GC leads to arthritis (usually monoarticular or pauciarticular) (see p. 572) and characteristic papular or pustular rash with an erythematous base in association with fever and malaise. It is more common in women.

Fig. 2.41 *Neisseria gonorrhoeae* – purulent urethral discharge. Courtesy of Dr B Goh.

Diagnosis

N. gonorrhoeae can be identified from infected areas by culture on selective media with a sensitivity of at least 95%. Microscopy of Gram-stained secretions may demonstrate intracellular, Gram-negative diplococci, allowing rapid diagnosis. The sensitivity ranges from 90% in urethral specimens from symptomatic men to 50% in endocervical specimens. Nucleic acid amplification tests (NAATs) using urine specimens are non-invasive and highly sensitive, although may give false positive results. Microscopy should not be used for pharyngeal specimens. Blood culture and synovial fluid investigations should be performed in cases of disseminated GC. Coexisting pathogens such as *Chlamydia*, *Trichomonas* and syphilis must be sought.

Treatment

Treatment is indicated in those patients who have a positive culture for GC, positive microscopy or a positive NAAT. Epidemiological treatment is given to patients who have had recent sexual intercourse with someone with confirmed GC infection. Although *N. gonorrhoeae* is sensitive to a wide range of antimicrobial agents, antibiotic-resistant strains have shown a recent significant increase in the UK. Up to 10% of strains show resistance to penicillins and ciprofloxacin and over 40% resistance to tetracyclines. Immediate therapy based on Gram-stained slides is usually initiated in the clinic, prior to culture and sensitivity results. Antibiotic choice is influenced by travel history or details known from contacts.

Single-dose oral therapy with either cefixime (400 mg), ceftriaxone i.m. (250 mg) or spectinomycin 2 g i.m. (not generally available in the UK) successfully treats uncomplicated anogenital infection. Single-dose amoxicillin 3 g with probenecid 1 g, ciprofloxacin (500 mg) or ofloxacin (400 mg) are recommended for use in areas with low prevalence of antibiotic resistance.

Longer courses of antibiotics are required for complicated infections. There should be at least one follow-up assessment, and culture tests should be repeated at least 72 hours after treatment is complete. All sexual contacts should be examined and treated as necessary.

Chlamydia trachomatis (CT)

Genital infection with CT is common, with up to 5% of sexually active women in the UK infected. It is regularly found in association with other pathogens: 20% of men and 40% of women with gonorrhoea have been found to have coexisting chlamydial infections. In men 40% of non-gonococcal and post-gonococcal urethritis is due to *Chlamydia*. As CT is often asymptomatic much infection goes unrecognized and untreated, which sustains the infectious pool in the population. The long-term complications associated with *Chlamydia* infection, especially infertility, impose significant morbidity in the UK. The organism has a world-wide distribution.

Clinical features

In men CT gives rise to an anterior urethritis with dysuria and discharge; infection is asymptomatic in up to 50% and detected by contact tracing. Ascending infection leads to epididymitis. Rectal infection leading to proctitis occurs in men practising anoreceptive intercourse. *In women* the most common site of infection is the endocervix where it may go unnoticed; up to 80% of infection in women is asymptomatic. Symptoms include vaginal discharge, post-coital or intermenstrual bleeding and lower abdominal pain. Ascending infection causes acute salpingitis. Reiter's disease (see p. 568) has been related to infection with *C. trachomatis*. Neonatal infection, acquired from the birth canal, can result in mucopurulent conjunctivitis and pneumonia.

Diagnosis

CT is an obligate intracellular bacterium, which complicates diagnosis. Cell culture techniques provide the 'gold standard' but are expensive and require considerable expertise. Indirect diagnostic tests include direct fluorescent antibody (DIF) tests, enzyme immunoassays (EIA) and

nucleic acid amplification techniques such as PCR or ligase chain reaction (LCR): none is diagnostic.

In men first-voided urine samples are tested, or urethral swabs obtained. In women endocervical swabs are the best specimens, and up to 20% additional positives will be detected if urethral swabs are also taken. Urine specimens are much less reliable than endocervical swabs in women and are not recommended. Specimen quality is critical and it must contain cellular material.

Treatment

Tetracyclines or macrolide antibiotics are most commonly used to treat *Chlamydia*. Doxycycline 100 mg 12-hourly for 7 days or azithromycin 1 g as a single dose are both effective for uncomplicated infection. Tetracyclines are contraindicated in pregnancy. Other effective regimens include erythromycin 500 mg four times daily. Routine test of cure is not necessary after treatment with doxycycline or azithromycin, although if symptoms persist or reinfection is suspected then further tests should be taken. Sexual contacts must be traced and treated, particularly as so many infections are clinically silent.

Urethritis

Urethritis is usually characterized in men by a discharge from the urethra, dysuria and varying degrees of discomfort within the penis. In 10–15% of cases there are no symptoms. A wide array of aetiologies can give rise to the clinical picture which are divided into two broad bands: gonococcal or non-gonococcal urethritis (NGU). NGU occurring shortly after infection with gonorrhoea is known as postgonococcal urethritis (PGU). Gonococcal urethritis and chlamydial urethritis (a major cause of NGU) are discussed above.

Trichomonas vaginalis, *Mycoplasma genitilium*, *Ureaplasma urealyticum* and *Bacteroides* spp. are responsible for a proportion of cases. HSV can cause urethritis in about 30% of cases of primary infection, considerably fewer in recurrent episodes. Other causes include syphilitic chancres and warts within the urethra. Non-sexually transmitted NGU may be due to urinary tract infections, prostatic infection, foreign bodies and strictures.

Clinical features

The urethral discharge is often mucoid and worse in the mornings. Crusting at the meatus or stains on underwear occur. Dysuria is common but not universal. Discomfort or itch within the penis may be present. The incubation period is 1–5 weeks with a mean of 2–3 weeks. Asymptomatic urethritis is a major reservoir of infection. Reiter's disease causing conjunctivitis and/or arthritis occurs, particularly in HLA B27-positive individuals.

Diagnosis

Smears should be taken from the urethra when the patient has not voided urine for at least 4 hours and should be Gram stained and examined under a high-power (×1000) oil-immersion lens. The presence of five or more polymorphonuclear leucocytes per high-power field is diagnostic. Men who are symptomatic but have no objective evidence of urethritis should be re-examined and tested after holding urine overnight. Cultures for gonorrhoea must be taken together with specimens for *Chlamydia* testing.

Treatment

Therapy for NGU is with either doxycycline 100 mg 12-hourly or azithromycin 1 g orally as a single dose. Sexual intercourse should be avoided. The vast majority of patients will show partial or total response. Sexual partners must be traced and treated; *C. trachomatis* can be isolated from the cervix in 50–60% of the female partners of men with PGU or NGU, many of whom are asymptomatic. This causes long-term morbidity in such women, acts as a reservoir of infection for the community, and may lead to reinfection in the index case if not treated.

Recurrent/persistent NGU

This is a common and difficult clinical problem, and can occur in 20–60% of men treated for acute NGU. The usual time for patients to re-present is 2–3 weeks following treatment. Tests for organisms, e.g. *Mycoplasma*, *Chlamydia* and *Ureaplasma* are usually negative. It is necessary to document objective evidence of urethritis, check adherence to treatment and establish any possible contact with untreated sexual partners. Investigations should include wet preparation and culture of urethral material for *Trichomonas vaginalis*. Cultures should be taken for HSV. A mid-stream urine sample should be examined and cultured. A further 1 week's treatment with erythromycin 500 mg four times a day for 2 weeks plus metronidazole 400 mg twice daily for 5 days may be given, and any specific additional infection treated appropriately. If symptoms are mild and all partners have been treated, patients should be reassured and further antibiotic therapy avoided. In cases of frequent recurrence and/or florid unresponsive urethritis, the prostate should be investigated and urethroscopy or cystoscopy performed to investigate possible strictures, periurethral fistulae or foreign bodies.

Lymphogranuloma venereum (LGV)

Chlamydia trachomatis types LGV 1, 2 and 3 are responsible for this sexually transmitted infection. It is endemic in the tropics, with the highest incidences in Africa, India and South East Asia.

Clinical features

The primary lesion is a painless ulcerating papule on the genitalia occurring 7–21 days following exposure. It is frequently unnoticed. A few days to weeks after this heals, regional lymphadenopathy develops. The lymph nodes are painful and fixed and the overlying skin develops a dusky erythematous appearance. Finally, nodes may become fluctuant (buboes) and can rupture. Acute LGV also presents as proctitis with perirectal abscesses, the appearances sometimes resembling anorectal Crohn's disease. The destruction of local lymph nodes can lead to lymphoedema of the genitalia.

Diagnosis

The diagnosis is often made on the basis of the characteristic clinical picture after other causes of genital ulceration or inguinal lymphadenopathy have been excluded. Syphilis and genital herpes must be excluded.

- Isolation of *C. trachomatis* in tissue culture. The sensitivity is 75–85%.
- Antigen-detection methods with material from bubo aspirates or ulcer scrapes:
  - direct immunofluorescence using monoclonal antibodies
  - enzyme immunoassay (EIA).
- Sensitivity 70–80%.
- Positive *C. trachomatis* serology (complement fixation tests, L-type immunofluorescence or micro-immunofluorescence test, IF). A fourfold rise in antibody titre in the course of the illness is diagnostic. NB: Micro-IF is the only serological means of distinguishing different serotypes of CT.

Treatment

Early treatment is critical to prevent the chronic phase. Doxycycline (100 mg twice daily for 21 days) or erythromycin (500 mg four times daily for 21 days) is efficacious. Follow-up should continue until signs and symptoms have resolved, usually 3–6 weeks. Chronic infection may result in extensive scarring and abscess and sinus formation. Surgical drainage or reconstructive surgery is sometimes required. Sexual partners in the 30 days prior to onset should be examined and treated if necessary.

Syphilis

Syphilis is a chronic systemic disease, which is acquired or congenital. In its early stages diagnosis and treatment are straightforward but untreated it can cause complex sequelae in many organs and eventually lead to death.

The causative organism, *Treponema pallidum* (TP), is a motile spirochaete that is acquired either by close sexual contact or can be transmitted transplacentally. The organism enters the new host through breaches in squamous or columnar epithelium. Primary infection of non-genital sites may occasionally occur but is rare.

Both acquired and congenital syphilis have early and late stages, each of which has classic clinical features (Table 2.49).

Primary

Between 10–90 days (mean 21 days) after exposure to the pathogen a papule develops at the site of inoculation. This ulcerates to become a painless, firm chancre. There is usually painless regional lymphadenopathy in association. The primary lesion may go unnoticed, especially if it is on the cervix or within the rectum. Healing occurs spontaneously within 2–3 weeks.

Table 2.49 Classification and clinical features of syphilis

	Clinical features
Acquired	
Early stages	
Primary	Hard chancre Painless, regional lymphadenopathy
Secondary	*General*: Fever, malaise, arthralgia, sore throat and generalized lymphadenopathy *Skin*: Red/brown maculopapular non-itchy, sometimes scaly rash; condylomata lata *Mucous membranes*: Mucous patches, 'snail-track' ulcers in oropharynx and on genitalia
Late stages	
Tertiary	*Late benign*: Gummas (bone and viscera) *Cardiovascular*: Aortitis and aortic regurgitation *Neurosyphilis*: Meningovascular involvement, general paralysis of the insane (GPI) and tabes dorsalis
Congenital	Stillbirth or failure to thrive
Early stages	'Snuffles' (nasal infection with discharge) Skin and mucous membrane lesions as in secondary syphilis
Late stages	'Stigmata': Hutchinson's teeth, 'sabre' tibia and abnormalities of long bones Keratitis, uveitis, facial gummas and CNS disease

Fig. 2.42 **Rash of secondary syphilis on the palms.** Courtesy of Dr B Goh.

during a period known as early latency, a 2-year period in the UK (1 year in USA). Late latency is based on reactive syphilis serology with no clinical manifestations for at least 2 years. This can continue for many years before the late stages of syphilis become apparent.

Tertiary

Late benign syphilis, so called because of its response to therapy rather than its clinical manifestations, generally involves the skin and the bones. The characteristic lesion, the gumma (granulomatous, sometimes ulcerating, lesions), can occur anywhere in the skin, frequently at sites of trauma. Gummas are commonly found in the skull, tibia, fibula and clavicle, although any bone may be involved. Visceral gummas occur mainly in the liver (hepar lobatum) and the testes.

Cardiovascular and neurosyphilis are discussed on pages 810 and 1240.

Congenital syphilis

Congenital syphilis usually becomes apparent between the second and sixth week after birth, early signs being nasal discharge, skin and mucous membrane lesions, and failure to thrive. Signs of late syphilis generally do not appear until after 2 years of age and take the form of 'stigmata' relating to early damage to developing structures, particularly teeth and long bones. Other late manifestations parallel those of adult tertiary syphilis.

Investigations for diagnosis

Treponema pallidum is not amenable to in vitro culture – the most sensitive and specific method is identification by dark-ground microscopy. Organisms may be found in variable numbers, from primary chancres and the mucous patches of secondary lesions. Individuals with either primary or secondary disease are highly infectious.

Serological tests used in diagnosis are either treponemal-specific or non-specific (cardiolipin test) (Table 2.50):

- **Treponemal specific**. The *T. pallidum* enzyme immunoassay (EIA). *T. pallidum* haemagglutination or particle agglutination assay (TPHA/TPPA) and fluorescent treponemal antibodies absorbed (FTA-abs)

Secondary

Between 4–10 weeks after the appearance of the primary lesion constitutional symptoms with fever, sore throat, malaise and arthralgia appear. Any organ may be affected – leading, for example, to hepatitis, nephritis, arthritis and meningitis. In a minority of cases the primary chancre may still be present and should be sought.

Signs include:

- Generalized lymphadenopathy (50%)
- Generalized skin rashes involving the whole body including the palms and soles but excluding the face (75%) – the rash, which rarely itches, may take many different forms, ranging from pink macules, through coppery papules, to frank pustules (Fig. 2.42)
- Condylomata lata – warty, plaque-like lesions found in the perianal area and other moist body sites
- Superficial confluent ulceration of mucosal surfaces – found in the mouth and on the genitalia, described as 'snail track ulcers'
- Acute neurological signs in less than 10% of cases (e.g. aseptic meningitis).

Untreated early syphilis in pregnant women leads to fetal infection in at least 70% of cases and may result in stillbirth in up to 30%.

Latent

Without treatment, symptoms and signs abate over 3–12 weeks, but in up to 20% of individuals may recur

Table 2.50 Syphilis serology

Stage of infection	Results			
	EIA	FTA-abs	TPHA/TPPA	VDRL/RPR
Very early primary	−	−	−	−
Early primary	+ (IgM)	+	−	−
Primary	+ (IgM)	+	±	+
Secondary or latent	+	+	+	+
Late latent	+	+	+	±
Treated	+	+	+	±
Biological false–positive	−	−	−	+

EIA, enzyme immunoassay; FTA–abs, fluorescent *Treponema* antibodies absorbed; TPHA/TPPA, *Treponema pallidum* haemagglutination/particle agglutination assay; VDRL, Venereal Disease Research Laboratory; RPR, rapid plasma reagin

test are both highly specific for treponemal disease but will not differentiate between syphilis and other treponemal infection such as yaws. These tests usually remain positive for life, even after treatment.

- **Treponemal non-specific**. The Venereal Disease Research Laboratory (VDRL) and rapid plasma reagin (RPR) tests are non-specific, becoming positive within 3–4 weeks of the primary infection. They are quantifiable tests which can be used to monitor treatment efficacy and are helpful in assessing disease activity. They generally become negative by 6 months after treatment in early syphilis. The VDRL may also become negative in untreated patients (50% of patients with late-stage syphilis) or remain positive after treatment in late stage. False-positive results may occur in other conditions – particularly infectious mononucleosis, hepatitis, *Mycoplasma* infections, some protozoal infections, cirrhosis, malignancy, autoimmune disease and chronic infections.

The EIA is the screening test of choice and can detect both IgM and IgG antibodies. A positive test is then confirmed with the TPHA/TPPA and VDRL/RPR tests. All serological investigations may be negative in early primary syphilis; the EIA IgM and the FTA-abs being the earliest tests to be positive. The diagnosis will then hinge on positive dark-ground microscopy, and treatment should not be delayed if serological tests are negative in such situations.

In certain cases, examination of the CSF for evidence of neurosyphilis and a chest X-ray to determine the extent of cardiovascular disease will be indicated.

Treatment

Treponemocidal levels of antibiotic must be maintained in serum for at least 7 days in early syphilis to cover the slow division time of the organism (30 hours). In late syphilis treponemes may divide even more slowly requiring longer therapy.

Early syphilis (primary or secondary) should be treated with long-acting penicillin such as procaine benzyl-penicillin (procaine penicillin) (e.g. Jenacillin A which also contains benzylpenicillin) 600 mg intramuscularly daily for 10 days. For late-stage syphilis, particularly when there is cardiovascular or neurological involvement, the treatment course should be extended for a further week. For patients sensitive to penicillin, either

doxycycline 200 mg daily or erythromycin 500 mg four times daily is given orally for 2–4 weeks depending on the stage of the infection. Non-compliant patients can be treated with a single dose of benzathine penicillin G 2.4 g intramuscularly. These long-acting penicillins are not generally available in the UK but are imported directly by GUM clinics.

The *Jarisch–Herxheimer reaction*, which is due to release of TNF-α, IL-6 and IL-8, is seen in 50% of patients with primary syphilis and up to 90% of patients with secondary syphilis. It occurs about 8 hours after the first injection and usually consists of mild fever, malaise and headache lasting several hours. In cardiovascular or neurosyphilis the reaction, although rare, may be severe and exacerbate the clinical manifestations. Prednisolone given for 24 hours prior to therapy may ameliorate the reaction but there is little evidence to support its use. Penicillin should not be withheld because of the Jarisch–Herxheimer reaction; since it is not a dose-related phenomenon, there is no value in giving a smaller dose.

The prognosis depends on the stage at which the infection is treated. Early and early latent syphilis have an excellent outlook but once extensive tissue damage has occurred in the later stages the damage will not be reversed although the process may be halted. Symptoms in cardiovascular and neurosyphilis may therefore persist.

All patients treated for early syphilis must be followed up at regular intervals for the first year following treatment. Serological markers should be followed and a fall in titre of the VDRL/RPR of at least fourfold is consistent with adequate treatment for early syphilis. The sexual partners of all patients with syphilis and the parents and siblings of patients with congenital syphilis must be contacted and screened. Babies born to mothers who have been treated for syphilis in pregnancy are retreated at birth.

Chancroid

Chancroid or soft chancre is an acute STI caused by *Haemophilus ducreyi*. It is probably the commonest cause of genital ulceration world-wide, and is prevalent in parts of Africa and Asia. Epidemiological studies in Africa have shown an association between genital ulcer disease, frequently chancroid, and the acquisition of HIV infection. A new urgency to control chancroid has resulted from these observations.

Clinical features

The incubation period is 3–10 days. At the site of inoculation an erythematous papular lesion forms which then breaks down into an ulcer. The ulcer frequently has a necrotic base, a ragged edge, bleeds easily and is painful. Several ulcers may merge to form giant serpiginous lesions. Ulcers appear most commonly on the prepuce and frenulum in men and can erode through tissues. In women the most commonly affected site is the vaginal entrance and the perineum. The lesions in women sometimes go unnoticed.

At the same time, inguinal lymphadenopathy develops (usually unilateral) and can progress to form large buboes which suppurate.

Diagnosis and treatment

Chancroid must be differentiated from other genital ulcer diseases (see Table 2.48). Co-infection with syphilis and herpes simplex is common. Isolation of *H. ducreyi* in specialized culture media is definitive but difficult. Swabs should be taken from the ulcer and material aspirated from the local lymph nodes for culture. Polymerase chain reaction (PCR) techniques are available. Gram stains of clinical material may show characteristic coccobacilli.

Single-dose regimens include azithromycin 1 g orally or ceftriaxone 250 mg i.m. Other regimens include ciprofloxacin 500 mg twice daily for 3 days, erythromycin 500 mg four times daily for 7 days. Clinically significant plasmid-mediated antibiotic resistance in *H. ducreyi* is developing.

Patients should be followed up at 3–7 days, when if treatment is successful ulcers will be responding.

Sexual partners should be examined and treated epidemiologically, as asymptomatic carriage has been reported.

HIV-infected patients should be closely monitored, as healing may be slower. Multiple-dose regimens are needed in HIV patients since treatment failures have been reported with single-dose therapy.

Donovanosis

Donovanosis is the least common of all STIs in North America and Europe, but is endemic in the tropics and subtropics, particularly the Caribbean, South East Asia and South India. Infection is caused by *Klebsiella granulomatis*, a short, encapsulated Gram-negative bacillus. The infection was also known as granuloma inguinale. Although sexual contact appears to be the most usual mode of transmission, the infection rates are low, even between sexual partners of many years' standing.

Clinical features

In the vast majority of patients, the characteristic, heaped-up ulcerating lesion with prolific red granulation tissue appears on the external genitalia, perianal skin or the inguinal region within 1–4 weeks of exposure. It is rarely painful. Almost any cutaneous or mucous membrane site can be involved, including the mouth and anorectal regions. Extension of the primary infection from the external genitalia to the inguinal regions produces the characteristic lesion, the 'pseudo-bubo'.

Diagnosis and treatment

The clinical appearance usually strongly suggests the diagnosis but *K. granulomatis* (Donovan bodies) can be identified intracellularly in scrapings or biopsies of an ulcer. Successful culture has only recently been reported and PCR techniques and serological methods of diagnosis are being developed, but none is routinely available.

Antibiotic treatment should be given until the lesions have healed. A minimum of 3 weeks' treatment is recommended. Regimens include doxycycline 100 mg twice daily, co-trimoxazole 960 mg twice daily, azithromycin 500 mg daily or 1 g weekly, or ceftriaxone 1 g daily.

Sexual partners should be examined and treated if necessary.

Herpes simplex (p. 43)

Genital herpes is one of the most common STIs worldwide. Between 1997 and 2002 there has been a 17% increase in diagnoses of genital herpes in the UK. The peak incidence is in 16- to 24-year-olds of both sexes. Infection may be either primary or recurrent. Transmission occurs during close contact with a person who is shedding virus. Most genital herpes is due to type 2. Genital contact with oral lesions caused by HSV-1 can also produce genital infection.

Susceptible mucous membranes include the genital tract, rectum, mouth and oropharynx. The virus has the ability to establish latency in the dorsal root ganglia by ascending peripheral sensory nerves from the area of inoculation. It is this ability which allows for recurrent attacks.

Clinical features

Asymptomatic infection has been reported but is rare. Primary genital herpes is usually accompanied by systemic symptoms of varying severity including fever, myalgia and headache. Multiple painful shallow ulcers develop which may coalesce (Fig. 2.43). Atypical lesions are common. Tender inguinal lymphadenopathy is usual. Over a period of 10–14 days the lesions develop crusts and dry. In women with vulval lesions the cervix is almost always involved. Rectal infection may lead to a florid proctitis. Neurological complications can include aseptic encephalitis and/or involvement of the sacral autonomic plexus leading to retention of urine.

Recurrent attacks occur in a significant proportion of people following the initial episode. Precipitating factors vary, as does the frequency of recurrence. A symptom prodrome is present in some people prior to the appearance of lesions. Systemic symptoms are rare in recurrent attacks.

The clinical manifestations in immunosuppressed patients (including those with HIV) may be more severe,

Fig. 2.43 **Herpes simplex rash on the penis.** Courtesy of Dr B Goh.

asymptomatic shedding increased, and recurrences occur with greater frequency. Systemic spread has been documented (see p. 139).

Diagnosis

Although the history and examination can be highly suggestive of HSV infection, a firm diagnosis can be made only on the basis of isolation of virus from lesions. Swabs should be taken from the base of lesions and placed in viral transport medium. Virus is most easily isolated from new lesions. Type-specific immune responses can be found 8–12 weeks following primary infection and may form the basis for newer serological assays, although these are not yet available in routine clinical practice.

Management

Primary

Saltwater bathing or sitting in a warm bath is soothing and may allow the patient to pass urine with some degree of comfort. Aciclovir 200 mg five times daily, famciclovir 250 mg three times daily or valaciclovir 500 mg twice daily, all for 5 days, are useful if patients are seen whilst new lesions are still forming. If lesions are already crusting, antiviral therapy will do little to change the clinical course. Secondary bacterial infection occasionally occurs and should be treated. Rest, analgesia and antipyretics should be advised. In rare instances patients may need to be admitted to hospital and aciclovir given intravenously, particularly if HSV encephalitis is suspected.

Recurrence

Recurrent attacks tend to be less severe and can be managed with simple measures such as saltwater bathing. Psychological morbidity is associated with recurrent genital herpes and frequent recurrences impose strains on relationships; patients need considerable support. Long-term suppressive therapy is given in patients with frequent recurrences. An initial course of aciclovir 400 mg twice daily or valaciclovir 250 mg twice daily for 6–12 months significantly reduces the frequency of attacks, although there may still be some breakthrough. Therapy should be discontinued after 12 months and the frequency of recurrent attacks reassessed.

HSV in pregnancy

The potential risk of infection to the neonate needs to be considered in addition to the health of the mother. Infection occurs either transplacentally or via the birth canal. If HSV is acquired for the first time during pregnancy, transplacental infection of the fetus may, rarely, occur. Management of primary HSV in the first or second trimester will depend on the woman's clinical condition and aciclovir can be prescribed in standard doses. Aciclovir therapy during the last 4 weeks of pregnancy may prevent recurrence at term.

Primary acquisition in the third trimester or at term with high levels of viral shedding usually leads to delivery by caesarean section.

For women with previous infection, concern focuses on the baby acquiring HSV from the birth canal. The risk is very low in recurrent attacks. For women with recurrent episodes, only those with genital lesions at the onset of labour are delivered by caesarean section. Sequential cultures during the last weeks of pregnancy to predict viral shedding at term are no longer indicated.

Prevention and control

Patients must be advised that they are infectious when lesions are present; sexual intercourse should be avoided during this time or during prodromal stages. Condoms may not be effective as lesions may occur outside the areas covered. Sexual partners should be examined and may need information on avoiding infection.

Warts

Anogenital warts are amongst the most common sexually acquired infections. The causative agent is human papillomavirus (HPV) especially types 6 and 11 (p. 48). HPV is acquired by direct sexual contact with a person with either clinical or subclinical infection. Genital HPV infection is common, with only a small proportion of those infected being symptomatic. Neonates may acquire HPV from an infected birth canal, which may result either in anogenital warts or in laryngeal papillomas. The incubation period ranges from 2 weeks to 8 months or even longer.

Clinical features

Warts develop around the external genitalia in women, usually starting at the fourchette, and involve the perianal region. The vagina may be infected. Flat warts may develop on the cervix and are not easily visible on routine examination. Such lesions are associated with cervical intraepithelial neoplasia. In men the penile shaft and subpreputial space are the most common sites, although warts involve the urethra and meatus. Perianal lesions are more common in men who practise ano-receptive intercourse but can be found in any patient. The rectum may become involved. Warts become more florid during pregnancy or in immunosuppressed patients.

Diagnosis

The diagnosis is essentially clinical. It is critical to differentiate condylomata lata of secondary syphilis.

Unusual lesions should be biopsied if the diagnosis is in doubt. Up to 30% of patients have coexisting infections with other STIs and a full screen must be performed.

Treatment

Significant failure and relapse rates are seen with current treatment modalities. Choice of treatment will depend on the number and distribution of lesions. Local agents, including podophyllin extract (15–25% solution, once or twice weekly), podophyllotoxin (0.5% solution or 1.5% cream in cycles), and trichloroacetic acid, are useful for non-keratinized lesions. Those that are keratinized respond better to physical therapy, e.g. cryotherapy, electrocautery or laser ablation. Imiquimod (5% cream used three times a week) is indicated in both types. Podophyllin, podophyllotoxin and imiquimod are not advised in pregnancy.

Sexual contacts should be examined and treated if necessary. In view of the difficulties of diagnosing subclinical HPV, condoms should be used for up to 8 months after treatment. Because of the association of HPV with cervical intraepithelial neoplasia, women with warts and female partners of men with warts are advised to have regular cervical screening, i.e. every 3 years. Colposcopy may be useful in women with vaginal and cervical warts.

Hepatitis B

This is discussed in Chapter 7. Sexual contacts should be screened and given vaccine if they are not immune (see p. 366).

Trichomoniasis

Trichomonas vaginalis (TV) is a flagellated protozoon which is predominantly sexually transmitted. It is able to attach to squamous epithelium and can infect the vagina and urethra. *Trichomonas* may be acquired perinatally in babies born to infected mothers.

Infected women may, unusually, be asymptomatic. Commonly the major complaints are of vaginal discharge which is offensive and of local irritation. Men usually present as the asymptomatic sexual partners of infected women, although they may complain of urethral discharge, irritation or urinary frequency.

Examination often reveals a frothy yellowish vaginal discharge and erythematous vaginal walls. The cervix may have multiple small haemorrhagic areas which lead to the description 'strawberry cervix'. *Trichomonas* infection in pregnancy has been associated with preterm delivery and low birth-weight.

Diagnosis and treatment

Phase-contrast, dark-ground microscopy of a drop of vaginal discharge shows TV swimming with a characteristic motion in 40–80% of female patients. Similar preparations from the male urethra will only be positive in about 30% of cases. Many polymorphonuclear leuco-cytes are also seen. Culture techniques are good and confirm the diagnosis. *Trichomonas* is sometimes observed on cervical cytology with a 60–80% accuracy in diagnosis. New, highly sensitive and specific tests based on polymerase chain reactions are in development.

Metronidazole is the treatment of choice, either 2 g orally as a single dose or 400 mg twice-daily for 7 days. There is some evidence of metronidazole resistance and nimorazole may be effective in these cases. Topical therapy with intravaginal tinidazole can be effective, but if extravaginal infection exists this may not be eradicated and vaginal infection reoccurs. Male partners should be treated, especially as they are likely to be asymptomatic and more difficult to detect.

Candidiasis

Vulvovaginal infection with *Candida albicans* is extremely common. The organism is also responsible for balanitis in men. *Candida* can be isolated from the vagina in a high proportion of women of childbearing age, many of whom will have no symptoms.

The role of *Candida* as pathogen or commensal is difficult to disentangle and it may be changes in host environment which allow the organism to produce pathological effects. Predisposing factors include pregnancy, diabetes, and the use of broad-spectrum antibiotics and corticosteroids. Immunosuppression can result in more florid infection.

Clinical features

In women, pruritus vulvae is the dominant symptom. Vaginal discharge is present in varying degree. Many women have only one or occasional isolated episodes. Recurrent candidiasis (four or more symptomatic episodes annually) occurs in up to 5% of healthy women of reproductive age. Examination reveals erythema and swelling of the vulva with broken skin in severe cases. The vagina may contain adherent curdy discharge. Men may have a florid balanoposthitis. More commonly, self-limiting burning penile irritation immediately after sexual intercourse with an infected partner is described. Diabetes must be excluded in men with balanoposthitis.

Diagnosis

Microscopic examination of a smear from the vaginal wall reveals the presence of spores and mycelia. Culture of swabs should be undertaken but may be positive in women with no symptoms. *Trichomonas* and bacterial vaginosis must be considered in women with itch and discharge.

Treatment

Topical. Pessaries or creams containing one of the imidazole antifungals such as clotrimazole 500 mg single dose used intravaginally are usually effective. Nystatin is also useful.

Oral. The triazole drugs such as fluconazole 150 mg as a single dose or itraconazole 200 mg twice in 1 day are used systemically where topical therapy has failed or is inappropriate. Recurrent candidiasis may be treated with fluconazole 100 mg weekly for 6 months, or clotrimazole pessary 500 mg weekly for 6 months.

The evidence for sexual transmission of *Candida* is slight and there is no evidence that treatment of male partners reduces recurrences in women.

Bacterial vaginosis

Bacterial vaginosis (BV) is a disorder characterized by an offensive vaginal discharge. The aetiology and pathogenesis are unclear but a mixed flora of *Gardnerella vaginalis*, anaerobes including *Bacteroides, Mobiluncus* spp. and *Mycoplasma hominis*, replaces the normal lactobacilli of the vagina. Amines and their breakdown products from the abnormal vaginal flora are thought to be responsible for the characteristic odour associated with the condition. As vaginal inflammation is not part of the syndrome the term vaginosis is used rather than vaginitis. The condition has been shown to more common in black women than in white. It is not regarded as a sexually transmitted disease.

Clinical features

Vaginal discharge and odour are the most common complaints although a proportion of women are asymptomatic. A homogeneous, greyish white, adherent discharge is present in the vagina, the pH of which is raised (greater than 5). Associated complications are ill-defined but may include chorioamnionitis and an increased incidence of premature labour in pregnant women. Whether BV disposes non-pregnant women to upper genital tract infection is unclear.

Diagnosis

Different authors have differing criteria for making the diagnosis of BV. In general it is accepted that three of the following should be present for the diagnosis to be made:

- characteristic vaginal discharge
- the amine test: raised vaginal pH using narrow-range indicator paper (> 4.7)
- a fishy odour on mixing a drop of discharge with 10% potassium hydroxide
- the presence of clue cells on microscopic examination of the vaginal fluid.

Clue cells are squamous epithelial cells from the vagina which have bacteria adherent to their surface, giving a granular appearance to the cell. A Gram stain gives a typical reaction of partial stain uptake.

Treatment

Metronidazole given orally in doses of 400 mg twice daily for 5–7 days is usually recommended. A single dose of 2 g metronidazole is less effective. Topical 2% clindamycin cream 5 g intravaginally once daily for 7 days is effective.

Recurrence is high, with some studies giving a rate of 80% within 9 months of completing metronidazole therapy. There is debate over the treatment of asymp-

tomatic women who fulfil the diagnostic criteria for BV. The diagnosis should be fully discussed and treatment offered if the woman wishes. Until the relevance of BV to other pelvic infections is elucidated, the treatment of asymptomatic women with BV is not to be recommended. There is no convincing evidence that simultaneous treatment of the male partner influences the rate of recurrence of BV, and routine treatment of male partners is not indicated.

INFESTATIONS (see also p. 1326)

Pediculosis pubis

The pubic louse (*Phthirus pubis*) is a blood-sucking insect which attaches tightly to the pubic hair. They may also attach to eyelashes and eyebrows. It is relatively host-specific and is transferred only by close bodily contact. Eggs (nits) are laid at hair bases and usually hatch within a week. Although infestation may be asymptomatic the most common complaint is of itch.

Diagnosis

Lice may be seen on the skin at the base of pubic and other body hairs. They resemble small scabs or freckles but if they are picked up with forceps and placed on a microscope slide will move and walk away. Blue macules may be seen at the feeding sites. Nits are usually closely adherent to hairs. Both are highly characteristic under the low-power microscope.

As with all sexually transmitted infections, the patient must be screened for coexisting pathogens.

Treatment

Both lice and eggs must be killed with 0.5% malathion, 1% permethrin or 0.5% carbaryl. The preparation should be applied to all areas of the body from the neck down and washed off after 12 hours. In a few cases a further application after 1 week may be necessary. For severe infestations, antipruritics may be indicated for the first 48 hours. All sexual partners should be seen and screened.

Scabies

This is discussed on page 1325.

FURTHER READING

Adler M (2004) *The ABC of Sexually Transmitted Diseases*, 5th edn. London: BMA Books.

British Association of Sexual Health and HIV. Clinical effectiveness guidelines: http://www.bashh.org/guidelines/ceguidelines.htm August 2004.

Brown AE, Sadler KE, Tomkins SE et al. (2004) Recent trends in HIV and other STIs in the United Kingdom: data to the end of 2002. *Sexually Transmitted Infections* 80(3): 159–166.

Centers for Disease Control and Prevention (2002) Sexual assault and STDs. Sexually transmitted diseases treatment guidelines. *MMWR Recommendations and Reports* 51(RR-6): 69–74.

Donovan B (2004) Sexually transmissible infections other than HIV. *Lancet* **363**(9408): 545–556.

Health Protection Agency (2003). *Renewing the Focus: HIV and Other Sexually Transmitted Infections in the United Kingdom in 2002.* London: HPA.

Klausner JD, Kent CK (2004) HIV and sexually transmitted diseases. Latest views on synergy, treatment, and screening. *Postgraduate Medicine* **115**(4): 79–84.

Lacey, H (2001) *National Guidelines on the Management of Adult Victims of Sexual Assault.* Online. Available: http://www.bashh.org/guidelines/ceguidelines. htm (accessed August 2004).

HUMAN IMMUNE DEFICIENCY VIRUS (HIV) AND AIDS

Epidemiology

HIV, the cause of the acquired immune deficiency syndrome (AIDS), continues to spread, being described as a global health emergency by the World Health Organization (WHO) in 2003. UNAIDS estimates for 2002 are that 41 million people are infected with HIV worldwide, over 70% of whom are in sub-Saharan Africa. Approximately 16 000 new infections occur daily, the majority in young adults. HIV is now the leading single cause of death in adults, causing 5 million deaths in 2003. In sub-Saharan Africa 5000 men and women and 1000 children die of HIV every 24 hours. Dramatic rises in infection have been seen in SE Asia with eastern Europe and Russia having the most rapidly expanding epidemic in 2003.

The human and economic costs are huge – 33% of 15-year-olds in high-prevalence countries in Africa will die of HIV, life expectancy in African countries is falling with an inevitable impact on the fabric of society and on economic growth and stability. The advent of more effective therapy for HIV has brought geographical differences in the impact of the epidemic into stark relief, with falling mortality and morbidity in resource-rich settings that are unmatched in poorer parts of the world. Although in the UK and other wealthy countries deaths from HIV have fallen, new diagnoses are rising sharply. At least 5000 new diagnoses were recorded in the UK in 2003, a 20% increase over the preceding year, and the highest annual number since surveillance began, with the result that prevalence is rising. Demographics have varied greatly within different regions influenced by social, behavioural, cultural and political factors. Despite the fact that HIV can be isolated from a wide range of body fluids and tissues, the majority of infections are transmitted via semen, cervical secretions and blood. The character of the epidemic in different regions of the world has been influenced by the relative frequency of each of the routes of transmission.

Sexual intercourse (vaginal and anal)

Globally, heterosexual intercourse accounts for the vast majority of infections, and coexistent STIs, especially those causing genital ulceration, enhance transmission. Passage of HIV appears to be more efficient from men to women, and to the passive partner in anal intercourse, than vice versa.

In the UK, sex between men still accounts for over half the infections reported, but there is an increasing rate of heterosexual transmission. Between 2000 and 2003 53% of new diagnoses were a result of heterosexual exposure, frequently in high-endemicity countries. Of these infections, 67% were in women compared to 5% in the late 1980s. In central and sub-Saharan Africa the epidemic has always been heterosexual and more than half the infected adults in these regions are women. South East Asia and the Indian subcontinent are experiencing an explosive epidemic, driven by heterosexual intercourse and a high incidence of other sexually transmitted diseases.

Mother to child (parentally, perinatally, breast-feeding)

Vertical transmission is the most common route of HIV infection in children. European studies suggest that, without intervention, 15% of babies born to HIV-infected mothers are likely to be infected, although rates of up to 40% have been reported from Africa and the USA. Increased vertical transmission is associated with advanced disease in the mother, maternal viral load, prolonged and premature rupture of membranes, and chorioamnionitis. Transmission can occur in utero although the majority of infections take place perinatally. Breast-feeding has been shown to increase the risk of vertical transmission by up to 20%. In the developed world interventions to reduce vertical transmission, including the use of antiretroviral agents, delivery by caesarean section and the avoidance of breast-feeding have led to a dramatic fall in the numbers of infected children. The lack of access to these interventions in resource-poor countries in which 90% of infections occur is a major issue.

Contaminated blood, blood products and organ donations

Screening of blood and blood products was introduced in 1985 in Europe and North America. Prior to this, HIV infection was associated with the use of clotting factors (for haemophilia) and with blood transfusions. In some developing countries where blood is not screened or treated, and in areas where the rate of new HIV infections is very high, transfusion-associated transmission remains significant.

Contaminated needles (intravenous drug misuse, injections, needle-stick injuries)

The practice of sharing needles and syringes for intravenous drug use continues to be a major route of transmission of HIV in both developed countries and parts of South East Asia, Latin America and the states of the former Soviet Union. In some areas, including the UK, successful education and needle exchange schemes have reduced the rate of transmission by this route. Iatrogenic transmission from needles and syringes used in developing countries is reported. Healthcare workers have a risk of approximately 0.3% following a single needle-stick injury with known HIV infected blood.

There is no evidence that HIV is spread by social or household contact or by blood-sucking insects such as mosquitoes and bed bugs.

The virus

HIV belongs to the lentivirus group of the retrovirus family. There are at least two types, HIV-1 and HIV-2. HIV-2 is almost entirely confined to West Africa although there is evidence of some spread to the Indian subcontinent. HIV-2 is associated with an AIDS-type illness although it may be more indolent in nature. The structure of the virus is shown in Figure 2.44.

Retroviruses are characterized by the possession of the enzyme reverse transcriptase, which allows viral RNA to be transcribed into DNA, and thence incorporated into the host cell genome. Reverse transcription is an error-prone process with a significant rate of misincorporation of bases. This, combined with a high rate of viral turnover, leads to considerable genetic variation and a diversity of viral subtypes or clades. On the basis of DNA sequencing, HIV-1 is divided into two subtypes:

- *Group M (major) subtypes.* There are at least 10, which are denoted A–J. There is a predominance of subtype B in Europe, North America and Australia, but areas of

central and sub-Saharan Africa have multiple M subtypes.
- *Group O (outlier) subtypes.* These are highly divergent from group M and are confined to small numbers centred on the Cameroons.

Recombination of viral material generates an array of circulating recombinant forms (CRFs), which increases the genetic diversity that may be encountered.

Connections between genetic diversity and biological effects, in particular pathogenicity, rates of transmission and response to therapy, are being sought.

Pathogenesis

The interrelationship between HIV and the host immune system is the basis of the pathogenesis of HIV disease. The host cellular receptor that is recognized by HIV surface glycoprotein is the CD4 molecule, which defines the cell populations that are susceptible to infection (Fig. 2.45). The interaction between CD4 and HIV surface glycoprotein together with chemokine co-receptors CCR5 and CXCR4 is responsible for HIV entry into cells. Mutations in the gene expressing the receptor for chemokine CCR5 may impair entry of HIV into cells and therefore confer some resistance to this infection. Auxiliary viral proteins such as those coded by the *Nef* gene have a role in influencing host cell membrane proteins and signal transduction pathways. CD4 receptors and HIV surface glycoprotein interactions mediate the process of syncytium formation, which is a cytopathic effect of HIV infection.

Studies of viral turnover in HIV-infected individuals have demonstrated a virus half-life in the circulation of about 6 hours. To maintain observed levels of plasma viraemia, 10^8–10^9 virus particles need to be released and cleared daily. Virus production by infected cells lasts for about 2 days and is probably limited by the death of the cell, owing to direct HIV effects, linking HIV replication to the process of CD4 destruction and depletion. Studies suggest that immunopathogenesis is a result of defective T cell homeostasis in HIV infection. The progressive and severe depletion of CD4 helper lymphocytes has profound repercussions for the functioning of the immune system (see p. 1218). Cell-mediated immunodeficiency, which is the major consequence, leaves the host open to infections with intracellular pathogens, whilst the co-existing antibody abnormalities predispose to infections with capsulated bacteria. HIV also has a direct effect on certain tissues, notably the nervous system.

Diagnosis and natural history (Fig. 2.46)

HIV infection is diagnosed either by the detection of virus-specific antibodies (anti-HIV) or by direct identification of viral material.

Detection of IgG antibody to envelope components (gp120 and its subunits). This is the most commonly used marker of infection. The routine tests used for screening are based on ELISA techniques, which may be confirmed with Western blot assays. Up to 3 months

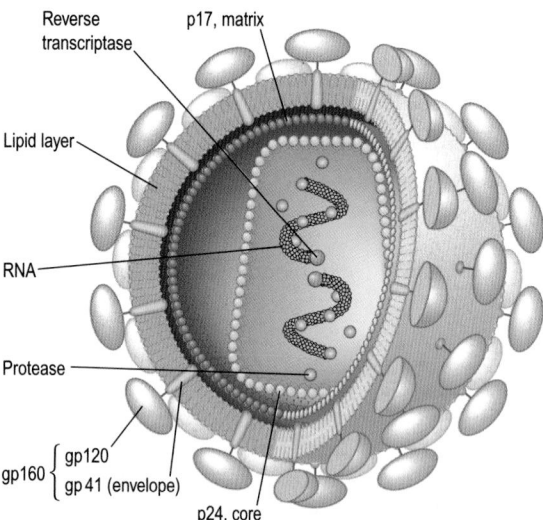

Fig. 2.44 **Structure of HIV.** Two molecules of single-stranded RNA are shown within the nucleus. The reverse transcriptase polymerase converts viral RNA into DNA (a characteristic of retroviruses). The protease includes integrase (p32 and p10). The p24 (core protein) levels can be used to monitor HIV disease. p17 is the matrix protein. gp120 is the outer envelope glycoprotein which binds to cell surface CD4 molecules. gp41, a transmembrane protein, influences infectivity and cell fusion capacity.

Reverse transcriptase
p17, matrix
Lipid layer
RNA
Protease
gp160 { gp120
gp 41 (envelope)
p24, core

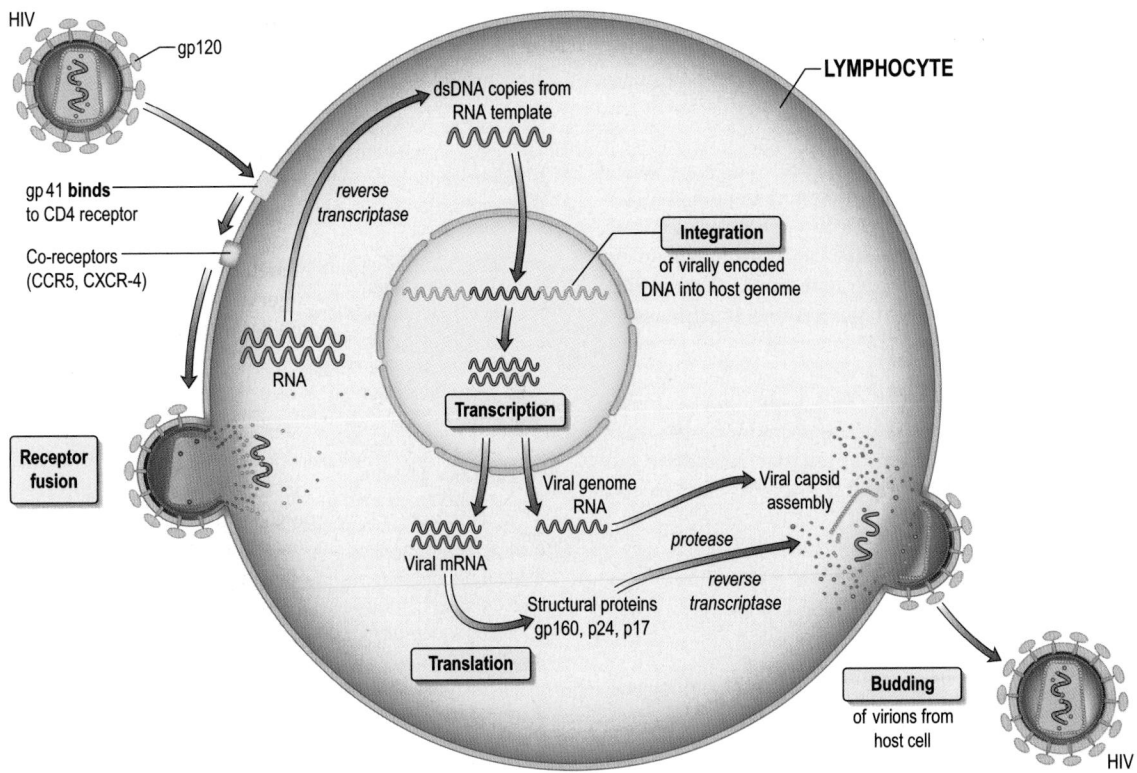

Fig. 2.45 **HIV entry and replication in CD4 T lymphocytes.** The human immune deficiency virus binds to the host CD4 inoculate via the envelope glycoprotein gp120. gp41 binds to the cell chemokine causing receptor fusion and uncoating of RNA. DNA copies are made from both RNA templates (reverse transcriptase). The enzyme polymerase from the host cell leads to formation of dsDNA. In the nucleus the virally encoded DNA is inserted into the host genome (integration). Regulatory proteins control transcription (a process in which an RNA molecule is synthesized from a DNA template). The virus is reassembled in the cytoplasm and budded out from the host cell.

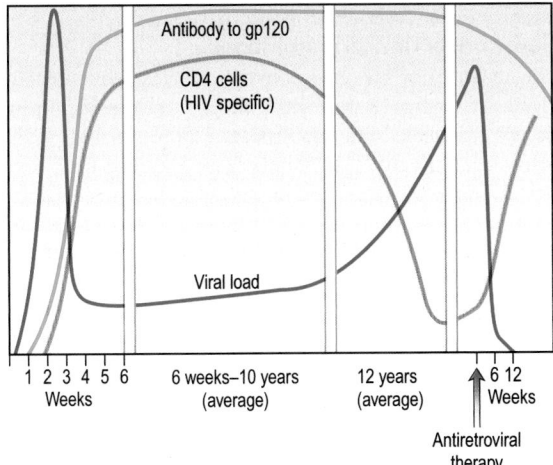

Fig. 2.46 **The immune response to HIV (seroconversion).**

may elapse from initial infection to antibody detection (serological latency, or window period). These antibodies to HIV have no protective function and persist for life. As with all IgG antibodies, anti-HIV will cross the placenta. All babies born to HIV-infected women will thus have the antibody at birth. In this situation, anti-HIV antibody is not a reliable marker of active infection, and in uninfected babies will be gradually lost over the first 18 months of life.

Other than in exceptional circumstances, HIV antibody testing should be carried out only after full discussion of the implications with the patient and with the patient's express consent.

Simple and rapid HIV antibody assays are increasingly available, giving results within hours. Such assays are easy to perform and require little or no additional equipment. They are designed for use with individual or a limited number of samples, Assays that can utilize alternative body fluids to serum/plasma such as saliva, whole blood and urine are becoming accessible.

A serologic testing algorithm for recent HIV seroconversions (STARHS) can be used to identify recently acquired infection. A highly sensitive ELISA that is able to detect HIV antibodies 6–8 weeks after infection is paired with a less sensitive (detuned) test that identifies later HIV antibodies within 130 days. A positive result on the sensitive test and a negative 'detuned' test are indicative of recent infection, whilst positive results on both tests point to an infection that is more than 130 days old. The major application of this is in epidemic surveillance and monitoring.

IgG antibody to p24 (anti-p24). This can be detected from the earliest weeks of infection and through the asymptomatic phase. It is frequently lost as disease progresses.

Antigen assays. Nucleic acid-based assays are available which amplify and test for components of the HIV genome. These assays are used to aid diagnosis of HIV in the babies of HIV-infected mothers or in situations where serological tests may be inadequate, such as subtyping HIV variants for medicolegal reasons. (See the discussion of viral load monitoring, p. 143.)

Viral p24 antigen (p24ag). This is detectable shortly after infection but has usually disappeared by 8–10 weeks after exposure. It can be a useful marker in individuals who have been infected recently but have not had time to mount an antibody response.

Isolation of virus in culture. This is a specialized technique available in some laboratories to aid diagnosis and as a research tool.

CLINICAL FEATURES OF HIV INFECTION

The spectrum of illnesses associated with HIV infection is broad and is the result of both direct HIV effects and the associated immune dysfunction. Several classification systems exist, the most widely used being the 1993 Centers for Disease Control (CDC) classification (Box 2.16). This classification depends to a large extent on definitive diagnoses of infection, which makes it more difficult to use in those areas of the world without sophisticated laboratory support. As immunosuppression progresses the patient is susceptible to an increasing range of opportunistic infections and tumours, certain of which meet the criteria for the diagnosis of AIDS (Box 2.17).

Since 1993 the definition of AIDS has differed between the USA and Europe. The USA definition includes individuals with CD4 counts below 200 in addition to the clinical classification based on the presence of specific indicator diagnoses shown in Box 2.17. In Europe the definition remains based on the diagnosis of specific clinical conditions with no inclusion of CD4 lymphocyte counts.

> **Box 2.17 AIDS-defining conditions**
>
> - Candidiasis of bronchi, trachea or lungs
> - Candidiasis, oesophageal
> - Cervical carcinoma, invasive
> - Coccidioidomycosis, disseminated or extrapulmonary
> - Cryptococcosis, extrapulmonary
> - Cryptosporidiosis, chronic intestinal (1-month duration)
> - Cytomegalovirus (CMV) disease (other than liver, spleen or nodes)
> - CMV retinitis (with loss of vision)
> - Encephalopathy, HIV-related
> - Herpes simplex, chronic ulcers (1-month duration); or bronchitis, pneumonitis or oesophagitis
> - Histoplasmosis, disseminated or extrapulmonary
> - Isosporiasis; chronic intestinal (1-month duration)
> - Kaposi's sarcoma
> - Lymphoma, Burkitt's
> - Lymphoma, immunoblastic (or equivalent term)
> - Lymphoma (primary) of brain
> - *Mycobacterium avium-intracellulare* complex or *M. kansasii*, disseminated or extrapulmonary
> - *Mycobacterium tuberculosis*, any site
> - *Mycobacterium*, other species or unidentified species, disseminated or extrapulmonary
> - *Pneumocystis carinii* pneumonia
> - Pneumonia, recurrent
> - Progressive multifocal leucoencephalopathy
> - *Salmonella* septicaemia, recurrent
> - Toxoplasmosis of brain
> - Wasting syndrome, due to HIV

Incubation

The 2–4 weeks immediately following infection are usually silent both clinically and serologically.

Seroconversion/primary illness

The majority of HIV seroconversions are also clinically silent. In a proportion, a self-limiting non-specific illness occurs 6–8 weeks after exposure. Symptoms include fever, arthralgia, myalgia, lethargy, lymphadenopathy, sore throat, mucosal ulcers and occasionally a transient faint pink maculopapular rash. Neurological symptoms are common, including headache, photophobia, myelopathy, neuropathy and in rare cases encephalopathy. The illness lasts up to 3 weeks and recovery is usually complete.

> **Box 2.16 Summary of CDC classification of HIV infection**
>
> | Absolute CD4 count (/mm³) | A: Asymptomatic OR persistent generalized lymphadenopathy OR acute seroconversion illness | B: HIV-related conditions,* not A or C | C: Clinical conditions listed in AIDS surveillance case definition (see Box 2.17) |
> |---|---|---|---|
> | > 500 | A1 | B1 | C1 |
> | 200–499 | A2 | B2 | C2 |
> | < 200 | A3 | B3 | C4 |
>
> * Examples of category B conditions include: bacillary angiomatosis, candidiasis (oropharyngeal), constitutional symptoms, oral hairy leucoplakia, herpes zoster involving more than one dermatome, idiopathic thrombocytopenic purpura, listeriosis, pelvic inflammatory disease especially if complicated by tubo-ovarian abscess, peripheral neuropathy

Laboratory abnormalities include lymphopenia with atypical reactive lymphocytes noted on blood film, thrombocytopenia and raised liver enzymes. CD4 lymphocytes may be markedly depleted and the CD4 : CD8 ratio reversed. Antibodies to HIV may be absent during this early stage of infection, although the level of circulating viral RNA is high and p24 core protein may be detectable. Patients experiencing a seroconversion illness may have a more rapidly progressive course of infection.

Clinical latency

The majority of people with HIV infection are asymptomatic for a substantial but variable length of time. However, the virus continues to replicate and the person is infectious. Studies suggest a median time of 10 years from infection to development of AIDS, although some patients progress much more rapidly and others have remained symptom-free for up to 15 years. Older age is associated with more rapid progression, and the influence of putative protective genetic factors is under scrutiny. Gender and pregnancy per se do not appear to influence the rate of progression, although women may fare less well for a variety of reasons. A subgroup of patients with asymptomatic infection have persistent generalized lymphadenopathy (PGL), defined as lymphadenopathy (> 1 cm) at two or more extrainguinal sites for more than 3 months in the absence of causes other than HIV infection. The nodes are usually symmetrical, firm, mobile and non-tender. There may be associated splenomegaly. The architecture of the nodes shows hyperplasia of the follicles and proliferation of the capillary endothelium. Biopsy is rarely indicated. Similar disease progression has been noted in asymptomatic patients with or without PGL. Nodes may disappear with disease progression.

Symptomatic HIV infection

As HIV infection progresses the viral load rises, the CD4 count falls, and the patient develops an array of symptoms and signs. The clinical picture is the result of direct HIV effects and of the associated immunosuppression.

In an individual patient the clinical consequences of HIV-related immune dysfunction will depend on at least three factors:

- *The microbial exposure of the patient throughout life.* Many clinical episodes represent reactivation of previously acquired infection, which has been latent. Geographical factors determine the microbial repertoire of an individual patient. Those organisms requiring intact cell-mediated immunity for their control are most likely to cause clinical problems.
- *The pathogenicity of organisms encountered.* High-grade pathogens such as *Mycobacterium tuberculosis*, *Candida* and the herpesviruses are clinically relevant even when immunosuppression is mild, and will thus occur earlier in the course of the disease. Less virulent organisms occur at later stages of immunodeficiency.
- *The degree of immunosuppression of the host.* When patients are severely immunocompromised (CD4 count < $100/mm^3$) disseminated infections with organisms of very low virulence such as *M. avium-intracellulare* (MAI) and *Cryptosporidium* are able to establish themselves. These infections are very resistant to treatment, mainly because there is no functioning immune response to clear organisms. This hierarchy of infection allows for appropriate intervention with prophylactic drugs.

EFFECTS OF HIV INFECTION

Neurological disease

Infection of the nervous tissue occurs at an early stage but clinical neurological involvement increases as HIV advances. This includes AIDS dementia complex (ADC), sensory polyneuropathy and aseptic meningitis (see p. 1241). These conditions are much less common since the introduction of HAART (highly active antiretroviral therapy). The pathogenesis is thought to be due both to the release of neurotoxic products by HIV itself and to cytokine abnormalities secondary to immune dysregulation.

ADC has varying degrees of severity, ranging from mild memory impairment and poor concentration through to severe cognitive deficit, personality change and psychomotor slowing. Changes in affect are common and depressive or psychotic features may be present. The spinal cord may show vacuolar myelopathy histologically. In severe cases brain CT scan shows atrophic change of varying degrees. MRI changes consist of white matter lesions of increased density on T2-weighted sections. EEG may show non-specific changes consistent with encephalopathy. The CSF is usually normal, although the protein concentration may be raised. Patients with mild neurological dysfunction may be unduly sensitive to the effects of other insults such as fever, metabolic disturbance or psychotropic medication, any of which may lead to a marked deterioration in cognitive functioning.

Sensory polyneuropathy is seen frequently in HIV infection, most commonly in the legs and feet, although hands may be affected in advanced disease. In its most severe form it causes intense pain, usually in the feet, which may disrupt sleep, impair mobility and generally reduce the quality of life.

Autonomic neuropathy may also occur with postural hypotension and diarrhoea. Autonomic nerve damage is found in the small bowel. Zalcitabine, didanosine and stavudine produce a similar neuropathy as a major toxic side-effect and must be used with caution in patients with HIV neuropathy.

HAART has a beneficial effect on HIV neurological disease, with startling improvement in cognitive function in many patients with ADC. It may also have a neuroprotective role.

Eye disease

Eye pathology is a regular finding in HIV infection, usually in the later stages. The most serious is cytomegalovirus retinitis (see p. 138), which is sight-threatening. Retinal cotton wool spots due to HIV per se are rarely troublesome but they may be confused with CMV retinitis. Anterior uveitis can present as acute red eye associated with rifabutin therapy for mycobacterial infections in HIV. Steroids used topically are usually effective but modification of the dose of rifabutin is required to prevent relapse. Pneumocystis, toxoplasmosis, syphilis and lymphoma can all affect the retina and the eye may be the site of first presentation.

Mucocutaneous manifestations (see Table 2.52)

The skin is a common site for HIV-related pathology as the function of dendritic and Langerhans' cells, both target cells for HIV, is disrupted. Delayed-type hypersensitivity (p. 226), a good indicator of cell-mediated immunity, is frequently reduced or absent even before clinical signs of immunosuppression appear. Pruritus is a common complaint at all stages of HIV. Generalized dry, itchy, flaky skin is typical and the hair may become thin and dry. An intensely pruritic papular eruption favouring the extremities may be found, particularly in patients from sub-Saharan Africa. Eosinophilic folliculitis presents with urticarial lesions particularly on the face, arms and legs.

Drug reactions with cutaneous manifestations are extremely frequent, with rashes developing notably to sulphur-containing drugs amongst others (see Fig. 23.39, p. 1359). Recurrent aphthous ulceration, which is severe and slow to heal is common and can impair the patient's ability to eat. Biopsy may be indicated to exclude other causes of ulceration. Topical steroids are useful and resistant cases may respond to thalidomide.

In addition to the above the skin is a common site of opportunistic infections (see below).

Haematological complications

Anaemia, neutropenia and thrombocytopenia are all common in advanced HIV infection.

- *Lymphopenia* – this progresses as the CD4 count falls.
- *Anaemia of chronic HIV infection* is usually mild, normochromic and normocytic.
- *Neutropenia* is common and usually mild.
- *Isolated thrombocytopenia* may occur early in infection and be the only manifestation of HIV for some time. Platelet counts are often moderately reduced but can fall dramatically to $10–20 \times 10^9/L$ producing easy bleeding and bruising. Circulating antiplatelet antibodies lead to peripheral destruction. Megakaryocytes are increased in the bone marrow but their function is impaired. Effective antiretroviral therapy usually produces a rise in platelet count. Thrombocytopenic patients undergoing dental, medical or surgical procedures may need therapy with human immunoglobulin, which gives a transient rise in platelet count, or be given platelet transfusion. Steroids are best avoided.
- *Pancytopenia* occurs because of underlying opportunistic infection or malignancies, in particular *Mycobacterium avium-intracellulare*, disseminated cytomegalovirus and lymphoma.

- *Other complications.* Myelotoxic drugs include zidovudine (megaloblastic anaemia, red cell aplasia, neutropenia), lamivudine (anaemia, neutropenia), ganciclovir (neutropenia), systemic chemotherapy (pancytopenia) and co-trimoxazole (agranulocytosis).

Gastrointestinal effects (see p. 335)

Weight loss and diarrhoea are extremely common in HIV-infected patients. Wasting is a common feature of advanced HIV infection, which although originally attributed to direct HIV effects on metabolism, is usually a consequence of anorexia. There is a small increase in resting energy expenditure in all stages of HIV, but weight and lean body mass usually remain normal during periods of clinical latency when the patient is eating normally.

HIV enteropathy is a term that has been used to describe a syndrome of diarrhoea, malabsorption and weight loss for which no other pathology has been found. HIV infection of the lymphocytes (in the lamina propria) which are distributed throughout both the large and small bowel, with disturbance of cytokine production, may be responsible. Villous atrophy is a common histological finding in the small bowel.

Hypochlorhydria is reported in patients with advanced HIV disease and may have consequences for drug absorption and bacterial overgrowth in the gut.

Rectal lymphoid tissue cells are the targets for HIV infection during penetrative anal sex and may be a reservoir for infection to spread through the body.

Renal complications

HIV-associated nephropathy (HIVAN) (see p. 635), although rare, can cause significant renal impairment, particularly in more advanced disease. It is most frequently seen in black male patients and can be exacerbated by heroin use.

Nephrotic syndrome subsequent to *focal glomerulosclerosis* is the usual pathology, which may be a consequence of HIV cytopathic effects on renal tubular epithelium. The course is usually relentlessly progressive and dialysis may be required.

Many nephrotoxic drugs are used in the management of HIV-associated pathology, particularly foscarnet, amphotericin B, pentamidine, sulfadiazine and indinavir.

Respiratory complications

The upper airway and lungs serve as a physical barrier to airborne pathogens and any damage will decrease the efficiency of protection, leading to an increase in upper and lower respiratory tract infections. The sinus mucosa may also function abnormally in HIV infection and is frequently the site of chronic inflammation. Response to antibacterial therapy and topical steroids is usual but some patients require surgical intervention. A similar process is seen in the middle ear, which can lead to chronic otitis media.

Lymphoid interstitial pneumonitis (LIP) is well described in paediatric HIV infection but is uncommon in adults. There is an infiltration of lymphocytes, plasma cells and lymphoblasts in alveolar tissue. Epstein–Barr virus may be present. The patient presents with dyspnoea, and a dry cough, which may be confused with pneumocystis infection (see p. 136). Reticular nodular shadowing is seen on chest X-ray. Therapy with steroids may produce clinical and histological benefit in some patients.

Endocrine complications

Various endocrine abnormalities have been reported, including reduced levels of testosterone and abnormal adrenal function. The latter assumes clinical significance in more advanced disease when intercurrent infection superimposed upon borderline adrenal function precipitates clear adrenal insufficiency requiring replacement doses of gluco- and mineralocorticoid. CMV is also implicated in adrenal-deficient states.

Cardiac complications

Cardiomyopathy, although rare associated with HIV, may lead to congestive cardiac failure. Lymphocytic and necrotic myocarditis have been described. Ventricular biopsy should be performed to ensure other treatable causes of myocarditis are excluded. Antiretrovirals therapy may be helpful.

CONDITIONS ASSOCIATED WITH IMMUNODEFICIENCY

Immunodeficiency allows the development of opportunistic infections (OI) (Table 2.51). These are diseases caused by organisms that are not usually considered pathogenic, unusual presentations of known pathogens, and the occurrence of tumours that may have an oncogenic viral aetiology. Susceptibility increases as the patient becomes more immunosuppressed. CD4 T lymphocyte numbers are used as markers to predict the risk of

Table 2.51 Major HIV-associated pathogens

Protozoa	Bacteria
Toxoplasma gondii	*Salmonella* spp.
Cryptosporidium parvum	*Mycobacterium tuberculosis*
Microsporidia spp.	*M. avium-intracellulare*
Leishmania donovani	*Streptococcus pneumoniae*
Isospora belli	*Staphylococcus aureus*
	Haemophilus influenzae
Viruses	*Moraxella catarrhalis*
Cytomegalovirus	*Rhodococcus equii*
Herpes simplex	*Bartonella quintana*
Varicella zoster	*Nocardia*
Human papillomavirus	
Papovavirus	
Fungi and yeasts	
Pneumocystis carinii	
Cryptococcus neoformans	
Candida spp.	
Dermatophytes (*Trichophyton*)	
Aspergillus fumigatus	
Histoplasma capsulatum	
Coccidioides immitis	

infection. Patients with CD4 counts above 200 are at low risk for the majority of AIDS-defining OIs. A hierarchy of thresholds for specific infectious risks can be constructed. Mechanisms include defective T cell function against protozoa, fungi and viruses, impaired macrophage function against intracellular bacteria such as mycobacteria and salmonella and defective B cell immunity against capsulated bacteria such as *Strep. pneumoniae* and *Haemophilus*. Many of the organisms causing clinical disease are ubiquitous in the environment or are already carried by the patient.

Diagnosis in an immunosuppressed patient may be complicated by a lack of typical signs, as the inflammatory response is impaired. Examples are lack of neck stiffness in cryptococcal meningitis or minimal clinical findings in early *Pneumocystis carinii* pneumonia (PCP). Multiple pathogens may coexist. Indirect serological tests are frequently unreliable. Specimens must be obtained from the appropriate site for examination and culture in order to make a diagnosis.

Opportunistic infections in the HAART era

In many developed countries the mortality and morbidity associated with HIV infection have declined dramatically since the introduction of potent antiretroviral therapy. In the USA the age-adjusted death rate from AIDS fell 48% between 1996 and 1997 and death rates across Europe fell fivefold between 1995 and 1998. European data showed a fall in AIDS defining illnesses (ADI) from 30.7 per 100 patient years of observation to 2.5 per 100 patient years between 1994 and 1998, with patients on HAART having a lower rate of ADIs than patients not on HAART. This trend has continued – recent data from Europe demonstrate a 50% lower incidence of AIDS in 1998–2001 than in 1996–1998, irrespective of CD4 count. Potential long-term adverse effects associated with HAART have not altered its effectiveness in treating AIDS. However the decline has been steeper for some OIs than others, suggesting that the immune reconstitution due to HAART may not be functionally equal against all HIV-associated complications. Importantly not all patients have adequate responses to these medications, even if they are available and tolerable. Immune reconstitution with HAART may produce unusual responses to opportunistic pathogens and confuse the clinical picture. Thus prevention and treatment of OIs remains an integral part of the management of HIV infection.

Prevention of opportunistic infection in HIV-infected patients

Avoid infection

Exposure to certain organisms can be avoided in those known to be HIV infected. Attention to food hygiene will reduce exposure to salmonella, toxoplasmosis and *Cryptosporidium*, and protected sexual intercourse will reduce exposure to herpes simplex virus (HSV), hepatitis B and papillomaviruses. Cytomegalovirus (CMV)-negative patients should be given CMV-negative blood products.

Immunization strategies

Immunization may not be as effective in HIV-infected individuals. Live virus vaccines should not be used (e.g. yellow fever, live polio).

Hepatitis A and B vaccines should be given for those without natural immunity who are at risk, particularly if there is coexisting liver pathology, e.g. hepatitis C.

Chemoprophylaxis

In the absence of a normal immune response, many OIs are hard to eradicate using antimicrobials, and the recurrence rate is high. Primary and secondary chemoprophylaxis has reduced the incidence of many OIs. Advantages must be balanced against the potential for toxicity, drug interactions and cost, with each medication added to what are often complex drug regimens.

Primary prophylaxis has been shown to be effective in reducing the risk of *Pneumocystis carinii*, toxoplasmosis and *Mycobacterium avium-intracellulare*.

Primary prophylaxis is not normally recommended against cytomegalovirus, herpesviruses or fungi.

With the introduction of HAART and immune reconstitution, ongoing chemoprophylaxis for previously life-threatening conditions (e.g. *Pneumocystis carinii*, cytomegalovirus retinitis, cryptococcus, toxoplasmosis, MAI) can be discontinued in those patients with CD4 counts that remain consistently above 200 and who have a low viral load. American guidelines for stopping and restarting prophylaxis have been published. It is necessary to review such decisions as clinical and laboratory parameters change. In developing countries unable to obtain HAART, long-term secondary prophylaxis is advocated. Other less severe but recurrent infections may also warrant prophylaxis (e.g. herpes simplex, candidiasis).

SPECIFIC CONDITIONS ASSOCIATED WITH HIV INFECTION

Fungal infections

Pneumocystis carinii (see p. 95)

This organism most commonly causes pneumonia (PCP) but can cause disseminated infection. It is not usually seen until patients are severely immunocompromised with a CD4 count below 200. The infection remains common although the use of primary prophylaxis in patients with CD4 < 200 has reduced the incidence. The organism damages alveolar epithelium, which impedes gas exchange and reduces lung compliance.

The onset is often insidious over a period of weeks, with a prolonged period of increasing shortness of breath (usually on exertion), non-productive cough, fever and malaise. Clinical examination reveals tachypnoea, tachycardia, cyanosis and signs of hypoxia. Fine crackles are heard on auscultation, although in mild cases there may be no auscultatory abnormality. In early infection the chest X-ray is normal but the typical appearances are of bilateral perihilar interstitial infiltrates, which can pro-

gress to confluent alveolar shadows throughout the lungs. High-resolution CT scans of the chest demonstrate a characteristic ground-glass appearance even when there is little to see on the chest X-ray. The patient is usually hypoxic and desaturates on exercise. Definitive diagnosis rests on demonstrating the organisms in the lungs via bronchoalveolar lavage. As the organism cannot be cultured in vitro it must be directly observed either with silver staining or immunofluorescent techniques.

Treatment should be instituted as early as possible. First-line therapy is with intravenous co-trimoxazole (100 mg/kg per day sulfamethoxazole and 20 mg/kg per day trimethoprim in divided doses) for 21 days. Up to 40% of patients receiving this regimen will develop some adverse drug reaction, including a typical allergic rash. Mutations in the gene for dihydropteroate synthetase in *P. carinii*, which may theoretically lead to co-trimoxazole resistance, have been reported. There is, however, no evidence that co-trimoxazole is becoming less efficacious clinically. If the patient is sensitive to co-trimoxazole, intravenous pentamidine (4 mg/kg per day) or dapsone and trimethoprim are given for the same duration. Atovaquone or a combination of clindamycin and primaquine is also used. In severe cases (P_aO_2 less than 9.5 kPa), systemic corticosteroids have been shown to reduce mortality and should be added. Continuous positive airways pressure (CPAP) or mechanical ventilation (see p. 982) may be required if the patient remains severely hypoxic or becomes too tired. Pneumothorax not uncommonly complicates the clinical course in an already severely hypoxic patient.

Long-term secondary prophylaxis is required in developing countries *without* HAART in patients whose CD4 count remains below 200, and to prevent relapse, the usual regimen being co-trimoxazole 960 mg three times a week. Patients sensitive to sulphonamide are given either dapsone or pyrimethamine or nebulized pentamidine. The latter only protects the lungs and does not penetrate the upper lobes particularly efficiently; hence if relapses occur on this regimen they may be either atypical or extrapulmonary.

Cryptococcus (see p. 93)

The most common presentation of cryptococcus in the context of HIV is meningitis, although pulmonary and disseminated infections can also occur. The organism, *C. neoformans*, is widely distributed – often in bird droppings – and is usually acquired by inhalation. The onset may be insidious with non-specific fever, nausea and headache. As the infection progresses the conscious level is impaired and changes in affect may be noted. Fits or focal neurological presentations are uncommon. Neck stiffness and photophobia may be absent as these signs depend on the inflammatory response of the host, which in this setting is abnormal.

The diagnosis is made on examination of the CSF (a CT scan must be carried out before lumbar puncture to exclude space-occupying pathology). Indian ink staining shows the organisms directly and CSF cryptococcal antigen is positive at variable titre. It is unusual for the cryptococcal antigen to become negative after treatment, although the levels should fall substantially. Cryptococci can also be cultured from CSF and/or blood.

Factors associated with a poor prognosis include a high organism count in the CSF, a low white cell count in the CSF, and an impaired consciousness level at presentation.

Treatment.   Initial treatment is usually with intravenous amphotericin B (0.7 mg/kg per day), although intravenous fluconazole (400 mg daily) is useful if renal function is impaired or if amphotericin side-effects are troublesome. Oral fluconazole can be substituted if the organism is shown to be fully sensitive and the patient is responding.

The mortality from a first episode of cryptococcal meningitis is up to 20%. Relapse is very common, possibly from a prostatic reservoir in men. Lifelong secondary prophylaxis is required in the absence of HAART.

Candida (see p. 91)

Mucosal infection with *Candida* is very common in HIV-infected patients. Oral *Candida* is one of the most common conditions. *C. albicans* is the usual organism, although *C. krusei* and *C. glabrata* occur. Pseudomembranous candidiasis consisting of creamy plaques in the mouth and pharynx is the best recognized. *Erythematous Candida* is more subtle and appears as reddened areas on the hard palate or as atypical areas on the tongue. Angular cheilitis can occur in association with either form or more rarely alone. Vulvovaginal *Candida* is often problematic.

Oesophageal Candida infection produces dysphagia with retrosternal discomfort (see p. 279). Barium swallow or endoscopy shows multiple areas of ulceration throughout the length of the oesophagus. Fluconazole or itraconazole are the agents of choice. With prolonged exposure to these agents in HIV-infected patients, azole-resistant *C. albicans* is becoming an increasing problem. Switching azoles may produce a response. Symptom relief may require intravenous amphotericin. *Disseminated Candida* is uncommon in the context of HIV infection. *C. krusei* may colonize patients who have been treated with fluconazole, as it is fluconazole-resistant. Amphotericin is useful in the treatment of this infection and an attempt to type *Candida* from clinically azole-resistant patients should be made.

Aspergillus (see p. 93)

Infection with *Aspergillus fumigatus* occurs in advanced HIV disease. *Aspergillus* is controlled by functioning neutrophils, and patients with long-standing neutropenia (often due to chemotherapy) and those on ganciclovir therapy for CMV and myelotoxic antiretrovirals, are prone to this infection. Spores are airborne and ubiquitous. Following inhalation, lung infection proceeds to haematogenous spread to other organs. Sinus infection occurs.

The prognosis is very poor, with amphotericin B being the mainstay of therapy. Itraconazole is also effective. It is almost impossible to deal effectively with *Aspergillus*

Table 2.52 Some mucocutaneous manifestations of HIV infection (see also Ch. 23)	
Skin	**Mucous membranes**
Dry skin and scalp	Candidiasis:
Onychomycosis	oral
Seborrhoeic dermatitis	vulvovaginal
Tinea:	Oral hairy leucoplakia
cruris	Aphthous ulcers
pedis	Herpes simplex:
Pityriasis:	genital
versicolor	oral
rosea	labial
Folliculitis	Periodontal disease
Acne	Warts:
Molluscum contagiosum	oral
Warts	genital
Herpes zoster:	
mutidermatomal	
disseminated	
Papular pruritic eruption	
Scabies	
Icthyosis	
Kaposi's sarcoma	

unless the neutrophil count can be sustained, and neutropenic patients should be supported with granulocyte colony-stimulating factors.

Histoplasmosis (see p. 92)

This infection is a well-recognized complication of HIV in the USA where it is endemic in soil. The most common manifestation is with pneumonia, which may be confused with *Pneumocystis carinii* in its presentation (see above).

Superficial dermatophyte infections

These are common. Nail infection with *Tricophyton rubrum* causes onychomycosis (see p. 1323 and Table 2.52).

Protozoal infections

Toxoplasmosis (see p. 103)

Toxoplasma gondii most commonly causes encephalitis and cerebral abscess in the context of AIDS, usually as a result of reactivation of previously acquired infection. The incidence depends on the rate of seropositivity to toxoplasmosis in the particular population. High levels are found in France where up to 90% of the adult population is seropositive. About 25% of the adult UK population is toxoplasmosis seropositive. AIDS patients who have these antibodies may develop cerebral toxoplasmosis.

The clinical presentation is of a focal neurological lesion with convulsions, fever, headache and possible confusion. Examination reveals focal neurological signs in more than 50% of cases. Eye involvement with chorioretinitis may also be present. In most but not all cases toxoplasmosis serology is positive. Typically CT scan of the brain shows multiple ring-enhancing lesions. A single lesion on CT may be found to be one of several on MRI. A solitary lesion on MRI, however, makes a diagnosis of toxoplasmosis unlikely.

The definitive method of diagnosis is brain biopsy, but in most cases an empirical trial of anti-toxoplasmosis therapy is instituted and if this leads to radiological improvement within 3 weeks this is considered diagnostic. The differential diagnosis includes cerebral lymphoma, tuberculoma or focal cryptococcal infection.

Treatment is with pyrimethamine for at least 6 weeks (loading dose 200 mg, then 50 mg daily) combined with sulfadiazine and folinic acid. Clindamycin and pyrimethamine may be used in patients allergic to sulphonamide. Anticonvulsants should be given. Lifelong maintenance is required to prevent relapse unless the CD4 count can be restored by HAART. There is some evidence to suggest that co-trimoxazole as PCP prophylaxis has some ability to reduce the incidence of toxoplasmosis.

Cryptosporidiosis (see p. 105)

Cryptosporidium parvum can cause a self-limiting acute diarrhoea in an immunocompetent individual. In HIV infection it can cause severe and progressive watery diarrhoea which may be associated with anorexia, abdominal pain, nausea and vomiting. Cysts attach to the epithelium of the small bowel wall, causing secretion of fluid into the gut lumen and failure of fluid absorption. It is associated with sclerosing cholangitis (see p. 404). The cysts are seen on stool specimen microscopy using Kinyoun acid-fast stain. The organism is readily identified in small bowel biopsy specimens.

Treatment is largely supportive, as there are no effective antimicrobial agents available other than a non-absorbable aminoglycoside, paromamycin, which may have a limited effect on diarrhoea.

Microsporidiosis

Enterocytozoon bieneusi and *Septata intestinalis* are associated with diarrhoeal illness in HIV infection. Spores can be detected in stools using a trichrome or fluorescent stain that attaches to the chitin of the spore surface. Albendazole eradicates the infection with amelioration of symptoms.

Leishmaniasis (see p. 101)

This is a cause of illness in immunosuppressed HIV-infected individuals who have been in endemic areas, which include South America, tropical Africa and much of the Mediterranean. Symptoms are frequently non-specific with fever, malaise, diarrhoea and weight loss. Splenomegaly, anaemia and thrombocytopenia are significant findings. Amastigotes may be seen on bone marrow biopsy or from splenic aspirates. Serological tests exist for *Leishmania* but they are not reliable in this setting.

Treatment is based on sodium stibogluconate (pentavalent antimony) but in HIV infection the response may be better to liposomal amphotericin. Relapse without HAART is common unless long-term secondary prophylaxis is given.

Viral infections

Hepatitis virus B and C (see pp. 364 and 367)

Because of the comparable routes of transmission of hepatitis viruses and HIV, co-infection is common, particularly in drug users and those infected by blood products. A higher prevalence of hepatitis viruses is found in those with HIV infection than in the general population. With the striking improvement in prognosis in HIV since the introduction of HAART, morbidity and mortality of hepatitis co-infection has become increasingly significant and may limit life expectancy in HIV. In co-infected patients the hepatotoxicity associated with certain antiretroviral agents may be potentiated.

Hepatitis B infection does not appear to influence the natural history of HIV; however, in HIV co-infected patients there is a significantly reduced rate of hepatitis B e antigen (HBeAg) clearance, and the risk of developing chronic infection is increased. HBV reactivation and reinfection is also seen. Liver disease occurs most commonly in those with high HBV DNA levels indicative of continuing replication.

It has been suggested that hepatitis C is associated with more rapid progression of HIV infection, and the CD4 responses to HAART in co-infected patients may be blunted. Hepatitis C progression is both more likely and more rapid in the presence of HIV infection, and the levels of hepatitis C viral activity tend to be elevated. The hepatotoxicity associated with HAART is worse in those with HCV co-infection.

Assessment of co-infected patients requires full clinical and laboratory evaluation and staging of both infections. For HCV both viral load and genotype will influence therapeutic decision-making. In HBV infection, detection and quantification of HBV DNA acts as a marker of viral activity, whilst the significance of viral genotype is still uncertain. Liver biopsy is useful to obtain a histological staging of disease.

There are limited treatment options for HBV. The ideal time to start treatment is not clear; however, response rates for co-infected patients may be better at higher CD4 counts. Treatments for HBV include some agents with concomitant anti-HIV activity, including lamivudine and tenofovir. These must be used within an effective anti-HIV regimen.

In HCV co-infection, criteria for treatment are similar for those infected with HCV alone, depending on stage of disease and HCV genotype. Pegylated interferon has greater efficacy than standard interferon in this situation and is combined with ribavirin. In HIV/HCV co-infected patients those with a CD4 count above 200 have a better chance of success. In general it is preferable to treat HCV first if HIV infection is stable, as this minimizes hepatotoxicity associated with HAART. However, if the CD4 count is low or the patient is at risk of HIV progression, HIV therapy should be instituted first.

Cytomegalovirus (see p. 46)

CMV can be a cause of considerable morbidity in HIV-infected individuals, especially in the later stages of disease. The major problems encountered are retinitis, colitis, oesophageal ulceration, encephalitis and pneumonitis. CMV infection is associated with an arteritis, which may be the major pathogenic mechanism. CMV also causes polyradiculopathy and adrenalitis.

CMV retinitis
This tends to occur once the CD4 count is below 100 and is found in up to 30% of AIDS cases. It is the most common cause of eye disease and blindness. Although usually unilateral to begin with, the infection frequently progresses to involve both eyes. Presenting features depend on the area of retina involved (loss of vision being most common with macular involvement) and include floaters, loss of visual acuity, field loss and scotomata, orbital pain and headache.

Examination of the fundus (Fig. 2.47) reveals haemorrhages and exudates, which follow the vasculature of the retina (so called 'pizza pie' appearances). The features are highly characteristic and the diagnosis is made clinically. Retinal detachment and papillitis may occasionally occur. If untreated, retinitis spreads within the eye, destroying the retina within its path. Routine fundoscopy should be carried out on all HIV-infected patients to look for evidence of early infection. Any patient with symptoms of visual disturbance should have a thorough examination with pupils dilated, and if no evident pathology is seen a specialist ophthalmologic opinion should be sought.

Treatment for CMV should be started as soon as possible with either ganciclovir (10 mg/kg daily) or foscarnet (60 mg/kg 8-hourly) given intravenously for at least 3 weeks, or until retinitis is quiescent. Reactivation is common, leading to blindness. The major side-effect of ganciclovir is myelosuppression, and foscarnet is nephrotoxic. Maintenance therapy requires long-term vascular access through either a Hickman line or subcutaneous reservoir device. An oral form of ganciclovir is available which has some long-term benefit when used as maintenance therapy, but has a lower efficacy than

intravenous ganciclovir. Ganciclovir can be given directly into the vitreous cavity but regular injections are required. A sustained-release implant of ganciclovir can be surgically inserted into the affected eye. Cidofovir is available for use when the above drugs are contraindicated. It has renal toxicity.

CMV colitis
The usual presenting features include abdominal pain, often generalized or left iliac, diarrhoea which may be bloody, generalized abdominal tenderness with rebound in some cases, and a low-grade fever. Loops of dilated large bowel may be seen on abdominal X-ray. Sigmoidoscopy shows a friable or ulcerated mucosa, which should be biopsied. The diagnosis is made on the histological appearances with characteristic 'owls eye' cytoplasmic inclusion bodies (see Fig. 2.16).

Treatment with either intravenous ganciclovir or foscarnet for 3 weeks improves symptoms and the histological changes are reversed. However, relapse is common once therapy is stopped, unless HAART is available. The issue of long-term maintenance therapy in this situation is controversial since, unlike CMV retinitis, repeated attacks of colitis do not necessarily have significant long-term sequelae of the sort associated with retinitis. Given the complications associated with maintenance anti-CMV therapy there may be no overall benefit.

Other sites along the gastrointestinal tract also are prone to CMV infection. Solitary ulceration of the oesophagus, usually in the lower third, causes painful dysphagia. CMV can also cause hepatitis.

CMV neurological conditions
CMV polyradiculopathy usually affects the lumbosacral roots, leading to paraparesis and sphincter disturbance. The CSF has an increase in white cells, which surprisingly are almost all neutrophils. Although progression may be arrested by anti-CMV medication, functional recovery may not occur. The encephalopathy of CMV has clinical similarities to that caused by HIV itself. It tends to respond poorly to therapy.

Herpesviruses (see pp. 43 and 1321)
Herpes simplex infection occurs with greater frequency and severity, presenting in an ulcerative rather than vesicle form in profoundly immunosuppressed individuals. Genital, oral and occasionally disseminated infection is seen. Viral shedding may be prolonged in comparison with immunocompetent patients.

Varicella zoster can occur at any stage of HIV but tends to be more aggressive and longer-lasting in the more immunosuppressed patient. Multidermatomal zoster may occur.

Therapy with aciclovir is usually effective. Frequent recurrences need suppressive therapy. Aciclovir-resistant strains (usually due to thymidine kinase-deficient mutants) in HIV-infected patients have become more common. Such strains may respond to foscarnet.

Fig. 2.47　**Untreated CMV retinitis.**

Herpesvirus 8 (HHV-8) is associated with Kaposi's sarcoma (see p. 48).

Epstein–Barr virus (see p. 47)

Patients with HIV have been shown to have high levels of EBV colonization. There are increased EBV titres in oropharyngeal secretions and high levels of EBV-infected B cells. The normal T cell response to EBV is depressed in HIV. EBV is strongly associated with primary cerebral lymphoma and non-Hodgkin's lymphoma (see below). Oral hairy leucoplakia caused by EBV is a sign of immunosuppression first noted in HIV but now also recognized in other conditions. It appears intermittently on the lateral borders of the tongue or the buccal mucosa as a pale ridged lesion. Although usually asymptomatic, patients may find it unsightly and occasionally painful. The virus can be identified histologically and on electron-microscopy. There is a variable response to aciclovir.

Human papillomavirus (see p. 48)

HPV produces genital, plantar and occasionally oral warts, which may be slow to respond to therapy and recur repeatedly. HPV is associated with the more rapid development of cervical and anal intraepithelial neoplasia, which in time may progress to squamous cell carcinoma of the cervix or rectum in HIV-infected individuals.

Papovavirus (see p. 48)

JC virus, a member of the papovavirus family, which infects oligodendrocytes, causes progressive multifocal leucoencephalopathy (PML). This leads to demyelination particularly within the white matter of the brain. The features are of progressive neurological and/or intellectual impairment, often including hemiparesis or aphasia. The course is usually inexorably progressive but a stuttering course may be seen. Radiologically the lesions are usually multiple and confined to the white matter. They do not enhance with contrast and do not produce a mass effect. MRI (Fig. 2.48) is more sensitive than CT and reveals enhanced signal on T2-weighted images of the lesions. Definitive diagnosis is made on

Fig. 2.48 **MRI scans showing progressive multifocal leucoencephalopathy.**

histological and viral examination of brain tissue obtained at biopsy. There is no specific therapy. HAART which enhances the immune response has, however, produced both clinical and radiological remission in a number of cases. Addition of cidofovir to HAART may improve outcome in some patients.

Bacterial infections

Bacterial infection in HIV is common and frequently disseminated. Cell-mediated immune responses normally control infection against intracellular bacteria, e.g. *Mycobacterium*. The abnormalities of B cell function associated with HIV lead to infections with encapsulated bacteria, as reduced production of IgG_2 cannot protect against the polysaccharide coat of such organisms. These functional abnormalities may be present well before there is a significant decline in CD4 numbers and so bacterial sepsis may be seen at early stages of HIV infection. *Streptococcus pneumoniae, Haemophilus influenzae* and *Moraxella catarrhalis* infections are examples. Bacterial infection is often disseminated and, although usually amenable to standard antibiotic therapy, may reoccur. Long-term prophylaxis is required if recurrent infection is frequent.

Skin conditions such as folliculitis, abscesses and cellulitis are common and are usually caused by *Staph. aureus*. Periodontal disease, which may be necrotizing, causes pain and damage to the gums. It is more common in smokers, but no specific causative agent has been identified. Therapy is with local debridement and systemic antibiotics.

Salmonella (non-typhoidal) (see p. 68) is a frequent pathogen in HIV infection. Salmonellas are able to survive within macrophages, this being a major factor in their pathogenicity. Organisms are usually acquired orally and frequently result in disseminated infection. Gastrointestinal disturbance may be disproportionate to the degree of dissemination, and once the pathogen is in the bloodstream any organ may be infected. Salmonella osteomyelitis and cystitis have been reported. Diagnosis is from blood and stool cultures.

Response to standard antibiotic therapy, depending on laboratory sensitivities, is usually good. Recurrent infection is, however, common and long-term prophylaxis may be required.

Education on food hygiene should be provided.

Mycobacteria
Mycobacterium tuberculosis (see p. 86)

The interaction between HIV and TB has several particular characteristics. Many parts of the world with a high prevalence of TB also have high rates of HIV infection. The respiratory transmission of TB means both HIV-positive and negative people are being infected. Although more common in immunosuppressed patients, TB can cause disease when there is only minimal immunosuppression and thus often appears early in the course of HIV infection. In many countries where HIV is spreading and TB is endemic there has been a substantial increase in the incidence of tuberculosis. HIV-related TB frequently represents reactivation of latent TB, but there is also clear evidence of newly acquired infection and nosocomial spread in HIV-infected populations.

The pattern of disease differs with immuno-suppression. Patients with relatively well preserved CD4 counts have a clinical picture similar to that seen in HIV-negative patients with pulmonary infection.

In more advanced HIV disease, atypical pulmonary presentations without cavitation and prominent hilar lymphadenopathy, or extrapulmonary TB affecting lymph nodes, bone marrow or liver occur. Bacteraemia may be present.

The diagnosis depends on demonstrating the organisms in appropriate tissue specimens. The response to tuberculin testing is blunted in HIV-positive individuals and is unreliable. Sputum microscopy may be negative even in pulmonary infection and culture techniques are the best diagnostic tool.

M. tuberculosis infection usually responds well to standard treatment regimens, although the duration of therapy may be extended, especially in extrapulmonary infection. Multidrug resistance is becoming a problem, particularly in the USA where it is becoming a nosocomial danger. Cases from HIV units in the UK have been reported. Compliance with antituberculous therapy needs to be emphasized. Treatment of TB in the HIV-infected individual is not curative and long-term isoniazid prophylaxis may be given. In patients from TB endemic areas, primary prophylaxis may prevent emergence of infection. Immune reconstitution phenomenon as a result of HAART occurs (p. 149).

Mycobacterium avium-intracellulare

Atypical mycobacteria, particularly *M. avium-intracellulare* (MAI), generally appear only in the later stages of HIV infection when patients are profoundly immuno-suppressed. It is a saprophytic organism of low pathogenicity that is ubiquitous in soil and water. Entry may be via the gastrointestinal tract or lungs with dissemination via infected macrophages.

The major clinical features are fevers, malaise, weight loss, anorexia and sweats. Dissemination to the bone marrow causes anaemia. Gastrointestinal symptoms may be prominent with diarrhoea and malabsorption. At this stage of disease patients frequently have other concurrent infections, so differentiating MAI is difficult on clinical grounds. Direct examination and culture of blood, lymph node, bone marrow or liver give the diagnosis most reliably.

MAI is typically resistant to standard antituberculous therapies, although ethambutol may be useful. Drugs such as rifabutin in combination with clarithromycin or azithromycin reduce the burden of organisms and in some ameliorate symptoms. A common combination is ethambutol, rifabutin and clarithromycin. Addition of amikacin to a drug regimen may produce a good symptomatic response. Primary prophylaxis with rifabutin or azithromycin may delay the appearance of MAI, but no corresponding increase in survival has been shown.

Treatment of mycobacteria in the age of HAART (see pp. 144 and 149)

Treatment of TB in HIV co-infected patients presents specific challenges and requires input from a specialist physician. Treatment is similar to that for HIV-negative patients, although intermittent and short-course regimens are not advised. Therapy should be initiated with four drugs, isoniazid, rifampicin, pyrazinamide and ethambutol for 2 months. Once sensitivities are confirmed, pyrazinamide and ethambutol may be withdrawn and the other two drugs continued for 4 months, although this may be extended in some circumstances. The drug–drug interactions between antiretroviral and anti-tuberculous medications are complex and are a consequence of enzyme induction or inhibition. Rifampicin is a potent inducer of cytochrome P450, which is also the route for metabolism of HIV protease inhibitors. Using both drugs together results in a reduction in circulating protease inhibitor with reduced efficacy and increased potential for drug resistance. Some protease inhibitors themselves block cytochrome P450, which leads to potentially toxic levels of rifampicin and problems such as uveitis and hepatotoxicity. The non-nucleoside reverse transcriptase class also interacts variably with rifamycins, requiring dose alterations. Additionally, there are overlapping toxicities between HAART regimens and anti-tuberculous drugs, in particular hepatotoxicity, peripheral neuropathy and gastrointestinal side-effects. Rifabutin has a weaker effect on cytochrome P450 and may be substituted for rifampicin. Dose adjustments must be made for drugs used in this situation to take account of these interactions.

Paradoxical inflammatory reactions (immune reconstitution inflammatory syndrome, IRIS) which can include exacerbation of symptoms, new or worsening clinical signs and deteriorating radiological appearances have been associated with the improvement of immune function seen in HIV-infected patients starting HAART in the face of *M. tuberculosis* infection. They are most commonly seen in the first few weeks after initiation of HAART in patients recovering from TB and can last several weeks or months. The syndrome does not reflect inadequate TB therapy and is not confined to any particular combination of antiretroviral agents. It is vital to exclude new pathology in this situation. Given these complexities, in certain circumstances it may be preferable to delay the initiation of HAART until TB is under control.

Infections due to other organisms

Strongyloides (see p. 111), a nematode found in tropical areas, may produce a hyperinfection syndrome in HIV-infected patients. Larvae are produced which invade through the bowel wall and migrate to the lung and occasionally to the brain. Albendazole or ivermectin may be used to control infection. Gram-negative septicaemia can develop (see p. 967).

Scabies (see p. 1325) may be much more severe in HIV infection. It may be widely disseminated over the body and appear as atypical, crusted papular lesions known as 'Norwegian scabies', from which mites are readily demonstrated. Superadded staphylococcal infection may occur. Treatment with conventional agents such as lindane may fail, and ivermectin has been used to good effect in some patients.

Neoplasms

The mortality and morbidity associated with neoplasia in HIV is substantial, non-Hodgkin's lymphoma being the most significant tumour now, ahead of Kaposi's sarcoma.

Kaposi's sarcoma (see p. 1353)

Kaposi's sarcoma (KS) in association with HIV (epidemic KS) behaves more aggressively than that associated with HIV-negative populations (endemic KS). The incidence has fallen significantly since the introduction of HAART. The tumour is most common in homosexual men and others who have acquired HIV sexually, particularly from a partner who has KS, implicating a sexually transmitted cofactor in the pathogenesis. Human herpesvirus 8 (HHV-8) is involved in pathogenesis. KS skin lesions are characteristically pigmented, well circumscribed and occur in multiple sites. It is a multicentric tumour consisting of spindle cells and vascular endothelial cells, which together form slit-like spaces in which red blood cells become trapped. This process is responsible for the characteristic purple hue of the tumour. In addition to the skin lesions, KS affects lymphatics and lymph nodes, the lung and gastrointestinal tract, giving rise to a wide range of symptoms and signs. Most patients with visceral involvement also have skin or mucous membrane lesions. Visceral KS carries a worse prognosis than that confined to the skin. Kaposi's sarcoma is seen around the eye (Fig. 2.49), particularly in the conjunctivae, which can lead to periorbital oedema.

Treatment with local radiotherapy gives good results in skin lesions and is helpful in lymph node disease. Initiation of HAART may cause regression of lesions and

prevent new ones emerging. For patients with aggressive disease, systemic chemotherapy is indicated using combinations of vincristine and bleomycin or the newer liposomal preparations of doxorubicin. Response is often very good although of uncertain duration. Alpha-interferon is also effective.

Lymphoma

A significant proportion of patients with HIV develop lymphoma, mostly of the non-Hodgkin's, large B cell type. These are frequently extranodal, often affecting the brain, lung and gastrointestinal tract. Many of these tumours are strongly associated with Epstein–Barr virus (EBV), with evidence of expression of latent gene nuclear antigens such as EBNA 1–6, some of which are involved in the immortalization of B cells and drive a neoplastic pathway.

HIV-associated lymphomas are frequently very aggressive. Patients often present with systemic 'B' syndromes and progress rapidly despite chemotherapy. Primary cerebral lymphoma is variably responsive to radiotherapy but overall carries a poor prognosis. Lymphomas occurring early in the course of HIV infection tend to respond better to therapy and carry a better prognosis, occasionally going into complete remission.

Squamous cell carcinoma

Squamous cell carcinoma, especially of the cervix and anus, is associated with HIV. Human papillomavirus may have a role in the pathogenesis of these malignancies. Women with HIV infection should have yearly cervical cytology for detection of premalignant change.

INVESTIGATIONS AND MONITORING

Initial assessment

A full history should be taken, followed by examination. Baseline investigations will depend on the clinical setting, but those for an asymptomatic person in the UK are shown in Box 2.18.

Monitoring

Patients are regularly monitored to assess the progression of the infection. Clinical examination will identify signs of immunosuppression (such as oral hairy leucoplakia) and detect early evidence of major opportunistic events. Decisions about appropriate intervention can be made.

Immunological monitoring

CD4 lymphocytes. The absolute CD4 count and the percentage of total lymphocytes that this represents falls as HIV progresses. These figures bear a relationship to the risk of the occurrence of HIV-related pathology, with patients with counts below 200 cells at greatest risk. Rapidly falling CD4 counts and those below 350 are an indication to consider HAART. Routine assays measure numbers of circulating CD4 lymphocytes but are unable to assess cellular function, which may be abnormal, even when numbers are relatively well preserved. Factors

Fig. 2.49   **Kaposi's sarcoma of the eyelid.**

Box 2.18 Baseline investigations in a newly diagnosed asymptomatic patient with HIV infection

Haematology
Full blood count, differential count and film
Erythrocyte sedimentation rate

Biochemistry
Serum, liver and renal function
Serum lipid profile
Blood glucose

Immunology
Lymphocyte subsets
Virology
HIV antibody (confirmatory)
HIV viral load
Hepatitis serology (A, B and C)
Cytomegalovirus antibody

Microbiology
Toxoplasmosis serology
Syphilis serology
Screen for other sexually transmitted infections

Other
Cervical cytology

other than HIV (e.g. smoking, exercise, intercurrent infections and diurnal variation) also affect CD4 numbers. CD4 counts are performed at approximately 3-monthly intervals unless values are approaching critical levels for intervention, in which case they are performed more frequently.

Virological monitoring
Viral load (HIV RNA)
The replication of HIV continues at a high rate throughout the course of infection, with many billion new virus particles being produced daily. The rate of viral clearance is relatively constant in any individual and thus the level of viraemia is a reflection of the rate of virus replication. This has both prognostic and therapeutic value.

The commonly used term 'viral load' has been coined to encompass viraemia and HIV RNA levels. Three HIV RNA assays for viral load are in current use:

- branched-chain DNA (bDNA)
- reverse transcription polymerase chain reaction (RT-PCR)
- nucleic acid sequence-based amplification (NASBA).

Results are given in copies of viral RNA per millilitre of plasma, or converted to a logarithmic scale, and there is good correlation between tests. The most sensitive test is able to detect as few as 20 copies of viral RNA per millilitre. Transient increases in viral load are seen following immunizations (e.g. for influenza and *Pneumococcus*) or during episodes of acute intercurrent infection (e.g. tuberculosis); and viral load measurements should not be carried out within a month of these events.

By about 6 months after seroconversion to HIV, the viral set-point for an individual is established and there is

a correlation between HIV RNA levels and long-term prognosis, independent of the CD4 count. Those patients with a viral load consistently greater than 10 000 copies/mL have a 10 times higher risk of progression to AIDS over the ensuing 5 years than those consistently below 10 000 copies/mL. Although a correlation exists between viral load and CD4 cell numbers, the viral load appears to be the best predictor of the long-term prognosis, whilst the CD4 count will give warning of the risks of immediate or shorter-term problems.

HIV RNA is the standard marker of treatment efficacy, with levels falling in response to the introduction of effective antiretroviral medication (see below). Both duration and magnitude of virus suppression are pointers to clinical outcome. None of the currently available therapies is able to suppress viral replication indefinitely, and a rising viral load indicates drug failure.

Various guidelines exist for viral load monitoring in clinical practice. Baseline measurements are followed by repeat estimations at intervals of 3–4 months, ideally in conjunction with CD4 counts to allow both pieces of evidence to be used together in decision-making. Following initiation of antiretroviral therapy or changes in therapy, effects on viral load should be seen by 4 weeks, reaching a maximum at 10–12 weeks, when repeat viral load testing should be carried out (see Fig. 2.46).

Phenotype determination
Two phenotypes of HIV, syncytium-inducing (SI) and non-syncytium-inducing (NSI), exist and appear to correlate with disease progression. This is a specialized technique that is currently available only as a research tool.

Genotype determination
Clear genotype variations exist within HIV and there are increasing numbers of well-identified point mutations associated with antiretroviral drugs. Viral genotype has now entered routine practice to guide therapy, particularly in treatment-experienced patients and women who are pregnant.

MANAGEMENT OF THE HIV-INFECTED PATIENT (Box 2.19)

The possibility of understanding HIV as a chronic controllable condition came with the advent of highly active antiretroviral therapy (HAART). Since then management in the resource-rich world has moved away from treating opportunistic conditions in immunosuppressed patients towards delivering long-term, effective suppressive therapy. The emphasis on using treatments to sustain life has shifted in favour of managing life with the current therapies.

Nonetheless there is still no cure for HIV and patients must live with a chronic, infectious and unpredictable condition. Limitations to efficacy include the inability of current drugs to clear HIV from certain intracellular pools, the occurrence of serious side-effects, strict adherence

Box 2.19 An approach to sick HIV-positive patients

Potential problems include
Adverse drug reactions
Acute opportunistic infections
Presentation or complication of malignancy
Immune reconstitution phenomenon
Infection in an immunocompromised host
Organic or functional brain disorders
Non-HIV-related pathology must not be forgotten

Full medical history
Remember:
- Antiretroviral drugs, prophylaxis, travel, previous HIV-related pathology, potential source of infectious agents (food hygiene, pets, contacts with acute infections, contact with TB, sexually transmitted infections)
- Secure confidentiality. Check with patient who is aware of HIV diagnosis.

Full physical examination
Remember:
- Signs of adverse drug reactions, e.g. skin rashes, oral ulceration
- Signs of disseminated sepsis
- Clinical evidence of immunosuppression, e.g. oral candida, oral hairy leucoplakia
- Focal neurological signs and/or meningism
- Evidence of altered mental state – organic or functional

- Examine:
  - the genitalia, e.g. herpes simplex, syphilis, gonorrhoea
  - the fundi, e.g. CMV retinitis
  - the mouth
- Lymphadenopathy.

Immediate investigations
Full blood count and differential count
Liver and renal function tests
Plasma glucose
Blood gases including acid–base balance
Blood cultures, including specimens for mycobacterial culture
Microscopy and culture of available/appropriate specimens: stool, sputum, urine, CSF
Malaria screen in recent travellers from malaria areas
Serological tests for cryptococcal antigen, toxoplasmosis: save serum for viral studies
Chest X-ray
CT/MR scan of brain if focal neurological signs, and ALWAYS before lumbar puncture

NB: Lymphocyte subsets and HIV viral load assays may yield misleading results during intercurrent illness.

---

requirements, complex drug–drug interactions, and the ongoing emergence of resistant viral strains.

The aims of management in HIV infection are to maintain physical and mental health, to avoid transmission of the virus, and to provide appropriate palliative support as needed. The complexity of HIV infection means that it is best managed via a multidisciplinary team approach. Confidentiality must be strictly observed and care taken over establishing who is aware of the patient's diagnosis and who is excluded from that knowledge. Psychological support is needed not only for the patient but also for family, friends and carers. Dietary assessment and advice should be freely accessible. Clear advice on reducing the risk of HIV transmission must be provided and future sexual practices discussed. Information must be available to allow people to make informed choices about childbearing. The implications for existing family members should be considered. General health promotion advice on smoking, alcohol, diet, drug misuse and exercise should be given, particularly in the light of the emerging cardiovascular, metabolic and hepatotoxicity risks associated with HAART (see p. 149).

Antiretroviral drugs (ARVs)

The complexity of treatment regimens against HIV infection increases with the rising number of available compounds and the growth in new information about their use. Drugs of five different classes (Table 2.53) are currently available in the UK, with several others close to release. Various events in the HIV life cycle have been identified as potential targets for antiretroviral therapy. Inhibitors of HIV reverse transcriptase and of HIV

protease are so far the most developed. Newer agents of these classes with improved pharmacokinetic, side-effect and resistance profiles are coming into production.

Reverse transcriptase inhibitors are of three types: nucleoside analogues (nucleoside reverse transcription inhibitors, NRTIs), nucleotide analogues (nucleotide reverse transcriptase inhibitors, NtRTIs) and non-nucleoside analogues (non-nucleoside reverse transcriptase inhibitors NNRTIs).

- *Nucleoside analogues (NRTIs)* inhibit reverse transcription by binding to viral DNA and also act as DNA chain terminators. NRTIs need to be phosphorylated intracellularly for activity to occur. These were the first group of agents to be used against HIV, initially as monotherapy and later as dual drug combinations. Usually two drugs of this class are combined to provide the 'backbone' of a HAART regimen. Zidovudine and lamivudine have been combined into a single tablet, (Combivir), and zidovudine, lamivudine and abacavir into Trizivir, which helps reduce the pill burden. NRTIs have been associated with mitochondrial toxicity, a consequence of their effect on the human mitochondrial DNA polymerase. Lactic acidosis is a recognized complication of this group of drugs.
- *Nucleotide analogues (NtRTIs)* have a similar mechanism of action but do not require intracellular phosphorylation for activity. Tenofovir, a monophosphorylated thymidine derivative, is the only licensed compound of this group.
- *Non-nucleoside analogues (NNRTIs)* interfere with reverse transcriptase by direct binding to the enzyme.

Table 2.53 Antiretroviral drugs available in the UK

Drug	Daily dose and pill burden	Metabolism/food	Side-effects
Nucleoside reverse transcriptase inhibitors (NRTIs) (nucleoside analogues)			
Abacavir	300 mg × 2 tablets/day	No food restrictions	Hypersensitivity reaction, fever, rash, vomiting. Association with mitochondrial dysfunction and lactic acidosis
Didanosine/DDI	400 mg o.d. (> 60 kg), 250 mg o.d. (< 60 kg) 1 capsule/day	30–60 minutes before food	Nausea, diarrhoea, peripheral neuropathy, pancreatitis. Association with mitochondrial dysfunction and lactic acidosis
Emtricitabine (PTC)	200 mg o.d.	No food effects. Renal excretion. Modify dose if creatinine clearance is < 50 mL/min	Headache, nausea, skin pigmentation
Lamivudine/3TC	150 mg × 2 2 tablets/day	No food effects, well absorbed with high bioavailability	Nausea, headache, rash, peripheral neuropathy, myelosuppression. Association with mitochondrial dysfunction and lactic acidosis
Stavudine/D4T	40 mg × 2 2 capsules/day × 3 Reduce to 30 mg × 2 for persons less than 60 kg	High bioavailability. Competes with zidovudine for phosphorylation so do not use together	Polyneuropathy. May be able to tolerate reduced dosage. Megaloblastic changes. Association with mitochondrial dysfunction and lactic acidosis
Zalcitabine/DDC	0.75 mg × 3 3 tablets/day	No food effects	Polyneuropathy, aphthous ulceration. Association with mitochondrial dysfunction and lactic acidosis
Zidovudine/AZT	250–300 mg × 2 2 capsules/day	Well absorbed with good bioavailability. No food effects	Nausea, headache, insomnia, skin and nail pigmentation, myelosuppression, megaloblastic changes. Myelopathy with extended use. Association with mitochondrial dysfunction and lactic acidosis
Combivir (AZT plus 3TC)	1 tablet twice daily		As for component drugs
Kivexa abacavir/3TC	1 tablet daily o.d.		
Triizivir (abacavir/AZT/3TC)	1 tablet twice daily		As for component drugs
Nucleotide reverse transcriptase inhibitor (NtRTI)			
Tenofovir	245 mg o.d. 1 tablet daily	After food	Hypophosphataemia, renal toxicity
Non-nucleoside reverse transcriptase inhibitors (NNRTIs)			
Efavirenz	600 mg o.d. 1 capsule at night	Metabolized by cytochrome P450 (3A mixed inducer and inhibitor). Do not take with high-fat foods	Rash, Stevens–Johnson syndrome, central nervous system effects (vivid dreams, agitation, hallucinations, and depression amongst others). Contraindicated in pregnancy
Nevirapine	200 mg o.d. for first 14 days then 200 mg × 2 2 tablets/day	High bioavailability, long half-life, wide tissue distribution. Induces its own metabolism, hence dose escalation. No food effects	Rash, Stevens–Johnson syndrome, hepatic toxicity
Protease inhibitors (single drugs)			
Amprenavir	1200 mg × 2 16 capsules/day May be used in lower doses boosted with ritonavir	Cytochrome P450 inhibitor High-fat meals lead to reduced plasma drug levels	Diarrhoea, nausea, rash, oral paraesthesia, abnormal liver function, body fat redistribution and abnormal plasma lipids
Atazanavir*	400 mg o.d. 2 tablets/day Can boost with ritonavir	Fewer lipid abnormalities than other protease inhibitors	Hyperbilirubinaemia

Cont'd

Drug	Daily dose and pill burden	Metabolism/food	Side-effects
Table 2.53 (Cont'd) Antiretroviral drugs available in the UK			
Protease inhibitors (single drugs)			
Indinavir	800 mg × 3 6 capsules/day	Food reduces plasma levels. Take 1 hour before or 2 hours after food. Drink additional 1.5 L water/day	Nephrolithiasis and crystalluria, dry skin, nail dystrophy, alopecia, hyperbilirubinaemia, fat redistribution, raised plasma lipids, hyperglycaemia
Nelfinavir	1250 mg × 2 10 tablets/day	Take with food. Cytochrome P450 3A inhibitor	Diarrhoea, fat redistribution, raised plasma lipids, hyperglycaemia
Ritonavir	600 mg × 2 12 capsules/day Most commonly taken at lower doses to boost other compounds	Take with meals. Potent cytochrome P450 3A4 inhibitor	Nausea/vomiting, diarrhoea, taste distortion, perioral paraesthesia, fat redistribution, hepatotoxicity, hyperglycaemia, pancreatitis
Saquinavir (soft gel)	1200 mg × 3 or 1800 mg × 2 18 capsules/day	Take with food	Nausea, diarrhoea, abdominal pain, fat redistribution, abnormal plasma lipids, hyperglycaemia
Protease inhibitors boosted with ritonavir			
Lopinavir R	3 capsules × 2 6 capsules/day	Take with food	Diarrhoea, nausea, fat redistribution, abnormal plasma lipids
Fosamprenavir	700 mg plus ritonavir 100 mg × 2	Pro-drug of amprenavir No food effect	Similar to amprenavir
Ritonavir/indinavir	100 mg/800 mg × 2 6 capsules/day	With a light meal/snack	As ritonavir and indinavir
Ritonavir/saquinavir	400 mg/400 mg × 2 12 capsules/day	With a light meal	As ritonavir and saquinavir
Tipranavir*/ritonavir	500 mg/200 mg × 2		Nausea, abnormal LFT
Fusion inhibitors			
Enfurvitide (T20)	90 mg × 2 – subcutaneous injection		Reaction at the injection site

* Not yet licensed in the UK

They are generally small molecules that are widely disseminated throughout the body and have a long half-life. NNRTIs affect cytochrome P450. They are ineffective against HIV-2. The level of cross-resistance across the class is very high. All have been associated with rashes and elevation of liver enzymes.

Protease inhibitors (PIs) act competitively on the HIV aspartyl protease enzyme, which is involved in the production of functional viral proteins, and enzymes. In consequence, viral maturation is impaired and immature dysfunctional viral particles are produced. Most of the protease inhibitors are active at very low concentrations and in vitro are found to have synergy with reverse-transcriptase inhibitors. However there are marked differences in toxicity, pharmacokinetics and resistance patterns which influence prescribing. Cross-resistance is common across the PI group, which makes it difficult to use the drugs sequentially. There appears to be no activity against human aspartyl proteases (e.g. renin), although there are clinically significant interactions with the

cytochrome P450 system. This is used to therapeutic advantage, boosting blood levels of PI by blocking drug metabolism with small doses of ritonavir. PIs have been linked with abnormalities of fat metabolism and control of blood sugar, and some have been associated with deterioration in clotting function in haemophiliacs.

Fusion inhibitors. Enfurvitide (T20) is the only licensed compound in this class of agents. It is a peptide derived from HIV GP41 that inhibits GP41-mediated fusion of HIV with the target cell. It is synergistic with NRTIs and PIs. Although resistance to enfurvitide has been described, there is no evidence of cross-resistance with other drug classes Because it has an extracellular mode of action there are few drug–drug interactions. Side-effects relate to the subcutaneous route of administration in the form of injection site reactions.

Newer drugs NRTIs include alovudine (MIV-310) and SPD-756 which appear to have activity against NRTI-resistant strains. New NNRTIs include capravirine in phase III trials. New PIs include tipranavir with activity against PI-resistant viral isolates and TMC 114, also with a good activity against resistant isolates. Entry inhibitors in development include compounds that block CD4 attachment and inhibitors of chemokine co-receptors CXCR4 and CCR5. Early studies of HIV integrase and maturation inhibitors are now in progress.

Starting therapy

Treatment regimens for HIV infection are complicated and require a long-term commitment to high levels of adherence. Risks of therapy include serious side-effects, drug interactions and the potential for development of resistant viral strains. The full involvement of patients in therapeutic decision-making is essential for success. Various national guidelines and treatment frameworks exist (e.g. BHIVA Guidelines, DHHS Guidelines, and IAS Recommendations). A combination of clinical assessment and laboratory marker data, including viral load and CD4 counts, together with individual circumstances, should guide therapeutic decision-making. The current UK recommendations are shown in Table 2.54. In situations where therapy is recommended but the patient elects not to start, then more intensive clinical and laboratory monitoring is advisable.

Clear clinical benefit has been demonstrated with the use of antiretroviral drugs in advanced HIV disease. Treatment should be recommended for all patients with symptomatic HIV disease, AIDS or a CD4 count that is consistently below 200 cells/mm^3. In such situations there is a significant risk of serious HIV-associated morbidity and mortality.

In asymptomatic patients the absolute CD4 count is the key investigation used to guide treatment decisions. A count below 200 cells/mm^3 is associated with disease progression and death. The outcome for patients initiating therapy below 200 CD4 cells/mm^3 is less good than for those who start at higher counts. *The UK recommendation is that therapy should be started before the count falls below 200.*

The risk of disease progression for individuals with a count greater than 350 is low, and treatment may be deferred. Therapy should be considered for people with a CD4 count between 350 and 201 cells/mm^3. Those who may have a higher risk of disease progression, e.g. those with high viral loads (> 60 000 copies/mL) or rapidly falling CD4 count (losing more than > 80 cells/year) may consider earlier intervention. Co-infection with hepatitis C virus may call for earlier intervention (see p. 372).

Treatment for primary HIV infection is only recommended either within a clinical trial or to alleviate symptoms.

Special situations (seroconversion, pregnancy, post-exposure prophylaxis) in which antiretrovirals may be used are described on page 151.

Choice of drugs

The drug regimen used for starting therapy must be individualized to suit each patient's needs. Treatment is initiated with three drugs, two NRTIs in combination, with either a boosted protease inhibitor or NNRTI (Tables 2.53 and 2.55).

The choice of which drugs to include in initial therapy is governed by effectiveness, adherence issues, side-effect profile, potential drug reactions, availability and the resistance and cross-resistance patterns of the drugs. Given that long-term patient adherence is essential to gain the most enduring viral suppression and to impede the emergence of drug resistance, it is crucial that patients be fully involved in therapeutic decision-making throughout and be treated with drug regimens that are manageable as part of their day-to-day lives. Current UK guidance (BHIVA 2003) prioritises ease of adherence and minimization of toxicity over the likely development of resistant mutations following failure of therapy.

Selection of the two NRTIs to form a backbone is increasingly influenced by ease of administration as no conclusive comparative efficacy data exist. Abacavir, didanosine, lamivudine, tenofovir and zidovudine are all licensed for use in naive patients. Stavudine has become associated with lipodystrophy and is not recommended.

Of the NNRTIs, efavirenz and nevirapine are both recommended options and comparable in potency. Efavirenz has the advantage of once-daily dosing but is associated with CNS side-effects such as dysphoria and insomnia. Nevirapine is taken twice daily and has a higher incidence of rash and hepatotoxicity.

The protease inhibitor class have demonstrated excellent efficacy in clinical practice. PIs combined with a low dose of ritonavir to provide a pharmacokinetic advantage are now most commonly used in naive patients. Using this approach, the half-life of the active drug is increased, which may allow simplification of dosing regimens, potency may be enhanced and the risk of resistance minimized.

Table 2.54	UK recommendations for starting therapy*	
Clinical presentation	Laboratory markers	Treatment recommendation
Symptomatic HIV infection, AIDS	Any CD4 count or viral load	Treat
Established, asymptomatic infection	CD4 < 200, any viral load	Treat
	CD4 201–350	Consider treatment based on viral load, rate of CD4 decline, coexisting clinical conditions, patient preference
	CD4 > 350	Defer treatment
Primary HIV infection		Treatment only recommended in a clinical trial or for severe symptoms.

*After British HIV Association (BHIVA) guidelines for the treatment of HIV-infected adults with antiretroviral therapy, 2003

Table 2.55	Initial HAART regimens – choice of initial therapy*		
Regimen	**Recommendation**	**Advantages**	**Disadvantages**
2 NRTIs + NNRTI	Recommended	Equivalent/superior surrogate marker trials compared with PI-based regimens at 104 weeks of follow-up Easier adherence	No randomized clinical trial (RCT) end-point data Shorter follow-up Single mutations may lead to cross class resistance
2 NRTIs + boosted PI	Recommended	Evidence of improved surrogate end-point efficacy for lopinavir/ritonavir compared to a single PI Better PK Easier adherence Less resistance at virological failure	No RCT clinical end-point data Possible increased toxicity and drug interactions
3 NRTIs	Not usually recommended except for patients with low viral load and major adherence concerns	Spares PI and NNRTI classes	No RCT clinical end-point data Short-term surrogate marker data suggest less potent than NNRTI or PI Less effective at high viral loads

* After British HIV Association (BHIVA) guidelines for the treatment of HIV-infected adults with antiretroviral therapy, 2003

Although previous studies have suggested that three NRTIs were able to produce good levels of viral suppression in ARV-naive patients, more recent comparative data show this approach to be less efficacious than combining two NRTIs with either an NNRTI or a PI. The combination is no longer recommended unless there are other pressing individual issues. Recent clinical trail data have shown early virological failure of the combinations of tenofovir + abacavir + lamivudine and tenofovir + didanosine + lamivudine. These combinations should not be offered.

Monitoring therapy (Box 2.20)

Virological success of HAART is a viral load of less than 50 copies/mL within 3–6 months of therapy. This is feasible for those starting therapy for the first time but may not be a realistic objective for heavily pretreated patients. Once ARV has been initiated the viral load should be measured at 4 weeks to assess efficacy. A viral load of 1000 copies/mL should be achievable by this stage if treatment is to be considered adequate. The durability of the virological response is linked both to the rate of viral load fall and the absolute nadir attained. Viral load and CD4 count should be measured at 12 weeks and then at 3-monthly intervals. Regular clinical assessment should include weight, blood pressure and urinalysis.

Box 2.20 Monitoring patients on highly active antiretroviral therapy (HAART)

- Clinical history and examination
- Weight
- HIV viral load
- Lymphocyte subsets
- Full blood count
- Liver and renal function
- Fasting lipid profile
- Blood glucose

Patients should be monitored for drug toxicity, including full blood count, liver and renal function and fasting lipids and glucose levels.

Drug resistance

Resistance to ARVs results from mutations in the protease and reverse transcriptase genes of the virus. HIV has a rapid turnover with 10^8 replications occurring per day. The error rate is high, resulting in genetic diversity within the population of virus in an individual. This mixture will include drug-resistant mutants. When drugs only partially inhibit virus replication there will be a selection pressure for the emergence of drug-resistant strains. The rate at which resistance develops depends on the frequency of pre-existing variants and the number of mutations required. Resistance to zidovudine occurs with an accumulation of mutations, whilst a single-point mutation will confer high-level resistance to all three NNRTIs.

HIV antiretroviral drug resistance testing has become routine clinical management of the HIV patient. Genotypic assays to determine the genetic structure of the RT and protease genes of HIV are available. The tests are based on PCR amplification of virus and give an indirect measure of drug susceptibility in the predominant variants. Such assays are limited both by the starting concentration of virus, most assays requiring at least 1000 copies/mL of blood, and by their poor ability to detect minority strains. For results to be useful, samples must be analysed when the patient is on therapy, as once the selection pressure of therapy is withdrawn, wild type virus becomes the predominant strain and resistance mutations present earlier may no longer be detectable.

The use of genotypic assays with appropriate interpretation in patients for whom therapy is failing has shown significant virological benefits. Phenotypic assays provide a more direct measure of susceptibility but the complexity of the assays limits availability and no additional advantage has been demonstrated. In the UK, increasing numbers of patients are infected with viral strains originating in sub-Saharan Africa, which may require modification of the assay and the interpretation of the results.

There is evidence for the transmission of HIV strains that are resistant to all or some classes of drugs. Studies of primary HIV infection have shown prevalence rates between 2–20%. Prevalence of primary mutations associated with drug resistance in chronically infected patients not on treatment ranges from 3% to 10% in various studies. Advantages exist for genotypic analysis prior to initiating treatment.

Drug interactions

Drug therapy in HIV is highly complex and the potential for clinically relevant drug interactions is substantial. Both PIs and NNRTIs are metabolized through cytochrome P450 dependent pathways. However both classes of drug are able to variably inhibit and induce cytochrome P450, influencing both their own and other drug metabolic rates. Situations occur where both inducers and inhibitors of cytochrome P450 are prescribed simultaneously. Induction of metabolism may result in sub-therapeutic antiretroviral drug levels with the risk of treatment failure and development of viral resistance, whilst inhibition can raise drug levels to toxic values and precipitate adverse reactions. Additionally, conventional (e.g. rifamycins) and complementary therapies (e.g. St John's Wort) affect cytochrome P450 activity and may precipitate substantial drug interactions. Therapeutic drug monitoring (TDM) indicating peak and trough plasma levels may be useful in certain settings.

Complications of antiretroviral therapy

Side-effects are a common problem in HAART (see Table 2.53). Some are acute and associated with initiation of medication, whilst others emerge after longer-term exposure to drugs. As increasing numbers of patients start antiretroviral therapy, adverse drug events are an important clinical presentation.

Allergic reactions

Allergic reactions occur with greater frequency in HIV infection and have been documented to all the anti-retroviral drugs. Abacavir is associated with a hyper-sensitivity reaction, usually within the first 6 weeks of treatment, in up to 4% of patients, which can be fatal. There may be a discrete rash and often a fever coupled with general malaise and gastrointestinal and respiratory symptoms. The diagnosis is clinical and symptoms resolve when abacavir is withdrawn. Rechallenge with abacavir can be fatal and is contraindicated. Allergies to NNRTIs (often in the second or third week of treatment) usually present with a widespread maculopapular pruritic rash, often with a fever and disordered liver function tests. Reactions may resolve in the face of continuing therapy but drugs should be stopped immediately in any patient with mucous membrane involvement or severe hepatic dysfunction.

Lipodystrophy

A syndrome of lipodystrophy in patients with HIV on HAART comprising characteristic morphological changes and metabolic abnormalities is now well described. It is a major complication for patients, being highly stigmatizing, and is a cause of drug discontinuation. The main charac-teristics, which may be found individually or in combination, are a loss of subcutaneous fat in the arms, legs and face (lipoatrophy), deposition of visceral, breast and local fat, raised total cholesterol, HDL cholesterol and triglycerides, and insulin resistance with hyperglycaemia. The syndrome is potentially associated with increased cardiovascular morbidity. A clinical case definition has been developed to attempt to standardize the definition of the syndrome. The aetiology is still unclear although PIs and NRTIs have been implicated. The highest incidence occurs in those taking combinations of NRTIs and PIs. Stavudine seems to be associated with the lipoatrophy component of the process. The syndrome is difficult to treat, and switching or stopping therapy may not always reverse the processes, although switching away from a stavudine and/or PI-based therapy is recommended. Dietary advice and increasing exercise may improve some of the metabolic problems and help body shape. The introduction of glitazones, metformin and growth hormone has been investigated with variable outcomes. Statins and fibrates are recommended to reduce circulating lipids. Pravastatin has a low likelihood of interactions with protease inhibitors. On the other hand, simvastatin is contraindicated as it has high levels of drug interactions with PIs. Surgical approaches are useful in improving facial appearance following lipoatrophy. Polylactic acid injections (New-Fill) have provided improvement in some patients.

Mitochondrial toxicity and lactic acidosis

Mitochondrial toxicity, mostly involving the nucleoside analogue class leads to raised lactate and lactic acidosis, which has in some cases been fatal. NRTIs inhibit gamma DNA polymerase, and other enzymes that are important for normal mitochondrial function. Different NRTIs affect different cell lines and so a variety of clinical syndromes may be observed. Lactic acidosis, occasionally fatal, has been seen. Symptoms are often vague and insidious and may include anorexia, nausea, abdominal pain and general malaise. Venous lactate is raised, and the anion gap is typically widened. This is a serious condition requiring immediate cessation of antiretroviral therapy and provision of appropriate supportive measures until normal biochemistry is restored. All patients should be alerted to possible symptoms and encouraged to attend hospital promptly.

Reports of osteopenia, osteoporosis and avascular necrosis of bone have also been described.

IRIS

Paradoxical inflammatory reactions (immune reconstitution inflammatory syndrome, IRIS) may occur on initiating HAART. This occurs usually in people who have been profoundly immunosuppressed and begin therapy. As their immune system recovers, they are able to mount an inflammatory response to a range of pathogens, which can include exacerbation of symptoms, new or worsening of clinical signs. Examples include unusual mass lesions or lymphadenopathy associated with mycobacteria, including deteriorating radiological appearances associated with MTB infection. Inflammatory retinal lesions in association with cytomegalovirus, deterioration in liver function in chronic hepatitis B carriers and vigorous vesicular eruptions with herpes zoster have also been described.

Adherence

Adherence to treatment is pivotal to success. Levels of adherence below 95% have been associated with poor virological and immunological responses. Many of the drugs used have a short half-life and require frequent dosing. Poor absorption and low bioavailability mean that for some compounds trough levels are barely adequate to suppress viral replication. For some regimens missing even a single dose will result in plasma drug levels falling dangerously low. Patchy adherence facilitates the emergence of drug-resistant variants, which in time will lead to virological treatment failure. Even with the development of more potent and sophisticated antiretroviral compounds, success will only be possible if patients adhere adequately to the dosing schedules.

Factors implicated in poor adherence may be associated with the medication, with the patient or with the provider. The former include side-effects associated with medications, the degree of complexity and pill burden and inconvenience of the regimen. Patient factors include the level of motivation and commitment to the therapy, psychological well-being, the level of available family and social support, and health beliefs. Supporting adherence is a key part of clinical care and specific guidelines are available (BHIVA 2004). Education of patients about their condition and treatment is a fundamental requirement for good adherence, as is education of clinicians in adherence support techniques. Provision of acute and ongoing multidisciplinary support for adherence within clinical settings should be universal. Medication-alert devices may be useful for some patients.

Treatment failure

Failure of antiretroviral treatment, i.e. persistent viral replication causing immunological deterioration and eventual clinical evidence of disease progression, is caused by a variety of factors. HAART drug regimens have limited potency. Food or other medication may compromise drug absorption. Drug interactions may interfere with metabolism and elimination of medication. There may be limited penetration of drug into sanctuary sites such as the CNS, permitting viral replication. Side-effects and other patient-related elements might contribute to poor adherence.

Changing therapy

A rise in viral load, a falling CD4 count or new clinical events that imply progression of HIV disease are all reasons to review therapy. Intolerance or adverse drug reactions may occur. Reasons for treatment failure include the emergence of resistant viral strains or poor patient adherence. New data in this rapidly changing field may lead to therapeutic changes.

Virological failure, i.e. two consecutive viral loads of greater than 400 copies/mL in a previously fully suppressed patient requires investigation. All possible factors including adherence, drug interactions affecting ARV metabolism or absorption and the viral genotype must be considered before therapy is changed. Following failure of initial therapy, viral genotype should be used to help select future therapy. If a new treatment option is available that is likely to lead to complete viral suppression then treatment should be switched as soon as possible. At least one or two different classes of drug should be used wherever practical. Failure consequent upon poor adherence may require simplification of the regimen as well as a change of drug class.

In a situation where a patient has been exposed to a wide variety of drugs, the likelihood of complete inhibition of viral replication is small and the CD4 count is stable there may be a rationale to continue with current therapy.

Treatment failure in highly treatment-experienced patients poses considerable challenges. The term salvage therapy may be applied in this situation. Reasons for treatment failure should be investigated and adherence optimized. As many drugs as possible should be changed, including new agents if there is a realistic chance of success. In some situations it may be better to hold back a new drug and await development of another new agent to give the maximum chance of success. In this situation, success may be better estimated by a rise in CD4 count or an improvement in clinical condition than by complete suppression of viral replication. However, even modest reductions in viral load have been shown to correlate with improved clinical outcome.

If the patient has a viral load below the limit of detection and a change needs to be made because of intolerance of a particular drug, then a switch to another drug within the same class may resolve the problem. Simplification of complex regimens may be considered if adherence is problematic.

Stopping therapy

Stopping antiretroviral drugs may be the proper course of action in a number of circumstances. Examples are cumulative toxicity, or potential drug interactions with medications needed to deal with another more pressing problem. In situations where adherence is poor, stopping completely may be preferable to continuing with inadequate dosing, in order to reduce the risk of the development of viral resistance. Poor quality of life and the view of the patient on the matter must be considered.

NNRTIs efavirenz and nevirapine have long half-lives. If all drugs in an NNRTI-containing regimen are stopped at the same time, there will be a period of time when only sub-therapeutic levels of NNRTI monotherapy are in the bloodstream. Even this period may be enough to allow drug-resistant mutations to emerge. The NNRTI component should be stopped approximately 1 week before the other drugs in the mixture to reduce this risk.

Structured treatment interruptions (STIs) have been studied as a means of enhancing HIV-specific immune responses to HIV or to reduce the exposure to drugs and limit adverse events. Treatment interruption leads to rapid viral rebound. The adverse effects of viral rebound on the immune system, the CD4 count falling within weeks of stopping, give cause for concern in already immunosuppressed patients, although there may be more room to manoeuvre in patients with higher CD4 counts. 'Drug holidays' in those who are virologically failing therapy and have multidrug-resistant viral strains may be considered. There is a suggestion that wild type virus may re-emerge in such patients. Current British guidance does not support treatment interruption as a standard of care.

Specific therapeutic situations

Acute seroconversion
Antiretroviral therapy in patients presenting with an acute seroconversion illness is controversial. This stage of disease may represent a unique opportunity for therapy as there is less viral diversity, and the host immune capacity is still intact. There is evidence to show that the viral load can be reduced substantially by aggressive therapy at this stage, although it rises when treatment is withdrawn. The longer-term clinical sequelae of treatment at this stage remain uncertain. People with severe symptoms during primary HIV infection may gain a clinical improvement on antiretrovirals. If treatment is contemplated in this situation, entry into a clinical trial may be considered. If patients are treated outside a clinical trial then a standard regimen is likely to be most appropriate, although the risk of limiting future options must be assessed.

Pregnancy
Management of HIV-infected pregnant women requires close collaboration between obstetric, medical and paediatric teams. The aim of HIV management is to deliver a healthy, uninfected baby to a healthy mother without prejudicing the future treatment options of the mother. Although considerations of pregnancy must be factored into clinical decision-making, pregnancy per se should not be considered a contraindication to providing optimum HIV-related care for the woman. HIV-positive women should be advised against breast-feeding, which doubles the risk of vertical transmission. Delivery by caesarean section reduces the risk of transmission. For women who would be eligible for treatment of their own HIV disease, whether pregnant or not, triple therapy is the regimen of choice. The specific drug choices will be based on both maternal and fetal considerations. Risk of vertical transmission increases with viral load. Although the fetus will be exposed to more drugs, the chances of reducing the viral load and hence preventing infection are greatest with a potent triple therapy regimen in the mother. The regimen should contain zidovudine, as this is the only agent shown to have an effect on vertical transmission. Treatment may start from 12–14 weeks of pregnancy and continue during delivery. The baby should receive zidovudine for 6 weeks postpartum. The woman should remain on treatment with appropriate monitoring and support. Women who do not need treatment for themselves may consider short-course triple therapy or zidovudine monotherapy to reduce vertical transmission. Treatment of the mother with zidovudine monotherapy is at variance with the data on combination therapy for adults as described above. This may have longer-term implications for the course of the mother's HIV infection, particularly with regard to the possible emergence of zidovudine-resistant virus.

Post-exposure prophylaxis
Healthcare workers following occupational exposure to HIV may need antiretroviral therapy. The British recommendation is zidovudine, lamivudine and either indinavir or nelfinavir for 4 weeks. Prophylaxis after sexual exposure may be appropriate in certain situations, in particular rape or in HIV-discordant relationships. The choice of drugs will depend on the clinical setting and what is known of the HIV source.

PREVENTION AND CONTROL

Antiretroviral drugs are not a cure and are accessible only to a privileged minority of the world's population. Vaccine development has been hampered by the genetic variability of the virus and the complex immune response that is required from the host. Prevention of new infection is fundamental to the control of the epidemic. Strategies that have been shown to be effective include treatment of sexually transmitted infections, consistent use of condoms, use of clean needles and syringes for drug users and antiretroviral drugs to reduce mother-to-child transmission. Topical microbicides for intravaginal use are in development.

Screening of blood products has reduced iatrogenic infection in developed countries but is expensive and not globally available.

Partner notification schemes are developing but are sensitive and controversial. Availability and accessibility of confidential HIV testing provides an opportunity for individual health education and risk reduction to be discussed.

Understanding and changing behaviour is crucial but notoriously difficult, especially in areas that carry as many taboos as sex, HIV and AIDS. Poverty, social unrest and war all contribute to the spread of HIV. Political will, not always readily available, is required if progress in these areas is to occur.

FURTHER READING

AIDS 2003 – a year in review (2003) *AIDS* **17** (Suppl 4).

Antman K, Chang Y (2000) Kaposi's sarcoma. *New England Journal of Medicine* **342**: 1027–1038.

Benson CA, Kaplan JE, Masur H et al. on behalf of CDC, National Institutes of Health, HIV Medicine Association/ID Society of America (2004) Treating opportunistic infections amongst HIV infected adults and adolescents. *Morbidity and Mortality Weekly Report* **53**: 1–112.

Brook MG, Gilson R, Wilkins EL (2003). BHIVA guidelines: coinfection with HIV and chronic hepatitis B infection. *HIV Medicine* **4** (Suppl 1): 42–51.

Centers for Disease Control and Prevention (April 2001) *Guidelines for the Use of Antiretroviral Agents in HIV – Infected Adults and Adolescents (the Living Document).* Atlanta, GA: HIV/AIDS Treatment Information Service (ATIS). Online. Available: http://www.hivatis.org.

EuroGuidelines Group for HIV Resistance (2001) Clinical and laboratory guidelines for the use of HIV-1 drug resistance testing as part of treatment management: recommendations for the European setting. *AIDS* **15**: 309–320.

Expert Advisory Group on AIDS (2004) *Guidelines on Post-exposure Prophylaxis for HIV.* London: Department of Health. www.dh.gov.uk/publications

Health Protection Agency (2003) *Renewing the Focus: HIV and Other Sexually Transmitted Infections in the UK 2002. An Update.* London: HPA.

Kovacs, JA, Masur H (2000) Prophylaxis against opportunistic infections in patients with human immunodeficiency virus infection. *New England Journal of Medicine* **342**(19): 1416–1429.

Lyall EGH, Blott M, de Ruiter A et al. (2001) Guidelines for the management of HIV in pregnant women and the prevention of mother to child transmission. British HIV Association. *HIV Medicine* **2**: 314–334.

Mocroft A, Ledergerber B, Katlama C et al.; EuroSIDA Study Group (2003) Decline in the AIDS and death rates in the EuroSIDA study: an observational study. *Lancet* **362**(9377): 22–29.

Mocroft, A, Katlama C, Johnson AM et al. (2000) AIDS across Europe 1994–1998: The EuroSIDA Study. *Lancet* **356**: 291–296.

Nelson MR, Matthews G, Brook MG, Main J (2003) BHIVA guidelines: coinfection with HIV and chronic hepatitis C virus infection. *HIV Medicine* **4** (Suppl 1): 52–62.

Panel on Clinical Practices for Treatment of HIV Infection (2004) *Guidelines for the Use of Antiretroviral Agents in HIV-infected Adults and Adolescents.* London: Department of Health and Human Services (DHHS), 29 October 2004. Available online: http://AIDSinfo.nih.gov.

Piscitelli SC, Gallicano KD (2001) Interaction among drugs for HIV and opportunistic infections. *New England Journal of Medicine* **344**: 984–996.

Poppa A, Davidson O, Deutsch J et al. (2004) British HIV Association (BHIVA)/British Association for Sexual Health and HIV (BASHH) guidelines on provision of adherence support to individuals receiving antiretroviral therapy (2003). *HIV Medicine* **5** (Suppl 2): 46–60.

Pozniak A, Gazzard B, Anderson J et al.; BHIVA Writing Committee BHIVA Executive Committee (2003) British HIV Association (BHIVA) guidelines for the treatment of HIV-infected adults with antiretroviral therapy. *HIV Medicine* **4** (Suppl 1): 1–41.

Rogstad KE (2004) HIV testing for patients attending general medical services: concise guidelines. *Clinical Medicine* **4**: 136–139.

Soriano V, Puoti M, Sulkowski M et al. (2004) Care of patients with hepatitis C and HIV co-infection. *AIDS* **18**(1): 1–12.

World AIDS Series (2000) Supplement to *Lancet* **356**: WA1–WA40.

Yeni PG, Hammer SM, Hirsch MS et al. (2004) Treatment for adult HIV infection: 2004 recommendations of the International AIDS Society – USA Panel. *Journal of the American Medical Association* **292**: 251–265.

SIGNIFICANT WEBSITES

http://www.hiv-druginteractions.org

http://www.rbm.who.int
Roll Back Malaria Global Partnership

Cell and molecular biology, and genetic disdorders

3

THE CELL AND CELL BIOLOGY

The cell (Fig. 3.1) is a highly organized structure and consists of various common organelles held by an adaptive internal scaffolding (the cytoskeleton), which radiates from the nuclear membrane to the cell plasma membrane. The number and finer detail of these common organelles varies according to the specialized function a

Fig. 3.1 **Diagrammatic representation of the cell, illustrating the major organelles.**

cell might perform. For example, the mitochondria of muscle cells contain many infolded cristae; they produce large amounts of ATP (from the electron transport chain that sits on the inner membrane), whereas the mitochondria of liver cells are smaller and rounded as they produce low levels of ATP, but many products from the inner matrix feed other metabolic pathways. Each cell is a component unit but can 'talk' to an adjacent cell via specific channels and receptors. Within a cell there is a constant flow of traffic between the organelles.

THE CELL MEMBRANE

The plasma cell membrane interfaces between the cell's internal mechanisms and the extracellular environment. It is a bilayer of amphipathic phospholipids that consist of a polar hydrophilic head (e.g. phosphatidyl choline) and an insoluble non-polar lipid hydrophobic tail (commonly two long-chain fatty acids). The phospholipids spontaneously form bilayers (as complete circular structures) that form an effective barrier that is impermeable to most water-soluble molecules. This barrier defines the interior environment of the cell. The exchanges across the plasma membrane are regulated by various proteins that are embedded in the lipid bilayer (Fig. 3.2). The lipids' hydrophobic structure means that relatively weak bonds hold the plasma membrane together. However, this strongly opposes the transverse movement of hydrophilic molecules but allows considerable freedom for lateral 'fluid' movement by molecules such as membrane proteins that are embedded in it. The plasma membrane is thus a very dynamic structure. Cell-to-cell communication is the key to many diseases and chemotherapeutic interventions.

The membrane proteins embedded in the lipid bilayer either traverse the whole membrane or are associated only with the outer or inner leaflet of the bilayer (Fig. 3.2). These proteins are responsible for the cell's interaction with its external environment. The molecules involved are either *channels*, *receptors* or *cell adhesion molecules* (see below).

Cell dynamics

Like all systems, the component proteins – and even organelles – of the cell are continually being formed and degraded. Most of the degradation steps involve ATP-dependent multienzyme complexes. Old cellular proteins are mopped up by a small cofactor molecule called '*ubiquitin*', which interacts with these worn proteins via their exposed hydrophobic residues. Ubiquitin acts as a signal for destruction or repair, and a complex containing more than five ubiquitin molecules is rapidly degraded by a large proteolytic multienzyme array termed '26S proteasome'. The failure to remove worn proteins can result in the development of chronic debilitating disorders. Alzheimer and frontotemporal dementias are associated with the accumulation of ubiquinated proteins (prion-like proteins), which are resistant to ubiquitin-mediated proteolysis. Similar proteolytic-resistant ubiquinated proteins give rise to inclusion bodies found in myositis and myopathies. This resistance can be due to point mutation in the target protein itself (e.g. mutant p53 in cancer; see p. 189) or as a result of an external factor altering the conformation of the normal protein to create a proteolytic-resistant shape, as in the prion protein of variant Creutzfeldt–Jakob disease (vCJD). Nuclear factor kappa B (NFκB) is bound by inhibitory factor IκB. Upon phosphorylation, NFκB, is released and IκB is degraded by the proteasome. Failure to do so results in an accumulation of IκB.

Phagocytosis, pinocytosis and exocytosis

Specialized cells such as macrophages and neutrophils can engulf about 20% of their surface area in the pursuit of large particles such as bacteria. Lysosomes rapidly fuse with phagosomes, giving equally rapid digestion of the contents, and recycling as much of the internalized membrane as possible. *Phagocytosis* is only triggered when specific cell surface receptors – such as the macrophage Fc receptor – are occupied by their ligand. *Pinocytosis* is a much smaller-scale model of phagocytosis

Fig. 3.2 **Cell membrane showing lipid structures and main types of integral proteins** such as receptors, G-proteins, channels, secondary messenger enzyme complexes and cell adhesion molecules.

and is continually occurring in all cells. In contrast to phagocytosis, receptors for smaller molecular complexes, such as low-density lipoprotein (LDL) (Fig. 3.3) result in surface clumping and the internal accumulation of a protein called *clathrin*. Clathrin-coated pits pinch inwards as clathrin-coated vesicles. Clathrin prevents fusion of lysosomes, and thus its removal will result in lysosomal fusion and degradation of the contents. Maintenance of a clathrin coat can result in transcellular transit of the contents and their *exocytosis* at another side of the plasma membrane, i.e. apical-to-basal surface transcytosis. Similarly, cell organelles bud off vesicles coated in clathrin to prevent lysosomal fusion and degradation. Some of these vesicles rapidly fuse with the plasma membrane and exocytose their contents. Other vesicles do not immediately fuse with the plasma membrane (or indeed any other organelle). The clathrin-coated vesicles have additional lipid bilayer-embedded proteins called v-SNAREs (signal and response elements), which interact with target organelle membrane proteins called t-SNAREs. Vesicle fusion is therefore specific, comprising fusion in the correct place (at a particular organelle or part of the plasma membrane) at the correct time (e.g. the fusion of neuronal transmitter vesicles and release of the transmitter at the synaptic membrane when stimulated).

Membrane transport and ion channels

The plasma membrane is freely permeable to gases such as O_2, CO_2 and N_2, and to small uncharged molecules such as H_2O (*not* H^+ and OH^-) and urea. Whilst larger hydrophobic lipid-soluble molecules – like steroids – also pass freely through the membrane, large uncharged molecules (glucose, amino acids and nucleotides) and small charged ions (K^+, Na^+, Ca^{2+}, Cl^-, Mg^{2+} and HCO_3^-) cannot pass unless via a specific transport protein embedded in the plasma membrane. Two structural types of transport molecules/complexes exist (Fig. 19.2):

- *Channel proteins* literally open a channel in the lipid membrane to allow a specific solute to pass through.
- *Carrier proteins* are slower in action, shuttling the solute across and either facilitating diffusion down a gradient across the membrane, or actively pumping solutes against the gradient using ATP as an energy source.

Active carrier pumps and gated ion channels work together in neural transmission (see Fig. 21.1). These carrier proteins pump Na^+ and K^+ across the neuronal cell membrane to create a differential gradient, but ion channels open in response to stimuli to cause a rapid depolarization, allowing the ions to flow back. At synaptic junctions these ion channels open in response to chemical signals such as the release of glutamate, epinephrine (adrenaline) or acetylcholine.

ATP-dependent transport molecules (ATPases) belong to a superfamily called the '*ABC transporter superfamily*'. These include the multidrug-resistance protein (MDR), which pumps out hydrophobic drugs and is overexpressed by tumour cells, and the chloride ion pump coded by the

Fig. 3.3 **Intracellular transport. (a)** Receptor-mediated pinocytosis. **(b)** Trafficking of vesicles containing synthesized proteins to the cell surface (e.g. hormones). **(c)** Traffic between organelles is also mediated by v- and t-SNARE-containing organelles. v-SNARE, vesicle-specific SNARE; t-SNARE, target-specific SNARE.

cystic fibrosis gene (see Fig. 3.23). All share a common structure of six transmembrane domains interrupted by a cytoplasmic ATPase domain, followed by a further six transmembrane domains and another cytoplasmic ATPase. The cystic fibrosis chloride ion channel is unusual in that it requires the binding and hydrolysis of both ATP and cAMP for activation.

Receptors

Membrane surface receptors pass their extracellular signal across the plasma membrane to cytoplasmic secondary signalling molecules. Examples of these receptors include the non-lipid-soluble ligands such as growth hormone (GH), insulin, insulin-like growth factor (IGF) and luteinizing hormone (LH). These membrane-bound receptors can be subclassified according to the mechanism by which they activate signalling molecules:

- ion channel linked (see above)
- G-protein linked
- enzyme linked.

Structurally these plasma membrane receptors can be:

- serpentine (seven transmembrane domains, e.g. the LH receptor)
- transmembrane with large extra- and intracellular domains (e.g. the epidermal growth factor (EGF) receptor)
- transmembrane with a large extracellular domain only
- entirely linked onto the outer membrane leaflet by a lipid moiety known as a GPI (glycan phosphatidylinositol) anchor (e.g. T-cell receptor).

The function of these membrane receptors is to initiate a secondary message that ultimately results in activation of a specific enzyme or a DNA-binding protein. This may involve translocation to the nucleus and initiation of transcription of a specific set of genes.

G-protein-linked receptors

The G-protein-linked receptor, once activated by a ligand, binds a trimeric complex (α, β, γ) which is anchored to the inner surface of the plasma membrane. This complex is a GTP-binding protein, or G-protein. The G-protein binds GTP rather than GDP, and then interacts with enzyme complexes anchored into the inner leaflet of the membrane. These complexes in turn activate one or all three of the secondary messengers:

- cyclic AMP (cAMP)
- Ca^{2+} ions
- inositol 1,4,5-trisphosphate/diacylglycerol (IP_3/DAG).

Enzyme-linked surface receptors

These receptors usually have a single transmembrane-spanning region, and a cytoplasmic domain that has intrinsic enzyme activity or will bind and activate other membrane-bound or cytoplasmic enzyme complexes. Four classes of enzymes have been designated:

- *Guanylyl cyclase-linked receptors* (e.g. the atrial natriuretic peptide receptor), which produce cyclic GMP. This in turn activates a cGMP-dependent kinase (G-kinase), which binds to and phosphorylates serine and threonine residues of specific secondary messengers.
- *Tyrosine kinase receptors* (e.g. the platelet-derived growth factor (PDGF) receptor), which either specifically phosphorylate kinases on a small set of intracellular signalling proteins, or associate with proteins that have tyrosine kinase activity.
- *Tyrosine phosphatase receptors* (e.g. CD45), which remove phosphates from tyrosine residues of specific intracellular signalling proteins.
- *Serine/threonine kinase receptors* (e.g. the transforming growth factor-beta (TGF-β) receptor), which phosphorylate specific serine and threonine residues of intracellular signalling proteins.

There are many intracellular receptors that bind lipid-soluble ligands such as steroid hormones (e.g. progesterone, cortisol, T_3 and T_4). These cytoplasmic receptors often change shape in response to binding their ligands, form dimers, enter the nucleus and interact directly with specific DNA sequences (see DNA-binding proteins, p. 167).

CYTOPLASM

This is the fluid component inside the cell membrane and contains many specialized organelles (see Fig. 3.1). It contains a scaffolding or cytoskeleton that regulates the passage and direction in which the interior solutes and storage granules flow. The cytoplasm contains:

- *Endoplasmic reticulum (ER)*. This consists of interconnecting tubules or flattened sacs (cisternae) of lipid bilayer membrane. It may contain ribosomes on the surface (termed rough endoplasmic reticulum (RER) when present, or smooth endoplasmic reticulum (SER) when absent). The ER is involved in the processing of proteins: the ribosomes translate mRNA into a primary sequence of amino acids of a protein peptide chain (see Fig. 3.4). This chain is synthesized into the ER where it is first folded and modified into mature peptides. ER is the major site of drug metabolism.
- *Golgi apparatus*. This consists of flattened cisternae similar to the ER. It is characterized as a stack of cisternae from which vesicles bud off from the thickened ends. The primary processed peptides of the ER are exported to the Golgi apparatus for maturation into functional proteins (e.g. glycosylation of proteins which are to be excreted occurs here) before packaging into secretory granules and cellular vesicles that bud off the end (see Fig. 3.3).
- *Lysosomes*. These are dense cellular vesicles containing acidic digestive enzymes. They fuse with phagocytotic vesicles from the outer cell membrane, digesting the contents into small biomolecules that can cross the lysosomal lipid bilayer into the cell cytoplasm. Lysosomal enzymes can also be released outside the

cell by fusion of the lysosome with the plasma membrane. Lysosomal action is crucial to the function of macrophages and polymorphs in killing and digesting infective agents, tissue remodelling during development and osteoclast remodelling of bone. Not surprisingly, many metabolic disorders result from impaired lysosomal function (p. 1146).

- *Peroxisomes.* These are dense cellular vesicles so named because they contain enzymes that catalyse the breakdown of hydrogen peroxide. They are involved in the metabolism of bile and fatty acids, and are primarily concerned with detoxification, e.g. D-amino acid oxidase and H_2O_2 catalase. The inability of the peroxisomes to function correctly can lead to rare metabolic disorders such as Zellweger's syndrome and rhizomelic dwarfism.

- *Mitochondria.* These organelles are the powerhouse of the cell. Each mitochondrion comprises two lipid bilayer membranes and a central matrix. It also possesses several copies of its own DNA in a circular genome. The *outer membrane* contains many gated receptors responsible for the import of raw materials like pyruvate and ADP, and the export of products such as oxaloacetate (precursor of amino acids and sugars) and ATP. An interesting caveat to our symbiotic relationship is that proteins of the *Bcl-2/Bax* family are incorporated in this outer membrane and can release mitochondrial enzymes that trigger apoptosis (see p. 162). The *inner membrane* is often highly infolded to form cristae to increase its effective surface area. It contains transmembrane enzyme complexes of the electron transport chain, which generate an H^+ ion gradient. This gradient then drives the adjacent transmembrane ATPase complex to form ATP from ADP and P_i. *The inner matrix* contains the enzymes of the Krebs cycle that generate the substrates of both the electron transport chain ($FADH_2$ and NADH) and central metabolism (e.g. succinyl CoA, α-oxoglutarate, oxaloacetate).

SECONDARY MESSENGERS

Secondary messengers are molecules that transduce a signal from a bound receptor to its site of action (e.g. the nucleus). There are essentially four mechanisms by which secondary messengers act but they cross talk and are rarely activated independently of each other (Fig. 3.4). These mechanisms are cyclic AMP, IP_3/DAG, Ca^{2+} ions and protein phosphorylation.

Cyclic AMP, IP_3/DAG and Ca^{2+} ions

The generation of cAMP by G-protein-linked receptors results in an increase in cellular cAMP (Fig. 3.4(ia)), which binds and activates specific cAMP-binding proteins. These dimerize and enter the cell nucleus to interact with set DNA sequences (the cAMP response elements). In addition, cofactors in the cAMP-binding proteins are co-activated and interact with the phosphorylation pathway.

Other G-protein complexes activate inner membrane-bound phospholipase complexes. These in turn cleave membrane phospholipid-polyphosphoinositide (PIP_2) into two components (Fig. 3.4(ib)). The first is the water-soluble molecule inositol trisphosphate, IP_3. This floats off into the cytoplasm and interacts with gated ion channels in the endoplasmic reticulum (or sarcoplasmic reticulum in muscle cells), causing a rapid release of Ca^{2+}. The lipid-soluble component diacylglycerol (DAG) (Fig. 3.4(ic)) remains at the membrane, but activates a serine/threonine kinase, protein kinase C (see phosphorylation section below).

Although the cellular calcium-binding proteins and ion pumps rapidly remove Ca^{2+} from the cytoplasm back into a storage compartment (such as the endoplasmic reticulum), free Ca^{2+} interacts with target proteins in the cytoplasm, inducing a phosphorylation/dephosphorylation cascade, resulting in activated DNA-binding proteins entering the nucleus.

Protein phosphorylation

Although phosphorylation of the cytoplasmic secondary messengers is often a consequence of secondary activation of cAMP, Ca^{2+} and DAG, the principal route for the protein phosphorylation cascades is from the dimerization of surface protein kinase receptors, which have bound their ligands. The tyrosine kinase receptors phosphorylate each other when ligand binding brings the intracellular receptor components into close proximity (see Fig. 3.4(ii)). The inner membrane and cytoplasmic targets of these activated receptor complexes are *ras*, protein kinase C and ultimately the MAP (mitogen activated protein) kinase, Janus-Stat pathways or phosphorylation of IκB causing it to release its DNA-binding protein, nuclear factor kappa B (NFκB). These intracellular signalling proteins usually contain conserved non-catalytic regions called SH2 and SH3 (serc homology regions 2 and 3). The SH2 region binds to phosphorylated tyrosine. The SH3 domain has been implicated in the recruitment of intermediates that activate *ras* proteins. Like G-proteins, *ras* (and its homologous family members *rho* and *rac*) switches between an inactive GDP-binding state and an active GTP-binding state. This starts a phosphorylation cascade of the MAP kinase, Janus-Stat protein pathways, which ultimately activate a DNA-binding protein (NFκB). NFκB undergoes a conformational change, enters the nucleus and initiates transcription of specific genes.

Lipid-soluble ligands (e.g. steroids) do not need secondary messengers; their cytoplasmic receptors, once activated, enter the nucleus as DNA-binding proteins and alter gene expression directly.

THE CYTOSKELETON

This is a complex network of structural proteins which regulates not only the shape of the cell, but also its ability to traffic internal cell organelles and even move in response to external stimuli (see Fig. 3.2). The major components are microtubules, intermediate filaments and microfilaments.

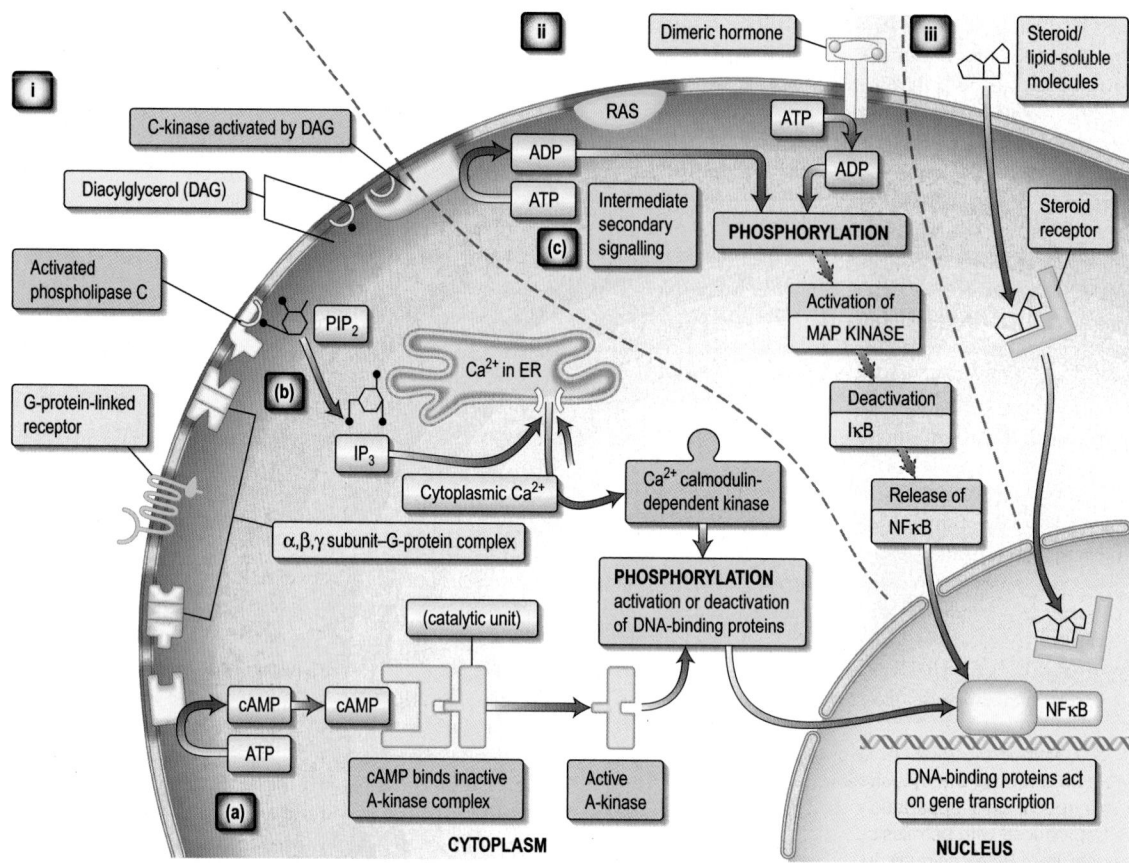

Fig. 3.4 Receptor and secondary messengers. (i) G-protein receptor binds ligand (e.g. hormone) and activates G-protein complex. The G-protein complex can activate three different secondary messengers: (a) cAMP generation; (b) inositol 1,4,5-trisphosphate (IP3) and release of Ca^{2+}; (c) diacylglycerol (DAG) activation of C-kinase and subsequent protein phosphorylation. **(ii) Dimeric hormone** binds receptor subunits bringing them into close association. Intracellular domains cross-phosphorylate and link to the phosphorylation cascades via molecules such as RAS. **(iii) Lipid-soluble molecules,** e.g. steroids, pass through the cell membrane and bind to cytoplasmic receptors, which enter the nucleus and bind directly to DNA. ER, endoplasmic reticulum; IκB, inhibitory factor kappa B; NFκB, nuclear factor kappa B.

- *Microtubules* (Fig. 3.5). These are made up of two protein subunits, α and β tubulin (50 kDa), and are continuously changing length. They form a 'highway', transporting organelles through the cytoplasm. There are two motor microtubule-associated proteins – dynein and kinesin – allowing antegrade and retrograde movement. Dynein is also responsible for the beating of cilia. During interphase the microtubules are rearranged by the microtubule-organizing centre (MTOC), which consists of centrosomes containing tubulin and provides a structure on which the daughter chromosomes can separate. Another protein involved in the binding of organelles to microtubules is the cytoplasmic linker protein (CLIP). Drugs that disrupt the microtubule assembly (e.g. colchicine and vinblastine) affect the positioning and morphology of the organelles. The anticancer drug paclitaxel causes cell death by binding to microtubules and stabilizing them so much that organelles cannot move, and thus mitotic spindles cannot form.
- *Intermediate filaments.* These form a network around the nucleus and extend to the periphery of the cell.

They make cell-to-cell contacts with the adjacent cells via desmosomes, and with basement matrix via hemidesmosomes (Fig. 3.6). Their function appears to be in structural integrity; they are prominent in cellular tissues under stress. The intermediate filament fibre proteins are specific to the embryonic lineage of the cell concerned, for example keratin intermediate fibres are only found in epithelial cells whilst vimentin is only found in mesothelial (fibroblastic) cells.
- *Microfilaments.* Muscle cells contain a highly ordered structure of actin (a globular protein, 42–44 kDa) and myosin filaments, which form the contractile system. These filaments are also present throughout the non-muscle cells as truncated myosins (e.g. myosin 1), in the cytosol (forming a contractile actomyosin gel), and beneath the plasma membrane. Cell movement is mediated by the anchorage of actin filaments to the plasma membrane at adherent junctions between cells (Fig. 3.6). This allows a non-stressed coordination of contraction between adjacent cells of a tissue. Similarly, vertical contraction of tissues is anchored across the cell membrane to the basement matrix at focal adhesion

epithelial cells (e.g. intestinal and renal cells) and form a barrier to the movement of ions and solutes across the epithelium, although they can be variably 'leaky' to certain solutes. The proteins responsible for the intercellular tight junction closure are called *claudins*. They show selective expression within tissue and regulate what small ions may pass through the gaps between cells. For example, the kidney displays a differential expression of these claudin proteins. Mutations of claudin-16 (which is expressed in the distal convoluted tubule in the kidney, where magnesium is reabsorbed) are responsible for some forms of Gitelman's syndrome (p. 706). Since magnesium reabsorption is paracellular, tight junctions (which contain claudin-16) prevent these divalent ions rapidly diffusing back between the cells into renal tubules.

Adherent junctions

Adherent junctions (zonula adherens) are continuous on the basal side of cells. They contain cadherins and are the major site of attachment of intracellular microfilaments. Intermediate filaments attach to *desmosomes*, which are apposed areas of thickened membranes of two adjacent cells. *Hemidesmosomes* attach cells to the basal lamina and are also connected to intermediate filaments. Transmembrane *integrins* link the extracellular matrix to microfilaments at focal areas where cells also attach to their basal laminae. In blistering dermatological disorders autoantibodies cause damage by attacking tight junction desmosomal proteins such as desmoglein-3 in *pemphigus vulgaris* and desmoglein-1 in *pemphigus foliaceus* (p. 1347).

Gap junctions

Gap junctions allow substances to pass directly between cells without entering the extracellular fluids. Protein channels (*connexons*) are lined up between two adjacent cells and allow the passage of solutes up to molecular weight 1000 kDa (e.g. amino acids and sugars), as well as ions, chemical messengers and other factors. The diameter of these channels is regulated by intracellular Ca^{2+}, pH and voltage. Connexons are made up of six subunits surrounding a channel and their isoforms in tissues are encoded by different genes. Mutant connexons can cause disorders, such as the X-linked form of Charcot–Marie–Tooth disease (p. 1263).

CELL ADHESION MOLECULES (see also p. 198)

Adhesion molecules and adhesion receptors are essential for tissue structural organization. Differential expression of such molecules is implicit in the processes of cell growth and differentiation, such as wound repair and embryogenesis. There are four major families of cell adhesion molecules: cadherins, integrins, the immunoglobulin superfamily and selectins (Fig. 3.6).

Cadherins

The cadherins establish molecular links between adjacent cells. They form zipper-like structures at 'adherens junctions', areas of the plasma membrane where cells make

Fig. 3.5 Immunofluorescent micrograph of dividing fibroblasts showing the cytoskeleton. Microtubules are shown in green, Golgi apparatus in yellow and the nuclei in blue. Reproduced with permission of Dr Philip Huie, Stanford University, from *Biotechniques* July/August 1995.

junctions where actin fibres converge (Fig. 3.6). Actin-binding proteins (e.g. fimbria) modulate the behaviour of microfilaments, and their effects are often calcium-dependent. The actin-associated proteins can be tissue type specific, for example actin-binding troponin is a complex of three subunits and two of these have isomers which are only found in cardiac muscle. Cardiac troponin I and T are released into the blood circulation after the onset of a myocardial infarction (p. 809).

Alterations in the cell's actin architecture are also controlled by the activation of small *ras*-like GTP-binding proteins *rho* and *rac*. These are involved in rearrangement of the cell during division, and thus dysfunctions of these proteins are associated with malignancy.

INTERCELLULAR CONNECTIONS

The cytoskeleton and plasma membrane interconnect, and extracellular domains form junctions between cells to form tissues. There are three types of junction between cells: tight junctions, adherent junctions and gap junctions (Fig. 3.6).

Tight junctions

Tight junctions (zonula occludens) hold cells together. They are situated at the ends of margins adjacent to

a | Homophilic interaction | | Heterophilic interaction |

CAM, e.g. VCAM-1

Matrix
— Fibronectin
— Fibrinogen
— RGD sequence

α_4 — β_1 α_5 — β_2

Glycosylation

Ca²⁺
Ca²⁺

| Cadherin | | Immunoglobulin superfamily cell adhesion molecule | | Integrin | | Selectin | Mucin | | Desmosome |

Intermediate microtubules, e.g. keratin, vimentin

Cadherins

Tight/gap junction
Claudins, occludins, or connexins

b

Adherent junction
Cadherins

Actin fibres

Plaque

c

| Focal adherent junction | | Hemidesmosome |

Actin fibres
Plaques
Integrins
Basal lamina

Fig. 3.6 **Cell adhesion molecules and cellular junctions. (a) Five main groups of adhesion molecules**. The cadherins have a Ca²⁺-dependent homodimer homophilic interaction and their intracellular domains link to the cytoskeleton. Immunoglobulin superfamily cell adhesion molecules (CAMs) have both homophilic and heterophilic (integrin) interactions. Binding is Ca²⁺ independent and the intracellular domains are cell signalling. Integrins have heterophilic interactions mostly with basement matrix components. They have an α–β chain structure and their intracellular domains are predominantly cell signalling but can directly interact with cytoskeletal complexes. Selectins have a weak binding affinity for specific sugar molecules found on mucins. Mucins are long tandem-repeat peptides which protrude from the cell membrane and are covered in glycosylation moieties. **(b) Adjacent cells form focal adhesion junctions**. *Desmosomes* are where the membrane forms a proteinaceous plaque containing molecules like desmoglein, from which cadherins protrude and bind cadherins of the adjacent cell. Intracellularly the plaque binds loops of cytoskeleton intermediate filaments, e.g. keratin in epithelial cells and vimentin in fibroblasts. *Tight junctions* are mediated by integral membrane proteins, claudins and diclaudins, which associate to form subunits bridging the intercellular gap. *Gap junctions* consists of connexin subunits that form a regulated hollow tube. *Adherent junctions* are similar to desmosomes in that cell-to-cell adhesion is mediated by cadherins but the membrane proteinaceous plaque components are different and bind contractile cytoskeletal fibres like actin at the terminus. **(c) Basement membrane adhesion**. This is similar to desmosomes and adherent junctions in that membrane plaques link intercellular intermediate filaments (e.g. keratin or vimentin) in *hemidesmosomes* and contractile cytoskeleton actin in *focal adherent junctions* to the basement matrix. However, integrins replace cadherins as the surface adhesion molecules.

contact with other cells. Through these junctions, bundles of actin filaments run from cell to cell. Related molecules such as desmogleins form the main constituents of desmosomes, the intercellular contacts found abundantly between epithelial cells. Desmosomes serve as anchoring sites for intermediate filaments of the cytoskeleton. When dissociated embryonic cells are grown in a dish, they tend to cluster according to their tissue of origin. The homophilic (like with like) interaction of cadherins is the basis of this separation, and has a key role in segregating embryonic tissues. The expression of specific adhesion molecules in the embryo is crucial for the migration of cells and the differentiation of tissues. For example, when neural crest cells stop producing N-CAM (see below) and N-cadherin and start to display integrin receptors they can separate, and begin to migrate on the extracellular matrix. Changes in cadherin expression are often associated with tumour metastatic potential.

Integrins

These are membrane glycoproteins with α and β subunits which exist in active and inactive forms. The integrins principally bind to extracellular matrix components such as fibrinogen, elastase and laminin. The amino acid sequence arginine–glycine–aspartic acid (RGD) is a potent recognition sequence for integrin binding, and

integrins replace cadherins in the focal membrane anchorage of hemidesmosomes and focal adhesion junctions (Fig. 3.6). A feature of integrins is that the active form can come about as a result of a cytoplasmic signal that causes a conformational change in the extracellular domain, increasing affinity for its ligand. This 'inside-out' signalling occurs when leucocytes are stimulated by bacterial peptides, rapidly increasing leukocyte integrin affinity for immunoglobulin superfamilies structures such as the Fc portion of immunoglobulin. The 'outside-in' signalling follows the binding of the ligand to the integrin and stimulates secondary signals resulting in diverse events such as endocytosis, proliferation and apoptosis. Defective integrins are associated with many immunological and clotting disorders such as Bernard–Soulier syndrome and Glanzmann's thrombasthenia (p. 472).

Immunoglobulin superfamily cell adhesion molecules (CAMs)

These molecules contain domain sequences which are immunoglobulin-like structures. The neural-cell adhesion molecule (N-CAM) is found predominantly in the nervous system. It mediates a homophilic (like with like) adhesion. When bound to an identical molecule on another cell, N-CAM can also associate laterally with a fibroblast growth factor receptor and stimulate the tyrosine kinase activity of that receptor to induce the growth of neurites. Thus adhesion molecules can trigger cellular responses by indirect activation of other types of receptors. The placenta and gastrointestinal tract also express immunoglobulin superfamily members, but their function is not completely understood.

Selectins

Unlike most adhesion molecules (which bind to other proteins), the selectins interact with carbohydrate-ligands or *mucin* complexes on leucocytes and endothelial cells (vascular and haematological systems). Selectins were named after the tissues in which they were first identified. *L-selectin* is found on leucocytes and mediates the homing of lymphocytes to lymph nodes. *E-selectin* appears on endothelial cells after they have been activated by inflammatory cytokines; the small basal amount of E-selectin in many vascular beds appears to be necessary for the migration of leucocytes. *P-selectin* is stored in the alpha granules of platelets and the Weibel–Palade bodies of endothelial cells, but it moves rapidly to the plasma membrane upon stimulation of these cells. All three selectins play a part in leucocyte rolling (p. 199).

THE NUCLEUS AND ITS RESPONSES

A nucleus is present in all eukaryotic cells that divide. It contains the human genome and is bound by two bilayer lipid membranes. The outer of the two is continuous with the endoplasmic reticulum. Nuclear pores are present in the membranes, allowing the passage of nucleotides and DNA interacting proteins in, and mRNA out (see Fig. 3.4). The genome consists of DNA and all the apparatus for replication and transcription into RNA (see p. 164). There are two types of cell division – meiosis and mitosis. In *meiosis*, which occurs only in germ cells, the chromosome complement is halved (haploid) and, at fertilization, the union of two cells restores the full complement of 46 chromosomes. *Mitosis* occurs in dividing cells after fertilization, and results in two identical daughter cells. It is only during cell division that chromosomes (see p. 171) become visible.

A nucleolus is a dense area within the nucleus. It is rich in proteins and RNA and is chiefly concerned with the synthesis of ribosomal RNA (rRNA) and ribosomes.

The cell cycle (Fig. 3.7)

Cells in the quiescent G0 phase (G, gap) of the cycle are stimulated by the receptor-mediated actions of growth factors (e.g. EGF, epithelial growth factor; PDGF, platelet-derived growth factor; IGF, insulin-like growth factor) via intracellular second messengers. Stimuli are transmitted to the nucleus (see below) where they activate transcription factors and lead to the initiation of DNA synthesis, followed by mitosis and cell division. Cell cycling is modified by the cyclin family of proteins that activate or deactivate proteins involved in DNA replication by phosphorylation (via kinases and phosphatase domains). Thus from G0 the cell moves on to G1 (gap 1) when the chromosomes are prepared for replication. This is followed by the synthetic (S) phase, when the 46

Fig. 3.7 **The cell cycle.** Cells are stimulated to leave non-cycle **G0** to enter **G1** phase by growth factors. During **G1**, transcription of the DNA synthesis molecules occurs. Rb is a 'checkpoint' (inhibition molecule) between G1 and S phases and must be removed for the cycle to continue. This is achieved by the action of the cyclin-dependent kinase produced during G1. During the **S phase** any DNA defects will be detected and p53 will halt the cycle (see p. 189). Following DNA synthesis (S phase) cells enter **G2**, a preparation phase for cell division. Mitosis takes place in the **M phase**. The new daughter cells can now either enter G0 and differentiate into specialized cells, or re-enter the cell cycle.

chromosomes are duplicated into chromatids, followed by another gap phase (G2), which eventually leads to mitosis (M).

Apoptosis (programmed cell death)

Apoptosis or physiological cell death occurs through the deliberate activation of constituent genes whose function is to cause their own demise.

Necrotic cell death, in contrast is where some external factor (e.g. hypoxia, chemical toxins) damages the cell's physiology and results in the disintegration of the cell. Characteristically there is an influx of water and ions, after which cellular organelles swell and rupture. Cell lysis induces acute inflammatory responses in vivo owing to the release of lysosomal enzymes into the extracellular environment.

Apoptotic cell death has characteristic morphological features:

- chromatin aggregation, with nuclear and cytoplasmic condensation into distinct membrane-bound vesicles which are termed apoptotic bodies
- organelles remain intact
- cell 'blebs' (which are intact membrane vesicles)
- there is no inflammatory response
- cellular 'blebs' and remains are phagocytosed by adjacent cells and macrophages.

This process requires energy (ATP), and several Ca^{2+}- and Mg^{2+}-dependent nuclease systems are activated which specifically cleave nuclear DNA at the inter-histone residues. An endonuclease destroys DNA following apoptosis. This involves the enzyme caspase (cysteine-containing aspartase-specific protease) which activates the CAD (caspase-activated DNase)/ICAD (inhibitor of CAD) system which can destroy DNA. Regulated apoptosis is essential for many life processes, from tissue structure formation in embryogenesis and wound healing to normal metabolic processes such as autodestruction of the thickened endometrium to cause menstruation in a non-conception cycle. In oncology, chemotherapy and radiotherapy regimens only work if they can trigger the tumour cells' own apoptotic pathways. Failure to do so in resistant tumours can result in the accumulation of further genetic damage to the surviving cells. Several factors initiate apoptosis but in general there are two signalling pathways: the extrinsic apoptotic pathway triggered by death receptors on the cell surface and the intrinsic pathway initiated at the mitochondrial level. Death receptors are all members of the TNF receptor superfamily and include CD95 (APO-1/Fas), TRAIL (TNF-related apoptosis ligand)-R1, TRAIL-R2, TNF-R1, DR3 and DR6.

The *extrinsic pathway* is involved in processes such as tissue remodelling and induction of immune self-tolerance. Activated receptors with internal death domain complexes multiply pro-caspase 8 molecules whose autocatalytic activity results in release of the initiator caspase 8 (Fig. 3.8). In turn caspase 8 cleaves pro-caspase 3 and caspase 3, in combination with the other effector

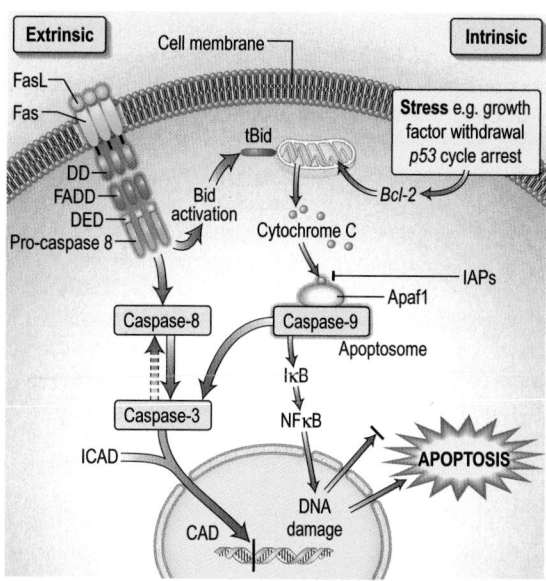

Fig. 3.8 Diagrammatic representation of the extrinsic and intrinsic apoptotic signalling network. The Fas protein and Fas ligand (FasL) are two proteins that interact to activate one of the best-defined apoptotic pathways.

Fas and **FasL** are both members of the TNF (tumour necrosis factor) family – Fas is part of the transmembrane receptor family and FasL is part of the membrane-associated cytokine family. When the homotrimer of FasL binds to Fas, it causes Fas to trimerize and brings together the **death domains (DD)** on the cytoplasmic tails of the protein. The adaptor protein, **FADD (Fas-associating protein with death domain)**, binds to these activated death domains and they bind to pro-caspase 8 through a set of **death effector domains (DED)**.
When pro-caspase 8s are brought together, they transactivate and cleave themselves to release **caspase 8**, a protease that cleaves protein chains after aspartic acid residues. Caspase 8 then cleaves and activates other caspases which eventually leads to activation of caspase 3. **Caspase 3** cleaves **ICAD**, the inhibitor of CAD (caspase activated DNase), which frees **CAD** to enter the nucleus and cleave DNA. Although caspase 3 is the pivotal execution caspase for apoptosis, the processes can be initiated by intrinsic signalling which always involves mitchondrial release of cytochrome C and activation of **caspase 9**.
The release of **cytochrome C** and mitochondrial inhibitor of IAPs is mediated via Bcl-2 family proteins (including Bax, Bak) forming pores in the mitochondrial membrane. Interestingly, the extrinsic apoptotic signal is aided and amplified by activation of **tBid** which recruits Bcl-2 family members and hence also activates the intrinsic pathway.
Apaf1, apoptotic protease activating factor 1; Bid, family member of Bcl-2 protein; IAPs, inhibitor of apoptosis proteins.

caspases, activating DNA cleavage, cell condensation and fragmentation.

The *intrinsic pathway* centres on the release of cytochrome C from the mitochondria. Cellular stress, such as growth factor withdrawal and p53 cell cycle arrest induces the expression of the pro-apoptotic Bcl-2 family of proteins, Bax and Bak. These form tetrameric complexes,

which imbed into the outer mitochondrial membrane forming permissive pores. Cytochrome C, released from the mitochondria, binds Apaf1, forming a complex known as the apoptosome, which then activates an initiator caspase, in this case caspase 9. Caspase 9, then activates the effector caspase, caspase 3. Other proteins released from damaged mitochondria, Smac/DIABLO and Omi/HtrA2, counteract the effect of IAPs (inhibitor of apoptosis proteins), which normally bind and prevent activation of pro-caspase 3. Anti-apoptotic Bcl-2 protein, when incorporated as a member of the Bak/Bax pore complex, renders the mitochondrial pore non-permissive to release of cytochrome C and the anti-IAPs.

There is an amplification link between the extrinsic and intrinsic apoptotic pathways in that caspase 8 cleaves a Bcl-2 family member, tBid, which then aids formation of the Bcl-2/Bax/Bak pore complexes. If this complex is predominately formed from pro-apoptotic members of the Bcl-2 family of proteins then apoptosome/caspase 9, along with mitochondrial anti-IAPs, amplifies the apoptotic activation of effector caspases 3 (Fig. 3.8). Conversely, overexpression of anti-apoptotic Bcl-2 will not only inhibit intrinsic, but also dampen down extrinsic apoptotic signalling.

FURTHER READING

Ashcroft FM (2000) *Ion Channels and Disease*. San Diego: Academic Press.

Blobe GC, Schiemann WP, Lodish HF (2000) Role of transforming growth factor-β in human disease. *New England Journal of Medicine* **342**: 1350–1358.

Cooper, GM (2000). *The Cell – A Molecular Approach*, 2nd edn. Sunderland (MA): Sinauer Associates.

Donaldson KM, Li W, Ching KA et al. (2003) Ubiquitin-mediated sequestration of normal cellular proteins into polyglutamine aggregates. *Proceedings of the National Academy of Sciences USA* **100**: 8892–8897.

Friedlander RM (2003) Apoptosis and caspases in neurodegenerative diseases. *New England Journal of Medicine* **348**: 1365–1375.

Friedman J, Xue D (2004) To live or die by the sword: the regulation of apoptosis by the proteasome. *Developmental Cell* **6**(4): 460–461.

Huber O (2003) Structure and function of desmosomal proteins and their role in development and disease. *Cellular and Molecular Life Sciences* **60**(9): 1872–1890.

Micheau O, Tschopp J (2003) Induction of TNF receptor I – mediated apoptosis via two sequential signaling complexes. *Cell* **114**: 181–190.

Wheelock MJ, Johnson KR (2003) Cadherins as modulators of cellular phenotype. *Annual Review of Cell and Developmental Biology* **19**: 207–235.

Wyllie AH (ed) (1997) Apoptosis: an overview. *British Medical Bulletin* **53**: 451–465.

MOLECULAR BIOLOGY AND GENETIC DISORDERS

Over 200 genetic disorders have been identified, and the role of molecular biology in the diagnosis of monogenic disease is clear cut. The interaction of 'at risk' genes in multifactorial diseases has also increased the role of genetics in rheumatology, cancer and schizophrenia.

DNA STRUCTURE AND FUNCTION

Genetic information is stored in the form of double-stranded deoxyribonucleic acid (DNA). Each strand of DNA is made up of a deoxyribose–phosphate backbone and a series of purine (adenine (A) and guanine (G)) and pyrimidine (thymine (T) and cytosine (C)) bases of the nucleic acid. For practical purposes the length of DNA is generally measured in numbers of base-pairs (bp).

The monomeric unit in DNA (and in RNA) is the nucleotide, which is a base joined to a sugar–phosphate unit (Fig. 3.9a). The two strands of DNA are held together by hydrogen bonds between the bases. There are only four possible pairs of nucleotides – TA, AT, GC and CG (Fig. 3.9b). The two strands twist to form a double helix with major and minor grooves, and the large stretches of helical DNA are coiled around histone proteins to form nucleosomes and further condensed into the chromosomes that are seen at metaphase (Fig. 3.9c, d).

GENES

A gene is a portion of DNA that contains the codes for a polypeptide sequence. Three adjacent nucleotides (a codon) code for a particular amino acid, such as AGA for arginine, and TTC for phenylalanine. There are only 20 common amino acids, but 64 possible codon combinations that make up the genetic code. This means that most amino acids are encoded for by more than one triplet; other codons are used as signals for 'initiating' or 'terminating' polypeptide-chain synthesis.

Genes consist of lengths of DNA that contain sufficient nucleotide triplets to code for the appropriate number of amino acids in the polypeptide chains of a particular protein. Genes vary greatly in size: most extend over 20–40 kbp, but a few (such as the gene for the muscle protein dystrophin) can extend over millions of base-pairs. In bacteria the coding sequences are continuous, but in higher organisms these coding sequences (exons) are interrupted by intervening sequences that are non-coding (introns) at various positions (see Fig. 3.10). Some genes code for RNA molecules which will not be further translated into proteins. These code for functional

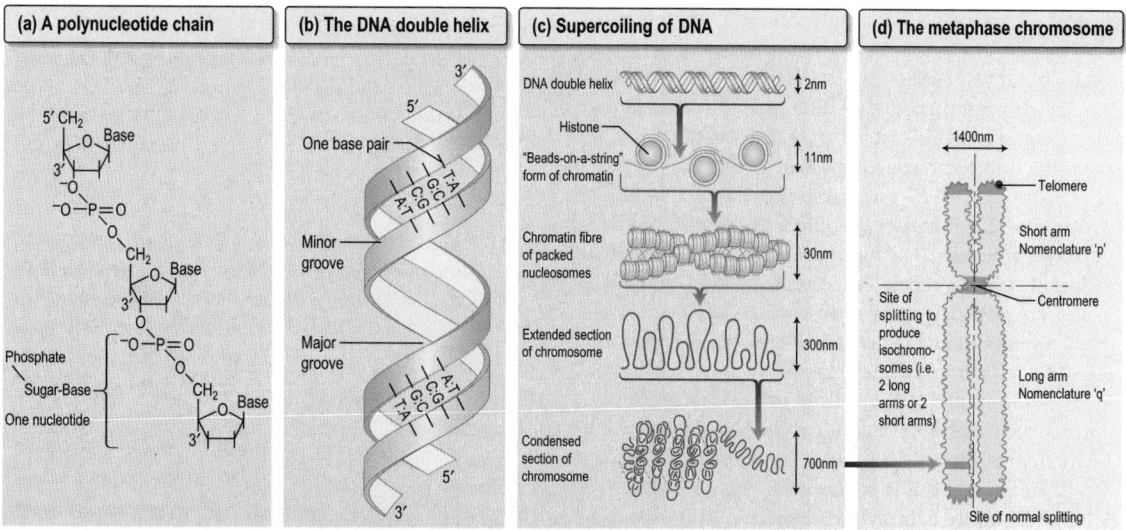

Fig. 3.9 **DNA and its structural relationship to human chromosomes.**
(a) A polynucleotide strand with the position of the nucleic bases indicated. Individual nucleotides form a polymer linked via the deoxyribose sugars. The 5′ carbon of the heterocyclic sugar structure links to the 3′ carbon of the next via a phosphate molecule forming the sugar–phosphate backbone of the nucleic acid. The 5′–3′ linkage gives an orientation to a sequence of DNA.
(b) Double-stranded DNA. The two strands of DNA are held together by hydrogen bonds between the bases. As T always pairs with A, and G with C, there are only four possible pairs of nucleotides – TA, AT, GC and CG. The orientation of the complementary single strands of DNA (ssDNA) is always opposite; i.e. one will be 5′–3′ whilst the partner will be 3′–5′. CG base-pairs form three hydrogen bonds whilst the AT bonds form only two. Thus, CG bonds are stronger than AT bonds, which affects the biophysical nature of different sequences of DNA. In a random sequence of DNA with equal proportions of CG and AT base-pairs, complementary strands form a helical 3D structure. This helix will have major and minor grooves and a complete turn of the helix will contain 12 base-pairs. These grooves are structurally important, as DNA-binding proteins predominantly interact with the major grooves. DNA sequences rich in repetitive CG base-pairs distort the helical shape whereby the minor grooves become more equal in size to the major grooves, giving a Z-like structure. These CG-rich regions are sites were DNA-binding proteins are likely to bind.
(c) Supercoiling of DNA. In humans, and other higher organisms, the large stretches of helical DNA are coiled to form nucleosomes and further condensed into the chromosomes that can be seen at metaphase. DNA is first packaged by winding around nuclear proteins – histones – every 180 bp. This can then be coiled and supercoiled to compact nucleosomes and eventually visible chromosomes.
(d) At the end of the metaphase DNA replication will result in a twin chromosome joined at the centromere. This picture shows the chromosome, its relationship to supercoiling, and the positions of structural regions: centromeres, telomeres and sites where the double chromosome can split.
Nomenclature of chromosomes. This is the assigned number or X or Y, plus short arm (p) or long arm (q). The region or subregion is defined by the transverse light and dark bands observed when staining with Giemsa (hence G-banding) or quinacrine and numbered from the centromere outwards.
Chromosome constitution = chromosome number + sex chromosomes + abnormality; e.g.
46XX = normal female
47XX+21 = Down's syndrome (trisomy 21)
46XYt (2;19) (p21;p12) = male with a normal number of chromosomes but a translocation between chromosome 2 and 19 with breakages at short-arm bands 21 and 12 of the respective chromosomes.

ribosomal RNA (rRNA) and transfer RNA (tRNA), which play vital roles in polypeptide synthesis.

TRANSCRIPTION AND TRANSLATION
(Fig. 3.10)

The conversion of genetic information to polypeptides and proteins relies on the transcription of sequences of bases in DNA to messenger RNA molecules; mRNAs are found mainly in the nucleolus and the cytoplasm, and are polymers of nucleotides containing a ribose–phosphate unit attached to a base. The bases are adenine, guanine, cytosine and uracil (U) (which replaces the thymine found in DNA). RNA is a single-stranded molecule but it can hybridize with a complementary sequence of single-stranded DNA (ssDNA). Genetic information is carried from the nucleus to the cytoplasm by mRNA, which in turn acts as a template for protein synthesis.

Each base in the mRNA molecule is lined up opposite to the corresponding base in the DNA: C to G, G to C, U to A and A to T. A gene is always read in the 5′–3′ orientation and at 5′ promoter sites which specifically bind the enzyme RNA polymerase and so indicate where transcription is to commence. Eukaryotic genes have two AT-rich promoter sites. The first, the TATA box, is located about 25 bp upstream of (or before) the transcription start site, while the second, the CAAT box, is 75 bp upstream of the start site. The initial or primary mRNA is a

complete copy of one strand of DNA and therefore contains both introns and exons. While still in the nucleus, the mRNA undergoes post-transcriptional modification whereby the 5' and 3' ends are protected by the addition of an inverted guanidine nucleotide (CAP) and a chain of adenine nucleotides (Poly A) (see Fig. 3.10). In higher organisms, the primary transcript mRNA is further processed inside the nucleus whereby the introns are spliced out. Splicing is achieved by small nuclear RNA in association with specific proteins. Furthermore, alternative splicing is possible whereby an entire exon can be omitted. Thus more than one protein can be coded from the same gene. The processed mRNA then migrates out of the nucleus into the cytoplasm. Polysomes (groups of ribosomes) become attached to the mRNA; the ribosomes consist of subunits composed of small RNA molecules (rRNA) and proteins. The rRNA components are key to the binding and translation of the genetic code. Held by the ribosomes, triplets of adjacent bases on the mRNA called codons are exposed and recognized by complementary sequences, or anti-codons, in transfer RNA (tRNA) molecules. Each tRNA molecule carries an amino acid that is specific to the anti-codon. As the ribosome passes along the mRNA in the 5'–3' direction, amino acids are transferred from tRNA molecules and sequentially linked by the ribosome in the order dictated by the order of codons. The ribosome, in effect, moves along the mRNA like a 'zipper', linking the assembled amino acids to form a polypeptide chain. The first 20 or more nucleotides are recognition and regulatory sequences and are untranslated but necessary for translation and possibly earlier transcription. Translation begins when the triplet AUG (methionine) is encountered. All proteins start with methionine but this is often lost as the leading sequence of amino acids of the native peptides are removed during protein folding and post-translational modification into a mature protein. Similarly the Poly A tail is not translated (3' untranslated region) and is preceded by a stop codon, UAA, UAG or UGA.

THE CONTROL OF GENE EXPRESSION

Gene expression can be controlled at many points in the steps between the translation of DNA to proteins. Proteins and RNA molecules are in a constant state of turnover; as soon as they are produced, processes for their destruction are at work. For many genes, transcriptional control is the key point of regulation. Deleterious, even oncogenic, changes to a cell's biology may arise through no fault in the expression of a particular gene. Apparent overexpression may be due to non-breakdown of mRNA or protein product. Conversely, a recent paper suggests the existence of a pathway that stops gene expression by promoting degradation of RNA (RNA interference, RNAi).

Transcriptional control

Gene transcription (DNA to mRNA) is not a spontaneous event and is possible only as a result of the interaction of a number of DNA-binding proteins with genomic DNA.

Fig. 3.10 Transcription and translation (DNA to RNA to protein).

RNA polymerase creates an **RNA copy** of the DNA gene sequence. This **primary transcript** is processed: capping of the 5' free end of the mRNA precursor involves the addition of an inverted guanine residue to the 5' terminal which is subsequently methylated, forming a 7-methylguanosine residue. (The corresponding position on the gene is thus called the CAP site.)

The 3' end of an mRNA defined by the sequence AAUAAA acts as a cleavage signal for an endonuclease, which cleaves the growing transcript about 20 bp downstream from the signal. The 3' end is further processed by a Poly A polymerase forming a Poly A tail (polyadenylation), which adds about 250 adenosine residues to the 3' end.

Without these additions, the mRNA sequence will be rapidly degraded 5'–3' but the inverted cap nucleotide prevents nuclease attachment. The activity of specific 5' mRNA nucleases to remove the cap is further regulated by the Poly A tail which must first be removed by other degradation enzymes.

Splicing out of the introns then produces the mature mRNA (prokaryote genes do not contain introns). This then moves out of the nucleus via nuclear pores and aligns on endoplasmic reticulum.

Ribosomal subunits assemble on the mRNA moving along 5' to 3'. With the transport of amino acids to their active sites by specific tRNAs, the complex translates the code, producing the peptide sequence. Once formed, the peptide is released into the cytoplasmic reticulum for post-translational modification into a mature protein.

Regulation of a gene's expression must first start with the opening up of the double helix of DNA in the correct region of the chromosome. In order to do this, a class of protein molecules that recognize the outside of the DNA helix have evolved. These DNA-binding proteins preferentially interact with the major groove of the DNA double helix (see Fig. 3.9). The base-pair composition of the DNA sequence can change the geometry of a DNA helix to facilitate the fit of a DNA-binding protein with its target region: CG-rich areas form the Z-structure DNA helix; sequences such as AAAANNN cause a slight bend, and if this is repeated every 10 nucleotides it produces pronounced curves. DNA-binding proteins that recognize these distorted helices result either in the opening up of the helix so that the gene may be transcribed, or in the prevention of the helix being opened.

Structural classes of DNA-binding proteins

There are four basic classes of DNA-binding protein, classified according to their structural motifs (see Fig. 3.11 and Table 3.1).

Control regions and proteins

DNA-binding proteins act as regulators of gene expression in three different ways. They are the promoters, the operators and the enhancers. The primary gene expression regulators are the *promoters*. The RNA polymerases bind to a promoter region, normally adjacent to the transcribed sequence of DNA. In eukaryotes active transcription is possible only when a number of DNA-binding and associated proteins come together and interact. Known as 'general transcription factors', these proteins are thought to assemble at promoter sites used by RNA polymerases (e.g. Pol II) that are characterized by specific motifs such as the TATA sequence.

Other DNA regulator proteins operate in close proximity to the site of promoter binding. These are called operator proteins/regions and act either as repressors by binding to DNA sequences within the promoter site or as positive regulators facilitating RNA polymerase binding. The third class of regulator proteins operate as enhancer sequences which are at least 200 bp away from the site of transcription initiation. Binding of regulator proteins to enhancer regions, several hundred bases from the promoter site, upregulates the expression. This turns out to be a distance favourable for DNA to loop back on itself without straining the backbone bonds of the DNA double helix.

The GAL4 enhancer of yeast physically aids the binding of transcription factors to the TATA region of the promoter, and thus acts like a catalyst for general transcription factor assembly, and consequently also the rate of RNA polymerase activity. In mammals, it is frequently a region termed the 'cyclic AMP response element' (CRE) that acts in this manner. Increasing intracellular cAMP levels cause activation and release of CRE-binding protein (CREB). This binds to the CRE sequence and enhances the transcription rate.

These relatively remote regulatory regions need not just enhance gene expression but may also repress transcription. Indeed, loops can be formed from regulatory regions downstream as well as upstream of the gene's coding sequence. Repressors can inhibit the transcription of a given gene by binding to the regulatory sequence and blocking positive regulators, binding and thus inactivating the positive regulator, or by interfering with the promoter protein assembly. Multiple regulatory regions and DNA-binding proteins can surround a given gene and precisely control its expression at a basal level and in response to a cellular stimulus (Table 3.1).

CHROMOSOMES, INTRONS AND THE SIZE OF THE HUMAN GENOME

Human genetics differs from that of bacteria in structural components of the genetic code and in the way DNA is packaged. The fact that humans have chromosomes and introns affects how much DNA we require to code for all our proteins in an unusual way. We have far more DNA $(3 \times 10^9$ bp) than protein-coding genes (32 000), whereas simple bacteria appear to have a much more economical DNA to gene ratio. Simple organisms like bacteria that have circular genomes, that are not contained within a membrane-bound organelle (the nucleus), are termed 'prokaryotes'. Higher eukaryotic organisms have their linear genomic packages – chromosomes – separated from the general cytoplasm by the nuclear envelope. In eukaryotes, genomic DNA is associated with nuclear proteins called histones.

Coiling around histones and structural regions such as the centromeres and telomeres, requires regions of DNA devoted specifically to the purpose of packaging (see Fig. 3.9c). Ten per cent of human DNA is highly repetitive (or 'satellite' DNA), consisting of long arrays of tandem

Table 3.1 Examples of DNA-binding proteins

Class of DNA-binding protein	Examples
Helix–turn–helix	CREB (cAMP response element binding protein)
Zinc finger	Steroid and thyroid hormone receptors Retinoic acid and vitamin D receptors Bcl-6 oncogene product (lymphoma) WT1 oncogene product (Wilms' tumour) GATA-1 erythrocyte differentiation and Hb expression factor
Leucine zippers	c-jun cell replication oncogene c-fos cell replication oncogene
Helix–loop–helix	myc oncogene mad oncogene max oncogene

(a) Helix-turn-helix

(i)

NH₂

DNA-binding
recognition
helix

COOH

(ii)

(iii)

2

1   3

(b) Zinc finger

(i)

HOOC

His 23

Zn

Cys 6

Cys 3

His 19

H₂N

(ii)

COOH

Zn

Zn

Zn

NH₂

(c) Leucine zipper

(i)

SUBUNIT DIMERIZATION REGION

DNA-BINDING REGION

+NH₂
H H

+NH₂
H H

Hydrophobic
region rich
in leucine
residues

Hydrophilic
region rich in
residues like
asparagine

(ii)

Leucine
residue

Hydrophobic
interaction

(d) Helix-loop-helix

(i)

Subunit
dimerization
helix

DNA-binding
helix

(ii)

---

repeats. These regions tend to be supercoiled around histones in condensed regions termed *heterochromatin*, even when the cell is not undergoing division. In contrast, most other DNA regions are relatively uncondensed and constitute the euchromatin. This remaining DNA is either moderately repetitive, accounting for about 30% of the genome, or codes for unique genes and gene families, occupying some 2% of the genome.

Although supercoiling of DNA around histones, intronic spacing (all giving tighter control of specific gene expression) and packaging into functional chromosomes accounts for some 40% of our total DNA, at least 60% is random and has no apparent function. However, life

Fig. 3.11 The four classes of DNA-binding proteins.
(a) Helix–turn–helix (HTH) motifs. The simplest and most common, it consists of a helix connected by a fixed angle to a second helix. **(i)** This represents the 'core' motif of HTH DNA-binding proteins but considerable modifications occur. **(ii)** Like all DNA-binding proteins they interact as dimers, binding at exactly one turn of the double helix (3.4 nm or 12 bp) apart. The homeodomain HLH DNA-binding proteins are a special class of HTH proteins. Discovered in the 1980s during investigation of the gene controlling *Drosophila* development, they contain an almost identical stretch of 60 amino acids. They have a third helix which holds the DNA-binding region in a fixed orientation. Indeed, all homeodomain proteins appear to have specific conserved amino acid positions and residues which interact with DNA. **(iii)** Furthermore, random orientation extension chains at the N-terminal can interact with the minor groove.
(b) Zinc finger motifs, characterized by the incorporation of zinc, in some form, into the protein's quartenary structure.
(i) The term originated from the structural model of a *Xenopus laevis* protein which uses a zinc ion to hold a loop in a 'finger'-shape by cross-linking two histidine residues with two cysteine residues. The Cys–Cys–His–His family of zinc finger DNA regulator proteins typically consists of an anti-parallel sheet forming a tight tertiary association with its own helix by zinc interaction with Cys and His residues within each of the two secondary structures. **(ii)** Several clusters of zinc fingers are found together and form a repeating structure which can interact with repetitive sequences in DNA.
(c) Leucine zipper motif. (i) This consists of a long α-helix which has many hydrophobic leucine residues at one end, responsible for dimer formation, whilst the opposite hydrophilic ends interact with DNA across the major groove of the double helix. **(ii)** The quaternary structure of the leucine zippers need not be homodimeric, and indeed heterodimers are extremely common. Thus multiple sequences may be recognized by two or three DNA leucine zipper proteins depending on the type of dimer formed.
(d) Helix–loop–helix (HLH) motifs. (i) These consist of a DNA-binding a-helix joined to a protein dimerization secondary α-helix via a loop. **(ii)** These combine leucine zipper properties with those of helix motif DNA-binding proteins. A helix interacting with DNA is linked via a loop to a large second helix which non-covalently binds to a similar HLH protein. Homo- and heterodimers can form, but the loop gives flexibility in the orientation of the given DNA-binding α-helix domain.

outside of the sea is exposed to increased DNA damage by radiations and chemicals. This additional genomic mass of terrestrial animals, compared to deep-sea creatures, may be there to absorb the increased risk of DNA damage.

FURTHER READING

NCBI *Genes and Disease*. (An eBook) Bethesda (MD): National Library of Medicine (US).

Stevenson M (2004) Therapeutic potential of RNA interference. *New England Journal of Medicine* **351**: 1772–1777.

Strachan T, Read AP (1999) *Human Molecular Genetics 2*, 2nd edn. Oxford: BIOS Scientific Publishers.

TOOLS FOR MOLECULAR BIOLOGY

Preparation of genomic DNA

The first step in studying the DNA of an individual involves preparation of genomic DNA. This is a simple procedure in which any cellular tissue including blood (the nucleated cells are isolated from the erythrocytes) can be used. The cells are lysed in order to open their cell and nuclear membranes, releasing chromosomal DNA. Following digestion of all cellular protein by the addition of proteolytic enzymes, the genomic DNA is isolated by chemical extraction with phenol. DNA is stable and can be stored for years.

Restriction enzymes and gel electrophoresis

Genomic DNA can be cut into a number of fragments by enzymes called 'restriction enzymes', which are obtained from bacteria. Restriction enzymes recognize specific DNA sequences and cut double-stranded DNA at these sites. For example, the enzyme EcoRI will cut DNA wherever it reads the sequence GAATTC, and so human genomic DNA is cut into hundreds of thousands of fragments. Whenever the genomic DNA from an individual is cut with EcoRI, the same 'restriction fragments' are produced. As DNA is a negatively charged molecule, the genomic DNA that has been digested with a restriction enzyme can be separated according to its size and charge, by electrophoresing the DNA through a gel matrix. The DNA sample is loaded at one end of the gel, a voltage is applied across the gel, and the DNA migrates towards the positive anode. The small fragments move more quickly than the large fragments, and so the DNA fragments separate out. Fragment size can be determined by running fragments of known size on the same gel.

Pulsed-field gel electrophoresis (PFGE) can be used to separate very long pieces of DNA (hundreds of kilobases) which have been cut by restriction enzymes that cut at rare sites in the genome. In this technique, DNA molecules are subjected to two perpendicular electric fields that are switched on alternately. The DNA molecules are separated on the basis of molecular size, and this technique can be used for long-range mapping of the genome to detect major deletions and rearrangements.

Southern blotting and DNA probes

This technique allows the visualization of individual DNA fragments (Fig. 3.12). A DNA probe is used to indicate where the fragment of interest lies. DNA probes are useful because a fundamental property of DNA is that when two strands are separated, for example by heating, they will always reassociate and stick together again because of their complementary base sequences. Therefore the presence or position of a particular gene can be identified using a gene 'probe' consisting of DNA with a base sequence that is complementary to that of the sequence of interest. A DNA probe is thus a piece of single-stranded DNA that can be labelled with a radioactive isotope (usually ^{32}P) or a fluorescent signal. The probe is added to a hybridization solution into which the membrane with the DNA is also placed. The single-stranded probe will locate and bind to its complementary

Fig. 3.12 **Southern blotting and DNA probes.**

sequence on the blot and can be identified by autoradiography or fluorescence.

A similar technique for blotting RNA fragments (which are not cut by restriction enzymes, but which are blotted as full-length mRNAs) on to membranes is called Northern blotting, and one for blotting proteins is called Western blotting.

The polymerase chain-reaction (PCR)

Minute amounts of DNA can be amplified over a million times within a few hours using this in vitro technique (Fig. 3.13). The exact DNA sequence to be amplified needs to be known because the DNA is amplified between two short (generally 17–25 bp) single-stranded DNA fragments ('oligonucleotide primers') which are complementary to the sequences at each end of the DNA of interest.

The technique has three steps. First, the double-stranded genomic DNA is denatured by heat into single-stranded DNA. The reaction is then cooled to favour DNA annealing, and the primers bind to their target DNA. Finally, a DNA polymerase is used to extend the primers in opposite directions using the target DNA as a template. After one cycle there are two copies of double-stranded DNA, after two cycles there are four copies, and this number rises exponentially with the number of cycles. Typically a polymerase chain-reaction is set for 25–30 cycles, allowing millions of amplifications, i.e. 2^n where n = number of cycles.

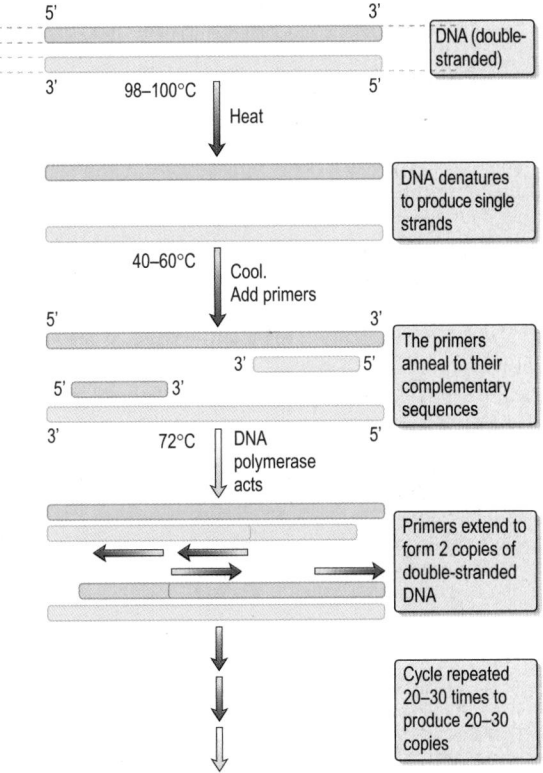

5'
3'

DNA (double-stranded)

3'   98–100°C   5'

Heat

DNA denatures to produce single strands

40–60°C   Cool. Add primers

5'   3'
        3'   5'
5'   3'

The primers anneal to their complementary sequences

3'   72°C   DNA polymerase acts   5'

Primers extend to form 2 copies of double-stranded DNA

Cycle repeated 20–30 times to produce 20–30 copies

Fig. 3.13 **Polymerase chain reaction.**

This technique has revolutionized genetic research because minute amounts of DNA not previously amenable to analysis can be amplified, such as from buccal cell scrapings, blood spots, or single embryonic cells.

DNA cloning

A particular DNA fragment of interest can be isolated and inserted into the genome of simple self-replicating organisms or organelles such as viruses and plasmids. When used for this purpose they are referred to as vectors. Replication by the million of the vector results in multiple copies or clones of the inserted sequence. Thus, after removal from the host vector, cloned gene sequences can be prepared in large quantities independently of other sequences. Vectors include: bacteriophage viruses; plasmids, which are self-replicating episomal circular DNA molecules found in bacteria that carry antibody resistance genes; and 'yeast artificial chromosomes' (YACs), which are derived from centromeric and telomeric DNA sequences found in yeast. Each vector takes an optimum size of cloned DNA insert. Typically, viruses can accommodate only small sequences up to a maximum of a kilobase, larger fragments of 2–10 kilobases can be inserted into a plasmid, and sequences of several hundred kilobases can be inserted into a YAC. Each has its relative merits – viruses being very efficient, but the vectors which take large clones being considerably less so. A hybrid between a plasmid and a bacteriophage (called a cosmid) has been constructed artificially. This has the ability to clone reasonably large sequences as plasmids within a host bacteria. However, cosmids trick bacteriophages into packaging them into a viral body, and this viral body is then able to infect the target bacteria, giving efficient transfection rates.

The DNA fragment of interest is inserted into the vector DNA sequence using an enzyme called a ligase. This takes place in vitro. The next step, cloning, creates many copies of the 'recombinant DNA molecule' and takes place in vivo when the plasmid or other vector is placed back into the bacterial (or yeast) host. Bacteria that have successfully taken up the recombinant plasmid can be selected if the plasmid also carries an antibiotic resistance gene (so bacteria without the plasmid die in the presence of antibiotic) (Fig. 3.14).

The DNA fragment of interest to be cloned may be a restriction fragment. Alternatively it could be cDNA which has been copied from an mRNA sequence. mRNA provides the template from which a viral enzyme called reverse transcriptase (RT) can synthesize a complementary single-stranded DNA copy (cDNA). A DNA polymerase may then be used to produce a double-stranded copy by PCR. A cDNA molecule contains all the sequences necessary for a functional gene, but unlike genomic DNA it lacks introns.

DNA libraries

These are pools of isolated and cloned DNA sequences that form a permanent resource for further experiments. Two types of library are used:

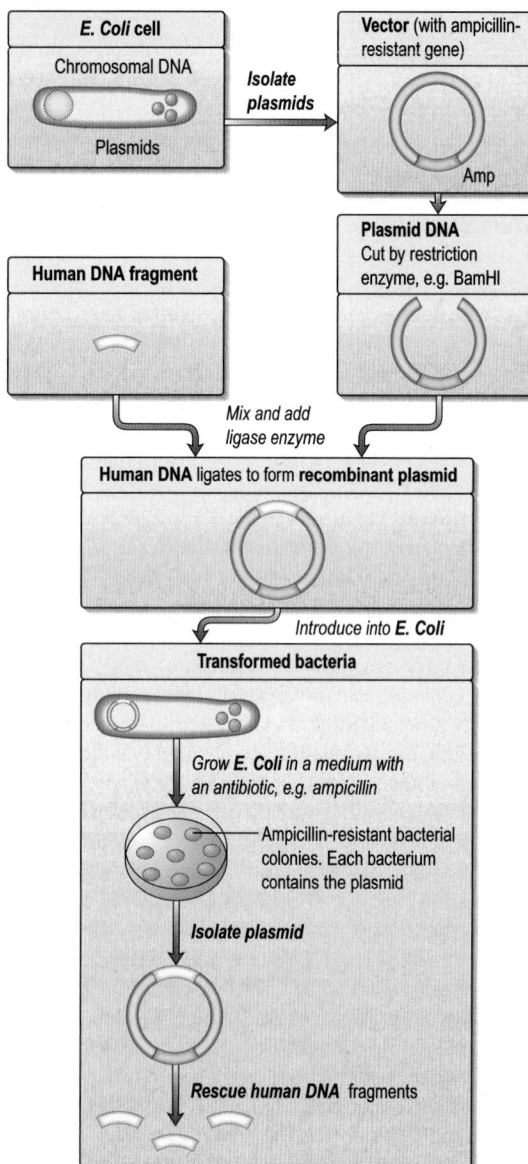

Fig. 3.14 DNA cloning. Recombinant DNA technique, showing incorporation of foreign DNA into a plasmid. The ampicillin-resistant genes can be used to distinguish transformed *Escherichia coli* cells.

- Genomic libraries are prepared from genomic DNA that has been digested with restriction enzymes, ligated into a vector and each individual clone passed into a bacterial (plasmid, bacteriophage, cosmid) or yeast (YAC) host. A genomic library usually contains almost every sequence in the genome.
- cDNA libraries are prepared from the total mRNA of a tissue, which is copied into cDNA by reverse transcriptase. The cDNA is ligated into a vector and passed into a host as above. A cDNA library should contain sequences derived from all the mRNAs expressed in that tissue type.

DNA sequencing

A chemical process known as dideoxy-sequencing allows the identification of the exact nucleotide sequence of a piece of DNA. As in PCR an oligonucleotide primer is annealed adjacent to the region of interest. This primer acts as the starting point for a DNA polymerase to build a new DNA chain that is complementary to the sequence under investigation. Chain extension can be prematurely interrupted when a dideoxynucleotide becomes incorporated (because they lack the necessary 3'-hydroxyl group). As the dideoxynucleotides are present at a low concentration, not all the chains in a reaction tube will incorporate a dideoxynucleotide in the same place; so the tubes contain sequences of different lengths but which all terminate with a particular dideoxynucleotide. Each base dideoxynucleotide (G, C, T, A) has a different fluorochrome attached, and thus each termination base can be identified by its fluorescent colour. As each strand can be separated efficiently by capillary electrophoresis according to its size/length, simply monitoring the fluorescence as the reaction products elute from the capillary will give the gene sequence (see Fig. 3.15).

Expression microarrays/gene chips

This is a methodology developed to examine the relative abundance of mRNA for thousands of genes present in cells/tissue of different types or conditions. For example, to examine the changes in gene expression from normal colonic tissue to that of malignant colonic polyps. The basic technology is the ability to immobilize sequences of DNA complementary to specific genes or different regions of known genes, onto a solid surface in precise microdot arrays. Total mRNA is extracted from one tissue and labelled with fluorescent tag Cy3-green, and the mRNA from the second tissue with fluorescent tag Cy5-red. The two fluorescent-tagged total mRNA samples are mixed in a 1:1 ratio and washed over the DNA gene chips. The mRNA for specific genes will bind to their complementary microdot and can be detected by laser-induced excitation of the fluorescent tag and the position and light wavelength and intensity recorded by a scanning confocal microscope. The relative intensity of Cy5-red : Cy3-green is a reliable measure of the relative abundance of specific mRNAs in each sample. Yellow results from equal binding of both fluorescent-tagged mRNAs. If no hybridization occurs on a dot then the area is black. The power of the system is that many thousands of genes can be screened for not only their expression but relative expression in normal and diseased tissue. A considerable amount of computing power and analysis is

FURTHER READING
Ding C, Cantor CR (2004) Quantitative analysis of nucleic acids – the last few years of progress. *Journal of Biochemistry and Molecular Biology* **37**: 1–10.
Suzuki DT et al. (2004). *Introduction to Genetic Analysis*, 8th edn. New York: WH Freeman.

Fig. 3.15 **Gene sequencing**. Sequence profile of **(a)** part of the normal luteinizing hormone beta chain gene and **(b)** that from a polymorphic variant. The base changes and consequential alterations in amino acid residues are indicated.

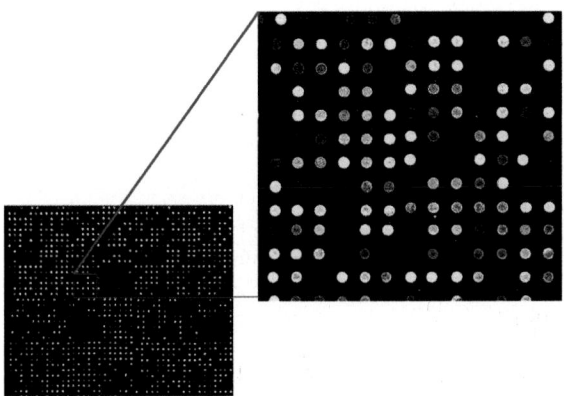

Fig. 3.16 **Expression microarray**. Example of part of a gene chip with hundreds of DNA sequences in micro-spots. The enlarged area shows the colour coding of no expression (black), overexpression (red), underexpression (green) and equal expression (yellow) of detected mRNA in two related samples.

required to interpret the thousands of dots on a microarray chip (Fig. 3.16).

THE BIOLOGY OF CHROMOSOMES

HUMAN CHROMOSOMES

The nucleus of each diploid cell contains 6×10^9 bp of DNA in long molecules called *chromosomes*. Chromosomes are massive structures containing one linear molecule of DNA that is wound around histone proteins into small units called nucleosomes, and these are further wound to make up the structure of the chromosome itself. Diploid human cells have 46 chromosomes, 23 inherited from each parent; thus there are 23 'homologous' pairs of chromosomes (22 pairs of 'autosomes' and two 'sex chromosomes'). The sex chromosomes, called X and Y, are not homologous but are different in size and shape. Males have an X and a Y chromosome; females have two

X chromosomes. (Primary male sexual characteristics are determined by the *SRY* gene – sex determining region, Y chromosome).

The chromosomes can be classified according to their size and shape, the largest being chromosome 1. The constriction in the chromosome is the centromere, which can be in the middle of the chromosome (metacentric) or at one extreme end (acrocentric). The centromere divides the chromosome into a short arm and a long arm, which are referred to as the p arm and the q arm respectively (see Fig. 3.9d). In addition, chromosomes can be stained when they are in the metaphase stage of the cell cycle and are very condensed. The stain gives a different pattern of light and dark bands that is diagnostic for each chromosome. Each band is given a number, and gene mapping techniques allow genes to be positioned within a band within an arm of a chromosome. For example, the *CFTR* gene (in which a defect gives rise to cystic fibrosis) maps to 7q21; that is, on chromosome 7 in the long arm in band 21.

During cell division (mitosis), each chromosome divides into two so that each daughter nucleus has the same number of chromosomes as its parent cell. During gametogenesis, however, the number of chromosomes is halved by meiosis, so that after conception the number of chromosomes remains the same and is not doubled. In the female, each ovum contains one or other X chromosome but, in the male, the sperm bears either an X or a Y chromosome.

Chromosomes can only be seen easily in actively dividing cells. Typically, lymphocytes from the peripheral blood are stimulated to divide and are processed to allow the chromosomes to be examined. Cells from other tissues can also be used – for example amniotic fluid, placental cells from chorionic villus sampling, bone marrow and skin (see Box 3.1).

THE X CHROMOSOME AND INACTIVATION

Although female chromosomes are XX, females do not have two doses of X-linked genes (compared with just one dose for a male XY), because of the phenomenon of

Box 3.1 Indications for chromosomal analysis

Chromosome studies may be indicated in the following circumstances.

Antenatal
- Pregnancies in women over 35 years
- Positive maternal serum screening test for aneuploid pregnancy
- Ultrasound features consistent with an aneuploid fetus
- Severe fetal growth retardation
- Sexing of fetus in X-linked disorders

In the neonate
- Congenital malformations
- Suspicion of trisomy or monosomy
- Ambiguous genitalia

In the adolescent
- Primary amenorrhoea or failure of pubertal development
- Growth retardation

In the adult
- Screening parents of a child with a chromosomal abnormality for further genetic counselling
- Infertility or recurrent miscarriages
- Learning difficulties
- Certain malignant disorders (e.g. leukaemias and Wilms' tumour)

X inactivation or Lyonization (after its discoverer, Dr Mary Lyon). In this process, one of the two X chromosomes in the cells of females becomes transcriptionally inactive, so the cell has only one dose of the X-linked genes. Inactivation is random and can affect either X chromosome.

TELOMERES AND IMMORTALITY

The ends of chromosomes, telomeres (see Fig. 3.9d) do not contain genes but many repeats of a hexameric sequence TTAGGG. Replication of linear chromosomes starts at coding sites (origins of replication) within the main body of chromosomes and not at the two extreme ends. The extreme ends are therefore susceptible to single-stranded DNA degradation back to double-stranded DNA. Thus cellular ageing can be measured as a genetic consequence of multiple rounds of replication with consequential telomere shortening. This leads to chromosome instability and cell death.

Stem cells have longer telomeres than their terminally differentiated daughters. However, germ cells replicate without shortening of their telomeres. This is because they express an enzyme called telomerase, which protects against telomere shortening by acting as a template primer at the extreme ends of the chromosomes. Most somatic cells (unlike germ and embryonic cells) switch off the activity of telomerase after birth and die as a result of apoptosis. Many cancer cells, however, reactivate telomerase, contributing to their immortality. Conversely, cells from patients with progeria (premature ageing syndrome) have extremely short telomeres. Recent research has shown transient expression of telomerase in

various stem and daughter cells as part of their normal biology. The inability to activate telomerase in cells such as those of the immune system can produce disease pathologies, in addition to overexpression.

THE MITOCHONDRIAL CHROMOSOME

In addition to the 23 pairs of chromosomes in the nucleus of every diploid cell, the mitochondria in the cytoplasm of the cell also have their own genome. The mitochondrial chromosome is a circular DNA (mtDNA) molecule of approximately 16 500 bp, and every base-pair makes up part of the coding sequence. These genes principally encode proteins or RNA molecules involved in mitochondrial function. These proteins are components of the mitochondrial respiratory chain involved in oxidative phosphorylation (OXPHOS) producing ATP. They also have a critical role in apoptotic cell death. Every cell contains several hundred mitochondria, and therefore several hundred mitochondrial chromosomes. Virtually all mitochondria are inherited from the mother as the sperm head contains no (or very few) mitochondria. Disorders are shown in Figure 3.17 (p. 176).

FURTHER READING
Buys C (2000) Telomeres, telomerase and cancer. *New England Journal of Medicine* **342**: 1282–1283.
Wong JMY, Collins K (2003) Telomere maintenance and disease. *Lancet* **362**: 983–988.

HUMAN GENETIC DISORDERS

The spectrum of inherited or congenital genetic disorders can be classified as the chromosomal disorders, including mitochondrial chromosome disorders, the Mendelian and sex-linked single-gene disorders, a variety of non-Mendelian disorders, and the multifactorial and polygenic disorders (Table 3.2 and Box 3.2). All are a result of a mutation in the genetic code. This may be a change of a single base-pair of a gene, resulting in functional change in the product protein (e.g. thalassaemia) or gross rearrangement of the gene within a genome (e.g. chronic myeloid leukaemia). These mutations can be congenital (inherited at birth) or somatic (arising during a person's life). The latter are responsible for the collective disease known as cancer, and the principles underlying Mendelian inheritance act in a similar manner to produce dominant and recessive traits. Both gross chromosomal and point mutations occur in somatic genetic disease.

CHROMOSOMAL DISORDERS

Chromosomal abnormalities are much more common than is generally appreciated. Over half of spontaneous abortions have chromosomal abnormalities, compared with only 4–6 abnormalities per 1000 live births. Specific chromosomal abnormalities can lead to well-recognized and severe clinical syndromes, although autosomal aneuploidy (a differing from the normal diploid number)

Box 3.2 Genetic disorders

Mendelian

- Inherited or new mutation
- Mutant allele or pair of mutant alleles at single locus
- Clear pattern of inheritance (autosomal or sex-linked) dominant or recessive
- High risk to relatives

Chromosomal

- Loss, gain or abnormal rearrangement of one or more of 46 chromosomes in diploid cell
- No clear pattern of inheritance
- Low risk to relatives

Multifactorial

- Common
- Interaction between genes and environmental factors
- Low risk to relatives

Mitochondrial

- Due to mutations in mitochondrial genome
- Transmitted through maternal line
- Different pattern of inheritance from Mendelian disorders

Somatic cell

- Mutations in somatic cells
- Somatic event is not inherited
- Often give rise to tumours

is usually more severe than the sex-chromosome aneuploidies. Abnormalities may occur in either the number or the structure of the chromosomes.

Abnormal chromosome numbers

If a chromosome or chromatids fail to separate ('non-disjunction') either in meiosis or mitosis, one daughter cell will receive two copies of that chromosome and one daughter cell will receive no copies of the chromosome. If this non-disjunction occurs during meiosis it can lead to an ovum or sperm having either (i) an extra chromosome, so resulting in a fetus that is 'trisomic' and has three instead of two copies of the chromosome; or (ii) no chromosome, so the fetus is 'monosomic' and has one instead of two copies of the chromosome. Non-disjunction can occur with autosomes or sex chromosomes. However, only individuals with trisomy 13, 18 and 21 survive to birth, and most children with trisomy 13 and trisomy 18 die in early childhood. Trisomy 21 (Down's syndrome) is observed with a frequency of 1 in 650 live births regardless of geography or ethnic background. This should be reduced with widespread screening (p. 191). Full autosomal monosomies are extremely rare and very deleterious. Sex-chromosome trisomies (e.g. Klinefelter's syndrome, XXY) are relatively common. The sex-chromosome monosomy in which the individual has an X chromosome only and no second X or Y chromosome is known as Turner's syndrome and is estimated to occur in 1 in 2500 live-born girls.

Occasionally, non-disjunction can occur during mitosis shortly after two gametes have fused. It will then result in the formation of two cell lines, each with a different chromosome complement. This occurs more often with the sex chromosome, and results in a 'mosaic' individual.

Very rarely the entire chromosome set will be present in more than two copies, so the individual may be triploid rather than diploid and have a chromosome number of 69. Triploidy and tetraploidy (four sets) result in spontaneous abortion.

Table 3.2 Prevalence of genetic disease	
Genetic disease	**Congenital malformation**
0.5% of all newborns have a chromosomal abnormality	3–5% of all births result in congenital malformations
7% of all stillborns have a chromosomal abnormality	
20–30% of all infant deaths are due to genetic disorders	30–50% of post-neonatal deaths are due to congenital malformations
11% of paediatric hospital admissions are for children with genetic disorders	18% of paediatric hospital admissions are for children with congenital malformations
12% of adult hospital admissions are for genetic causes	
15% of all cancers have an inherited susceptibility	
10% of chronic diseases of the adult population (heart, diabetes, arthritis) have a significant genetic component	

European incidences per 1000 births				
Single gene disorders:	**10**	Congenital malformations:	**31**	
Dominant	7.0	Genetically determined	0.6	
Recessive	1.66	Multifactorial	30	
X-linked	1.33	Non-genetic	~ 0.4	
Chromosomal disorders:	**3.5**			
Autosomes	1.69			
Sex chromosomes 10	1.80			

Although individual genetic diseases are rare, regional variation is enormous – the incidence of Down's syndrome varies from 1/1000 to 1/100 world-wide. Single gene diseases collectively comprise over 15 500 recognized genetic disorders. The global prevalence of all single gene diseases at birth is approximately 10/1000

Abnormal chromosome structures

As well as abnormal numbers of chromosomes, chromosomes can have abnormal structures, and the disruption to the DNA and gene sequences may give rise to a genetic disease.

- *Deletions.* Deletions of a portion of a chromosome may give rise to a disease syndrome if two copies of the genes in the deleted region are necessary, and the individual will not be normal with just the one copy remaining on the non-deleted homologous chromosome. Many deletion syndromes have been well described. For example, Prader–Willi syndrome (p. 252) is the result of cytogenetic events resulting in deletion of part of the long arm of chromosome 15, Wilms' tumour is characterized by deletion of part of the short arm of chromosome 11, and microdeletions in the long arm of chromosome 22 give rise to the DiGeorge syndrome.
- *Duplications.* Duplications occur when a portion of the chromosome is present on the chromosome in two copies, so the genes in that chromosome portion are present in an extra dose. A form of the neuropathy, Charcot–Marie–Tooth disease (p. 1263), is due to a small duplication of a region of chromosome 17.
- *Inversion.* Inversions involve an end-to-end reversal of a segment within a chromosome; e.g. abcdefgh becomes abcfedgh, for example, haemophilia (p. 472).
- *Translocations.* Translocations occur when two chromosome regions join together, when they would not normally. Chromosome translocations in somatic cells may be associated with tumorigenesis (see p. 485).

Translocations can be very complex, involving more than two chromosomes, but most are simple and fall into one of two categories. Reciprocal translocations occur when any two non-homologous chromosomes break simultaneously and rejoin, swapping ends. In this case the cell still has 46 chromosomes but two of them are rearranged. Someone with a balanced translocation is likely to be normal (unless a translocation breakpoint interrupts a gene); but at meiosis, when the chromosomes separate into different daughter cells, the translocated chromosomes will enter the gametes and any resulting fetus may inherit one abnormal chromosome and have an unbalanced translocation, with physical manifestations.

Robertsonian translocations occur when two acrocentric chromosomes join and the short arm is lost, leaving only 45 chromosomes. This translocation is balanced as no genetic material is lost and the individual is healthy. However, any offspring have a risk of inheriting an unbalanced arrangement. This risk depends on which acrocentric chromosome is involved. Clinically relevant is the 14/21 Robertsonian translocation. A woman with this karyotype has a 1 in 8 risk of delivering a baby with Down's syndrome (a male carrier has a 1 in 50 risk). However, they have a 50% risk of producing a carrier like themselves, hence the necessity for genetic family studies. Relatives should be alerted to the increased risk of Down's syndrome in their offspring, and should have their chromosomes checked.

Table 3.3 shows some of the syndromes resulting from chromosomal abnormalities.

Mitochondrial chromosome disorders (Fig. 3.17)

The mitochondrial chromosome (p. 172) carries its genetic information in a very compact form; for example there are no introns in the genes. Therefore any mutation has a high chance of having an effect. However, as every cell contains hundreds of mitochondria, a single altered mitochondrial genome will not be noticed. As mitochondria divide there is a statistical likelihood that there will be more mutated mitochondria, and at some point this will give rise to a mitochondrial disease.

Most mitochondrial diseases are myopathies and neuropathies with a maternal pattern of inheritance. Other abnormalities include retinal degeneration, diabetes mellitus and hearing loss. Many syndromes have been described. Myopathies include chronic progressive external ophthalmoplegia (CPEO); encephalomyopathies include myoclonic epilepsy with ragged red fibres (MERRF) and mitochondrial encephalomyopathy, lactic acidosis and stroke-like episodes (MELAS) (see p. 1271). Kearus–Sayre syndrome includes ophthalmoplegia, heart block, cerebellar ataxia, deafness and mental deficiency due to long deletions and rearrangements. Leber's hereditary optic neuropathy (LHON) is the commonest cause of blindness in young men, with bilateral loss of central vision and cardiac arrhythmias, and is an example of a mitochondrial disease caused by a point mutation in one gene. Multisystem disorders include Pearson's syndrome (sideroblastic anaemia, pancytopenia, exocrine pancreatic failure, subtotal villous atrophy, diabetes mellitus and renal tubular dysfunction). In some families, hearing loss is the only symptom, and one of the mitochondrial genes implicated may predispose patients to aminoglycoside ototoxicity.

Analysis of chromosome disorders

The cell cycle can be arrested at mitosis with colchicines and, following staining, the chromosomes with their characteristic banding can be seen and any abnormalities identified (Fig. 3.18).

YAC-cloned probes are also available and cover large genetic regions of individual chromosomes. These probes can be labelled with fluorescently tagged nucleotides and used in in situ hybridization of the nucleus of isolated tissue from patients. These tagged probes allow rapid and relatively unskilled identification of metaphase chromosomes, and allow the identification of chromosomes dispersed within the nucleus. Furthermore, tagging two chromosome regions with different fluorescent tags allows easy identification of chromosomal translocations (Fig. 3.19).

GENE DEFECTS

Mendelian and sex-linked single-gene disorders are the result of mutations in coding sequences and their control elements. These mutations can have various effects on the

Table 3.3 Chromosomal abnormalities: examples of a few syndromes

Syndrome	Chromosome karyotype	Incidence and risks	Clinical features	Mortality
Autosomal abnormalities				
Trisomy 21 (Down's syndrome)	47, +21 (95%) Mosaicism Translocation 5%	1 : 650 (overall) (risk with 20- to 29-year-old mother 1 : 1000; > 45-year-old mother 1 : 30)	Flat face, slanting eyes, epicanthic folds, small ears, simian crease, short stubby fingers, hypotonia, variable learning difficulties, congenital heart disease (up to 50%)	High in first year, but many survive to adulthood
Trisomy 13 (Patau's syndrome)	47, +13	1 : 5000	Low-set ears, cleft lip and palate, polydactyly, micro-ophthalmia, learning difficulties	Rarely survive for more than a few weeks
Trisomy 18 (Edward's syndrome)	47, +18	1 : 3000	Low-set ears, micrognathia, rocker-bottom feet, learning difficulties	Rarely survive for more than a few weeks
Sex chromosome abnormalities				
Fragile X syndrome	46, XX, fra (X) 46, XY, fra (X)	1 : 2000	Most common inherited cause of learning difficulties predominantly in male Macro-orchidism	
Female				
Turner's syndrome	45, XO	1 : 2500	Infantilism, primary amenorrhoea, short stature, webbed neck, cubitus valgus, normal IQ	
Triple X syndrome	47, XXX	1 : 1000	No distinctive somatic features, learning difficulties	
Others	48, XXXX 49, XXXXX	Rare	Amenorrhoea, infertility, learning difficulties	
Male				
Klinefelter's syndrome	47, XXY (or XXYY)	1 : 1000 (more in sons of older mothers)	Decreased crown–pubis : pubis–heel ratio, eunuchoid, testicular atrophy, infertility, gynaecomastia, learning difficulties (20%; related to number of X chromosomes)	
Double Y syndrome	47, XYY	1 : 800	Tall, fertile, minor mental and psychiatric illness, high incidence in tall criminals	
Others	48, XXXY 49, XXXXY		Learning difficulties, testicular atrophy	

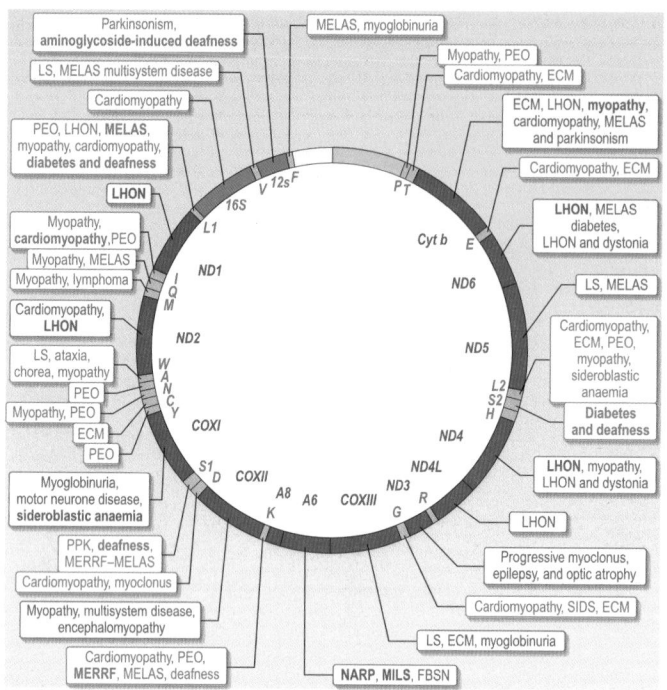

Fig. 3.17 **Mitochondrial chromosome abnormalities**. Disorders that are frequently or prominently associated with mutations in a particular gene are shown in bold. Diseases due to mutations that impair mitochondrial protein synthesis are shown in blue. Diseases due to mutations in protein-coding genes are shown in red.
ECM, encephalomyopathy; FBSN familial bilateral striatal necrosis; LHON, Leber's hereditary optic neuropathy; LS Leigh's syndrome; MELAS, mitochondrial encephalomyopathy, lactic acidosis, and stroke-like episodes; MERRF, myoclonic epilepsy with ragged-red fibres; MILS, maternally inherited Leigh's syndrome; NARP, neuropathy, ataxia and retinitis pigmentosa; PEO progressive external ophthalmoplegia; PPK, palmoplantar keratoderma; SIDS, sudden infant death syndrome.

(a)

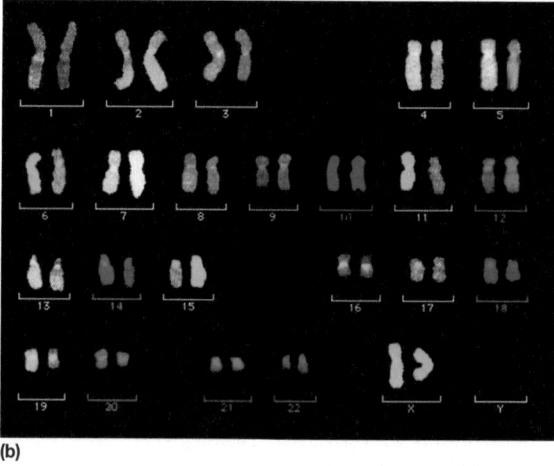

(b)

Fig. 3.18 **Karyotyping. (a)** G-banded spread of metaphase chromosomes, showing trisomy 21 (arrowed) Down's syndrome. **(b)** Whole chromosome painting probes labeled with different fluorochromes or fluorochrome combinations on 24 colour or mFISH analysis is based on a DNA probe kit. Digital image analysis software analyses the colour information and identifies the chromosomal origin of each individual pixel within the image. Inter-chromosomal rearrangements will show up as colour changes within the aberrant chromosome. Courtesy of D Lillington, Medical Oncology Unit, St Bartholomew's Hospital.

expression of the gene, as explained below, but all cause a dysfunction of the protein product.

Mutations

Although DNA replication is a very accurate process, occasionally mistakes occur to produce changes or mutations. These changes can also occur owing to other factors such as radiation, ultraviolet light or chemicals. Mutations in gene sequences or in the sequences which regulate gene expression (transcription and translation) may alter the amino acid sequence in the protein encoded by that gene. In some cases protein function will be maintained; in other cases it will change or cease, perhaps

Fig. 3.19 **Fluorescence in situ hybridization (FISH).** Two-coloured FISH using a red paint for the *ABL* gene on chromosome 9 and a green paint for the *BCR* gene on chromosome 22 in the anaphase cell nucleus. Where a translocation has occurred the two genes become juxtaposed on the Philadelphia chromosome and a hybrid yellow fluorescence can be seen only in the affected cell nucleus on the right. Courtesy of D Lillington, Medical Oncology Unit, St. Bartholomew's Hospital.

producing a clinical disorder. Many different types of mutation occur.

Point mutation

This is the simplest type of change and involves the substitution of one nucleotide for another, so changing the codon in a coding sequence. For example, the triplet AAA, which codes for lysine, may be mutated to AGA, which codes for arginine. Whether a substitution produces a clinical disorder depends on whether it changes a critical part of the protein molecule produced. Fortunately, many substitutions have no effect on the function or stability of the proteins produced as several codons code for the same amino acid. However, some mutations may have a severe effect; for example, in sickle cell disease a mutation within the globin gene changes one codon from GAG to GTG, so that instead of glutamic acid, valine is incorporated into the polypeptide chain, which radically alters its properties.

Insertion or deletion

Insertion or deletion of one or more bases is a more serious change, as it results in the alteration of the rest of the following sequence to give a frame-shift mutation. For example, if the original code was:

TAA GGA GAG TTT

and an extra nucleotide (A) is inserted, the sequence becomes:

TAA AGG AGA GTT T

Alternatively, if the third nucleotide (A) is deleted, the sequence becomes:

TAG GAG AGT TT

In both cases, different amino acids are incorporated into the polypeptide chain. This type of change is responsible for some forms of thalassaemia (p. 440). Insertions and deletions can involve many hundreds of base-pairs of DNA. For example, some large deletions in the dystrophin gene remove coding sequences and this results in Duchenne muscular dystrophy. Insertion/deletion (ID) polymorphism in the angiotensin-converting enzyme (ACE) gene has been shown to result in the genotypes II, ID and DD. The deletion is of a 287 bp repeat sequence, and DD is associated with higher concentrations of circulating ACE and possibly cardiac disease (see p. 802).

Splicing mutations

If the DNA sequences which direct the splicing of introns from mRNA are mutated, then abnormal splicing may occur. In this case the processed mRNA which is translated into protein by the ribosomes may carry intron sequences, so altering which amino acids are incorporated into the polypeptide chain.

Termination mutations

Normal polypeptide chain termination occurs when the ribosomes processing the mRNA reach one of the chain termination or 'stop' codons (see above). Mutations involving these codons will result in either late or premature termination. For example, Haemoglobin Constant Spring is a haemoglobin variant where instead of the 'stop' sequence, a single base change allows the insertion of an extra amino acid (see p. 442).

Single-gene disease

Monogenetic disorders involving single genes can be inherited as dominant, recessive or sex-linked characteristics. Although classically divided into autosomal dominant, recessive or X-linked disorders (see Tables 3.5–3.7), many syndromes show multiple forms of inheritance pattern. This is predominately because multiple defects can occur within a given disease-associated gene or in separate genes which all contribute to a particular molecular/cellular pathway and thus give rise to the same phenotype. For example in Ehlers–Danlos syndrome we find autosomal dominant, recessive and X-linked inheritance. In addition there is a spectrum between autosomal recessive and autosomal dominance in that having just one defective allele gives a mild form of the disease whilst having both alleles with the mutation results in a more severe form of the syndrome. In some cases, such as factor V Leiden disease, the boundary between dominant and recessive forms is very blurred.

Tables 3.4 and 3.5 list some autosomal dominant and autosomal recessive genetic diseases with their chromosomal localization. Some diseases show a racial or geographical prevalence. Thalassaemia (see p. 440) is seen mainly in Greeks, South East Asians and Italians, porphyria variegata occurs more frequently in the South African white population, and Tay–Sachs (p. 1147) disease particularly occurs in Ashkenazi Jews. The most common

Table 3.4 Examples of autosomal dominant disorders with chromosome location and gene defect

Syndrome	Disease prevalence	Gene (Product)	Gene location	Genetic test detection rate
Achondroplasia	1/15 000–1/40 000	FGFR3 (Fibroblast growth factor receptor-3)	4p16.3	99%
Alexander disease	Very rare	GFAPP (Glial fibrillary acidic protein)	17q21	95%
Alagille syndrome (AGS)	1/70 000	JAG1 (Jagged 1 protein)	20p12	77%
Alzheimer's disease (early onset)	41/10 000 at risk	PSENI (Presenilin 1)	14q24.3	30–70%
		PSENII (Presenilin 2)	1q31–q42	< 5%
		APP (Amyloid beta A4 protein)	21q21	10–15%
Aniridia	1–2/100 000	PAX6 (Paired box protein Pax-6)	11p13	90%
Breast cancer (familial early onset)	1/300–1/800	BRAC-1 (Breast cancer type 1 susceptibility protein)	17q21	50–75%
		BRAC-2 (Breast cancer type 2 susceptibility protein)	13q12.3	15–30%
Charcot–Marie–Tooth disease subtypes:	(30/100 000)			
CMT1	15/100 000	PMP22 (Peripheral myelin protein 22)	17p11.2	~ 50%
		MPZ (Myelin P_0 protein)	1q22	< 20%
		LITAF (Lipopolysaccharide-induced tumour necrosis factor-alpha factor)	16p13.1–12.3	Unknown
		EGR2 (Early growth response protein 2)	10q21.1–q22.1	Unknown
CMT2	6–12/100 000	KIF1B (Kinesin-like protein KIF1B)	1p36.2	Unknown
		RAB7 (Ras-like protein RAB-7)	3q21	Unknown
		GARS (Glycyl-tRNA synthetase)	7p15	Unknown
		NEFL (Neurofilament triplet L protein)	8p21	Unknown
				Unknown
		Unknown	12q23–24	Unknown
		Unknown	7q21–22	Unknown
Cerebral cavernous malformation (familial) subtypes:	Rare			
CM1	(40% of cases)	CCM1 (Krit-1 protein)	7q21–22	~ 70%
CM2	(20% of cases)	Unknown	7p15–13	Unknown
CM3	(40% of cases)	Unknown	3q25.2–27	Unknown
22q11.2 Deletion syndrome (includes DiGeorge syndrome)	1/5000	Multiple known and unknown sequences	22q11.2	100%
Dystrophia myotonica	1/20 000	DMPK (Myotonin – protein kinase)	19q13.2–13.3	100%
Ehlers–Danlos Syndrome				
Classic type	1/20 000	COL5A1 (Collagen alpha 1 (V) chain)	9q34–34.3	50–75%
		COL5A2 (collagen alpha 2 (V) chain)	2q31	50–75%
Vascular type	1/50 000	COL3A1 (Type III collagen chains)	2q31	98–99%
Epidermolysis bullosa simplex	1/50 000	KRT5 (Keratin 5)	12q13	50–70%
		KRT14 (Keratin 14)	17q12–21	50–70%
Facioscapulohumoral muscular dystrophy	6/100 000	D4Z4 (Repeat motif domain)	4q35 9	5%
Familial adenomatous polyposis	3/100 000	APC (Adenomatous polyposis coli protein)	5q21–22	95%
Familial hypercholesterolaemia	1–2/500 (95–98% of cases)	LDLR (Low-density lipoprotein receptor)	19p13.2	Unknown
	(2–5% of cases)	APOB (Apolipoprotein B100)	2p23–24	Unknown

Cont'd

Table 3.4 (Cont'd)   **Examples of autosomal dominant disorders with chromosome location and gene defect**

Syndrome	Disease prevalence	Gene (Product)	Gene location	Genetic test detection rate
Familial periodic fever/ TRAPS	Rare	*TNFRSF1A* (Serum/soluble TNF receptor)	12p13	Unknown
Haemorrhagic telangiectasia (hereditary)	1–4/50 000	*ENG* (Endoglin)	9q34.1	50–80%
		ACVRL1 (Activin – serine/ threonine-protein kinase receptor R3)	12q11–14	50–80%
Hirschsprung's disease (congenital intestinal aganglionosis)	1/5000	Multiple syndromes and chromosomal deletions give rise to Hirschsprung's disease		
		RET (Tyrosine-protein kinase receptor)	10q11.2	10–80%
		GDNF (Glial cell line-derived neutrotrophic factor)	5p13.1–12	< 1%
		NRTN (Neurturin)	19p13.3	< 1%
		EDNRB (Endothelin B receptor)	13q22	3–5%
		EDN3 (Endothelin-3)	20q13.2–13.3	5%
		ECE1 (Endothelin-converting enzyme)	1p36.1	< 1%
Li Fraumeni syndrome	Rare	*TP53* (p53)	17p13.1	95%
		CHEK2 (Serine/threonine-protein kinase Chk2)	22q12.1	Unknown
Malignant hyperthermia	1–5/50 000	*RYR1* (Ryanodine receptor type 1)	19q13.1	70%
		CACNA1S (Voltage-dependent L-type calcium channel alpha-1S subunit)	1q32	Unknown
		Unknown	17q11.2–24	Unknown
		Unknown	7q21–q22	Unknown
		Unknown	3q13.1	Unknown
		Unknown	5p	Unknown
Marfan's syndrome	1–2/10 000	*FBN1* (Fibrillin 1)	15q21.1	70–90%
MEN type 2 (multiple endocrine neoplasia)	1/30 000	*RET* (Tyrosine-protein kinase receptor)	10q11.2	88–95%
Neurofibromatosis:				
Type 1	1/4000	*NF1* (Neurofibromin)	17q11.2	80–95%
Type 2	1/40 000	*NF2* (Merlin)	22q12.2	~ 65%
Peutz–Jeghers syndrome	1–10/250 000	*STK11* (Serine/threonine-protein kinase 11)	19p13.3	65–75%
Polycystic kidney kidney disease (AD)	1–2/1000 (~ 85% of cases)	*PKD1* (Polycystin 1)	16p13.3–13.12	50–75%
Retinitis pigmentosa (AD)	(~ 15% of cases)	*PKD2* (Polycystin 2)	4q21–23	75%
	4–7/100 000			
	(25–30% of cases)	*RHO* (Rhodopsin)	3q22.1	Unknown
	(15–20% of cases)	*PRPF31* (Pre-mRNA splicing factor 31)	19q3.4	Unknown
	(5–10% of cases)	*RP1* (Oxygen-regulated protein 1)	8q12.1	Unknown
	(5–10% of cases)	*RDS* (Peripherin 2)	6p21.2	Unknown
	(3–5% of cases)	*IMPDH1* (Inosine monophosphate dehydrogenase 1)	7q14.3	Unknown
	(3% of cases – Japan)	*FSCN2* (Retinal fascin homologue 2, actin bundling protein)	17q25	Unknown
Retinoblastoma	~ 1/20 000	*RB1* (Retinoblastoma-associated protein)	13q14.1–14.2	~ 80%
Tuberous sclerosis (TS)	~ 1/6000	*TSC1* (Hamartin protein)	9q34	10–30%
		TSC2 (Tuberin)	16p13.3	50–70%
von Hippel–Lindau syndrome	1/40 000	*VHL* (von Hippel–Lindau disease tumour suppressor)	3p25–26	~ 75%
von Willebrand's disease (types 1 and 2)	Up to 3/100	*vWF* (von Willebrand factor)	12p13.2	Unknown
Wilms' tumour	1/10 000	*WT1* (Wilms' tumour protein)	11p13	Unknown

Table 3.5 Examples of autosomal recessive disorders with chromosome location and gene defects

Syndrome	Disease prevalence	Gene (Product)	Gene location	Genetic test detection rate
Alpha mannosidosis	0.5–2/million	MAN2B1 (Lysosomal alpha-mannosidase)	19cen–q12	100%
Alström syndrome	Rare	ALMS1 (ALMS1 protein)	2p13	Unknown
Ataxia telangiectasia	1–3/100 000	ATM (Serine-protein kinase ATM)	11q22.3 >	95%
Alkaptonuria	1/500 000	HGD (Homogentisic acid dioxygenase)	3q21–q23	90%
Charcot–Marie–Tooth (CMT) disease subtype CMT4	< 1/100 000	GDAP1 (Ganglioside-induced differentiation-associated protein-1)	8q13–12.1	Unknown
		MTMR2 (Myotubularin-related protein 2)	11q22	Unknown
		MTMR13 (Myotubularin-related protein 13)	11p15	Unknown
		KIAA1985 (Unknown)	5q32	Unknown
		NDRG1 (NDRG1 protein)	8q24.3	Unknown
		EGR2 (Early growth response protein 2)	10q21.1–22.1	Unknown
		PRX (Periaxin)	19q13.1–13.2	Unknown
Cockayne syndrome	< 1/100 000			
Type A	(25% of cases)	CKN1 (Cockayne syndrome WD-repeat protein/EECC-6 associated protein)	Ch5	Unknown
Type B	(75% of cases)	ERCC6 (Transcription coupled excision DNA repair protein ERCC-6)	10q11	Unknown
Cystic fibrosis	1–10/30 000	CTFR (Cystic fibrosis transmembrane conductance regulator)	7q31.2	50–95%
Cystinosis	1/20 000	CTNS (Cystinosin)	17p13	40–65%
Congenital adrenal hyperplasia 21-Hydroxylase deficiency (21-OHD)	1/15 000	CYP21A2 (Cytochrome P450 XXIB)	6p21.3	90–95%
Congenital icthyosis	1–2/200 000	TGM1 (Transglutaminase-K)	14q11.2	90%
Familial Mediterranean fever (FMF)	Rare	MEFV (Pyrin)	16p13.3	70–95%
Dysferlinopathy	Rare	DYSF (Dysferlin)	2p13.3–13.1	80%
Ehlers–Danlos – kyphoscoliotic form	1/100 000	PLOD (Procollagen-lysine, 2-oxoglutarate 5-dioxygenase 1)	1p36.3–36.2	20%
Fanconi anaemia	1/100 000			
	(66% of cases)	FRANCA (Fanconi anaemia group A protein)	16q24.3	Unknown
	(10% of cases)	FANCC (Fanconi anaemia group C protein)	9q22.3	Unknown
	(10% of cases)	FANCE (Fanconi anaemia protein E)	6p22–21	Unknown
	(10% of cases)	FANCG (Fanconi anaemia group G protein)	9p13	Unknown
	(Rare)	FANCD2 (Fanconi anaemia group D2 protein)	3p25.3	Unknown
	(Rare)	FANCF (Fanconi anaemia complementation group F)	11p15	Unknown

Cont'd

Table 3.5 (Cont'd) **Examples of autosomal recessive disorders with chromosome location and gene defects**

Syndrome	Disease prevalence	Gene (Product)	Gene location	Genetic test detection rate
Free sialic acid storage disorders	Rare	*SLC17A5* (Sialin)	6q14–q15	91%
Galactosaemia	1/30 0000	*GALT* (Galactose-phosphate uridyl transferase)	9p13	95–100%
Gaucher's disease	1–2/100 000	*GBA* (Glucocerebrosidase)	1q21	95–100%
Glycine encephalopathy	1/50 000			
	(80% of cases)	*GLDC* (Glycine dehydrogenase)	9p22	84%
	(10–15% of cases)	*AMT* (Amino methyl transferase)	3p21.2–21.1	10–30%
		GCSH (Glycine cleavage system H protein)	6q24	Unknown
Hereditary haemochromatosis	1/3000	*HFE* (Hereditary haemochromatosis protein)	6p21.3	60–98%
Homocystinuria type I	1/200 000	CBS (Cystathionine β synthetase)	21q22.3	95%
Mucopolysaccharidosis type I (Hurler's syndrome)	1–5/500 000	*IDUA* (α-l-iduronidase)	4p16.3	95%
Niemann–Pick disease:	1/150 000			
Type 1	(90% of cases)	*NPC1* (Niemann–Pick C1 protein)	18q11–12	95%
Type 2	(4% of cases)	*NPC2* (Epididymal secretory protein E1)	14q24.3	100%
Oculocutaneous albinism:				
Type 1	1/40 000	*TYR* (tyrosinase)	11q14–21	71%
Type 2	1/40 000	*OCA2* (P protein)	15q11.2–12	80–90%
Phenylalanine hydroxylase deficiency (phenylketonuria – PKU)	1–55/150 000	*PAH* (Phenylalanine hydroxylase)	12q23.2	99%
Peroxisome biogenesis disorders (Zellweger's syndrome and Refsum's disease)	1/50 000			
	(65% of cases)	*PEX1* (Peroxisome biogenesis factor-1)	7q21–22	80%
	(11% of cases)	*PEX6* (Peroxisome assembly factor-2)	6p21.1	Unknown
	(7% of cases)	*PEX26* (PEX26 protein)	22q11.2	Unknown
	(4% of cases)	*PEX10* (Peroxisome assembly protein 10)	Ch1	Unknown
	(4% of cases)	*PEX12* (Peroxisome assembly protein 12)	17q21.1	Unknown
	(1–2% of cases)	*PEX3* (Peroxisomal assembly protein PEX3)	6q23–24	Unknown
	(1–2% of cases)	*PXR1* (Peroxisomal targeting signal 1 receptor)	12p13.3	Unknown
	(Rare)	*PXMP3* (Peroxisome assembly factor-1)	8q21.1	Unknown
	(Rare)	*PEX13* (Peroxisomal membrane protein PEX13)	2p15	Unknown
	(Rare)	*PEX16* (Peroxisomal membrane protein PEX16)	11p12–11.2	Unknown
	(Rare)	*PXF* (Peroxisomal farnesylated protein)	1q22	Unknown
Retinitis pigmentosa (AR)	4–5/100 000			
	(10–20% of cases)	*Unknown*	6q14–15	Unknown
	(4–5% of cases)	*USH2A* (Usherin protein)	1q41	Unknown
	(3–4% of cases)	*PDE6B* (Rod cGMP-specific 3′,5′ cyclic phosphodiesterase β)	4p16.3	Unknown
	(3–4% of cases)	*PDE6A* (Rod cGMP-specific 3′,5′ cyclic phosphodiesterase α)	5q33.1	Unknown
	(2% of cases)	*RPE65* (Retinal pigment epithelium 61 kDa protein)	1p31.2	Unknown
	At least 16 other gene and gene loci have been found associated with autosomal recessive (AR) retinitis pigmentosa			

Cont'd

Table 3.5 (Cont'd) Examples of autosomal recessive disorders with chromosome location and gene defects				
Syndrome	**Disease prevalence**	**Gene (Product)**	**Gene location**	**Genetic test detection rate**
Sickle cell disease	Rare (1–2/10 000 in Africa)	HBB (β-globin)	11p15	100%
β-Thalassaemia	Rare (1–2/100 Cyprus)	HBB (β-globin)	11p15	99%
α-Thalassaemia	Complex	HBA1 (Haemoglobin, alpha 1)	16p13.3	
		HBA2 (Haemoglobin, alpha 2)	16p13.3	
Hexosaminidase A deficiencies (Tay–Sachs disease)	Rare	HEXA (Beta-hexosaminidase alpha chain)	15q23–24	40–98%
Wilson's disease	1/30 000	ATP7B (Copper transporting ATPase 2)	13q14.3–12.1	Unknown
Xeroderma pigmentosum	1–10/million			
	(25% of cases)	XPA (DNA-repair protein complementing XP-A cells)	9q22.3	Unknown
	(25% of cases)	XPC (DNA-repair protein complementing XP-C cells)	3p25	Unknown
	(21% of cases)	POLH (Error-prone DNA photoproduct bypass polymerase)	6p21.1–12	Unknown
	(15% of cases)	ERCC2 (TFIIH basal transcription factor complex helicase subunit)	19q13.2–13.3	Unknown
	(6% of cases)	ERCC4 (DNA-repair protein complementing XP-F cells)	16p13.3–13.13	Unknown
	(6% of cases)	ERCC5 (DNA-repair protein complementing XP-G cells)	13q33	Unknown
	(Rare)	ERCC3 (TFIIH basal transcription factor complex helicase XPB subunit)	2q21	Unknown
	(Rare)	DDB2 (DNA damage binding protein 2)	11p12–11	Unknown

recessive disease in the UK is cystic fibrosis (see pp. 192 and 909). Thus the worldwide prevalence of a disease may be low (as detailed in Tables 3.4–3.6) but much higher in specific populations. Some disorders are rare to the extent that the prevalence is counted in the total number of cases ever reported. Molecular biology has enabled the subclassification of some syndromes according to which gene is giving rise to the disease (e.g. polycystic kidney disease) and the proportion of cases arising from defects in that particular gene can be estimated from linkage analysis. However, this may not be reflected in the detection rate of a given clinical genetic test, since a single test cannot detect all the possible mutations arising at a particular locus.

Autosomal dominant disorders (Fig. 3.20 and Table 3.4)

Each diploid cell contains two copies of all the autosomes. An autosomal dominant disorder occurs when one of the two copies has a mutation and the protein produced by the normal form of the gene cannot compensate. In this case a heterozygous individual who has two different forms (or alleles) of the same gene will manifest the disease. The offspring of heterozygotes have a 50% chance of inheriting the chromosome carrying the disease allele, and therefore also of having the disease. However,

estimation of risk to offspring for counselling families can be difficult because of three factors:

- These disorders have a great variability in their manifestation. 'Incomplete penetrance' may occur if patients have a dominant disorder but it does not manifest itself clinically in them. This gives the appearance of the gene having 'skipped' a generation.
- Dominant traits are extremely variable in severity (variable expression) and a mildly affected parent may have a severely affected child.
- New cases in a previously unaffected family may be the result of a new mutation. If it is a mutation, the risk of a further affected child is negligible. Most cases of achondroplasia are due to new mutations.

The overall incidence of autosomal dominant disorders is 7 per 1000 live births.

Autosomal recessive disorders (Fig. 3.20 and Table 3.5)

These disorders manifest themselves only when an individual is homozygous for the disease allele, i.e. both chromosomes carry the mutated gene. In this case the parents are generally unaffected, healthy carriers (heterozygous for the disease allele). There is usually no family history, although the defective gene is passed from

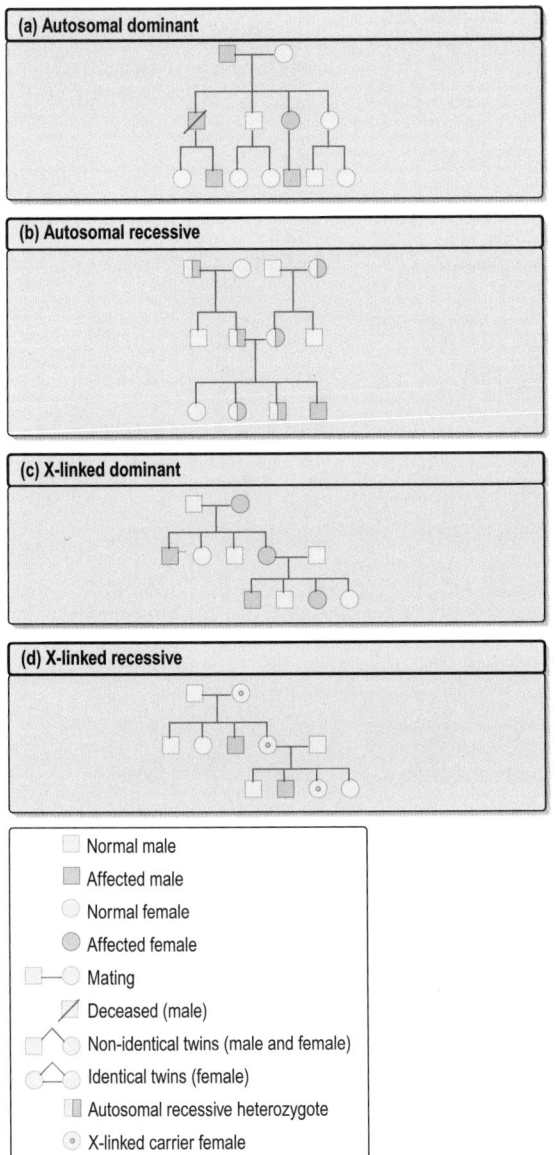

(a) Autosomal dominant

(b) Autosomal recessive

(c) X-linked dominant

(d) X-linked recessive

☐ Normal male
■ Affected male
○ Normal female
● Affected female
☐— Mating
⧄ Deceased (male)
Non-identical twins (male and female)
Identical twins (female)
▯ Autosomal recessive heterozygote
⊙ X-linked carrier female

Fig. 3.20 **Modes of inheritance of simple gene disorders**, with a key to the standard pedigree symbols.

generation to generation. The offspring of an affected person will be healthy heterozygotes unless the other parent is also a carrier. If carriers marry, the offspring have a 1 in 4 chance of being homozygous and affected, a 1 in 2 chance of being a carrier, and a 1 in 4 chance of being genetically normal. Consanguinity increases the risk. The clinical features of autosomal recessive disorders are usually severe; patients often present in the first few years of life and have a high mortality. The overall incidence of autosomal recessive disorders is about 2.5 per 1000 live births.

Sex-linked disorders (Fig. 3.20 and Table 3.6)

Genes carried on the X chromosome are said to be 'X-linked', and can be dominant or recessive in the same way as autosomal genes. As females have two X chromosomes they will be unaffected carriers of X-linked recessive diseases. However, since males have just one X chromosome, any deleterious mutation in an X-linked gene will manifest itself because no second copy of the gene is present.

X-linked dominant disorders

These are rare. Vitamin D-resistant rickets is the best-known example. Females who are heterozygous for the mutant gene and males who have one copy of the mutant gene on their single X chromosome will manifest the disease. Half the male or female offspring of an affected mother and all the female offspring of an affected man will have the disease. Affected males tend to have the disease more severely than the heterozygous female.

X-linked recessive disorders

These disorders present in males and present only in homozygous females (usually rare). X-linked recessive diseases are transmitted by healthy female carriers or affected males if they survive to reproduce. An example of an X-linked recessive disorder is haemophilia A (see p. 472), which is caused by a mutation in the X-linked gene for factor VIII. It has been shown that in 50% of cases there is an intrachromosomal rearrangement (inversion) of the tip of the long arm of the X chromosome (one break point being within intron 22 of the factor VIII gene).

Of the offspring from a carrier female and a normal male:

- 50% of the girls will be carriers as they inherit a mutant allele from their mother and the normal allele from their father; the other 50% of the girls inherit two normal alleles and are themselves normal
- 50% of the boys will have haemophilia as they inherit the mutant allele from their mother (and the Y chromosome from their father); the other 50% of the boys will be normal as they inherit the normal allele from their mother (and the Y chromosome from their father).

The male offspring of a male with haemophilia and a normal female will not have the disease as they do not inherit his X chromosome. However, all the female offspring will be carriers as they all inherit his X chromosome.

Y-linked genes

Genes carried on the Y chromosome are said to be Y-linked and only males can be affected. However, there are no known examples of Y-linked single-gene disorders which are transmitted.

Sex-limited inheritance

Occasionally a gene can be carried on an autosome but manifests itself only in one sex. For example, frontal baldness is an autosomal dominant disorder in males but behaves as a recessive disorder in females.

Other single-gene disorders

These are disorders which may be due to mutations in

Table 3.6 Examples of X-linked disorders with chromosome location and gene defects

Syndrome	Disease prevalence	Gene (Product)	Gene location	Genetic test detection rate
Recessive				
Alport's syndrome	1/50 000	COL4A5 (Collagen alpha 5(IV) chain)	Xq22	60%
Adrenal hypoplasia (congenital) – X-linked	1/13 000	NR0B1 (Orphan nuclear receptor DAX-1)	Xp21.3–21.2	70–100%
Adrenoleucodystrophy – X-linked	1–3/50 000	ABCD1 (Adrenoleucodystrophy protein)	Xq28	98%
Agammaglobulinaemia – X-linked	3–6/million	BTK (Tyrosine-protein kinase BTK)	Xq21.3–22	98–99%
Androgen insensitivity syndrome	2–5/100 000	AR (Androgen receptor)	Xq11–q12	90%
Dystrophinopathies (Becker's and Duchenne muscular dystrophies)	1–4/20 000 (UK)	DMD (Dystrophin)	Xp21.2	65–85%
Charcot–Marie–Tooth disease subtype CMX	3–6/100 000	GJB1 (Gap junction beta-1 protein)	Xq13.1	90%
Fabry's disease	1–2/100 000	GLA (α-galactosidase A)	Xq22	100%
Haemophilia A	1/4000	F8 (Factor VIII)	Xq28	98%
Haemophilia B	1/20 000	F9 (Factor IX)	Xq27.1–27.2	99%
Myotubular myopathy – X-linked	1/50 000	MTM1 (Myotubularin)	Xq28 8	0–85%
Nephrogenic diabetes insipidus	Rare	AVPR2 (Vasopressin V2 receptor)	Xq28	97%
α-Thalassaemia – X-linked (mental retardation syndrome)	Rare	ATRX (Transcriptional regulator ATRX)	Xq13	90%
X-linked severe combined immunodeficiency (X-SCID)	1–2/100 000	IL2RG (Cytokine receptor common gamma chain)	Xq13.1	99%
Dominant				
Coffin–Lowry syndrome	1/50 000	RPS6KA3 (Ribosomal protein S6 kinase alpha 3)	Xp22.2–22.1	35–40%
Incontinentia pigmenti	Rare	IKBKG (NF-kappaB essential modulator)	Xq28	80%
Oral–facial–digital syndrome type-1	1–5/250 000	OFD1 (Oral–facial–digital syndrome 1 protein)	Xp22.3–p22.2	Unknown
Periventricular heterotopia – X-linked	Unknown	FLNA (Filamin 1)	Xq28	83%
Retinitis pigmentosa – X-linked	1–4/100 000 (70% of cases)	RPGR (Retinitis pigmentosa GTPase regulator)	Xp21.1	Unknown
	(8% of cases)	RP2 (XRP2 protein)	Xp11.2	Unknown
Rett syndrome	1/10 000	MECP2 (Methyl-CpG-binding protein 2)	Xq28	80%

single genes but which do not manifest as simple monogenic disorders. They can arise from a variety of mechanisms, including the following.

Triplet repeat mutations (Table 3.7)

In the gene responsible for dystrophia myotonica (p. 1270), the mutated allele was found to have an expanded 3'UTR region in which three nucleotides, CTG, were repeated up to about 200 times. In families with dystrophia myotonica, people with the late-onset form of the disease had 20–40 copies of the repeat, but their children and grandchildren who presented with the disease from birth had vast increases in the number of repeats, up to 2000 copies. It is thought that some mechanism during meiosis causes this 'triplet repeat expansion' so that the offspring inherit an increased number of triplets. The number of triplets affects mRNA and protein function. See also page 191 for the phenomenon of 'anticipation'.

Table 3.7 Examples of trinucleotide repeat genetic disorders

Syndrome inheritance pattern	Disease prevalence	Gene, product, location and disorder	Genetic test detection rate
Friedreich's ataxia – AR	2–4/100 000	*FRDA* (Frataxin) 9q13 – GAA trinucleotide repeat expansion disorder in intron 1 of *FRDA*	96%
Fragile X syndrome – X-linked	16–25/100 000	*FMR1* (Fragile X mental retardation 1 protein) Xq27.3 – CGG trinucleotide repeat expansion and methylation changes in the 5′ untranslated region of *FMR1* exon 1	99%
Huntington's disease – AD	3–15/100 000	*HD* (Huntingtin protein) 4p16.3 – CAG trinucleotide repeat expansion within the translated protein giving rise to long tracts of repeat glutamine residues in HD	98%
Dystrophia myotonica – AD	1/20 000	*DMPK* (Myotonin-protein kinase) 19q13.2–13.3 – CTG trinucleotide repeat expansion in the 3′ untranslated region of the *DMPK* gene	100%

AD, autsomal dominant; AR, autsomal recessive

Mitochondrial disease (Fig. 3.17)

As discussed on pages 74 and 76 various mitochondrial gene mutations can give rise to complex disease syndromes with incomplete penetrance maternal inheritance.

Imprinting

It is known that normal humans need a diploid number of chromosomes of 46. However, the maternal and paternal contributions are different and, in some way which is not yet clear, the fetus can distinguish between the chromosomes inherited from the mother and the chromosomes inherited from the father, although both give 23 chromosomes. In some way the chromosomes are 'imprinted' so that the maternal and paternal contributions are different. Imprinting is relevant to human genetic disease because different phenotypes may result depending on whether the mutant chromosome is maternally or paternally inherited. A deletion of part of the long arm of chromosome 15 (15q11–q13) will give rise to the Prader–Willi syndrome (PWS) if it is paternally inherited. A deletion of a similar region of the chromosome gives rise to Angelman's syndrome (AS) if it is maternally inherited. Recently the affected gene has been identified as ubiquitin (*UBE3A*). Significantly, maternal chromosome 15 *UBE3A* is expressed in the brain and hypothalamus. Defective maternal ubiquitin in Angelman's syndrome is thus responsible for accumulation of undegraded protein, and hence neuronal damage.

Complex traits: multifactorial and polygenic inheritance

Characteristics resulting from a combination of genetic and environmental factors are said to be multifactorial; those involving multiple genes can also be said to be polygenic.

Measurements of most biological traits (e.g. height) show a variation between individuals in a population, and a unimodal, symmetrical (Gaussian) frequency distribution curve can be drawn. This variability is due to vari-ation in genetic factors and environmental factors. Environmental factors may play a part in determining some characteristics, such as weight, whilst other characteristics such as height may be largely genetically determined. This genetic component is thought to be due to the additive effects of a number of alleles at a number of loci, many of which can be individually identified using molecular biological techniques, for example studying identical twins in different environments.

A common genetic variation in the 3′ untranslated region of the prothrombin gene is associated with elevated prothrombin (up to fourfold) and an increased risk of venous thrombosis (thrombophilia, see p. 477), and myocardial infarction. Presumably the 3′ mutation induces overexpression of the prothrombin gene by increasing mRNA stability. In some pedigree studies those homozygous for this mutation and heterozygous for factor V Leiden mutation have an even greater risk of thrombotic events (p. 477). Conversely, downregulation of the α_1-antitrypsin gene (due to similar mutation in the 3′ and 5′ untranslated regions) is associated with emphysema and cirrhosis (p. 388). There are sex differences. Congenital pyloric stenosis is most common in boys, but if it occurs in girls the latter have a larger number of affected relatives. This difference suggests that a larger number of the relevant genes are required to produce the disease in girls than in boys. Most human diseases, such as heart disease, diabetes and common mental disorders, are multifactorial traits (Table 3.8).

FURTHER READING

Brown LY, Brown SA (2004) Alanine tracts: the expanding story of human illness and trinucleotide repeats. *Trends in Genetics* **20**: 51–58.

Leonard JV, Shapira AHV (2000) Mitochondrial respiratory chain disorders I and II. *Lancet* **355**: 299–304, 389–394.

Sybert VP, McCauley E (2004) Turner's syndrome. *New England Journal of Medicine* **351**: 1227–1238.

Table 3.8 Examples of disorders that may have a polygenic inheritance

Disorder	Frequency (%)	Heritability (%)*
Hypertension	5	62
Asthma	4	80
Schizophrenia	1	85
Congenital heart disease	0.5	35
Neural tube defects	0.5	60
Congenital pyloric stenosis	0.3	75
Ankylosing spondylitis	0.2	70
Cleft palate	0.1	76

* Percentage of the total variation of a trait which can be attributed to genetic factor

ANALYSIS OF MUTATIONS AND GENETIC DISEASE

Tracking a disease gene

Of the estimated 3400 inherited genetic disorders, only a small number have been characterized in terms of their biochemistry and genetics. Their clinical phenotype may have been described extensively but the identity of the culpable gene is still unknown. However, it is not necessary to identify the gene because two genes that are situated close together on a chromosome are nearly always co-inherited. Only on rare occasions do they segregate during meiosis when the two chromosomes of a diploid pair crossover and exchange parts (recombination) – even then the crossover point must be between the two genes. The closer the genes, the less chance of a segregating crossover, such that two genes that are one million base-pairs apart will only have a 1% chance of being separated by recombination. This might be an enormous distance in molecular terms, but for clinical genetic analysis this is acceptable for diagnosis. If a known gene or non-coding repetitive DNA sequence is within this one million base-pairs of the disease gene, it will act as the tag or marker probe for the disease.

The large amount of non-coding DNA between genes, like all DNA, accumulates random base-pair changes throughout many generations. If these changes occur within genes, then they cause inherited disorders. The rate of mutation in some genes is quite low as there is a strong genetic selection against variants, but this is not true of non-coding DNA where a base-pair change has no deleterious effect. The frequency of change can approach 1 in 100 base-pairs. These changes occur randomly throughout the non-coding DNA, as do restriction enzyme sites. Sometimes a base-pair change will create or destroy a particular restriction site. Generally two members of a chromosome pair (homologues) will have broadly the same restriction patterns at any one point (Fig. 3.21a). However, owing to a random base-pair change, one chromosome will show a different restriction pattern for one enzyme (BamHI in Fig. 3.21a) compared

Fig. 3.21 **(a) Restriction fragment length polymorphism.** Diagrammatic representation of two allelic sections of DNA from a chromosome pair. The restriction site map of the two is identical except for a BamHI sequence which has been mutated by environmental radiation, resulting in a restriction fragment length polymorphism (RFLP). The blue area represents a cloned sequence which acts as a marker probe or tag for the polymorphism. This polymorphism is within one million base pairs of a disease gene and co-segregates with the disease. **(b) RFLP and disease tracking.** A family with four children whose parents are heterozygous for the polymorphism shown in (a). The bands below show DNA fragments (large, L, and small, S) on a Southern blot of DNA. If the RLFP which gives the L fragment is on the chromosome carrying the defective gene then only the fetus which is homozygous for the large fragment (LL) will be affected. The fetus homozygous for the small fragment (SS) will not be a sufferer. The heterozygous fetuses (LS and SL) will also be unaffected but will be carriers.

with its homologue. These differences in restriction pattern are inherited, and are known as polymorphisms. Because they are observable as differences in length of particular restriction fragments, they are known as *restriction fragment length polymorphisms* (RFLPs).

The inheritance of RFLPs

The blue area in Figure 3.21a shows a cloned area of DNA from two chromosomes. If this is used as a probe, it will detect any restriction fragment that contains an identical piece of DNA sequence, and thus it can be used to detect the BamHI polymorphism shown. A person with these two chromosomes will be heterozygous for the BamHI polymorphism, as the two chromosomes are different. The person will produce gametes that have only one of these chromosomes: 50% of the cells will have one type, 50% the other. If the mate of this person is also heterozygous for the same polymorphism, he or she will produce gametes that are 50% of one type and 50% the other. At fertilization there is a random chance that any one gamete will fuse with any gamete from the other parent, and thus four types of progeny will be produced. Two will be heterozygous for the polymorphism (Fig. 3.21b), one will be homozygous for the large BamHI fragment, the other will be homozygous for the small BamHI fragment.

If the chromosome carrying the BamHI polymorphism has a closely linked gene that when defective causes an inherited disorder, then by studying the family pedigree, the inheritance of both the disorder and the RFLP can be monitored. Generally, inherited disorders are caused by recessive genes. Both parents can therefore be carriers without being affected. If both parents come from families that have affected relatives, or they themselves have produced affected children, then they may wish to know if any subsequent children will also be sufferers. Suppose that the large BamHI fragment of the polymorphism is on the same chromosome as the defective gene, the small fragment being on the same chromosome as the normal allele. This can be checked by showing that any sufferers of the condition must be homozygous for the defective gene and thereby homozygous for the large BamHI fragment. To determine if any subsequent children are likely sufferers, DNA from a chorionic villus or amniocentesis sample can be digested with BamHI and electrophoresed on an agarose gel. It can then be probed with a cloned fragment using a Southern blot.

DNA can be amplified from very small tissue samples using PCR. If a polymorphism is reasonably well characterized, PCR across the RFLP will yield a suitable fragment to test for its presence. Other markers used to trace disease genes are simple sequence repeats. More common and more polymorphic (i.e. having greater variability) than RFLPs, these are short di-, tri-, tetra- or pentanucleotide repeats (such as (CA)n) which are present throughout the genome and have highly variable lengths. By designing primers to the sequence either side of one of these repeats, the repeat can be amplified by PCR. The amplified product is electrophoresed on a gel and different-sized products are produced from different people. If the mutant gene is close by, then a particular size repeat in that region will always segregate with the disease allele.

The likelihood of recombination between the marker under study and the disease allele must be taken into account. This measure of likelihood is known as the 'lod score' (the logarithm of the odds) and is a measure of the statistical significance of the observed co-segregation of the marker and the disease gene, compared with what would be expected by chance alone. Positive lod scores make linkage more likely; negative lod scores make it less likely. By convention a lod score of +3 is taken to be definite evidence of linkage because this indicates 1000 to 1 odds that the co-segregation of the DNA marker and the disease did not occur by chance alone.

Linkage analysis has provided many breakthroughs in mapping the positions of genes that cause genetic diseases, such as the gene for cystic fibrosis which was found to be tightly linked to a marker on chromosome 7, or the gene for Friedreich's ataxia which is tightly linked to a marker on chromosome 9.

Gene hunting

Two approaches to the identification of a disease gene are possible – functional or positional cloning (Fig. 3.22).

Functional cloning
Extracted mRNA from tissue expressing the disease gene (from both normal and affected individuals) is cloned into a vector. The clones are engineered such that the gene product is expressed by the host organism (i.e. bacteria) which may then be screened by antibodies or functional (enzyme–substrate) assay for those clones producing the desired gene product. The selected clones are isolated, propagated and the insert sequenced. The isolated cDNA insert can then be used as a probe to identify the location of the gene on a chromosome by in situ hybridization and to identify the genomic sequence from genome libraries. As already stated, the biochemistry of most genetic disease is unknown and positional cloning is required.

Positional cloning
The first step in this cloning approach is to study the pattern of inheritance. This may provide valuable clues about whether a single gene is affected, and whether this gene is likely to be autosomal or on the sex chromosomes or the mitochondrial chromosome. Gross chromosome analysis can be useful and geneticists look for chromosomal

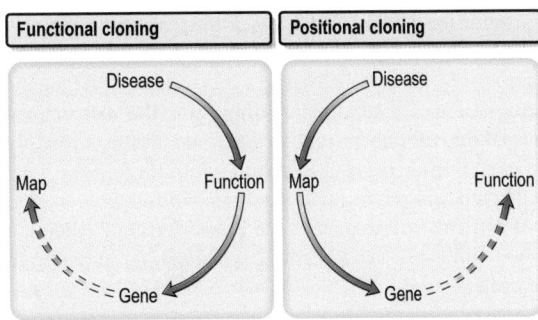

Fig. 3.22 Diagrammatic representation of two classic approaches to gene cloning.

Functional cloning requires a working knowledge of the biochemistry of the disease such that the defective protein/enzyme has previously been characterized in some way. From this the gene can be isolated and then its chromosomal location found.

Positional cloning is used to isolate genes whose protein products are not known, but whose existence can be inferred from a disease phenotype. The process involves narrowing the search to a chromosome, then to a region of the chromosome, and finally to a gene in which a mutation is always present in affected individuals and absent in normal individuals.

aberrations (for example deletions), which are present at an unusually high frequency in individuals affected with the disease, compared with the normal population. If there are no further clues, often the next stage in locating the gene that is mutated in the disease is to look for genetic markers as described earlier. Once polymorphic markers from across the genome have been tested, it should be possible by linkage analysis to see if any segregate with the disease allele in a family. If the position of the polymorphic marker is known, then the affected gene is likely to be close by and is therefore mapped to a region of the genome (i.e. a specific band on a chromosome arm).

Isolating the gene

Once linkage analysis has established which chromosome and which region of the chromosome contains the disease gene, the next step is to identify the gene. The region of DNA which contains the gene may span several million base-pairs, and a variety of techniques exist for cloning cDNAs and gene sequences from such regions. Genes which have been cloned and are very tightly linked to a genetic disease may be 'candidate genes' for that disease, and researchers have to show that a mutation in the gene is likely to give rise to the disease.

However, most are unknown and markers which span the disease gene's physical location on the chromosome are traced through the affected families' genetic samples. These markers define the target interval of genetic code – often several million base-pairs – within which the disease gene lies. Essentially the whole target interval is cloned and partially or entirely sequenced by 'chromosome walking' or searching cDNA libraries for uncharacterized sequences which hybridize to regions of the target interval. Sequencing approaches require searching for motif sequences, such as areas rich in repetitive cytosine and guanidine base-pairs, which are characteristic of a gene. A further criterion for candidacy is that the gene is expressed in the affected tissues. It is unlikely that a gene giving rise to a liver disease might give the instructions for making protein purely in neuronal tissue. Probably the most useful criterion is to find a mutation in the gene in affected and not in unaffected individuals.

When candidate genes have been identified, they are cloned and expressed in order to establish the function of the protein product.

THE GENETIC BASIS OF CANCER

Cancers are genetic diseases and involve changes to the normal function of cellular genes. However, multiple genes interact during oncogenesis and an almost stepwise progression of defects leads from an overproliferation of a particular cell to the breakdown of control mechanisms such as apoptosis (programmed cell death). This would be triggered if a cell were to attempt to survive in an organ other than its tissue of origin. For the vast majority of cancer cases (especially those in older people) the multiple genetic changes which occur are somatic. However, it is clear that susceptibility to the development of a particular form of cancer can be inherited. Indeed for some rare cancers a dominant single-gene defect can give rise to an almost Mendelian trend. In some other cancers (e.g. forms of breast cancer) the mode of inheritance is much more complex. In these cases close relatives may have an increased susceptibility to cancer (Table 9.3), and the genetics are clearly those of a multifactorial trait.

- Cancer tissues are clonal, and tumours arise from changes in only one cell, which then proliferates in the body.
- The genes that are primarily damaged by the genetic changes which lead to cancer fall into two categories: oncogenes and tumour suppressor genes.
- Oncogenesis is a multistep process in that a number of mutations or alterations to key genes are required before a malignant phenotype is expressed.
- Once mutations have begun to cause unchecked clonal expansion of the primary tumour cells, further mutations occur within the subsequent generations of daughter cells that give rise to clones which are invasive and/or form metastases.

ONCOGENES (see p. 485)

The genes coding for proteins which are either growth factors, growth factor receptors, secondary messengers or even DNA-binding proteins would act as promoters of abnormal cell growth if mutated. This concept was verified when viruses were found to carry genes which, when integrated into the host cell, promoted oncogenesis. These were originally termed viral or 'v-oncogenes', and later their normal cellular counterparts, c-oncogenes, were found. Thus, oncogenes encode proteins that are known to participate in the regulation of normal cellular proliferation e.g. *erb-A* on chromosome 17q11–q12 encodes for the thyroid hormone receptor. See also Table 9.4.

Activation of oncogenes

Non-activated oncogenes which are functioning normally have been referred to as 'proto-oncogenes'. Their transformation to oncogenes can occur by three routes.

Mutation

Carcinogens such as those found in cigarette smoke, ionizing radiation and ultraviolet light can cause point mutations in genomic DNA. By chance some of these point mutations will occur in regions of the oncogene which lead to activation of that gene. Not all bases in an oncogene cause cancer if mutated, but some (e.g. those in the coding region) do.

Chromosomal translocation

If during cell division an error occurs and two chromosomes translocate, so that a portion swaps over, the translocation breakpoint may occur in the middle of two genes. If this happens then the end of one gene is translocated on to the beginning of another gene, giving rise to a 'fusion gene'. Therefore sequences of one part of the fusion gene are inappropriately expressed because they are under the control of the other part of the gene.

An example of such a fusion gene (the Philadelphia chromosome) occurs in chronic myeloid leukaemia (CML, see p. 501). Similarly in Burkitt's lymphoma a translocation causes the regulatory segment of the *myc* oncogene to be replaced by a regulatory segment of an unrelated immunoglobulin.

Viral stimulation

When viral RNA is transcribed by reverse transcriptase into viral cDNA and in turn is spliced into the cellular DNA, the viral DNA may integrate within an oncogene and activate it. Alternatively the virus may pick up cellular oncogene DNA and incorporate it into its own viral genome. Subsequent infection of another host cell might result in expression of this viral oncogene. For example, the Rous sarcoma virus of chickens was found to induce cancer because it carried the *ras* oncogene.

After the initial activation event other changes occur within the DNA. A striking example of this is amplification of gene sequences, which can affect the *myc* gene for example. Instead of the normal two copies of a gene, multiple copies of the gene appear either within the chromosomes (these can be seen on stained chromosomes as homogeneously staining regions) or as extra-chromosomal particles (double minutes). N-*myc* sequences are amplified in neuroblastomas as are N-*myc* or L-*myc* in some lung small-cell carcinomas.

TUMOUR SUPPRESSOR GENES

These genes restrict undue cell proliferation (in contrast to oncogenes), and induce the repair or self-destruction (apoptosis) of cells containing damaged DNA. Therefore mutations in these genes which disable their function lead to uncontrolled cell growth in cells with active oncogenes. An example is the germline mutations in genes found in non-polyposis colorectal cancer which are responsible for repairing DNA mismatches (p. 328).

The first tumour suppressor gene to be described was the *RB* gene. Mutations in *RB* lead to retinoblastoma which occurs in 1 in 20000 young children and can be sporadic or familial. In the familial variety, the first mutation is inherited and by chance a second somatic mutation occurs with the formation of a tumour. In the sporadic variety, by chance both mutations occur in both the *RB* genes in a single cell. Since the finding of *RB*, other tumour suppressor genes have been described, including the gene *p53*. Mutations in *p53* have been found in almost all human tumours, including sporadic colorectal carcinomas, carcinomas of breast and lung, brain tumours, osteosarcomas and leukaemias. The protein, encoded by *p53*, is a cellular 53 kDa nuclear phosphoprotein that plays a role in DNA repair and synthesis, in the control of the cell cycle and cell differentiation and programmed cell death – apoptosis. p53 is a DNA-binding protein which activates many gene expression pathways but it is normally only short-lived. In many tumours, mutations that disable p53 function also prevent its cellular catabolism. Although in some cancers there is a loss of *p53* from both chromosomes, in most cancers (particularly colorectal carcinomas; see Fig. 6.40) such long-lived mutant *p53* alleles can disrupt the normal alleles' protein. As a DNA-binding protein, p53 is likely to act as a tetramer. Thus, a mutation in a single copy of the gene can promote tumour formation because a hetero-tetramer of mutated and normal p53 subunits would still be dysfunctional.

How tumour suppressor genes work

Tumour suppressor gene products are intimately involved in control of the cell cycle (see Fig. 3.7). Progression through the cell cycle is controlled by many molecular gateways, which are opened or blocked by the cyclin group of proteins that are specifically expressed at various stages of the cycle. The RB and p53 proteins control the cell cycle and interact specifically within many cyclin proteins. The latter are affected by INK 4α acting on p16 proteins. The general principle is that being held at one of these gateways will ultimately lead to programmed cell death. p53 is a DNA-binding protein which induces the expression of other genes and is a major player in the induction of cell death. Its own expression is induced by broken DNA. The induction of p53 by damage initially causes the expression of DNA repair enzymes. If DNA repair is too slow or cannot be effected, then other proteins that are induced by p53 will effect programmed cell death.

One gateway event that has been largely elucidated is that between the G1 and the S phase of the cell cycle. The transcription factor dimer E2F-DP1 causes progression from the G1 to the S phase. However, the RB protein binds to the E2F transcription factor, preventing its induction of DNA synthesis. Other, cyclin D-related molecules inactivate the RB protein, thus allowing DNA synthesis to proceed. This period of rapid DNA synthesis is susceptible to mutation events and will propagate a pre-existing DNA mistake. Damaged DNA-induced p53 expression rapidly results in the expression of a variety of closely related (and possibly tissue-specific) proteins WAF-1/p21, p16, p27. These inhibit the inactivation of RB by cyclin D-related molecules. As a result RB, the normal gate which stops the cell cycle, binds to the E2F-DP1 transcription factor complex, halting S phase DNA synthesis. If the DNA damage is not repaired apoptosis ensues.

Viral inactivation of tumour suppressors

The suppression of normal tumour suppressor gene function can be achieved by disabling the normal protein once it has been transcribed, rather than by mutating the gene. Viruses have developed their own genes which produce proteins to do precisely this. The main targets of these proteins are RB and p53 to which they bind and thus disable. The best understood are the adenovirus E1A and human papillomavirus (HPV) E7 gene products which bind RB, whilst the adenovirus E1B and HPV E6 gene products bind p53. The SV40 virus large T antigen binds both RB and p53.

Microsatellite instability

Microsatellites are short (50–300 bp) sequences composed of tandemly repeated segments of DNA two to five nucleotides in length (dinucleotide/trinucleotide/tetranucleotide repeats). Scattered throughout the genome in the non-coding regions between genes or within genes (introns), many of these microsatellites are highly polymorphic. Often used as markers for linkage analysis because of high variability in repeat number between individuals, these regions are inherently unstable and susceptible to mutations. Somatic microsatellite instability (MSI) has been detected in a number of tumours. Detecting MSI involves comparing the length of microsatellite alleles amplified from tumour DNA with the corresponding allele in normal tissue from the same individual. Recent studies indicate that MSI can be detected in approximately 90% of tumours from individuals with hereditary non-polyposis colorectal cancer (HNPCC). The presence of these additional microsatellite alleles (repeated segments) in tumour cells, results from the inherent susceptibility of these areas to such alterations and from mutations in the DNA mismatch repair mechanism that would normally correct these errors.

Tumour angiogenesis

Once a nest of cancer cells reaches 1–2 mm in diameter, it must develop a blood supply in order to survive and grow larger, as diffusion is no longer adequate to supply the cells with oxygen and nutrients. As with all tissues, solid tumour cancer cells secrete substances that promote the formation of new blood vessels – a process called angiogenesis. Over a dozen substances have been identified that promote angiogenesis (e.g. angiopoietin-1, basic fibroblast growth factor (bFGF) and vascular endothelial growth factor (VEGF)). This has led to the discovery of a number of inhibitors of angiogenesis and some have already advanced to clinical trials as part of a cancer treatment strategy such as:

- angiostatin – a polypeptide of approximately 200 amino acids, produced by the cleavage of plasminogen; it binds to subunits of ATP synthase exposed at the surface of the cell embedded in the plasma membrane
- endostatin – a polypeptide of 184 amino acids which is derived from the globular domain found at the C-terminal of type XVIII collagen (a specific collagen of blood vessels) cleaved from the parent molecule.

Several therapeutic vaccine preparations are under development to produce a range of host immunity responses (humoral, cellular) against pro-angiogenic factors and their receptors in tumours. One approach has been directed at cell adhesion molecules found in tumour blood vessels. It turns out that the new blood vessels in tumours express a vascular integrin – designated alpha-v/beta-3 – that is not found on the old blood vessels of normal tissues. Vitaxin, a monoclonal antibody directed against the alpha-v/beta-3 vascular integrin, shrinks tumours in mice without harming them. In Phase II clinical trials in humans, Vitaxin has shown some promise in shrinking solid tumours without harmful side-effects.

CANCER AETIOLOGY: INHERITANCE OR ENVIRONMENT?

It is clear that a mutation causing the dysfunction of a single oncogene or tumour suppressor gene is not sufficient to induce unregulated clonal expansion. The Knudson multi-hit hypothesis elegantly unites the genetics of familial and sporadic tumour development: an inherited mutation in one gene allele may be insufficient to cause a tumour but will cause a significant susceptibility to the development of a particular cancer. Subsequent lifetime exposure to environmental carcinogens (viral, chemical, radiation), along with simple mistakes during cell division, may deregulate the normal allele. Other mutations which accumulate in a similar manner then lead to tumour development. Research has clearly shown that germline mutations in particular genes, such as *p53* and *RB*, have a much stronger influence on the chance of subsequent tumour development than others.

FURTHER READING

Carmeliet P (2004) Manipulating angiogenesis in medicine. *Journal of Internal Medicine* **255**: 538–561.
Charames GS, Bapat B (2003) Genomic instability and cancer. *Current Molecular Medicine* **3**: 589–596.
Eichhorst ST, Krammer PH (2001) Derangement of apoptosis in cancer. *Lancet* **358**: 345–346.
Slee EA, O'Connor DJ, Lu X (2004) To die or not to die: how does p53 decide? *Oncogene* **23**: 2809–2818.

POPULATION GENETICS

The genetic constitution of a population depends on many factors. The Hardy–Weinberg equilibrium is a concept, based on a mathematical equation, that describes the outcome of random mating within populations. It states that 'in the absence of mutation, non-random mating, selection and genetic drift, the genetic constitution of the population remains the same from one generation to the next'.

This genetic principle has clinical significance in terms of the number of abnormal genes in the total gene pool of a population. The Hardy–Weinberg equation states that:

$$p^2 + 2pq + q^2 = 1$$

where p is the frequency of the normal gene in the population, q is the frequency of the abnormal gene, p^2 is the frequency of the normal homozygote, q^2 is the frequency of the affected abnormal homozygote, $2pq$ is the carrier frequency, and $p + q = 1$.

Example. The equation can be used, for example, to find the frequency of heterozygous carriers in cystic fibrosis. The incidence of cystic fibrosis is 1 in 2000 live births. Thus $q^2 = 1/2000$, and therefore $q = 1/44$. Since $p = 1 - q$, then $p = 43/44$. The carrier frequency is represented by $2pq$, which in this case is 1/22. Thus 1 in 22 individuals in the whole population is a heterozygous carrier for cystic fibrosis.

CLINICAL GENETICS AND GENETIC COUNSELLING

Genetic disorders pose considerable health and economic problems because often there is no effective therapy. In any pregnancy the risk of a serious developmental abnormality is approximately 1 in 30 pregnancies; approximately 15% of paediatric inpatients have a multifactorial disorder with a predominantly genetic element.

People with a history of a congenital abnormality in a member of their family often seek advice as to why it happened and about the risks of producing further abnormal offspring. Interviews must be conducted with great sensitivity and psychological insight, as parents may feel a sense of guilt and blame themselves for the abnormality in their child.

Genetic counselling should have the following aims:

- *Obtaining a full history.* The pregnancy history, drug and alcohol ingestion during pregnancy and maternal illnesses (e.g. diabetes) should be detailed.
- *Establishing an accurate diagnosis.* Examination of the child may help in diagnosing a genetically abnormal child with characteristic features (e.g. trisomy 21) or whether a genetically normal fetus was damaged in utero.
- *Drawing a family tree is essential.* Questions should be asked about abortions, stillbirths, deaths, marriages, consanguinity and medical history of family members. Diagnoses may need verification from other hospital reports.
- *Estimating the risk of a future pregnancy being affected or carrying a disorder.* Estimation of risk should be based on the pattern of inheritance. Mendelian disorders (see earlier) carry a high risk; chromosomal abnormalities carry a low risk. Empirical risks may be obtained from population or family studies.
- *Information giving.* On prognosis and management.
- *Continued support and follow-up.* Explanation of the implications for other siblings and family members.
- *Genetic screening.* This includes prenatal diagnosis if requested, carrier detection and data storage in genetic registers. A growing number of molecular genetic tests are now available (http://www.geneclinics.org).

Genetic counselling should be non-directive, with the couple making their own decisions on the basis of an accurate presentation of the facts and risks in a way they can understand.

GENETIC ANTICIPATION

It has been noted that successive generations of patients with, for example, dystrophia myotonica and Huntington's chorea, present earlier and with progressively worse symptoms. This 'anticipation' is due to unstable mutations occurring within the disease gene. Trinucleotide repeats such as CTG (dystrophia myotonica) and CAG (Huntington's chorea) expand within the disease gene with each generation, and somatic expansion with cellular replication is also observed. This novel type of genetic mutation can occur within the translated region or untranslated (and presumably regulatory) regions of the target genes. This genetic distinction has been used to subclassify a number of genetic diseases which have now been shown to be caused by trinucleotide repeat expansion and display phenotypic 'anticipation' (Table 3.7).

PRENATAL DIAGNOSIS

This is offered to all pregnant women in the UK. Practice varies in different maternity units, with some only offering screening to high-risk mothers. Prediction factors for high-risk include women who are older than 35 years and those with a history or family history of chromosomal abnormalities.

Investigations

First trimester

- Ultrasound (high resolution) for nuchal translucency to exclude major chromosomal abnormalities (e.g. trisomies and Turner's syndrome).
- Maternal serum for pregnancy-associated plasma protein-A (PAPP-A from the syncytial trophoblast) for trisomy 21. This is more accurate than the triple test at 16 weeks.

Second trimester

- Ultrasound for structural abnormalities (e.g. neural tube defects, congenital heart defects). Serum screening has been superseded by high-resolution ultrasound (above) in specialist centres.
- Triple test (used by some) for chromosomal abnormalities. This consists of a serum α-fetoprotein (low), unconjugated oestradiol (low) and human chorionic gonadotrophin (high). α-Fetoprotein (high for neural tube defects).

All markers are corrected for gestational ages, a multiple of the mean (MOM) value for the appropriate week of gestation. If abnormalities are detected, it is necessary to continue investigations with chorionic villus sampling (CVS) at 11–13 weeks, or amniocentesis at 15 weeks, under ultrasound control to sample amniotic fluid and fetal cells necessary for cytogenetic testing.

These tests may well be superseded by salvage of fetal cells from the maternal blood sample at 12 weeks.

FURTHER READING

Finsterer J (2004) Mitochondriopathies. *European Journal of Neurology* **11**: 163–186.

Guetta E, Simchen MJ, Mammon-Daviko K et al. (2004) Analysis of fetal blood cells in the maternal circulation: challenges, ongoing efforts, and potential solutions. *Stem Cells and Development* **13**: 93–99.

Kumar S, O'Brien A (2004) Recent developments in fetal medicine. *British Medical Journal* **328**: 1002–1006.

Morris K (2004) Prenatal screening for birth defects: an update. *Molecular Medicine* **101**: 121–124.

Stojilkovic-Mikic T, Rodeck CH (2003) Screening for chromosomal anomalies: first or second trimester, biochemical or ultrasound? *Annals of the Academy of Medicine, Singapore* **32**: 583–589.

APPLICATIONS OF MOLECULAR GENETICS

The use of molecular biological techniques in genetics is having a massive impact on the investigation, diagnosis, treatment and control of genetic disorders.

The avoidance and control of genetic disease

Some genetic disorders, such as phenylketonuria or haemophilia, can be managed by diet or replacement therapy, but most have no effective treatment. By understanding what causes genetic damage, potential mutagens such as radiation, environmental chemicals, viruses or drugs (e.g. thalidomide) can be avoided.

GENE THERAPY

There are many technical problems to overcome in gene therapy, particularly in finding delivery systems to introduce DNA into a mammalian cell. Very careful control and supervision of gene manipulation will be necessary because of its potential hazards and the ethical issues.

Gene therapy entails placing a normal copy of a gene into the cells of a patient who has a defective copy of the gene.

Experiments have concentrated on recessive disorders, such as cystic fibrosis where the disease is due to the absence of a normal gene product. In dominant disorders the pathogenic potential of the mutant allele is normally expressed in the presence of a normal allele. This requires gene correction, whereby the mutant sequence is replaced by an equivalent sequence from a normal allele, or the mutant allele is inactivated. Such procedures are more difficult.

Two major factors are involved in gene therapy:

- the introduction of the functional gene sequence into target cells
- the expression and permanent integration of the transfected gene into the host cell genome.

Suitable diseases for current gene therapy experiments include cystic fibrosis, adenosine deaminase deficiency, and familial hypercholesterolaemia.

Cystic fibrosis (see also p. 909 and p. 413)

The gene responsible for cystic fibrosis was first localized to chromosome 7 by linkage analysis. The cystic fibrosis transmembrane regulator gene (*CFTR*) was then isolated by chromosome-mediated gene transfer, chromosome walking and jumping. The *CFTR* gene spans about 250 kbp and contains 27 exons. The DNA sequence analysis predicts a polypeptide sequence of 1480 amino acids. The *CFTR* gene also encodes a simple chloride ion channel within the cystic fibrosis transmembrane regulator (Fig. 3.23). The commonest is a single mutation with a 3 bp deletion in exon 10 resulting in the removal of a codon specifying phenylalanine (F508del). There are also over 1000 different minor mutations of the *CFTR* gene with most mapping to the ATP-binding domains.

Fig. 3.23 **Model of cystic fibrosis transmembrane regulator (CFTR).** This is an integral membrane glycoprotein, consisting of two repeated elements. The cylindrical structures represent six membrane-spanning helices in each half of the molecule. The nucleotide-binding folds (NBFs) are in the cytoplasm, and the dots in these shaded areas represent the means of entry by the nucleotide. The regulatory (R) domain links the two halves and contains charged individual amino acids and protein kinase phosphorylation sites (black triangles). N and C are the N and C terminals. The branched structure on the right half represents potential glycosylation sites. The chloride channel is shown.

Gene therapy experiments are still under way in trying to restore *CFTR* function by transfection of cells with wild type receptor. Two different routes have been tried, either placing the *CFTR* gene in an adenovirus vector (Fig. 14.30) or into a liposome. The latter can be conveyed to the lung using an aerosol spray, and the fatty surface of the liposome fuses with the cell membrane to deliver the *CFTR* DNA into the cell, where the gene should function normally. However, neither is yet a treatment option. An alternative method is to suppress premature termination codons and thus permit translation to continue; topical nasal gentamicin (an aminoglycoside antibiotic) has been shown to result in the expression of functional *CFTR* channels.

Adenosine deaminase (ADA) deficiency

Gene therapy for this rare immunodeficiency disease entails introducing a normal human *ADA* gene into the patient's lymphocytes to reconstitute the function of the cellular and humoral immune system in severe combined immunodeficiency (SCID). Lymphocytes have been tried for short-term therapy, but for longer-term treatment bone marrow transplantation would be the definitive approach (see p. 496).

Familial hypercholesterolaemia

This disorder is a result of a defective low-density lipoprotein (LDL) receptor gene. In therapy, a receptor gene is inserted into hepatocytes, removed by liver biopsy from the patient. Gene-corrected hepatocytes are then reinjected into the portal circulation of the patient. These cells migrate back to the liver where they are reincorporated and should start to produce LDL receptor protein, which would dramatically lower the patient's cholesterol level.

Muscle-cell-mediated gene therapy

Much of the problem associated with gene therapy of chronic genetic disease is how long the transfected cells will survive. Isolated myoblasts transfected with a retrovirus have been shown to function and live for the lifetime of mouse models (2 years). The myoblasts fuse with the animal's muscle fibres and express the transfected protein. The long life of the muscle fibres and their rich blood supply make them an ideal site for treatment of diseases in which functional serum-born factors are missing (e.g. human growth hormone, coagulation factors and erythropoietin).

Obviously, myoblast transfection would appear to be the best option for the treatment of Duchenne muscular dystrophy. However, the Duchenne gene is far too large to fit into any current viral vector, and reimplanted myoblasts do not colonize muscles fibres distant from the site of injection.

Treatment of somatic disease

Gene therapy which requires only a transient expression of the transfected genetic material circumvents the problems currently plaguing gene therapy of inherited disorders. This may also prove to be the front-line of gene therapy.

Vascular disease

The ideal therapy in heart disease would be neovascularization to increase blood flow and the repair of cardiac tissue after a myocardial infarction. In fact, any vascular disease might require regeneration or new blood vessel growth. Temporary expression of angiogenic factors at the site of a blockage would induce new blood vessels. Alternatively, local temporary expression of clot-disintegrating enzymes such as streptokinase and lipases may repair damaged and diseased arteries. It is quite possible to deliver liposomes loaded with DNA or, in fact, directly inject DNA plasmids into the tissue, and the protein will be expressed by the cells which take it up. Only 1–3% will do so, but this is sufficient for the local effect required and it is a transient expression. This gives a controllable gene therapy.

Neuronal disease

Neurotrophic factors can be transiently expressed as described above for vascular diseases. The local expression of neurotrophins is essential for nerve cell regeneration and maintenance. It is possible to extend the expression period of the neurotrophin by injecting transfected myocytes into the damaged area. They will fuse with any adjacent muscle tissue to give a prolonged expression of the factor gene.

Cancer

Cancer is a genetic disease and many genes are deregulated. *p53* is a tumour suppressor gene; the reintroduction and overexpression of a functional *p53* in tumours is being investigated with some success. Since *p53* will induce apoptosis in cells with damaged genetic material, the transient expression of high levels in a tumour cell with *p53* pathway defects should induce its own (apoptotic) demise. Since this is only likely to occur in rapidly dividing cells, this is a perfect target for cancer gene therapy. Transient expression induced by repeat exposure to vectors such as retroviruses, liposomes and naked DNA plasmids is all relatively straightforward. Trials using aerosols of these vectors in patients with lung cancer are being performed.

Tumour growth depends on the development of new blood vessels (angiogenesis), and inhibitors of this process are also being used in trials.

Creating and using animal models

There is a need for model systems in which to test gene therapies prior to use in patients. To some extent gene 'knock-out' experiments in mice are providing new animal models of disease. In these experiments the normal gene of interest in a mouse is targeted using recombinant DNA techniques so that gene function is impaired, in analogy to the situation in the particular gene of a human patient. However, mice and humans are different and it will not be possible to mimic some human genetic diseases in mice. Transgenic mice are created when exogenous DNA carrying a gene of interest is injected into a mouse egg. If this egg is fertilized then all the cells of the resulting animal will carry the extra gene sequences. Transgenic mice have also been used as animal models of human diseases in which new therapies may be tested.

Other animal models have paved the way for gene therapy techniques. For example, some of the first experiments in the transfer of globin genes (which will be useful for gene therapy for sickle cell disease and thalassaemia) have taken place in mice. These include transplanting normal donor cells with normal genes into lethally irradiated mice, which results in engraftment of the donor cells.

The human genome project (HGP)

On 14 April 1983 the entire human genome, all 3×10^9 bp on the 24 different chromosomes was sequenced (www.genome.gov 11006929). Now that the entire genome has been sequenced to an accuracy of 99.99%, finding genes that are co-located with a genetic disease marker takes a matter of hours instead of years and is in fact a database or adapted 'in silico' cloning exercise.

Only 2% of the genome codes for actual proteins; some 30 000 genes in the human genome of 300 million bases. However, many genetic disorders are the result of deregulation of expression, and it is the control elements surrounding the coding that are deregulated. The complete sequence also gives rise to an understanding of how genes are packaged as euchromatin or heterochromatin and why the genome is organized in the way it is.

The human proteome project

A more direct route to understanding genetic and somatic disease is by studying the protein expression characteristics of normal and diseased cells – the proteome. This relies on the separation of proteins expressed by a given tissue by molecular size and charge on a simple two-dimensional display and is achieved by using two-dimensional gel electrophoresis. The pattern of dots corresponds to the different proteins expressed. With the improvement in technology, the patterns are reproducible and can be stored as electronic images. Non-, over- and underexpression of a given protein can be detected by a corresponding change on the proteome two-dimensional electrophoresis image. As can be seen in Figure 3.24, the protein profile of synovial fluid from a diseased joint shows a new protein arising with disease. Such proteins have been identified as inflammatory cytokines. Furthermore, post-translational modifications of the protein show up as a change in either size or charge on the proteome picture. In order to positively identify the altered protein and the post-translational modification it may contain, these protein spots are eluted and subjected to modern mass spectrometry techniques such matrix-assisted laser desorption (MALDI) and electrospray ionization (ESI) time of flight (TOF), which not only give the precise mass of the protein, up to ~ 500 000 Da, but can also sequence its amino acid, phosphorylation and glycosylation structure. This cannot be detected by genome analysis. Looking for such changes has already led to the discovery of new protein markers for the diagnosis of Creutzfeldt–Jakob disease, multiple sclerosis, schizophrenia, Parkinson's disease (spinal fluid protein) and Alzheimer's disease (blood and brain proteins). In 2000, the Swiss Institute of Bioinformatics (SIB) and the European Bioinformatics Institute (EBI) announced a major effort to annotate, describe and provide highly accurate information concerning human protein sequences, effectively launching the Human Proteomics Initiative (HPI).

Metabolomics

In the post-genomic era, computing power, statistical software, separation science and modern mass spectrometry have allowed the analysis of a complex mixture as a complete entity, and not merely the fluctuation in concentration of one analyte within it. Metabolomics is the study of the repertoire of non-proteinaceous, endogenously synthesized small molecules present in an organism. Such small molecules include well-known compounds like glucose, cholesterol, ATP and lipid signalling molecules. These molecules are the ultimate product of cellular metabolism, and the metabolome refers to the catalogue of those molecules in a specific organism, e.g. the human metabolome. In terms of clinical biochemistry, the analysis of the pattern of change of such molecules in urine samples of individuals with and without a particular disease and those treated with specific drugs represents a change in the metabolome. It is very likely that, in the future, medicine-regulating authorities will require metabolomic studies on all new drugs.

Ethical considerations

Ethical considerations must be taken into account in any discussion of clinical genetics. For example, prenatal diagnosis with the option of termination may be unacceptable on moral or religious grounds. With diseases for which there is no cure and currently no treatment (e.g. Huntington's), genetic tests can predict accurately which family members will be affected; however, many people would rather not know this information. One very serious outcome of the new genetic information is that disease susceptibility may be predictable, for example in Alzheimer's disease, so the medical insurance companies can decline to give policies for individuals at high risk.

Society has not yet decided who should have access to an individual's genetic information and to what extent privacy should be preserved.

○ Peaks lost from SF   ○ New peak in SF

Fig. 3.24 Two-dimensional gel electrophoresis comparing paired serum and synovial fluid in a patient with rheumatoid arthritis. Biofluids were first separated according to isoelectric point on a linear immobilized pH gradient followed by SDS-PAGE in a 10% gel. The circled proteins indicate major proteins which differ between the two biofluids. Although serum contained many proteins not found in synovial fluid, one major protein was found to be present in the synovial fluid electropherogram but not in the serum electropherogram. This indicates that synovial fluid is not a simple transudate of serum. Courtesy of Prof. D Perrett and Dr R Bevan, Department of Medicine, Barts and The London School of Medicine.

FURTHER READING

Guttmacher AE, Collins FS (2002) Genomic medicine – a primer. *New England Journal of Medicine* **347**: 1512–1520.

Holt I (ed.) (2003) *Genetics of Mitochondrial Diseases.* Oxford: Oxford University Press

Kiechle FL, Holland-Staley CA (2003) Genomics, transcriptomics, proteomics, and numbers. *Archives of Pathology and Laboratory Medicine* **127**: 1089–1097.

Onyango P (2004) The role of emerging genomics and proteomics technologies in cancer drug target discovery. *Current Cancer Drug Targets* **4**: 111–124.

Super M (2000) CFTR and disease: implications for drug development. *Lancet* **355**: 1840–1842.

Wang S, El-Deiry WS (2004) The p53 pathway: targets for the development of novel cancer therapeutics. *Cancer Treatment and Research* **119**: 175–187.

CHAPTER BIBLIOGRAPHY

McKusick VA (1998) *Mendelian Inheritance in Man*, 12th edn. London: Johns Hopkins Press.

Nabel GJ (2004) Genetic, cellular and immune approaches to disease therapy: past and future. *Nature Medicine* **10**: 135–141.

Scott MP et al (2003) *Molecular Cell Biology*, 5th edn. WH Freeman.

Watson JD et al (2003) *Molecular Cell Biology*, 5th edn. WH Freeman.

Weatherall DJ (1996) *Basic Molecular and Cell Biology*, 3rd edn. London: BMJ Publishing.

SIGNIFICANT WEBSITES

http://www.genetichealth.com
  US e-health company

Clinical immunology

4

THE IMMUNE SYSTEM IN HEALTH

HOST DEFENCE

Throughout life we are exposed to millions of organisms which are inhaled, swallowed or in contact with our skin or mucous membranes. Whether these organisms invade and cause disease is determined by the balance of the pathogenicity of the organism (i.e. the virulence factors that it has at its disposal) and the integrity of the host defence mechanisms. Immunity is often divided into two types termed innate and adaptive (acquired or specific), although in practice these overlap and interlink.

INNATE IMMUNITY

Innate immunity provides the immediately active, first line, non-specific host defence mechanisms. It includes physical (e.g. epithelial cells) and chemical (e.g. 'natural' antimicrobial substances like defensins at surface barriers) as well as immune mechanisms (Table 4.1). The latter consist of cells such as phagocytic cells (neutrophils, and monocytes in the blood; macrophages including dendritic cells in tissues), eosinophils, mast cells and basophils, as well as humoral components (e.g. complement, acute-phase reactants, cytokines). These are directly activated by infectious agents, tissue damage or tumours via surface receptors, e.g. for complement factors when antibody molecules bind through immunoglobulin fc receptors (p. 206). Cells also possess pattern recognition receptors (PRRs) (p. 202) which can recognize structures on micro-organisms collectively. These 'structures' recognized by PRRs are called pathogen-associated molecular patterns (PAMPs) (p. 204). PAMPs include, for example, bacterial lipopolysaccharides, bacterial DNA, double-stranded RNA, peptidoglycans.

Despite the lack of specificity, innate immunity is very effective. Stimulation of either innate or adaptive immunity can also enhance each other's responses.

These non-specific immune responses illustrate normal mechanisms of cell production, recruitment and activation used by all cells of the immune system. The

Table 4.1   Non-immunological host defence mechanisms

Normal barriers	Examples of defects leading to infection
Physical barriers	
Skin and mucous membranes	Breach, e.g. trauma, burns, eczema, cannulae
Cough reflex	Suppression, e.g. by opiates, neurological disease
Mucociliary escalator	Ciliary paralysis (smoking, primary ciliary dyskinesis syndromes)
	Increased mucus production (asthma)
	Abnormally viscid secretions (cystic fibrosis)
Washing, tears, saliva, urine	Decreased fluid, e.g. sicca syndromes, drugs
	Urinary stasis, e.g. prostatic hypertrophy
Chemical barriers, e.g. gastric acid	Gastric acid secretion inhibitors
Colonization resistance provided by non-pathogenic commensal organisms of skin and gut	Use of broad-spectrum antibiotics

mechanisms that lead to protective inflammation are the same as those which cause extensive damage if not regulated.

Initiation of the inflammatory response

The neutrophil (polymorphonuclear, or PMN cell) is a specialized microbicidal (microbe-killing) phagocyte. The human body contains over 10^{11} polymorphonuclear leucocytes/kg, most of which are in the bone marrow. A series of events leads to the recruitment and activation of these cells at the site of tissue damage.

Adhesion molecules (Table 4.2)

Neutrophils, like most of the cells involved in immune responses, are not static within a particular tissue. Neutrophils travel within the blood, either flowing freely as part of the circulating pool or rolling along the vascular endothelium as the marginating pool (see below).

Table 4.2 Adhesion molecules		
Adhesion molecule	**Tissue distribution**	**Ligand**
Immunoglobulin superfamily		
ICAM-1 (CD54)	Endothelial cells, monocytes, T and B cells, dendritic cells, keratinocytes, chondrocytes, epithelial cells	LFA-1
ICAM-2 (CD102)	Endothelial cells, monocytes, dendritic cells, subpopulations of lymphocytes	LFA-1
ICAM-3	Lymphocytes	LFA-1, Mac-1
VCAM-1 (CD106)	Endothelial cells, kidney epithelium, macrophages, dendritic cells, myoblasts, bone marrow fibroblasts	VLA-4
PECAM-1	Platelets, T cells, endothelial cells, monocytes, granulocytes	Unknown
MAdCAM-1	Endothelial venules in mucosal lymph nodes	$\alpha 4\beta 7$ integrin and L-selectin
Selectin family		
E-selectin (CD62E)/ELAM-1	Endothelial cells	Unknown
L-selectin (CD62L)	Lymphocytes, neutrophils, monocytes	CD34
P-selectin (CD62P)	Megakaryocytes, platelets and endothelial cells	Unknown
Integrin family		
VLA subfamily		
VLA-1 to VLA-4	Endothelial cells, resting T cells, monocytes, platelets and epithelial cells	Various molecules including laminin, fibronectin, collagen and VCAM-1
VLA-5 (fibronectin receptor)	Endothelial cells, monocytes and platelets	Laminin
VLA-6 (laminin receptor)	Endothelial cells, monocytes and platelets	Laminin
$\beta 1\alpha 7$	Endothelial cells	Laminin
$\beta 1\alpha 8$	Endothelial cells	Unknown
$\beta 1\alpha$	Platelets and megakaryocytes	Fibronectin
$\beta 2$	Widely distributed	Collagen, laminin, vitronectin
Leucam subfamily		
LFA-1	Lymphocytes	ICAMs 1 to 3
Mac-1	Endothelial cells	ICAM-1, fibrinogen, C3bi
Cytoadhesin subfamily		
Vitronectin receptor	Platelets and megakaryocytes	Vitronectin, fibrinogen, laminin, fibronectin, von Willebrand factor, thrombospondin
$\beta 4\alpha 6$	Endothelial cells, thymocytes and platelets	Laminin
$\beta 5\alpha$	Platelets and megakaryocytes	Vitronectin, fibronectin
$\beta 6\alpha$	Platelets and megakaryocytes	Fibronectin
$\beta 7\alpha 4$/LPAM-1	Endothelial cells, thymocytes, monocytes	Fibronectin, VCAM-1
$\beta 8\alpha$	Platelets and megakaryocytes	Unknown

E-selectin or ELAM, endothelial leucocyte adhesion molecule; ICAM, intercellular adhesion molecule; LFA, leucocyte function antigen; LPAM, lymphocyte Peyer's patch adhesion molecule; MAdCAM-1, mucosal addressin; PECAM, platelet/endothelial cell adhesion molecule; VCAM vascular cell adhesion molecule; VLA, very late antigen

Recruitment of cells of the immune system (phagocytes and lymphocytes) to tissue sites involves cellular adhesion molecules (CAM) (p. 160, Fig. 3.6). The main ones are the intercellular adhesion molecules (ICAM), integrins, selectins and cadherins (calcium-dependent adherins). Adhesion molecules associate with cytoskeletal components to cause cytoskeletal reorganization, resulting in migration and spreading, allowing the cells to move. The binding of adhesion molecules to their ligand also causes signal transduction with increased expression of other receptors, altered gene expression and effects on protein synthesis and cell survival. This often leads to cell activation.

Cell recruitment

Cells move towards the site of inflammation in response to chemoattractants (chemicals which attract cells) at sites of infection or tissue damage. The main chemoattractants for neutrophils in vivo are N-formyl-methionyl-leucylphenylalanine (FMLP) from bacterial cell walls, which in turn causes the release of another chemoattractant, leukotriene B_4 (LTB$_4$) from tissue mast cells; the chemokine (chemoattractant cytokine) interleukin-8 (from macrophages); and C5a from the activation of complement. These substances cause migration of neutrophils by three mechanisms:

- *Upregulation of neutrophil adhesion molecules*, L-selectin and the integrin LFA-1 (leucocyte function antigen), which increases the stickiness of the cells.
- *Increase in local vascular endothelial cell expression of the adhesion molecules* E-selectin and ICAM-1, which causes increased stickiness of the endothelium. The selectin expression causes the circulating neutrophil to be tethered and roll along the endothelium slowly (margination), whereas the reaction between the integrins LFA-1 and ICAM-1 is much stronger, causing the cells to stop moving.
- *Stimulation of neutrophil chemotaxis* (directed movement along the chemoattractant gradient towards the stimulus).

The cells pass between endothelial cells into the tissues by the formation of foot-like processes (pseudopodia) that push through the intercellular spaces; this is called diapedesis. The cells continue to move along the chemoattractant gradient to the site of infection (Fig. 4.1). When the cells reach the highest concentration of chemoattractant, the receptor on the cell surface is downregulated, ensuring that the phagocytes remain at the site of inflammation.

The exodus of neutrophils leads to the inflammatory response and if it involves large numbers causes the formation of pus, the characteristic yellow colour being due to the cytochromes within the cells. Patients with congenital deficiencies of adhesion molecules or those on systemic corticosteroids who have acquired adhesion molecule defects (steroids reduce ICAM-1 expression on endothelial cells) cannot target their neutrophils to sites of infection. As a result of this they suffer recurrent infections. The peripheral blood characteristically shows a leucocytosis as the cells cannot leave the circulation.

Similar mechanisms of cell recruitment and trafficking

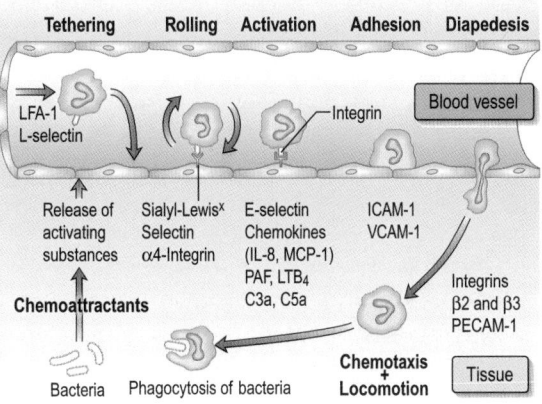

Fig. 4.1 **Neutrophil migration**. Neutrophils arrive at the site of the inflammation, attracted by chemoattractants. They *roll* along the blood-vessel wall and their progress is halted by L-selectin, on their surface, binding to a carbohydrate structure, e.g. sialyl-Lewis^x, an adhesion molecule. On *activation*, the L-selectin is replaced by another cell surface adhesion molecule, e.g. integrin which binds to E-selectin. Various other chemokines, e.g. interleukin-8 (IL-8), macrophage chemoattractant factor (MCP), TNF-α and other inflammatory mediators are involved. These inflammatory markers attract the activated neutrophil into the tissue where it phagocytoses and destroys C3b-coated bacteria. The inflammation releases activating substances, attracting more neutrophils.
LFA, leucocyte function antigen; PAF, platelet-activating factor, LTB4, leukotriene B4; ICAM, intracellular adhesion molecule; VCAM, vascular cell adhesion molecule; PECAM, platelet/endothelial cell adhesion molecule.

by the use of adhesion molecules are described for other cells within the immune system, for example L-selectin facilitates 'homing' of lymphocytes to lymph nodes.

Phagocytosis and intracellular killing

Once the neutrophils have been recruited, phagocytosis (ingestion) and intracellular killing of microbes begins. Phagocytosis occurs by the formation of pseudopodia (projections of cytoplasmic membrane) around the organism or particle to be ingested (see Fig. 4.11a). Owing to the fluidity of the cell membrane, the tips eventually fuse to form a membrane-bound vesicle called a phagosome. This fuses with the neutrophil cytoplasmic granules (Table 4.3) to form a phagolysosome. Within this localized environment, killing occurs, the cytoplasm being protected. There are two major mechanisms:

- O_2-*dependent response* or 'respiratory burst', in which there is production of reactive oxygen metabolites, such as hydrogen peroxide, hydroxyl radicals and singlet oxygen, via the reduction of oxygen by a cytochrome-dependent NADPH oxidase.
- O_2-*independent response*, due to the toxic action of preformed cationic proteins and enzymes contained within the cytoplasmic granules.

Ingestion and killing of organisms is much more effective if the particle is first coated or opsonized ('made ready to

Table 4.3 Neutrophil granule proteins (there are two types distinguished by staining characteristics)

Primary granule (azurophilic)
Defensins
Lysozyme
Elastase
Bactericidal/permeability-increasing factor
Cathepsin G
Myeloperoxidase
Acid glycolases
Collagenase

Secondary granule (specific)
Lysozyme
Lactoferrin
Collagenase
Cytochrome B
Vitamin B_{12}-binding protein

eat') with specific antibody and complement. This is because neutrophils have receptors for the Fc portion of antibody molecules (FcR), and complement (CR). Binding of cell-surface receptors to complement and antibody on the particle both increases the strength of adhesion and causes transduction of intracellular signals, which activate the cell to promote phagocytic and killing activity.

Granulocyte and granulocyte–macrophage colony-stimulating factors (G-CSF and GM-CSF) are cytokines released by activated endothelial cells and macrophages and act on the bone marrow to release more neutrophils into the circulation. This causes the characteristic neutrophil leucocytosis observed in infectious or inflammatory disease. Interleukin-6 is also produced and induces the liver synthesis of the acute-phase reactants, particularly complement components, C-reactive protein (CRP), mannan-binding lectin and fibrinogen (Table 4.4). Many of these are opsonins. CRP and fibrinogen (the main factor which affects the ESR reading) are measured diagnostically to monitor infection and inflammatory conditions.

Neutrophils can only ingest particles smaller than themselves and are only able to detect extracellular infections, particularly bacteria and some fungi. Monocytes and macrophages act in the same way using similar types of receptors. Phagocytes also remove particles of foreign material and tissue debris. Once the stimulus is controlled, the neutrophils undergo apoptosis (programmed cell death) and are themselves phagocytosed by macrophages, limiting the inflammatory reaction.

Table 4.4 Acute-phase proteins

Pentraxins – C-reactive protein, serum amyloid P protein
Complement components
Fibrinogen
Haptoglobulin
Caeruloplasmin
α_1-Antitrypsin
Mannan-binding lectin
Ferritin

Eosinophils in host defence

In developed countries eosinophils are most commonly associated with allergic disease, but their physiological function is in parasite control. Eosinophils have receptors for IgE which is the major antiparasite antibody, particularly against nematodes. Eosinophils bind IgE via the FcεR, and toxic metabolites are released from the eosinophil granules directly onto the parasite surface. Examples are major basic protein (MBP), which produces ballooning and detachment of the helminth tegumental membrane, and eosinophil cationic protein (ECP), which is present in smaller amounts but is eight to ten times more toxic than MBP, producing complete fragmentation and disruption of the parasites.

Mast cells and basophils

Mast cells consist of two populations, which are distinguished by their enzyme content. The T mast cells contain trypsin alone (also termed mucosal mast cells owing to their location). The TC mast cells contain both trypsin and chymotrypsin and are called connective tissue mast cells. Mast cell function appears to be in the initiation of inflammatory responses (increased vascular permeability, bronchoconstriction) by the release (following degranulation) of pro-inflammatory mediators such as histamine, leukotrienes, platelet-activating factor (PAF), prostaglandins and some cytokines (e.g. IL-4). Basophils are morphologically similar to mast cells but are found in very small numbers in the blood. These cells bear high-affinity IgE receptors FcεR1 (CD23) which rapidly absorb any local IgE and participate in immediate-type hypersensitivity reactions (see p. 220).

Dendritic cells/Langerhans' cells

These are derived from the lymphoid and myeloid cell lines; dendritic cells in the skin are called Langerhans' cells. Their major function is to present antigen to T cells when stimulated. Dendritic cells link innate immunity to the adaptive immune system (p. 204) by being the only cell that can activate naive T cells to initiate an adaptive immune response. They are activated by signals from PAMP, heat shock proteins and TNF-α, and IFN-α (secreted from host cells) reacting to injury. When activated, dendritic cells can change their expression of chemokine receptors and migrate from tissue to the T cell zones of lymph nodes.

Complement

The complement system comprises a series of at least 20 glycoproteins that are activated in a cascade sequence, with proenzymes that undergo sequential proteolytic cleavage to their active forms. It is a major part of the innate immune system.

Three main pathways of complement activation exist, termed the classical, alternative and mannan-binding lectin (MBL) pathways (Fig. 4.2). The terminology of the

MBL Pathway	Classical Pathway	Alternative Pathway
Started by: MBL binding to mannan residues on surface of bacterial cell	Started by: C1 complex (C1q, C1r, C1s) antibody binding to antigen	Started by: C3b binding to hydroxyl groups on surface of cell, carbohydrates and proteins on organisms

C4/C2 cleavage

−ve control C1INH

Alternative pathway +ve feedback loop

C3 cleavage by C3 convertases

C3a

Anaphylatoxins
Smooth muscle contraction
Vascular permeability
Mast cell degranulation

−ve control
C3 convertase inhibitors CR1, C4BP, DAF, MCP, factor H, factor I
+ve control
C3 convertase stabilization Properdin

Opsonization stimulates phagocytosis and APC and B cell endocytosis

C3b

C5 cleavage by C5 convertases

C5a

Neutrophil, monocyte chemotactic agent

C5b

MAC assembly + C6–C9

−ve control Protectin (CD59)

Cell lysis

Fig. 4.2 **Complement pathway**. The three activation pathways (mannan-binding lectin (MBL), classical and alternative) converge at the central C3 component. This leads to a final common pathway with the assembly of C5 to C9 forming a transmembrane pore (membrane attack complex MAC) in the cell surface and death by osmotic lysis. C1INH, C1 esterase inhibitor; factors H and I, regulatory factors; DAF (CD55), decay-accelerating factor; MCP, macrophage chemoattractant protein; APC, antigen-presenting cell; CR1, complement receptor 1; C4BP, C4 binding protein.

complement proteins is that components of the classical pathway are named by 'C' followed by a number (the numbering sequence is in order of their discovery not position in the sequence). Alternative pathway components are called factors followed by a specific letter. During activation some components are initially cleaved into fragments. The smaller fragment, designated 'a', is released; the larger 'b' fragment is usually deposited on the surface of the activating cell. Further fragmentation may occur to 'c', 'd' and 'g' fragments.

The complement pathways are triggered by different factors:

- *Classical pathway* by antigen–antibody immune complexes, apoptotic cells, C-reactive protein bound to ligand and certain viruses and bacteria.
- *Alternative pathway* by bacterial endotoxin, fungal cell walls, viruses and tumour cells.

- *Mannan-binding lectin (MBL) pathway* is activated by microbes with terminal mannose groups. MBL has a similar structure to C1q and activates through the classical pathway without the requirement for antibody.

The pathways converge in the activation of C3 (by the formation of either classical or alternative C3 convertase). This leads into a final common pathway with the assembly of components C5–C9 to form the membrane attack complex (MAC) which assembles into a 'doughnut-like' transmembrane channel leading to cell lysis by osmotic shock.

Complement activation is focused at cell membranes. Host cells are protected from complement-mediated lysis by inhibitory surface molecules, for example decay accelerating factor (DAF). Most organisms lack any protective molecules and are therefore susceptible to complement.

Functions of complement

- *Anti-infective function:*
  - opsonization by C3b and C4b
  - chemotaxis – attraction of phagocytes by chemo-attractant activation products
  - activation of leucocytes by anaphylatoxins (C5a, C3a and C4a); via receptors on leucocytes
  - lysis of bacteria and cells (C5b–C9).
- *Interplay between innate and adaptive immune system.* Immunomodulation of B-cell responses to specific antigen through binding of complement receptors on B-cell surface, thus augmenting antibody responses and immunological memory.
- *Clearance of:*
  - immune complexes (C1q, C3 and C4)
  - apoptotic cells (C1q, C3 and C4).

Other cells or factors active in non-specific immunity

Natural killer (NK) cells

These non-phagocytic cells have the morphology of lymphocytes but do not bear the markers for T or B cells. They are distinguished by the presence of numerous cytoplasmic granules. They have non-specific antiviral and antitumour activity, causing lysis of cells with which they react.

NK cells recognize abnormal cells in two ways. Firstly, they bear immunoglobulin receptors (FcR) and bind antibody-coated targets leading to antibody-dependent cellular cytotoxicity (ADCC). Secondly, they have surface receptors for MHC (major histocompatibility complex) class I. If these MHC receptors are not bound on interaction with a cell, the NK cell is programmed to lyse this target cell. It does this by making holes in its cell membrane by secreting 'perforins'; granzymes are injected through these pores and cause the induction of apoptosis. As normal host cells are MHC class I positive, the 'death pathway' is inhibited by the NK cell binding to this receptor. However, tumours on affected cells and viruses often cause downregulation of class I and thus it leaves them open to NK cell attack.

NK cells may also shape the adaptive T cell responses to Th1 or Th2 type depending on the balance of the NK receptor activation during the early stage of an immune response.

Cytokines

Cytokines are small soluble intercellular messengers that exert their effect by binding to specific receptors on target cells. They act as autocrine, paracrine or endocrine messengers. Cytokines are produced by any cell. Their biological effect varies according to the cytokine and the cell involved (Table 4.5), but typically these molecules will signal certain cell populations to activate, divide or home in on a particular site in the body. Cytokines include:

- *Interleukins* produced by and signal between white cells.
- *Chemokines* have a chemoattractant function.
- *Colony-stimulating factors* cause differentiation and proliferation of stem cells.
- *Interferons* (see below).
- *Tumour necrosis factors*. TFN-α increases phagocyte function.

Interferons (IFN) are a major class of cytokine. They are divided into type I (alpha and beta) and type II (gamma or 'immune' interferon). Type I interferons are antiviral agents produced mainly by fibroblasts, monocytes and infected cells as a reaction to viral infection. *Alpha* and *beta IFN* bind the same cellular receptor and protect uninfected cells by inducing the intracellular production of molecules that inhibit viral RNA and DNA production. They also increase the expression of MHC class I molecules, leading to enhanced lysis of virally infected cells by specific cytotoxic T lymphocytes. Type I interferons also have antiproliferative function. IFN-α is used in the treatment of chronic hepatitis B and C infections as well as in some forms of leukaemia. IFN-β reduces the relapse rate in some forms of multiple sclerosis.

Gamma-interferon has different functions, acting mainly on the immune response. It activates macrophage and neutrophil intracellular killing, stimulates natural killer cells and enhances T-cell responses by increasing MHC class II expression on antigen-presenting cells. IFN-γ uses a separate receptor from the type I interferons. It is used therapeutically in the congenital neutrophil defect (chronic granulomatous disease), in patients with defects in IFN-γ production or receptor expression, and in the adjunct therapy of some infections (leishmaniasis, atypical mycobacterial disease).

Other cytokines are also involved in innate immunity. Interleukin-6 mediates the acute-phase reaction through hepatic induction. Interleukin-8 is a powerful chemoattractant. Granulocyte and macrophage– granulocyte colony-stimulating factors (G- and GM-CSF) increase phagocyte numbers.

Heat-shock proteins (HSP)

Heat-shock proteins are a family of highly conserved proteins which act as immunodominant antigens in many infections. They are molecular chaperones, housekeeping proteins within cells, preserving the cell's protein structure. They are similar in configuration to antigens found on certain microorganisms and may induce auto-immunity through molecular mimicry.

HSPs are also released and may act on cells to modulate function by inducing cytokines, adhesion molecules and maturation signals.

Pattern recognition receptors (PRRs) (Fig. 4.3)

The innate immune response is essential for host survival as it is immediately active. It is not antigen specific but can detect tissue damage and discriminate foreign molecules from 'self' (sometimes called 'danger–stranger' recognition). Phagocytic cells (macrophages, dendritic and B cells – antigen-presenting cells) bear pattern-recognition receptors with lectin-like activity which recognize *pathogen-associated molecular patterns* (PAMPs) present on microbes but not host cells. PRRs include:

- Mannan-binding lectin, which initiates complement activity inducing *opsonization* (p. 201).
- *Endocytic pattern recognition receptors*, which act by enhancing antigen presentation on macrophages, by recognizing microorganisms with mannose-rich carbohydrates on their surface or by binding to bacterial cell walls and scavenging bacteria from the circulation. All lead to *phagocytosis*.
- *Signalling receptors* that initiate nuclear factor kappa B induction (e.g. toll-like receptors) and immune response genes leading to *cell activation*. These may have some specificity, e.g. TLR4 binds Gram-negative bacterial endotoxin and TLR2 binds Gram-positive bacterial lipoteichoic acid. TLR3 and TLR9 detect nucleic acid. TLR5 recognizes a protein on bacterial flagella. Innate immunity critically depends on toll-like receptor signalling. These receptors act through a critical adaptor molecule, myeloid differentiation factor 88 (MyD88), to regulate the activity of NFκB pathways and the expression of many of the cytokines necessary to mount an innate defence response.
- *TREM-1* (triggering receptor expressed on myeloid cells), a member of the aminoglobulin superfamily, is a cell surface receptor which, when bound to its ligand, triggers secretion of proinflammatory cytokines. It is upregulated by bacterial lipopolysaccharides (e.g. pseudomonas), but not in non-infective disorders. It is a mechanism that links bacteria on the outside of the cell membrane with gene transcription of cytokines in the cell nucleus.

Nuclear factor kappa B (NFκB)

NFκB is a pivotal transcription factor in chronic inflammatory diseases. It is a heterodimer of two proteins (p. 157) and is found in the cytoplasm bound to an inhibitor (IκB), which prevents it from entering the nucleus. It is released from IκB on stimulation of the cell and passes

Table 4.5 Origins and biological functions of cytokines (including chemokines)

Cytokine	Source	Mode of action
Haemopoietins		
IL-1	Macrophages/monocytes	Immune activation: induces an inflammatory response
IL-2	Primarily Th1 cells	Activates T (and NK) cells and supports their growth
IL-3	T cells	Primarily promotes growth of haemopoietic cells
IL-4	Th2 cells	Lymphocyte growth factor; involved in IgE responses
IL-5	Th2 cells	Promotes growth of B cells and acute phase response eosinophils
IL-6	Th2 cells and macrophages	Promotes B-cell growth and antibody production
IL-7	Stromal cells	Lymphocyte growth factor, important in the growth of immature cells
IL-10	CD4 cells, activated monocytes	Inhibits the production of IFN-γ, IL-1, IL-6, TNF-α and antigen presentation
IL-11	Macrophage	Maintains epithelial integrity of gastrointestinal tract and megakaryocyte differentiation
IL-12	Monocytes/macrophages	Augments Th1 responses and induces IFN-γ
IL-13	Activated T cells	Stimulates B cells
IL-15	Many tissues, not T cells	Similar action to IL-2
G-CSF	Primarily monocytes	Promotes growth of myeloid cells
M-CSF	Primarily monocytes	Promotes growth of macrophages
GM-CSF	Primarily T cells	Promotes growth of monomyelocytic cells
Interferons		
IFN-α	Leucocytes	Immune activation and modulation (following viral infection)
IFN-β	Fibroblasts	Immune activation and modulation (following viral infection)
IFN-γ	Th1 and NK cells	Immune activation and modulation (inhibits Th2 cells, activates macrophages)
Tumour necrosis factors		
TNF-α	Macrophages, NK, T, B and mast cells	Stimulates generalized immune activation as well as tumour necrosis; formerly known as cachectin
TNF-β	T and B cells, macrophages, mast cells	Stimulates immune activation and generalized vascular effects; also known as lymphotoxin
TGF-β	Platelets	Immunoinhibitory but stimulates tumorigenesis, angiogenesis and fibrosis
Chemokines*		
'CC chemokines'		
MCP1–MCPS	Monocytes, macrophages, fibroblasts, keratinocytes	Attracts monocytes and memory T cells to inflammatory sites
MIP-1α	Macrophages	Attracts monocytes and T cells
MIP-1β	Monocytes, macrophages, endothelial cells, T and B cells	Attracts monocytes and CD8$^+$ T cells
Eotaxin	Macrophages, activated leucocytes, endothelial cells	Attracts eosinophils, basophils
RANTES	Platelets and T cells	Attracts monocytes, T cells, eosinophils
'CXC chemokines'		
IL-8	Macrophages	Attracts neutrophils, naive T cells
CINC	Macrophages	Attracts neutrophils
MIP2	Kupffer cells	Attracts neutrophils
ENA78	Epithelial cells, Kupffer cells	Activates neutrophils
GROα	Macrophages, hepatocytes, endothelial cells	Unknown
IP10	Hepatocytes, endothelium	Unknown
MIG	Monocytes/macrophages, hepatocytes	Attracts lymphocytes

* Refers to a double cysteine amino acid structure (-CC-) within the cytokine; in some cases this is interspersed with another amino acid (-CXC-) CINC, cytokine-induced neutrophil chemoattractant; ENA78, epithelial neutrophil activating protein 78; G-CSF, granulocyte colony-stimulating factor; GM-CSF, granulocyte–macrophage colony-stimulating factor; GROα, growth-related oncogene; IFN, interferon; IL, interleukin; IP10, interferon-gamma-inducible protein 10; MCP, monocyte chemoattractant protein; M-CSF, monocyte colony-stimulating factor; MIG, monokine induced by interferon gamma; MIP, macrophage inflammatory protein; MIP2, macrophage inflammatory protein; RANTES, regulated on activation, normal T-cell expressed and secreted; TGF, transforming growth factor; TNF, tumour necrosis factor

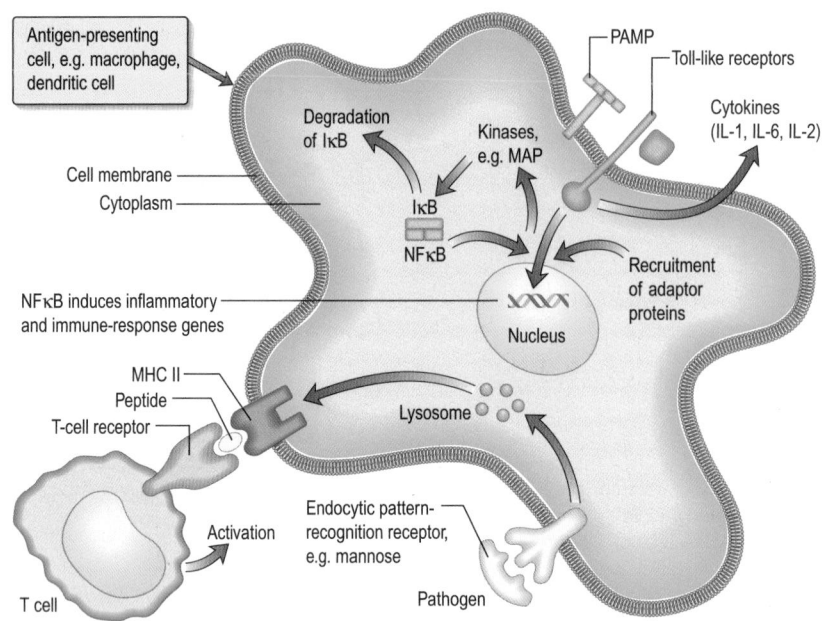

Fig. 4.3 Pattern recognition receptors in the innate and adaptive immune systems. The innate immune system has pattern-recognition receptors, e.g. toll-like receptors, which recognize microbial products by their pathogen-associated molecular pattern (PAMP). This leads to activation of kinases (e.g. mitogen-activated protein – MAP), which in turn leads to degradation of inhibitory κB (IκB) and release of NFκB. NFκB induces inflammatory and immune-response genes in the nucleus and is activated by the recognition of PAMP. An antigen-presenting cell, e.g. macrophage, dendritic cell, has endocytic pattern-recognition receptors (e.g. macrophage mannose receptor) through which it binds to and phagocytoses pathogens. These are processed by lysosomes to produce peptides which form a complex with the major histocompatibility complex (MHC) on the surface. These are recognized by T-cell receptors leading to activation of this cell. NF, nuclear factor.

into the nucleus where it binds to specific sequences in the promoter regions of target genes. It is stimulated by, for example, cytokines, protein C activators and viruses, and itself regulates various proteins (e.g. pro-inflammatory cytokines, chemokines, adhesion molecules, inflammatory enzymes and receptors).

The importance of regulation of the inflammatory response is demonstrated in sepsis when overwhelming activation, by for example, endotoxin, leads to induction of a 'cytokine storm' with organ failure, shock and death as a result. Proteosome inhibitors are being developed which inhibit the degradation of ubiquinated proteins including the cell cycle regulating proteins like cyclins and cyclin-dependent kinases. For example, bortezomib, a proteosome inhibitor (p. 518) inhibits activation of NFκB.

Dysregulated chronic inflammation is also associated with clinical disease, in particular an increased risk of cardiovascular complication in conditions with chronically elevated CRP such as rheumatoid arthritis. The inflammatory process is thought to contribute to the atheromatous lesions.

ADAPTIVE (SPECIFIC OR ACQUIRED) IMMUNITY

Specific or 'adaptive' immunity is the hallmark of the immune system of higher animals. Innate immunity is a

rapid non-specific response whereas adaptive immunity gives a targetted attack against, for example, a pathogen. The characteristic of this response is the use of antigen-specific receptors on T lymphocytes (T-cell receptor, TCR) and B lymphocytes (surface and secreted antibody) to direct the response. Specificity is achieved by an unusual mechanism involving multiple rearrangements of original (germline) DNA in T and B lymphocytes. The altered DNA codes for proteins with hypervariable regions and creates the specific antigen-binding T-cell receptor and antibody sites. This diversity allows the production, for example, of over 10^8 different antibodies and 10^7 distinct TCRs, enough to cover the spectrum of pathogenic antigens encountered by man. T and B cells do not recognize exactly the same part of any antigen. T-cell receptors recognize peptide fragments, whereas antibody identifies the shape of epitopes. This increases the ability of the immune system to recognize a wider range of antigens and provides back-up for each system. The response takes time to develop so that although specific immunity has the benefit of being very focused it cannot provide immediate protection on first meeting an antigen. However, another characteristic is the development of memory so that subsequent exposure leads to a more rapid response. The role of T and B lymphocytes in specific immunity is shown in Figure 4.4.

T and B cell immunity extends the ability to combat infection and tumours. Phagocytes only recognize extra-

Specific immunity

Fig. 4.4 **Components of the immune response**. Antigen is presented to T-helper cells (Th cells) by an antigen-presenting cell. Th cells secrete lymphokines, which activate cytotoxic T cells (Tc cells) that are involved in antiviral and anti-tumour activity. The lymphokines also activate NK cells, which are involved in tumour surveillance. B cells are activated when the antigen binds to the surface immunoglobulins in the presence of cytokines. This leads to secretion of antibodies. Antibody and complement coat the antigen (opsonize), leading to phagocytosis by phagocytes via binding to the complement receptor and Fc receptor (FcR). NK, natural killer cell.

cellular organisms, mostly bacteria. In contrast, T cells are able to combat intracellular infections, such as viruses, as well as the organisms that parasitize macrophages such as facultative intracellular bacteria (mycobacteria, legionella, listeria, brucella, salmonella), many fungi and protozoa. Such intracellular infections are controlled by two separate T-cell mechanisms.

- *Cytotoxic T cells* recognize tiny fragments of foreign antigen (virus or tumour antigen) that are expressed on the surface of affected cells and are able to destroy the cell and pathogen within it. Cytotoxic cells usually bear CD8.
- *Helper T cells* are unable to destroy pathogens or cells directly, but through cytokine production are able to activate macrophages to kill organisms within them and further activate cytotoxic T cells and NK cells. Helper T-cells are usually CD4 positive.

Antibody enhances the innate response by opsonizing foreign particles, neutralizing viruses and toxins, and plays a part in antigen presentation.

ORGANIZATION OF THE LYMPHOID SYSTEM

Most lymphocyte maturation and activation occurs within the lymphoid tissue/organs located throughout the body. Populations of lymphoid cells of different types originate from pluripotent stem cells in the bone marrow (Fig. 4.5). Immature B lymphocytes remain in the bone marrow to mature. Lymphoid precursors destined to be T cells move to the thymus for maturation. These are termed the primary lymphoid tissues. Once cells have matured, they are released into the circulation and populate secondary lymphoid tissue such as lymph nodes, tonsils and spleen where they are ready to respond to foreign antigens.

Mucosa-associated lymphoid tissue (MALT)

Lymphoid tissue is frequently found in mucosal surfaces in non-encapsulated patches. This is termed mucosa-associated lymphoid tissue (MALT), consisting of genito-urinary and gut-associated lymphoid tissue (GALT, mainly Peyer's patches), bronchus-associated lymphoid tissue (BALT, found in the lobes of the lungs along the main bronchi) and skin-associated lymphoid tissue (SALT).

B cells

These cells comprise approximately 25% of lymphocytes. In response to antigen binding to the B-cell receptor (BCR) and usually with T-cell help, B cells divide and are activated to become plasma cells which secrete large amounts of antibody (Fig. 4.5).

Antibody molecules (immunoglobulins)

Antibodies are glycoproteins. They consist of two heavy chains and two light chains (either κ or λ polypeptides) (Fig. 4.6). The heavy chain determines the antibody *isotype* or class, i.e. IgG, A, M, D or E. The major regions of immunoglobulin are as follows:

Variable 'V' domains have variation in the amino acid sequence between immunoglobulins, with short segments of hypervariable regions. Antigen binding occurs in the area where the loops bearing the hypervariable regions of the light and heavy chains come together, called the *Fab* (*fragment antigen binding*) region. The shape of the binding site determines the 'goodness of fit' or affinity/avidity of any particular antibody for an antigen.

Idiotypes are markers found in the hypervariable region and are associated with the antigen-binding site. The idiotype is antigenic, and idiotypes and anti-idiotypes are

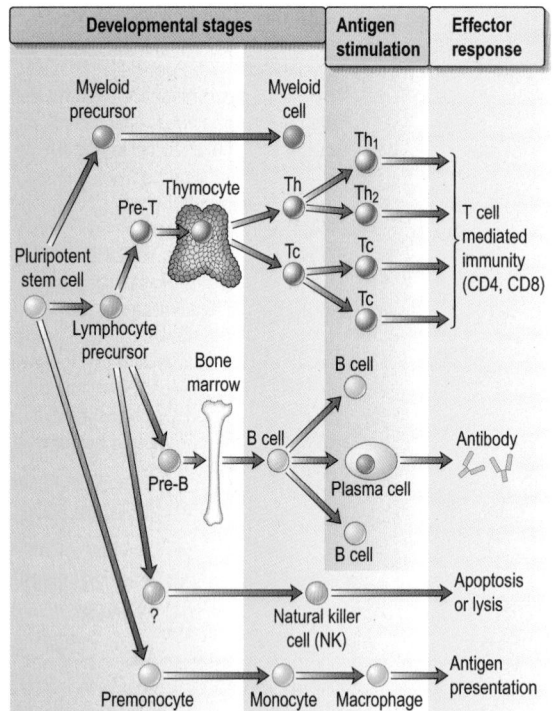

Fig. 4.5 Development of cells involved in immune responses. Cells destined to be lymphocytes or myeloid cells are derived from a common pluripotent stem cell in the bone marrow.

Immature T cells leave the bone marrow to enter the thymus as thymocytes. Gene rearrangement takes place to form the antigen-specific T-cell receptor; positive and negative selection occur to ensure that functional cells that are non-autoreactive survive and differentiate to CD4+ or CD8+ cells. These antigen-naive T cells leave the thymus to populate peripheral lymphoid tissue. On encountering their specific antigen, proliferation and activation occur, having either helper (CD4+ cell) or cytotoxic (CD8+ cell) function.

B cells undergo development to maturity within the bone marrow, including gene rearrangement for production of antigen-specific antibody molecules. The mature cells are released and populate the follicles of lymph nodes. On meeting their specific antigen, B cells proliferate and differentiate to antibody-secreting plasma cells.

Cells of the myeloid lineage develop within the marrow under the influence of colony-stimulating factors to become monocytes, neutrophils, eosinophils and basophils (Fig. 8.1).

thought to make a network regulating the production of antibody.

The Fc (fragment crystalline) region is formed from the constant domains in which the amino acid sequences are relatively conserved. This is the part that binds to cell-surface immunoglobulin receptors (FcR) or causes complement fixation; hence it controls the effects of the antibody molecule after it has bound its antigen.

Genetics of antibody production

Rearrangement of the germline DNA occurs within

Fig. 4.6 Immunoglobulin structure. **(a) Basic subunit** consisting of two heavy and two light chains. **(b) Schematic diagram of the same molecule.** C and V, constant and variable domains; H and L, heavy and light chains; Fab, fragment antigen binding; Fc fragment crystalline. **(c) Genes on the Fab and Fc regions of an immunoglobulin.** The chain is made up of a V (variable) gene which is translocated to the J (joining) chain. The VJ segment is then spliced to the C (constant) gene. Heavy chains have an additional D (diversity) segment which forms the VDJ segment that bears the antigen-binding site determinants.

immature B cells in the bone marrow, leading to production of antibodies with many different antigen-binding sites or *clonal diversity* (Fig. 4.6). There are three main areas of the gene called the variable (V), diversity (D) and joining (J) regions which need to be spliced together to form the final sequence from which protein will be transcribed to form the antibody molecule. It is during this splicing that much of the variability occurs. Firstly, there is a multiplicity of all these regions within the DNA (V = 25–100 genes, D = 10 genes and J = 5–6 genes). Any one of the multiple genes within a region can join any other (called *combinational freedom*) to form the final VDJ sequence. Secondly, splicing of the genes together is frequently inaccurate and 'frame-shift' in base-pairs leads to misreading and production of the 'wrong' amino acid (junctional diversity). Thirdly, somatic mutation in the genes may occur during cell division.

Once the VDJ region is spliced it combines successively to the IgM, IgD, IgG, IgA, and IgE constant genes to cause progressive switching in the isotype of the antibody. However, as the Fab gene is not further altered the same antigen-binding region is maintained. Thus, a mature but naive B cell that has rearranged its VDJ gene will initially make an IgM response on antigen stimulation, as this is the first to be translocated. The primary immune response is therefore of the IgM isotype with IgG and other isotype responses developing later and usually requiring additional T-cell help (T-independent responses are restricted to polysaccharide antigens and usually do not progress from the IgM isotype). However, once the 'switch' from IgM to another isotype has occurred, memory B cells remain in the body for many years. These react rapidly to any re-challenge with the same antigen, and the characteristic IgG production of the secondary or late primary response occurs. Knowledge of the timing of primary and secondary antibody responses is used in the serological diagnosis of infections, the presence of IgM suggesting acute infection.

Immunoglobulin isotypes and their functions

The main biological features of the human antibodies are summarized in Table 4.6. Different classes of antibody tend to predominate at different sites. The major functions of antibody are:

- elimination of infective organisms by:
  - binding to prevent adhesion and invasion of organisms (e.g. preventing the entry of poliovirus and other enteroviruses)
  - opsonization of particles for phagocytosis
  - lysis (in combination with complement)
- antitoxin activity (e.g. in prevention of tetanus)
- sensitization of cells for antibody-dependent cell cytotoxicity (ADCC)
- immune regulation, acting as the antigen receptor on B cells and presenting the antigen to helper T cells.

IgM

The antibody is confined mainly to the intravascular pool. It is a large pentameric molecule, bound together by the joining 'J' chain. It does not cross the placenta, and is not normally produced in the child until after birth. Therefore, if present in the newborn infant, antigen-specific IgM is a good marker for intrauterine infection. It is usually a sign of acute infections.

IgG

This is the most abundant immunoglobulin in serum, present as a monomer. IgG is the antibody of secondary response, and has high antigen affinity. It is the only antibody to cross the placenta in significant quantities. There are four subclasses: IgG_1, IgG_2, IgG_3 and IgG_4. IgG_1 and IgG_3 are produced mainly in response to protein antigens, such as viruses. These subclasses are good opsonins, binding Fc receptors on neutrophils and activating complement. IgG_2 and IgG_4 are produced in response to polysaccharide antigen (e.g. the capsule of bacteria such as pneumococcus and *Haemophilus influenzae*) and are the major opsonins for such organisms. IgG antibody is involved in resistance to infection, as patients who are lacking in IgG suffer with recurrent, even life-threatening bacterial infections. Those with isolated IgA or IgM deficiency have much less severe problems.

IgA

This is mainly the antibody of secretions, being present in the respiratory, gastrointestinal and urinary tracts. There are two subclasses, IgA_1 and IgA_2; their functions appear to be similar. IgA is mainly monomeric in the serum, but dimeric in secretions, the two molecules being complexed

Table 4.6	**Characteristics of the immunoglobulins**				
	IgG Dominant class of antibody	**IgM** Produced first in immune response	**IgA** Found in mucous membrane secretions	**IgE** Responsible for symptoms of allergy; used in defence against nematode parasites	**IgD** Found almost solely on lymphocyte membrane
Heavy chain	γ	μ	α	ε	δ
Mean adult serum levels (mg/mL):	IgG (total) = 8–16 G_1 = 6.5 G_2 = 2.5 G_3 = 0.7 G_4 = 0.3	0.5–2	IgA (total) = 1.4–4 A_1 = 1.5 A_2 = 0.2	17–450 ng/mL	0–0.4
Half-life (days)	21	10	6	2	3
Complement fixation					
Classical	++	+++	–	–	–
Alternative	–	–	+	–	–
Binding to mast cells	–	–	–	+	–
Crosses placenta	+	–	–	–	–

by a joining (J) chain. The mechanism for transport from serum to intestinal mucosal surface is well established. IgA in serum binds to a poly-Fc receptor for IgA and IgM on the basal surface of enterocytes and hepatocytes. Transcellular transport delivers the immunoglobulin to the luminal surface where it is secreted still bound to the receptor, which is termed the *secretory component* (SC). For IgA responses, localized antigen exposure gives rise to generalized mucosal immunity, which is of importance in vaccination. This is because after encountering antigen, IgA precursor B cells in the mucosal lymphoid follicles journey to regional lymph nodes. After clonal expansion the cells return to the systemic circulation via the thoracic duct and circulate to settle widely in the mucosa-associated lymphoid tissue (MALT; see p. 205), not just the area where antigen exposure occurred.

IgD

Serum levels are very low and its function at this site is uncertain. IgD is present on the surface of B lymphocytes, and may have an immunoregulatory role. Levels are high in conditions with B-cell activation such as systemic lupus erythematosus (SLE), HIV infection and Hodgkin's disease.

IgE

IgE is a monomer that is normally present in very low levels in serum, as most is membrane-bound to the high-affinity receptors on mast cells and basophils. Its main physiological role is its antinematode activity, but its most common clinical relevance is in the pathogenesis of type 1 hypersensitivity (atopic or allergic) disease.

T lymphocytes

T cells are classified into CD4 (mainly cytokine-secreting helper cells, making up about 75% of peripheral blood T cells) and CD8 (mainly cytotoxic suppressor cells, which account for the remainder). These cell types are indistinguishable morphologically, but can be separated by the presence of cell-surface molecules detected by monoclonal antibodies detecting cluster of differentiation or CD molecules.

Cytotoxic/suppressor cells

The cytotoxic/suppresser lymphocyte can be recognized by the presence of the CD8$^+$ cell surface molecule and its ability to recognize antigen only when presented with MHC class I molecules. Cytotoxic T cells kill other cells, either by inserting perforins into target cell membranes, producing pores through which granzyme is inserted and causing the action of granule-associated osmotic lysis of the cell (similar to the membrane attack complex of complement) or via activation of caspases to induce apoptosis (programmed cell death, p. 162) in the target. This kind of response is used in controlling viral infections and possibly malignancies. The suppressor cell down-regulates immune responses. It may function by releasing soluble factors which act on B lymphocytes to reduce their output of antibodies. CD8 cells can also mount a

non-cytotoxic antiviral response (NCAR) that blocks viral replication through the secretion of CD8 antiviral factor (CAF); this has been demonstrated in HIV infection.

Helper/inducer cells

T-helper cells can be distinguished by the presence of the CD4 protein on their surface and the ability to recognize antigen only when expressed with MHC class II on antigen-presenting cells. Whereas the cytotoxic response is a simple recognition system for foreign invasion, the CD4-cell system is more elaborate, involving a limited number of cells to produce an even more specific series of reactions. T-helper cells are viewed as orchestrating the immune response. They cannot directly destroy their target, but recognize specific foreign antigen and proceed to activate other parts of the system which can eradicate it (Fig. 4.7).

T-helper cells have been categorized into two major functional subpopulations based on their pattern of cytokine production. A single clone of T cells can differentiate to either type, depending on antigen route, dose, the cytokine environment in which the response occurs and hereditary tendency. The *T-helper 1 (Th1)* class produces IL-2, IL-3 and gamma-interferon. These cytokines will promote immune responses that are primarily cell-mediated/inflammatory by activating cytotoxic T cells, NK cells and macrophages. Cells in the *T-helper 2 (Th2)* category produce cytokines that favour induction of antibody responses by B cells, i.e. IL-4, IL-5, IL-6, IL-10, and are thought to be involved in the development of allergic disease.

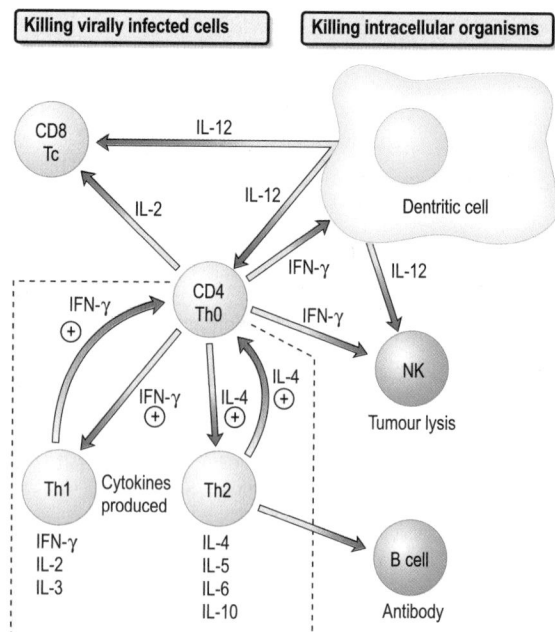

Fig. 4.7 **CD4$^+$ orchestration of the immune response.** CD4 T helper cells (Th0) differentiate into either Th1 or Th2. The type of cell produced depends on the cytokine environment. The presence of IFN-γ leads to production of Th1 cells; IL-4 leads to Th2 predominance. Stimulation of B cells leads to antibody production and NK cells to tumour lysis.

Cluster of differentiation (CD) classification

The CD nomenclature classifies over 300 molecules both within and outside the immune system, using monoclonal antibodies. As the surface molecule has many different epitopes (antibody-binding sites), several different antibodies may react (a cluster). As initially most of the surface molecules defined the stage of development of the cell, they were termed 'differentiation' molecules. The term CD therefore refers to a specific target molecule on a cell that is recognized by one or more antibodies and defines a particular cell type or function. A list of CD molecules that are commonly mentioned is given in Table 4.7

Antigen recognition – the T-cell receptor complex

Antigen recognition by T cells is accomplished by a mechanism similar to that employed by immunoglobulin. Essentially, a limited set of gene segments can recombine to encode a highly diverse set of receptor specificities; however, unlike B cells, the receptor is not released. The T-cell receptor (TCR) is on the surface of all thymus-derived lymphocytes. It comprises two transmembrane glycoprotein chains, termed α and β ($\alpha\beta$ cells) (although analogous structures named γ and δ ($\gamma\delta$ cells) can be found on some immature T cells). The $\alpha\beta$ cells play a role in adaptive immune responses, whereas the $\gamma\delta$ cells are

Table 4.7 **Major CD antigens and their cellular distribution***

Cluster designation	Tissue distribution	Function
CD1	Cortical thymocytes	
CD2	All T cells and NK cells	Ligand for CD58; pair (e.g. between T cell and antigen-presenting cell)
CD3	Found on all mature T cells Intimately associated with the T cell receptor	Signal transduction following antigen presentation
CD4	T-helper/inducer lymphocytes comprise {2/3} circulating T cells	Interacts with class II MHC molecules associated with processed antigen fragments
CD5	T cells; also B cells	Ligand for CD72
CD8	Cytotoxic/suppressor T cells	Interacts with class I MHC molecules associated with processed antigen fragments
CD11a	Lymphocytes (especially memory T cells), granulocytes, monocytes and macrophages	Part of adhesion molecule LFA-1
CD14	Macrophages	Receptor for bacterial lipopolysaccharide
CD15 (also known as Lewis X)	Granulocytes	Ligand for selectins
CD16	Natural killer cells and macrophages	CD16 is a low-affinity Fc receptor involved in signal transduction
CD18	Leucocytes	Common β-chain of LFA family (beta integrins)
CD19	All mature B cells	Signal transduction
CD20	All mature B cells	Involved in cell activation; may be a calcium channel
CD21	Mature B cells, follicular dendritic cells, pharyngeal and cervical epithelial cells	Complement C3d receptor
CD23	B cells, macrophages, eosinophils	Low-affinity receptor for IgE
CD25	T, B cells, macrophages	IL-2 receptor
CD28	Activated T cells and some B cells	Activation of naive T cells
CD34	Precursors of haemopoietic cells	Unknown
CD36	Monocytes, platelets	GPIIIb
CD40	B cells	B-cell activation, induced by T-cell interaction
CD44	Leucocytes, RBCs, endothelium	Cell adhesion and migration, removal of apoptotic neutrophils by macrophages
CD45	All cells of a haemopoietic origin; also called leucocyte common antigen	Two isoforms, RO and RA. RO is associated with memory. Functions by cell signalling through the T-cell receptor; RA identifies naive cell
CD56	NK cell marker	Mediates cell adhesion
CD62	Endothelial cells, leucocytes and platelets (E-, L-, P-selectin)	Adhesion
CD72	All mature B cells	Ligand for CD5; involved in signalling
CD80/86	Antigen-presenting cells	Costimulatory ligands for CD28
CD95 (Fas Ag, APO-1)	Multiple cells	Induction of programmed cell death
CD103	Intraepithelial lymphocytes	Binds to E-cadherin

*This list is far from exhaustive and has been confined to CD types most commonly encountered in a clinical immunology setting

involved in epithelial defence (see p. 302). As with antibody, the polypeptide chains have both a variable (V) and a constant region (C) of amino acid residues. In the β chain the variable region is encoded by V-, D- and J-like elements. The α chain is made up of V- and J-like elements (Fig. 4.6). The polypeptide chains of the receptor are linked by disulphide bridges. The molecule is arranged on the T-cell membrane as a complex with another structure known as CD3. This association is necessary for the antigen receptor to be expressed at the cell surface. The receptor also has a transmembrane tail. When an antigenic peptide is received by the receptor, either in association with MHC class 1 for cytotoxic T cell activation or MHC class II for T-helper cell activation, a signal, manifesting as a series of enzyme phosphorylation reactions, is transmitted to the nucleus and the cell then responds accordingly by becoming activated, releasing cytokines and/or proliferating.

Antigen presentation

The term antigen means any structure that can be recognized by the specific immune response and is not restricted to microbial pathogens and toxins but includes antigens from foreign tissues (i.e. following organ transplantation) and certain tumour-associated structures. The immune system has the ability to discriminate between 'self' and 'non-self' antigens. This process is facilitated by a recognition system called the *major histocompatibility complex* (MHC) which dictates the way antigen is processed and recognized as foreign. In man, the products of MHC are termed human leucocyte antigens (HLA).

HUMAN LEUCOCYTE ANTIGENS
(Fig. 4.8)

The HLA cluster of genes is located on the short arm of chromosome 6. The system comprises six genetic loci –

HLA-A, -B, -C, -D, -DR and -DQ. Each locus may be one of many polymorphic forms or alleles, which number over 40 in the case of HLA-B. The combination or segregation of the A, B, C, D, DR and DQ alleles in any one individual is called the haplotype. A list of the main HLA antigens is presented in Table 4.8. The HLA molecules are distributed throughout the body tissues and it is through differences in HLA that cells are classified as self or non-self. The possibility of two different individuals having the same combination of HLA molecules is very remote. Although it is this that enables the immune system to recognize foreign cells and molecules, it is also the aspect of the immune system that presents problems for organ transplantation. Unless the HLA types of the donor and the recipient are virtually identical, the organ graft will be recognized as non-self and rejected by the immune system of the host. Thus donors and recipients have to be tissue typed to find the best-matched organ or bone marrow. Some diseases show a close association with HLA type.

Genetic linkage
The genes at a given locus are inherited as co-dominants, so that each individual expresses both alleles, one from the mother and the other from the father. Because of the close linkage between the loci, all the genes in the MHC tend to be inherited together. 'Crossing over' can occur within the HLA region. However, certain alleles occur more frequently in the same haplotype than expected by chance and this is known as 'linkage disequilibrium'; for example, the haplotype A1 B8 occurs more frequently than would be expected from the individual gene frequencies of A1 or B8. There is a wide inter-racial variation in HLA antigens.

Products of the HLA genes
The HLA genes code for cell-surface glycoproteins that extend from the plasma membrane to the cytoplasm and are known as class I and class II molecules. These

Fig. 4.8 **The major histocompatibility complex**, showing the regions, genes and gene products on the short arm of chromosome 6. GLO, glyoxalase; TNF, tumour necrosis factor.

Table 4.8   HLA – associations with disease

A1, B8, DR3	Polymyositis and dermatomyositis
A3, B14	Hereditary haemochromatosis
A28	Schizophrenia
B5	Behçet's syndrome
	Polycystic kidney disease
	Ulcerative colitis
B8	Tuberculoid leprosy (Asians)
B8, DR3	Autoimmune hepatitis
	Dermatitis herpetiformis
	Graves' disease
	Idiopathic membranous glomerulonephritis
	Myasthenia gravis (without thymoma)
	Addison's disease
	Sjögren's syndrome
	Systemic lupus erythematosus
B8, DR3, DR7, DQ2	Coeliac disease
B18	Hodgkin's disease
B27	Acute anterior uveitis
	Ankylosing spondylitis
	Psoriatic arthropathy
	Reiter's syndrome
	Juvenile arthritis
B47	Congenital adrenal hyperplasia
C6, B13, 17	Psoriasis
DR7, DR2	Goodpasture's syndrome (anti-GBM)
	Multiple sclerosis
	Narcolepsy (100% association)
DR4	Rheumatoid arthritis
	Vitiligo
DR4, DR6	Pemphigus vulgaris
DR4, DR3 (B8, 15 [62] 18)	Diabetes mellitus (insulin-dependent)
DR5	Hashimoto's thyroiditis
	Systemic sclerosis
DR5, DQ3	Associated with spontaneous clearance of hepatitis C virus
DR7	Minimal change disease (nephrotic)
MHC class III	C4A associated with SLE

GBM, glomerular basement membrane

glycoproteins consist of two chains of unequal size (α and β chains). The chains form a groove in which an antigenic peptide sits ready for presentation to T cells.

Class I molecules

Class I (HLA-A, -B and -C) antigens are expressed on all cell types except erythrocytes and trophoblasts. Striated muscle cells and liver parenchymal cells are normally negative but become strongly positive in inflammatory reactions. Class I molecules interact with CD8 T cells during antigen presentation and therefore are involved in driving mainly cytotoxic reactions.

Class II molecules

Class II antigens (HLA-D and -DR, D-related) are constitutively expressed only on professional antigen-presenting cells (B cells, monocytes/macrophages, Langerhans' cells, dendritic cells) and activated T cells. Other cells do not normally express this antigen but may

be induced to do so in the presence of gamma-interferon at sites of inflammation and can then become antigen-presenting cells. Class II antigens link with CD4 molecules during antigen presentation and the reaction induced by cells bearing this molecule is therefore of the helper type.

Regulation of antigen-specific responses

Activation of antigen-specific cells is closely regulated. This is essential as the receptors on T cells are very sensitive and a cell can be activated by interaction with a very few molecules of the relevant antigen, leading to the potential for inappropriate and excessive responses. The antigen-presentation system ensures that only antigens that have invaded far enough to be within cells, or those which are recognized and engulfed by antigen-presenting cells, are presented to T lymphocytes.

Antigen presentation to T cells (Fig. 4.9)

For T-cell activation to occur, several interactions between the antigen and the T-cell receptor have to take place. Firstly, the antigen must be presented to the T cell as a peptide fragment within the groove of the MHC molecules on the antigen-presenting cell. This is necessary as the TCR only recognizes the combined shape of the foreign antigen together with self-MHC. Free antigen will have no effect. The combination of T-cell receptor, MHC molecule and antigen fragment is known as the *trimolecular complex*. The antigen gains access to the MHC molecule during intracellular processing in which the peptide enters the MHC cleft during the assembly of this molecule. The whole molecule is then expressed on the surface of the cell. CD8$^+$ cells recognize antigen with class I MHC. As this molecule is present on nearly all nucleated cells, most cells can present to cytotoxic cells. Antigen expressed with class I is endogenous, i.e. the molecules are produced from within the cell, such as viral proteins and tumour antigens. CD4 cells are more limited as they can only be stimulated by cells that bear MHC class II. Such cells are mainly cells of the immune system that have the specific function of antigen presentation, sometimes termed *accessory cells*. These cells take up exogenous antigen by endocytosis and degrade it intracellularly. The processed antigen is then re-expressed on the cell surface with class II.

As there are differences in the three-dimensional shape of the MHC molecules owing to genetic variation, some antigens may be more effective than others in inducing immune responses, because they present an optimum shape or conformation to the T cells. Immune responses that only occur with certain antigen–MHC combinations are called MHC restricted. The host MHC reacts with either CD4 (MHC class II) (Fig. 4.10) or CD8 accessory molecules (MHC class I) on the T cell. These interactions stabilize the TCR/MHC/antigen reaction and act as costimulatory molecules to further activate the T cell through intracellular signalling cascades.

The interaction of another molecule, B7 on antigen-presenting cells with its ligand CD28 on T cells is also a

Fig. 4.9 **Antigen presentation**. Antigen processing is different for endogenous antigens compared to exogenous antigens which have to be taken up by antigen-presenting cells prior to processing. **Endogenous antigen** peptide fragments are transported into the endoplasmic reticulum, where they are picked up in the peptide-binding groove of MHC class I molecules. The antigen-bearing MHC molecules are then expressed on the surface of the cell. All nucleated cells produce class I molecules. **Exogenous antigen** is internalized by specialized antigen-presenting cells. Acidification occurs within the endosome, causing breakdown of the protein to peptide fragments. MHC class II molecules made within the endoplasmic reticulum are transported to the endosome via the Golgi apparatus. The peptides bind to the class II molecules, which are then expressed on the cell surface. The restriction of MHC class II molecule expression to antigen-presenting cells means that only a few cells can perform this process.

ER, endoplasmic reticulum. Modified from a figure in *Immunology Today* **14**, Raychaudhuri S, Morrow WJW pp. 344–348. © 1993, with permission from Elsevier.

Fig. 4.10 **Activation of T cells**. This figure shows the complex interaction of the antigen-presenting cell with the CD4[+] T lymphoctye. Cross-linking of the T-cell receptor (TCR) causes aggregation with the CD3 complex containing ε, δ and γ chains together with the three dimers. This leads to activation of phosphorylation and differentiation. If the costimulatory molecules are not activated at the same time, a different sequence of signals is activated, leading to cell death and apoptosis.

Lck, lymphocyte cytoplasmic kinase; ZAP, zeta-associated protein; DAG, diacyl glycerol; Ras, rous adenosarcoma; Sos, son of sevenless; Raf, raf-associated factor; Mek, mitogenic extracellular kinase; MAPK, mitogenic-associated proliferation kinase; PKC, protein kinase C; PLC, phospholipase C. From *Lancet* (2001) **357**: 1786. Courtesy of Dr Keith Nye.

major costimulating interaction. Cytokines produced during the reaction by the antigen-presenting cell (interleukins-1 and -12) and the early activation steps of the T cells (interleukin-2) enhance the reaction by decreasing the threshold for T-cell activation.

Antigen-presenting cells

The main antigen-presenting cells are macrophages (which are widely distributed throughout the tissues), Langerhans' cells (found in skin) and dendritic or veiled cells (found in the mucosa, lymph and blood). These cells (p. 200) are of the same lineage. Follicular dendritic cells are of a different lineage and are located in the germinal centres of lymph nodes (follicles). They are surrounded by B lymphocytes to which they present antigen, usually complexed with antibody, on the surface of their dendrites. Their surfaces are rich in Fc and C3b receptors to facilitate antigen trapping. B cells are also class II positive and trap antigen in immune complexes through their Fc receptors. They are able to present to T cells.

Antibody-dependent cytotoxic cells (ADCC)

These are populations of lymphocytes that are not characterized by their surface molecules, but by function. ADCC are NK cells that bear Fc receptors on their surface, and recognize target cells coated with immunoglobulin. They may have a role in eradicating virus-infected and tumour cells.

Lymphokine-activated killer (LAK) cells

Incubation of lymphocytes with interleukin-2 (IL-2) causes them to become highly cytotoxic (hence 'lymphokine activated') particularly to tumour cells. These artificially stimulated cells have been used in the treatment of malignancies, where patients' blood lymphocytes have been harvested, cultured with IL-2 and then re-infused to target tumours.

THE IMMUNE SYSTEM IN CONCERT

The immune system is not fixed, but dynamic. Cells traffic to different sites within the body via blood and lymphatic vessels, using adhesion molecules and chemokines/chemoattractants. Following an antigenic stimulus, the components of the immune system cooperate to meet and eliminate the challenge. The cells return to lymphoid tissue, bringing antigen to these specialized processing and presenting sites. Activated lymphocytes proliferate and leave the lymphoid tissue as armed effector cells to return to the site of infection. The immune system communicates intimately with, and is regulated by the neuroendocrine axis. Corticosteroids inhibit T-cell responses by reducing IL-2 and other pro-inflammatory cytokine production. Reduction in adhesion molecule expression by steroids also affects neutrophil function. Neuropeptides such as prolactin, which antagonizes corticosteroids and activates T cells, B cells

and macrophages, are produced by both the pituitary and peripheral blood mononuclear cells. Another cytokine, macrophage inhibitory factor (MIF), which was thought to be exclusively a product of the immune system, has also been found to be produced by the pituitary. Substance P, produced by sensory nerves on stimulation, binds to receptors on endothelial cells and lymphocytes and induces an inflammatory reaction.

Therefore, infection, tumour, autoimmune disease, pain or other stress, may induce immune reaction and a change in hypothalamic–pituitary–adrenal hormone production which prepares the body to repair tissues and regulates the inflammatory response.

IMMUNODEFICIENCY – CONGENITAL AND ACQUIRED

General principles

While many specific congenital immunodeficiencies are relatively rare, HIV infection and the widespread use of corticosteroid and immunosuppressive therapies mean that immunosuppression is a major aspect of clinical practice in many fields. Prompt recognition, appropriate management and referral of patients with suspected immunodeficiency are vital. Furthermore, the occurrence of infections in the context of specific immune defects can illuminate the physiological role of those parts of immune defence in the normal control of infection.

The main categories of immunodeficiency, by host mechanism, are:

- reduced neutrophil (and monocyte/macrophage) numbers and/or function
- deficiencies of individual complement components
- B cell defects, causing antibody deficiency
- T cell defects, impairing cell-mediated immunity
- combined T and B cell defects.

Congenital immunodeficiencies (Table 4.9)

These are usually due to specific genetic defects, leading to abnormalities in defined molecular and cellular mechanisms; most are rare. They usually present in childhood, but some types and the less severe forms may not become apparent until adult life. Abnormalities can be restricted to the immune system, but in others the immune defects are part of a wider range of congenital defects.

Acquired immunodeficiencies (Table 4.9)

These are much more common, but often less-precisely defined in terms of immunological mechanisms. They can result from malnutrition, splenectomy, some infections and autoimmune disorders, tumours of the immune system, immunosuppressive therapy or drug side-effects (Table 4.9). The most common infective cause is HIV infection,

Table 4.9 Congenital and acquired immunodeficiencies

Congenital	Acquired
Phagocytes	
Congenital neutropenia	Neutropenia due to
Cyclical neutropenia	myelosuppression
Leucocyte adhesion defects	Hypersplenism
Hyper-IgE syndrome	Autoimmune neutropenia
Shwachman's syndrome	Corticosteroid therapy
Chronic granulomatous	Diabetes mellitus
disease	Hypophosphataemia
Other intrinsic killing defects	Myeloid leukaemias
Storage diseases	Influenza
Chediak–Higashi syndrome	
Complement deficiency	
C3, C1q, I, H deficiencies	
C5, 6, 7, 8, 9, deficiencies	
Mannan-binding lectin deficiency	
Complement-dependent opsonization defects	
Antibody deficiency (B-cell defects)	
X-linked	Myeloma, lymphoma
hypogammaglobulinaemia	Splenectomy
Common variable	Congenital rubella
immunodeficiency	
IgA (± IgG$_2$) deficiency	
Specific antibody	
deficiencies	
T-cell deficiencies	
DiGeorge anomaly	
IL-2 deficiency	Measles
Signal transduction defect	Corticosteroid therapy
	Calcineurin inhibitors
	(e.g. ciclosporin, tacrolimus)
Combined T and B cell immunodeficiencies	
Severe combined immunodeficiency:	
X-linked severe combined	Protein–calorie malnutrition
immunodeficiency	Immunodeficiency of
syndrome	prematurity
Adenosine deaminase	AIDS
deficiency	
Purine nucleoside	
phosphorylase deficiency	
Non-expression of	
MHC class II	
Reticular dysgenesis	
Wiskott–Aldrich syndrome	
Ataxia telangiectasia	
EBV-associated immunodeficiency	
Hyper-IgM syndrome	

which leads to the acquired immunodeficiency syndrome (AIDS); this is covered in some detail (see p. 129).

Opportunist infections

Infection is the result of microbial virulence on the one hand and weakness of host defence on the other. Pathogenic organisms have mechanisms of evading normal defence mechanisms. Organisms of low virulence can only cause disease if the host defence mechanisms

that normally control them are defective. Organisms taking advantage of the opportunity of impaired host defence mechanisms are called *opportunists*. Different host defence defects cause increased susceptibility to different groups of organisms. Therefore, recognizing a pattern of infections can provide the best clinical clue to the type of underlying defence defect.

Patterns of opportunist infection

Examples of opportunist organisms in the setting of non-immunological innate defence defects include: staphylococci and *Pseudomonas* in burns patients; *Haemophilus influenzae* and pneumococci in smokers; *Pseudomonas* in cystic fibrosis patients; Gram-negative infections where there is urinary obstruction; staphylococcal and candidal infections with indwelling venous catheters and other foreign bodies; *Candida* and pathogenic *Escherichia coli* following elimination of gut flora after antibiotic therapy.

Table 4.10 shows the main infecting organisms for the principal classes of immunodeficiency. In broad terms, the following principles apply:

- *Neutrophil defects*. Extracellular infections mainly consist of bacterial diseases (e.g. staphylococci, Gram-negative organisms) and systemic fungal infections. These organisms are able to survive and replicate in the extracellular environment. The main defence against such infections is through neutrophil phagocytosis and intracellular killing, which is enhanced

Table 4.10 Immune defects and some opportunist organisms

Neutropenia and defective neutrophil function	Lytic complement pathway defects (C5–9)
Staphylococcus aureus	Meningococcus
Staphylococcus epidermidis	Gonococcus (disseminated)
Escherichia coli	
Klebsiella pneumoniae	**Cell-mediated**
Proteus mirabilis	**immunodeficiency**
Pseudomonas aeruginosa	*Listeria monocytogenes*
Serratia marcescens	*Legionella pneumophila*
Bacteroides spp.	*Salmonella* spp. (non-typhi)
Aspergillus fumigatus	*Nocardia asteroides*
Candida spp. (systemic)	*Mycobacterium tuberculosis*
Mucor spp.	Atypical mycobacteria,
	especially *M. avium-*
Opsonin defects	*intracellulare*
(antibody/complement	*Candida* spp.
deficiency, splenectomy)	(mucocutaneous)
Pneumococcus	*Cryptococcus neoformans*
Haemophilus influenzae	*Histoplasma capsulatum*
Meningococcus	*Pneumocystis carinii*
Streptococcus spp.	*Toxoplasma gondii*
(capsulated)	Herpes simplex
	Herpes zoster
Antibody deficiency only	Cytomegalovirus
Campylobacter spp.	Epstein–Barr virus
Mycoplasma spp.	Measles virus
Ureaplasma spp.	Papovaviruses
Echovirus	

Fig. 4.11 Control of infection. (a) Control of extracellular infection. Neutrophils phagocytose and kill antibody- and complement (C′)-coated antigens, e.g. bacteria. **(b) Control of intracellular infection by two immune mechanisms.** Intracellular viral proteins are complexed with MHC class I molecules and expressed on the surface of the virally infected cell. Antigen-specific CD8+ cytotoxic T cells (Tc) lyse the infected cells. Infected macrophages activate specific CD4+ helper T cells (Th) that produce gamma-interferon (IFN) which activates macrophages to kill the intracellular infection.

100-fold by coating (opsonization) of organisms by complement and antibody to specific receptors on the neutrophil surface (Fig. 4.11a). Failure of neutrophils to eradicate these extracellular organisms leads to infection.

- *Opsonic defects* due to antibody deficiencies or defects of the main complement pathways, and splenectomy lead to infection with capsulated organisms. These cannot be eliminated by neutrophils alone, as the capsule prevents phagocytosis unless opsonized by either antibody or complement.
- *Defects of the lytic pathway of complement* cause susceptibility to disseminated infections with Gram-negative cocci (mainly *Neisseria*, meningococcal meningitis).
- *Cell-mediated immune defects.* Neutrophils, antibody and complement react with the surface of the organism and therefore cannot detect intracellular infections. These are mainly due to viruses which require the intracellular environment for their replication, as well as fungi and protozoa which often parasitize macrophages. Some bacteria, especially mycobacteria, are facultative intracellular parasites that can also live within macrophages. The immune system has two mechanisms to eradicate such pathogens (Fig. 4.11b). Virally infected cells produce endogenous viral proteins that are complexed with MHC class I molecules and expressed on the cell surface. These are recognized by antigen-specific CD8+ cytotoxic T cells, which lyse the infected cell. Organisms within macrophages are killed through a different mechanism. This involves activation of specific CD4+ helper T cells that produce gamma-interferon locally. This activates the macrophages to kill the intracellular infections. The different mechanisms of control explain why patients with neutrophil, complement or antibody deficiency tend to have bacterial infections, whereas those with T-cell defects have viral, fungal and protozoal disease.

PHAGOCYTE DEFECTS

Neutropenia

Congenital neutropenias are rare and, if severe, are often fatal at an early age. Most, however, are relatively mild and benign and may even be incidental findings. They generally reflect defects of maturation and release of neutrophils from bone marrow. A particular and typically benign variant is *cyclical neutropenia*, with cycles of 3–5 weeks.

Acquired neutropenias are due to myelosuppression by disease, such as the leukaemias, or due to drug therapy. Myelosuppressive drugs used in the treatment of tumours, for prevention or treatment of transplant rejection, and in severe autoimmune disease are common causes. A number of other drugs, such as some antiviral drugs (e.g. zidovudine, ganciclovir) are myelosuppressive and can cause neutropenia; agranulocytosis can also be an idiosyncratic side-effect (e.g. chloramphenicol). Neutropenia due to an increased rate of destruction of neutrophils is seen in hypersplenism and in autoimmune neutropenia.

The risk of infection rises steeply once the neutrophil count falls below $0.5 \times 10^9/L$, regardless of cause. The risk is less if the monocyte count is preserved, as these cells can serve as a back-up phagocyte population. (In cyclical neutropenia, monocytes usually have cycles of opposite phase, which is probably why serious infections are uncommon.) Infections are typically disseminated, with septicaemia, fungaemia and deep abscess formation. Colonization of the gut with pathogens can readily lead to septicaemia. Local infections often affect the mouth, perianal area and sites of skin damage, including indwelling vascular catheters, and these can readily lead to systemic infection. Pus, which largely comprises neutrophils, may be scanty and may appear serous.

If myelosuppressive agents are being used, the dose should be reduced, or the drug stopped. The duration of neutropenia can be reduced by the use of G-CSF or GM-CSF, which appear to reduce infective episodes. Antibiotic or antifungal prophylaxis may be valuable. Otherwise, prompt antimicrobial therapy for febrile episodes during neutropenia is essential, using agents with broad cover for the common organisms encountered (see p. 30).

Defects of neutrophil function

Defects of neutrophil function (some of which also affect monocyte/macrophage function) interfere with migration into the tissues through vascular endothelium, locomotion in tissues, phagocytosis or intracellular killing.

Clinical features

Mucocutaneous sepsis in the mouth and perianal areas is common and local infections often lead to chronic abscess formation in the tissues or draining lymph nodes. Granulomas may be seen, because of failure of neutrophils to degrade microbes effectively. Systemic spread is less common than with neutropenia. Congenital causes may first present with infection or delayed separation of the umbilical stump.

Congenital

Leucocyte adhesion defect

This is an autosomal recessive disorder caused by abnormal synthesis of the β-chain CD18 that is shared by the CD11a, b and c molecules to form leucocyte function antigen (LFA) LFA-1, the C3bi (inactivated C3b) receptor and the C3dg receptor (p150/95). There is impaired leucocyte tissue localization, locomotion and endocytosis. Bone marrow transplantation has been successful in a few cases.

Hyper-IgE syndrome

The syndrome is characterized by very high levels of IgE (much of it anti-staphylococcal), impaired neutrophil locomotion and severe eczema, with frequent staphylococcal secondary infections and abscesses. Other immune defects may be seen, causing a wider spectrum of pyogenic and fungal infections.

Shwachman's syndrome

This may resemble cystic fibrosis clinically, with exocrine pancreatic insufficiency and pyogenic infections, in which mild neutropenia is associated with a defect of neutrophil migration.

Chronic granulomatous disease (CGD)

This is the prototype congenital defect of neutrophil (and monocyte) killing.

Pathogenesis

In this disorder, the oxidative pathway of microbial killing is severely impaired, either owing to a defective cytochrome b558 (X-linked CGD) or components of the associated NADPH oxidase (autosomal recessive CGD). Production of superoxide is abnormal, this being the first of a cascade of microbicidal oxygen radicals, including hydrogen peroxide, hypohalites, hydroxyl radicals and singlet oxygen. Impaired production of oxygen radicals can also affect the efficiency of non-oxidative killing.

Clinical features

Patients have chronic suppurative granulomas or abscesses affecting skin, lymph nodes and sometimes lung and liver, as well as osteomyelitis. They may present during early or late childhood years, depending on the severity of the defect. Most of the typical infections associated with neutrophil defects can be seen, particularly those that produce catalase, which inactivates any endogenous microbial peroxide that can kill organisms inside the phagocytic vacuole. Because macrophages are also affected, cell-mediated opportunist infections may also be seen, such as atypical mycobacteria, *Nocardia* and salmonellae.

Diagnosis

Diagnosis is made with the nitroblue tetrazolium (NBT) test, which uses a coloured dye reaction to assay the oxidative pathway; it can also be used to screen carriers.

Treatment

Infections respond to appropriate antimicrobial therapy and surgical measures as needed; in some patients prophylaxis may be merited. Regular gamma-interferon can reduce the frequency of infections, probably through enhanced monocyte/macrophage killing.

Chédiak–Higashi syndrome

This autosomal recessive disorder is characterized by giant granules in myeloid cells and large granular lymphocytes. Abnormal microbial killing, and hence recurrent infections, are due to defective phagolysosome fusion; NK cell activity is similarly impaired. Similar fusion abnormalities in melanocytes cause partial oculocutaneous albinism.

A wide variety of other rare disorders can impair microbial killing, including other inborn errors in microbicidal mechanisms, such as leucocyte G6PD deficiency (much less common than that affecting red cells) and myeloperoxidase deficiency. Storage diseases, such as Gaucher's and glycogen storage diseases, can impair phagocyte function.

Acquired

The commonest of these is corticosteroid therapy, which also affects T cell–macrophage cooperation, causing cell-mediated immunodeficiency. The main effect of corticosteroids on neutrophils is to impair leucocyte–endothelial adhesion. This reduces the marginated pool of leucocytes and impairs their attachment to endothelium at the site of tissue injury or infection. Corticosteroids thus prevent neutrophils reaching the tissues. The corollary of reduced margination is a rise in the neutrophil count; this can be deceptive if its significance is not appreciated.

The effect of corticosteroid therapy on neutrophil function is reflected by increased focal and systemic infections with staphylococci and Gram-negative bacteria. The effect is usually apparent above doses of 15 or 20 mg prednisolone daily or equivalent, and can be substantially reduced (as can other side-effects) by alternate-day therapy.

An infective cause of acquired neutrophil dysfunction is influenza, which causes a specific transient impairment of phagosome–lysosome fusion. This is the main reason for the high risk of staphylococcal pneumonia in influenza epidemics.

Myeloid leukaemias can cause defective neutrophil function, as well as causing neutropenia. Neutrophil and macrophage function can also be impaired in abnormal metabolic states, such as uncontrolled diabetes mellitus and hypophosphataemia. The latter may be seen during intravenous feeding of critically ill patients. Inhibitors of endogenous chemotactic factors for neutrophils may be seen in Hodgkin's disease and alcoholic cirrhosis, and may be responsible for their increased pyogenic infections.

COMPLEMENT DEFICIENCIES

There are two major patterns of infection associated with complement deficiencies:

- *Deficiencies of C3, C1q or of factors H or I* cause increased susceptibility to capsulated bacteria. These patients may also develop immune complex disorders and SLE-like disorders, as do patients with deficiencies of other classical pathway components of complement.
- *Deficiencies of the lytic complement pathway, C5–9*, cause susceptibility to disseminated neisserial infections, meningococcaemia and gonococcaemia; the latter has also been seen in association with disorders of complement function.

These complement deficiencies are rare, but functional defects of complement deposition on microbial surfaces are common. These are responsible for increased infections with *Haemophilus* and pneumococcal infections, especially in the early childhood years before a sufficiently wide specific antibody repertoire is acquired.

A common and well-defined opsonization defect is caused by *mannan-binding lectin* (*MBL*) deficiency. MBL is a member of the *collectin* family, which is in the serum in the form of multimers of the basic 32 kDa peptide. It activates the classical complement C1 complex in the absence of other activating factors. Mutations in codons 52, 54 or 57 prevent the formation of the multimers, leading to intracellular degradation or defective function. The defect is present in up to 5% of Caucasian populations, but appears to be associated with recurrent viral and pyogenic infections in children.

The C3 depletion caused by C3nef, an autoantibody that stabilizes the alternative pathway convertase and is seen in association with partial lipodystrophy, may also increase the risk of pyogenic infection.

C1 esterase inhibitor deficiency (see p. 1335) is not associated with infection but with hereditary angio-oedema, with episodes of localized oedema in skin of limbs or face, and the mucosa of the larynx or gut; the latter can cause life-threatening respiratory obstruction or severe episodes of abdominal pain.

ANTIBODY DEFICIENCIES

Congenital

X-linked hypogammaglobulinaemia

There is a profound reduction in all immunoglobulin classes; B cells and plasma cells are reduced. The defect is in the differentiation of pre-B cells into B cells; T cells are normal. The specific gene defect has now been shown to be in the *btk* gene for a tyrosine kinase signal transducing molecule involved in the maturation of B cells; the gene is at a position Xq 21.2-22 on the long arm of the X chromosome. It typically presents with infections, e.g. meningitis, mycoplasmal infections, after the first 3–6 months of life, when the protection from passively transferred maternal antibody has largely been lost. Immunoglobulin replacement therapy is very successful

and is now generally given intravenously. Many patients treat themselves at home.

Common variable immunodeficiency (CVI)

This is a late-onset antibody deficiency, which may present in childhood or adult life. IgG levels are especially low. B-cell numbers are usually normal; the defect appears to result from failure of their further differentiation. Some tests of T-cell function may be abnormal but few clinical manifestations of T-cell immunodeficiency are documented. CVI is probably a heterogeneous group of disorders in its cellular and molecular origins, reflecting defective interactions between T and B cells, with arrested maturation of B cells.

The patients have similar infections to those with the X-linked variety. However, a particular feature is follicular hyperplasia of lymph nodes, which in the gut takes the form of nodular lymphoid hyperplasia, and there may be splenomegaly. CVI patients may develop autoimmune disease and there is also an increased risk of lymphoreticular malignancy. The finding of reduced immunoglobulin levels and normal B-cell numbers indicates the diagnosis. Most of the manifestations are satisfactorily prevented by regular immunoglobulin replacement therapy.

IgA deficiency

This is an extremely common disorder (affecting 1 in 600 of the UK population) but is often symptomless. Only a small proportion have an increased risk of pyogenic infection and many of these have another defect, such as IgG_2 subclass deficiency. Some have allergic disorders or gluten hypersensitivity, and autoimmune disorders may also occur.

Other rare deficiencies

Isolated IgG_2 subclass deficiency. This is a rare cause of increased infection with capsulated organisms, for which it is the main immunoglobulin subclass; intravenous immunoglobulin replacement provides effective restoration.

Hypogammaglobulinaemia with raised IgM. There is a defect in isotype switching; the genetic basis has been shown to be due to the mutations in the gene for CD40 ligand, which is at Xq26 on the long arm of the X chromosome. Patients have recurrent bacterial infections and are susceptible to *Pneumocystis carinii* pneumonia.

Functional dysgammaglobulinaemia. Patients have increased bacterial infections with apparently normal levels of immunoglobulin but fail to produce specific antibodies to certain organisms.

Acquired

Hypogammaglobulinaemia is seen in the immune paresis of patients with myeloma and chronic lymphocytic leukaemia or lymphoma. Infection with capsulated bacteria may be seen, especially with myeloma. Splenectomy

these regimens, many patients show a marked improvement in CD4 cell numbers within a matter of 4–8 weeks, mainly due to redistribution of lymphocytes from the tissues and proliferation of pre-existing memory T-cells. Functional improvement with regeneration of T cells showing the naive phenotype, and antigen-specific responses (immune reconstitution) takes about 6 months to be established and continues to improve slowly thereafter. Immune reconstitution disorders due to intensive lymphocyte reactions may occur. For the presentation and management of HIV infection and AIDS, see p. 132.

Measles

Measles can cause a transient T-cell immunodeficiency, but it is rarely long-lasting enough for severe clinical problems to ensue.

Immunosuppressive therapy

Immunosuppressive therapy with cytotoxic agents such as cyclophosphamide and azathioprine tends to cause predominant T-cell immunosuppression. Ciclosporin and tacrolimus are potent immunosuppressive agents, which interfere with T-cell activation mechanisms at an intracellular level. Surprisingly, they are associated with only modest increases in infection, unless combined with corticosteroids or other agents. In such combinations, increased risk of Epstein–Barr virus (EBV)-associated lymphoma has been reported. Antilymphocyte immunoglobulin or monoclonal anti-CD3 antibody therapy also suppresses T-cell responses transiently. TNF-α inhibitors have good activity in controlling inflammatory conditions such as rheumatoid arthritis, inflammatory bowel disease and vasculitides. However, their use is associated with increased mycobacterial and other infections.

Corticosteroid therapy

This interferes with cell-mediated immunity, in particular T cell–macrophage cooperation. This is due to effects on T-cell traffic and impairment of macrophage responses to cytokines, together with impaired antigen presentation. Mucocutaneous candidiasis, *Pneumocystis carinii* pneumonia, cytomegalovirus infection, mycobacterial infection, *Nocardia*, non-typhi *Salmonella* septicaemia and cryptococcosis are some of the very many infections seen with prolonged high-dose steroid therapy.

COMBINED T AND B IMMUNODEFICIENCIES

The most severe immunodeficiencies are those that affect both B- and T-cell responses. These can stem from a variety of defective mechanisms in lymphocyte function, but tend to have rather similar clinical features, combining the opportunist infections of cell-mediated immunodeficiency with those of antibody deficiency.

Congenital

Severe combined immunodeficiency (SCID)

This typically presents in the first weeks of life. Failure to thrive, absent lymphoid tissue, lymphopenia and hypo-gammaglobulinaemia with multiple severe infections are characteristic.

There are primary X-linked and autosomal recessive variants of SCID. The X-linked defect has been mapped to Xq13 which leads to mutations in the gamma chain common to the IL-2, IL-4, IL-7, IL-11 and IL-15 receptors, leading to failure to respond to these growth factors in T and B cells. There is complete absence of CD3 and NK cells. Other causes include adenosine deaminase (ADA) deficiency, in which a defective purine salvage enzyme that is expressed in all cells, has a particular effect on lymphocytes because of the accumulation of substrates and metabolites that interfere with lymphocyte function. An analogous disorder is seen in purine nucleoside phosphorylase deficiency. Non-expression of MHC class II, owing to a variety of defects in class II transactivating proteins, and reticular dysgenesis cause similar syndromes. Milder expressions of these defects exist, some presenting in later life, and are sometimes termed *benign combined immunodeficiency* or *Nezelof's syndrome*.

Even with supportive and antimicrobial therapy, most of these conditions have a very poor prognosis without reconstitutive therapy. Immunoglobulin therapy is effective for the antibody deficiency, but the cell-mediated opportunists are the main determinant of outcome. Bone marrow transplantation is the definitive approach and has had significant success, especially if undertaken before extensive infection has set in. Recent approaches have included attempts to restore the defective enzymes in ADA deficiency, and gene therapy has had some success.

Hyper-IgM syndrome

This is usually an X-linked, but occasionally autosomal recessive, condition associated with mutation in the CD40L (ligand) gene. There is failure to switch from IgM to the other classes of antibody, leading to normal or high levels of IgM, and very low IgG and IgA. There is also a marked defect in T-cell function. Opportunistic infection (mainly due to this defect) occur with *Pneumocystis carinii*, *Cryptosporidium* (including sclerosing cholangitis), herpes virus infection and candidiasis or cryptococcosis.

Wiskott–Aldrich syndrome

This is an X-linked defect (at Xp11-23) with associated eczema and thrombocytopenia; a mainly cell-mediated defect with falling immunoglobulins is seen, and auto-immune manifestations and lymphoreticular malignancy may develop.

Ataxia telangiectasia

These patients have defective DNA repair mechanisms and have cell-mediated defects with low IgA and IgG$_2$; lymphoid malignancy is again common.

EBV-associated immunodeficiency (Duncan's syndrome)

Apparently normal, but genetically predisposed (usually X-linked) individuals develop overwhelming EBV infection, polyclonal EBV-driven lymphoproliferation, combined immunodeficiency, aplastic anaemia and lymphoid malignancy. EBV appears to act as a trigger for the expression of a hitherto silent immunodeficiency.

Acquired

Protein–calorie malnutrition

This is a very common cause of acquired combined immunodeficiency, with predominantly cell-mediated defects. Mechanisms are not fully established. Measles is a major cause of morbidity and mortality among children. *Pneumocystis carinii* is also a major pathogen, causing pneumonia, and this was first recognized in the Warsaw ghetto.

The immunodeficiency of prematurity

An immune response is not essential for normal fetal development and growth, but is necessary for survival after birth. Premature infants of 26 weeks' gestation and under are now surviving and have several immunological deficiencies and problems:

- *Antibody deficiency.* IgM synthesis does not occur before 30 weeks' gestation and IgG production occurs several weeks after birth. Active placental transfer of maternal antibody does not occur until the third trimester and therefore babies born before 28 weeks have hypogammaglobulinaemia, with antibody levels continuing to drop further after birth owing to loss of maternal IgG.
- *Neutropenia and impaired chemotaxis.*
- *Disruption of host defence barriers:*
  - insertion of foreign bodies, such as indwelling catheters and ventilator tubes
  - antibiotic therapy, which reduces resistance.

HYPERSENSITIVITY DISEASES

Allergy or hypersensitivity was initially defined by Von Pirquet in 1906 as: 'Specifically changed reactivity of an host to an agent on a second or subsequent occasion'. This definition would apply to all specific immune responses, and allergy is now taken to mean a damaging reaction. Hypersensitivity reactions underlie a number of autoimmune and allergic conditions. The immunological classification of these reactions is shown in Table 4.12. This scheme devised by Gell and Coombs is useful to group conditions with a similar underlying pathogenesis.

ALLERGIC DISEASE (TYPE I REACTION OR IMMEDIATE HYPERSENSITIVITY REACTIONS)

The type I reaction is an allergic response produced within 5–10 minutes of exposure to a specific allergen. Type I reactivity is mediated by IgE, although later in the reaction other mechanisms of inflammation including infiltration with eosinophils and lymphocytes may contribute. Allergens (antigens that evoke allergic responses), e.g. house-dust mite, pollens, animal danders or moulds,

only elicit significant IgE reactions in genetically predisposed individuals, who are said to be *atopic*. Atopic diseases include, extrinsic asthma, some forms of eczema, allergic rhinitis/conjunctivitis, food allergies, anaphylaxis and angio-oedema. The diagnosis is made by a typical clinical history and examination in conjunction with either skin-prick testing (when a type I wheal and flare reaction is elicited by pricking the skin through a solution of the test antigens) or by measuring specific IgE in the serum.

Susceptibility to atopic disease

In all cases of true allergic disease the individual must have been previously sensitized to the allergen. There is an inherited component, because if one parent is atopic the child has a 25–40% chance of also being atopic; if both parents are affected the risk rises to 50–75%. This is compared to a background incidence in the developed world of approximately 30% (this figure is continually rising). There is also an association with HLA-A1, B8, Dw3 and HLA-A3, Dw2, although no specific 'allergy gene' has been identified. However, not all individuals who make IgE antibody to environmental allergens suffer with atopic disease; other factors play a part:

Age. Exposure in the first few years of life is more likely to induce atopic disease. In addition, childhood atopic disease tends to improve with age.

Intercurrent infections. Viral infections may induce atopic disease, potentially by damaging the respiratory mucosa and allowing greater allergen penetration and sensitization.

Non-specific irritants. Pollutants such as diesel emission particles (DEPs) and cigarette smoke increase bronchial reactivity and may also damage the mucosa.

Immunodeficiency. Patients with underlying immunodeficiency are more susceptible to atopic disease. This may be due to greater allergen exposure after damage to the respiratory or gut mucosa by infection or due to decreased T cell regulation of IgE production.

Mechanisms of allergic disease

High-affinity FcϵRI on mast cells tightly bind locally produced allergen-specific IgE. On subsequent allergen exposure, cross-linkage of the surface IgE molecules causes *degranulation* of the mast cell and release of preformed (granule-derived) and newly formed (membrane-derived) mediators. These initiate the allergic response through increasing vascular permeability (causing swelling of the tissue), inducing chemotaxis of neutrophils and eosinophils and later lymphocytes (inflammation) and increasing airways hyperactivity (bronchoconstriction) (Box 4.1).

Arachidonic acid metabolites

Arachidonic acid is generated in sensitized cells from membrane lipids following the binding of specific allergen.

Table 4.12   Hypersensitivity reactions

	I (immediate)	II (cytotoxic)	III (immune complex)	IV (delayed)	V (stimulating/ blocking)*
Antigens	Pollens, moulds, mites, drugs, food and parasites	Cell surface or tissue bound	Exogenous (viruses, bacteria, fungi, parasites) Autoantigens	Cell/tissue bound	Cell surface receptors
Mediators	IgE and mast cells	IgG, IgM and complement and lymphokines	IgG, IgM, IgA and complement	Td, Tc, activated macrophages	IgG
Diagnostic tests	Skin-prick tests: wheal and flare Specific IgE in serum	Coombs' test Indirect immunofluorescence (antibodies) Red cell agglutination Precipitating antibodies ELISA	Immune complexes	Skin test: erythema induration (e.g. tuberculin test)	Indirect immuno-fluorescence
Time taken for reaction to develop	5–10 min	6–36 hours	4–12 hours	48–72 hours	Variable
Immuno-pathology	Oedema, vasodilatation, mast cell degranulation, eosinophils	Antibody-mediated damage to target cells	Acute inflammatory reaction, neutrophils, vasculitis	Perivascular inflammation, mononuclear cells, fibrin Granulomas Caseation and necrosis in TB	Hypertrophy or normal
Diseases and conditions produced	Asthma (extrinsic) Urticaria/oedema Allergic rhinitis Anaphylaxis Food allergies	Autoimmune haemolytic anaemia Transfusion reactions Haemolytic disease of newborn Goodpasture's syndrome Addisonian pernicious anaemia Myasthenia gravis	Autoimmune (e.g. SLE, glomerulonephritis, rheumatoid arthritis) Low-grade persistent infections (e.g. viral hepatitis) Disease caused by environmental antigens (e.g. farmer's lung)	Pulmonary TB Contact dermatitis Graft-versus-host disease Insect bites Leprosy	Neonatal hyperthyroidism Graves' disease Myasthenia gravis
Treatment	Antigen avoidance Antihistamines Corticosteroids (usually topical) Leukotriene receptor antagonists Sodium cromoglicate Epinephrine (adrenaline) for life-threatening anaphylaxis	Exchange transfusion Plasmapheresis Immunosuppressives/ cytotoxics	Corticosteroids Immunosuppressives/ cytotoxics Plasmapheresis Anti TNF antibody Anti B cell antibody Anti CTLA-4 antibody	Immunosuppressives Corticosteroids Removal of antigen	Treatment of individual disease

*Type V hypersensitivity may also be classified with type II reactions
RAST, radioallergosorbent test; SLE, systemic lupus erythematosus; TB, tuberculosis; Tc, T cytotoxic; Td, T delayed hypersensitivity

Preformed mediators
- Histamine and serotonin:
  - Bronchoconstriction
  - Increased vascular permeability
- Neutrophil and eosinophil chemotactic factors (NCF and ECF):
  - Induce inflammatory cell infiltration.

Newly formed mediators (membrane-derived)
- Leukotriene (LT) B4:
  - Chemoattractant
- LTC4, -D4, -E4 (slow-reacting substance of anaphylaxis, SRS-A):
  - Sustained bronchoconstriction and oedema
- Prostaglandins and thromboxanes:
  - Platelet-activating factor (PAF)
  - Prolonged airway hyperactivity

It is subsequently metabolized to produce prostaglandins (cyclo-oxygenase pathway), leukotrienes (lipoxygenase pathway) or platelet-activating factor (PAF acetylation), depending on which cell type is being activated. Leukotrienes and prostaglandins are together termed eicosanoids. The arachidonic acid metabolites involved in type 1 hypersensitivity reactions are PAF, leukotrienes (LT) B_4, C_4, D_4 and E_4 and prostaglandins (PG) D_2, E_2 and F_2. They have four main actions:

- *Inflammatory cell mucosal infiltration.* This is mediated by LTB_4 and PAF, which attract and activate neutrophils, eosinophils and monocytes/macrophages. LTB_4 is released by activated mast cells and macrophages, and PAF is released by mast cells, neutrophils and eosinophils.
- *Bronchoconstriction.* This is mediated by several metabolites including PAF, LTC_4, LTD_4, LTE_4, PGD_2 and PGF_2. LTC_4 and PGD_2 are the major arachidonic acid metabolites released by mast cells. The remaining eicosanoids are generated by human lung tissue and/or alveolar macrophages.
- *Bronchial mucosal oedema* is mediated by LTC_4, LTD_4 and PGE_2. PGE_2 is released from alveolar macrophages and human lung tissue.
- *Mucus hypersecretion* is mediated by LTC_4 and LTD_4.

This reaction is termed the *early-phase response*. The *late-phase reaction* comes 4–6 hours later and is characterized by inflammatory cell infiltrates with neutrophils, eosinophils and lymphocytes. It is likely that this reaction is involved in asthma pathogenesis.

Regulation of IgE production

The regulation of IgE production appears to be controlled by functional subsets of helper T lymphocytes termed *Th1* and *Th2*, which develop after antigen stimulation from an undifferentiated population termed *Th0* (p. 208).

Th1 cells produce the cytokines gamma-interferon and interleukin-2 and suppress IgE production by B cells. Th2 cells produce mainly IL-4 and IL-5. IL-4 is the switch factor for B cells to produce IgE. IL-5 drives eosinophil production. Thus Th2 cells drive an atopic response and Th1 cells suppress it. There appears to be a dysregulation towards a Th2 response in atopic individuals.

Therapeutic interventions

Various therapeutic agents act at different stages of the pathways described above to control allergic disease. Sodium cromoglicate stabilizes mast cell membranes to reduce degranulation, antihistamine-receptor (H_1) blockers reduce the effect of histamine release, corticosteroids reduce production of mediators and the inflammatory response. Leukotriene receptor blockers are used in asthma. All these agents, in conjunction with β-adrenergic drugs, help to control allergic disease but do not alter the underlying sensitivity. *Hyposensitization* is a technique used to reduce IgE responses. This involves the injection of gradually increasing doses of the allergen, starting at very tiny amounts. This leads to a switch from an IgE to an IgG response. However, there is the risk of anaphylaxis and its use is largely confined to the treatment of life-threatening allergy (e.g. that to bee or wasp venom) and only at specialist centres with on-site resuscitation facilities. Experimental approaches using anti-IL-4 agents and anti-IgE antibodies are under investigation.

AUTOIMMUNITY (TYPE II HYPERSENSITIVITY)

An autoimmune disease occurs when the immune system fails to recognize the body's own tissues and attacks itself. Autoimmune disorders (Table 4.13) comprise some common diseases, such as rheumatoid arthritis, multiple sclerosis, insulin-dependent diabetes and thyroiditis. Illnesses are often divided into those that are organ specific and organ non-specific or multisystemic. The diseases are characterized by the presence of autoantibodies or autoreactive T cells. These autoreactive antibodies or cells may be directly pathogenic (for example the autoantibodies in autoimmune cytopenias and antiglomerular antibody in Goodpasture's disease). In other circumstances auto-antibodies may not directly cause damage (such as anti-nuclear antibodies in various connective tissue diseases) but are a marker of an autoimmune state.

Mechanism of development of autoimmune disease

In the healthy individual the immune system is made tolerant to self-antigens at an early stage of immune development (tolerance is a state in which the immune system fails to respond to a given antigen). On occasions when tolerance fails or is incomplete, autoimmunity can result.

Several factors influence the balance between the development of either tolerance or immunity. Continuous antigenic stimulation over several days, e.g. by self-antigens, usually transmits tolerogenic stimuli. A sudden increase in antigens, e.g. infection, usually transmits an

Table 4.13 Autoimmune diseases and their antigens

Disease	Antigens
Graves' disease	Thyroid-stimulating hormone receptor
Hashimoto's thyroiditis	Thyroid peroxidase, thyroglobulin
Pernicious anaemia	H/+K+-ATPase, intrinsic factor
Addison's disease	21-Hydroxylase
Diabetes mellitus type 1	GAD
Goodpasture's syndrome	Type IV collagen
Myasthenia gravis	Acetylcholine receptor
Pemphigus vulgaris	Desmoglein-3
Multiple sclerosis	Myelin basic protein Myelin oligodendritic glycoprotein
Primary biliary cirrhosis	PDC.E2
Coeliac disease	Tissue transglutaminase
Wegener's granulomatosis	ANCA+
Sjögren's syndrome	Ro/La ribonuclear particle
Rheumatoid arthritis	Citrullinated cyclic peptide IgM
Polymyositis/ dermatomyositis	tRNA synthases
Scleroderma	Topoisomerase
Systemic lupus erythematosus	Sm/RNP, Ro/La (SS-A/SS-B) histone and native DNA

ANCA, antinuclear cytoplasmic antibodies; GAD, glutamic acid decarboxylase; PDC.E2, pyruvate dehydrogenase complex, E2 component

immunologenic signal. Binding of antigens during immature lymphocyte formation in the bone marrow/thymus produces tolerance, whereas binding of mature lymphocytes produces immunity.

Tolerance

Positive and negative selection (central tolerance) (see Fig. 4.5)
There are several mechanisms of T-cell tolerance. One occurs in the thymus by means of a complicated, multistep selection mechanism. In the first stage of this process, immature T cells which do not bear either of the CD4 and CD8 molecules (double-negative cells) enter the subcapsular region of the thymus, divide and proliferate. T-cell receptors, CD4 and CD8 molecules, are then co-expressed simultaneously; these cells are termed 'double-positive'. Maturing cells migrate towards the cortex of the thymus where the selection process occurs. T cells that can engage with MHC class I or II molecules on the epithelium of the thymic cortex are said to be 'positively selected' and they undergo further processing. They will lose either the CD4 or CD8 co-receptor, depending on which particular MHC molecule they engage. Cells that do not interact with the MHC undergo programmed cell death (apoptosis). Thus after positive selection, only cells that can recognize MHC molecules (and thus antigenic peptides presented in association with these structures) remain.

However, another step is necessary to remove cells that can react with self-peptides, and this occurs through negative selection. This part of the selection process occurs in the corticomedullary junction, which is rich in dendritic cells and macrophages. If either CD4 or CD8 cells engage with cells bearing MHC class I or II molecules containing self-peptide (i.e. autoreactive T cells) they undergo apoptosis and are clonally deleted. The remaining cells pass through the thymus and become part of the mature T-cell pool. Negative selection is probably the most significant aspect of tolerance induction. The loss of thymocytes through the positive and negative selection process is high, with over 90% of cells undergoing apoptosis.

Peripheral tolerance
Self-reactive cells occasionally escape the elimination process in the thymus and become part of the circulating pool of T cells. While these lymphocytes may become auto-aggressive there are other forms of tolerance that occur outside the thymus. Although poorly understood, processes exist to eliminate (by specialized cytotoxic T cells) or inactivate (anergize) both self-reactive T and B lymphocytes. In the case of B cells, anti-idiotypic antibodies (which bind to the idiotype marker on the autoreactive B cell) may also play a part.

Mechanism of loss of tolerance

There are several mechanisms proposed to account for a change from tolerance to immunity.

Immune dysregulation
T cells regulate any autoreactive T and B cells that have survived clonal deletion. It is hypothesized that dysregulation of T-cell function could therefore lead to loss of control and the development of autoimmune disease. This is backed up by the observation that immunodeficiency diseases such as hypogammaglobulinaemia and HIV infection are commonly associated with autoimmune phenomena. However, most patients with autoimmune disease do not have obvious immune deficiency.

Tissue damage
There are some autoantigens to which the developing immune system is not usually exposed because these antigens are 'hidden' within the cells or tissues. Therefore clonal deletion of self-reactive cells does not occur. Normally these self-antigens remain hidden, so no autoimmune disease develops. If, however, the tissue is damaged by trauma, infection or tumour, the antigens may be released and evoke an autoimmune response. Examples of this in clinical practice are Dressler's syndrome in which patients with myocardial infarction develop acute pericarditis secondary to the production of antimyocardial antibodies, or the association of Coxsackie virus infection with the development of insulin-dependent diabetes. The presence of inflammatory cytokines at the site of injury may enhance the expression of costimulatory molecules on local antigen-presenting cells and increase the likelihood of an autoreactive T-cell response still

further. This hypothesis may be supported by the observation that patients given alpha-interferon (which upregulates class I expression) develop thyroid autoantibodies on therapy.

T-cell bypass

This is a mechanism by which T cells are tricked into providing help to autoreactive B cells rather than suppressing them. For this to occur the self-antigen needs to be attached to a foreign antigen that is recognized by the T cell. T-cell activation will occur with the production of cytokines such as IL-4. If an autoreactive B cell has also bound the self-antigen it will then receive the signals to proliferate and produce autoantibody. There are several examples of this in drug-induced autoimmune responses. Quinine binds to platelets, creating a foreign epitope for T cells and inducing autoreactive B cells to make antiplatelet antibodies with sometimes fatal thrombocytopenia developing. Methyldopa or infection with mycoplasma causes changes in red cell epitopes to induce a similar autoantibody response to red cells with haemagglutination or lysis.

Molecular mimicry

This occurs when an organism has a similar antigenic structure to self-molecules. The infection generates antigen-specific T cells and antibodies that cross-react with host tissues and cause autoimmune disease. Examples where there is known cross-reaction between an infective agent and host antigen include the production of anticardiac antibodies (antimyosin) after streptococcal infection leading to rheumatic fever, Klebsiella and HLA-B27 in ankylosing spondylitis, and Coxsackie and glutamic acid decarboxylase in insulin-dependent diabetes.

The development of autoimmune disease can be viewed as either a loss of tolerogenic signals to lymphocytes, or an increase in immunogenic signals. The underlying mechanism appears to be the activation of lymphocytes by different pathways.

HLA and autoimmunity

There is a strong association between certain HLA types and the development of (or sometimes protection from) autoimmune diseases (Table 4.8). These may represent linkage-disequilibrium with a true disease-susceptibility gene that has not yet been identified (this seems particularly likely in those conditions such as narcolepsy that are not immunologically mediated but where there is a strong HLA association). The other possibilities are that HLA types determine the degree of immune response to antigens (the polymorphisms of HLA will determine how well a particular antigen fits within the cleft for presentation) and therefore the ease of autoimmune reactions ('high-reactor' status).

Immunopathology of autoimmune disease
(Fig. 4.12)
Formation of autoantibodies may be a normal physio-

logical process and help to remove tissue debris. Many autoantibodies are detectable at low levels in normal individuals or may rise temporarily in inflammatory conditions without any evidence of pathogenicity. However, excessive and persistent production of such antibodies can be harmful. Antibodies may directly react with a specific tissue, resulting in inflammation and tissue damage by complement activation, neutrophil, mast cell, or antibody-dependent cellular cytotoxic attack (Fig. 4.12a). Autoantibodies in some situations do not damage the tissue but block or stimulate function, type V hypersensitivity which in turn leads to disease (Fig. 4.12b). The activation of autoantigen-specific T cells causes infiltration of the tissues with lymphocytes and damage.

A third type of hypersensitivity reaction is caused by immune complex formation. The immune complexes may either be formed from antibody binding pathogen or autoantigen.

IMMUNE COMPLEX DISEASE (TYPE III HYPERSENSITIVITY)

Immune complexes are often found in healthy individuals; for example after eating, circulating complexes with food antigens are normal. However, if the complexes are persistent, disease may develop. Immune complexes are normally removed from the circulation attached to receptors on red blood cells and removed by the liver or spleen. Complexes with antibody or antigen excess are either easily removed or remain soluble but those at around equivalence are more difficult to remove, yet precipitate easily.

Immune complexes can be formed in tissues causing a local (Arthus) reaction, or in the circulation, causing systemic disease. Examples of the former are extrinsic allergic alveolitis (e.g. farmer's lung) where repeated inhaled exposure to an antigen such as mouldy hay leads to the production of high levels of specific antibody in the lung. Further exposure causes local immune complex production and inflammatory responses leading to chronic progressive lung fibrosis. Examples of diseases where systemic immune complexes play a major role are listed in Table 4.13, and include the major vasculitides such as systemic lupus erythematosus and other connective tissue diseases, as well as accounting for the vasculitic component of rheumatoid arthritis and other conditions. Serum sickness used to be common in patients receiving horse antisera for the treatment of tetanus and diphtheria (before effective vaccination programmes) as they made anti-horse immunoglobulin antibodies which formed immune complexes with the antiserum. A similar reaction is once again being observed as an adverse effect of the newly developed mouse-derived monoclonal antibodies under investigation as immunosuppressants (owing to anti-mouse immunoglobulin antibodies) and in patients receiving streptokinase post-myocardial infarction (who may have unsuspected high circulating antistreptococcal antibody levels because of intercurrent streptococcal infections).

Fig. 4.12 **Mechanisms of autoimmunity (type II and V hypersensitivity).**
(a) Type II hypersensitivity occurs when a cell-bound autoantigen is recognized by the immune system. Damage occurs in several different ways. Antibody binding to the autoantigen leads to local complement activation and lysis of the cells. Complement activation products recruit neutrophils, which bind to the IgG and release their granules directly onto the surface of the cell. Lymphocytes binding antigen-specific Ig (killer cells) can bind to the autoantigens on cells and induce their killing by apoptosis.
(b) Type V hypersensitivity. Some autoantibodies do not cause tissue destruction, but affect cellular regulation. In myasthenia gravis an anti-acetylcholine-receptor antibody binds to the receptors at the neuromuscular junction and blocks any further activation. In Graves' disease the autoantibody, thyroid-stimulating immunoglobulin (TSI), binds to TSH receptors on thyrocytes and causes prolonged excess thyroid hormone secretion. Modified from an original figure courtesy of Bryony Cohen, Barts and The London NHS Trust.

Immunopathogenesis of immune complex disease (Fig. 4.13)

Immune complexes activate the classical pathway of complement, releasing C3a and C5a, which cause increased adhesion molecule expression on the vascular endothelial cells and on circulating neutrophils. This causes the circulating neutrophils to adhere to the vascular endothelial cells. The neutrophils bind the immune complexes via their Fc and C' receptors and are activated, leading to the release of toxic oxygen metabolites through the respiratory burst, which results in tissue damage. The inflammatory mediators cause separation of the vascular endothelial cells and immune complexes and neutrophils

Fig. 4.13 Mechanisms of immune complex (IC) disease (type III hypersensitivity). LFA, leucocyte function antigen; ICAM, intercellular adhesion molecule; FcR, receptor for Fc antibody; CR, complement receptor. Modified from an original figure courtesy of Bryony Cohen, Barts and The London NHS Trust.

pass into the tissues. Immune complexes also activate *platelets* with release of vasoactive amines and clumping, resulting in microthrombus formation and tissue infarction. Immune complexes tend to be deposited in the walls of vessels at sites of turbulence (such as bifurcations), at hydrostatic pressure gradients (such as in the glomerulus and synovium), or where the complex contains an antigen that binds to tissue (such as in the presence of DNA in immune complexes in SLE, which is attracted by charge differences to the glomerular basement membrane). Inflammation in larger vessels causes weakening of the blood vessel wall and microaneurysm formation (e.g. in polyarteritis nodosa, PAN). In smaller vessels the inflammation and thrombus formation leads to infarction and necrosis of tissue.

DELAYED TYPE (TYPE IV HYPERSENSITIVITY)

This is mediated by macrophages and T-cell responses to antigens, often after chronic stimulation. It is the cause of granulomatous reactions to foreign particles (e.g. silicosis in lungs) as well as some forms of allergic drug reaction and eczema. It is also the basis of the 'patch' test for contact sensitivity skin testing.

PRINCIPLES OF IMMUNOSUPPRESSIVE THERAPY

Treatment to suppress the inflammation caused by autoimmune reactions includes systemic steroids to suppress neutrophil-driven inflammation, and cytotoxics, such as methotrexate, azathioprine and cyclophosphamide, to suppress lymphocyte numbers and function, including antibody production. More intense lymphocyte suppression is provided by ciclosporin A, tacrolimus, mycophenolate and monoclonal antilymphocyte immunoglobulin and anti-TNF. Opportunist infection and tumours are major side-effects of these therapies. Where the antibody is known to be directly damaging (e.g. Goodpasture's syndrome), plasmapheresis can be used to reduce the levels rapidly.

Immunological interventions

A number of products of the immune response can now be produced for therapeutic use by purification from blood (immunoglobulins and C1 esterase inhibitor), cell culture (e.g. fibroblast interferons) and molecular techniques (recombinant interferons, interleukin-2, colony-stimulating factors).

Others such as monoclonal antibodies can be produced to inhibit or enhance immune responses. Some have proven to be very effective, such as the success of anti-TNF in rheumatoid arthritis, inflammatory bowel disease and psoriasis. However, there are also complications of modulating the immune response; for example, the increased rate of infection with anti-TNF therapy and the development of autoimmune conditions with inter-feron. Gene therapy has been used in the management of severe immunodeficiences (SCID) to replace the defective gene in lymphocytes in a few patients. Although significant immune reconstitution has been observed, there has also been development of T-cell leukaemia in relation to retroviral gene insertion.

Some are still in trials (Table 4.14).

Table 4.14   Immunological interventions

Intravenous immunoglobulin
Replacement (e.g. in hypogammaglobulinaemic states)
Fc-receptor blockade (e.g. in autoimmune cytopenias; idiopathic thrombocytopenic purpura)
Immunomodulation in autoimmune disease
Guillain–Barré syndrome
Chronic inflammatory demyelinating polyneuropathies
Lambert–Eaton myasthenic syndrome
Adult dermatomyositis

Cytokines
Interferons
Antiproliferative agents (e.g. in hairy cell leukaemia; Kaposi's sarcoma)
Antiviral and immunomodulatory agents (e.g. in chronic hepatitis B and C infection; multiple sclerosis)
Immunomodulation (e.g. gamma-interferon in chronic granulomatous disease)

Interleukins
Interleukin-2 to enhance CD4 reconstitution in HIV treatment

Colony-stimulating factors
e.g. Granulocyte and granulocyte–monocyte colony-stimulating factors (G-CSF and GM-CSF) in neutropenia

Monoclonal antibodies
Immunosuppressives (e.g. anti-T-cell antibody to prevent graft-versus-host disease
Anti-inflammatory agents (e.g. anti-TNF, anti-IL-1, anti-CD20 B cell in rheumatoid arthritis, inflammatory bowel disease, psoriasis and Behçet's disease

Gene therapy
Treatment of ADA deficiency by insertion of gene into bone marrow stem cell
X-linked SCID

Adoptive immunotherapy
Growth ex vivo of specific lymphocyte clones for subsequent reinjection to treat disease, e.g. management of CMV infection after bone marrow transplant

Immune modulation
Anti-IgE antibodies in suppressing IgE response in peanut-allergic individuals

---

CHAPTER BIBLIOGRAPHY

Kamradt T, Mitchison NA (2001) Advances in immunology: tolerance and autoimmunity. *New England Journal of Medicine* **344**: 655–664.

Kay AB (2001) Advances in immunology: allergy and allergic diseases (Parts I and II). *New England Journal of Medicine* **344**: 30–37, 109–113.

Lancet (2001) Immunology series. *Lancet* **357**: June.

Medzhitov R, Janeway C (2000) Advances in immunology: innate immunity. *New England Journal of Medicine* **343**: 338–344.

Scofield RM (2004) Autoantibodies as predictors of disease. *Lancet* **363**: 1544–1546.

von Andrian UH, Mackay CR (2000) Advances in immunology: T-cell function and migration – two sides of the same coin. *New England Journal of Medicine* **343**: 1020–1034.

Walport MJ (2001) Advances in immunology: complement (Parts I and II). *New England Journal of Medicine* **343**: 1058–1066, 1140–1144.

SIGNIFICANT WEBSITES

http://www-micro.msb.le.ac.uk/MCQs/MCQ.html
http://www-micro.msb.le.ac.uk/MBChB/ImmGloss.html
MCQs and immunology glossary (University of Leicester)

http://www.antibodyresource.com/
Source of antibody resources for educators and researchers

Nutrition

GENERAL ASPECTS

In developing countries, lack of food and poor usage of the available food can result in protein–energy malnutrition (PEM); 50 million pre-school African children have PEM. In developed countries, excess food is available and the most common nutritional problem is obesity.

Diet and disease are interrelated in many ways. Excess energy intake, particularly when high in animal (saturated) fat content, is thought to contribute to a number of diseases, including ischaemic heart disease and diabetes. A relationship between food intake and cancer has been found in many epidemiological studies; an excess of energy-rich foods (i.e. fat and sugar containing), often with physical inactivity, plays a role in the development of certain cancers, while diets high in vegetables and fruits reduce the risk of most epithelial cancers. Numerous carcinogens, either intentionally added to food (e.g. nitrates for preserving foods) or accidental contaminants (e.g. moulds producing aflatoxin and fungi), may also be involved in the development of cancer.

The proportion of processed foods eaten may affect the development of disease. A number of processed convenience foods have a high sugar and fat content and therefore predispose to dental caries and obesity respectively. They also have a low fibre content, and dietary fibre is possibly necessary in the prevention of a number of diseases (see p. 234). Some epidemiological data suggest that there are long-term effects of undernutrition; low growth rates in utero being associated with high death rates from cardiovascular disease in adult life.

In 1991 the Department of Health published the dietary reference values for food and energy and nutrients for the United Kingdom. Values were based on all of the available information including data from the 1985 Food and Agriculture Organization (FAO–WHO), United Nations University (UNU) expert committee, so that there is broad agreement on the reference values given. In the UK recommended daily amounts (RDAs) are no longer used, but have been replaced by the *reference nutrient intake* (RNI) to provide more help in interpreting dietary surveys.

The RNI is roughly equivalent to the previous RDA, and is sufficient or more than sufficient to meet the nutritional needs of 97.5% of healthy people in a population. Most people's daily requirements are less than this, and so an *estimated average requirement* (EAR) is also given, which will certainly be adequate for most. A lower reference nutrient intake (LRNI) which fails to meet the requirement of 97.5% of the population is also given. The RNI figures quoted in this chapter are for the age group 19–50 years. These represent values for healthy subjects and are not always appropriate for patients with disease.

> **FURTHER READING**
> Panel on Dietary Reference Values of the Committee on Medical Aspects of Food Policy (1991) *Dietary Reference for Food Energy and Nutrients for the United Kingdom* (Report 41DOH). London: HMSO.

WATER AND ELECTROLYTE BALANCE

Water and electrolyte balance is dealt with fully in Chapter 12. About 1 L of water is required in the daily diet to balance insensible losses, but much more is usually drunk, the kidneys being able to excrete large quantities. The daily RNI for sodium is 70 mmol (1.6 g) but daily sodium intake varies in the range 90–440 mmol (2–10 g). These are needlessly high intakes of sodium which are thought by some to play a role in causing hypertension (see p. 858).

DIETARY REQUIREMENTS

Energy

Food is necessary to provide the body with energy (Fig. 5.1). The SI unit of energy is the joule (J), and 1 kJ = 0.239 kcal. The conversion factor of 4.2 kJ, equivalent to 1 kcal, is used in clinical nutrition.

Energy balance

Energy balance is the difference between energy intake and energy expenditure. Weight gain or loss is a simple, but accurate, way of indicating differences in energy balance.

Energy requirements

There are two approaches to assessing energy requirements for subjects who are weight stable and close to energy balance:

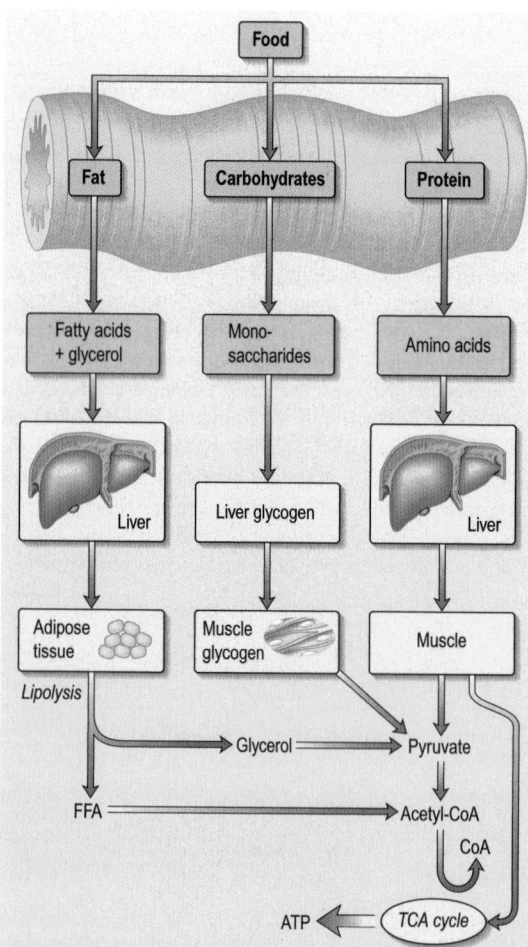

Fig. 5.1 The production of energy from the main constituents of food. Alcohol produces up to 5% of total calories, but the variation between individuals is wide. 1 mol of glucose produces 36 mol of ATP. FFA, free fatty acids; ATP, adenosine triphosphate.

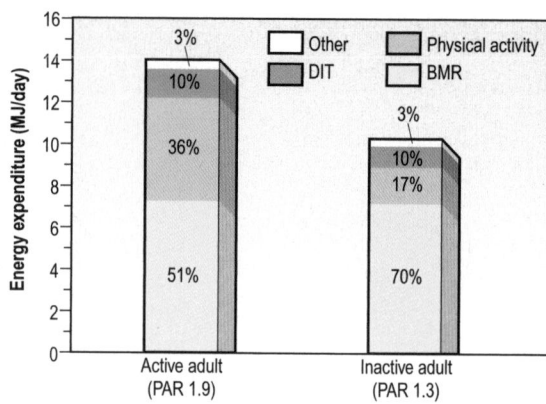

Fig. 5.2 Daily energy expenditure in an active and a sedentary 70 kg adult. BMR, basal metabolic rate; DIT, dietary induced thermogenesis; PAR, physical activity ratio.

- assessment of energy intake
- assessment of total energy expenditure.

Energy intake

This can be estimated from dietary surveys and in the past has been used to decide daily energy requirements. However, measurement of energy expenditure gives a more accurate assessment of requirements.

Energy expenditure

Daily energy expenditure (Fig. 5.2) is the sum of:

- the basal metabolic rate (BMR)
- the thermic effect of food eaten
- occupational activities
- non-occupational activities.

Total energy expenditure can be measured using a double-labelled water technique. Water containing the stable isotopes ^{2}H and ^{18}O is given orally. As energy is expended carbon dioxide and water are produced. The difference between the rates of loss of the two isotopes is used to calculate the carbon dioxide production, which is then used to calculate energy expenditure. This can be done on urine samples over a 2- to 3-week period with the subject ambulatory. The technique is accurate, but it is expensive and requires the availability of a mass spectrometer. An alternative tracer technique for measuring total energy expenditure is to estimate CO_2 production by isotopic dilution. A subcutaneous infusion of labelled bicarbonate is administered continuously by minipump, and urine is collected to measure isotopic dilution by urea, which is formed from CO_2. Other methods for estimating energy expenditure, such as heart rate monitors or activity monitors, are also available but are less accurate.

Basal metabolic rate. The BMR can be calculated by measuring oxygen consumption and CO_2 production, but it is more usually taken from standardized tables (Table 5.1) that require knowledge of the subject's age, weight and sex.

Table 5.1 Equations for the prediction of basal metabolic rate (in MJ per day)		
Age range (years)	Prediction equation (BMR =)	95% confidence limits
Men		
10–17	0.074 (wt)* + 2.754	± 0.88
18–29	0.063 (wt)* + 2.896	± 1.28
30–59	0.048 (wt)* + 3.653	± 1.40
60–74	0.0499 (wt)* + 2.930	N/A
75+	0.0350 (wt)* + 3.434	N/A
Women		
10–17	0.056 (wt)* + 2.898	± 0.94
18–29	0.062 (wt)* + 2.036	± 1.00
30–59	0.034 (wt)* + 3.538	± 0.94
60–74	0.0386 (wt)* + 2.875	N/A
75+	0.0410 (wt)* + 2.610	N/A

*Bodyweight (wt) in kilograms
Data reproduced with permission of Department of Health, 1991

Table 5.2 Physical activity ratio (PAR) for various activities (expressed as multiples of BMR)	
	PAR
Occupational activity	
Professional/Housewife	1.7
Domestic helper/Sales person	2.7
Labourer	3.0
Non-occupational activity	
Reading/Eating	1.2
Household/Cooking	2.1
Gardening/Golf	3.7
Jogging/Swimming/Football	6.9

Physical activity. The physical activity ratio (PAR) is expressed as multiples of the BMR for both occupational and non-occupational activities of varying intensities (Table 5.2).

$$\begin{array}{l} \text{Total daily} \\ \text{energy} \\ \text{expenditure} \end{array} = \begin{array}{l} \text{BMR} \times [\text{Time in bed} + \\ (\text{Time at work} \times \text{PAR}) + \\ (\text{Non-occupational time} \times \text{PAR})]. \end{array}$$

Thus, for example, to determine the daily energy expenditure of a 63-year-old, 50 kg female doctor, with a BMR of 4805 kJ per day spending one-third of a day sleeping, working or engaged in non-occupational activities, the latter at a PAR of 2.1, the following calculation ensues:

(4805 kJ/day) × [0.3 + (0.3 × 1.7) + (0.3 × 2.10)]
= 6919 kJ or 1655 kcal/day.

In the UK the estimated 'average' daily requirement is:

- for a 55-year-old female – 8100 kJ (1940 kcal)
- for a 55-year-old male – 10 600 kJ (2550 kcal).

This is at present made up of 50% carbohydrate, 35% fat, 15% protein plus or minus 5% alcohol. In developing countries, however, carbohydrate may be more than 75% of the total energy input, and fat less than 15% of the total energy input.

Energy requirements increase during the growing period, with pregnancy and lactation, and sometimes following infection or trauma. In general, the increased BMR associated with inflammatory or traumatic conditions is counteracted or more than counteracted by a decrease in physical activity, so that total energy requirements are not increased.

In the basal state, energy demands for resting muscle are 20% of the total energy required, abdominal viscera 35–40%, brain 20% and heart 10%. There can be more than a 50-fold increase in muscle energy demands during exercise.

Energy stores
Although virtually all body fat and glycogen are available for oxidation, less than half the protein is available for oxidation. Figure 5.3 shows that fat accounts for the largest reserves of energy in both lean and obese subjects. The size of the stores determines survival during starvation.

Bodyweight
Bodyweight depends on energy balance. Intake depends not only on food availability but also on a number of complex interrelationships that include the stimulus of good food, the role of hunger, metabolic changes (e.g. hypoglycaemia), and the pleasure and habit of eating. Some people are able to keep their bodyweight constant

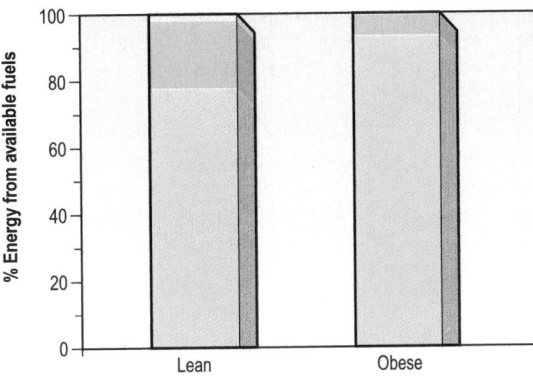

Fig. 5.3 Available energy reserves from different fuels expressed in MJ (upper) and as a percentage of total (lower) in a lean hypothetical 70 kg adult and an obese 140 kg adult.

within a few kilograms for many years, but most gradually increase their weight owing to a small but continuous increase of intake over expenditure. A gain or loss of energy of 25–29 MJ (6000–7000 kcal) would respectively increase or decrease bodyweight by approximately 1 kg.

Protein

In the UK the adult daily RNI for protein is 0.75 g/kg, with protein representing at least 10% of the total energy intake. Most affluent people eat more than this, consuming 80–100 g of protein per day. The total amount of nitrogen excreted in the urine represents the balance between protein breakdown and synthesis. In order to maintain nitrogen balance, at least 40–50 g of protein are needed. The amount of protein oxidized can be calculated from the amount of nitrogen excreted in the urine over 24 hours using the following equation:

Grams of protein required = Urinary nitrogen × 6.25 (most proteins contain about 16% of nitrogen).

In practice, urinary urea is more easily measured and forms 80–90% of the total urinary nitrogen (N). In healthy individuals urinary nitrogen excretion reflects protein intake. However, urine N excretion does not match intake either in catabolic conditions (negative N balance) or during growth or repletion following an illness (positive N balance).

Protein contains many amino acids, of which nine are indispensable (essential): trytophan, histidine, methionine, threonine, isoleucine, valine, phenylalanine, lysine, leucine. These amino acids cannot be synthesized and must be provided in the diet. The dispensable (non-essential) amino acids can be synthesized in the body, but some may still be needed in the diet unless adequate amounts of their precursors are available. Animal proteins, such as in milk, meat and eggs, are of high nutritional value as they contain all indispensable amino acids. Conversely, many proteins from vegetables are deficient in at least one indispensable amino acid.

In developing countries, adequate protein intake is achieved mainly from vegetable proteins. By combining foodstuffs with different low concentrations of indispensable amino acids (e.g. maize with legumes), protein intake can be adequate provided enough vegetables are available.

Loss of protein from the body (negative N balance) occurs not only because of inadequate protein intake, but also owing to inadequate energy intake. When there is loss of energy from the body, more protein is directed towards oxidative pathways and eventually gluconeogenesis for energy. Of all the amino acids, glutamine is quantitatively the most significant in the circulation and in inter-organ exchange. Alanine is released from muscle; it is deaminated and converted into pyruvic acid before entering the citric acid cycle. Homocysteine is a sulphur-containing amino acid which is derived from methionine in the diet. A raised plasma concentration is an independent risk factor for vascular disease (see p. 802).

Amino acids may be utilized to synthesize products other than protein or urea. For example:

- haem requires glycine
- melanin and thyroid hormones require tyrosine
- nucleic acid bases require glutamine, aspartate and glycine
- glutathione, which is part of the defence system against free radicals, requires glutamate, cysteine and glycine.

Fat

Dietary fat is chiefly in the form of triglycerides, which are esters of glycerol and free fatty acids. Fatty acids vary in chain length and in saturation (Table 5.3). Unsaturated fatty acids are monounsaturated or polyunsaturated. The hydrogen molecules related to these double bonds can be in the *cis* or the *trans* position, most natural fatty acids in food being in the *cis* position (Box 5.1).

The essential fatty acids (EFAs) are linoleic and α-linolenic acid, both of which are precursors of prostaglandins (see Fig. 14.32). Eicosapentaenoic and docosahexaenoic are also necessary, but can be made to a limited extent in the tissues from linoleic and linolenic, and thus a dietary supply is not essential.

Table 5.3   The main fatty acids in foods

Saturated
Lauric C12:0
Myristic C14:0
Palmitic C16:0
Stearic C18:0

Monosaturated
Oleic C18:1 (n-9)
Elaidic C18:1 (n-9 *trans**)

Polyunsaturated
Linoleic C18:2 (n-6)
α-Linolenic C18:3 (n-3)
Arachidonic C20:4 (n-6)
Eicosapentaenoic C20:5 (n-3)
Docosahexaenoic C22:6 (n-3)

The number of carbon atoms is indicated before the colon; the number of double bonds after the colon. In parentheses the positions of the double bonds (designated either n as here or ω) are shown counted from the methyl end of the molecule. All double bonds are in the *cis* position except that marked with an asterisk (*)

 Box 5.1 Dietary sources of fatty acids

Type of acid	Sources
Saturated fatty acids	Mainly animal fat
n-6 fatty acids	Vegetable oils and other plant foods
n-3 fatty acids	Vegetable foods, rapeseed oil, fish oils
trans fatty acids	Hydrogenated fat or oils, often in margarine

Synthesis of triglycerides, sterols and phospholipids is very efficient, and even with low-fat diets subcutaneous fat stores can be normal.

Dietary fat provides 37 kJ (9 kcal) of energy per gram. A high fat intake has been implicated in the causation of:

- cardiovascular disease
- cancer (e.g. breast, colon and prostate)
- obesity
- type 2 diabetes.

The data on causation are largely epidemiological and disputed by many. Nevertheless, it is often suggested that the consumption of saturated fatty acids should be reduced, accompanied by an increase in monounsaturated fatty acids (the 'Mediterranean diet') or polyunsaturated fatty acids. Any increase in polyunsaturated fats should not, however, exceed 10% of the total food energy, particularly as this requires a big dietary change.

Increased consumption of hydrogenated vegetable and fish oils in margarines has led to an increased *trans* fatty acid consumption and their intake should not, on present evidence, increase more than the current estimated average of 5 g per day or 2% of the dietary energy. This is because *trans fatty acids* (also called *trans* fats) behave as if they were saturated fatty acids, increasing circulating low-density lipoprotein (LDL) cholesterol concentration, which in turn increases the risk of cardiovascular disease. For this reason, the US Food and Drug Administration recommended in 2003 that in nutritional labelling, *trans* fatty acids should be listed separately under saturated fatty acids.

The *n-6 polyunsaturated fatty acids* (PUFA) are components of membrane phospholipids, influencing membrane fluidity and ion transport. They also have anti-arrhythmic, anti-thrombotic and anti-inflammatory properties, all of which are potentially helpful in preventing cardiovascular disease. In addition, n-3 PUFA increase circulating high-density lipoprotein (HDL) cholesterol and lower triglycerides, both of which might reduce cardiovascular risk. Some of the actions of n-3 PUFA are mediated by a range of leukotrienes and eicosanoids, which differ in pattern and functions from those produced from n-6 PUFA. A number of epidemiological studies and clinical intervention studies suggest that n-3 PUFA may have effects in the *secondary* prevention of cardiovascular disease and 'all-cause mortality' (e.g. 20–30% reduction in mortality from cardiovascular disease according to some studies). The benefits, which have been noted as early as 4 months after intervention, have been largely attributed to the anti-arrhythmic effects of n-3 PUFA, but recent work suggests that n-3 PUFA administered as capsules, can be rapidly incorporated into atheromatous plaques, stabilizing them and preventing rupture. Whether these effects are due directly to n-3 PUFA or other changes in the diet is still debated. To answer this, the GISSI Prevention Trial, which followed over 11 000 patients for 3.5 years after a myocardial infarction, administered the fish oils (eicosopentanoic acid (EPA) and decohexanoic acid (DHA)) in the form of capsules and demonstrated a striking benefit. The effects

of vitamin E (300 mg α-tocopherol/day) were also studied, but no benefit was found.

The British Nutrition Foundation and the American Heart Association presently recommend a two-fold increase of the current intake of total n-3 PUFA (several fold increase in the intake of fish oils, and a 50% increase in the intake of α-linolenic acid). Implementing this recommendation will mean either a major change in the dietary habits of populations that eat little fish, or ingestion of capsules containing fish oils. Some government agencies have warned of the hazards of eating certain types of fish, which increase the risk of mercury poisoning and possibly other toxicities.

The current recommendations for fat intake for the UK are as follows:

- saturated fatty acids should provide approximately 10% of the dietary energy
- *cis*-monounsaturated acids (mainly oleic acid) should continue to provide approximately 12% of the dietary energy
- *cis*-polyunsaturated acids should provide 6% of dietary energy, and are derived from n-6 and n-3 polyunsaturated fatty acids, which should provide ~ 0.5% of total energy intake
- total fat intake should be no more than 35% of the total dietary energy, and restriction to 30% is desirable.

Cholesterol is found in all animal products. Eggs are particularly rich in cholesterol, which is virtually absent from plants. The average daily intake in the UK is 300–500 mg. Cholesterol is also synthesized (see p. 350) and only very high or low dietary intakes will significantly affect blood levels.

Essential fatty acid deficiency

Essential fatty acid deficiency may accompany protein–energy malnutrition (PEM), but it has been clearly defined as a clinical entity only in patients on long-term parenteral nutrition given glucose, protein and no fat. Alopecia, thrombocytopenia, anaemia and a dermatitis occur within weeks with an increased ratio of triene (n-9) to tetraene (n-6) in plasma fatty acids.

Carbohydrate

Carbohydrates are readily available in the diet, providing 17 kJ (4 kcal) per gram of energy (15.7 kJ (3.75 kcal) per gram monosaccharide equivalent).

Carbohydrate intake comprises the polysaccharide starch, the disaccharides (mainly sucrose) and monosaccharides (glucose and fructose). Carbohydrate is cheap compared with other foodstuffs; a great deal is therefore eaten, usually more than required.

Dietary fibre, which is largely *non-starch polysaccharide* (NSP) (entirely NSP according to some authorities), is often removed in the processing of food. This leaves highly refined carbohydrates such as sucrose which contribute to the development of dental caries and obesity. Lignin is included in dietary fibre in some classification systems, but it is not a polysaccharide. It is only a minor component of the human diet.

The principal classes of NSP are:

- cellulose
- hemicelluloses
- pectins
- gums.

None of these is digested by gut enzymes. However, NSP is partly broken down in the gastrointestinal tract, mainly by colonic bacteria, producing gas and volatile fatty acids, e.g. butyrate.

All plant food, when unprocessed, contains NSP, so that all unprocessed food eaten will increase the NSP content of the diet. *Bran*, the fibre from wheat, provides an easy way of adding additional fibre to the diet: it increases faecal bulk and is helpful in the treatment of constipation.

The average daily intake of NSP in the diet is approximately 16 g. *NSP deficiency* is accepted as an entity by many authorities in the UK. It is suggested that the total NSP be increased to up to 30 g daily. This could be achieved by increased consumption of bread, potatoes, fruit and vegetables, with a reduction in sugar intake in order not to increase total calories. Each extra gram of fibre daily adds approximately 5 g to the daily stool weight.

Pectins and gums have been added to food to slow down monosaccharide absorption, particularly in type 2 diabetes. A high intake of dietary fibre reduces blood lipids (p. 1139). A high intake of fruits and vegetables probably reduces the risk of cancer, although this is controversial. Recently, however, a large scale multi-ethnic study in the USA (Prostate, Lung, Colorectal, and Ovarian screening study; PCLO) and the European Prospective Investigation into Cancer and Nutrition (EPIC), which operated across 10 European countries, showed an association between a high-fibre diet and protection against colonic adenomas or colonic cancer, and partly because of this, eating a diet rich in plant foods (fruits, vegetables, cereals and whole grain) is still generally recommended for general health promotion, including protection against colorectal cancer.

Health promotion

Many chronic diseases – particularly obesity, diabetes mellitus and cardiovascular disease – cause premature mortality and morbidity and are potentially preventable by dietary change.

Box 5.2 suggests the composition of the 'ideal healthy diet'. The values given are based on the principle of:

- reducing total fat in the diet, particularly saturated fat
- increasing consumption of fish which contain n-3 (or ω-3) polyunsaturated fatty acids
- increasing intake of whole-grain cereals, green and orange vegetables and fruits, leading to an increase in fibre and antioxidants.

Reductions in dietary sodium and cholesterol have also been suggested. There would be no disadvantage in this, and most studies have suggested some benefit.

Fortification of foods with specific nutrients is common. In the UK *margarine* and *milk* are fortified with vitamins A and D, *flour* with calcium, iron, thiamin and niacin, and *breakfast cereals* with several vitamins and iron. Not all substances used in fortification have nutritive value. For example, *Olestra* is a polymer of sucrose and six or more triglycerides which has been introduced to combat obesity. It is not absorbed and is therefore used particularly in savoury snack foods (where it has FDA approval) as a 'fake fat'. Therefore, it results in a reduction in total calories. It has side-effects (mainly in the gut) and its use is being carefully monitored.

The interests of the individual are often different from those associated with government policy. A distinction needs to be made about nutrient goals and dietary guidelines. Nutrient goals refer to the national intakes of nutrients that are considered appropriate for optimal health in the population, whereas dietary guidelines refer to the dietary methods used to achieve these goals. Since dietary habits in different countries vary, dietary

---

Box 5.2 Recommended healthy dietary intake

Dietary component	Approximate amounts (% of total energy unless otherwise stated)*	General hints
Total carbohydrate	55 (55–75)	Increase fruit vegetables, beans, pasta, bread
Free sugar	10 (< 10)	Decrease sugary drinks
Protein	15 (10–15)	Decrease red meat (see fat below)
Total fat	30 (15–30)	Increase vegetable (including olive oil) and fish oil and
Saturated fat	10 (< 10)	decrease animal fat
Unsaturated fat	20	
Cholesterol	< 300 (< 300) mg/day	Decrease meat and eggs
Salt	< 6 (< 5) g/day	Decrease prepared meats and do not add extra salt to food
Total dietary fibre	30 (> 25) g/day	Increase fruit and vegetables and wholegrain foods

* Values in parentheses are goals for the intake of populations, as given by the WHO (including populations who are already on low-fat diets). Some of the extreme ranges are not realistic short-term goals for developed countries, e.g. 75% of total energy from carbohydrate and 15% fat.

guidelines may also differ, even when the nutrient goals are the same. Nutrient goals are based on scientific information that links nutrient intake to disease. Although the information is incomplete, it includes evidence from a wide range of sources, including experimental animal studies, clinical studies and both short-term and long-term epidemiological studies.

FURTHER READING

Ferguson LR, Harris PJ (2003) The dietary fibre debate. *Lancet* **361**: 1487–1488.

Lee KW, Lip GYH (2003) The role of omega-3 fatty acids in the secondary prevention of cardiovascular disease. *Quarterly Journal of Medicine* **96**: 465–480.

Royal College of Physicians (2002) *Nutrition and Patients: a Doctor's Responsibility. A Report of a Working Party of the Royal College of Physicians.* London: RCP.

Thies F, Garry JMC, Yaqoob P et al. (2003) Association of n-3 polyunsaturated fatty acids with stability of atherosclerotic plaques: a randomised controlled trial. *Lancet* **361**: 477–485.

WHO/FAO Expert Consultation (2003) *Diet, Nutrition and the Prevention of Chronic Diseases.* Geneva: WHO.

PROTEIN–ENERGY MALNUTRITION (PEM)

IN DEVELOPED COUNTRIES

Starvation uncomplicated by disease is relatively uncommon in developed countries, although some degree of undernourishment is seen in very poor areas. Most nutritional problems occurring in the population at large are due to eating wrong combinations of foodstuffs, such as an excess of refined carbohydrate or a diet low in fresh vegetables. Undernourishment associated with disease is common in hospitals and nursing homes, and Table 5.4 gives a list of conditions in which malnutrition is often seen. Surgical complications, with sepsis, are a common cause. Many patients are admitted to hospital undernourished, and a variety of chronic conditions predispose to this state (Table 5.5).

The majority of the weight loss, leading to malnutrition, *is due to poor intake secondary to the anorexia associated with the underlying condition.* Disease may also contribute by causing malabsorption and increased catabolism, which is mediated by complex changes in cytokines, hormones, side-effects of drugs, and immobility. The elderly are particularly at risk of malnutrition because they often suffer from diseases and psychosocial problems such as social isolation or bereavement (Table 5.5).

Pathophysiology of starvation (Fig. 5.4)

In the first 24 hours following low dietary intake, the body relies for energy on the breakdown of hepatic glycogen to glucose. Hepatic glycogen stores are small and therefore gluconeogenesis is soon necessary to

Table 5.4 Common conditions associated with protein–energy malnutrition

Sepsis	Dementia
Trauma	Malignancy
Surgery, particularly of GI tract with complications	Any very ill patient
	Severe chronic inflammatory diseases
GI disease, particularly involving the small bowel	Psychosocial: poverty, social isolation, anorexia nervosa, depression

Table 5.5 Nutritional consequences of disease and the underlying risk factors (physical/psychosocial problems)

Risk factors	Consequence
Underlying disease Almost any moderate/severe chronic disease Recovery from severe acute/subacute disease	Anorexia, increased requirements for some nutrients, and *other effects indicated below (depending on condition)*
Physical problems Muscle weakness (respiratory and peripheral muscles) and/or incoordination Severe arthritis in hands and arms Swallowing problem (neurological causes), painful or obstructive conditions of mouth and gastrointestinal tract (GIT) GIT symptoms (e.g. nausea, vomiting, diarrhoea, jaundice) Sensory deficit (e.g. impaired sight, hearing and other deficits)	Problems with shopping, cooking and eating Inadequate food intake, and/or risk of aspiration pneumonia Food aversion, malabsorption (small bowel disease), anorexia Difficulties in shopping, cooking and/or decreased intake of food
Psychosocial problems Loneliness, depression, bereavement, confusion, living alone, poverty, alcoholism, drug addiction	Self-neglect, inadequate intake of food or quality of food
Multiple drug use (polypharmacy)	Indicates severe disease or multiple physical and psychosocial problems; drugs may lead to confusion, sedation, depression and GIT side-effects (including malabsorption of nutrients)

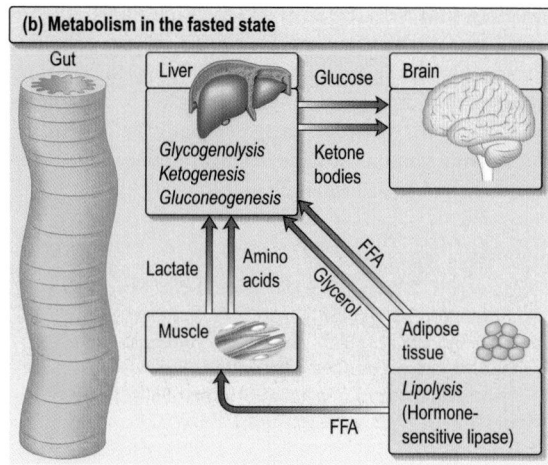

Fig. 5.4 **Metabolism in (a) the fed and (b) the fasted state.** FFA, free fatty acids.

maintain glucose levels. Gluconeogenesis takes place mainly from pyruvate, lactate, glycerol and amino acids, especially alanine and glutamine. The majority of protein breakdown takes place in muscle, with eventual loss of muscle bulk.

Lipolysis, the breakdown of the body's fat stores, also occurs. It is inhibited by insulin, but the level of this hormone falls off as starvation continues. The stored triglyceride is hydrolysed by lipase to glycerol, which is used for gluconeogenesis, and also to non-esterified fatty acids that can be used directly as a fuel or oxidized in the liver to ketone bodies.

As starvation continues, *adaptive processes* take place lest the body's available protein be completely utilized. There is a decrease in metabolic rate and total body energy expenditure. Central nervous metabolism changes from glucose as a substrate to ketone bodies, which now become the main source of energy for the brain. Gluconeogenesis in the liver decreases as does protein breakdown in muscle, both of these processes being inhibited directly by ketone bodies, which are derived from fat. Most of the energy at this stage comes from adipose tissue, with some gluconeogenesis from amino acids, particularly from alanine in the liver, and glutamine in the kidney.

The metabolic response to prolonged starvation differs between lean and obese individuals. One of the major differences concerns the proportion of energy derived from protein oxidation, which determines the proportion of weight loss from lean tissues. This proportion may be up to three times smaller in obese subjects than lean subjects. It can be regarded as an adaptation which depends on the compensation of the initial reserves (Fig. 5.3). This means that deterioration in body function is more rapid in lean subjects. Furthermore, survival time is much less in lean subjects (~ 2 months), compared to the obese (can be at least several months).

Following trauma or shock, some of the adaptive changes do not take place. Glucocorticoids and cytokines (see below) stimulate the ubiquitin–proteasome pathway in muscle, which is responsible for accelerated proteolysis in muscle in many catabolic illnesses. In starvation there is a

decrease in BMR, whilst in inflammatory and traumatic disease, the BMR is often increased. These changes all result in continuing gluconeogenesis with massive muscle breakdown, and further reduction in survival time.

Regulation of metabolism

Tissue metabolism is regulated by multiple coordinated processes. Some are rapid, involving nerves, whilst others are slower involving circulating substrates and hormones. The availability of substrates (e.g. glucose, non-esterified fatty acids (NEFA), and ketone bodies) in the circulation can have major effects on tissue metabolism, as a result of mass action effects that are *independent of hormones.* For example, the markedly elevated circulating ketone body concentration during starvation (up to 5 or more mmol/L), leads to increased uptake and metabolism of tissues such as the brain. The liver that produces these ketone bodies can be regarded as controlling the metabolism of the brain. Adipose tissue, which releases NEFA, controls hepatic metabolism, which in turn depends on this substrate for ketogenesis. Substrates may also compete with each other, again independently of hormones. Tissue triglyceride and glycogen (which produce NEFA and glucosyl units on hydrolysis) also compete for uptake and metabolism in muscle and heart.

Blood flow to a tissue can also influence metabolism by affecting the delivery of substrates to the tissue or their release into the circulation. NEFA are bound to two or three high affinity sites on albumin, and when these high affinity sites become nearly saturated, the efflux of NEFA would be limited. During starvation or prolonged exercise, when there is increased demand for NEFA, there is a major increase in the blood flow to adipose tissue, which supplies more albumin with unsaturated binding sites.

In many tissues there is coupling between metabolic activity and blood flow with the arterioles regulating blood flow to the tissue according to demand.

Hormonal signals also regulate intracellular metabolism.

The activation of lipoprotein lipase, which hydrolyses circulating triglycerides so that NEFA can enter adipose tissue for storage is delayed several hours after a meal to coincide with the rise in circulating triglycerides, which occurs later than the changes of other metabolites such as glucose, NEFA and amino acids.

In the fed state, insulin/glucagon ratios are high. Insulin promotes synthesis of glycogen, protein and fat, and inhibits lipolysis and gluconeogenesis.

In the fasted state, the insulin/glucagon ratios are low. Glucagon acts mainly on the liver and has no action on muscle. It increases glycogenolysis and gluconeogenesis, as well as increasing ketone body production from fatty acids. It also stimulates lipolysis in adipose tissue. Catecholamines have a similar action to glucagon but also affect muscle metabolism. Both these agents act via cyclic adenosine monophosphate (cAMP) to stimulate lipolysis, producing free fatty acids that can then act as a major source of energy.

Cytokines, such as interleukin-1, interleukin-6 and tumour necrosis factor (TNF), have also been shown to play a role in regulating metabolism. In acute diseases they contribute to the catabolic process, glycogenolysis, and acute-phase protein synthesis. TNF, which inhibits lipoprotein lipase, is the 'cachexia factor' in patients with cancer.

It is now recognized that the metabolic response to trauma, injury and inflammation depends on the balance between pro-inflammatory and anti-inflammatory cytokines (e.g. IL-10) and that the production of many of these cytokines is influenced by genetic polymorphisms. Since many chronic diseases, including atherosclerosis, have an inflammatory component, these considerations have wide-reaching metabolic implications.

It is unclear how these cytokines interact with central feeding pathways to cause anorexia. However, in animal models of both cancer and inflammatory bowel disease, many peripheral and central mediators of appetite are involved. For example, neuropeptide Y levels in the hypothalamus are often inappropriately low, so there is a reduced drive to feeding.

Clinical features

Patients are sometimes seen with loss of weight or malnutrition as the primary symptom (failure to thrive in children). Mostly, however, malnourishment is only seen as an accompaniment of some other disease process, such as malignancy. Severe malnutrition is seen mainly with advanced organic disease or after surgical procedures followed by complications. Three key features which help in the detection of chronic protein–energy malnutrition (PEM) in adults are:

1. *The body mass index (BMI):*

   - Probable chronic PEM: < 18.5 kg/m^2
   - Possible chronic PEM: 18.5–20 kg/m^2
   - Little or no risk of chronic PEM: > 20 kg/m^2.

   In patients with oedema or dehydration the BMI may be somewhat misleading.

2. *Weight loss in previous 3–6 months:* > 10%, high risk; 5–10%, possible risk; < 5% low/no risk of developing PEM.

3. *Acute disease effect:* Diseases that have resulted or are likely to result in no dietary intake for more than 5 days are associated with a high risk of malnutrition (e.g. prolonged unconsciousness, persistent swallowing problems after a stroke, or prolonged ileus after abdominal surgery).

Other factors:
- History of decreased food intake/loss of appetite
- Clothes becoming loosely fitting (weight loss) and a general appearance indicating obvious wasting
- Physical and psychosocial disturbances likely to have contributed to the weight loss.

These factors act as a link between detection and management (Fig. 5.5). If the underlying physical or psychosocial problems are not adequately addressed, treatment may not be successful.

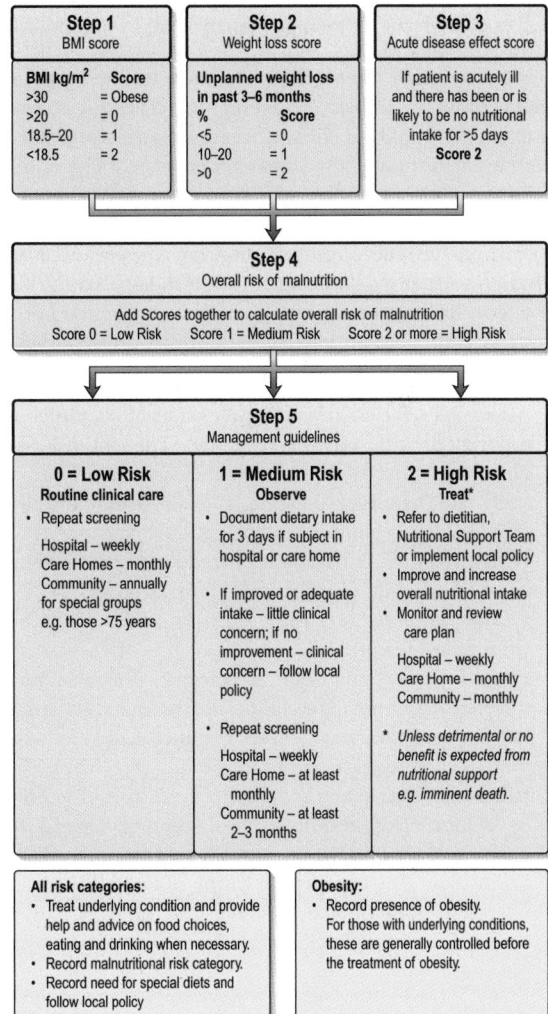

Fig. 5.5 Malnutrition Universal Screening Tool (MUST). Reproduced with permission from the Malnutrition Advisory Group – A Standing Committee of British Association of Parenteral and Enteral Nutrition (BAPEN): http://www.bapen.org.uk.

PEM leads to a depression of the immunological defence mechanism, resulting in a decreased resistance to infection. It also detrimentally affects muscle strength and fatigue, reproductive function (e.g. in anorexia nervosa, which is common in adolescent girls; p. 1310), wound healing, and psychological function (depression, anxiety, hypochondriasis, loss of libido).

Treatment (see also pp. 257 and 260)

When malnutrition is obvious and the underlying disease cannot be corrected at once, some form of nutritional support is necessary. Nutrition should be given enterally if the gastrointestinal tract is functioning adequately. This can most easily be done by encouraging the patient to eat more often and by giving a high-calorie supplement. If this is not possible, a liquefied diet may be given intragastrically via a fine-bore tube or by a percutaneous endoscopic gastrostomy (PEG). If both of these measures fail, parenteral nutrition is given.

IN DEVELOPING COUNTRIES

In many areas of the world, people are on the verge of malnutrition. In addition, if events such as drought, war or changes in political climate occur, millions suffer from starvation. Although the basic condition of PEM is the same in all parts of the world from whatever cause, malnutrition resulting from long periods of near-total starvation produces unique clinical appearances in children virtually never seen in high-income countries. The term 'protein–energy malnutrition' covers the spectrum of clinical conditions seen in adults and children. Children under 5 years may present with:

- *Marasmus* is the childhood form of starvation, which is associated with obvious wasting. The child looks emaciated, there is obvious muscle wasting and loss of body fat. There is no oedema. The hair is thin and dry (Fig. 5.6a). The child is not so apathetic or anorexic as with kwashiorkor. Diarrhoea is frequently present and signs of infection must be looked for carefully.
- *Kwashiorkor* occurs typically in a young child displaced from breast-feeding by a new baby. It is often precipitated by infections such as measles, malaria and diarrhoeal illnesses. The child is apathetic and lethargic with severe anorexia. There is generalized oedema with skin pigmentation and thickening (Fig. 5.6b). The hair is dry, sparse and may become reddish or yellow in colour. The abdomen is distended owing to hepatomegaly and/or ascites. The serum albumin is always low. The exact cause is unknown, but theories related to diet (low in protein, and high in carbohydrate) and free radical damage in the presence of inadequate antioxidant defences have been proposed.

A recent classification of severe malnutrition by the World Health Organization (Table 5.6) makes no distinction between kwashiorkor and marasmus, because their approach to treatment is similar.

The World Health Organization (WHO) classification of chronic undernutrition in children is based on standard deviation (SD) scores. Thus, children with an SD score

(a)

(b)

Fig. 5.6 **Malnourished children: (a) marasmus and (b) kwashiorkor.** Courtesy of Dr Paul Kelly.

between −2 and −3 (between 3 and 2 standard deviation scores below the median – corresponding to a value between 0.13 and 2.3 centile) can be regarded as being at moderate risk of undernutrition, and below an SD score of −3, of severe malnutrition. A low weight-for-height is a measure of thinness (wasting when pathological), and a low height-for-age is a measure of shortness (stunting when pathological). Those with oedema and clinical signs of severe malnutrition are classified as having oedematous malnutrition.

Table 5.6 Classification of childhood malnutrition

	Moderate malnutrition	Severe malnutrition*
Symmetrical oedema	No	Yes (oedematous malnutrition)[†]
Weight-for-height	SD score –3 to –2 (70–79%)[‡]	SD score below –3 (< 70%)[‡] (severe wasting)[§]
Height-for-age	SD score –3 to –2 (85–89%)[‡]	SD score below –3 (< 85%)[‡] (severe stunting)

*The diagnoses are not mutually exclusive
[†]This includes kwashiorkor and marasmic-kwashiorkor in the older classifications. To avoid confusion with the clinical syndrome of kwashiorkor, which includes other features (see text), the term oedematous malnutrition is preferred
[‡]Percentage of the median National Centre for Health Statistics/WHO reference
[§]This corresponds to marasmus (without oedema) in the Wellcome classification and to grade II in the Gomez classification. To avoid confusion the term 'severe' wasting is preferred

Starvation in adults may lead to extreme loss of weight depending upon the severity and duration. They may crave for food, are apathetic and complain of cold and weakness with a loss of subcutaneous fat and muscle wasting. Infections such as gastrointestinal or bronchopneumonia are common. The WHO classification is based on body mass index, with a value less than 18.5 kg/m² indicating malnutrition (severe malnutrition if less than 16.0 kg/m².

Severely malnourished adults and children are very susceptible to respiratory and gastrointestinal infections, leading to an increased mortality in these groups.

Investigation

It must be realized that this is not always practicable.

- **Blood tests**
  - (a) Anaemia due to folate, iron and copper deficiency is often present, but the haematocrit may be high owing to dehydration.
  - (b) Eosinophilia suggests parasitic infestation.
  - (c) Electrolyte disturbances are common.
  - (d) Malarial parasites should be looked for.
  - (e) HIV tests.
- **Stools** should be examined for parasitic infestations.
- **Chest X-ray** – tuberculosis is common and is easily missed if a chest X-ray is not performed.

Treatment

Treatment must involve the provision of protein and energy supplements and the control of infection.

Resuscitation and stabilization

The severely ill child will require correction of fluid and electrolyte abnormalities, but intravenous therapy should be avoided if possible because of the danger of fluid overload. Treatment of shock may require oxygen. Treatment should also focus on hypoglycaemia (blood glucose < 3 mmol/L), hypothermia (reduce heat loss, and provide additional heat if necessary) and infection (antibiotics), which often coexist. The standard WHO oral hydration solution has a high sodium and low potassium content and is not suitable for severely malnourished children. Instead, the rehydration solution for malnutrition (ReSoMal) is recommended. It is commercially available but can be produced by modification of the standard WHO oral hydration solution.

Diarrhoea is often due to bacterial or protozoal overgrowth; metronidazole is very effective and is often given routinely. Parasites are also common and, as facilities for stool examination are usually not available, mebendazole 100 mg twice daily should be given for 3 days. In high-risk areas, antimalarial therapy is given. Large doses of vitamin A are also given because deficiency of this vitamin is common. After the initial resuscitation, further stabilization over the next few days is undertaken, as indicated in Table 5.7.

Refeeding

This needs to be planned carefully. During the initial treatment of the acute situation, a balanced diet with

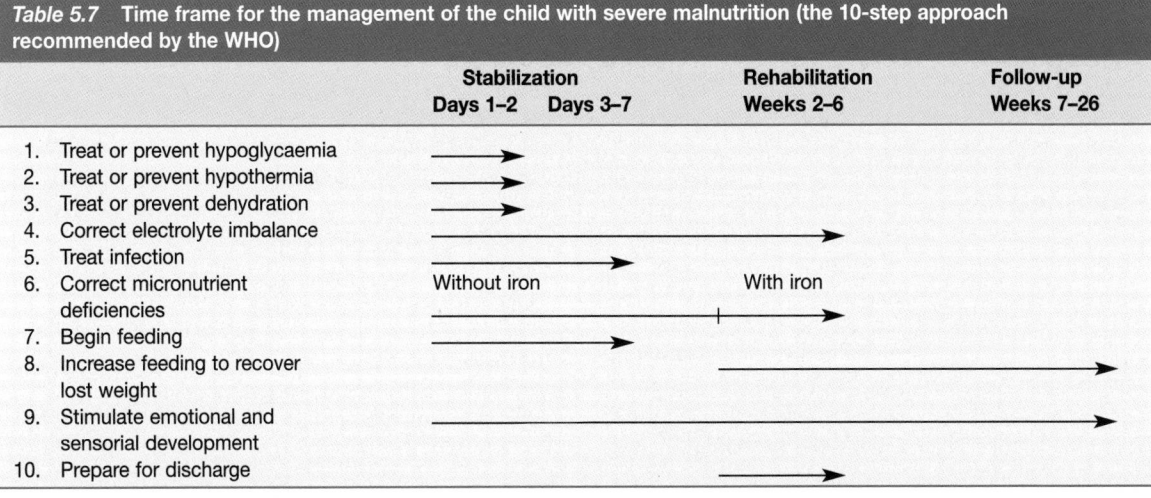

Table 5.7 Time frame for the management of the child with severe malnutrition (the 10-step approach recommended by the WHO)

	Stabilization Days 1–2	Days 3–7	Rehabilitation Weeks 2–6	Follow-up Weeks 7–26
1. Treat or prevent hypoglycaemia	→			
2. Treat or prevent hypothermia	→			
3. Treat or prevent dehydration	→			
4. Correct electrolyte imbalance		→		
5. Treat infection		→		
6. Correct micronutrient deficiencies	Without iron		With iron	
7. Begin feeding		→		
8. Increase feeding to recover lost weight			→	→
9. Stimulate emotional and sensorial development			→	→
10. Prepare for discharge			→	

sufficient protein and energy is given to maintain a steady state. Large increases in energy lead to heart failure, circulatory collapse and death (refeeding syndrome). Initial feeding involves administration of feeds of low osmolarity and low in lactose (WHO recommendations: 100 kcal/kg/day, 1.0–1.5 g protein/kg/day and 130 mL liquid/kg/day (100 mL/kg/day if the child has marked oedema). Attempts should be made to give the feeds slowly and frequently (e.g. 2-hourly during days 1–2; 3-hourly during days 3–5; and 4-hourly thereafter), although anorexia is often a problem and can be exacerbated by excessive feeding. If necessary, fluids and food should be given by nasogastric tube. The child is then gradually weaned to liquids and then solids by mouth. All severely malnourished children have vitamin and mineral deficiencies. Although anaemia is common, the WHO recommends to give iron only after the child develops a good appetite and starts gaining weight, because of concern about making the infection worse (iron is a pro-oxidant). The child should be given daily micronutrient supplements for at least 2 weeks. These should include a multivitamin supplement with folic acid, zinc and copper.

Rehabilitation

Gradually, as the child improves, more energy can be given, and during rehabilitation weight gain is achieved by providing extra energy and protein ('catch-up weight gain'). Children who have been severely ill need constant attention right through the convalescent period, as often home conditions are poor and feeds are refused. Sensory stimulation and emotional support is a major component of management during both the stabilization and rehabilitation phases.

Adults do not usually suffer such severe malnutrition, but the same general principles of treatment should be followed.

Prognosis

Children with extreme malnutrition have a mortality of over 50%. By careful management this can be reduced significantly to 1–2%, depending on the availability of facilities. Brain development takes place in the first years of life, a time when severe PEM frequently occurs. There is evidence that intellectual impairment and behavioural abnormalities occur in severely affected children. Physical growth is also impaired. Probably both of these effects can be alleviated if it is possible to maintain a high standard of living with a good diet and freedom from infection over a long period.

Prevention

Prevention of PEM depends not only on adequate nutrients being available but also on education of both governments and individuals in the importance of good nutrition and immunization (Box 5.3). Short-term programmes are useful for acute shortages of food, but long-term programmes involving improved agriculture are equally necessary. Bad feeding practices and infections are more prevalent than actual shortage of food in many

Box 5.3 Prevention of protein–energy malnutrition – GOBIF (a WHO priority programme)

- **G**rowth monitoring: The WHO has a simple growth chart that the mother keeps
- **O**ral rehydration, particularly for diarrhoea
- **B**reast-feeding supplemented by food after 6 months
- **I**mmunization: against measles, tetanus, pertussis, diphtheria, polio and tuberculosis
- **F**amily planning

areas of the world. However, good surveillance is necessary to avoid periods of famine.

Food supplements (and additional vitamins) should be given to 'at-risk' groups by adding high-energy food (e.g. milk powder, meat concentrates) to the diet. Pregnancy and lactation are times of high energy requirement and supplements have been shown to be beneficial.

FURTHER READING

Ashworth A et al (2004) WHO guidelines for management of severe malnutrition in rural South African hospitals. *Lancet* **363**: 1110–1115.

Bhan MK, Bhandari N, Bhal R (2003) Management of the severely malnourished child: perspective from developing countries. *British Medical Journal* **326**: 146–151.

Elia M (2001) Metabolic response to starvation, injury and sepsis. In: Payne-James J, Grimble G, Silk D (eds) *Artificial Nutritional Support in Clinical Practice*, 2nd edn. London: Greenwich Medical Media.

Stratton RJ, Green CJ, Elia M (2003) *Disease-related Malnutrition. An Evidence-based Approach to Treatment*. Oxford: CABI Publishing (CAB International).

WHO (1999) *Management of Severe Malnutrition: A Manual for Physicians and Other Senior Health Workers*. Geneva: WHO.

WHO (2000) *Management of the Child with Serious Infection or Severe Malnutrition*. Geneva: WHO.

VITAMINS

Deficiencies due to inadequate intake associated with PEM (Table 5.8) are commonly seen in the developing countries. This is not, however, invariable. For example, vitamin A deficiency is never seen in Jamaica, but is common in PEM in Hyderabad, India. In the West, deficiency of vitamins is rare except in the specific groups shown in Table 5.9. The widespread use of vitamins as 'tonics' is unnecessary and should be discouraged. Toxicity from excess fat-soluble vitamins is occasionally seen.

FAT-SOLUBLE VITAMINS

Vitamin A

Vitamin A (retinol) is part of the family of retinoids which is present in food and the body as esters combined with

Table 5.8 Fat-soluble and water-soluble vitamins: reference nutrient intake (RNI) and lower reference nutrient intake (LRNI)

Vitamin	RNI/day (sufficient)	LRNI/day (insufficient)	Major clinical features of deficiency
Fat-soluble			
A (retinol)	700 µg	300 µg	Xerophthalmia, night blindness, keratomalacia, follicular hyperkeratosis
D (cholecalciferol)	No dietary intake required	10 µg (living indoors)	Rickets, osteomalacia
K	1 µg/kg bodyweight		Coagulation defects
E (α-tocopherol)	10°*		Neurological disorders, e.g. ataxia
Water-soluble			
B$_1$ (thiamin)	0.4 mg per 1000 kcal[†]	0.23 mg per 1000 kcal[†]	Beriberi, Wernicke–Korsakoff syndrome
B$_2$ (riboflavin)	1.3 mg	0.8 mg	Angular stomatitis
Niacin	6.6 mg per 1000 kcal	4.4 mg per 1000 kcal	Pellagra
B$_6$ (pyridoxine)	15 µg per g of dietary protein	11 µg per g of dietary protein	Polyneuropathy
B$_{12}$ (cobalamin)	1.5 µg	1.0 µg	Megaloblastic anaemia, neurological disorders
Folate	200 µg	100 µg	Megaloblastic anaemia
C (ascorbic acid)	40 mg	10 mg	Scurvy

*No official RNI because amount varies depending upon polyunsaturated fatty acid content of diet
[†]Thiamin requirements are related to energy metabolism

Table 5.9 Some causes of vitamin deficiency in developed countries

Decreased intake
Alcohol dependency: chiefly B vitamins (e.g. thiamin)
Small bowel disease: chiefly folate, occasionally fat-soluble vitamins
Vegans: vitamin D (if no exposure to sunlight), vitamin B$_{12}$
Elderly with poor diet: chiefly vitamin D (if no exposure to sunlight), folate
Anorexia from any cause: chiefly folate

Decreased absorption
Ileal disease/resection: only vitamin B$_{12}$
Liver and biliary tract disease: fat-soluble vitamins
Intestinal bacterial overgrowth: vitamin B$_{12}$
Oral antibiotics: vitamin K

Miscellaneous
Long-term enteral or parenteral nutrition: usually vitamin supplements are given
Renal disease: vitamin D
Drug antagonists (e.g. methotrexate interfering with folate metabolism

long-chain fatty acids. The richest food source is liver, but it is also found in milk, butter, cheese, egg yolks and fish oils. Retinol or carotene is added to margarine in the UK and other countries.

Beta-carotene is the main carotenoid found in green vegetables, carrots and other yellow and red fruits. Other carotenoids, lycopene and lutein, are probably of little quantitative importance as dietary precursors of vitamin A.

Beta-carotene is cleaved in the intestinal mucosa by carotene dioxygenase, yielding retinaldehyde which can be reduced to retinol. Between a quarter and a third of dietary vitamin A in the UK is derived from retinoids. Nutritionally, 6 µg of β-carotene is equivalent to 1 µg of preformed retinol; vitamin A activity in the diet is given as retinol equivalents.

Function

Retinol is stored in the liver and is transported in plasma bound to an α-globulin, retinol-binding protein (RBP). Vitamin A has several metabolic roles:

- Retinaldehyde in its *cis* form is found in the opsin proteins in the rods (rhodopsin) and cones (iodopsin) of the retina. Light causes retinaldehyde to change to its *trans* isomer, and this leads to changes in membrane potentials that are transmitted to the brain.
- Retinol and retinoic acid are involved in the control of cell proliferation and differentiation.
- Retinyl phosphate is a cofactor in the synthesis of most glycoproteins containing mannose.

Deficiency

Vitamin A deficiency and xerophthalmia (see below) is the major cause of blindness in young children despite intensive preventative programmes. The WHO estimates that between six and seven million new cases of xerophthalmia occur each year, with 20% of survivors being totally blind and 50–56% partially blind. South and East Asia, parts of Africa and Latin America as well as the Middle East are the most severely affected.

Xerophthalmia has been classified by the WHO (Table 5.10). Impaired adaptation followed by night blindness is the first effect. There is dryness and thickening of the conjunctiva and the cornea (xerophthalmia occurs as a result of keratinization). Bitot's spots – white plaques of keratinized epithelial cells – are found on the conjunctiva of young children with vitamin A deficiency. These spots can, however, be seen without vitamin A deficiency, possibly caused by exposure. Corneal softening, ulceration and dissolution (keratomalacia) eventually occur; superimposed infection is a frequent accompaniment and both lead to blindness.

Table 5.10 Classification of xerophthalmia by ocular signs

Night blindness (XN)
Conjunctival xerosis (XIA)
Bitot's spot (X2)
Corneal xerosis (X2)
Corneal ulceration/keratomalacia < $^1/_3$ corneal surface (X3A)
Corneal ulceration/keratomalacia = $^1/_3$ corneal surface (X3B)
Corneal scar (XS)
Xerophthalmic fundus (XF)

X, xerophthalmia
Reproduced with permission from WHO/UNICEF/IVACG 1988

In PEM, retinol-binding protein along with other proteins is reduced. This suggests vitamin A deficiency, although body stores are not necessarily reduced.

Vitamin A in malnourished children

Vitamin A supplementation appears to improve morbidity and mortality from measles. It has also been suggested that supplementation reduces morbidity and/or mortality from diarrhoeal diseases and respiratory infections and improves growth. However, despite the large number of studies in both developed and developing countries over the last two decades, the results remain controversial. Furthermore, although low circulating concentrations of vitamin A in HIV-infected individuals are associated with increased risk of vertical transmission of HIV, vitamin A supplementation during pregnancy and the interpartum period is unlikely to reduce vertical transmission to the child.

Diagnosis

In parts of the world where the deficiency is common, diagnosis is made on the basis of the clinical features, and deficiency should always be suspected if any degree of malnutrition is present. Blood levels of vitamin A will usually be low, but the best guide to the diagnosis is a response to replacement therapy.

Treatment

Urgent treatment with retinol palmitate 30 mg orally should be given on 2 successive days. In the presence of vomiting and diarrhoea, 30 mg of vitamin A is given intramuscularly. Associated malnutrition must be treated, and superadded bacterial infection should be treated with antibiotics. Referral for specialist ophthalmic treatment is necessary in severe cases.

Prevention

Most western diets contain enough dairy products and green vegetables, but vitamin A is added to foodstuffs (e.g. margarine) in some countries. Vitamin A is not destroyed by cooking.

In some developing countries vitamin A supplements are given at the time the child attends for measles vaccination. Food fortification programmes are another approach. Education of the population is necessary and people should be encouraged to grow their own vegetables. In particular, pregnant women and children should be encouraged to eat green vegetables.

Other effects of vitamin A

The effect of β-carotene in cardiovascular and other diseases is discussed below in the section entitled 'Dietary antioxidants'. Retinoic acid and some synthetic retinoids are used in dermatology (p. 1338).

Possible adverse effects

- *High intakes of vitamin A.* Chronic ingestion of retinol can cause liver and bone damage, hair loss, double vision, vomiting, headaches and other abnormalities. Single doses of 300 mg in adults or 100 mg in children can be harmful.
- *Retinol is teratogenic.* The incidence of birth defects in infants is high with vitamin A intakes of more than 3 mg a day during pregnancy. In pregnancy, extra vitamin A or consumption of liver is not recommended in the UK. However, β-carotene is not toxic.

Vitamin D

See page 592.

Vitamin K

Vitamin K is found as phylloquinone (vitamin K_1) in green leafy vegetables, dairy products, rape seed and soya bean oils. Intestinal bacteria can synthesize the other major form of vitamin K, menaquinone (vitamin K_2), in the terminal ileum and colon. Vitamin K is absorbed in a similar manner to other fat-soluble substances in the upper small gut. Some menaquinones must also be absorbed as this is the major form found in the human liver.

Function

Vitamin K is a cofactor necessary for the production not only of blood clotting factors (p. 475), but also for proteins necessary in the formation of bone.

Vitamin K is a cofactor for the post-translational carboxylation of specific protein-bound glutamate residues in γ-carboxyglutamate (Gla). Gla residues bind calcium ions to phospholipid templates, and this action on factors II, VII, IX and X, and on proteins C and S, is necessary for coagulation to take place.

Bone osteoblasts contain three vitamin K-dependent proteins, osteocalcin, matrix Gla protein and protein S, which have a role in bone matrix formation. Osteocalcin contains three Gla residues which bind tightly to the hydroxyapatite matrix depending on the degree of carboxylation; this leads to bone mineralization. There is, however, no convincing evidence that vitamin K deficiency or antagonism affects bone other than rapidly growing bone.

Vitamin K deficiency

Vitamin K deficiency results in inadequate synthesis of clotting factors (p. 475), which leads to an increase in the prothrombin time and haemorrhage. Deficiency occurs in the following circumstances:

The newborn

Deficiency occurs in the newborn owing to:

- poor placental transfer of vitamin K
- little vitamin K in breast milk
- no hepatic stores of menaquinone (no intestinal bacteria in the neonate).

Deficiency leads to a haemorrhagic disease of the newborn, which can be prevented by prophylactic vitamin K. The Chief Medical and Nursing Officers (England) recommend administration of vitamin K to all neonates after risks have been discussed with parents and consent obtained.

Cholestatic jaundice

When bile flow into the intestine is interrupted, malabsorption of vitamin K occurs as no bile salts are available to facilitate absorption and the prothrombin time increases. This can be corrected by giving 10 mg of phytomenadione intramuscularly. (Note that an increased prothrombin time because of liver disease does not respond to vitamin K injection, there being no shortage of vitamin K, just bad liver function.) In patients with chronic cholestasis (e.g. primary biliary cirrhosis) oral therapy using a water-soluble preparation, menadiol sodium phosphate 10 mg daily, is used.

Concomitant vitamin K antagonists

Oral anticoagulants antagonize vitamin K (p. 480). Antibacterial drugs also interfere with the bacterial synthesis of vitamin K.

Vitamin E

Vitamin E includes eight naturally occurring compounds divided into tocopherols and tocotrienoles. The most active compound and the most widely available in food is the natural isomer d- (or RRR) α-tocopherol, which accounts for 90% of vitamin E in the human body. Vegetables and seed oils, including soya bean, saffron, sunflower, cereals and nuts, are the main sources. Animal products are poor sources of the vitamin.

Vitamin E is absorbed with fat, transported in the blood largely in low-density lipoproteins (LDL).

An individual's vitamin E requirement depends on the intake of polyunsaturated fatty acids (PUFAs). Since this varies widely, no daily requirement is given in the UK. The requirement stated in the USA is approximately 7–10 mg per day, but average diets contain much more than this. If PUFAs are taken in large amounts, more vitamin E is required.

Function

The biological activity of vitamin E results principally from its antioxidant properties. In biological membranes it contributes to membrane stability. It protects cellular structures against damage from a number of highly reactive oxygen species, including hydrogen peroxide, superoxide and other oxygen radicals. Vitamin E may also affect cell proliferation and growth.

Vitamin E deficiency

The first deficiency to be demonstrated was a haemolytic anaemia described in premature infants. Infant formulations now contain vitamin E.

Deficiency is seen only in children with abetalipoproteinaemia (p. 308) and in patients on long-term parenteral nutrition. The severe neurological deficit (gross ataxia) can be prevented by vitamin E injection.

Plasma or serum levels of α-tocopherol can be measured and should be corrected for the level of plasma lipids by expressing the value as per milligram of plasma lipid or cholesterol.

WATER-SOLUBLE VITAMINS

Water-soluble vitamins are non-toxic and relatively cheap and can therefore be given in large amounts if a deficiency is possible. The daily requirements of water-soluble vitamins are given in Table 5.8.

Thiamin (vitamin B₁)

Thiamin consists of pyrimidine and thiazole rings. The alcohol side-chain is esterified with one, two or three phosphates (Fig. 5.7a).

Function

Thiamin diphosphate, often called thiamin pyrophosphate (TPP), is an essential cofactor, particularly in carbohydrate metabolism.

TPP is involved in the oxidative decarboxylation of acetyl CoA in mitochondria. In the Krebs cycle, TPP is the key enzyme for the decarboxylation of α-ketoglutarate to succinyl CoA. TPP is also the cofactor for transketolase, a key enzyme in the hexose monophosphate shunt.

Thiamin is found in many foodstuffs, including cereals, grains, beans, nuts, as well as pork and duck. It is often added to food (e.g. in cereals) in developed countries. The dietary requirement (see Table 5.8) depends on energy intake, more being required if the diet is high in carbohydrates.

Following absorption, thiamin is found in all body tissues, the majority being in the liver. Body stores are small and signs of deficiency quickly develop with inadequate intake.

There is no evidence that a high oral intake is dangerous, but ataxia has been reported after high parenteral therapy.

Thiamin deficiency

Thiamin deficiency is seen:

- as beriberi, where the only food consumed is polished rice
- in chronic alcohol-dependent patients who are consuming virtually no food at all

(a)

(b)

Fig. 5.7 **(a) Thiamin. (b) Pellagra.** A child with pellagra showing chronic thickening and pigmentation of the skin, particularly on the backs of hands. Courtesy of Professor David Warrell.

- rarely in starved patients (e.g. with carcinoma of the stomach), and in severe prolonged hyperemesis gravidarum, especially when treated by intravenous fluids alone.

Beriberi

This is now confined to the poorest areas of South East Asia. It can be prevented by eating undermilled or parboiled rice, or by fortification of rice with thiamine. Probably the most important factor in the reduction of beriberi is the general increase in overall food consumption so that the staple diet is varied and contains legumes and pulses, which contain a large amount of thiamin. There are two main clinical types of beriberi, which, surprisingly, only rarely occur together.

Dry beriberi usually presents insidiously with a symmetrical polyneuropathy. The initial symptoms are heaviness and stiffness of the legs, followed by weakness, numbness, and pins and needles. The ankle jerk reflexes are lost and eventually all the signs of polyneuropathy that may involve the trunk and arms are found (p. 1262). Cerebral involvement occurs, producing the picture of the Wernicke–Korsakoff syndrome (p. 1263). In endemic areas, mild symptoms and signs may be present for years without unduly affecting the patient.

Wet beriberi causes oedema. Initially this is of the legs, but it can extend to involve the whole body, with ascites and pleural effusions. The peripheral oedema may mask the accompanying features of dry beriberi.

Thiamin deficiency impairs pyruvate dehydrogenase with accumulation of lactate and pyruvate, producing peripheral vasodilatation and eventually oedema. The heart muscle is also affected and heart failure occurs, causing a further increase in the oedema. Initially there are warm extremities, a full, fast, bounding pulse and a raised venous pressure ('high-output state'), but eventually heart failure advances and a poor cardiac output ensues. The electrocardiogram may show conduction defects.

Infantile beriberi occurs, usually acutely, in breast-fed babies at approximately 3 months of age. The mothers show no signs of thiamin deficiency but presumably their body stores must be virtually nil. The infant becomes anorexic, develops oedema and has some degree of aphonia. Tachycardia and tachypnoea develop and, unless treatment is instituted, death occurs quickly.

Diagnosis

In endemic areas the diagnosis of beriberi should always be suspected and if in doubt treatment with thiamine should be instituted. A rapid disappearance of oedema after thiamine (50 mg i.m.) is diagnostic. Other causes of oedema must be considered (e.g. renal or liver disease), and the polyneuropathy is indistinguishable from that due to other causes. The diagnosis is confirmed by measurement of the circulating thiamin concentration or transketolase activity in red cells using fresh heparinized blood. This enzyme is dependent on TPP. The assay is performed with and without added TPP; an increase in activity of 25% with TPP indicates deficiency.

Treatment

Thiamine 50 mg i.m. is given for 3 days, followed by 25 mg of thiamine daily by mouth. The response in wet beriberi occurs in hours, giving dramatic improvement, but in dry beriberi improvement is often slow to occur. In most cases all the B vitamins are given because of multiple deficiency. Infantile beriberi is treated by giving thiamine to the mother, which is then passed on to the infant via the breast milk.

Thiamin deficiency in patients with alcohol dependence or acute illness

In the western world alcohol-dependent patients and those with severe acute illness receiving high carbohydrate infusions without vitamins are the only major groups to suffer from thiamin deficiency. Rarely they develop wet beriberi, which must be distinguished from alcoholic cardiomyopathy. More usually, however, thiamin deficiency presents with polyneuropathy or with the Wernicke–Korsakoff syndrome.

This syndrome, which consists of dementia, ataxia, varying ophthalmoplegia and nystagmus (see p. 1263), presents acutely and should be suspected in all heavy drinkers. If treated promptly it is reversible; if left it becomes irreversible. It is a major cause of dementia in the USA.

Urgent treatment with thiamine 250 mg i.m. or i.v. twice daily is given for 3 days, often combined with other B-complex vitamins. Anaphylaxis can occur. Thiamine must always be given before any intravenous glucose infusion.

Riboflavin

Riboflavin is widely distributed throughout all plant and animal cells. Good sources are dairy products, offal and leafy vegetables. Riboflavin is not destroyed appreciably by cooking, but is destroyed by sunlight. Riboflavin is a flavoprotein that is a cofactor for many oxidative reactions in the cell.

There is no definite deficiency, although many communities have low dietary intakes. Studies in volunteers taking a low riboflavin diet have produced:

- angular stomatitis or cheilosis (fissuring at the corners of the mouth)
- a red, inflamed tongue

- seborrhoeic dermatitis, particularly involving the face (around the nose) and the scrotum or vulva.

Conjunctivitis with vascularization of the cornea and opacity of the lens has also been described. It is probable, however, that many of the above features are due to multiple deficiencies rather than the riboflavin itself.

Riboflavin 5 mg daily can be tried for the above conditions, usually given as the vitamin B complex.

Niacin

This is the generic name for the two chemical forms, nicotinic acid and nicotinamide, the latter being found in the two pyridine nucleotides, nicotinamide adenine dinucleotide (NAD) and nicotinamide adenine dinucleotide phosphate (NADP). Both act as hydrogen acceptors in many oxidative reactions, and in their reduced forms (NADH and NADPH) act as hydrogen donors in reductive reactions. Many oxidative steps in the production of energy require NAD, and NADP is equally necessary in the hexose monophosphate shunt (p. 446) for the generation of NADPH, which is necessary for fatty-acid synthesis.

Niacin is found in many foodstuffs, including plants, meat (particularly offal) and fish. Niacin is lost by removing bran from cereals but is added to processed cereals and white bread in many countries.

Niacin can be synthesized in humans from tryptophan, 60 mg of tryptophan being converted to 1 mg of niacin. The amount of niacin in food is given as the 'niacin equivalent', which is equal to the amount of niacin plus one-sixtieth of the tryptophan content. Eggs and cheese contain tryptophan.

Kynureninase and kynurenine hydroxylase are both B_6 and riboflavin dependent, and deficiency of these B vitamins can also produce pellagra.

Pellagra

This is rare and is found in people who eat virtually only maize, for example in parts of Africa. Maize contains niacin in the form of niacytin, which is biologically unavailable, and has a low content of tryptophan. In central America, pellagra has always been rare because maize (for the cooking of tortillas) is soaked overnight in calcium hydroxide, which releases niacin. Many of the features of pellagra can be explained purely by niacin deficiency; but some are probably due to multiple deficiencies, including deficiencies of proteins and of other vitamins.

Clinical features

The classical features are of dermatitis (5.7b), diarrhoea and dementia. Although this is an easily remembered triad, not all are always present and the mental changes are not a true dementia.

- *Dermatitis*. In the areas of skin exposed to sunlight, initially there is redness followed by cracks with occasional ulceration. Chronic thickening, dryness and pigmentation develop. The lesions are always symmetrical and often affect the dorsal surfaces of the hands. The perianal skin and vulva are frequently involved. Casal's necklace or collar is the term given to the skin lesion around the neck, which is confined to this area by the clothes worn.

- *Diarrhoea*. This is often a feature but constipation is occasionally seen. Other gastrointestinal manifestations include a painful, red, raw tongue, glossitis and angular stomatitis. Recurring mouth infections occur.
- *Dementia*. This occurs in chronic disease. In milder cases there are symptoms of depression, apathy and sometimes thought disorders. Tremor and an encephalopathy frequently occur. Hallucinations and acute psychosis are seen with more severe cases.

Pellagra may also occur in the following circumstances:

- Isoniazid therapy can lead to a deficiency of vitamin B$_6$, which is needed for the synthesis of nicotinamide from tryptophan. Vitamin B$_6$ is now given concomitantly with isoniazid.
- In Hartnup's disease, a rare inborn error, in which basic amino acids including tryptophan are not absorbed by the gut. There is also loss of this amino acid in the urine.
- In generalized malabsorption (rare).
- In alcohol-dependent patients who do not eat.
- Very low protein diets given for renal disease or taken as a food fad.
- In the carcinoid syndrome and phaeochromocytomas, tryptophan metabolism is diverted away from the formation of nicotinamide to form amines.

Diagnosis and treatment

In endemic areas this is based on the clinical features, remembering that other vitamin deficiencies can produce similar changes (e.g. angular stomatitis). Nicotinamide (approximately 300 mg daily by mouth) with a maintenance dose of 50 mg daily is given with dramatic improvement in the skin and diarrhoea. Mostly, however, vitamin B complex is given, as other deficiencies are often present.

An increase in the protein content of the diet and treatment of malnutrition and other vitamin deficiencies is essential.

Vitamin B$_6$

Vitamin B$_6$ exists as pyridoxine, pyridoxal and pyridoxamine, and is found widely in plant and animal foodstuffs. Pyridoxal phosphate is a cofactor in the metabolism of many amino acids. Dietary deficiency is extremely rare. Some drugs (e.g. isoniazid, hydralazine and penicillamine) interact with pyridoxal phosphate, producing B$_6$ deficiency. The polyneuropathy occurring after isoniazid usually responds to vitamin B$_6$.

Sideroblastic anaemia occasionally responds to vitamin B$_6$ (see p. 429). A polyneuropathy has occurred after high doses (> 200 mg) given over many months. Vitamin B$_6$ is used for premenstrual tension: a daily dose of 10 mg should not be exceeded.

Biotin and pantothenic acid

Biotin is involved in a number of carboxylase reactions. It occurs in many foodstuffs and the dietary requirement is small. Deficiency is extremely rare and is confined to a few people who consume raw eggs, which contain an antagonist (avidin) to biotin. It has also been reported in patients receiving long-term parenteral nutrition without adequate amounts of biotin. It causes a dermatitis that responds to biotin replacements.

Pantothenic acid is widely distributed in all foods and deficiency in humans has not been described.

Vitamin C

Ascorbic acid is a simple sugar and a powerful reducing agent, its main role being to control the redox potential within cells. It is involved in the hydroxylation of proline to hydroxyproline, which is necessary for the formation of collagen. The failure of this biochemical pathway in vitamin C deficiency accounts for virtually all of the clinical effects seen.

Humans, along with a few other animals (e.g. primates and the guinea-pig), are unusual in not being able to synthesize ascorbic acid from glucose.

Vitamin C is present in all fresh fruit and vegetables. Unfortunately, ascorbic acid is easily leached out of vegetables when they are placed in water and it is also oxidized to dehydro-ascorbic acid during cooking or exposure to copper or alkalis. Potatoes are a good source as many people eat a lot of them, but vitamin C is lost during storage.

It has been suggested that ascorbic acid in high dosage (1–2 g daily) will prevent the common cold. While there is some scientific support for this, clinical trials have shown no significant effect. Vitamin C supplements have also been advocated to prevent atherosclerosis and cancer, but again a clear benefit has not been demonstrated.

Vitamin C deficiency is seen mainly in infants fed boiled milk and in the elderly and single people who do not eat vegetables. In the UK it is also seen in Asians eating only rice and chapattis, and in food faddists.

Scurvy

In adults the early symptoms may be non-specific, with weakness and muscle pain. Other features are shown in Table 5.11. In infantile scurvy there is irritability, painful legs, anaemia and characteristic subperiosteal haemorrhages, particularly into the ends of long bones.

Table 5.11 **Clinical features of vitamin C deficiency**
Keratosis of hair follicles with 'corkscrew' hair
Perifollicular haemorrhages
Swollen, spongy gums with bleeding and superadded infection, loosening of teeth
Spontaneous bruising
Spontaneous haemorrhage
Anaemia
Failure of wound healing

Diagnosis

The anaemia is usually hypochromic but occasionally a normochromic or megaloblastic anaemia is seen. The type of anaemia depends on whether iron deficiency (owing to decreased absorption or loss due to haemorrhage) or folate deficiency (folate being largely found in green vegetables) is present.

Plasma ascorbic acid is very low in obvious deficiency and a vitamin C level of less than 11 μmol/L (0.2 mg per 100 mL) indicates vitamin C deficiency. The leucocyte–platelet layer (buffy coat) of centrifuged blood corresponds to vitamin C concentrations in other tissues. The normal level of leucocyte ascorbate is 1.1–2.8 pmol per 10^6 cells.

Treatment

Initially the patient is given 250 mg of ascorbic acid daily and encouraged to eat fresh fruit and vegetables. Subsequently, 40 mg daily will maintain a normal exchangeable body pool of about 900 mg (5.1 mmol).

Prevention

Orange juice should be given to bottle-fed infants. The intake of breast-fed infants depends on the mother's diet. In the elderly, eating adequate fruit and vegetables is the best way to avoid scurvy. Careful surveillance of the elderly, particularly those who live alone, is necessary. Ascorbic acid supplements should only be necessary occasionally.

Vitamin B_{12} and folate

These are dealt with on page 430 and daily requirements are shown in Table 5.8. In many developed countries, up to 15% of the population have a partial deficiency of 5,10-methylene tetrahydrofolate reductase, a key folate-metabolizing enzyme. This is due to a point mutation and is associated with an increase in neural tube defects and hyperhomocysteinaemia, which may lead to cardiovascular damage. Autoantibodies against folate receptors have been found in women who have had a pregnancy complicated by neural tube defects.

In the USA and some other countries, enriched cereals are fortified with 1.4 mg/kg grain of folic acid to increase daily requirements.

Dietary antioxidants

Free radicals are generated during inflammatory processes, radiotherapy, and smoking, and during the course of a wide range of diseases. They may cause uncontrolled damage of multiple cellular components, the most sensitive of which are unsaturated lipids, proteins and DNA and they also disrupt the normal replication process. They have been implicated as a cause of a wide range of diseases, including malignant, acute inflammatory and traumatic diseases, cardiovascular disease, neurodegenerative conditions such as Alzheimer's disease, senile macular degeneration, and cataract. The defence against uncontrolled damage by free radicals is provided by antioxidant enzymes (e.g. catalase, super-oxide dismutase) and antioxidants, which may be endogenous (e.g. glutathione) or exogenous (e.g. vitamins C and E, carotenoids). A possible causal link between antioxidant and cardiovascular disease has emerged from epidemiological studies although several RCTs have not confirmed this.

Epidemiological studies
Dietary intake
- A high intake of fruits and vegetables has been linked to reduced risk of heart disease, cerebrovascular disease and total cardiovascular morbidity and mortality.
- A high intake of nuts (rich in vitamin E) and dietary components, e.g. red wine, onions, apples (rich in flavonoids), which are strong scavengers of free radicals, have also been linked to reduced risk of cardiovascular disease.
- The seasonal variation in cardiovascular disease, which is higher in winter, has been related to decreased intake of fresh fruit and vegetables.
- The decline in cardiovascular disease in the USA since the 1950s has been associated with a simultaneous increase in the intake of fresh fruit and vegetables.

Status of antioxidant nutrients.
The level of antioxidant nutrients in the circulation, has been reported to be inversely related to cardiovascular morbidity and mortality, extent of atherosclerosis assessed by ultrasound, and clinical signs of ischaemic heart disease. The tissue content of lycopene, a marker of vegetable intake, has been reported to be low in patients with myocardial infarction.

Antioxidants, especially vitamin E, have been shown to prevent the initiation and progression of atherosclerotic disease in animals. They also reduce the oxidation of low-density lipoprotein (LDL) in the arterial wall in vitro. Oxidation of LDL is an initial event in the atherosclerotic process (p. 798).

Randomized controlled trials (RCT) (see also p. 998)
For primary or secondary prevention of cardiovascular disease, intervention with β-carotene, α-tocopherol (vitamin E) and ascorbic acid (vitamin C) has demonstrated no significant benefit. Similarly, intervention with vitamin E or β-carotene in particular conditions, such as stroke and fatal and non-fatal myocardial infarction, has also not yielded benefits. Therefore the initial optimism, based on epidemiological studies, is not borne out by RCT evidence. Indeed, healthy individuals given carotene and tocopherol showed an increased risk of intracerebral and subarachnoid haemorrhage, and a meta-analysis has shown a small increased risk of cardiovascular death and all-cause mortality. An increase in the risk of developing lung cancer has also been established from a systematic analysis of administering large doses of β-carotene to smokers. However, there are limitations to published RCTs. For example, some RCTs have used single rather than multiple antioxidants, the ratios of vitamin E and C combinations may have been different from normal dietary intakes, the doses given may have been insufficient

or too large, the duration may not have been long enough, and the correct metabolic effects may not have been measured. In addition, some of the trials were not set up to primarily assess the cardiovascular risk, some trials have only been in smokers and, lastly, the conditions may have been unsuitable for antioxidants to manifest their properties.

It is also possible that epidemiological studies are confounded by other associated variables, e.g. eating a low-fat diet or undertaking more exercise. The latter may be more valuable in the causal pathway than the intake of antioxidants. Diets rich in fresh fruit and vegetables also contain a range of antioxidants that were not tested in the clinical trials. Therefore, the results of large-scale randomized controlled trials using various combinations and doses of antioxidant nutrients are currently awaited. In the meantime, the policy of encouraging 'healthy' behaviour, which includes increased physical activity, and a varied diet rich in fresh fruit and vegetables, and nuts, is still generally recommended both for the population as a whole and for those at risk of cardiovascular disease.

Homocysteine, cardiovascular disease and B vitamins

The circulating concentration of the amino acid homocysteine is an independent risk factor for cardiovascular disease. A high concentration is related to ischaemic heart disease, stroke, thrombosis, pulmonary embolism, coronary artery restenosis, and heart failure. The strength of the association is similar to that with smoking or hyperlipidaemia. An elevation in homocysteine concentration by 5 μmol/L has been estimated to double the risk of death in patients with coronary heart disease. The risk of cardiovascular disease is *low* when serum homocysteine is < 10 μmol/L, *mildly increased* at 10–15 μmol/L, and *high* above 15 μmol/L (p. 802).

It is estimated that 5–20% of the population have a homocysteine concentration > 15 μmol/L. Factors that increase the plasma homocysteine concentration include physiological factors (male gender, menopause, and increasing age), lifestyle (smoking, high coffee and alcohol intake, and inactivity), vitamin deficiencies (or a low intake of folate, B_{12}, B_6, B_2) and organ dysfunction (liver and kidney dysfunction). It may also result from prescription of some drugs and from genetic causes (see below).

Proposed mechanisms, based on experimental evidence, by which homocysteine detrimentally affects vascular function, include (a) the direct damaging effects of homocysteine on epithelial cells of blood vessels, (b) an increase in blood vessel stiffness, and (c) an increase in blood coagulation. Homocysteine is not found in food and its formation within the body is dependent on enzymatic reactions that involve folic acid, vitamin B_{12} and vitamin B_6 (Fig. 5.8).

A large meta-analysis of the genotypes of the enzyme methylene tetrahydrofolate reductase showed that the presence of cytosine instead of thymidine in the gene coding for this enzyme, increases the plasma homocysteine concentration, and at the same time the risk of

Fig. 5.8 **Homocysteine metabolism.**

cardiovascular disease. Since there is no relationship between this mutation and other cardiovascular risk factors, it appears that a direct causal link between homocysteine concentrations and the cardiovascular risk is more likely. In the rare autosomal recessive genetic disorder, homocysteinuria, high homocysteine concentrations are associated with premature cardiovascular problems and a thrombotic tendency.

It has been estimated that a reduction in concentration by as little as 3 μmol/L, reduces the risk of ischaemic heart disease by 16%, of deep vein thrombosis by 25% and of stroke by 24%. A reduction in homocysteine concentration following administration of three B vitamins (folic acid, vitamin B_{12} and vitamin B_6) reduced the rate and severity of coronary artery restenosis 6–12 months after angioplasty compared to control patients receiving a placebo. However, a recent trial using the same therapy after coronary stenting showed an increased risk of restenosis and further studies are awaited.

Prevalence

Deficiencies of these vitamins are common, especially in the elderly. The National Diet and Nutrition Survey for people aged 65 years and over in the UK revealed that in free-living individuals folate deficiency was present in 29% of subjects (severe deficiency in 8%), and vitamin B_{12} deficiency in 8%. The values for pyridoxine deficiency are not clearly established in the elderly; about half the values were outside the normal range for younger adult populations.

Prevention

Administration of these vitamins, especially folic acid, reduces the circulating concentration of homocysteine, depending on the genotype of the enzyme methylene tetrahydrofolate reductase. Finally, the administration of these vitamins is relatively simple and inexpensive. Folic acid fortification of food is already practised in some countries, including the USA, but not in the UK. There are now a large number of intervention trials assessing the effects of folate, B_{12} and pyridoxine on cardiovascular risk.

FURTHER READING

Asplund K (2002) Antioxidant vitamins in the prevention of cardiovascular disease: a systematic review. *Journal of Internal Medicine* **251**: 372–392.

Carmel R, Jacobsen DW (2001) *Homocysteine in Health and Disease*. New York: Cambridge Academic Press.

Herrmann MC (2004) Prevention of cardiovascular events after percutaneous coronary intervention. *New England Journal of Medicine* **350**: 2708–2710.

Institute of Medicine (2000) *Dietary Reference Intakes for Thiamin, Riboflavin, Niacin, Vitamin B_6, Folate, Vitamin B_{12}, Pantothenic Acid, Biotin, and Choline*. Washington DC: National Academic Press.

Vivekananthan DP, Penn MS, Sapp SK et al. (2003) Use of antioxidant vitamins for the prevention of cardiovascular disease: meta-analysis of randomised trials. *Lancet* **361**: 2017–2023.

Wald DS, Law M, Morris JK (2002) Homocysteine and cardiovascular disease: evidence on causality from meta-analysis. *British Medical Journal* **325**: 1202–1206.

MINERALS

A number of minerals have been shown to be essential in animals, and an increasing number of deficiency syndromes are becoming recognized in humans. Long-term total parenteral nutrition allowed trace element deficiency to be studied in controlled conditions; now trace elements are always added to long-term parenteral nutrition regimens. It is highly probable (but difficult to study because of multiple deficiencies) that trace-element deficiency is also a frequent accompaniment of all PEM states. Sodium (RNI 70 mmol/day), potassium (RNI 90 mmol/day), magnesium (RNI 12.3 mmol/day for men and 10.9 for women) and chloride are discussed in Chapter 12.

Iron (see also p. 426)

The daily RNI for men is 160 μmol (8.7 mg) and for women 260 μmol (14.8 mg). Iron deficiency is common world-wide, affecting both developing and developed countries. It is particularly prevalent in women of a reproductive age. Dietary iron overload is seen in South African men who cook and brew in iron pots.

Copper

The daily RNI of copper is 1.2 mg (19 μmol). Shellfish, legumes, cereals and nuts are good dietary sources.

Deficiency

Menkes' kinky hair syndrome is a rare condition caused by malabsorption of copper. The Menkes' disease gene (*ATP7A*) encodes a copper-transporting ATPase and has a homology to the gene in Wilson's disease. Infants with this sex-linked recessive abnormality develop growth failure, mental retardation, bone lesions and brittle hair. Anaemia and neutropenia also occur. This condition,

which serves as a model for copper deficiency, supports the idea that some of the clinical features seen in PEM are due to copper deficiency. Breast and cow's milk are low in copper, and supplementation is occasionally necessary when first treating PEM.

Copper toxicity

This occurs in Wilson's disease; see page 387.

Zinc

The daily RNI of zinc is 9.5 mg (145 μmol) for men, 7 mg (110 μmol) for women and it is widely available in food. Zinc is involved in many metabolic pathways, often acting as a coenzyme; it is essential for the synthesis of RNA and DNA.

Deficiency

Acrodermatitis enteropathica is an inherited disorder caused by malabsorption of zinc. Infants develop growth retardation, severe diarrhoea, hair loss and associated *Candida* and bacterial infections. This condition provides a model for zinc deficiency. Zinc supplementation results in a complete cure. Deficiency probably also plays a role in PEM.

Zinc levels have been shown to be low in some patients with malabsorption or skin disease, and in patients with AIDS, but the exact role of zinc in these situations is disputed. Zinc has low toxicity, but high zinc levels from water stored in galvanized containers interfere with iron and copper metabolism. Wound healing is impaired with moderate zinc deficiency and is improved by zinc supplements. Impaired taste and smell, hair loss and night blindness are also features of severe zinc deficiency.

Iodine

The daily RNI of iodine is 140 μg (1.1 μmol) for men and women, and it is found in milk, meat and seafoods.

It exists in foodstuffs as inorganic iodides which are efficiently absorbed. Iodine is a constituent of the thyroid hormones (p. 1069).

Deficiency

Many mountainous areas throughout the world lack iodine in the soil, and so iodine deficiency, which impairs brain development, is a WHO priority. Endemic goitre occurs in remote areas where the daily intake is below 70 μg, and in those parts 1–5% of babies are born with cretinism. In these areas, iodized oil should be given intramuscularly to all reproductive women every 3–5 years. In developed countries, salt is iodized and endemic goitre has disappeared.

Fluoride

In areas where the level of fluoride in drinking water is less than 1 p.p.m. (0.7–1.2 mg/L), dental caries is relatively more prevalent. Fluoridation of the water provides 1–2 mg daily, resulting in a reduction of about 50% of tooth decay in children. There is little fluoride in food except for seafish and tea, the latter providing 70% of the daily intake. Fluoride-containing toothpaste may add up to 2 mg a day.

Excessive fluoride intake in areas where the water fluoride level is above 3 mg/L can result in fluorosis, in which there is infiltration into the enamel of the teeth, producing pitting and discoloration.

Selenium

Clinical deficiency of selenium is rare except in areas of China where Keshan disease, a selenium-responsive cardiomyopathy, occurs. Selenium deficiency may also cause a myopathy. Toxicity has been described with very high intakes.

Calcium (see also p. 591)

In the UK, the daily RNI of calcium is 700 mg (17.5 mmol), but substantially higher values are now recommended in the USA. It is found in many foodstuffs, with two-thirds of the intake coming from milk and milk products, only 5% from vegetables. In the UK most flour is fortified. Calcium absorption from the gastrointestinal tract is vitamin D-dependent. Ninety-nine per cent of body calcium is in the skeleton.

Increased calcium is required in pregnancy and lactation, when dietary intake must be increased. Calcium deficiency is usually due to vitamin D deficiency.

Phosphate (see also p. 711)

The daily RNI of phosphate is the same as that of calcium, i.e. 17.5 mmol. Phosphates are present in all natural foods, and dietary deficiency has not been described. Patients taking large amounts of aluminium hydroxide can, however, develop phosphate deficiency owing to binding in the gut lumen. It can also be seen in total parenteral nutrition. Symptoms include anorexia, weakness and osteoporosis.

Other trace elements

The possible significance of cadmium, chromium, cobalt, manganese, molybdenum, nickel and vanadium is shown in Table 5.12.

Table 5.12	Other trace elements (see text)
Element	**Deficiency**
Cadmium	?
Chromium	Glucose intolerance
Cobalt	Anaemia (vitamin B_{12})
Manganese	Skin rash, ? osteoporosis, ? mood
Molybdenum	? (case study involving parenteral nutrition)
Nickel	? Animals only
Vanadium	?

FURTHER READING
Institute of Medicine (2001) *Dietary Reference Intakes for Vitamin A, Vitamin K, Arsenic, Chromium, Copper, Iodine, Iron, Manganese, Molybdenum, Silicon, Vanadium, and Zinc.* Washington DC: IOM.

NUTRITION AND AGEING

Many animal studies have shown that life expectancy can be extended by restricting food intake. It is, however, not known whether the ageing process in humans can be altered by nutrition.

The ageing process

The process of ageing is not well understood. While wear and tear may play a role, it is an insufficient explanation for the causation of ageing. The 'programmed' theories depend on inbuilt biological clocks that regulate lifespan, and involve genes that are responsible for controlling signals that influence various body systems. The 'error' theories involve environmental stressors that induce damage (e.g. mitochondrial DNA damage or cross-linking).

The search for a single cause of ageing, e.g. a single gene defect, has been replaced by the view that ageing is a complex multifactorial process that involves an interaction between genetic, environmental, and stochastic (random damage to essential molecules) causes. The following theories have been suggested:

Molecular theories
- *Gene regulation* – ageing, for example, results from changes in expression of genes that regulate both development and ageing. An insulin-like signalling pathway has been linked to the lifespan of worms, flies and mice (activation of a transcription factor in response to reduced insulin-like signalling prolongs lifespan).
- *Codon restriction* – inadequate mRNA translation resulting from inadequate decoding of codons in mRNA.
- *Error catastrophe* – errors in gene expression result in abnormal proteins.
- *Somatic mutation* – cumulative molecular damage mainly to genetic material.
- *Dysdifferentiation* – cumulative random molecular damage detrimentally affects gene expression.

Cellular theories
- *Cellular senescence-telomere* – an increase in senescent cells occurs from:
  (a) Loss of telomeres, which is known to occur with ageing (with each cell division a small amount of DNA is necessarily lost at each end of the chromosome). Activation of the telomerase enzyme regenerates telomeres, prevents senescence (replicative senescence) and immortalizes cell cultures. Cancer cells are known to activate telomerase.

(b) Damage due to a variety of other factors, including DNA damage (stress-induced senescence).

- *Free radical* – production of free radicals during oxidative metabolism which damages fat, protein and DNA.
- *Wear and tear* – cumulative damage from normal injury/stress which is unable to repair itself.
- *Apoptosis theory* – programmed cell death due to genetic events

System theories

These theories involve loss in the function of neuro-endocrine or immune systems with consequent age-related physiological changes and an increase in autoimmunity.

Whole body metabolism and energy expenditure theory proposes that there is a fixed limit to the cumulative energy expenditure and metabolism during a lifetime, so that if this limit is reached quickly the lifespan is short. Energy restriction in rodents reduces energy expenditure and prolongs lifespan, but there is a lack of studies in primates or humans.

Evolutionary theories

- *Cumulative mutation* – mutations that accumulate during the lifetime act in older age rather than during the active reproductive period (for which there is evolutionary selection), producing pathology and senescence. The theory was initially based on the observation that Huntington's disease, a dominant lethal mutation which typically manifests itself between 35 and 55 years, allows affected individuals to reproduce.
- *Disposable soma* – the somatic body is maintained to ensure reproductive success, after which it is disposable. Factors that may enhance reproductive success may have detrimental effects on ageing – a possible example being androgen secretion, which may be beneficial to reproduction but potentially detrimental with development of prostatic cancer and cardiovascular disease in later life.

Several of these theories have strong nutritional components. *Disability and dependency* in older humans are at least partly due to poor nutrition, and correction of deficiencies or nutrient imbalances can prevent the decline in function from falling below the disability threshold (Fig. 5.9). In this way some loss of function may be prevented or reversed, especially if other measures, such as physical activity, which increases muscle mass and strength are undertaken.

Early origins of health and disease in older adults

A low birth weight (and or length) is associated with reduced height, as well as reduced mass and fat-free mass in adult life. These relationships can occur independently of genetic factors, since the smaller of identical twins becomes a shorter and lighter adult. Relationships have also been reported between growth of the fetus and a variety of diseases and risk factors for disease in adults and older people. These include cardiovascular disease, especially ischaemic heart disease, hypertension, and diabetes, and even obesity and fat distribution. However, the strength of association for some of these conditions is in some cases weak. Animal studies involving dietary modifications during pregnancy or early postnatal life (e.g. protein, zinc), even within the normal range of intakes, have clearly demonstrated effects, such as hypertension, which persist through the lifetime of the offspring, and even their offspring. The extent to which these apply to humans is uncertain, and the mechanisms are poorly understood. Since relationships with cardiovascular disease in old age have also been related to growth in the first few years of life as well as starvation during puberty, it is likely that cumulative environmental stresses, including nutritional, from the time of implantation of the fertilized egg, to fetal and postnatal growth and development, and adult life, summate to produce an overall disease risk (Fig. 5.9).

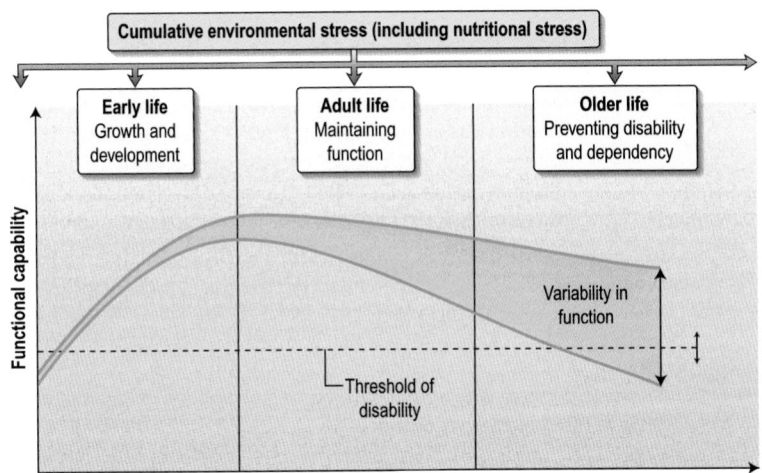

Fig. 5.9 **Nutrition and ageing.** Nutrition is a contributory cause of the variability in function during the lifespan. Appropriate nutrition may improve function, or delay deterioration below the threshold of disability and dependence.

Nutritional requirements in the elderly

These are qualitatively similar to the requirements of younger adults, but as energy expenditure is less, there is a lower energy requirement. However, maintaining physical activity is required for the overall health of the elderly.

The daily energy requirement of 'elderly people' (aged 60 and above, irrespective of age) has been set to be approximately $1.5 \times$ BMR. The BMR is reduced, owing to a fall in the fat-free mass, from an average of 60 kg to 50 kg in men and from 40 kg to 35 kg in women. In disease, physical activity is usually decreased. The diet should contain approximately the same *proportions* of nutrients, and essential nutrients are still required. Although disabilities and diseases are common in older people, the RNIs are intended for healthy people without disease. The nutrient requirements for those with disease are less well defined.

Nutritional deficits in the elderly are common and may be due to many factors, such as dental problems, lack of cooking skills (particularly in widowers), depression and lack of motivation. Significant malnourishment in developed countries is usually secondary to social problems or disease. In the elderly who are institutionalized, multiple nutrient deficiencies are common. Vitamin D supplements may be required because often these people do not go into the sunlight. Owing to the high prevalence of osteoporosis in elderly people, daily calcium intake of 1–1.5 g/day is often recommended.

FURTHER READING

Finch S, Doyle W, Lowe C et al. (1998) *National Diet and Nutrition Survey: People Aged 65 Years and Over.* London: The Stationery Office.

O' Brien PMS, Wheeler T, Barker DPJ (1999) Fetal Programming. *Influences on Development and Disease in Later Life.* London: Royal College of Obstetricians and Gynaecologists Press.

Schurch B, Scrimshaw NS (2000) Impact of human ageing on energy and protein metabolism and requirements. Proceeding of an IDECG workshop, Boston USA, May 3–6, 1999. *European Journal of Clinical Nutrition* **54** (Suppl 3): S1–S165.

Sohal RS (2002) The role of oxidative stress and protein oxidation in the aging process. *Free Radical Biology and Medicine* **33**: 37–44.

Tatar M, Bartle A, Antebi A (2003) The endocrine regulation of aging by insulin-like signals. *Science* **299**: 1346–1351.

Vijg J, Suh Y (2003) Functional genomics of ageing. *Mechanisms of Ageing and Development* **124**: 3–8.

Weinert BT, Timiras PS (2003) Physiology of aging. Invited review: theories of aging. *Journal of Applied Physiology* **95**: 1706–1716.

WHO (2002) Active Aging: A Policy Framework. Geneva: WHO.

OBESITY

Obesity is almost invariable in developing countries and almost all people accumulate some fat as they get older.

Table 5.13 Conditions in which obesity is an associated feature

Genetic syndromes associated with hypogonadism (e.g. Prader–Willi syndrome, Laurence–Moon–Biedl syndrome)
Hypothyroidism
Cushing's syndrome
Stein–Leventhal syndrome
Drug-induced (e.g. corticosteroids)
Hypothalamic damage (e.g. due to trauma, tumour)

The World Health Organization also acknowledges that obesity (body mass index $> 30 \text{ kg/m}^2$) is a worldwide problem which also affects many developing countries. Obesity implies an excess storage of fat, and this can most easily be detected by looking at the undressed patient.

Most patients suffer from *simple obesity*, but in certain conditions obesity is an associated feature (Table 5.13). Even in the latter situation, the intake of calories must have exceeded energy expenditure over a prolonged period of time. Hormonal imbalance is often incriminated in women (e.g. postmenopause or when taking contraceptive pills), but most weight gain in such cases is usually small and due to water retention.

Not all obese people eat more than the average person, but all obviously eat more than they need.

Suggested mechanisms
Genetic and environmental factors

These have always been difficult to separate when studying obesity. However, refeeding experiments in both monozygotic and dizygotic twins, reared together or apart, suggest that genetic influences account for 70% of the difference in body mass index (BMI) later in life, and that the childhood environment has little or no influence.

These refeeding experiments also showed that weight gain did not occur in all pairs of twins, suggesting that in some a facultative increase in thermogenesis occurred so that part of their extra dietary energy was expended inefficiently. Genetic factors have led to the discovery of a putative gene, firstly in the obese (*ob ob*) mouse and now in humans. The *ob* gene was shown to be expressed solely in both white and brown adipose tissue. The *ob* gene is found on chromosome 7 and produces a 16 kDa protein called leptin. In the *ob ob* mouse a mutation in the *ob* gene leads to production of a non-functioning protein. Administration of normal leptin to these obese mice reduces food intake and corrects the obesity. A similar situation has been described in a very rare genetic condition causing obesity in humans, in which leptin is not expressed.

In massively obese subjects, leptin mRNA in subcutaneous adipose tissue is 80% higher than in controls. Plasma levels of leptin are also very high, correlating with the BMI. Weight loss due to food restriction decreases plasma levels of leptin. However, in contrast to the *ob ob* mouse, the leptin structure is normal, and abnormalities in leptin are not the prime cause of human obesity.

Leptin secreted from fat cells was thought to act as a feedback mechanism between the adipose tissue and the brain, acting as a 'lipostat' (adipostat), controlling fat stores by regulating hunger and satiety (see below). However, many other signals are involved. It is interesting that obesity is largely restricted to humans, and animals that are domesticated or in zoos.

Food intake

Many factors related to the home environment, such as finance and the availability of sweets and snacks, will affect food intake. Some individuals eat more during periods of heavy exercise or during pregnancy and are unable to get back to their former eating habits. The increase in obesity in social class 5 can usually be related to the type of food consumed (i.e. food containing sugar and fat). Psychological factors and how food is presented may override complex biochemical interactions.

It has been shown that obese patients eat more than they admit to eating, and over the years a very small daily excess can lead to a large accumulation of fat. For example, a 44 kJ (10.5 kcal) daily excess would lead to a 10 kg weight gain over 20 years.

Control of appetite

Appetite is the desire to eat and this usually initiates food intake. Following a meal, satiation occurs. This depends on gastric and duodenal distension and the release of many substances peripherally and centrally.

Following a meal, cholecystokinin (CCK), bombesin, glucagon-like peptide 1 (GLP1), enterostatin, and somatostatin are released from the small intestine, and glucagon and insulin from the pancreas. All of these hormones have been implicated in the control of satiety. Centrally, the hypothalamus – particularly the lateral hypothalamic area, and paraventricular and arcuate nuclei – plays a key role in integrating signals involved in appetite and bodyweight regulation (Fig. 5.10). There are two main pathways in the arcuate nucleus (see Fig. 5.10):

- *The central appetite-stimulating (orexogenic) pathway* in the ventromedial part of the arcuate nucleus, which expresses NPY (neuropeptide Y) and AgRP (agouti-related protein). Animal studies suggest that this pathway also decreases energy expenditure.

- *The central appetite-suppressing (anorexogenic pathway, or leptin–melanocortin pathway)* in the dorsolateral part of the arcuate nucleus, which expresses POMC/CART (pro-opiomelanocortin/cocaine-and-amfetamine-regulated transcript). In this pathway, α-MSH (α-melanocyte-stimulating hormone), formed by cleavage of POMC by PC1 (prohormone convertase), exerts its appetite-suppressing effect via the Mc4R (melanocortin-4 receptors) in areas of the brain that regulate food intake and autonomic activity. Animal studies suggest that this pathway also increases energy expenditure.

These pathways interact with each other and feed into the lateral hypothalamus, which communicates with other parts of the brain, and influence the autonomic nervous system and ingestive behaviour. These central pathways are in turn influenced by a variety of peripheral signals

Fig. 5.10 **Peripheral signals and central pathways (central nervous system) involved in the control of food intake.**
(i) the stimulatory and suppressive peripheral signals and central pathways are identified (NPY/AgRP (neuropeptide Y/agouti-related protein) involved in the stimulatory pathway) and POMC/CART (pro-opiomelanocortin/cocaine-and-amfetamine-regulated transcript) involved in the suppressive pathway). POMC is converted to melanocortins including α-MSH (α-melanocyte-stimulating hormone) through the action of prohormone convertase (PC1).
(ii) The solid red areas represent receptors for a variety of signals (GhR, ghrelin receptor; LepR, leptin receptor; InsR, insulin receptor; Mc3R, melanocortin 3 receptor; Mc4R, melanocortin 4 receptor; Y1R, Y1 subtype of neuropeptide Y (NPY) receptor).
(iii) Asterisks (*) indicate mutations that have resulted in human obesity.
CCK, cholecystokinin; CRH, corticotrophin-releasing hormone; GLP1, glucagon-like peptide; PVN, paraventricular nucleus; PYY, peptide YY; TRH, thyrotrophin-releasing hormone.

which can also be classified as appetite stimulating or appetite suppressing.

- *Peripheral appetite-suppressing: Leptin* and *insulin* act centrally to activate the appetite-suppressing pathway (whilst also inhibiting the appetite-stimulating pathway). Since these hormones circulate in proportion to adipose tissue mass, they can be regarded as long-term signals, although they probably also modulate short-term signals (insulin also responds acutely to meal ingestion). Peptide YY (PYY) is produced by the L cells of the large bowel and distal small bowel in proportion to the energy ingested. The release of this rapidly responsive (short-acting) signal begins shortly after food intake, suggesting that the initial response involves neural pathways, before ingested nutrients reach the site of PYY production. PYY is thought to reduce appetite, at least partly through inhibition of the appetite-stimulating pathway (NPY/AgRP-expressing neurones).

- *Peripheral appetite-stimulating:* Ghrelin is a *28-amino-acetylated peptide* produced by the oxyntic cells of the fundus of the stomach. It is the first known gastrointestinal tract peptide that stimulates appetite by activating the central appetite-stimulating pathway. The circulatory concentration is high before a meal and is reduced rapidly by ingestion of a meal or glucose (cf. peptide YY, which increases after a meal). It may also act as a long-term signal, as its circulating concentration in weight-stable individuals is inversely related to body mass index over a wide range (cf. insulin and leptin which are positively related to BMI (see below)). It is also increased in several situations in which there is a negative energy balance, e.g. long-term exercise, very low-calorie diets, anorexia nervosa and both cancer and cardiac cachexia (an exception is vertical banded gastric bypass surgery, where its concentration is low rather than high).

The single gene mutations affecting this pathway in humans, e.g. leptin, leptin receptor, *POMC*, *Mc4R*, *PC1*, and *SIM1*, are rare and recessive, with the exception of the *Mc4R*, which is common and dominant with incomplete penetrance. It appears that the *Mc4R mutation* accounts for 2–6% of human obesity. Affected individuals are obese without disturbances in pituitary function or resting energy expenditure, although children tend to be tall. However, these mutations are of little significance as obesity is predominantly polygenetic in origin (the human obesity gene map has already identified several hundreds of candidate genes).

The recent obesity epidemic is mainly due to behaviour and lifestyle changes (although it may be that individuals with certain genes are affected more than others) with a trebling in the prevalence of obesity in the UK over the last 25 years.

The control of appetite is extremely complex. For example, if one considers only one signal, i.e. leptin, there can be leptin resistance where obese individuals have high circulating leptin but with no reduction of appetite. Alternatively in starvation there may be inappropriate correlation between leptin release and loss of adipose tissue. It is known that cytokines, such as TNF and IL-2, which are elevated in a wide range of inflammatory and traumatic conditions, also suppress appetite, although the exact pathways involved are not entirely clear. Finally, there are a range of transmitters in the central nervous system, some of which appear to inhibit appetite (dopamine, serotonin, γ-aminobutyric acid) and others which stimulate appetite (e.g. opioids).

Energy expenditure
Basal metabolic rate (BMR). BMR in obese subjects is higher than in lean subjects, which is not surprising since obesity is associated with an increase in lean body mass.

Physical activity. Obese patients tend to expend more energy during physical activity as they have a larger mass to move. On the other hand, many obese patients decrease their amount of physical activity. The energy expended on walking at 3 miles per hour is only 15.5 kJ/min (3.7 kcal/min) and therefore increasing exercise plays only a small part in losing weight. Nevertheless, because increased body fat develops insidiously over many years, any change in energy balance is helpful.

Thermogenesis
About 10% of ingested energy is dissipated as heat and is unconnected with physical activity. This dietary induced thermogenesis has been reported to be lower in obese and post-obese subjects than in lean subjects.

This would tend to favour energy deposition in obesity and those predisposed to obesity. However, other workers have found no difference in dietary induced thermogenesis between lean and obese subjects.

Brown adipose tissue in animals, when stimulated by cold or food, dissipates the energy derived from ingested food into heat. This can be a major component of overall energy balance in small mammals. However, the importance of brown adipose tissue thermogenesis in adult humans is likely to be very small, and of doubtful clinical significance. β_3-Adrenergic receptors are the principal receptors mediating catecholamine-stimulated lipolysis in brown adipose tissue and to a lesser extent at other sites. Drugs with β_3-adrenergic activities have been developed, but side-effects have limited their use.

Morbidity and mortality
Obese patients are at risk of early death, mainly from diabetes, coronary heart disease and cerebrovascular disease. The greater the obesity the higher the morbidity and mortality rates. For example, men who are 10% overweight have a 13% increased risk of death, while the increase in mortality for those 20% overweight is 25%. The rise is less in women, and in men over 65 obesity is not an independent risk factor. Weight reduction reduces this mortality and therefore should be strongly encouraged. The benefits are probably greater in more obese subjects (Table 5.14).

Clinical features
Most patients recognize their own problems, although often they are unaware of the main foods that cause obesity. Many symptoms are related to psychological problems or social pressures, such as the woman who cannot find fashionable clothes to wear.

The degree of obesity can be assessed by comparison with tables of ideal weight for height, from the BMI (Box 5.4), and by measuring skinfold thickness. The latter should be measured over the middle of the triceps muscle; normal values are 20 mm in a man and 30 mm in a woman. A central distribution of body fat (a waist/hip

Box 5.4 Ranges of body mass index (BMI) used to classify degrees of overweight and associated risk of co-morbidities

WHO classification	BMI (kg/m²)	Risk of co-morbidities
Overweight	25–30	Mildly increased
Obese	> 30	
Class I	30–35	Moderate
Class II	35–40	Severe
Class III	> 40	Very severe

Table 5.14 Potential benefits that may result from the loss of 10 kg in patients who are initially 100 kg and suffer from co-morbidities

Mortality	20–25% fall in total mortality 30–40% fall in diabetes-related deaths 40–50% fall in obesity-related cancer deaths
Blood pressure	Fall of about 10 mmHg (systolic and diastolic)
Diabetes	Reduces risk of developing diabetes by > 50% Fall of 30–50% in fasting blood glucose Fall of 15% in HbA_{1c}
Serum lipids	Fall of 10% in total cholesterol Fall of 15% in LDL cholesterol Fall of 30% in triglycerides Increase of 8% in HDL cholesterol

circumference ratio of > 1.0 in men and > 0.9 in women) is associated with a higher risk of morbidity and mortality than is a more peripheral distribution of body fat (waist/hip ratio < 0.85 in men and < 0.75 in women). This is because fat located centrally, especially inside the abdomen, is more sensitive to lipolytic stimuli, with the result that the abnormalities in circulating lipids are more severe.

Table 5.15 shows the conditions and complications that are associated with obesity.

The metabolic syndrome (syndrome X) is a cluster of cardiovascular risk factors associated with excess fat. A commonly used definition (NCEP ATP III) defines the syndrome as the coexistence of three or more of the following five abnormalities: high blood pressure (> 130/85 mmHg); elevated serum triglycerides

Table 5.15 Conditions and complications associated with obesity

Psychological	Hypertension
Osteoarthritis of knees and hips	Breathlessness
Varicose veins	Ischaemic heart disease
Hiatus hernia	Stroke
Gallstones	Diabetes mellitus (type 2)
Postoperative problems	Hyperlipidaemia
Back strain	Menstrual abnormalities
Accident proneness	Increased morbidity and mortality
Obstructive sleep apnoea	Increased cancer risk
	Heart failure

(> 1.5 g/L); serum LDL cholesterol > 0.4 g/L (men) or > 0.5 g/L (women); increased abdominal circumference > 102 cm (men) or > 88 cm (women); and impaired fasting glucose (> 1.1 g/L or > 6.1 mmol/L). It is estimated that it affects up to about a quarter of adults in the USA.

The relationship between cardiovascular disease (hypertension or ischaemic heart disease), hyperlipidaemia, smoking, physical exercise and obesity is complex. Difficulties arise in interpreting mortality figures because of the number of factors involved. Many studies do not differentiate between the types of physical exercise taken or take into account the cuff-size artefact in the measurement of blood pressure (an artefact will occur if a large cuff is not used in patients with a large arm). Nevertheless, obesity almost certainly plays a part in all of these diseases and should be treated. An exception is that stopping smoking, even if accompanied by weight gain, is more beneficial than any of the other factors. Physical fitness is also helpful, and there is some evidence to suggest that a fit obese person may have similar or even lower cardiovascular risk than a leaner unfit person.

Treatment

Dietary control

This largely depends on a reduction in calorie intake.

The most common diets allow a daily intake of approximately 4200 kJ (1000 kcal), although this may need to be nearer 6300 kJ (1500 kcal) for someone engaged in physical work. Very low calorie diets are also advocated by some, usually over shorter periods of time, but unless they are accompanied by changes in lifestyle, weight regain is likely. Patients must realize that prolonged dieting is necessary for large amounts of fat to be lost. Furthermore, a permanent change in eating habits is required to maintain the new low weight. It is relatively easy for most people to lose the first few kilograms, but long-term success in moderate obesity is poor, with an overall success rate of no more than 10%.

Many dietary regimens aim to produce a weight loss of approximately 1 kg per week. Weight loss will be greater initially owing to accompanying protein and glycogen breakdown and consequent water loss. After 3–4 weeks, incremental weight loss may be very small because only adipose tissue is broken down and there is less accompanying water loss.

Patients must understand the principles of energy intake and expenditure, and the best results are obtained in educated, well-motivated patients. Constant supervision by healthcare professionals, by close relatives or through membership of a slimming club helps to encourage compliance. It is essential to establish realistic aims. A 10% weight loss, which is regarded by some as a 'success' (see Table 5.14) is a realistic initial aim.

An increase in exercise will increase energy expenditure and should be encouraged – provided there is no contraindication – since weight control is usually not achieved without exercise. The effects of exercise are complex and not entirely understood. However, exercise alone will usually produce little long-term benefit. On the other hand there is evidence to suggest that in combination with dietary therapy, it can prevent weight being regained. In addition, regular exercise (30 min daily) will improve general health.

The diet should contain adequate amounts of protein, vitamins and trace elements. A diet of 4200 kJ (1000 kcal) per day should be made up of more than 50 g protein, approximately 100 g of carbohydrate, and 40 g of fat. The carbohydrate should be in the form of complex carbohydrates such as vegetables and fruit rather than simple sugars. Alcohol contains 29 kJ/g (8 kcal/g) and should be discouraged. It can be substituted for other foods in the diet, but it often reduces the willpower. With a varied diet, vitamins and minerals will be adequate and supplements are not necessary.

A balanced diet, attractively presented, is of much greater value and safer than any of the slimming regimens often advertised in magazines.

Most obese people oscillate in weight; they often regain the lost weight, but many manage to lose weight again. This 'cycling' in bodyweight may play a role in the development of coronary artery disease.

A wide range of diets are available, including low-fat or low-carbohydrate diets, and some suit certain individuals better than others. The following general statements can be made about them.

- All low-calorie diets produce loss of bodyweight and fat, irrespective of dietary composition. Short-term weight loss is faster on low-carbohydrate diets, as a result of greater loss of body water, which is regained after the end of dietary therapy.
- Very low-fat diets are low in vitamins E, B_{12}, and zinc. Very low-carbohydrate diets are also nutritionally inadequate, and may lead to deficiencies.
- Low-fat diets decrease LDL triglycerides and increase HDL, whereas low-carbohydrate diets produce a greater decrease in HDL and triglyceride, with no change in LDL.
- There are some potential long-term concerns with low-carbohydrate diets (high in fat and protein), including increased risk of osteoporosis, renal stones and atheroma (due to high saturated fat, high *trans* fat and cholesterol and the lack of fruits, vegetables and whole grains), but long-term studies are lacking.

Behavioural modification

The aim of behavioural modification is to encourage the patient to take personal responsibility for changing lifestyle, which will determine dietary habits and physical activity. Family therapy may also be useful, especially when it involves obese children. It can be time-consuming and expensive. Cognitive behavioural therapy is even more time-consuming and expensive.

Drug therapy

Drugs can be used in the short term (up to 3 months) as an adjunct to the dietary regimen, but they do not substitute for strict dieting.

Centrally acting drugs:
- Drugs acting on the noradrenergic pathways do suppress appetite but all have been withdrawn in the UK because of cardiovascular side-effects.
- Drugs acting on both serotoninergic and noradrenergic pathways, e.g. sibutramine.

Peripherally acting drugs. Orlistat is an inhibitor of pancreatic and gastric lipases. It reduces dietary fat absorption and aids weight loss. Weight regain occurs after the drug is stopped. It has been used continuously in a large-scale trial for up to 2 years. The patients may complain of diarrhoea during treatment and to avoid this take a low-fat diet resulting in weight loss.

A recent systematic review on long-term pharmacotherapy concluded that there was a paucity of long-term studies with antiobesity agents, and that in weight loss trials of 1-year duration, orlistat and sibutramine appear to be only modestly effective in promoting weight loss (2.7 and 4.3 kg greater weight loss respectively than the control group).

Surgical treatment

Surgery is used in some cases of morbid obesity (BMI > 40 kg/m^2) or patients with a BMI > 35 kg/m^2 and obesity-related complications, after conventional medical treatments have failed. A variety of gastrointestinal surgical procedures have been used. They fall into two main groups;

- restrictive procedures, which restrict the ability to eat
- malabsorptive procedures, which reduce the ability to absorb nutrients.

A systematic analysis of bariatric surgical procedures concluded that in comparison to non-surgical treatments, they produced significantly more weight loss (23–37 kg), which was maintained to 8 years and associated with improvement in quality of life and co-morbidities.

- *Roux-en-Y gastric bypass.* This procedure incorporates both restrictive and malabsorptive elements (gastro-jejunostomy). This procedure, like other malabsorptive procedures, may result in nutrient deficiencies requiring careful long-term follow-up.
- *Bilio-pancreatic diversion (including the duodenal switch variation).* This is another malabsorptive procedure that requires long-term evaluation.
- *Laparoscopic adjustable gastric banding.* This is a restrictive procedure, in which a band is placed around the upper stomach to produce a small proximal pouch and a large distal remnant. It has a perioperative mortality of < 0.5%, and results in loss of about 60% (43–78%) of the excess weight after 3 years, although longer-term follow-up studies are required. Laparoscopic adjustable gastric banding has been reported to produce greater weight loss, fewer side-effects (e.g. vomiting) and operative revisions than with vertical banded gastroplasty.
- *Liposuction.* The removal of large amounts of fat by suction (liposuction) does not deal with the

underlying problem and weight regain frequently occurs. There is no reduction in cardiovascular risk factors.

- *Jaw wiring.* This procedure, which permits liquid feeds only, requires good dental hygiene. It is only a temporary measure, since weight regain usually occurs after the wires have been removed, and therefore it is rarely practiced.

Prevention

Preventing obesity must always be the goal because most obese people find it difficult to maintain any weight loss they have managed to achieve. All health professionals must be aware of the dangers of obesity and encourage children, young as well as older adults, from gaining too much weight. A small gain each year over a long period produces an obese individual for whom treatment is difficult. Public health policies should consider creation of public places to encourage physical activity and fitness, education about the benefits of losing weight or not gaining it through healthy eating and physical activity, and changes in food composition (alternatives to high-fat high-energy dense foods).

FURTHER READING
Bloom S et al (2005) Gut feeling – the secret of satiety? *Clinical Medicine* 5: 147–152.
Bonow RO, Eckel RH (2003) Diet, obesity and cardiovascular risk. *New England Journal of Medicine* 348: 2057–2058.
Colquitt JAC, Sidhu M, Royle P (2003) Surgery for morbid obesity. *Cochrane Database of Systematic Reviews* CD003641.
Cummings DE, Schwartz MW (2002) Genetics and pathophysiology of human obesity. *Annual Review of Medicine* 54: 453–471.
Freedman MR, King J, Kennedy E (2001) Popular diets: a scientific review. *Obesity Research* 9 (Suppl 1): 1S–40S.
Korner J, Leibel RL (2003) To eat or not to eat – how the gut talks to the brain. *New England Journal of Medicine* 10: 926–929.
Padwal R, Li S, Lau DC (2003) Long-term pharmacotherapy for overweight and obesity: a systematic review and meta-analysis of randomized controlled trials. *International Journal of Obesity and Related Disorders* 27: 1437–1446.
Royal College of Physicians (2003) *Anti-obesity Drugs: Guidance on Appropriate Prescribing and Management. A report of the Nutrition Committee of the Royal College of Physicians.* London: Royal College of Physicians.

NUTRITIONAL SUPPORT IN THE HOSPITAL PATIENT

Nutritional support is recognized as being necessary in many hospitalized patients. The pathophysiology and hallmarks of malnutrition have been described earlier (p. 237); here the forms of nutritional support that are available are discussed, along with special nutritional requirements in some diseases.

Principles

Some form of nutritional supplementation is required in those patients who cannot eat, should not eat, will not eat or cannot eat enough. It is usually necessary to provide nutritional support for:

- all severely malnourished patients on admission to hospital
- moderately malnourished patients who, because of their physical illness, are not expected to eat for more than 3–5 days
- normally nourished patients expected not to eat for more than 5 days or to eat less than half their intake for more than 8–10 days.

Enteral rather than parenteral nutrition should be used if the gastrointestinal tract is functioning normally.

Nutritional requirements for adults

- *Water.* Typical requirements are ~ 2–3 L/day. Increased requirements occur in patients with large-ouput fistulae, nasogastric aspirates and diarrhoea. Reduced requirements occur in patients with oedema, hepatic failure, renal failure (oliguric and not dialysed) and brain oedema.
- *Energy.* Typical requirements are ~ 7.5–10.0 MJ/day (1800–2400 kcal/day). Disease increases resting energy expenditure but decreases physical activity. Extra energy is given for repletion and reduced energy for obesity.
- *Protein.* Typically 10–15 g N/day (62–95 g protein/day) or 0.15–0.25 g N/kg/day (0.94–1.56 g protein/kg/day). Extra protein may be needed in severely catabolic conditions, such as extensive burns.
- *Major minerals.* Typical requirements for sodium and potassium are 70–100 mmol/day. Increased requirements occur in patients with gastrointestinal effluents. The excretion of these minerals in various effluents can provide an indication of the additional requirements (Table 12.9, p. 702). Low requirements may be necessary in those with fluid overload (or patients with hypernatraemia and hyperkalaemia). The requirements of calcium and magnesium are higher for enteral than for parenteral nutrition because only a proportion of these minerals is absorbed by the gut.
- *Trace elements.* For trace elements such as iodide, fluoride, and selenium that are well absorbed, the requirements for enteral and parenteral nutrition are similar. For other trace elements, such as iron, zinc, manganese and chromium, the requirements for parenteral nutrition are substantially lower than for enteral nutrition (Fig. 5.11).
- *Vitamins.* Many vitamins are given in greater quantities in patients receiving parenteral nutrition than in those receiving enteral nutrition (Fig. 5.12). This is because patients on parenteral nutrition may have increased requirements, partly because of severe disease, partly because they may already have depleted pools of vitamins, and partly because some vitamins

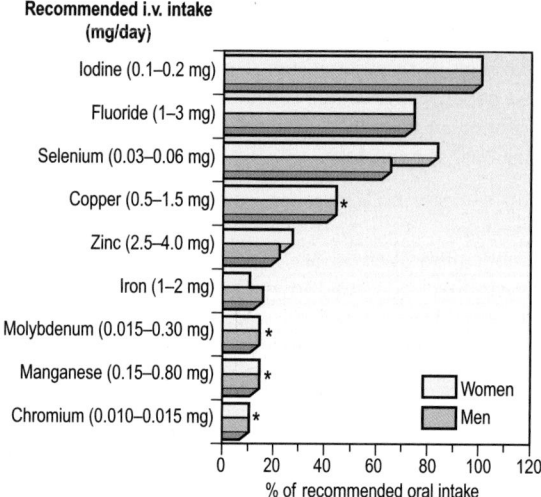

Recommended i.v. intake (mg/day)

Iodine (0.1–0.2 mg)
Fluoride (1–3 mg)
Selenium (0.03–0.06 mg)
Copper (0.5–1.5 mg) *
Zinc (2.5–4.0 mg)
Iron (1–2 mg)
Molybdenum (0.015–0.30 mg) *
Manganese (0.15–0.80 mg) *
Chromium (0.010–0.015 mg) *

☐ Women
■ Men

0 20 40 60 80 100 120
% of recommended oral intake

Fig. 5.11 Recommended intravenous intake of trace elements in absolute values and as a percentage of recommended oral intake. Trace elements marked with an asterisk are those for which there was too little information to establish recommended value for dietary oral intake: therefore the midpoint of estimated safe and adequate oral intake is used for comparison.

Recommended i.v. intake (mg/day)

Pantothenic acid (15 mg) *
Vitamin B$_{12}$ (0.005 mg)
Riboflavin (3.6 mg)
Niacin (40 mg)
Thiamine (3 mg)
Pyridoxine (4 mg)
Folic acid (0.4 mg)
Vitamin C (100 mg)
Vitamin E (10 mg)
Vitamin A (1 mg)
Vitamin D (0.005 mg)
Biotin (0.060 mg) *

☐ Women
■ Men

0 100 200 300
% of recommended oral intake

Fig. 5.12 Recommended intravenous intake of vitamins in absolute values and as a percentage of recommended oral intake. Vitamins marked with an asterisk are those for which there was too little information to establish recommended dietary oral intake: therefore the midpoint of estimated safe and adequate oral intake is used for comparison.

degrade during storage. Vitamin K is usually absent from parenteral nutrition regimens and therefore it may need to be administered separately.

Enteral nutrition (EN) (Practical box 5.1)

Feeds can be given by various routes:

- By mouth.
- By fine-bore nasogastric tube.
- Percutaneous endoscopic gastrostomy (PEG) is useful for patients who need enteral nutrition for a prolonged period (e.g. more than 30 days), such as those with swallowing problems following a head injury or in elderly people after a stroke. A catheter is placed percutaneously into the stomach under endoscopic control.
- With needle catheter jejunostomy, a fine catheter is inserted into the jejunum at laparotomy and brought out through the abdominal wall.

Diet formulation (see Table 5.16)

A polymeric diet with whole-protein and fat can be used, except in patients with severely impaired gastrointestinal

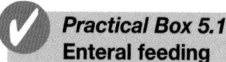

> **Practical Box 5.1**
> **Enteral feeding**
>
> **Procedure**
> - Insert fine-bore tube intranasally with wire stylet.
> - Confirm position of tube in stomach by aspiration of gastric contents and auscultation of the epigastrium.
> - Check by X-ray if aspiration or auscultation is unsuccessful.
>
> **Problems**
> No satisfactory way of keeping nasogastric tubes in place (up to 60% come out).
>
> **Main complications**
> - Regurgitation and aspiration into bronchus.
> - Blockage of the nasogastric tube.
> - Gastrointestinal side-effects, the most common being diarrhoea.
> - Metabolic complications including hyperglycaemia and hypokalaemia, as well as low levels of magnesium, calcium and phosphate, occur.

Table 5.16 Standard enteric diet, providing 8.4 MJ per day (= 2000 kcal)

Energy
Carbohydrate as glucose polymers (49–53% of total energy)
Fat as triglycerides (30–35% of total energy)

Nitrogen
Whole protein (10–14 g of nitrogen/day)
Additional electrolytes, vitamins and trace elements

Features
Ratio of energy to nitrogen kJ : g = 620 : 1 (kcal : g = 150 : 1)
Osmolality = 285–300 mOsm/kg

function who may require a predigested (i.e. elemental) diet. In these patients, the nitrogen source is purified low-molecular-weight peptides or amino acid mixtures, with sometimes the fat being given partly as medium-chain triglycerides.

Management

Daily amounts of diet vary between 2 and 2.5 L and the full amount can be started immediately.

Hypercatabolic patients require a high supply of nitrogen (15 g daily) and often will not achieve positive nitrogen balance until the primary injury is resolved.

The success of enteral feeding depends on careful supervision of the patient, with monitoring of weight, biochemistry and diet charts.

Total parenteral nutrition (TPN)

Peripheral parenteral nutrition

Specially formulated mixtures for peripheral use are available, with a low osmolality and containing lipid emulsions. Heparin and corticosteroids can be added to the infusion and local application of glyceryl trinitrate patches reduces the occurrence of thrombophlebitis and prolongs catheter life. Peripheral parenteral nutrition is often preferred initially (each catheter will last for about 5 days), allowing time to consider the necessity for having to insert a central venous catheter.

Parenteral nutrition via a central venous
catheter (see Practical box 5.2)
A silicone catheter is placed into a central vein, usually using the infraclavicular approach to the subclavian vein. The skin-entry site should be dressed carefully and not disturbed unless there is a suggestion of catheter-related sepsis.

Complications of catheter placement include central vein thrombosis, pneumothorax and embolism, but the major problem is catheter-related sepsis. Organisms, mainly staphylococci, enter along the side of the catheter, leading to septicaemia. Sepsis can be prevented by careful and sterile placement of the catheter, by not removing the dressing over the catheter entry site, and by not giving other substances (e.g. blood products, antibiotics) via the central vein catheter.

Sepsis should be suspected if the patient develops fever and leucocytosis. In two-thirds of cases, organisms can be grown from the catheter tip. Treatment involves removal of the catheter and appropriate systemic antibiotics.

Nutrients

With TPN it is possible to provide sufficient nitrogen for protein synthesis and calories to meet energy requirements. Electrolytes, vitamins and trace elements are also necessary. All of these substances are infused simultaneously.

Nitrogen source

Most patients receive at least 11–15 g N per day, in the form of synthetic L-amino acids.

Practical Box 5.2
Central catheter placement for parenteral nutrition

This should be performed only by experienced clinicians under aseptic conditions in an operating theatre. Give an explanation and obtain consent from the patient.

- The patient is placed supine with 5° of head-down tilt to avoid air embolism.
- The skin below the midpoint of the left clavicle is infiltrated with 1–2% lidocaine (lignocaine) and a 1 cm skin incision is made.
- A 20-gauge needle on a syringe is inserted beneath the clavicle and first rib and angled towards the tip of a finger held in the suprasternal notch.
- When blood is aspirated freely, the needle is used as a guide to insert the cannula through the skin incision and into the subclavian vein.
- The catheter is advanced so that its tip lies in the distal part of the superior vena cava.
- A skin tunnel is created under local anaesthetic using an introducer inserted through a point about 10 cm below and medial to the incision and passed upwards to the incision.
- The proximal end of the catheter (with hub removed) is passed backwards through the introducer to emerge 10 cm below the clavicle, where it is sutured to the chest wall.
- The original infraclavicular entry incision is now sutured.

Energy source

This is provided by glucose, with additional calories provided by a fat emulsion. Fat infusions provide a greater number of calories in a smaller volume than can be provided by carbohydrate. Fat infusions are not hypertonic and they also prevent essential fatty acid deficiency.

Essential fatty acid deficiency has been reported in long-term parenteral nutritional regimens without fat emulsions. It causes a scaly skin, hair loss and a delay in healing.

Electrolytes and trace elements

(see Figs 5.11 and 5.12)
Initially, the electrolyte status should be monitored on a daily basis and electrolyte solutions given as appropriate. Water-soluble vitamins can be given daily but fat-soluble vitamins should be given weekly, as overdose can occur. A trace-metal solution is available for patients on long-term parenteral nutrition, but if the patient requires blood transfusions trace-metal supplements are not needed.

Administration and monitoring

Peripheral parenteral nutrition is administered via 3-L bags over 24 hours, with the constituents being premixed under sterile conditions by the pharmacy. Table 5.17 shows the composition which provides 9 g of nitrogen and 1700 calories in 24 hours.

For a central venous TPN regimen, most hospitals now use premixed 3-L bags. A standard parenteral nutrition

Table 5.17 Examples of total parenteral nutrition regimens

CENTRAL: all mixed in 3 L bags and infused over 24 hours		
Nitrogen	L-Amino acids 14 g/L	1 L
Energy	Glucose 50%	0.5 L
	Glucose 20%	0.5 L
	plus	
	Lipid 10%	0.5 L
	as either Intralipid	Fractionated soya
	or Lipofundin	oil 100 g/L
		Soya oil 50 g,
		medium-chain
		triglycerides 50 g/L
+ Electrolytes, water-soluble vitamins, fat-soluble vitamins, trace elements, heparin and insulin may be added if required. Nitrogen 14 g, non-protein calories 9305 kJ (2250 kcal)		
PERIPHERAL: all mixed in 3 L bags and infused over 24 hours		
Nitrogen	L-Amino acids 9 g/L	1 L
Energy	Glucose 20%	1 L
	Lipid 20%	0.5 L
+ Trace elements, electrolytes, and water-soluble and fat-soluble vitamins, heparin 1000 UL and hydrocortisone 100 mg; insulin is added if required. Nitrogen 9 g, non-protein calories 7206 kJ (1700 kcal)		

regimen which provides 14 g of nitrogen and 2250 calories over 24 hours is given in Table 5.17.

Essential monitoring includes daily plasma electrolytes and weekly assessments of nutritional status (weight and skinfold thickness if appropriate callipers are available). Nitrogen balance could also be assessed but complete collections of urine are necessary.

Complications
- Catheter-related (see above)
- Metabolic (e.g. hyperglycaemia – insulin therapy is usually necessary)
- Fluid and electrolyte disturbances
- Hypercalcaemia
- Liver dysfunction.

NUTRITIONAL SUPPORT IN THE HOME PATIENT

In both high- and low-income countries there is considerably more undernutrition in the community than in hospital. However, the principles are very similar: detection of malnutrition and the underlying risk factors; treatment of underlying disease processes and disabilities; correction of specific nutrient deficiencies and provision of appropriate nutritional support. This typically begins with dietary advice, and may involve the provision of 'meals on wheels' by social services. A systematic review of the use of nutritional supplements in the community came to the following conclusions:

- Supplements are generally of more value in patients with a BMI < 20 kg/m^2 and children with growth failure (weight for height < 85% of ideal) than in those with better anthropometric indices. They are likely to be of little or no value in patients with little weight loss and a BMI > 20 kg/m^2. The supplemental energy intake in such subjects largely replaces oral food intake.
- Supplements may be of value in weight-losing patients (e.g. > 10% weight loss compared to pre-illness) with a BMI > 20 kg/m^2, and in children with deteriorating growth performance without chronic protein–energy undernutrition.
- The functional benefits varied according to the patient group. In patients with chronic obstructive airways disease the functional benefits were increased respiratory muscle strength, increase in handgrip strength, and an increase in walking distance/duration of exercise. In the elderly the benefits were reduced number of falls, or increase in activities of daily living, and reduced pressure sore surface area. In patients with HIV/AIDS there were changes in immunological function and improved cognition. Patients with liver disease experienced a lower incidence of severe infections and had a lower frequency of hospitalization.
- Acceptability and compliance are likely to be better when a choice of supplements (of type, flavour, consistency) and schedule is decided in conjunction with the patient and/or carer. Changes in these may be necessary when there is a change in patterns of daily activities, disease status, and 'taste fatigue' with prolonged use of the same supplement.
- Nutritional counselling and monitoring are recommended before and after the start of supplements (see also below).

Some patients receive enteral tube feeding and parenteral nutrition at home. At any one point in time in developed countries enteral tube feeding occurs more frequently at home than in hospital. In adults the commonest reason for starting home tube feeding is for swallowing difficulties. This involves patients with neurological disorders, such as motor neurone disease, multiple sclerosis and Parkinson's disease, but the commonest single diagnosis is cerebrovascular disease. In 1998 it was estimated that almost 2% of patients who had a stroke in the UK received home enteral tube feeding (HETF). The outcome of this is indicated in Table 5.18. Fifteen per cent of patients were able to resume full oral nutrition after a year. It is therefore necessary to intermittently assess the swallowing capabilities of patients in order to avoid unnecessary tube feeding. The patients and/or carers should have adequate training, contacts with appropriate health professions, and a reliable delivery service for feeds and ancillary equipment. They should also be clear about how to manage simple problems associated with the feeding tube, which is usually a gastrostomy tube rather than a nasogastric tube.

Home parenteral nutrition is practised much less frequently, usually under the supervision of specialist centres. The potential value of intestinal transplantation in patients with long-term intestinal failure is still being assessed.

Table 5.18 Outcome of patients at 1 year after starting home enteral tube feeding (HETF)*

	All patients (n = 15 143) %	Cerebrovascular disease (n = 5660) %	Motor neurone disease (n = 874) %	Multiple sclerosis (n = 856) %
Continuing on HETF	50.2	53.0	35.8	81.0
Returned to oral feeding	14.2	12.9	1.1	3.7
Died	33.5	32.6	62.1	13.7
Other†	2.2	1.5	1.0	1.6

*Based on the British Artificial Nutrition Survey (1996–2000). Patients who returned to oral feeding or refused/withdrew from HETF may have died subsequently
†Withdrew or refused HETF, or in hospital

FURTHER READING

Elia M, Russell C, Stratton R (2001) *Trends in Artificial Nutrition Support in the UK During 1996–2000. A Report by the British Artificial Nutrition Survey (BANS)*. Redditch: BAPEN.

Payne-James J, Grimble G, Silk D (2001) *Artificial Nutritional Support*, 2nd edn. London: Greenwich Medical Media.

Stratton RJ, Green CJ, Elia M (2003) *Disease-related Malnutrition. An Evidence-based Approach to Treatment*. Oxford: CABI Publishing (CAB International).

Stroud M, Duncan H, Nightingale J (2003) Guidelines for enteral feeding in adult hospital patients. *Gut* **52** (Suppl VII): vii1–vii12.

FOOD ALLERGY AND FOOD INTOLERANCE

Many people ascribe their various symptoms to food, and many such sufferers are seen and started on exclusion diets. The scientific evidence that food does harm in most instances is weak, although adverse reactions to food certainly exist. These can be divided into those that involve immune mechanisms (food allergy) and those that do not (food intolerance).

Food allergy

Food allergy, which is estimated to affect up to about 5% of young children and about 1–2% of adults, may be IgE mediated or non-IgE mediated (T-cell mediated). The IgE-mediated reactions tend to occur early after a food challenge (within minutes to an hour). Adults tend to be allergic to fish, shellfish and peanuts, while children tend to be allergic to cow's milk, egg white, wheat, and soy. Peanuts are very allergenic and peanut allergy persists throughout life. The following conditions can result from food allergy:

- *Acute hypersensitivity*. An example is urticaria, vomiting or diarrhoea after eating nuts, strawberries or shellfish. These IgE-mediated reactions do not usually produce clinical problems as the patients have already learned to avoid the suspected food. Inadvertent ingestion of the incriminating food can sometimes occur, leading to angioneurotic oedema (p. 1334).
- *Eczema and asthma*. These tend to affect young children and are often due to egg and are IgE mediated.
- *Rhinitis and asthma*. These have been produced by foods such as milk and chocolate, mainly in atopic subjects.
- *Chronic urticaria*. This has been treated successfully by an exclusion diet.
- *Food-sensitive enteropathy*. This may manifest itself as coeliac disease (gluten (wheat) sensitive enteropathy), and cow's milk enteropathy (in infants) and is T-cell mediated.

Food intolerance

- *Migraine*. This sometimes follows the intake of foods such as chocolate, cheese and alcohol, which are rich in certain amines, such as tyramine. Patients on monoamine oxidase inhibitors, which are involved in the metabolism of these amines, are particularly vulnerable.
- *Irritable bowel syndrome*. In some patients this seems to be related to ingestion of certain food items, such as wheat, but the mechanisms are not clearly defined (p. 1283).
- *Chinese restaurant syndrome*. Monosodium glutamate, a flavour enhancer used in cooking Chinese food, may produce dizziness, faintness, nausea, sweating and chest pains.
- *Lactose intolerance*. Patients develop abdominal bloating and diarrhoea following ingestion of lactose, which is present in milk (p. 300). This is probably the commonest form of food intolerance world-wide, and may be genetic in origin.
- *Phenylketonuria*. This can also be classified as a form of food intolerance, and is due to lack of phenylalanine hydroxylase, which is necessary for the metabolism of phenylalanine present in dietary protein.

A number of other inborn errors of metabolism can also be regarded as forms of food intolerance.

Food intolerance may be due to a constituent of food (e.g. the histamine in mackerel or canned food, or the tyramine in cheeses), chemical mediators released by food (e.g. histamine may be released by tomatoes or strawberries), or toxic chemicals found in food (e.g. the food additive tartrazine).

Many other additives and compounds with certain E numbers have been implicated as causing reactions, but here the evidence for this is poor.

There is little or no evidence to suggest that diseases such as arthritis, behaviour and affective disorders and Crohn's disease are due to ingestion of a particular food.

Multiple vague symptoms such as tiredness or malaise are also not due to food allergy. Most of the patients in this group are suffering from a psychiatric disorder (p. 1283).

Management

- A careful history may help to delineate the causative agent, particularly when the effects are immediate.
- Skin-prick testing with allergen and measurement in the serum of antigen or antibodies have not correlated with symptoms and are usually misleading. 'Fringe' techniques such as hair analysis, although widely advertised, are of limited value.
- Diagnostic exclusion diets are sometimes used, but they are time-consuming. They can occasionally be of value in identifying a particular food causing problems.
- Dietary challenge consists of the food and the test being given sublingually or by inhalation in an attempt to reproduce the symptoms. Again this may be helpful in a few cases.
- Most people who have acute reactions to food realize it and stop the food, and do not require medical attention. In the remainder of patients, a small minority seem to be helped by modifying their diet, but there is no good scientific evidence to support these exclusion diets.

FURTHER READING

American Gastroenterology Association. American Gastroenterological Association medical position statement: guidelines for the evaluation of food allergy (2001). *Gastroenterology* **120**: 1023–1025.

American Gastroenterology Association. Review on the evaluation of food allergy in GI disorder, official recommendation of American Gastroenterology Association (2001). *Gastroenterology* **120**: 1026–1040.

Kimber I, Dearman RJ (2002) Factors affecting the development of food allergy. *Proceedings of the Nutrition Society* **6**: 435–439.

Lack G, Fox D, Northstone K, Golding J (2003) Factors associated with the development of peanut allergy in childhood. *New England Journal of Medicine* **348**: 977–985.

Box 5.5 The main pathways of ethanol oxidization

- Alcohol dehydrogenase:

$$CH_3CH_2OH + NAD^+ \xrightarrow{ADH} CH_3CHO + NADH + H^+$$
(ethanol)   (acetaldehyde)

- The liver microsomal enzyme oxidizing system (MEOS) including the specific P450 enzyme, CYP2EI, which is induced by ethanol:

$$CH_3CH_2OH + NADPH + H^+ + O_2$$

$$\xrightarrow{MEOS} CH_3CHO + NADP + 2H_2O$$

ALCOHOL

Alcohol is a popular 'nutrient' consumed in large quantities all over the world. In many countries, alcohol consumption is becoming a major problem (see p. 1302).

Ethanol (ethyl alcohol) is oxidized, in the steps shown in Box 5.5, to acetaldehyde. Acetaldehyde is then converted to acetate, 90% in the liver mitochondria. Acetate is released into the blood and oxidized by peripheral tissues to carbon dioxide, fatty acids and water.

Alcohol dehydrogenases are found in many tissues and it has been suggested that enzymes present in the gastric mucosa may contribute substantially to ethanol metabolism.

Ethanol itself produces 29.3 kJ/g (8 kcal/g), but many alcoholic drinks also contain sugar, which increases their calorific value. For example, one pint of beer provides 1045 kJ (250 kcal), so the heavy drinker will be unable to lose weight if he or she continues to drink.

Effects of excess alcohol consumption

Excess consumption of alcohol leads to two major problems, both of which can be present in the same patient:

- alcohol dependence syndrome (p. 1303)
- physical damage to various tissues.

Each unit of alcohol (defined as one half pint of normal beer, one single measure of spirit, or one small glass of wine) contains 8 g of ethanol (Fig. 5.13). All the long-term effects of excess alcohol consumption are due to excess

1 unit of alcohol (8 g)

½ pint of beer   1 single measure (25 ml spirit)   1 glass of wine   1 glass of sherry

Fig. 5.13 **Measures of 1 unit of alcohol.**

Box 5.6 Guide to sensible drinking of alcohol

Daily maximum
3 units for men
2 units for women

To help achieve this
Use a standard measure.
Do not drink during the daytime.
Have alcohol-free days each week.

Remember
Health can be damaged without being 'drunk'.
Regular heavy intake is more harmful than occasional binges.
Do not drink to 'drown your problems'.
In the UK the drink-before-driving limit of alcohol in the blood is 800 mg/L (80 mg%).
One unit of alcohol is eliminated per hour, therefore spread drinking time.
Food decreases absorption and therefore results in a lower blood alcohol level.
4–5 units are sufficient to put the blood alcohol level over the legal driving limit in a 70 kg man (less in a lighter person).

ethanol, irrespective of the type of alcoholic beverage; i.e. beer and spirits are no different in their long-term effects. Short-term effects, such as hangovers, depend on additional substances, particularly other alcohols such as isoamyl alcohol, which are known as congeners. Brandy and bourbon contain the highest percentage of congeners.

The amount of alcohol that produces damage varies and not everyone who drinks heavily will suffer physical damage. For example, only 20% of people who drink heavily develop cirrhosis of the liver. The effect of alcohol on different organs of the body is not the same; in some patients the liver is affected, in others the brain or muscle. The differences may be genetically determined.

Thiamin deficiency contributes to both neurological (confusion, Wernicke–Korsakoff syndrome; see p. 1263) and some of the non-neurological manifestations (cardiomyopathy). Susceptibility to damage of different organs is variable and the figures in Box 5.6 are given only as a guide. Heavy persistent drinkers for many years are at greater risk than heavy sporadic drinkers.

Liver disease

In general the effects of a given intake of alcohol seem to be worse in women. The following figures are for men and should be reduced by 50% for women:

- 160 g ethanol per day (20 single drinks) carries a high risk
- 80 g ethanol per day (10 single drinks) carries a medium risk
- 40 g ethanol per day (five single drinks) carries little risk.

Alcohol consumption in pregnancy

Women are advised not to drink alcohol at all during pregnancy because even small amounts of alcohol consumed can lead to 'small babies'. The *fetal alcohol syndrome* is characterized by mental retardation, dysmorphic features and growth impairment; it occurs in fetuses of alcohol-dependent women.

Summary

A summary of the physical effects of alcohol is given in Table 5.19. Details of these diseases are discussed in the relevant chapters. The effects of alcohol withdrawal are discussed on page 1304.

Table 5.19 Physical effects of excess alcohol consumption

Central nervous system Epilepsy Wernicke–Korsakoff syndrome Polyneuropathy	**Respiratory system** Chest infections
Muscles Acute or chronic myopathy	**Gastrointestinal system** Acute gastritis Carcinoma of the oesophagus or large bowel Pancreatic disease Liver disease
Cardiovascular system Cardiomyopathy Beriberi heart disease Cardiac arrhythmias Hypertension	**Haemopoiesis** Macrocytosis (due to direct toxic effect on bone marrow or folate deficiency) Thrombocytopenia Leucopenia
Metabolism Hyperuricaemia (gout) Hyperlipidaemia Hypoglycaemia Obesity	**Bone** Osteoporosis Osteomalacia
Endocrine system Pseudo-Cushing's syndrome	

FURTHER READING
Lieber CS (1995) Medical disorders of alcoholism. *New England Journal of Medicine* 333: 1058–1063.

CHAPTER BIBLIOGRAPHY
Elia M (1995) Changing concepts of nutrient requirements in disease: implications for artificial nutritional support. *Lancet* 345: 1279–1284.
Elia M, Stubbs RE, Henry CJK (1999) Differences in fat carbohydrate, and protein metabolism between lean and obese subjects undergoing total starvation. *Obesity Research* 7: 597–604.
Stratton RJ, Elia M (1999) A critical systematic analysis of the use of oral nutritional supplements in the community. *Clinical Nutrition* 18 (Suppl 2): 29–84.
Wisepan M ed. (2004) Nutrition series. Continuing Medical Education. *Clinical Medicine* 4 (5): 397–414.

SIGNIFICANT WEBSITES

http://www.who.int/nutgrowthdb/
World Health Organization site, provides information on world-wide nutritional issues, resources and research

http://www.fao.org/
Food and Agriculture Organization (FAO) – autonomous body within the United Nations, aims to improve health through nutrition and agricultural productivity, especially in rural populations

http://www.ific.org/
International Food Information Council (IFIC) – non-profit organization providing access to health and nutrition resources to improve communication of health and nutrition information to consumers

http://www.ag.uiuc.edu/~food-lab/nat/
Free analysis of the nutrient content of food available to anyone (at University of Illinois, USA)

http://www.ama-assn.org/ama/pub/category/10931.html
American Medical Association: Assessment and management of adult obesity

http://www.nhlbi.nih.gov/health/public/heart/obesity/lose_wt/profmats.htm
National Heart, Lung and Blood Institute: Aim for a healthy weight

http://www.hda-online.org.uk/downloads/pdfs/obesity_evidence_briefing.pdf
Health Development Agency: Management of obesity and overweight

Selected nutrition journals (for more extensive website addresses see Journal of Nutrition 1997; **127**:1527–1532):

http://www.faseb.org/ajcn
American Journal of Clinical Nutrition

http://www.nutrition.org/
The Journal of Nutrition

http://www.nature.com/ijo
International Journal of Obesity

http://www.cabi-publishing.org/JOURNALS/BJN/Index.asp
The British Journal of Nutrition

http://www.ilsi.org/publications/reviews.html
Nutrition Reviews

http://clinnutr.org/
Journal of Parenteral and Enteral Nutrition

http://www.naturesj.com/ejcn/
European Journal of Clinical Nutrition

Gastrointestinal disease

6

In developed countries gastrointestinal problems are a common reason for attendance at the primary care clinic as well as the outpatient clinic of the hospital. Many of these consultations (approximately 75%) are for symptoms related to non-organic disease. The clinician's main task is therefore to separate out the patients who require investigation, remembering that 20% of all cancers occur in the gastrointestinal tract (Fig. 6.1).

In developing countries, poor hygiene and malnutrition allow the spread of infective organisms. The clinician's main role here is to treat infections promptly and to help with prevention by encouraging improved sanitation and education.

In this chapter, the essential anatomy and principles of physiology are divided and discussed under the relevant sections.

CLINICAL APPROACH TO GASTROINTESTINAL SYMPTOMS AND SIGNS

Dyspepsia and indigestion

Dyspepsia is the term used by healthcare workers to describe upper abdominal symptoms, e.g. nausea, heartburn, acidity, pain or discomfort, wind, fullness or belching. Patients seldom use the term 'dyspepsia'; they are more likely to refer to indigestion to describe any symptom that is food related. Indigestion is common; 80% of the population will have had indigestion at some time.

'Alarm' features suggestive of serious disease are:

- dysphagia
- weight loss
- protracted vomiting
- anorexia
- haematemesis or melaena.

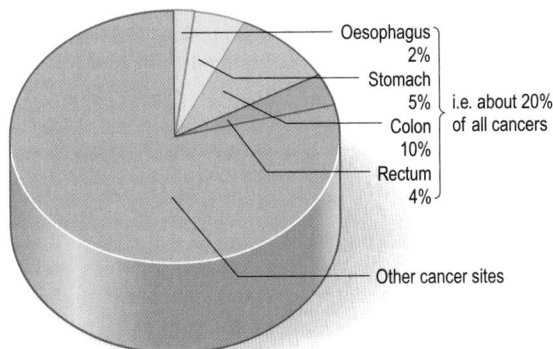

Fig. 6.1   Incidence (approximate) of cancers at various sites of the gastrointestinal tract.

Oesophagus 2%
Stomach 5%
Colon 10%
Rectum 4%
i.e. about 20% of all cancers
Other cancer sites

Table 6.1   Causes of vomiting

Any gastrointestinal disease	Drugs, e.g.
Acute infections, e.g.	digoxin toxicity
influenza	levodopa
pertussis	opiates
urinary tract infection	antibiotics
Central nervous disease, e.g.	chemotherapy
raised intracranial	immunotherapy
pressure	Reflex, e.g.
vestibular disturbances	severe pain: myocardial
migraine	infarction
Metabolic causes, e.g.	Psychogenic
uraemia	Pregnancy
diabetes: ketoacidosis	Alcohol excess
or gastroparesis	
hypercalcaemia	

Nausea and vomiting

There are three phases:

- nausea – a feeling of wanting to vomit, often associated with autonomic effects including hypersalivation, pallor and sweating
- retching – a strong involuntary effort to vomit
- vomiting – the expulsion of gastric contents through the mouth.

The vomiting centres are located in the lateral reticular formation of the medulla and are stimulated by the chemoreceptor trigger zones (CTZs) in the floor of the fourth ventricle, and also by vagal afferents from the gut. These zones are directly stimulated by drugs, motion sickness and metabolic causes.

Many gastrointestinal conditions are associated with vomiting (Table 6.1), but nausea and vomiting without pain are frequently non-gastrointestinal in origin.

Haematemesis is vomiting blood or 'coffee-grounds' from the stomach.

Large volumes of vomit suggest intestinal obstruction; *faeculent vomit* suggests low intestinal obstruction or the presence of a gastrocolic fistula, while *projectile vomiting* is due to gastric-outflow obstruction.

Chronic nausea ± vomiting with no other abdominal symptoms is usually due to a psychological cause (p. 337).

Early-morning vomiting is seen in pregnancy, alcohol dependence and some metabolic disorders (e.g. uraemia).

Flatulence

This is the term used to describe excessive wind. It includes belching, abdominal distension, 'wind' or the passage of flatus per rectum. Swallowing air (aerophagia) is described on page 337. Some of the swallowed air is passed into the intestine where most of it is absorbed. Intestinal bacterial breakdown of food also produces a small amount of gas. Flatus consists of nitrogen, carbon dioxide, hydrogen and methane. Flatus is normally passed 13–20 times per day.

Diarrhoea and constipation

These are common complaints which are not usually due to serious disease. They are described in detail on pages 320 and 331 respectively.

A single episode of diarrhoea can be due to dietary indiscretion or anxiety. Watery stools of large volume are always due to organic disease. Bloody diarrhoea usually implies colonic disease.

Acute diarrhoea lasting 2–5 days is often due to an infective cause, and stool cultures are necessary.

Patients often consider themselves constipated if their bowels are not open on most days. The difficult passage of hard stool is also regarded as constipation, irrespective of stool frequency.

Abdominal pain

Pain is stimulated mainly by the stretching of smooth muscle or organ capsules. Severe acute abdominal pain can be due to a large number of gastrointestinal conditions, and normally presents as an emergency (p. 340). An 'acute abdomen' can occasionally be due to referred pain from the chest, as in pneumonia, or to metabolic causes, such as diabetic ketoacidosis.

In patients with abdominal pain the following should be ascertained:

- the site, intensity, character, duration and frequency of the pain
- the aggravating and relieving factors
- associated symptoms, including non-gastrointestinal symptoms.

Upper abdominal pain

Epigastric pain is very common; it is often a dull ache, but sometimes sharp and severe. Its relationship to food intake should be ascertained. It is a common feature of peptic ulcer disease, but also occurs in functional dyspepsia. In biliary tract disease, the pain is often epigastric.

Right hypochondrial pain is usually from the gall bladder or biliary tract. Hepatic congestion (e.g. in hepatitis) and sometimes peptic ulcer can present with pain in the right hypochondrium. Chronic, often persistent, pain in the right hypochondrium is a frequent symptom in healthy females suffering from functional bowel disorders. This chronic pain is not due to gall bladder disease (p. 399).

Lower abdominal pain

Acute pain in the left iliac fossa is usually colonic in origin (e.g. acute diverticulitis). *Chronic pain* is most commonly associated with functional bowel disorders.

In females, lower abdominal pain occurs in a number of gynaecological disorders and the differentiation from GI disease is often difficult.

Persistent pain in the right iliac fossa over a long period is not due to chronic appendicitis.

Proctalgia is a severe pain deep in the rectum that comes on suddenly but lasts only for a short time. It is not due to organic disease.

Abdominal wall pain

Recurrent localized abdominal pain with local tenderness can very rarely arise from the abdominal wall itself. Causes are thought to include nerve entrapment, external hernias and entrapment of internal viscera (commonly omentum) within traumatic ruptures of abdominal wall musculature.

Weight loss

This is due to anorexia (loss of appetite) and is a frequent accompaniment of all gastrointestinal disease. Anorexia is also common in systemic disease and may be seen in psychiatric disorders, particularly anorexia nervosa. Anorexia often accompanies carcinoma but it is a late symptom and not of diagnostic help. Weight loss with a normal or increased dietary intake occurs with hyperthyroidism. Malabsorption is never so severe as to cause weight loss without anorexia. Weight loss should be assessed objectively as patients often 'think' they have lost weight. Appetite and satiety are described on page 253.

CLINICAL EXAMINATION

A general examination is performed, with particular emphasis on the examination of all lymph nodes and noting the presence of anaemia or jaundice. Detailed examination of the gastrointestinal tract starts with the mouth and tongue, before examining the abdomen with the patient lying flat.

EXAMINATION OF THE ABDOMEN

Inspection
Abdominal distension, whether due to flatus, fat, fetus, fluid or faeces, must be looked for. Lordosis may give the appearance of a distended abdomen; it is a common feature of the 'abdominal distension' seen in functional bowel disorders.

Palpation
The abdominal organs may be felt in some normal subjects (Fig. 6.2) but this is not common and such organs are usually only just palpable. A Reidel's lobe is an extension of the lateral portion of the right lobe of the liver and can occasionally be palpated. Figure 6.3 shows a normal CT scan at the T12 level.

Any palpable mass is carefully felt to decide which organ is involved and also to evaluate its size, shape and consistency and whether it moves with respiration.

The hernial orifices should be examined if intestinal obstruction is suspected.

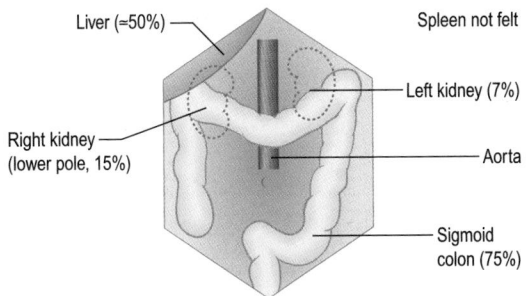

Fig. 6.2 **The organs sometimes palpable in thin subjects.**

Fig. 6.3 **CT scan of the normal abdomen at the level of T12.** 1, aorta; 2, spine; 3, top of right kidney; 4, liver; 5, gall bladder; 6, stomach (containing air); 7, pancreas; 8, spleen.

A succussion splash suggests gastric outlet obstruction if the patient has not drunk for 2–3 hours; the splash of fluid in the stomach can be heard with a stethoscope laid on the abdomen when the patient is moved.

Percussion
This is performed in the usual way to detect the area of dullness caused by the liver and spleen, and possibly bladder enlargement. The presence of fluid in the peritoneal cavity (i.e. ascites) is detected by shifting dullness. The percussion note changes from resonance to dullness when the patient is moved from one side to the other. It is a good physical sign, but 1–2 L of fluid must be present to elicit it. A large ovarian cyst can sometimes produce an enlarged abdomen, but the dullness is more centrally placed than in ascites.

Auscultation
Auscultation is not of great value in gastrointestinal disease, apart from in the evaluation of the acute abdomen (see p. 341). Abdominal bruits are often present in normal subjects, but these are not clinically significant.

EXAMINATION OF THE RECTUM AND SIGMOID COLON

Digital examination of the rectum should be performed in all patients with a change in bowel habit and rectal bleeding.

Rigid sigmoidoscopy (Practical box 6.1) should, in hospital, be part of the routine examination in all cases of diarrhoea and in patients with lower abdominal symptoms such as a change in bowel habit or rectal bleeding.

Proctoscopy (Practical box 6.1) is performed in all patients with a history of bright red blood per rectum; the narrow sigmoidoscope does not distend the lumen and haemorrhoids can be missed.

Flexible sigmoidoscopy

The rigid sigmoidoscope allows inspection of only the lower 20–25 cm of the bowel. A 60 cm flexible sigmoidoscope can be readily used in the outpatient department after minimal bowel preparation (a disposable enema). Specialist nurse practitioners use this technique in many outpatient clinics. At least 50% of colonic neoplasms occur within the range of the flexible sigmoidoscope (see Fig. 6.42).

 Practical Box 6.1
Sigmoidoscopy and proctoscopy

Sigmoidoscopy

- The technique using a 25 cm rigid sigmoidoscope is easy to learn, provides valuable information and is safe in competent hands.
- No bowel preparation is required.
- Explain to the patient the nature of the procedure.
- The technique is relatively painless. In the irritable bowel syndrome, the patient's pain is often reproduced by air insufflation

1. Rectal examination is initially performed.
2. The sigmoidoscope is passed into the anus, pointing towards the symphysis pubis. The obturator is removed, and the instrument passed under direct vision to the rectosigmoid junction and beyond if possible (using air insufflation).
3. The mucosa of the anus and rectum is inspected. The normal mucosa is shiny with superficial vessels and no contact bleeding.
4. Biopsies can be taken of any lesions that are seen or from apparently normal-looking mucosa, which occasionally shows histological evidence of inflammation.

Proctoscopy

1. The proctoscope is passed into the anus directed towards the symphysis pubis and the obturator is removed.
2. The patient strains down as the proctoscope is removed.
3. Haemorrhoids are seen as purplish veins in the left lateral, right posterior or right anterior positions.
4. Fissures may also be seen, but pain often prevents the procedure from being performed.

It is used to biopsy lesions in the sigmoid area seen on barium enema and for the follow-up of patients with distal colitis. It is useful as an initial test for patients with left-sided colonic symptoms and rectal bleeding but a full colonoscopy will be needed if no pathology is found.

Stool examination

This can be useful occasionally to confirm the patient's symptoms (e.g. passing of blood or steatorrhoea). The shape and size may be helpful (e.g. rabbity stools in the irritable bowel syndrome). Stool charts for recording volume and frequency of defecation are useful in inpatients to follow the progress of diarrhoea.

INVESTIGATIONS

Radiology and endoscopy are the principal investigations. These are usually preceded by routine haematology and biochemistry. The investigation of small bowel disease is discussed in more detail on page 299. Manometry is mainly used in oesophageal disease (p. 274) and rectal disorders (p. 320).

Barium contrast studies (Box 6.1)

Most examinations are performed after an overnight fast. The radiologist should be given sufficient clinical information and directed to the particular area under suspicion. X-rays should be reviewed with the radiologist, if possible.

- **Barium swallow**. The oesophagus is visualized as barium is swallowed in both the upright and prone positions. Motility abnormalities as well as anatomical lesions can then be observed. Reflux, as demonstrated by the retrograde flow of barium from the stomach into the oesophagus, is best observed with the patient tipped head down. It can be more effectively demonstrated by asking the patient to drink water (water siphon test) or by distension of the stomach with gas by an effervescent agent. Swallowing a lump of bread or a marshmallow coated in barium can be useful in evaluating patients with dysphagia.
- **Double-contrast barium meal**. This is performed to examine the stomach and duodenum. A small amount of barium is given together with effervescent granules to produce carbon dioxide so that a double contrast between air and barium is obtained. This test has a high accuracy rate for the detection of significant pathology – ulcers and cancer – but requires good technique to achieve high-quality pictures. Gastroscopy is a more sensitive test for small superficial mucosal lesions and for bleeding and enables biopsy of any suspicious area.
- **Small bowel follow-through**. This is used to examine the small bowel and ideally should be performed separately from a barium meal as a different technique is employed. Barium is swallowed and X-rays are

Box 6.1 **The use of barium contrast studies**

Barium contrast study	Main use	Comments
Barium swallow	Dysphagia	Particularly useful in motility disorders
Barium meal	Epigastric pain Vomiting	Gastroscopy has replaced barium meal in most centres as biopsy and histology is possible for *Helicobacter pylori* and carcinoma
Small bowel follow-through	Diarrhoea Abdominal pain	Only practical way of studying gross small bowel anatomy
Barium enema	Altered bowel habit Abdominal pain	Colonoscopy has largely replaced this examination for rectal bleeding, inflammatory bowel disease and polyp follow-up

taken as the barium passes through the jejunum and ileum into the right colon, which usually takes about 1 hour. The fold pattern and calibre of the small bowel can be assessed, and specific views of the terminal ileum are obtained using compression to separate the loops of bowel and particularly to identify early changes in patients with suspected Crohn's disease.

- **Small bowel enema (enteroclysis).** A tube is passed through the duodenum and a large volume of dilute barium is introduced. In some centres this is the examination of choice for the assessment of small bowel disease. It is particularly useful when there is suspicion of intermittent bowel obstruction to demonstrate strictures or adhesions.
- **Barium enema.** Patients are given a low-fibre diet for 3 days and the colon thoroughly cleansed with oral laxative preparations. Barium and air are insufflated via a rectal catheter and double-contrast views obtained of the entire colon. Rectal examination and sigmoidoscopy should precede this examination. Some patients find the examination rather difficult to tolerate – particularly the elderly, frail or immobile in whom other tests such as CT should be used. An 'instant' barium enema involving no bowel preparation is very occasionally used in colitis .

Plain X-rays

Plain X-rays of the chest and abdomen are chiefly used in the investigation of an acute abdomen (see p. 341) including patients presenting with acute colitis (p. 317). Analysis of gas shadows gives information about the bowel. Areas of calcification can be seen in chronic pancreatitis. Faecal loading is seen in constipation.

Ultrasound, computed tomography (CT) and magnetic resonance imaging (MRI)

These techniques are used to define the intra-abdominal organs (e.g. liver, spleen, pancreas) but also to detect thickened bowel, masses, abscesses or fistulae. Ultrasound is often performed first as it is cheap and easy to perform although very operator dependent.

- **Ultrasound.** This involves no exposure to radiation and is the first-line investigation for the liver, gall bladder, spleen and pancreas. It will show dilated fluid-filled loops of bowel where there is obstruction, and thickening of the bowel wall when inflamed or infiltrated. It is valuable when ascites is suspected or when there is suspicion of abscess when it can be used to guide percutaneous drainage. In the acute abdomen, ultrasound can diagnose cholecystitis, appendicitis, enlarged mesenteric glands and other inflammatory conditions.
- **Endoscopic ultrasound (EUS).** A gastroscope incorporating a high-frequency ultrasound probe at the tip is used to assess abnormalities arising in the oesophageal or gastric wall. It is particularly valuable in the detailed staging of oesophageal/gastric cancer, including detection of local lymph nodes. It is also a sensitive technique for detection of small pancreatic tumours.
- **Endoanal ultrasonography** involves the passage of a transducer into the rectum. It is used to define the anatomy of the anal sphincters (p. 323), to detect perianal disease and to stage rectal carcinomas.
- **Computed tomography.** CT, particularly thin-section spiral CT, gives excellent anatomical definition. Modern multi-slice fast scanners are also able to evaluate the vascularity of an abnormality using intravenous contrast. The bowel wall and mesentery are well seen, together with the retroperitonal structures. It is used as a first-line investigation for the acute abdomen in many centres. Small volumes of gas from a perforated viscus can be detected as well as leakage of contrast from the gut lumen. Abscesses, appendicitis, diverticulitis, Crohn's disease and its complications can be demonstrated as well as the presence and cause of high-grade bowel obstruction. It is widely used in cancer staging and as guidance for fine-needle biopsy of tumour or lymph nodes. CT pneumocolon/CT colonography (virtual colonoscopy) involves air insufflation into the colon after colon preparation and provides a valuable alternative for evaluation of colon mass lesions. It is being used as a screening test for colon cancer with sensitivities of over 90% for > 10 mm polyps (see p. 334)
- **Magnetic resonance imaging.** MRI has the advantage of using no ionizing radiation. It is particularly useful in the evaluation of abscesses and fistulae in the perianal region and its use is evolving in the evaluation of luminal gut disease. MRI is used more in hepatobiliary and pancreatic disease (see p. 354).

- **Positron emission tomography (PET)** after fludeoxy-glucose F18 is used for staging oesophageal, gastric and colorectal cancer and in the detection of metastatic and recurrent disease.

Radioisotope imaging

Radionuclides are used to a varying degree depending on local enthusiasm and expertise. Indications are:

- to demonstrate oesophageal reflux using [^{99m}Tc] technetium–sulphur colloid
- to determine the rate of gastric emptying using [^{99m}Tc] technetium–sulphur colloid or ^{111}In-DTPA (indium-labelled diethylene triamine penta-acetic acid)
- to demonstrate a Meckel's diverticulum using [^{99m}Tc] pertechnetate, which has an affinity for gastric mucosa
- to show the extent of inflammation and the presence of any inflammatory collections in inflammatory bowel disease using ^{99m}Tc HMPAO (hexamethylpropylene amine oxime) labelled white cells
- neuroendocrine tumours using radiolabelled octreotide and whole-body scanning.

Isotopes can also be used for assessing:

- gastrointestinal loss of red cells by giving ^{51}Cr red cells and measuring radioactivity in the faeces, or by labelling red cells with ^{99m}Tc and scanning the abdomen, e.g. Meckel's diverticulum
- albumin loss in the stools in protein-losing enteropathy by giving ^{51}CrCl$_3$ intravenously (p. 306)
- bile salt malabsorption by whole-body scanning and counting the activity in the faeces following oral ^{75}Se-homochoyl taurine (SeHCAT)
- urea breath test (p. 248)
- bacterial overgrowth by measuring ^{14}CO$_2$ in the breath following ^{14}C glycocholic acid orally.

Endoscopy (Practical box 6.2)

Video endoscopes have largely replaced the old fibreoptic types. They have three chips (for blue, green and red light) mounted at the tip of the instrument. These chips relay colour images via an image processor to a television monitor. A permanent record of the procedure can be obtained.

The tip of the endoscope can be angulated in all directions. Channels are present in the endoscope for air insufflation, water injection, suction and for the passage of biopsy forceps or brushes for obtaining tissue. These latter channels can also be used for other therapeutic interventions (e.g. injection of varices).

- **Oesophagogastroduodenoscopy (OGD).** This is often used as the investigation of choice for upper GI disorders by gastroenterologists because of easy access, the possibility of interventional therapy and obtaining mucosal biopsies. Relative contraindications include severe chronic obstructive pulmonary disease, a recent myocardial infarction, or instability of the atlanto-axial joints. The mortality for diagnostic endoscopy is

Practical Box 6.2
Gastroscopy and colonoscopy

- Explain to the patient the nature of the procedure (pamphlets are available).
- Get written consent.
- Tell the patient that i.v. sedation may be given.

Gastroscopy
1. The patient is fasted for at least 4 hours.
2. The throat is sprayed with lidocaine.
3. Intravenous sedation is usually not given except to the very anxious patient or for additional procedures.
4. Oxygen saturation is monitored.
5. Oxygen via nasal prongs is given to elderly patients.
6. The instrument is passed into the pharynx under direct vision, then down the oesophagus into the stomach and duodenum.
7. The patient must be 'nil by mouth' for approximately 1½ hours following the procedure and may complain of a sore throat and abdominal discomfort.
8. Complications include local perforation and aspiration pneumonia.

Colonoscopy
1. *Two days before* the procedure, start a low-residue diet.
2. *One day before* the procedure:
   - Light lunch followed by clear fluids only.
   - In the morning take one sachet of sodium picosulfate with 1 pint of water.
   - In the afternoon take second sachet of sodium picosulfate with water.
   - In the evening take bisacodyl tablets with 1 pint of water.
3. *Day of procedure* take clear fluids only early morning, then nothing until after the test.
4. *Procedure:*
   - Intravenous sedation with a benzodiazepine and pethidine is required.
   - Oxygen saturation is monitored.
   - The instrument is passed under direct vision and manoeuvred around to the caecum and into the terminal ileum.
   - Observation is required for approximately 2 hours following the procedure.
   - Complications include perforation or haemorrhage following a biopsy or polypectomy.

0.001% with significant complications in 1:1000, usually when performed as an emergency (e.g. GI haemorrhage).

- **Colonoscopy.** This allows good visualization of the whole colon and terminal ileum. Biopsies can be obtained and polyps removed. The success rate for reaching the terminal ileum is approximately 90%. Perforation occurs in 1:2500 examinations and in 2% after polypectomy. The mortality is 0.02% for diagnostic colonoscopy.
- **Enteroscopy.** The small bowel from the duodenum to the ileum can be visualized by enteroscopes. The indications for this technique are limited (mainly gastrointestinal blood loss); the instruments are expensive, and consequently they are used only in a few centres.

- **Wireless capsule endoscopy** is now being used for the evaluation of gastroscopy- and colonoscopy-negative GI bleeding and for the detection of small bowel tumours.

FURTHER READING

Mallery S, Van Dam J (2000) Endoscopic practice at the start of the new millennium. *Gastroenterology* **118**: 5129–5147.

Pickhardt P J et al. (2003) Screening virtual colonoscopy. *New England Journal of Medicine* **349**: 2191–2201.

THE MOUTH

The oral cavity extends from the lips to the pharynx and contains the tongue, teeth and gums. Its primary functions are mastication, swallowing and speech.

Problems in the mouth are extremely common and, although they may be trivial, they can produce severe symptoms. Poor dental hygiene is often a factor.

Stomatitis is inflammation in the mouth from any cause, such as ill-fitting dentures. Angular stomatitis is inflammation of the corners of the mouth.

The burning mouth syndrome consists of a burning sensation with a clinically normal oral mucosa. It occurs more commonly in middle-aged and elderly females. It is probably psychogenic in nature. Halitosis is a common symptom; causes are shown in Box 6.2.

Oral ulceration

Recurrent ulceration

Recurrent aphthous ulceration of unknown aetiology is a common oral mucosa disorder affecting 20% of the population. It consists of recurrent bouts of one or more rounded, shallow, painful ulcers recurring at intervals of days to a few months.

Minor aphthous ulcers are the most common. They are less than 10 mm diameter, have a grey/white centre with a thin erythematous halo and heal within 14 days without scarring. *Major aphthous ulcers* are larger (more than 20 mm diameter), often persist for weeks or months and heal with scarring.

Most patients with recurrent ulcers are otherwise well. Various nutritional deficiencies of iron, folic acid or vitamin B_{12} (with or without gastrointestinal disorders) are occasionally found.

There are no specific, effective therapies. Corticosteroids may lessen the duration and severity of the attacks.

Box 6.2 Causes of halitosis

- Poor oral hygiene
- Anxiety when halitosis is more imaginary than real
- Rare causes:
    - oesophageal stricture
    - pulmonary sepsis

Chlorhexidine gluconate mouthwash, dapsone, colchicine, systemic steroids and azathioprine have all been used with variable effect.

Ulceration associated with systemic disorders

Oral ulceration is seen in gastrointestinal disorders, such as Crohn's disease, ulcerative colitis and coeliac disease in approximately 10–20% of cases. Other diseases associated with oral ulceration include lupus erythematosus (systemic and discoid), Behçet's disease, neutropenia (p. 464) and immunodeficiency disorders. In Reiter's disease, ulceration occurs in approximately 25–30% of patients.

Ulceration associated with dermatological disorders

These include erythema multiforme major, toxic epidermal necrolysis, lichen planus, pemphigus vulgaris, bullous pemphigoid, 'epidermolysis bullosa' and dermatitis herpetiformis.

Ulceration associated with viral infection

Herpes simplex virus. Primary herpes simplex (usually type I but rarely type II) presents with fever and widespread confluent painful ulcers. After resolution, the virus remains latent and recurs as herpes labialis ('cold sores', see p. 44).

Coxsackie. Hand, foot and mouth disease and herpangina, due to a different Coxsackie A, or rarely B, infection are described on page 50.

Other viruses. Herpes zoster and cytomegalovirus are among many viruses that can produce mouth ulceration, usually during the acute infective phase.

Ulceration associated with bacterial infection

Syphilis and tuberculosis can rarely cause oral ulcerations and are seen mainly in developing countries.

Ulceration associated with drugs

Certain drugs can cause oral lichenoid eruptions. They include antimalarials, methyldopa, tolbutamide, penicillamine and gold salts.

Trauma

Traumatic ulcers may be due to ill-fitting dentures, tooth brushing or lacerations by sharp teeth.

Neoplastic lesions (squamous cell carcinoma)

Malignant tumours of the mouth account for 1% of all malignant tumours in the UK. The majority develop on the floor of the mouth or lateral borders of the tongue. Early tumours may be painless, but advanced tumours are easily recognizable as indurated aphthous ulcers with raised and rolled edges. Aetiological agents include tobacco, heavy alcohol consumption and the areca nut. Intra-oral lesions which undergo malignant transformation include leucoplakia, lichen planus, submucous fibrosis and erythroplakia (a red patch). The previous male predominance has declined. Treatment is by surgical excision and/or radiotherapy.

Oral white patches

White lesions may be transient or persistent. Transient white patches are either due to *Candida* infection or are very occasionally seen in systemic lupus erythematosus. Oral candidiasis in adults is seen in seriously ill or immunocompromised patients, or following therapy with broad-spectrum antibiotics or inhaled steroids.

Local causes include mechanical, irritative or chemical trauma from drugs (e.g. aspirin).

Leucoplakia describes white patches for which no local cause can be found. It is associated with alcohol and (particularly) smoking, and is regarded as a premalignant condition. A biopsy should always be undertaken; histology shows alteration in the keratinization and dysplasia of the epithelium; aneuploidy is associated with a very high risk of cancer. Treatment is unsatisfactory. Isotretinoin possibly reduces disease progression. Oral *lichen planus* presents as white striae.

Oral pigmented lesions

Non-neoplastic lesions

Racial pigmentation is scattered and symmetrically distributed. Amalgam tattoo is the most common form of localized oral pigmentation and consists of blue-black macules involving the gingivae and results from the dental amalgam sequestering into the tissues. Diseases causing pigmentation include Peutz–Jeghers syndrome, Addison's disease and lichen planus. Heavy metals, such as lead, bismuth and mercury, and drugs (e.g. phenothiazines and antimalarials) all cause gingival pigmentation.

Neoplastic lesions

These include melanotic naevi on the hard palate and buccal mucosa. These are rarer in the mouth than on the skin. Malignant melanomas are rare, more common in males, and occur mainly on the upper jaw. The 5-year survival is only 5%.

The tongue

The tongue may be involved in a generalized stomatitis with similar lesions to those described above. *Glossitis* is a red, smooth, sore tongue seen in anaemia due to B$_{12}$, folate or iron deficiency. It is also seen in infections due to *Candida* and in riboflavin and nicotinic acid deficiency.

A *black hairy tongue* is due to a proliferation of chromogenic microorganisms causing brown-staining of elongated filiform papillae. The causes are unknown, but heavy smoking and the use of antiseptic mouthwashes have been implicated. A *geographic tongue* is an idiopathic condition occurring in 1–2% of the population and may be familial. There are erythematous areas surrounded by well-defined, slightly raised irregular margins. The lesions are usually painless and the patient should be reassured.

The gums

The gingivae consist of the mucous membranes covering the alveolar process of the mandible and the maxilla.

Chronic gingivitis is the most common cause of bleeding gums and is an inflammation following the accumulation of bacterial plaque. It resolves when the plaque is removed.

Acute (necrotizing) ulcerative gingivitis (Vincent's gingivitis) is characterized by the proliferation of spirochaete and fusiform bacteria. Young male smokers with poor oral hygiene are predominantly affected. It responds to oral metronidazole 200 mg three times daily for 3 days, used with chlorhexidine gluconate mouthwash.

Desquamatous gingivitis is a clinical description of smooth, red atrophic gingivae caused by lichen planus or mucous membrane pemphigoid. The diagnosis is confirmed by biopsy.

Gingival swelling is due to fibrous hyperplasia or is a result of inflammatory changes. Fibrous gingival hyperplasia is a result of hereditary gingival fibromatosis or associated with drugs (e.g. phenytoin, ciclosporin, nifedipine). Inflammatory swellings are seen in pregnancy, gingivitis and scurvy. Swelling due to infiltration is seen in acute leukaemia and Wegener's granulomatosis.

The teeth

Streptococcus mutans is the main bacterial cause of dental caries in man. These bacteria are cariogenic only in the presence of dietary sugar. Dental caries can progress to pulpitis and pulp necrosis, and spreading infection can cause dentoalveolar abscesses. If there is soft tissue swelling, antibiotics (e.g. amoxicillin or metronidazole) should be prescribed prior to dental intervention. Erosion of the teeth can also result from exposure to acid (e.g. in bulimia nervosa – p. 1311) or, very occasionally, in patients with gastro-oesophageal reflux disease.

Oral manifestations of HIV infection

In the UK, 60% of HIV-infected patients have characteristic oral lesions. Lesions strongly associated with HIV infection include candidiasis (with erythema and/or white exudates), erythematous candidiasis, oral hairy leucoplakia, Kaposi's sarcoma, non-Hodgkin's lymphoma, necrotizing ulcerative gingivitis, and necrotizing ulcerative periodontitis.

Oral hairy leucoplakia is almost pathognomonic of HIV infection and may be an early sign. It is more common in HIV-infected homosexual men than in any other high-risk group. It is characterized by white vertical corrugations on the lateral borders of the tongue, and immunostaining shows Epstein–Barr virus (p. 47).

Kaposi's sarcoma presents as a red, purple or blue macule or nodule, most commonly on the palate. It is diagnostic of AIDS. The lesion is associated with herpesvirus 8 (p. 48).

All lesions are much less common since the introduction of HAART (p. 143).

FURTHER READING
Lehner T (2003) The mouth and salivary glands. In: Cox TM, Firth JD, Warrell DA (eds) *Oxford Textbook of Medicine*, 4th edn. Oxford: Oxford University Press, 526–544.
Rees TD (2000) Orofacial granulomatosis and related conditions. *Periodontology* 21: 145–157.

THE SALIVARY GLANDS

Ptyalism (excessive salivation)

Ptyalism occurs prior to vomiting, but may be secondary to other intra-oral pathology. It can be psychogenic.

Xerostomia (dry mouth)

This can result from:

- Sjögren's syndrome
- drugs (e.g. antimuscarinic, antiparkinsonian, antihistamines, lithium, monoamine oxidase inhibitors, tricyclic and related antidepressants, and clonidine)
- radiotherapy
- psychogenic causes
- dehydration, shock and renal failure.

The principles of management are to preserve what flow remains, stimulate flow and replace saliva (glycerine and lemon mouthwash and artificial saliva).

Sialadenitis

Acute sialadenitis is due to mumps (parotitis) or bacteria. Bacteria include *Staphylococcus aureus*, *Streptococcus pyogenes* and *Strep. pneumoniae*. There is an ascending infection, usually secondary to secretory failure. Pus can be expressed from the affected duct.

Salivary duct obstruction due to calculus

Obstruction to salivary flow is usually due to a calculus. There is a painful swelling of the submandibular gland after eating and stones can sometimes be felt in the floor of the mouth. Sialography and plain X-ray films will show the calculus. Removal of the obstruction gives complete relief.

Sarcoidosis (see also p. 935)

Sarcoidosis can involve the major salivary glands and forms part of Heerfordt's syndrome (parotitis, uveitis, low-grade fever). When combined with lacrimal gland enlargement it is known as the Mikulicz syndrome.

Neoplasms

Salivary gland neoplasms account for 3% of all tumours world-wide. The majority occur in the parotid gland. The pleomorphic adenoma is the most common and 15% of these undergo malignant transformation. Recurrence following surgical excision is common. Malignant tumours classically result in 7th cranial nerve lower motor neurone signs.

THE PHARYNX AND OESOPHAGUS

Structure and function

The oesophagus is a muscular tube, approximately 25 cm long, connecting the pharynx to the stomach. The muscle coat has two layers – an outer longitudinal layer and an inner circular layer of fibres. In the upper portion both muscle layers are striated. They gradually change to smooth muscle in the lower oesophagus, where they are continuous with the muscle layer of the stomach. The oesophagus joins to the stomach, just below the diaphragm after a short intra-abdominal segment (the gastro-oesophageal junction).

The oesophagus is lined by stratified squamous epithelium; the squamo-columnar junction lies 2 cm above the gastro-oesophageal junction and is recognized endoscopically by an irregular white Z line.

The oesophagus is separated from the pharynx by the *upper oesophageal sphincter*, which is normally closed by the continuous contraction of the cricopharyngeus muscle. The *lower oesophageal sphincter* (LOS) consists of an area of the distal end of the oesophagus that has a high resting tone and is largely responsible for the prevention of gastric reflux. The reduction in tone and relaxation of the LOS that occurs with swallowing is under the control of cholinergic excitatory neurones and non-adrenergic non-cholinergic (NANC) inhibitory neurones as well as hormonal mechanisms. The presynaptic neurotransmitter is acetylcholine. The postsynaptic neurotransmitter is nitric oxide (NO), with vasoactive intestinal peptide (VIP) and other peptides playing a role.

During swallowing, the bolus of food is moved from the mouth to the pharynx voluntarily. Immediately, the upper sphincter relaxes and food enters the oesophagus. A primary peristaltic wave starts in the pharynx at the onset of swallowing and sweeps down the whole oesophagus (Fig. 6.4). Secondary peristalsis occurs locally in response to direct stimulation (e.g. distension by the bolus) and helps to clear food residue from the oesophagus. Non-peristaltic, non-propulsive tertiary waves are frequent in the elderly. The LOS relaxes when swallowing is initiated, before the arrival of the peristaltic wave.

Symptoms of oesophageal disorders

Major oesophageal symptoms are:

- dysphagia
- substernal discomfort/heartburn
- acid regurgitation
- painful swallowing (odynophagia).

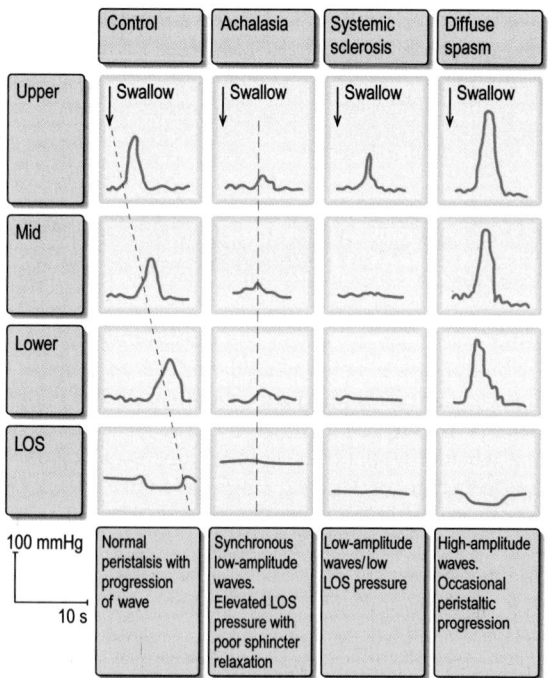

Fig. 6.4 **Oesophageal manometric patterns in normals and diseased states.** LOS, lower oesophageal sphincter. Dotted line shows peristaltic wave.

Dysphagia

This is difficulty in swallowing which is due to a local lesion or is part of a generalized disease. Patients will complain of something sticking in their throat or chest during swallowing or immediately afterwards. It is always a serious symptom and the cause must be found (Table 6.2); benign and malignant oesophageal strictures are the most common causes seen in hospital practice. *Globus* is described on page 337

Substernal discomfort/heartburn (see p. 275)

This is a common symptom of acid reflux. It is usually a retrosternal burning pain that can spread to the neck, across the chest, and can be difficult to distinguish from the pain of ischaemic heart disease. It can occur at night when the patient lies flat or after bending or stooping.

Table 6.2 **Causes of dysphagia**

Disease of mouth and tongue (e.g. tonsillitis)	Extrinsic pressure: Mediastinal glands
Neuromuscular disorders:	Goitre
Pharyngeal disorders	Enlarged left atrium
Bulbar palsy (e.g. motor neurone disease)	Intrinsic lesion: Foreign body
Myasthenia gravis	Stricture:
Oesophageal motility disorders:	benign – peptic,
Achalasia	corrosive
Scleroderma	malignant – carcinoma
Diffuse oesophageal spasm	Lower oesophageal rings
Presbyoesophagus	Oesophageal web
Diabetes mellitus	Pharyngeal pouch
Chagas' disease	

Acid regurgitation

Acid regurgitation is the effortless reflux of gastric contents into the mouth and pharynx. It occurs infrequently in normal subjects but frequently in patients with gastro-oesophageal reflux disease.

Painful swallowing

Painful swallowing without real difficulty occurs with infections (p. 279). Ingestion of tablets such as bisphosphonates and potassium (slow release) will produce local ulceration if they lodge in the gullet when swallowed lying down and without water.

Signs of oesophageal disorders

There are very few signs associated with oesophageal disease, the main one being of weight loss as a consequence of dysphagia.

Investigation of oesophageal disorders

- **Barium swallow and meal**.
- **Oesophagoscopy**.
- **Manometry** (Fig. 6.4) is performed by passing a catheter through the nose into the oesophagus and measuring the pressures generated within the region of the lower oesophageal sphincter (LOS) and body of oesophagus either for a short fixed time period (static) or up to 24 hours (ambulatory).
- **pH monitoring** – 24-hour ambulatory monitoring using a pH-sensitive probe positioned in the lower oesophagus is used to identify reflux episodes (pH < 4) and when combined with manometry is a valuable means of correlating episodes of acid reflux and oesophageal dysmotility with patients' symptoms (see Fig. 6.6).
- **Radioisotope studies** with technetium–sulphur colloid incorporated into food can also be used to study reflux. It is not widely used in the UK.
- **The Bernstein test** (alternate dilute acid and alkali infused into the oesophagus to reproduce the pain) is hardly ever used. A positive test suggests oesophagitis, but there are many false negatives.

HIATUS HERNIA

This describes the 'herniation' of part of the stomach into the chest.

In a *sliding hiatus hernia,* the gastro-oesophageal junction 'slides' through the hiatus so that it lies above the diaphragm. This type of hernia occurs in approximately 30% of people of 50 years of age and by itself is of no diagnostic significance. It does not produce symptoms on its own; symptoms occur because of the presence of associated reflux (see below).

A *para-oesophageal or rolling hernia* is when a small part of the fundus of the stomach rolls up through the hernia alongside the oesophagus. The sphincter remains below the diaphragm and remains competent. Occasionally a rolling para-oesophageal hernia will produce severe pain and require surgical treatment for gastric volvulus or strangulation.

- **Hiatus hernia** – anatomical abnormality with part of the stomach in the chest, usually asymptomatic.
- **Gastro-oesophageal reflux** – reflux of gastric contents which can occur normally with no symptoms.
- **Gastro-oesophageal reflux disease (GORD)** – patient with reflux who has persistent symptoms.
- **Reflux oesophagitis** – inflammation of the lower oesophagus produced by persistent episodes of reflux. Patients may be asymptomatic.
- **Barrett's oesophagus** – presence of intestinal metaplastic columnar epithelium which has replaced squamous epithelium as a consequence of acid reflux.

Table 6.3 Factors associated with gastro-oesophageal reflux

Pregnancy or obesity
Fat, chocolate, coffee or alcohol ingestion
Large meals
Cigarette smoking
Drugs – antimuscarinic, calcium-channel blockers, nitrates
Systemic sclerosis
After treatment for achalasia
Hiatus hernia

GASTRO-OESOPHAGEAL REFLUX DISEASE (GORD)

Gastro-oesophageal reflux occurs as a normal event, and the clinical features of GORD occur only when the antireflux mechanisms fail sufficiently to allow gastric contents to make prolonged contact with the lower oesophageal mucosa. Definitions of terms used in oesophageal disease are shown in Box 6.3.

Antireflux mechanisms (Fig. 6.5)
The lower oesophageal sphincter (LOS) is formed by the distal 4 cm of oesophageal smooth muscle. It rapidly regains its normal tone (following relaxation to allow a bolus to enter the stomach) and thereby prevents reflux. It is capable of increasing tone in response to rises in intra-abdominal and intragastric pressures.

Other antireflux measures involve the intra-abdominal segment of the oesophagus, which acts as a flap valve, and the mucosal rosette formed by folds of the gastric mucosa also helps to occlude the gastro-oesophageal junctional lumen. In addition, contraction of the crural diaphragm exerts a 'pinchcock-like' action at the LOS.

The oesophagus is normally rapidly cleared of any reflux contents by secondary peristalsis.

Pathogenesis
The following mechanisms have been implicated:

Fig. 6.5 The main antireflux mechanisms.

- Transient LOS relaxations.
- Low resting LOS tone which fails to increase when the patient is lying flat, as occurs normally.
- The LOS tone fails to increase when intra-abdominal pressure is increased by tight clothing or pregnancy.
- There is increased oesophageal mucosal sensitivity to acid.
- There is reduced oesophageal clearance of acid because of poor oesophageal peristalsis. The reduced acid clearance is exacerbated with a hiatus hernia, owing to trapping of acid within the hernial sac.
- A large hiatus hernia can impair the 'pinchcock' mechanism of the crural diaphragm.
- Delayed gastric emptying occurs, which may increase the chance of reflux.
- Prolonged episodes of gastro-oesophageal reflux occurring at night and postprandially.

Factors associated with increased gastro-oesophageal reflux are shown in Table 6.3. All or some of these features play a role in the individual patient and can occur whether or not a hiatus hernia is present. GORD often occurs without a hiatus hernia.

Clinical features
Heartburn is the major feature of GORD. Pain is mainly due to direct stimulation of the hypersensitive oesophageal mucosa, but is also partly due to spasm of the distal oesophageal muscle. The burning is aggravated by bending, stooping or lying down and may be relieved by antacids. The patient may complain of pain on drinking hot liquids or alcohol. The correlation between heartburn and oesophagitis is poor. Some patients have mild oesophagitis, but severe heartburn; others have severe oesophagitis without symptoms, and present with a haematemesis or an iron deficiency anaemia from chronic blood loss.

Regurgitation of food and 'acid' into the mouth occurs, particularly when the patient is bending or lying flat. Aspiration into the lungs, producing pneumonia, is unusual without an accompanying stricture, but cough and nocturnal asthma from regurgitation and aspiration can occasionally occur. The differential diagnosis of the retrosternal pain from angina can be difficult; 20% of cases admitted to a coronary care unit have GORD (Box 6.4).

> **Box 6.4** Features of gastro-oesophageal reflux and myocardial ischaemia
>
> **Gastro-oesophageal reflux**
> Burning pain produced by bending, stooping or lying down
> Pain seldom radiates to the arms
> Pain precipitated by drinking hot liquids or alcohol
> Relieved by antacids
>
> **Myocardial ischaemia**
> Gripping or crushing pain
> Pain radiates into neck, shoulders and both arms
> Pain produced by exercise
> Accompanied by dyspnoea

Fig. 6.7 **Endoscopic picture, showing oesophagitis.** Courtesy of Dr Geoff Smith.

Diagnosis and investigations

GORD is a clinical diagnosis and in many patients the diagnosis can be made without investigation. Under the age of 45 years, all patients should be treated initially without investigations, unless there are alarm symptoms (see p. 265).

Documenting reflux

■ Barium swallow when combined with the water siphon test is a reliable way of assessing the potential severity of reflux. It will also show the presence of a hiatus hernia.
■ 24-Hour intraluminal pH monitoring combined with manometry (see p. 274), which should always be performed to confirm GORD before considering surgery. There should be a good correlation between reflux (pH < 4.0) and symptoms (Fig. 6.6). It is also necessary to exclude oesophageal dysmotility as the cause of symptoms.
■ Radiolabelled technetium (see p. 270) is used in some centres to demonstrate reflux.

Assessing oesophagitis (Fig. 6.7)

Fibreoptic oesophagoscopy is used to confirm the presence of oesophagitis, i.e. a red friable mucosa with ulceration in severe cases (erosive oesophagitis). The technique is also used to diagnose Barrett's oesophagus (p. 277).

Fig. 6.6 **24-hour intraluminal pH monitoring.** Five reflux episodes (pH < 4) occurred, but only three gave symptoms (arrows).

Treatment

Many patients with reflux symptoms (approximately 50%) can be treated successfully with simple antacids, loss of weight, and raising the head of the bed at night. Precipitating factors should be avoided, with a reduction in alcohol consumption and cessation of smoking. These measures are simple to say, difficult to carry out, but are useful in mild cases.

Drugs

Simple antacids magnesium trisilicate and aluminium hydroxide are readily available and are often used initially by patients. The former tends to cause diarrhoea whilst the latter causes constipation. Many antacids contain sodium which may exacerbate fluid retention; aluminium hydroxide has less sodium than magnesium trisilicate.

Alginate-containing antacids (10 mL three times daily) are the most frequently prescribed agents for GORD. They form a gel or 'foam raft' with gastric contents and thereby reduce reflux. They are available over the counter and are often used by the patient before consultation.

H_2-receptor antagonists (e.g. cimetidine, ranitidine, famotidine and nizatadine) are used for acid suppression if the above measures fail and as they can be obtained over the counter in the UK they are frequently used.

Proton pump inhibitors (PPIs) (e.g. omeprazole, rabeprazole, lansoprazole, pantoprazole, esomeprazole) inhibit gastric hydrogen/potassium-ATPase (see Fig. 6.10). PPIs reduce gastric acid secretion by 90% and are the drugs of choice for all but mild cases. Patients with severe symptoms need prolonged treatment, often for years. Sometimes a lower dose, e.g. omeprazole 10 mg, is sufficient for maintenance. Rebound increased acid secretion lasting approximately 2 months occurs after 2 months' omeprazole therapy (40 mg daily).

The prokinetic agents metoclopramide and domperidone are dopamine antagonists. They are occasionally helpful as they enhance peristalsis and speed gastric emptying. Cisapride increases the QT_c interval and has been withdrawn because of the risk of arrhythmias.

Helicobacter pylori eradication in GORD has little effect on the symptoms but is usually advised (p. 285).

Using the above treatments, most patients can be kept symptom-free, but symptoms usually return when treatment is stopped and long-term therapy is then required.

Surgery

Surgery should never be performed for a hiatus hernia alone. The properly selected case with severe reflux symptoms confirmed by pH monitoring and with oesophagitis on oesophagoscopy responds well to surgery. Repair of the hernia and some sort of additional antireflux surgery (e.g. a modified Nissen fundoplication) is performed laparoscopically. Results show an improvement in symptoms in up to 80% of cases. The indications for surgery are not always clear as medical therapy with PPIs is so effective; the young patient needing years of drug treatment is one common indication.

Patients with oesophageal dysmotility unrelated to acid reflux tend to do less well as do those with underlying functional bowel disease.

Management of reflux oesophagitis

There is a poor correlation between GORD symptoms and the presence of endoscopic oesophagitis.

Many gastroenterologists treat severe oesophagitis (even in the absence of symptoms) with long-term PPIs with regular surveillance oesophagoscopy in an attempt to reduce the risk of complications. Long-term PPI therapy appears very safe.

Complications

Peptic stricture usually occurs in patients over the age of 60. The symptoms are those of intermittent dysphagia over a long period. Treatment is by dilatation of the stricture and management of the reflux usually medically with a proton-pump inhibitor to achieve anacidity. Occasionally surgery is required.

Barrett's oesophagus. This occurs from long-standing reflux. It consists of columnar epithelium with intestinal metaplasia extending upwards into the lower oesophagus replacing normal squamous epithelium. It is seen in up to 20% of patients undergoing endoscopy for gastro-oesophageal reflux disease. Endoscopically, Barrett's may be seen as a continual sheet, a finger like projection extending upwards from the squamo-columnar junction or as islands of columnar mucosa interspersed in areas of residual squamous mucosa. It is very common in middle-aged men. Barrett's oesophagus (even a short segment < 3 cm) is premalignant for adenocarcinoma. An indocarmine spray down the endoscope can detect intestinal metaplasia and possibly dysplasia. The dysplasia is patchy, and biopsies from all four quadrants (every 2 cm) of the Barrett's segment must be performed. There is no evidence that treatment with PPIs or antireflux surgery leads to Barrett's regression. Surveillance – looking for severe dysplasia/cancer – is costly and subject to observer error. Current recommendations are still controversial but the consensus view is that patients without dysplasia do not require surveillance gastroscopy. With low-grade dysplasia, 6-monthly endoscopy for 1 year, followed by endoscopy at 2- to 3-yearly intervals (along with intensive medical therapy) has been suggested. There is much controversy over high-grade dysplasia, as approximately a quarter do not progress to cancer; oesophagectomy is associated with a mortality of 3–10% and high morbidity. There are no current randomized controlled trials for guidance but laser mucosal ablation and photodynamic therapy are being tried.

Adenocarcinoma. Patients with weekly reflux symptoms are nearly eight times more likely to develop adenocarcinoma compared with those without symptoms. The greater the frequency, severity and the duration of reflux symptoms, the greater the risk.

MOTILITY DISORDERS

Achalasia

Achalasia is a disease characterized by aperistalsis in the body of the oesophagus and failure of relaxation of the lower oesophageal sphincter on initiation of swallowing. In the majority of cases the aetiology is unknown (idiopathic). The disease can present at any age but is rare in childhood. The incidence is about 1 per 100 000 per year in all ages. A similar clinical picture is seen in chronic Chagas' disease (American trypanosomiasis, p. 101) where there is damage to the neural plexus of the gut.

Pathogenesis

Degenerative lesions are found in the vagus as well as a decrease in ganglionic cells in the myenteric nerve plexus of the oesophageal wall. NANC inhibitory neurones are affected more than the cholinergic nerves, and thus the relaxation of the sphincter is impaired in the absence of nitric oxide. Some patients have autoantibodies to a dopamine-carrying protein on the surface of the cells in the myenteric plexus.

Clinical features

Patients usually have a long history of intermittent dysphagia for both liquids and solids. Regurgitation of food from the dilated oesophagus may be induced by the patient or may occur spontaneously, particularly at night, and aspiration pneumonia can occur. Occasionally food gets stuck but patients often learn to overcome this by drinking large quantities, thereby increasing the head of pressure in the oesophagus and forcing the food through. Severe retrosternal chest pain occurs particularly in younger patients with vigorous non-peristaltic contraction of the oesophagus. The dysphagia in these patients can be mild and the pain misdiagnosed as cardiac in origin. Weight loss is usually not marked.

Investigations

- **Chest X-ray** may show a dilated oesophagus, sometimes with a fluid level seen behind the heart. The fundal gas shadow is not present.

- **Barium swallow** will show dilatation of the oesophagus, lack of peristalsis and often synchronous contractions. The lower end gradually narrows ('swan neck deformity'); this appearance is due to failure of the sphincter to relax (Fig. 6.8).
- **Oesophagoscopy** is necessary to exclude a carcinoma at the lower end of the oesophagus, as an intramucosal carcinoma can produce a similar X-ray appearance. When there is marked dilatation, extensive cleansing is necessary to remove food debris in order to obtain a clear view. In achalasia the oesophagoscope easily flops through the apparent narrowing without resistance.
- **CT scan**. This is helpful, particularly in detecting an intramucosal carcinoma.
- **Manometry** shows aperistalsis of the oesophagus as well as the failure of relaxation of the lower oesophageal sphincter (see Fig. 6.4).

Treatment

The treatment of choice is endoscopic dilatation of the LOS using a pneumatic bag (passed under X-ray control). This weakens the sphincter and is successful in 80% of cases. Endoscopic injection of botulinum toxin into the LOS has been used with variable success. If these measures fail, surgical division of the muscle at the lower end of the oesophagus (cardiomyotomy or Heller's operation) is performed laparoscopically. Reflux oesophagitis complicates all procedures and the aperistalsis of

Fig. 6.8 **Barium swallow showing achalasia** with atonic body of the oesophagus and a narrowed distal end. Note food residue in dilated oesophagus.

the oesophagus remains. In older patients, nifedipine (20 mg sublingually) or sildenafil can be tried initially.

Complications

There is a slight increase in the incidence of squamous carcinoma of the oesophagus in both treated and untreated cases (7% after 25 years).

Systemic sclerosis (see also p. 577)

There is oesophageal involvement in 90% or more of patients with this disease. Diminished peristalsis, detected manometrically (see Fig. 6.4) or by barium swallow, is due to replacement of the smooth muscle layers by fibrous tissue. The lower oesophageal sphincter pressure is also decreased, allowing reflux; mucosal damage occurs as a consequence. Strictures may develop. Initially there are no symptoms, but dysphagia and heartburn occur as the oesophagus becomes severely involved.

Similar motility abnormalities may be found in other connective-tissue disorders, particularly if Raynaud's phenomenon is present. Treatment is as for reflux (see p. 276) and stricture formation.

Diffuse oesophageal spasm

This is a severe form of abnormal oesophageal motility that can sometimes produce retrosternal chest pain and dysphagia. It can accompany GORD. Swallowing is accompanied by bizarre and marked contractions of the oesophagus without propagation of the waves (see Fig. 6.4). On barium swallow the appearance may be that of a 'corkscrew'. However, changes in oesophageal motility 'dysmotility' are not infrequent, particularly in patients over the age of 60 years (presbyoesophagus). Care must therefore be taken that the symptoms, the manometry and X-ray findings of oesophageal spasm are not falsely correlated; functional dyspepsia is commoner than oesophageal spasm.

A variant of diffuse oesophageal spasm is the 'nutcracker' oesophagus, which is characterized by finding very high-amplitude peristalsis (pressures > 200 mmHg) within the oesophagus. Chest pain and dysphagia occur.

Treatment

True oesophageal spasm producing severe symptoms is uncommon and treatment is often difficult. When the spasm is due to GORD, acid suppression is given. Antispasmodics, nitrates, or calcium-channel blockers – such as sublingual nifedipine 10 mg three times daily – may be tried. Occasionally, balloon dilatation or even myotomy is necessary.

Miscellaneous motility disorders

Abnormalities of motility that are mostly asymptomatic but occasionally produce dysphagia are found in the elderly, in diabetes mellitus, myotonia dystrophica and myasthenia gravis, as well as neurological disorders involving the brainstem.

OTHER OESOPHAGEAL DISORDERS

Oesophageal diverticulum

This is a pouch lined with epithelium that can produce dysphagia and regurgitation. It is usually asymptomatic and often detected accidentally on a barium swallow performed for other reasons. Diverticula can occur:

- immediately above the upper oesophageal sphincter (pharyngeal pouch) (p. 1161)
- near the middle of the oesophagus (traction diverticulum produced by extrinsic inflammation)
- just above the lower oesophageal sphincter (epiphrenic diverticulum).

Only when symptoms are severe should surgery be undertaken.

Rings and webs

A number of rings and webs have been described throughout the oesophagus.

Upper oesophageal web

This is a constriction near the upper oesophageal sphincter in the post-cricoid region and appears radiologically as a web. The web may be asymptomatic or may produce dysphagia. In the Plummer–Vinson syndrome (Paterson–Brown–Kelly syndrome) this web is associated with iron deficiency anaemia, glossitis and angular stomatitis. This rare syndrome affects mainly women and its aetiology is not understood. At oesophagoscopy the web may be difficult to see. Dilatation of the web is rarely necessary. Iron is given for the iron deficiency.

Cricopharyngeal dysfunction

There is poor relaxation of the cricopharyngeal muscle during swallowing so that a prominent indentation or 'bar' is seen on a barium swallow. It occurs in the elderly. Dysphagia is treated with dilatation but surgical myotomy may be necessary.

Lower oesophageal or Schatzki ring

This is a narrowing of the lower end of the oesophagus due to a ridge of mucosa or a fibrous membrane. The ring may be asymptomatic, but it can very occasionally produce dysphagia after swallowing a large bolus of bread or meat. A barium swallow (with the oesophagus well distended with barium) often shows the narrowing; barium-coated bread will lodge at the narrowing. Treatment is with reassurance and dietary advice, but dilatation is occasionally necessary.

Benign oesophageal stricture

Peptic stricture secondary to reflux is the most common cause of benign strictures (for treatment, see p. 277). They also occur after the ingestion of corrosives, after radiotherapy, after sclerosis of varices, and following prolonged nasogastric intubation. All strictures give rise to dysphagia. They are usually treated by dilatation, but occasionally surgery is necessary.

Oesophageal infections

Infection is a cause of painful swallowing and is seen particularly in immunosuppressed debilitated patients and patients with AIDS. Infection can occur with:

- *Candida*
- herpes simplex
- cytomegalovirus.

It is occasionally difficult to distinguish between these either on barium swallow or oesophagoscopy, as only widespread ulceration is seen. In candidiasis the characteristic white plaques on top of friable mucosa are frequently found but oral candidiasis is not always present. The diagnosis of *Candida* infection can be confirmed by examining a direct smear taken at endoscopy, but often infections are mixed and cultures and biopsies must be performed.

Treatment

Most patients on large doses of immunosuppressive agents are treated prophylactically with nystatin or amphotericin. Other antifungal or antiviral treatment is given appropriately (see Ch. 2).

The Mallory–Weiss syndrome

This is described on page 293.

Oesophageal perforation or rupture

Oesophageal perforation usually occurs at the time of endoscopic dilatation or very occasionally following insertion of a nasogastric tube. Patients with a malignant, corrosive or post-radiotherapy stricture are more likely to perforate than those with a benign peptic stricture.

Management usually involves placement of an oesophageal stent (p. 281), which dilates the usually malignant stricture and seals the hole. A water-soluble contrast X-ray is performed after 2–3 days to check the perforation has sealed.

Oesophageal rupture occurs with violent vomiting, producing severe chest pain and collapse. It may follow alcohol ingestion. A chest X-ray shows a hydropneumothorax. The diagnosis is made radiologically using water-soluble contrast. Treatment is surgical; mortality is high.

OESOPHAGEAL TUMOURS

Cancer of the oesophagus

This is the fifth most common cancer seen throughout the world. Approximately 40% occur in the middle third of the oesophagus and are squamous carcinomas. Adeno-carcinomas (approx 45%) occur in the lower third of the oesophagus and at the cardia. Tumours of the upper third are rare (15%).

Epidemiology and aetiological factors

Squamous cell carcinoma (SCC)

The incidence of this carcinoma varies throughout the world, being high in China, parts of Africa and in the Caspian regions of Iran (where the incidence is the highest observed for any type of cancer anywhere in the world). In the UK the incidence is 5–10 per 100 000 and represents 2.2% of all malignant disease. The variation in incidence throughout the world is greater than for any other carcinoma and is unusual in that sharp differences occur in regions very close to one another. The incidence of SCC is decreasing, in contrast to adenocarcinoma.

SCC of the oesophagus is more common in men (2 : 1); risk factors are shown in Table 6.4. Monotonous diets very high in cereals and *N*-nitroso compounds in preserved food, possibly increase the risk. Diets high in carotenoids and vitamin C (vegetables and fruit) possibly decrease the risk.

Adenocarcinoma

These tumours arise in the columnar-lined epithelium of the lower oesophagus (Barrett's oesophagus, p. 277). This columnarization results from long-standing reflux, although some patients will have no preceding symptoms. This premalignant lesion increases the chances of developing an adenocarcinoma 30–40-fold. The incidence rate of this tumour is increasing (fivefold in Europe and the USA). Extension of an adenocarcinoma of the gastric cardia into the oesophagus can present with the same symptoms.

Clinical features

Carcinoma of the oesophagus occurs mainly in those aged 60–70 years, although it is now occurring in younger age groups. Dysphagia is the most common single

Table 6.4	Risk factors for cancer of the oesophageal
Squamous cell carcinoma	**Adenocarcinoma**
Tobacco smoking	Long-standing weekly GORD
High alcohol intake	Barrett's oesophagus
Plummer–Vinson	Tobacco smoking
syndrome	Obesity
Achalasia	Breast cancer treated
Corrosive strictures	with radiotherapy
Coeliac disease	
Breast cancer treated with	
radiotherapy	
Tylosis*	
Diet deficient in vitamins;	
high dietary carotenoids	
and vitamin C possibly	
decrease the risk	

* Tylosis is an autosomal dominant condition with hyperkeratosis of the palms and soles

symptom and is progressive and unrelenting. Initially there is difficulty in swallowing solids, but eventually dysphagia for liquids also occurs. Benign strictures, on the other hand, initially produce intermittent dysphagia. Impaction of food causes pain, but more persistent pain implies infiltration.

The lesion is usually ulcerative, extending around the wall of the oesophagus to produce a stricture. Direct invasion of the surrounding structures occurs rather than widespread metastases. Weight loss, due to the dysphagia as well as to anorexia, frequently occurs. The oesophageal obstruction eventually causes difficulty in swallowing saliva, and coughing and aspiration into the lungs is common.

Signs are often absent. Weight loss, anorexia and lymphadenopathy are occasionally found.

Investigation

Diagnostic

Endoscopy/barium swallow. Many gastroenterologists like to go directly to oesophagoscopy, which provides histological or cytological proof of the carcinoma; 90% of oesophageal carcinomas can be confirmed with this technique. Barium swallow (Fig. 6.9a) is also a very sensitive technique and is useful in the younger patient with dysphagia where the differential diagnosis includes a motility disorder.

Staging for surgery

The TNM staging system is used (p. 490). Extent of tumour invasion (T), presence of tumour in lymph nodes (N) or metastases (M) are combined into stage categories.

- **CT scan and MRI** of the thorax and upper abdomen will show the volume of the tumour, local invasion and lymph node involvement.
- **Endoscopic ultrasound** (Fig. 6.9b) has an accuracy rate of nearly 90% for assessing depth of tumour and infiltration and 80% for staging lymph node involvement.
- **Positron emission tomography (PET)** after fludeoxyglucose F18 is being used. Its specificity is high with a similar sensitivity to CT and MRI for distant metastases.

Treatment

This depends on the age and performance status of the patient and the stage of the disease. Five-year survival with stage 1 is 80% (T_1/T_2, N_0, M_0), stage 2 is 30%, stage 3 is 18% and stage 4 is 4%. Seventy per cent of patients present with stage 3 disease, so that overall survival is 27% at 1 year and 14% at 5 years. Management should be undertaken by multidisciplinary teams.

Surgery

Surgery provides the best chance of a cure and should be used only when imaging (see above) has shown that the tumour has not infiltrated outside the oesophageal wall. Surgery in this group shows an 80% 5-year survival rate if the postoperative pathology confirms the staging. The patients must be carefully evaluated preoperatively,

(a)

(b)

Fig. 6.9 **Carcinoma of the oesophagus. (a) Barium swallow**, showing an irregular narrowed area (arrows) at the lower end of the oesophagus. **(b) Endoscopic ultrasound.** The central concentric circles are the probe. The arrow points to a break in the muscle layer and the soft tissue mass of the carcinoma.

particularly with regard to performance status (p. 490), and surgery undertaken in designated units.

Radiotherapy

This is now seldom used on its own for squamous or adenocarcinoma except for palliation.

Chemotherapy/chemoradiation

5FU, cisplatinum and combined chemoradiation are being used for squamous carcinoma (see p. 521) before and after surgical resection (neo-adjuvant) in some centres, with some prolongation of survival.

Palliative therapy (see also p. 524)

This is often the only realistic possibility. Repeated dilatation or dilatation of the stricture with the insertion of an expanding metal stent to keep the oesophageal lumen open is performed via an endoscope. This allows liquids and soft foods to be eaten. Fizzy drinks are recommended to keep the tubes from blocking. Additional chemoradiation improved survival from 9 months to 14.9 months in one study. Brachytherapy has also been shown to give long-term relief.

Tumours can be photocoagulated using a laser beam delivered through an endoscope, or necrosed using alcohol injections. This relieves the dysphagia, but repeated treatments are necessary. Photodynamic therapy is being tried to reduce the tumour bulk.

Nutritional support, as well as support for the patient and their family, is vital in this distressing condition.

Other oesophageal tumours

Most other tumours are rare. Gastrointestinal stromal tumours (p. 290) are found usually by chance. Ten per cent cause dysphagia or bleeding. Surgical removal is performed for symptomatic lesions.

Kaposi's sarcoma is found in the oesophagus as well as the mouth (see p. 272) and hypopharynx in patients with AIDS.

FURTHER READING
Allum WH (2002) Guidelines for the management of oesophageal and gastric cancer. *Gut* **50** (Suppl. V): 1–17.
Enzinger PC, Mayer RJ (2003) Esophageal cancer. *New England Journal of Medicine* **349**: 2241–2252.
Fiorica F et al. (2004) Preoperative chemoradiotherapy for oesophageal cancer – meta-analysis. *Gut* **53**: 925–930.
Katzha DA, Rustgi AK (2000) Gastro-oesophageal reflux disease and Barrett's oesophagus. *Medical Clinics of North America* **84**: 1137–1161.
Lagergreen J et al. (1999) Symptomatic gastro-oesophageal reflux as a risk factor for oesophageal adenocarcinoma. *New England Journal of Medicine* **340**: 825–831.
Mittal RK, Balaban DH (1997) The esophago-gastric junction. *New England Journal of Medicine* **336**: 924–932.
Richter JE (2001) Oesophageal motility disorders. *Lancet* **358**: 823–828.

THE STOMACH AND DUODENUM

Structure

The stomach, which varies considerably in size, is divided into a small area immediately distal to the oesophagus (the cardia), the upper region (the fundus which lies under the left diaphragm), the mid-region or body, and the antrum, which extends into the pyloric region.

There are two sphincters, the gastro-oesophageal sphincter and the pyloric sphincter; the latter is largely made up of a thickening of the circular muscle layer. The muscle wall of the stomach has three layers – an outer longitudinal, an inner circular, and an innermost oblique layer of smooth muscle.

The duodenum has outer longitudinal and inner smooth muscle layers. It is C-shaped and the pancreas sits in the concavity. It terminates in the jejunum at the duodenojejunal flexure.

The mucosal lining of the stomach, particularly in the greater curvature, is thrown into thick folds or rugae. The upper two-thirds of the stomach contains parietal cells, which secrete hydrochloric acid, and chief cells, which secrete pepsinogen (which initiates proteolysis). The junction between the body and the antrum of the stomach can often be seen macroscopically, but can be confirmed by measuring surface pH. The antrum contains mucus-secreting and G cells, which secrete gastrin. There are two major forms of gastrin, G17 and G34, depending on the number of amino-acid residues. G17 is the major form found in the antrum. Mucus-secreting cells are present throughout the stomach and secrete mucus and bicarbonate which is trapped in the mucus gel. The mucus is made of glycoproteins called mucins. Somatostatin is also produced by specialized antral cells (D cells).

The mucosal barrier, made up of the surface membranes of mucosal cells and the mucus, protects the gastric epithelium from damage by, for example, alcohol, aspirin, NSAIDs, and bile salts. Prostaglandins stimulate secretion of mucus, and their synthesis is inhibited by aspirin and NSAIDs, which inhibit cyclo-oxygenase (see Fig. 14.32).

The duodenal mucosa contains Brunner's glands, which secrete alkaline mucus. This, along with the pancreatic and biliary secretions, helps to neutralize the acid secretion from the stomach when it reaches the duodenum.

Function

The factors controlling acid secretion are shown in Figure 6.10. Secretion is under neural and hormonal control. Both stimulate acid secretion through the direct release of histamine on the parietal cell. Acetylcholine and gastrin also release histamine via the enterochromaffin cells. Somatostatin inhibits both histamine and gastrin release and therefore acid secretion.

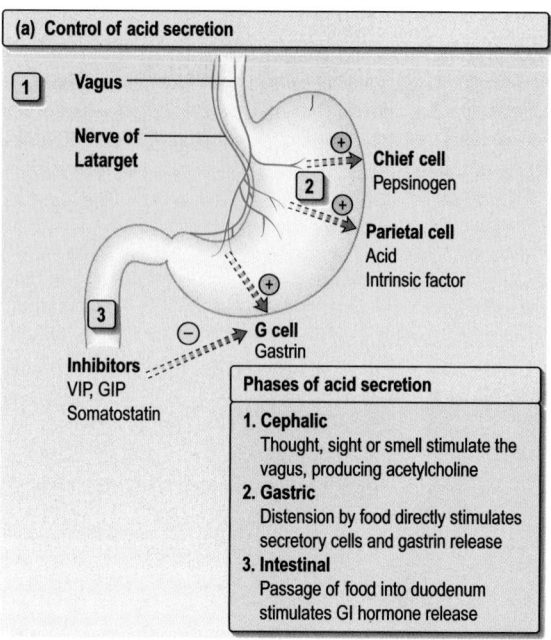

(a) **Control of acid secretion**

Phases of acid secretion

1. **Cephalic**
   Thought, sight or smell stimulate the vagus, producing acetylcholine
2. **Gastric**
   Distension by food directly stimulates secretory cells and gastrin release
3. **Intestinal**
   Passage of food into duodenum stimulates GI hormone release

(b) **Mechanisms involved in acid secretion**

Fig. 6.10 **(a) Control of acid secretion.**
(b) Mechanisms involved in acid secretion.

- *Gastrin* acts via the gastrin receptor, increasing the intracellular free calcium, and the ECL cell stimulating histamine.
- *Acetylcholine* (ACh) acts via the M_3 receptors and is vagally stimulated.
- ACh and gastrin also act via the enterochromaffin cell.
- *Histamine* stimulates G_s via the H_2 receptors and acts via cyclic AMP.
- *Prostaglandin E_2* activates the G_i protein and INHIBITS acid secretion.

G_s and G_i, stimulating and inhibiting G-proteins; ECL, enterochromaffin cells.

Other major gastric functions are:

- acting as a reservoir for food
- the emulsification of fat and mixing of gastric contents
- the secretion of intrinsic factor
- absorption (of only minimal importance).

Gastric emptying depends on many factors. There are osmoreceptors in the duodenal mucosa that control gastric emptying by local reflexes and the release of gut hormones. In particular, intraduodenal fat delays gastric emptying by negative feedback through duodenal receptors.

HELICOBACTER PYLORI INFECTION

H. pylori is a spiral-shaped Gram-negative urease-producing bacterium (Fig. 6.11). Its complete genomic sequence is known. It is found in the gastric antrum and in areas of gastric metaplasia in the duodenum. *H. pylori* is found in greatest numbers under the mucus layers in gastric pits, where it adheres specifically to gastric epithelial cells.

(a)

(b)

Fig. 6.11   Helicobacter pylori.
(a) Organisms (arrowed) are shown on the gastric mucosa (cresyl fast violet (modified Giemsa) stain). Courtesy of Dr Alan Phillips, Department of Paediatric Gastroenterology, Royal Free Hospital.
(b) Scanning electron microscopy, showing the spiral-shaped bacterium.

Colonization in the acid environment of the gastric mucosa occurs because:

- Sheathed flagella allow the organisms to move quickly from the acidic lumen of the stomach through the mucus layer where the pH is higher. (Mutant strains that are non-motile do not colonize.)
- Acute infection produces transient hypochlorhydria.
- *H. pylori* produces urease (see Fig. 6.12). The ammonia produced neutralizes the acid.
- It possesses a proton pump.

Epidemiology

The exact mode of transmission is unclear, but intra-familial clustering suggests person-to-person spread, either oral–oral or faeco-oral mainly in childhood. The prevalence of *H. pylori* is high in developing countries (80–90% of the population) and its presence is associated with lower socio-economic status world-wide. Between one- and two-thirds of the western populations have this infection and the prevalence is high in the older population – presumably acquired in their childhood when hygiene was less good than today.

Pathogenesis

H. pylori infection produces a gastritis mainly in the antrum of the stomach. The mucosa appears reddened endoscopically, and histologically there is epithelial cell damage from local release of cytokines such as IL-6 and IL-8. This leads to recruitment and activation of an inflammatory infiltrate in the lamina propria. This consists of polymorphonuclear leucocytes, eosinophils, lymphocytes, monocytes and plasma cells.

In some individuals this chronic superficial gastritis can involve the body of the stomach and this leads to atrophic gastritis. Intestinal metaplasia, which is a pre-malignant pathological change, occurs in some of these areas (see Fig. 6.15).

Duodenal ulcer (DU) disease

H. pylori is causally associated with DU disease because in patients with DU:

- 95% are infected with *H. pylori*
- cure of the infection stops duodenal ulcer recurrence.

The precise mechanism of how duodenal ulceration occurs is unclear, as only 15% of patients infected with *H. pylori* (approximately 50–60% of the adult population world-wide) develop duodenal ulcers. Factors that have been implicated include:

- Increased acid secretion because of:
  – increased parietal cell mass
  – increased gastrin secretion.
- Smoking impairing gastric mucosal healing.
- Virulence factors: *H. pylori* produces toxins, Vac A (vacuolating toxin) and Cag A (cytotoxic associated protein) as well as urease and adherence factors. There is controversy over their role in producing duodenal ulcer disease.

- Decreased inhibition of acid secretion; *H. pylori*-induced gastritis reduces somatostatin production in the antrum with loss of the negative feedback on gastrin secretion.
- Genetic susceptibility may play a role. DUs are more common in patients who have blood group O and are non-secretors of blood group substances in saliva.
- These factors lead to an increased acid load to the duodenum, which precipitates bile salts which would normally inhibit the growth of *H. pylori*.

Bicarbonate secretion is decreased in the duodenum by *H. pylori* inflammation and the damage and repair leads to gastric metaplasia which *H. pylori* colonizes, causing local release of cytokines and further damage.

Gastric ulcers (GU)

Gastric ulcers are associated with a gastritis affecting the body as well as the antrum of the stomach (pangastritis). Parietal cell damage occurs so that acid production is normal or low. The ulcers occur because of local epithelial damage by cytokines released by *H. pylori* and also because of abnormal mucus production.

Clinical syndromes

H. pylori gastritis

This is usually asymptomatic; whether *H. pylori* gastritis itself produces epigastric discomfort, i.e. functional dyspepsia, is controversial.

Peptic ulcer disease

Epidemiology

DUs are very common and are two to three times more common than gastric ulcers (GUs). Approximately 10–15% of the population will suffer from a DU.

Ulcer rates are declining rapidly for younger men and increasing for older individuals, particularly women. Both DUs and GUs are common in the elderly. There is a considerable geographical variation; for example, DUs are more common in northern England and Scotland than in other parts of the UK.

Pathology

Gastric ulcers are found in any part of the stomach, but are most commonly seen on the lesser curve. Most duodenal ulcers are found in the duodenal cap; the surrounding mucosa appears inflamed, haemorrhagic or friable (duodenitis). Erosions are superficial mucosal defects, whereas in a peptic ulcer there is a break in the superficial epithelial cells penetrating down to the muscularis mucosa at the site of the ulcer; there is a fibrous base and an increase in inflammatory cells. *H. pylori*-induced gastritis is present, confined to the antrum in DU disease but also involving the body in gastric ulcer disease. Occasionally peptic ulcers are seen without *H. pylori*, e.g. Zollinger–Ellison syndrome (p. 416).

Clinical features

The characteristic feature is epigastric pain. It has been shown that if a patient points to the epigastrium as the site of the pain this has a high discriminatory value for diagnosis. The relationship of the pain to food is variable and on the whole not helpful in the diagnosis. The pain of a DU classically occurs at night (as well as during the day) and is worse when the patient is hungry. Both gastric and duodenal ulcers are helped by antacids.

Nausea may accompany the pain; vomiting is infrequent but often relieves the pain. Heartburn occurs owing to acid regurgitation. Anorexia and weight loss may occur, particularly with gastric ulcers. If the patient complains of persistent and severe pain, complications such as penetration into other organs may have occurred. Back pain suggests a penetrating posterior duodenal ulcer. Severe ulceration can occasionally be symptomless, as 50% of patients who have died from the complications of peptic ulceration were unaware of the diagnosis prior to the final event. Patients can present for the first time with either a haematemesis or melaena or a perforation.

Untreated, the symptoms of a DU are periodic with spontaneous relapses and remissions. The natural history is for the disease to remit over many years with the onset of atrophic gastritis and a decrease in acid secretion.

Examination. This is usually unhelpful; epigastric tenderness is quite common in non-ulcer dyspepsia.

Diagnosis of *Helicobacter pylori* infection

Non-invasive methods

- ^{13}C *Urea breath test* (Fig. 6.12). This is a quick and easy way of detecting the presence of *H. pylori* and is used as a screening test. The measurement of $^{13}CO_2$ in the breath, after ingestion of ^{13}C urea, requires a mass spectrometer, which is expensive, but the test is very

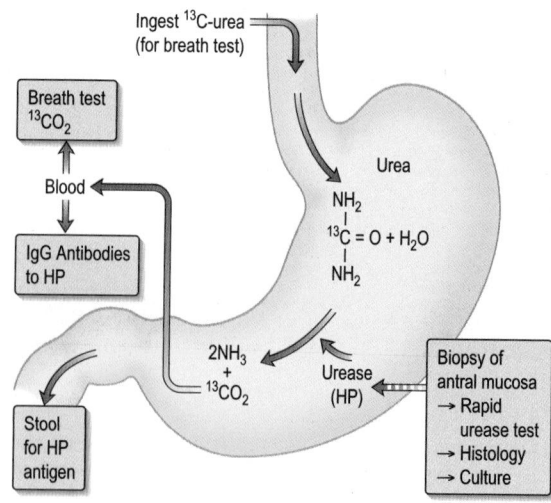

Fig. 6.12 Metabolism of urea by *Helicobacter pylori* (HP), showing the different tests that are available for the detection of *H. pylori*.

sensitive (97%) and specific (96%). The breath test is also used to demonstrate eradication of the organism following treatment.

- *Serological tests* detect IgG antibodies and are reasonably sensitive (90%) and specific. They are used in the diagnosis and in epidemiological studies. IgG titres may take up to 1 year to fall by 50% after eradication therapy and therefore are not useful for confirming eradication or the presence of a current infection. Antibodies can also be found in the saliva, but tests are not as sensitive or specific as serology.
- *Stool test.* A specific immunoassay using monoclonal antibodies for the qualitative detection of *H. pylori* antigen is widely available. The overall sensitivity is 96% with a specificity of 97%. It is useful in the diagnosis of *H. pylori* infection and for monitoring efficacy of eradication therapy. (Patients should be off PPIs for 1 week but can continue with H_2 blockers.)

Invasive (endoscopy)

- *Rapid urease test.* Gastric biopsies are added to a urea solution containing phenol red. If *H. pylori* are present, the urease enzyme splits the urea to release ammonia which raises the pH of the solution and causes a rapid colour change.
- *Culture.* Biopsies obtained can be cultured on a special medium, and sensitivities to antibiotics can be ascertained.
- *Histology.* *H. pylori* can be detected histologically on routine (Giemsa) stained sections of gastric mucosa obtained at endoscopy.

Investigation of suspected peptic ulcer disease

- *Patients under 55 years of age* with typical symptoms of peptic ulcer disease who are *H. pylori* positive require no further investigation and can start eradication therapy.
- *In older patients*, confirmation of peptic ulcer is required. Endoscopy is the preferred investigation (Fig. 6.13). All gastric ulcers must be biopsied. A duodenal ulcer is shown in Figure 6.14.
- *In all patients* with 'alarm symptoms', (p. 265) endoscopy is required.

Eradication therapy

Current recommendations are that all patients with duodenal and gastric ulcers should have *H. pylori* eradication therapy.

Many patients, however, are tested for *H. pylori* (see above). Some of these patients will have incidental *H. pylori* infection with no gastric/duodenal lesion, and whether all such patients should have eradication therapy is controversial (see Functional dyspepsia, p. 337). There has been an increase in the prevalence of GORD and adenocarcinoma of the lower oesophagus in the last few years and some gastroenterologists thought this might be linked to eradication of *H. pylori*. This is unlikely and eradication of *H. pylori* is often advised in the hope that symptoms will be reduced and because of the link between *H. pylori* and gastric cancer.

Fig. 6.13 **Endoscopic picture of a benign gastric ulcer.** Courtesy of Dr P.D. Fairclough.

Fig. 6.14 **Duodenal ulcer**. Endoscopic view showing the ulcer with inflamed duodenal folds. Courtesy of Dr P.D. Fairclough.

All eradication therapies are successful in approximately 90% of patients.

Reinfection is very uncommon (1%) in developed countries. In developing countries, where compliance with treatment may be poor and metronidazole resistance is high (> 50%) failure of eradication is common.

There are several regimens for eradication, but all regimens must take into account the following factors:

- the necessity of good compliance with the chosen treatment regimen
- the high incidence of antibiotic resistance to metronidazole (25%+)
- the side-effects of treatment with oral metronidazole
- bismuth chelate is unpleasant to take, even as tablets.

Currently favoured regimens are triple therapy with a PPI along with two antibiotics for 1 week. For example:

- omeprazole 20 mg + metronidazole 400 mg and clarithromycin 500 mg (all twice daily)
- omeprazole 20 mg + clarithromycin 500 mg and amoxicillin 1 g (all twice daily).

Resistance to amoxicillin has not yet been demonstrated.

Tripotassium dicitratobismuthate (bismuth chelate) binds to the ulcer crater and stimulates prostaglandin secretion. It is effective against *H. pylori* and is used in some eradication therapies with two antibiotics. It blackens the tongue and stools.

In some regimens, H_2-receptor antagonists, e.g. ranitidine or ranitidine bismuth citrate, are included instead of a PPI.

General measures

Stopping smoking should be strongly encouraged as smoking slows mucosal healing. Patients with peptic ulcers usually require 3–4 weeks' further treatment with a proton pump inhibitor after eradication therapy.

The effectiveness of treatment should be assessed symptomatically. If symptoms persist, a ^{13}C urea breath test or stool test for *H. pylori* should be performed to check eradication. Patients with complications, i.e. haemorrhage or perforation, should always be tested to be sure eradication is successful.

A patient with a gastric ulcer should be re-endoscoped at 6 weeks to exclude a malignant tumour.

Complications of peptic ulcer

Haemorrhage

This is discussed on page 291.

Perforation (Box 6.5; see also p. 342)

The frequency of perforation of peptic ulceration is decreasing; this is partly attributable to better medical therapy. Duodenal ulcers perforate more commonly than gastric ulcers, usually into the peritoneal cavity; perforation into the lesser sac also occurs.

Management of perforation

Detailed management is described on page 342. Surgery is performed to close the perforation and drain the abdomen. Conservative management using nasogastric suction, intravenous fluids and antibiotics is occasionally used in elderly and very sick patients.

Gastric outlet obstruction

The obstruction may be prepyloric, pyloric or in the duodenum. The obstruction occurs either because of an active ulcer with surrounding oedema or because the healing of an ulcer has been followed by scarring.

Box 6.5 Suspected perforated peptic ulcer

Look for:
- other acute gastrointestinal conditions (e.g. cholecystitis, pancreatitis – check serum amylase)
- non-GI conditions (e.g. myocardial infarction)
- silent perforation in the elderly or patients on steroids.

Remember:
- There is harm in leaving an undiagnosed perforation.
- Avoid laparotomy if pancreatitis is diagnosed.

Obstruction is now rare with peptic ulcer disease and gastric malignancy; Crohn's disease or external compression from a pancreatic carcinoma are more common causes. Adult hypertrophic pyloric stenosis is a rare cause.

The main symptom of this condition is vomiting, usually without pain as the characteristic ulcer pain has abated owing to healing.

Vomiting is projectile and huge in volume, and the vomitus contains particles of yesterday's food. On examination of the abdomen the patient may have a succussion splash.

Severe or persistent vomiting causes loss of acid from the stomach and a metabolic alkalosis occurs (see p. 720).

The diagnosis is made by endoscopy but can be suspected when large quantities of fluid are removed by gastric intubation in the fasting state. Fluid and electrolyte replacement is necessary, together with the regular removal of gastric contents via a nasogastric tube. In some patients the symptoms will settle with this regimen and acid suppression therapy. Endoscopic dilatation is useful and 70% of patients can be managed without surgery.

Surgical treatment and its long-term consequences

Surgery in peptic ulceration disease is used only for the complications:

- recurrent uncontrolled haemorrhage, when the bleeding vessel is ligated
- perforation, which is oversewn.

For both of these conditions no other procedure, such as a gastrectomy or vagotomy, is required.

Two types of operation were performed:

- *partial gastrectomy*
- *vagotomy:* usually highly selective vagotomy or proximal gastric vagotomy, in which only the nerves supplying the parietal cells were transected, and therefore no drainage of the stomach was required.

Long-term complications of surgery are still seen occasionally.

- *A recurrent ulcer.* Check for *H. pylori*. Rule out the Zollinger–Ellison syndrome (see p. 416).
- *Dumping.* This is the term used to describe a number of upper abdominal symptoms (e.g. nausea and distension associated with sweating, faintness and palpitations) that occur in patients following gastrectomy or gastroenterostomy. It is due to 'dumping' of food into the jejunum, which is followed by rapid fluid dilution of the high osmotic load. A number of patients had mild symptoms of dumping but learned to cope with them. It was rare for it to be a clinical problem and, if it was, the symptoms had a functional element.
- *Diarrhoea.* This was chiefly seen after vagotomy with occasional urgency and recurrent severe episodes (1%). Treatment is with antidiarrhoeals.

- *Nutritional complications*:
  - anaemia – mainly iron deficiency due to poor absorption
  - occasionally folate deficiency due to poor intake
  - vitamin B_{12} deficiency due to intrinsic factor deficiency
  - patients often fail to gain weight owing to anorexia after gastric surgery.

Other *H. pylori*-associated diseases

Gastric adenocarcinoma

The incidence of gastric cancer parallels that of *H. pylori* infection in countries with a high incidence of gastric cancer. Serological studies show that people infected with *H. pylori* have a higher incidence of gastric carcinoma. For further discussion, see page 288.

Gastric B cell lymphoma

Over 70% of patients with gastric B cell lymphomas (mucosal-associated lymphoid tissue – MALT) have *H. pylori*. *H. pylori* gastritis has been shown to contain the clonal B cell that eventually gives rise to the MALT lymphoma (p. 290).

GASTROPATHY AND GASTRITIS

Gastropathy is the term used when there is epithelial/endothelial damage in the mucosa but there is little or no accompanying inflammation. Erosions and subepithelial haemorrhage are most commonly seen at endoscopy.

Gastritis is inflammation of the gastric mucosa.

The terms are often used loosely, particularly at endoscopy when any redness of the gastric mucosa may be described as 'gastritis'. Gastritis (as opposed to gastropathy) can only be readily diagnosed histologically.

The Sydney classification of gastritis was introduced in 1990 but has not been widely adopted because of the poor correlation between histological and endoscopic findings.

The commonest cause of *gastropathy* is mucosal damage associated with the use of aspirin and other NSAIDs and alcohol.

The commonest cause of *gastritis* is *H. pylori* infection (80%) and this is fully discussed on page 283. Autoimmune gastritis is seen in 5% while the remaining causes include viruses (e.g. CMV and herpes simplex), disorders of duodenogastric reflux and specific causes, e.g. Crohn's.

Erosive and haemorrhagic gastropathy

Aspirin and other NSAIDs deplete mucosal prostaglandins by inhibiting the cyclo-oxygenase (COX) pathway, which leads to mucosal damage. Cyclo-oxygenase occurs in two main forms: COX-1, the constitutive enzyme, and COX-2, the inducible form which is produced by cytokine stimulation in areas of inflammation. NSAIDs more specific for COX-2 are still available but see page 550, and these drugs have less effect on the COX-1 enzyme in the gastric mucosa. They still produce gastric mucosal damage but less than with COX-1 drugs.

Fifty per cent of patients on regular NSAIDs will develop gastric mucosal damage and approximately 30% will have ulcers on endoscopy. Only a small proportion of patients have symptoms (about 5%) and only 1–2% have a major problem, i.e. GI bleed. Because of the large number of patients on NSAIDs including low-dose aspirin for vascular prophylaxis, this is still a significant problem, particularly in the elderly.

H. pylori and NSAIDs are independent risk factors for the development of ulcers. There is little evidence to suggest that *H. pylori* infection increases the risk of ulceration in NSAID users.

Alcohol in high concentration damages the gastric mucosal barrier and is associated with acute gastric mucosal erosions and subepithelial haemorrhage which can lead to upper GI bleeding.

Acute erosive/haemorrhagic gastropathy can also be seen after severe stress (stress ulcers) and secondary to burns (Curling ulcers), trauma, shock, renal or liver (called portal gastropathy) disease. The underlying mechanism for these ulcers is unknown but may be related to an alteration in mucosal blood flow.

Management

In patients who develop problems, NSAIDs or alcohol should be stopped. Patients who are found to have mucosal damage and continuing symptoms are usually given an H_2-receptor antagonist or a PPI as a therapeutic trial. For established ulcers, a PPI is the best treatment. There is a little evidence that *H. pylori* eradication is helpful but if found, eradication therapy is usually given.

In many patients with severe arthritis, stopping NSAIDs may not be possible. Use:

- an NSAID with low GI side-effects at lowest dose possible (p. 549)
- prophylactic cytoprotective therapy, e.g. PPI or misoprostol (a synthetic analogue of prostaglandin E_1) for all high-risk patients, i.e. over 65 years; those with a peptic ulcer history, particularly with complications, and patients on therapy with corticosteroids or anticoagulants

Autoimmune gastritis

This affects the fundus and body of the stomach (pangastritis), leading to atrophic gastritis with loss of parietal cells.

This leads to achlorhydria and intrinsic factor deficiency causing pernicious anaemia. Autoantibodies to gastric parietal cells and intrinsic factor are found in the serum (see p. 432).

Ménétrier's disease

This is a rare condition consisting of giant gastric folds, mainly in the fundus and the body of the stomach. Histologically there is hyperplasia of the gastric pits, atrophy of glands and an overall increase of mucosal thickness. Hypochlorhydria is usually present.

The patient may complain of epigastric pain and occasionally peripheral oedema may occur because of hypoalbuminaemia resulting from protein loss through the gastric mucosa. It is possibly premalignant. Treatment is unclear as some patients improve spontaneously. Anti-secretory drugs are usually given. A few patients will require surgery.

Management of dyspepsia in the community

Dyspepsia (or indigestion) is very common in the general population. Over-the-counter antacids and H_2-receptor antagonists are available and are widely used.

Some patients' history is very suggestive of gastro-oesophageal reflux disease (GORD) and this subgroup of dyspepsia patients should be treated (see p. 277).

In young people (< 45 years) with dyspepsia, significant gastrointestinal pathology is very uncommon. Investigation with endoscopy is therefore not necessary. Their *H. pylori* status can be assessed serologically and, if positive, eradication therapy instituted. Further investigation should be reserved for those who remain symptomatic after successful eradication (p. 285). Patients who are *H. pylori*-negative on testing should be treated as for functional dyspepsia (p. 337), which is much commoner than organic disease.

Older people (> 45 years) with new-onset dyspepsia and all patients with 'alarm symptoms' (p. 265) must be investigated with endoscopy to exclude significant organic disease. Even in this age group, functional dyspepsia is very common and management of symptoms must reflect life event problems.

Therapies

Antacids are described on page 276.

H_2-receptor antagonists have molecular structures that fit the H_2-receptors on the parietal cells. They can produce up to 80% reduction in nocturnal acid production. They are useful in the management of dyspepsia and are part of some *H. pylori* eradication regimens. There is little difference between the several H_2-receptor antagonists available, but some have side-effects and cross-react with other medication, such as warfarin.

Proton pump inhibitors (p. 276) are also widely used. They are very effective for reflux symptoms and are also used in functional dyspepsia despite their cost, as many find them helpful.

GASTRIC TUMOURS

Adenocarcinoma

Carcinoma of the stomach (see Fig. 6.17) is the eighth most common fatal cancer in the UK. The frequency varies throughout the world, being high in Japan and Chile and relatively low in the USA.

In the UK, 15 per 100 000 males are affected per year. Although the overall world-wide incidence of gastric carcinoma appears to be falling, even in Japan, proximal gastric cancers are increasing in the West. The incidence increases with age (peak incidence 50–70 years), being rare under the age of 30 years, and more men than women are affected.

Epidemiology and pathogenesis

There is a strong link between *H. pylori* infection and gastric cancer. *H. pylori* infection results in chronic gastritis which eventually leads to atrophic gastritis and intestinal metaplasia – a premalignant pathological change (Fig. 6.15). Much of the earlier epidemiological data (i.e. the increase of cancer in lower socio-economic groups) can be explained by the intrafamilial spread of *H. pylori*. *H. pylori* is recognized by WHO as a Class 1 gastric carcinogen.

Dietary factors may still be involved, as both initiators and promoters may have separate roles in carcinogenesis. Diets high in salt probably increase the risk. Dietary nitrates can be converted into nitrosamines by bacteria at neutral pH, and nitrosamines are known to be carcinogenic in animals. Nitrosamines are also present in the stomach of patients with achlorhydria, who have an increased cancer risk. Consumption of diets high in vegetables and

Fig. 6.15 Flow diagram showing the development of gastric cancer associated with *H. pylori* infection.

fruits, and low in salt, protect against cancer. Smoking is also associated with an increased incidence of stomach cancer.

The commonest genetic abnormality is a loss of heterozygosity (LOH) of tumour suppressor genes such as *p53* (in 70% of cancers as well as in pre-cancerous states) and the *APC* gene (in over a third of gastric cancers). These abnormalities are similar to those found in colorectal cancers (see p. 392). Some families with diffuse gastric cancer have been shown to have mutations in the E-cadherin gene. There is a higher incidence of gastric cancer in blood group A patients. First-degree relatives of patients with gastric cancer have two- to three-fold increased relative risk of developing the disease.

Benign gastric ulcers (see Fig. 6.13) have not been shown to develop into gastric cancer. It can, however, be difficult to differentiate a benign ulcer from a malignant ulcer, as even malignant ulcers can partially heal on medical treatment. For these reasons it was originally thought that gastric ulcers could become malignant.

Pernicious anaemia carries a small increased risk of developing gastric carcinoma. Atrophic gastritis present in the body and fundus of the stomach of these patients may be a precancerous lesion.

There is an increased risk of gastric cancer after a partial gastrectomy (postoperative stomach) whether performed for a gastric or a duodenal ulcer. This may be a reflection of *H. pylori* causing the original ulceration.

(a)

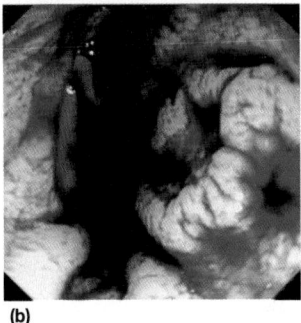

(b)

Fig. 6.16   Early gastric cancer:
(a) endoscopic view – showing subtle changes in mucosa;
(b) same view following an ink spray. By courtesy of Dr Peter Fairclough.

Screening

Gastric cancer has an appalling prognosis despite treatment, and earlier diagnosis has been advocated in an attempt to improve this. Screening is discussed on page 488; it has had no effect on overall mortality in gastric cancer. Similarly, early investigation of dyspepsia has had little effect on mortality.

Early gastric cancer

In Japan, mass screening with mobile X-ray units has increased the proportion of early gastric cancers diagnosed. Early gastric cancer is defined as a carcinoma that is confined to the mucosa or submucosa. It is associated with 5-year survival rates of approximately 90%. In a large series of patients with gastric cancer from the UK, only 0.7% were identified as having early gastric cancer and they are usually detected by chance (Fig. 6.16).

Pathology

Most gastric cancers occur in the antrum and are almost invariably adenocarcinomas. The common type is 'intestinal' and the tumours are polypoid or ulcerating lesions with heaped-up, rolled edges. Intestinal metaplasia is seen in the surrounding mucosa, often with *H. pylori*. The diffuse type is composed of scattered or small clusters of cells, often with extensive submucosal spread which may result in the picture of 'linitis plastica', where the stomach appears rigid on X-ray.

Clinical features

Symptoms

The most common symptom is epigastric pain, which is indistinguishable from the pain of peptic ulcer disease, both being relieved by food and antacids. The pain can vary in intensity, but may be constant and severe. Most patients with carcinoma of the stomach have advanced disease at the time of presentation, and also have nausea, anorexia and weight loss. Vomiting is frequent and can be severe if the tumour is near the pylorus. Dysphagia can occur with tumours involving the fundus. Gross haematemesis is unusual, but anaemia from occult blood loss is frequent. No pattern of symptoms is suggestive of early gastric cancer.

Patients can present with metastases causing abdominal swelling due to ascites or jaundice due to liver involvement. Metastases also occur in bone, brain and lung, producing appropriate symptoms.

Signs

Nearly 50% of patients have a palpable epigastric mass with abdominal tenderness. Often weight loss is the only feature. A palpable lymph node is sometimes found in the supraclavicular fossa (Virchow's node) and signs of metastases are present in up to one-third of patients. Carcinoma of the stomach is the cancer most frequently associated with dermatomyositis (p. 580) and acanthosis nigricans.

Fig. 6.17 **Carcinoma of the stomach.** Endoscopic picture showing a large irregular ulcer with rolled edges.

Investigations

- **Routine full blood count and liver biochemistry**.
- **Gastroscopy** (Fig. 6.17). Gastroscopy is usually performed as the primary procedure and has the advantage that biopsies can be performed for histological assessment and to exclude lymphoma. Positive biopsies can be obtained in almost all cases of obvious carcinoma, but a negative biopsy does not necessarily rule out the diagnosis. For this reason, 8–10 biopsies should be taken from around the ulcer margin and its base. Superficial brushings for cytology will further improve the diagnostic rate.
- **Barium meal**. This has largely been replaced by gastroscopy; however, a good-quality double-contrast barium meal has a diagnostic accuracy of up to 90%. The carcinoma is usually seen as a filling defect or an irregular ulcer with rolled edges. With a diffuse (linitis plastica) infiltrating type, the X-ray may show a rigid stomach.

Staging

Imaging. CT can demonstrate gastric wall thickening, but has limited value in determining tumour invasion into adjacent tissues. Ultrasound can demonstrate masses and wall thickening. Liver secondaries can be detected. Endoscopic ultrasound can demonstrate the penetration of the cancer through the gastric wall and extension into lymph nodes. It complements CT and ultrasound.

The TNM classification is used (p. 490). The tumour (T) indicates depth of tumour invasion, N denotes the presence or absence of lymph nodes, M indicates presence or absence of metastases.

TNM classification is then combined with stage categories 0–4. At presentation, two-thirds of patients are at stage 3 or 4, i.e. advanced disease.

Treatment

The 5-year survival rate of patients operated on for early gastric cancer (EGC) in Japan is 90%, but outside Japan EGC is rare. Surgery remains the best form of treatment if the patient is operable. Better preoperative staging has reduced the numbers undergoing surgery and has improved the overall surgical 5-year survival rates to around 30%. Five-year survival rates in 'curative' operations are as high as 50%. Surgery and combined chemo-radiotherapy and treatment of advanced disease is described on page 521. Despite the improved results, the overall survival rate for a patient with gastric carcinoma has not dramatically improved, with a 10% 5-year survival.

Palliative care with relief of pain, and counselling are essential, as described on page 524.

Stromal tumour

These tumours were known as leiomyomas or leiomyosarcomas. They are not of smooth muscle origin but are from the stroma and are thought to share a common ancestry with the interstitial cells of Cajal. They have a varying pattern of differentiation. There is a mutation in the cellular proto-oncogene *KIT* which leads to activation and cell-surface expression of the tyrosine kinase KIT (CD 117). They are usually asymptomatic and found by chance but they can occasionally ulcerate and produce a haematemesis.

Treatment is surgical. These tumours grow slowly and were thought to be benign, but histologically, tumours with more than 10 mitoses per 10 high-power fields are malignant and recurrences occur. Imatinib, a tyrosine kinase inhibitor, is being used for unresectable or metastatic disease.

Primary lymphoma

Lymphoma of the stomach can account for 10% of all gastric malignancies in the developed world. It is a non-Hodgkin's lymphoma of the B cell type. Gastric lymphomas in mucosal-associated lymphoid tissue (MALT) are caused by *H. pylori* (p. 287). The clinical presentation is the same as with gastric carcinoma. Some lymphomas due to *H. pylori* can be treated successfully by eradication therapy. Chemotherapy ± radiotherapy is the usual treatment for other lymphomas (p. 512). Prognosis is good, with a 75% 5-year survival depending on the type of lymphoma.

Gastric polyps

These are uncommon and again are found usually by chance. They produce no symptoms. The most common are regenerative or hyperplastic polyps, which are often multiple and require no treatment. Rarely adenomatous polyps are found and endoscopic removal is recommended because of possible malignant potential. Most gastric cancers appear not to arise from pre-existing adenomas (in contrast to colonic carcinomas).

FURTHER READING

Delaney et al. (2000) Cost effectiveness of initial endoscopy for dyspepsia in patients over 50 years of age. *Lancet* **356**: 1965–1969.

Fox JG, Wang TC (2001) *Helicobacter pylori* – not a good bug after all. *New England Journal of Medicine* **345**: 829–831.

Graham DY (2001) Therapy of *H. pylori*: current status and issues. *Gastroenterology* **118**: 52–58.

Hohenberger P, Gretschel S (2003) Gastric cancer. *Lancet* **362**: 305–315.

Kelson DP (2004) Esophageal and gastric cancer. *Seminars in Oncology* **31**: 441–554.

Laine L (2001) Approaches to nonsteroidal anti-inflammatory drug use in the high-risk patient. *Gastroenterology* **120**: 594–606.

ACUTE AND CHRONIC GASTROINTESTINAL BLEEDING

This section should be read in conjunction with the descriptions of the specific conditions mentioned.

Acute upper gastrointestinal bleeding

Haematemesis is the vomiting of blood from a lesion proximal to the distal duodenum.

Melaena is the passage of black tarry stools; the black colour is due to blood altered by bacteria – 50 mL or more is required to produce this. Melaena can occur with bleeding from any lesion from areas proximal to and including the caecum. Following a massive bleed from the upper GI tract, unaltered blood (owing to rapid transit) can appear per rectum, but this is rare. The colour of the blood appearing per rectum is dependent not only on the site of bleeding but also on the time of transit through the gut.

Aetiology

Peptic ulceration is the commonest cause of serious and life threatening gastrointestinal bleeding. This and other causes are shown in Figure 6.18. The relative incidences of these causes vary depending on the patient population; overall the incidence has fallen. In the developing world; haemorrhagic viral infections (see Table 2.23) can cause significant gastrointestinal bleeding.

Drugs. Aspirin (even 75 mg a day) and other NSAIDs can produce gastric lesions. These agents are also responsible for GI haemorrhage from both duodenal and gastric ulcers, particularly in the elderly. Remember, these drugs are available over the counter and detailed questioning is necessary. Corticosteroids in the usual therapeutic doses probably have no influence on GI haemorrhage. Anticoagulants do not cause acute GI haemorrhage per se but bleeding from any cause is greater if the patient is anticoagulated.

Clinical approach to the patient

All cases with a recent (i.e. within 48 hours) significant

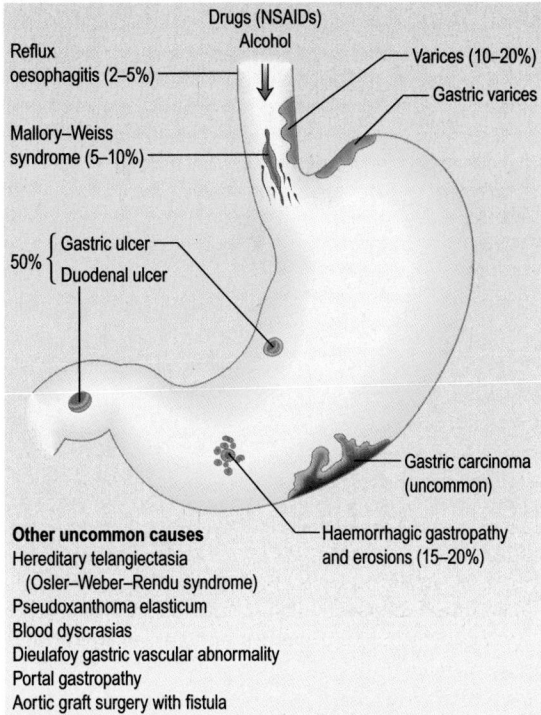

Fig. 6.18   Causes of upper gastrointestinal haemorrhage. The approximate frequency is also given.

gastrointestinal bleed should be seen in hospital. In many, no immediate treatment is required as often there has been only a small amount of blood loss and the patient's cardiovascular system can compensate for this. Approximately 85% of patients stop bleeding spontaneously within 48 hours.

The following factors affect the management:

- age (see below)
- the amount of blood lost, which may give some guide to the severity
- continuing visible blood loss
- signs of chronic liver disease on examination
- evidence of co-morbidity, e.g. cardiac failure, ischaemic heart disease, renal disease and malignant disease
- presence of the classical clinical features of shock (pallor, cold nose, tachycardia and low blood pressure – see Emergency box 6.1).

With liver disease, the bleeding is often severe and recurrent if it is from varices. Splenomegaly suggests portal hypertension but its absence does not rule out oesophageal varices. Liver failure can develop.

With shock, remember that the peripheral arterial constriction that occurs may keep the blood pressure falsely high.

Immediate management

- Rapid history and examination.
- Note age of patient.
- Rapid assessment of haemodynamic state.
- Look for evidence of co-morbidity.

Emergency Box 6.1
Management of acute gastrointestinal bleeding

- History and examination.
- Monitor the pulse and blood pressure half-hourly.
- Take blood for haemoglobin, urea, electrolytes, grouping and crossmatching (2 units initially).
- Establish intravenous access – central line if brisk bleed.
- Give blood transfusion/colloid if necessary. *Indications for blood transfusion are:*
  - (a) SHOCK (pallor, cold nose, systolic PB below 100 mmHg, pulse > 100 b.p.m.)
  - (b) haemoglobin < 10 g/dL in patients with recent or active bleeding.
- Oxygen therapy for shocked patients.
- Urgent endoscopy in shocked patients/liver disease.
- Continue to monitor pulse and BP.
- Re-endoscope for continued bleeding/hypovolaemia.
- Surgery if bleeding persists.

- Take blood for haemoglobin, urea, electrolytes, liver function, coagulation studies and for grouping and crossmatching.
- Stop drugs, e.g. NSAIDs, warfarin (see p. 481).

Urgent resuscitation is required in patients with large bleeds and the clinical signs of shock. Details of the management of shock are given in Figure 15.21. Many hospitals have multidisciplinary specialist teams with agreed protocols and these should be followed carefully. Such patients should be managed in high-dependency beds. Oxygen should be given by face mask and the patient should be kept nil by mouth until endoscopy has been performed.

Blood volume

The major principle is to rapidly restore the blood volume to normal. This can be best achieved by transfusion of whole blood via one or more large-bore intravenous cannulae; physiological saline is given until the blood becomes available (p. 974).

The rate of blood transfusion must be monitored carefully to avoid overtransfusion and consequent heart failure. The pulse rate and venous pressure are the best guides to transfusion rates. All patients with organ failure and requiring blood transfusion, as well as patients with severe hypotension, should have a central venous pressure line.

Anaemia does not develop immediately as haemodilution has not taken place, and therefore the haemoglobin level is a poor indicator of the need to transfuse. If the level is low (less than 10 g/dL) and the patient has either bled recently or is actively bleeding, transfusion may be necessary. In most patients the bleeding stops, albeit temporarily, so that further assessment can be made.

Endoscopy

Endoscopy should be performed within 24 hours in most patients. Early endoscopy helps to make a diagnosis and to make decisions regarding discharge from hospital, particularly in patients with minor bleeds and under 60 years of age. Clinical risk scores are used in some centres to identify patients at low risk who do not require endoscopy.

Urgent endoscopy (i.e. after resuscitation) should be performed in patients with shock, suspected liver disease or with continued bleeding. Endoscopy can detect the cause of the haemorrhage in 80% or more of cases. In patients with a peptic ulcer, if the stigmata of a recent bleed are seen (i.e. a spurting artery, active oozing, fresh or organized blood clot or black spots) the patient is more likely to re-bleed.

At first endoscopy:

- varices should be injected – see page 379 for management of varices
- all bleeding ulcers should be either injected with epinephrine (adrenaline), the vessel coagulated either with a heater probe or with laser therapy or metallic clips applied.

These methods reduce the incidence of re-bleeding, although they do not significantly improve mortality as re-bleeding still occurs in 20% within 72 hours. Intravenous omeprazole 80 mg followed by infusion 8 mg/h for 72 hours should be given to all patients in this group, as it reduces re-bleeding rates and the need for surgery.

Drug therapy

There is little evidence that H_2-receptor antagonists or proton-pump inhibitors (PPIs) affect the mortality rate of GI haemorrhage, but PPIs are usually given to all patients with ulcers because of their longer-term benefits. Somatostatin (which reduces the splanchnic blood flow as well as acid secretion) can be given as an infusion if the bleeding is difficult to stop, although a meta-analysis of clinical trials has shown no clear benefit.

Reassessment/risk factors

- Age is clearly significant. Below the age of 60 years mortality from GI bleeding is small, < 0.1%, but above the age of 80 the mortality is greater than 20%.
- Patients with recurrent haemorrhage have an increased mortality.
- Most re-bleeds (approximately 20% of all cases) occur within 48 hours.
- Co-morbidity invariably increases mortality.
- Melaena is usually less hazardous than haematemesis.
- Presence of shock at *any time* increases mortality.

Uncontrolled or repeat bleeding

Endoscopy should be repeated to assess the bleeding site and to treat, if possible. Surgery is necessary only if bleeding is persistent and/or uncontrollable and should be limited to controlling the haemorrhage.

Discharge policy

The patient's age, diagnosis on endoscopy, co-morbidity and the presence or absence of shock should be taken into consideration. In general, all patients who are dynamically stable and have no stigmata of recent haemorrhage on endoscopy, can be discharged from hospital within 24 hours. All shocked patients and patients with co-morbidity need inpatient observation.

Specific conditions

Chronic peptic ulcer. Eradication of *H. pylori* is started as soon as possible (see p. 285). A proton-pump inhibitor is continued for 4 weeks to ensure ulcer healing. Eradication of *H. pylori* should always be checked in a patient who has bled. If necessary to control haemorrhage, surgery with ligation of the bleeding vessel is performed, but no other surgical procedure is undertaken.

Gastric carcinoma. Most patients do not have large bleeds with this condition but surgery is occasionally necessary for uncontrolled or repeat bleeding. Usually surgery can be delayed until the patient has been fully evaluated (p. 290).

Oesophageal varices. These are discussed on page 379.

Mallory–Weiss tear. This is a linear mucosal tear occurring at the oesophagogastric junction and produced by a sudden increase in intra-abdominal pressure. It often occurs after a bout of coughing or retching and is classically seen after an alcohol binge. There may, however, be no antecedent history of retching. The haemorrhage may be large but most patients stop spontaneously. Early endoscopy confirms diagnosis and allows early discharge from the hospital (within 24 hours). Rarely, surgery with oversewing of the tear will be required.

Prognosis

The mortality from gastrointestinal haemorrhage has not changed from 5 to 12% over the years, despite many changes in management, mainly because more patients are elderly and have more co-morbidity. The lowest mortality rates are achieved in dedicated medical/surgical GI units. Early therapeutic endoscopy has not so far reduced the mortality, although bleeding episodes are reduced.

Acute lower gastrointestinal bleeding

Massive bleeding from the lower GI tract is rare. On the other hand, small bleeds from haemorrhoids occur very commonly. Massive bleeding is usually due to diverticular disease or ischaemic colitis. The causes of lower gastrointestinal bleeding are shown in Figure 6.19.

Management

Most acute lower GI bleeds start spontaneously. The few patients that continue bleeding and are haemodynamically unstable need resuscitation using the same principles as for upper GI bleeding (p. 291). Surgery is rarely required. A diagnosis is made using the history, and the following investigations as appropriate:

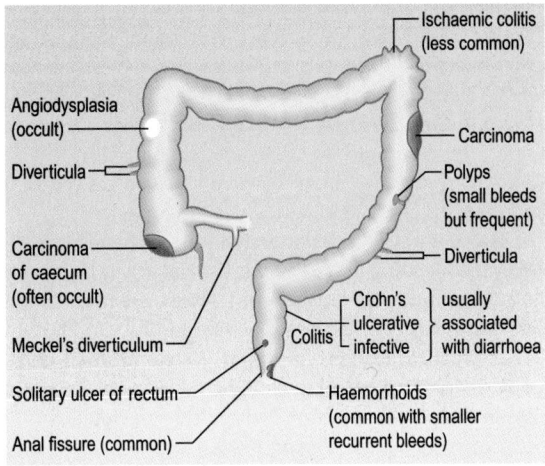

Fig. 6.19 **Causes of lower gastrointestinal bleeding.** The sites shown are illustrative – many of the lesions can be seen in other parts of the colon.

- rectal examination (e.g. carcinoma)
- proctoscopy (e.g. anorectal disease, particularly haemorrhoids)
- sigmoidoscopy (e.g. inflammatory bowel disease)
- barium enema – ischaemic colitis
- colonoscopy – for any mucosal lesion and removal of polyps
- angiography – vascular abnormality (e.g. angiodysplasia, which can be sometimes treated with argon plasma coagulation).

Isolated episodes of rectal bleeding in the young (< 45 years) only require rectal examination and sigmoidoscopy. Colorectal cancer is rare in this age group without a strong family history.

Individual lesions are treated as appropriate.

Chronic gastrointestinal bleeding

Patients with chronic bleeding usually present with iron-deficiency anaemia (see Ch. 8).

Chronic blood loss producing iron deficiency anaemia in all men and all women after the menopause is always due to bleeding from the gastrointestinal tract, often from a right-sided colonic neoplasm which must be excluded. Occult blood tests are not necessary (Box 6.6).

 Box 6.6 Measurement of faecal occult blood

This is frequently performed *unnecessarily*. It is *only* of value in:

- premenopausal women – if a history of menorrhagia is uncertain and the cause of iron deficiency is unclear
- mass population screening for large bowel malignancy.
  Advantages: cheap and easy to perform.
  Disadvantages: high false-positive rate, leading to unnecessary investigations.

Diagnosis

Chronic blood loss can occur with any lesion of the gastrointestinal tract that produces acute bleeding (see Figs 6.18 and 6.19). It is, however, usual for oesophageal varices to bleed severely and rarely to present as chronic blood loss. It should be remembered that, world-wide, hookworm is the most common cause of chronic gastrointestinal blood loss.

History and examination may indicate the most likely site of the bleeding, but if no clue is available it is usual to investigate both the upper and lower gastrointestinal tract endoscopically at the same session ('top and tail').

For practical reasons an upper gastrointestinal endo-scopy is performed first as this takes only minutes, followed by colonoscopy when any lesion can be removed or biopsied. A barium enema is performed only if colonoscopy is unavailable.

A small bowel follow-through is the next investi-gation, but the diagnostic yield is very low.

Following negative investigations, a coeliac axis and mesenteric angiography may show the site of bleeding, although the yield is low. Occasionally, intravenous technetium-labelled colloid may be used to demonstrate the bleeding site in a Meckel's diverticulum. Endoscopes to visualize the whole of the small bowel (enteroscopy) are available at specialist centres. Wireless capsule endo-scopy is useful, particularly with melaena of obscure origin (90% of causes were found in a recent study).

Treatment

The cause of the bleeding should be treated, if found. Oral iron is given to treat anaemia (see p. 429).

FURTHER READING

BSG endoscopy committee guidelines on non-gastro-intestinal haemorrhage (2002) Gut **51** Suppl 4 (October).

Lau JY et al. (2000) Effect of intravenous omeprazole on recurrent bleeding of peptic ulcers. *New England Journal of Medicine* **343**: 310–316.

Pennazlo M et al. (2004). Outcome of patients with obscure GI bleeding after capsule endoscopy. *Gastroenterology* **126**: 643–653.

Rockall TA et al. (1996) National audit for acute upper gastrointestinal haemorrhage. *Lancet* **347**: 1138–1140.

Rockall TA, Logan RFA, Devlin HB, Northfield TC (1995) Incidence of and mortality from upper gastrointestinal haemorrhage in the UK. *British Medical Journal* **311**: 222–226.

THE SMALL INTESTINE

Structure

The small intestine extends from the duodenum to the ileocaecal valve. It is approximately 6 m in length, the upper 40% – the jejunum; the remainder – the ileum. Its surface area is enormously increased by mucosal folds. In addition, the mucosa has numerous finger-like pro-jections called villi and the surface area is further increased by microvilli (Fig. 6.20). Each villus consists of a

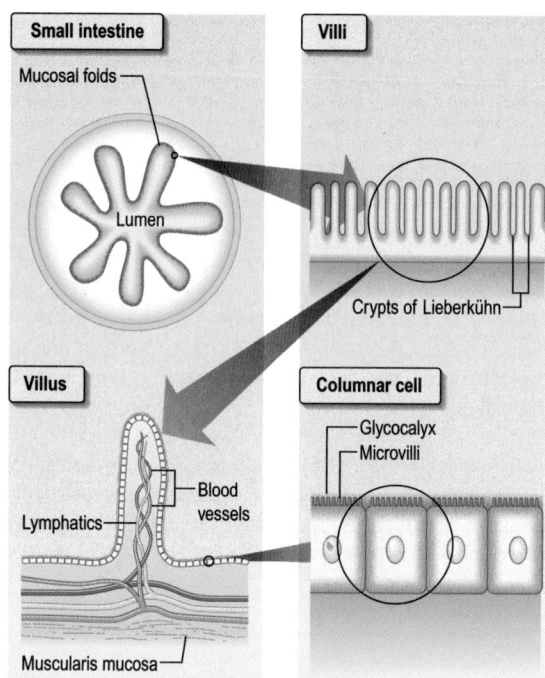

Fig. 6.20 **Structure of the small intestine.**

core containing blood vessels, lacteals (lymphatics) and cells (e.g. plasma cells and lymphocytes), and is covered by epithelial columnar cells that are absorptive. The crypts of Lieberkühn open into the lumen, between the villi.

The epithelial cells are formed at the bottom of these crypts and migrate to the tops of the villi, from where they are shed. This process takes 3–4 days. On its luminal side the epithelial cell has a brush border of microvilli that is covered by the glycocalyx. The lamina propria contains plasma cells, lymphocytes, macrophages, eosinophils and mast cells. Scattered throughout the gut are peptide-secreting cells.

Most of the blood supply to the small intestine is via branches of the superior mesenteric artery. The terminal branches are end arteries – there are no local anastomotic connections.

The *enteric nervous system* is linked to the central nervous system via the autonomic. The nerve plexuses in the mucosa, submucosa and muscularis propria are of three types:

- cholinergic parasympathetic (with muscarinic or nicotinic receptors)
- adrenergic sympathetic (with both α and β receptors)
- non-cholinergic non-adrenergic (NANC).

For NANC, the transmitters are thought to be either cyclic nucleotides and ATP (the purinergic system) or intestinal hormones (e.g. VIP – the peptidergic hypo-thesis) or nitric oxide.

Functions (Table 6.5)

The epithelial cells form a physical barrier permeable to ions, small molecules and macromolecules. The small

Table 6.5   Functions of the small intestine

Digestion and absorption
Continuous cell renewal and cell death
Defence against antigen entry:
   Structural
   Immunological:
      innate (see p. 197), e.g. antimicrobial peptides, trefoil
         peptides
      acquired (see p. 204)
Neuroendocrine peptide production
Motor function – transit of nutrients

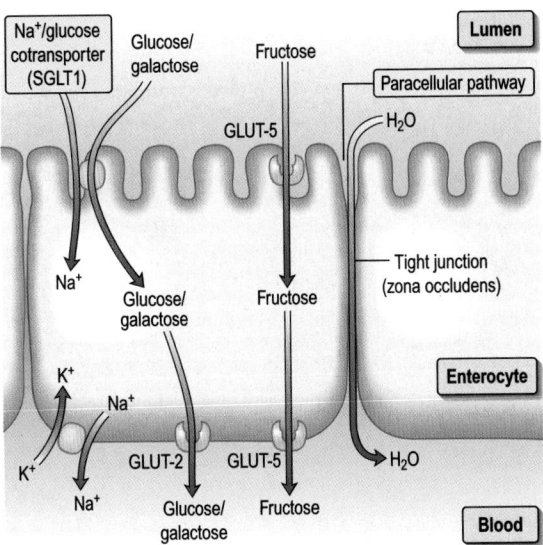

Fig. 6.21   Solute (glucose, galactose, fructose) transport across the apical membrane (glucose and galactose are transported via the sodium/glucose cotransporter – SGLT1). Fructose is transported by the facilitative transporter GLUT-5 across the apical and basolateral membranes. Water absorption is mainly cellular but paracellular absorption also occurs. The tight junction is a network of strands and is a dynamic structure. The sodium/potassium-ATPase pump is located in the basolateral membrane.

intestine is concerned with the digestion and absorption of nutrients, salt and water. Digestive enzymes (e.g. proteases, disaccharidases) are produced by intestinal cells; some of these enzymes are membrane-bound whilst others (e.g. lipases produced by the pancreas) are associated with the glycocalyx. Nutrients can be absorbed throughout the small intestine, but vitamin B_{12} and bile salts have specific receptors in the terminal ileum.

General principles of absorption
Simple diffusion
This process requires no energy and takes place if there is a concentration gradient from the intestinal lumen (high concentration) to the bloodstream (low concentration).

Active transport
This requires energy and can work against a concentration gradient. A carrier protein is required and the process in the enterocyte is sodium-dependent. For example, glucose enters the enterocyte on the luminal side via a sodium-dependent carrier molecule (sodium/glucose cotransporter I, SGLTI) and leaves on the serosal side via a sodium-independent carrier (GLUT-2) that is found in the basolateral membrane. A Na^+ gradient is maintained across the membrane by an energy-dependent sodium pump (Na^+/K^+-ATPase) that keeps the intracellular sodium concentration low (Fig. 6.21).

Facilitated diffusion
This is an energy-independent carrier-mediated transport system (GLUT-5) that allows a faster absorption rate than simple diffusion (e.g. fructose absorption). GLUT-5 has a very low affinity for glucose.

Absorption in the small intestine
Carbohydrate
Dietary carbohydrate consists mainly of starch with some sucrose and a small amount of lactose. Starch is a polysaccharide made up of numerous glucose units. Its hydrolysis begins in the mouth by salivary amylase. The majority of hydrolysis takes place in the upper intestinal lumen by pancreatic amylase. This hydrolysis is limited by the fact that amylases have no specificity for some glucose–glucose branching links.

   The breakdown products of starch digestion, together with sucrose and lactose, are hydrolysed on the brush border membrane by their appropriate oligo- and disaccharidases to form the monosaccharides glucose, galactose and fructose. These monosaccharides are transported into the cells (Fig. 6.21).

Protein
Dietary protein is digested by pancreatic enzymes prior to absorption. These proteolytic enzymes are secreted by the pancreas as proenzymes and transformed to active enzymes in the lumen. The presence of protein in the lumen stimulates the release of enterokinase, which activates trypsinogen to trypsin, and this in turn activates the other proenzymes, chymotrypsin and elastase. These enzymes break down protein into oligopeptides. Some di- and tripeptides are absorbed intact by a carrier-mediated process, while the remainder are broken down into free amino acids by peptidases on the microvillus membranes of the cell, prior to absorption in a similar way to disaccharides. These amino acids are transported into the cell by a variety of carrier systems.

Fat (Fig. 6.22)
Dietary fat consists mainly of triglycerides with some cholesterol and fat-soluble vitamins. Emulsification of fat occurs in the stomach and is followed by hydrolysis of triglycerides in the duodenum by pancreatic lipase to yield fatty acids and monoglycerides.

   Bile enters the duodenum following gall bladder contraction. Bile contains phospholipids and bile salts, both of which are partially water-soluble and act as detergents.

(a) The pathophysiology of fat absorption

Absorption

Malabsorption (steatorrhoea)

Bile salts synthesized in liver

Dietary fat (mainly triglycerides)

Liver disease

Cholestatic jaundice

Emulsification in stomach

Pancreatic disease
Drugs – e.g. orlistat

Hydrolysis by pancreatic lipase

Small bowel disease
Mucosal lesion,
 e.g Coeliac disease
  Tropical sprue
Bacterial overgrowth
 (deconjugation of bile salts)
Parasites, e.g. *Giardia*
Intestinal resection
Ileal disease – Crohn's
Abetalipoproteinaemia
Drugs

Formation of mixed micelles

Chylomicrons

Lymphatics

Bile salts reabsorbed

(b) The formation of mixed micelles

Pancreatic lipase

Triglyceride   2-Monoglyceride Bile salts micelle   Mixed micelle

Fig. 6.22 **(a) The pathophysiology of fat absorption. (b) Diagram showing the formation of mixed micelles.**

They aggregate together to form micelles with their hydrophilic ends on the outside. Trapped in the hydrophobic centre of the micelles are the monoglycerides, fatty acids and cholesterol; these are then transported to the intestinal cell membrane.

At the cell membrane the lipid contents of the micelles are absorbed, while the bile salts remain in the lumen. Inside the cell the monoglycerides and fatty acids are re-esterified to triglycerides. The triglycerides and other fat-soluble molecules (e.g. cholesterol, phospholipids) are then incorporated into chylomicrons to be transported into the lymph.

Medium-chain triglycerides (which contain fatty acids of chain length 6–12) as well as a small amount of long-chain fatty acids are transported via the portal vein.

Bile salts are not absorbed in the jejunum, so that the intraluminal concentration in the upper gut is high. They pass down the intestine to be absorbed in the terminal ileum and are transported back to the liver. This enterohepatic circulation prevents excess loss of bile salts (see p. 351).

The pathophysiology of fat absorption is shown in Figure 6.22. Interference with absorption can occur at all stages, as indicated, giving rise to steatorrhoea (> 17 mmol (6 g) of fat per day).

Water and electrolytes

A large amount of water and electrolytes, partly dietary, but mainly from intestinal secretions, are absorbed coupled with monosaccharides, amino acids and bicarbonate in the upper jejunum. Water and electrolytes are also absorbed paracellularly down electrochemical and osmotic gradients. Additional water and electrolytes are absorbed in the ileum and right side of the colon, where active sodium transport occurs that is not coupled to solute absorption. Intestinal secretion also takes place and abnormalities of this mechanism cause secretory diarrhoea (see p. 331).

Water-soluble vitamins, essential metals and trace elements

These are all absorbed in the small intestine. Vitamin B_{12} (see p. 431) is the only substance other than bile salts that is specifically absorbed in the terminal ileum, and malabsorption of both these substances will always occur following ileal resection.

Calcium absorption

Calcium absorption is discussed on page 592.

Iron absorption

Iron absorption is discussed on page 426.

Defence against antigens (see also p. 197)

Several strategies are used by the small bowel to prevent pathogenic invasion:

- the *physical barrier*, e.g. the epithelial and mucous layers
- *innate and adaptive immune mechanisms* – these interact to ensure maximum protection while at the same time tolerating harmless commensal organisms and dietary antigens.

All cell populations in the GI tract, including enterocytes, goblet cells and myofibroblasts, actively participate in the innate immune response. Enzymes such as lysozyme and phospholipase A_2 secreted by the goblet cells help ensure an infection-free environment in the gut, even in the presence of commensal bacteria. Antimicrobial peptides (e.g. defensins) are secreted in response to pathogenic bacteria, enterocytes and Paneth cells. These peptides exhibit potent activity against various classes of pathogens including Gram-positive and -negative bacteria, fungi and viruses. Enterocytes and Paneth cells also secrete cytokines (including IL-1 and TNF) critical for activating innate immune mechanisms.

The secretory immunoglobulin (sIg) system plays a major role in mucosal immunity. There are approximately 10^{10} Ig-producing immunocytes (plasma cells and plasmablasts) per metre of human small bowel, of which 70–90% are IgA immunocytes. Dimeric and polymeric IgA (pIgA), which contains a disulphide-linked polypeptide called 'J' (or 'joining') chain, and IgM are transported through the glandular epithelium via the transmembrane pIg receptor called 'secretory component' (SC) into the gut lumen. These antibodies are the first-line defence antigens in the lumen and may also take part in maintaining immunological homeostasis within the mucosa (e.g. damping T-cell-mediated hypersensitivity responses against harmless absorbed luminal antigens). SC expression can be upregulated by cytokines, including IFN-γ and TNF-α, secreted by activated T cells and macrophages respectively, thus promoting the transport of IgA and IgM into the lumen.

An additional source of long-term host defence is provided by T lymphocytes that initiate, activate and regulate adaptive immune responses. Intestinal T cells occur principally in three major compartments: (a) organized gut-associated lymphoid tissue (GALT) such as the Peyer's patches; (b) the mucosal lamina propria and (c) the surface epithelium where they are referred to as intraepithelial lymphocytes (IELS) (Fig. 6.23). GALT is the major site of antigen priming as it is dominated by a population of naive T and B cells. Specialized epithelial cells above the Peyer's patches (called 'M' or 'membrane' cells) lack digestive enzymes and SC but express class II molecules and allow non-selective inward transport of luminal antigens and presentation of antigen to Peyer's patch T cells. Antigen is also transported to mesenteric lymph nodes by mucosal dendritic cells where T cell priming is initiated. Antigens may also be taken up by other class II expressing epithelial cells (expressing HLA-DR) and may subsequently be presented to primed (memory) T lymphocytes.

In contrast to GALT, the lamina propria and the surface epithelium are effector compartments that receive primed T cells. CD4$^+$ T cells dominate in the lamina propria where they are significant secretors of cytokines. CD8$^+$ T cells including significant populations of gamma/

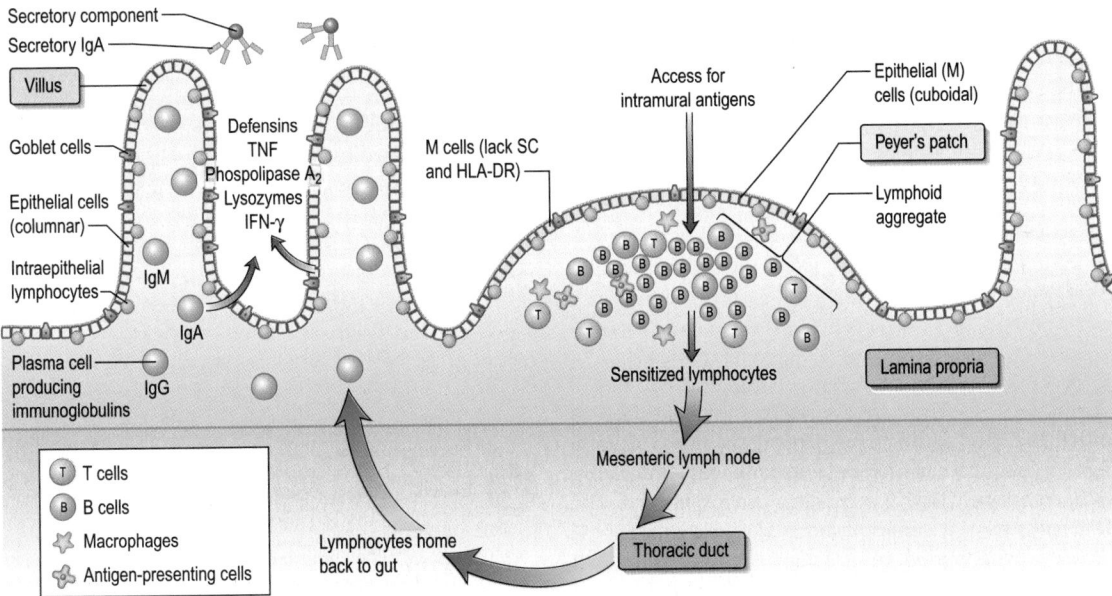

Fig. 6.23 **Small intestinal mucosa with a Peyer's patch, showing the gut-associated lymphoid tissue (GALT).**
SC, secretory component; HLA-DR, human lymphocyte antigen-DR; TNF, tumour necrosis factor; IFN-γ, gamma-interferon; M cells, membrane cells.

delta TCR$^+$ cells predominate in the latter where they have a cytotoxic role. At present, identification of the exact function of various T cell subsets in the pathogenesis of inflammatory gut diseases is being actively pursued.

Neuroendocrine peptide production

The hormone-producing cells of the gut are scattered diffusely throughout its length and also occur in the pancreas. The cells that synthesize hormones are derived from neural ectoderm and are known as APUD (amine precursor uptake and decarboxylation) cells. Many of these hormones have very similar structures. Although they can be detected by radioimmunoassay in the circulation, their action is often local.

Table 6.6 shows some gut neuroendocrine peptides and their possible physiological actions. Many are also found in other tissues, particularly the brain. A number do not act as true hormones but act as neurotransmitters or have local effects on adjacent cells only (paracrine effects).

The exact physiological role of these peptides continues to be evaluated. They may be secreted in excess, particularly in neuroendocrine tumours of the pancreas (see p. 416).

Trefoil peptides

The trefoil factor family (TFF) of small proteins each consist of a three-loop structure. They help to protect the lining of the gastrointestinal tract by stabilizing the mucus in normal conditions and by upregulating and stimulating the repair process (e.g. epithelial restitution) in acute injury. TFF1 is produced predominantly by mucin-secreting cells of the stomach, small and large intestine. TFF2 is produced by mucus-producing cells of the stomach and by Brunner's glands and goblet cells in the small intestine, and is absent in the colon. TFF3 is absent from the stomach but secreted in the small intestine and colon. All three trefoil peptides can also be secreted ectopically in the cells around damaged areas (e.g. in inflammatory bowel disease and peptic ulceration).

Gut motility

The contractile patterns of the small intestinal muscular layers are primarily determined by integrated neural circuits within the gut wall – the enteric nervous system. The CNS and gut hormones also have a modulatory role on motility. The interstitial cells of Cajal lie within the smooth muscle. These mesenchymal cells appear to govern rhythmic contractions. During fasting, a distally migrating sequence of motor events termed the migrating motor complexes (MMC) occurs in a cyclical fashion. The MMC consists of a period of motor quiescence (phase I) followed by a period of irregular contractile activity (phase II), culminating in a short (5–10 min) burst of regular phasic contractions (phase III). Each MMC cycle lasts for approximately 90 minutes. In the duodenum, phase III is associated with increased gastric, pancreatic and biliary secretions. The role of the MMC is unclear, but the strong phase III contractions propel secretions, residual food and desquamated cells towards the colon, acting as an 'intestinal housekeeper'.

After a meal, the MMC pattern is disrupted and replaced by irregular contractions. This seemingly chaotic-fed pattern lasts typically for 2–5 hours, depending on the size and nutrient content of the meal. The irregular contractions of the fed pattern have a mixing function, moving intraluminal contents to and fro, aiding the digestive process.

Presenting features of small bowel disease

Regardless of the cause, the common presenting features of small bowel disease are:

- *Diarrhoea.* This is a common feature of small bowel disease but approximately 10–20% of patients will have no diarrhoea or any other gastrointestinal symptoms. Steatorrhoea is occasionally present (Box 6.7).
- *Abdominal pain and discomfort.* Abdominal distension can cause discomfort and flatulence. The pain has no specific character or periodicity and is not usually severe.
- *Weight loss.* Weight loss is due to the anorexia that invariably accompanies small bowel disease. Although malabsorption occurs, the amount is small relative to intake.
- *Nutritional deficiencies.* Deficiencies of iron, B$_{12}$, folate or all of these, leading to anaemia, are the only common deficiencies. Occasionally malabsorption of other vitamins or minerals occurs, causing bruising (vitamin K deficiency), tetany (calcium deficiency), osteomalacia (vitamin D deficiency), or stomatitis, sore tongue and aphthous ulceration (multiple vitamin deficiencies). Ankle oedema may be seen and is partly nutritional and partly due to intestinal loss of albumin.

Physical signs of small bowel disease

These are few and non-specific. If present they are associated with anaemia and the nutritional deficiencies described above.

Abdominal examination is often normal, but sometimes distension and, rarely, hepatomegaly or an abdominal mass are found. In the severely ill patient, gross malnutrition with muscle wasting is seen. A neuropathy, not always due to B$_{12}$ deficiency, can be present.

 Box 6.7 Steatorrhoea

The stools:
- are pale, bulky, offensive and contain fat (> 17 mmol/day)
- float in the lavatory pan because of their increased air content
- are difficult to flush away.

Table 6.6 Gut regulatory peptides

Hormone	Physiological action	Main gut localization
Gastrin/cholecystokinin family		
Cholecystokinin (CCK)	Stimulates gall bladder contraction and has trophic effects on duodenum and pancreas	Duodenum and jejunum (I cells)
	Pancreatic secretion (minor role)	Enteric nerves
	Role in satiety	
Gastrin	Stimulates acid secretion	Gastric antrum, duodenum (G cells)
	Trophic effect on gut mucosa	
Secretin and related peptides (all possess structural homology with secretin)		
Secretin	Pancreatic bicarbonate secretion	Duodenum and jejunum (S cells)
Vasoactive intestinal polypeptide (VIP)	Intestinal secretion of water and electrolytes	Enteric nerves
	Splanchnic vasodilatation, stimulates insulin release	
Peptide-histidine methionine	As for VIP	Enteric nerves
Glucose-dependent insulinotropic peptide (GIP)	Facilitates insulin release by islets	Duodenum (K cells)
		Gastric antrum
		Ileum
Glucagon-like peptide-1 (GLP-1)	Increases insulin secretion	Pancreas (A cells)
Glucagon-like peptide-2 (GLP-2)	Enterocyte-specific growth hormone	Ileum and colon (L cells)
Growth hormone-releasing factor (GHRF)	Unclear	Small gut
Pancreatic polypeptide family		
Pancreatic polypeptide	Inhibitor of pancreatic and biliary secretion	Pancreas (PP cells)
Peptide YY	Inhibition of pancreatic exocrine secretion; slows gastric and small bowel transit ('ileal brake'); reduces food intake and appetite	Ileum and colon (L cells)
Neuropeptide Y	Regulation of intestinal blood flow	Enteric nerves
Other		
Motilin	Increases gastric emptying and small bowel contraction	Whole gut
Ghrelin	Appetite stimulation, increases gastric emptying	Stomach
Bombesin (gastrin releasing-polypeptide in humans)	Stimulates pancreatic exocrine secretion and gastric acid secretion	Whole gut and pancreas
Somatostatin	Inhibits secretion and action of most hormones	Stomach and pancreas (D cells)
		Small and large intestine
Galanin	Inhibits insulin secretion	Enteric nerves
Pancreastatin	Inhibits pancreatic exocrine and endocrine secretion	Pancreas, whole gut
Substance P	Enhances gastric acid secretion, smooth muscle contraction	Enteric nerves
Calcitonin gene-related peptide	Vasodilatation. Inhibits gastric and pancreatic secretion	Enteric nerves
Neurotensin	Affects gut motility. Increases jejunal and ileal fluid secretion	Ileum
Insulin	Increases glucose utilization	Pancreas B cells
Chromogranin family	Process regulatory peptides and prohormones	Neuroendocrine cells

Investigation of small bowel disease
(Fig. 6.24)

Blood tests
- **Full blood count and film**. Anaemia can be microcytic (low mean corpuscular volume – MCV) or macrocytic (high MCV). The blood film may therefore be dimorphic and also show other abnormal cells (e.g. Howell–Jolly bodies which are seen in splenic atrophy associated with coeliac disease).

- If the MCV is low, serum ferritin and the serum soluble transferrin receptor are measured (p. 428).
- If the MCV is high, serum B$_{12}$, and serum and red cell folate are measured. However, with mixed deficiencies, the MCV may be normal. The red cell folate is a good indicator of the presence of small bowel disease. It is frequently low in both coeliac disease and Crohn's disease, which are the two most common causes of small bowel disease in developed countries.

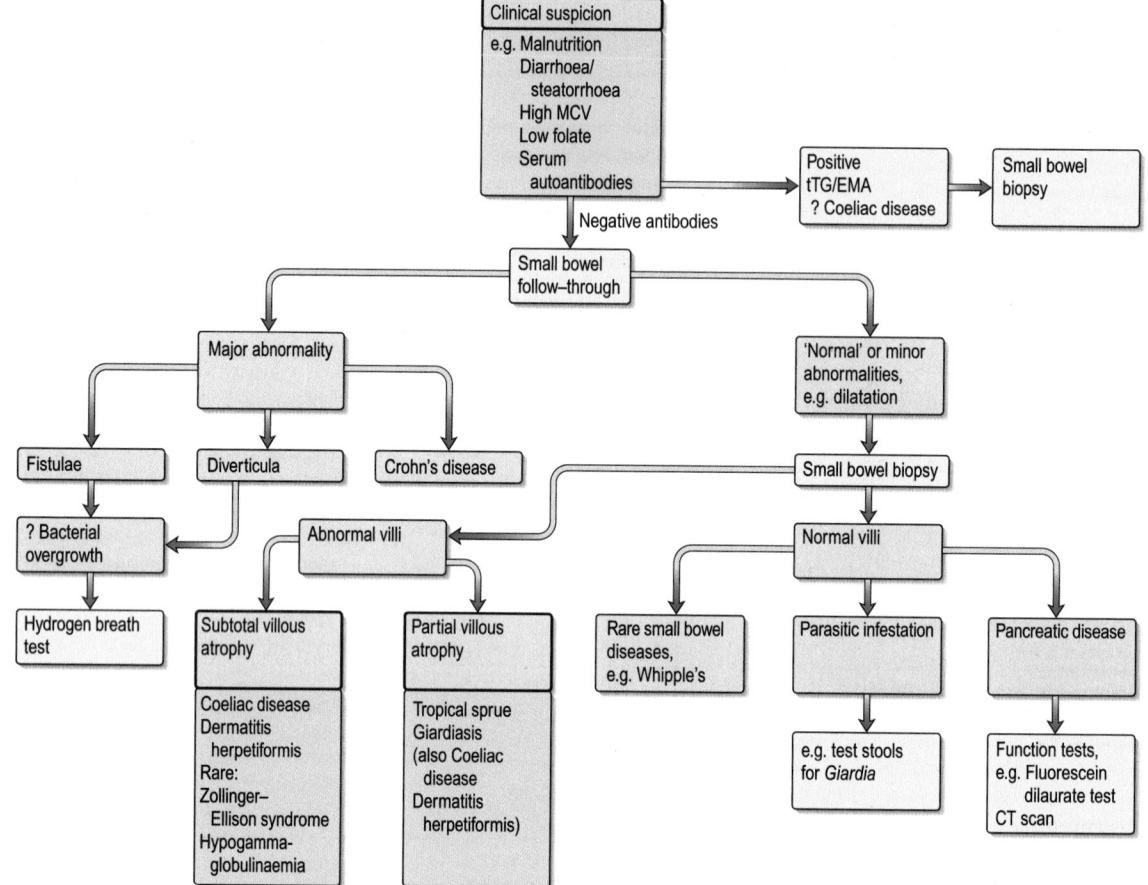

Fig. 6.24 **Flow diagram for investigation of patients with suspected small bowel disease.** EMA, endomysial antibody; tTG, tissue transglutaminase.

- **Serum albumin** gives some indication of the nutritional status.
- **Low serum calcium and raised alkaline phosphatase.** These may indicate the presence of osteomalacia.
- **Autoantibodies.** Measurement in the serum of antibodies to endomysium and tissue transglutaminase are useful for the diagnosis of coeliac disease.

Small bowel anatomy

The macroscopic and microscopic appearances of the small bowel are studied unless the diagnosis has already been made (e.g. the presence of endomysial antibodies in coeliac disease).

- **Small bowel follow-through** (see p. 268). This detects gross anatomical defects such as diverticula, strictures and Crohn's disease. Dilatation of the bowel and a changed fold pattern may suggest malabsorption but, as these are not specific findings, the diagnosis should not be based on these alone. Gross dilatation is seen in myopathic pseudo-obstruction.
- **Small bowel biopsy.** This is used to assess the micro-anatomy of the small bowel. Biopsies are usually obtained via an endoscope passed into the duodenum using large forceps and should be well-orientated for

correct evaluation. The histological appearances are described in the sections on individual diseases.

A smear of the jejunal juice or a mucosal impression can also be made and is helpful in the diagnosis of *Giardia intestinalis* (see p. 105).

Tests of absorption

These are required only in *complicated* cases.

- **Fat malabsorption.** The confirmation of the presence of steatorrhoea is only occasionally necessary. Three-day faecal fat analysis, breath tests and serum β carotene are now rarely performed. In the rare cases when it is really necessary to confirm steatorrhoea, Sudan III staining of a faecal sample can be used.
- **Lactose tolerance test.** This involves the oral ingestion of 50 g of lactose and the measurement of blood glucose. The test is of little use in adults as lactose intolerance is not a clinical problem since these patients avoid milk by choice. There is a high incidence of lactase deficiency in many parts of the world (e.g. the Mediterranean countries, and parts of Africa and Asia). It should be remembered that a glass of milk contains only approximately 11 g of lactose.

- **B$_{12}$ absorption studies** are no longer performed in the UK (see p. 432).

Other tests

- **Hydrogen breath test**. This is frequently used as a screening test to detect bacterial overgrowth. Oral lactulose or glucose is metabolized by bacteria with the production of hydrogen. An early rise in the breath hydrogen will indicate bacterial breakdown in the small intestine. Rapid transit of the lactulose to the large intestine will also produce a rise in breath hydrogen. As bacteria are present in the oral cavity, the mouth should be rinsed out with an antiseptic mouthwash prior to the test being performed. This test is simple to perform and it does not involve radioisotopes. However, interpretation is often difficult with a low sensitivity and specificity.
- **^{14}C-glycocholic acid breath test**. This was performed to look for bacterial overgrowth. Bacteria deconjugate the bile salts, releasing [^{14}C]-glycine, which is metabolized and appears in the breath as $^{14}CO_2$. It has largely been replaced by the hydrogen breath test.
- **Direct intubation**. Aspiration of intestinal juices is another method by which bacterial contamination can be detected, but is seldom used. Bacterial counts are performed on aerobic and anaerobic cultures. Chromatography of bile salts can also be performed on the aspirate to detect evidence of deconjugation by bacteria.
- **Pancreatic tests** (see p. 408). These are used in the differential diagnosis of steatorrhoea.
- **Other blood tests**. Serum immunoglobulins are measured to exclude immune deficiencies. Gut peptides (e.g. vasoactive intestinal peptide – VIP) are measured in high-volume secretory diarrhoea, and chromogranins A and B are raised in endocrine tumours.
- **Test for protein-losing enteropathy**. Intravenous radioactive chromium chloride ($^{51}CrCl_3$) is used to label circulating albumin. In excess gastrointestinal protein loss, the faeces will contain radioactivity. This test is rarely required unless a low serum albumin is a major clinical feature.
- **Bile salt loss**. This can be demonstrated by giving oral ^{75}Se-homochoyl taurine (SeHCAT – a synthetic taurine conjugate) and measuring the retention of the bile acid by whole-body counting at 7 days.

MALABSORPTION

In many small bowel diseases, malabsorption of specific substances occurs, but these deficiencies do not dominate the clinical picture. An example is Crohn's disease, in which malabsorption of vitamin B$_{12}$ can be demonstrated, but this is not usually a problem and diarrhoea and general ill-health are the major features.

Steatorrhoea – malabsorption of fat – is discussed on page 298.

The major disorders of the small intestine that cause malabsorption are shown in Table 6.7.

Table 6.7 Disorders of the small intestine causing malabsorption

Coeliac disease
Dermatitis herpetiformis
Tropical sprue
Bacterial overgrowth
Intestinal resection
Whipple's disease
Radiation enteritis
Parasite infestation (e.g. *Giardia intestinalis*)

Coeliac disease (gluten-sensitive enteropathy)

Coeliac disease is a condition in which there is an inflammation of the jejunal mucosa that improves when the patient is treated with a gluten-free diet and relapses when gluten is reintroduced. Gluten is contained in the cereals wheat, rye and barley. Pure oats are not harmful.

It is closely related to dermatitis herpetiformis, a skin disorder that has an associated gluten-sensitive enteropathy (see below).

Incidence

Coeliac disease is common in Northern Europe and epidemiological studies have shown a prevalence of 1 in 100 to 1 in 6500 in different temperate countries. It occurs throughout the world, but is rare in the black African.

There is an increased incidence of coeliac disease within families but the exact mode of inheritance is unknown; 10–15% of first-degree relatives will have the condition, although it may be asymptomatic. DQ2 (DQA*0501, DQB1*0201) and DQ8 (DQA1*0301, DQB1*0302) are associated with coeliac disease. Over 90% of patients will have DQ2, compared with 20–30% of the general population. Non-HLA regions linked to coeliac disease are chromosome 5q31–33, possibly 11q, and others are being identified. However, the fact that not all patients have these haplotypes, and that as many as 30% of identical twins are discordant for the condition, suggests an additional factor, e.g. environmental.

Aetiology

Gluten is a high-molecular-weight, heterogeneous compound that can be fractionated to produce α-, β-, γ- and ω-gliadin peptides. α-Gliadin is the main damaging peptide to the small intestinal mucosa although the other smaller peptides are also 'toxic'. T cells play a central role in the aetiopathogenesis and react with the enzyme tissue transglutaminase (the main antigen of the endomysial antibody). This enzyme is one of the targets of the auto-immune response; it modifies gliadin and enhances gliadin-specific T cell response in genetically predisposed individuals. An environmental factor, such as a viral infection, may play a role (e.g. adenovirus 12 which shows a sequence homology with gliadin). There are many other immunological abnormalities that revert to normal on treatment.

Pathology

The mucosa of the proximal small bowel is predominantly affected, the mucosal damage decreasing in severity towards the ileum as the gluten is digested into smaller 'non-toxic' fragments.

There is an absence of villi, making the mucosal surface flat. Histological examination shows crypt hyperplasia with chronic inflammatory cells in the lamina propria and villous atrophy (Marsh type III) (Fig. 6.25). The lesion is described as subtotal villus atrophy, although true atrophy of the mucosa is not present because the crypt hyperplasia compensates for villus atrophy and the total mucosal thickness remains normal. A partial villus atrophy (Marsh type II) can also be found.

The surface cells become cuboidal. There is an increase in the number of intraepithelial lymphocytes (IELs) which show an increased expression of the γ/δ T-cell receptor, instead of the α/β receptor, and this is specific to coeliac disease and remains after treatment. In the lamina propria there is an increase in lymphocytes and plasma cells. A few patients just show an increase in IELs (latent coeliac disease Marsh type 0 and I) and others, e.g. relatives, a coeliac-like antibody pattern (potential coeliac disease). The most severe form with atrophy and hypoplasia (Marsh type IV) is thought to be associated with non-response to a gluten-free diet and its complications (p. 303).

Clinical features

Coeliac disease can present at any age. In infancy it appears after weaning on to gluten-containing foods. The peak incidence in adults is in the fifth decade, with a female preponderance. The symptoms are very variable and often non-specific with tiredness and malaise often associated with an anaemia. Many patients are asymptomatic (silent) and picked up on incidental findings, e.g. a raised MCV. Common GI symptoms include diarrhoea or steatorrhoea, abdominal discomfort, bloating or pain and weight loss. Mouth ulcers and angular stomatitis are frequent and can be intermittent. Infertility and neuropsychiatric symptoms of anxiety and depression occur. Osteoporosis is common and occurs even in patients on long-term gluten-free diets. Rare complications include tetany, osteomalacia, or gross malnutrition with peripheral oedema. Neurological symptoms such as paraesthesia, ataxia (due to cerebellar calcification), muscle weakness or a polyneuropathy occur; the prognosis for these symptoms is variable.

There is an increased incidence of atopy and autoimmune disease, including thyroid disease, insulin-dependent diabetes, primary biliary cirrhosis and Sjögren's syndrome. Other associated diseases include inflammatory bowel disease, chronic liver disease, fibrosing allergic alveolitis and epilepsy. IgA deficiency is more common than in the general population.

(a)

(c)

(b)

(d)

Fig. 6.25 **Small bowel mucosal appearances – macroscopic and microscopic. (a)** Normal mucosa under the dissecting microscope (DM). **(b)** Normal mucosal histology. **(c)** Coeliac disease (DM) – flattened mucosa. **(d)** Coeliac disease – showing subtotal villous atrophy.

Physical signs are usually few and non-specific and are related to anaemia and malnutrition.

Investigations

- **Endomysial (EMA) and tissue transglutaminase (tTG) antibodies (IgA).** These antibodies have a high sensitivity and specificity for the diagnosis of untreated coeliac disease and can also be used as screening tests. They are the investigation of first choice. An immunofluorescent test for endomysial antibodies (EMA) can be performed on umbilical cord tissue or monkey oesophagus and the antigen for EMA is tissue transglutaminase. Anti-tissue transglutaminase antibodies are measured using an ELISA. In the presence of a typical clinical picture and the presence of these antibodies, a confirmatory small bowel biopsy may not always be required although most doctors prefer to have one performed.
- **Anti-reticulin antibodies (ARA)** are also very sensitive but not so specific, as they are seen in other gastrointestinal conditions (e.g. Crohn's disease). Anti-gliadin antibodies (AGA) are less sensitive and are not used.
- **Duodenal/jejunal biopsy.** The mucosal appearance (Fig. 6.25) of a small bowel biopsy specimen is diagnostic and regarded as the 'gold standard' although errors occur, particularly with poorly orientated specimens. Other causes of a flat mucosa in adults are rare and are shown in Figure 6.24. At endoscopy, the duodenal folds look effaced and a dye can be sprayed on to the duodenal mucosa to accentuate the smoothness of the mucosa (positive dye test) before the biopsy is taken.
- **Haematology.** A mild or moderate anaemia is present in 50% of cases. Folate deficiency is almost invariably present in coeliac disease, giving rise in most instances to a high MCV. B_{12} deficiency is rare but iron deficiency due to malabsorption of iron and increased loss of desquamated cells is common. A blood film may therefore show microcytes and macrocytes as well as hypersegmented polymorphonuclear leucocytes and Howell–Jolly bodies due to splenic atrophy found in most patients.
- **Absorption tests** are often abnormal (see p. 300) but are seldom performed.
- **Radiology.** A small bowel follow-through may show dilatation of the small bowel with a change in fold pattern. Folds become thicker and in the severer forms total effacement is seen. Radiology is now mainly used when a complication, e.g. lymphoma, is suspected.
- **Wireless capsule endoscopy** (p. 271) is used to look for gut abnormalities when a complication is suspected.
- **Bone densitometry** (DXA) should be performed on all patients because of the risk of osteoporosis.
- **Biochemistry.** *In the severely ill patient*, biochemical abnormalities, e.g. hypoalbuminaemia, low calcium and high phosphate (osteomalacia) are seen.

Treatment and management

Treatment with a gluten-free diet usually produces a rapid clinical and morphological improvement. Replacement haematinics, e.g. iron, folic acid, calcium, are given initially to replace body stores. The usual cause for failure to respond to the diet is poor compliance. Dietary adherence can be monitored by serial tests for EMA and tTG. If clinical progress is suboptimal then a repeat intestinal biopsy should be taken. If the diagnosis is equivocal a gluten challenge, i.e. reintroduction of gluten with evidence of jejunal morphological change, confirms the diagnosis, but is only performed if the diagnosis is equivocal. A transient gluten intolerance can occur in early childhood.

Despite advice, many patients do not keep to a strict diet but nevertheless maintain good health. The long-term effects of this low gluten intake are uncertain but osteoporosis is seen even in the treated case.

Patients should have pneumococcal vaccinations (because of splenic atrophy) once every 5 years (p. 457).

Complications

A few patients do not improve on a strict diet (unresponsive 'coeliac disease'). Often no cause for this is found, but intestinal lymphoma, ulcerative jejunitis or carcinoma are sometimes responsible. The incidence of enteropathy-associated T-cell lymphoma (EATCL) (see p. 309) is increased in coeliac disease. Ulcerative jejunitis may present with fever, abdominal pain, perforation and bleeding. Diagnosis for these conditions is with barium studies but laparotomy with full-thickness biopsies is often required. Steroids and immunosuppressive agents, e.g. azathioprine, are used. Carcinoma of the small bowel and oesophagus as well as extragastrointestinal cancers are also seen. Malignancy seems to be unrelated to the duration of the disease but the incidence is reduced by a gluten-free diet.

Dermatitis herpetiformis (see also p. 1348)

This is an uncommon blistering subepidermal eruption of the skin associated with a gluten-sensitive enteropathy. Rarely there may be gross malabsorption, but usually the jejunal morphological abnormalities are not as severe as in coeliac disease. The inheritance and immunological abnormalities are the same as for coeliac disease. The skin condition responds to dapsone but both the gut and the skin will improve on a gluten-free diet.

Tropical sprue

This is a condition presenting with malabsorption that occurs in residents or visitors to a tropical area where the disease is endemic.

Malabsorption of a mild degree, sometimes following an enteric infection, is quite common and is usually asymptomatic. This is sometimes called tropical malabsorption. The term tropical sprue is reserved for severe malabsorption (of two or more substances) that is usually accompanied by diarrhoea and malnutrition. Tropical sprue is endemic in most of Asia, some Caribbean islands, Puerto Rico and parts of South America. Epidemics occur, lasting up to 2 years, and in some areas repeated epidemics occur at varying intervals of up to 10 years.

Aetiology

The aetiology is unknown, but is likely to be infective because the disease occurs in epidemics and patients improve on antibiotics.

A number of agents have been suggested but none has been shown to be unequivocally responsible. Different agents could be involved in different parts of the world.

Clinical features

These vary in intensity and consist of diarrhoea, anorexia, abdominal distension and weight loss. The onset is sometimes acute and occurs either a few days or many years after being in the tropics. Epidemics can break out in villages, affecting thousands of people at the same time. The onset can also be insidious, with chronic diarrhoea and evidence of nutritional deficiency.

The clinical features of tropical sprue vary in different parts of the world, particularly as different criteria are used for diagnosis.

Diagnosis

Acute infective causes of diarrhoea must be excluded (see p. 333), particularly *Giardia*, which can produce a syndrome very similar to tropical sprue.

Malabsorption should be demonstrated, particularly of fat and B_{12}.

The jejunal mucosa is abnormal, showing some villous atrophy (partial villous atrophy). In most cases the lesion is less severe than that found in coeliac disease, although it affects the whole small bowel. Mild changes can be seen in asymptomatic individuals in the tropics, so jejunal mucosal changes must be interpreted carefully.

Treatment and prognosis

Many patients improve when they leave the sprue area and take folic acid (5 mg daily). Most patients also require an antibiotic (usually tetracycline 1 g daily) to ensure a complete recovery; it may be necessary to give this for up to 6 months.

The severely ill patient requires resuscitation with fluids and electrolytes for dehydration; any nutritional deficiencies should be corrected. Vitamin B_{12} (1000 µg) is also given to all acute cases.

The prognosis is excellent. Mortality is usually associated with water and electrolyte depletion, particularly in epidemics.

Bacterial overgrowth

The gut contains many resident bacteria with anaerobic bacteria, e.g. *Bacteroides*, bifidobacteria, being 100–1000 times more abundant than aerobic (facultative anaerobes), e.g. *Escherichia, Enterobacter, Enterococcus*. This gut microflora has major functions including metabolic, e.g. fermentation of non-digestible dietary residues into short chain fatty acids as an energy source in the colon. Bacteria also initiate vitamin K production. They control

epithelial cell proliferation and are involved in the development and maintenance of the immune system. They protect the gut mucosa from colonization by pathogenic bacteria.

The upper part of the small intestine is almost sterile, containing only a few organisms derived from the mouth. Gastric acid kills most organisms and intestinal motility keeps the jejunum empty. The normal terminal ileum contains faecal-type organisms, mainly *Escherichia coli* and anaerobes and the colon has abundant bacteria

Bacterial overgrowth is normally only found associated with a structural abnormality of the small intestine, although it can occur occasionally in the elderly without such abnormality. *E. coli* and/or *Bacteroides*, both in concentrations greater than $10^6/mL$ are found as part of a mixed flora. These bacteria are capable of deconjugating and dehydroxylating bile salts, so that unconjugated and dehydroxylated bile salts can be detected in aspirates by chromatography. The *clinical features* are chiefly diarrhoea and steatorrhoea. Steatorrhoea (see p. 298) occurs as a result of conjugated bile salt deficiency.

The bacteria are able to metabolize vitamin B_{12} and interfere with its binding to intrinsic factor, thereby leading to B_{12} deficiency (p. 431). Conversely some bacteria produce folic acid giving a high serum folate.

Bacterial overgrowth has only minimal effects on other substances absorbed from the small intestine. The vitamin B_{12} deficiency is not so severe as to produce a neurological deficit. Confirmation of bacterial overgrowth is with the hydrogen breath test (p. 301); aspiration studies are not routinely performed.

Although bacterial overgrowth may be responsible for the presenting symptoms, it must be remembered that many of the symptoms may be due to the underlying small bowel pathology.

Treatment

If possible, the underlying lesion should be corrected (e.g. a stricture should be resected). With multiple diverticula, grossly dilated bowel, or in Crohn's disease, this may not be possible and rotating courses of antibiotics are necessary, such as metronidazole, a tetracycline, or ciprofloxacin.

Intestinal resection (Fig. 6.26)

Intestinal resection is usually well tolerated, but massive resection is followed by the short-bowel syndrome. The effects of resection depend on the extent and the areas involved. Because the gut is long, a 30–50% resection can usually be tolerated without undue problems. Residual jejunum shows less capacity for structural and functional adaptation than residual ileum.

Ileal resection

The ileum has specific receptors for the absorption of bile salts and vitamin B_{12}, so that relatively small resections will lead to malabsorption of these substances. Removal of the ileocaecal valve increases the incidence of diarrhoea. The following occur in ileal resection:

- Bile salts and fatty acids enter the colon and cause malabsorption of water and electrolytes leading to diarrhoea (p. 334).
- Increased bile salt synthesis can compensate for loss of approximately one-third of the bile salts in the faeces. Greater loss than this results in decreased micellar formation and steatorrhoea, and lithogenic bile and gallstone formation.
- Increased oxalate absorption is caused by the presence of bile salts in the colon. This gives rise to renal oxalate stones.
- There is a low serum B_{12} and macrocytosis.
- Glucagon-like peptide 2 (GLP-2) is low following ileal resection. GLP-2 is a specific growth hormone for the enterocyte and this deficiency may explain the lack of adaptation with an ileal resection.

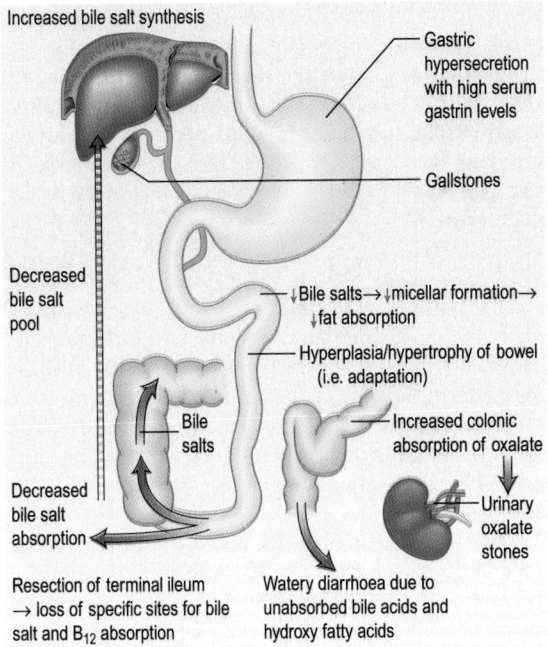

Increased bile salt synthesis

Gastric hypersecretion with high serum gastrin levels

Gallstones

Decreased bile salt pool

↓Bile salts→↓micellar formation→↓fat absorption

Hyperplasia/hypertrophy of bowel (i.e. adaptation)

Bile salts

Increased colonic absorption of oxalate

Decreased bile salt absorption

Urinary oxalate stones

Resection of terminal ileum → loss of specific sites for bile salt and B_{12} absorption

Watery diarrhoea due to unabsorbed bile acids and hydroxy fatty acids

Fig. 6.26 **The effects of resection of distal small bowel.**

Investigations include a small bowel follow-through, measurement of B_{12}, bile salts and occasionally fat absorption (see p. 300). A hydrogen breath test will show rapid transit (p. 301). Many patients require B_{12} replacement and some need a low-fat diet if there is steatorrhoea. If diarrhoea is a problem, colestyramine, which binds bile salts, often helps.

Jejunal resection

The ileum can take over the jejunal absorptive function. Jejunal resection may lead to gastric hypersecretion with high gastrin levels; the exact mechanism of this is unclear. Structural and functional intestinal adaptation take place over the course of a year, with an increase in the absorption per unit length of bowel.

Massive intestinal resection (short-bowel syndrome)

This most often occurs following resection for Crohn's disease, mesenteric vessel occlusion (p. 307), radiation enteritis (see p. 306) or trauma. There are two types of short-bowel syndrome:

Shortened small intestine ending at a terminal stoma

The major problem is of sodium and fluid depletion and the majority of patients with 100 cm or less of jejunum remaining will require parenteral supplements of fluid and electrolytes, often with nutrients. Sodium losses can be minimized by increasing salt intake, restricting clear fluids between meals and administering oral glucose– electrolyte mixture with a sodium concentration > 90 mmol/L. Jejunal transit time can be increased and stomal effluent loss of fluids and electrolytes reduced by treatment with the somatostatin analogue octreotide, and to a much lesser extent, with loperamide, codeine phosphate or co-phenotrope. There is no benefit of a low-fat diet, but fat assimilation can be increased on treatment with colestyramine and synthetic bile acids.

Shortened small intestine in continuity with colon

Only a small proportion of these patients require parenteral supplementation of fluid, electrolytes and nutrients because of the absorptive capacity of the colon for fluid and electrolytes. Unabsorbed fat results in impairment of colonic fluid and electrolyte absorption so patients should be on a low-fat diet. A high carbohydrate intake is advised as unabsorbed carbohydrate is metabolized anaerobically to short-chain fatty acids (SCFAs). SCFAs are absorbed and act as an energy source (1.6 kcal/g) and stimulate fluid and electrolyte absorption in the colon. Patients are often treated with colestyramine, which binds dihydroxy bile acids which otherwise have a deleterious effect on colonic fluid and electrolyte absorption and increase colonic oxalate absorption to form renal stones.

Whipple's disease

This is a rare disease usually affecting males. It presents with steatorrhoea and abdominal pain along with systemic symptoms of fever and weight loss. Peripheral lymphadenopathy, arthritis and involvement of the heart, lung and brain may occur. Histologically, in the small bowel, the villi are stunted and contain diagnostic periodic acid–Schiff (PAS)-positive macrophages. On electron microscopy, bacilli can be seen 'within' the macrophages. The organism was identified by the polymerase chain reaction and can be cultured; it is classified as an actinobacterium and has been given the name *Tropheryma whippeii*. A dramatic improvement occurs with antibiotic therapy, which should include an antibiotic that crosses the blood–brain barrier (e.g. co-trimoxazole) for 6 months.

Radiation enteritis

Radiation of more than 40 Gy will damage the intestine. The ileum and rectum are the areas most often involved, as pelvic irradiation is frequently used for gynaecological and urinary tract malignancies. There may be nausea, vomiting, diarrhoea and abdominal pain at the time of the irradiation. These symptoms usually improve within 6 weeks after completion of therapy. Chronic radiation enteritis is diagnosed if symptoms persist for 3 months or more. The prevalence is more than 15%. Many patients suffer from an increased bowel frequency.

Radiation produces muscle fibre atrophy, ulcerative changes due to ischaemia, and obstruction due to strictures produced by radiation-induced fibrosis. Abdominal pain is the main symptom due to the obstruction, which is usually partial but eventually may be complete. Malabsorption due to mucosal damage as well as bacterial overgrowth in dilated segments can occur. Treatment is symptomatic, although often unsuccessful in chronic enteritis. Surgery should be avoided if at all possible, being reserved for life-threatening situations such as complete obstruction or occasionally perforation. Radiation damage to the rectum produces a radiation proctitis with diarrhoea, with or without blood and tenesmus. Local steroids sometimes help initially. The telangiectasia that form and cause persistent bleeding can be treated with argon plasma coagulation or by placing a formalin-soaked swab in the rectum (for 2 min), both of which heal the lesions.

Parasite infestation

Giardia intestinalis (see p. 105) not only produces diarrhoea but can produce malabsorption with steatorrhoea. Minor changes are seen in the jejunal mucosa and the organism can be found in the jejunal fluid or mucosa.

Cryptosporidiosis (see p. 105) can also produce malabsorption.

Patients with HIV infection are particularly prone to parasitic infestation (see Table 6.20).

Other causes of malabsorption

- Drugs that bind bile salts (e.g. colestyramine) and some antibiotics (e.g. neomycin) produce steatorrhoea.
- Orlistat (p. 256) inhibits gastric and pancreatic lipase, reducing fat absorption. It is used in obesity; its side-effect is diarrhoea and steatorrhoea. Hence patients restrict their fat intake, which is the main reason why they lose weight.
- Diarrhoea, rarely with steatorrhoea, occurs in thyrotoxicosis owing to increased gastric emptying and increased motility. Steatorrhoea occurs in the Zollinger–Ellison syndrome (see p. 416).
- Intestinal lymphangiectasia produces diarrhoea and rarely steatorrhoea (see p. 308).
- Lymphoma that has infiltrated the small bowel mucosa causes malabsorption.
- In some patients with diabetes mellitus, diarrhoea, malabsorption and steatorrhoea occur, sometimes due to bacterial overgrowth from bowel stasis.
- Hypogammaglobulinaemia, which is seen in a number of conditions including lymphoid nodular hyperplasia, causes steatorrhoea due either to an abnormal jejunal mucosa or to secondary infestation with *Giardia intestinalis*.

MISCELLANEOUS INTESTINAL DISEASES

Protein-losing enteropathy

Protein-losing enteropathy is seen in many gastrointestinal and systemic conditions. Increased protein loss across an abnormal mucosa causes hypoalbuminaemia. Causes include inflammatory or ulcerative lesions (e.g. Crohn's disease), tumours, Ménétrier's disease, coeliac disease and lymphatic disorders (e.g. lymphangiectasia). Usually protein-losing enteropathy forms a minor part of the generalized disorder, but occasionally hepatic synthesis of albumin cannot compensate for the hypoalbuminaemia, and the peripheral oedema produced may dominate the clinical picture. The investigations are described on page 301 and treatment is that of the underlying disorder.

Meckel's diverticulum

This is the most common congenital abnormality of the GI tract, affecting 2–3% of the population. The diverticulum projects from the wall of the ileum approximately 60 cm from the ileocaecal valve. It is usually symptomless, but 50% contain gastric mucosa that secretes hydrochloric acid. Peptic ulcers can occur and may bleed (see p. 291) or perforate.

Acute inflammation of the diverticulum also occurs and is indistinguishable clinically from acute appendicitis. Obstruction from an associated band rarely occurs. Treatment is surgical removal, often laparoscopically.

Tuberculosis

Tuberculosis (TB) can affect the intestine as well as the peritoneum (see p. 344).

Intestinal tuberculosis is due to reactivation of primary disease caused by *M. tuberculosis*. Bovine TB occurs in areas where milk is unpasteurized and is very rare in the UK. The ileocaecal area is most commonly affected, but the colon, and rarely other parts of the gastrointestinal tract, can be involved too.

Tuberculosis is being seen more frequently in patients with HIV infection.

Clinical features

These are chiefly diarrhoea and abdominal pain with generalized systemic manifestations, including fever, anorexia and weight loss. One-third of patients present acutely with intestinal obstruction or generalized peritonitis.

ment. Abdominal pain, nausea and vomiting and upper GI bleeding occur. Eosinophilia occurs in only 20% of patients. Radiology or endoscopy will demonstrate the lesion. Steroids are used for the widespread infiltration, particularly if peripheral eosinophilia is present.

In some adults the condition appears to be allergic (allergic gastroenteritis) and is associated with peripheral eosinophilia and high levels of blood and tissue IgE.

Intestinal lymphangiectasia

Dilatation of the lymphatics may be primary or secondary to lymphatic obstruction, such as occurs in malignancy or constrictive pericarditis. In the rare primary form it may be detected incidentally as dilated lacteals on a jejunal biopsy or it can produce steatorrhoea of varying degrees. Hypoproteinaemia with ankle oedema is the other main feature. Serum immunoglobulin levels are reduced, with low circulating lymphocytes. Treatment is with a low-fat diet.

Abetalipoproteinaemia

In this rare condition, there is failure of apo B-100 synthesis in the liver and apo B-48 in the intestinal cell, so that chylomicrons are not formed. This leads to fat accumulation in the intestinal cells, giving a characteristic histological appearance to the jejunal mucosa. Clinical features include acanthocytosis (spiky red cells owing to membrane abnormalities), a form of retinitis pigmentosa, and mental and neurological abnormalities. The latter can be prevented by vitamin E injections.

GI problems in patients with HIV infection

See Table 6.20.

TUMOURS OF THE SMALL INTESTINE

The small intestine is relatively resistant to the development of neoplasia and only 3–6% of all GI tumours and fewer than 1% of all malignant lesions occur here. The reasons for the rarity of tumours is unknown. Explanations include the fluidity and relative sterility of small bowel contents and the rapid transit time, reducing the time of exposure to potential carcinogens. It is also possible that the high population of lymphoid tissue and secretion of IgA in the small intestine protect against malignancy.

Adenocarcinoma of the small intestine is rare and found most frequently in the duodenum (in the peri-ampullary region) and in the jejunum. It is the most common tumour of the small intestine, accounting for up to 50% of primary tumours.

Lymphomas are most frequently found in the ileum. These are of the non-Hodgkin's type and must be distinguished from peripheral or nodal lymphomas involving the gut secondarily.

In developed countries, the most common type of lymphoma is the B-cell type arising from MALT (see p. 205). These lymphomas tend to be annular or polypoid masses in the distal or terminal ileum, whereas most T-cell lymphomas are ulcerated plaques or strictures in the proximal small bowel.

A tumour similar to Burkitt's lymphoma also occurs and commonly affects the terminal ileum of the children in North Africa and the Middle East.

Predisposing factors for adenocarcinoma and lymphoma

Coeliac disease

There is an increased incidence of lymphoma of the T-cell type and adenocarcinoma of the small bowel in coeliac disease, as well as an unexplained increase in all malignancies both in the GI tract and elsewhere. The reason for the local development of malignancy is unknown. It is now accepted that coeliac disease is a premalignant condition, but there is no association with the length of the symptoms. Treatment of coeliac disease with a gluten-free diet reduces the risk of both lymphoma and carcinoma.

Crohn's disease

There is a small increase in the incidence of adeno-carcinoma of the small bowel in Crohn's disease.

Immunoproliferative small intestinal disease (IPSID)

IPSID is a B cell disorder in which there is proliferation of plasma cells in the lamina propria of the upper small bowel. These cells produce truncated monoclonal heavy chains, but lack associated light chains. The α heavy chains are found in the gut mucosa on immuno-fluorescence and can also be detected in the serum. IPSID occurs usually in countries surrounding the Mediterranean, but it has also been found in other developing countries in South America and the Far East. IPSID predominantly affects people in lower socio-economic groups in areas with poor hygiene and a high incidence of bacterial and parasitic infection of the gut. IPSID presents itself as a malabsorptive syndrome associated with diffuse lymphoid infiltration of the small bowel and neighbouring lymph nodes. This then progresses in some cases to a lymphoma. The condition has also been documented in the developed world.

Clinical features

Patients present with abdominal pain, diarrhoea, anorexia, weight loss and symptoms of anaemia.

There may be a palpable mass, and a small bowel follow-through will detect most lesions. Ultrasound and CT will show bowel wall thickening and the involvement of lymph nodes, which is common with lymphoma. Wireless capsule endoscopy is also being used.

Treatment

Adenocarcinoma. Most patients are treated surgically with a segmental resection. The overall 5-year survival rate is 20–35%; this varies with the histological grade and the presence or absence of lymph node involvement. Radiotherapy and chemotherapy are used in addition.

IPSID. If there is no evidence of lymphoma, antibiotics, e.g. tetracycline, should be tried initially. In the presence of lymphoma, combination chemotherapy is used; in one series the 3- to 5-year survival was 58%.

Lymphoma. Most patients require surgery and radiotherapy with chemotherapy for more extensive disease. The prognosis varies with the type.

The 5-year survival rate for T-cell lymphomas is 25%, but is better for B-cell lymphomas, varying from 50% to 75%, depending on the grade of lymphoma.

Carcinoid tumours

These originate from the enterochromaffin cells (APUD cells) of the intestine. They make up 10% of all small bowel neoplasms, the most common sites being in the appendix, terminal ileum and the rectum. It is often difficult to be certain histologically whether a particular tumour is benign or malignant. Clinically most carcinoid tumours are asymptomatic until metastases are present. Ten per cent of carcinoid tumours in the appendix present as acute appendicitis, the inflammation being secondary to obstruction. Surgical resection of the tumour is usually performed.

Carcinoid syndrome occurs in only 5% of patients with carcinoid tumours and only when there are liver metastases. Patients complain of spontaneous or induced bluish-red flushing, predominantly on the face and neck. This can lead to permanent changes with telangiectasis. Gastrointestinal symptoms consist of abdominal pain and recurrent watery diarrhoea. Cardiac abnormalities are found in 50% of patients and consist of pulmonary stenosis or tricuspid incompetence. Examination of the abdomen reveals hepatomegaly.

The tumours secrete a variety of biologically active amines and peptides, including serotonin (5-hydroxytryptamine; 5-HT), bradykinin, histamine, tachykinins and prostaglandins.

The diarrhoea and cardiac complications are probably caused by 5-HT itself, but the cutaneous flushing is thought to be produced by one of the kinins, such as bradykinin, which is known to cause vasodilatation, bronchospasm and increased intestinal motility.

Diagnosis and treatment

Ultrasound examination confirms the presence of liver secondary deposits, and the major metabolite of 5-HT, 5-hydroxyindoleacetic acid (5-HIAA), is found in high concentration in the urine.

Octreotide and lanreotide are octapeptide somatostatin analogues that have been shown to inhibit the release of many gut hormones. They alleviate the flushing and diarrhoea and can control a carcinoid crisis. Octreotide is given subcutaneously in doses up to 200 μg three times daily initially; a depot preparation 30 mg every 4 weeks can then be used. Lanreotide 30 mg is given every 7–10 days, or as a gel 60 mg every 28 days.

Long-acting octreotide also sometimes inhibits tumour growth and, since its introduction, other therapy is usually unnecessary. Interferon and other chemotherapeutic regimens occasionally reduce tumour growth, but have not been shown to increase survival. Most patients survive for 5–10 years after diagnosis.

Peutz–Jeghers syndrome

This consists of mucocutaneous pigmentation (circumoral, hands and feet) and gastrointestinal polyps and has an autosomal dominant inheritance. The gene *LKB1* responsible for Peutz–Jeghers is a serine protein kinase and can be used for genetic analysis. The brown buccal pigment is characteristic of this condition. The polyps, which are hamartomas, can occur anywhere in the GI tract but are most frequent in the small bowel. They may bleed or cause small bowel obstruction or intussusception. The polyps can occasionally contain areas of epithelial dysplasia which can become malignant. Treatment is by individual polypectomy. Multiple polypectomies may have to be performed, but bowel resection should be avoided. Follow-up is every 2 years with X-ray and endoscopy.

Other tumours

Adenomas, lipomas and stromal tumours (p. 290) are rarely found and are usually asymptomatic and picked up incidentally. They occasionally present with iron deficiency anaemia. In familial adenomatous polyposis the upper gut, particularly the duodenum, is affected in one-third of patients.

FURTHER READING

Brands LT, Boley ST (2000) Intestinal ischaemia. *Gastroenterology* **118**: 954–968.

Guarner F, Malagelada JR (2003) Gut flora in health and disease. *Lancet* **360**: 512–519.

James S (ed) (2005) Celiac disease – proceedings of NIH conference. *Gastroenterology* **128** (Suppl. 4).

Johnson LR (1994) *Physiology of the Gastrointestinal Tract.* New York: Raven Press.

Scott E M et al. (2000) Guidelines for osteoporosis in coeliac disease and inflammatory bowel disease. *Gut* **46** (Suppl. I): i1–i8.

INFLAMMATORY BOWEL DISEASE (IBD)

Two major forms of *non-specific* inflammatory bowel disease are recognized: Crohn's disease (CD), which can affect any part of the GI tract, and ulcerative colitis (UC), which affects only the large bowel.

There is overlap between these two conditions in their clinical features, histological and radiological abnormalities; in 10% of cases of colitis a definitive diagnosis of either UC or CD is not possible. Currently it is necessary to distinguish between these two conditions because of certain differences in their management. However, it is possible that these conditions represent two aspects of the same disease.

Three additional forms of non-specific inflammatory bowel disease are also recognized, namely microscopic ulcerative, microscopic lymphocytic and microscopic collagenous colitis (see p. 319).

Epidemiology

The incidence of Crohn's disease varies from country to country but is approximately 4–10 per 100 000 annually, with a prevalence of 27–106 per 100 000. The incidence of ulcerative colitis is stable at 6–15 per 100 000 annually, with a prevalence of 80–150 per 100 000.

Both conditions have a world-wide distribution but are more common in the West. The incidence is lower in the non-white races. Jews are more prone to inflammatory bowel disease than non-Jews, and the Ashkenazi Jews have a higher risk than the Sephardic Jews.

Crohn's disease is slightly commoner in females (M : F = 1 : 1.2) and occurs at a younger age (mean 26 years) than ulcerative colitis (M : F = 1.2 : 1; mean 34 years).

Aetiopathogenesis

Although the aetiology of IBD is unknown, it is becoming clear that IBD represents the outcome of three essential interactive co-factors: genetic susceptibility, environment and host immune response (Fig. 6.27), with the environmental factors representing both the local microenvironment (enteric microflora) and also the nutritional environment.

■ *Familial.* Both Crohn's disease (CD) and ulcerative colitis (UC) are more common amongst relatives of patients than in the general population. Thus 6–10% of patients affected with CD or UC have one or more relatives with the disease. The risk of CD in first-degree relatives of a CD patient is 10–14 times higher than in the general population, with the risk of UC being about 8. In CD, but not UC, affected patients are more likely to be siblings than first-degree relatives.

■ *Genetic.* A role for genetic factors in IBD was first suggested by epidemiological studies showing increased concordance for the disease (CD more than UC) in monozygotic twins in comparison with dizygotic twins who demonstrated familial aggregation. In 2001 three independent studies reported the identification of the first Crohn's disease susceptibility gene (IBD1) on chromosome 16q12, originally known as *NOD2* but subsequently renamed *CARD15* by the International Nomenclature Committee. In experimental studies, wild type *CARD15* protein activates NFκB in response to a bacterial peptidoglycan; this did not occur in a mutant form of *CARD15*. Three main independent mutations within *CARD15* have been found in association with CD. Ten to thirty per cent of CD patients are heterozygous for one of the three *CARD15* mutations, while 3–15% of patients are either homozygous or compound heterozygotes. The relative risks of developing CD from inheriting *CARD15* mutations can be estimated to be 1.5–3% in people carrying one mutation and 10–40% in people carrying two mutations. The contribution of *CARD15* mutations to disease susceptibility varies according to subpopulation, and they are not associated with CD in the Japanese population. While all clinically recognizable forms of CD can be found in patients with and without *CARD15* variants, *CARD15* variants are associated with younger age of onset, ileal (versus non-ileal) disease and a tendency to develop strictures. Since the *CARD15* mutations seem to account for less than 20% of CD, other candidate susceptibility genes have been searched for. Putative loci have been mapped to chromosome 12 (IBD2) 6 (IBD3) and 14 (IBD4).

Apart from susceptibility, HLA genes on chromosome 6 also have a role in modifying the disease. For example, the DRB1*0103 allele, which is uncommon, produces extensive and more severe disease; DRB1*0103 as well as MICA*010 are associated with perianal disease, DRB1*0701 with ileal disease (in the absence of *CARD15* alleles); and uveitis with HLA-B27 and DRB1*0103.

■ *Environmental factors.* Good domestic hygiene has been shown to be a risk factor for CD but not for UC – similarly *Helicobacter pylori* seroprevalence is reduced in CD but not in UC. In a 'clean' environment the intestinal immune system may not be exposed to pathogenic or non-pathogenic microorganisms, particularly helminthic parasites, and therefore be 'untrained' to confront minor infections without recruiting the full array of specific immune functions that lead to inflammation. Helminth infections are associated with a type 2 helper T cell response (Th₂), which would counterbalance the type-1 helper T cell response (Th₁) that is characteristic of CD. If such a mechanism is operative, it would explain why there is a frequent association of a recent intestinal infection

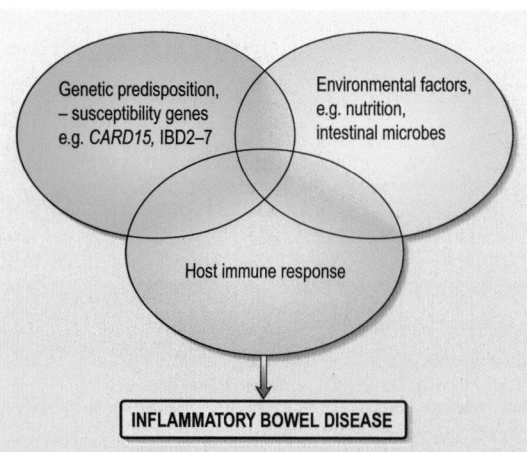

Fig. 6.27 Inflammatory bowel disease. Schematic diagram showing the aetiopathogenesis. Modified from Cashman KD, Shanahan F (2003) *European Journal of Gastroenterology and Hepatology* **15**: 607–613, with permission.

with the first presentation and subsequent flare-ups of CD.

■ *Nutritional factors.* Many foods and food components have been suggested to play a role in the aetiopathogenesis of IBD (e.g. high sugar and fat intake). Unfortunately the results of numerous studies have been equivocal so, as yet, there are no definitive data to support nutritional factors as a cause of either CD or UC.

■ *Smoking.* Patients with CD are more likely to be smokers, and smoking has been shown to exacerbate CD. In contrast, there is an increased risk of UC in non- or ex-smokers and nicotine has been shown to be an effective treatment of UC.

■ *Appendicectomy.* Appendicectomy is protective for the development of UC, particularly if performed before the age of 20 for appendicitis or mesenteric lymphadenitis. Appendicectomy also influences the clinical course of UC, with a lower incidence of colectomy and need for immunosuppressive therapy. In contrast, appendicectomy may increase the risk of development of CD and may result in more aggressive disease.

■ *Intestinal microflora.* The gut is colonized by 10 times more bacterial organisms than there are host cells, there being 300–400 distinct bacterial species. Evidence now supports a hypothesis that IBD is characterized by an overaggressive immune response to luminal bacterial antigens and other products, occurring against a background of genetic susceptibility.

 – *Bacterial flora.* There is an alteration in the bacterial flora, with an increase in anaerobic bacteria in CD and an increase in aerobic bacteria in UC.

 – *Bacterial antigens.* Bacteria may exert their pro-inflammatory influence by producing toll-like receptor ligands such as peptidoglycan-polysaccharides (PG-PS), lipopolysaccharides (LPS), bacterial DNA motifs or formylated oligopeptides, e.g. *N*-formyl-methionyl leucyl-phenylalanine (FMLP), which interact in the normal intestine with surface toll-like receptors (TLR). The disruption in TLR signalling could prevent the mucosa withstanding bacterial insult.

 – *Intestinal mucosal invasion.* The intestinal wall in IBD patients is contaminated by adherent and invading bacteria.

 – *Defective chemical barrier or intestinal defensins.* These cationic antimicrobial peptides normally protect the mucosa against adherent and invading bacteria. Evidence suggests a decrease in human β defensin-1 (HBD-1) in both CD and UC and lack of induction of HBD-2 and HBD-3 in CD.

 – *Impaired mucosal barrier function* may explain the presence of unusual and potentially pathogenic bacteria, e.g. *Mycobacterium paratuberculosis* (MAP), *Listeria*, mucosal adherent *E. coli*. Their presence does not necessarily imply causation of the disease. However, MAP has recently been found in the blood of patients with Crohn's disease and further studies are awaited.

 – *Measles virus* has been implicated as it was found in the vascular epithelium with associated vascular injury and focal enteritis. However, RT-PCR did not detect the virus from intestinal biopsies from patients. There may be antigen mimicry.

 – *Butyrate.* Sulphate-producing bacteria increase luminal levels of hydrogen sulphide (H_2S), which leads to a reduction of butyrate oxidation in colonic mucosa, producing an energy-deficient state and leading to mucosal inflammation. H_2S and methane-ethiol may produce the malodorous flatus that some patients complain of prior to a flare-up.

■ *Immunopathogenesis.* Many immunological abnormalities have been described. It is suggested that genetically susceptible patients with defective immunoregulation or barrier function/healing lack the ability to appropriately downregulate immune (antigen-specific) or antigen-non-specific inflammatory responses to endogenous luminal antigens. Specifically there is upregulation of macrophages and Th1 lymphocytes in Crohn's disease. This produces an excess of cytokines, interleukin-1β (IL-1β), IL-1 receptor antagonist (IL-1RA), IL-6, the chemokine IL-8 and TNF-α. UC is a modified Th$_2$ response with IL-5 and IL-10. Nuclear factor kappa B (NFκB) plays a central regulatory role by controlling the transcription of genes for these pro-inflammatory cytokines. There is also activation of other cells (eosinophils, mast cells, neutrophils and fibroblasts) which leads to excess production of chemokines (lymphokines, arachidonic acid metabolites, neuropeptides and free oxygen radicals), all of which can lead to tissue damage.

Pathology

■ *Crohn's disease* is a chronic inflammatory condition that may affect any part of the gastrointestinal tract from the mouth to the anus (see Table 6.10) but has a particular tendency to affect the terminal ileum and ascending colon (ileocolonic disease). The disease can involve one small area of the gut such as the terminal ileum, or multiple areas with relatively normal bowel in between (skip lesions). It may also involve the whole of the colon (total colitis) sometimes without small bowel involvement.

■ *Ulcerative colitis* can affect the rectum alone (proctitis), can extend proximally to involve the sigmoid and descending colon (left-sided colitis), or may involve the whole colon (total colitis). In a few of these patients there is also inflammation of the distal terminal ileum (backwash ileitis).

Macroscopic changes

In *Crohn's disease* the involved small bowel is usually thickened and narrowed. There are deep ulcers and fissures in the mucosa, producing a cobblestone appearance. Fistulae and abscesses may be seen in the colon. An early feature is aphthoid ulceration, usually seen at colonoscopy (Fig. 6.28); later, larger and deeper ulcers appear in a patchy distribution, again producing a cobblestone appearance.

In *ulcerative colitis* the mucosa looks reddened, inflamed and bleeds easily. In severe disease there is

(a)

(b)

Fig. 6.28 Crohn's disease. Colonoscopic appearances of **(a)** aphthoid ulcers typical of Crohn's disease, **(b)** cobblestone appearance.

extensive ulceration with the adjacent mucosa appearing as inflammatory polyps.

In fulminant colonic disease of either type, most of the mucosa is lost, leaving a few islands of oedematous mucosa (mucosal islands), and toxic dilatation occurs. On healing, the mucosa can return to normal, although there is usually some residual glandular distortion.

Microscopic changes

In *Crohn's disease* the inflammation extends through all layers (transmural) of the bowel, whereas in ulcerative colitis a superficial inflammation is seen. In Crohn's disease

Table 6.8   Histological differences between Crohn's disease and ulcerative colitis

	Crohn's disease	Ulcerative colitis
Inflammation	Deep (transmural) Patchy	Mucosal Continuous
Granulomas	++	Rare
Goblet cells	Present	Depleted
Crypt abscesses	+	++

there is an increase in chronic inflammatory cells and lymphoid hyperplasia, and in 50–60% of patients granulomas are present. These granulomas are non-caseating epithelioid cell aggregates with Langhans' giant cells.

In *ulcerative colitis* the mucosa shows a chronic inflammatory cell infiltrate in the lamina propria. Crypt abscesses and goblet cell depletion are also seen.

The differentiation between these two diseases can usually be made not only on the basis of clinical and radiological data but also on the histological differences seen in the rectal and colonic mucosa obtained by biopsy (Table 6.8).

It is occasionally not possible to distinguish between the two disorders, particularly if biopsies are obtained in the acute phase, and such patients are considered to have an indeterminate inflammatory colitis. Serological testing may be of value in differentiating the two conditions (p. 314).

Extragastrointestinal manifestations

These occur with both diseases. Joint complications are commonest, and the peripheral arthropathies are now classified as type 1 (pauci-articular) and type 2 (polyarticular). Type 1 attacks are acute, self-limiting (< 10 weeks) and occur with IBD relapses; they are associated with other extraintestinal manifestations of IBD activity. Type 2 arthropathy lasts longer (months to years), is independent of IBD activity and usually associated with uveitis. The incidence of joint and other extragastrointestinal manifestations is shown in Table 6.9. This is an association HLA DRB1*0103 with pauci-articular large joint arthritis in UC and CD and small joint symmetrical arthritis with HLA-B44. HLA B27 is associated with sacroileitis.

Differential diagnosis

All causes of diarrhoea should be excluded (see Table 6.18) and stool cultures are always performed. Crohn's disease should be considered in all patients with evidence of malabsorption, e.g. megaloblastic anaemia, or malnourishment, as well as in children with small stature. Ileocolonic tuberculosis (p. 306) is common in developing countries, e.g. India, and makes a diagnosis of Crohn's disease difficult. Microscopy and culture for TB of any available tissue is essential in these countries. A therapeutic trial of antituberculosis therapy may be required.

Lymphomas can occasionally involve the ileum and caecum.

Table 6.9 Extragastrointestinal manifestation of inflammatory bowel disease (percentage of cases)

	Ulcerative colitis	Crohn's disease
Eyes		
Uveitis	2	5
Episcleritis		
Conjunctivitis	5–8	3–10
Joints		
Type I (pauci-articular) arthropathy	4	6
Type II (polyarticular) arthropathy	2.5	4
Arthralgia	5	14
Ankylosing spondylitis	1	1.2
Inflammatory back pain	3.5	9
Skin		
Erythema nodosum	1	4
Pyoderma gangrenosum	1	2
Liver and biliary tree		
Sclerosing cholangitis	2.5–7.5	1–2
Fatty liver	Common	Common
Chronic hepatitis	Uncommon	Uncommon
Cirrhosis	Uncommon	Uncommon
Gallstones	As normal population	15–30
Nephrolithiasis	–	5–10 oxalate stones in patients with small bowel disease or after resection
Venous thrombosis	5	1

Crohn's disease

Clinical features

The major symptoms are diarrhoea, abdominal pain and weight loss. Constitutional symptoms of malaise, lethargy, anorexia, nausea, vomiting and low-grade fever may be present and in 15% of these patients there are no gastrointestinal symptoms. Despite the recurrent nature of this condition, many patients remain well and have an almost normal lifestyle. However, patients with extensive disease often have frequent recurrences, necessitating multiple hospital admissions.

The clinical features are very variable and depend partly on the region of the bowel that is affected. The disease may present insidiously or acutely. The abdominal pain can be colicky, suggesting obstruction but it usually has no special characteristics and sometimes in colonic disease only minimal discomfort is present. Diarrhoea is present in 80% of all cases and in colonic disease it usually contains blood, making it difficult to differentiate from ulcerative colitis. Steatorrhoea can be present in small bowel disease.

Crohn's disease can present as an emergency with acute right iliac fossa pain mimicking appendicitis. If laparotomy is undertaken, an oedematous reddened terminal ileum is found. There are other causes of an acute ileitis (e.g. infections such as *Yersinia*). Up to 30% of patients presenting with acute ileitis turn out eventually to have Crohn's disease. Crohn's disease can be complicated by anal and perianal disease and this is the presenting feature in 25% of cases, often preceding colonic and small intestinal symptoms by many years (Table 6.10).

Enteric fistulae, e.g. to bladder or vagina, occur in 20–40% of cases, equally divided between internal and external fistulae; the latter usually occurring after surgery.

Examination

Physical signs are few, apart from loss of weight and general ill-health. Aphthous ulceration of the mouth is often seen. Abdominal examination is often normal although tenderness and a right iliac fossa mass are occasionally found. The mass is due either to inflamed loops of bowel that are matted together or to an abscess. The anus should always be examined to look for oedematous anal tags, fissures or perianal abscesses.

Extragastrointestinal features of inflammatory bowel disease should be looked for (Table 6.9).

Sigmoidoscopy should always be performed in a patients with Crohn's disease. With small bowel involvement the rectum may appear normal, but a biopsy must be taken as non-specific histological changes can

Table 6.10 Anal and perianal complications of Crohn's disease

Fissure in ano (multiple and indolent)
Haemorrhoids
Skin tags
Perianal abscess
Ischiorectal abscess
Fistula in ano (may be multiple)
Anorectal fistulae

sometimes be found in the mucosa. Even with extensive colonic Crohn's disease the rectum may be spared and be relatively normal, but patchy involvement with an oedematous haemorrhagic mucosa can be present.

Investigations

Blood tests

- Anaemia is common and is usually the normocytic, normochromic anaemia of chronic disease. Deficiency of iron and/or folate also occurs. Despite terminal ileal involvement in Crohn's disease, megaloblastic anaemia due to B_{12} deficiency is unusual, although serum B_{12} levels can be below the normal range.
- Raised ESR and CRP and a raised white cell count.
- Hypoalbuminaemia is present in severe disease.
- Liver biochemistry may be abnormal.
- Blood cultures are required if septicaemia is suspected.
- Serological tests. *Saccharomyces cerevisiae* antibody is usually present while p-ANCA antibody is negative. The reverse is true in UC but the clinical value of these tests is limited.

Stool cultures

These should always be performed on presentation if diarrhoea is present.

Radiology and imaging

A *barium follow-through* examination should always be performed in patients suspected of having Crohn's disease. The findings include an asymmetrical alteration in the mucosal pattern with deep ulceration, and areas of narrowing or stricturing. Although commonly confined to the terminal ileum (Fig. 6.29), other areas of the small bowel can be involved and skip lesions with normal bowel are seen between affected sites.

Imaging of the small bowel may also be performed by magnetic resonance enteroclysis. Colonoscopy is performed if colonic involvement is suspected except in patients presenting with severe acute disease. The findings vary from mild patchy superficial (aphthoid) ulceration to more widespread larger and deeper ulcers producing a cobblestone appearance (see Fig. 6.28).

In patients presenting acutely with colonic symptoms plain abdominal X-ray, ultrasound or CT is used to outline the colon as for UC (p. 317).

High-resolution ultrasound and *spiral CT scanning* are both helpful techniques in defining thickness of the bowel wall and mesentery as well as intra-abdominal and para-intestinal abscesses. Rectal ultrasound and MRI are used to evaluate perianal disease.

Radionuclide scans with gallium-labelled polymorphs or indium- or technetium-labelled leucocytes are used in some centres to identify small intestinal and colonic disease and to localize extraintestinal abscesses.

Disease activity

This can be assessed using simple parameters such as Hb, white cell count, inflammatory markers (raised ESR, CRP and platelet count) and serum albumin. Formal clinical

Fig. 6.29 **Terminal ileum on small bowel follow-through in Crohn's disease,** showing narrowing and ulceration of the terminal ileum (arrow). Note the presence of deep 'rose thorn' type ulcers and 'cobblestoning' in the terminal ileum.

activity indices (e.g. Crohn's disease activity index) are used in research studies. Calprotectin is a calcium-binding protein and accounts for 60% of cytosolic protein of neutrophils. Faecal calprotectin has the potential as a simple cheap non-invasive marker of disease activity in IBD and may be of value in predicting response to and failure of treatment.

Medical management of Crohn's disease
(Box 6.8)

The aim of management is to induce and then maintain a remission. Patients with mild symptoms may require only symptomatic treatment. Cigarette smoking should be stopped. Diarrhoea can be controlled with loperamide, codeine phosphate or co-phenotrope. Diarrhoea in long-standing inactive disease may be due to bile acid malabsorption (p. 334) and should be treated with colestyramine. Anaemia, if due to vitamin B_{12}, folic acid or iron deficiency, should be treated with the appropriate haematinics. Anaemia in more active disease is usually normochromic and normocytic (anaemia of chronic disease, p. 430) and will usually improve as the patient gets

Box 6.8 Options for medical treatment of Crohn's disease

Induction of remission
- Oral or i.v. glucocorticosteroids
- Enteral nutrition
- Oral glucocorticosteroids + azathioprine or 6 mercaptopurine (6MP)

Maintenance of remission
- Aminosalicylates
- Azathioprine, 6MP, mycophenolate mofetil

Treatment of glucocorticosteroid/immunosuppressive therapy-resistant disease
- Methotrexate
- Intravenous ciclosporin
- Infliximab (TNF-α antibody)
- New biological agents

Perianal disease
- Ciprofloxacin and metronidazole

better. Patients with active (moderate/severe) attacks may have to be admitted to hospital. Patients with moderate to severe total *Crohn's colitis* are treated as for UC (p. 317).

Glucocorticosteroids are commonly used to induce remission in moderate and severe attacks of Crohn's disease (oral prednisolone 30–60 mg/day). In patients with ileocaecal, but not colonic, Crohn's disease, slow-release formulations of budesonide are as efficacious as oral prednisolone. Budesonide has high topical potency and because of its extensive hepatic inactivation has low systemic availability, which induces less suppression of endogenous cortisol and reduces frequency and intensity of steroidal side-effects. Overall remission/response rates vary from 60% to 90% depending on type, site and extent of disease.

Enteral nutrition is an underutilized means of inducing remission in moderate and severe attacks of Crohn's disease, and efficacy is independent of nutritional status. If enteral diets with a low fat (1.3% of total calories) and a low linoleic acid content are administered as the sole source of nutrition for 28 days, rates of induction of remission are similar to those obtained with steroids. Relapse rates are high, however, particularly in those with colonic involvement.

Flare-ups commonly occur after steroid dosages are tapered and/or enteral nutrition stopped, and alternative treatment strategies have to be introduced, e.g. steroid dosage may have to be temporarily increased, to re-induce and maintain remission. Aminosalicylates are particularly useful in Crohn's colitis. The immuno-suppressive agents azathioprine (AZA) and its metabolite 6-mercaptopurine (6MP) are both effective in inducing and maintaining remission and have steroid-sparing properties. Mycophenolate mofetil, which suppresses the proliferation of T and B lymphocytes, is also effective in maintaining remission.

Long-term treatment with AZA and 6MP is necessary as the rate of relapse on discontinuation of treatment is high (70%). Regular blood counts should be performed after commencing treatment as the key enzyme involved in AZA and 6MP metabolism (thiopurine methyltransferase, TPMT) has significant genetic variation in the population, with deficiencies resulting in high levels of active thioguanine nucleotides which result in immune and bone marrow suppression. Assays for TPMT are now available in some centres and early detection of a deficiency will alert clinicians to the potential dangers of AZA and 6MP therapy. In unresponsive patients, remission is sometimes induced and maintained by raising the dose of AZA to levels that make patients leucopenic.

In patients with corticosteroid/immunosuppressive therapy-resistant Crohn's disease, methotrexate or i.v. (but not oral) ciclosporin has been shown to be effective in inducing remission, but not in maintaining it. Biological treatments directed against specific inflammatory mediators, e.g. anti TNF-α antibody (infliximab), are now being used and the results of the first maintenance trials have been reported (Box 6.9). A single infusion of this agent has been shown to be effective in producing clinical improvement in up to 60% of patients with steroid-resistant disease.

In the future, other anti TNF-α agents currently under assessment may be approved for clinical use (e.g. CDP571, CDP870) as will other biological agents (e.g. natalizumab, basiliximab, visilizumab, RDP 58, MLN-02). Anti-interleukins, e.g. Anti-IL-12, are also being tested.

Surgical management of Crohn's disease

Approximately 80% of patients will require an operation at some time during the course of their disease. Nevertheless, surgery should be avoided if possible and only minimal resections undertaken, as recurrence (15% per year) is almost inevitable. The indications for surgery are:

Box 6.9 Tumour necrosis factor-α (TNF-α) in Crohn's disease

- TNF-α is a pro-inflammatory cytokine.
- It has a major role in the pathogenesis of Crohn's disease.
- Infliximab – a chimeric anti-TNF-α monoclonal antibody – binds with high affinity to TNF-α and neutralizes its biological activity.
- Infliximab 5 mg/kg i.v. as a single infusion can induce remission in patients with moderately to severely active Crohn's disease.
- Responders without fistulizing disease are more likely to remain in remission if repeat infusions are administered at weeks 2 and 6, and then every 8 weeks until week 46 (ACCENT I trial).
- Infliximab 5 mg/kg at 0, 2 and 6 weeks closes fistulae in patients with fistulizing Crohn's disease, with a median duration of response of 12 weeks.
- Added maintenance treatment (5 mg/kg) 8-weekly until week 46 increases the chances of not having a draining fistula at week 54 (36% vs placebo 19%; ACCENT II trial).
- Side-effects include the detection of antibodies to infliximab, anti-dsDNA and ANA and the development of lupus-like syndrome. Infusion reactions, serum sickness-like reactions and infections (e.g. tuberculosis) in up to a third of patients have been reported.

- failure of medical therapy, with acute or chronic symptoms producing ill-health
- complications (e.g. toxic dilatation, obstruction, perforation, abscesses, enterocutaneous fistula)
- failure to grow in children.

In patients with small bowel disease, some strictures can be widened (stricturoplasty), whereas others require resection and end-to-end anastomosis.

When colonic Crohn's disease involves the entire colon and the rectum is spared or minimally involved a subtotal colectomy and ileorectal anastomosis may be performed. An eventual recurrence rate of 60–70% in the ileum, rectum or both is to be expected; however, two-thirds of these patients retain a functional rectum for 10 years. If the whole colon and rectum are involved a panproctocolectomy with an end ileostomy is the standard operation. In this operation the colon and rectum are removed and the ileum is brought out through an opening in the right iliac fossa and attached to the skin. The patient wears an ileostomy bag, which is stuck on to the skin over the ileostomy spout. The bag needs to be emptied once or twice daily, so this is compatible with a near-normal lifestyle. Stoma care therapists are readily available with help and advice. Crohn's disease patients are not suitable for a pouch operation (p. 318) as recurrence in the pouch is high.

Problems associated with ileostomies include:

- mechanical problems
- dehydration, particularly in hot climates
- psychosexual problems
- infertility in men
- recurrence of Crohn's disease.

Ulcerative colitis

Clinical features

The major symptom in ulcerative colitis is diarrhoea with blood and mucus, sometimes accompanied by lower abdominal discomfort. General features include malaise, lethargy and anorexia. Aphthous ulceration in the mouth is seen. The disease can be mild, moderate or severe, and in most patients runs a course of remissions and exacerbations. Ten per cent of patients have persistent chronic symptoms, while some patients may have only a single attack.

When the disease is confined to the rectum (proctitis), blood mixed with the stool, urgency and tenesmus are common. There are normally few constitutional symptoms, but patients are nevertheless greatly inconvenienced by the frequency of defecation.

In an acute attack of UC, patients have bloody diarrhoea, passing up to 10–20 liquid stools per day. Diarrhoea also occurs at night, with urgency and incontinence that is severely disabling for the patient. Occasionally blood and mucus alone are passed.

The definition of a severe attack is given in Table 6.11. The patient is often very ill and needs urgent treatment in hospital.

Table 6.11 **Definition of a severe attack of ulcerative colitis**

Stool frequency	> 6 stools per day with blood +++
Fever	> 37.5°C
Tachycardia	> 90 per minute
ESR	> 30 mm per hour
Anaemia	< 10 g/dL haemoglobin
Albumin	< 30 g/L

Examination

In general there are no specific signs in ulcerative colitis. The abdomen may be slightly distended or tender to palpation. The anus is usually normal. Rectal examination will show the presence of blood. Rigid sigmoidoscopy is usually abnormal, showing an inflamed, bleeding, friable mucosa. Very occasionally rectal sparing occurs, in which case sigmoidoscopy will be normal.

Investigations

Blood tests

- In moderate to severe attacks an iron deficiency anaemia is commonly present and the white cell and platelet counts are raised.
- The ESR and CRP are often raised; liver biochemistry may be abnormal, with hypoalbuminaemia occurring in severe disease.
- pANCA may be positive. This is contrary to Crohn's disease, where pANCA is usually negative (p. 345).

Stool cultures

These should always be performed to exclude infective causes of colitis.

Imaging

A *plain abdominal X-ray* with an *abdominal ultrasound* are the key investigations in moderate to severe attacks. The extent of disease can be judged by the air distribution in the colon and the presence of colonic dilatation can be noted. Thickening of the colonic wall can be detected on ultrasound, as can the presence of free fluid within the abdominal cavity. CT is also valuable in acute attacks. An instant *unprepared barium enema* is sometimes performed.

Colonoscopy

A *colonoscopy* should not be performed in severe attacks of disease for fear of perforation. In more long-standing and chronic disease it is useful in defining extent and activity of disease, and in patients with total ulcerative colitis of 10 years' duration or more, *colonoscopy* and multiple biopsies should be performed to exclude dysplasia and carcinoma.

Radionuclide scans

These can be used to assess colonic inflammation (p. 270).

Medical management of ulcerative colitis (UC)

Wherever possible, patients with ulcerative colitis and Crohn's disease should be managed in patient-focused inflammatory bowel disease clinics. All patients with ulcerative colitis should be treated with an amino-salicylate. The active moiety of these drugs is 5-aminosalicylic acid (5-ASA). 5-ASA is absorbed in the small intestine (and may be nephrotoxic) so the design of the various aminosalicylate preparations is based on the binding of 5-ASA by an azo bond to sulfapyridine (sulfasalazine), 4-aminobenzoyl-β-alanine (balsalazide) or to 5-ASA itself (olsalazine), coating with a pH-sensitive polymer (Asacol) or packaging of 5-ASA in microspheres (Pentasa).

The azo bonds are broken down by colonic bacteria to release 5-ASA within the colon. The pH-dependent forms are designed to release 5-ASA in the terminal ileum. Luminal pH profiles in patients with inflammatory bowel disease are abnormal and in some patients capsules of 5-ASA coated with pH-sensitive polymer may pass through into the faeces intact. 5-ASA is released from microspheres throughout the small intestine and colon. The mode of action of 5-ASA in inflammatory bowel disease is unknown, but the aminosalicylates have been shown to be effective in inducing remission in mild to moderately active disease and maintaining remission in all forms of disease. Sulfasalazine is being used less frequently because of its wider side-effect profile.

Proctitis

Oral aminosalicylates plus a local rectal steroid prep-aration (10% hydrocortisone foam; prednisolone 20 mg enemas or foam) are the first-line treatment. Mesalazine enemas and budesonide enemas can be tried. Some cases of proctitis can be 'resistant' to treatment. In these, oral corticosteroids alone or in combination with azathioprine are used and in rare cases short-chain fatty acid enemas may help.

Left-sided proctocolitis

Oral aminosalicylates plus local rectal steroid preparations may be effective but in moderate to severe attacks oral prednisolone will be required. If patients do not respond within 2 weeks they should be admitted to hospital.

Total colitis (moderate to severe attacks) (Table 6.11)

Patients should be admitted to hospital and treated initially with hydrocortisone 100 mg i.v. 6-hourly with oral aminosalicylates. Full investigations (see above) should be performed initially and full supportive therapy administered (i.v. fluids, nutritional support via the enteral (not parenteral) route if required).

Patients who have been previously admitted within 2–3 years with moderate to severe attacks of total colitis can be started on azathioprine if not already on this treatment, as it takes time to work. The clinical status of patients should subsequently be monitored carefully (fever, tachycardia, abdominal signs) and daily FBC, ESR, CRP, electrolytes and urea, tests of liver function, including serum albumin, straight abdominal X-ray, and stool weights should be performed. Success or failure of medical treatment of a severe attack of ulcerative colitis must be judged by an experienced gastroenterologist.

Fig. 6.30 **Plain abdominal X-ray, showing toxic dilatation in ulcerative colitis.** The arrows indicate mucosal islands.

A persistent fever, tachycardia, falling Hb, rising white cell count, falling potassium, falling albumin and per-sistently raised stool weights (> 500 g/day) with loose blood-stained stool are all signs that the patient is not responding to treatment and that surgery may be indicated.

Toxic dilatation of the colon in which the plain abdominal X-ray shows a dilated thin-walled colon with a diameter of more than 5 cm that is gas filled and con-tains mucosal islands (Fig. 6.30) is a particularly dangerous stage of advanced disease with impending perforation and high mortality (15–25%). Urgent surgery is required in all patients in whom toxic dilatation has not resolved within 48 hours.

In patients responding to i.v. hydrocortisone treatment, oral prednisolone therapy should be substituted and doses slowly tailed off (5–10 mg weekly). Maintenance of remission is with aminosalicylates. In patients in whom it is not possible to reduce the dose of prednisolone without flare-up, azathioprine is used.

Surgical management of ulcerative colitis

While the treatment of ulcerative colitis remains primarily medical, surgery continues to have a central role because it may be life-saving, is curative and eliminates the long-term risk of cancer. The main indication for surgery is for a severe attack which fails to respond to medical therapy. Other indications are listed in Box 6.10.

In acute disease, subtotal colectomy with end ileostomy and preservation of the rectum is the operation of choice. At a later date a number of surgical options are available. These include proctectomy with a permanent ileostomy. To avoid a permanent ileostomy, ileorectal anastomosis can be performed; annual biopsies of the rectal mucosa must be carried out to exclude dysplasia, a

> **Box 6.10 Indications for surgery in ulcerative colitis**
>
> **Fulminant acute attack**
> - Failure of medical treatment
> - Toxic dilatation
> - Haemorrhage
> - Perforation
>
> **Chronic disease**
> - Incomplete response to medical treatment
> - Excessive steroid requirement
> - Non-compliance with medication
> - Risk of cancer

> **Box 6.11 Probiotic use in inflammatory bowel disease**
>
> Probiotics are live microorganisms which when ingested can modify the composition of enteric microflora. Commonly used probiotics are lactobacilli, bifidobacteria, non-pathogenic *E. coli*.
>
> **Rationale for use**
> - Germ-free animals are susceptible to gastrointestinal infections and inflammation.
> - Pseudomembranous colitis due to *C. difficile* follows antibiotic therapy.
> - In vitro isolates of normal bacteria inhibit growth of pathogenic bacteria.
> - Regulatory signals between bacterial flora and intestinal epithelial cells maintain mucosal integrity.
>
> **Use**
> - Pouchitis (p. 318) – they can prevent onset and maintain a remission, possibly by increasing tissue levels of IL-10 and reducing TH-1 cytokine production as well as normalizing colonic bacterial function.
> - May be useful in maintaining remissions in ulcerative colitis.

histological change that precedes the development of a rectal stump carcinoma. With an ileo-anal anastomosis (Fig. 6.31), a pouch of ileum is formed that acts as a reservoir. The pouch is anastomosed to the anus at the dentate line following endoanal excision of the mucosa of the distal rectum and anal canal. Continence is usually achieved. A third of patients, however, will experience 'pouchitis' in which there is inflammation of the pouch mucosa with clinical symptoms of diarrhoea, bleeding, fever and at times exacerbation of extracolonic manifestations (Fig. 6.32). The incidence of pouchitis is twice as high in patients with primary sclerosing cholangitis. Two-thirds of pouchitis cases will recur either as acute relapsing or chronic unremitting forms. Treatment is not always satisfactory and includes topical and oral 5-ASA, corticosteroids, metronidazole and ciprofloxacin. Probiotics (four strains of lactobacillus, three strains of bifidobacterium and one of streptococcus) have been shown to prevent the onset of pouchitis and to maintain remission in pouchitis patients. Probiotics have also been used as maintenance therapy in UC (Box 6.11). Finally, short-chain fatty acid enemas and alicaforsen (a selective inhibitor of intercellular adhesion molecule-1, ICAM-1, expression) enemas have shown promise in the treatment of pouchitis.

Course and prognosis

A third of patients with distal inflammatory proctitis due to ulcerative colitis will develop more proximal disease, with 5–10% developing total colitis. A third of patients with ulcerative colitis will have a single attack and the others will have a relapsing course. A third of patients with ulcerative colitis will undergo colectomy within 20 years of diagnosis.

Cancer in inflammatory bowel disease

Patients with extensive ulcerative colitis of more than 10 years' duration are at an increased risk of developing colorectal cancer. (Cumulative risk 5% after 20 years, 12% at 25 years.) Although patients with Crohn's colitis are also at risk, this is lower than with ulcerative colitis. Many centres recommend that colonoscopy and multiple biopsies should be undertaken at 1- to 2-year intervals in patients with extensive ulcerative colitis of more than 10 years' duration, and those with evidence of high-grade dysplasia should undergo colectomy. There is, however, no supportive evidence for this strategy. There is as yet insufficient evidence to support the use of a surveillance program in patients with Crohn's colitis.

Pregnancy and inflammatory bowel disease

Women with inactive IBD have normal fertility. Fertility, however, may be reduced in those with active disease, and patients with active disease are twice as likely to suffer spontaneous abortion than those with inactive disease.

Although the risk of an exacerbation of IBD is not increased in pregnancy, when exacerbations occur they do so most commonly in the first trimester and during the immediate postpartum period.

Aminosalicylates, steroids and azathioprine are safe at the time of conception and during pregnancy. The sulfapyiridine moiety of sulfasalazine impairs spermatogenesis, so the partners of women trying to conceive should be treated with an alternative aminosalicylate.

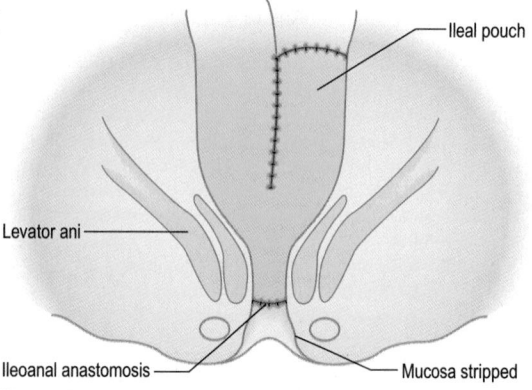

Fig. 6.31 An ileo-anal pouch for ulcerative colitis.

Ileal pouch

Levator ani

Ileoanal anastomosis

Mucosa stripped

(a)   **(b)**

Fig. 6.32 **Pouchitis.** Fibreoptic sigmoidoscopic appearances. **(a)** Mild changes. **(b)** Severe haemorrhagic ulceration.

Mortality in inflammatory bowel disease

Population based studies demonstrate a mortality in UC similar to that in the general population. The two exceptions are patients with severe colitis who have a slightly higher mortality in the first year after diagnosis and patients aged over 60 at the time of diagnosis. Although currently it is unclear whether there is a slightly higher overall mortality in patients with CD or not, those with extensive jejunal and ileal disease and those with gastric and duodenal disease have been shown to have a higher relative mortality.

Microscopic inflammatory colitis

Patients with this group of disorders present with chronic or fluctuating watery diarrhoea. Although the macroscopic features on colonoscopy are normal, the histopathological findings on biopsy are abnormal. There are three distinct forms of microscopic inflammatory colitis:

- microscopic ulcerative colitis
- microscopic lymphocytic colitis
- microscopic collagenous colitis.

In *microscopic ulcerative colitis*, there is a chronic inflammatory cell infiltrate in the lamina propria, with deformed crypt architecture, and goblet cell depletion with or without crypt abscesses. *Treatment* is as for ulcerative colitis; many patients respond to treatment with aminosalicylates alone.

In *microscopic lymphocytic colitis* there is surface epithelial injury, prominent lymphocytic infiltration in the surface epithelium and increased lamina propria mononuclear cells. It affects males and females equally and is associated with a high prevalence of antibiotic use.

In *microscopic collagenous colitis* there is a thickened subepithelial collagen layer (> 10 μm) adjacent to the basal membrane with increased infiltration of the lamina propria with lymphocytes and plasma cells and surface epithelial cell damage. It is predominantly a disorder of middle-aged or elderly females, and is associated with a variety of autoimmune disorders (arthritis, thyroid disease, CREST syndrome and primary biliary cirrhosis). The prevalence of collagenous colitis has been shown to be $15.7/10^5$ population with an annual incidence of

$1.8/10^5$ population. There are a number of reports linking drugs to the development of collagenous colitis (nonsteroidal anti-inflammatory drugs, simvastatin, H_2-receptor antagonists).

There are no controlled clinical trials of treatment in microscopic lymphocytic or collagenous colitis. Treatment is usually with aminosalicylates, budesonide, bismuth-containing preparations (tripotassium, dicitratobismuthate, peptobismol), prednisolone and azathioprine in that order. In general, patients with microscopic collagenous colitis are easier to treat than those with the lymphocytic form of the disease.

FURTHER READING
Carter MJ et al. (2004). Guidelines for the management of inflammatory bowel disease in adults. *Gut* **53** (Suppl. V): 1–16.
Farrell RJ, Peppercorn MA (2002) Ulcerative colitis. *Lancet* **359**: 331–340.
Gionchetti P et al. (2003) Prophylaxis of pouchitis onset with probiotic therapy: a double-blind, placebo-controlled trial. *Gastroenterology* **124**: 1202–1209.
Hanover SB et al. (2002) Maintenance infliximab for Crohn's disease: The ACCENT 1 randomized trial. *Lancet* **359**: 1541–1549.
Saitor RB, Mayer L (2004) Inflammatory bowel diseases: the paradigm for 21st century medicine. Special Issue *Gastroenterology* **126**: 1504–1648.
Sands BE et al. (2004) Infliximab maintenance therapy for fistulizing Crohn's disease. *New England Journal of Medicine* **350**: 876–885.
Scholmerich J (2003) New developments in aetiological mechanisms of inflammatory bowel disease. *European Journal of Gastroenterology and Hepatology* **15**: 585–634.
Shanahan F (2002) Crohn's disease. *Lancet* **359**: 62–69.

THE COLON AND RECTUM

Structure

The large intestine starts at the caecum, on the posterior medial wall of which is the appendix. The colon is made up of ascending, transverse, descending and sigmoid parts, which join the rectum at the rectosigmoid junction.

The muscle wall consists of an inner circular layer and an outer longitudinal layer. The outer layer is incomplete, coming together to form the taenia coli, which produce the haustral pattern seen in the normal colon.

The mucosa of the colon is lined with epithelial cells with crypts but no villi, so that the surface is flat. The mucosa is full of goblet cells. A variety of cells, mainly lymphocytes and macrophages, are found in the lamina propria.

The blood supply to the colon is from the superior and inferior mesenteric vessels. Generally there are good anastomotic channels, but the caecum and splenic flexure are areas where ischaemia can occur. The colon is innervated mainly by the enteric nervous system with input from the parasympathetic and sympathetic pathways. Spinal afferent neurones from the dorsal root ganglia innervate the entire colon.

The rectum is about 12 cm long. Its interior is divided by three crescentic circular muscles producing shelf-like folds. These are the rectal valves that can be seen at sigmoidoscopy. The anal canal has an internal and an external sphincter.

Physiology of the colon

The main roles of the colon are the absorption of water and electrolytes (Table 6.12) and the propulsion of contents from the caecum to the anorectal region. Approximately 1.5–2 L of fluid pass the ileocaecal valve each day. Absorption is stimulated by short-chain fatty acids which are produced predominantly in the right colon by the anaerobic metabolism of dietary fibre by bacterial polysaccharidase enzyme systems. Colonic contents are mixed, aiding absorption by non-propagative segmenting muscular contractions. High-amplitude propagative colonic contractions cause propulsion. Peristalsis is induced by the release of serotonin (5-HT) from neuroendocrine cells in response to luminal distension. Serotonin activates the HT_4 receptors, which in turn results in the activation of sensory (calcitonin gene-related peptide (CGRP)) neurones. Normal colonic transit time is 24–48 h with normal stool weights of up to 250 g/day.

Physiology of defecation

The role of the rectum and anus in defecation is complex. The rectum is normally empty. Stool is propelled into the rectum by propagated colonic contractions. Sensation of fullness, a desire to defecate and urgency to defecate are experienced with increasing volumes of rectal content (threshold 100 mL). The sensations are associated with rectal contraction and a relaxation of the internal anal sphincter, both of which serve to push the stool down into the proximal anal canal. This increases the defecatory urge, which can only be suppressed by vigorous contraction of the external sphincter and puborectalis. If conditions are appropriate for defecation the subject sits or squats, contracts the diaphragm and abdominal muscles and relaxes the pelvic floor muscles, including the puborectalis, and the anal sphincter muscles.

CONSTIPATION

'Constipation' is a very common symptom, particularly in women and the elderly. It is often more of a perception than a real entity. A consensus definition used in research (The Rome II criteria) defines constipation as having two or more of the following for at least 12 weeks: infrequent passage of stools (< 3/week), straining > 25% of time, passage of hard stools, incomplete evacuation and sensation of anorectal blockage. According to these definitions 'constipation' affects more than 1 in 5 of the population.

Many symptoms are attributed by patients to constipation and include headaches, malaise, nausea and a bad taste in the mouth. Other symptoms include abdominal bloating and/or discomfort (undistinguishable from the irritable bowel syndrome) as well as local and perianal pain. The causes of constipation are shown in Table 6.13.

Assessment of constipation

This relies on the history. When there has been a recent change in bowel habit in association with other symptoms (e.g. rectal bleeding) a barium enema or colonoscopy is indicated. A barium enema should always be preceded by a rectal examination and rigid sigmoidoscopy to exclude anorectal lesions that can otherwise be missed. By these means, gastrointestinal causes such as colorectal cancer and narrowed segments due to diverticular disease (Table 6.13) can be excluded.

Constipation can be classified into three broad categories but there is much overlap:

- normal transit through the colon (59%)
- defecatory disorders (25%)
- slow transit (13%).

Defecatory disorders with slow transit can occur together (3%).

Normal-transit constipation

In normal-transit constipation, stool traverses the colon at a normal rate, the stool frequency is normal and yet patients believe they are constipated. This is likely to be

Table 6.12 Input and output of water and electrolytes in the gastrointestinal tract over 24 hours			
	Water (mL)	Sodium (mmol)	Potassium (mmol)
Input			
Diet	1500	150	80
GI secretions	7500	1000	40
Totals	9000	1150	120
Output			
Faeces	150	5	12
Ileostomy (adapted)	500–1000	60–120	4

Table 6.13 Causes of constipation

General
Pregnancy
Inadequate fibre intake
Immobility

Metabolic/endocrine
Diabetes mellitus
Hypercalcaemia
Hypothyroidism
Porphyria

Functional
Irritable bowel syndrome
Idiopathic slow transit

Drugs
Opiates
Antimuscarinics
Calcium-channel blockers, e.g. verapamil
Antidepressants, e.g. tricyclics
Iron

Neurological
Spinal cord lesions
Parkinson's disease

Psychological
Depression
Anorexia nervosa
Repressed urge to defecate

Gastrointestinal disease
Intestinal obstruction and pseudo-obstruction
Colonic disease, e.g. carcinoma, diverticular disease
Aganglionosis, e.g. Hirschprung's disease, Chagas' disease
Painful anal conditions, e.g. anal fissure

Defecatory disorders
Rectal prolapse, mucosal prolapse intussusception and
    solitary rectal ulcer syndrome
Large rectocele
Pelvic floor dyssynergia/anismus
Megarectum

Fig. 6.33 **Slow-transit constipation.** Straight abdominal X-ray taken on day 6 after ingestion of capsules each containing 20 radio-opaque shapes, which were administered daily on days 1, 2 and 3. All the markers are retained, confirming the diagnosis of severe slow-transit constipation.

due to perceived difficulties of evacuation or the passage of hard stools. Patients may complain of abdominal pain or bloating.

Normal-transit constipation can be distinguished from slow-transit constipation by undertaking marker studies of colonic transit. Capsules containing 21 radio-opaque shapes are swallowed on days 1, 2 and 3 and an abdominal X-ray obtained 120 hours after ingestion of the first capsule. Each capsule contains shapes of different configuration and the presence of more than 4 shapes from the first capsule, 6 from the second and 12 from the third denotes moderate to severe slow transit (Fig. 6.33).

Slow-transit constipation

Slow-transit constipation occurs predominantly in young women who have infrequent bowel movements (usually less than once a week). The condition often starts at puberty and the symptoms are usually an infrequent urge to defecate, bloating, abdominal pain and discomfort, which can make the condition difficult to distinguish from constipation-predominant irritable bowel syndrome. Some patients with severe slow-transit constipation have delayed emptying of the proximal colon and others a failure of 'meal-stimulated' colonic motility. Histopathological abnormalities have been demonstrated in the colons of some patients with severe slow-transit constipation, and some patients have coexisting disorders of small intestinal motility, consistent with a diagnosis of chronic idiopathic intestinal pseudo-obstruction (p. 343).

Defecatory disorders

A 'paradoxical' contraction rather than the normal relaxation of the puborectalis and external anal sphincter and associated muscles during straining may prevent evacuation (pelvic floor dyssynergia, anismus). These are mainly due to dysfunction of the anal sphincter and pelvic floor. An anterior rectocele is a common problem where there is a weakness of the rectovaginal septum, resulting in protuberance of the anterior wall of the rectum with trapping of stool if the diameter is > 3 cm. In some patients the mucosa of the anterior rectal wall prolapses downwards during straining (see p. 326)

Fig. 6.34 **Evacuating proctogram** showing the presence of an anterior rectocele (arrowed).

 Box 6.12 Laxatives and enemas

Bulking-forming laxatives
Dietary fibre
Wheat bran
Methylcellulose
Mucilaginous gums – sterculia
Mucilaginous seeds and seed coats, e.g. ispaghula husk

Stimulant laxatives (stimulate motility and intestinal secretion)
Phenolphthalein
Bisacodyl
Anthraquinones – senna and dantron (only for the terminally ill)
Docusate sodium

Osmotic laxatives
Magnesium sulphate
Lactulose
Macrogols

Suppositories
Bisacodyl
Glycerol

Enemas
Arachis oil
Docusate sodium
Hypertonic phosphate
Sodium citrate

impeding the passage of stool, whilst in others there may be a higher mucosal intussusception.

In some patients the rectum can become unduly sensitive to the presence of small volumes of stool, resulting in the urge to pass frequent amounts of small-volume stool and the sensation of incomplete evacuation..

The defecatory disorders can often be characterized by performing evacuation proctography (Fig. 6.34) and tests of anorectal physiology.

Treatment

Any underlying cause should be treated. In patients with normal and slow-transit constipation the main focus should be directed to increasing the fibre content of the diet in conjunction with increasing fluid intake. Fibre intake should be increased by dietary means rather than by prescribing commercially available fibre sources in order to avoid substrate inducibility of colonic bacterial polysaccharidase enzyme systems. These patients should therefore be referred to a dietitian.

The use of laxatives should be restricted to severe cases. Types of laxatives available are listed in Box 6.12. Osmotic laxatives act by increasing colonic inflow of fluid and electrolytes; this acts not only to soften the stool but to stimulate colonic contractility. Magnesium sulphate 5–10 g dissolved in a glass of hot water should be taken before breakfast; it works in 2–4 hours. The polyethylene glycols (Macrogols) have the advantage over the synthetic disaccharide lactulose in that they are not fermented anaerobically in the colon to gas which can distend the colon to cause pain. The osmotic laxatives are preferred to the stimulatory laxatives, which act by stimulating colonic contractility and by causing intestinal secretion. The use of irritant suppositories can be helpful in some patients with defecatory disorders. The use of enemas should be restricted to the management of elderly, infirm and immobile patients and those with neurological disorders.

Patients with defecatory disorders should be referred to a specialist centre as surgery may be indicated for, for example, anterior rectocele or internal anal mucosal intussusception. Anterior mucosal prolapse can be treated by injection, and those with pelvic floor dyssynergia (anismus) can benefit from biofeedback therapy.

FURTHER READING
Lembo A, Camilleri M (2003) Chronic constipation. *New England Journal of Medicine* **349**: 1360–1368.
Maddoff RD et al. (2004) Faecal incontinence in adults. *Lancet* **364**: 621–632.

MISCELLANEOUS COLONIC CONDITIONS

Megacolon

The term 'megacolon' is used to describe a number of congenital and acquired conditions in which the colon is dilated. In many instances it is secondary to chronic constipation and in some parts of the world Chagas' disease is a common cause.

All young patients with megacolon should have Hirschsprung's disease excluded. In this disease, which presents in the first years of life, an aganglionic segment of the rectum (megarectum) gives rise to constipation and subacute obstruction. Occasionally Hirschsprung's disease affecting only a short segment of the rectum can be missed in childhood. A preliminary rectal biopsy is performed and stained with special stains for ganglion cells in the submucosal plexus. In doubtful cases full-thickness biopsy, under anaesthesia, should be obtained.

A frozen section is stained for acetylcholinesterase, which is elevated in Hirschsprung's disease. Manometric studies show failure of relaxation of the internal sphincter, which is diagnostic of Hirschsprung's disease. This disease can be successfully treated surgically.

Treatment of other causes of a megacolon is similar to that of slow-transit constipation, but saline washouts and manual removal of faeces are sometimes required.

Faecal incontinence

Seven per cent of the healthy population over the age of 65 experience incontinence at least weekly. Incontinence occurs when the intrarectal pressure exceeds the intra-anal pressure and is classified as minor (inability to control flatus or liquid stool, causing soiling) or major (frequent and inadvertent evacuation of stool of normal consistency). The common causes of incontinence are shown in Table 6.14. Obstetric injury is a common cause and sphincter defects have been found in up to 30% of primiparous women. A faecal incontinence rate of over 25% has been described and this gets more severe with increasing age. Endoanal ultrasonography with enhancing per vaginal views is the investigation of choice in the assessment of anal sphincter damage (Fig. 6.35). Neurophysiological investigation of pudendal nerve function, anal sensation and anal sphincter function may be required to elicit the cause of the problem. In the future static and dynamic pelvic magnetic resonance imaging may become the investigation of choice in faecal incontinence.

Initial management of minor incontinence is bowel habit regulation. Loperamide is the most potent antidiarrhoeal agent which also increases internal sphincter tone.

Biofeedback is effective in some patients with faecal incontinence associated with impaired function of the puborectalis muscle and the external anal sphincter. Sacral spinal nerve stimulation has been shown to be effective in the treatment of patients with a functionally deficient but morphologically intact external anal sphincter.

Surgery may be required for anal sphincter trauma and should be carried out in specialist centres.

Ischaemic disease of the colon (ischaemic colitis)

Occlusion of branches of the superior mesenteric (SMA) or inferior mesenteric arteries (IMA), often in the older age group, commonly presents with sudden onset of abdominal pain and the passage of bright red blood per rectum, with or without diarrhoea. There may be signs of shock and evidence of underlying cardiovascular disease. The majority of cases affect the splenic flexure and left colon. This condition has also been described in women taking the contraceptive pill and in patients with thrombophilia (p. 477) and small- or medium-vessel vasculitis (p. 581).

On examination the abdomen is distended and tender. A straight abdominal X-ray often shows thumb-printing

Table 6.14 Aetiology of faecal incontinence

Congenital
e.g. imperforate anus

Anal sphincter dysfunction
Structural damage:
Surgery – anorectal, vaginal hysterectomy
Obstetric injury during childbirth
Trauma
Radiation
Perianal Crohn's disease
Pudendal nerve damage:
Childbirth
Perineal descent:
Prolonged straining at stool

Rectal prolapse

Faecal impaction with overflow diarrhoea

Severe diarrhoea
e.g. ulcerative colitis

Neurological and psychological disorders
Spinal trauma (S2–S4)
Spina bifida
Stroke
Multiple sclerosis
Diabetes mellitus (with autonomic involvement)
Dementia
Psychological illness
Irritable bowel syndrome

Fig. 6.35 Endoanal ultrasound scan, axial mid canal image, showing a large tear between 10 and 1 o'clock (arrows) following vaginal delivery, involving the external (EAS) and internal anal sphincters (IAS) and resulting in faecal incontinence. Courtesy of Professor Clive Bartram, Princess Grace Hospital, London.

(a characteristic sign of ischaemic disease) at the site of the splenic flexure.

The differential diagnosis is of other causes of acute colitis. A rigid sigmoidoscopy (normal mucosal appearances often with presence of blood) and a gentle instant enema is preferred to colonoscopy (to avoid perforation) in cases where the diagnosis is in doubt. A barium enema should be performed when the patient recovers, to exclude the formation of a stricture at the site of disease. Patients without evidence of underlying cardiovascular disease should be screened for thrombophilia and vasculitis.

Treatment

Most patients settle on symptomatic treatment. A few develop gangrene and perforation and require urgent surgery.

Pneumatosis cystoides intestinalis

This is a rare condition in which multiple gas-filled cysts are found in the submucosa of the intestine, chiefly the colon. The cause is unknown but some cases are associated with chronic obstructive pulmonary disease. Patients are usually asymptomatic, but abdominal pain and diarrhoea do occur and occasionally the cysts rupture to produce a pneumoperitoneum. This condition is diagnosed on X-ray of the abdomen, barium enema or sigmoidoscopy when cysts are seen.

Treatment is often unnecessary but continuous oxygen therapy will help to disperse the largely nitrogen-containing cysts. Metronidazole may help.

DIVERTICULAR DISEASE

Diverticula are frequently found in the colon and occur in 50% of patients over the age of 50 years. They are most frequent in the sigmoid, but can be present over the whole colon.

The term *diverticulosis* indicates the presence of diverticula; *diverticulitis* implies that these diverticula are inflamed. It is perhaps better to use the more general term *diverticular disease*, as it is often difficult to be sure whether the diverticula are inflamed. The precise mechanism of diverticula formation is not known. There is thickening of the muscle layer and, because of high intraluminal pressures, pouches of mucosa extrude through the muscular wall through weakened areas near blood vessels to form diverticula. An alternative explanation is cholinergic denervation with increasing age which leads to hypersensitivity and increased un-coordinated muscular contraction. Diverticular disease seems to be related to the low-fibre diet eaten in developed countries.

Diverticulitis occurs when faeces obstruct the neck of the diverticulum causing stagnation and allowing bacteria to multiply and produce inflammation. This can then lead to bowel perforation (peridiverticulitis), abscess formation, fistulae into adjacent organs, or even generalized peritonitis.

Clinical features and management

Diverticular disease is asymptomatic in 95% of cases and is usually discovered incidentally on a barium enema examination. No treatment other than dietary advice is required in those patients. In symptomatic patients intermittent left iliac fossa pain or discomfort and an erratic bowel habit commonly occur. In severe disease luminal narrowing can occur in the sigmoid colon, giving rise to severer pain and constipation. In the absence of clinical signs of acute diverticulitis a barium enema is the investigation of choice (Fig. 6.36), combined with an abdominal ultrasound scan to assess bowel wall thickness and to exclude paracolic inflammatory disease. Technically it is sometimes difficult to obtain adequate views of the sigmoid region in diverticular disease and if this is the case a fibreoptic sigmoidoscopy may be required. Treatment of uncomplicated symptomatic disease is with a well-balanced (*soluble* and *insoluble*, see p. 234) fibre diet (20 g/day) with smooth muscle relaxants if required.

Acute diverticulitis

This most commonly affects diverticula in the sigmoid colon. It presents with severe pain in the left iliac fossa, often accompanied by fever and constipation. These symptoms and signs are similar to appendicitis but on the left side. On examination the patient is often febrile with a tachycardia. Abdominal examination shows tenderness, guarding and rigidity on the left side of the abdomen. A palpable tender mass is sometimes felt in the left iliac fossa.

Investigations

- **Blood tests**. A polymorphonuclear leucocytosis is often present. The ESR and CRP are raised.
- **Spiral CT of the lower abdomen** (Fig. 6.37) will show colonic wall thickening, diverticula and often pericolic collections and abscesses. There is usually a streaky increased density extending into the immediate pericolic fat with thickening of the pelvic fascial planes. These findings are diagnostic of acute diverticulitis and differ from those of malignant disease.

Ultrasound examination is often more readily available and is cheaper. It can demonstrate thickened bowel and large pericolic collections, but is less sensitive than CT.

Treatment

Acute attacks can be treated on an outpatient basis using a cephalosporin and metronidazole. Patients who are more ill will require admission for bowel rest, intravenous fluids and antibiotic therapy (e.g. gentamicin, or a cephalosporin) and metronidazole.

Complications of diverticular disease

- Perforation, which usually, but not always, occurs in association with acute diverticulitis, can lead to formation of a paracolic or pelvic abscess or generalized peritonitis. Surgery is usually required.

(a)

(b)

Fig. 6.36 **Diverticular disease. (a) Double-contrast enema showing diverticular (arrows).** The barium is black on these films. **(b) Diverticula (arrows) seen on colonoscopy.**

- Fistula formation into the bladder, causing dysuria or pneumaturia, or into the vagina, causing discharge.
- Intestinal obstruction (see p. 343) usually after repeated episodes of acute diverticulitis.
- Bleeding, which is sometimes massive. In most cases the bleeding stops and the cause of the bleeding can be established by colonoscopy and sometimes angiography. In rare cases emergency segmental colectomy is required.
- Mucosal inflammation in areas of diverticula occurs, giving the appearance of a segmental colitis at endoscopy.

FURTHER READING
Golder M et al. (2003) Smooth muscle cholinergic denervation hypersensitivity in diverticular disease. *Lancet* **361**: 1945–1951.
Stouman N (2004) Diverticular disease. *Lancet* **363**: 631–639.

ANORECTAL DISORDERS

Pruritus ani

Pruritus ani, or an itchy bottom, is common. Perianal excoriation results from scratching. Usually the condition results from seepage from haemorrhoids or overactivity of sweat glands. Treatment consists of salt baths, keeping the area dry with powder; the use of all creams should be avoided. Secondary causes include threadworm (*Enterobius vermicularis*) infestation, fungal infections (e.g.

Fig. 6.37 **Spiral CT of lower abdomen, showing acute diverticulitis** (arrow). The bowel wall is thickened and there is loss of clarity of the pericolic fat. A narrow segment of bowel is seen to the left of the diseased segment.

candidiasis) and perianal eczema, which should be treated appropriately.

Haemorrhoids

Haemorrhoids (primary, internal, second degree, prolapsing, third degree prolapsed) usually cause rectal bleeding, discomfort and pruritus ani. Patients may notice red blood on their toilet paper and blood on the outside of their stools. They are the most common cause of rectal bleeding (see Fig. 6.19). *Diagnosis* is made by inspection, rectal examination and proctoscopy. If symptoms are minor no treatment is required; depending on severity of symptoms, treatment is with injection of sclerosant, rubber band ligation or surgery.

Anal fissures

An anal fissure is a tear in the sensitive skin-lined lower anal canal distal to the dentate line which produces pain on defecation. It can be an isolated primary problem in young to middle-aged adults or occur in association with Crohn's disease or ulcerative colitis, in which case perianal abscesses and anal fistulae can complicate the fissure. Diagnosis can usually be made on the history alone and the fissures can be seen usually posteriorly. Rectal examination is often not possible because of pain and sphincter spasm. The spasm not only causes pain but impairs wound healing. In severe cases proctoscopy and sigmoidoscopy should be performed under anaesthesia to exclude other anorectal disease. Initial treatment is with local anaesthetic gel and stool softeners. Use of 0.2% glyceryl trinitrate and 2% diltiazem ointments are of benefit. Botulinum toxin is used in chronic fissures but lateral subcutaneous internal sphincterotomy may be required in severe cases.

Fistula in ano

Subcutaneous, low and high anal fistulae are the commonest types (Fig. 6.38). Anorectal fistulae are rarer forms. The fistulae usually present as abscesses and heal after the abscess is incised. In other cases a small discharging sinus may be noted by the patient. Endoanal ultrasonography magnetic resonance and/or examination under anaesthetic is usually required to define the primary and any secondary tracks and detect any associated disease. Management is usually surgical with approximately 90% of fistulae being laid open or excised.

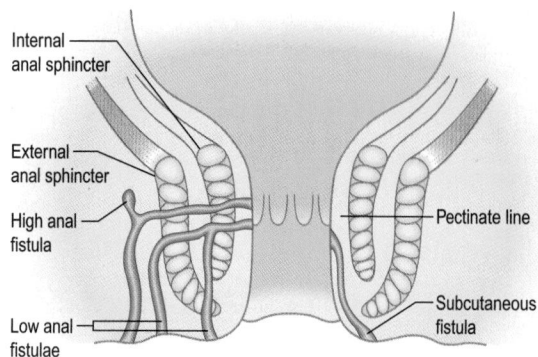

Fig. 6.38 **Common sites of anal fistulae. Note** subcutaneous fistulae do not traverse the sphincters, whereas low and high fistulae do.

Anorectal abscesses

Anorectal abscesses are a common cause of admission to hospital. They are two to three times commoner in men, particularly in homosexual men who indulge in penetrative anal sex. They may be the first manifestation of Crohn's disease, ulcerative colitis and tuberculosis. Perianal and ischiorectal abscess, the commonest forms, present with painful, tender swellings and discharge. Examination under anaesthetic, MRI and endoanal ultrasound are used for evaluation. Treatment is with surgical incision and drainage with antibiotics.

Rectal prolapse, intussusception and solitary rectal ulcer syndrome (SRUS)

All these conditions are thought to be related, with rectal prolapse being the unifying pathology. Some patients with SRUS do not have prolapse but strain excessively and ulcerate the anterior rectal wall, which is forced into the anus during futile straining efforts.

Rectal prolapse starts as an intussusception of the upper rectum which passes into the lower part of the viscus, and progression results in its protrusion through the anal canal to emerge as an external prolapse. Constipation and chronic straining are the likely causes. In addition, the presence of an intussuscepting rectum will mimic presence of stool in the rectum and lead to straining efforts to evacuate the prolapse. In some patients repeated straining leads to traumatic ulceration of the mucosa and formation of SRUS, commonly on the anterior wall of the rectum within 13 cm of the anal verge. Sometimes difficult to distinguish from cancer and Crohn's disease during endoscopic examination, SRUS has typical histological features of non-specific inflammatory changes with bands of smooth muscle extending into the lamina propria.

Patients commonly present with slight bleeding and mucus on defecation, tenesmus and sensation of anal obstruction. Asymptomatic SRUS should not be treated. Symptomatic patients should be advised to stop straining and measures taken to soften the stool. If rectal prolapse can be demonstrated during defecation, this should be repaired; in severe cases surgical treatment by resection rectopexy may be indicated. Surgical treatment for complete rectal prolapse is also required.

COLONIC TUMOURS

Colon polyps and polyposis syndromes

A polyp is an elevation above the mucosal surface. The majority of colorectal polyps are adenomas with malignant potential. Polyps range in size from a few millimetres to several centimetres in diameter. They may be single or multiple and in the polyposis syndromes hundreds may be found.

Larger polyps in the rectum and 70–80% of all polyps in the colon are adenomas, and 5% of these may contain invasive carcinoma at discovery. Most polyps are asymptomatic and found by chance when patients are investigated for pain, altered bowel habit, rectal bleeding or some other cause.

Table 6.15 Classification of colorectal polyps

Type of polyp	Pathogenesis	Polyposis syndrome
Adenoma	Neoplastic	Familial adenomatous polyposis
Juvenile	Hamartoma	Juvenile polyposis
Peutz–Jeghers	Hamartoma	Peutz–Jeghers syndrome
Metaplastic	Unknown	Metaplastic polyposis
Lymphoid	Hyperplasia	Lymphoid polyposis
Inflammatory	Inflammation	Inflammatory polyposis

Fig. 6.39 **Colonoscopic appearance of a large peduncular polyp.** Courtesy of Dr PD Fairclough.

Classification of colorectal polyps (Table 6.15)

Non-neoplastic polyps

Hamartomatous polyps are commonly large and stalked.

Juvenile polyps (occurring in children and teenagers) are confined mainly to the colon and histologically show mucus retention cysts. *Juvenile polyposis* (more than 10 colonic polyps) is inherited in an autosomal dominant fashion and the relevant gene has been identified (Box 6.13). The polyps are a cause of bleeding and intussusception in the first decade of life. There is also an increased risk of colonic cancer, and surveillance and removal of polyps must be undertaken.

Peutz–Jeghers syndrome is considered on page 309.

Cowden syndrome is an autosomal dominant disease associated with skin stigmata and intestinal polyps regarded as hamartomas but with a mixture of cell types. These patients have an increased risk of various extra-intestinal malignancies (thyroid, breast, uterine and ovarian).

Metaplastic polyps. These are frequently found in the rectum and sigmoid colon. These pale, sessile mucosal nodules usually measure < 5 mm and are non-neoplastic lesions without significant malignant potential. *Metaplastic polyposis* is defined as the presence of more than 10 colonic metaplastic polyps. These phenotypes are rare but appear to exhibit an increased risk of colon cancer.

Neoplastic polyps

Posrt-mortem studies have shown the incidence of adenomas to be 30–40% in western populations, and most colorectal cancers develop from sporadic adenomatous polyps. Flat adenomas, which were first described in Japan, may be difficult to detect at endoscopy (see below).

Polyps rarely produce symptoms and most are diagnosed on X-ray or on colonoscopy performed for other reasons. Large polyps (Fig. 6.39) may bleed intermittently and cause anaemia. Large sessile villous adenomas of the rectum can present with profuse diarrhoea and hypokalaemia.

Several factors influence the risk of cancer developing in an adenoma (see Box 6.14). Flat adenomas were thought to account for 10% of all adenomas but using dye spraying and extra magnification at colonoscopy, many more are being detected. The natural history is unclear but some of these flat lesions show malignant progression without any polyp formation. This increases the problem of surveillance and screening.

Once a polyp has been found it is usually possible to remove it endoscopically. The National Polyp Study conducted in the USA showed that colonoscopic polypectomy with surveillance reduced colorectal cancer incidence by 76–90%. Recent guidelines recommend a surveillance colonoscopy following polypectomy at 3 years in patients with 1–3 polyps > 1 cm. Screening at 1 year is recommended for more than 4 polyps and 5 years for small polyps < 1 cm. If any doubt exists about

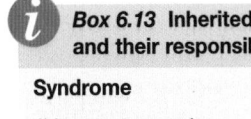

Box 6.13 Inherited syndromes of colonic polyps and their responsible genes

Syndrome	Responsible gene
Adenomatous polyps	
FAP	*APC*
Attenuated FAP	*APC (MUTYH)*
HNPCC	*MMR*
Hamartomatous polyps	
Peutz–Jeghers syndrome	*STK11 (LKB1)*
Juvenile polyposis	*SMAD4/DPC4*
Cowden syndrome	*PTEN*

Box 6.14 Factors affecting risk of malignant change in an adenoma

	Higher risk	Lower risk
Size	> 1.5 cm	< 1 cm
Type	Sessile or flat	Pedunculated
Histology	Severe dysplasia	Mild dysplasia
	Villous architecture	Tubular architecture
	Squamous metaplasia	
Number	Multiple polyps	Single polyp

the excision margins of any polyp then an earlier repeat examination is suggested.

Familial adenomatous polyposis (FAP) arises from germline mutations of the *APC* gene located on chromosome 5q and is inherited in an autosomal dominant fashion. The disease is characterized by the presence of hundreds to thousands of colorectal adenomas. The mean age of adenoma development is 16 years, whereas the average age for developing colorectal cancer is 39 years. Tracing and screening of relatives is essential (usually after 12 years of age) and affected individuals should be offered a prophylactic colectomy, often before the age of 20. Surgical options include colectomy and ileorectal anastomosis, which requires life-long surveillance of the rectal stump or a restorative proctocolectomy or pouch procedure.

Attenuated FAP may be missed as it presents in later life (44 years average age) and has fewer polyps (< 100), which tend to occur more on the right side of the colon than on the left; it may be indistinguishable from sporadic cases but the gene mutation is in the *APC* germ line. A recessive form of FAP has recently been described due to a mutation in the MutY homologue (*MUTYH*) gene in a patient with multiple colonic adenomas.

Gastric fundic gland polyps and duodenal adenomas are frequently found in FAP, as well as other extra-intestinal lesions such as osteomas, epidermoid cysts and desmoid tumours. *Congenital hypertrophy of the retinal pigment epithelium* (CHRPE) occurs in many families with FAP. Other cancers that are observed in FAP include thyroid, pancreatic and hepatoblastomas.

APC gene mutations can be found on screening in about 80% of families with FAP. Once the disease-causing mutation has been identified in an index case known to have FAP, other family members can be tested for the mutation and screening can then be directed at mutation carriers. If a mutation cannot be found in a known FAP case, then all family members should undergo clinical screening with regular endoscopy.

Colorectal carcinoma

Colorectal cancer (CRC) is the second most common cause of cancer death in the UK. Each year over 30 000 new cases are diagnosed in England and Wales (68% colon, 32% rectal cancer) and it is registered as the underlying cause of death in about half this number. The prevalence rate per 100 000 (all ages) is 53.5 for men and 36.7 for women. The incidence increases with age, the average age at diagnosis being 60–65 years. The disease is much more common in westernized countries than in Asia or Africa.

Increased risk:

- Western diets are low in dietary fibre which increase faecal bulk and reduce transit time.
- Fat and meat consumption correlates with risk of CRC.

Decreased risk:

- Fruit and vegetables consumption has a protective effect.
- Increase fibre intake in the diet.

- Exercise reduces the risk of CRC.
- Aspirin and other NSAIDs reduce the risk of developing both adenomas and cancers.
- Hormone-replacement therapy (combined oestrogen and progesterone) may reduce the risk of colorectal cancer.

Genetics

Most colorectal cancers develop as a result of a stepwise progression from normal mucosa to adenoma to invasive cancer. This progression is controlled by the accumulation of alterations or mutations in a number of critical growth-regulating genes. Germline mutations of the *APC* gene are responsible for FAP (see above), but inactivation of this tumour suppressor gene and β-catenin (a transcription activator) is also seen in up to 70% of sporadic colorectal cancers. A cytoplasmic complex consisting of the APC protein, β-catenin, connexon/axin and glycogen synthase kinase-3β (GSK-3β) ensures the tight control of β-catenin. GSK-3β is a serine–threonine kinase which destroys β-catenin. Other factors which regulate β-catenin include cyclin D_1, gastrin and peroxisome, proliferator-activated receptor β (PPARβ) which mediates transcription of prostaglandins and fatty acids. Inactivation of *APC* appears to occur at an early stage in the development of an adenoma, which has led to it being described as a 'gatekeeper' gene. The sequence is usually followed by K-*ras* mutations which appear to facilitate the growth of adenomatous tissue and then by *DCC* (deleted in colon cancer) and *p53* gene mutations which occur around the adenoma–carcinoma transition (Fig. 6.40). The exact order of these mutations may vary. Around 15% of sporadic colorectal cancers appear to follow a different pathway. In these there are insertions or deletions of nucleotides within repeated sequences of DNA – microsatellite instability (MSI) due to defective repair of mismatched nucleotides. Sporadic tumours with MSI tend to occur on the right side of the colon, have greater lymphocytic infiltration and are often poorly differentiated. MSI seems to be associated with increased survival. Revised Bethesda guidelines for patients who should be tested for MSI are available.

Cancer families

A family history of colon cancer confers an increased risk to relatives. Family history is, next to age, the most common risk factor for colon cancer. FAP (Fig. 6.41) is the best-recognized syndrome predisposing to colorectal cancer but represents less than 1% of all colorectal cancers. *Hereditary non-polyposis colorectal cancer* (HNPCC) arises from germline mutations in any one of five mismatch repair (MMR) genes. Mutations in two of these, *hMLH1* and *hMSH2*, account for > 95% of HNPCC families. Mutations in these genes lead to genomic instability in the tumours of affected individuals. Other cancers frequently occur in HNPCC, including endometrial, gastric, biliary tract, urinary tract, ovarian and small bowel malignancies. Diagnostic criteria, based on family history, were devised to help identify those affected and have subsequently been modified to include non-colonic tumours (Box 6.15).

Fig. 6.40 **Genetic model for colorectal tumorigenesis, showing the progression from adenoma to carcinoma.** The stages are shown at which mutations occur in the genes: *APC* (adenomatous polyposis coli), K-*ras*, *DCC*, *p53*, *hMSH2*, and *hMLH1*.

Patients with HNPCC tend to develop right-sided cancers at an early age, and regular surveillance with colonoscopy is recommended.

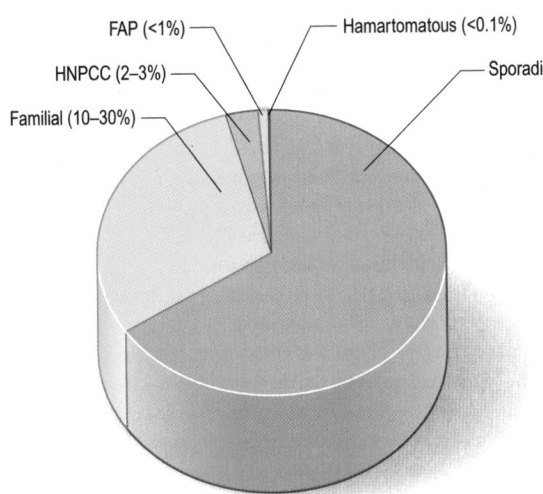

Fig. 6.41 **Percentages of colon cancer according to family risk.** HNPCC, hereditary non-polyposis colorectal cancer; FAP, familial adenomatous polyposis.

> ### Box 6.15 Modified Amsterdam Criteria for hereditary non-polyposis colorectal cancer
>
> - There are more cases of colorectal cancer in a minimum of two generations.
> - One affected individual must be a first-degree relative of the other two (or more) cases.
> - One case must be diagnosed at age < 50.
> - Colorectal cancer can be replaced by endometrial or small bowel cancer.
> - Familial adenomatous polyposis (FAP) should be excluded.
> - Tumours should be verified by pathological examination.

In addition to the above syndromes are some colon cancers that arise, at least in part, from an inherited predisposition, so-called *familial risk* (Table 6.16). Estimates of their frequency range from 10% to 30% of all CRC but the genes involved have yet to be identified. The risk of CRC can be estimated from a careful family history matched with empirical risk tables so that appropriate advice regarding screening can then be offered.

Most colorectal cancers are, however, sporadic and occur in individuals without a strong family history. Approximately half these familial cancers arise in the rectosigmoid area (Fig. 6.42) but there is evidence to suggest that there is an increase in right-sided tumours.

Pathology

CRC, which is usually a polypoid mass with ulceration, spreads by direct infiltration through the bowel wall. It involves lymphatics and blood vessels with subsequent spread, most commonly to the liver. Synchronous tumours are present in 2% of cases. *Histology* is adenocarcinoma with moderately to well differentiated glandular epithelium with mucin production. 'Signet ring' cells in which mucin displaces the nucleus to the side of the cell are characteristic.

Clinical features

Alteration in bowel habit, with or without abdominal pain, is a common symptom of left-sided colonic lesions.

Table 6.16 Lifetime risk of colorectal cancer in first-degree relatives of a patient with colorectal cancer

Population risk	1 in 50
One first-degree relative affected (any age)	1 in 17
One first-degree and one second-degree relative affected	1 in 12
One first-degree relative affected (age < 45)	1 in 10
Two first-degree relatives affected	1 in 6
Autosomal dominant pedigree	1 in 2

Houlston et al. (1990) *British Medical Journal* **301**: 366–368

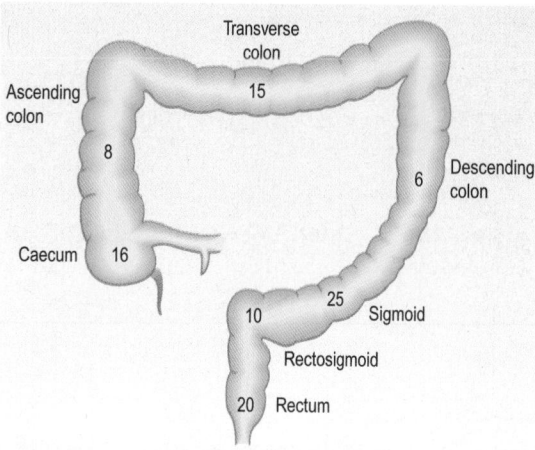

Fig. 6.42 **Distribution of sporadic colorectal cancer.** Only 60% are in the range of flexible sigmoidoscopy.

Fig. 6.43 **Colonoscopic appearance of a carcinoma in the ascending colon** – a large irregular ulcer. Courtesy of Dr PD Fairclough.

Rectal and sigmoid cancers often bleed, blood being mixed in with the stool. Cancers arising in the caecum and right colon are often asymptomatic and present as an iron deficiency anaemia. The elderly often present with intestinal obstruction.

Patients aged greater than 35–40 presenting with new large bowel symptoms should be investigated. *The alarm symptoms*, suggestive of colorectal cancer, include change in bowel habit, rectal bleeding, anorexia and weight loss, faecal incontinence, tenesmus and passing mucus per rectum.

Examination is usually unhelpful but a mass may be palpable. Hepatomegaly may be found with liver metastases. Digital examination of the rectum is essential and rigid sigmoidoscopy should be performed in all cases.

Investigations

- **Blood count and routine biochemistry**.
- **Serum carcinoembryonic antigen** level is related to outcome.
- **Colonoscopy** (Fig. 6.43) is the gold standard for investigation and allows biopsies and polypectomies to obtain specimens for histological examination.
- **Double-contrast barium enema** can visualize the large bowel but is now being superseded by CT pneumocolon.
- **Endoanal ultrasound and pelvic MRI** are used for staging rectal cancer.
- **CT and PET scanning** (p. 270) help to evaluate tumour size, local and secondary spread and hepatic metastases.

Faecal occult blood tests have been used for mass screening but are of no value in hospital practice.

Treatment

This should involve multidisciplinary teams working in designated centres. About 80% of patients with colorectal cancer undergo surgery, though fewer than half survive more than 5 years. The operative procedure depends on the cancer site and long-term survival relates to the stage of the primary tumour and the presence of metastatic disease (see Table 6.17). There has been a gradual move from using Dukes' classification to using the TNM classification system.

Long-term survival is only likely when the cancer is completely removed. Total mesorectal excision (TME) is an approach to rectal surgery in which meticulous care is taken to remove all the tissue surrounding the cancer. TME combined with preoperative chemo-radiotherapy reduces local recurrence rates in rectal cancer to less than 5% and improves survival. Radiotherapy for colonic cancers is not helpful because of difficulties delivering a sufficient dose without excess toxicity to the small bowel. Adjuvant postoperative chemotherapy will improve disease-free survival and overall survival in stage III (Dukes' C) colon cancer (p. 331). Those with Duke's B tumours with advanced features such as vascular invasion may also benefit.

Advanced colorectal cancer treatment is discussed on p. 521.

Follow-up

All patients who have surgery should have a colonoscopy performed before (or soon afterwards) to look for additional lesions. Patients with stage II or III disease should have serum carcinoembryonic antigen (CEA) measured every 3 months and colonoscopy every 3 years.

Prevention and screening

Healthcare agencies advocate a low-fat, high-fibre diet for the prevention of sporadic colorectal cancer, and endoscopic screening is a recommendation for high-risk patients with inherited syndromes (e.g. FAP, HNPCC). NSAIDs or aspirin may play a role in prevention. Faecal occult blood (FOB) tests have been studied as a screening test for

Table 6.17 Staging and survival of colorectal cancers

TNM classification			Modified Dukes' classification	5-Year survival (%)
Stage I (N0, M0)	Tumours invade submucosa	T1	A	80–95
	Tumours invade muscularis propria	T2		
Stage IIA (N0, M0)	Tumours invade into subserosa	T3	B	72–85
IIB	Tumours invade directly into other organs	T4		65–66
Stage III (M0)	T1, T2 + 1–3 regional lymph nodes involved	N1		55–65
IIIB	T3, T4 + 1–3 regional lymph nodes involved	N1	C	35–42
IIIC	Any T + 4 or more regional lymph nodes	N2		25–27
Stage IV	Any T, any N + distant metastases	M1	D	5–7

colorectal cancer. Several large randomized studies have demonstrated a reduction in cancer-related mortality of 15–33%. The disadvantage of screening with FOB is its relatively low sensitivity, which means many unnecessary colonoscopies. In a recent study of those who screened positive, 11.5% had cancer and 16.8% had large adenomas.

A once-only flexible sigmoidoscopy at 55–65 years has been shown to reduce overall CRC mortality by a third and is recommended in the USA. A multicentre trial of this strategy has been undertaken in the UK. Initial results suggest that such a screening regimen is acceptable, feasible and safe.

Colonoscopy is the gold-standard technique for the examination of the colon and rectum and is the investigation of choice for high-risk patients. Its expense, the need for full bowel preparation and sedation, and the small risk of perforation obviate its use as a population screening tool at present, though trials are underway in the USA. CT colonoscopy (or 'virtual colonoscopy') and the refinement of genetic testing may contribute to screening programmes. Universal screening strategies have been recommended in the USA. There are two large-scale pilot studies of FOB screening in the UK at present and it is anticipated that some form of colorectal screening will be introduced in the NHS in due course.

FURTHER READING

Atkins WS, Saunders BP (2002) Surveillance guidelines after removal of colorectal adenomatous polyps. *Gut* **51** (Suppl. 5): V6–9.

Giardiello FM, Brensinger JD (2001) AGA technical review of hereditary colorectal cancer and genetic testing. *Gastroenterology* **121**: 198–213.

Meyerhardt JA, Mayer RJ (2005) Systemic therapy for colorectal cancer. *New England Journal of Medicine* **352**: 476–487.

Schoenfield MD et al (2005) Colonoscopic screening for average risk women for colorectal neoplasia. *New England Journal of Medicine* **352**: 2061–2068.

Weitz J, Koch M, Debus J et al (2005) Colorectal cancer. *Lancet* **365**: 153–165.

Winawer S (2003) Colorectal cancer: screening and surveillance. *Gastroenterology* **124**: 544–560.

DIARRHOEA

Diarrhoea is a common clinical problem and there is no uniformly accepted definition of diarrhoea. Organic causes (stool weights > 250 g per day) have to be distinguished from 'functional causes', and is the first step in the assessment of the history. Sudden onset of bowel frequency associated with crampy abdominal pains, and a fever will point to an infective cause; bowel frequency with loose blood-stained stools to an inflammatory basis; and the passage of pale offensive stools that float, often accompanied by loss of appetite and weight loss, to steatorrhoea. Nocturnal bowel frequency and urgency usually point to an organic cause. Passage of frequent small-volume stools (often formed) points to a functional cause (see Functional gastrointestinal disorders, p. 335).

Mechanisms
Osmotic diarrhoea

The gut mucosa acts as a semipermeable membrane and fluid enters the bowel if there are large quantities of non-absorbed hypertonic substances in the lumen. This occurs because:

- the patient has ingested a non-absorbable substance (e.g. a purgative such as magnesium sulphate or magnesium-containing antacid)
- the patient has generalized malabsorption so that high concentrations of solute (e.g. glucose) remain in the lumen
- the patient has a specific absorptive defect (e.g. disaccharidase deficiency or glucose–galactose malabsorption).

The volume of diarrhoea produced by these mechanisms is reduced by the absorption of fluid by the ileum and colon. The diarrhoea stops when the patient stops eating or the malabsorptive substance is discontinued.

Secretory diarrhoea

In this disorder, there is both active intestinal secretion of fluid and electrolytes as well as decreased absorption. The mechanism of intestinal secretion is shown in Figure 6.44a.

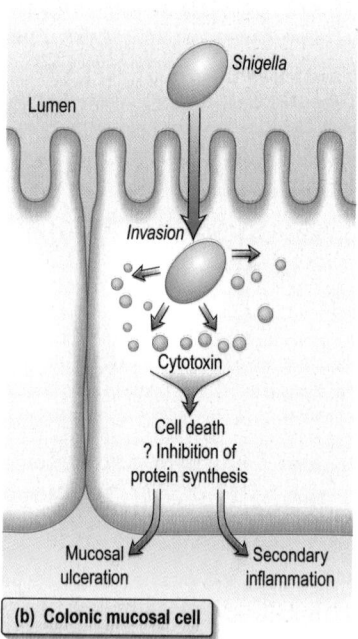

Fig. 6.44 Mechanisms of diarrhoea.
(a) Small intestinal secretion of water and electrolytes.

- *Cholera toxin* binds to its receptor (monosialoganglioside G_i) via fimbria (toxin co-regulated pilus) on its β subunit. This activates the α_s subunit (of the G_s protein), which in turn dissociates and activates cyclic AMP (cAMP). The increase in cAMP activates intermediates (e.g. protein kinase and Ca^{2+}) which then act on the apical membrane causing Cl^- secretion (with water) and inhibition of Na^+ and Cl^- absorption.
- *E. coli*. Heat-labile *E. coli* enterotoxin shares a receptor with cholera toxin. Heat-stable (HS) *E. coli* toxin binds to its own receptor and activates guanylate cyclase (cGMP), producing the same effect on secretion.
- *C. difficile* activates the protein kinases via Ca^{2+}/calmodulin (Ca^{2+}/CM).
- *Zona occludens toxin*. This toxin is the product of the *ZOT* gene, which is the gene required for the *CTX* gene which encodes for cholera toxin. It has enterotoxic activity, producing secretion.

Cholera and *E. coli* cause these effects without invasion of the cell.
G, G protein consisting of subunits α, β, γ; i, inhibitory; s, stimulatory; ATP, adenosine triphosphate; GTP, guanosine triphosphate; GMP, guanosine monophosphate; GC, guanyl cyclase; PKC, protein kinase C; VIP, vasoactive intestinal polypeptide.
(b) Colonic mucosal cell. This demonstrates one of the mechanisms by which an invasive pathogen (e.g. *Shigella*) acts. Following penetration, the pathogens generate cytotoxins which lead to mucosal ulceration and cell death.

Common causes of secretory diarrhoea are:

- enterotoxins (e.g. cholera, *E. coli* – thermolabile or thermostable toxin)
- hormones (e.g. vasoactive intestinal peptide in the Verner–Morrison syndrome, p. 416)
- bile salts (in the colon) following ileal resection
- fatty acids (in the colon) following ileal resection
- some laxatives (e.g. docusate sodium).

Inflammatory diarrhoea (mucosal destruction)

Diarrhoea occurs because of damage to the intestinal mucosal cell so that there is a loss of fluid and blood (Fig. 6.44b). In addition, there is defective absorption of fluid and electrolytes. Common causes are infective conditions (e.g. dysentery due to *Shigella*), and inflammatory conditions (e.g. ulcerative colitis and Crohn's disease).

Abnormal motility

Diabetic, post-vagotomy and hyperthyroid diarrhoea are all due to abnormal motility of the upper gut. In many of these cases the volume and weight of the stool is not all that high, but frequency of defecation occurs; this therefore is not true diarrhoea.

Causes of diarrhoea are shown in Table 6.18. It should be noted that the irritable bowel syndrome, colorectal cancer, diverticular disease and faecal impaction with overflow in the elderly do not cause 'true' organic diarrhoea (i.e. > 250 g/day), even though the patients may complain of diarrhoea. World-wide, infection and infestation are a major problem and these are discussed under the causative organisms in Chapter 2.

Acute diarrhoea (excluding cholera, discussed on p. 67)

Diarrhoea of sudden onset is very common, often short-lived and requires no investigation or treatment. This type of diarrhoea is seen after dietary indiscretions, but diarrhoea due to viral agents also lasts 24–48 hours (see p. 51). The causes of other infective diarrhoeas are shown on page 61. Travellers' diarrhoea, which affects people travelling outside their own countries, particularly to developing countries, usually lasts 2–5 days; it is discussed on page 70. Clinical features associated with the acute diarrhoeas include fever, abdominal pain and vomiting. If the diarrhoea is particularly severe, dehydration can be a problem; the very young and very old are at special risk from this. Investigations are necessary if the diarrhoea has lasted more than 1 week. Stools (up to three) should be sent immediately to the laboratory for culture and examination for ova, cysts and parasites. If the diagnosis has still not been made, a sigmoidoscopy and rectal biopsy should be performed and radiological studies should be considered.

Oral fluid and electrolyte replacement is of prime importance in the treatment. Special oral rehydration solutions (e.g. sodium chloride and glucose powder) are available for use in severe episodes of diarrhoea, particularly in infants. Antidiarrhoeal drugs are thought to impair the clearance of any pathogen from the bowel but may be necessary for short-term relief (e.g. codeine phosphate 30 mg four times daily, or loperamide 2 mg three times daily). Antibiotics are sometimes given (see p. 71) depending on the organism.

Chronic diarrhoea

This always needs investigation. All patients should have a sigmoidoscopy and rectal biopsy. The flow diagram in Figure 6.45 is illustrative; whether the large or the small bowel is investigated first will depend on the clinical story of, for example, bloody diarrhoea or steatorrhoea. The investigations and treatment are described in detail under the individual diseases.

When difficulties exist in distinguishing between functional and organic causes of diarrhoea, hospital admission for a formal 72-hour assessment of stool weights is helpful and will also lead to the diagnosis of factitious causes of diarrhoea.

Table 6.18 Causes of diarrhoea

Infective causes
Bacterial, e.g.
  Campylobacter jejuni
  Salmonella sp.
  Shigella
  Escherichia coli (particularly enterohaemorrhagic *E. coli* 0157:H7)
  Staphylococcal enterocolitis
  Bacillus cereus
  Clostridium perfringens
  Clostridium botulinum
  gastrointestinal tuberculosis
Viral, e.g.
  rotavirus
Fungal, e.g.
  histoplasmosis
Parasitic, e.g.
  amoebic dysentery (*Entamoeba histolytica*)
  schistosomiasis
  Giardia intestinalis

Non-infective causes of diarrhoea
Inflammatory bowel disease
Pseudomembranous colitis
Radiation proctitis or colitis
Behçet's disease
Diverticular disease
Ischaemic colitis
Gastrointestinal lymphoma
Carcinoma of the colon (change in bowel habit)
Malabsorption
Gut resection
Bile acid malabsorption
Drugs – many, including
  laxatives
  metformin
  anticancer drugs
Faecal impaction with overflow
Irritable bowel syndrome and functional diarrhoea

Endocrine
Zollinger–Ellison syndrome
Vipoma
Somatostatinoma
Glucagonoma
Carcinoid syndrome
Thyrotoxicosis
Medullary carcinoma of thyroid
Diabetic autonomic neuropathy

Factitious diarrhoea (4%)
Purgative abuse
Dilutional diarrhoea

Antibiotic-associated diarrhoea (pseudomembranous colitis) (see p. 69)

Pseudomembranous colitis may develop following the use of any antibiotic. Diarrhoea occurs in the first few

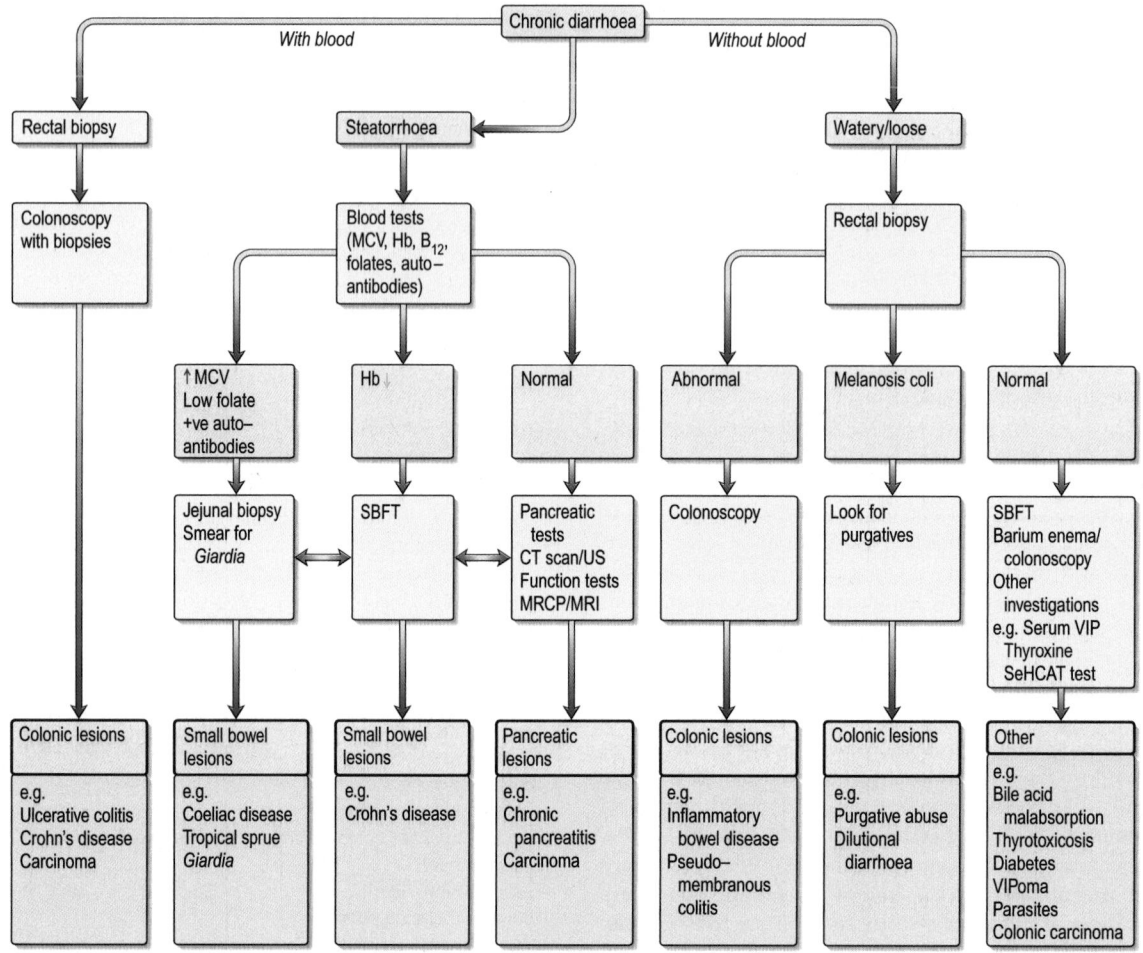

Fig. 6.45 **Flow diagram for the investigation of chronic diarrhoea.** NB: All patients should have had stool cultures. SBFT, small bowel follow-through; VIP, vasoactive intestinal polypeptide; ERCP, endoscopic retrograde cholangiopancreatography; SeHCAT, ^{75}Se-homochoyl taurine.

days after taking the antibiotic or even up to 6 weeks after stopping the drug. The causative agent is *Clostridium difficile* (p. 69).

Bile acid malabsorption

Bile acid malabsorption is an underdiagnosed cause of chronic diarrhoea and many patients with this disorder are assumed to have irritable bowel syndrome. Bile acid diarrhoea occurs when the terminal ileum fails to reabsorb bile acids. Bile acids (particularly the dihydroxy bile acids – deoxycholate and chenodeoxycholate) when present in increased concentrations in the colon lead to diarrhoea by reducing absorption of water and electrolytes and, at higher concentrations, inducing secretion as well as increasing colonic motility. A variety of causes of bile acid malabsorption are recognized (Table 6.19).

Bile acid malabsorption should be considered not only in patients with chronic diarrhoea of unknown cause but also in patients with diarrhoea and associated disease who are not responding to standard therapy (e.g. patients with terminal ileal Crohn's disease, microscopic inflammatory colitis).

Diagnosis is made using the SeHCAT test in which a radiolabelled bile acid analogue is administered and percentage retention at 7 days calculated (< 19% retention abnormal). Treatment is with colestyramine, a resin which binds and inactivates the action of bile acids in the

Table 6.19 **Causes of bile acid malabsorption**

Increased small intestinal transit
Ileal resection
Ileal disease, e.g. active or inactive Crohn's disease
Idiopathic or primary bile acid malabsorption (structurally normal ileum)
Postinfective gastroenteritis
Associated with:
   post-cholecystectomy diarrhoea
   diabetic diarrhoea
   post-vagotomy diarrhoea
   chronic pancreatitis
   cystic fibrosis
   coeliac disease
   microscopic inflammatory colitis
   drugs (e.g. colchicine, metformin)

colon. The best results of treatment are obtained in patients with a SeHCAT retention of < 5%.

Factitious diarrhoea

Factitious diarrhoea accounts for up to 4% of new patients with diarrhoea attending gastroenterology clinics.

Purgative abuse

This is most commonly seen in females who surreptitiously take high-dose purgatives and are often extensively investigated for chronic diarrhoea. The diarrhoea is usually of high volume (> 1 L daily) and patients may have a low serum potassium. Sigmoidoscopy may show pigmented mucosa, a condition known as melanosis coli. Histologically the rectal biopsy shows pigment-laden macrophages in patients taking an anthraquinone purgative (e.g. senna). Melanosis coli is also seen in people regularly taking purgatives in normal doses.

In advanced cases a barium enema may show a dilated colon and loss of haustral pattern.

Phenolphthalein laxatives can be detected by pouring an alkali (e.g. sodium hydroxide) on the stools, which then turn pink; a magnesium-containing purgative will give a high faecal magnesium content. Anthraquinones can also be measured in the urine. If the diagnosis is suspected, a locker or bed search (while the patient is out of the ward) is occasionally necessary. Management is difficult as most patients deny purgative ingestion. Purgative abuse often occurs in association with eating disorders and all patients needs psychiatric help.

Dilutional diarrhoea

In this condition raised stool weights occur as a consequence of patients deliberately diluting their stool with urine or tap water. The diagnosis is made by measuring stool osmolality and electrolyte concentrations in order to calculate the faecal osmolar gap. Measurement of stool creatinine content is helpful in excluding dilution of stools with urine, and early admission to hospital for formal assessment of stool weights may avoid unnecessary invasive investigations being carried out.

Diarrhoea in patients with HIV Infection

Chronic diarrhoea is a common symptom in HIV infection, but HIV's role in the pathogenesis of diarrhoea is unclear. *Cryptosporidium* (see p. 105) is the pathogen most commonly isolated. *Isospora belli* and microsporidia have also been found.

The cause of the diarrhoea is often not found and treatment is symptomatic. Table 6.20 shows the conditions affecting the gastrointestinal tract in patients with AIDS.

FURTHER READING
Thapar N, Sanderson IR (2004) Diarrhoea in children: an interface between developing and developed countries. *Lancet* **363**: 641–653.
Thomas PD et al. (2003) Guidelines for the investigation of chronic diarrhoea, 2nd edition. *Gut* **52** (Suppl.): 1V–15V.

Table 6.20 Gastrointestinal problems in patients with AIDS

Site	Symptoms	Causes
Mouth/ oesophagus	Dysphagia Candidiasis Retrosternal discomfort Oral ulceration	Herpes simplex virus (HSV) Cytomegalovirus (CMV)
Small bowel/ colon	Chronic diarrhoea Steatorrhoea Weight loss	Parasites: *Entamoeba histolytica* *Giardia intestinalis* *Cryptosporidium* *Blastocystis hominis* *Isospora belli* Microsporidia *Cyclospora cayetanensis* Viruses: CMV/HSV, adenovirus Bacteria: *Salmonella* *Campylobacter* *Shigella* *Mycobacterium avium-intracellulare* Non-infective enteropathy – cause unknown
Rectum/ colon	Bloody diarrhoea	Bacterial infection (e.g. *Shigella*)
Any	Weight loss Diarrhoea	Neoplasia: Kaposi's sarcoma Lymphoma Squamous carcinoma Infection – disseminated, e.g. *Mycobacterium avium-intracellulare* HAART therapy

FUNCTIONAL GASTROINTESTINAL DISORDERS

There is a large group of gastrointestinal disorders that are termed 'functional' because symptoms occur in the absence of any demonstrable abnormalities in the digestion and absorption of nutrients, fluid and electrolytes and no structural abnormality can be identified in the gastrointestinal tract.

Table 6.21 lists some of the symptoms that are suggestive of a functional gastrointestinal disorder; modern classification systems (e.g. Rome II 1999, p. 338) are based on the premise that for each disorder there is a symptom cluster that 'breeds true' across clinical and population groups. There is inevitably overlap, with some symptoms being common to more than one disorder.

Table 6.21 Chronic gastrointestinal symptoms suggestive of a functional gastrointestinal disorder (FGID)

Nausea alone
Vomiting alone
Belching
Chest pain unrelated to exercise
Postprandial fullness
Abdominal bloating
Abdominal discomfort/pain (right or left iliac fossa)
Passage of mucus per rectum
Frequent bowel actions with urgency first thing in morning

Table 6.22 Common functional gastrointestinal disorders

Functional oesophageal disorders
Globus
Rumination syndrome
Chest pain of presumed oesophageal origin

Functional gastroduodenal disorders
Functional dyspepsia
Aerophagia
Vomiting

Functional bowel disorders
Irritable bowel syndrome (IBS)
Pain/gas/bloat syndrome
Functional diarrhoea

Fig. 6.46 **A biopsychosocial conceptualization of the pathogenesis and clinical expression of functional gastrointestinal disorders (FGID)**, showing how genetic, environmental and psychological factors may interact to cause dysregulation of brain–gut function. Modified from *Gut* **45** (Suppl.) 1999.

Table 6.22 lists the common functional gastrointestinal disorders. These conditions are extremely common world-wide, making up to 80% of patients seen in the gastroenterology clinic.

Pathophysiology and brain–gut interactions

People with functional gastrointestinal disorders (FGID), are characterized by having a greater gastrointestinal motility response to life events than normal subjects. There is, however, a poor association between measured gastrointestinal motility changes and pain in many of the FGIDs. Patients with FGID have been shown to have abnormalities in visceral sensation and have a lower pain threshold when tested with balloon distension (visceral hyperalgesia). Visceral hypersensitivity possibly relates to:

■ altered receptor sensitivity at the viscus itself
■ increased excitability of the spinal cord dorsal horn neurones
■ altered central modulation of sensations.

Symptoms are likely to be generated as a consequence of disturbed gastrointestinal motility that leads to distension with visceral hyperalgesia accentuating the pain. In a group of patients who developed IBS symptoms following an acute enteric infection, inflammatory changes were demonstrated in the enteric mucosa with serotonin-producing enteroendocrine cell hyperplasia, the excessive release of serotonin being thought to contribute to symptom development.

The brain–gut axis describes a combination of intestinal motor, sensory and CNS activities (Fig. 6.46). Thus extrinsic (e.g. vision, smell) and intrinsic (e.g., emotion, thought) information can affect gastrointestinal sensation because of the neural connections from higher centres. Conversely, viscerotropic events can affect central pain perception, mood and behaviour.

Psychological stress can exacerbate gastrointestinal symptoms, and psychological disturbances are more common in patients with FGIDs. These disturbances alter attitude to illness, promote healthcare seeking, and often lead to a poor clinical outcome. They have psychosocial consequences with poor quality of life at home and work. Early in life, genetic and environmental influences (e.g. family attitudes towards bowel training, verbal or sexual abuse, exposure to an infection) may affect psychosocial development (susceptibility to life stress, psychological state, coping skills, development of social support) or the development of gut dysfunction (abnormal motility or visceral hypersensitivity).

FGID should be regarded as a dysregulation of brain–gut function.

FUNCTIONAL OESOPHAGEAL DISORDERS

The criteria for diagnosis rest mainly on compatible symptoms. However, *pathological gastro-oesophageal reflux and other causes may need full investigation*, particularly in the elderly with a short history.

Globus

Diagnostic criteria

- Persistent or intermittent sensation of a lump or foreign body in the throat.
- Occurrence of the sensation between meals.
- The absence of dysphagia and pain on swallowing (odynophagia).

Treatment

Reassurance and a trial of antireflux therapy are the mainstays of treatment.

Rumination syndrome

Diagnostic criteria

- Persistent or recurrent effortless regurgitation of recently ingested food into the mouth with subsequent re-mastication and re-swallowing.
- Absence of nausea and vomiting, abdominal discomfort, heartburn.
- Cessation of the process when the regurgitated material becomes acidic.

Central factors contribute significantly to the occurrence of rumination, and the disorder is common in individuals with learning difficulties. A range of medical, behavioural and nutritional approaches have been attempted in these patients, with varying success.

Functional chest pain, of presumed oesophageal origin

This is characterized by episodes of mainly midline chest pain, not burning in nature, that are potentially of oesophageal origin and which occur in the absence of a cardiological cause, gastro-oesophageal reflux and achalasia.

More than half of patients will respond to high-dose acid-suppression therapy in the first week; some will respond to nitrates and calcium-channel blockers. A history of psychiatric disorder is found in more than 60% of patients and low-dose antidepressant therapy, e.g. amitriptyline 10 mg, has been shown to be effective.

FUNCTIONAL GASTRODUODENAL DISORDERS

Functional dyspepsia

This is the second most common functional gastrointestinal disorder (after irritable bowel syndrome). Patients can present with a spectrum of symptoms including upper abdominal pain/discomfort, fullness, early satiety, bloating and nausea.

These patients have no structural abnormality as an explanation for their symptoms.

Functional dyspepsia subgroups

Two subgroups based on the predominant (or most bothersome) single symptoms are suggested:

- *Ulcer-like dyspepsia* with pain centred in the upper abdomen as the predominant (most bothersome) symptom.
- *Dysmotility-like dyspepsia* with an unpleasant or troublesome non-painful sensation (discomfort) centred in the upper abdomen being the predominant symptom. This sensation may be associated with upper abdominal fullness, early satiety, bloating and nausea.

There is considerable overlap between these two groups.

Investigations

Many young patients (< 50) require no investigation. Older patients or those with alarm symptoms require endoscopy (p. 265). Gastroscopy often shows gastritis but whether this is the cause of the symptoms is doubtful.

Treatment

The range of therapies prescribed for functional dyspepsia reflects the uncertain pathogenesis and the lack of satisfactory treatment options. Management is further confounded by high placebo response rates (20–60%). A proportion of patients will respond satisfactorily to reassurance, explanations and lifestyle changes, but antisecretory or prokinetic agents are used for patients with ulcer-like and dysmotility-like dyspepsia respectively. Reducing intake of fat, coffee, alcohol and cigarette smoking may help.

H. pylori eradication therapy is often used in functional dyspepsia but there is little evidence to recommend its use. Most gastroenterologists usually try such therapy if only for its possible long-term benefit.

In one study omeprazole produced symptomatic relief in patients with *H. pylori* and did not help *H. pylori*-negative patients.

Aerophagia

Aerophagia refers to a repetitive pattern of swallowing or ingesting air and belching. It is usually an unconscious act unrelated to meals. Usually no investigation is required. Explanation that the symptoms are due to swallowed air and reassurance are necessary, as is treatment of associated psychiatric disease.

Functional vomiting

Functional vomiting is a rare condition in clinical practice. Chronic nausea is a frequent accompaniment in all functional gastrointestinal disorders. Clinically functional vomiting is characterized by:

- frequent episodes of vomiting, occurring on at least 3 separate days in a week
- absence of criteria for an eating disorder, rumination, or major psychiatric disease

- absence of self-induced and medication-induced vomiting
- absence of abnormalities in the gut or central nervous system and metabolic disease to explain the recurrent vomiting.

Investigation is often not required but always exclude non-GI disorders (Table 6.1).

Treatment is with anti-nausea drugs and anti-depressants; behavioural and psychotherapy are helpful. Dietary changes occasionally help.

FUNCTIONAL BOWEL DISORDERS

Irritable bowel syndrome (IBS)

IBS is the commonest FGID. In western populations, up to 1 in 5 people report symptoms consistent with IBS. Only approximately 50% will consult their doctors and of these up to 30% will be referred by their GP to a hospital specialist. Up to 40% of all patients seen in specialist gastroenterology clinics will have IBS. Estimates in the UK put the annual cost of IBS to healthcare resources as £45.6 million; in the US the cost is higher at $8 billion. In the UK approximately a quarter of IBS patients lose time off work for periods ranging from 7 to 13 days each year.

The factors that determine whether an IBS sufferer in the community seeks medical advice include the demonstration that consulters have higher illness attitude scores and higher anxiety and depression scores than non-consulters. Consulters perceive that their symptoms are severer than non-consulters, and consulting behaviour may be determined by the number of presenting symptoms. Female consulters outnumber male consulters by a factor of 2–3. Reasons for this include the fact that anxiety and depression scores are higher in women than in men and the gut may be more sensitive to various stimuli in women. It is likely that men and women perceive internal events in the abdomen differently and that women may be more focused on these events. Food and eating are of more special psychological significance for women, as evidenced by a much higher incidence of eating disorders in women. The whole pelvic region carries a more specific significance for women, being associated not only with defecation, urination and sexuality but additionally with menstruation, pregnancy and childbirth. Finally, women in western society in general seem more willing than men to seek medical attention for a whole variety of disorders.

IBS – a multisystem disorder

IBS patients suffer from a number of non-intestinal symptoms (Table 6.23). The non-intestinal symptoms of IBS can be more intrusive than the classical features of IBS. IBS coexists with chronic fatigue syndrome (see p. 1281), fibromyalgia (see p. 1282) and temporomandibular joint dysfunction.

The biopsychosocial conceptualization of the pathogenesis and clinical expression of FGIDs (Fig. 6.46) is particularly relevant to IBS and Box 6.16 lists some com-

Table 6.23 Non-gastrointestinal features of irritable bowel syndrome

Gynaecological symptoms
Painful periods (dysmenorrhoea)
Pain following sexual intercourse (dyspareunia)
Premenstrual tension

Urinary symptoms
Frequency
Urgency
Passing urine at night (nocturia)
Incomplete emptying of bladder

Other symptoms
Back pain
Headaches
Bad breath, unpleasant taste in the mouth
Poor sleeping
Fatigue

mon factors that have been shown to trigger IBS symptoms. Infectious diarrhoea precedes the onset of IBS symptoms in 7–30% of patients. Whether this is a factor for all patients or just a small subgroup remains controversial. Risk factors in these patients have been shown to include female gender, severity and duration of diarrhoea, pre-existing life events and high hypochondriacal anxiety and neurotic scores at the time of the initial illness. Symptoms of anxiety and depression are more common in IBS patients and stress or life events often precedes the onset of chronic bowel symptoms.

Box 6.16 Some factors that can trigger onset of irritable bowel symptoms

- Gastrointestinal infection
- Antibiotic therapy
- Pelvic surgery
- Psychological stress
- Psychological trauma
- Sexual, physical, verbal abuse
- Mood disturbances
- Anxiety, depression
- Eating disorders
- Food intolerance

Diagnostic criteria (Rome II 1999)

These criteria state that, in the preceding 12 months there should be at least 12 weeks (consecutive) of abdominal discomfort or pain that has two of three of the following features:

- relieved with defecation; and/or
- onset associated with a change in frequency of stool; and/or
- onset associated with a change in form (appearance) of stool.

The following symptoms cumulatively support the diagnosis of IBS:

- abnormal stool frequency ('abnormal' may be defined as > 3/day and < 3/week)
- abnormal stool form (lumpy/hard or loose/watery stool)
- abnormal stool passage (straining, urgency, or feeling of incomplete evacuation)
- passage of mucus
- bloating or feeling of abdominal distension.

These symptoms can be used to subclassify patients into diarrhoea- and constipation-predominant forms of IBS. In practice a third subgroup of alternating IBS exists, in which constipation and diarrhoea alternate. The three forms have equal frequency. Many patients with constipation (p. 320) have abdominal discomfort or pain with bloating or distension so there is considerable overlap with constipation-predominant IBS.

The decision as to whether to investigate and if so what choice of investigations is required should be based on clinical judgement. Pointers to the need for thorough investigation are the presence of the above symptoms in association with rectal bleeding, nocturnal pain, fever and weight loss.

Treatment

Current strategies for treatment of IBS are based on the biopsychosocial conceptualization of IBS (Fig. 6.46) with targeting of central and end-organ therapies (Box 6.17). End-organ and central approaches to treatment should not be mutually exclusive and can be used in sequence and in combinations. Hydroxytryptamine (HT_3)-receptor antagonists for diarrhoea-predominant IBS, HT_4-receptor agonists for constipation-predominant IBS as well as kappa opioid agonists for use in patients in whom visceral hyperalgesia plays a predominant role in the pathogenesis of their symptoms may become available.

Pain/gas/bloat syndrome

There exist a group of patients with functional bowel disease whose abdominal pain and other clinical features are likely to occur as a consequence of disordered motility and visceral sensation that predominantly affects the small intestine or midgut. The symptom-based diagnostic criteria are *abdominal pain,* often exacerbated by eating and not relieved by opening the bowels and not associated with the passage of more frequent or looser stools than normal and not associated with constipation. Other symptoms include *abdominal distension.* Abdominal distension that is not restricted to the upper abdomen occurs, as well as postprandial fullness, nausea and, on occasions, anorexia and weight loss.

Some patients with pain/gas/bloat syndrome have particularly severe and chronic symptoms, that may also be nocturnal. A subgroup of these have been shown to have manometric features consistent with a diagnosis of chronic idiopathic intestinal pseudo-obstruction (CIIP), and specifically of an enteric neuropathy. Full-thickness small intestinal biopsies have confirmed the diagnosis in some patients, while in others a deficiency of α actin staining in the inner circular layer of smooth muscle has been demonstrated.

Treatment of patients with pain/gas/bloat syndrome is not easy; and in some, pain can be chronic and severe. Narcotics should always be avoided. Central and end-organ targeted treatment approaches should be combined, e.g. selective serotonin reuptake inhibitor paroxetine combined with a prokinetic agent domperidone or smooth muscle relaxant, e.g. mepeverine. In the future, consideration should be given to treating these patients with a 5-HT_4-receptor agonist.

 Box 6.17 Approaches to management of irritable bowel syndrome

End organ treatment	Action
Explore dietary triggers	Refer to dietitian
High-fibre diet ± fibre supplements for constipation	Refer to dietitian ± prescribe ispaghula husk
Anti-diarrhoeal drugs for bowel frequency	Loperamide
	Codeine phosphate
	Co-phenotrope
Smooth muscle relaxants for pain	Mebeverine hydrochloride
	Dicycloverine hydrochloride
	Peppermint oil

Central treatment	Action
Physiological explanation and symptoms	At consultation (leaflets with diagrams help)
Psychotherapy	Refer to clinical psychologist (see p. 1282)
Hypnotherapy	
Cognitive behavioural therapy	
Antidepressants	Clomipramine in functional diarrhoea; tricyclic group, e.g. nortriptyline 75 mg daily in diarrhoea-predominant IBS; selective serotonin reuptake inhibitors in constipation-predominant IBS, e.g. paroxetine 20 mg daily

Functional diarrhoea

In this form of functional bowel disease, symptoms occur in the absence of abdominal pain and commonly are:

- The passage of several stools in rapid succession usually first thing in the morning. No further bowel action may occur that day or defecation only after meals.
- The first stool of the day is usually formed, the later ones mushy, looser or watery.
- Urgency of defecation.
- Anxiety, uncertainty about bowel function with restriction of movement (e.g. travelling).
- Exhaustion after the 'morning rush'.

Chronic diarrhoea without pain is caused by many diseases indistinguishable by history from functional diarrhoea (p. 333). Features atypical for a functional disorder (e.g. large-volume stools, rectal bleeding, nutritional deficiency, and weight loss) call for more extensive studies of intestinal structure and function. In cases where it proves difficult to distinguish between functional and organic causes of diarrhoea, patients should be admitted to hospital for a formal 3-day analysis of stool weights and faecal fat estimation, and a purgative screen together with stool osmolality and creatinine contents to exclude factitious causes of diarrhoea (see p. 335). Outpatient analysis of stool weights is unreliable as brain–gut dysrhythmia may result in increased stool weights in the normal home environment.

Treatment of functional diarrhoea is usually with loperomide and a tricyclic antidepressant at night (e.g. clomipramine 10–30 mg).

FURTHER READING

Camilleri M (2001) Management of the irritable bowel syndrome. *Gastroenterology* **120**: 652–668.

Castle MZD, Silk DBA, Libby GW (2004) Review article: the rationale for antidepressant therapy in functional gastrointestinal disorders. *Alimentary Pharmacology & Therapeutics* **19**: 969–979.

Knowles CH, Silk DB, Darzi A et al. (2004) Deranged smooth muscle α-actin as a biomarker of intestinal pseudo-obstruction: a controlled multinational case series. *Gut* **53**(11): 1583–1589.

Mertz HR (2003) Irritable bowel syndrome. *New England Journal of Medicine* **349**: 2136–2146.

Rome II (1999) A multinational consensus document on functional gastrointestinal disorder. *Gut* **45** (Suppl. II): II1–II81.

Spiller RC (2003) Postinfectious irritable bowel syndrome. *Gastroenterology* **124**: 1662–1671.

Wingate D, Hongo M, Kellow J et al. (2002) Disorders of gastrointestinal motility: towards a new classification. *Journal of Gastroenterology and Hepatology* **17** (Suppl.): S1–S14.

THE ACUTE ABDOMEN

This section deals with the acute abdominal conditions that cause the patient to be hospitalized within a few hours of

Table 6.24	Common causes of acute abdominal pain
Diagnosis	**No. of patients**
Non-specific abdominal pain	466
Acute appendicitis	449
Renal colic	61
Gynaecological disorders	44
Intestinal obstruction	32
Urinary tract infection	30
Gall bladder disease	12
Perforated ulcer/dyspepsia	10
Diverticular disease	6
Other diagnoses	58
No diagnosis established	39

Data drawn from a series of 1204 patients reported by Dixon et al. 1991. *British Medical Journal* **302**: 386–388

the onset of pain (Table 6.24). The diagnosis when made quickly reduces morbidity and mortality. Although a specific diagnosis should be attempted, the immediate problem in management is to decide whether an 'acute abdomen' exists and whether surgery is required.

History

This should include previous operations, any gynaecological problems and whether any concurrent medical condition is present.

Pain

The onset, site, type and subsequent course of the pain should be determined as accurately as possible. In general, the pain of an acute abdomen can either be constant (usually owing to inflammation) or colicky because of a blocked 'tube'. The inflammatory nature of a *constant pain* will be supported by a raised temperature, tachycardia and/or a raised white cell count. If these are normal, then other causes (e.g. musculoskeletal, aortic aneurysm) or rare causes (e.g. porphyria) should be considered. Colicky pain can be due to an obstruction of the gut, biliary system, urogenital system or the uterus. These will probably initially require conservative management along with analgesics. If a colicky pain becomes a constant pain, then inflammation of the organ may have supervened (e.g. strangulated hernia, ascending cholangitis or salpingitis).

A *sudden onset of pain* suggests:

- a perforation (e.g. of a duodenal ulcer)
- a rupture (e.g. of an aneurysm)
- torsion (e.g. of an ovarian cyst)
- acute pancreatitis.

Back pain suggests:

- pancreatitis
- rupture of an aortic aneurysm
- renal tract disease.

Inflammatory conditions (e.g. appendicitis) produce a more gradual onset of pain. With peritonitis the pain is continuous and may be made worse by movement.

Vomiting

Vomiting may accompany any acute abdominal pain but, if persistent, it suggests an obstructive lesion of the gut. The character of the vomit should be asked – does it contain blood, bile or small bowel contents?

Other symptoms

Any change in bowel habit or of urinary frequency should be documented and, in females, a gynaecological history should be taken.

Physical examination

The general condition of the person should be noted. Does the patient look ill? Is he or she shocked? Large volumes of fluid may be lost from the vascular compartment into the peritoneal cavity or into the lumen of the bowel, giving rise to hypovolaemia, i.e. a pale cold skin, a weak rapid pulse and hypotension.

The abdomen

■ **Inspection**. Look for the presence of scars, distension or masses.
■ **Palpation**. The abdomen should be examined gently for sites of tenderness and the presence or absence of guarding. Guarding is involuntary spasm of the abdominal wall and it indicates peritonitis. This can be localized to one area or it may be generalized, involving the whole abdomen.
■ **Bowel sounds**. Increased high-pitch tinkling bowel sounds indicate fluid obstruction; this occurs because of fluid movement within the large dilated bowel lumen. Absent bowel sounds suggest peritoneal involvement. In an obstructed patient, absent bowel sounds suggest strangulation ischaemia or ileus. It is essential that the hernial orifices be examined if intestinal obstruction is suspected.

Pelvic and rectal examination

Pelvic examination can be very helpful, particularly in diagnosing gynaecological causes of an acute abdomen (e.g. a ruptured ectopic pregnancy). Rectal examination is less helpful as localized tenderness may be due to any cause; it may show blood on the finger stall.

Sigmoidoscopy

If diarrhoea is present, sigmoidoscopy is indicated to aid exclusion of infective, inflammatory and ischaemic causes of acute pain. A specimen of stool should be taken for stool culture for bacterial pathogens (e.g. campylobacter, salmonella, shigella) when diarrhoea is present – stool should also be tested for *Clostridium difficile* toxin if antibiotic therapy precedes onset of diarrhoea and acute abdominal pain (see p. 69).

Other observations

■ *Mouth*. The tongue is furred in some cases and a fetor is present.
■ *Temperature*. Fever is more common in acute inflammatory processes.

Table 6.25 Medical causes of acute abdomen

Referred pain
Pneumonia
Myocardial infarction

Functional gastrointestinal disorders

Renal causes
Pelviureteric colic
Acute pyelonephritis

Metabolic causes
Diabetes mellitus
Acute intermittent porphyria
Lead poisoning

Haematological causes
Haemophilia and other bleeding disorders
Henoch–Schönlein purpura
Sickle cell crisis
Polycythaemia vera

Vasculitis
Embolic

■ *Urine*. Examine for:
  – blood – suggests urinary tract infection or renal colic
  – glucose and ketones – ketoacidosis can present with acute pain
  – protein and white cells – to exclude acute pyelonephritis.
■ Think of medical causes (Table 6.25).

Investigations

■ **Blood count**. A raised white cell count occurs in inflammatory conditions.
■ **Serum amylase**. High levels (more than five times normal) indicate acute pancreatitis. Raised levels below this can occur in any acute abdomen and should not be considered diagnostic of pancreatitis.
■ **Serum electrolytes**. These are not particularly helpful for diagnosis but useful for general evaluation of the patient.
■ **Pregnancy**. A urine dipstick is used with women of child-bearing age.
■ **X-rays.** A chest X-ray is useful to detect air under the diaphragm owing to a perforation. Dilated loops of bowel or fluid levels are suggestive of obstruction (supine abdominal X-ray).
■ **Ultrasound**. This is useful in the diagnosis of acute cholangitis, cholecystitis and aortic aneurysm, and in expert hands is reliable in the diagnosis of acute appendicitis. Gynaecological and other pelvic causes of pain can be detected.
■ **CT scan**. Spiral CT is the most accurate investigation in most acute emergencies. It should be used more often to avoid unnecessary laparotomies.
■ **Laparoscopy**. This has gained increasing importance as a diagnostic tool prior to proceeding with surgery, particularly in men and women over the age of

50 years. In addition, therapeutic manoeuvres, such as appendicectomy, can be performed.

Acute appendicitis

This is the most common surgical emergency. It affects all age groups. Appendicitis should always be considered in the differential diagnosis if the appendix has not been removed.

Acute appendicitis mostly occurs when the lumen of the appendix becomes obstructed with a faecolith; however, in some cases there is only generalized acute inflammation. If the appendix is not removed at this stage, gangrene occurs with perforation, leading to a localized abscess or to generalized peritonitis.

Clinical features and management

Most patients present with abdominal pain; in many it starts vaguely in the centre of the abdomen, becoming localized to the right iliac fossa in the first few hours. Nausea, vomiting, anorexia and occasional diarrhoea can occur.

Examination of the abdomen usually reveals tenderness in the right iliac fossa, with guarding due to the localized peritonitis. There may be a tender mass in the right iliac fossa. Laboratory tests are unhelpful, except that the white cell count may be raised. An ultrasound scan is accurate for the detection of an inflamed appendix and will also indicate an appendix mass or other localized lesion. CT is highly sensitive and specific, and reduces the incidence of removing the 'normal' appendix.

Differential diagnosis

- Non-specific mesenteric lymphadenitis – may mimic appendicitis.
- Acute terminal ileitis due to Crohn's disease or *Yersinia* infection.
- Acute salpingitis – should be considered in women; there is usually a vaginal discharge and on vaginal examination, adnexal tenderness is found.
- Inflamed Meckel's diverticulum.
- Functional bowel disease.

It should be noted that 45% of women aged 15–45 years who have an appendicectomy have a normal appendix removed.

Treatment

The appendix is removed by open surgery or laparoscopically. If an appendix mass is present, the patient is usually treated conservatively with intravenous fluids and antibiotics. The pain subsides over a few days and the mass usually disappears over a few weeks. Interval appendicectomy is recommended at a later date to prevent further acute episodes.

Gynaecological causes

Ruptured ectopic pregnancy. The fallopian tube is the commonest extrauterine site of implantation. Delayed diagnosis is the major cause of morbidity. Most patients will present with recurrent low abdominal pain associated with vaginal bleeding. Diagnosis is usually made with abdominal and transvaginal ultrasound. Most patients can be managed by laparoscopic salpingostomy or salpingectomy.

Ovarian:
- Rupture of 'functional' ovarian cysts in the middle of the cycle (Mittelschmerz).
- Torsion or rupture of ovarian cysts.

Acute salpingitis. Most cases are associated with sexually transmitted infection. Patients commonly present with bilateral low abdominal pain, a fever and vaginal discharge. In the Fitz-Hughes–Curtis syndrome the chlamydia infection tracks up the right paracolic gutter to cause a perihepatitis. Patients can present with acute right hypochondrial pain, fever and mildly abnormal liver biochemistry.

Acute peritonitis

Localized peritonitis

There is virtually always some degree of localized peritonitis with all acute inflammatory conditions of the gastrointestinal tract (e.g. acute appendicitis, acute cholecystitis). Pain and tenderness are largely features of this localized peritonitis. The treatment is for the underlying disease.

Generalized peritonitis

This is a serious condition resulting from irritation of the peritoneum owing to infection (e.g. perforated appendix), or from chemical irritation due to leakage of intestinal contents (e.g. perforated ulcer). In the latter case, superadded infection gradually occurs; *E. coli* and *Bacteroides* are the most common organisms.

The peritoneal cavity becomes acutely inflamed, with production of an inflammatory exudate that spreads throughout the peritoneum, leading to intestinal dilatation and paralytic ileus.

Clinical features and management

In perforation, the onset is sudden with acute severe abdominal pain, followed by general collapse and shock. The patient may improve temporarily, only to become worse later as generalized toxaemia occurs.

When the peritonitis is secondary to inflammatory disease, the onset is less rapid with the initial features being those of the underlying disease.

Investigations should always include an erect chest X-ray to detect free air under the diaphragm, and a serum amylase to diagnose acute pancreatitis, which is treated conservatively. Imaging with ultrasound and/or CT should also be performed for diagnosis.

Peritonitis is always treated surgically after adequate resuscitation with the re-establishment of a good urinary output. This includes insertion of a nasogastric tube, intravenous fluids and antibiotics. Surgery has a twofold objective:

- peritoneal lavage of the abdominal cavity
- specific treatment of the underlying condition.

Complications

Any delay in treatment of peritonitis produces more profound toxaemia and septicaemia. In addition, local abscess formation occurs and should be suspected if a patient continues to remain unwell postoperatively with a swinging fever, high white cell count and continuing pain. Abscesses are commonly pelvic or subphrenic and can be localized and drained using ultrasound and CT scanning techniques.

Intestinal obstruction

Most intestinal obstruction is due to a mechanical block. Sometimes the bowel does not function, leading to a paralytic ileus. This occurs temporarily after most abdominal operations and with peritonitis. Some causes of intestinal obstruction are shown in Table 6.26.

Obstruction of the bowel leads to bowel distension above the block, with increased secretion of fluid into the distended bowel. Bacterial contamination occurs in the distended stagnant bowel. In strangulation the blood supply is impeded, leading to gangrene, perforation and peritonitis unless urgent treatment of the condition is undertaken.

Clinical features

The patient complains of abdominal colic, vomiting and constipation without passage of wind. In upper gut obstruction the vomiting is profuse but in lower gut obstruction it may be absent.

Examination of the abdomen reveals distension with increased bowel sounds. Marked tenderness suggests strangulation, and urgent surgery is necessary. Examination of the hernial orifices and rectum must be performed. X-ray of the abdomen reveals distended loops of bowel proximal to the obstruction. Fluid levels are seen in small bowel obstruction on an erect film. In large bowel obstruction, the caecum and ascending colon are distended. An instant water-soluble gastrografin enema without air insufflation may help to demonstrate the site of the obstruction. CT can localize the lesion accurately.

Management

Initial management is by resuscitation with intravenous fluids (mainly isotonic saline with potassium) and decompression. Many cases will settle on conservative management, but an increasing temperature, raised pulse rate, increasing pain and a rising white cell count require exploratory laparotomy.

Laparotomy with removal of the obstruction will be necessary in some cases of *small bowel obstruction*. If the bowel is gangrenous owing to strangulation, gut resection will be required. A few patients (e.g. those with Crohn's disease) may have recurrent episodes of incomplete intestinal obstruction that can be managed conservatively. In *large bowel obstruction* due to malignancy, colorectal stents are being used, followed by elective surgery. In critically ill patients, a defunctioning colostomy may be required. Volvulus of the sigmoid colon can be managed by the passage of a flexible sigmoidoscope or a rectal tube to un-kink the bowel, but recurrent volvulus may require sigmoid resection.

Intestinal pseudo-obstruction

It is now recognized that a clinical picture mimicking mechanical obstruction may develop in patients who do not have a mechanical cause. Colonic pseudo-obstruction is the commonest form. In more than 80% of cases it complicates other clinical conditions, for example:

- intra-abdominal trauma, pelvic spinal and femoral fractures
- postoperatively (abdominal, pelvic, cardiothoracic, orthopaedic, neurosurgical)
- intra-abdominal sepsis
- pneumonia
- metabolic (e.g. electrolyte disturbances, malnutrition, diabetes mellitus, Parkinson's disease)
- drugs – opiates (particularly after orthopaedic surgery) antidepressants, antiparkinsonian drugs.

Patients present with rapid and progressive abdominal distension and pain. X-ray shows a gas-filled large bowel. Management is of the underlying problem (e.g. withdraw opiate analgesia) together with a trial of i.v. neostigmine therapy (Box 6.18). Patients should be monitored care-

Table 6.26 Some causes of intestinal obstruction
Small intestinal obstruction
Adhesions (80% in adults)
Hernias
Crohn's disease
Intussusception
Obstruction due to extrinsic involvement by cancer
Colonic obstruction
Carcinoma of the colon
Sigmoid volvulus
Diverticular disease

Box 6.18 Treatment of acute colonic pseudo-obstruction

- Neostigmine 2.0 mg i.v. over 3–5 min in presence of doctor with ECG monitor.
- 0.3–1 mg atropine if symptomatically bradycardic. Nurse the patient supine for 60 min.
- Monitor abdominal circumference and the diameter of the caecum, ascending, transverse and descending colon on straight abdominal X-ray.

fully and consideration should be given to surgery if the diameter of the caecum exceeds 14 cm.

Small intestinal pseudo-obstruction is a rare chronic condition that can occur in association with systemic sclerosis, systemic lupus erythematosus (SLE), Sjögren's syndrome, thyroid disease, amyloidosis and paraneoplastic syndromes. Primary myopathic and neuropathic forms also exist, with the former sometimes being familial. There are other patients with clinical and manometric features of small intestinal pseudo-obstruction who have normal full-thickness biopsies of smooth muscle but α actin deficiency in the inner circular layer of the smooth muscle. Myopathic forms can present with attacks of non-mechanical obstruction and/or functional small intestinal failure with dilated non-propulsive intestines and coexisting bacterial overgrowth. These patients are managed in specialist centres with facilities to manage home total parenteral nutrition (p. 259). The other patients, including those with enteric neuropathies, often present with a long history of abdominal pain and other intractable midgut symptoms. Many have extraintestinal symptoms, and a multidisciplinary approach to management is required, including, in a number, access to facilities to provide needle catheter jejunostomy enteral feeding as well as home TPN.

FURTHER READING

Silk DBA (2004) Chronic idiopathic intestinal pseudo-obstruction: the need for a multidisciplinary approach to management. *Proceedings of the Nutrition Society* **63**: 1–8.

Steinbrook RA (2001) An opioid antagonist for postoperative ileus. *New England Journal of Medicine* **345**: 988–989.

THE PERITONEUM

The peritoneal cavity is a closed sac lined by mesothelial cells, which produce surfactant that acts as a lubricant within the peritoneal cavity. The cavity contains less than 100 mL of serous fluid containing less than 30 g/L of protein.

The mesothelial cells lining the diaphragm have gaps that allow communication between the peritoneum and the diaphragmatic lymphatics. Approximately one-third of fluid drains through these lymphatics, the remainder through the parietal peritoneum. These mechanisms allow particulate matter to be removed rapidly from the peritoneal cavity.

Complement activation is an early defence mechanism followed rapidly by upregulation of the peritoneal mesothelial cells and migration of polymorphonuclear neutrophils and macrophages into the peritoneum.

Mast cells release potent mediators of inflammation and interact with T cells to generate an immune response.

The peritoneal-associated lymphoid tissue includes the omental milky spots, the lymphocytes within the peritoneal cavity and the draining lymph nodes. B cells

Table 6.27 Disease of the peritoneum

Infective (bacterial) peritonitis
Secondary to gut disease, e.g.
  appendicitis
  perforation of any organ
Chronic peritoneal dialysis
Spontaneous, usually in ascites with liver disease
Tuberculosis

Neoplasia
Secondary deposits (e.g. from ovary, stomach)

Primary mesothelioma

Vasculitis
Connective tissue disease
Polyserositis (e.g. familial Mediterranean fever)

with a unique CD5$^+$ are common. This defence system plays a major role in localizing peritoneal infection. Some conditions that can affect the peritoneum are shown in Table 6.27.

Peritonitis can be acute or chronic, as seen in tuberculosis. Most cases of infective peritonitis are secondary to gastrointestinal disease, but it occurs occasionally without intra-abdominal sepsis in ascites due to liver disease. Very rarely, fungal and parasitic infections can also cause primary peritonitis (e.g. amoebiasis, candidiasis). Peritonitis is discussed further on page 342.

The peritoneum can be involved by *secondary malignant deposits*, and the most common cause of ascites in a young to middle-aged woman is an ovarian carcinoma.

A *subphrenic abscess* is usually secondary to infection in the abdomen and is characterized by fever, malaise, pain in the right or left hypochondrium and shoulder-tip pain. An erect chest X-ray shows gas under the diaphragm, impaired movement of the diaphragm on screening and a pleural effusion. Ultrasound is usually diagnostic. Percutaneous catheter drainage inserted under CT or ultrasound guidance and antibiotics is highly successful therapy.

Ascites is associated with all diseases of the peritoneum. The fluid that collects is an exudate with a high protein content. It is also seen in liver disease. The mechanism, causes and investigation of ascites are discussed on page 381.

Retroperitoneal fibrosis (periaortitis)

This is a rare condition in which there is a marked fibrosis over the posterior abdominal wall and retroperitoneum. It is described on p. 656.

Tuberculous peritonitis

This is the second most common form of abdominal TB.

Three subgroups can be identified: wet, dry and fibrous.

- In patients with the wet type, ascitic fluid should be examined for protein concentration (> 20 g/L) and tubercle bacilli (rarely found).
- In the dry form, patients present with subacute intestinal obstruction which is due to tuberculous small bowel adhesions.
- In the fibrous form, patients present with abdominal pain, distension and ill-defined irregular tender abdominal masses.

The diagnosis of peritoneal TB can be supported by findings on ultrasound or CT screening (mesenteric thickening and lymph node enlargement). A histological diagnosis is not always required before instituting treatment. In some patients careful laparoscopy (to avoid perforation) may have to be performed, and rarely laparotomy.

Treatment

Drug treatment is similar to that for pulmonary TB (see p. 932) and should be supervised by chest physicians who have experience in dealing with contacts.

FURTHER READING

Gastrointestinal cancer mechanisms, diagnosis and treatment. *Gastroenterology* (2005) **128**: 153–1764.
Hall JC et al. (1998) The pathobiology of peritonitis. *Gastroenterology* 114: 188–196.

CHAPTER BIBLIOGRAPHY

Feldman M et al. (2002) *Sleisenger and Fordtran's Gastrointestinal and Liver Disease*, 7th edn. Philadelphia: WB Saunders.

SIGNIFICANT WEBSITES

http://www.graylab.ac.uk/cancernet/100025.html
   Gastric cancer
http://www.jr2.ox.ac.uk/bandolier/band27/b27-7.html
band38/b38-4.html
   Gastric ulcer and GORD
http://www.nacc.org.uk
   UK National Association for colitis and Crohn's Disease
http://www.digestivedisorders.org.uk/leaflets/ibs.html
   Irritable bowel syndrome
http://www.coeliac.co.uk
   Coeliac disease
http://www.bsg.org.uk
   British Society of Gastroenterology

Liver, biliary tract and pancreatic disease

7

In many countries alcohol is the major cause of liver disease, followed by hepatitis C virus infection. Hepatitis B virus is still a significant factor but widespread vaccination will reduce its prevalence. Health education and the improvement in public health should help to stop the spread of viral infections.

Imaging techniques enable the liver, biliary tree and pancreas to be visualized with precision, resulting in earlier diagnosis. Therapeutic endoscopy, laparoscopic and minimally invasive surgery are now widely available for biliary tract and pancreatic disease. Finally, liver transplantation is established therapy for both acute and chronic liver disease.

THE LIVER

STRUCTURE OF THE LIVER AND BILIARY SYSTEM

The liver

The liver is the largest internal organ in the body and is situated in the right hypochondrium. Functionally, it is divided into right and left lobes by the middle hepatic vein. The right lobe is larger and contains the caudate and quadrate lobes. The liver is further subdivided into a total of eight segments (Fig. 7.1) by divisions of the right, middle and left hepatic veins. Each segment receives its own portal pedicle, permitting individual segment resection at surgery.

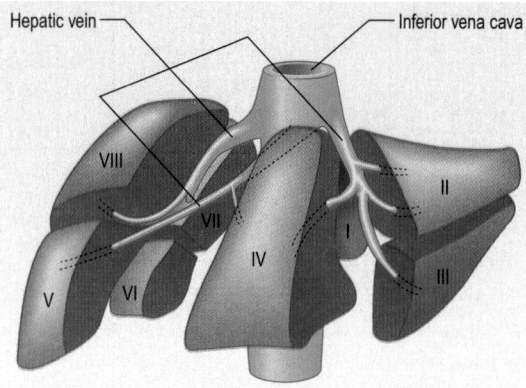

Fig. 7.1 **Segmental anatomy of the liver showing the eight hepatic segments.** I, caudate lobe; II–IV the left

Fig. 7.2 **Diagram of an acinus.** Zones 1, 2 and 3 represent areas supplied by blood, with zone 1 being best oxygenated. Zone 3 is supplied by blood remote from afferent vessels and is in the microcirculatory periphery of the acinus. The perivascular area (star shaped green area around THV) is formed by the most peripheral parts of zone 3 of several adjacent acini and is the least well oxygenated. THV, terminal hepatic venule; PT, portal triad.

The blood supply to the liver constitutes 25% of the resting cardiac output and is via two main vessels:

- The *hepatic artery*, which is a branch of the coeliac axis, supplies 25% of the total blood flow. Autoregulation of blood flow by the hepatic artery ensures a constant total liver blood flow.
- The *portal vein* drains most of the gastrointestinal tract and the spleen. It supplies 75% of the blood flow. The normal portal pressure is 5–8 mmHg; flow increases after meals.

Both vessels enter the liver via the hilum (porta hepatis). The blood from these vessels is distributed to the segments and passes into the sinusoids via the portal tracts.

Blood leaves the sinusoids, entering branches of the hepatic vein which join into three main branches before entering the inferior vena cava.

The caudate lobe is an autonomous segment as it receives an independent blood supply from the portal vein and hepatic artery, and its hepatic vein drains directly into the inferior vena cava.

Lymph, formed mainly in the perisinusoidal space, is collected in lymphatics which are present in the portal tracts. These small lymphatics enter larger vessels which eventually drain into the hepatic ducts.

The functional unit of the liver is the acinus. This consists of parenchyma supplied by the smallest portal tracts containing portal vein radicles, hepatic arterioles and bile ductules (Fig. 7.2). The hepatocytes near this triad (zone 1) are well supplied with oxygenated blood and are more resistant to damage than the cells nearer the terminal hepatic (central) veins (zone 3).

The sinusoids lack a basement membrane and are loosely surrounded by specialist fenestrated endothelial cells and Kupffer cells (phagocytic cells). Sinusoids are separated by plates of liver cells (hepatocytes). The subendothelial space that lies between the sinusoids and hepatocytes is the space of Disse, which contains a matrix of basement membrane constituents and stellate cells. (See Fig. 7.21).

Stellate cells store retinoids in their resting state and contain the intermediate filament, desmin. When activated (to myofibroblasts) they are contractile and probably regulate sinusoidal blood flow. Endothelin and nitric oxide play a major role in modulating stellate cell contractility. Stellate cells, after activation, produce collagen types I, III and IV (see p. 375).

The biliary system

Bile canaliculi form a network between the hepatocytes. These join to form thin bile ductules near the portal tract, which in turn enter the bile ducts in the portal tracts. These then combine to form the right and left hepatic ducts that leave each liver lobe. The hepatic ducts join at the porta hepatis to form the common hepatic duct. The cystic duct connects the gall bladder to the lower end of the common hepatic duct. The gall bladder lies under the right lobe of the liver and stores and concentrates hepatic bile; it has a capacity of approximately 50 mL. The common bile duct is formed by the combination of the cystic and hepatic ducts and is approximately 8 mm in diameter, narrowing at its distal end to pass into the duodenum. The common bile duct and pancreatic duct open into the second part of the duodenum through a common channel at the ampulla of Vater. The lower end of the common bile duct contains the muscular sphincter of Oddi, which contracts rhythmically and prevents bile from entering the duodenum in the fasting state.

FURTHER READING
Sherlock S, Dooley J (2002) *Anatomy and Function in Diseases of the Liver and Biliary System*, 11th edn. Oxford: Blackwell Science.

FUNCTIONS OF THE LIVER

Protein metabolism (see also p. 232)

Synthesis

The liver is the principal site of synthesis of all circulating proteins apart from γ-globulins, which are produced in the reticuloendothelial system. The liver receives amino acids from the intestine and muscles and, by controlling the rate of gluconeogenesis and transamination, regulates levels in the plasma. Plasma contains 60–80 g/L of protein, mainly in the form of albumin, globulin and fibrinogen.

Albumin has a half-life of 16–24 days and 10–12 g are synthesized daily. Its main functions are first to maintain the intravascular oncotic (colloid osmotic) pressure, and second to transport water-insoluble substances such as bilirubin, hormones, fatty acids and drugs. Reduced synthesis of albumin over prolonged periods produces hypoalbuminaemia and is seen in chronic liver disease and malnutrition. Hypoalbuminaemia is also found in hypercatabolic states (e.g. trauma with sepsis) and in diseases where there is an excessive loss (e.g. nephrotic syndrome, protein-losing enteropathy).

Transport or carrier proteins such as transferrin and caeruloplasmin, acute-phase and other proteins (e.g. α_1-antitrypsin and α-fetoprotein) are also produced in the liver.

The liver also synthesizes all factors involved in coagulation (apart from one-third of factor VIII) – that is, fibrinogen, prothrombin, factors V, VII, IX, X and XIII, proteins C and S and antithrombin (see Ch. 8) as well as components of the complement system.

Degradation (nitrogen excretion)

Amino acids are degraded by transamination and oxidative deamination to produce ammonia, which is then converted to urea and excreted by the kidneys. This is a major pathway for the elimination of nitrogenous waste. Failure of this process occurs in severe liver disease.

Carbohydrate metabolism

Glucose homeostasis and the maintenance of the blood sugar is a major function of the liver. It stores approximately 80 g of glycogen. In the immediate fasting state, blood glucose is maintained either by glucose released from the breakdown of glycogen (glycogenolysis) or by newly synthesized glucose (gluconeogenesis). Sources for gluconeogenesis are lactate, pyruvate, amino acids from muscles (mainly alanine and glutamine) and glycerol from lipolysis of fat stores. In prolonged starvation, ketone bodies and fatty acids are used as alternative sources of fuel and the body tissues adapt to a lower glucose requirement (see Ch. 5).

Lipid metabolism

Fats are insoluble in water and are transported in the plasma as protein–lipid complexes (lipoproteins). These are discussed in detail on page 1135.

The liver has a major role in the metabolism of lipoproteins. It synthesizes very-low-density lipoproteins (VLDLs) and high-density lipoproteins (HDLs). HDLs are the substrate for lecithin–cholesterol acyltransferase (LCAT), which catalyses the conversion of free cholesterol to cholesterol ester (see below). Hepatic lipase removes triglyceride from intermediate-density lipoproteins (IDLs) to produce low-density lipoproteins (LDLs) which are degraded by the liver after uptake by specific cell-surface receptors (see Fig. 19.19).

Triglycerides are mainly of dietary origin but are also formed in the liver from circulating free fatty acids (FFAs) and glycerol and incorporated into VLDLs. Oxidation or de novo synthesis of FFA occurs in the liver, depending on the availability of dietary fat.

Cholesterol may be of dietary origin but most is synthesized from acetyl-CoA mainly in the liver, intestine, adrenal cortex and skin. It occurs either as free cholesterol or is esterified with fatty acids; this reaction is catalysed by LCAT. This enzyme is reduced in severe liver disease, increasing the ratio of free cholesterol to ester, which alters membrane structures. One result of this is the red cell abnormalities (e.g. target cells) seen in chronic liver disease. Phospholipids (e.g. lecithin) are synthesized in the liver.

The complex interrelationships between protein, carbohydrate and fat metabolism are shown in Figure 7.3.

Formation of bile

Bile secretion

Bile consists of water, electrolytes, bile acids, cholesterol, phospholipids and conjugated bilirubin. Two processes are involved in bile secretion across the canalicular membrane of the hepatocyte – a *bile salt-dependent* and a *bile salt-independent* process – each contributing about 230 mL per day. The remainder of the bile (about 150 mL daily) is produced by the epithelial cells of the bile ductules.

Bile formation requires firstly the uptake of bile acids and other organic and inorganic ions across the basolateral (sinusoidal) membranes by multiple transport proteins. This process is driven by Na^+–K^+-ATPase in the basolateral membrane. Intracellular transport across the hepatocyte is partly through microtubules and partly by cytosol transport proteins. The canalicular membrane contains additional transporters, mainly ATPase-dependent, which carry molecules into the biliary canaliculi against a concentration gradient. The canalicular multi-specific organic anion transporter (cMOAT) also known as multidrug-resistance protein 2 (MRP2) mediates transport of a broad range of compounds including

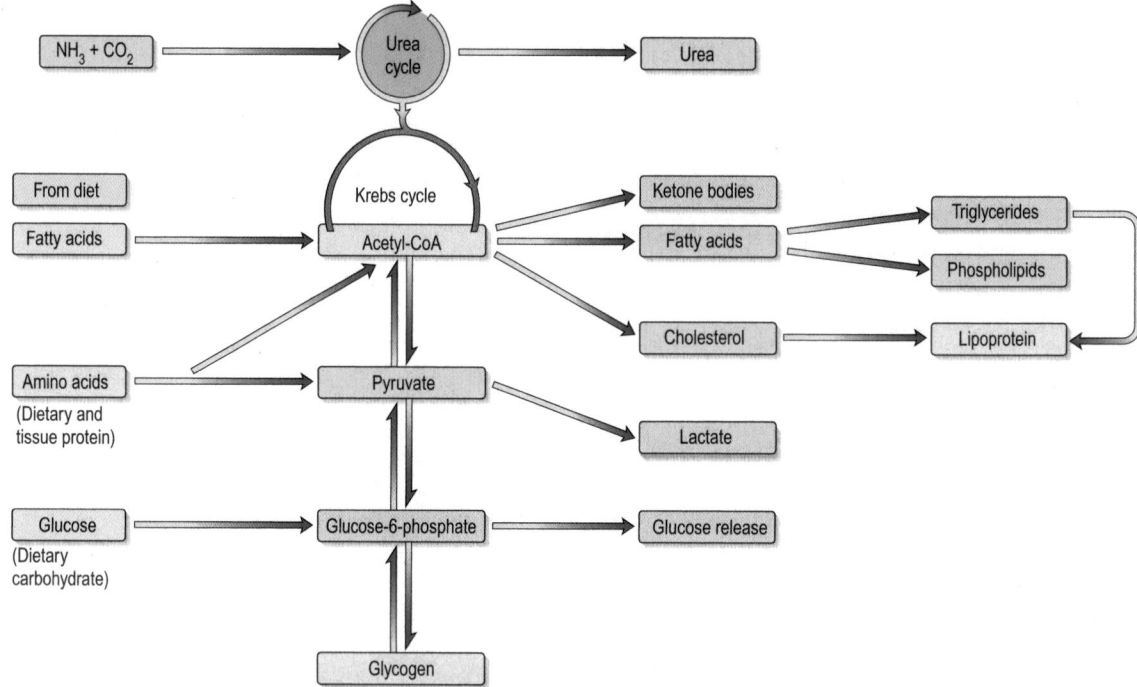

Fig. 7.3 Interrelationships of protein, carbohydrate and lipid metabolism in the liver.

bilirubin diglucuronide, glucuronidated and sulphated bile acids and other organic anions. Na^+ and water follow the passage of bile salts into the biliary canaliculus by diffusion across the tight junction between hepatocytes (a bile salt-dependent process). In the bile salt-independent process water flow is due to other osmotically active solutes such as glutathione and bicarbonate.

Secretion of a bicarbonate-rich solution is stimulated mainly by secretin and is inhibited by somatostatin. In this process several membrane proteins are involved, including the Cl^-/HCO_3^- exchanger and the cystic fibrosis transmembrane conductance regulator which controls Cl^- secretion, as well as water channels (aquaporins) in cholangiocyte membranes.

The average total bile flow is approximately 600 mL per day. In the fasted state half of the bile flows directly into the duodenum and half is diverted into the gall bladder. The mucosa of the gall bladder absorbs 80–90% of the water and electrolytes, but is impermeable to bile acids and cholesterol. Following a meal, cholecystokinin is secreted by the I cells of the duodenal mucosa and stimulates contraction of the gall bladder and relaxation of the sphincter of Oddi, so that bile enters the duodenum. An adequate bile flow is dependent on bile salts being returned to the liver by the enterohepatic circulation.

Bile acid metabolism

Bile acids are synthesized in hepatocytes from cholesterol. The rate-limiting step in their production is that catalysed by cholesterol-7α-hydroxylase. They are excreted into the bile and then pass into the duodenum. The two primary bile acids – cholic acid and chenodeoxycholic acid (Fig. 7.4) – are conjugated with glycine or taurine (in a ratio of 3 : 1 in humans) and this process increases their solubility. Intestinal bacteria convert these acids into secondary bile acids, deoxycholic and lithocholic acid. Figure 7.5 shows the enterohepatic circulation of bile acids.

Bile acids act as detergents; their main function is lipid solubilization. Bile acid molecules contain both a hydrophilic and a hydrophobic end. In aqueous solutions they aggregate to form micelles, with their hydrophobic (lipid-soluble) ends in the centre. Micelles are expanded by cholesterol and phospholipids (mainly lecithin), forming mixed micelles.

Bilirubin metabolism

Bilirubin is produced mainly from the breakdown of mature red cells in the Kupffer cells of the liver and in the reticuloendothelial system; 15% of bilirubin comes from the catabolism of other haem-containing proteins, such as myoglobin, cytochromes and catalases.

Normally, 250–300 mg of bilirubin are produced daily. The iron and globin are removed from the haem and are reused. Biliverdin is formed from the haem and this is reduced to form bilirubin. The bilirubin produced is unconjugated and water-insoluble, and is transported to the liver attached to albumin. Bilirubin dissociates from albumin and is taken up by the hepatic cell membrane and transported to the endoplasmic reticulum by cytoplasmic proteins, where it is conjugated with glucuronic acid and excreted into bile. The microsomal enzyme, uridine diphosphoglucuronosyl transferase, catalyses the formation of bilirubin monoglucuronide and then diglucuronide. This conjugated bilirubin is water-soluble and is actively secreted into the bile canaliculi and excreted into the intestine within the bile (Fig. 8.5). It is not absorbed from the small intestine because of its large

Fig. 7.4 **Cholesterol synthesis and its conversion to primary and secondary bile acids.** All bile acids are normally conjugated with glycine or taurine.

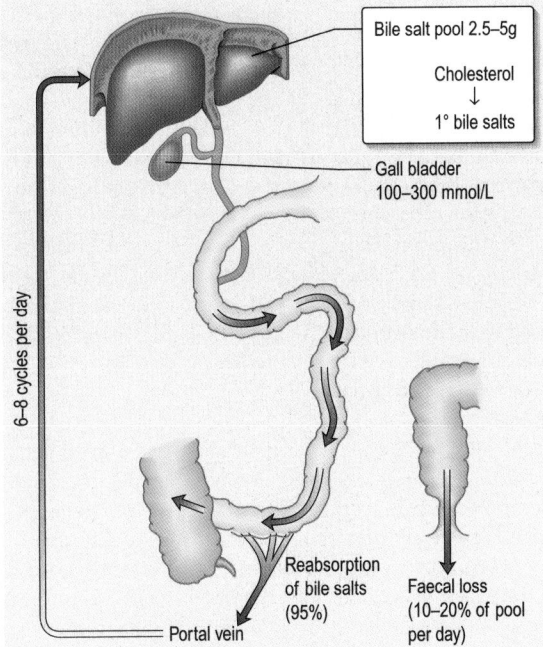

Fig. 7.5 **Recirculation of bile acids.** The bile salt pool is relatively small and the entire pool recycles six to eight times via the enterohepatic circulation. Up to 40 g are excreted daily into the bile and the synthesis of new bile acids only compensates for faecal loss.

molecular size. In the terminal ileum, bacterial enzymes hydrolyse the molecule, releasing free bilirubin, which is then reduced to urobilinogen. Some of this is excreted in the stools as stercobilinogen. The remainder is absorbed by the terminal ileum, passes to the liver via the enterohepatic circulation, and is re-excreted into the bile. Urobilinogen bound to albumin enters the circulation and is excreted in the urine via the kidneys. When hepatic excretion of conjugated bilirubin is impaired, a small amount of conjugated bilirubin is found strongly bound to serum albumin. It is not excreted by the kidneys and accounts for the continuing hyperbilirubinaemia for a short time after cholestasis has resolved.

Hormone and drug inactivation

The liver catabolizes hormones such as insulin, glucagon, oestrogens, growth hormone, glucocorticoids and parathyroid hormone. It is also the prime target organ for many hormones (e.g. insulin). It is the major site for the metabolism of drugs (see p. 993) and alcohol (see p. 262). Fat-soluble drugs are converted to water-soluble substances that facilitate their excretion in the bile or urine. Cholecalciferol is converted to 25-hydroxycholecalciferol.

Immunological function

The reticuloendothelial system of the liver contains many immunologically active cells. The liver acts as a 'sieve' for the bacterial and other antigens carried to it via the portal tract from the gastrointestinal tract. These antigens are phagocytosed and degraded by Kupffer cells, which are macrophages attached to the endothelium. Kupffer cells have specific membrane receptors for ligands and are activated by several factors, such as infection. They secrete interleukins, tumour necrosis factor (TNF), collagenase and lysosomal hydrolases. Antigens are degraded without the production of antibody, as there is very little lymphoid tissue. They are thus prevented from reaching other antibody-producing sites in the body and thereby prevent generalized adverse immunological reactions. The reticuloendothelial system plays a role in tissue repair, T and B lymphocyte interaction, and cytotoxic activity in disease processes. Following stimulation by, for example, endotoxin, the Kupffer cells release IL-6, IL-8 and TNF-α. These cytokines stimulate the sinusoidal cells, stellate cells and natural killer cells to release pro-inflammatory cytokines. The stimulated hepatocytes themselves express adhesion molecules and release IL-8, which is a potent neutrophil chemoattractant. Homing of mucosal lymphocytes (enterohepatic circulation) has been proposed. These exogenous leucocytes again release more cytokines – all damaging the function of the hepatocyte, including hepatocellular bile formation which leads to cholestasis. Cytokines also stimulate hepatic apoptosis.

INVESTIGATIONS

Investigative tests can be divided into:

- **Blood tests**
  - **(a)** Liver 'function' tests:
    - (i) serum albumin
    - (ii) prothrombin time
  - **(b)** Liver biochemistry:
    - (i) serum aspartate and alanine aminotransferases – reflecting hepatocellular damage
    - (ii) serum alkaline phosphatase, γ-glutamyl transpeptidase – reflecting cholestasis
    - (iii) total protein
  - **(c)** Viral markers
  - **(d)** Additional blood investigations; haematological, biochemical, immunological and genetic
- **Urine tests** – for bilirubin and urobilinogen
- **Imaging techniques** – to define gross anatomy
- **Liver biopsy** – for histology.

Most routine 'liver function tests' sent to the laboratory will be processed by an automated multichannel analyser to produce serum levels of bilirubin, aminotransferases, alkaline phosphatase, γ-glutamyl transpeptidase (γ-GT) and total proteins. These routine tests are markers of liver damage, but not actual tests of 'function' per se. Subsequent investigations are often based on these tests.

Blood tests

Useful blood tests for certain liver diseases are shown in Table 7.1.

Table 7.1 Useful blood tests for certain liver diseases

Test	Disease
Antimitochondrial antibody	Primary biliary cirrhosis
Antinuclear, smooth muscle (actin), liver/kidney microsomal antibody	Autoimmune hepatitis
Raised serum immunoglobulins:	
IgG	Autoimmune hepatitis
IgM	Primary biliary cirrhosis
Viral markers	Hepatitis A, B, C, D and others
α-Fetoprotein	Hepatocellular carcinoma
Serum iron, transferrin saturation, serum ferritin	Hereditary haemochromatosis
Serum and urinary copper, serum caeruloplasmin	Wilson's disease
α₁-Antitrypsin	Cirrhosis (± emphysema)
Antinuclear cytoplasmic antibodies	Primary sclerosing cholangitis
Genetic analyses	e.g. *HFE* gene (hereditary haemochromatosis)

Liver function tests
Serum albumin

This is a marker of synthetic function and is a valuable guide to the severity of chronic liver disease. A falling serum albumin in liver disease is a bad prognostic sign. In acute liver disease initial albumin levels may be normal.

Prothrombin time (PT)

This is also a marker of synthetic function. Because of its short half-life, it is a sensitive indicator of both acute and chronic liver disease. Vitamin K deficiency should be excluded as the cause of a prolonged PT by giving an intravenous bolus (10 mg) of vitamin K. Vitamin K deficiency commonly occurs in biliary obstruction, as the low intestinal concentration of bile salts results in poor absorption of vitamin K.

Prothrombin times vary in different laboratories depending upon the thromboplastin used in the assay. The International Normalized Ratio (INR) is therefore used in many countries (see p. 480).

Liver biochemistry
Bilirubin

In the serum, bilirubin is normally almost all unconjugated. In liver disease, increased serum bilirubin is usually accompanied by other abnormalities in liver biochemistry. Determination of whether the bilirubin is conjugated or unconjugated is only necessary in congenital disorders of bilirubin metabolism (see below) or to exclude haemolysis.

Aminotransferases

These enzymes (often referred to as transaminases) are present in hepatocytes and leak into the blood with liver cell damage. Two enzymes are measured:

- *Aspartate aminotransferase* (AST) is primarily a mitochondrial enzyme (80%; 20% in cytoplasm) and is also present in heart, muscle, kidney and brain. High levels are seen in hepatic necrosis, myocardial infarction, muscle injury and congestive cardiac failure.

- *Alanine aminotransferase* (ALT) is a cytosol enzyme, more specific to the liver so that a rise only occurs with liver disease.

Alkaline phosphatase (ALP)

This is present in the canalicular and sinusoidal membranes of the liver, but is also present in many other tissues, such as bone, intestine and placenta. If necessary, its origin can be determined by electrophoretic separation of isoenzymes or bone-specific monoclonal antibodies. Alternatively, if there is also an abnormality of, for example, the γ-GT, the ALP can be presumed to come from the liver.

Serum ALP is raised in cholestasis from any cause, whether intrahepatic or extrahepatic disease. The synthesis of ALP is increased and this is released into the blood. In cholestatic jaundice, levels may be four to six times the normal limit. Raised levels may also occur in conditions with infiltration of the liver (e.g. metastases) and in cirrhosis, frequently in the absence of jaundice. The highest serum levels due to liver disease (> 1000 IU/L) are seen with hepatic metastases and primary biliary cirrhosis.

γ-Glutamyl transpeptidase

This is a microsomal enzyme that is present in many tissues as well as the liver. Its activity can be induced by such drugs as phenytoin and by alcohol. If the ALP is normal, a raised serum γ-GT is a good guide to alcohol intake and can be used as a screening test (see p. 1303). Mild elevation of the γ-GT is common even with a small alcohol consumption and does not necessarily indicate liver disease if the other liver biochemical tests are normal. In cholestasis the γ-GT rises in parallel with the ALP as it has a similar pathway of excretion. This is also true of the 5-nucleotidase, another microsomal enzyme that can be measured in blood.

Total proteins

This measurement, in itself, is of little value. Serum albumin is discussed above. The globulin fraction consists of many proteins that can be separated on electrophoresis. A raised globulin fraction, seen in liver disease, is usually due to increased circulating immunoglobulins and is polyclonal (see below).

Viral markers

Viruses are a major cause of liver disease. Virological studies have a key role in diagnosis; markers are available for most common viruses that cause hepatitis.

Additional blood investigations

Haematological

A full blood count is always performed. Anaemia may be present. The red cells are often macrocytic and can have abnormal shapes – target cells and spur cells – owing to membrane abnormalities. Vitamin B_{12} levels are normal or high, while folate levels are often low owing to poor dietary intake. Other changes are caused by the following:

- Bleeding produces a hypochromic, microcytic picture.
- Alcohol causes macrocytosis, sometimes with leucopenia and thrombocytopenia.
- Hypersplenism results in pancytopenia.
- Cholestasis can often produce abnormal-shaped cells and also deficiency of vitamin K.
- Haemolysis accompanies acute liver failure and jaundice.
- Aplastic anaemia is present in up to 2% of patients with acute viral hepatitis.
- A raised serum ferritin with transferrin saturation (> 60%) is seen in hereditary haemochromatosis.

Biochemical

- $α_1$-*Antitrypsin*. A deficiency of this enzyme can produce cirrhosis.
- *α-Fetoprotein*. This is normally produced by the fetal liver. Its reappearance in increasing and high concentrations in the adult indicates hepatocellular carcinoma. Increased concentrations in pregnancy in the blood and amniotic fluid suggest neural-tube defects of the fetus. Blood levels are also slightly raised with regenerative liver tissue in patients with hepatitis, chronic liver disease and also in teratomas.
- Serum and urinary copper and serum caeruloplasmin – for Wilson's disease (see p. 387).

Immunological tests

There are no specific antibodies to the liver itself that are measured routinely.

Serum immunoglobulins

Increased γ-globulins are thought to be due to reduced phagocytosis by sinusoidal and Kupffer cells of the antigens absorbed from the gut. These antigens then stimulate antibody production in the spleen, lymph nodes and lymphoid and plasma cell infiltrate in the portal tracts. In primary biliary cirrhosis, the predominant serum immunoglobulin that is raised is IgM, while in autoimmune hepatitis it is IgG.

Serum autoantibodies

- *Antimitochondrial antibody* (AMA) is found in the serum in over 95% of patients with primary biliary cirrhosis (p. 385). Many different AMA subtypes have been described, depending on their antigen specificity. AMA is demonstrated by an immunofluorescent technique and is neither organ- nor species-specific. Some subtypes are occasionally found in autoimmune hepatitis and other autoimmune diseases.
- *Nucleic, smooth muscle (actin), liver/kidney microsomal antibodies* can be found in the serum in high titre in patients with autoimmune hepatitis. These antibodies can be found in the serum in other autoimmune conditions and other liver diseases.
- *Antinuclear cytoplasmic antibodies* (ANCA) are present in primary sclerosing cholangitis.

Genetic analysis

These tests are performed routinely for haemochromatosis (*HFE* gene). Markers are also available for Wilson's disease (see p. 387).

Bromsulphthalein (BSP) clearance test

This is now very rarely performed. The liver normally clears BSP from the blood. The level of BSP in the blood after an intravenous injection of BSP is a sensitive guide to hepatocellular damage. A second recirculation peak occurs in the congenital hyperbilirubinaemia of the Dubin–Johnson syndrome. Anaphylactic reactions may occur.

Urine tests

Dipstick tests are available for bilirubin and urobilinogen. Bilirubinuria is due to the presence of conjugated (soluble) bilirubin. It is found in the jaundiced patient with hepatobiliary disease; its absence implies that the jaundice is due to increased unconjugated bilirubin. Urobilinogen in the urine is, in practice, of little value but suggests haemolysis or hepatic dysfunction of any cause.

Imaging techniques

Ultrasound examination

This is a non-invasive, safe and relatively cheap technique. It involves the analysis of the reflected ultrasound beam detected by a probe moved across the abdomen. The normal liver appears as a relatively homogeneous structure. The gall bladder, common bile duct, pancreas, portal vein and other structures in the abdomen can be visualized. Abdominal ultrasound is useful in:

- a jaundiced patient (p. 358)
- hepatomegaly/splenomegaly
- the detection of gallstones (Fig. 7.6)
- focal liver disease – lesions > 1 cm
- general parenchymal liver disease
- assessing portal and hepatic vein patency
- lymph node enlargement.

Other abdominal masses can be delineated and biopsies obtained under ultrasonic guidance. Colour Doppler ultrasound will demonstrate the vascularity of a lesion and the direction of blood flow in the portal and hepatic veins. The introduction of ultrasound contrast agents, most of which are based on the production of micro-bubbles within the flowing blood, may enhance the vascularity within a lesion, allowing abnormal circulation to be detected within liver nodules, giving a more specific diagnosis of hepatocellular carcinoma.

Computed tomography (CT) examination

This technique is complementary to ultrasound, which should usually be performed first. It provides excellent visualization of the liver, pancreas, spleen, lymph nodes and lesions in the porta hepatis. CT allows assessment of the size, shape and density of the liver and can

Fig. 7.6 Gall bladder ultrasound with multiple echogenic gallstones causing well-defined acoustic shadowing. 1, gall bladder; 2, gallstones; 3, echogenic shadow.

characterize focal lesions in terms of their vascularity. CT is more sensitive in detecting calcification than plain X-rays. Ultrasound is usually more valuable for lesions in the bile duct and gall bladder, CT has advantages in obese subjects.

Spiral CT involves rapid acquisition of a volume of data during or immediately after i.v. contrast injection. Data can thus be acquired in both arterial and portal venous phases of enhancement, enabling more precise characterization of a lesion and its vascular supply (Fig. 7.7). Retrospective analysis of data allows multiple overlapping slices to be obtained with no increase in the radiation dose. Multi-planar and three-dimensional reconstruction in the arterial phase can create a CT angiogram, often making formal invasive angiography unnecessary. CT also provides guidance for biopsy. In general lesions over 2 cm can usually be biopsied under ultrasound guidance, which is quicker and more cost-effective.

Magnetic resonance imaging (MRI)

(see also p. 1202)

MRI produces cross-sectional images in any plane within the body. Diffuse liver disease alters the T1 and T2 characteristics, and MRI is probably the most sensitive investigation of focal liver disease. Other fat-suppression modes such as STIR allow good differentiation between haemangiomas and other lesions. Contrast agents such as intravenous gadolinium allow further characterization of lesions, and are suitable for those with iodine allergy and provide angiography and venography of the splanchnic circulation. This has superseded direct arteriography.

Magnetic resonance cholangiopancreatography (MRCP)

This technique involves the manipulation of a volume of data acquired by MRI. A heavily T2-weighted sequence

(a) Unenhanced.

(b) Arterial phase (note high density contrast in the aorta).

(c) Portal venous phase scan through the right lobe of the liver.

Fig. 7.7 **Use of contrast-enhanced spiral CT.**
There is an irregular mass (arrow) in the posterior aspect of the right lobe of the liver which is only well seen on the early arterial phase enhanced scan **(b)**.

enhances visualization of the 'water-filled' bile ducts and pancreatic ducts to produce high-quality images of ductal anatomy. This non-invasive technique is replacing diagnostic (but not therapeutic) ERCP (see below).

Plain X-rays of the abdomen

These are rarely requested but may show:

- gallstones – 10% contain enough calcium to be seen
- air in the biliary tree owing to its recent instrumentation, surgery or to a fistula between the intestine and the gall bladder
- pancreatic calcification
- rarely, calcification of the gall bladder (porcelain gall bladder).

Cholecystogram

This test is rarely required as it has been almost universally replaced by ultrasound but may be useful as a test of gall bladder function. Oral iopanoic acid is absorbed from the gut, conjugated in the liver, secreted in bile and concentrated in the gall bladder, which opacifies homogeneously. A fatty meal is given to make the gall bladder contract. The dye is excreted by the liver via the same mechanism as bilirubin, so that non-visualization will occur in the jaundiced patient and in the patient with liver disease.

Radionuclide imaging – scintiscanning

In a technetium-99m (^{99m}Tc) colloid scan, the colloid is injected intravenously to be taken up by the reticulo-endothelial cells of the liver and spleen. In chronic liver disease there is poor intake in the liver and most of the colloid is taken up in the spleen and bone marrow. Ultrasound has largely replaced this technique.

In a ^{99m}Tc-Iodida scan, technetium-labelled iododiethyl IDA is taken up by the hepatocytes and excreted rapidly into the biliary system. Its main uses are in the diagnosis of:

- acute cholecystitis
- jaundice due to either biliary atresia or hepatitis in the neonatal period.

Endoscopy

Upper GI endoscopy is used for the diagnosis and treatment of varices, for the detection of portal hypertensive gastropathy, and for associated lesions such as peptic ulcers. Colonoscopy may show portal hypertensive colopathy.

Endoscopic ultrasound (EUS)

In this technique, a small high-frequency ultrasound probe is mounted on the tip of an endoscope and placed by direct vision into the duodenum. The close proximity of the probe to the pancreas and biliary tree permits high-resolution ultrasound imaging. It allows accurate staging of small, potentially operable, pancreatic tumours and offers a less-invasive method for bile duct imaging. It has a high accuracy in detection of small neuroendocrine tumours of the pancreas. EUS-guided fine-needle aspiration of tumours provides cytological/histological tissue for confirmation of malignancy. EUS is also used to place transmural tubes to drain pancreatic and peri-pancreatic fluid collections.

Endoscopic retrograde cholangiopancreatography (ERCP)

This technique is used to outline the biliary and pancreatic ducts. It involves the passage of an endoscope into the second part of the duodenum and cannulation of the ampulla. Contrast is injected into both systems and the patient is screened radiologically. Contrast medium with a low iodine content of 1.5 mg/mL is used for the common bile duct so that gallstones are not obscured; a higher iodine content of 2.8 mg/mL is used for the pancreatic duct. In addition, other diagnostic and therapeutic procedures can be carried out:

- Common bile duct stones can be removed after a diathermy cut to the sphincter has been performed to facilitate their withdrawal (p. 403). Sphincterotomy has a serious morbidity rate of 3–5%: acute pancreatitis is the commonest, severe haemorrhage is rare. There is an overall mortality of 0.5–1%.
- The biliary system can be drained by passing a tube (stent) through an obstruction, or placement of a nasobiliary drain.
- Brachytherapy can be administered after placement at ERCP for therapy of cholangiocarcinoma.

The complication rate in diagnostic ERCP is 2–3%.

A raised serum amylase is often seen and pancreatitis is the most common complication. Cholangitis is also seen, and broad-spectrum antibiotics (e.g. 500 mg ciprofloxacin × 2) should be given prophylactically to all patients with suspected biliary obstruction, or a history of cholangitis.

Percutaneous transhepatic cholangiography (PTC)

Under a local anaesthetic, a fine flexible needle is passed into the liver. Contrast is injected slowly until a biliary radicle is identified and then further contrast is injected to outline the whole of the biliary tree. In patients with dilated ducts, the success rate is near 100%. ERCP is the preferred first investigation because therapy (e.g. stone removal) can be undertaken at the same time.

In difficult cases the two techniques are sometimes combined, PTC showing the biliary anatomy above the obstruction, with ERCP showing the more distal anatomy. If an obstruction in the bile ducts is seen, a bypass stent can sometimes be inserted, draining either externally or, for long-term use, internally. Contraindications are as for liver biopsy (see below). The main complications are bleeding and cholangitis with septicaemia, and prophylactic antibiotics should be given as for ERCP.

Angiography

This is performed by selective catheterization of the coeliac axis and hepatic artery. It detects the abnormal vasculature of hepatic tumours, but spiral CT and magnetic resonance angiography (MRA) have replaced this in many cases. The portal vein can be demonstrated with increased definition using subtraction techniques, and splenoportography (by direct splenic puncture) is rarely performed. In digital vascular imaging (DVI), contrast given intravenously or intra-arterially can be detected in the portal system using computerized subtraction analysis. Hepatic venous cannulation allows abnormal hepatic veins to be diagnosed in patients with Budd–Chiari syndrome and also serves as an indirect measurement of portal pressure. There is a 1 : 1 relationship of occluded (by balloon) hepatic venous pressure with portal pressure in patients with alcoholic or viral-related cirrhosis. The height of portal pressure has been shown to have prognostic value for survival and a reduced portal pressure 20% from baseline values has been associated with protection from rebleeding. Retrograde CO_2 portography is used when there is doubt about portal vein patency and can be combined with transjugular biopsy and hepatic venous pressure measurement.

Liver biopsy (see Practical box 7.1)

Histological examination of the liver is valuable in the differential diagnosis of diffuse or localized parenchymal disease. Liver biopsy can be performed on a day-case or overnight-stay basis. The indications and contraindications are shown in Table 7.2. The mortality rate is less than 0.02% when performed by experienced operators.

Practical Box 7.1
Needle biopsy of the liver

This should be performed only by experienced doctors and with sterile precautions. Patient consent must be obtained following explanation of the procedure.

- The patient's coagulation status (prothrombin time, platelets) is checked.
- The patient's blood group is checked and serum saved for crossmatching.
- The patient lies on his back at the edge of the couch.
- The liver margins are delineated using percussion. *Alternatively* ultrasound examination can be used to confirm liver margins and position of the gall bladder.
- Local anaesthetic is injected at the point of maximum dullness in the mid-axillary line through the intercostal space during expiration. Anaesthetic (1% lidocaine), approximately 5 mL) should be injected down to the liver capsule.
- A tiny cut is made in the skin with a scalpel blade.
- A special needle (Menghini, Trucut or Surecut) is used to obtain the liver biopsy whilst the patient holds his breath in expiration.
- The biopsy is laid on filter paper and placed in 10% formalin. If a culture of the biopsy is required it should be placed in a sterile pot.
- The patient should be observed, with pulse and blood pressure measurements taken regularly for at least 6 h.

Table 7.2 Indications and contraindications for liver biopsy

Indications
Liver disease
  Unexplained hepatomegaly
  Some cases of jaundice
  Persistently abnormal liver biochemistry
  Occasionally in acute hepatitis
  Chronic hepatitis
  Cirrhosis
  Drug-related liver disease
  Infiltrations
  Tumours: primary or secondary
  Infections (e.g. tuberculosis)
  Storage disease (e.g. glycogen storage)
Pyrexia of unknown origin

Usual contraindications to percutaneous needle biopsy
Uncooperative patient
Prolonged prothrombin time (by more than 3 s)
Platelets $< 80 \times 10^9$/L
Ascites
Extrahepatic cholestasis

Liver biopsy guided by ultrasound or CT is also performed particularly when specific lesions need to be biopsied. Laparoscopy with guided liver biopsy is performed through a small incision in the abdominal wall under local anaesthesia (general anaesthesia is preferred in some centres). A transjugular approach is used when liver histology is essential for management but coagulation abnormalities prevent the percutaneous approach.

Most complications of liver biopsy occur within 24 hours (usually in the first 2 hours). They are often minor and include abdominal or shoulder pain which settles with analgesics. Minor intraperitoneal bleeding can occur, but this settles spontaneously. Rare complications include major intraperitoneal bleeding, haemothorax and pleurisy, biliary peritonitis, haemobilia and transient septicaemia. Haemobilia produces biliary colic, jaundice and melaena within 3 days of the biopsy.

FURTHER READING
Baillie J et al (2003) Biliary imaging. *Gastroenterology* **124**: 1696–1699.
British Society of Gastroenterology (2004) Guidelines on the use of liver biopsy in clinical practice. bsg.org.uk/clinical-prac/guidelines/liver-biop.htm
Green RM, Flamm S (2002) AGA technical revew on the evaluation of liver chemistry tests. *Gastroenterology* **123**: 1367–1384.

SYMPTOMS OF LIVER DISEASE

Acute liver disease
This may be asymptomatic and anicteric. Symptomatic disease, which is often viral, produces generalized symptoms of malaise, anorexia and fever. Jaundice may appear as the illness progresses.

Chronic liver disease
Patients may be asymptomatic or complain of non-specific symptoms, particularly fatigue. Specific symptoms include:

- right hypochondrial pain due to liver distension
- abdominal distension due to ascites
- ankle swelling due to fluid retention
- haematemesis and melaena from gastrointestinal haemorrhage
- pruritus due to cholestasis – this is often an early symptom of primary biliary cirrhosis
- breast swelling (gynaecomastia), loss of libido and amenorrhoea due to endocrine dysfunction
- confusion and drowsiness due to neuropsychiatric complications (portosystemic encephalopathy).

SIGNS OF LIVER DISEASE

Acute liver disease
There may be few signs apart from jaundice and an enlarged liver. Jaundice is a yellow coloration of the skin and mucous membranes and is best seen in the conjunctivae and sclerae. In the cholestatic phase of the illness, pale stools and dark urine are present. Spider naevi and liver palms usually indicate chronic disease but they can occur in severe acute disease.

Chronic liver disease
The physical signs are shown in Figure 7.8. However, it is possible for the physical examination to be normal in patients with advanced chronic liver disease.

The skin
The chest and upper body may show spider naevi. These are telangiectases that consist of a central arteriole with radiating small vessels. They are found in the distribution of the superior vena cava (i.e. above the nipple line). They are also found in pregnancy. In haemochromatosis the skin may have a slate-grey appearance.

The hands may show palmar erythema, which is a non-specific change indicative of a hyperdynamic circulation; it is also seen in pregnancy, thyrotoxicosis or rheumatoid arthritis. Clubbing occasionally occurs, and a Dupuytren's contracture is often seen in alcoholic cirrhosis.

Xanthomas (cholesterol deposits) are seen in the palmar creases or above the eyes in primary biliary cirrhosis.

The abdomen
Initial hepatomegaly will be followed by a small liver in well-established cirrhosis. Splenomegaly is seen with portal hypertension.

The endocrine system
Gynaecomastia (occasionally unilateral) and testicular atrophy may be found in males. The cause of

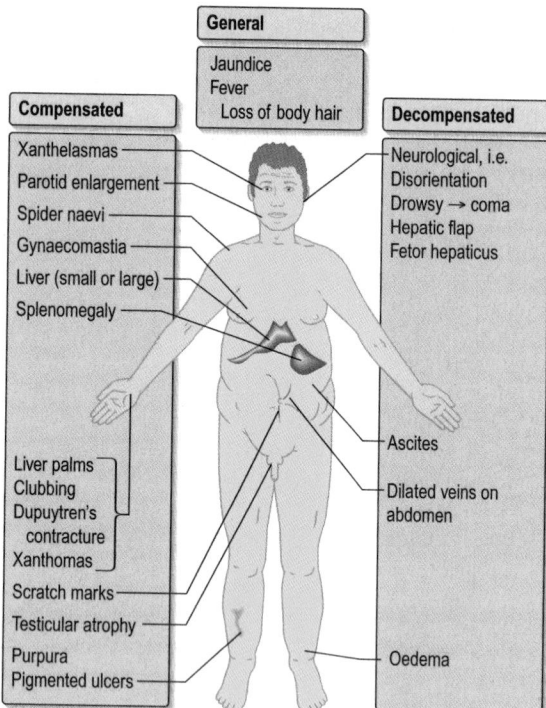

General
- Jaundice
- Fever
- Loss of body hair

Compensated
- Xanthelasmas
- Parotid enlargement
- Spider naevi
- Gynaecomastia
- Liver (small or large)
- Splenomegaly

- Liver palms
- Clubbing
- Dupuytren's contracture
- Xanthomas
- Scratch marks
- Testicular atrophy
- Purpura
- Pigmented ulcers

Decompensated
- Neurological, i.e.
- Disorientation
- Drowsy → coma
- Hepatic flap
- Fetor hepaticus

- Ascites
- Dilated veins on abdomen
- Oedema

Fig. 7.8   **Physical signs in chronic liver disease.**

gynaecomastia is complex, but it is probably related to altered oestrogen metabolism or to treatment with spironolactone.

In decompensated cirrhosis, additional signs that can be seen are shown in Figure 7.8.

JAUNDICE

Jaundice (icterus) is detectable clinically when the serum bilirubin is greater than 50 µmol/L (3 mg/dL). The usual division of jaundice into prehepatic, hepatocellular and obstructive (cholestatic) is an oversimplification as in hepatocellular jaundice there is invariably cholestasis and the clinical problem is whether the cholestasis is intrahepatic or extrahepatic. Jaundice will therefore be considered under the following headings:

- haemolytic jaundice – increased bilirubin load for the liver cells
- congenital hyperbilirubinaemias – defects in conjugation
- cholestatic jaundice, including hepatocellular (parenchymal) liver disease and large duct obstruction.

Haemolytic jaundice

The increased breakdown of red cells (see p. 424) leads to an increase in production of bilirubin. The resulting jaundice is usually mild (serum bilirubin of 68–102 µmol/L or 4–6 mg/dL) as normal liver function can easily handle the increased bilirubin derived from excess haemolysis.

Unconjugated bilirubin is not water-soluble and therefore will not pass into the urine; hence the term 'acholuric jaundice'. Urinary urobilinogen is increased.

The causes of haemolytic jaundice are those of haemolytic anaemia (p. 438). The clinical features depend on the cause; anaemia, jaundice, splenomegaly, gallstones and leg ulcers may be seen.

Investigations show features of haemolysis (p. 437). The level of unconjugated bilirubin is raised but the serum ALP, transferases and albumin are normal. Serum haptoglobulins are low. The differential diagnosis is from other forms of jaundice.

Congenital hyperbilirubinaemias (non-haemolytic)

Unconjugated
Gilbert's syndrome

This is the most common familial hyperbilirubinaemia and affects 2–7% of the population. It is asymptomatic and is usually detected as an incidental finding of a slightly raised bilirubin (17–102 µmol/L or 1–6 mg/dL) on a routine check. All the other liver biochemistry is normal and no signs of liver disease are seen. There is a family history of jaundice in 5–15% of patients. Hepatic glucuronidation is approximately 30% of normal, resulting in an increased proportion of bilirubin monoglucuronide in bile. Most patients have reduced levels of UDP-glucuronosyl transferase (UGT-1) activity, the enzyme that conjugates bilirubin with glucuronic acid. Mutations occur in the gene (*HUG-Br1*) encoding this enzyme, with an expanded nucleotide repeat consisting of two extra bases in the upstream 5′ promoter element. This abnormality appears to be necessary for the syndrome, but is not in itself sufficient for the phenotypic expression of the syndrome.

The major importance of establishing this diagnosis is to inform the patient that this is not a serious disease and to prevent unnecessary investigations. The raised unconjugated bilirubin rises on fasting and during a mild illness. The reticulocyte count is normal, excluding haemolysis and no treatment is necessary.

Crigler–Najjar syndrome

This is very rare. Only patients with type II (autosomal dominant) with a decrease rather than absence (type I – autosomal recessive) of UDP-glucuronosyl transferase can survive into adult life. Mutation of the *HUG-Br1* gene for UDP-glucuronosyl transferase has been demonstrated in the coding region. Liver histology is normal. Transplantation is the only effective treatment.

Conjugated

Dubin–Johnson (autosomal recessive) and *Rotor's* (possibly autosomal dominant) *syndromes* are due to defects in bilirubin handling in the liver. The prognosis is good in both. In the Dubin–Johnson syndrome there are mutations in both *MRP2* (p. 349) transporter genes.

The liver is black owing to melanin deposition.

Recurrent familial intrahepatic cholestasis (FIC1), benign recurrent intrahepatic cholestasis

This is rare. Recurrent attacks of acute cholestasis occur without progression to chronic liver disease. Jaundice, severe pruritus, steatorrhoea and weight loss develop. Serum γ-GT is normal. The gene has been mapped to the FIC1 locus, but the precise relation to cholestasis is unclear.

Progressive familial intrahepatic cholestasis syndromes

These are autosomal recessive. In *type 1*, with cholestasis in infancy (previously known as Byler's disease), γ-GT is normal. The gene is also on the FIC1 locus, but has been mapped to a region encoding P type ATPases. *Type 2* has been mapped to the bile salt export pump gene (*BSEP*). The protein is located in the canalicular domain of the plasma membrane of the hepatocyte. The phenotypic expression frequently presents as a non-specific giant cell hepatitis progressing to cholestasis. *Type 3* is due to *PGY3* gene mutation leading to deficient canalicular phosphatidylcholine transport and thus toxic bile causing liver damage. Liver transplantation is the only cure for these syndromes.

Intrahepatic cholestasis of pregnancy

This has been associated with mutations in the genes of the progressive familial intrahepatic cholestasis syndromes. It is described on page 393.

FURTHER READING
Jansen PLM, Muller M (2000) The molecular genetics of familial intrahepatic cholestasis. *Gut* **47**: 1–5.

Cholestatic jaundice (acquired)

This can be divided into extrahepatic and intrahepatic cholestasis. The causes are shown in Figure 7.9.

■ Extrahepatic cholestasis is due to large duct obstruction of bile flow at any point in the biliary tract distal to the bile canaliculi.

■ Intrahepatic cholestasis occurs owing to failure of bile secretion. A number of cellular mechanisms in cholestasis have been described in animal models, including inhibition of the Na^+–K^+-ATPase in the basolateral membranes, decreased fluidity of the sinusoidal plasma membrane, disruption of the microfilaments responsible for canalicular tone, and damage to the tight junctions. In addition, inflammatory change in ductular cells interferes with bile flow.

Clinically in both types there is jaundice with pale stools and dark urine, and the serum bilirubin is conjugated. However, intrahepatic and extrahepatic cholestatic jaundice must be differentiated as their clinical management is entirely different.

Differential diagnosis of jaundice

A careful history may give a clue to the diagnosis. Certain causes of jaundice are more likely in particular categories of people. For example, a young person is more likely to have hepatitis, so questions should be asked about drug and alcohol use, and sexual behaviour. An elderly person with gross weight loss is more likely to have a carcinoma. All patients may complain of malaise. Abdominal pain occurs in patients with biliary obstruction by gallstones and, sometimes with an enlarged liver there is pain resulting from distension of the capsule.

Questions should be appropriate to the particular situation, and the following aspects of the history should be covered.

■ *Country of origin.* The incidence of hepatitis B virus (HBV) infection is increased in many parts of the world (p. 364).
■ *Duration of illness.* A history of jaundice with prolonged weight loss in an older patient suggests malignancy. A short history, particularly with a prodromal illness of malaise, suggests a hepatitis.
■ *Recent outbreak of jaundice.* An outbreak in the community suggests hepatitis A virus (HAV).

Fig. 7.9 Causes of jaundice.

Types	HAEMOGLOBIN	Causes
Prehepatic	↓ BILIRUBIN	Haemolysis
Cholestatic	↓ CONJUGATION	Viral hepatitis Drugs Alcoholic hepatitis Cirrhosis – any type Pregnancy Recurrent idiopathic cholestasis Some congenital disorders Infiltrations
Intrahepatic		

Extrahepatic	GALL BLADDER
	PANCREAS
		Common duct stones
		Carcinoma
		    – bile duct
		    – head of pancreas
		    – ampulla
		Biliary stricture
		Sclerosing cholangitis
		Pancreatitis pseudocyst

- *Recent consumption of shellfish.* This suggests HAV infection.
- *Intravenous drug abuse, or recent injections or tattoos.* These all increase the chance of HBV and hepatitis C virus (HCV) infection.
- *Male homosexuality.* This increases the chance of HBV infection.
- *Female prostitution.* This increases the chance of HBV infection.
- *Blood transfusion or infusion of pooled blood products.* Increased risk of HBV and HCV. In developed countries all donors are screened for HBV and HCV.
- *Alcohol consumption.* A careful history of drinking habits should be taken, although many patients often understate the actual amount they drink.
- *Drugs taken* (particularly in the previous 2–3 months). Many drugs cause jaundice (see p. 396).
- *Travel.* Certain areas have an increased risk of HAV infection as well as hepatitis E (HEV) infection (this has a high mortality in pregnancy).
- *A recent anaesthetic.* Halothane (see p. 396) and occasionally enflurane, isoflurane, for example, may cause jaundice, particularly in those already sensitive to halogenated anaesthetics. The risk with desflurane appears remote.
- *Family history.* Patients with, for example, Gilbert's disease may have family members who get recurrent jaundice.
- *Recent surgery* on the biliary tract or for carcinoma.
- *Environment.* People engaged in recreational activities in rural areas, as well as farm and sewage workers, are at risk for leptospirosis.
- *Fevers or rigors.* These are suggestive of cholangitis or possibly a liver abscess.

Clinical features

The signs of acute and chronic liver disease should be looked for (p. 358). Certain additional signs may be helpful:

- **Hepatomegaly.** A smooth tender liver is seen in hepatitis and with extrahepatic obstruction, but a knobbly irregular liver suggests metastases. Causes of hepatomegaly are shown in Table 7.3.
- **Splenomegaly.** This indicates portal hypertension in patients when signs of chronic liver disease are present. The spleen can also be 'tipped' occasionally in viral hepatitis.
- **Ascites.** This is found in cirrhosis but can also be due to carcinoma (particularly ovarian) and many other causes (see Table 7.14).

A palpable gall bladder can suggest a carcinoma of the pancreas obstructing the bile duct. Generalized lymphadenopathy suggests a lymphoma.

Cold sores may suggest a herpes simplex virus hepatitis.

Investigations

Jaundice is not itself a diagnosis and the cause should always be sought. The two most useful tests are

---

Table 7.3 Causes of hepatomegaly

Apparent	Haematological
Low-lying diaphragm	Leukaemias
Reidel's lobe	Lymphoma
	Myeloproliferative disorders
Cirrhosis (early)	Thalassaemia
Inflammation	**Tumours: primary and**
Hepatitis	**secondary carcinoma**
Schistosomiasis	
Abscesses (pyogenic or	**Venous congestion**
amoebic)	Heart failure
	Hepatic vein occlusion
Cysts	
Hydatid	**Biliary obstruction**
Polycystic	**(particularly extrahepatic)**
Metabolic	
Fatty liver	
Amyloid	
Glycogen storage disease	

---

the viral markers for HAV, HBV and HCV (in high-risk groups), plus an ultrasound examination. Liver biochemistry confirms the jaundice and may help in the diagnosis.

An ultrasound examination should always be performed to exclude an extrahepatic obstruction, and to diagnose any features compatible with chronic liver disease except when hepatitis A is strongly suspected in a young patient. Ultrasound will demonstrate:

- the size of the bile ducts, which are dilated in extrahepatic obstruction (Fig. 7.10)
- the level of the obstruction
- the cause of the obstruction in virtually all patients with tumours and in 75% of patients with gallstones.

The pathological diagnosis of any mass lesion can be made by fine-needle aspiration cytology (sensitivity approximately 60%) or by needle biopsy using a spring-loaded device (sensitivity approximately 90%).

A flow diagram for the general investigation of the jaundiced patient is shown in Figure 7.11.

Liver biochemistry

In hepatitis, the serum AST or ALT tends to be high early in the disease with only a small rise in the serum ALP. Conversely, in extrahepatic obstruction the ALP is high with a smaller rise in aminotransferases. These findings cannot, however, be relied on alone to make a diagnosis in an individual case. The prothrombin time (PT) is often prolonged in long-standing liver disease, and the serum albumin is also low.

Haematological tests

In haemolytic jaundice the bilirubin is raised and the other liver biochemistry is normal (p. 358). A raised white cell count may indicate infection (e.g. cholangitis). A leucopenia often occurs in viral hepatitis, while abnormal mononuclear cells suggest infectious mononucleosis and a Monospot test should be performed.

(a)　　　　　　　　　　　　　　　　　　　(b)

Fig. 7.10 **Liver ultrasound showing (a) dilated intrahepatic bile ducts (arrow), (b) common bile duct (arrow).** The normal bile duct measures 6 mm at the porta hepatis.

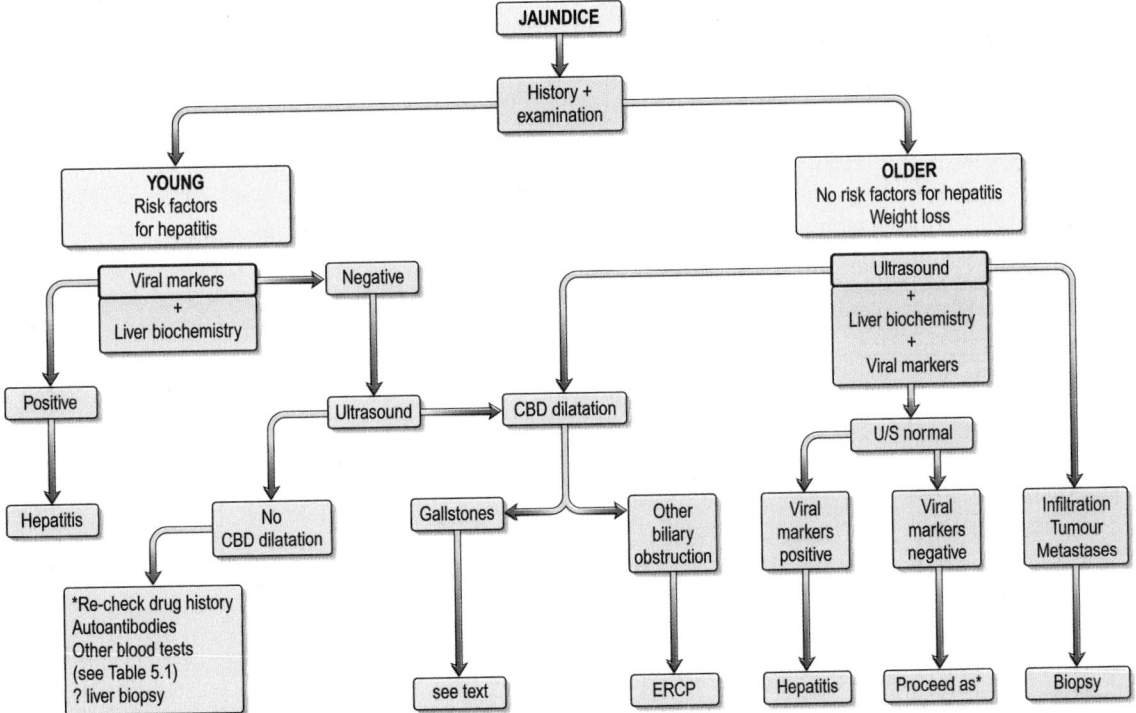

Fig. 7.11 **Approach to patient with jaundice.** ERCP, endoscopic retrograde cholangiopancreatography; CBD, common bile duct; US, ultrasound; MRCP, magnetic resonance cholangiopancreatography.

Other blood tests

These include tests to exclude unusual causes of liver disease (e.g. cytomegalovirus antibodies), autoimmune antibodies, e.g. antimitochondrial antibodies (AMA) for the diagnosis of primary biliary cirrhosis, and α-fetoprotein for a hepatocellular carcinoma.

ACUTE HEPATITIS

Acute parenchymal liver damage can be caused by many agents (Fig. 7.12).

Pathology

Although some histological features are suggestive of the aetiological factor, most of the changes are essentially

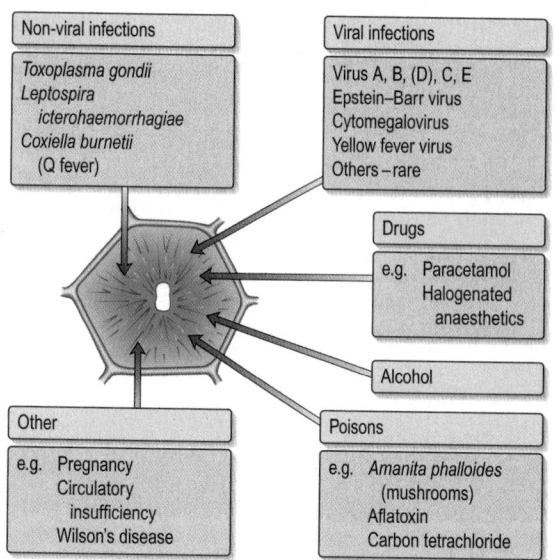

Fig. 7.12 Some causes of acute parenchymal damage.

Non-viral infections

Toxoplasma gondii
Leptospira
  icterohaemorrhagiae
Coxiella burnetii
  (Q fever)

Viral infections

Virus A, B, (D), C, E
Epstein–Barr virus
Cytomegalovirus
Yellow fever virus
Others –rare

Drugs

e.g. Paracetamol
      Halogenated
      anaesthetics

Alcohol

Other

e.g. Pregnancy
      Circulatory
      insufficiency
      Wilson's disease

Poisons

e.g. Amanita phalloides
      (mushrooms)
      Aflatoxin
      Carbon tetrachloride

similar whatever the cause. Hepatocytes show degenerative changes (swelling, cytoplasmic granularity, vacuolation), undergo necrosis (becoming shrunken, eosinophilic Councilman bodies) and are rapidly removed. The distribution of these changes varies somewhat with the aetiological agent, but necrosis is usually maximal in zone 3. The extent of the damage is very variable between individuals affected by the same agent: at one end of the spectrum, single and small groups of hepatocytes die (spotty or focal necrosis), while at the other end there is multiacinar necrosis involving a substantial part of the liver (massive hepatic necrosis) resulting in fulminant hepatic failure. Between these extremes there is limited confluent necrosis with collapse of the reticulin framework resulting in linking (bridging) between the central veins, the central veins and portal tracts, and between the portal tracts. The extent of the inflammatory infiltrate is also variable, but portal tracts and lobules are infiltrated mainly by lymphocytes. Other variable features include cholestasis in zone 3 and fatty change, the latter being prominent in hepatitis that is due to alcohol or certain drugs.

Management

This is discussed below under the individual aetiological factors.

VIRAL HEPATITIS

The differing features of the common forms of viral hepatitis are summarized in Table 7.4.

Hepatitis A

Hepatitis A virus (HAV)

HAV is a picornavirus, having the structure shown in Figure 7.13. It has a single serotype as only one epitope is immunodominant. It replicates in the liver, is excreted in

Table 7.4   Some features of hepatitis viruses

	A	B	D	C	E
Virus	RNA	DNA	RNA	RNA	RNA
	27 nm	42 nm	36 nm	approx. 50 nm	27 nm
			(with HBsAg coat)		
	Picorna	Hepadna	Unclassified	Flavi	Calici
Spread					
Faeco-oral	Yes	No	No	No	Yes
Blood/blood products	Rare	Yes	Yes	Yes	No
Vertical	No	Yes	Rare	Occasional	No
Saliva	Yes	Yes	Yes	? No	?
Sexual	Rare	Yes	Yes (rare)	Uncommon	No
Incubation	Short (2–3 weeks)	Long (1–5 months)	Long	Intermediate	Short
Age	Young	Any	Any	Any	Any
Carrier state	No	Yes	Yes	?	No
Chronic liver disease	No	Yes	Yes	Yes	No
Liver cancer	No	Yes	Yes	Yes	No
Mortality (acute)	< 0.5%	< 1%	Rare	< 1%	1–2% (pregnant women 10–20%)
Immunization:					
Passive	Normal immunoglobulin serum i.m. (0.04–0.06 mL/kg)	Hepatitis B immunoglobulin (HBIg)	No	No	No
Active	Vaccine	Vaccine	HBV vaccine	No	No

Fig. 7.13 **(a)** The hepatitis A (HAV) virion consists of four polypeptides (VP1–VP4) which form a tight protein shell, or capsid, containing the RNA. The major antigenic component is associated with VP1. **(b)** Arrangement of HAV genome.

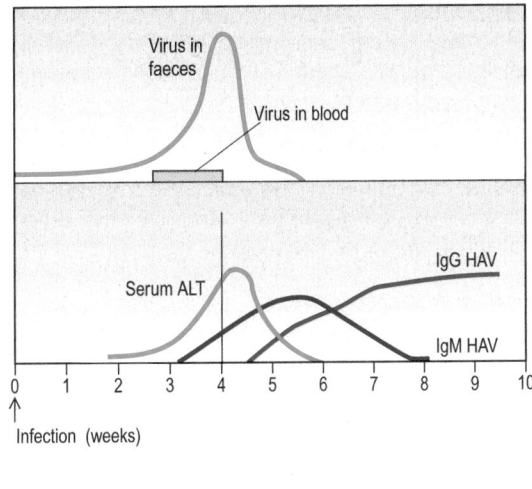

Fig. 7.14 HAV – sequence of events after exposure.

Occasionally, tender lymphadenopathy is seen, with a transient rash in some cases. Thereafter the jaundice lessens and in the majority of cases the illness is over within 3–6 weeks. Extrahepatic complications are rare but include arthritis, vasculitis, myocarditis and renal failure. A biphasic illness occasionally occurs, with the return of jaundice. Rarely the disease may be very severe with fulminant hepatitis, liver coma and death. The typical sequence of events after HAV exposure is shown in Figure 7.14.

Investigations

Liver biochemistry
In the prodromal stage the serum bilirubin is usually normal. However, there is bilirubinuria and increased urinary urobilinogen. A raised serum AST or ALT, which can sometimes be very high, precedes the jaundice.

In the icteric stage the serum bilirubin reflects the level of jaundice. Serum AST reaches a maximum 1–2 days after the appearance of jaundice, and may rise above 500 IU/L. Serum ALP is usually less than 300 IU/L.

After the jaundice has subsided, the aminotransferases may remain elevated for some weeks and occasionally for up to 6 months.

Haematological tests
There is leucopenia with a relative lymphocytosis. Very rarely there is a Coombs'-positive haemolytic anaemia or an associated aplastic anaemia. The prothrombin time (PT) is prolonged in severe cases. The erythrocyte sedimentation rate (ESR) is raised.

Viral markers: antibodies to HAV
IgG antibodies are common in the general population over the age of 50 years, but an anti-HAV IgM means an acute infection. In areas of high prevalence most children have antibodies by the age of 3 years following asymptomatic infection.

bile and is then excreted in the faeces of infected persons for about 2 weeks before the onset of clinical illness and for up to 7 days after. The disease is maximally infectious just before the onset of jaundice. HAV particles can be demonstrated in the faeces by electron microscopy.

Epidemiology

Hepatitis A is the most common type of viral hepatitis occurring world-wide, often in epidemics. The disease is commonly seen in the autumn and affects children and young adults. Spread of infection is mainly by the faeco-oral route and arises from the ingestion of contaminated food or water (e.g. shellfish). Overcrowding and poor sanitation facilitate spread. There is no carrier state. In the UK it is a notifiable disease.

Clinical features

The viraemia causes the patient to feel unwell with non-specific symptoms that include nausea, anorexia and a distaste for cigarettes. Many recover at this stage and remain anicteric.

After 1 or 2 weeks some patients become jaundiced and symptoms often improve. As the jaundice deepens, the urine becomes dark and the stools pale owing to intrahepatic cholestasis. The liver is moderately enlarged and the spleen is palpable in about 10% of patients.

Other tests

Further tests are not necessary in the presence of an IgM antibody, but liver biochemistry must be followed to establish a return to normal levels.

Differential diagnosis

Clinically the differential diagnosis is from all other causes of jaundice – but in particular from other types of viral and drug-induced hepatitis.

Course and prognosis

The prognosis is excellent, with most patients making a complete recovery. The mortality in young adults is 0.1% but it increases with age. Death is due to fulminant hepatic necrosis. During convalescence, 5–15% of patients may have relapse of the hepatitis but this settles spontaneously. Occasionally a more severe jaundice with cholestasis will run a prolonged course of 7–20 weeks and is called 'cholestatic viral hepatitis'.

There is no reason to stop alcohol consumption other than for the few weeks when the patient is ill. Patients may complain of debility for several months following resolution of the symptoms and biochemical parameters. This is known as the post-hepatitis syndrome; it is a functional illness. Treatment is by reassurance. HAV hepatitis never progresses to chronic liver disease.

Treatment

There is no specific treatment, and rest and dietary measures are unhelpful. Corticosteroids have no benefit. Admission to hospital is not usually necessary.

Prevention and prophylaxis

Control of hepatitis depends on good hygiene. The virus is resistant to chlorination but is killed by boiling water for 10 minutes.

Active immunization

A formaldehyde-inactivated HAV vaccine is given to people travelling frequently to endemic areas, patients with chronic liver disease, people with haemophilia, and workers in frequent contact with hepatitis cases (e.g. in residential institutions for patients with learning difficulties). Community outbreaks can be interrupted by vaccination. A single dose produces antibodies that persist for at least 1 year, with immunity lasting beyond 10 years. This obviates the need for a booster injection in healthy individuals. Universal vaccination has been suggested.

Passive immunization

Normal human immunoglobulin (0.04–0.06 mL/kg i.m.) gives protection for 3–4 months but is not used routinely. It is used for close contacts of patients with hepatitis A.

Hepatitis B

Hepatitis B virus (HBV)

The complete infective virion or Dane particle is a 42 nm particle comprising an inner core or nucleocapsid (27 nm) surrounded by an outer envelope of surface protein (HBsAg). This surface coat is produced in excess by the infected hepatocytes and can exist separately from the whole virion in serum and body fluid as 22 nm particles or 22 nm tubules.

HBsAg contains a major 'a' antigenic determinant as well as several subtypes: 'd', 'y', 'w' and 'r'. Combinations of these subdeterminants (e.g. adr, adw, ayw and ayr) are used to classify HBV genotypes A–G, of which 35% are type A, 22% B, 31%C and 10% D. There is a strong correlation between genotypes and ethnicity.

The core or nucleocapsid is formed of core protein (HBcAg) containing incompletely double-stranded circular DNA and the DNA polymerase/reverse transcriptase. One strand is almost a complete circle and contains overlapping genes that encode both structural proteins (pre-S, surface (S), core (C)) and replicative proteins (polymerase and X). The other strand is variable in length (Fig. 7.15).

HBeAg is a protein formed via specific self-cleavage of the pre-core/core gene product which is secreted separately by the cell.

Pre-S_1 and pre-S_2 regions are involved in attachment to the specific HBV receptor on the hepatocyte. After penetration, the virus core is transported to the nucleus without processing, with transcription of HBV into mRNA taking place.

Translation into HBV proteins (Table 7.5) as well as replication of the genome takes place in the endoplasmic reticulum; they are then packaged together and exported from the cell. During the period of replication, the viral genome may integrate into the chromosomal DNA of the hepatocyte.

The HBV is not directly cytopathic and the liver damage produced is by the cellular immune response of the host. Specific failure of T cells to recognize HBV antigens leads to viral persistence.

Fig. 7.15 Hepatitis B virus (HBV) genome. The viral DNA is partially double-stranded (red incomplete circle and blue circle). The long strand (blue) encodes seven proteins from four overlapping reading frames (S, surface (Pre-S_1, Pre-S_2, S); C, core (Pre-C, C) P, polymerase (P) and X gene (X)). EcoRI restriction-enzyme-binding site is included as a reference point.

Table 7.5	HBV proteins
HBV protein	**Significance**
Core	Protein of core particle; kinase activity (role in replication?)
Pre-core (HBeAg)	Pre-core/core cleaves to HBeAg; good marker of active replication and role in inducing immunotolerance
Surface (HBsAg)	Envelope protein of HBV; basis of current vaccine
Pre-S$_2$ Pre-S$_1$ }	HBV binding and entry into hepatocytes
Polymerase	Viral replication
X protein	Transcriptional and transactivator activity

(a) Acute infection

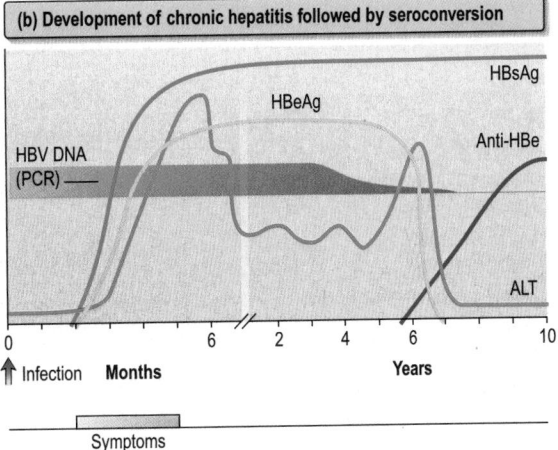

(b) Development of chronic hepatitis followed by seroconversion

Fig. 7.16 Time course of the events and serological changes seen following infection with hepatitis B virus.

(a) Acute infection

Antigens

HBsAg appears in the blood from about 6 weeks to 3 months after an acute infection and then disappears.

HBeAg rises early and usually declines rapidly.

Antibodies

Anti-HBs appears late and indicates immunity.

Anti-HBc is the first antibody to appear and high titres of IgM anti-HBc suggest an acute and continuing viral replication. It persists for many months. IgM anti-HBc may be the only serological indicator of recent HBV infection in a period when HBsAg has disappeared and anti-HBs is not detectable in the serum.

Anti-HBe appears after the anti-HBc and its appearance relates to a decreased infectivity, i.e. a low risk.

(b) Development of chronic hepatitis followed by seroconversion.

HBsAg persists and indicates a chronic infection (or carrier state).

HBeAg persists and correlates with increased severity and infectivity and the development of chronic liver disease. When anti-HBe develops (seroconversion) the Ag disappears and there is a rise in ALT.

HBV DNA suggests continual viral replication.

For **mutants** – see text.

Hepatitis B mutants

Mutations occur in the various reading frames of the HBV genome (see Fig. 7.15). These mutants can emerge in chronic HBV carriers or can be acquired by infection. Patients have HBsAg and HBV DNA but not the e antigen itself: anti-HBe is present in almost all cases. The amino acid sequence of the e antigen protein is almost identical to that of the core antigen which is involved in viral replication. Separate messenger RNAs have not been described for the two antigens, but HBeAg is initiated several nucleotides upstream of HBcAg. A guanosine (G) to adenosine (A) mutation in the pre-core region of the genome creates a stop codon (TAG) that prevents the production of HBeAg, but the synthesis of HBcAg is unaffected. Different mutants have also been seen following interferon or lamivudine therapy and in patients with fulminant and fatal hepatitis. Their existence means that serological markers such as the HBeAg are less useful in detecting infectivity and HBV DNA must be always measured.

Epidemiology

The hepatitis B virus is present world-wide with an estimated 300 million carriers. The UK and the USA have a low carrier rate (0.5%), but it rises to 10–15% in parts of Africa, the Middle and the Far East.

Spread of this virus is either by the intravenous route (e.g. by transfusion of infected blood or blood products, or by contaminated needles used by drug addicts, tattooists or acupuncturists), or by close personal contact, such as during sexual intercourse, particularly in male homosexuals. The virus can be found in semen and saliva. Vertical transmission from mother to child during parturition or soon after birth is the usual means of transmission world-wide. There is no evidence that HBV replicates in insect vectors but the virus has been detected in mosquitoes and bed bugs.

Clinical features

The sequence of events following acute HBV infection is shown in Figure 7.16. In many cases, however, the infection is subclinical. The clinical picture is the same as that found in HAV infection, although the illness may be more severe. In addition, a serum sickness-like immunological syndrome may be seen. This consists of rashes (e.g. urticaria or a maculopapular rash) and poly-arthritis affecting small joints occurring in up to 25% of cases in the prodromal period. Fever is usual. Extra-hepatic immune complex-mediated conditions such as an arteritis or glomerulonephritis are occasionally seen.

Investigations

These are generally the same as for hepatitis A.

Specific tests

The markers for HBV are shown in Table 7.6. HBsAg is looked for initially; if it is found, a full viral profile is then performed. In acute infection, as HBsAg may be cleared rapidly, anti-HBc IgM is diagnostic. HBV DNA is the most sensitive index of viral replication and is found without e antigen in hepatitis due to mutants. HBV DNA has been shown to persist (using PCR techniques) even when the e antibody has developed.

Course

The majority of patients recover completely, fulminant hepatitis occurring in up to 1%. Some patients go on to develop chronic hepatitis (p. 370) and hepatocellular carcinoma (p. 394) or become asymptomatic carriers (Fig. 7.17). The outcome depends upon several factors, including the virulence of the virus and the immuno-competence and age of the patient as well as some genetic factors, while abnormalities in mannan-binding protein (p. 200) may alter host defence to HBV.

Treatment

There is no specific treatment apart from symptomatic therapy.

Prevention and prophylaxis

Prevention depends on avoiding risk factors, such as shared needles, multiple male homosexual partners, and

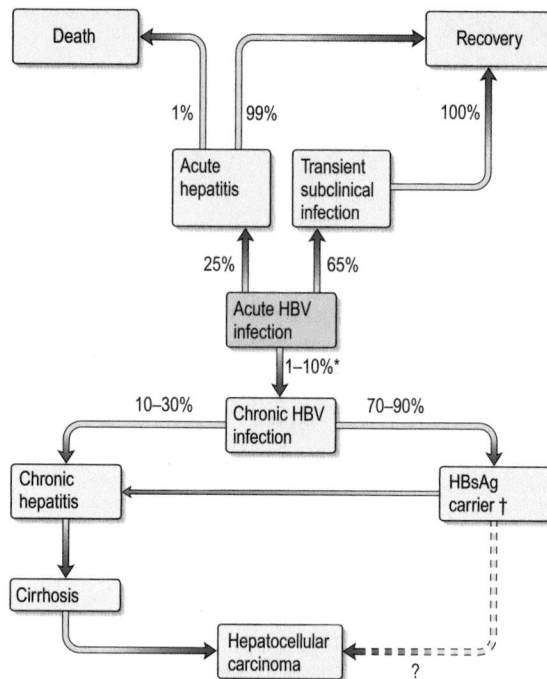

Fig. 7.17 **Clinical course of hepatitis B infection.**
*, percentage variable world-wide; † have normal liver biochemistry – a minority, having acquired infection at birth or in childhood, are HBeAg and HBV-DNA-positive. They may develop hepatitis as the immune system recognizes infected hepatocytes.

prostitutes. Infectivity is highest in those with the e antigen and/or HBV DNA in their blood. These patients should be counselled about their infection. In developing countries, blood and blood products are still a hazard. Standard safety precautions in laboratories and hospitals must be enforced strictly to avoid accidental needle punctures and contact with infected body fluids.

Passive and active immunization

Vaccination is universal in most developed countries as well as countries with high endemicity. Groups at high risk are: all healthcare personnel; members of emergency and rescue teams; morticians and embalmers; children in high-risk areas; people with haemophilia; patients in some psychiatric units; patients with chronic renal failure/on dialysis units; long-term travellers; homosexual and bisexual men and prostitutes; intravenous drug abusers.

Combined prophylaxis (i.e. vaccination and immuno-globulin) should be given to: staff with accidental needle-stick injury; all newborn babies of HBsAg-positive mothers; regular sexual partners of HBsAg-positive patients, who have been found to be HBV-negative.

To adults give 500 IU of specific hepatitis B immuno-globulin (HBIG) (200 IU to newborns) and the vaccine i.m. at another site.

Active immunization

This is with a recombinant yeast vaccine produced by

Table 7.6 Significance of viral markers in hepatitis B	
Antigens	
HBsAg	Acute or chronic infection
HBeAg	Acute hepatitis B
	Persistence implies:
	continued infectious state
	development of chronicity
	increased severity of disease
HBV DNA	Implies viral replication
	Found in serum and liver
Antibodies	
Anti-HBs	Immunity to HBV; previous exposure
Anti-HBe	Seroconversion
Anti-HBc	
IgM	Acute hepatitis B (high titre)
	Chronic hepatitis B (low titre)
IgG	Past exposure to hepatitis B (HBsAg-negative)

insertion of a plasmid containing the gene of HBsAg into a yeast.

Dosage regimen. Three injections (at 0, 1 and 6 months) are given into the deltoid muscle; this gives short-term protection in over 90% of patients. People who are over 50 years of age or clinically ill and/or immuno-compromised (including those with HIV infection or AIDS) have a poor antibody response; more frequent and larger doses are required. Antibody levels should be measured at 7–9 months after the initial dose in all at-risk groups. Antibody levels fall steadily after vaccination and booster doses may be required after approximately 3–5 years. It is not cost-effective to check antibody levels prior to active immunization. There are few side-effects from the vaccine; soreness at the site of injection may occur, with very occasionally a fever, rash or a 'flu-like' illness. Vaccines containing pre-S components which have a greater immunogenicity are being developed.

Chronic asymptomatic subjects with HBV

Following an acute HBV infection which may be sub-clinical, approximately 1–10% of patients will not clear the virus and most will become carriers of HBsAg. This occurs more readily with neonatal or childhood infection than when HBV is acquired in adult life. There is a vast geographical variation in the incidence of carriers. In the UK, asymptomatic carriers are usually discovered incidentally on blood tests, such as when they are screened for donating blood for transfusion or when attending genital medicine or antenatal clinics. Asymptomatic carriers have HBsAg in their serum and are HBeAg-negative, HBe antibody-positive with no HBV DNA in the serum. They have no evidence of active liver disease and are not highly infective. Most remain HBsAg-positive, but do not develop active liver disease; there is an annual spontaneous clearance rate of HBsAg of 1–2%.

There are also asymptomatic people who have the e antigen and HBV DNA in the serum. They may have normal liver function tests for many years; liver disease develops when the immune balance changes, and lymphocytes recognize infected hepatocytes causing hepatitis. These patients need to be followed up.

Hepatitis D

This is caused by the hepatitis D virus (HDV or delta virus). It is an incomplete RNA particle enclosed in a shell of HBsAg. It is unable to replicate on its own but is activated by the presence of HBV. It is particularly seen in intravenous drug abusers but can affect all risk groups for HBV infection. Active HBV synthesis is reduced by delta infection and patients are usually negative for HBeAg and HBV DNA. Hepatitis D viral infection can occur either as a co-infection with HBV or as a superinfection in an HBsAg-positive patient.

Co-infection of HDV and HBV is clinically indistinguishable from an acute icteric HBV infection, but a biphasic rise of serum aminotransferases may be seen. *Diagnosis* is confirmed by finding serum IgM anti-delta in the presence of IgM anti-HBc. IgM anti-delta appears at 1 week and disappears by 5–6 weeks (occasionally 12 weeks) when serum IgG anti-delta is seen. The infection may be transient but the clinical course is variable.

Superinfection results in an acute flare-up of previously quiescent chronic HBV infection. A rise in serum AST or ALT may be the only indication of infection. Diagnosis is by finding serum IgM anti-delta at the same time as IgG anti-HBc; patients are usually negative for IgM anti-HBc.

Fulminant hepatitis can follow both types of infection but is more common after co-infection. HDV RNA in the serum and liver can be measured and is found in acute and chronic HDV infection.

Hepatitis C

Hepatitis C virus (HCV)

HCV is a single-stranded RNA virus of the Flaviviridae family. The RNA genome is approximately 10 Kb in length, encoding a polyprotein product consisting of structural (capsid and envelope) and non-structural viral proteins (Fig. 7.18). Comparisons of subgenomic regions, such as E1, NS4 or NS5, have allowed variants to be classified into at least six genotypes. Variability is distributed throughout the genome with the non-structural gene of different genotypes showing only 65–70% nucleotide sequence similarity. Genotypes 1a or 1b account for 70–80% of cases in the USA and Europe. There is a rapid change in envelope proteins, making it difficult to develop a vaccine. Antigens from the nucleo-capsid regions have been used to develop enzyme-linked immunosorbent assays (ELISA). The current assay, ELISA-3, incorporates antigens NS3, NS4 and NS5 regions.

Epidemiology

The prevalence rate of infection in healthy blood donors is about 0.02% in Northern Europe, 1–3% in Southern Europe, possibly linked to intramuscular injections of vaccines or other medicines; 6% in Africa and with rates as high as 19% in Egypt, owing to parenteral antimony treatment for schistosomiasis. The virus is transmitted by blood and blood products and it is postulated that 80% of people with haemophilia in the UK may have been infected. The incidence in intravenous drug abusers is high, up to 90%. The low rate of HCV infection in high-

Fig. 7.18 **Hepatitis C virus.** Diagram showing a single-stranded RNA virus with viral proteins. C, core; NS, non-structural; E, envelope.

risk groups, such as homosexuals, prostitutes and attendees at STI clinics, suggests a limited role for sexual transmission. Vertical transmission from healthy mother to child can occur, but is very rare. Other routes of community-acquired infection (e.g. close contact) are unlikely. In 20% of cases the exact mode of transmission is unknown. An estimated 240 million people are infected with this virus world-wide.

Clinical features

Most acute infections are asymptomatic with about 10% of patients having a mild flu-like illness with jaundice and a rise in serum aminotransferases. Most patients will not be diagnosed until they present, years later, with evidence of abnormal transferase values at health checks or with chronic liver disease. Extrahepatic manifestations are seen, including arthritis, glomerulonephritis associated with cryoglobulinaemia, and porphyria cutanea tarda. There is a higher incidence of diabetes, and associations with lichen planus, sicca syndrome, and non-Hodgkin's lymphoma are under investigation.

Diagnosis

This is frequently by exclusion in a high-risk individual with negative markers for HAV, HBV and other viruses. A drug cause for hepatitis should be excluded if possible. HCV RNA can be detected 1 or 2 weeks after infection. Anti-HCV is usually positive 6 weeks from infection.

Treatment

Interferon has been used in acute cases to prevent chronic disease. Needle-stick injuries must be followed and treated early if there is evidence of HCV viraemia.

Course

At least 85% of patients go on to develop chronic liver disease (p. 372). Cirrhosis develops in about 15–20% within 10–30 years and of these patients between 7% and 15% will develop hepatocellular carcinoma. The course is adversely affected by alcohol consumption, which should be discouraged. Male patients and patients acquiring the infection over 40 years and those with genotype 1 or 4 have a more rapid development of fibrosis.

Hepatitis E

Hepatitis E virus (HEV) is an RNA virus (Calicivirus) (Fig. 7.19) which causes a hepatitis clinically very similar to hepatitis A. It is enterally transmitted, usually by contaminated water, with 30% of dogs, pigs and rodents carrying the virus. Epidemics have been seen in many developing countries. It has a mortality from fulminant hepatic failure of 1–2% which rises to 20% in pregnant women. There is no carrier state and it does not progress to chronic liver disease. An ELISA for IgG and IgM anti-HEV is available for diagnosis, although this ELISA is not always reliable. HEV RNA can be detected in the serum or stools by PCR (polymerase chain reaction). Prevention and control depend on good sanitation and hygiene; vaccination may soon be available.

Fig. 7.19 Hepatitis E genome – showing a single-stranded RNA genome with three open reading frames (ORF).

Non-A–E hepatitis

Approximately 10–15% of acute viral hepatitides cannot be typed. GB agent (HGV hepatitis G virus) and TTV (transfusion-transmitted virus) agents have not been documented as causing disease in humans. Hepatitis non-A–E is the best term to label this cryptogenic group.

FULMINANT HEPATIC FAILURE (FHF)

This is defined as severe hepatic failure in which encephalopathy develops in under 2 weeks in a patient with a previously normal liver (occasionally in some patients with previous liver damage; e.g. D virus superinfection in a previous carrier of HBsAg and in Wilson's disease). Cases that evolve at a slower pace (2–12 weeks) are called subacute or subfulminant hepatic failure. FHF is a rare but often life-threatening syndrome that is due to acute hepatitis from many causes (Table 7.7). The causes vary throughout the world; the majority are due to viral hepatitis, but paracetamol overdose is commonly implicated in the UK (50% of cases). HCV does not cause

Table 7.7   Causes of fulminant hepatic failure

Viruses A, B, (D), E	**Toxins** *Amanita* poisoning Halohydrocarbons
Other viruses	
Drugs (examples) Analgesics (e.g. paracetamol) Monoamine oxidase inhibitors Halogenated anaesthetics Antituberculosis (e.g. isoniazid) Antiepileptic (e.g. valproate) 'Social' drugs (e.g. 'Ecstasy')	**Miscellaneous** Wilson's disease Acute fatty liver of pregnancy Reye's syndrome Budd–Chiari syndrome Autoimmune hepatitis

FHF although exceptional cases have been reported from Japan.

Histologically there is multiacinar necrosis involving a substantial part of the liver. Severe fatty change is seen in pregnancy (p. 394), Reye's syndrome (p. 395), or following tetracycline administration intravenously.

Clinical features

Examination shows a jaundiced patient with a small liver and signs of hepatic encephalopathy. The mental state varies from slight drowsiness, confusion and disorientation (grades I and II) to unresponsive coma (grade IV) with convulsions. Fetor hepaticus is common, but ascites and splenomegaly are rare. Fever, vomiting, hypotension and hypoglycaemia occur. Neurological examination shows spasticity and extension of the arms and legs; plantar responses remain flexor until late. Cerebral oedema develops in 80% of patients with FHF but is far less common with subacute failure and its consequences of intracranial hypertension and brain herniation are the most common causes of death. Other complications include bacterial and fungal infections, gastrointestinal bleeding, respiratory arrest, renal failure (hepatorenal syndrome and acute tubular necrosis) and pancreatitis.

Investigations

There is hyperbilirubinaemia, high serum aminotransferases and low levels of coagulation factors, including prothrombin and factor V. Aminotransferases are not useful indicators of the course of the disease as they tend to fall along with the albumin with progressive liver damage. An EEG is sometimes helpful in grading the encephalopathy. Ultrasound will define liver size and any evidence of underlying liver pathology.

Treatment

There is no specific treatment, but patients should be managed in a specialized unit. Transfer criteria to such units are shown in Box 7.1. Supportive therapy as for hepatic encephalopathy is necessary (see p. 383). When signs of raised intracranial pressure (which is sometimes measured directly) are present, 20% mannitol (1 g/kg bodyweight) should be infused intravenously; this dose may need to be repeated. Dexamethasone is of no value. Hypoglycaemia, hypokalaemia, hypomagnesaemia, hypophosphataemia and hypocalcaemia should be anticipated and corrected with 10% dextrose infusion (checked by 2-hourly Dextrostix testing), potassium, calcium, phosphate, and magnesium. Coagulopathy is managed with intravenous vitamin K, platelets, blood or

 Box 7.1 Transfer criteria to specialized units for patients with acute liver injury

- INR > 3.0
- Presence of hepatic encephalopathy
- Hypotension after resuscitation with fluid
- Metabolic acidosis
- Prothrombin time (seconds) > interval (hours) from overdose (paracetamol cases)

 Box 7.2 Poor prognostic variables in fulminant hepatic failure indicating a need for liver transplantation

Non-paracetamol (three of following five)
- Drug or non-A–E hepatitis
- Age < 10 and > 40 years
- Interval from onset of jaundice to encephalopathy > 7 days
- Serum bilirubin > 300 µmol/L
- Prothrombin time > 50 s (or > 100 s in isolation)

Paracetamol
- Arterial pH < 7.3 (after resuscitation, 7.25 on *N*-acetylcysteine)

Or
- Serum creatinine > 300 µmol/L and
- PT > 100 s and
- Grade III–IV encephalopathy

fresh frozen plasma. Haemorrhage may be a problem and patients are given H_2-receptor antagonists to prevent gastrointestinal bleeding. Prophylaxis against bacterial and fungal infection is routine, and suspected infection should be treated immediately with suitable antibiotics. Renal and respiratory failure should be treated as necessary. Liver transplantation has been a major advance for patients with FHF. It is difficult to judge the timing or the necessity for transplantation, but there are guidelines based on validated prognostic indices of survival (see below).

Course and prognosis

In mild cases (grades I and II encephalopathy with drowsiness and confusion), two-thirds of the patients will survive. The outcome of severe cases (grades III and IV encephalopathy with stupor or deep coma) is related to the aetiology. In special units, 70% of patients with paracetamol overdosage and grade IV coma survive, as do 30–40% patients with HAV or HBV hepatitis. Poor prognostic variables indicating a need to transplant the liver are shown in Box 7.2.

ACUTE HEPATITIS DUE TO OTHER VIRUSES

Infectious mononucleosis (see also p. 47)
This is due to the Epstein–Barr (EB) virus. Mild jaundice associated with minor abnormalities of liver biochemistry is extremely common, but 'clinical' hepatitis is rare. Hepatic histological changes occur within 5 days of onset; the sinusoids and portal tracts are infiltrated with large mononuclear cells but the liver architecture is preserved. A Paul–Bunnell or Monospot test is usually positive, and atypical lymphocytes are present in the peripheral blood. Treatment is of the symptoms.

Cytomegalovirus (CMV) (see also p. 46)
This can cause acute hepatitis, particularly in a patient with an impaired immune response. The virus may be isolated from the urine. The liver biopsy shows intranuclear inclusions and giant cells.

Yellow fever (see also p. 53)

This viral infection is carried by the mosquito *Aedes aegypti* and can cause acute hepatic necrosis. There is no specific treatment.

Herpes simplex (see also p. 43)

Very occasionally the herpes simplex virus causes a generalized acute infection, particularly in the immunosuppressed patient, and occasionally in pregnancy. Aminotransferases are usually massively elevated. Liver biopsy shows extensive necrosis. Aciclovir is used for treatment.

OTHER INFECTIOUS AGENTS

Abnormal liver biochemistry is frequently found in a number of acute infections. The abnormalities are usually mild and have no clinical significance.

Toxoplasmosis (see also p. 103)

This produces a clinical picture similar to that of infectious mononucleosis, with abnormal liver biochemistry, but the Paul–Bunnell test is negative.

FURTHER READING

Craig AS, Schaffner W (2004) Prevention of hepatitis A with the hepatitis A vaccine. *New England Journal of Medicine* **350**: 476–481.

Ganem D, Prince AM (2004) Hepatitis B virus infection. *New England Journal of Medicine* **350**: 118–129.

Murphy N, Wendon J (2004) Fulminant hepatic failure: treatment. In: McDonald H, Burroughs AK, Feagan B (eds) *Evidence Based Gastroenterology and Hepatology*, 2nd edn. London: BMJ Books.

Poland GA, Jacobson RM (2004) Clinical practice: prevention of hepatitis B with the hepatitis B vaccine. *New England Journal of Medicine* **351**: 2832–2838.

Skidmore SS (1999) Factors in spread of hepatitis E. *Lancet* **354**: 1049–1050.

CHRONIC HEPATITIS

Clinically this is defined as any hepatitis lasting for 6 months or longer. Chronic hepatitis is best classified according to the aetiology (Table 7.8):

- due to viral disease
- due to autoimmune disease
- drug-induced
- unknown cause.

Table 7.8 Causes of chronic hepatitis

Viral	Hereditary
Hepatitis B ± hepatitis D	Wilson's disease
Hepatitis C	
	Others
Autoimmune	Inflammatory bowel disease – ulcerative colitis
Drugs	Alcohol (rarely)
(e.g. methyldopa, isoniazid, ketoconazole, nitrofurantoin)	

Chronic viral hepatitis is the principal cause of chronic liver disease, cirrhosis and hepatocellular carcinoma in the world.

Pathology

Chronic inflammatory cell infiltrates comprising lymphocytes, plasma cells and sometimes lymphoid follicles are usually present in the portal tracts. The amount of inflammation varies from mild to severe. In addition, there may be:

- loss of definition of the portal/periportal limiting plate – interface hepatitis (damage is due to apoptosis rather than necrosis)
- lobular change, focal lytic necrosis, apoptosis and focal inflammation
- confluent necrosis
- fibrosis which may be mild, bridging (across portal tracts) or severe cirrhosis.

The overall severity of the hepatitis is judged by the degree of the hepatitis and inflammation (grading) and the severity of the fibrosis or cirrhosis (staging) using various scoring systems.

Terms such as 'chronic persistent' or 'chronic active' hepatitis should no longer be used.

CHRONIC HEPATITIS DUE TO VIRAL DISEASE

Two main viruses (HBV and HCV) that cause chronic hepatitis (CH) can produce similar clinical features, biochemical abnormalities and histological characteristics, although some features are more suggestive of one virus than the other being involved.

Chronic hepatitis B infection

This is common in developing countries where vertical transmission still frequently occurs. In the UK it is mainly confined to high-risk groups (see p. 360) and immigrants from developing countries. The outcome of HBV infection is shown in Figure 7.17.

Pathogenesis

Cytotoxic T cells recognize the viral antigen via HLA class I molecules on the infected hepatocytes; Th1 responses (interleukin-2, gamma-interferon) are thought to be associated with the clearance of the virus and Th2 (interleukins 4, 5, 6, 10, 13) responses with the development of chronic infection and severity of the disease. Viral persistence in patients with a very poor cell-mediated response leads to a healthy carrier state. A better response, however, results in continuing hepatocellular damage with the development of CH.

Chronic HBV infection goes through a replicative and an integrated phase. In the former there is active viral replication with hepatic inflammation and the patient is highly infectious with HBeAg and HBV DNA positivity. At some stage the viral genome becomes integrated into the host DNA and the viral genes are then transcribed along with those of the host. At this stage, the level of HBV DNA in the serum is low and the patient is HBeAg-negative and HBe antibody-positive. The amino-transferases are now normal or only slightly elevated and liver histology shows little inflammation, often with cirrhosis. Hepatocellular carcinoma (HCC) develops in patients with this late-stage disease, but the mechanism is still unclear. Integration of the viral DNA with the host-cell chromosomal DNA does appear to have a major role in carcinogenesis. There is evidence to implicate in-activation of p53-induced apoptosis by protein X (Table 7.5), allowing accumulation of abnormal cells and, eventually, carcinogenesis.

Clinical features and investigations

Chronic hepatitis is more frequent in men and it is often not preceded by an acute attack. The condition may be asymptomatic or may present as a mild, slowly pro-gressive hepatitis; 50% present with established chronic liver disease. Clinical relapses occur, sometimes associ-ated with seroconversion (see below) of HBeAg to anti-HBe or vice versa.

Investigations show a moderate rise in amino-transferases and a slightly raised ALP. The serum bilirubin is often normal. HBsAg and HBV DNA are found in the serum, usually with HBe antigen, unless a mutant virus is involved (see p. 365).

Histologically, there is a full spectrum of changes from near normal with only a few lymphocytes and interface hepatitis to a full-blown cirrhosis. HBsAg may be seen as a 'ground-glass' appearance in the cytoplasm on haematoxylin and eosin staining, and this can be confirmed on orcein staining or more specifically with immunohistochemical staining. HBcAg can also be demonstrated in hepatocytes by appropriate immuno-histochemical staining.

Treatment

Patients with HBsAg, HBeAg and HBV DNA in the serum with abnormal serum aminotransferases and chronic hepatitis on liver biopsy should be treated. Patients with normal aminotransferases and those with decompensated liver disease should not be treated with interferon (see below).

The main aim of treatment is to eliminate the HBeAg and HBV DNA from the serum with consequent reduction in inflammatory necrosis of the hepatocyte. This seroconversion occurs spontaneously at a rate of 10–15% per year, and this varies in different populations.

In patients in whom HBeAg disappears, remission is usually sustained. The patient remains a carrier with HBsAg present, although some will eventually become HBsAg-negative.

Antiviral agents

Interferon, lamivudine and adefovir dipivoxil (p. 144) have been shown to be effective. Pegylated α-2b interferon (100 µg once a week subcutaneously) gives response rates of 25–45% (depending on genotype – A and B respond best) after 6 months of treatment.

Side-effects of treatment are many, with an acute flu-like illness occurring 6–8 hours after the first injection. This usually disappears after subsequent injections, but malaise, headaches and myalgia, are common and depression, diarrhoea, reversible hair loss and bone marrow depression and infection may occur. The platelet count should be monitored. These drug reactions occur in up to 30% of patients, and the dose may have to be lowered; in 10% the treatment has to be discontinued.

Overall, the response rate with disappearance of HBeAg is 25–40%. The success rate depends on factors shown in Table 7.9.

Those with chronic hepatitis with no HBeAg (i.e. a mutant HBV, see p. 365) generally do not respond to interferon, and HDV-infected patients only respond with prolonged high-dose courses; patients with concomitant HIV infection also have a poor response. Patients with decompensated liver disease often have severe side-effects and should not be routinely treated with this drug but could be treated with lamivudine.

Lamivudine 100 mg/day can be given orally and is well-tolerated. It appears more effective than interferon, particularly in HBV-DNA-positive individuals who have acquired the infection perinatally or in childhood. At 1 year, 50–70% of patients have normalization of their serum ALT, 30% have lost their HBe antigen with seroconversion in 15–20%. However, there is a complication of a mutant escape virus (YMDD mutant –

Table 7.9	Factors predictive of a sustained response to treatment in patients with chronic hepatitis	
	Chronic hepatitis B	**Chronic hepatitis C**
Duration of disease	Short	Short
Liver biochemistry	High serum aminotransferase concentrations	
Histology	Active liver disease	Absence of cirrhosis or minimal amounts of hepatic fibrosis
Viral levels	Low HBV DNA levels	Low HCV RNA levels
		Genotype 2 or 3
Other	Absence of immunosuppression	Low hepatic iron stores
	Female gender	Young age
	Adult acquired	Non-obese
	Delta virus negative	Low body weight

tyrosine, methionine, aspartate), which in itself causes hepatitis (15% per year of therapy), but usually less severe than that due to the wild type infection. These mutants respond to adefovir dipivoxil 10 mg/day. The latter is also effective in HBeAg-positive and HBeAg-negative naive patients. Adefovir mutants are to date extremely rare.

The duration of all treatment, and which combination of antivirals is optimal, is still being assessed. Currently, treatment is with alpha-interferon (4 months), lamivudine and adefovir (12 months).

Prognosis

The progression is slow and remission may occur. Established cirrhosis is associated with a poor prognosis. Hepatocellular carcinoma is a frequent association and is one of the most common carcinomas in HBV endemic areas such as the Far East. This incidence is being reduced by routine HBV vaccination of all children.

Chronic hepatitis C infection
(see also p. 367)

Pathogenesis

As with hepatitis B infection, cytokines in the Th2 phenotypes are profibrotic and lead to the development of chronic infection. A dominant CD4 Th2 response with a weak CD8 gamma-interferon response may lead to rapid fibrosis. Th1 cytokines are anti-fibrotic and thus a dominant CD4 Th1 and CD8 cytolytic response may cause less fibrosis. Variability may be related to the genetic phenotype; persistence of HCV infection has been shown to be associated with HLA-DRB1*0701 and DRB4*0101. Other factors also have an effect on the development of fibrosis, particularly fatty liver, and diabetes (p. 368).

Clinical features

Patients with chronic hepatitis C infection are usually asymptomatic, the disease being discovered only following a routine biochemical test when mild elevations in the aminotransferases (usually ALT) are noticed (50%). The elevation in ALT may be minimal and fluctuating, and some patients have a persistently normal ALT (25%) – the disease being detected by checking HCV antibodies (e.g. in blood donors).

Despite this, severe chronic hepatitis (25%) and even cirrhosis can be present with only minimal elevation in aminotransferases, but progression is very uncommon in those with a persistently normal ALT. Those with severe inflammation may have fatigue. A few patients present with the symptoms and signs found in cirrhosis.

Diagnosis

This is made by finding HCV antibody in the serum using third-generation ELISA-3 tests. HCV RNA should be assayed using quantitative HCV-RNA PCR. The viraemia is usually variable; less than 2×10^6 genome equivalents/mL signifies a greater likelihood of response to antiviral therapy.

The HCV genotype should be characterized in patients who are to be given treatment (see below).

Liver biopsy is indicated if active treatment is being considered. The changes on liver biopsy are highly variable. Sometimes only minimal inflammation is detected, but in most cases the features of CH are present, as previously described (p. 370). Lymphoid follicles are often present in the portal tracts, and fatty change is frequently seen.

Treatment (Fig. 7.20)

Treatment is appropriate for patients with chronic hepatitis on liver histology who have HCV RNA in their serum and who have raised serum aminotransferases for more than 6 months. Patients with persistently normal aminotransferases are also treated if they have abnormal histology. The presence of cirrhosis is not a contraindication, but therapeutic responses are less likely. Patients with decompensated cirrhosis should be considered for transplantation. The aim of treatment is to eliminate the HCV RNA from the serum in order to:

Fig. 7.20 **Approach to a patient with hepatitis C.** ALT, alanine aminotransferase; PCR, polymerase chain reaction. Adapted from Dhumeaux D et al. (2003) Treatment of hepatitis C. The 2002 French consensus. *Gut* **52**.

- stop the progression of active liver disease
- prevent the development of hepatocellular carcinoma.

Antiviral agents

Current treatment is combination therapy with pegylated interferon, which is interferon with a polyethyleneglycol tail (α2a 180 µg/week or α2b 1.5 µg/kg/week) and ribavirin (1000–1200 mg/day for genotype 1, 800 mg/day for genotype 2 or 3); in divided doses for 12 months for genotype 1, and 6 months for other genotypes. Efficacy is also determined by viral load with HCV RNA > 2×10^6 genome equivalents per mL less likely to respond.

Side-effects of interferon. (p. 371) are less than for the treatment of HBV infection because of the lower dose. Ribavirin is usually well tolerated but side-effects include a dose-related haemolysis, pruritus and nasal congestion. Pregnancy should be avoided as it is teratogenic.

Monitoring results. The effects of treatment are monitored by measurement of the aminotransferases, with measurement of the PCR HCV RNA at 3 months. If the aminotransferases remain abnormal and HCV RNA is present in the serum above a 2 log drop in concentration from pre-treatment values, treatment is stopped because a response to further treatment is then unlikely.

A sustained response is achieved in 40–50% at 12 months with genotype 1 and 80% in genotype 2 or 3. Best results are obtained in patients with the predictive factors shown in Table 7.9. If PCR HCV RNA remains negative 6 months after the end of treatment relapse is unlikely and histological progression is halted.

Chronic D hepatitis

This is a relatively infrequent chronic hepatitis, but spontaneous resolution is rare. Between 60% and 70% of patients will develop cirrhosis and more rapidly than with HBV infection alone. In 15% the disease is rapidly progressive with development of cirrhosis in only a few years. The diagnosis is made by finding anti-delta antibody in a patient with chronic liver disease who is HBsAg-positive. It can be confirmed by finding HDV in the liver or HDV RNA in the serum by reverse transcription – polymerase reaction. Treatment is with alpha-interferon, usually at the high dose of 10M units three times weekly for 12 months, but response is poor. Lamivudine and adefovir appear to be unhelpful.

AUTOIMMUNE HEPATITIS

This condition occurs most frequently in women. In type I (see below) there is an association with other auto-immune diseases (e.g. pernicious anaemia, thyroiditis and Coombs'-positive haemolytic anaemia), and 60% of cases are associated with HLA, DR3, DR52a loci, HLADRB3*0101 and HLADRB*0401. In Asians, the condition is associated with HLADR4.

Pathogenesis

The cause is unknown. It is proposed, in a genetically predisposed person, that an environmental agent causes an autoimmune process to develop against liver antigens, producing a progressive necroinflammatory process which results in fibrosis and cirrhosis. In vitro observations have shown that there is a defect of suppressor (regulatory) T cells which may be primary or secondary. However, no clear mechanism causing the inflammation has been found.

Clinical features

There are two peaks in presentation. In the peri- and postmenopausal group, patients may be asymptomatic or present with fatigue, the disease being discovered by abnormalities in liver biochemistry or because of signs of chronic liver disease on routine examination. In the teens and early twenties the disease (often type II) presents as an acute hepatitis with jaundice and very high amino-transferases, which do not improve with time. This age group often has clinical features of cirrhosis with hepatosplenomegaly, cutaneous striae, acne, hirsuties, bruises and, sometimes, ascites. An ill patient can also have features of an autoimmune disease with a fever, migratory polyarthritis, glomerulonephritis, pleurisy, pulmonary infiltration or fibrosing alveolitis.

There are overlap syndromes with primary biliary cirrhosis and primary sclerosing cholangitis.

Investigations

Liver biochemistry

The serum aminotransferases are high, with lesser elevations in the ALP and bilirubin. The serum γ-globulins are high, frequently twice normal, particularly the IgG. The biochemical pattern is the same with all three types.

Haematology

A mild normochromic normocytic anaemia with thrombocytopenia and leucopoenia is present, even before portal hypertension and splenomegaly. The prothrombin time is often high.

Autoantibodies

Three types of autoimmune hepatitis have been recognized:

- Type I with antibodies:
  (a) antinuclear
  (b) anti-smooth muscle (anti-actin).
- Type II with antibodies: anti-liver/kidney microsomal (anti-LKM1). The main target is cytochrome P4502D6 (CYP2D6) on liver cell plasma membranes.
- Type III with soluble liver antigen (now designated anti SLP/LP) but this group behaves as type I.

Type II occurs most frequently in girls and young women. Approximately 13% of patients lack the above auto-antibodies.

Liver biopsy

This shows the changes of CH described previously. The amount of interface hepatitis is variable, but tends to be high in untreated patients. Lymphoid follicles are less often seen than in hepatitis C, and plasma cell infiltration is frequent. Approximately one-third of patients have cirrhosis at presentation.

Treatment

Prednisolone 30 mg is given daily for 2 weeks, followed by a slow reduction and then a maintenance dose of 10–15 mg daily; azathioprine should be added, 1–2 mg/kg daily, as a steroid-sparing agent and in some patients as sole long-term maintenance therapy. Mycophenalate, ciclosporin, and tacrolimus have been used in resistant cases.

Course and prognosis

Steroid and azathioprine therapy induce remission in over 80% of cases. The length of treatment is lifelong in most cases. Those with initial cirrhosis are more likely to relapse following treatment withdrawal and require indefinite therapy. Liver transplantation is performed if treatment fails, although the disease may recur.

DRUG-INDUCED CHRONIC HEPATITIS

Several drugs can cause a CH which clinically bears many similarities to autoimmune hepatitis (see Table 7.8). Patients are often female, present with jaundice and hepatomegaly, have raised serum aminotransferases and globulin levels, and LE cells and anti-LKM1 antibodies may be detected. Improvement follows drug withdrawal but exacerbations can occur with drug reintroduction. Isoniazid, amiodarone and methotrexate can lead to chronic histological changes. With rare exceptions patients with pre-existing chronic liver disease are not more susceptible to drug injury.

Chronic alcoholic liver disease can occasionally have histological appearances more like a chronic hepatitis.

NON-ALCOHOLIC FATTY LIVER DISEASE (NAFLD)

This is an increasingly recognized condition that can lead to cirrhosis (in 1%) and hepatocellular carcinoma. NAFLD progression accounts for the majority of cases of cryptogenic cirrhosis, and obesity is a risk factor for the development of hepatocellular carcinoma. The histological changes are similar to those of alcohol-induced hepatic injury and range from simple fatty change to fat and inflammation (steatohepatitis) and fibrosis. Inflammation can lead to fibrosis, probably via an oxidative stress injury leading to lipid peroxidation in the presence of fatty infiltrations; the latter causes insulin resistance, which in turn switches on connective tissue growth factor leading to fibrosis. Risk factors for NAFLD are obesity, hypertension, type 2 diabetes, hyperlipidaemia. NAFLD is estimated to affect 3–6% of the population in the USA and of these, 1–3% have steatohepatitis (NASH). Most patients are asymptomatic; hepatomegaly may be present. Mild increases in serum transferases are frequently the sole abnormality in the liver biochemistry. Liver biopsy allows staging the disease but when this should be performed is unclear. Most would biopsy if the ALT is persistently over

twice normal. Currently weight loss, strict control of hypertension, diabetes, and lipid levels are the only treatments in the early stages, but the disease may still progress. Liver transplantation is reserved for end-stage cirrhosis, but the condition may recur. Regular follow-up is indicated, particularly for steatohepatitis.

CHRONIC HEPATITIS OF UNKNOWN CAUSE

As more and more people are having routine blood tests, mild elevations in the serum aminotransferases and γ-GT are found. Many of these patients have no symptoms and no evidence of liver disease clinically. All known aetiological agents should be excluded (see above), as well as tests to exclude primary biliary cirrhosis, primary sclerosing cholangitis, Wilson's disease, haemochromatosis and α_1-antitrypsin deficiency. Risk factors for NAFLD should be evaluated.

Liver biopsy should be performed if the elevation in the aminotransferases continues for over a year, to confirm the presence of chronic hepatitis, although this is often unhelpful.

FURTHER READING

Czaja AJ, Freese DK (2002) Diagnosis and treatment of autoimmune hepatitis. *Hepatology* **36**: 479–497.

Dhumeaux D, Marcellin P, Lerebours E (2003) Treatment of hepatitis C. The 2002 French consensus. *Gut* **52**: 1784–1787.

Emerson SV, Purcell RH (2004) The omnipresence of hepatitis E. *New England Journal of Medicine* **351**: 2367–2368.

Ishak K, Baptista A, Bianchi L et al. (1995) Histological grading and staging of chronic hepatitis. *Journal of Hepatology* **22**: 696–699.

Kita H et al. (2001) The lymphoid liver: considerations on pathways to autoimmune injury. *Gastroenterology* **120**: 1485–1501.

Lai CL et al. (2003) Viral hepatitis B. *Lancet* **362**: 2089–2094.

Malnick SDM et al. (2003) Non alcoholic fatty liver. *Quarterly Journal of Medicine* **96**: 699–709.

Neuschwander-Tetri BA, Caldwell SH (2003) Non-alcoholic steatohepatitis: summary of an AASLD Single Topic Conference. *Hepatology* **37**(5): 1202–1219.

Poynard T et al. (2003) Viral hepatitis C. *Lancet* **362**: 2095–2100.

CIRRHOSIS

Cirrhosis results from the necrosis of liver cells followed by fibrosis and nodule formation. The liver architecture is diffusely abnormal and this interferes with liver blood flow and function. This derangement produces the clinical features of portal hypertension and impaired liver cell function.

Aetiology

The causes of cirrhosis are shown in Table 7.10. Alcohol is now the most common cause in the West, but viral

Table 7.10 Causes of cirrhosis

Common	Others
Alcohol	Biliary cirrhosis:
Hepatitis B ± D	primary
Hepatitis C	secondary
? Other viruses	Autoimmune hepatitis
	Hereditary haemochromatosis
	Hepatic venous congestion
	Budd–Chiari syndrome
	Wilson's disease
	Drugs (e.g. methotrexate)
	α_1-Antitrypsin deficiency
	Cystic fibrosis
	Non-alcoholic fatty liver disease (NAFLD)
	Galactosaemia
	Glycogen storage disease
	Veno-occlusive disease
	Idiopathic (cryptogenic)

infection is the most common cause world-wide. With the identification of HCV, idiopathic (cryptogenic) cirrhosis is diagnosed less commonly. Young patients with cirrhosis must be investigated carefully as the cause may be treatable (e.g. Wilson's disease).

Pathogenesis

Chronic injury to the liver results in inflammation, necrosis and, eventually, fibrosis (Fig. 7.21). Fibrosis is initiated by activation of the stellate cells (see p. 348). Kupffer cells seem to have a role in their activation, but hepatocytes and other cells are probably involved. Stellate cells are activated by many cytokines and their receptors, reactive oxygen intermediates and other paracrine and autocrine signals.

In the early stage of activation the stellate cells become swollen and lose retinoids with upregulation of receptors for proliferative and fibrogenic cytokines, such as platelet-derived growth factor (PDGF), and possibly transforming growth factor β_1 (TGF-β_1). TGF-β_1 is the most potent fibrogenic mediator identified so far.

In the space of Disse, the normal matrix is replaced by collagens, predominantly types 1 and 3, and fibronectin. Subendothelial fibrosis leads to loss of the endothelial fenestrations (ports), and this impairs liver function. Collagenases (matrix metalloproteinases, MMP) are able to degrade this collagen but are inhibited by tissue inhibitors of metalloproteinases (TIMPs), which are increased in human liver fibrosis. There is accumulating evidence that liver fibrosis is reversible.

Pathology

The characteristic features of cirrhosis are regenerating nodules separated by fibrous septa and loss of the normal lobular architecture within the nodules (Fig. 7.22a). Two types of cirrhosis have been described which give clues to the underlying cause:

- *Micronodular cirrhosis*. Regenerating nodules are usually less than 3 mm in size and the liver is involved uniformly. This type is often caused by ongoing alcohol damage or biliary tract disease.

(a)

(b)

Fig. 7.22 **(a) Pathology of cirrhosis.** Histological appearance showing nodules of liver tissue of varying size surrounded by fibrosis.
(b) CT scan showing an irregular lobulated liver. There is splenomegaly and enlargement of collateral vessels beneath the anterior abdominal wall (arrows) as a result of portal hypertension.

Fig. 7.21 **Pathogenesis of fibrosis.** Activation of the stellate cell is followed by proliferation of fibroblasts and the deposition of collagen.

Macronodular cirrhosis. The nodules are of variable size and normal acini may be seen within the larger nodules. This type is often seen following previous hepatitis, such as HBV infection.

A mixed picture with small and large nodules is sometimes seen.

Symptoms and signs are described on page 357.

Investigations

These are performed to assess the severity and type of liver disease.

Severity

- **Liver function.** Serum albumin and prothrombin time are the best indicators of liver function: the outlook is poor with an albumin level below 28 g/L. The prothrombin time is prolonged commensurate with the severity of the liver disease (Box 7.3).
- **Liver biochemistry.** This can be normal depending on the severity of cirrhosis. In most cases there is at least a slight elevation in the serum ALP and serum aminotransferases. In decompensated cirrhosis all biochemistry is deranged.
- **Serum electrolytes.** A low sodium indicates severe liver disease due to a defect in free water clearance or to excess diuretic therapy.

In addition, serum α-fetoprotein if > 400 ng/mL is strongly suggestive of the presence of a hepatocellular carcinoma.

Type

This can be determined by:

- viral markers
- serum autoantibodies
- serum immunoglobulins
- iron indices and ferritin
- copper, caeruloplasmin (p. 387)
- α_1-antitrypsin (p. 388).

Serum copper and serum α_1-antitrypsin should always be measured in young cirrhotics. Total iron-binding capacity (TIBC) and ferritin should be measured to exclude hereditary haemochromatosis; genetic markers are also available (p. 386)

Imaging

- **Ultrasound examination.** This can demonstrate changes in size and shape of the liver. Fatty change and fibrosis produce a diffuse increased echogenicity. In established cirrhosis there may be marginal nodularity of the liver surface and distortion of the arterial vascular architecture. The patency of the portal and hepatic veins can be evaluated. It is useful in detecting hepatocellular carcinoma.
- **CT scan** (see p. 354). Figure 7.22b shows hepatosplenomegaly and dilated collaterals seen in chronic liver disease. Arterial phase-contrast-enhanced scans are useful in the detection of hepatocellular carcinoma.

- **Endoscopy** is performed for the detection and treatment of varices, and portal hypertensive gastropathy. Colonoscopy is occasionally performed for colopathy.
- **MRI scan.** This is useful in the diagnosis of benign tumours such as haemangiomas. MR angiography can demonstrate the vascular anatomy and MR cholangiography the biliary tree. However, intrahepatic bile duct damage is poorly identified by current MR technology.

Liver biopsy

This is necessary to confirm the severity and type of liver disease. The core of liver often fragments and sampling errors may occur in macronodular cirrhosis. Special stains may be required for iron and copper, and various immunocytochemical stains can identify viruses, bile ducts and angiogenic structures. Chemical measurement of iron and copper are necessary to confirm diagnosis of iron overload or Wilson's disease.

Management

Management is that of the complications seen in decompensated cirrhosis. Patients should have 6-monthly ultrasound and serum α-fetoprotein measurements to detect the development of a hepatocellular carcinoma as early as possible (see p. 394), as all therapeutic strategies work best with small and single tumours.

There is no treatment that will arrest or reverse the cirrhotic changes although progression may be halted by correcting the underlying cause (see below). Patients with compensated cirrhosis should lead a normal life. The only dietary restriction is to reduce salt intake. Aspirin and NSAIDs should be avoided. Alcohol should be avoided, although if the cirrhosis is not due to alcohol and not due to viral hepatitis, small amounts not taken on a regular basis are probably not harmful.

Course and prognosis

This is extremely variable, depending on many factors, including the aetiology and the presence of complications. Poor prognostic indicators are given in Table 7.11. Development of any complication usually worsens the prognosis. In general, the 5-year survival rate is approximately 50%, but this also varies depending on the aetiology and the stage at which the diagnosis is made.

There are a number of prognostic classifications based on modifications of Child's grading (A, B and C; see Box 7.3). Surgical procedures carry an overall operative mortality of 30% in non-bleeding cirrhotics.

LIVER TRANSPLANTATION

This is an established treatment for a number of liver diseases. Shortage of donors is a major problem in all developed countries and in some such as Japan living related donors form the majority of transplant operations where there has been only one donor death, but in Europe, mortality has been between 0.4 to 0.9%.

Table 7.11 Poor prognostic indicators in cirrhosis

Blood tests
Low albumin (< 28 g/L)
Low serum sodium (< 125 mmol/L)
Prolonged prothrombin time > 6 seconds above normal value
Raised creatinine > 160 µmol/L

Clinical
Persistent jaundice
Failure of response to therapy
Ascites
Haemorrhage from varices, particularly with poor liver function
Neuropsychiatric complications developing with progressive liver failure
Small liver
Persistent hypotension
Aetiology (e.g. alcoholic cirrhosis, if the patient continues drinking)

Box 7.3 Modified Child's–Pugh classification

Score	1	2	3
Ascites	None	Mild	Moderate/severe
Encephalopathy	None	Mild	Marked
Bilirubin (µmol/L)	< 34	34–50	> 50
Albumin (g/L)	> 35	28–35	< 28
Prothrombin time (seconds over normal)	< 4	4–6	> 6

Add above scores for your patient for survival figures below

		% survival	
Grade (scores)	1 year	5 years	10 years
Child's A (< 7)	82	45	25
Child's B (7–9)	62	20	7
Child's C (10+)	42	20	0

Indications include the following:

Acute liver disease. Patients with fulminant hepatic failure of any cause, including acute viral hepatitis (p. 362), may be considered.

Chronic liver disease. The indications for transplantation vary and the timing of the transplant is often difficult. All patients with end-stage (Child's grade C) cirrhosis should be referred to a transplant centre and also those with debilitating symptoms.

- *Primary biliary cirrhosis.* Patients with this disease should be transplanted when their serum bilirubin is persistently > 100 µmol/L or symptoms such as itching are intolerable.
- *Chronic hepatitis B if HBV-DNA-negative.* Following transplantation, recurrence of the hepatitis can occur despite use of hepatitis B immunoglobulin and lamivudine, because of escape mutants (see p. 365).
- *Chronic hepatitis C.* In end-stage disease the 5-year prognosis of the graft is good, despite universal HCV

reinfection. However, cirrhosis occurs in 10–20% at 5 years and there is progressive disease. Antiviral agents may delay this progression and trials continue.
- *Autoimmune hepatitis.* In patients who have failed to respond to medical treatment or have major side-effects of corticosteroid therapy. It can reoccur.
- *Alcoholic liver disease.* Well-motivated patients who have stopped drinking without improvement of liver disease are offered a transplant.
- *Primary metabolic disorders.* Examples are Wilson's disease, hereditary haemochromatosis and α_1-antitrypsin deficiency.
- *Other conditions*, such as sclerosing cholangitis.

Contraindications

Absolute contraindications include active sepsis outside the hepatobiliary tree, malignancy outside the liver, liver metastases (except neuroendocrine), and if the patient is not psychologically committed.

Relative contraindications are mainly anatomical considerations that would make surgery more difficult, such as extensive splanchnic venous thrombosis. With exceptions, patients aged 65 years or over are not usually transplanted. In hepatocellular carcinoma the recurrence rate is high unless there are fewer than three small (< 3 cm) lesions, or a solitary nodule of < 5 cm.

Surgical procedure

Pretransplant work-up includes confirmation of the diagnosis, ultrasound and cross-sectional imaging, radiological demonstration of the hepatic arterial and biliary tree as well as assessment of cardiorespiratory and renal status. Because of the ethical and financial implications of this operation, regular psychosocial support is vital, and psychiatric counselling may be necessary in some cases.

The donor should be ABO-compatible. He or she should ideally be under 50 years of age and have no evidence of sepsis, malignancy, HIV, HBV or HCV infection. The liver is cooled and stored on ice; its preservation time can be up to 20 hours. The recipient operation takes approximately 8 hours and may require a large blood transfusion, but sometimes none at all.

The operative mortality is low. Most postoperative deaths occur in the first 3 months. Sepsis and haemorrhage can be serious complications. Opportunistic infections (see p. 29) are still a problem owing to immunosuppression. Various immunosuppressive agents have been used, but microemulsified ciclosporin, tacrolimus in combination with either azathioprine or mycophenolate mofetil, steroids and sirolimus are the most common. A pretransplant serum creatinine above 160 µmol/L (2 mg/dL) is the best predictor of post-transplant death.

Rejection

Acute or cellular rejection is usually seen 5–10 days post-transplant; it can be asymptomatic or there may be a fever. Histologically, there is a pleomorphic portal infiltrate with prominent eosinophils, bile duct damage and endothelialitis of the blood vessels. This type of rejection responds to immunosuppressive therapy.

Chronic ductopenic rejection is seen from 6 weeks to 9 months post-transplant, with disappearing bile ducts (vanishing bile duct syndrome, VBDS) and an arteriopathy with narrowing and occlusion of the arteries. Early ductopenic rejection may rarely be reversed by immunosuppression, but often requires retransplantation.

Graft-versus-host disease is extremely rare.

Prognosis

Elective liver transplantation in low-risk patients has a 90% 1-year survival. Five-year survivals are as high as 70–85% largely owing to the introduction of ciclosporin and tacrolimus. Patients require lifelong immunosuppression, although the doses can be reduced over time without significant problems.

COMPLICATIONS AND EFFECTS OF CIRRHOSIS

These are shown in Table 7.12.

Portal hypertension

The portal vein is formed by the union of the superior mesenteric and splenic veins. The pressure within it is normally 5–8 mmHg with only a small gradient across the liver to the hepatic vein in which blood is returned to the heart via the inferior vena cava. Portal hypertension can be classified according to the site of obstruction:

- *prehepatic* – due to blockage of the portal vein before the liver
- *intrahepatic* – due to distortion of the liver architecture, which can be presinusoidal (e.g. in schistosomiasis) or postsinusoidal (e.g. in cirrhosis)
- *posthepatic* – due to venous blockage outside the liver (rare).

As portal pressure rises above 10–12 mmHg, the compliant venous system dilates and collaterals occur within the systemic venous system. The main sites of the collaterals are at the gastro-oesophageal junction, the rectum, the left renal vein, the diaphragm, the retroperitoneum and the anterior abdominal wall via the umbilical vein.

The collaterals at the gastro-oesophageal junction (varices) are superficial in position and tend to rupture. Portosystemic anastomoses at other sites seldom give rise to symptoms. Rectal varices are found frequently (30%) if

carefully looked for and can be differentiated from haemorrhoids, which are lower in the anal canal.

Pathophysiology

Portal vascular resistance is increased in chronic liver disease. During liver injury, stellate cells are activated (see p. 348) and transform into myofibroblasts. In these cells there is de novo expression of the specific smooth muscle protein α-actin. Under the influence of mediators, such as endothelin, nitric oxide or prostaglandins, the contraction of these activated cells contributes to abnormal blood flow patterns and increased resistance to blood flow. In addition the balance of fibrogenic and fibrolytic factors is shifted towards fibrogenesis. This increased resistance leads to portal hypertension and opening of portosystemic anastomoses in both precirrhotic and cirrhotic livers. Patients with cirrhosis have a hyperdynamic circulation. This is thought to be due to the release of mediators, such as nitric oxide and glucagon, which leads to peripheral and splanchnic vasodilatation. This effect is followed by plasma volume expansion due to sodium retention (see the discussion on ascites, p. 381), and this has a significant effect in maintaining portal hypertension.

Causes (see Table 7.13)

The most common cause is cirrhosis. Other causes include the following.

Prehepatic causes

Extrahepatic blockage is due to portal vein thrombosis. The cause is often unidentified, but some cases are due to portal vein occlusion secondary to congenital portal venous abnormalities or neonatal sepsis of the umbilical vein. Many are due to inherited defects causing prothrombotic conditions, e.g. factor V Leiden. Patients usually present with bleeding, often at a young age. They have normal liver function and, because of this, their prognosis following bleeding is excellent. The portal vein blockage can be identified by ultrasound or Doppler imaging. Splenectomy is only performed if there is isolated splenic vein thrombosis. Treatment is usually repeated endoscopic therapy or non-selective beta-blockade.

Table 7.12 Complications and effects of cirrhosis

Portal hypertension and gastrointestinal haemorrhage
Ascites
Portosystemic encephalopathy
Renal failure
Hepatocellular carcinoma
Bacteraemias, infections
Malnutrition

Table 7.13 Causes of portal hypertension

Prehepatic	Posthepatic
Portal vein thrombosis	Budd–Chiari syndrome
	Veno-occlusive disease
Intrahepatic	Right heart failure (rare)
Cirrhosis	Constrictive pericarditis
Hepatitis (alcoholic)	
Idiopathic non-cirrhotic portal hypertension	
Schistosomiasis	
Partial nodular transformation	
Congenital hepatic fibrosis	
Myelosclerosis (extramedullary haemopoiesis)	
Granulomata	

Intrahepatic causes

Although cirrhosis is the most common intrahepatic cause of portal hypertension, there are other causes:

- *Non-cirrhotic portal hypertension.* Patients present with portal hypertension and variceal bleeding but without cirrhosis. Histologically, the liver shows mild portal tract fibrosis. The aetiology is unknown, but arsenic, vinyl chloride and other toxic agents have been implicated. A similar disease is found frequently in India. The liver lesion does not progress and the prognosis is therefore good.
- *Schistosomiasis* with extensive pipe-stem fibrosis is the commonest cause, but is confined to endemic areas such as Egypt and Brazil. However, often there may be concomitant liver disease such as HCV infection.
- Other causes include congenital hepatic fibrosis, nodular regenerative hyperplasia, and partial nodular transformation. The last two conditions are rare. They share the common features of hyperplastic liver cell growth in the form of nodules, but in contrast to cirrhosis, fibrosis is typically absent. A wedge liver biopsy is usually required to establish the diagnosis. In none of these conditions are hormones implicated in aetiology or progression.

Posthepatic causes

Prolonged severe heart failure with tricuspid incompetence and constrictive pericarditis can both lead to portal hypertension. The Budd–Chiari syndrome is described on page 390.

Clinical features

Patients with portal hypertension are often asymptomatic and the only clinical evidence of portal hypertension is splenomegaly. Clinical features of chronic liver disease are usually present (see p. 357). Presenting features may include:

- haematemesis or melaena from rupture of gastro-oesophageal varices or portal hypertensive gastropathy
- ascites
- encephalopathy.

Variceal haemorrhage

Approximately 90% of patients with cirrhosis will develop gastro-oesophageal varices, over 10 years, but only one-third of these will bleed from them. Bleeding is likely to occur with large varices, red signs on varices (diagnosed at endoscopy) and in severe liver disease.

Management

Management can be divided into the active bleeding episode, the prevention of rebleeding, and prophylactic measures to prevent the first haemorrhage. Despite all the therapeutic techniques available, the prognosis depends on the severity of the underlying liver disease, with an overall mortality from variceal haemorrhage of 25% – reaching 50% in Child's grade C.

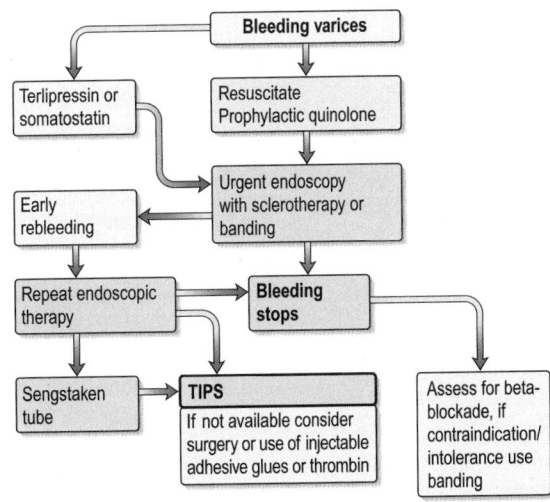

Fig. 7.23 **Management of gastrointestinal haemorrhage due to oesophageal varices.** TIPS, transjugular intrahepatic portosystemic shunt.

Initial management of acute variceal bleeding
(Fig. 7.23)
See also the discussion of the general management of gastrointestinal haemorrhage on page 291.

Resuscitation

- Assess the general condition of the patient – pulse and blood pressure.
- Insert an intravenous line and obtain blood for grouping and crossmatching, haemoglobin, PT/INR, urea, electrolytes, creatinine, liver biochemistry and blood cultures.
- Restore blood volume with plasma expanders or, if possible, blood transfusion. These measures are discussed in more detail in the treatment of shock (p. 972). Prompt correction of hypovolaemia is necessary in patients with cirrhosis as their baroreceptor reflexes are diminished.
- Ascitic tap.
- Monitor for alcohol withdrawal. Give thiamine.

Urgent endoscopy

Endoscopy should be performed to confirm the diagnosis of varices (Fig. 7.24) and to exclude bleeding from other sites (e.g. gastric ulceration). Portal hypertensive (or congestive) gastropathy is the term used for chronic gastric congestion, punctate erythema and gastric erosions and is a source of bleeding. Varices may or may not be present. Propranolol (see below) is the best treatment for this.

Injection sclerotherapy or variceal banding

The varices should be injected with a sclerosing agent that may arrest bleeding by producing vessel thrombosis. A needle is passed down the biopsy channel of the endoscope and a sclerosing agent is injected into the varices. Alternatively, the varices can be banded by mounting a band on the tip of the endoscope, sucking the varix just

Fig. 7.24 Endoscopic picture of oesophageal varices, showing blood spurting from a varix.

into the end of the scope and dislodging the band over the varix using a trip-wire mechanism.

Acute variceal sclerotherapy and banding are the treatment of choice; they arrest bleeding in 80% of cases and reduce early rebleeding. Between 15% and 20% of bleeding comes from gastric varices and here results of endoscopic therapy are poor.

Other measures available

Vasoconstrictor therapy

The main use of this is for emergency control of bleeding whilst waiting for endoscopy and in combination with endoscopic techniques. The aim of vasoconstrictor agents is to restrict portal inflow by splanchnic arterial constriction.

- *Terlipressin*. This is the only vasoconstrictor which has been shown to reduce mortality, albeit in small trials. Dose is 2 mg 6-hourly, reducing to 1 mg 4-hourly after 48 hours if a prolonged dosage regimen is used. It should not be given to patients with ischaemic heart disease. The patient will complain of abdominal colic, will defecate and have facial pallor owing to the generalized vasoconstriction.
- *Somatostatin*. This drug has few side-effects. An infusion of 250–500 µg/h appears to reduce bleeding, but has no effect on mortality. It should be used if there are contraindications to terlipressin, although the data on efficacy are less convincing than with terlipressin.

Balloon tamponade

This procedure is used mainly to control bleeding if endoscopic therapy or vasoconstrictor therapy has failed or is contraindicated or if there is exsanguinating haemorrhage. The tube should be left in place for up to 12 hours and removed in the endoscopy room prior to the endoscopic procedure. The usual tube is a four-lumen Sengstaken–Blakemore. The tube is passed into the stomach and the gastric balloon is inflated with air and pulled back. It should be positioned in close apposition to the gastro-oesophageal junction to prevent the cephalad variceal blood flow to the bleeding point. The oesophageal balloon should be inflated only if bleeding is not controlled by the gastric balloon alone.

This technique is successful in up to 90% of patients and is very useful in the first few hours of bleeding. However, it can have serious complications such as aspiration pneumonia, oesophageal rupture and mucosal ulceration, which lead to a 5% mortality. The procedure is very unpleasant for the patient.

Additional management of acute episode

- *Prophylactic antibiotics*. These have been shown to reduce infection and reduce mortality. Both oral and intravenous quinolones are used, e.g. ciprofloxacin 500 mg twice daily.
- *Measures to prevent encephalopathy*. Portosystemic encephalopathy (PSE) can be precipitated by a large bleed (since blood contains protein). The management is described on page 384.
- *Nursing*. Patients require high-dependency/intensive-care nursing. They should be nil by mouth until bleeding has stopped.
- *Sucralfate*. 1 g four times daily is given to reduce oesophageal ulceration following endoscopic therapy.

Management of an acute rebleed

Thirty per cent of patients rebleed within 5 days after a single therapeutic endoscopy. The source of the rebleed should be established by endoscopy. It is sometimes due to an ulcer produced by previous sclerotherapy and this is difficult to manage. Management starts with repeat endoscopic therapy – once only to control rebleeding (further sessions of sclerotherapy or banding are not advisable).

Transjugular intrahepatic portocaval shunt (TIPS)

TIPS is used in cases where the bleeding cannot be stopped after two sessions of endoscopic therapy within 5 days. In this technique, a guidewire is passed from the jugular vein into the liver and an expandable metal shunt is forced over it into the liver substance to form a channel between the systemic and portal venous systems. It reduces the hepatic sinusoidal and portal vein pressure by creating a total shunt, but without the risks of general anaesthesia and major surgery. TIPS is useful in the short term, but recurrent portal hypertension owing to stent stenosis or thrombosis occurs, although this has been reduced by the use of covered stents. Collaterals arising from the splenic or portal veins can be selectively embolized.

Emergency surgery

This is used when other measures fail or if TIPS is not available and, particularly, if the bleeding is from gastric fundal varices. Oesophageal transection and ligation of the feeding vessels to the bleeding varices is the most common surgical technique. Acute portosystemic shunt surgery (see below) is infrequently performed.

Prevention of recurrent variceal bleeding

Following an episode of variceal bleeding, the risk of recurrence is 60–80% over a 2-year period with an approximate mortality of 20% per episode. These facts justify the use of measures to prevent rebleeding.

Long-term measures

Non-selective beta-blockade. Oral propranolol in a dose sufficient to reduce resting pulse rate by 25% has been shown to decrease portal pressure. Portal inflow is reduced by two mechanisms: by a decrease in cardiac output (β_1), and by the blockade of β_2 vasodilator receptors on the splanchnic arteries, leaving an unopposed vasoconstrictor effect. This has been shown to decrease the frequency of rebleeding, and is as effective as sclerotherapy and ligation as it also prevents bleeding from portal hypertensive gastropathy. It is the treatment of first choice, but a substantial number of patients have either contraindications or are intolerant of treatment. Monitoring target reductions of portal pressure by hepatic venous pressure measurements is being evaluated.

Endoscopic treatment. The use of repeated courses of banding at 2-weekly intervals leads to obliteration of the varices. This markedly reduces rebleeding, most occurring before the varices have been fully obliterated. Between 30% and 40% of varices return per year, so that follow-up endoscopy with ablation should be performed. Banding is superior to sclerotherapy.

Although a reduction in bleeding episodes occurs, the effect on survival is controversial and probably small. Complications include oesophageal ulceration, mediastinitis and rarely strictures.

Transjugular portosystemic stent shunts. These reduce rebleeding rates compared to endoscopic techniques but do not improve survival, and increase encephalopathy. They are used if endoscopic or medical therapy fails. Covered stents are being evaluated.

Surgical procedures

Surgical portosystemic shunting is associated with an extremely low risk of rebleeding, but the diversion of portal blood away from the liver produces significant encephalopathy. Operative mortality is low in patients with Child's grade A (0–5%) but encephalopathy still occurs. Child's grade C has a very poor prognosis. The 'shunts' performed are usually an end-to-side portocaval anastomosis or a selective distal splenorenal shunt (Warren shunt), which maintains hepatic blood flow via the superior mesenteric vein.

Devascularization procedures including oesophageal transection do not produce encephalopathy, and can be used when there is splanchnic venous thrombosis.

Liver transplantation (p. 376) is the best option when there is poor liver function.

Prophylactic measures

Patients with cirrhosis and varices, who have not bled, should be prescribed non-selective beta-blockers (e.g. propranolol). This reduces the chances of upper GI bleeding, may increase survival and is cost-effective. If there are contraindications or intolerance, variceal banding is an option.

Ascites

Ascites is the presence of fluid within the peritoneal cavity and is a common complication of cirrhosis of the liver. The pathogenesis of the development of ascites in liver disease is controversial, but is probably secondary to renal sodium and water retention. Several factors are involved.

- *Sodium and water retention* occur as a result of peripheral arterial vasodilatation and consequent reduction in the effective blood volume. Nitric oxide has been postulated as the putative vasodilator, although other substances (e.g. atrial natriuretic peptide and prostaglandins) may be involved. The reduction in effective blood volume activates various neurohumoral pressor systems such as the sympathetic nervous system and the renin–angiotensin system, thus promoting salt and water retention (Fig. 12.3).
- *Portal hypertension* exerts a local hydrostatic pressure and leads to increased hepatic and splanchnic production of lymph and transudation of fluid into the peritoneal cavity.
- *Low serum albumin* (a consequence of poor synthetic liver function) may further contribute by a reduction in plasma oncotic pressure.

In patients with ascites, urine sodium excretion rarely exceeds 5 mmol in 24 hours. Loss of sodium from extra-renal sites accounts for approximately 30 mmol in 24 hours. The normal daily dietary sodium intake may vary between 120 and 200 mmol, resulting in a positive sodium balance of approximately 90–170 mmol in 24 hours (equivalent to 600–1300 mL of fluid retained).

Clinical features

The abdominal swelling associated with ascites may accumulate over many weeks or as rapidly as a few days. Precipitating factors include a high sodium diet or the development of a hepatocellular carcinoma or splanchnic vein thrombosis. Mild generalized abdominal pain and discomfort are common but, if more severe, should raise the suspicion of spontaneous bacterial peritonitis (see below). Respiratory distress accompanies tense ascites, and also causes difficulty in eating.

The presence of fluid is confirmed by the demonstration of shifting dullness. Many patients will also have peripheral oedema. A pleural effusion (usually on the right side) may infrequently be found and is believed to arise from the passage of ascitic fluid through congenital defects in the diaphragm.

Table 7.14 Causes of ascites divided according to the type of ascitic fluid

Straw-coloured	Chylous
Malignancy (most common cause)	Obstruction of main lymphatic duct (e.g. by carcinoma) – chylomicrons are present
Cirrhosis	
Infective	Cirrhosis
Tuberculosis	
Following intra-abdominal perforation – any bacteria may be found (e.g. *E. coli*)	**Haemorrhagic**
Spontaneous in cirrhotics	Malignancy
Hepatic vein obstruction (Budd–Chiari syndrome) protein level high in fluid	Ruptured ectopic pregnancy
	Abdominal trauma
	Acute pancreatitis
Chronic pancreatitis	
Congestive cardiac failure	
Constrictive pericarditis	
Meigs' syndrome (ovarian tumour)	
Hypoproteinaemia, (e.g. nephrotic syndrome)	

Investigations

A diagnostic aspiration of 10–20 mL of fluid should be obtained and the following performed:

- **Cell count.** A neutrophil count above 250 cells/mm^3 is indicative of an underlying (usually spontaneous) bacterial peritonitis.
- **Gram stain and culture** – for bacteria and acid-fast bacilli.
- **Protein.** The ascitic protein level enables a division into transudative and exudative ascites. For this division the serum albumin must be used as a reference point. An ascitic albumin of 11 g/L or more below the serum albumin level suggests a transudate. The level of ascitic protein provides an indirect estimate of opsonization capacity, and thereby the risk of developing spontaneous bacterial peritonitis. Patients at most risk are those with ascitic protein levels below 10 g/L.
- **Cytology** – for malignant cells.
- **Amylase** – to exclude pancreatic ascites.

The differential diagnosis of ascites is listed in Table 7.14.

Management

The aim is to both reduce sodium intake and increase renal excretion of sodium – and by doing so produce a net reabsorption of fluid from the ascites back into the circulating volume. The maximum rate at which ascites can be mobilized is 500–700 mL in 24 hours (see below). The management is as follows:

- Check serum electrolytes and creatinine at the start and every other day; weigh patient and measure urinary output daily.
- Bed rest alone will lead to a diuresis in a small proportion of people by improving renal perfusion, but in practice is not helpful.

- By dietary sodium restriction it is possible to reduce sodium intake to 40 mmol in 24 hours and still maintain an adequate protein and calorie intake with a palatable diet.
- Drugs. Remember, many contain significant amounts of sodium (could be up to 50 mmol daily). Examples include antacids, antibiotics (particularly the penicillins and cephalosporins) and effervescent tablets. Sodium-retaining drugs (non-steroidals, corticosteroids) should be avoided if possible.
- Fluid restriction is probably not necessary unless the serum sodium is under 128 mmol/L (see below).
- The diuretic of first choice is the aldosterone antagonist spironolactone, staring at 100 mg daily. Chronic administration produces gynaecomastia; amiloride, 5–15 mg daily, is then substituted.

The aim of diuretic therapy should be to produce a net loss of fluid approaching 700 mL in 24 hours (0.7 kg weight loss or 1.0 kg if peripheral oedema is present). Although 60% of patients respond with this regimen, diuresis is often poor and the spironolactone can be increased gradually to 500 mg daily providing there is no hyperkalaemia. A loop diuretic, such as furosemide 20–40 mg or bumetanide 1 mg daily, may be added if response is poor. These loop diuretics have several potential disadvantages, including hyponatraemia, hypokalaemia and volume depletion.

Ascitic fluid is mobilized more slowly than interstitial fluid, and diuretics should be given with great care in those without peripheral oedema.

Diuretics should be temporarily discontinued if a rise in serum creatinine level occurs, representing over-diuresis and hypovolaemia. Hyponatraemia occurring during therapy almost always represents haemodilution secondary to a failure to clear free water (usually a marker of reduced renal perfusion) and should be treated by stopping the diuretics if the sodium level falls below approximately 128 mmol/L as well as introducing water restriction. Diuretics should also be stopped if there is hyperkalaemia or the development of precoma.

Paracentesis

This is used to relieve symptomatic tense ascites. It is also used as a means of rapid therapy in patients with ascites and peripheral oedema, thus avoiding prolonged hospital stay. The main danger of this approach is the production of hypovolaemia as the ascites reaccumulates at the expense of the circulating volume. In patients with normal renal function and in the absence of hyponatraemia, this has largely been overcome by the administration of albumin (8 g per litre of ascitic fluid removed). In practice, up to 20 L can be removed over 4–6 hours. This procedure has more complications in end-stage cirrhosis or if the patient has renal failure.

Shunts

A transjugular intrahepatic portosystemic shunt (TIPS) is useful for resistant ascites providing there is inactive cirrhosis and minimal disturbance of renal function; as renal function improves, diurectic use is reduced and sodium excretion increases, but survival is unchanged. The use of a peritoneo-venous shunt has been abandoned in most centres as there is a high rate of blockage.

Spontaneous bacterial peritonitis (SBP)

This condition represents one of the more serious complications of ascites and occurs in approximately 8% of cirrhotics with ascites. The infecting organisms are believed to gain access to the peritoneum by haematogenous spread. The most frequently incriminated bacteria are *Escherichia coli*, *Klebsiella* and enterococci. The condition should be suspected in any patient with ascites with evidence of clinical deterioration. Features such as pain and pyrexia are frequently absent. Diagnostic aspiration should always be performed in patients with ascites (see above). A raised neutrophil count in ascites is alone sufficient evidence to start treatment immediately. A third-generation cephalosporin, such as cefotaxime or ceftazidime, is used and is modified on the basis of culture results. Recurrence is common (70% within a year) and an oral quinolone, e.g. norfloxacin, 400 mg twice daily is prescribed to prevent it. This also prolongs the survival.

Today the mortality has decreased to 10–15% depending on the severity of the liver disease. SBP is an indication for referral to a liver transplant centre.

Portosystemic encephalopathy

The term 'portosystemic encephalopathy' (PSE) refers to a chronic neuropsychiatric syndrome secondary to chronic liver disease. This condition occurs with cirrhosis, but a similar acute encephalopathy can occur in acute fulminant hepatic failure (see p. 368). PSE is seen in patients with portal hypertension that is due to spontaneous 'shunting', or in patients following a portosystemic shunt procedure, e.g. TIPS. Encephalopathy is potentially reversible.

Pathogenesis

The mechanism is unknown but several factors are thought to play a part. In cirrhosis, the portal blood bypasses the liver via the collaterals and the 'toxic' metabolites pass directly to the brain to produce the encephalopathy.

Many 'toxic' substances have been suggested as the causative factor, including ammonia, free fatty acids, mercaptans and accumulation of false neurotransmitters (octopamine) or activation of the γ-aminobutyric acid (GABA) inhibitory neurotransmitter system. Increased blood levels of aromatic amino acids (tyrosine and phenylalanine) and reduced branched-chain amino acids (valine, leucine and isoleucine) also occur. Nevertheless, ammonia seems to have a major role, and ammonia-induced alteration of brain neurotransmitter balance – especially at the astrocyte–neurone interface – is the leading concept of the causation. Ammonia is produced by the breakdown of protein by intestinal bacteria, and a high blood ammonia is seen in most patients. The factors that can precipitate PSE are shown in Table 7.15.

Table 7.15 Factors precipitating portosystemic encephalopathy

High dietary protein
Gastrointestinal haemorrhage
Constipation
Infection, including spontaneous bacterial peritonitis
Fluid and electrolyte disturbance due to:
  diuretic therapy
  paracentesis
Drugs (e.g. any CNS depressant)
Portosystemic shunt operations, TIPS
Any surgical procedure
Progressive liver damage
Development of hepatocellular carcinoma

TIPS, transjugular intrahepatic portocaval shunt

Clinical features

An acute onset often has a precipitating factor (Table 7.15). The patient becomes increasingly drowsy and comatose.

Chronically, there is a disorder of personality, mood and intellect, with a reversal of normal sleep rhythm. These changes may be fluctuating and a history from a relative must be obtained. The patient is irritable, confused, disorientated and has slow slurred speech. General features include nausea, vomiting and weakness. Coma occurs as the encephalopathy becomes more marked, but there is always hyperreflexia and increased tone. Convulsions are so very rare that other causes must be looked for.

Signs include:

- fetor hepaticus (a sweet smell to the breath)
- a coarse flapping tremor seen when the hands are outstretched and the wrists hyperextended (asterixis)
- constructional apraxia, with the patient being unable to write or draw, for example, a five-pointed star
- decreased mental function, which can be assessed by using the serial-sevens test (see p. 1277). A trail-making test (the ability to join numbers and letters with a pen within a certain time – a standard psychological test for brain dysfunction) is prolonged and is a useful bedside test to assess encephalopathy.

Diagnosis is clinical. Routine liver biochemistry merely confirms the presence of liver disease, not the presence of encephalopathy.

Additional investigations

- Electroencephalography (EEG) shows a decrease in the frequency of the normal α-waves (8–13 Hz) to δ-waves of 1.5–3 Hz. These changes occur before coma supervenes.
- Visual evoked responses (see p. 1203) also detect subclinical encephalopathy.
- Arterial blood ammonia is occasionally useful in the differential diagnosis of the cause of the coma and to follow the course of the PSE, but is not readily available.

Management

Management consists of evacuation of the bowels and sterilizing the bowel. Restriction of protein intake is reserved for resistant cases.

Immediate management

- Identify and remove the possible precipitating cause, such as drugs with cerebral depressant properties, constipation or electrolyte imbalance due to overdiuresis.
- Give purgation and enemas to empty the bowels of nitrogenous substances. Lactulose (10–30 mL three times daily) is an osmotic purgative that reduces the colonic pH and limits ammonia absorption. Lactilol (β-galactoside sorbitol 30 g daily) is metabolized by colonic bacteria and is comparable in efficacy to lactulose. The value of both agents has been questioned.
- Maintain nutrition with adequate calories, given if necessary via a fine-bore nasogastric tube, and do not restrict protein for more than 48 hours.
- Give antibiotics. Rifaximin is mainly unabsorbed and well tolerated long term. Metronidazole (200 mg four times daily) is also effective in the acute situation. Neomycin should not be used. Stop or reduce diuretic therapy.
- Give intravenous fluids as necessary (beware of too much sodium).
- Treat any infection.
- Increase protein in the diet to the limit of tolerance as the encephalopathy improves.

Course and prognosis

Acute encephalopathy, often seen in FHF, has a very poor prognosis as the disease itself has a high mortality. In cirrhosis, chronic PSE is very variable and the prognosis is that of the underlying liver disease. Very rarely an organic syndrome with cerebellar signs, or choreoathetosis can develop in long-standing cases. Hepatic myelopathy leading to a spastic paraparesis due to demyelination also occurs. Both conditions are associated with chronic portosystemic shunting. Patients should be referred to a live transplant centre.

Renal failure (hepatorenal syndrome)

The hepatorenal syndrome occurs typically in a patient with advanced cirrhosis with jaundice and ascites. The urine output is low with a low urinary sodium concentration, a maintained capacity to concentrate urine (i.e. tubular function is intact) and an almost normal renal histology. The renal failure is described as 'functional'. It is sometimes precipitated by overvigorous diuretic therapy, diarrhoea or paracentesis, but often no precipitating factor is found. Advanced cases may progress beyond the 'functional' stage to produce an acute tubular necrosis.

The mechanism is similar to that producing ascites. The initiating factor is thought to be extreme peripheral vasodilatation possibly due to nitric oxide, leading to an extreme decrease in the effective blood volume and hypotension (p. 665). This activates the homeostatic mechanisms, causing a rise in plasma renin, aldosterone, norepinephrine (noradrenaline) and vasopressin, leading to vasoconstriction of the renal vasculature. There is an increased preglomerular vascular resistance causing the blood flow to be directed away from the renal cortex. This leads to a reduced glomerular filtration rate and plasma renin remains high. Salt and water retention occur with reabsorption of sodium from the renal tubules.

A number of other mediators have been incriminated in the pathogenesis of the hepatorenal syndrome, in particular the eicosanoids. This has been supported by the precipitation of the syndrome by inhibitors of prostaglandin synthetase such as non-steroidal anti-inflammatory agents.

Diuretic therapy should be stopped and intravascular hypovolaemia corrected. Terlipressin has been used as a short-term measure with improvement, but the overall prognosis is poor. Studies of TIPS are in progress. Liver transplantation is the best option.

Hepatopulmonary syndrome

This is defined as a hypoxaemia occurring in patients with advanced liver disease. It is due to intrapulmonary vascular dilatation with no evidence of primary pulmonary disease. The patients have features of cirrhosis with spider naevi and clubbing as well as cyanosis. Most patients have no respiratory symptoms but with more severe disease are breathless on standing. Transthoracic ECHO shows intrapulmonary shunting, and arterial blood gases confirm the arterial oxygen desaturation. These changes are improved with liver transplantation.

This condition must be distinguished from pulmonary hypertension (1–2% in association with cirrhosis) which is often a contraindication for transplantation.

Primary hepatocellular carcinoma

This is discussed on page 394.

REFERENCES

Benyon RC, Iredale JP (2000) Is liver fibrosis reversible? *Gut* **46**: 443–446.

Ginès P et al. (2004) Management of cirrhosis and ascites. *New England Journal of Medicine* **350**: 1646–1654.

Ginès P et al. (2003) Hepatorenal syndrome. Lancet **362**: 1819-1827

Hoeper MM et al. (2004) Portopulmonary hypertension and hepatopulmonary syndrome. *Lancet* **363**: 1401–1468.

Keefe FB (2001) Liver transplantation. *Gastroenterology* **120**: 749–762.

Lewis M, Howdle PD (2003) The neurology of liver failure. *Quarterly Journal of Medicine* **96**: 623–633.

Moore KP et al. (2003) Management of ascites in cirrhosis. *Hepatology* **38**: 258–266.

Sharara AI, Rockey DC (2001) Gastro-oesophageal variceal haemorrhage. *New England Journal of Medicine* **345**: 669–681.

Shawcross DL, Jalan R (2005) Dispelling myths in the treatment of hepatic encephalopathy. *Lancet* **365**: 431–433.

TYPES OF CIRRHOSIS

Alcoholic cirrhosis

This is discussed in the section on alcoholic liver disease (p. 389).

Primary biliary cirrhosis

Primary biliary cirrhosis (PBC) is a chronic disorder in which there is a progressive destruction of bile ducts, eventually leading to cirrhosis. Ninety per cent of those affected are women in the age range 40–50 years. PBC was thought to be rare but is now being diagnosed frequently in its milder forms. The prevalence is approximately 7.5 per 100 000, with a 1–6% increase in first-degree relatives. PBC has been called 'chronic non-suppurative destructive cholangitis'; this term is more descriptive of the early lesion and emphasizes that true cirrhosis occurs only in the later stages of the disease.

Aetiology

The aetiology is unknown, but immunological mechanisms play a part. Serum antimitochondrial antibodies are found in almost all patients with PBC, and of the mitochondrial proteins involved, the antigen M2 is specific to PBC.

Five M2-specific antigens have been further defined using immunoblot techniques, of which the E2 component of the pyruvate dehydrogenase complex (PDC) is the major M2 autoantigen. The five antigens are a 72 kDa E2 subunit (PDC.E2), the 52 kDa protein X, the 50 kDa branched-chain 2-oxo-acid dehydrogenase complex (BCOADC.E2), the 48 kDa 2-oxo-glutarate dehydrogenase complex (OGDC.E2), and the 41 kDa E1 α-subunit of PDC.

The presence of AMA in high titre is unrelated to the clinical or histological picture and its role in pathogenesis is unclear.

It seems likely that an environmental factor acts on a genetically predisposed host. *E. coli* and other entero-bacteria, as well as retroviruses have been proposed as the triggering infective agent.

Although damage to bile ducts is a feature, antibodies to bile ductules are not specific to PBC. Biliary epithelium from patients with PBC expresses aberrant class II HLAs, but it is not known whether this expression is the cause or result of the inflammatory response. Cell-mediated immunity is impaired (demonstrated both in vitro and by skin testing), suggesting that sensitized T lymphocytes might be involved in producing damage. There may be a defect in immunoregulation, or a decrease in T suppressor cells which allows cytotoxic T cells to produce damage to the bile ducts. There is also evidence to suggest that lymphokine secretion and cell activation by T lymphocytes is impaired at the site of tissue destruction. There is an increased synthesis of IgM, thought to be due to a failure of the switch from IgM to IgG antibody synthesis. No specific associated Class 2 MHC loci have been found but DQA1*0102 haplotype has been associated with disease resistance.

Clinical features

Asymptomatic patients are discovered on routine examination or screening to have hepatomegaly, a raised serum alkaline phosphatase or autoantibodies.

Pruritus is often the earliest symptom, preceding jaundice by a few years. Fatigue may accompany pruritus, particularly in progressive cases. When jaundice appears, hepatomegaly is usually found. In the later stages, patients are jaundiced with severe pruritus. Pigmented xanthelasma on eyelids or other deposits of cholesterol in the creases of the hands may be seen.

Associations

Autoimmune disorders (e.g. Sjögren's syndrome, scleroderma, rheumatoid arthritis) occur with increased frequency. Keratoconjunctivitis sicca (dry eyes and mouth) is seen in 70% of cases. Renal tubular acidosis and membranous glomerulonephritis occur.

Investigations

- **Mitochondrial antibodies** – measured routinely by ELISA (in titres > 1 : 160) – are present in over 95% of patients; M2 antibody is specific. Other non-specific antibodies (e.g. antinuclear factor and smooth muscle) may also be present.
- **High serum alkaline phosphatase** is often the only abnormality in the liver biochemistry.
- **Serum cholesterol** is raised.
- **Serum IgM** may be very high.
- **Ultrasound** can show a diffuse alteration in liver architecture.
- **Liver biopsy** shows characteristic histological features of a portal tract infiltrate mainly of lymphocytes and plasma cells; approximately 40% have granulomas. Most of the early changes are in zone 1. Later, there is damage to and loss of small bile ducts with ductular proliferation. Portal tract fibrosis and, eventually, cirrhosis is seen.

Hepatic granulomas are not specific and are also seen in sarcoidosis, tuberculosis, schistosomiasis, drug reactions, brucellosis, parasitic infestation (e.g. strongyloidiasis) and other conditions.

Differential diagnosis

The classical picture presents little difficulty with diagnosis (high serum alkaline phosphatase and the presence of AMA); this can be confirmed by the characteristic features on liver biopsy although this is not necessary except in doubtful cases. There is a group of patients with the histological changes of PBC, but the serology of autoimmune hepatitis (i.e. positive antinuclear and smooth muscle antibodies but negative AMA). This has been given the name of autoimmune cholangitis and responds to steroids and azathioprine.

In the jaundiced patient, extrahepatic biliary obstruction should be excluded by ultrasound and, if there is doubt about the diagnosis, MRCP (or ERCP) should be performed to make sure that the bile ducts are normal.

Treatment

Ursodeoxycholic acid (10–15 mg/kg) improves bilirubin and aminotransferase values. It is not clear if prognosis is altered. Symptoms are not improved. Steroids improve biochemical and histological disease but may lead to increased osteoporosis and other side-effects and should not be used.

Malabsorption of fat-soluble vitamins (A, D and K) occurs and supplementation is required when deficiency is detected and in the jaundiced patient prophylactically. Bisphosphonates are required for osteoporosis. Hyperlipidaemia should be treated (see p. 1139).

Pruritus is difficult to control, but colestyramine, one 4 g sachet three times daily, can be helpful, although it is unpalatable. Rifampicin as well as naloxone hydrochloride and naltrexone (opioid antagonists) have been shown to be of benefit. Intractable pruritus can be relieved by a molecular absorbent re-circulating system (MARS).

The lack of effective medical therapy has made PBC a major indication for orthotopic liver transplantation (p. 376).

Complications

The complications are those of cirrhosis. In addition, osteoporosis, and rarely osteomalacia and a polyneuropathy can also occur.

Course and prognosis

This is very variable. Asymptomatic patients and those presenting with pruritus will survive for more than 20 years. Symptomatic patients with jaundice have a more rapidly progressive course and die of liver failure or bleeding varices in approximately 5 years. Liver transplantation should therefore be offered when the serum bilirubin reaches 100 µmol/L. Transplantation has a 5-year survival of at least 80%.

Secondary biliary cirrhosis

Cirrhosis can result from prolonged (for months) large duct biliary obstruction. Causes include bile duct strictures, gallstones and sclerosing cholangitis. An ultrasound examination, followed by ERCP or PTC, is performed to outline the ducts and any remedial cause is dealt with.

Hereditary haemochromatosis

Hereditary haemochromatosis (HH) is an inherited disease characterized by excess iron deposition in various organs leading to eventual fibrosis and functional organ failure.

Prevalence and aetiology

HH is transmitted by an autosomal recessive gene with a prevalence in Caucasians of homozygotes (affected) of 1 in 400 and a heterozygote (carrier) frequency of 1 in 10. It is the most common single gene disorder in Caucasians. It is associated with HLA-A3 (72% versus 28% of the general population); in addition HLA-B14 is increased in France and HLA-B7 in Australia. The most common form of HH has been shown to be due to a mutation in a gene, *HFE* – on the short arm of chromosome 6, but the clinical phenotype varies greatly between homozygous individuals.

Between 85% and 90% of patients with overt HH are homozygous for the Cys 282 Tyr; C282Y mutation. A second mutation (His 63 Asp; H63D) occurs in about 25% of the population and is in complete linkage disequilibrium with Cys 282 Tyr. A third, different form of haemochromatosis occurs in Southern Europe, and is associated with TfR2, a transferrin receptor isoform.

Dietary intakes of iron and chelating agents (ascorbic acid) may be relevant. Iron overload may be present in alcoholics, but alcohol excess per se does not cause HH although there is a history of excess alcohol intake in 25% of patients.

Mechanism of damage. This is still unclear. The *HFE* gene protein interacts with the transferrin receptor 1, which is a mediator in intestinal iron absorption (see Fig. 8.8). Iron is taken up by the mucosal cells inappropriately, exceeding the binding capacity of transferrin. Hepatic expression of the hepcidin gene is decreased in HFE haemochromatosis, facilitating liver iron overload. Excess iron is then taken up by the liver and other tissues gradually over a long period. It seems likely that it is the iron itself that precipitates fibrosis.

Pathology

In symptomatic patients the total body iron content is 20–40 g, compared with 3–4 g in a normal person. The iron content is particularly increased in the liver and pancreas (50–100 times normal) but is also increased in other organs (e.g. the endocrine glands, heart and skin).

In established cases the liver shows extensive iron deposition and fibrosis. Early in the disease, iron is deposited in the periportal hepatocytes (in pericanalicular lysosomes). Later it is distributed widely throughout all acinar zones, biliary duct epithelium, Kupffer cells and connective tissue. Cirrhosis is a late feature.

Clinical features

The course of the disease depends on a number of factors, including sex, dietary iron intake, presence of associated hepatotoxins (especially alcohol) and genotypes. Overt clinical manifestations occur more frequently in men; the reduced incidence in women is probably explained by physiological blood loss and a smaller dietary intake of iron. Most affected individuals present in the fifth decade. The classic triad of bronze skin pigmentation (due to melanin deposition), hepatomegaly and diabetes mellitus is only present in cases of gross iron overload.

Hypogonadism secondary to pituitary dysfunction is the most common endocrine feature. Deficiency of other pituitary hormones is also found, but symptomatic endocrine deficiencies, such as loss of libido, are very rare. Cardiac manifestations, particularly heart failure and arrhythmias, are common, especially in younger patients.

Calcium pyrophosphate is deposited asymmetrically in both large and small joints (chondrocalcinosis) leading to an arthropathy. The exact relationship of chondrocalcinosis to iron deposition is uncertain.

Complications

Thirty per cent of patients with cirrhosis will develop primary hepatocellular carcinoma (HCC). HCC has only very rarely been described in non-cirrhotic patients in whom the excess iron stores have been removed. Early diagnosis is vital.

Investigations

Homozygotes

- **Serum iron** is elevated (> 30 µmol/L) in 90% with a reduction in the TIBC and a transferrin saturation of (> 60%) or more.
- **Serum ferritin** is elevated (usually > 500 µg/L or 240 nmol/L).
- **Liver biochemistry** is often normal, even with established cirrhosis.

Heterozygotes

Heterozygotes may have normal biochemical tests or modest increases in serum iron transferrin saturation (> 45%) or serum ferritin (usually > 400 µg/L).

Genetic testing

If abnormal iron studies are found, genetic testing is performed. Liver biopsy is now not usually required.

Liver biopsy

This can define the extent of tissue damage, assess tissue iron, and the hepatic iron concentration can be measured (> 180 µmol/g dry weight of liver indicates haemochromatosis) but it is now not required for diagnosis.

Mild degrees of parenchymal iron deposition in patients with alcoholic cirrhosis can often cause confusion with true homozygous HH. It is highly likely that many of this former group are heterozygotes for the haemochromatosis gene.

Magnetic resonance imaging

MRI shows dramatic reduction in the signal intensity of the liver and pancreas owing to the paramagnetic affect of ferritin and haemosiderin. A highly T2 weighted gradient recalled echo (GRE) technique detects all clinically relevant liver iron overload (> 60 µmol/g of liver). In secondary iron overload (haemosiderosis), which involves the reticuloendothelial cells, the pancreas is spared – enabling distinction between these two conditions.

Treatment and management

Venesection

This prolongs life and may reverse tissue damage; the risk of malignancy still remains if cirrhosis is present. All patients should have excess iron removed as rapidly as possible. This is achieved using venesection of 500 mL performed twice-weekly for up to 2 years; i.e. 160 units with 250 mg of iron per unit, equals 40 g removed. During venesection, serum iron and ferritin and the mean corpuscular volume (MCV) should be monitored. These fall only when available iron is depleted. Three or four venesections per year are required to prevent reaccumulation of iron. Serum ferritin should remain within the normal range. Liver biopsy can show the removal of iron to assess progress but is now seldom used.

Manifestations of the disease usually improve or disappear, except for diabetes, testicular atrophy and chondrocalcinosis. The requirements for insulin often diminish in diabetic patients. Testosterone replacement is often helpful.

Chelation therapy

In the rare patient who cannot tolerate venesection (because of severe cardiac disease or anaemia), chelation therapy with desferrioxamine either intermittently or continuously by infusion has been successful in removing iron.

Screening

In all cases of HH, all first-degree family members must be screened to detect early and asymptomatic disease. HFE mutation analysis is performed with measurement of transferrin saturation and serum ferritin.

In the general population, the serum iron and transferrin saturation are the best and cheapest tests available.

Wilson's disease (hepatolenticular degeneration)

Dietary copper is normally absorbed from the stomach and upper small intestine. It is transported to the liver loosely bound to albumin. Here it is incorporated into caeruloplasmin, a glycoprotein synthesized in the liver, and secreted into the blood. Copper is normally excreted in the bile.

Wilson's disease is a very rare inborn error of copper metabolism that results in copper deposition in various organs, including the liver, the basal ganglia of the brain and the cornea. It is potentially treatable and all young patients with liver disease must be screened for this condition.

Aetiology

It is an autosomal recessive disorder with a molecular defect within a copper-transporting ATPase encoded by a gene (designated *ATP7B*) located on chromosome 13. Over 60 mutations have been identified, the most frequent being His1069 Gly found in approximately 50% of cases in the USA and Europe. It occurs world-wide, particularly in countries where consanguinity is common. There is a failure of both incorporation and biliary excretion of copper. In the liver, copper is incorporated into caeruloplasmin and then excreted with bile. There is a low serum caeruloplasmin in over 80% of patients owing to poor synthesis, but the precise mechanism for the failure of copper excretion is not known.

Pathology

The liver histology is not diagnostic and varies from that of chronic hepatitis to macronodular cirrhosis. Stains for copper show a periportal distribution but this can be unreliable (see below). The basal ganglia are damaged and show cavitation, the kidneys show tubular degeneration, and erosions are seen in bones.

Clinical features

Children usually present with hepatic problems, whereas young adults have more neurological problems, such as tremor, dysarthria, involuntary movements and eventually dementia. The liver disease varies from episodes of acute hepatitis, especially in children, which can go on to fulminant hepatic failure to chronic hepatitis or cirrhosis.

Typical signs are of chronic liver disease with neurological signs of basal ganglia involvement (p. 1231). A specific sign is the Kayser–Fleischer ring, which is due to copper deposition in Descemet's membrane in the cornea. It appears as a greenish brown pigment at the corneoscleral junction just within the cornea. Identification of this ring frequently requires slit-lamp examination. It may be absent in young children.

Investigations

- **Serum copper and caeruloplasmin** are usually reduced but can be normal.
- **Urinary copper** is usually increased (100–1000 mg in 24 hours; normal levels < 40 mg in 24 hours).
- **Liver biopsy.** The diagnosis depends on measurement of the amount of copper in the liver, although high levels of copper are also found in the liver in chronic cholestasis. Measurement of ^{64}Cu incorporation into the liver may be helpful.
- **Haemolysis and anaemia** may be present.
- **Genetic analysis** is limited as already over 200 mutations have been identified at the ATP7B locus.

Treatment

Lifetime treatment with penicillamine, 1–1.5 g daily, is effective in chelating copper. If treatment is started early, clinical and biochemical improvement can occur. Urine copper levels should be monitored and the drug dose adjusted downwards after 2–3 years. Serious side-effects of the drug occur in 10% and include skin rashes, leucopenia and renal damage. All siblings and children of patients should be screened and treatment given even in the asymptomatic if there is evidence of copper accumulation.

Prognosis

Early diagnosis and effective treatment have improved the outlook. Neurological damage is, however, permanent. Fulminant hepatic failure or decompensated cirrhosis should be treated by liver transplantation.

α_1-Antitrypsin deficiency (see also p. 902)

A deficiency of α_1-antitrypsin (α_1AT) is sometimes associated with liver disease and pulmonary emphysema (particularly in smokers). α_1AT is a glycoprotein, part of a family of serine protease inhibitors, or serpin, superfamily. α_1AT-deficiency is inherited as an autosomal dominant and 1 in 10 northern Europeans carries an abnormal gene.

The protein is a 394-amino acid 52 kDa acute-phase protein that is synthesized in the liver and constitutes 90% of the serum α_1-globulin seen on electrophoresis. Its main role is to inhibit the proteolytic enzyme, neutrophil elastase.

The gene is located on chromosome 14. The genetic variants of α_1AT are characterized by their electrophoretic mobilities as medium (M), slow (S) or very slow (Z). The normal genotype is protease inhibitor MM (PiMM), the homozygote for Z is PiZZ, and the heterozygotes are PiMZ and PiSZ. S and Z variants are due to a single amino acid replacement of glutamic acid at positions 264 and 342 of the polypeptide, respectively. This results in decreased synthesis and secretion of the protein by the liver as protein–protein interactions occur between the reactive centre loop of one molecule and the β-pleated sheet of a second (loop sheet polymerization).

How this causes liver disease is uncertain. It is postulated that the failure of secretion of the abnormal protein leads to an accumulation in the liver, causing liver damage.

Clinical features

The majority of patients with clinical disease are homozygotes with a PiZZ phenotype. Some may present in childhood and a few require transplantation. Approximately 10–15% of adult patients will develop cirrhosis, usually over the age of 50 years, and 75% will have respiratory problems. Approximately 5% of patients die of their liver disease. Heterozygotes (e.g. PiSZ or PiMZ) may develop liver disease, but the risk is small.

Investigations

- **Serum α_1-antritrypsin** is low, at 10% of the normal level in the PiZZ phenotypes, 60% of normal in the S variant.

On liver biopsy periodic acid–Schiff (PAS)-positive, diastase-resistant globules are seen in periportal hepatocytes. These can be shown to be α_1AT using specific antiserum. Fibrosis and cirrhosis can be present.

Treatment

There is no treatment apart from dealing with the complications of liver disease. Patients with hepatic decompensation should be considered for liver transplantation. Patients should stop smoking (see p. 893).

FURTHER READING

Carrell RW, Lomas DA (2002) Alpha-1 antitrypsin deficiency. *New England Journal of Medicine* **346**: 45–53.

Pietrangelo A (2004) Hereditary hemochromatosis. *New England Journal of Medicine* **350**: 2383–2397.

Talwalkar JA, Lindor KD (2003) Primary biliary cirrhosis. *Lancet* **362**: 53–61.

ALCOHOLIC LIVER DISEASE

This section gives the pathology and clinical features of alcoholic liver disease. The amounts needed to produce liver damage, alcohol metabolism, and other clinical effects of alcohol are described on page 263.

Ethanol is metabolized in the liver by two pathways (see p. 262), resulting in an increase in the NADH/NAD ratio. The altered redox potential results in increased hepatic fatty acid synthesis with decreased fatty acid oxidation, both events leading to hepatic accumulation of fatty acid that is then esterified to glycerides.

The changes in oxidation–reduction also impair carbohydrate and protein metabolism and are the cause of the centrilobular necrosis of the hepatic acinus typical of alcohol damage.

Acetaldehyde is formed by the oxidation of ethanol and its effect on hepatic proteins may well be a factor in producing liver cell damage. The exact mechanism of alcoholic hepatitis and cirrhosis is unknown, but since only 10–20% of people who drink heavily will suffer from cirrhosis, a genetic predisposition is suggested. Immunological mechanisms have also been proposed.

Alcohol can enhance the effects of toxic metabolites of drugs (e.g. paracetamol) on the liver, as it induces microsomal metabolism via the microsomal ethanol oxidizing system (MEOS) (p. 262).

Pathology

Alcohol can produce a wide spectrum of liver disease from fatty change to hepatitis and cirrhosis.

Fatty change

The metabolism of alcohol invariably produces fat in the liver, mainly in zone 3. This is minimal with small amounts of alcohol, but with larger amounts the cells become swollen with fat (steatosis) giving, eventually, a Swiss-cheese effect on haematoxylin and eosin stain. Steatosis can also be seen in obesity, diabetes, starvation and occasionally in chronic illness (p. 374) There is no liver cell damage. The fat disappears on stopping alcohol.

In some cases collagen is laid down around the central hepatic veins (perivenular fibrosis) and this can sometimes progress to cirrhosis without a preceding hepatitis. Alcohol directly affects stellate cells, transforming them into collagen-producing myofibroblast cells. Cirrhosis might then develop if there is an imbalance between degradation and production of collagen.

Alcoholic hepatitis

In addition to fatty change there is infiltration by polymorphonuclear leucocytes and hepatocyte necrosis mainly in zone 3. Dense cytoplasmic inclusions called Mallory bodies are sometimes seen in hepatocytes and giant mitochondria are also a feature. Mallory bodies are suggestive of, but not specific for, alcoholic damage as they can be found in other liver disease, such as Wilson's disease and PBC. If alcohol consumption continues, alcoholic hepatitis may progress to cirrhosis.

Alcoholic cirrhosis

This is classically of the micronodular type, but a mixed pattern may also be seen accompanying fatty change, and evidence of pre-existing alcoholic hepatitis may be present.

Clinical features

Fatty liver

There are often no symptoms or signs. Vague abdominal symptoms of nausea, vomiting and diarrhoea are due to the more general effects of alcohol on the gastrointestinal tract. Hepatomegaly, sometimes huge, can occur together with other features of chronic liver disease.

Alcoholic hepatitis

The clinical features vary in degree:

- The patient may be well, with few symptoms, the hepatitis only being apparent on the liver biopsy in addition to fatty change.
- Mild to moderate symptoms of ill-health, occasionally with mild jaundice, may occur. Signs include all the features of chronic liver disease. Liver biochemistry is deranged and the diagnosis is made on liver histology.
- In the severe case, usually superimposed on patients with alcoholic cirrhosis, the patient is ill, with jaundice and ascites. Abdominal pain is frequently present, with a high fever associated with the liver necrosis. On examination there is deep jaundice, hepatomegaly, sometimes splenomegaly, and ascites with ankle oedema. The signs of chronic liver disease are also present.

Alcoholic cirrhosis

This represents the final stage of liver disease from alcohol abuse. Nevertheless, patients can be very well with few symptoms. On examination, there are usually signs of chronic liver disease. The diagnosis is confirmed by liver biopsy.

Usually the patient presents with one of the complications of cirrhosis. In many cases there are features of alcohol dependency (see p. 1302) as well as evidence of involvement of other systems, such as polyneuropathy.

Investigations

Fatty liver

An elevated MCV often indicates heavy drinking. Liver biochemistry shows mild abnormalities with elevation of both serum aminotransferase enzymes. The γ-GT level is a sensitive test for determining whether the patient is taking alcohol. With severe fatty infiltration, marked changes in all liver biochemical parameters can occur. Ultrasound or CT will demonstrate fatty infiltration, as will liver histology.

Alcoholic hepatitis

Investigations show a leucocytosis with markedly deranged liver biochemistry with elevated:

- serum bilirubin
- serum AST and ALT

- serum alkaline phosphatase
- prothrombin time (PT).

A low serum albumin may also be found. Rarely, hyperlipidaemia with haemolysis (Zieve's syndrome) may occurs.

Liver biopsy, if required, is performed by the transjugular route because of prolonged PT.

Alcoholic cirrhosis

Investigations are as for cirrhosis in general.

Management and prognosis

General management

Patients should be advised to stop drinking. Delirium tremens (a withdrawal symptom) may be treated with diazepam. Intravenous thiamine should be given empirically to prevent Wernicke–Korsakoff encephalopathy. Bed rest with a diet high in protein and vitamin supplements is given. Dietary protein may have to be limited because of encephalopathy. Follow-up of patients with alcoholic liver disease shows, however, that – apart from highly motivated groups – most patients continue to drink alcohol.

Fatty liver

In all but the mildest cases the patient is advised to stop drinking alcohol; the fat will disappear and the liver biochemistry usually returns to normal. Small amounts of alcohol can be drunk subsequently as long as patients are aware of the problems and can control their consumption.

Alcoholic hepatitis

In severe cases the patient is confined to bed. Treatment for encephalopathy and ascites is commenced. Patients should be fed preferably via a fine-bore nasogastric tube or sometimes intravenously. Vitamins B and C should be given by injection. Corticosteroids should be given providing infection is absent, or following a course of antibiotics. Antifungal prophylaxis should also be used.

Patients are advised to stop drinking for life, as this is undoubtedly a precirrhotic condition. The prognosis is variable and, despite abstinence, the liver disease is progressive in many patients. Conversely, a few patients continue to drink heavily without developing cirrhosis.

In severe cases the mortality is at least 50%, and with a PT twice the normal, progressive encephalopathy and renal failure, the mortality approaches 90%.

Alcoholic cirrhosis

The management of cirrhosis is described on page 376. Again, all patients are advised to stop drinking for life. Abstinence from alcohol results in an improvement in prognosis, with a 5-year survival of 90%, but with continued drinking this falls to 60%. With advanced disease (i.e. jaundice, ascites and haematemesis) the 5-year survival rate falls to 35%, with most of the deaths occurring in the first year. Liver transplantation is being used widely in some countries with good survival figures.

A trial of abstention to establish if liver disease can improve is mandatory, but transplantation should not be denied if the patient continues to deteriorate.

Hepatocellular carcinoma is a complication particularly in men.

> **FURTHER READING**
> Lieber C (1995) Medical disorders of alcoholism. *New England Journal of Medicine* **133**: 1058–1065.
> Tilg H, Diehl AM (2000) Cytokines in alcoholic steatohepatitis. *New England Journal of Medicine* **343**: 1467–1476.

BUDD–CHIARI SYNDROME

In this condition there is obstruction to the venous outflow of the liver owing to occlusion of the hepatic vein. In one-third of patients the cause is unknown, but specific causes include hypercoagulability states, such as polycythaemia vera, taking the contraceptive pill, or leukaemia. Other causes include occlusion of the hepatic vein owing to posterior abdominal wall sarcomas, renal or adrenal tumours, hepatocellular carcinoma, hepatic infections (e.g. hydatid cyst), congenital venous webs, radiotherapy, or trauma to the liver.

The acute form presents with abdominal pain, nausea, vomiting, tender hepatomegaly and ascites (a fulminant form occurs particularly in pregnant women). In the chronic form there is enlargement of the liver (particularly the caudate lobe), mild jaundice, ascites, a negative hepatojugular reflex, and splenomegaly with portal hypertension.

Investigations

Investigations show a high protein content in the ascitic fluid and characteristic liver histology with centrizonal congestion, haemorrhage, fibrosis and cirrhosis. Ultrasound, CT or MRI will demonstrate hepatic vein occlusion with diffuse abnormal parenchyma on contrast-enhancement, which spares the caudate lobe because of its independent blood supply and venous drainage. There may be compression of the inferior vena cava. Pulsed Doppler sonography or a colour Doppler are useful as they show abnormalities in the direction of flow in the hepatic vein. Investigations to identify a cause are also performed, such as blood tests and coagulation studies.

Differential diagnosis

A similar clinical picture can be produced by inferior vena caval obstruction, right-sided cardiac failure or constrictive pericarditis, and appropriate investigations should be performed.

Treatment

In the acute situation, thrombolytic therapy should be given. Ascites should be treated as well as any underlying cause (e.g. polycythaemia). Congenital webs should be treated radiologically or resected surgically. A side-to-side portocaval or splenorenal anastomosis may decompress the congested liver providing there is no caval obstruction, with considerable improvement in the clinical state of the patient. Transjugular intrahepatic portosystemic shunts (TIPS) instead of portocaval shunts are being increasingly used, as caval compression does not prejudice the efficacy of TIPS. Liver transplantation is the treatment of choice for chronic Budd–Chiari syndrome and for the fulminant form, followed by lifelong anticoagulation.

Prognosis

The prognosis depends on the aetiology, but some patients can survive for several years.

REFERENCE
Menom KVN et al. (2004) The Budd-Chiari syndrome. *New England Journal of Medicine* **350**: 578–585.

VENO-OCCLUSIVE DISEASE

This is due to injury of the hepatic veins and presents clinically like the Budd–Chiari syndrome. It was originally described in Jamaica, where the ingestion of toxic pyrrolizidine alkaloids in bush tea (made from plants of the genera *Senecio, Heliotropium* and *Crotolaria*) caused damage to the hepatic veins. It can be seen in other parts of the world. It is also seen as a complication of chemotherapy and total body irradiation before allogeneic bone marrow transplantation. The development of veno-occlusive disease after transplantation carries a high mortality. Treatment is supportive with control of ascites and hepatocellular failure. Defibrotide has been tried and TIPS has been used in a few cases.

FIBROPOLYCYSTIC DISEASES

These diseases are usually inherited and lead to the presence of cysts or fibrosis in the liver, kidney and occasionally the pancreas, and other organs.

Polycystic disease of the liver

Multiple cysts can occur in the liver as part of autosomal dominant polycystic disease of the kidney (p. 681). These cysts are usually asymptomatic but occasionally cause abdominal pain and distension. Liver function is normal and complications such as oesophageal varices are very rare. The prognosis is excellent and depends on the kidney disease.

Solitary cysts

These are usually found by chance during imaging and are mainly asymptomatic.

Congenital hepatic fibrosis

In this rare condition the liver architecture is normal but there are broad collagenous fibrous bands extending from the portal tracts. It is often inherited as an autosomal recessive condition but can also occur sporadically. It usually presents in childhood with hepatosplenomegaly, and portal hypertension is common. It may present later in life and can be misdiagnosed as cirrhosis.

A wedge biopsy of the liver may be required to confirm the diagnosis. The outlook is good and the condition should be distinguished from cirrhosis. Patients who bleed do well after endoscopic therapy of varices or a portocaval anastomosis because of their good liver function.

Congenital intrahepatic biliary dilatation (Caroli's disease)

In this rare, non-familial disease there are saccular dilatations of the intrahepatic or extrahepatic ducts. It can present at any age (although usually in childhood) with fever, abdominal pain and recurrent attacks of cholangitis with Gram-negative septicaemia. Jaundice and portal hypertension are absent. Diagnosis is by ultrasound, PTC, ERCP or MRCP.

LIVER ABSCESS

Pyogenic abscess

These abscesses are uncommon, but may be single or multiple. The most common is a portal pyaemia from intra-abdominal sepsis (e.g. appendicitis or perforations), but now in many cases the aetiology is not known. In the elderly, biliary sepsis is a common cause. Other causes include trauma, bacteraemia and direct extension from, for example, a perinephric abscess.

The organism found most commonly is *E. coli. Streptococcus milleri* and anaerobic organisms such as *Bacteroides* are often seen. Other organisms include *Enterococcus faecalis, Proteus vulgaris* and *Staphylococcus aureus*. Often the infection is mixed. Failure to culture an organism may be due to previous antibiotic therapy or inadequate anaerobic culture.

Clinical features

Some patients are not acutely ill and present with malaise lasting several days or even months. Others can present with fever, rigors, anorexia, vomiting, weight loss and abdominal pain. In these patients a Gram-negative septicaemia with shock can occur. On examination there may be little to find. Alternatively, the patient may be toxic, febrile and jaundiced. In such patients, the liver is tender and enlarged and there may be signs of a pleural effusion or a pleural rub in the right lower chest.

Investigations

Patients who are not acutely ill are often investigated as a 'pyrexia of unknown origin' (PUO) and most investigations will be normal. Often the only clue to the diagnosis is a raised serum alkaline phosphatase.

- **Serum bilirubin** is raised in 25% of cases.
- **Normochromic normocytic anaemia** may occur, usually accompanied by a polymorphonuclear leucocytosis.
- **Serum alkaline phosphatase and ESR** are often raised.
- **Serum B_{12}** is very high, as vitamin B_{12} is stored in and subsequently released from the liver.
- **Blood cultures** are positive in only 30% of cases.

Imaging

Ultrasound is useful for detecting abscesses. A CT scan may be of value in complex and multiple lesions. A chest X-ray will show elevation of the right hemidiaphragm with a pleural effusion in the severe case. Depending on age, imaging of the colon may be necessary to find the source of the infection.

Management

Aspiration of the abscess should be attempted under ultrasound control. Antibiotics should initially cover Gram-positive, Gram-negative and anaerobic organisms until the causative organism is identified.

Further drainage via a large-bore needle under ultrasound control or surgically may be necessary if resolution is difficult or slow. Any underlying cause must also be treated.

Prognosis

The overall mortality depends on the nature of the underlying pathology and has been reduced to approximately 16% with needle aspiration and antibiotics. A unilocular abscess in the right lobe has the better prognosis. Scattered multiple abscesses have a very high mortality, with only one in five patients surviving.

Amoebic abscess (see also p. 104)

This condition occurs world-wide and must be considered in patients travelling from endemic areas. *Entamoeba histolytica* (p. 104) can be carried from the bowel to the liver in the portal venous system. Portal inflammation results, with the development of multiple microabscesses and eventually single or multiple large abscesses.

Clinically the onset is usually gradual but may be sudden. There is fever, anorexia, weight loss and malaise. There is often no history of dysentery. On examination the patient looks ill and has tender hepatomegaly and signs of an effusion or consolidation in the base of the right side of the chest. Jaundice is unusual.

Investigations

These are as for pyogenic abscess, plus:

- Serological tests for amoeba (e.g. haemagglutination, amoebic complement-fixation test, ELISA). These are always positive, particularly if there are bowel symptoms, and remain positive after a clinical cure and therefore do not indicate current disease. A repeat negative test, however, is good evidence against an amoebic abscess.
- Diagnostic aspiration of fluid looking like anchovy sauce.

Treatment

Metronidazole 800 mg three times daily is given for 10 days. Aspiration is used in patients failing to respond, in multiple and sometimes large abscesses, and in those with abscesses in the left lobe of the liver or impending rupture.

Complications

Complications include rupture, secondary infection and septicaemia.

OTHER INFECTIONS OF THE LIVER

Schistosomiasis (see also p. 112)

Schistosoma mansoni and *S. japonicum* affect the liver, but *S. haematobium* rarely does so. During their life cycle the ova reach the liver via the venous system and obstruct the portal branches, producing granulomas, fibrosis and inflammation but not cirrhosis.

Clinically there is hepatosplenomegaly and portal hypertension, which is particularly severe with *S. mansoni*.

Investigations show a raised serum alkaline phosphatase and ova can be found in the stools (centrifuged deposits) and in rectal and liver biopsies. Skin tests and other immunological tests often have false results and may also be positive because of past infection.

Treatment is with praziquantel, but fibrosis still remains with a potential risk of portal hypertension, characteristically pre-sinusoidal due to intense portal fibrosis.

Hydatid disease (see also p. 116)

Cysts caused by *Echinococcus granulosus* are single or multiple. They usually occur in the lower part of the right lower lobe. The cyst has three layers: an outside layer derived from the host, an intermediate laminated layer, and an inner germinal layer that buds off brood capsules to form daughter cysts.

Clinically there may be no symptoms or a dull ache and swelling in the right hypochondrium. Investigations show a peripheral eosinophilia in 30% of cases and usually a positive hydatid complement-fixation test or haemagglutination (85%). Plain abdominal X-ray may show calcification of the outer coat of the cyst. Ultrasound and CT scan demonstrate cysts and may show diagnostic daughter cysts within the parent cyst (Fig. 7.25).

Medical treatment (e.g. with albendazole 10 mg/kg, which penetrates into large cysts) can result in reduction

Fig. 7.25 **CT scan of liver showing a large hydatid cyst (arrow) with 'daughter' cysts lying within it.**

of cyst size. Puncture, aspiration, injection, reaspiration (PAIR) has been used since the 1980s. Fine-needle aspiration is undertaken under ultrasound control with chemotherapeutic cover. Surgery can be performed with removal of the cyst intact if possible after first sterilizing the cyst with alcohol, saline or cetrimide. Chronic calcified cysts can be left. There have been no well-designed clinical trials for any modality.

Complications include rupture into the biliary tree, other organs or intraperitoneally, with spread of infection. The prognosis without any complications is good, although there is always the risk of rupture. Preventative measures include deworming of pet dogs and prevention of pets from eating infected carcasses, as well as veterinary control programmes.

Echinococcus multilocularis causes alveolar echino-coccosis and is almost exclusively a hepatic disease, with a high mortality if not treated. Early diagnosis would enable radical surgery and then continued chemosuppression.

Acquired immunodeficiency syndrome

(see also p. 129)

The liver is often involved but rarely causes significant morbidity or mortality. HIV itself is probably not the cause of the liver abnormalities. The following are seen:

- pre-existing/coincidental viral hepatitis – the hepatitis progresses more rapidly (HBV, HCV, HDV)
- neoplasia: Kaposi's sarcoma and non-Hodgkin's lymphoma
- opportunistic infection (e.g. *Mycobacterium tuberculosis*, *M. avium-intracellulare*, *Cryptococcus*, *Candida albicans*, toxoplasmosis)
- drug hepatotoxicity
- sclerosing cholangitis (see p. 404).

Clinical hepatomegaly is common (60% of patients).

LIVER DISEASE IN PREGNANCY

Liver function is not impaired in pregnancy. Any liver disease from whatever cause can occur incidentally and coincide with pregnancy. For example, viral hepatitis accounts for 40% of all cases of jaundice during pregnancy. Pregnancy does not necessarily exacerbate established liver disease, but it is uncommon for women with advanced liver disease to conceive.

The following changes take place:

- Plasma and blood volumes increase during pregnancy but the hepatic blood flow remains constant.
- The proportion of cardiac output delivered to the liver therefore falls from 35% to 29% in late pregnancy; drug metabolism can thus be affected.
- The size of the liver remains constant.
- Liver biochemistry remains unchanged apart from a rise in serum alkaline phosphatase from the placenta (up to three to four times) and a decrease in total protein owing to increased plasma volume.
- Triglycerides and cholesterol levels rise, and caeruloplasmin, transferrin, α_1-antitrypsin and fibrinogen levels are elevated owing to increased hepatic synthesis.
- Postpartum there is a tendency to hypercoagulability, and acute Budd–Chiari syndrome can occur.

There are a number of liver diseases that complicate pregnancy.

Hyperemesis gravidarum

Pathological vomiting during pregnancy can be associated with liver dysfunction and jaundice. Liver dysfunction resolves when vomiting subsides.

Intrahepatic cholestasis of pregnancy

This condition of unknown aetiology presents usually with pruritus alone in the third trimester. It has a familial tendency and there is a higher prevalence in Scandinavia, Chile and Bolivia.

Liver biochemistry shows a cholestatic picture with high serum ALP (up to four times normal) and raised aminotransferases which occasionally can be very high. The serum bilirubin is slightly raised with jaundice in 60% of cases. Liver biopsy is not indicated but would show centrilobular cholestasis.

Treatment is symptomatic with ursodeoxycholic acid 15 mg/kg. *Prognosis* is usually excellent for the mother but there is increased fetal loss and the condition resolves after delivery. Recurrent cholestasis may occur during subsequent pregnancies or with the ingestion of oestrogen-containing oral contraceptive pills.

Pre-eclampsia and eclampsia

Pre-eclampsia is characterized by hypertension, proteinuria

and oedema occurring in the second or third trimester. Eclampsia is marked by seizures or coma in addition. Hepatic complications include subcapsular haematoma and infarction, and occasionally fulminant hepatic failure. The HELLP syndrome – a combination of haemolysis, elevated liver enzymes and a low platelet count – can occur in association with severe pre-eclampsia. In the HELLP syndrome, there is epigastric pain, nausea and vomiting, with jaundice in 5% of patients. Delivery is the best treatment for eclampsia.

Acute fatty liver of pregnancy (AFLP)

This is a rare, serious condition of unknown aetiology. There is an association between acute fatty liver and long-chain 3-hydroxylacyl-CoA-dihydroxyl (LCHAD) deficiency. The mechanism is unclear, but abnormal fatty acid metabolites produced by the homozygous or hetero-zygous fetus enter the circulation and overcome maternal hepatic mitochondrial oxidation systems in a hetero-zygote mother. It presents in the last trimester with symptoms of fulminant hepatitis – jaundice, vomiting, abdominal pain, occasionally haematemesis and coma.

Investigations show hepatocellular damage, hyper-uricaemia, thrombocytopenia, and rarely DIC. CT scanning shows a low density of the liver owing to the high fat content. It can sometimes be difficult to differentiate from the HELLP syndrome and as LCHAD deficiency has also been shown in HELLP there is a view that there is a spectrum of HELLP to AFLP. Liver biopsy shows fine droplets of fat (microvesicles) in the liver cells with little necrosis, but is not necessary for diagnosis.

Immediate delivery of the child may save both baby and mother. Early diagnosis and treatment has reduced the mortality to less than 20%. Treatment is as for acute liver failure.

FURTHER READING
Koux TA, Olans LB (1996) Liver disease in pregnancy. *New England Journal of Medicine* **335**: 569–576.

LIVER TUMOURS

The most common liver tumour is a secondary (metastatic) tumour (Fig. 7.26), particularly from the gastrointestinal tract, breast or bronchus. Clinical features are variable but usually include hepatomegaly. Ultrasound is the primary investigation, with CT or MRI used when available; MRI is comparable to CT at detecting metastases. Primary liver tumours may be benign or malignant, but the most common are malignant.

MALIGNANT TUMOURS

Hepatocellular carcinoma (HCC)

Hepatocellular carcinoma (HCC) is one of the 10 most common cancers world-wide.

(a)

(b)

Fig. 7.26 Liver MRI. **(a)** T1- and **(b)** T2-weighted sequences showing multiple liver metastases. Structures of fluid density have high signal on T2 images. Note the central tumour necrosis in **(b)** (arrows).

Aetiology

Carriers of HBV and HCV have an extremely high risk of developing HCC. In areas where HBV is prevalent, 90% of patients with this cancer are positive for the hepatitis B virus. Cirrhosis is present in over 80% of these patients. The development of HCC is related to the integration of viral HBV DNA into the genome of the host hepatocyte (see p. 364) and possibly the degree of viral replication. The risk of HCC in HCV is as high as or higher than in HBV despite no viral integration. Primary liver cancer is also associated with other forms of cirrhosis, such as alcoholic cirrhosis and haemochromatosis. Males are affected more than females; this may account for the high incidence seen in haemochromatosis and low incidence in PBC. Other suggested aetiological factors are aflatoxin (a metabolite of a fungus found in groundnuts) and androgenic steroids, and there is a weak association with the contraceptive pill.

Pathology

The tumour is either single or occurs as multiple nodules throughout the liver. Histologically it consists of cells resembling hepatocytes. It can metastasize via the hepatic or portal veins to the lymph nodes, bones and lungs.

Clinical features

The clinical features include weight loss, anorexia, fever, an ache in the right hypochondrium, and ascites. The rapid development of these features in a cirrhotic patient is suggestive of HCC. On examination, an enlarged, irregular, tender liver may be felt. Increasingly due to surveillance, HCC is found without symptoms in cirrhotics.

Investigations

Serum α-fetoprotein may be raised, but is normal in at least a third of patients. Ultrasound scans show filling defects in 90% of cases. A liver biopsy, particularly under ultrasonic guidance may be performed for diagnosis, but is increasingly less used as imaging techniques show characteristic appearances and because seeding along the biopsy tract can occur.

Treatment and prognosis

Surgical resection is occasionally possible. Small tumours in patients with cirrhosis do well with liver transplantation. Chemotherapy and radiotherapy are unhelpful, but chemoembolization and probably embolization alone in selected patients prolong survival.

Survival, except in very selected groups, is seldom more than 6 months.

Prevention

Persistent HBV infection, usually acquired after perinatal infection, is a high risk factor for HCC in many parts of the world, such as South East Asia. Widespread vaccination against HBV is being used and this has shown a reduction in the annual incidence of HCC in Taiwan.

Cholangiocarcinoma

Cholangiocarcinomas can be extrahepatic (see p. 405) or intrahepatic. Intrahepatic adenocarcinomas arising from the bile ducts account for approximately 10% of primary tumours. They are not associated with cirrhosis or hepatitis B. In the Far East they may be associated with infestation with *Clonorchis sinensis* or *Opisthorchis viverrini*. The clinical features are similar to primary HCC except that jaundice is frequent with hilar tumours, and cholangitis is more frequent.

Surgical resection is rarely possible and patients usually die within 6 months. Transplantation is contraindicated.

BENIGN TUMOURS

The most common benign tumour is a *haemangioma*. It is usually small and single but can be multiple and large. They are usually found incidentally on ultrasound, CT or MRI and have characteristic appearances. They require no treatment.

Hepatic adenomas are associated with oral contraceptives. They can present with abdominal pain or intraperitoneal bleeding. Resection is only required for symptomatic patients, or in those in whom discontinuation of the oral contraception does not result in shrinkage of the tumour.

FURTHER READING

Seef LB, Hoofnagle JH, McLaughlin A (2004) Hepatocellular carcinoma. *Gastroenterology* (Suppl.) **127**: S1–S323

Wands JR (2004) Prevention of hepatocellular carcinoma. *New England Journal of Medicine* **351**: 1567–1570.

MISCELLANEOUS CONDITIONS OF THE LIVER

Hepatic mitochondrial injury syndromes

These syndromes – in which there is mitochondrial damage with inhibition of β-oxidation of fatty acids – can be categorized as follows:

- *Genetic*, with abnormalities which include medium-chain acyl-coenzyme A dehydrogenase deficiency leading to microsteatosis.
- *Toxins* leading to liver failure include aflatoxin and cerulide (produced by *Bacillus cereus*) which causes food poisoning (see p. 69).
- *Drugs* (e.g. i.v. tetracycline, valproic acid and nucleoside reverse-transcriptase inhibitors) can produce a fatal microsteatosis.
- *Idiopathic*, the best known being fatty liver of pregnancy (p. 394) and Reye's syndrome. This condition, due to inhibition of β-oxidation and uncoupling of oxidative phosphorylation in mitochondria, leads in children to an acute encephalopathy and diffuse microvesicular fatty infiltration of the liver. Aspirin ingestion and viral infections have been implicated as precipitating agents. Mortality is about 50%, usually due to cerebral oedema.

Idiopathic adult ductopenia

This unexplained condition is characterized by pruritus and cholestatic jaundice. Histology of the liver shows a decrease in intrahepatic bile ducts in at least 50% of the portal tract, together with the features of cholestasis and marked fibrosis or cirrhosis. In most the disease is progressive and the only treatment is liver transplantation.

Indian childhood cirrhosis

This condition of children is seen in the Indian subcontinent. The cause is unknown. Eventually there is development of a micronodular cirrhosis with excess copper in the liver.

Hepatic porphyrias

These are dealt with on page 1148.

Cystic fibrosis (see also p. 909)

This disease affects mainly the lung and pancreas, but patients can develop fatty liver, cholestasis and cirrhosis. The aetiology of the liver involvement is unclear.

DRUGS AND THE LIVER

Drug metabolism

The liver is the major site of drug metabolism. Drugs are converted from fat-soluble to water-soluble substances that can be excreted in the urine or bile. This metabolism of drugs is mediated by a group of mixed-function enzymes (p. 993).

Drug hepatotoxicity

Many drugs impair liver function, and drugs should always be considered as a cause when mildly abnormal liver tests are found. Damage to the liver by drugs is usually classified as being either predictable (or dose-related) or non-predictable (not dose-related) (see p. 996). This classification should not be used rigidly, as there is considerable overlap and at least six mechanisms may be involved in the production of damage: (1) disruption of intracellular calcium homeostasis; (2) disruption of bile canalicular transport mechanisms; (3) formation of non-functioning adducts (enzyme–drug) which may then (4) present on the surface of the hepatocyte as new immunogens (attacked by T cells); (5) induction of apoptosis; (6) inhibition of mitochondrial function, which prevents fatty acid metabolism, and accumulation of both lactate and reactive oxygen species. The predominant mechanism or combination of mechanisms determines the type of liver injury, i.e. hepatitic, cholestatic or immunological (skin rashes, fever and arthralgia (serum-sickness syndrome)). Eosinophilia and circulating immune complexes and antibodies may occasionally be detected.

When a small amount of hepatotoxic drug whose effect is dose-dependent (e.g. paracetamol) is ingested, a large proportion of it undergoes conjugation with glucuronide and sulphate, whilst the remainder is metabolized by microsomal enzymes to produce toxic derivatives that are immediately detoxified by conjugation with glutathione. If larger doses are ingested, the former pathway becomes saturated and the toxic derivative is produced at a faster rate. Once the hepatic glutathione is depleted, large amounts of the toxic metabolite accumulate and produce damage (p. 1017).

The 'predictability' of drugs to produce damage can, however, be affected by metabolic events preceding their ingestion. For example, chronic alcohol abusers may become more susceptible to liver damage because of the enzyme-inducing effects of alcohol, or ill or starving patients may become susceptible because of the depletion of hepatic glutathione produced by starvation. Many other factors such as environmental or genetic effects may be involved in determining the 'susceptibility' of certain patients to certain drugs.

Hepatitic damage

The type of damage produced by various drugs is shown in Table 7.16. The diagnosis of these conditions is usually by exclusion of other causes. Most reactions occur within 3 months of starting the drug. Monitoring liver biochemistry in patients on long-term treatment, such as antituberculosis therapy, is advisable. If a drug is suspected of causing hepatic damage it should be stopped immediately. Liver biopsy is of limited help in confirming the diagnosis, but occasionally hepatic eosinophilia or granulomas may be seen. Diagnostic challenge with subtherapeutic doses of the drug is sometimes required after the liver biochemistry has returned to normal, to confirm the diagnosis.

Individual drugs

Paracetamol

In high doses paracetamol produces liver cell necrosis (see above). The toxic metabolite binds irreversibly to liver cell membranes. Overdosage is discussed on page 1017.

Halothane and other volatile liquid anaesthetics

Halothane produces a hepatitis in patients having repeated exposures. The mechanism is thought to be a hypersensitivity reaction. An unexplained fever occurs approximately 10 days after the second or subsequent halothane anaesthetic and is followed by jaundice, typically with a hepatitic picture. Most patients recover spontaneously but there is a high mortality in severe cases. There are no chronic sequelae. Both enflurane and isoflurane also cause hepatotoxicity in those sensitized to halogenated anaesthetics but the risk is smaller than with halothane.

Steroid compounds

Cholestasis is caused by natural and synthetic oestrogens as well as methyltestosterone. These agents interfere with canalicular biliary flow and cause a pure cholestasis. Cholestasis is rare with the contraceptive pill because of the low dosage used. However, the contraceptive pill is associated with an increased incidence of gallstones, hepatic adenomas (rarely HCCs), the Budd–Chiari syndrome and peliosis hepatis. The latter condition, which also occurs with anabolic steroids, consists of dilatation of the hepatic sinusoids to form blood-filled lakes.

Phenothiazines

Phenothiazines (e.g. chlorpromazine) can produce a cholestatic picture owing to a hypersensitivity reaction. It occurs in 1% of patients, usually within 4 weeks of starting the drug. Typically it is associated with a fever and eosinophilia. Recovery occurs on stopping the drug.

Antituberculous chemotherapy

Isoniazid produces elevated aminotransferases in 10–20% of patients. Hepatic necrosis with jaundice occurs in a

Table 7.16 Some drugs causing types of liver damage

Types of liver damage	Drugs	Types of liver damage	Drugs
Zone 3 necrosis	Carbon tetrachloride	Chronic hepatitis	Methyldopa
	Amanita mushrooms		Nitrofurantoin
	Paracetamol		Fenofibrate
	Salicylates		Isoniazid
	Piroxicam	General hypersensitivity	Sulphonamides e.g.
	Cocaine		Sulfasalazine
Zone 1 necrosis	Ferrous sulphate		Co-trimoxazole
Microvesicular fat	Sodium valproate		Fansidar
	Tetracyclines		Penicillins, e.g.
Steatohepatitis	Amiodarone		Flucloxacillin
	Synthetic oestrogens		Ampicillin
	Nifedipine		Amoxicillin
Fibrosis	Methotrexate		Co-amoxiclav
	Other cytotoxic agents		NSAIDs e.g.
	Arsenic		Salicylates
	Vitamin A		Diclofenac
	Retinoids		Allopurinol
Vascular			Antithyroid e.g.
Sinusoidal dilatation	Contraceptive drugs		Propylthiouracil
	Anabolic steroids		Carbimazole
	Azathioprine		Quinine e.g.
Pelioses hepatis	Oral contraceptives		Quinidine
	Anabolic steroids, e.g.		Diltiazem
	Danazol		Anticonvulsants e.g.
	Azathioprine		Phenytoin
Veno-occlusive	Pyrrolizidine alkaloids	Canalicular cholestasis	Sex hormones
	(*Senecio* in bush tea)		Ciclosporin A
	Cytotoxics – cyclophosphamide,	Hepatocanalicular cholestasis	Chlorpromazine
Acute hepatitis	Isoniazid		Haloperidol
	Rifampicin		Erythromycin
	Methyldopa		Cimetidine/ranitidine
	Atenolol		Nitrofurantoin
	Enalapril		Imipramine
	Verapamil		Azathioprine
	Ketoconazole		Oral hypoglycaemics
	Cytotoxic drugs		Dextropropoxyphene
	Clonazepam	Biliary sludge	Ceftriaxone
	Disulfiram	Sclerosing cholangitis	Hepatic arterial infusion
	Niacin		of 5-fluorouracil
	Volatile liquid anaesthetics, e.g.	Hepatic tumours	Pills with high hormone
	Halothane		content (adenomas)
		Hepatocellular carcinoma	Contraceptive pill
			Danazol

NSAID, non-steroidal anti-inflammatory drug

smaller percentage. The hepatotoxicity of isoniazid appears to be related to acetylator status, as the damage is due to the metabolites.

Rifampicin produces a hepatitis, usually within 3 weeks of starting the drug, particularly in patients on high doses.

Pyrazinamide produces abnormal liver biochemical tests and, rarely, liver cell necrosis.

Amiodarone

This leads to a steatohepatitis histologically and liver failure if the drug is not stopped in time.

Drug prescribing for patients with liver disease

The metabolism of drugs is impaired in severe liver disease (with jaundice and ascites) as the removal of many drugs depends on liver blood flow and the integrity of the hepatocyte. In general, therefore, the effect of drugs is prolonged by liver disease and also by cholestasis. This is further accentuated by portosystemic shunting, which diminishes the first-pass extraction of drugs. With hypoproteinaemia there is decreased protein binding of some drugs, and bilirubin competes with many drugs for the binding sites on serum albumin. In patients with portosystemic encephalopathy, care must be taken in prescribing drugs with a central depressant action.

FURTHER READING
Lee WM (2003) Drug-induced hepatotoxicity. *New England Journal of Medicine* **349**: 474–485.

GALL BLADDER AND BILIARY SYSTEM

The structure, formation and function of bile is discussed on page 349.

GALLSTONES

Prevalence of gallstones

Gallstones may be present at any age but are unusual before the third decade. The prevalence of gallstones is strongly influenced both by age and sex. There is a progressive increase in the presence of gallstones with age but the prevalence is two to three times higher in women than in men, although this difference is less marked in the sixth and seventh decade. At this age the prevalence ranges between 25–30%. There are considerable racial differences, gallstones being more common in Scandinavia, South America and Native North Americans.

Types of gallstones

Two principal types of gallstone disease occur. In the western world 80% of gallstones contain cholesterol. The second less frequent type of gallstone is 'pigment stones', being predominantly composed of calcium bilirubinate or polymer-like complexes with calcium, copper and some cholesterol.

Cholesterol gallstones

The formation of cholesterol stones is the consequence of cholesterol crystallization from gall bladder bile. This is dependent upon three factors:

- cholesterol supersaturation of bile
- crystallization-promoting factors within bile
- motility of the gall bladder.

Cholesterol is derived partly from dietary sources, but in addition is synthesized within the liver. The rate-limiting step in cholesterol synthesis is beta-hydroxy-beta methyl glutaryl Co-A (HMG-CoA) reductase, which catalyses the first step, i.e. the conversion of acetate to mevalonate (see Fig. 7.4). The cholesterol formed is co-secreted with phospholipids into the biliary canaliculus as unilamellar vesicles. Cholesterol will only crystallize into stones when the bile is supersaturated with cholesterol relative to the bile salt and phospholipid content. This can occur as a consequence of excess cholesterol secretion into bile which, in some instances, has been shown to be due to an increase in HMG-CoA reductase activity. Recently, leptin (p. 253) has been shown to increase cholesterol secretion

into bile. Elevated levels of leptin during rapid weight loss may account for the increased incidence of cholesterol gallstones. An alternative mechanism of supersaturation is a decreased *bile salt content* which may be genetically predetermined or occur as a consequence of bile salt loss (e.g. terminal ileal Crohn's disease).

The *composition* of the bile salt pool may also influence the ability to maintain cholesterol in solution. There is evidence that an increased proportion of the secondary hydrophobic bile acid (deoxycholic acid) in the bile acid pool may predispose to cholesterol stone formation. This has been linked with slow colonic transit during which the primary bile acid cholic acid may undergo microbial enzyme metabolism yielding deoxycholic acid which is then absorbed back into the bile salt pool (see Fig. 7.4).

Whilst cholesterol supersaturation of bile is essential for cholesterol stone formation, many individuals in whom such supersaturation occurs will never develop stones. It is the balance between cholesterol crystallizing and solubilizing factors that determine whether cholesterol will crystallize out of solution. A number of lipoproteins have been reported as putative crystallizing factors.

Gall bladder motility represents a further factor that may influence the cholesterol crystallization from supersaturated bile. There is evidence from animal models that gall bladder stasis leads to cholesterol crystallization mediated by hypersecretion of mucin.

Abnormalities of gall bladder motility have been suggested as factors in such circumstances as pregnancy, multiparity and diabetes as well as octreotide-related gall bladder stones (p. 1069). Recognized risk factors for gallstones are shown in Table 7.17.

Bile pigment stones

The pathogenesis of pigment stones is entirely independent of cholesterol gallstones. There are two main types of pigment gallstones, black and brown.

Black pigment gallstones are composed of calcium bilirubinate and a network of mucin glycoproteins that interlace with salts such as calcium carbonate and/or

Table 7.17 Risk factors for cholesterol gallstones

Increasing age	Drugs (e.g. contraceptive pill)
Sex (F > M)	Ileal disease or resection
Multiparity	Diabetes mellitus
Obesity	Acromegaly treated with octreotide
Rapid weight loss	Liver cirrhosis
Diet (e.g. high in animal fat)	

calcium phosphate. These stones range in colour from deep black to very dark brown and have a glass-like cross-sectional surface on fracturing. Black pigment stones are seen in 40–60% of patients with haemolytic conditions such as sickle cell disease and hereditary spherocytosis in which there is chronic excess bilirubin production. However, the majority of pigment stones occur without haemolysis. These black stones have been shown to contain bacteria, many of which produce glucuronidase and phospholipase, factors that are known to facilitate stone formation. It is speculated that this subclinical bacterial colonization of the bile duct is responsible for the pigment stone formation.

Brown stones are usually of a muddy hue and on cross-section seem to have alternating brown and tan layers. These stones are composed of calcium salts of fatty acids as well as calcium bilirubinate. They are almost always found in the presence of bile stasis and/or biliary infection. Brown stones are a common cause of recurrent bile duct stones following cholecystectomy and may also be found in the intrahepatic ducts in circumstances of duct disease such as Caroli's syndrome and primary sclerosing cholangitis. In the Far East such brown stones are identified within both the intra- and extrahepatic biliary tree and have been linked with chronic parasitic infection.

Clinical presentation of gallstones
(Fig. 7.27)

The majority of gallstones are asymptomatic and remain so during a person's lifetime. Gallstones are increasingly detected as an incidental finding at the time of either abdominal radiography or ultrasound scanning. Over a 10- to 15-year period approximately 20% of these stones will be the cause of symptoms with 10% having severe complications. Once gallstones have become symptomatic there is a strong trend towards recurrent complications, often of increasing severity. Gallstones do not cause dyspepsia, fat intolerance, flatulence or other vague upper abdominal symptoms. The chances of a fair, fat, female of 40 having gallstones is the same as in the general population.

Biliary or gallstone colic

Biliary colic is the term used for the pain associated with the temporary obstruction of the cystic or common bile duct by a stone usually migrating from the gall bladder. Despite the term 'colic' the pain of stone-induced ductular obstruction is one of a severe but constant pain, which has a crescendo characteristic. Many sufferers can relate the symptoms to over-indulgence with food, particularly when this has a high fat content. The most common time of day for such an episode is in the mid-evening and lasting until the early hours of the morning. The initial site of pain is usually in the epigastrium but there may be a right upper quadrant component. Radiation may occur over the right shoulder and right subscapular region. Nausea and vomiting frequently accompany the more severe attacks. The cessation of attack may be spontaneous after a number of hours or terminated by the administration of opiate analgesia. More protracted pain, particularly when associated with fevers and rigors, suggests secondary complications such as cholecystitis, cholangitis or gallstone-related pancreatitis (see below).

Acute cholecystitis

The initial event in acute cholecystitis is obstruction to gall bladder emptying. In 95% of cases a gall bladder stone can be identified as the cause. Such obstruction results in an increase of gall bladder glandular secretion leading to progressive distension which in turn may compromise the vascular supply to the gall bladder. There is also an inflammatory response secondary to retained bile within the gall bladder. Infection is a secondary phenomenon following the vascular and inflammatory events described above.

The initial clinical features of an episode of chole-cystitis are similar to those of biliary colic described above. However, over a number of hours there is progression with severe localized right upper quadrant abdominal pain corresponding to parietal peritoneal involvement in the inflammatory process. The pain is associated with tenderness and muscle guarding or rigidity. Occasionally the gall bladder can become distended by pus (an empyema) and rarely an acute gangrenous cholecystitis develops which can perforate, with generalized peritonitis.

Investigations

Biliary colic as a consequence of a stone in the neck of the gall bladder or cystic duct is unlikely to be associated with significant abnormality of laboratory tests. Acute cholecystitis is usually associated with a moderate leucocytosis and raised inflammatory markers (e.g. C-reactive protein).

- **The serum bilirubin, alkaline phosphatase and aminotransferase** levels may be marginally elevated

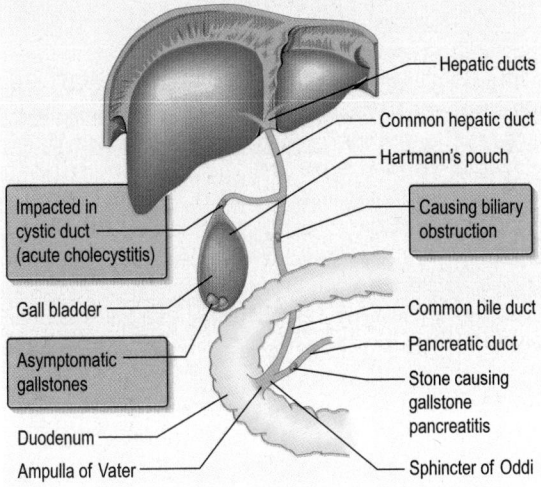

Fig. 7.27 **Clinical presentation of gallstones.**

Labels in figure:
- Hepatic ducts
- Common hepatic duct
- Hartmann's pouch
- Impacted in cystic duct (acute cholecystitis)
- Causing biliary obstruction
- Gall bladder
- Common bile duct
- Pancreatic duct
- Asymptomatic gallstones
- Stone causing gallstone pancreatitis
- Duodenum
- Ampulla of Vater
- Sphincter of Oddi

Fig. 7.28 **Ultrasound scan in a patient with acute cholecystitis.** There is a stone (casting an acoustic shadow – thin arrow) impacted in the gall bladder neck, with a distended gall bladder (thick arrow) and thickening and oedema of the gall bladder wall.

in the presence of cholecystitis alone, even in the absence of bile duct obstruction. More significant elevation of the bilirubin and alkaline phosphatase is in keeping with bile duct obstruction.

- **A plain abdominal X-ray** may provide evidence of gall bladder disease in the form of radio-opaque stones or calcification of the gall bladder. In severe cases of acute cholecystitis there may be gas within the gall bladder lumen and wall due to either gas-forming organisms or fistulation of a gallstone into the bowel.
- **An abdominal ultrasound scan** is the single most useful investigation for the diagnosis of gallstone-related disease (Fig. 7.28). Look for:
  (a) *gallstones* within the gall bladder, particularly when these are obstructing the gall bladder neck or cystic duct
  (b) *focal tenderness* over the underlying gall bladder
  (c) *thickening of the gall bladder wall.* This may also be seen with hypoalbuminaemia, portal hypertension and acute viral hepatitis.
  Gallstones are a common finding in an ageing population, and in the absence of specific symptoms great care should be taken as to whether the gallstones are responsible for the symptoms.
- **Biliary scintigraphy using technetium derivatives of iminodiacetate.** These isotopes are taken up by hepatocytes and excreted into bile. They delineate the extrahepatic biliary tree. The absence of cystic duct and gall bladder filling provides evidence towards acute cholecystitis although the findings must be closely correlated with the presenting symptoms.

Differential diagnosis

Typical cases of biliary colic are usually suspected by a careful clinical history. The differential diagnosis includes the irritable bowel syndrome (spasm of the hepatic flexure), carcinoma of the right side of the colon, atypical peptic ulcer disease, renal colic and pancreatitis.

The differential diagnosis of acute cholecystitis includes a number of other conditions marked by severe right upper quadrant pain and fever, e.g. acute episodes of pancreatitis, perforated peptic ulceration or an intra-hepatic abscess. Conditions above the right diaphragm such as basal pneumonia as well as myocardial infarction may on occasions mimic the clinical picture.

MANAGEMENT OF GALL BLADDER STONES

Cholecystectomy

Cholecystectomy is the treatment of choice for virtually all patients with *symptomatic* gall bladder stones. Cholecystectomy should not be performed in the absence of typical symptoms just because stones are found on investigation. The laparotomy approach to cholecystectomy has now been largely replaced by the laparoscopic technique. Postoperative pain is minimized with only a short period of ileus and the early ability to mobilize the patient. Laparoscopic cholecystectomy has been carried out on a day-care basis but more commonly requires a 48-hour admission. This has considerable cost benefits over open cholecystectomy, which is now reserved for a small proportion of patients with contraindications such as extensive previous upper abdominal surgery, ongoing bile duct obstruction or portal hypertension.

In approximately 5% of cases a laparoscopic cholecystectomy is converted to an open operation because of technical difficulties, in particular adhesions in the right upper quadrant or difficulty in identifying the biliary anatomy.

Acute cholecystitis. The initial management is conservative, consisting of nil by mouth, intravenous fluids, opiate analgesia and intravenous antibiotics (e.g. cefotaxime).

Cholecystectomy is usually delayed for a few days to allow the symptoms to settle but can then be carried out quite safely in the majority of cases.

When the clinical situation fails to respond to this conservative management, particularly if there is increasing pain and fever, an empyema or gangrene of the gall bladder may have occurred. Urgent ultrasound is performed and urgent surgery will be required if these complications have developed.

Specific complications of cholecystectomy include a biliary leak either from the cystic duct or from the gall bladder bed. Injury to the bile duct itself occurs in up to 0.5% of laparoscopic operations and may have serious long-term sequelae in the form of biliary sepsis and secondary biliary liver injury. There is an overall mortality of 0.2%.

Stone dissolution and shock wave lithotripsy

These *non-surgical techniques* for the management of gall bladder stones are infrequently used but are used in a highly selected group of patients who may not be fit for laparoscopic cholecystectomy.

Dissolution Pure or near-pure cholesterol stones can be solubilized by increasing the bile salt content of bile. Chenodeoxycholic acid and ursodeoxycholic acid are used. For dissolution to occur there must be a functioning gall bladder and optimally the stones should be almost pure cholesterol with a diameter of less than 10 mm. Using these criteria, only 20% of patients with gallstones will be eligible and even under such circumstances the time to achieve dissolution is often a matter of several months. There is also a high relapse rate when the drugs are discontinued. These limitations have restricted the application of this approach. Further benefit may be attained by the addition of an HMG-CoA reductase inhibitor (e.g. simvastatin) to a regimen of ursodeoxycholic acid. This will then combine reduced cholesterol content of bile as well an enhanced bile salt concentration but uses are still limited.

Extracorporeal shock wave lithotripsy. A shock wave can be directed either radiologically or by ultrasound on to gall bladder stones. This technique was highly successful but in only a restricted patient population. Fragmentation was limited to a small number of stones only and these had to be greater than 10 mm in diameter. The greater the calcium content of the stone the less likely the success of fragmentation. Gall bladder function has to be intact so the stone fragments can clear via the cystic duct.

The post-cholecystectomy syndrome

This refers to right upper quadrant pain often biliary in type which occurs a few months after the cholecystectomy but it may be delayed for a number of years. The patients often comment that the pain is identical to that for which the original operation was carried out. In many cases this syndrome is related to functional large bowel disease with colonic spasm at the hepatic flexure (hepatic flexure syndrome). In a small proportion of patients the pain is a result of a retained common bile duct stone. In a further minority of patients, hypertension of the sphincter of Oddi is a potential cause. This is most likely in patients with abnormal liver biochemistry and dilatation of the common bile duct (on ultrasound) during episodes of pain (and in the absence of a documented retained stone). The diagnosis is confirmed by pressure measurements of the sphincter of Oddi, and the condition can be successfully managed by endoscopic sphincterotomy (see below).

COMMON BILE DUCT STONES

The classical features of common bile duct (CBD) stones are biliary colic, fever and jaundice (acute cholangitis). This triad is only present in the minority of patients. Abdominal pain is the most common symptom and has the typical features of biliary colic (see above). Jaundice is a variable accompaniment and is almost always preceded by abdominal pain. A patient with bile duct stones may experience sequential episodes of pain, only some of which are accompanied by jaundice. In contrast to malignant bile duct obstruction, the level of jaundice associated with CBD stones characteristically tends to fluctuate.

Fever is only present in a minority of cases but indicates biliary sepsis and sometimes an associated septicaemia. The presence of such biliary sepsis is a significant adverse prognostic factor.

A minority of patients with bile duct stones are discovered incidentally during imaging for gall bladder disease. Fifteen per cent of patients undergoing cholecystectomy will have stones within the bile duct only detected at the time of operative cholangiography.

Physical examination

If the patient is examined between episodes there may be no abnormal physical finding. During a symptomatic episode the patient may be jaundiced with a fever and associated tachycardia. There is tenderness in the right upper quadrant varying from mild to extremely severe.

More widespread abdominal tenderness extending from the epigastrium to the left upper quadrant, associated with distension, may indicate associated stone-related pancreatitis (see below).

Investigations
Laboratory tests
- *Full blood count* is usually normal in the presence of uncomplicated bile duct stones.
- *An elevated neutrophil count* as well as raised inflammatory markers (ESR and CRP) are frequent accompaniments of cholangitis.
- *The raised serum bilirubin* tends to be mild and often transient. Very high concentrations of bilirubin (= 200 μmol/L) almost always reflect complete bile duct obstruction.
- *Serum alkaline phosphatase and gamma glutamyl transpeptidase* are similarly elevated in proportion to the degree of hyperbilirubinaemia.
- *Aminotransferase levels* are usually mildly elevated but with complete bile duct obstruction they may rise to 10–15 times the normal value.
- *Serum amylase levels* are often mildly elevated in the presence of bile duct obstruction but are markedly so if stone-related pancreatitis has occurred.
- *Prothrombin time* may be prolonged if bile duct obstruction has occurred; this reflects decreased absorption of vitamin K.

Trans-abdominal ultrasound

This is the initial imaging technique of choice and in many cases the only imaging technique required.

Bile duct obstruction is characterized by dilatation of intrahepatic biliary radicals, which are usually easily detected by the ultrasound scan. It may, however, not be possible to identify the cause of obstruction. Stones situated in the distal common bile duct are poorly visualized by trans-abdominal ultrasound and up to 50% are missed. The detection of stones within the gall bladder is poorly predictive as to the cause of bile duct obstruction. Asymptomatic gallstones are common (up to 15%) in patients in the cancer age group (65 years and older). Conversely, in 5–10% of patients with bile duct stones no calculi can be seen within the gall bladder.

Other imaging techniques

Magnetic resonance cholangiography (MRC) delineates the fluid column within the biliary tree and is the technique of choice to supplement trans-abdominal ultrasound (Fig. 7.29).

Spiral CT scanning is an alterative way to detect bile duct dilatation. Opaque stones are more readily identifiable within the bile duct than radiolucent cholesterol stones. CT scanning provides a means of excluding other causes of bile duct obstruction such as carcinoma of the head of the pancreas.

Endoscopic ultrasound scanning (Fig. 7.30) has enabled high-resolution imaging of the common bile duct, gall bladder and pancreas, although unlike the preceding imaging techniques it is an invasive procedure. The endoscopic ultrasound probe can be brought into close proximity with the distal common bile duct and hence identify the majority of stones at this level.

This technique may be particularly useful for identifying small calculi (microcalculi).

Endoscopic retrograde cholangiography (ERC)

The endoscopic technique of ERC (p. 356) enables good visualization of the common bile duct. In experienced hands this will be successful in 98% of cases, providing

Fig. 7.30 **An endoscopic ultrasound scan** with the probe within the duodenum (upper margin of the figure) clearly demonstrating the gall bladder (GB) with multiple small stones within.

Fig. 7.31 **An ERCP in a patient presenting with abdominal pain, jaundice and fever.** Several stones can be seen within the dilated common bile duct (arrows).

good documentation of bile duct stones (Fig. 7.31). However, microcalculi can still be missed.

ERC gives the therapeutic opportunity for sphincterotomy and stone extraction (see below).

Differential diagnosis

Cholangitis may occur independently of gallstones in conditions such as primary sclerosing cholangitis and

Fig. 7.29 **A magnetic resonance cholangiogram in a patient presenting with abdominal pain and jaundice.** This shows evidence of a distal common bile duct stricture (arrows) with a large gallstone proximal to this in the mid common bile duct (top arrow).

Caroli's syndrome. On occasions cholangitis may accompany malignant bile duct obstruction. Jaundice may also be a feature of acute cholecystitis in the absence of bile duct stones when there is pressure on the common bile duct by a gallstone in the cystic duct (Mirizzi's syndrome). Common bile duct stones may produce pain, but in the absence of jaundice, the differential diagnosis is that of biliary colic (see above).

Management

Acute cholangitis has a high morbidity and mortality, particularly in the elderly age group. Successful management depends on intravenous antibiotics (e.g. i.v. cefotaxime), and urgent bile duct drainage by an endoscopic retrograde approach (Fig. 7.31). Access to the bile duct is achieved by sphincterotomy, and thereafter the stones can be removed either by balloon or basket catheters. In the severely ill patient a piece of plastic tubing (termed a stent) can be inserted into the bile duct to maintain bile drainage without the need to remove the stones, hence minimizing the time period to complete the procedure. The residual stones can then be removed endoscopically when the patient has recovered from the episode. In the presence of acute cholangitis surgical drainage has been associated with a high mortality and is now limited to those very few cases which cannot be managed by the endoscopic approach.

Endoscopic bile duct clearance is also the treatment of choice for patients with acute gallstone pancreatitis as well as patients who have retained common bile duct stones after a previous cholecystectomy.

Patients shown to have common bile duct stones as well as gall bladder stones may be treated by two different approaches:

■ *Laparoscopic cholecystectomy* which can also include exploration of the CBD via the cystic duct or by direct choledochotomy. By using these techniques the laparoscopist can extract stones from the common bile duct. This, however, prolongs the procedure, particularly in the presence of large stones or biliary sepsis.
■ *Endoscopic approach* either immediately before or after the cholecystectomy. Removal of CBD stones by this method is the preferred way in the UK.

COMPLICATIONS OF GALLSTONES

■ Acute cholecystitis and acute cholangitis have been discussed (p. 399).
■ Gallstone-related pancreatitis is discussed on page 409.
■ Gallstones can occasionally erode through the wall of the gall bladder into the intestine giving rise to a biliary enteric fistula. Passage of a gallstone through into the small bowel can give rise to an ileus or true obstruction.
■ There is some evidence that gallstones are associated with an increased risk of adenocarcinoma of the gall bladder (p. 405).

MISCELLANEOUS CONDITIONS OF THE BILIARY TRACT

GALL BLADDER

There are a number of non-calculous conditions of the gall bladder, some of which have been associated with symptoms.

Non-calculous cholecystitis

Almost 10% of gall bladders removed for biliary symptoms are shown to have chronic inflammation within the wall but an absence of gallstones. Such cases are described as non-calculous cholecystitis. In many instances the gall bladder inflammation is minor and of doubtful significance. In a minority of cases non-calculous cholecystitis is characterized by severe inflammation frequently associated with gall bladder perforation. This condition is characteristically found in an elderly and critically ill group of patients.

Chemical inflammation of the gall bladder may also occur from reflux of pancreatic enzymes back into the biliary tree, usually through the common channel at the ampulla of Vater.

Bacterial infection of the gall bladder has occasionally been recognized as a cause of chronic inflammation.

The decision to carry out cholecystectomy in the absence of defined gall bladder stones should be guided by the specific features of the history and whether there is evidence of diseased gall bladder wall on ultrasound scanning.

Cholesterolosis of the gall bladder

In cholesterolosis, cholesterol and other lipids are deposited in macrophages within the lamina propria of the gall bladder. These may be diffusely situated giving a granular appearance to the gall bladder wall or on occasions more discrete, giving a polypoid appearance (see below). Cholesterolosis of the gall bladder may coexist with gallstones but occurs independently. Some degree of cholesterolosis may be found in up to 25% of autopsies in an elderly population. It is doubtful whether this is a cause of symptoms.

Adenomyomatosis of the gall bladder

Adenomyomatosis is a gall bladder abnormality characterized by hyperplasia of the mucosa, thickening of the muscle wall and multiple intramural diverticulae (the so-called Rokitansky–Aschoff sinuses).

The condition is usually detected as an incidental finding during investigation for possible gall bladder disease. It has been suggested that this condition is secondary to increased intraluminal gall bladder pressure but this is not proven. Gallstones may frequently coexist but there is no evidence to support a direct relationship. It is unlikely that adenomyomatosis alone is a cause of biliary symptoms.

Chronic cholecystitis

There are no symptoms or signs that can conclusively be shown to be due to chronic cholecystitis. Symptoms attributed to this condition are vague, such as indigestion, upper abdominal discomfort or distension. There is no doubt that gall bladders studied histologically can show signs of chronic inflammation, and occasionally a small, shrunken gall bladder is found either radiologically or on ultrasound examination. However, these findings can be seen in asymptomatic people and therefore this clinical diagnosis should not be made. Most patients with chronic right hypochondrial pain suffer from functional bowel disease (p. 335).

EXTRAHEPATIC BILIARY TREE

Primary sclerosing cholangitis

Primary sclerosing cholangitis (PSC) is a chronic cholestatic liver disease characterized by fibrosing inflammatory destruction of both the intra- and extrahepatic bile ducts. In 75% of patients PSC is associated with inflammatory bowel disease (usually ulcerative colitis) but it is not unusual for the PSC to predate the onset of the inflammatory bowel disease. The causes are unknown but genetic susceptibility to PSC is associated with the HLA A1-B8-DR3 haplotype. The autoantibody p-ANCA (anti-neutrophil cytoplasmic antibody) is found in serum of 60% of cases. Seventy per cent of patients are men with an average age of onset of approximately 40 years.

With increasing screening of patients with inflammatory bowel disease PSC is detected at an asymptomatic phase with abnormal liver biochemistry, usually a raised serum alkaline phosphatase. Symptomatic presentation is usually with fluctuating pruritus, jaundice and cholangitis. The typical biliary changes associated with PSC may usually be identified by MRC scanning. This technique may not identify minor, but still clinically significant, intrahepatic duct abnormalities and this may require endoscopic retrograde cholangiography (ERC). The cholangiogram characteristically shows irregularity of calibre of both intra- and extrahepatic ducts, although either may be involved alone (see Fig. 7.32).

Confirmation of the diagnosis comes from liver histology, which shows inflammation of the intrahepatic biliary radicals with associated scar tissue classically described as being onion skin in appearance. The histological changes may range from minor inflammatory infiltrates to the level of established cirrhosis. The presence of cirrhosis has prognostic implications.

PSC is a slowly progressive lesion (symptoms and biochemical tests may fluctuate), ultimately leading to liver cirrhosis and associated decompensation. Cholangiocarcinoma occurs in up to 20% of patients.

The only proven treatment is liver transplantation. The bile acid ursodeoxycholic acid has been evaluated extensively in the treatment of PSC, with some transient improvement in liver function but no evidence of proven

Fig. 7.32 Primary sclerosing cholangitis. An endoscopic cholangiogram showing the typical features of primary sclerosing cholangitis. There are calibre irregularities of the intra-hepatic ducts (IHD). There is also minor stricturing of the extra-hepatic ducts at the confluence between the common bile duct (CBD) and the common hepatic duct (CHD).

long-term benefit. In a small minority of patients with PSC the dominant lesion is of the extrahepatic ducts. Such lesions may be amenable to endoscopic biliary intervention with balloon dilatation and temporary stent placement.

Choledochal cyst

Congenital cystic disease of the bile ducts may occur at all levels of the biliary tree, although the majority are extrahepatic. The dilatation may be saccular, diverticular or of fusiform configuration. The majority of symptomatic cases present in childhood with features of cholangitis. In adult life choledochal cysts may be a differential diagnosis in patients presenting with symptoms suggestive of bile duct stones. The cyst must be fully resected to avoid the recurrent biliary complications as well as averting the risk (approximately 15%) of subsequent cholangiocarcinoma.

Haemobilia

Haemobilia is the term used to describe bleeding into the biliary tree. This may be as a consequence of liver trauma or as a complication of liver surgery. Biopsy of the liver is also a well-recognized cause. The end result is a fistula between a branch of the hepatic artery and an intrahepatic bile duct.

Haemobilia may be a cause of significant gastrointestinal blood loss and should be suspected when melaena is accompanied by right-sided upper abdominal pain and jaundice. However, the bleeding may occur without any overt biliary symptoms. If the diagnosis is suspected, bleeding may be managed by occlusion of the feeding artery by thrombosis performed radiologically. Some patients will require surgery to control the bleeding point.

TUMOURS OF THE BILIARY TRACT

Gall bladder polyps

Polyps of the gall bladder are a common finding, being seen in approximately 4% of all patients referred for hepatobiliary ultrasonography. The vast majority of these are small (less than 5 mm), are non-neoplastic and are inflammatory in origin or composed of cholesterol deposits (see above). Adenomas are the most common benign neoplasm of the gall bladder. Only a proportion of these have a cancerous potential. The only reliable means of defining those at risks is by polyp size. Cholecystectomy is recommended for any polyp approximating to 1 cm in diameter or larger.

Primary cancer of the gall bladder

Adenocarcinoma of the gall bladder represents 1% of all cancers. The mean age of occurrence is in the early sixties with a ratio of 3 women to 1 man. Gallstones have been suggested as an aetiological factor but this relationship remains unproven. Diffuse calcification of the gall bladder (porcelain gall bladder), considered to be the end stage of chronic cholecystitis, has also been associated with cancer of the gall bladder and is an indication for early cholecystectomy. Adenomatous polyps of the gall bladder in excess of 1 cm in diameter are also recognized as premalignant lesions (see above).

Carcinoma of the gall bladder is often detected at the time of planned cholecystectomy for gallstones and in such circumstances resection of an early lesion may be curative. Early lymphatic spread to the liver and adjacent biliary tract precludes curative resection in more advanced lesions. There are no proven chemotherapeutic agents for carcinoma of the gall bladder. A small proportion of cases are sensitive to radiotherapy but the overall 5-year survival is less than 5%.

Cholangiocarcinoma (see also p. 395)

Cancer of the biliary tree may be intra- or extrahepatic. These malignancies represent approximately 1% of all cancers. A number of associations have been identified such as that with choledochal cyst (see above), and chronic infection of the biliary tree with, for example, *Clonorchis sinensis*. There are also associations with auto-immune disease processes such as primary sclerosing cholangitis. The bile duct malignancy usually presents with jaundice and may be suspected by imaging, initially ultrasound and thereafter spiral CT and in particular magnetic resonance cholangiopancreatography (MRCP). The disease spread is usually by local lymphatics or by local extension. Cholangiocarcinoma of the common bile duct may be resectable at presentation but local extension precludes such management in the majority of more proximal lesions. Localized disease justifies an aggressive surgical approach including partial hepatic resection.

Secondary malignant involvement of the biliary tree

Carcinoma of the head of the pancreas frequently presents with common bile duct obstruction and jaundice. Metastases to the bile ducts from distant cancers are uncommon. Melanoma is the most frequent neoplasm to do so.

Other carcinomas that have caused bile duct metastases, in order of frequency, are those arising in the lung, breast and colon as well as those from the pancreas (metastatic as compared to direct infiltration). Infiltration of the bile duct is not uncommon in disseminated lymphomatous disease.

Palliation of malignant bile duct obstruction

A small proportion of cholangiocarcinomas are surgically resectable, more commonly those in the distal bile duct as compared to the hilar region. All patients must be fully screened for operability using the imaging techniques described above. However, in the greater proportion of patients the treatment is palliative. The response to chemotherapy and radiation is poor in these tumours. Relief of bile duct obstruction has been shown to improve quality of life considerably and with pain control is the major end point of palliation. In recent years endoscopic techniques have allowed the insertion of stents into the biliary tree to re-establish bile flow. The initial use of plastic stents has largely been replaced by self-expanding metal stents which have considerably longer periods of patency (Fig. 7.33). In the small proportion of patients in whom bile duct drainage is not possible endoscopically, the percutaneous route offers an alternative method of stent placement. There is some evidence of benefit from the use of photodynamic therapy in those patients in whom biliary drainage has been achieved. This technique involves the use of a porphyrin derivative to sensitize the malignant cells prior to activation by an endoscopically placed laser probe. The aim is to provide local tumour destruction and maintain bile duct patency.

(a) (b)

Fig. 7.33 **Stents.**
(a) An endoscopic cholangiogram showing a distal stricture of the common bile duct (CBD) (arrow). This is secondary to a carcinoma of the head of pancreas. The CBD and intra-hepatic ducts (IHD) are dilated. A guide wire has been passed across the stricture.
(b) In the same patient a self-expanding metal stent (arrow) has been inserted re-establishing drainage of the biliary tree.

FURTHER READING
Bree RL, Ralls PW, Balfe DM (2000) Evaluation of patients with acute right upper quadrant pain. American College of Radiology. ACR Appropriateness Criteria. *Radiology* **215** (Suppl): 153–157.
Dowling RH (2000) Review: pathogenesis of gallstones. *Alimentary Pharmacology and Therapeutics* **14** (Suppl 2): 39–47.

Freeman ML, Nelson DB, Sherman S et al. (1995) Complications of endoscopic biliary sphincterotomy. *New England Journal of Medicine* **225**: 909–917.
Grant AJ et al. (2002) Homing of mucosal lymphocytes to the liver in the pathogenesis of hepatic complications of inflammatory bowel disease. *Lancet* **359**: 150–157.

THE PANCREAS

STRUCTURE AND FUNCTION

Structure

The pancreas extends retroperitoneally across the posterior abdominal wall from the second part of the duodenum to the spleen. The head is encircled by the duodenum; the body, which forms the main bulk of the organ, ends in a tail that lies in contact with the spleen. The pancreas consists of exocrine and endocrine cells making up 98% of the human pancreas.

The pancreatic acinar cells are grouped into lobules forming the ductal system which eventually joins into the main pancreatic duct.

The main pancreatic duct has many tributary ductules and gradually tapers towards the tail of the pancreas. The main pancreatic duct itself usually joins the common bile duct to enter the duodenum as a short single duct at the ampulla of Vater.

Exocrine function

The pancreatic acinar cells are responsible for production of digestive enzymes. These include amylase, lipase, colipase, phospholipase and the proteases (trypsinogen and chymotrypsinogen). These enzymes are stored within the acinar cells in secretory granules and are released by exocytosis (Fig. 7.34).

After ingestion of a meal pancreatic exocrine secretion is regulated by cephalic, gastric, and intestinal stimuli. The cephalic phase is mediated by the central nervous system and is stimulated by behavioural cues related to the sight and smell of food. With ingestion of food, the gastric phase commences and in response to distension of

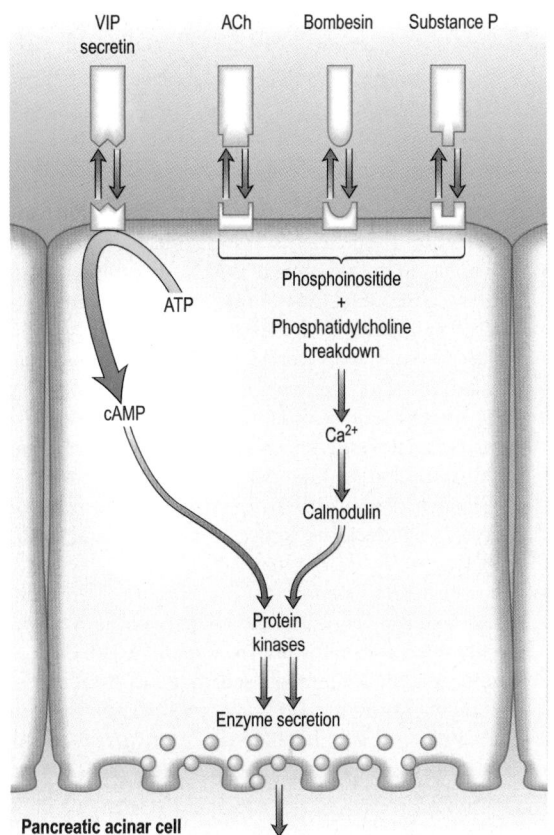

Fig. 7.34 Diagram showing stimulus–secretion coupling of pancreatic cell protein secretion. There is no CCK receptor in humans; stimulation is probably via neural fibres. VIP, vasoactive intestinal polypeptide; CCK, cholecystokinin; ACh, acetylcholine.

the stomach a neural pathway involving the central nervous system stimulates pancreatic secretion. Both these phases are under vagal control.

Finally, the presence of protein, fat and gastric acid within the small intestine further augments pancreatic secretion by both hormonal and neurotransmitter activity which produces local enteropancreatic control of secretion. Feedback regulatory events eventually terminate pancreatic secretion.

Cholecystokinin (CCK) is produced in specialized gut endocrine cells (I cells) of the mucosa of the small intestine and is secreted in response to intraluminal food. In animals, it exerts its biological activity by binding to specific G-protein-coupled receptors on target cells in the pancreas. Activated G-proteins lead to the activation of phospholipases. This in turn leads to calcium release from intracellular stores, which in turn results in the fusion of the digestive enzyme granules to the apical plasma membrane and enzyme release. There are no CCK receptors in pancreatic cells in humans and CCK acts via receptors on vagal afferent fibres to stimulate pancreatic secretion. Of the enzymes produced by the pancreatic acinar cells, the proteases and colipase are secreted as inactive precursors and require duodenal enterokinase to initiate activity.

Secretin is also released from specialized entero-endocrine cells of the small intestine during a meal and in particular during duodenal acidification. Secretin has a direct effect on the pancreatic acinar cells as well as the ductal cells. There is also a vagal-mediated secretory response. Secretin action is mediated via G-coupled receptors and calcium-mediated enzyme release. Secretin results in a bicarbonate-rich pancreatic secretion.

Completion of the postprandial secretory phase involves both neural and hormonal control.

Central neuronal inhibition of pancreatic secretion acts through dopamine and somatostatin receptors mediated by noradrenergic nerves. The islet cell hormone pancreatic polypeptide is released from the pancreas in response to a meal and has an inhibitory effect upon acinar enzyme secretion both by a local effect and via central receptors.

Somatostatin, present within the pancreas, stomach and central nervous system, is released in response to food. Its effect is mediated both by direct pancreatic acinar inhibition and by a central nervous system effect. Two other mechanisms of inhibition have been described. Proteases within the duodenal lumen have a negative feedback on acinar secretion. Secondly, nutrients within the ileum inhibit pancreatic secretion by means of local hormone release (peptide YY and glucagon-like peptide) acting on the acinar cells themselves as well as centrally.

There is now increasing evidence that the gut-related peptides, leptin and ghrelin, as well as influencing appetite behaviour, are also regulatory factors in the exocrine function of the pancreas. This effect is believed to occur via hypothalamic centres.

The endocrine pancreas

This consists of hormone-producing cells arranged in nests or islets (islets of Langerhans). The hormones produced are secreted directly into the circulation and there is no access to the pancreatic ductular system. There are *five main types of islet cell* corresponding to different secretory components. The beta-cells are the most common and are responsible for insulin production. The alpha-cells produce glucagon. The D cells produce somatostatin, PP-cells produce pancreatic polypeptide and enterochromaffin cells produce serotonin.

A number of other hormones have been identified within the endocrine pancreas including gastrin-releasing peptide, neuropeptide Y and galanin. These are believed to be neurotransmitters active in the neuro-gastrointestinal axis.

INVESTIGATION OF THE PANCREAS

Assessment of exocrine function

Overt fat malabsorption does not occur until approximately 85–90% of the function has been lost. This large reserve of pancreatic function means that any pancreatic function test based upon the measurement of either the pancreatic enzymes or their breakdown products is insensitive, particularly in mild to moderate disease.

Duodenal sampling and pancreatic function tests
These tests rely upon the analysis of a duodenal aspirate following pancreatic stimulation.

The original test involved the oral administration of a specified meal (Lundh meal). Pancreatic stimulation is now achieved by intravenous secretin and cholecystokinin. The aspirate is assessed for pancreatic enzymes and bicarbonate production.

The procedure is time-consuming and requires a meticulous technique. There is a good correlation with moderate to severe pancreatic function loss, but not for mild damage. These tests are not widely available.

Non-invasive test of pancreatic function
Serum biochemistry Serum lipase, trypsin–trypsinogen and amylase can all be measured. Serum trypsin is the most useful although diminished levels are only detected after pancreatic insufficiency is clinically detectable by overt malabsorption. Their main use is in acute pancreatitis.

Faecal tests
- *Faecal fat estimation* (see p. 300).
- *Faecal chymotrypsin.* The test is not useful until severe impairment of pancreatic function is present.
- *Faecal elastase.* This pancreatic specific enzyme is not degraded in the intestine and has high concentrations within the faeces. Diminished levels may be detected in moderate as well as severe pancreatic insufficiency, and this is probably more sensitive than other serum and faecal tests.

Oral pancreatic function tests
- *PABA-test.* Oral N-benzoyl-L-tyrosyl-p-aminobenzoic acid is hydrolysed by chymotrypsin to release p-aminobenzoic acid (PABA), which is then absorbed, conjugated and excreted in the urine where it can be measured. The test is time-consuming but is specific for pancreatic insufficiency, with a 65–80% sensitivity.
- *Fluorescein dilaurate test.* Oral fluorescein dilaurate is digested by pancreatic esterase to release the fluorescein which is then absorbed and excreted in the urine. This test is relatively inexpensive and commercially available as the 'Pancreolauryl test'. This is highly sensitive and specific in severe pancreatic insufficiency but has only a 50% sensitivity in mild to moderate disease.

Clinical application of pancreatic function tests
Whilst the invasive duodenal aspiration tests represent the most sensitive and specific means of assessing pancreatic function, these are very rarely used outside specialized centres. The Pancreolauryl and PABA tests are non-invasive and are widely available but are only highly sensitive in the detection of severe pancreatic insufficiency. The faecal elastase test (in a commercially available form) provides similar sensitivity and specificity and is the test

of choice as a screening tool for pancreatic insufficiency, but again detection of mild disease is problematic.

Pancreatic imaging (see p. 354)
This can detect structural abnormalities even when functional tests are still within normal limits.

- A *plain abdominal radiograph* may show pancreatic calcification, particularly when alcohol is the aetiology.
- *Ultrasound* of the pancreas is a useful screening investigation for inflammation and neoplasia. Views may be limited by overlying bowel gas.
- *Spiral CT scan* with contrast enhancement is more reliable.
- *MRI scanning* represents an alternative to CT. Magnetic resonance cholangiopancreatography (MRCP) gives clear definition of the pancreatic duct as well as the biliary tree. Gallstones (including microcalculi) may also be identified in the biliary tree using MRI/MRCP.
- *Endoscopic ultrasound* is very useful for identifying distal common bile duct stones as well as a microcalculi either within the duct or within the gall bladder. Endoscopic ultrasound is a sensitive means of detecting small pancreatic tumours, particularly those of neuroendocrine origin. There is also an increasing role for this technique to stage the operability of pancreatic adenocarcinoma.
- *Endoscopic retrograde cholangiopancreatography (ERCP)* was considered the gold standard for diagnosing pancreatic disease. However, with MRCP and endoscopic ultrasound, ERCP is restricted to therapeutic intervention.

Summary An initial transabdominal ultrasound supplemented by spiral CT provides sufficient diagnostic information for most inflammatory and neoplastic conditions of the pancreas. MRI and MRCP are now widely available and provide additional information, particularly with respect to pancreatic ductular and biliary anatomy.

Endoscopic ultrasound is available in specialized centres if diagnostic information is still lacking.

PANCREATITIS

Classification
Pancreatitis is divided into acute and chronic. By definition acute pancreatitis is a process that occurs on the background of a previously normal pancreas and can return to normal after resolution of the episode. In chronic pancreatitis there is continuing inflammation with irreversible structural changes.

In practice the differentiation between acute and chronic pancreatitis may be extremely difficult, particularly in the setting of recurrent acute episodes which may represent true acute pancreatitis or may be an acute manifestation of underlying chronic disease.

Table 7.18 Causes of pancreatitis

Acute	Chronic
Gallstones	Alcohol
Alcohol	Tropical (nutritional)
Infections (e.g. mumps, Coxsackie B)	Hereditary
Pancreatic tumours	Trypsinogen and inhibitory protein defects
Drugs (e.g. azathioprine, oestrogens, corticosteroids)	Cystic fibrosis
Iatrogenic (e.g. post-surgical, ERCP)	Idiopathic
Hyperlipidaemias	Trauma
Miscellaneous	Hypercalcaemia
Trauma	
Scorpion bite	
Cardiac surgery	
Idiopathic	

Fig. 7.35 Complications of acute pancreatitis in relation to time after presentation.

Acute pancreatitis

The causes of acute pancreatitis are listed in Table 7.18.

In the western world gallstones and alcohol account for the vast majority of episodes. Alcohol also causes chronic pancreatitis (see below). The severity of the pancreatitis may range from mild and self-limiting to extremely severe with extensive pancreatic and peripancreatic necrosis as well as haemorrhage. In its most severe form the mortality rises to between 40–50%.

Pathogenesis

Mechanisms by which pancreatic necrosis occurs remain speculative. Any theory must take into account how a very diverse group of aetiological factors can produce the same end point. There is some suggestion that the final common pathway is a marked elevation of intracellular calcium which in turn leads to activation of intracellular proteases. It is these activated enzymes which are responsible for cellular necrosis.

In the case of gallstone-related pancreatitis it is believed stones occlude the pancreatic drainage at the level of the ampulla leading to pancreatic ductular hypertension. Such ductular hypertension has been shown in animal models to increase cytosolic free ionized calcium. There is also evidence that alcohol interferes with calcium homeostasis in pancreatic acinar cells.

Clinical features

Acute pancreatitis is a differential diagnosis in any patient with upper abdominal pain. The pain usually begins in the epigastrium accompanied by nausea and vomiting. As inflammation spreads throughout the peritoneal cavity the pain becomes more intense. Involvement of the retroperitoneum frequently leads to back pain.

The patient may give a history of previous similar episodes or be known to have gallstones. An attack may follow an alcoholic binge. However, in many cases there are no obvious aetiological factors.

Physical examination at the time of presentation may show little more than a patient in pain with some upper abdominal tenderness but no systemic abnormalities. In more severe disease the patient may have a tachycardia, hypotension and be oliguric. Abdominal examination may show widespread tenderness with guarding as well as reduced or absent bowel sounds. Specific clinical signs that support a diagnosis of severe necrotizing pancreatitis include periumbilical (Cullen's sign) and flank bruising (Grey Turner's sign). In patients with a gallstone aetiology the clinical picture may also include the features of cholangitis. The complications are shown in Figure 7.35.

Diagnosis

Blood tests

- *Serum amylase level* is the standard laboratory test carried out to confirm the diagnosis. If this is measured within 24 hours of the onset of pain an elevation of three times the upper limit of normal is an extremely sensitive test. A number of other conditions may occasionally cause a very elevated amylase (see Table 7.19). Amylase levels gradually fall back towards normal over the next 3–5 days. With a late presentation the serum amylase level may give a false-negative result.
- *Urinary amylase levels* may be diagnostic as these remain elevated over a longer period of time.
- *Serum lipase levels* are also raised in acute pancreatitis and these remain elevated for a longer period of time

Table 7.19 Elevation of serum amylase unrelated to pancreatitis

Leakage of upper gastrointestinal contents into the peritoneum
Upper gastrointestinal perforation
Biliary peritonitis
Intestinal infarction

Inherited abnormalities of amylase
Macroamylasaemia

than those of amylase. However, overall, the accuracy of serum lipase is not significantly greater than amylase and it is technically more difficult to measure.

■ *Other baseline investigations* include a full blood count and CRP, urea and electrolytes, blood glucose, liver biochemistry, plasma calcium and arterial blood gases. These are documented at presentation and then repeated at 24 and 48 hours and provide a basis for assessing the severity of an attack (see below).

Radiology

■ An erect *chest X-ray* is mandatory to exclude gastro-duodenal perforation, which also raises the serum amylase (Table 7.19). A supine abdominal film may show gallstones or pancreatic calcification.

■ An *abdominal ultrasound scan* is used as a screening test to identify a possible biliary (gallstone) cause of pancreatitis. Gallstones are difficult to detect in the distal common bile duct but dilated intrahepatic ducts may be present in the presence of bile duct obstruction. Stones within the gall bladder are not sufficient to justify a diagnosis of gallstone-related pancreatitis. The ultrasound may also demonstrate pancreatic swelling and necrosis as well as peripancreatic fluid collections if present. In severe pancreatitis the pancreas may be difficult to visualize because of gas-filled loops of bowel.

■ *Contrast-enhanced spiral CT scanning* is essential in all but the most mild attacks of pancreatitis (Fig. 7.36). Carried out within 2–3 days of presentation, it allows the extent of pancreatic necrosis to be assessed. This provides very valuable prognostic information. Later in the course of the disease, repeated CT scans may be used to detect other complications including fluid collections, abscess formation and pseudocyst development.

■ *MRI (MRCP)* can assess the degree of pancreatic damage and identify gallstones within the biliary tree. MRI is particularly useful to differentiate between fluid and solid inflammatory masses.

Fig. 7.36 **CT scan in patient with acute pancreatitis** showing necrosis of the pancreatic parenchyma (arrow) and a fluid collection extending outside the gland with inflammatory thickening of the colon.

■ *ERCP* is used as a treatment measure to remove bile duct stones in the presence of gallstone-related pancreatitis (see below).

Assessment of disease severity

The majority of cases of acute pancreatitis are mild but approximately 25% run a more complicated course which may result in haemodynamic instability and multiple organ failure. The early prediction of such a severe attack allows appropriate monitoring and intensive care to be in place.

Early clinical assessment has been shown to have poor sensitivity for predicting a severe attack. Similarly, individual laboratory tests have very limited value. Elevations of CRP have been associated with severe episodes, although the sensitivity and specificity remains to be defined. To improve the predictive value multiple factors have been used to develop scoring systems (see Table 7.20). The Ranson and Glasgow scoring systems are based on such parameters and have been shown to have an 80% sensitivity for predicting a severe attack, although only after 48 hours following presentation. The acute physiology and chronic health evaluation score (APACHE) currently has been extensively adopted as a means of assessing the severity of a wide spectrum of illness. The APACHE scoring system is based on common physiological and laboratory values and adjusted for age as well as the presence or absence of a number of other chronic health problems (see Table 7.21). This scoring system

Table 7.20 Factors during the first 48 hours that indicate severe pancreatitis and a poor prognosis (three or more factors present predict a severe episode)

Age	> 55 years
WBC	> 15 × 10^9/L
Blood glucose	> 10 mmol/L
Serum urea	> 16 mmol/L
Serum albumin	< 30 g/L
Serum aminotransferase	> 200 U/L
Serum calcium	< 2 mmol/L
Serum LDH	> 600 U/L
P_aO_2	< 8.0 kPa (60 mmHg)

LDH, lactate dehydrogenase

Table 7.21 The APACHE II scoring system parameters

Physiological	Laboratory
Temperature	Oxygenation (P_aO_2)
Heart rate	Arterial pH
Respiratory rate	Serum:
Mean arterial pressure	sodium
Glasgow Coma Scale	potassium
	creatinine
	Haematocrit
	White blood cell count

Score 0–4 (normal–abnormal)
Adjust for age and severe organ insufficiency or for immunocompromised. BMI is an additional parameter

appears to have a high sensitivity as early as 24 hours after onset of symptoms.

There is evidence that obesity predicts the outcome from an episode of pancreatitis as the excessive adipose tissue is a substrate for activated enzyme activity. This will in turn generate an extensive inflammatory reaction.

Even modest obesity (basal metabolic index (BMI) between 25–30) has an adverse affect. This is incorporated as an adverse factor in the APACHE score (p. 410) for acute pancreatitis and other variables have also been added.

Treatment

The initial management of acute pancreatitis is similar, whatever the cause. A multiple factor scoring system (ideally APACHE II with a modification for obesity) should be carried out at the end of the first 24 hours after presentation to allow identification of the 25% of patients with a predicted severe attack. This should be repeated at 48 hours to identify a further subgroup who appear to be moving into the severe category. These patients should then be managed on a high-dependency or intensive care unit. Even patients outside of the severe category may require considerable supportive care.

Early fluid losses in acute pancreatitis may be large, requiring well-maintained intravenous access as well as a central line and urinary catheter to monitor circulating volume and renal function.

- *Nasogastric suction* prevents abdominal distension and vomitus and hence the risk of aspiration pneumonia.
- *Baseline arterial blood gases* determine the need for continuous oxygen administration.
- *Prophylactic antibiotics.* Broad-spectrum antibiotics, e.g. cefuroxime or aztreonam, reduce the risk of infective complications and are given from the outset.
- *Analgesia requirements.* Pethidine and tramadol are the drugs of choice, usually administered by a patient control system. The morphine derivatives should be avoided because they can cause sphincter of Oddi contraction.
- *Feeding.* In patients with a severe episode there is little likelihood of oral nutrition for a number of weeks. Total parenteral nutrition has been associated with a high risk of infection and has been replaced by enteral nutrition. This is administered via a nasojejunal tube, which is well tolerated and can maintain adequate nutritional input. The nasojejunal position of the feeding tube placed endoscopically overcomes the frequent problem of gastric paresis and there is less likelihood of pancreatic stimulation.

In a small proportion of patients, multiorgan failure will develop in the first few days after presentation reflecting the extent of pancreatic necrosis. Such patients will require positive-pressure ventilation and often renal support. The mortality in this group is extremely high (in excess of 80%).

Gallstone-related pancreatitis

In patients with gallstone-related pancreatitis and associated cholangitis, endoscopic intervention with sphincterotomy and stone extraction is of proven benefit and is the treatment of choice. In the absence of cholangitis, sphincterotomy and stone extraction is only of proven benefit when the episode of pancreatitis is predicted as severe. In less severe cases of gallstone-related pancreatitis intervention can be deferred until full recovery is obtained (an approximate 6-week period).

Late complications of acute pancreatitis

Within the first 7 days the morbidity and mortality of acute pancreatitis reflect the systemic inflammatory response which in turn results in multiple organ failure. After this initial period the prognosis thereafter is most closely related to the extent of pancreatic necrosis. This can be most accurately assessed by contrast-enhanced CT, which should be carried out in all patients with severe disease after the first week. Extensive necrosis (greater than 50% of the pancreas) is associated with high risk of further complicated disease frequently requiring surgical intervention.

It is infection of the necrotic pancreas which is of most concern and which may rapidly lead to overwhelming sepsis. Prophylactic antibiotics have been used to prevent this but do not reliably do so. If there is evidence of incipient infection monitored by a rising neutrophil count and CRP level, an aspirate of the necrotic pancreas is taken and cultured. The vast majority of patients with a positive culture should be considered for surgical resection of the necrotic pancreas. In the most severe cases multiple operations are required to fully resect the areas of necrosis.

Peripancreatic fluid collections are common in the early stages of acute pancreatitis, the vast majority of which will resolve spontaneously.

Some fluid collections will be surrounded by granulation tissue producing the so-called *pseudocyst.* These by definition are not found until 6 weeks after the onset of the illness. The smaller pseudocysts (less than 6 cm in diameter) frequently resolve on their own but others may persist in the long term, giving rise to potential complications such as infection and intra-peritoneal bleeding. Larger pseudocysts persisting for longer than 6 weeks are usually actively managed by either percutaneous (or endoscopic) drainage or by surgical intervention.

Long-term outcome

The vast majority of patients with a mild to moderate episode of acute pancreatitis will make a full recovery with no long-term sequelae. Recurrent episodes of pancreatitis may occur, particularly if there has been any long-term pancreatic ductular damage. Patients with more severe acute pancreatitis may become pancreatic insufficient both with respect to exocrine (malabsorption) and endocrine function (diabetes).

Chronic pancreatitis

Aetiology

In developed countries by far the most common cause of

chronic pancreatitis is alcohol, accounting for 60–80% of cases (see Table 7.18).

In developing countries malnutrition and associated dietary factors have been implicated. In a small group of patients chronic pancreatitis has been shown to be hereditary, inherited as an autosomal dominant condition with variable penetrance. Almost all patients with cystic fibrosis (p. 413) have established chronic pancreatitis, usually from birth. Cystic fibrosis gene mutations have also been identified in patients with chronic pancreatitis but in whom there were no other manifestations of cystic fibrosis.

Obstruction of the pancreatic duct because of either a benign or malignant process may result in chronic pancreatitis. Congenital abnormalities of the pancreatic duct, in particular pancreas divisum, have been implicated.

Pathogenesis

A possible common pathway for pancreatic damage is the inappropriate activation of enzymes within the pancreas. This has been well demonstrated in the case of hereditary pancreatitis where genetic abnormalities of cationic trypsinogen and its inhibitory proteins have led to unopposed trypsin activity within the pancreas itself. Chronic alcohol intake is also believed to increase the level of trypsinogen relative to its inhibitor. Human trypsinogen has a propensity to autoactivate, and any relative impairment or deficiency of inhibitor proteins will lead to unopposed enzyme activity and possible pancreatic damage.

It is believed that the intrapancreatic enzyme activity leads to the precipitation of proteins within the duct lumen in the form of plugs. These then form a nidus for calcification but are also the cause of ductal obstruction leading to ductal hypertension and further pancreatic damage. Cytokine activation and oxygen stress are thought to play a role in perpetuating this process.

Clinical features

Pain is the most common presentation of chronic pancreatitis and is usually epigastric and often radiating through into the back. The pattern of pain may be episodic with short periods of severe pain or chronic unremitting. Exacerbations of the pain may follow further alcohol excess although this is not a uniform relationship. During periods of abdominal pain anorexia is common and weight loss may be severe. This is particularly so in those patients with chronic unremitting symptoms.

Exocrine and endocrine insufficiency may develop at any time, and occasionally malabsorption or diabetes are the presenting features in the absence of abdominal pain.

Jaundice secondary to common bile duct obstruction during its course through the fibrosed head of pancreas, may also occur and may be a presenting feature in a small proportion of patients.

Investigations

The extent to which investigations are required is dependent upon the clinical setting. In a patient with known alcohol abuse and typical pain few confirmatory tests are required.

Fig. 7.37 Contrast-enhanced CT scan demonstrating multiple calcific densities (arrow) along the line of the main pancreatic duct in a patient with chronic pancreatitis.

- *Serum amylase and lipase* levels are rarely significantly elevated in established chronic pancreatitis.
- *Faecal elastase* level will be abnormal in the majority of patients with moderate to severe pancreatic disease.
- *PABA and Pancreolauryl tests* (see p. 408).
- *Transabdominal ultrasound scan* is used for initial assessment.
- *Contrast-enhanced spiral CT scan* provides a more detailed assessment. In the presence of pancreatic calcification and a dilated pancreatic duct the diagnosis of chronic pancreatitis can be easily established (Fig. 7.37). This may be much more difficult when these features are not present and in particular with an atypical presentation such as with steatorrhoea alone.
- *MRI with MRCP* is increasingly utilized to define more subtle abnormalities of the pancreatic duct which may be seen in non-dilated chronic pancreatitis.
- *Endoscopic ultrasound* is used in a small proportion of patients in whom the diagnosis is not confirmed with the above imaging or specifically for assessing complications of chronic pancreatitis including pseudocyst formation.
- *Diagnostic ERCP* has been replaced by MRCP.

Differential diagnosis

The differential diagnosis is that of pancreatic malignancy. Carcinoma of the pancreas can reproduce many of the symptoms and imaging abnormalities that are commonly seen with chronic pancreatitis. The diagnosis of malignancy should be considered in patients with a short history and in whom there is a localized ductular abnormality. Considerable difficulties may arise when a malignancy develops on the background of established chronic pancreatitis (the latter being a recognized premalignant lesion).

High-quality imaging is able to define malignant features with a localized mass lesion, local invasion and lymph node enlargement. Endoscopic ultrasound may provide the most accurate assessment of a potential mass lesion.

Treatment

In patients with alcohol-related chronic pancreatitis long-term abstinence is likely to be of benefit although this has been difficult to prove.

Abdominal pain. For short-term flare-ups of pain a combination of a non-steroidal anti-inflammatory drug and an opiate (tramadol) is usually sufficient for symptomatic relief. In patients with chronic unremitting pain this may be inadequate and also risk opiate addiction.

Tricyclic antidepressants (e.g. amitriptyline) are used for chronic pain and reduce the need for opiates. Oral pancreatic enzyme supplements reduce pancreatic stimulation (by a negative-feedback mechanism) and hence the intensity of pain. Antioxidant use awaits evidence of benefit. Coeliac axis nerve block may produce good pain relief but is unreliable in its extent and duration of action.

In the majority of patients some spontaneous improvement in pain control occurs with time. After a 6- to 10-year period some 60% of patients will become pain-free. For patients with debilitating pain, surgical intervention is justified. Both duct drainage and limited resection procedures have been carried out with total or partial pain relief in approximately 80% of patients but with a mortality of 5%.

Other endoscopic techniques used to improve pancreatic drainage as well as managing intraductal stones have been tried with reported success.

Steatorrhoea. The steatorrhoea associated with pancreatic insufficiency may be high, with up to 30 mmol of fat lost per 24 hours. This will usually improve with pancreatic enzymes supplements and a low fat diet. Current preparations are presented in the form of microspheres which reduce the problems of acid degradation in the stomach. An acid suppressor (H_2-receptor antagonist or proton pump inhibitor) is also given. Despite this, a proportion of patients continue to malabsorb, usually reflecting the inadequate mixing of the pancreatic supplements with the food as well as the low pH in the duodenum secondary to inadequate pancreatic bicarbonate production.

Diabetes associated with pancreatic endocrine failure may be difficult to control with a rapid progression from oral hypoglycaemic agents to an insulin requirement. Brittle control is a common problem secondary to inadequate glucagon production from the damaged pancreas.

Complications

The most common structural complication of chronic pancreatitis is a pancreatic pseudocyst, a fluid collection surrounded by granulation tissue (see p. 411). These usually occur in relationship to a period of enhanced inflammatory activity within the pancreas giving abdominal pain but may develop silently during what would appear to be a stable phase. Intra- or retroperitoneal rupture, bleeding or cyst infection occur. The larger cysts may occlude nearby structures including the duodenum and the bile duct. In pseudocysts less than 6 cm in diameter, spontaneous resolution can be anticipated. In larger cysts that have been present for a period in excess of 6 weeks, resolution is uncommon and a long-term complication rate of approximately 30% can be anticipated. Many pseudocysts are closely apposed to the posterior wall of the stomach or duodenum and can be successfully drained endoscopically using endoscopic ultrasound to identify the optimum drainage site. A direct fistula is created between the pseudocyst lumen and the gastric or duodenal lumen which is then kept patent by the insertion of plastic stents. This approach will be successful in approximately 75% of cases. Surgical drainage is required for failures of endoscopic therapy or in circumstances in which the pseudocyst anatomy does not allow endoscopic access.

Ascites and occasionally pleural effusions can be a direct consequence of chronic pancreatitis when there has been disruption of the main pancreatic duct. A high ascites or pleural fluid amylase will confirm the aetiology. Such disruptions of the main pancreatic duct require surgical intervention.

Cystic fibrosis (see pp. 909 and 192)

This common cause of pancreatic disease in childhood is inherited as an autosomal recessive. A specific gene mutation ΔF_{508} is present in 70% of cases. The gene(s) code for a membrane protein in epithelial cells which regulates chloride transport (the cystic fibrosis transmembrane regular, CFTR). Defective chloride channel transport secondarily leads to a failure to hydrate pancreatic secretion. The increased viscosity of such secretions then leads to ductular obstruction and secondary pancreatic damage. Ninety per cent of patients with cystic fibrosis will have pancreatic failure, and in the majority of these this will be present from the perinatal period.

It has recently been recognized that a small proportion of patients with chronic pancreatitis of unknown aetiology are homozygous for cystic fibrosis genes but have no other overt manifestation of cystic fibrosis.

Clinical features and diagnosis

Clinical features and diagnostic tests are described on page 910; pancreatic function tests and imaging are described on p. 407.

Treatment

In the vast majority of patients with cystic fibrosis, pulmonary complications dominate the clinical picture. However, the management of pancreatic insufficiency is necessary to optimize the growth and overall nutrition. Pancreatic supplements are closely titrated against the level of steatorrhoea. To obtain optimal enzyme mixing with food, the supplements are taken throughout the meal. These are most commonly administered in an enteric coated form to minimize degradation within the acid milieu of the stomach. A daily lipase intake of up to 10 000 units/kg bodyweight may be required. High-dose enteric-coated preparations are available but have been implicated in right-sided colon stricture formation in children with cystic fibrosis. The exact mechanism by which this occurred has not been fully defined but these preparations are no longer recommended in children.

Despite appropriate enzyme dosage, up to 20% of patients continue to have significant fat malabsorption. In many cases this is secondary to poor compliance. Other mechanisms include acid degradation of the enzyme preparations, and this can be ameliorated by acid suppression, either with H_2-receptor antagonists or proton pump inhibitors. Coeliac disease (which has an increased prevalence in cystic fibrosis) should be excluded as a possible cause of continued malabsorption.

There is documented evidence of an age-related deterioration in glucose tolerance in patients with cystic fibrosis. Ten per cent of patients will develop clinically significant diabetes mellitus. It is extremely important to detect this at the earliest opportunity to prevent the adverse nutritional effects. In the large proportion of cases, management will be insulin dependent. Restriction of dietary fat helps the steatorrhoea but leads to malnourishment.

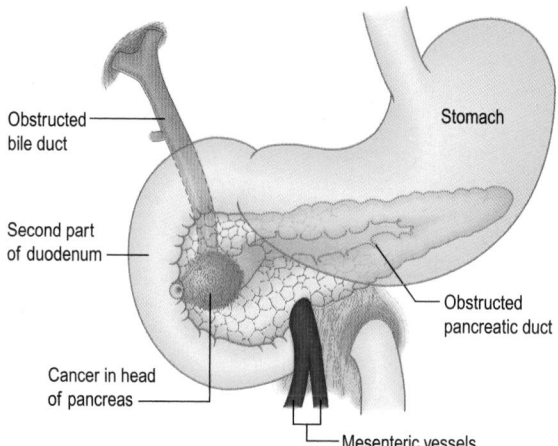

Fig. 7.38 **Carcinoma of the head of the pancreas.** A diagrammatic representation of the close relationship of a carcinoma of the head of pancreas to the surrounding structures.

CARCINOMA OF THE PANCREAS

The incidence of pancreatic cancer in the West has been estimated at approximately 9 cases per 100 000 with no increase over the last 20 years. Pancreatic cancer is now the fifth most common cause of cancer death in the western world. The incidence increases with age and the majority of cases occur in patients over the age of 60. Approximately 60% of patients with this condition are male. Ninety-six per cent of pancreatic cancers are adenocarcinoma in type and the large majority are of ductal origin. It has proved difficult to identify environmental risk factors but smoking is associated with a twofold increase. Other possible environmental factors include the petroleum product, naphthalamine. Chronic pancreatitis has been documented as a potential precancerous lesion. There is increasing evidence that pancreatic ductal adenocarcinoma is a result of accumulated genetic alterations. Subtle changes in an oncogene and both mutations and deletions of tumour suppressor genes are the most common forms of genetic alteration. The best known among the oncogenes is K-*ras*, present in 90% of human ductal adenocarcinomas. Other oncogenes include β-*catenin*. Tumour suppressor genes include *p16*, *p53* and *DPC4* (or SMAD4). The latter is a key transcription factor in growth regulation and is inactivated in over 50% of cases.

Clinical picture

Pancreatic adenocarcinoma may be viewed clinically as two diseases – the lesions of the head and lesions of the body and tail.

Symptoms

Carcinoma of the head of pancreas or the ampulla of Vater tends to present earlier with obstruction to the bile duct

as this passes through the head of pancreas giving jaundice (Fig. 7.38). These more localized lesions are usually painless, although pain may become a feature with tumour progression.

Carcinoma localized to the body or tail of the pancreas is much more likely to present with abdominal pain as well as non-specific symptoms such as anorexia and weight loss. The pain is often dull in character with radiation through into the back. A characteristic feature is partial relief of pain by sitting forward. Bile duct obstruction and jaundice may infrequently be a late phenomena.

Physical signs

With *carcinoma of the head of pancreas* the patient is jaundiced with the characteristic scratch marks secondary to cholestasis. In a proportion of cases the gall bladder will be palpable (Courvoisier's sign). A central abdominal mass may be palpable as well as hepatomegaly if metastatic disease is present. With *carcinoma of the body and tail*, there are often no physical signs.

Other presenting physical signs include thromboembolic phenomena, polyarthritis and skin nodules. The latter are secondary to localized fat necrosis and associated inflammation. These manifestations, distant to the tumour itself, have not been fully explained but may precede the overt presentation of pancreatic cancer by months to years.

Investigations

- *Transabdominal ultrasound* is the initial investigation in the majority of patients. In the presence of bile duct obstruction this will confirm dilated intrahepatic bile ducts as well as a mass in the head of the pancreas. Ultrasound is less reliable when the cancer is found in the body and tail of the pancreas because of overlying bowel gas, with a sensitivity of detection of 60%.
- *Contrast-enhanced spiral CT scan* should confirm the presence of a mass lesion (Fig. 7.39). It is also necessary prior to possible surgical resection with contrast

Fig. 7.39 **A contrast-enhanced CT scan showing a cancer of the body of the pancreas.** There is retroperitoneal tumour extension enclosing the branches of the coeliac axis (arrow).

providing vascular definition to exclude tumour invasion as well as local lymph node involvement and distant metastases.

- *Laparoscopy* is also used for preoperative assessment.
- *ERCP* is usually restricted to palliative treatment but may provide a source of cytology to confirm the diagnosis when this is in question.
- *Percutaneous needle biopsy* is discouraged in potentially operable cases as this may be a source of tumour cell spread within the peritoneum. If palliative chemotherapy is considered, a histological diagnosis is essential prior to treatment.
- *MRI scanning and endoscopic ultrasound* are techniques that are useful in a small proportion of patients in whom the tumour has not been adequately defined.
- *Several tumour markers* have been evaluated for the diagnosis and monitoring of pancreatic cancer. The CA19-9 has a high sensitivity (80%) but a high false-positive rate. In individual patients single values of these tumour markers may be of little help but a progressive elevation over time is often diagnostic, and in such circumstances tumour marker levels can be used to monitor response to treatment.

Differential diagnosis

The diagnosis should not be difficult in the presence of painless jaundice or epigastric pain radiating into the back with progressive weight loss.

Unfortunately many patients present with very minor symptoms including pain, change in bowel habit and weight loss. Imaging, particularly abdominal CT should be performed if pancreatic cancer is suspected. Pancreatic cancer may rarely present with recurrent episodes of typical acute pancreatitis.

Management

The 5-year survival rate for carcinoma of the pancreas is approximately 2% with surgical intervention representing the only chance of long-term survival. Approximately 20% of all cases have a localized tumour suitable for resection but in an elderly population many of these have co-morbid factors that preclude such major surgery. To optimize the percentage of patients undergoing possible surgical resection it is necessary to review each case in a multidisciplinary meeting. This approach also allows formulation of treatment strategies for those considered unsuitable for surgery.

In the majority of cases the management is *palliative*. Jaundice is a debilitating complication, often associated with severe pruritus but also the cause of non-specific malaise, lethargy and anorexia. Endoscopic placement of endoprostheses (stents) offers excellent palliation with a low associated procedural morbidity and mortality.

Palliative surgery has a role in duodenal obstruction (a complication seen in 10% of cases) but in advanced disease self-expanding metal stents can be placed across the duodenal obstruction with excellent short-term results.

The results of radiotherapy have been disappointing but there is now increasing evidence of benefit from a number of chemotherapeutic agents. 5-Fluorouracil and gemcitabine have been shown to improve survival in advanced disease and have also demonstrated survival benefit as an adjuvant therapy to pancreatic resection.

With disease progression, abdominal pain is a frequent complicating factor which may prove extremely difficult to treat.

This is best managed by experienced palliative care teams which offer a multidisciplinary approach. Endocrine and exocrine pancreatic failure occur and are managed as described on page 413.

CYSTIC TUMOURS OF THE PANCREAS

Cystic lesions of the pancreas are not uncommon. Seventy-five per cent of these lesions will be pseudocysts (see above) but of the remainder the majority are true cystic neoplasms. These neoplastic lesions can be divided into the serous and mucinous cyst adenomata. Serous cyst adenomata are composed of multiple small cystic cavities lined by cuboidal glycogen-rich, mucin-poor cells. These lesions tend to occur in an elderly age group and are often an asymptomatic finding. Malignant transformation in a serous cystadenoma is extremely rare. Mucinous cyst adenomata are almost exclusively found in women in the 5th and 6th decade and are sited in the pancreatic body and tail. Multiloculor cysts are lined by tall mucin-synthesizing cells. Twenty per cent of these lesions are malignant at the time of presentation and the majority appear to have a malignant potential. As a consequence they are much more likely to produce symptoms.

The importance of cystic lesions of the pancreas is to identify those at high risk of malignancy who should then undergo resection. Pseudocysts can usually be confirmed by the history of pancreatitis and features of the diagnosis upon imaging.

The differentiation between serous and mucinous cyst adenomata may be difficult, even when multiple imaging techniques are applied. Increasingly endoscopic ultrasound scanning and fine-needle aspiration have been applied to confirm the underlying diagnosis. The measurement of cyst fluid CEA and CA19-9 may help to identify malignant change.

NEUROENDOCRINE TUMOURS OF THE PANCREAS

The islets of Langerhans (p. 1101) have the capacity to synthesize more than one hormone. They also synthesize ectopic hormones that are not usually found in the pancreas such as gastrin, adrenocorticotrophin, vasoactive intestinal peptide and growth hormone. Whilst many pancreatic endocrine tumours are multihormonal, one peptide tends to predominate and is responsible for the clinical syndrome. Other tumours, whilst containing peptide hormone, are functionally inactive.

These tumours are rare with an incidence of less than 1 in 100 000 of the population. Insulinomas are the commonest variant and account for approximately 50% of cases, gastrinomas account for 20% and the rarer functioning tumours 5%. The remaining 25% are non-functioning tumours. Approximately 25% of islet cell tumours are associated with a multiple endocrine syndrome (type I) (see p. 1099). The majority of the endocrine pancreatic tumours are malignant in their behaviour.

The presentation of pancreatic neuroendocrine tumours is most commonly related to the actions of ectopic hormone secretion. Chromogranin A is a secretory protein present in 80% of neuroendocrine tumours and has been used as a tumour marker, although the specificity is poor. Identification of the primary and possibly metastatic lesions may be difficult despite multiple-imaging techniques. Endoscopic ultrasound may be the most sensitive means of detecting small tumours. Many of these tumours have somatostatin receptors, and radiolabelled somatostatin analogues (such as octreotide) scanning provide a means of tumour localization.

Treatment options for pancreatic neuroendocrine tumours requires a multidisciplinary approach and is dependent upon the presence or absence of metastatic (usually hepatic) disease. Surgical resection of the pancreatic lesion is the only potential curative approach. Aggressive surgical intervention including a resection of the primary lesion as well as liver resection for metastasis has been used in selected cases. Somatostatin analogues such as octreotide and lanreotide have been used specifically for the control of symptoms secondary to the hormonal secretion.

There is some evidence that the somatostatin analogues combined with alpha-interferon also control tumour proliferation. The chemotherapeutic agents streptozotocin, 5-fluorouracil and doxorubicin produce partial remission in approximately 40% of cases. In patients with extensive liver metastasis, occlusion of the arterial blood flow by hepatic arterial embolization may control hormone-related symptoms. In most cases the tumours are slowly progressive and may allow a reasonable quality of life for many years.

Clinical syndromes

Insulinoma is described on page 1133.

A *gastrinoma* accounts for approximately 1 : 1000 cases of duodenal ulcer disease. This results from hypersecretion of gastric acid secondary to ectopic gastrin secretion within the endocrine pancreas (*Zollinger–Ellison*). Recurrent severe duodenal ulceration occurs with only a partial response to acid suppression. The diagnosis is confirmed by an elevated gastrin level. High-dose proton pump inhibitors are used to suppress symptoms.

A *VIPoma* is an endocrine pancreatic tumour producing vasoactive intestinal polypeptide (VIP). This causes a severe secretory diarrhoea secondary to the stimulation of adenyl cyclase within the enterocyte (*Verner–Morrison syndrome*). The clinical syndrome is one of profuse watery diarrhoea, hypokalaemia and a metabolic acidosis. To produce the syndrome, the tumours are usually in excess of 3 cm in diameter. The clinical syndrome can be controlled by either glucocorticoids, long-acting octreotide or lanreotide.

Glucagonomas are rare alpha-cell tumours which are responsible for the syndrome of migratory necrolytic dermatitis, weight loss, diabetes mellitus, deep vein thrombosis, anaemia and hypoalbuminaemia. The diagnosis is made by measuring pancreatic glucagon in the serum. Metastases are common at presentation but if the tumour is localized, pancreatic resection may be curative.

Somatostatinomas are rare malignant D cell tumours of the pancreas and 30% occur in the duodenum and small bowel. These tumours cause diabetes mellitus, gallstones and diarrhoea/steatorrhoea. They can be diagnosed by high serum somatostatin levels, CT/MR scans or octreotide scintiscans. Treatment is by resection, where possible, and octreotide therapy.

Non-functioning neuroendocrine tumours usually present by the local mass effect with pain, weight loss and the occasional bile duct obstruction. At the time of presentation the tumours are frequently large with distant metastases. Curative resection is possible in only a small proportion. Palliative surgery may be indicated to alleviate mass-related symptoms.

FURTHER READING

Brand R (2001) The diagnosis of pancreatic cancer. *Cancer Journal* **7**(4): 287–297.

Etemad B, Whitcomb DC (2001) Chronic pancreatitis: diagnosis, classification, and new genetic developments. *Gastroenterology* **120**: 682–707.

Lowenfels AB, Lankisch PG, Maisonneuve P (2000) What is the risk of biliary pancreatitis in patients with gallstones? *Gastroenterology* **119**(3): 879.

Sharma VK, Howden CW (1999) Metaanalysis of randomized controlled trials of endoscopic retrograde cholangiography and endoscopic sphincterotomy for the treatment of acute biliary pancreatitis. *American Journal of Gastroenterology* **94**: 3211–3214.

Tamm E, Charnsangavej C (2001) Pancreatic cancer: current concepts in imaging for diagnosis and staging. *Cancer Journal* **7**(4): 298–311.

UK Working Party on Acute Pancreatitis (2005) Guidelines for the management of acute pancreatitis. *Gut* **54**: Suppl. iii.

SIGNIFICANT WEBSITES

http://www.gastrohep.com
Resources for gastroenterology, hepatology and endoscopy

http://www.micro.msb.le.ac.uk/335/Hepatitis.html
Viral hepatitis

http://www.emedicine.com/emerg/topic98.htm
Cholecystitis, cholelithiasis

Haematological disease

8

INTRODUCTION AND GENERAL ASPECTS

Blood consists of

- red cells
- white cells
- platelets
- plasma, in which the above elements are suspended.

Plasma is the liquid component of blood, which contains soluble fibrinogen. Serum is what remains after the formation of the fibrin clot.

The formation of blood cells (haemopoiesis)

The haemopoietic system includes the bone marrow, liver, spleen, lymph nodes and thymus. The turnover of cells is enormous; red cells survive 120 days, platelets around 7 days but granulocytes only 7 hours. The production of as many as 10^{13} new myeloid cells (all blood cells except for lymphocytes) per day in the normal healthy state obviously requires to be tightly regulated according to the needs of the body.

Blood islands are formed in the yolk sac in the third week of gestation and produce primitive blood cells which migrate to the liver and spleen. These organs are the chief sites of haemopoiesis from 6 weeks to 7 months, when the bone marrow becomes the main source of blood cells. The bone marrow is the only source of blood cells during normal childhood and adult life.

At birth, haemopoiesis is present in the marrow of nearly every bone. As the child grows the active red marrow is gradually replaced by fat (yellow marrow) so that haemopoiesis in the adult becomes confined to the central skeleton and the proximal ends (trabecular area) of the long bones. Only if the demand for blood cells increases and persists do the areas of red marrow extend. Pathological processes interfering with normal haemopoiesis may result in resumption of haemopoietic activity in the liver and spleen, which is referred to as *extramedullary haemopoiesis*.

All blood cells are derived from pluripotent stem cells. These stem cells are supported by stromal cells (see below) which also influence haemopoiesis. The stem cell has two properties – the first is *self-renewal*, i.e. the production of more stem cells, and the second is its proliferation and differentiation into progenitor cells, committed to one specific cell line.

There are two major ancestral cell lines derived from the pluripotential stem cell: lymphocytic and myeloid (non-lymphocytic) cells (Fig. 8.1). The former gives rise to T and B cells. The myeloid stem cell gives rise to the progenitor CFU-GEMM (colony-forming unit, granulocyte–erythrocyte–monocyte–megakaryocyte). The progenitor cells such as CFU-GEMM cannot be recognized in bone marrow biopsies but are recognized by their ability to form colonies when haemopoietic cells are immobilized in a soft gel matrix. The CFU-GEMM can go on to form CFU-GM, CFU-Eo, and CFU-Meg, each of which can produce a particular cell type (for example, neutrophils, eosinophils and platelets) under appropriate growth conditions. Haemopoiesis is under the control of

growth factors and inhibitors, and the microenvironment of the bone marrow also plays a role in its regulation.

Haemopoietic growth factors

Haemopoietic growth factors are glycoproteins which regulate the differentiation and proliferation of haemopoietic progenitor cells and the function of mature blood cells. They act on receptors expressed on haemopoietic cells at various stages of development to maintain the haemopoietic progenitor cells and to stimulate increased production of one or more cell lines in response to stresses such as blood loss and infection (Fig. 8.1).

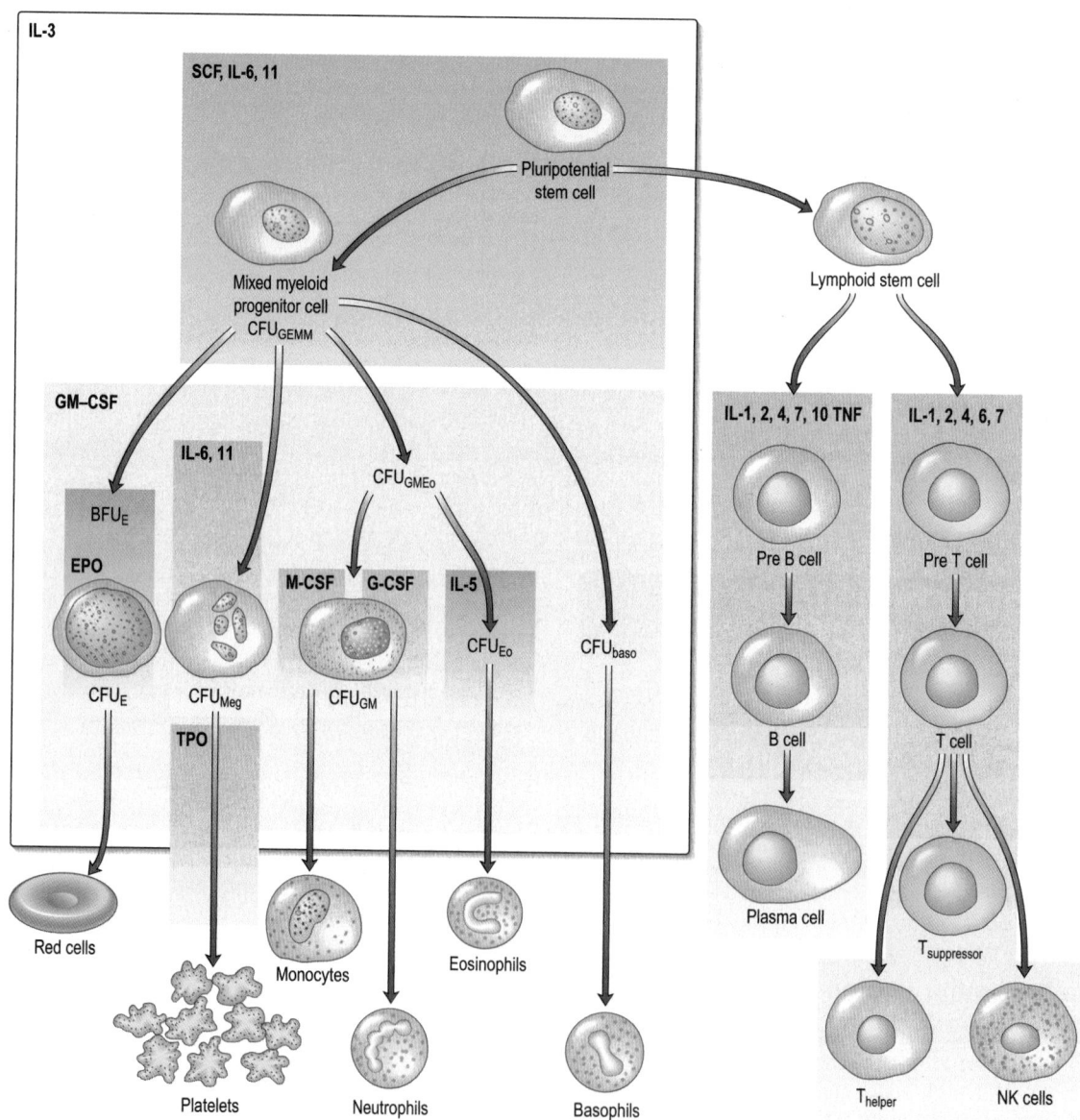

Fig. 8.1 **Role of growth factors in normal haemopoiesis.** Some of the multiple growth factors acting on stem cells and early progenitor cells are shown. BFU, burst-forming unit; CFU, colony-forming unit; CSF, colony-stimulating factor; E, erythroid; Eo, eosinophil; EPO, erythropoietin; G, granulocyte; GEMM, mixed granulocyte, erythroid, monocyte, megakaryocyte; GM, granulocyte, monocyte; IL, interleukin; M, monocyte; Meg, megakaryocyte; SCF, stem cell (Steel) factor or C-kit ligand; TNF, tumour necrosis factor; TPO, thrombopoietin.

The pluripotential stem cells are under the influence of a number of haemopoietic growth factors including interleukin-3 (IL-3), IL-6, -7, -11, β-catenin and stem cell factor (SCF, Steel factor or C-kit ligand). Colony-stimulating factors (CSFs, the prefix indicating the cell type, see Fig. 8.1), as well as interleukins and erythropoietin (EPO) regulate the lineage committed progenitor cells. Thrombopoietin (TPO, which, like erythropoietin, is produced in the kidneys and the liver) along with IL-6 and IL-11 control platelet production. In addition to these factors stimulating haemopoiesis, other factors inhibit the process and include tumour necrosis factor (TNF) and transforming growth factor-β (TGF-β). Many of the growth factors are produced by activated T cells, monocytes and bone marrow stromal cells such as fibroblasts, endothelial cells and macrophages; these cells are also involved in inflammatory responses.

Many growth factors have been produced by recombinant DNA techniques and are being used clinically. Examples include G-CSF, which is used to accelerate haemopoietic recovery after chemotherapy and haemopoietic cell transplantation, and erythropoietin, which is used to treat anaemia in patients with chronic renal failure. Thrombopoietin is undergoing clinical trials in patients with idiopathic thrombocytopenic purpura.

Peripheral blood

Automated cell counters are used to measure the level of haemoglobin (Hb) and the number and size of red cells, white cells and platelets (Table 8.1). Other indices can be derived from these values. The mean corpuscular volume (MCV) of red cells is the most useful of the indices and is used to classify anaemia (see p. 425).

The white cell count (WCC, or WBC, white blood count) gives the total number of circulating leucocytes, and many automated cell counters produce differential counts as well.

Normally, less than 2% of the red cells are reticulocytes (p. 422). The reticulocyte count gives a guide to the erythroid activity in the bone marrow. An increased count is seen with increased marrow maturity, e.g. following haemorrhage or haemolysis, and during the response to treatment with a specific haematinic. A low count in the presence of anaemia indicates an inappropriate response by the bone marrow and may be seen in bone marrow failure (from whatever cause) or where there is a deficiency of a haematinic.

A carefully evaluated blood film is still an essential adjunct to the above, as definitive abnormalities of cells can be seen.

Erythrocyte sedimentation rate (ESR)
This is the rate of fall of red cells in a column of blood and is a measure of the acute-phase response. The pathological process may be immunological, infective, ischaemic, malignant or traumatic. A raised ESR reflects an increase in the plasma concentration of large proteins, such as fibrinogen and immunoglobulins. These proteins cause rouleaux formation, when cells clump together like a stack of coins, and therefore fall more rapidly. The ESR increases with age, and is higher in females than in males. It is low in polycythaemia vera, owing to the high red cell concentration, and increased in patients with severe anaemia.

Plasma viscosity
Plasma viscosity measurement is used instead of the ESR in many laboratories. As with the ESR, the level is dependent on the concentration of large molecules such as fibrinogen and immunoglobulins. There is no difference between levels found in males and females, and viscosity increases only slightly in the elderly. It is not affected by the level of Hb and the result may be obtained within 15 minutes.

C-reactive protein
C-reactive protein is a pentraxin, one of the proteins produced in the acute-phase response (see Table 4.4). It is synthesized exclusively in the liver and rises within 6 hours of an acute event. It rises with fever (possibly triggered by IL-1, IL-6 and TNF-α and other cytokines) and in inflammatory conditions and after trauma. It follows the clinical state of the patient much more rapidly than does the ESR and is unaffected by the level of Hb, but it is less helpful than the ESR or plasma viscosity in monitoring chronic inflammatory diseases. Its measurement is easy and quick to perform using an immunoassay that can be automated. High-sensitivity assays have shown that increased levels predict future cardiovascular disease (p. 802).

Table 8.1 Normal values for peripheral blood		
	Male	**Female**
Hb (g/dL)	13.5–17.5	11.5–16
PCV (haematocrit; L/L)	0.4–0.54	0.37–0.47
RCC (10^{12}/L)	4.5–6.0	3.9–5.0
MCV (fL)		80–96
MCH (pg)		27–32
MCHC (g/dL)		32–36
WBC (10^9/L)		4.0–11.0
Platelets (10^9/L)		150–400
ESR (mm/h)		< 20
Reticulocytes		0.5–2.5% (50–100 × 10^9/L)

ESR, erythrocyte sedimentation rate; Hb, haemoglobin; MCH, mean corpuscular haemoglobin; MCHC, mean corpuscular haemoglobin concentration; MCV, mean corpuscular volume of red cells; PCV, packed cell volume; RCC, red cell count; WBC, white blood count.

THE RED CELL

Erythropoiesis

Red cell precursors pass through several stages in the bone marrow. The earliest morphologically recognizable cells are pronormoblasts. Smaller normoblasts result from cell divisions, and precursors at each stage progressively contain less RNA and more Hb in the cytoplasm. The nucleus becomes more condensed and is eventually lost from the late normoblast in the bone marrow, when the cell becomes a reticulocyte.

Reticulocytes contain residual ribosomal RNA and are still able to synthesize Hb. They remain in the marrow for about 1–2 days and are released into the circulation, where they lose their RNA and become mature red cells (erythrocytes) after another 1–2 days. Mature red cells are non-nucleated biconcave discs.

Nucleated red cells (*normoblasts*) are not normally present in peripheral blood, but are present if there is extramedullary haemopoiesis and in some marrow disorders (see leucoeryothroblastic anaemia, p. 464).

About 10% of erythroblasts die in the bone marrow even during normal erythropoiesis. Such ineffective erythropoiesis is substantially increased in some anaemias such as thalassaemia major and megaloblastic anaemia.

Erythropoietin is a hormone which controls erythropoiesis. The gene for erythropoietin is on chromosome 7 and codes for a heavily glycosylated polypeptide of 165 amino acids. Erythropoietin has a molecular weight of 30 400 and is produced in the peritubular cells in the kidneys (90%) and in the liver (10%). Its production is regulated mainly by tissue oxygen tension. Production is increased if there is hypoxia from whatever cause – for example, anaemia or cardiac or pulmonary disease. The erythropoietin gene is one of a number of genes that is regulated by the hypoxic sensor pathway. The 3'-flanking region of the erythropoietin gene has a hypoxic response element which is necessary for the induction of transcription of the gene in hypoxic cells. Hypoxia-inducible factor 1 (HIF-1) is a transcription factor which binds to the hypoxia response element and acts as a master regulator of several genes that are responsive to hypoxia. Erythropoietin stimulates an increase in the proportion of bone marrow precursor cells committed to erythropoiesis, and CFU-E are stimulated to proliferate and differentiate. Increased 'inappropriate' production of erythropoietin is also seen in patients with renal disease and neoplasms in other sites which result in polycythaemia (see Table 8.16).

Haemoglobin synthesis

Haemoglobin performs the main functions of red cells – carrying O_2 to the tissues and returning CO_2 from the tissues to the lungs. Each normal adult Hb molecule (Hb A) has a molecular weight of 68 000 and consists of two α and two β globin polypeptide chains ($\alpha_2\beta_2$) which have 141 and 146 amino acids respectively. HbA comprises about 97% of the Hb in adults. Two other types, Hb A_2 ($\alpha_2\delta_2$) and Hb F ($\alpha_2\gamma_2$), are found in adults in small amounts (1.5–3.2% and < 1%, respectively) (p. 440).

Haemoglobin synthesis occurs in the mitochondria of the developing red cell (Fig. 8.2). The major rate-limiting step is the conversion of glycine and succinic acid to δ-aminolaevulinic acid (ALA) by ALA synthase (also see Fig. 19.22). Vitamin B_6 is a coenzyme for this reaction, which is inhibited by haem and stimulated by erythro-

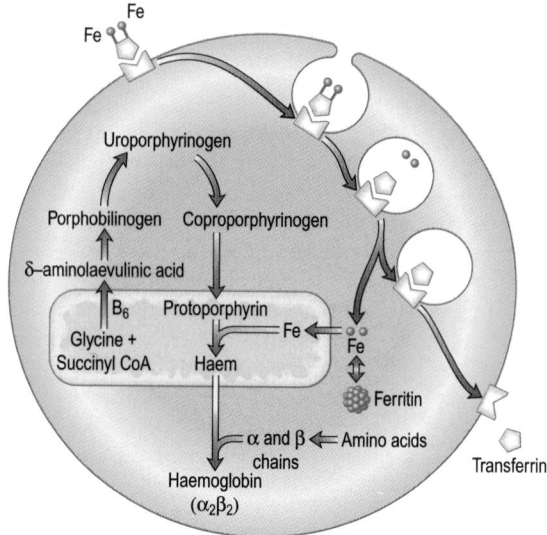

Fig. 8.2 Haemoglobin synthesis. Transferrin attaches to a surface receptor on developing red cells. Iron is released and transported to the mitochondria, where it combines with protoporphyrin to form haem. Protoporphyrin itself is manufactured from glycine and succinyl-CoA. Haem combines with α and β chains (formed on ribosomes) to make haemoglobin.

poietin. Two molecules of δ-ALA condense to form a pyrrole ring (porphobilinogen). These rings are then grouped in fours to produce protoporphyrins. Finally, iron is inserted to form haem. Haem is then inserted into the globin chains to form Hb. The structure of Hb is shown in Figure 8.3.

Fig. 8.3 Model of the haemoglobin molecule showing α (pink) and β (blue) chains. 2,3-BPG (bisphosphoglycerate) binds in the centre of the molecule and stabilizes the deoxygenated form by cross-linking the β chains (also see Fig. 8.4). M, methyl; P, propionic acid; V, vinyl.

Haemoglobin function

The biconcave shape of red cells provides a large surface area for the uptake and release of oxygen and carbon dioxide. Haemoglobin becomes saturated with oxygen in the pulmonary capillaries where the partial pressure of oxygen is high and Hb has a high affinity for oxygen. Oxygen is released in the tissues where the partial pressure of oxygen is low and Hb has a low affinity for oxygen.

In adult haemoglobin (Hb A), a haem group is bound to each of the four globin chains; the haem group has a porphyrin ring with a ferrous atom which can reversibly bind one oxygen molecule. The haemoglobin molecule exists in two conformations, R and T. The T (taut) conformation of deoxyhaemoglobin is characterized by the globin units being held tightly together by electrostatic bonds (Fig. 8.4). These bonds are broken when oxygen binds to haemoglobin, resulting in the R (relaxed) conformation in which the remaining oxygen-binding sites are more exposed and have a much higher affinity for oxygen than in the T conformation. The binding of one oxygen molecule to deoxyhaemoglobin increases the oxygen affinity of the remaining binding sites – this property is known as 'cooperativity' and is the reason for the sigmoid shape of the oxygen dissociation curve. Haemoglobin is, therefore, an example of an allosteric protein. The binding of oxygen can be influenced by secondary effectors – hydrogen ions, carbon dioxide and red-cell 2,3-bisphosphoglycerate (2,3-BPG, formerly called 2,3-diphosphoglycerate (2,3-DPG)). Hydrogen ions and carbon dioxide added to blood cause a reduction in the oxygen-binding affinity of haemoglobin (the Bohr effect) (Fig. 15.5). Oxygenation of haemoglobin reduces its affinity for carbon dioxide (the Haldane effect). These effects help the exchange of carbon dioxide and oxygen in the tissues.

Red cell metabolism produces 2,3-BPG from glycolysis. 2,3-BPG accumulates because it is sequestered by binding to deoxyhaemoglobin. The binding of 2,3-BPG stabilizes the T conformation and reduces its affinity for oxygen. The P_{50} is the partial pressure of oxygen at which the haemoglobin is 50% saturated with oxygen. P_{50} increases with 2,3-BPG concentrations (right-hand shift in Fig. 15.5), which increase when oxygen availability is reduced in conditions such as hypoxia or anaemia. P_{50} also rises with increasing body temperature, which may be beneficial during prolonged exercise. Haemoglobin regulates oxygen transport as shown in the oxyhaemoglobin dissociation curve. When the primary limitation to oxygen transport is in the periphery, e.g. heavy exercise, anaemia, the P_{50} is increased to enhance oxygen unloading. When the primary limitation is in the lungs, e.g. lung disease, high altitude exposure, the P_{50} is reduced to enhance oxygen loading.

A summary of normal red cell production and destruction is given in Figure 8.5.

FURTHER READING
Pepys MB, Berger A (2001) The renaissance of C reactive protein. *British Medical Journal* **322**: 4–5.

Prychal JT (2003) Delivery on demand – a new era of gene therapy. *New England Journal of Medicine* **348**: 1282–1283.

Rosenthal N (2003) Prometheus's vulture and the stem-cell promise. *New England Journal of Medicine* **349**: 267–274.

Weatherall D, Provan D (2000) Red cells I: inherited anaemias. *Lancet* **355**: 1169–1175.

ANAEMIA

Anaemia is present when there is a decrease in the level of haemoglobin in the blood below the reference level for the age and sex of the individual (Table 8.1). Alterations in the level of Hb may occur as a result of changes in the plasma volume, as shown in Figure 8.6. A reduction in the plasma volume will lead to a spuriously high Hb – this is seen with dehydration and in the clinical condition of apparent polycythaemia (see p. 455). A raised plasma volume produces a spurious anaemia, even when combined with a small increase in red cell volume as occurs in pregnancy. After a major bleed, anaemia may not be apparent for several days until the plasma volume returns to normal.

The various types of anaemia, classified in terms of the red cell indices, particularly the MCV, are shown in Figure 8.7, p. 425. There are three major types:

- hypochromic microcytic with a low MCV
- normochromic normocytic with a normal MCV
- macrocytic with a high MCV.

Clinical features

Patients with anaemia may be asymptomatic. A slowly falling level of Hb allows for haemodynamic compen-

***Fig. 8.4* Oxygenated and deoxygenated haemoglobin molecule.** The haemoglobin molecule is predominantly stabilized by α–β chain bonds rather than α–α and β–β chain bonds. The structure of the molecule changes during O_2 uptake and release. When O_2 is released, the β chains rotate on the $\alpha_1\beta_2$ and $\alpha_2\beta_1$ contacts, allowing the entry of 2,3-BPG which causes a lower affinity of haemoglobin for O_2 and improved delivery of O_2 to the tissues. From Hoffbrand AV, Pettit JE (1993) *Essential Haematology*, 3rd edn. Oxford: Blackwell Scientific Publications, with permission.

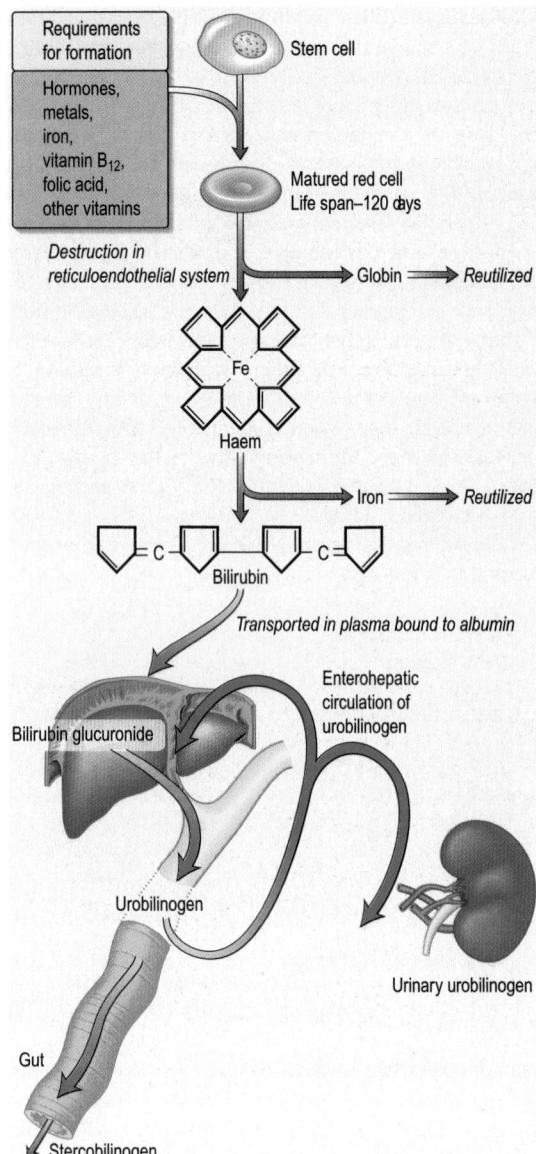

Fig. 8.5 **Red cell production and breakdown** (see p. 350).

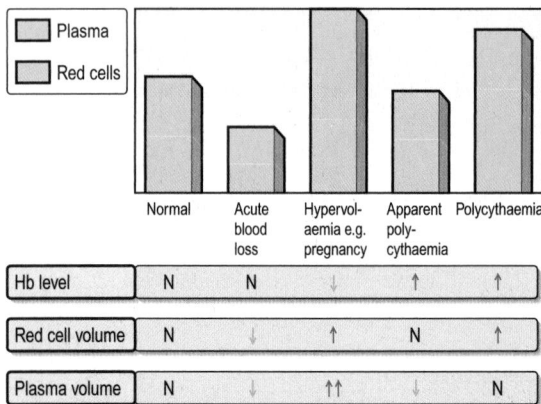

Fig. 8.6 **Alterations of haemoglobin in relation to plasma.**

sation and enhancement of the oxygen-carrying capacity of the blood. A rise in 2,3-BPG causes a shift of the oxygen dissociation curve to the right, so that oxygen is more readily given up to the tissues. Where blood loss is rapid, more severe symptoms will occur, particularly in elderly people.

Symptoms (all non-specific)
- Fatigue
- Headaches
- Faintness

(The above three symptoms are all very common in the general population.)

- Breathlessness
- Angina
- Intermittent claudication
- Palpitations.

Signs
- Pallor
- Tachycardia
- Systolic flow murmur
- Cardiac failure
- Rarely papilloedema and retinal haemorrhages after an acute bleed (can be accompanied by blindness).

Specific signs of the different types of anaemia will be discussed in the appropriate sections. Examples include:

- koilonychia – spoon-shaped nails seen in iron deficiency anaemia
- jaundice – found in haemolytic anaemia
- bone deformities – found in thalassaemia major
- leg ulcers – occur in association with sickle cell disease.

It must be emphasized that anaemia is not a diagnosis, and a cause must be found.

Investigations

Peripheral blood
A low haemoglobin should always be considered in relation to:

- the white blood cell (WBC) count
- the platelet count
- the reticulocyte count (as this indicates marrow activity)
- the blood film, as abnormal red cell morphology (see Fig. 8.8) may indicate the diagnosis.

Where two populations of red cells are seen, the blood film is said to be dimorphic. This may, for example, be seen in patients with 'double deficiencies' (e.g. combined iron and folate deficiency in coeliac disease, or following treatment of anaemic patients with the appropriate haematinic).

Bone marrow
Examination of the bone marrow is performed to further investigate abnormalities found in the peripheral blood

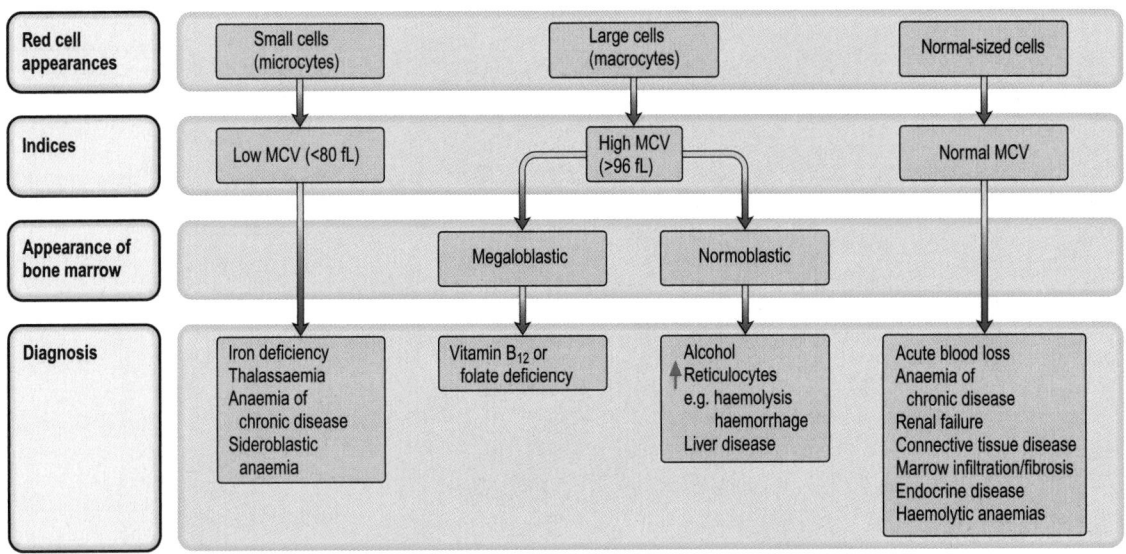

Red cell appearances	Small cells (microcytes)		Large cells (macrocytes)		Normal-sized cells
Indices	Low MCV (<80 fL)		High MCV (>96 fL)		Normal MCV
Appearance of bone marrow			Megaloblastic	Normoblastic	
Diagnosis	Iron deficiency Thalassaemia Anaemia of chronic disease Sideroblastic anaemia	Vitamin B$_{12}$ or folate deficiency		Alcohol ↑Reticulocytes e.g. haemolysis haemorrhage Liver disease	Acute blood loss Anaemia of chronic disease Renal failure Connective tissue disease Marrow infiltration/fibrosis Endocrine disease Haemolytic anaemias

Fig. 8.7 Classification of anaemia. MCV, mean corpuscular volume.

(Practical box 8.1). Aspiration provides a film which can be examined by microscopy for the morphology of the developing haemopoietic cells. The trephine provides a core of bone which is processed as a histological specimen and allows an overall view of the bone marrow architecture, cellularity and presence/absence of abnormal infiltrates.

The following are assessed:

- cellularity of the marrow
- type of erythropoiesis (e.g. normoblastic or megaloblastic)
- cellularity of the various cell lines
- infiltration of the marrow
- iron stores.

Special tests may be performed: cytogenetic, immunological, cytochemical markers, biochemical analyses (e.g. deoxyuridine suppression test), microbiological culture.

MICROCYTIC ANAEMIA

Iron deficiency is the most common cause of anaemia in the world, affecting 30% of the world's population equivalent to 500 million people. This is because of the body's limited ability to absorb iron and the frequent loss of iron owing to haemorrhage. Although iron is abundant, most is in the insoluble ferric (Fe^{3+}) form, which has poor bioavailability. Ferrous (Fe^{2+}) is more readily absorbed. Free iron is toxic, and it is bound to various proteins for transport and storage.

The other causes of a microcytic hypochromic anaemia are anaemia of chronic disease, sideroblastic anaemia, and thalassaemia. In thalassaemia (p. 440) there is a defect in globin synthesis, in contrast to the other three causes of

Practical Box 8.1
Techniques for obtaining bone marrow

The technique should be explained to the patient and consent obtained

Aspiration
Site – usually iliac crest
Give local anaesthetic injection
Use special bone marrow needle (e.g. Salah)
Aspirate marrow
Make smear with glass slide
Stain with:
    Romanowsky technique
    Perls' reaction (acid ferrocyanide) for iron.

Trephine
Indications include:
    'Dry tap' obtained with aspiration
    Better assessment of cellularity, e.g. aplastic anaemia
    Better assessment of presence of infiltration or
        fibrosis.

Technique
Site – usually posterior iliac crest
Give local anaesthetic injection
Use special needle (e.g. Jamshidi – longer and wider
    than for aspiration)
Obtain core of bone
Fix in formalin; decalcify – this takes a few days
Stain with:
    Haematoxylin and eosin
    Reticulin stain.

microcytic anaemia where the defect is in the synthesis of haem.

Iron

Dietary intake
The average daily diet in the UK contains 15–20 mg of

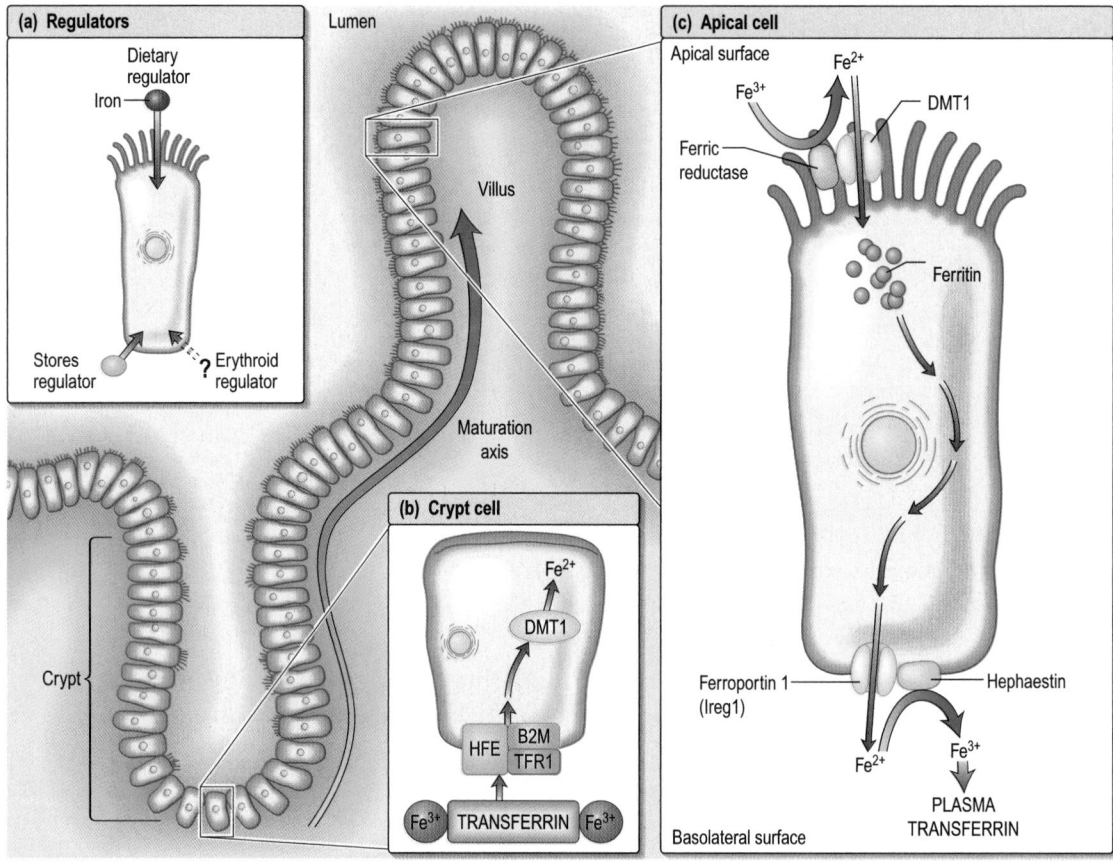

Fig. 8.8 **(a) Regulation of the absorption of intestinal iron.** The iron-absorbing cells of the duodenal epithelium originate in the intestinal crypts and migrate toward the tip of the villus as they differentiate (maturation axis). Absorption of intestinal iron is regulated by at least three independent mechanisms. First, iron absorption is influenced by recent dietary iron intake (dietary regulator). After a large dietary bolus, absorptive cells are resistant to iron uptake for several days. Second, iron absorption can be modulated considerably in response to body iron stores (stores regulator). Third, a signal communicates the state of bone marrow erythropoiesis to the intestine (erythroid regulator). **(b) Duodenal crypt cells** sense body iron status through the binding of transferrin to the HFE/B2 microglobulin/TFR1 complex. Cytosolic enzymes change the oxidative state of iron from ferric (Fe^{3+}) to ferrous (Fe^{2+}). A decrease in crypt cell iron concentration upregulates the divalent metal transporter (DMT1). This increases as crypt cells migrate up the villus and become mature absorptive cells. **(c) Apical cell.** Dietary iron is reduced from the ferrous to the ferric state by the brush border ferrireductase. DMT1 facilitates iron absorption from the intestinal lumen. The export proteins, e.g. ferroportin 1 (Ireg1) and hephaestin, transfer iron from the enterocyte into the circulation. HFE, hereditary haemochromatosis gene; B2M, β_2-microglobulin.

iron, although normally only 10% of this is absorbed. Absorption may be increased to 20–30% in iron deficiency and pregnancy.

Non-haem iron is mainly derived from cereals, which are commonly fortified with iron; it forms the main part of dietary iron. Haem iron is derived from haemoglobin and myoglobin in red or organ meats. Haem iron is better absorbed than non-haem iron, whose availability is more affected by other dietary constituents.

Absorption (Fig. 8.8(a),(b))

Factors influencing iron absorption are shown in Table 8.2. Haem iron is partly broken down to non-haem iron, but some haem iron is absorbed intact into mucosal cells.

Iron absorption occurs primarily in the duodenum. Non-haem iron is dissolved in the low pH of the stomach and reduced from the ferric to the ferrous form by a brush border ferrireductase. Cells in duodenal crypts are able to sense the body's iron requirements and retain this information as they mature into cells capable of absorbing iron at the tips of the villi. A protein, divalent metal transporter 1 (DMT1), (formerly called divalent cation transporter [DCT1] or natural resistance-associated macrophage protein [NRAMP2]) transports iron (and other metals) across the apical (luminal) surface of the mucosal cells in the small intestine. Haem iron is absorbed in a separate less-well-characterized process.

Once inside the mucosal cell, iron may be transferred across the cell to reach the plasma, or be stored as ferritin; the body's iron status at the time the absorptive cell developed from the crypt cell is probably the crucial deciding factor. Iron stored as ferritin will be lost into the gut lumen when the mucosal cells are shed; this regulates iron balance. The mechanism of transport of iron across

Haem iron is absorbed better than non-haem iron

Ferrous iron is absorbed better than ferric iron

Gastric acidity helps to keep iron in the ferrous state and soluble in the upper gut

Formation of insoluble complexes with phytate or phosphate decreases iron absorption

Iron absorption is increased with low iron stores and increased erythropoietic activity, e.g. bleeding, haemolysis, high altitude

There is a decreased absorption in iron overload, except in hereditary haemochromatosis, where it is increased

the basolateral surface of mucosal cells involves a transporter protein, ferroportin 1 (Ireg1). This transporter protein requires an accessory, multicopper protein, hephaestin (see Fig. 8.9c).

The iron content of the body is kept within narrow limits and its loss and intake are normally finely balanced. Its absorption is closely related to the total iron stores of the body; in iron deficiency, absorption of iron may increase to 3–4 mg daily. The body is unable to excrete iron once it has been absorbed so the regulation of iron absorption is critical. Iron absorption is regulated in several ways (see Fig. 8.9) by dietary, stores and erythroid regulators. The liver peptide hepcidin may be the store and/or erythroid regulator. The hereditary haemochromatosis gene (*HFE*) plays a role in iron absorption, although the mechanism is not fully understood. It is not the prime regulator since iron absorption also responds to the stores of iron and erythroid regulators when *HFE* is either mutated or absent.

Anaemias with increased rates of erythropoiesis do not cause equal increases in iron absorption; for example, conditions with 'ineffective erythropoiesis' such as thalassaemia stimulate greater iron absorption than haemolytic anaemias such as hereditary spherocytosis and autoimmune haemolytic anaemia where red cell destruction occurs in the periphery.

Transport in the blood

The normal serum iron level is about 13–32 µmol/L; there is a diurnal rhythm with higher levels in the morning. Iron is transported in the plasma bound to transferrin, a β-globulin that is synthesized in the liver. Each transferrin molecule binds two atoms of ferric iron and is normally one-third saturated. Most of the iron bound to transferrin comes from macrophages in the reticuloendothelial system and not from iron absorbed by the intestine. Transferrin-bound iron becomes attached by specific receptors to erythroblasts and reticulocytes in the marrow and the iron is removed (see Fig. 8.2).

In an average adult male, 20 mg of iron, chiefly obtained from red cell breakdown in the macrophages of the reticuloendothelial system, is incorporated into Hb every day.

Iron stores

About two-thirds of the total body iron is in the circulation as haemoglobin (2.5–3 g in a normal adult man).

Iron is stored in reticuloendothelial cells, hepatocytes and skeletal muscle cells (500–1500 mg). About two-thirds of this is stored as ferritin and one-third as haemosiderin in normal individuals. Small amounts of iron are also found in plasma (about 4 mg bound to transferrin), with some in myoglobin and enzymes.

Ferritin is a water-soluble complex of iron and protein. It is more easily mobilized than haemosiderin for Hb formation. It is present in small amounts in plasma.

Haemosiderin is an insoluble iron–protein complex found in macrophages in the bone marrow, liver and spleen. Unlike ferritin, it is visible by light microscopy in tissue sections and bone marrow films after staining by Perls' reaction.

Requirements

Each day 0.5–1.0 mg of iron is lost in the faeces, urine and sweat. Menstruating women lose 30–40 mL of blood per month, an average of about 0.5–0.7 mg of iron per day. Blood loss through menstruation in excess of 100 mL will usually result in iron deficiency as increased iron absorption from the gut cannot compensate for such losses of iron. The demand for iron also increases during growth (about 0.6 mg per day) and pregnancy (1–2 mg per day). In the normal adult the iron content of the body remains relatively fixed. Increases in the body iron content (haemochromatosis) are classified into:

- hereditary haemochromatosis (p. 386), where a mutation in the *HFE* gene causes upregulation of DMT1 and increased iron absorption
- secondary haemochromatosis (transfusion siderosis; see p. 441). This is due to iron overload in conditions where repeated transfusion is the only therapy.

Iron deficiency

Iron deficiency anaemia develops when there is inadequate iron for haemoglobin synthesis. A normal level of Hb is maintained for as long as possible after the iron stores are depleted; latent iron deficiency is said to be present during this period.

Causes

- Blood loss
- Increased demands such as growth and pregnancy
- Decreased absorption (e.g. postgastrectomy)
- Poor intake.

Most iron deficiency is due to blood loss, usually from the uterus or gastrointestinal tract. Premenopausal women are in a state of precarious iron balance owing to menstruation. Iron deficiency affects more than a quarter of the world's population, but isolated nutritional iron deficiency is rare in developed countries. The most common cause of iron deficiency world-wide is blood loss from the gastrointestinal tract resulting from hookworm infestation. The poor quality of the diet, predominantly containing vegetables, also contributes to the high prevalence of iron deficiency in developing countries. Even in developed countries, iron deficiency is not uncommon in infancy where iron intake is insufficient for the demands of growth. It is more prevalent in infants born prematurely or where the introduction of mixed feeding is delayed.

Clinical features

The symptoms of anaemia are described on page 424. Other clinical features occur as a result of tissue iron deficiency. These are mainly epithelial changes induced by the effect of inadequate iron in the cells:

- brittle nails
- spoon-shaped nails (koilonychia)
- atrophy of the papillae of the tongue
- angular stomatitis
- brittle hair
- a syndrome of dysphagia and glossitis (Plummer–Vinson or Paterson–Brown–Kelly syndrome; see p. 279).

The diagnosis of iron deficiency anaemia relies on a good clinical history with questions about dietary intake, regular self-medication with non-steroidal anti-inflammatory drugs (which may give rise to gastrointestinal bleeding), and the presence of blood in the faeces (which may be a sign of haemorrhoids or carcinoma of the lower bowel). In women, a careful enquiry about the duration of periods, the occurrence of clots and the number of sanitary towels or tampons (normal 3–5/day) used should be made.

Investigations

Blood count and film

A characteristic blood film is shown in Figure 8.9. The red cells are microcytic (MCV < 80 fL) and hypochromic (MCH < 27 pg). There is poikilocytosis (variation in shape) and anisocytosis (variation in size). Target cells are seen.

Serum iron and iron-binding capacity

The serum iron falls and the total iron-binding capacity (TIBC) rises in iron deficiency compared with normal. Iron deficiency is regularly present when the transferrin saturation (i.e. serum iron divided by TIBC) falls below 19% (Table 8.3).

Fig. 8.9 Hypochromic microcytic cells (arrow) on a blood film. Poikilocytosis and anisocytosis are seen.

Serum ferritin

The level of serum ferritin reflects the amount of stored iron. The normal values for serum ferritin are 30–300 µg/L (11.6–144 nmol/L) in males and 15–200 µg/L (5.8–96 nmol/L) in females. In simple iron deficiency, a low serum ferritin confirms the diagnosis. However, ferritin is an acute-phase reactant, and levels increase in the presence of inflammatory or malignant diseases. In these cases, measurement of serum iron/TIBC, serum ferritin and soluble transferrin receptors is used.

Serum soluble transferrin receptors

The number of transferrin receptors increases in iron deficiency. The results of this immunoassay compares well with results from bone marrow aspiration at estimating iron stores.

This assay can help to distinguish between iron deficiency and anaemia of chronic disease (see Table 8.3), and may avoid the need for bone marrow examination even in complex cases.

Bone marrow

Erythroid hyperplasia with ragged normoblasts is seen in the marrow in iron deficiency. Staining using Perls' reaction (acid ferrocyanide) does not show the characteristic Prussian-blue granules of stainable iron in the bone marrow fragments or in the erythroblasts.

Examination of the bone marrow is not essential for the diagnosis of iron deficiency but it may be helpful in

Table 8.3 Microcytic anaemia: the differential diagnosis

	Iron deficiency	Anaemia of chronic disease	Thalassaemia trait (α or β)	Sideroblastic anaemia
MCV	Reduced	Low normal or normal	Very low for degree of anaemia	Low in inherited type but often raised in acquired type
Serum iron	Reduced	Reduced	Normal	Raised
Serum TIBC	Raised	Reduced	Normal	Normal
Serum ferritin	Reduced	Normal or raised	Normal	Raised
Serum soluble transfer receptors	Increased	Normal	Normal or raised	Normal or raised
Iron in marrow	Absent	Present	Present	Present
Iron in erythroblasts	Absent	Absent or reduced	Present	Ring forms

TIBC, total iron binding capacity

the investigation of complicated cases of anaemia, e.g. to determine if iron deficiency is present in a patient with anaemia of chronic disease.

Other investigations

These will be indicated by the clinical history and examination. Investigations of the gastrointestinal tract are often required to determine the cause of the iron deficiency (see p. 293).

Differential diagnosis

The presence of anaemia with microcytosis and hypochromia does not necessarily indicate iron deficiency. The most common other causes are thalassaemia, sideroblastic anaemia and anaemia of chronic disease, and in these disorders the iron stores are normal or increased. The differential diagnosis of microcytic anaemia is shown in Table 8.3.

Treatment

Iron deficiency is not a diagnosis per se. The correct management of iron deficiency is to find and treat the underlying cause, and to give iron to correct the anaemia and replace iron stores. The response to iron therapy can be monitored using the reticulocyte count and Hb level, with an expected rise in haemoglobin of 1 g/dL per week.

Oral iron is all that is required in most cases. The best preparation is ferrous sulphate (200 mg three times daily, a total of 180 mg ferrous iron) which is absorbed best when the patient is fasting. If the patient has side-effects such as nausea, diarrhoea or constipation, taking the tablets with food or reducing the dose using a preparation with less iron such as ferrous gluconate (300 mg twice daily, only 70 mg ferrous iron) is all that is usually required to reduce the symptoms. The use of expensive iron compounds, particularly the slow-release ones which release iron beyond its main sites of absorption, is unnecessary.

In developing countries, distribution of iron tablets is the main approach for the alleviation of iron deficiency. However, iron supplementation programmes have been ineffective, probably mainly because of poor compliance.

Oral iron should be given for long enough to correct the Hb level and to replenish the iron stores. This can take 6 months. The commonest causes of failure of response to oral iron are:

- lack of compliance
- continuing haemorrhage
- incorrect diagnosis, e.g. thalassaemia trait.

These possibilities should be considered before parenteral iron is used. However, parenteral iron is required by occasional patients, including those who have general intolerance of oral preparations even at low dose, those with severe malabsorption, and those who have chronic gastrointestinal diseases such as ulcerative colitis or Crohn's disease. Iron stores are replaced much faster with parenteral iron than with oral iron, but the haematological response is no quicker. Parenteral iron can be given as repeated deep intramuscular injections of iron–sorbitol (1.5 mg of iron per kg bodyweight) or by slow intravenous infusion of iron–sucrose.

Anaemia of chronic disease

One of the most common types of anaemia, particularly in hospital patients, is the anaemia of chronic disease, occurring in patients with chronic infections such as infective endocarditis or tuberculosis and osteomyelitis in developing countries. Other causes include chronic inflammatory diseases such as Crohn's disease, rheumatoid arthritis, systemic lupus erythematosus (SLE), polymyalgia rheumatica, and malignant disease. There is decreased release of iron from the bone marrow to developing erythroblasts, an inadequate erythropoietin response to the anaemia, and decreased red cell survival. The exact mechanisms responsible for these effects are not clear, but they seem to be mediated by inflammatory cytokines such as IL-1, tumour necrosis factor and interferons.

The serum iron and the TIBC are low, and the serum ferritin is normal or raised because of the inflammatory process. The serum soluble transferrin receptor level is normal (Table 8.3). Stainable iron is present in the bone marrow, but iron is not seen in the developing erythroblasts. Patients do not respond to iron therapy, and treatment is, in general, that of the underlying disorder. Recombinant erythropoietin therapy is used in the anaemia of renal disease (p. 673), inflammatory disease (rheumatoid arthritis, inflammatory bowel disease) and is being trialled in, for example, myelodyplasia).

Sideroblastic anaemia

Sideroblastic anaemias are inherited or acquired disorders characterized by a refractory anaemia, a variable number of hypochromic cells in the peripheral blood, and excess iron and ring sideroblasts in the bone marrow. The presence of ring sideroblasts is the diagnostic feature of sideroblastic anaemia. There is accumulation of iron in the mitochondria of erythroblasts owing to disordered haem synthesis forming a ring of iron granules around the nucleus that can be seen with Perls' reaction. The blood film is often dimorphic; ineffective haem synthesis is responsible for the microcytic hypochromic cells. Sideroblastic anaemias are classified as shown in Table 8.4. A structural defect in δ-aminolaevulinic acid (ALA) synthase, the pyridoxine-dependent enzyme responsible for the first step in haem synthesis (see Fig. 8.2), has been identified in one form of inherited sideroblastic anaemia. Primary acquired sideroblastic anaemia is one of the myelodysplastic syndromes (see p. 455). Lead toxicity is described on p. 1014.

Treatment

Some patients respond when drugs or alcohol are withdrawn, if these are the causative agents. In occasional cases, there is a response to pyridoxine. Treatment with folic acid may be required to treat accompanying folate deficiency.

Table 8.4 Classification of sideroblastic anaemia

Inherited
X-linked disease – transmitted by females

Acquired
Myelodysplasia
Myeloproliferative disorders
Myeloid leukaemia
Drugs, e.g. isoniazid
Alcohol abuse
Lead toxicity
Other disorders, e.g. rheumatoid arthritis, carcinoma, megaloblastic and haemolytic anaemias

FURTHER READING
Bomford A (2002) Genetics of haemochromatosis. *Lancet* **360**: 1673–1681.
Fleming RE, Bacon BR (2005) Orchestration of iron homeostasis. *New England Journal of Medicine* **352**: 1741–1744.
Provan D, Weatherall D (2000) Red cells II: acquired anaemias. *Lancet* **355**: 1260–1268.
Spivak JL (2000) The blood in systemic disorders. *Lancet* **355**: 1707–1712.

NORMOCYTIC ANAEMIA

Normocytic, normochromic anaemia is seen in anaemia of chronic disease, in some endocrine disorders (e.g. hypopituitarism, hypothyroidism and hypoadrenalism) and in some haematological disorders (e.g. aplastic anaemia and some haemolytic anaemias) (see Fig. 8.7). In addition, this type of anaemia is seen acutely following blood loss.

MACROCYTIC ANAEMIAS

These can be divided into megaloblastic and non-megaloblastic types, depending on bone marrow findings.

MEGALOBLASTIC ANAEMIA

Megaloblastic anaemia is characterized by the presence in the bone marrow of erythroblasts with delayed nuclear maturation because of defective DNA synthesis (megaloblasts). Megaloblasts are large and have large immature nuclei. The nuclear chromatin is more finely dispersed than normal and has an open stippled appearance (Fig. 8.10). A characteristic abnormality of white cells, giant metamyelocytes, is frequently seen in megaloblastic anaemia. These cells are about twice the size of normal cells and often have twisted nuclei. Megaloblastic changes occur in:

- vitamin B_{12} deficiency or abnormal vitamin B_{12} metabolism
- folic acid deficiency or abnormal folate metabolism

Fig. 8.10 Megaloblasts (arrowed) in the bone marrow.

- other defects of DNA synthesis, such as congenital enzyme deficiencies in DNA synthesis (e.g. orotic aciduria), or resulting from therapy with drugs interfering with DNA synthesis (e.g. hydroxycarbamide (hydroxyurea), azathioprine, zidovudine – AZT)
- myelodysplasia due to dyserythropoiesis.

Haematological values
Anaemia may be present. The MCV is characteristically > 96 fL unless there is a coexisting cause of microcytosis when there may be a dimorphic picture with a normal/low average MCV. The peripheral blood film shows macrocytes with hypersegmented polymorphs with six or more lobes in the nucleus (see Fig. 8.11). If severe, there may be leucopenia and thrombocytopenia.

Biochemical basis of megaloblastic anaemia
The key biochemical problem common to both vitamin B_{12} and folate deficiency is a block in DNA synthesis owing to an inability to methylate deoxyuridine monophosphate to deoxythymidine monophosphate, which is then used to build DNA (Fig. 8.12). The methyl group is supplied by the folate coenzyme, methylene tetrahydrofolate.

Deficiency of folate reduces the supply of this coenzyme; deficiency of vitamin B_{12} also reduces its supply by slowing the demethylation of methyltetrahydrofolate (methyl THF) and preventing cells receiving tetrahydrofolate for synthesis of methylene tetrahydrofolate polyglutamate.

Other congenital and acquired forms of megaloblastic anaemia are due to interference with purine or pyrimidine synthesis causing an inhibition in DNA synthesis.

Deoxyuridine suppression test
This is a useful method for rapidly determining the nature and severity of the vitamin B_{12} or folate deficiency in severe or complex cases of megaloblastic anaemia.

Fig. 8.11 Macrocytes and a hypersegmented neutrophil (arrowed) on a peripheral blood film.

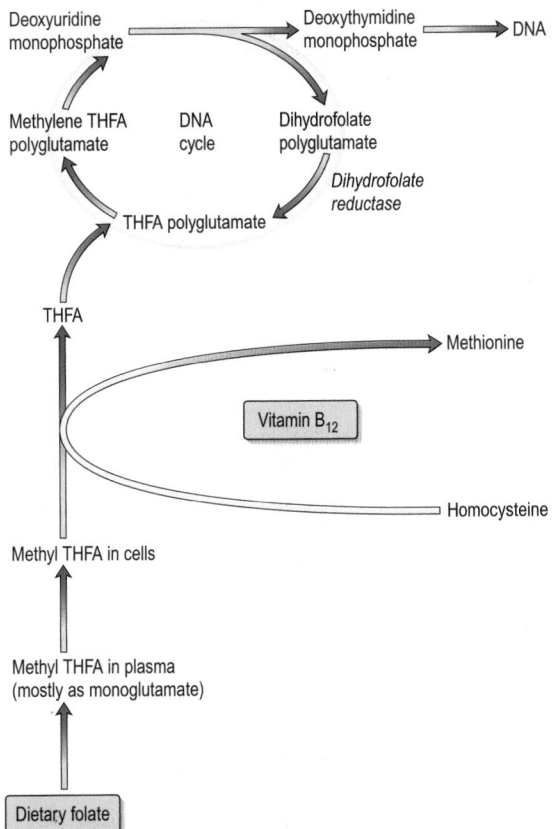

Fig. 8.12 Biochemical basis of megaloblastic anaemia.
The metabolic relationship between vitamin B$_{12}$ and folate and
their role in DNA synthesis. THF, tetrahydrofolate.

Tritiated thymidine is added to the patient's bone
marrow in vitro. In a normoblastic marrow, the thymidine
requirement is supplied by the methylation of deoxyuridine and this 'suppresses' the requirement for preformed
tritiated thymidine to less than 5%. In a megaloblastic
marrow, however, much more tritiated thymidine is used
(5–50%). If the addition of B$_{12}$ corrects the abnormality, it
suggests that B$_{12}$ is the cause of the deficiency. The
addition of folate corrects the abnormality in both
vitamin B$_{12}$ and folate deficiency.

Vitamin B$_{12}$

Vitamin B$_{12}$ is synthesized by certain microorganisms,
and humans are ultimately dependent on animal sources.
It is found in meat, fish, eggs and milk, but not in plants.
Vitamin B$_{12}$ is not usually destroyed by cooking. The
average daily diet contains 5–30 μg of vitamin B$_{12}$, of
which 2–3 μg is absorbed. The average adult stores some
2–3 mg, mainly in the liver, and it may take 2 years or
more after absorptive failure before B$_{12}$ deficiency
develops, as the daily losses are small (1–2 μg).

Structure and function

Cobalamins consist of a planar group with a central
cobalt atom (corrin ring) and a nucleotide set at right-

Fig. 8.13 Methylcobalamin structure. This is the main
form of vitamin B$_{12}$ in the plasma.

angles (Fig. 8.13). Vitamin B$_{12}$ was first crystallized as
cyanocobalamin, but the main natural cobalamins have
deoxyadenosyl-, methyl- and hydroxocobalamin groups
attached to the cobalt atom.

The main function of B$_{12}$ is the methylation of homocysteine to methionine with the demethylation of methyl
THF polyglutamate to THF. THF is a substrate for folate
polyglutamate synthesis.

Deoxyadenosylcobalamin is a coenzyme for the conversion of methylmalonyl CoA to succinyl CoA. Measurement of methylmalonic acid in urine was used as a test for
vitamin B$_{12}$ deficiency but it is no longer carried out
routinely.

Absorption and transport

Vitamin B$_{12}$ is liberated from protein complexes in
food by gastric enzymes and then binds to a vitamin
B$_{12}$-binding protein ('R' binder) related to plasma
transcobalamin I (TC I), derived from saliva. Vitamin B$_{12}$
bound to 'R' binder is released by pancreatic enzymes
and becomes bound to intrinsic factor.

Intrinsic factor is a glycoprotein with a molecular
weight of 45 000. It is secreted by gastric parietal cells
along with H$^+$ ions. It combines with vitamin B$_{12}$ and
carries it to specific receptors on the surface of the mucosa
of the ileum. Vitamin B$_{12}$ enters the ileal cells and intrinsic
factor remains in the lumen. Vitamin B$_{12}$ is transported
from the enterocytes to the bone marrow and other
tissues by the glycoprotein *transcobalamin II* (TC II).
Although TC II is the essential carrier protein for vitamin
B$_{12}$, the amount of B$_{12}$ on TC II is low; it has a rapid
clearance and is able to deliver cobalamin to all cells of
the body. Vitamin B$_{12}$ in plasma is mainly bound to TC I
(70–90%), but the functional role of this protein is
unknown. About 1% of an oral dose of B$_{12}$ is absorbed

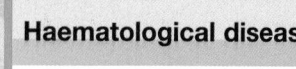

Table 8.5 Vitamin B_{12} deficiency and abnormal B_{12} utilization: further causes (see text)

Low dietary intake	Abnormal utilization
Vegans	Congenital transcobalamin II deficiency
	Nitrous oxide (inactivates B_{12})
Impaired absorption	
Stomach	
Pernicious anaemia	
Gastrectomy	
Congenital deficiency of intrinsic factor	
Small bowel	
Ileal disease or resection	
Bacterial overgrowth	
Tropical sprue	
Fish tapeworm (*Diphyllobothrium latum*)	

'passively' without the need for intrinsic factor, mainly through the duodenum and ileum.

Vitamin B_{12} deficiency

There are a number of causes of B_{12} deficiency and abnormal B_{12} metabolism (Table 8.5). The most common cause of vitamin B_{12} deficiency in adults is pernicious anaemia. Malabsorption of vitamin B_{12} because of pancreatitis, coeliac disease or treatment with metformin is mild and does not usually result in significant vitamin B_{12} deficiency.

Pernicious anaemia

Pernicious anaemia (PA) is an autoimmune disorder in which there is atrophic gastritis with loss of parietal cells in the gastric mucosa with consequent failure of intrinsic factor production and vitamin B_{12} malabsorption.

Pathogenesis of pernicious anaemia

This disease is common in the elderly, with 1 in 8000 of the population aged over 60 years being affected in the UK. It can be seen in all races, but occurs more frequently in fair-haired and blue-eyed individuals, and those who have the blood group A. It is more common in females than males.

There is an association with other autoimmune diseases, particularly thyroid disease, Addison's disease and vitiligo. Approximately one-half of all patients with PA have thyroid antibodies. There is a higher incidence of gastric carcinoma with PA than in the general population; the incidence in PA is 1–3%.

Parietal cell antibodies are present in the serum in 90% of patients with PA – and also in many older patients with gastric atrophy. Conversely, intrinsic factor antibodies, although found in only 50% of patients with PA, are specific for this diagnosis. Two types of intrinsic factor antibodies are found: a blocking antibody, which inhibits binding of intrinsic factor to B_{12}, and a precipitating antibody, which inhibits the binding of the B_{12}–intrinsic factor complex to its receptor site in the ileum.

B_{12} deficiency may rarely occur in children from a congenital deficiency or abnormality of intrinsic factor, or as a result of early onset of the adult autoimmune type.

Pathology

Autoimmune gastritis (see p. 287) affecting the fundus is present with plasma cell and lymphoid infiltration. The parietal and chief cells are replaced by mucin-secreting cells. There is achlorhydria and absent secretion of intrinsic factor. The histological abnormality can be improved by corticosteroid therapy, which supports an autoimmune basis for the disease.

Clinical features

The onset of PA is insidious, with progressively increasing symptoms of anaemia. Patients are sometimes said to have a lemon-yellow colour owing to a combination of pallor and mild jaundice caused by excess breakdown of haemoglobin. A red sore tongue (glossitis) and angular stomatitis are sometimes present.

The neurological changes, if left untreated for a long time, can be irreversible. These neurological abnormalities occur only with very low levels of serum B_{12} (less than 60 ng/L) and occasionally occur in patients who are not clinically anaemic. The classical neurological features are those of a polyneuropathy progressively involving the peripheral nerves and the posterior and eventually the lateral columns of the spinal cord (subacute combined degeneration; p. 1263). Patients present with symmetrical paraesthesiae in the fingers and toes, early loss of vibration sense and proprioception, and progressive weakness and ataxia. Paraplegia may result. Dementia, psychiatric problems, e.g. depression, hallucinations, delusions, and optic atrophy also occur from vitamin B_{12} deficiency.

Investigations

- **Haematological findings** show the features of a megaloblastic anaemia as described on page 430.
- **Bone marrow** shows the typical features of megaloblastic erythropoiesis (Fig. 8.10), although it is frequently not performed in cases of straightforward macrocytic anaemia and a low serum vitamin B_{12}.
- **Serum bilirubin** may be raised as a result of ineffective erythropoiesis. Normally a minor fraction of serum bilirubin results from premature breakdown of newly formed red cells in the bone marrow. In many megaloblastic anaemias, where the destruction of developing red cells is much increased, the serum bilirubin can be increased.
- **Serum vitamin B_{12}** is usually well below 160 ng/L, which is the lower end of the normal range. Serum vitamin B_{12} can be assayed using radioisotope dilution or immunological assays.
- **Serum folate level** is normal or high, and the red cell folate is normal or reduced owing to inhibition of normal folate synthesis.

Absorption tests

Vitamin B_{12} absorption tests are performed only occasionally when the underlying cause of the B_{12} deficiency is not obvious. They cannot be performed in the UK as radioactive B_{12} is not available. However, the principle of the absorption test is useful.

Schilling test. Radioactive B_{12} is given orally followed by an i.m. injection of non-radioactive B_{12} to saturate B_{12} binding proteins and to flush out $^{58}Co\text{-}B_{12}$. The urine is collected for 24 hours and > 10% of the oral dose would be excreted in a normal person. If this is abnormal, the test is repeated with the addition of oral intrinsic factor capsules. If the excretion is now normal, the diagnosis is pernicious anaemia or gastrectomy. If the excretion is still abnormal, the lesion must be in the terminal ileum or there may be bacterial overgrowth. The latter could be confirmed by repeating the test after a course of antibiotics.

Gastrointestinal investigations

In PA there is achlorhydria. Intubation studies can be performed to confirm this but are rarely carried out in routine practice. Endoscopy or barium meal examination of the stomach is performed only if gastric symptoms are present.

Differential diagnosis

Vitamin B_{12} deficiency must be differentiated from other causes of megaloblastic anaemia, principally folate deficiency, but usually this is quite clear from the blood level of these two vitamins.

Pernicious anaemia should be distinguished from other causes of vitamin B_{12} deficiency (see Table 8.5). Any disease involving the terminal ileum or bacterial overgrowth in the small bowel can produce vitamin B_{12} deficiency (see p. 304). Gastrectomy can lead, in the long term, to vitamin B_{12} deficiency. Vegans are strict vegetarians and eat no meat or animal products. A careful dietary history should be obtained.

Treatment

See page 434.

Folic acid

Folic acid monoglutamate is not itself present in nature but occurs as polyglutamates (extra glutamic acid residues).

Folates are present in food as polyglutamates in the reduced dihydrofolate or tetrahydrofolate (THF) forms (Fig. 8.14), with methyl (CH_3), formyl (CHO) or methylene (CH_2) groups attached to the pteridine part of the molecule. Polyglutamates are broken down to monoglutamates in the upper gastrointestinal tract, and during the absorptive process these are converted to methyl THF monoglutamate, which is the main form in the serum. The methylation of homocysteine to methionine requires both methylcobalamin and methyl THF as coenzymes. This reaction is the first step in which methyl THF entering cells from the plasma is converted into folate polyglutamates. Intracellular polyglutamates are the active forms of folate and act as coenzymes in the transfer

Fig. 8.14 Folic acid structure. This is formed from three building blocks as shown. Tetrahydrofolate has additional hydrogen atoms at positions 5, 6, 7 and 8.

of single carbon units in amino acid metabolism and DNA synthesis (see Fig. 8.12).

Dietary intake

Folate is found in green vegetables such as spinach and broccoli, and offal, such as liver and kidney. Cooking causes a loss of 60–90% of the folate. The minimal daily requirement is about 100 μg.

Folate deficiency

The causes of folate deficiency are shown in Table 8.6. The main cause is poor intake, which may occur alone or in combination with excessive utilization or malabsorption. The body's reserves of folate, unlike vitamin B_{12}, are low (about 10 mg). On a deficient diet, folate deficiency develops over the course of about 4 months, but folate deficiency may develop rapidly in patients who have both a poor intake and excess utilization of folate (e.g. patients in intensive care units).

There is no simple relationship between maternal folate status and fetal abnormalities but folic acid supplements at the time of conception and in the first

Table 8.6 Causes of folate deficiency	
Nutritional (major cause)	**Excess utilization**
Poor intake	*Physiological*
Old age	Pregnancy
Poor social conditions	Lactation
Starvation	Prematurity
Alcohol excess (also causes impaired utilization)	*Pathological*
	Haematological disease with excess red cell production, e.g. haemolysis
Poor intake due to anorexia	Malignant disease with increased cell turnover
Gastrointestinal disease, e.g. partial gastrectomy, coeliac disease, Crohn's disease	Inflammatory disease
	Metabolic disease, e.g. homocystinuria
Cancer	Haemodialysis or peritoneal dialysis
Antifolate drugs	
Anticonvulsants:	*Malabsorption*
phenytoin	Occurs in small bowel
primidone	disease, but the effect is
Methotrexate	minor compared with that
Pyrimethamine	of anorexia
Trimethoprim	

12 weeks of pregnancy reduce the incidence of neural tube defects. A high incidence of a partial deficiency in a key enzyme in folate metabolism, methyl THF reductase, has been found in parents of fetuses with neural tube defects. The 5% of individuals with this abnormality have increased levels of homocysteine (Fig. 8.12), which may be the mechanism underlying the increased incidence of neural tube defects. Autoantibodies to the folate receptor have also been found in some women with a pregnancy complicated by a neural tube defect.

Clinical features

Patients with folate deficiency may be asymptomatic or present with symptoms of anaemia or of the underlying cause. Glossitis can occur. Unlike with B_{12} deficiency, neuropathy does not occur.

Investigations

The haematological findings are those of a megaloblastic anaemia as discussed on page 430.

Blood measurements

Serum and red cell folate are assayed by radioisotope dilution or immunological methods. Normal levels of serum folate are 4–18 μg/L (5–63 nmol/L). The amount of folate in the red cells is a better measure of tissue folate; the normal range is 160–640 μg/mL.

Further investigations

In many cases of folate deficiency the cause is not obvious from the clinical picture or dietary history. Occult gastro-intestinal disease should then be suspected and appropriate investigations, such as small bowel biopsy, should be performed (p. 300).

Treatment and prevention of megaloblastic anaemia

Treatment depends on the type of deficiency. Blood transfusion is not indicated in chronic anaemia; indeed, it is dangerous to transfuse elderly patients, as heart failure may be precipitated. Folic acid may produce a haematological response in vitamin B_{12} deficiency but may aggravate the neuropathy. Large doses of folic acid alone should not be used to treat megaloblastic anaemia unless the serum vitamin B_{12} level is known to be normal. In severely ill patients, it may be necessary to treat with both folic acid and vitamin B_{12} while awaiting serum levels.

Treatment of vitamin B_{12} deficiency

Hydroxocobalamin 1000 μg can be given intramuscularly to a total of 5–6 mg over the course of 3 weeks; 1000 μg is then necessary every 3 months for the rest of the patient's life. Alternatively, it is now recommended that oral B_{12} 2 mg per day is given, as 1–2% of an oral dose is absorbed by diffusion and therefore does not require intrinsic factor.

Compliance with an oral daily regimen may be a problem, particularly in elderly patients. The use of sublingual nuggets of B_{12} (2 × 1000 μg daily) has been suggested to be an effective and more convenient option.

Clinical improvement may occur within 48 hours and a reticulocytosis can be seen some 2–3 days after starting therapy, peaking at 5–7 days. Improvement of the poly-neuropathy may occur over 6–12 months, but long-standing spinal cord damage is irreversible. Hypokalaemia can occur and, if severe, supplements should be given. Iron deficiency often develops in the first few weeks of therapy. Hyperuricaemia also occurs but clinical gout is uncommon. In patients who have had a total gastrectomy or an ileal resection, vitamin B_{12} should be monitored; if low levels occur, prophylactic vitamin B_{12} should be given.

Treatment of folate deficiency

Folate deficiency can be corrected by giving 5 mg of folic acid daily; the same haematological response occurs as seen after treatment of vitamin B_{12} deficiency. Treatment should be given for about 4 months to replace body stores. Any underlying cause, e.g. coeliac disease, should be treated.

Prophylactic folic acid (400 μg daily) is recommended for all women planning a pregnancy. Many authorities also recommend prophylactic administration of folate throughout pregnancy. Whether this can be achieved by increased consumption of foods with a high folate content or whether women should take folate supplements is under debate. The US Food and Drugs Administration has introduced a requirement for the fortification with folic acid of grain products such as bread, flour and rice (p. 247).

Women who have had a child with a neural tube defect should take 5 mg folic acid daily before and during a subsequent pregnancy.

Prophylactic folic acid is also given in chronic haematological disorders where there is rapid cell turnover. A dose of 5 mg each week is probably sufficient.

MACROCYTOSIS WITHOUT MEGALOBLASTIC CHANGES

A raised MCV with macrocytosis on the peripheral blood film can occur with a normoblastic rather than a megaloblastic bone marrow.

A common *physiological* cause of macrocytosis is pregnancy. Macrocytosis may also occur in the newborn.

Common *pathological* causes are:

- alcohol excess
- liver disease
- reticulocytosis
- hypothyroidism
- some haematological disorders (e.g. aplastic anaemia, sideroblastic anaemia, pure red cell aplasia)
- drugs (e.g. cytotoxics – azathioprine)
- spurious (agglutinated red cells measured on red cell counters)
- cold agglutinins due to autoagglutination of red cells (see p. 449) (the MCV decreases to normal with warming of the sample to 37°C).

In all these conditions, normal serum levels of vitamin B_{12} and folate will be found. The exact mechanisms in each case are uncertain, but in some there is increased lipid deposition in the red cell membrane.

An increased number of reticulocytes leads to a raised MCV because they are large cells.

Alcohol is a frequent cause of a raised MCV in an otherwise normal individual. A megaloblastic anaemia can also occur in people who abuse alcohol; this is due to a toxic effect of alcohol on erythropoiesis or to dietary folate deficiency.

FURTHER READING

Chanarin I, Metz J (1997) Diagnosis of cobalamin deficiency: the old and the new. *British Journal of Haematology* **97**: 695–700.

Kuzminski AM et al. (1998) Effective treatment of cobalamin deficiency with oral cobalamin. Blood **92**: 1191–1198.

Mills JL (2000) Fortification of foods with folic acid. *New England Journal of Medicine* **342**: 1442–1445.

Toh BH, van Driel IR, Gleeson PA (1997) Pernicious anaemia. *New England Journal of Medicine* **337**: 1441–1448.

Wharton B, Booth I (2001) Fortification of flour with folic acid. *British Medical Journal* **323**: 1198–1199.

ANAEMIA DUE TO MARROW FAILURE (APLASTIC ANAEMIA)

Aplastic anaemia is defined as pancytopenia with hypocellularity (aplasia) of the bone marrow; there are no leukaemic, cancerous or other abnormal cells in the peripheral blood or bone marrow. It is an uncommon but serious condition that may be inherited but is more commonly acquired.

Aplastic anaemia is due to a reduction in the number of pluripotential stem cells (see Fig. 8.1) together with a fault in those remaining or an immune reaction against them so that they are unable to repopulate the bone marrow. Failure of only one cell line may also occur, resulting in isolated deficiencies such as the absence of red cell precursors in pure red cell aplasia. Evolution to myelodysplasia, paroxysmal nocturnal haemoglobinuria (PNH) or acute myeloblastic leukaemia occurs in some cases, probably owing to the emergence of an abnormal clone of haemopoietic cells.

Causes

A list of causes of aplasia is given in Table 8.7. Immune mechanisms are probably responsible for most cases of idiopathic acquired aplastic anaemia and play a part in at least the persistence of many secondary cases. Activated cytotoxic T cells in blood and bone marrow are responsible for the bone marrow failure.

Many drugs may cause marrow aplasia, including cytotoxic drugs such as busulfan and doxorubicin, which are expected to cause transient aplasia as a consequence

Table 8.7 Causes of aplastic anaemia

Primary
Congenital, e.g. Fanconi's anaemia
Idiopathic acquired (67% of cases)

Secondary
Chemicals, e.g. benzene
Drugs:
  chemotherapeutic
  idiosyncratic reactions
Insecticides
Ionizing radiation
Infections:
  viral, e.g. hepatitis, EBV, HIV, parvovirus
  other, e.g. tuberculosis
Paroxysmal nocturnal haemoglobinuria
Miscellaneous, e.g. pregnancy

of their therapeutic use. However, some individuals develop aplasia due to sensitivity to non-cytotoxic drugs such as chloramphenicol, gold, carbimazole, chlorpromazine, phenytoin, tolbutamide, non-steroidal anti-inflammatory agents, and many others which have been reported to cause occasional cases of aplasia.

Congenital aplastic anaemias are rare. Gene mutations are being identified, e.g. the telomerase RNA component, and have also been seen in one third of aplastic anaemias. Fanconi's anaemia is inherited as an autosomal recessive and is associated with skeletal, renal and central nervous system abnormalities. It usually presents between the ages of 5 and 10 years.

Clinical features

The clinical manifestations of marrow failure from any cause are anaemia, bleeding and infection. Bleeding is often the predominant initial presentation of aplastic anaemia with bruising with minimal trauma or blood blisters in the mouth. Physical findings include ecchymoses, bleeding gums and epistaxis. Mouth infections are common. Lymphadenopathy and hepatosplenomegaly are rare in aplastic anaemia.

Investigations

- pancytopenia
- the virtual absence of reticulocytes
- a hypocellular or aplastic bone marrow with increased fat spaces (Fig. 8.15).

Differential diagnosis

This is from other causes of pancytopenia (Table 8.8). A bone marrow trephine is essential for assessment of the bone marrow cellularity.

Treatment and prognosis

The treatment of aplastic anaemia depends on providing supportive care while awaiting bone marrow recovery and specific treatment to accelerate marrow recovery.

The main danger is infection and stringent measures should be undertaken to avoid this (see also p. 495). Any suspicion of infection in a severely neutropenic patient

Fig. 8.15 Bone marrow trephine biopsies in low-power view. **(a)** Normal cellularity. **(b)** Hypocellularity in aplastic anaemia.

Table 8.8   Causes of pancytopenia

Aplastic anaemia (see Table 8.7)
Drugs
Megaloblastic anaemia
Bone marrow infiltration or replacement
   Hodgkin's and non-Hodgkin's lymphoma
   Acute leukaemia
   Myeloma
   Secondary carcinoma
   Myelofibrosis
Hypersplenism
Systemic lupus erythematosus
Disseminated tuberculosis
Paroxysmal nocturnal haemoglobinuria
Overwhelming sepsis

---

should lead to immediate institution of broad-spectrum parenteral antibiotics. Supportive care including transfusions of red cells and platelets should be given as necessary. The cause of the aplastic anaemia must be eliminated if possible.

The course of aplastic anaemia can be variable, ranging from a rapid spontaneous remission to a persistent increasingly severe pancytopenia, which may lead to death through haemorrhage or infection. The most reliable determinants for the prognosis are the number of neutrophils, reticulocytes, platelets, and the cellularity of the bone marrow.

A bad prognosis (i.e. severe aplastic anaemia) is associated with the presence of two of the following three features:

- neutrophil count of $< 0.5 \times 10^9/L$
- platelet count of $< 20 \times 10^9/L$
- reticulocyte count of $< 40 \times 10^9/L$.

In severe aplastic anaemia, there is a very poor outcome without treatment. Bone marrow transplantation is the treatment of choice for patients under 40 years of age who have an HLA-identical sibling donor, which gives a 75–90% chance of long-term survival and restoring the blood count to normal. Patients over the age of 40 are not eligible for bone marrow transplantation whether an HLA-identical donor is available or not, because of the high risk of graft-versus-host disease as a complication of bone marrow transplantation. Immunosuppressive therapy is used for patients without HLA-matched siblings and those over the age of 40 years; antilymphocyte globulin (ALG) and ciclosporin in combination give a response rate of 60–80%.

For the patients under the age of 40 who fail to respond to immunosuppression, bone marrow transplantation using unrelated donors is an option, but the results are poor (5-year survival of only 30%) owing to a high incidence of graft rejection, graft-versus-host disease and viral infections.

Levels of haemopoietic growth factors (Fig. 8.1) are normal or increased in most patients with aplastic anaemia, and are ineffective as primary treatment.

Androgens (e.g. oxymethalone) are sometimes useful in patients not responding to immunosuppression and in patients with moderately severe aplastic anaemia.

Steroids have little activity in severe aplastic anaemia but are used for serum sickness due to ALG. They are also used to treat children with congenital pure red cell aplasia (Diamond–Blackfan syndrome). Adult pure red cell aplasia is associated with a thymoma in 30% of cases and thymectomy may induce a remission. It may also be associated with autoimmune disease or may be idiopathic. Steroids and ciclosporin are effective treatment in some cases.

FURTHER READING
British Committee for Standards in Haematology (2003) Guidelines for the diagnosis and management of acquired aplastic anaemia. *British Journal of Haematology* **123**: 782–801.
Brodsky RA, Jones RJ (2005) Aplastic anaemia. *Lancet* **365**: 1647–1656.
Young NS (2002) Acquired aplastic anaemia. *Annals of Internal Medicine* **136**: 534–546.

HAEMOLYTIC ANAEMIAS: AN INTRODUCTION

Haemolytic anaemias are caused by increased destruction of red cells. The red cell normally survives about 120 days, but in haemolytic anaemias the red cell survival times are considerably shortened.

Breakdown of normal red cells occurs in the macrophages of the bone marrow, liver and spleen (see Fig. 8.5).

Consequences of haemolysis

Shortening of red cell survival does not always cause anaemia as there is a compensatory increase in red cell production by the bone marrow. If the red cell loss can be contained within the marrow's capacity for increased output, then a haemolytic state can exist without anaemia (*compensated haemolytic disease*). The bone marrow can increase its output by six to eight times by increasing the proportion of cells committed to erythropoiesis (*erythroid hyperplasia*) and by expanding the volume of active marrow. In addition, immature red cells (*reticulocytes*) are released prematurely. These cells are larger than mature cells and stain light blue on a peripheral blood film (the description of this appearance on the blood film is *polychromasia*). Reticulocytes may be counted accurately as a percentage of all red cells on a blood film using a supra-vital stain for residual RNA (e.g. new methylene blue).

Sites of haemolysis

Extravascular haemolysis

In most haemolytic conditions red cell destruction is extravascular. The red cells are removed from the circulation by macrophages in the reticuloendothelial system, particularly the spleen.

Intravascular haemolysis

When red cells are rapidly destroyed within the circulation, haemoglobin is liberated (Fig. 8.16). This is initially bound to plasma haptoglobins but these soon become saturated.

Excess free plasma Hb is filtered by the renal glomerulus and enters the urine, although small amounts are reabsorbed by the renal tubules. In the renal tubular cell, Hb is broken down and becomes deposited in the cells as *haemosiderin*. This can be detected in the spun sediment of urine using Perls' reaction. Some of the free plasma Hb is oxidized to *methaemoglobin*, which dissociates into *ferrihaem* and globin. *Plasma haemopexin* binds ferrihaem; but if its binding capacity is exceeded, ferrihaem becomes attached to albumin, forming *methaemalbumin*. On spectro-photometry of the plasma, methaemalbumin forms a characteristic band; this is the basis of *Schumm's test*.

The *liver* removes Hb bound to haptoglobin and *haemopexin* and any remaining free Hb.

Evidence for haemolysis

Increased red cell breakdown leads to:

- elevated serum bilirubin (unconjugated)
- excess urinary urobilinogen (resulting from bilirubin breakdown in the intestine, Fig. 8.5)
- reduced plasma haptoglobin
- raised serum lactic dehydrogenase (LDH).

Increased red cell production leads to:

- reticulocytosis
- erythroid hyperplasia of the bone marrow.

There may be evidence of abnormal red cells in some haemolytic anaemias:

- spherocytes (see Fig. 8.18)
- sickle cells (see Fig. 8.23)
- red cell fragments.

Demonstration of shortened red cell lifespan

Red cell survival can be estimated from ^{51}Cr-labelled red cells given intravenously but is rarely performed.

Intravascular haemolysis

This is suggested by raised levels of plasma Hb, haemosiderinuria, very low or absent haptoglobins, and the presence of methaemalbumin (positive Schumm's test).

Various laboratory studies will be necessary to determine the exact type of haemolytic anaemia present. The causes of haemolytic anaemias are shown in Table 8.9.

INHERITED HAEMOLYTIC ANAEMIA

RED CELL MEMBRANE DEFECTS

The normal red cell membrane consists of a lipid bilayer crossed by integral proteins with an underlying lattice of proteins (or cytoskeleton), including spectrin, actin, ankyrin and protein 4.1, attached to the integral proteins (Fig. 8.17).

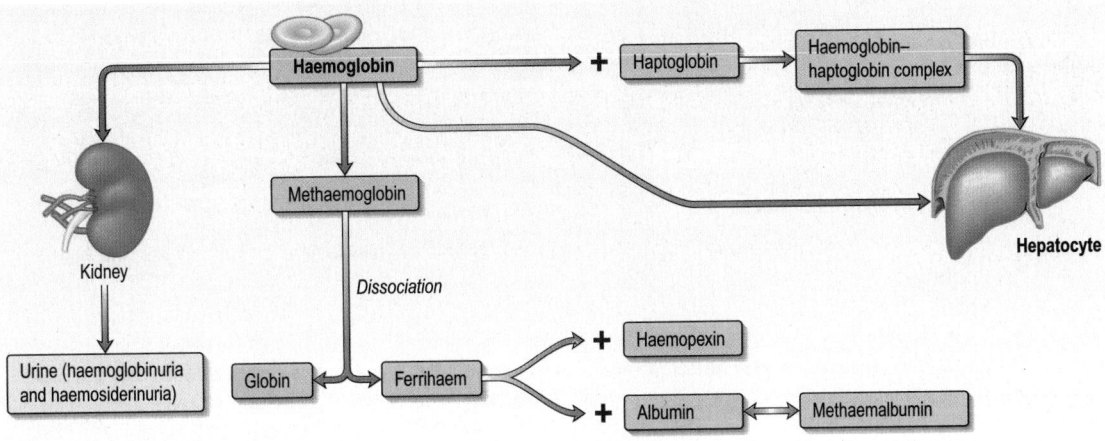

Fig. 8.16 **The fate of haemoglobin in the plasma following haemolysis.**

Table 8.9 Causes of haemolytic anaemia

Inherited	Acquired
Red cell membrane defect	**Immune**
Hereditary spherocytosis	Autoimmune (see Table 8.15)
Hereditary elliptocytosis	Warm
	Cold
Haemoglobin abnormalities	Alloimmune
Thalassaemia	Haemolytic transfusion reactions
Sickle cell disease	Haemolytic disease of the newborn
Metabolic defects	After allogeneic bone
Glucose-6-phosphate	marrow or organ
dehydrogenase	transplantation
deficiency	Drug-induced
Pyruvate kinase deficiency	
	Non-immune
Miscellaneous	Acquired membrane defects
Infections, e.g. malaria,	Paroxysmal nocturnal
mycoplasma	haemoglobinuria
Clostridium welchii,	Mechanical
generalized sepsis	Microangiopathic
Drugs and chemicals	haemolytic anaemia
causing damage to the	Valve prosthesis
red cell membrane or	March haemoglobinuria
oxidative haemolysis	Secondary to systemic
Hypersplenism	disease
Burns	Renal and liver failure

Hereditary spherocytosis (HS)

HS is the most common inherited haemolytic anaemia in northern Europeans, affecting 1 in 5000. It is inherited in an autosomal dominant manner, but in 25% of patients neither parent is affected and it is presumed that HS has occurred by spontaneous mutation. HS is due to defects in the red cell membrane, resulting in the cells losing part of the cell membrane as they pass through the spleen, possibly because the lipid bilayer is inadequately supported by the membrane skeleton. The best-characterized defect is a deficiency in the structural protein spectrin, but quantitative defects in other membrane proteins have been identified (Fig. 8.17), with ankyrin defects being the most common. The abnormal red cell membrane in HS is associated functionally with an increased permeability to sodium, and this requires an increased rate of active transport of sodium out of the cells which is dependent on ATP produced by glycolysis. The surface-to-volume ratio decreases, and the cells become spherocytic. Spherocytes are more rigid and less deformable than normal red cells. They are unable to pass through the splenic microcirculation and they die.

Clinical features

The condition may present with jaundice at birth. However, the onset of jaundice can be delayed for many years and some patients may go through life with no symptoms and are detected only during family studies. The patient may eventually develop anaemia, splenomegaly and ulcers on the leg. As in many haemolytic anaemias, the course of the disease may be interrupted by aplastic, haemolytic and megaloblastic crises. Aplastic anaemia usually occurs after infections, particularly with parvovirus, whereas megaloblastic anaemia is the result of folate depletion owing to the hyperactivity of the bone marrow. Chronic haemolysis leads to the formation of pigment gallstones (see p. 398).

Investigations

- **Anaemia.** This is usually mild, but occasionally can be severe.
- **Blood film.** This shows spherocytes (Fig. 8.18) and reticulocytes.
- **Haemolysis** is evident (e.g. the serum bilirubin and urinary urobilinogen will be raised).

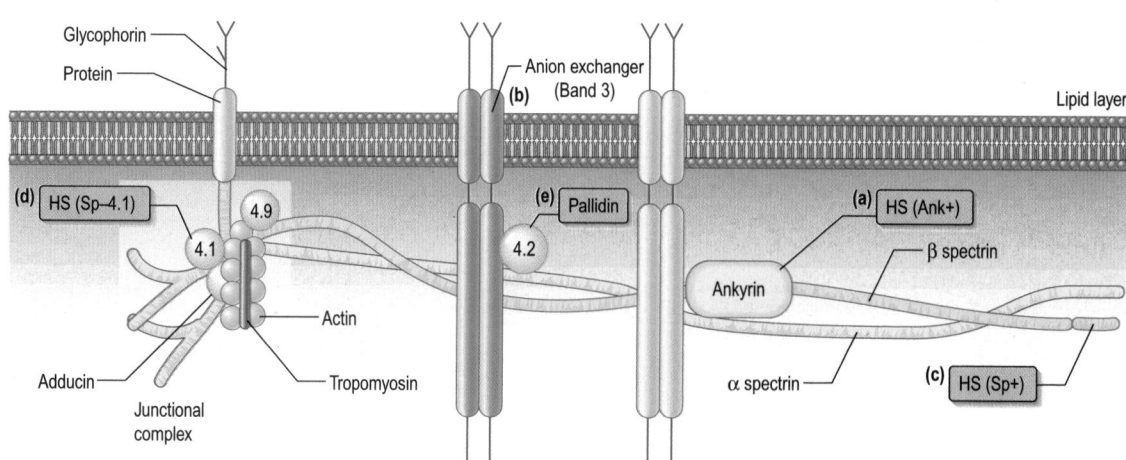

Fig. 8.17 **Hereditary spherocytosis (HS) and hereditary elliptocytosis (HE): red cell membrane showing the sites (purple) of the principal defects.** *Vertical interactions producing HS:* (a) ankyrin mutation, HS (Ank+) producing deficiency (45% of cases); (b) HS band 3 deficiency (20%); (c) β spectrin deficiency, HS (Sp+) (< 20%); (d) abnormal spectrin/protein 4.1 binding, HS (Sp–4.1); (e) protein 4.2 (pallidin) deficiency (Japanese). These produce various autosomal dominant and recessive forms of the disease. *Horizontal interactions producing HE:* α spectrin (80%), protein 4.1 (15%), β spectrin (5%).

Fig. 8.18 Spherocytes (arrowed). This blood film also shows reticulocytes, polychromasias and a nucleated erythroblast.

- **Osmotic fragility.** When red cells are placed in solutions of increasing hypotonicity, they take in water, swell, and eventually lyse. Spherocytes tolerate hypotonic solutions less well than do normal biconcave red cells. Osmotic fragility tests are infrequently carried out in routine practice, but may be useful to confirm a suspicion of spherocytosis on a blood film.
- **Direct antiglobulin (Coombs') test** is negative in spherocytosis, virtually ruling out autoimmune haemolytic anaemia where spherocytes are also commonly present.

Treatment

The spleen, which is the site of cell destruction, should be removed in all but the mildest cases. The decision about splenectomy in symptomless patients is difficult, but a raised bilirubin and especially the presence of gallstones should encourage splenectomy.

It is best to postpone splenectomy until after childhood, as sudden overwhelming fatal infections, usually due to encapsulated organisms such as pneumococci, may occur (see p. 457). Splenectomy should be preceded by appropriate immunization and followed by lifelong penicillin prophylaxis (see Box 2.9).

Following splenectomy, the spherocytes persist but the Hb level usually returns to normal as the red cells are no longer destroyed.

Folate deficiency often occurs in chronic haemolysis with rapid cell turnover. Folate levels should be monitored, or folic acid can be given prophylactically.

Hereditary elliptocytosis

This disorder of the red cell membrane is inherited in an autosomal dominant manner and has a prevalence of 1 in 2500 in Caucasians. The red cells are elliptical due to deficiencies of protein 4.1 or the spectrin/actin/4.1 complex which leads to weakness of the horizontal protein interaction and to the membrane defect (Fig. 8.17). Clinically it is a similar condition to HS but milder. Only a minority of patients have anaemia and only occasional patients require splenectomy.

Rarely, hereditary spherocytosis or elliptocytosis may be inherited in a homozygous fashion giving rise to a severe haemolytic anaemia sometimes necessitating splenectomy in early childhood.

Hereditary stomatocytosis

Stomatocytes are red cells in which the pale central area

appears slit-like. Their presence in large numbers may occur in a hereditary haemolytic anaemia associated with a membrane defect, but excess alcohol intake is also a common cause.

HAEMOGLOBIN ABNORMALITIES

In early embryonic life, haemoglobins Gower 1, Gower 2 and Portland predominate (Fig. 8.19). Later, fetal haemoglobin (Hb F), which has two α and two γ chains, is produced. There is increasing synthesis of β chains from 13 weeks of gestation and at term there is 80% Hb F and 20% Hb A. The switch from Hb F to Hb A occurs after birth when the genes for γ chain production are further suppressed and there is rapid increase in the synthesis of β chains. The exact mechanism responsible for the switch remains unknown. There is little Hb F produced (normally less than 1%) from 6 months after birth. The δ chain is synthesized just before birth and Hb A_2 ($\alpha_2\delta_2$) remains at a level of about 2% throughout adult life (Table 8.10).

Globin chains are synthesized in the same way as any protein (see Ch. 3). Four globin chain genes are required to control α-chain production (Fig. 8.19). Two are present on each haploid genome (genes derived from one parent). These are situated close together on chromosome 16. The genes controlling the production of ε, γ, δ and β chains are close together on chromosome 11. The globin genes are arranged on chromosomes 16 and 11 in the order in which they are expressed and combine to give different haemoglobins. Normal haemoglobin synthesis is discussed on page 422.

Abnormal haemoglobins

Abnormalities occur in:

- globin chain production (e.g. thalassaemia)
- structure of the globin chain (e.g. sickle cell disease)
- combined defects of globin chain production and structure, e.g. sickle cell β-thalassaemia.

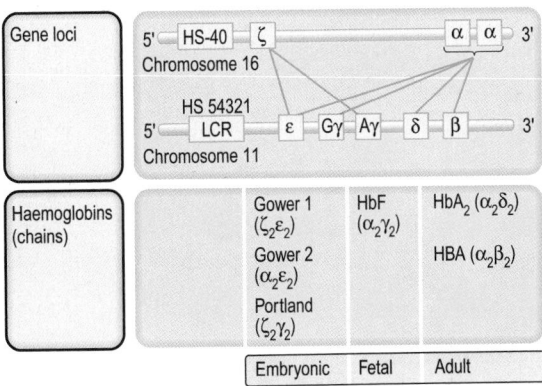

Fig. 8.19 Loci of genes on chromosomes 16 and 11 and the combination of various chains to produce different haemoglobins. HS-40 (for α genes) and locus control region (LCR) HS1–5 (for β genes) are regulatory control elements.

Table 8.10 Some types of haemoglobin

	Haemoglobin	Structure	Comment
Normal	A	$\alpha_2\beta_2$	Comprises 97% of adult haemoglobin
	A_2	$\alpha_2\delta_2$	Comprises 2% of adult haemoglobin
			Elevated in β-thalassaemia
	F	$\alpha_2\gamma_2$	Normal haemoglobin in fetus from 3rd to 9th month
			Increased in β-thalassaemia
			Comprises < 1% of haemoglobin in adult
Abnormal chain production	H	β_4	Found in α-thalassaemia
			Biologically useless
	Barts	γ_4	Comprises 100% of haemoglobin in homozygous α-thalassaemia
			Biologically useless
Abnormal chain structure	S	$\alpha_2\beta_2{}^S$	Substitution of valine for glutamine acid in position 6 of β chain
	C	$\alpha_2\beta_2{}^C$	Substitution of lysine for glutamic acid in position 6 of β chain

Genetic defects in haemoglobin are the most common of all genetic disorders.

THE THALASSAEMIAS

The thalassaemias (Greek *thalassa* = sea) affect people throughout the world (Fig. 8.20). Normally there is balanced (1:1) production of α and β chains. The defective synthesis of globin genes in thalassaemia leads to 'imbalanced' globin chain production, leading to precipitation of globin chains within the red cell precursors and resulting in ineffective erythropoiesis. Precipitation of globin chains in mature red cells leads to haemolysis.

β-Thalassaemia

In *homozygous* β-thalassaemia, either no normal β chains are produced (β^0), or β-chain production is very reduced (β^+). There is an excess of α chains, which precipitate in erythroblasts and red cells causing ineffective erythropoiesis and haemolysis. The excess α chains combine with whatever β, δ and γ chains are produced, resulting in increased quantities of Hb A_2 and Hb F and, at best, small amounts of Hb A. In *heterozygous* β-thalassaemia there is usually symptomless microcytosis with or without mild anaemia. Table 8.11 shows the findings in the homozygote and heterozygote for the common types of β-thalassaemia.

Molecular genetics

The molecular errors accounting for over 200 genetic defects leading to β-thalassaemia have been characterized. Unlike in α-thalassaemia, the defects are mainly point mutations rather than gene deletions. The mutations result in defects in transcription, RNA splicing and modification, translation via frame shifts and nonsense codons producing highly unstable β-globin which cannot be utilized.

Clinical syndromes

Clinically, β-thalassaemia can be divided into the following:

Fig. 8.20 Major haemoglobin abnormalities: geographical distribution.

Legend: Sickle cell | HbC | Thalassaemia | HbD | HbE

Table 8.11 β-Thalassaemia: common findings

Type of thalassaemia	Findings in homozygote	Findings in heterozygote
β^+	Thalassaemia major	Thalassaemia minor
	Hb A + F + A_2	Hb A_2 raised
β^0	Thalassaemia major	Thalassaemia minor
	Hb F + A_2	Hb A_2 raised
$\delta\beta$	Thalassaemia intermedia	Thalassaemia minor
		Hb F 5–15%
	Hb F only	Hb A_2 normal
$\delta\beta^+$ **(Lepore)**	Thalassaemia major or intermedia	Thalassaemia minor
		Hb Lepore 5–15%
	Hb F and Lepore	Hb A_2 normal

Hb Lepore is a cross fusion product of δ and β globin genes
Adapted with permission from Weatherall DJ (2003) Disorders of the synthesis of function of haemoglobin. In: Weatherall DJ, Warrell DA, Cox TM, Firth JD (eds) *Oxford Textbook of Medicine*, 4th edn. Oxford: Oxford University Press.

- thalassaemia minor (or trait), the symptomless heterozygous carrier state
- thalassaemia intermedia, with moderate anaemia, rarely requiring transfusions
- thalassaemia major, with severe anaemia requiring regular transfusions.

Thalassaemia minor (trait)

This common carrier state (heterozygous β-thalassaemia) is asymptomatic. Anaemia is mild or absent. The red cells are hypochromic and microcytic with a low MCV and MCH, and it may be confused with iron deficiency. However, the two are easily distinguished, as in thalassaemia trait the serum ferritin and the iron stores are normal (see Table 8.3). Hb electrophoresis usually shows a raised Hb A_2 and often a raised Hb F (Fig. 8.21). Iron should not be given to these patients unless they develop coincidental iron deficiency.

Thalassaemia intermedia

Thalassaemia intermedia includes patients who are symptomatic with moderate anaemia (Hb 7–10 g/dL) and who do not require regular transfusions. That is, it is more severe than in β-thalassaemia trait but milder than in transfusion-dependent thalassaemia major.

Thalassaemia intermedia may be due to a combination of homozygous mild β⁺- and α-thalassaemia, where there is reduced α-chain precipitation and less ineffective erythropoiesis and haemolysis. The inheritance of hereditary persistence of Hb F with homozygous β-thalassaemia also results in a milder clinical picture than unmodified β-thalassaemia major because the excess α chains are partially removed by the increased production of γ chains.

Patients may have splenomegaly and bone deformities. Recurrent leg ulcers, gallstones and infections are also seen.

Thalassaemia major (Cooley's anaemia)

Most children affected by homozygous β-thalassaemia present during the first year of life with:

- failure to thrive and recurrent bacterial infections
- severe anaemia from 3–6 months when the switch from γ- to β-chain production should normally occur
- extramedullary haemopoiesis that soon leads to hepatosplenomegaly and bone expansion, giving rise to the classical thalassaemic facies (Fig. 8.22a).

Skull X-rays in these children show the characteristic 'hair on end' appearance of bony trabeculation as a result of expansion of the bone marrow into cortical bone (Fig. 8.22b). The expansion of the bone marrow is also shown in an X-ray of the hand (Fig. 8.22c).

The classic features of untreated thalassaemia major are only observed in patients from countries without good blood transfusion support.

Management

The aims of treatment are to suppress ineffective erythropoiesis, prevent bony deformities and allow normal activity and development. Long-term folic acid supplements are required, and regular transfusions should be given to keep the Hb above 10 g/dL. Blood transfusions may be required every 4–6 weeks.

If transfusion requirements increase, splenectomy should be considered, although this is usually delayed until after the age of 6 years because of the risk of infection. Prophylaxis against infection is required for patients undergoing splenectomy (see p. 457).

Iron overload caused by repeated transfusions (transfusion haemosiderosis) may lead to damage to the endocrine glands, liver, pancreas and the myocardium by the time patients reach adolescence. The iron-chelating agent of choice remains desferrioxamine, although it has to be administered parenterally. The oral iron-chelating agent ICL670 appears to be safe and effective but long-term studies are awaited. Desferrioxamine is given as an overnight subcutaneous infusion on 5–7 nights each week. Ascorbic acid 200 mg daily is given, along with desferrioxamine, as it increases the urinary excretion of iron in response to desferrioxamine.

With current therapy, normal growth and sexual development occur but compliance may be a problem, especially in teenagers. Intensive treatment with desferrioxamine has been reported to reverse damage to the heart in patients with severe iron overload, but excessive doses of desferrioxamine may cause cataracts, retinal damage and nerve deafness. Infection with *Yersinia enterocolitica* occurs in iron-loaded patients treated with desferrioxamine. Iron overload should be periodically assessed by measuring the serum ferritin and by measurement of hepatic iron stores.

Bone marrow transplantation has been used in young patients with HLA-matched siblings. It has been successful in cases in good clinical condition with a 3-year mortality of less than 5%, but there is a high mortality (> 50%) in patients in poor condition with iron overload and liver dysfunction.

Fig. 8.21 **Patterns of haemoglobin electrophoresis.**

Fig. 8.22 **Thalassaemia.**
(a) A child with thalassaemia, showing the typical facial features.
(b) Skull X-ray of a child with β-thalassaemia, showing the 'hair on end' appearance.
(c) X-ray of hand, showing expansion of the marrow and a thinned cortex.

Prenatal diagnosis and gene therapy are discussed on page 191.

α-Thalassaemia

Molecular genetics

In contrast to β-thalassaemia, α-thalassaemia is often caused by gene deletions, although mutations also occur. The gene for α chains is duplicated on both chromosomes 16, i.e. there are four genes. Deletion of one α-chain gene (α^+) or both α-chain genes (α^0) on each chromosome 16 may occur (Table 8.12). The former is the most common of these abnormalities.

- Four-gene deletion (deletion of both genes on both chromosomes); there is no α-chain synthesis and only Hb Barts (γ_4) is present. Hb Barts cannot carry oxygen and is incompatible with life (Tables 8.10 and 8.12). Infants are either stillborn at 28–40 weeks or die very shortly after birth. They are pale, oedematous and have enormous livers and spleens – a condition called hydrops fetalis.
- Three-gene deletion; there is moderate anaemia (Hb 7–10 g/dL) and splenomegaly (Hb H disease). The patients are not usually transfusion-dependent. Hb A, Hb Barts and Hb H (β_4) are present. Hb A_2 is normal or reduced.
- Two-gene deletion (α-thalassaemia trait); there is microcytosis with or without mild anaemia. Hb H bodies may be seen on staining a blood film with brilliant cresyl blue.
- One-gene deletion; the blood picture is usually normal.

Globin chain synthesis studies for the detection of a reduced ratio of α to β chains may be necessary for the definitive diagnosis of α-thalassaemia trait.

Less commonly, α-thalassaemia may result from genetic defects other than deletions, for example mutations in the stop codon producing an α chain with many extra amino acids (Hb Constant Spring). (See p. 177.)

SICKLE SYNDROMES

Sickle cell haemoglobin (Hb S) results from a single-base mutation of adenine to thymine which produces a substitution of valine for glutamine at the sixth codon of the β-globin chain ($\alpha_2\beta_2^{6\,glu \to val}$). In the homozygous state (*sickle cell anaemia*) both genes are abnormal (Hb SS), whereas in the heterozygous state (*sickle cell trait*, Hb AS) only one chromosome carries the gene. As the synthesis of Hb F is normal, the disease usually does not manifest itself until the Hb F decreases to adult levels at about 6 months of age.

The disease occurs mainly in Africans (25% carry the gene) but is also found in India, the Middle East and southern Europe (see Fig. 8.20).

Table 8.12 **The α-thalassaemias**

Gene deletion		Haemoglobin type	Clinical picture
4 genes	α^0 $--/--$	Hb Barts (γ4)	Hydrops fetalis
3 genes	α^0 $--/-\alpha$	Hb H (β4)	Moderate anaemia
			Splenomegaly
2 genes	α^0 $--/\alpha\,\alpha$ or	Some Hb H bodies	Mild anaemia
	$-\alpha/-\alpha$	Hb A	α-Thalassaemia trait
1 gene	α^+ $-\alpha/\alpha\,\alpha$	'Normal'	α-Thalassaemia trait

Pathogenesis

Deoxygenated Hb S molecules are insoluble and polymerize. The flexibility of the cells is decreased and they become rigid and take up their characteristic sickle appearance. This process is initially reversible but, with repeated sickling, the cells eventually lose their membrane flexibility and become irreversibly sickled. This is due to dehydration, partly caused by potassium leaving the red cells via calcium activated potassium channels called the Gados channel. These irreversibly sickled cells are dehydrated and dense and will not return to normal when oxygenated. Sickling can produce:

- a shortened red cell survival
- impaired passage of cells through the microcirculation, leading to obstruction of small vessels and tissue infarction.

Sickling is precipitated by infection, dehydration, cold, acidosis or hypoxia. In many cases the cause is unknown, but adhesion proteins on activated endothelial cells (VCAM-1) may play a causal role, particularly in vaso-occlusion when rigid cells are trapped, facilitating polymerization. Hb S releases its oxygen to the tissues more easily than does normal Hb (see Fig. 15.5), and patients therefore feel well despite being anaemic (except of course during crises or complications).

Depending on the type of haemoglobin chain combinations, three clinical syndromes occur:

- homozygous Hb SS have the most severe disease
- combined heterozygocity (Hb SC) for Hb S and C (see below) who suffer intermediate symptoms.
- heterozygous Hb AS (sickle cell trait) usually have no symptoms (see p. 445).

Sickle cell anaemia

Clinical features
Vaso-occlusive crises

The earliest presentation in the first few years of life is acute pain in the hands and feet (dactylitis) owing to vaso-occlusion of the small vessels. Severe pain in other bones, e.g. femur, humerus, vertebrae, ribs, pelvis, occurs in older children/adults. These attacks vary in frequency from daily to perhaps only once a year. Fever often accompanies the pain.

Anaemia

Chronic haemolysis produces a stable haemoglobin level, usually in the 6–8 g/dL range but an acute fall in the haemoglobin level can occur owing to:

- splenic sequestration
- bone marrow aplasia
- further haemolysis.

Splenic sequestration

Vaso-occlusion produces an acute painful enlargement of the spleen. There is splenic pooling of red cells and hypovolaemia, leading in some to circulatory collapse and death. The condition occurs in childhood before multiple infarctions have occured. The latter eventually leads to a fibrotic non-functioning spleen. Liver sequestration can also occur.

Bone marrow aplasia

This most commonly occurs following infection with parvovirus B_{19}, which invades proliferating erythroid progenitors. There is a rapid fall in haemoglobin with no reticulocytes in the peripheral blood, because of the failure of erythropoiesis in the marrow.

Haemolysis due to drugs, acute infection or associated G6PD deficiency also occurs. Anaemia can also result from folate deficiency.

Long-term problems

In adults, nearly every organ is involved eventually, as patients survive longer with better treatment.

Growth and development. Young children are short but regain their height by adulthood. However, they remain below the normal weight. There is often delayed sexual maturation which may require hormone therapy. (Splenectomy can also reverse this.)

Bones are a common site for vaso-occlusive episodes, leading to chronic infarcts. Avascular necrosis of hips, shoulders, compression of vertebrae and shortening of bones in the hands and feet occur. Pain is a major problem. Osteomyelitis is commoner in sickle cell disease and is caused by *Salmonella*, *Staphylococcus aureus* and *Staph. pneumoniae*. Antibiotic treatment is necessary (p. 573). Joint replacements therapy may be required.

Infections are common in tissues susceptible to vaso-occlusion, e.g. bones, lungs, kidneys.

Respiratory. The acute sickle chest syndrome occurs in up to 30%, and pulmonary hypertension and chronic lung disease are the commonest cause of death of adults with sickle cell disease. The acute chest syndrome is caused by infection, fat embolism from necrotic bone marrow or pulmonary infarction due to sequestration of sickle cells. It comprises shortness of breath, chest pain, hypoxia, and new chest X-ray changes due to consolidation. The presentation may be gradual or very rapid, leading to death in a few hours. Initial management is with pain relief, inspired oxygen, antibiotics and exchange transfusion to reduce the amount of Hb S to < 20%; occasionally ventilation may be necessary. Infections can be due to chlamydia and mycoplasma, as well as *Streptococcus pneumoniae*.

Leg ulcers occur spontaneously (vaso-occlusive episodes) or following trauma and are usually over the medial or lateral malleoli. They often become infected and are quite resistant to treatment.

Cardiac problems occur, with cardiomegaly, arrhythmias and iron overload cardiomyopathy. Myocardial infarctions occur due to thrombotic episodes which are not secondary to atheroma.

Neurological complications occur in 25% of patients, with transient ischaemic attacks, fits, cerebral infarction, cerebral haemorrhage and coma. Ischaemic strokes occur in children and it has been suggested that regular transcranial Doppler ultrasonography is performed annually and patients are transfused in order to avoid brain damage.

Cholelithiasis. Pigment stones occur as a result of chronic haemolysis.

Liver. Chronic hepatomegaly and liver dysfunction are caused by trapping of sickle cells.

Renal. Chronic tubulo-intestitial nephritis occurs (see p. 643).

Priapism. An unwanted painful erection occurs from vaso-occlusion and can be recurrent. This may result in impotence. Treatment is with an α-adrenergic blocking drug, analgesia and hydration.

Eye. Background retinopathy, proliferative retinopathy, vitreous haemorrhages and retinal detachments all occur. Regular yearly eye checks are required.

Pregnancy. Impaired placental blood flow causes spontaneous abortion, intrauterine growth retardation, pre-eclampsia and fetal death. Painful episodes, infections and severe anaemia occur in the mother. Prophylactic transfusion does not improve fetal outcome. Oral contraceptives with low-dose oestrogens are safe.

Investigations

- **Blood count.** The level of Hb is in the range 6–8 g/dL with a high reticulocyte count (10–20%).
- **Blood films** can show features of hyposplenism (see Fig. 8.28).
- **Sickling** of red cells on a blood film can be induced in the presence of sodium metabisulphite (see Fig. 8.23).
- **Sickle solubility test.** A mixture of Hb S in a reducing solution such as sodium dithionite gives a turbid appearance because of precipitation of Hb S, whereas normal Hb gives a clear solution. A number of commercial kits such as Sickledex are available for rapid screening for the presence of Hb S, for example before surgery in appropriate ethnic groups and in the A&E department.

- **Hb electrophoresis** (see Fig. 8.21) is always needed to confirm the diagnosis. There is no Hb A, 80–95% Hb SS, and 2–20% Hb F.
- **The parents** of the affected child will show features of sickle cell trait.

Management

Precipitating factors (see above) should be avoided or treated quickly. The complications requiring inpatient management are shown in Table 8.13.

Acute painful attacks require supportive therapy with intravenous fluids, oxygen, antibiotics and adequate analgesia. Crises can be extremely painful and require strong, usually narcotic, analgesia. Morphine is the drug of choice. Milder pain can sometimes be relieved by codeine, paracetamol and NSAIDs.

Prophylaxis is with penicillin 500 mg daily and vaccination with polyvalent pneumococcal and *Haemophilus influenzae* type B vaccine (see p. 42). Folic acid is given to all patients with haemolysis.

Anaemia

Transfusions should only be given for clear indications. Patient with steady state anaemia, those having minor surgery or having painful episodes without complications should not be transfused. Transfusions should be given for heart failure, TIAs, strokes, acute chest syndrome, acute splenic sequestration and aplastic crises. Before elective operations and during pregnancy, repeated transfusions may be used to reduce the proportion of circulating Hb S to less than 20% to prevent sickling. Exchange transfusions may be necessary in patients with severe or recurrent crises, or before emergency surgery. Transfusion and splenectomy may be life-saving for young children with splenic sequestration. A full compatibility screen should always be performed.

Hydroxycarbamide (hydroxyurea) is the first drug which has been widely used as therapy for sickle cell anaemia. It acts by increasing Hb F concentrations but the reduction in neutrophils may also help. Hydroxycarbamide has been shown in trials to reduce the episodes of pain, the acute chest syndrome, and the need for blood transfusions.

Fig. 8.23 Sickle cells (arrowed) and target cells.

Table 8.13 Complications requiring inpatient management
Pain uncontrolled by non-opiate analgesia
Swollen painful joints
Central nervous system deficit
Acute sickle chest syndrome or pneumonia
Mesenteric sickling and bowel ischaemia
Splenic or hepatic sequestration
Cholecystitis
Renal papillary necrosis resulting in colic or severe haematuria
Hyphema and retinal detachment

From Davies SC, Oni L (1997) Management of patients with sickle cell disease. *British Medical Journal* **315**: 656–660.

Inhaled nitric oxide inhibits platelet function, reduces vascular adhesion of red cells and is also a vasodilator. It has been shown to reduce opiate requirements in acute painful episodes.

Bone marrow transplantation has been used to treat sickle cell anaemia although in fewer numbers than for thalassaemia. Children and adolescents younger than 16 years of age who have severe complications (strokes, recurrent chest syndrome, or refractory pain) and have an HLA-matched donor are the best candidates for transplantation.

Counselling

A multidisciplinary team should be involved, with regular clinic appointments to build up relationships. Adolescents require careful counselling over psychosocial issues, drug and birth control.

Prognosis

Some patients with Hb SS die in the first few years of life from either infection or episodes of sequestration. However, there is marked individual variation in the severity of the disease and some patients have a relatively normal lifespan with few complications.

Sickle cell trait

These individuals have no symptoms unless extreme circumstances cause anoxia, such as flying in non-pressurized aircraft or problems with anaesthesia. Sickle cell trait protects against *Plasmodium falciparum* malaria (see p. 97), and consequently the sickle gene has been seen as an example of a balanced polymorphism (where the advantage of the malaria protection in the heterozygote is balanced by the mortality of the homozygous condition). Typically there is 60% Hb A and 40% Hb S. The blood count and film are normal. The diagnosis is made by a positive sickle test or by Hb electrophoresis (see Fig. 8.21).

Other structural globin chain defects

There are many Hb variants (e.g. Hb C, D), many of which are not associated with clinical manifestations.

Hb C ($\alpha_2\beta_2^{6Glu-lys}$) disease may be associated with Hb S (Hb SC disease). The clinical course is similar to that with Hb SS, but there is an increased likelihood of thrombosis, which may lead to life-threatening episodes of thrombosis in pregnancy, and retinopathy.

Combined defects of globin chain production and structure

Abnormalities of Hb structure (e.g. Hb S, C) can occur in combination with thalassaemia. The combination of β-thalassaemia trait and sickle cell trait (sickle cell β-thalassaemia) resembles sickle cell anaemia (Hb SS) clinically.

Hb E ($\alpha_2\beta_2^{26Glu-lys}$) is the most common Hb variant in South East Asia, and the second most prevalent haemoglobin variant world-wide. Hb E heterozygotes are asymptomatic; the haemoglobin level is normal, but red cells are microcytic. Homozygous Hb E causes a mild microcytic anaemia, but the combination of heterozygosity for Hb E and β-thalassaemia produces a variable anaemia which can be as severe as β-thalassaemia major.

Prenatal screening and diagnosis of severe haemoglobin abnormalities

Of the offspring of parents who both have either β-thalassaemia or sickle cell trait, 25% will have β-thalassaemia major or sickle cell anaemia, respectively. Recognition of these heterozygous states in parents and family counselling provide a basis for antenatal screening and diagnosis.

Prognosis

Pregnant women with either sickle cell trait or thalassaemia trait must be identified at antenatal booking either by selective screening of high-risk groups on the basis of ethnic origin or by universal screening of all pregnant women. β-Thalassaemia trait can always be detected by a low MCV and MCH and confirmed by haemoglobin electrophoresis. However, sickle cell trait is undetectable from a blood count and the laboratory need a specific request to screen for sickle cell trait.

If a pregnant woman is found to have a haemoglobin defect, her partner should be tested. Antenatal diagnosis is offered if both are affected as there is a risk of a severe fetal Hb defect, particularly β-thalassaemia major. Fetal DNA analysis can be carried out using amniotic fluid, chorionic villus or fetal blood samples. Abortion is offered if the fetus is found to be affected. Chorionic villus biopsy has the advantage that it can be carried out in the first trimester, thus avoiding the need for second trimester abortions.

Gene therapy would be the ultimate corrective therapy for severe Hb abnormalities. Normal Hb genes could be inserted into the patient's haemopoietic cells in vitro and these cells could be transplanted back into the patient after ablative bone marrow treatment.

METABOLIC DISORDERS OF THE RED CELL

Red cell metabolism

The mature red cell has no nucleus, mitochondria or ribosomes and is therefore unable to synthesize proteins. Red cells have only limited enzyme systems but they maintain the viability and function of the cells. In particular, energy is required in the form of ATP for the maintenance of the flexibility of the membrane and the biconcave shape of the cells to allow passage through small vessels, and for regulation of the sodium and potassium pumps to ensure osmotic equilibrium. In addition, it is essential that Hb be maintained in the reduced state.

The enzyme systems responsible for producing energy and reducing power are (Fig. 8.24):

- the glycolytic (Embden–Meyerhof) pathway, in which glucose is metabolized to pyruvate and lactic acid with production of ATP

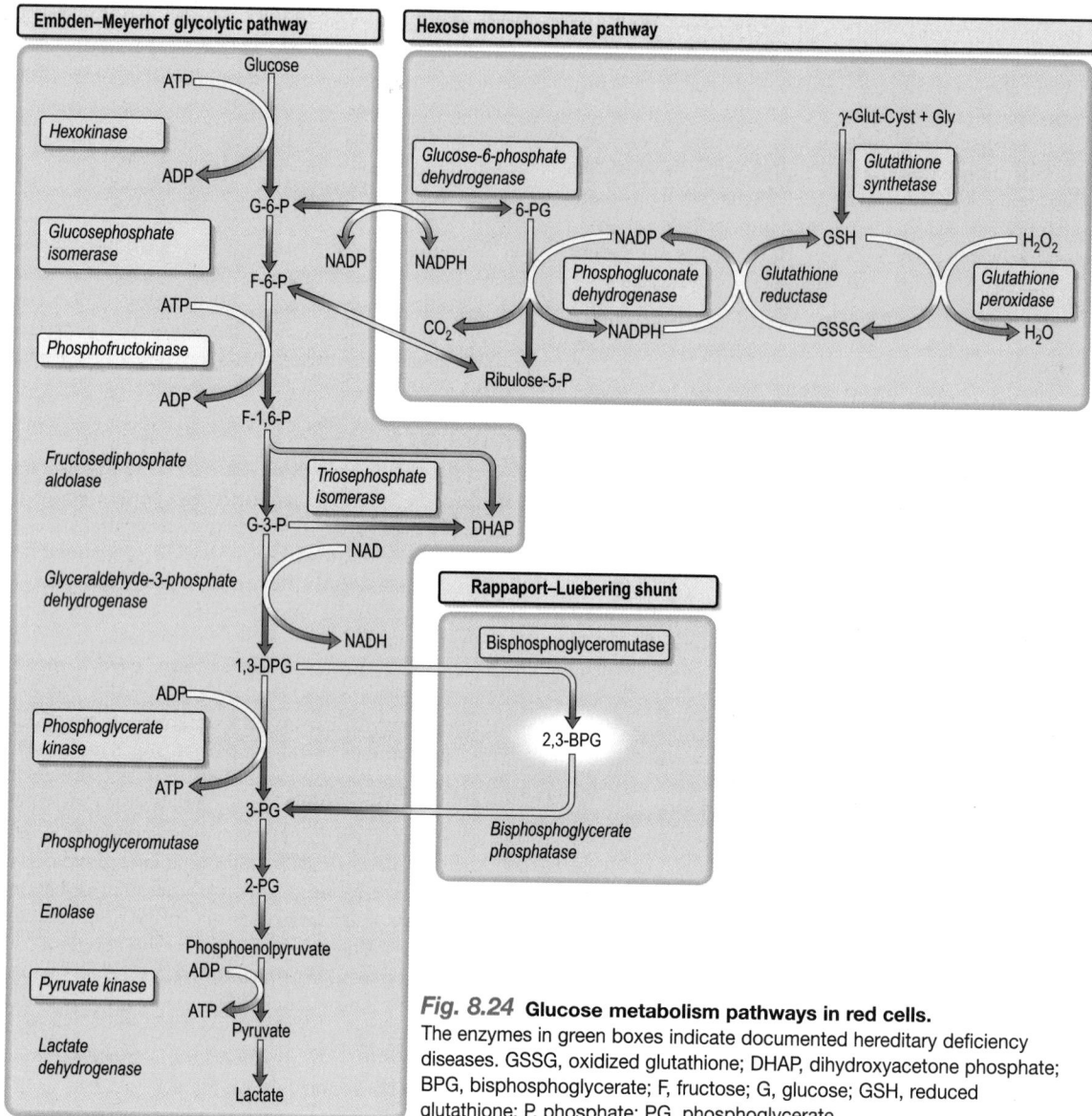

Fig. 8.24 Glucose metabolism pathways in red cells.
The enzymes in green boxes indicate documented hereditary deficiency diseases. GSSG, oxidized glutathione; DHAP, dihydroxyacetone phosphate; BPG, bisphosphoglycerate; F, fructose; G, glucose; GSH, reduced glutathione; P, phosphate; PG, phosphoglycerate.

- the hexose monophosphate (pentosephosphate) pathway, which provides reducing power for the red cell in the form of NADPH.

About 90% of glucose is metabolized by the former and 10% by the latter. The hexose monophosphate shunt maintains glutathione (GSH) in a reduced state. Glutathione is necessary to combat oxidative stress to the red cell, and failure of this mechanism may result in:

- rigidity due to cross-linking of spectrin, which decreases membrane flexibility (see Fig. 8.17) and causes 'leakiness' of the red cell membrane
- oxidation of the Hb molecule, producing methaemoglobin and precipitation of globin chains as Heinz bodies localized on the inside of the membrane; these bodies are removed from circulating red cells by the spleen.

2,3-BPG is formed from a side-arm of the glycolytic pathway (see Fig. 8.24). It binds to the central part of the Hb tetramer, fixing it in the low-affinity state (see Fig. 8.4). A decreased affinity with a shift in the oxygen dissociation curve to the right enables more oxygen to be delivered to the tissues (see Fig. 15.5).

In addition to the G6PD and pyruvate kinase deficiencies described below, there are a number of rare enzyme deficiencies that need specialist investigation.

Glucose-6-phosphate dehydrogenase (G6PD) deficiency

The enzyme G6PD holds a vital position in the hexose monophosphate shunt (Fig. 8.24), oxidizing glucose-6-phosphate to 6-phosphoglycerate with the reduction of NADP to NADPH. The reaction is necessary in red cells where it is the only source of NADPH, which is used via glutathione to protect the red cell from oxidative damage. G6PD deficiency is a common condition that presents with a haemolytic anaemia and affects millions of people throughout the world, particularly in Africa, around the Mediterranean, the Middle East (around 20%) and South East Asia (up to 40% in some regions).

The gene for G6PD is localized to chromosome Xq28 near the factor VIII gene. The deficiency is more common in males than in females. However, female heterozygotes can also have clinical problems due to lyonization, whereby because of random X-chromosome inactivation female heterozygotes have two populations of red cells – a normal one and a G6PD-deficient one.

There are over 400 structural types of G6PD, and mutations are mostly single amino acid substitutions. The most common types with normal activity are called type B$^+$, which is present in almost all Caucasians and about 70% of black Africans, and type A$^+$, which is present in about 20% of black Africans. There are many variants with reduced activity but only two are common. In the African, or A$^-$ type, the degree of deficiency is mild and more marked in older cells. Haemolysis is self-limiting as the young red cells newly produced by the bone marrow have nearly normal enzyme activity. However, in the Mediterranean type, both young and old red cells have very low enzyme activity. After an oxidant shock the Hb level may fall precipitously; death may follow unless the condition is recognized and the patient is transfused urgently.

Clinical syndromes

- Acute drug-induced haemolysis (Table 8.14) – usually dose related
- Favism (ingestion of fava beans)
- Chronic haemolytic anaemia
- Neonatal jaundice
- Infections and acute illnesses will also precipitate haemolysis in patients with G6PD deficiency.

Mothballs containing naphthalene can also cause haemolysis.

Table 8.14 Drugs causing haemolysis in glucose-6-phosphate deficiency

Analgesics, such as:	Antibacterials, such as:
Aspirin	Most sulphonamides
Phenacetin (withdrawn in the UK)	Dapsone
	Nitrofurantoin
Antimalarials, such as:	Chloramphenicol
Primaquine	Quinolones
Pyrimethamine	
Quinine	**Miscellaneous drugs, such as:**
Chloroquine	Vitamin K
Pamaquin	Probenecid
	Nalidixic acid
	Quinidine
	Dimercaprol
	Phenylhydrazine

Fig. 8.25 'Blister' cells (arrowed) in G6PD deficiency.

The clinical features are due to rapid intravascular haemolysis with symptoms of anaemia, jaundice and haemoglobinuria.

Investigations

- **Blood count** is normal between attacks.
- **During an attack** the blood film may show irregularly contracted cells, bite cells (cells with an indentation of the membrane), blister cells (cells in which the Hb appears to have become partially detached from the cell membrane; see Fig. 8.25), Heinz bodies (best seen on films stained with methyl violet) and reticulocytosis.
- **Haemolysis** is evident (see p. 437).
- **G6PD deficiency** can be detected using several screening tests, such as demonstration of the decreased ability of G6PD-deficient cells to reduce dyes. The level of the enzyme may also be directly assayed. There are two diagnostic problems. Immediately after an attack the screening tests may be normal (because the oldest red cells with least 6GPD activity are destroyed selectively). Secondly, the diagnosis of heterozygous females may be difficult because the enzyme level may range from very low to normal depending on lyonization. However, the risk of clinically significant haemolysis is minimal in patients with borderline G6PD activity.
- DNA analysis may also be performed.

Treatment

- Any offending drugs should be stopped.
- Underlying infection should be treated.
- Blood transfusion may be life-saving.
- Splenectomy is not usually helpful.

Pyruvate kinase deficiency

This is the most common defect of red cell metabolism after G6PD deficiency, affecting thousands rather than millions of people. The site of the defect is shown in Figure 8.24. There is reduced production of ATP, causing rigid red cells. Homozygotes have haemolytic anaemia and splenomegaly. It is inherited as an autosomal recessive.

Investigations

- **Anaemia** of variable severity is present (Hb 5–10 g/dL). The oxygen dissociation curve is shifted to the right as a result of the rise in intracellular 2,3-BPG (Fig. 15.5), and this reduces the severity of symptoms due to anaemia.

- **Blood film** shows distorted ('prickle') cells and a reticulocytosis.
- **Pyruvate kinase activity** is low (affected homozygotes have levels of 5–20%).

Treatment

Blood transfusions may be necessary during infections and pregnancy. Splenectomy may improve the clinical condition and is usually advised for patients requiring frequent transfusions.

FURTHER READING

Platt OS (2000) The acute chest syndrome of sickle cell disease. *New England Journal of Medicine* **342**: 1904–1907.

Porter JB (2001) Practical management of iron overload. *British Journal of Haematology* **115**: 239–252.

Steinberg MH et al. (2003) Effect of hydroxyurea on mortality and morbidity in adult sickle cell anaemia; risks and benefits up to 9 years of treatment. *Journal of the American Medical Association* **289**: 1645–1651.

Stuart M, Nagel RL (2004) Sickle cell disease. *Lancet* **364**: 1343–1360.

Vichinsky E (2002) New therapies in sickle cell disease. *Lancet* **360**: 629–631.

Weatherall DJ, Clegg JB (eds) (2001) The thalassaemic syndromes, 4th edn. Oxford: Oxford Blackwell Science.

Weatherall DJ, Provan AB (2000) Red cells I: inherited anaemias. *Lancet* **355**: 1169–1175.

ACQUIRED HAEMOLYTIC ANAEMIA

These anaemias may be divided into those due to immune, non-immune, or other causes (see Table 8.9).

Causes of immune destruction of red cells

- Autoantibodies
- Drug-induced antibodies
- Alloantibodies.

Causes of non-immune destruction of red cells

- Acquired membrane defects (e.g. paroxysmal nocturnal haemoglobinuria; see p. 452).
- Mechanical factors (e.g. prosthetic heart valves, or microangiopathic haemolytic anaemia; see p. 453).
- Secondary to systemic disease (e.g. renal and liver disease).

Miscellaneous causes

- Various toxic substances can disrupt the red cell membrane and cause haemolysis (e.g. arsenic, and products of *Clostridium welchii*).
- Malaria frequently causes anaemia owing to a combination of a reduction in red cell survival and reduced production of red cells.
- Hypersplenism (p. 457) results in a reduced red cell survival, which may also contribute to the anaemia seen in malaria.

- Extensive burns result in denaturation of red cell membrane proteins and reduced red cell survival.
- Some drugs (e.g. dapsone, sulfasalazine) cause oxidative haemolysis with Heinz bodies.
- Some ingested chemicals (e.g. weedkillers such as sodium chlorate) cause severe oxidative haemolysis leading to acute renal failure.

AUTOIMMUNE HAEMOLYTIC ANAEMIAS

Autoimmune haemolytic anaemias (AIHA) are acquired disorders resulting from increased red cell destruction due to red cell autoantibodies. These anaemias are characterized by the presence of a positive direct antiglobulin (Coombs') test, which detects the autoantibody on the surface of the patient's red cells (Fig. 8.26).

AIHA is divided into 'warm' and 'cold' types, depending on whether the antibody attaches better to the red cells at body temperature (37°C) or at lower temperatures. The major features and the causes of these two forms of AIHA are shown in Table 8.15. In warm AIHA, IgG antibodies predominate and the direct antiglobulin test is positive with IgG alone, IgG and complement, or complement only. In cold AIHA, the antibodies are usually IgM. They easily elute off red cells, leaving complement which is detected as C3d.

Immune destruction of red cells

IgM or IgG red cell antibodies which fully activate the complement cascade cause lysis of red cells in the circulation (intravascular haemolysis).

IgG antibodies frequently do not activate complement and the coated red cells undergo extravascular haemolysis (Fig. 8.27). They are either completely phagocytosed in the spleen through an interaction with Fc receptors on macrophages, or they lose part of the cell membrane through partial phagocytosis and circulate as spherocytes until they too become sequestered in the spleen. Some IgG antibodies partially activate complement, leading to deposition of C3b on the red cell surface, and this may enhance phagocytosis as macrophages also have receptors for C3b.

Non-complement-binding IgM antibodies are rare and have little or no effect on red cell survival. IgM antibodies which partially rather than fully activate complement cause adherence of red cells to C3b receptors on macrophages, particularly in the liver, although this is an ineffective mechanism of haemolysis. Most of the red cells are released from the macrophages when C3b is cleaved to C3d and then circulate with C3d on their surface.

'Warm' autoimmune haemolytic anaemias

Clinical features

These anaemias may occur at all ages and in both sexes, although they are most frequent in middle-aged females. They can present as a short episode of anaemia and

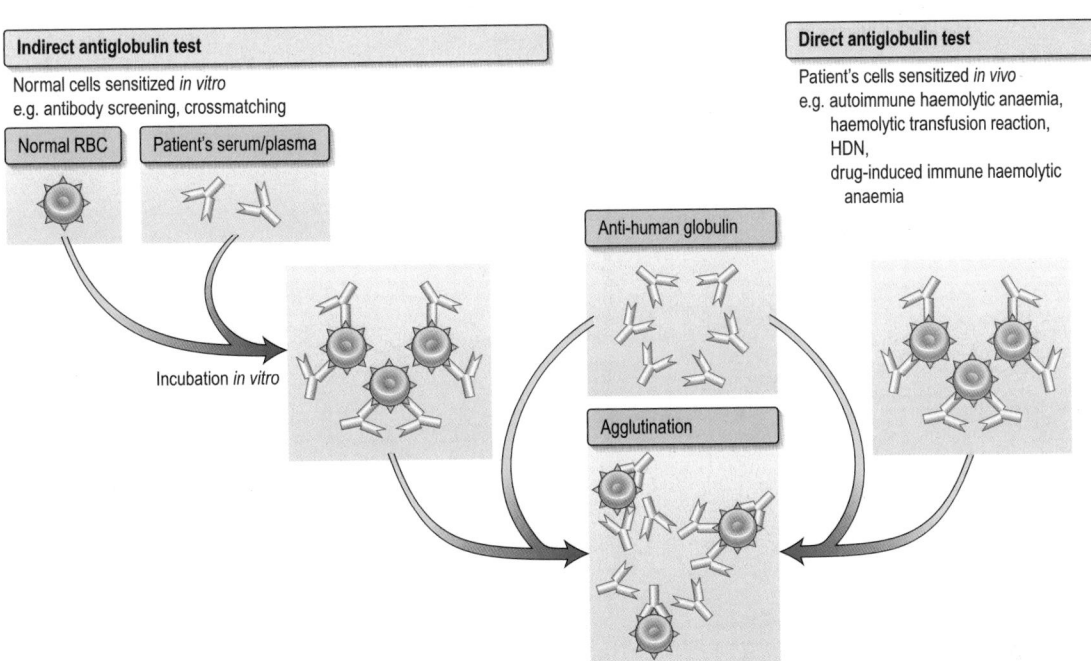

Normal cells sensitized *in vitro*
e.g. antibody screening, crossmatching

Normal RBC   Patient's serum/plasma

Incubation *in vitro*

Anti-human globulin

Agglutination

Direct antiglobulin test

Patient's cells sensitized *in vivo*
e.g. autoimmune haemolytic anaemia,
     haemolytic transfusion reaction,
     HDN,
     drug-induced immune haemolytic
     anaemia

Fig. 8.26 **Antiglobulin (Coombs') tests.** The anti-human globulin forms bridges between the sensitized cells causing visible agglutination. The direct test detects patients' cells sensitized in vivo. The indirect test detects normal cells sensitized in vitro. HDN, haemolytic disease of newborn.

Table 8.15   **Causes and major features of autoimmune haemolytic anaemias**

	Warm	Cold
Temperature at which antibody attaches best to red cells	37°C	Lower than 37°C
Type of antibody	IgG	IgM
Direct Coombs' test	Strongly positive	Positive
Causes of primary conditions	Idiopathic	Idiopathic
Causes of secondary condition	Autoimmune disorders, e.g. systemic lupus erythematosus Chronic lymphocytic leukaemia Lymphomas Hodgkin's lymphoma Carcinomas Drugs, e.g. methyldopa	Infections, e.g. infectious mononucleosis, *Mycoplasma* pneumoniae, other viral infections (rare) Lymphomas Paroxysmal cold haemoglobinuria (IgG)

jaundice but they often remit and relapse and may progress to an intermittent chronic pattern. The spleen is often palpable. Infections or folate deficiency may provoke a profound fall in the haemoglobin level.

In more than 30% of cases, the cause remains unknown. These anaemias may be associated with lymphoid malignancies or diseases such as rheumatoid arthritis and SLE or drugs (Table 8.15).

Investigations

- **Haemolytic anaemia** is evident (see p. 437).
- **Spherocytosis** is present as a result of red cell damage.
- **Direct antiglobulin test** is positive, with either IgG alone (67%), IgG and complement (20%), or complement alone (13%) being found on the surface of the red cells.
- **Autoantibodies** may have specificity for the Rh blood group system (e.g. for the e antigen).

- **Autoimmune thrombocytopenia** and/or neutropenia may also be present (Evans' syndrome).

Treatment and prognosis

Corticosteroids (e.g. prednisolone in doses of 1 mg/kg daily) are effective in inducing a remission in about 80% of patients. Steroids reduce both production of the red cell autoantibody and destruction of antibody-coated cells. Splenectomy may be necessary if there is no response to steroids or if the remission is not maintained when the dose of prednisolone is reduced. Other immunosuppressive drugs, such as azathioprine and cyclophosphamide, may be effective in patients who fail to respond to steroids and splenectomy.

'Cold' autoimmune haemolytic anaemias

Normally, low titres of IgM cold agglutinins reacting at

Fig. 8.27 Extravascular haemolysis is due to interaction of antibody-coated cells with cells in the reticuloendothelial system, predominantly in the spleen. **(a)** Spherocytosis results from partial phagocytosis. **(b)** Complete phagocytosis may occur and this is enhanced if there is complement as well as antibody on the cell surface. **(c)** Cells coated with complement only are ineffectively removed and circulate with C3d or C3b on their surface.

4°C are present in plasma and are harmless. At low temperatures these antibodies can attach to red cells and cause their agglutination in the cold peripheries of the body. In addition, activation of complement may cause intravascular haemolysis when the cells return to the higher temperatures in the core of the body.

After certain infections (such as *Mycoplasma*, cytomegalovirus, Epstein–Barr virus (EBV)) there is increased synthesis of polyclonal cold agglutinins producing a mild to moderate transient haemolysis.

Chronic cold haemagglutinin disease (CHAD)

This usually occurs in the elderly with a gradual onset of haemolytic anaemia owing to the production of monoclonal IgM cold agglutinins. After exposure to cold, the patient develops an acrocyanosis similar to Raynaud's (see p. 869) as a result of red cell autoagglutination.

Investigations

- **Red cells** agglutinate in the cold or at room temperature. Agglutination is sometimes seen in the sample tube after cooling but is more easily seen on the peripheral blood film made at room temperature. The agglutination is reversible after warming the sample. The agglutination may cause a spurious increase in the MCV (see p. 1425).
- **Direct antiglobulin test** is positive with complement alone.
- **Monoclonal IgM antibodies** with specificity for the Ii blood group system, usually for the I antigen but occasionally for the i antigen.

Treatment

The underlying cause should be treated, if possible. Patients should avoid exposure to cold. Treatment with steroids, alkylating agents and splenectomy is usually ineffective. Treatment with anti-CD20 (rituximab) has been successful in some cases.

Paroxysmal cold haemoglobinuria (PCH)

This is a rare condition associated with common childhood infections, such as measles, mumps and chickenpox. Intravascular haemolysis is associated with polyclonal IgG complement-fixing antibodies. These antibodies are biphasic, reacting with red cells in the cold in the peripheral circulation, with lysis occurring due to complement activation when the cells return to the central circulation. The antibodies have specificity for the P red cell antigen. The lytic reaction is demonstrated in vitro by incubating the patient's red cells and serum at 4°C and then warming the mixture to 37°C (Donath–Landsteiner test). Haemolysis is self-limiting but supportive transfusions of warmed blood may be necessary.

DRUG-INDUCED IMMUNE HAEMOLYTIC ANAEMIA

The interaction between a drug and red cell membrane produces a composite antigenic structure (or neoantigen), provoking two types of antibodies:

- *Drug-dependent antibodies*, which bind to both the drug and the cell membrane but not to either separately.

Clinically there is usually severe complement-mediated intravascular haemolysis, which resolves quickly after withdrawal of the drug.

- *Drug-independent antibodies*, which are induced by a subtle alteration of the red cell membrane. Such antibodies react with red cells in vitro in the absence of the drug and are indistinguishable from 'true' autoantibodies. There is extravascular haemolysis and the clinical course tends to be more protracted.

This concept for drug-induced immune haemolytic anaemia probably also applies to drug-induced thrombocytopenia and neutropenia.

ALLOIMMUNE HAEMOLYTIC ANAEMIA

Antibodies produced in one individual react with the red cells of another. This situation occurs in haemolytic disease of the newborn, haemolytic transfusion reactions (see p. 461) and after allogeneic bone marrow, renal, liver or cardiac transplantation when donor lymphocytes transferred in the allograft ('passenger lymphocytes') may produce red cell antibodies against the recipient and cause haemolytic anaemia.

Haemolytic disease of the newborn (HDN)

HDN is due to fetomaternal incompatibility for red cell antigens. Maternal alloantibodies against fetal red cell antigens pass from the maternal circulation via the placenta into the fetus, where they destroy the fetal red cells. Only IgG antibodies are capable of transplacental passage from mother to fetus.

The most common type of HDN is that due to ABO incompatibility, where the mother is usually group O and the fetus group A.

HDN due to ABO incompatibility is usually mild and exchange transfusion is rarely needed. HDN due to RhD incompatibility has become much less common in developed countries following the introduction of anti-D prophylaxis (see below). HDN may be caused by antibodies against antigens in many blood group systems (e.g. other Rh antigens such as c and E, and Kell, Duffy and Kidd; see p. 458).

Sensitization occurs as a result of passage of fetal red cells into the maternal circulation (which most readily occurs at the time of delivery), so that first pregnancies are rarely affected. However, sensitization may occur at other times, for example after a miscarriage, ectopic pregnancy or blood transfusion, or due to episodes during pregnancy which cause transplacental bleeding such as amniocentesis, chorionic villus sampling and threatened miscarriage.

Clinical features

These vary from a mild haemolytic anaemia of the newborn to intrauterine death from 18 weeks' gestation with the characteristic appearance of hydrops fetalis (hepatosplenomegaly, oedema and cardiac failure).

Kernicterus occurs owing to severe jaundice in the neonatal period, where the unconjugated (lipid-soluble) bilirubin exceeds 250 μmol/L and bile pigment deposition occurs in the basal ganglia. This can result in permanent brain damage, choreoathetosis, and spasticity. In mild cases it may present as deafness.

Investigations

Routine antenatal serology

All mothers should have their ABO and RhD groups determined and their serum tested for atypical antibodies after attending the antenatal booking clinic. Tests for red cell antibodies should be repeated at 28 weeks' gestation.

If an antibody is detected, its blood group specificity should be determined and the mother should be retested at least monthly. A rising antibody titre of IgG antibodies or a history of HDN in a previous pregnancy is an indication for referral to a specialist unit to determine the need for amniocentesis (to assess the level of bilirubin in the amniotic fluid) or fetal blood sampling to determine the severity of HDN and to guide further management.

Ultrasound

This shows changes in the fetal blood flow and cardiac function caused by compensated anaemia and can be demonstrated in utero before hydrops develops. Fetal DNA may be obtained by amniocentesis, chorionic villous sampling, or fetal blood sampling. Soluble fetal DNA in maternal plasma can also be used for this purpose, avoiding an invasive procedure.

At the birth of an affected infant

A sample of cord blood is obtained. This shows:

- anaemia with a high reticulocyte count
- a positive direct antiglobulin test
- a raised serum bilirubin.

Treatment

Management of the baby

In mild cases, phototherapy may be used to convert bilirubin to water-soluble biliverdin. Biliverdin can be excreted by the kidneys and this therefore reduces the chance of kernicterus.

In more severely affected cases, exchange transfusion may be necessary to replace the infant's red cells and to remove bilirubin. Indications for exchange transfusion include:

- a cord Hb of < 12 g/dL (normal cord Hb is 13.6–19.6 g/dL)
- a cord bilirubin of > 60 μmol/L
- a later serum bilirubin of > 300 μmol/L
- a rapidly rising serum bilirubin level.

Further exchange transfusions may be necessary to remove the unconjugated bilirubin.

The blood used for exchange transfusions should be ABO-compatible with the mother and infant, lack the antigen against which the maternal antibody is directed, be fresh (no more than 5 days from the day of collection), and be CMV-seronegative to prevent transmission of cytomegalovirus.

A severely affected fetus may need intrauterine blood transfusions carried out in a special unit.

An advance in the antenatal management of RhD alloimmunized women is the development of molecular methods for fetal RhD blood grouping in women with partners heterozygous for RhD. RhD-negative fetuses, who will be unaffected, can be distinguished from RhD-positive fetuses, who may be severely affected and require intensive monitoring.

Prevention of RhD immunization in the mother
Anti-D should be given after delivery when all of the following are present:

- the mother is RhD negative
- the fetus is RhD positive
- there is no maternal anti-D detectable in the mother's serum; i.e. the mother is not already immunized.

The dose is 500 i.u. of IgG anti-D intramuscularly within 48 hours of delivery. *The Kleihauer test* is used to assess the number of fetal cells in the maternal circulation. A blood film prepared from maternal blood is treated with acid, which elutes Hb A. Hb F is resistant to this treatment and can be seen when the film is stained with eosin. If large numbers of fetal red cells are present in the maternal circulation, a higher or additional dose of anti-D will be necessary.

It may be necessary to give prophylaxis to RhD-negative women at other times when sensitization may occur, for example after an ectopic pregnancy, threatened miscarriage or amniocentesis. The dose of anti-D is 250 i.u. before 20 weeks' gestation and 500 i.u. after 20 weeks.

Of previously non-immunized RhD-negative women carrying RhD-positive fetuses, 1–2% are immunized by the time of delivery. *Antenatal prophylaxis* with administration of 500 i.u. anti-D to RhD-negative women at both 28 and 34 weeks' gestation has been shown to reduce the incidence of immunization, and its routine use is being implemented in the UK. Monoclonal anti-D could in principle replace polyclonal anti-D, which is collected from RhD-negative women immunized in pregnancy and deliberately immunized RhD-negative males, but it is likely to be some years before trials have been completed and it is available in sufficient quantity.

FURTHER READING

Joint Working Party of the British Blood Transfusion Society and the Royal College of Obstetricians and Gynaecologists (1999) Guidelines for the use of anti-D immunoglobulin for Rh prophylaxis. *Transfusion Medicine* **9**: 93–97.
Urbaniak SJ, Greiss MA (2000) RhD haemolytic disease of the newborn. *Blood Reviews* **14**: 44–61.

NON-IMMUNE HAEMOLYTIC ANAEMIA

Paroxysmal nocturnal haemoglobinuria (PNH)

This is a rare acquired red cell defect in which a clone of red cells is particularly sensitive to destruction by activated complement. These cells are continually haemolysed intravascularly. Platelets and granulocytes are also affected and there may be thrombocytopenia and neutropenia.

The underlying defect is an inability of PNH cells to make glycosylphosphatidylinositol (GPI), which anchors surface proteins such as decay accelerating factor (DAF; CD55) and membrane inhibitor of reactive lysis (MIRL; CD59) to cell membranes. CD55 and CD59 and other proteins are involved in complement degradation (at the C3 and C5 levels), and in their absence the haemolytic action of complement continues. The molecular basis of PNH has been found to be mutations in the *pig*-A (phosphatidylinositol glycan protein A) gene responsible for synthesis of the GPI anchor.

Clinical features

The major clinical signs are intravascular haemolysis, venous thrombosis and haemoglobinuria. Haemolysis may be precipitated by infection, iron therapy or surgery. Characteristically only the urine voided at night and in the morning on waking is dark in colour, although the reason for this phenomenon is not clear. In severe cases all urine samples are dark. Urinary iron loss may be sufficient to cause iron deficiency.

Some patients present insidiously with signs of anaemia and recurrent abdominal pains.

Venous thrombotic episodes are very common in unusual places and severe thromboses may occur, for example in hepatic (Budd–Chiari syndrome), mesenteric or cerebral veins. The cause of the increased predisposition to thrombosis is not known, but may be due to complement-mediated activation of platelets deficient in CD55 and CD59.

Investigations

- **Intravascular haemolysis** is evident (see p. 437).
- **Flow cytometric analysis** of red cells with anti-CD55 and anti-CD59 has replaced the Ham's test.
- **Bone marrow** is sometimes hypoplastic (or even aplastic) despite haemolysis.

Treatment and prognosis

PNH is a chronic disorder requiring supportive measures such as blood transfusions, which are necessary for patients with severe anaemia. Leucocyte-depleted blood should be used in order to prevent transfusion reactions resulting in complement activation and acceleration of the haemolysis. Recently a recombinant humanized monoclonal antibody (eculizumab) that prevents the cleavage of C5 (and therefore the formation of the membrane attack complex) has been shown to reduce intravascular haemolysis, haemoglobinuria and the need for transfusion in PNH.

Long-term anticoagulation may be necessary for patients with recurrent thrombotic episodes. In patients with bone marrow failure, treatment options include immunosuppression with antilymphocyte globulin, ciclosporin, or bone marrow transplantation. Bone marrow transplantation has been successfully carried out using either HLA-matched sibling donors in patients under the age of 50 or matched unrelated donors in patients under the age of 25.

The course of PNH is variable. PNH may transform into aplastic anaemia or acute leukaemia, but it may remain stable for many years and the PNH clone may even disappear, which must be taken into account if considering potentially dangerous treatments such as bone marrow transplantation. The median survival is 10–15 years.

Gene therapy will perhaps be possible in the future.

MECHANICAL HAEMOLYTIC ANAEMIA

Red cells may be injured by physical trauma in the circulation. Direct injury may cause immediate cell lysis or be followed by resealing of the cell membrane with the formation of distorted red cells or 'fragments'. These cells may circulate for a short period before being destroyed prematurely in the reticuloendothelial system.

The causes of mechanical haemolytic anaemia include:

- damaged artificial heart valves
- march haemoglobinuria, where there is damage to red cells in the feet associated with prolonged marching or running
- microangiopathic haemolytic anaemia (MAHA), where fragmentation of red cells occurs in an abnormal microcirculation caused by malignant hypertension, eclampsia, haemolytic uraemic syndrome, thrombotic thrombocytopenic purpura, vasculitis or disseminated intravascular coagulation.

FURTHER READING
Rosse WF, Nishimura J (2003) Clinical manifestations of paroxysmal nocturnal haemoglobinuria. *International Journal of Haematology* **77**: 113–120.
Schwartz RS (2004) Paroxysmal nocturnal haemoglobinuria. *New England Journal of Medicine* **350**: 537–538.

MYELOPROLIFERATIVE DISORDERS

In these disorders there is uncontrolled clonal proliferation of one or more of the cell lines in the bone marrow, namely erythroid, myeloid and megakaryocyte lines. Myeloproliferative disorders include polycythaemia vera (PV), essential thrombocythaemia (ET), myelofibrosis and chronic myeloid leukaemia (CML). These disorders are grouped together as there can be transition from one disease to another; for example PV can lead to myelofibrosis. They may also transform to acute

---

Table 8.16 Causes of polycythaemia

Primary
Polycythaemia vera

Secondary

Due to an appropriate increase in erythropoietin	*Due to an inappropriate increase in erythropoietin*
High altitude	*Congenital:* Chuvasch polycythaemia
Lung disease	*Renal disease:* tumours, cysts
Cardiovascular disease (right-to-left shunt)	*Liver disease:* hepatocellular carcinoma, cirrhosis
Heavy smoking	*Endocrine:* adrenal tumours
Mutant high oxygen affinity haemoglobin, e.g. congenital polycythaemia	*Tumours:* cerebellar haemangioblastoma, massive uterine fibroma, bronchial carcinoma
Relative	*Drugs:* erythropoietin, androgens
'Apparent' polycythaemia	
Dehydration	
Burns	

---

myeloblastic leukaemia. The non-leukaemic myeloproliferative disorders (PV, ET and myelofibrosis) will be discussed in this section. Chronic myeloid leukaemia is described on page 505.

POLYCYTHAEMIA

Polycythaemia (or erythrocytosis) is defined as an increase in haemoglobin, PCV and red cell count. PCV is a more reliable indicator of polycythaemia than is Hb, which may be disproportionately low in iron deficiency. Polycythaemia can be divided into absolute erythrocytosis where there is a true increase in red cell volume, or relative erythrocytosis where the red cell volume is normal but there is a decrease in the plasma volume (see Fig. 8.6).

Absolute erythrocytosis is due to primary polycythaemia (PV) or secondary polycythaemia. Secondary polycythaemia is due to either an appropriate increase in red cells in response to anoxia, or an inappropriate increase associated with tumours, such as a renal carcinoma. The causes of polycythaemia are given in Table 8.16.

Primary polycythaemia: polycythaemia vera (PV)

PV is a clonal stem cell disorder in which there is an alteration in the pluripotent progenitor cell leading to excessive proliferation of erythroid, myeloid and megakaryocytic progenitor cells. This is partly due to a failure of apoptosis as a result of deregulation of the *Bcl-x* gene (opposes programmed cell death, p. 162), in addition a mutation in the JAK2 protein has been found; this stimulates low grade erythropoeisis.

Clinical features

The onset is insidious. It usually presents in patients aged over 60 years with tiredness, depression, vertigo, tinnitus and visual disturbance. It should be noted that these symptoms are also common in the normal population over the age of 60 and consequently PV is easily missed. These features, together with hypertension, angina, intermittent claudication and a tendency to bleed, are suggestive of PV.

Severe itching after a hot bath or when the patient is warm is common. Gout due to increased cell turnover may be a feature, and peptic ulceration occurs in a minority of patients. Thrombosis and haemorrhage are the major complications of PV.

The patient is usually plethoric and has a deep dusky cyanosis. Injection of the conjunctivae is commonly seen. The spleen is palpable in 70% and is useful in distinguishing PV from secondary polycythaemia. The liver is enlarged in 50% of patients.

Investigations

- **Hb and PCV** are increased. The WBC is raised in about 70% of cases of PV and the platelet count is elevated in about 50%.
- **Bone marrow** shows erythroid hyperplasia and increased numbers of megakaryocytes.
- **Red cell volume** measured using ^{51}Cr-labelled red cells is increased (> 36 mL/kg in males and 32 mL/kg in females).
- **Plasma volume** shows normal or increased values (normal range is 45 ± 5 mL/kg).
- **Serum uric acid** levels may be raised.
- **Leucocyte alkaline phosphatase** (LAP) score is usually high.
- **Serum vitamin B_{12} and vitamin B_{12}-binding protein** transcobalamin I (TC I) levels may be high, although these are not routinely measured.

Differential diagnosis

An increase in the red cell volume should be established. Raised WBC and platelet counts with splenomegaly makes a diagnosis of PV very likely. The principal secondary causes can often be excluded by the history and examination, but a renal ultrasound, an arterial Po_2 and carboxyhaemoglobin levels are of additional help.

The serum erythropoietin level is not diagnostic but may be helpful in distinguishing PV from secondary polycythaemia. In PV the level is low or normal, whereas in secondary polycythaemia the level may be raised, as expected, but also can be normal.

Course and management

Treatment is designed to maintain a normal blood count and to prevent the complications of the disease, particularly thromboses and haemorrhage. *Treatment is* aimed at keeping the PCV below 0.45 L/L and the platelet count below $400 \times 10^9/L$. There are three types of specific treatment:

- **Venesection**. This will successfully relieve many of the symptoms of PV. Iron deficiency limits erythropoiesis. Venesection is often used as the sole treatment and other therapy is reserved to control the thrombocytosis.

- **Chemotherapy**. Continuous or intermittent treatment with hydroxycarbmide (hydroxyurea) is used frequently because of the ease of controlling thrombocytosis and general safety in comparison to the alkylating agents such as busulfan, which carry an increased risk of acute leukaemia. Low-dose intermittent busulfan may be more convenient for elderly people, and this must be weighed against the potential risk of long-term complications.
- **Radioactive ^{32}P**. One dose may give control for up to 18 months, but the administration of ^{32}P carries an increased risk of transformation to acute leukaemia. ^{32}P is confined to the over-70 years age group.

General treatment

Allopurinol is given to block uric acid production. Low-dose aspirin (100 mg daily) can safely prevent thrombotic complications in treated patients. The pruritus is lessened by avoiding very hot baths. H_1-receptor antagonists have largely proved unsuccessful in relieving distressing pruritus, but H_2-receptor antagonists such as cimetidine are occasionally effective.

Patients with uncontrolled PV have a high operative risk; 75% of patients have severe haemorrhage following surgery and 30% of these patients die. Polycythaemia should be controlled before surgery. In an emergency, reduction of the haematocrit by venesection and appropriate fluid replacement must be carried out.

Prognosis

PV develops into myelofibrosis in 30% of cases and into acute myeloblastic leukaemia in 5% as part of the natural history of the disease.

Secondary polycythaemias

Many high-oxygen affinity haemoglobin mutants (HOAHM) have been described which lead to increased oxygen affinity but decreased oxygen delivery to the tissues, resulting in compensatory polycythaemia. A congenital (autosomal recessive disorder – Chuvasch polycythaemia) is due to a defect in the oxygen-sensing erythropoietin production pathway caused by a mutation of the von Hippel–Lindau (VHL) gene, resulting in an increased production of erythropoietin.

The causes of secondary polycythaemias are shown in Table 8.16.

The treatment is that of the precipitating factor; for example, renal or posterior fossa tumours need to be resected. Heavy smoking can produce as much as 10% carboxyhaemoglobin and this can produce polycythaemia because of a reduction in the oxygen-carrying capacity of the blood. Complications of secondary polycythaemia are similar to those seen in PV, including thrombosis, haemorrhage and cardiac failure, but the complications due to myeloproliferative disease such as progression to myelofibrosis or acute leukaemia do not develop. Venesection may be symptomatically helpful in the hypoxic patient, particularly if the PCV is above 0.55 L/L.

'Relative' or 'apparent' polycythaemia (Gaisböck's syndrome)

This condition was originally thought to be stress-induced. The red cell volume is normal, but as the result of a decreased plasma volume, there is a relative poly-cythaemia. 'Relative' polycythaemia is more common than PV and occurs in middle-aged men, particularly in smokers who are obese and hypertensive. The condition may present with cardiovascular problems such as myocardial or cerebral ischaemia. For this reason, it may be justifiable to venesect the patient. Smoking should be stopped.

Essential thrombocythaemia (ET)

ET is closely related to PV. The platelet count is usually $> 1000 \times 10^9/L$. It presents with bruising, bleeding and cerebrovascular symptoms. Initially splenic hypertrophy may be seen but, as the condition progresses, recurrent thromboses owing to the increased number of platelets reduce the size of the spleen and it may atrophy.

ET should be distinguished from secondary throm-bocytosis that is seen in haemorrhage, connective tissue disorders, malignancy, after splenectomy and in other myeloproliferative disorders.

Treatment is with hydroxycarbamide (hydroxyurea), anagrelide or busulfan to control the platelet count to less than $400 \times 10^9/L$.

α-Interferon is also effective but it is expensive and is administered by subcutaneous injection. ET may eventually transform into PV, myelofibrosis or acute leukaemia, but the disease may not progress for many years.

MYELOFIBROSIS (MYELOSCLEROSIS)

The terms myelosclerosis and myelofibrosis are inter-changeable. There is clonal proliferation of stem cells and myeloid metaplasia in the liver, spleen and other organs. Increased fibrosis in the bone marrow is caused by hyper-plasia of abnormal megakaryocytes which release fibroblast-stimulating factors such as platelet-derived growth factor. In about 25% of cases there is a preceding history of PV.

Clinical features

The disease presents insidiously with lethargy, weakness and weight loss. Patients often complain of a 'fullness' in the upper abdomen due to splenomegaly. Severe pain related to respiration may indicate perisplenitis secondary to splenic infarction, and bone pain and attacks of gout can complicate the illness. Bruising and bleeding occur because of thrombocytopenia or abnormal platelet function. Other physical signs include anaemia, fever and massive splenomegaly (for other causes, see p. 457).

Investigations

- **Anaemia** with leucoerythroblastic features is present (p. 464). Poikilocytes and red cells with characteristic tear-drop forms are seen. The WBC count may be over $100 \times 10^9/L$, and the differential WBC count may be

very similar to that seen in chronic myeloid leukaemia (CML); later leucopenia may develop.

- **The platelet count** may be very high, but in later stages, thrombocytopenia occurs.
- **Bone marrow aspiration** is often unsuccessful and this gives a clue to the presence of the condition. A bone marrow trephine is necessary to show the markedly increased fibrosis. Increased numbers of megakary-ocytes may be seen.
- **The Philadelphia chromosome** is absent; this helps to distinguish myelofibrosis from most cases of CML.
- **The leucocyte alkaline phosphatase (LAP) score** is normal or high.
- **A high serum urate** is present.
- **Low serum folate** levels may occur owing to the increased haemopoietic activity.

Differential diagnosis

The major diagnostic difficulty is the differentiation of myelofibrosis from CML as in both conditions there may be marked splenomegaly and a raised WBC count with many granulocyte precursors seen in the peripheral blood. The main distinguishing features are the appear-ance of the bone marrow and the absence of the Philadelphia chromosome in myelofibrosis.

Fibrosis of the marrow, often with a leucoerythroblastic anaemia, can also occur secondarily to leukaemia or lymphoma, tuberculosis or malignant infiltration with metastatic carcinoma, or to irradiation.

Treatment

This consists of general supportive measures such as blood transfusion, folic acid, analgesics and allopurinol. Drugs such as hydroxycarbamide (hydroxyurea) and busulfan are used to reduce metabolic activity and high WBC count and platelet levels; hydroxycarbamide is the most common drug used. Chemotherapy and radio-therapy are used to reduce splenic size. If the spleen becomes very large and painful, and transfusion require-ments are high, it may be advisable to perform splenectomy. Splenectomy may also result in relief of severe thrombocytopenia.

Prognosis

Patients may survive for 10 years or more; median survival is 3 years. Death may occur in 10–20% of cases from transformation to acute myeloblastic leukaemia. The most common causes of death are cardiovascular disease, infection and gastrointestinal bleeding.

MYELODYSPLASIA (MDS)

Myelodysplasia (MDS) describes a group of acquired bone marrow disorders that are due to a defect in stem cells. They are characterized by increasing bone marrow failure with quantitative and qualitative abnormalities of all three myeloid cell lines (red cells, granulocyte/monocytes and platelets). The natural history of MDS is variable, but there is a high morbidity and mortality owing to bone marrow failure, and transformation into

Table 8.17 Classification of myelodysplasia (based on WHO and FAB)

	Category	Peripheral blasts (%)	Bone marrow (%)	Median prognosis (months)
1a	Refractory anaemia (RA)	< 1	Blasts < 5 RS < 15	≃ 50
2a	RA and ring sideroblasts (RARS)	< 1	Blasts < 5 RS > 15	≃ 50
3a	RA with excess blasts (RAEB) I	1–4	Blasts 5–10	10
3b	(RAEB-t) II	5–19	Blasts 11–19	5

In all categories, monocytes in the peripheral blood < 1.0×10^9/L
RS, ring sideroblasts; RAEB-t (in transformation) also includes the 5q syndrome (deletion of 5q⁻) – usually elderly females but with good prognosis

acute myeloblastic leukaemia occurs in about 30% of cases. A classification of the myelodsyplastic syndrome is shown in Table 8.17.

Clinical and laboratory features

MDS occurs mainly in the elderly, and presents with symptoms of anaemia, infection or bleeding due to pancytopenia. Serial blood counts show evidence of increasing bone marrow failure with anaemia, neutropenia, monocytosis and thrombocytopenia, either alone or in combination. In contrast, in chronic myelomonocytic leukaemias (CMML), monocytes are $> 1 \times 10^9$/L and the WBC count may be $> 100 \times 10^9$/L.

The bone marrow usually shows increased cellularity despite the pancytopenia. Dyserythropoiesis is present, and granulocyte precursors and megakaryocytes also have abnormal morphology. Ring sideroblasts are present in all types. In RAEB and RAEB-t, the number of blasts in the bone marrow is increased, and the prognosis is worse than in those types with a low number of blast cells (< 5%).

Management

Patients with < 5% blasts in the bone marrow are usually managed conservatively with red cell and platelet transfusions and antibiotics for infections, as they are needed. Haemopoietic growth factors (e.g. erythropoietin, G-CSF) may be useful in some patients.

Patients with > 5% blasts have a less favourable prognosis, and a number of treatment options are available:

- **Supportive care** only is suitable for elderly patients with other medical problems.
- **'Gentle' chemotherapy** (low-dose or single-agent, e.g. azacytidine) may be useful in patients with high WBC counts.
- **Intensive chemotherapy** schedules used for acute myeloblastic leukaemia (see p. 504) may be tried in patients under the age of 60, but the remission rate is less, and prolonged pancytopenia may occur owing to poor haemopoietic regeneration because of the defect in stem cells.
- **Bone marrow transplantation** offers the hope of cure in the small proportion of MDS patients who are under the age of 50 and who have an HLA-identical sibling or an unrelated HLA-matched donor.

FURTHER READING
Cazzola M, Malcovati L (2005) Myelodysplastic syndromes. *New England Journal of Medicine* **352**: 536–538.
Provan D, Weatherall D (2000) Red cells II: acquired anaemias. *Lancet* **355**: 1260–1268.
Schwartz RC (1998) Polycythaemia vera – chance, death and mutability. *New England Journal of Medicine* **338**: 613–615.
Spirak J (2004) Daily aspirin – only half the answer (in polycythaemia vera). *New England Journal of Medicine* **350**: 99–101.

THE SPLEEN

The spleen is the largest lymphoid organ in the body and is situated in the left hypochondrium. There are two anatomical components:

- the red pulp, consisting of sinuses lined by endothelial macrophages and cords (spaces)
- the white pulp, which has a structure similar to lymphoid follicles.

Blood enters via the splenic artery and is delivered to the red and white pulp. During the flow the blood is 'skimmed', with leucocytes and plasma preferentially passing to white pulp. Some red cells pass rapidly through into the venous system while others are held up in the red pulp.

Functions

Sequestration and phagocytosis. Normal red cells, which are flexible, pass through the red pulp into the venous system without difficulty. Old or abnormal cells are damaged by the hypoxia, low glucose and low pH found in the sinuses of the red pulp and are therefore removed by phagocytosis along with other circulating foreign matter. Howell–Jolly and Heinz bodies and sideroblastic granules have their particles removed by 'pitting' and are then returned to the circulation. IgG-coated red cells are removed through their Fc receptors by macrophages.

Extramedullary haemopoiesis. Pluripotential stem cells are present in the spleen and proliferate during severe haematological stress, such as in haemolytic anaemia or thalassaemia major.

Immunological function. About 25% of the body's T lymphocytes and 15% of B lymphocytes are present in the spleen. The spleen shares the function of production of antibodies with other lymphoid tissues.

Blood pooling. Up to one-third of the platelets are sequestrated in the spleen and can be rapidly mobilized. Enlarged spleens pool a significant percentage (up to 40%) of the red cell mass.

SPLENOMEGALY

Causes

A clinically palpable spleen can have many causes.

- Infection:
  - **(a)** acute – e.g. septic shock, infective endocarditis, typhoid, infectious mononucleosis
  - **(b)** chronic – e.g. tuberculosis and brucellosis
  - **(c)** parasitic – e.g. malaria, kala-azar and schistosomiasis.
- Inflammation: rheumatoid arthritis, sarcoidosis, SLE.
- Haematological: haemolytic anaemia, haemoglobinopathies and the leukaemias, lymphomas and myeloproliferative disorders.
- Portal hypertension: liver disease.
- Miscellaneous: storage diseases, amyloid, primary and secondary neoplasias, tropical splenomegaly.

Massive splenomegaly is seen in myelofibrosis, chronic myeloid leukaemia, chronic malaria, kala-azar or, rarely, Gaucher's disease.

Hypersplenism

This can result from splenomegaly due to any cause. It is commonly seen with splenomegaly due to haematological disorders, portal hypertension, rheumatoid arthritis (Felty's syndrome) and lymphoma. Hypersplenism produces:

- pancytopenia
- haemolysis due to sequestration and destruction of red cells in the spleen
- increased plasma volume.

Treatment is often dependent on the underlying cause, but splenectomy is sometimes required for severe anaemia or thrombocytopenia.

Splenectomy

Splenectomy is performed mainly for:

- trauma
- idiopathic thrombocytopenic purpura (p. 470)
- haemolytic anaemias (p. 441)
- hypersplenism.

Problems after splenectomy

An immediate problem is an increased platelet count (usually $600–1000 \times 10^9/L$) for 2–3 weeks. Thromboembolic phenomena may occur. In the longer term there

Vaccinate 2–3 weeks before elective splenectomy.

- A 23-valent unconjugated pneumococcal polysaccharide vaccine repeated every 5 years
- Meningococcal group C conjugate vaccine
- Annual influenza vaccine
- *Haemophilus influenzae* type b (Hib) vaccine
- Long-term penicillin V 500 mg 12-hourly (if sensitive, use erythromycin)
- Meningococcal polysaccharide vaccine (ACWY) for travellers to Africa/Saudi Arabia, e.g. during Hajj and Umrah pilgrimages.

is an increased risk of overwhelming infections, particularly pneumococcal infections.

Prophylaxis against infection after splenectomy or splenic dysfunction (Box 8.1)

All patients should be educated about the risk of infection and the importance of its early recognition and treatment. They should be given an information leaflet and should carry a card or bracelet to alert health professionals to their risk of overwhelming infection.

Postsplenectomy haematological features

- *Thrombocytosis* persists in about 30% of cases.
- *The WBC count* is usually normal but there may be a mild lymphocytosis and monocytosis.
- *Abnormalities in red cell morphology* are the most prominent changes and include Howell–Jolly bodies, Pappenheimer bodies (contain sideroblastic granules), target cells and irregular contracted red cells (see Fig. 8.28). Pitted red cells can be counted.

Splenic atrophy

This is seen in sickle cell disease due to infarction. It is also seen in coeliac disease, in dermatitis herpetiformis, and occasionally in ulcerative colitis and essential thrombocythaemia. Postsplenectomy haematological features are seen.

Fig. 8.28 Postsplenectomy film with Howell–Jolly bodies (arrowed), target cells and irregularly contracted cells.

FURTHER READING
Davies JM, Barnes R, Milligan D (2003) Update of guidelines for the prevention and treatment of infection in patients with an absent or dysfunctional spleen. *Clinical Medicine* **2**: 440–443.

BLOOD TRANSFUSION

The cells and proteins in the blood express antigens which are controlled by polymorphic genes; that is, a specific antigen may be present in some individuals but not in others. A blood transfusion may immunize the recipient against donor antigens that the recipient lacks (alloimmunization), and repeated transfusions increase the risk of the occurrence of alloimmunization. Similarly, the transplacental passage of fetal blood cells during pregnancy may alloimmunize the mother against fetal antigens inherited from the father. Antibodies stimulated by blood transfusion or pregnancy, such as Rhesus antibodies, are termed *immune* antibodies and are usually IgG, in contrast to *naturally occurring* antibodies, such as ABO antibodies, which are made in response to environmental antigens present in food and bacteria and which are usually IgM.

BLOOD GROUPS

The blood groups are determined by antigens on the surface of red cells; more than 400 blood groups have been found. The ABO and Rh systems are the two major blood groups, but incompatibilities involving many other blood groups (e.g. Kell, Duffy, Kidd) may cause haemolytic transfusion reactions and/or haemolytic disease of the newborn (HDN).

ABO system

This blood group system involves naturally occurring IgM anti-A and anti-B antibodies which are capable of producing rapid and severe intravascular haemolysis of incompatible red cells.

The ABO system is under the control of a pair of allelic genes, *H* and *h*, and also three allelic genes, *A*, *B* and *O*, producing the genotypes and phenotypes shown in Table 8.18. The A, B and H antigens are very similar in structure; differences in the terminal sugars determine their

Table 8.18 The ABO system: antigens and antibodies

Phenotype	Genotype	Antigens	Antibodies	Frequency UK (%)
O	OO	None	Anti-A and anti-B	44
A	AA or AO	A	Anti-B	45
B	BB or BO	B	Anti-A	8
AB	AB	A and B	None	3

specificity. The *H* gene codes for enzyme *H*, which attaches fucose to the basic glycoprotein backbone to form H substance, which is the precursor for A and B antigens (Fig. 8.29).

The *A* and *B* genes control specific enzymes responsible for the addition to H substance of *N*-acetylgalactosamine for Group A and D-galactose for Group B. The *O* gene is amorphic and does not transform H substance and therefore O is not antigenic. The A, B and H antigens are present on most body cells. These antigens are also found in soluble form in tissue fluids such as saliva and gastric juice in the 80% of the population who possess secretor genes.

Rh system

There is a high frequency of development of IgG RhD antibodies in RhD-negative individuals after exposure to RhD-positive red cells. The antibodies formed are of major importance in causing HDN and haemolytic transfusion reactions.

This system is coded by allelic genes, *C* and *c*, *E* and *e*, *D* and no *D*, which is signified as *d*; they are inherited as triplets on each chromosome, one from each pair of genes (i.e. *CDE/cde*). The presence of the d antigen has not been demonstrated and the presence or absence of the D antigen determines whether an individual is characterized as RhD positive or negative.

Fig. 8.29 **Sugar chains in the ABO blood group system.** Reproduced from Fricker J (1996) Conversion of red blood cells to group O. *Lancet* **347**: 680, © The Lancet Ltd. 1996.

PROCEDURE FOR BLOOD TRANSFUSION

The safety of blood transfusion depends on meticulous attention to detail at each stage leading to and during the transfusion. Avoidance of simple errors involving patient and blood sample identification at the time of collection of the sample for crossmatching and at the time of transfusion would avoid most serious haemolytic transfusion reactions, almost all of which involve the ABO system.

Pretransfusion compatibility testing

This involves a number of steps, outlined below.

Blood grouping
The ABO and RhD groups of the patient are determined.

Antibody screening
The patient's serum or plasma is screened for atypical antibodies that may cause a significant reduction in the survival of the transfused red cells. The patient's serum or plasma is tested against red cells from at least two group O donors, expressing a wide range of red cell antigens, for detection of IgM red cell alloantibodies (using a direct agglutination test of cells suspended in saline) and IgG antibodies (using an indirect antiglobulin test, see p. 449). About 10% of patients have a positive antibody screening result; in which case, further testing is carried out using a comprehensive panel of typed red cells to determine the blood group specificity of the antibody (clinically significant red cell antibodies are detected in about 20% of patients with positive antibody screens).

Selection of donor blood and crossmatching
Donor blood of the same ABO and RhD group as the patient is selected. Matching for additional blood groups is carried out for patients with clinically significant red cell antibodies (see below), for patients who are likely to be multitransfused and at high risk of developing antibodies, e.g. sickle cell disease, and many centres routinely provide c-negative and Kell-negative blood for women of child-bearing age to minimize the risk of alloimmunization and subsequent HDN.

Crossmatching procedures
Patients without atypical red cell antibodies. The full crossmatch involves testing the patient's serum or plasma against the donor red cells suspended in saline in a direct agglutination test, and also using an indirect antiglobulin test. In some hospitals the *serological crossmatch* has been omitted as the negative antibody screen makes it highly unlikely that there will be any incompatibility with the donor units. A greater risk is that of a transfusion error involving the collection of the patient sample or a mix-up of samples in the laboratory. Laboratories can use the blood bank computer to check its records of the patient and the donor units and authorize the release of the donor units if a number of criteria are met (*computer* or *electronic crossmatching*), including:

- The system is automated for ABO and RhD grouping and antibody screening including positive sample identification and electronic transfer of results.
- The antibody screening procedure conforms to national recommendations.
- The patient's serum or plasma does not contain clinically significant red cell antibodies.
- The release of ABO incompatible blood must be prevented by conformation of laboratory computer software to the following requirements:
  - (a) the issue of blood is not allowed if the patient has only been grouped once
  - (b) the issue of blood is not allowed if the current group does not match the historical record
  - (c) the system must not allow the reservation and release of units which are ABO incompatible with the patient.
- The laboratory must assure the validity of the ABO and RhD group of the donor blood either by written verification from the National Blood Service or confirmatory testing in the laboratory; the UK National Blood Service guarantees that the blood group information is correct.

Alternatively, the crossmatch can be shortened to an immediate spin crossmatch where the patient's serum or plasma is briefly incubated with the donor red cells, followed by centrifugation and examination for agglutination; this rapid crossmatch is an acceptable method of excluding ABO incompatibility in patients known to have a negative antibody screen.

Patients with atypical red cell antibodies. Donor blood should be selected that lacks the relevant red cell antigen(s), as well as being the same ABO and RhD group as the patient. A full crossmatch should always be carried out.

Several other systems for blood grouping, antibody screening and crossmatching are available to hospital transfusion laboratories. They do not depend on agglutination of red cells in suspension, but rather on the differential passage of agglutinated and unagglutinated red cells through a column of dextran gel matrix (e.g. DiaMed, and Ortho Biovue systems), or on the capture of antibodies by red cells immobilized on the surface of a microplate well (e.g. Capture-R solid phase system).

Blood ordering

Elective surgery
Many hospitals have guidelines for the ordering of blood for elective surgery (maximum surgical blood ordering schedules). These are aimed at reducing unnecessary crossmatching and the amount of blood that eventually becomes outdated. Many operations in which blood is required only occasionally for unexpectedly high blood loss can be classified as 'group and save'; this means that, where the antibody screen is negative, blood is not reserved in advance but can be made available quickly if necessary, using serum or plasma saved in the laboratory.

If a patient has atypical antibodies, compatible blood should always be reserved in advance.

Emergencies

There may be insufficient time for full pretransfusion testing. The options include:

■ Blood required immediately – use of 2 units of O RhD negative blood ('*emergency stock*'), to allow additional time for the laboratory to group the patient.
■ Blood required in 10–15 minutes – use of blood of the same ABO and RhD groups as the patient.
■ Blood required in 45 minutes – most laboratories will be able to provide fully crossmatched blood within this time.

COMPLICATIONS OF BLOOD TRANSFUSION
(see Table 8.19)

In the United States, it has been mandatory to report transfusion-associated deaths to the Food and Drug Administration since 1975; such reports have provided useful data which have contributed to efforts to improve the safety of blood transfusion. Similar reporting schemes under the term '*haemovigilance*' have been set up in other countries, including the Serious Hazards of Transfusion (SHOT) scheme which produced its first report in the UK in 1997. Figure 8.30 shows the reports to SHOT in 2002/03, indicating that '*incorrect blood component transfused*' was the most frequent type of serious incident. Errors in collection and administration of blood were the commonest source of error followed by laboratory errors and mistakes in the prescription of blood or the collection of blood samples for compatibility testing. Death or serious morbidity can also be attributed to other complications of blood transfusion including transfusion-associated lung injury (TRALI), transfusion-associated graft-versus-host disease (TA-GvHD), and bacterial infection of blood components.

Table 8.19 Complications of blood transfusion	
Immunological	**Non-immunological**
Alloimmunization and incompatibility	***Transmission of infection***
Red cells	Viruses:
Immediate haemolytic transfusion reactions	HAV, HBV, HCV
	HIV
Delayed haemolytic transfusion reactions	CMV, EBV, HTLV-1, West Nile virus
Leucocytes and platelets	Parasites:
Non-haemolytic (febrile) transfusion reactions	malaria, trypanosomiasis
Post-transfusion purpura	toxoplasmosis
Poor survival of transfused platelets and granulocytes	Bacteria
	Prion – vCJD
	Circulatory failure due to volume overload
Graft-versus-host disease	***Iron overload*** due to multiple transfusions (see p. 441)
Lung injury (TRALI)	***Massive transfusion*** of stored blood may cause
Plasma proteins	bleeding reactions and
Urticarial and anaphylactic reactions	electrolyte changes
	Physical damage due to freezing or heating
	Thrombophlebitis
	Air embolism

Immunological complications

Alloimmunization and incompatibility

Blood transfusion carries a risk of alloimmunization to the many 'foreign' antigens present on red cells, leucocytes, platelets and plasma proteins. Alloimmunization may also occur during pregnancy – to fetal antigens inherited from the father and not shared by the mother (p. 451).

Alloimmunization does not usually cause clinical problems with the first transfusion but these may occur with subsequent transfusions. There may also be delayed consequences of alloimmunization, such as HDN and rejection of tissue transplants.

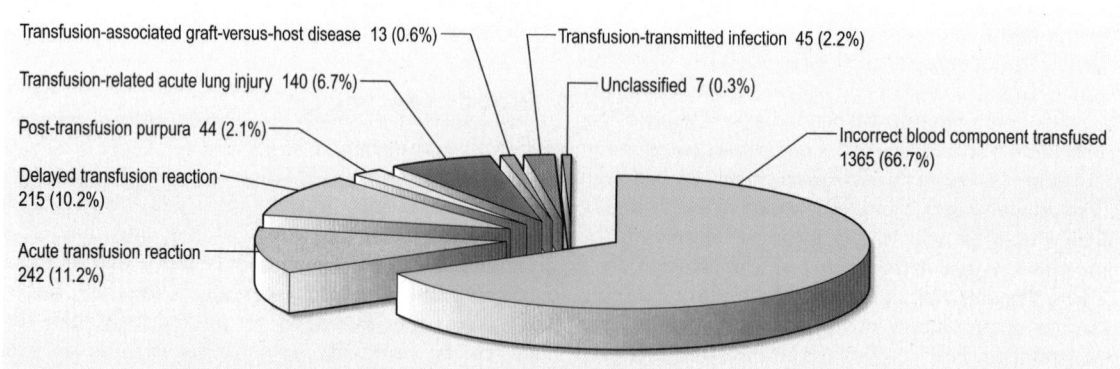

Fig. 8.30 Overview of 2191 cases reported to the Serious Hazards of Transfusion (SHOT) scheme between 1996 and 2003.

Incompatibility

This may result in poor survival of transfused cells, such as red cells and platelets, and also in the harmful effects of antigen–antibody reaction.

Red cells

Haemolytic transfusion reactions

Immediate reaction. This is the most serious complication of blood transfusion and is usually due to ABO incompatibility. There is complement activation by the antigen–antibody reaction, usually caused by IgM antibodies, leading to rigors, lumbar pain, dyspnoea, hypotension, haemoglobinuria and renal failure. The initial symptoms may occur a few minutes after starting the transfusion. Activation of coagulation may also occur and bleeding due to disseminated intravascular coagulation (DIC) is a bad prognostic sign. Emergency treatment may be needed to maintain the blood pressure and renal function.

Diagnosis

This is confirmed by finding evidence of haemolysis (e.g. haemoglobinuria), and incompatibility between donor and recipient. All documentation should be checked to detect errors such as:

- failure to check the identity of the patient when taking the sample for compatibility testing (i.e. sample from the wrong patient)
- mislabelling the blood sample with the wrong patient's name
- simple labelling or handling errors in the laboratory
- errors in the collection of blood, leading to delivery of the wrong blood to the ward/theatre
- failure to perform proper identity checks before the blood is transfused (i.e. blood transfused to the wrong patient).

The serious consequences of such failures emphasize the need for meticulous checks at all stages in the procedure of blood transfusion.

Investigations

To confirm where the error occurred, blood grouping should be carried out on:

- the patient's original sample (used for the compatibility testing)
- a new sample taken from the patient after the reaction
- the donor units.

At the first suspicion of any serious transfusion reaction, the transfusion should always be stopped and the donor units returned to the blood transfusion laboratory with a new blood sample from the patient to exclude a haemolytic transfusion reaction.

Delayed reaction. This may occur in patients alloimmunized by previous transfusions or pregnancies. The antibody level is too low to be detected by pretransfusion compatibility testing, but a secondary immune response occurs after transfusion, resulting in destruction of the transfused cells, usually by IgG antibodies.

Haemolysis is usually extravascular as the antibodies are IgG, and the patient may develop anaemia and jaundice about a week after the transfusion, although most of these episodes are clinically silent. The blood film shows spherocytosis and reticulocytosis. The direct antiglobulin test is positive and detection of the antibody is usually straightforward.

Leucocytes and platelets

Non-haemolytic (febrile) transfusion reactions

Febrile reactions are a common complication of blood transfusion in patients who have previously been transfused or pregnant. The usual causes are the presence of leucocyte antibodies in an alloimmunized recipient acting against donor leucocytes in red cell concentrates leading to release of pyrogens, or the release of cytokines from donor leucocytes in platelet concentrates. Typical signs are flushing and tachycardia, fever (> 38°C), chills and rigors. Aspirin may be used to reduce the fever, although it should not be used in patients with thrombocytopenia. The introduction of leucocyte-depleted blood in the UK, to minimize the risk of transmission of variant Creutzfeldt–Jakob disease (vCJD) by blood transfusion (see below), has reduced the incidence of febrile reactions.

Potent leucocyte antibodies in the plasma of donors, who are usually multiparous women, may cause severe pulmonary reactions (called transfusion-related acute lung injury or TRALI) characterized by dyspnoea, fever, cough, and shadowing in the perihilar and lower lung fields on the chest X-ray.

Plasma proteins

Urticaria and anaphylaxis

Urticarial reactions are often attributed to plasma protein incompatibility, but in most cases, they are unexplained. They are common but rarely severe; stopping or slowing the transfusion and administration of chlorphenamine (chlorpheniramine) 10 mg i.v. are usually sufficient treatment.

Anaphylactic reactions (see p. 997) occasionally occur; severe reactions are seen in patients lacking IgA who produce anti-IgA that reacts with IgA in the transfused blood. The transfusion should be stopped and epinephrine (adrenaline) 0.5 mg i.m. and chlorphenamine 10 mg i.v. should be given immediately; endotracheal intubation may be required. Patients who have had severe urticarial or anaphylactic reactions should receive either washed red cells, autologous blood, or blood from IgA-deficient donors for patients with IgA deficiency.

Non-immunological complications

Transmission of infection

Viral contamination: donor blood in the UK is currently tested for HBV, HCV, HIV-1 and HTLV-1. CMV-seronegative tested blood is given to immunosuppressed patients who are susceptible to acquiring CMV. Blood Services continue a vigilant search for new infectious agents. Donor questionnaires now record recent travel to exclude possible risks of West Nile virus (WNV) and severe acute respiratory syndrome (SARS). Recently, WNV has been the causal agent of meningoencephalitis transmitted by transfusion or transplantation in the USA.

The incidence of transmission of HBV is about 1 in 900 000 units transfused, and it is less than 1 in 30 million units transfused for HCV since the introduction of testing minipools of donor plasma (48 donations per pool) for viral DNA.

In the UK the incidence of transmission of HIV by blood transfusion is extremely low – under 1 in 8 million units transfused. Prevention is based on self-exclusion of donors in 'high-risk' groups and testing each donation for anti-HIV.

There is still a potential risk of viral transmission from coagulation factor concentrates prepared from large pools of plasma. Measures for inactivating viruses such as treatment with solvents and detergents are undertaken. Viral transmission via blood transfusion is still a major issue in the developing world.

Bacterial contamination of blood components is rare but it is one of the most frequent causes of death associated with transfusion. Some organisms such as *Yersinia enterocolitica* can proliferate in red cell concentrates stored at 4°C, but platelet concentrates stored at 22°C are a more frequent cause of this problem. Systems to avoid bacterial contamination include automated culture systems and bacterial antigen detection systems, but none are currently in routine use in the UK.

Transfusion-transmitted syphilis is very rare in the UK. Spirochaetes do not survive for more than 72 hours in blood stored at 4°C, and each donation is tested using the *Treponema pallidum haemagglutination assay* (TPHA).

There continues to be concern about the risk of transmitting the prion protein causing vCJD (p. 60) by transfusion: a possible transmission occurred following a transfusion in 2003. A number of measures have been taken in the UK, including universal leucocyte depletion of blood components (in 1999) because the prion protein is thought to be primarily associated with lymphocytes. UK donor plasma is not used for the manufacture of blood products; imported plasma from the US is used instead. For children born after January 1 1996, fresh frozen plasma (FFP) is sourced from plasma (from unremunerated donors) imported from the USA, on the basis that exposure to bovine spongiform encephalitis (BSE) from food was eliminated by 1 January 1996. FFP for this group is treated with methylthioninium chloride (methylene blue) to inactivate viruses. Blood donors must not have had a blood transfusion since 1980.

While stringent measures are being taken to minimize the risk of transfusion-transmitted infection in the UK, it may never be possible to guarantee that donor blood is absolutely 'safe'. The current approach to the safety of blood components and plasma in the UK is extremely cautious, but it is not an absolute guarantee of safety. Clinicians should always carefully consider the patient's requirement for transfusion, and only transfuse if clinically appropriate.

Immunosuppression

Ever since observations were made of the favourable effect of transfusion on survival of subsequent renal allografts, the basis of transfusion-induced immunomodulation has been the subject of debate. It is assumed that allogeneic leucocytes are required to cause transfusion-induced immunosuppression, but the underlying mechanisms remain uncertain. There has been considerable interest in other clinical effects caused by transfusion-induced immunosuppression, such as postoperative infection and tumour recurrence.

Strategies for avoiding or reducing the use of blood transfusion should be used. These include stopping drug therapy that may cause bleeding and treatment of anaemia prior to surgery.

Strict criteria for the use of blood components and blood products must be in place.

Artificial haemoglobin solutions and other blood substitutes are in clinical trial. They have a short intravascular half-life, and are likely to find their initial clinical application in trauma and surgery.

Autologous transfusion

An alternative to using blood from volunteer donors is to use the patient's own blood. There are three types of autologous transfusion:

- *Predeposit.* The patient donates 2–5 units of blood at approximately weekly intervals before elective surgery.
- *Preoperative haemodilution.* One or two units of blood are removed from the patient immediately before surgery and retransfused to replace operative losses.
- *Blood salvage.* Blood lost during or after surgery may be collected and retransfused. Several techniques of varying levels of sophistication are available. The operative site must be free of bacteria, bowel contents and tumour cells.

There is little demand for pre-deposit autologous transfusion in the UK as blood is generally perceived as being 'safe'. Blood salvage is increasingly being used as a way of avoiding the use of donor blood. In developing countries, autologous blood and blood from relatives are commonly used.

BLOOD, BLOOD COMPONENTS AND BLOOD PRODUCTS

Most blood collected from donors is processed as follows:

- **Blood components**, such as red cell and platelet concentrates, fresh frozen plasma (FFP) and cryoprecipitate, are prepared from a single donation of blood by simple separation methods such as centrifugation and are transfused without further processing.
- **Blood products**, such as coagulation factor concentrates, albumin and immunoglobulin solutions, are prepared by complex processes using the plasma from many donors as the starting material (UK donor plasma is not used, see above).

In most circumstances it is preferable to transfuse only the blood component or product required by the patient (component therapy) rather than use whole blood. This is the most effective way of using donor blood, which is a scarce resource, and reduces the risk of complications from transfusion of unnecessary components of the blood.

Whole blood
The average volume of blood withdrawn is 470 mL taken into 63 mL of anticoagulant. Blood stored at 4°C has a 'shelf-life' of 5 weeks when at least 70% of the transfused red cells should survive normally. Whole blood is rarely used; packed cells or red cell concentrates plus crystalloid or colloid solutions are acceptable alternatives even for the management of acute blood loss.

Red cell concentrates
Virtually all the plasma is removed and is replaced by about 100 mL of an optimal additive solution, such as SAG-M, which contains sodium chloride, adenine, glucose and mannitol. The mean volume is about 330 mL. The PCV is about 0.57 L/L, but the viscosity is low as there are no plasma proteins in the additive solution, and this allows fast administration if necessary. All blood components (red cell and platelet concentrates, and plasma) are leucocyte-depleted in the UK by filtration within 48 hours of collection of the donor blood.

Washed red cell concentrates
These are preparations of red cells suspended in saline, produced by cell separators to remove all but traces of plasma proteins. They are used in patients who have had severe recurrent urticarial or anaphylactic reactions.

Platelet concentrates
These are prepared either from whole blood by centrifugation or by plateletpheresis of single donors using cell separators. They may be stored for up to 5 days at 22°C. They are used to treat bleeding in patients with severe thrombocytopenia, and prophylactically to prevent bleeding in patients with bone marrow failure.

Granulocyte concentrates
These are prepared from single donors using cell separators and are used for patients with severe neutropenia with definite evidence of bacterial infection. The numbers of granulocytes are increased by treating donors with G-CSF and steroids.

Fresh frozen plasma
FFP is prepared by freezing the plasma from 1 unit of blood at −30°C within 6 hours of donation. The volume is approximately 200 mL. FFP contains all the coagulation factors present in fresh plasma and is used mostly for replacement of coagulation factors in acquired coagulation factor deficiencies. For children, see p. 462.

Cryoprecipitate
This is obtained by allowing the frozen plasma from a single donation to thaw at 4–8°C and removing the supernatant. The volume is about 20 mL and it is stored at −30°C. It contains factor VIII:C, von Willebrand factor (vWF) and fibrinogen, and may be useful in DIC and other conditions where the fibrinogen level is very low. It is no longer used for the treatment of haemophilia A and von Willebrand's disease because of the greater risk of virus transmission compared with virus-inactivated coagulation factor concentrates.

Factor VIII and IX concentrates
These are freeze-dried preparations of specific coagulation factors prepared from large pools of plasma. They are used for treating patients with haemophilia and von Willebrand's disease, where recombinant coagulation factor concentrates are unavailable. Recombinant coagulation factor concentrates, where they are available, are the treatment of choice for patients with inherited coagulation factor deficiencies (see p. 472).

Albumin
There are two preparations:

- *Human albumin solution 4.5%*, previously called plasma protein fraction (PPF), contains 45 g/L albumin and 160 mmol/L sodium. It is available in 50, 100, 250 and 500 mL bottles.
- *Human albumin solution 20%*, previously called 'salt-poor' albumin, contains approximately 200 g/L albumin and 130 mmol/L sodium and is available in 50 and 100 mL bottles.

Human albumin solutions are generally considered to be inappropriate fluids for acute volume replacement or for the treatment of shock because they are no more effective in these situations than synthetic colloid solutions such as polygelatins (Gelofusine) or hydroxyethyl starch (Haemaccel). However, albumin solutions are indicated for treatment of acute severe hypoalbuminaemia and as the replacement fluid for plasma exchange. The 20% albumin solution is particularly useful for patients with nephrotic syndrome or liver disease who are fluid overloaded and resistant to diuretics. Albumin solutions should not be used to treat patients with malnutrition or chronic renal or liver disease with low serum albumin.

Normal immunoglobulin
This is prepared from normal plasma. It is used in patients with hypogammaglobulinaemia, to prevent infections, and in patients with, e.g. idiopathic thrombocytopenia (p. 470).

Specific immunoglobulins
These are obtained from donors with high titres of antibodies. Many preparations are available, such as anti-D, anti-hepatitis B, and anti-varicella zoster.

FURTHER READING

Dodd RY (2003) Emerging infections, transfusion safety, and epidemiology. *New England Journal of Medicine* **349**: 1205–1206.

Goodnough LT, Shander A, Brecher ME (2003) Transfusion medicine: looking to the future. *Lancet* **361**: 161–169.

Klein HG (2000) The prospect for red cell substitutes. *New England Journal of Medicine* **342**: 1666–1668.

Murphy MF, Pamphilon D (eds) (2001) *Practical Transfusion Medicine*. Oxford: Blackwell Science.

Turner M (1999) The impact of new-variant Creutzfeldt–Jakob disease on blood transfusion practice. *British Journal of Haematology* **106**: 842–850.

THE WHITE CELL (see also Ch. 4)

The five types of leucocytes found in peripheral blood are neutrophils, eosinophils and basophils (which are all called *granulocytes*) and lymphocytes and monocytes. The development of these cells is shown in Figure 8.1.

NEUTROPHILS

The earliest morphologically identifiable precursors of neutrophils in the bone marrow are myeloblasts, which are large cells constituting up to 3.5% of the nucleated cells in the marrow. The nucleus is large and contains 2–5 nucleoli. The cytoplasm is scanty and contains no granules. Promyelocytes are similar to myeloblasts but have some primary cytoplasmic granules, containing enzymes such as myeloperoxidase. Myelocytes are smaller cells without nucleoli but with more abundant cytoplasm and both primary and secondary granules. Indentation of the nucleus marks the change from myelocyte to metamyelocyte. The mature neutrophil is a smaller cell with a nucleus with 2–5 lobes, with predominantly secondary granules in the cytoplasm which contain lysozyme, collagenase and lactoferrin.

Peripheral blood neutrophils are equally distributed into a circulating pool and a marginating pool lying along the endothelium of blood vessels. In contrast to the prolonged maturation time of about 10 days for neutrophils in the bone marrow, their half-life in the peripheral blood is extremely short, only 6–8 hours. In response to stimuli (e.g. infection, corticosteroid therapy) neutrophils are released into the circulating pool from both the marginating pool and the marrow. Immature white cells are released from the marrow when a rapid response (within hours) occurs in acute infection (described as a 'shift to the left' on a blood film).

Function

The prime function of neutrophils is to ingest and kill bacteria, fungi and damaged cells. Neutrophils are attracted to sites of infection or inflammation by chemotaxins. Recognition of foreign or dead material is aided by coating of particles with immunoglobulin and complement (opsonization) as neutrophils have Fc and C3b receptors (see p. 201). The material is ingested into vacuoles where it is subjected to enzymic destruction, which is either oxygen-dependent with the generation of hydrogen peroxide (myeloperoxidase) or oxygen-independent (lysosomal enzymes and lactoferrin). Leucocyte alkaline phosphatase (LAP) is an enzyme found in leucocytes. It is raised when there is a neutrophilia due to an acute illness. It is also raised in the polycythaemia and myelofibrosis and reduced in CML.

Neutrophil leucocytosis

A rise in the number of circulating neutrophils to $> 10 \times 10^9/L$ occurs in bacterial infections or as a result of tissue damage. This may also be seen in pregnancy, during exercise and after corticosteroid administration (Table 8.20). With any tissue necrosis there is a release of various soluble factors, causing a leucocytosis. Interleukin-1 is also released in tissue necrosis and causes a pyrexia. The pyrexia and leucocytosis accompanying a myocardial infarction are a good example of this and may be wrongly attributed to infection.

A leukaemoid reaction (an overproduction of white cells, with many immature cells) may occur in severe infections, tuberculosis, malignant infiltration of the bone marrow and occasionally after haemorrhage or haemolysis.

In leucoerythroblastic anaemia, nucleated red cells and white cell precursors are found in the peripheral blood. Causes include marrow infiltration with metastatic carcinoma, myelofibrosis, osteopetrosis, myeloma, lymphoma, and occasionally severe haemolytic or megaloblastic anaemia.

Neutropenia and agranulocytosis

Neutropenia is defined as a circulatory neutrophil count below $1.5 \times 10^9/L$. A virtual absence of neutrophils is called agranulocytosis. The causes are given in Table 8.21. It should be noted that black patients may have somewhat lower neutrophil counts. Neutropenia caused by viruses is probably the most common type. Chemotherapy

---

Table 8.20   Neutrophil leucocytosis

Bacterial infections
Tissue necrosis, e.g. myocardial infarction, trauma
Inflammation, e.g. gout, rheumatoid arthritis
Drugs, e.g. corticosteroids, lithium
Haematological:
   myeloproliferative disease
   leukaemoid reaction
   leucoerythroblastic anaemia
Physiological, e.g. pregnancy, exercise
Malignant disease, e.g. bronchial, breast, gastric
Metabolic, e.g. renal failure, acidosis
Congenital, e.g. leucocyte adhesion deficiency, hereditary
   neutrophilia

Table 8.21   Causes of neutropenia

Acquired
Viral infection
Severe bacterial infection, e.g. typhoid
Felty's syndrome
Immune neutropenia – autoimmune, autoimmune neonatal
  neutropenia
Pancytopenia from any cause, including drug-induced
  marrow aplasia (see p. 435)
Pure white cell aplasia

Inherited
Ethnic (neutropenia is common in black races)
Kostmann's syndrome (severe infantile agranulocytosis)
Cyclical (genetic defect with neutropenia every 2–3 weeks)
Others, e.g. Schwachman–Diamond syndrome,
  dyskeratosis congenita, Chédiak–Higashi syndrome

Table 8.22   Causes of eosinophilia

Parasitic infestations, such as:	Pulmonary disorders, such as:
Ascaris	Bronchial asthma
Hookworm	Tropical pulmonary
Strongyloides	eosinophilia
	Allergic bronchopulmonary
Allergic disorders, such as:	aspergillosis
Hayfever (allergic rhinitis)	Churg–Strauss syndrome
Other hypersensitivity reactions, including drug reactions	**Malignant disorders,** such as:
	Hodgkin's lymphoma
	Carcinoma
Skin disorders, such as:	Eosinophilic leukaemia
Urticaria	
Pemphigus	**Miscellaneous,** such as:
Eczema	Hypereosinophilic syndrome
	Sarcoidosis
	Hypoadrenalism
	Eosinophilic gastroenteritis

and radiotherapy predictably produce neutropenia; many other drugs have been known to produce an idiosyncratic cytopenia and a drug cause should always be considered.

Clinical features

Infections may be frequent, often serious, and are more likely as the neutrophil count falls. An absolute neutrophil count of less than $0.5 \times 10^9/L$ is regarded as 'severe' neutropenia and may be associated with life-threatening infections such as pneumonia and septicaemia. A characteristic glazed mucositis occurs in the mouth, and ulceration is common.

Investigations

The blood film shows marked neutropenia. The appearance of the bone marrow will indicate whether the neutropenia is due to depressed production or increased destruction of neutrophils. Neutrophil antibody studies are performed if an immune mechanism is suspected.

Treatment

Antibiotics should be given as necessary to patients with acute severe neutropenia (see p. 495).

If the neutropenia seems likely to have been caused by a drug, all current drug therapy should be stopped. Recovery of the neutrophil count usually occurs after about 10 days. G-CSF (see p. 421) is used to decrease the period of neutropenia after chemotherapy and haemopoietic transplantation. It is also used successfully in the treatment of chronic neutropenia.

Steroids and high-dose intravenous immunoglobulin are used to treat patients with severe autoimmune neutropenia and recurrent infections, and G-CSF has produced responses in some cases.

EOSINOPHILS

Eosinophils are slightly larger than neutrophils and are characterized by a nucleus with usually two lobes and large cytoplasmic granules that stain deeply red. The eosinophil plays a part in allergic responses (p. 200) and in the defence against infections with helminths and protozoa.

Eosinophilia is $> 0.4 \times 10^9/L$ eosinophils in the peripheral blood. The causes of eosinophilia are listed in Table 8.22.

BASOPHILS

The nucleus of basophils is similar to that of neutrophils but the cytoplasm is filled with large black granules. The granules contain histamine, heparin and enzymes such as myeloperoxidase. The physiological role of the basophil is not known. Binding of IgE causes the cells to degranulate and release histamine and other contents involved in acute hypersensitivity reactions (p. 220).

Basophils are usually few in number ($< 1 \times 10^9/L$) but are significantly increased in myeloproliferative disorders.

MONOCYTES

Monocytes are slightly larger than neutrophils. The nucleus has a variable shape and may be round, indented or lobulated. The cytoplasm contains fewer granules than neutrophils. Monocytes are precursors of tissue macrophages and spend only a few hours in the blood but can continue to proliferate in the tissues for many years.

A monocytosis ($> 0.8 \times 10^9/L$) may be seen in chronic bacterial infections such as tuberculosis or infective endocarditis, chronic neutropenia and patients with myelodysplasia, particularly chronic myelomonocytic leukaemia.

LYMPHOCYTES

Lymphocytes form nearly half the circulating white cells. They descend from pluripotential stem cells (see Fig. 8.1).

Circulating lymphocytes are small cells, a little larger than red cells, with a dark-staining central nucleus. There are two main types: T and B lymphocytes (see p. 205).

Lymphocytosis (lymphocyte count $> 5 \times 10^9/\text{L}$) occurs in response to viral infections, particularly EBV, CMV and HIV, and chronic infections such as tuberculosis and toxoplasmosis. It also occurs in chronic lymphocytic leukaemia and in some lymphomas.

FURTHER READING
Stock W, Hoffman R (2000) White blood cells 1: non-malignant disorders. *Lancet* **355**: 1351–1356.

HAEMOSTASIS AND THROMBOSIS

The integrity of the circulation is maintained by blood flowing through intact vessels lined by endothelial cells. Injury to the vessel wall exposes collagen and together with tissue injury sets in motion a series of events leading to haemostasis.

HAEMOSTASIS

Haemostasis is a complex process depending on interactions between the vessel wall, platelets and coagulation and fibrinolytic mechanisms. The formation of the haemostatic plug is shown in Figure 8.31.

Vessel wall
The vessel wall is lined by endothelium which, in normal conditions, prevents platelet adhesion and thrombus formation. This property is partly due to its negative charge but also to:

- thrombomodulin and heparan sulphate expression
- synthesis of prostacyclin (PGI_2) and nitric oxide (NO), which cause vasodilatation and inhibit platelet aggregation
- production of plasminogen activator.

Injury to vessels causes reflex vasoconstriction, while endothelial damage results in loss of antithrombotic properties, activation of platelets and coagulation and inhibition of fibrinolysis (Fig. 8.31).

Platelets
Platelet adhesion (Fig. 8.31a) to collagen is dependent on platelet membrane receptors: glycoprotein Ia (GPIa), which binds directly to collagen; and glycoprotein Ib (GPIb), which binds to von Willebrand factor (vWF) in the plasma, and vWF in turn adheres to collagen. Following adhesion, platelets undergo a shape change from a disc to a sphere, spread along the subendothelium and release the contents of their cytoplasmic granules, i.e. the dense bodies (containing ADP and serotonin) and the α-granules (containing platelet-derived growth factor, heparin antagonist (platelet factor 4), β-thromboglobulin, fibrinogen, vWF, fibronectin, thrombospondin and other factors).

Fig. 8.31 Formation of the haemostatic plug: sequential interactions between the vessel wall, platelets and coagulation factors.
(a) Contact of platelets with collagen, either via the platelet receptor GPIb and factor vWF in plasma, or directly via GPIa, activates platelet prostaglandin synthesis which stimulates release of ADP from the dense bodies. Vasoconstriction of the vessel occurs as a reflex and by release of serotonin and thromboxane A_2 (TXA_2) from platelets.
(b) Release of ADP from platelets induces platelet aggregation and formation of the platelet plug. The coagulation pathway is stimulated leading to formation of fibrin.
(c) Fibrin strands are cross-linked by factor XIII and stabilize the haemostatic plug by binding platelets and red cells. PF-3, platelet factor-3 (platelet phospholipid).

Platelet release: the release of ADP leads to a conformational change in the fibrinogen receptor, the glycoprotein IIb–IIIa complex (GPIIb–IIIa), on the surfaces of adherent platelets allowing it to bind to fibrinogen (see also Fig. 8.39).

Fig. 8.32 Prostaglandin synthesis.

Fig. 8.33 Coagulation mechanism. The in vivo pathway begins with the activation of factor IX by factor VIIa. Factor XI is activated by thrombin. TFPI, tissue factor pathway inhibitor.

Platelet aggregation (Fig. 8.31b): fibrinogen then binds platelets into activated aggregates (platelet aggregation) and further platelet release occurs. A self-perpetuating cycle of events is set up leading to formation of a platelet plug at the site of the injury.

Coagulation: further platelet membrane receptors, e.g. P_2Y_{12}, are exposed during aggregation, providing a surface for the interaction of coagulation factors; this platelet phospholipid activity is referred to as platelet factor 3 (PF-3). The presence of thrombin encourages fusion of platelets, and fibrin formation reinforces the stability of the platelet plug.

Central to normal platelet function is platelet *prostaglandin synthesis*, which is induced by platelet activation and leads to the formation of TXA_2 in platelets (Fig. 8.32). Thromboxane (TXA_2) is a powerful vasoconstrictor and also lowers cyclic AMP levels and initiates the platelet release reaction.

Prostacyclin (PGI_2) is synthesized in vascular endothelial cells and opposes the actions of TXA_2. It produces vasodilatation and increases the level of cyclic AMP, preventing platelet aggregation on the normal vessel wall as well as limiting the extent of the initial platelet plug after injury.

Coagulation and fibrinolysis

Coagulation involves a series of enzymatic reactions leading to the conversion of soluble plasma fibrinogen to fibrin clot (Fig. 8.33). Roman numerals are used for most of the factors, but I and II are referred to as fibrinogen and prothrombin respectively; III, IV and VI are redundant. The active forms are denoted by 'a'.

The coagulation factors are primarily synthesized in the liver and are either enzyme precursors (factors XII, XI, X, IX and thrombin) or cofactors (V and VIII), except for fibrinogen, which is degraded to form fibrin.

Coagulation pathway

This enzymatic amplification system is traditionally divided into 'extrinsic' and 'intrinsic' pathways. This concept remains very useful for the interpretation of clinical laboratory tests (see p. 469) but is an over-simplification. Coagulation is initiated by binding of activated factor VII (VIIa) in plasma to tissue factor (TF), a glycoprotein which is expressed on the surface of cells which are exposed after injury. The complex of VIIa and tissue factor (TF:VIIa) activates factor X but this reaction is opposed by tissue factor pathway inhibitor (TFPI), and the main role of TF:VIIa in vivo is to activate factor IX (Fig. 8.33). Activated factor IX then works with factor VIII to initiate the crucial activation of factor X. (It is this reaction which amplifies the generation of thrombin and which fails in haemophilia A and B. Factor XI is activated in vivo by thrombin and makes a limited contribution to haemostasis so that factor XI deficiency results in a rather mild bleeding disorder.)

Activated factor X induces the conversion of prothrombin to thrombin. Thrombin hydrolyses the peptide bonds of fibrinogen, releasing fibrinopeptides A and B, and allowing polymerization between fibrinogen molecules to form fibrin. At the same time, thrombin, in the presence of calcium ions, activates factor XIII, which stabilizes the fibrin clot by cross-linking adjacent fibrin molecules. The presence of thrombin helps in the activation of factors XI, V, VIII and XIII (and protein C; see limitation of coagulation below and Fig. 8.34).

Factor VIII consists of a molecule with coagulant activity (VIII:C) associated with von Willebrand factor. VWF's function here is to stabilize factor VIII:C and to promote platelet–endothelial interaction. VIII:C is a single-chain protein with a molecular weight of about 350 000.

Von Willebrand Factor (vWF) is a glycoprotein with a molecular weight of about 200 000 which readily forms multimers in the circulation with molecular weights of up to 20×10^6. It is synthesized by endothelial cells and megakaryocytes and stored in platelet and granules as well as the endothelial cells. The high-molecular-weight

Fig. 8.34 **Activation of protein C.** PAI-1, plasminogen activator inhibitor 1.

Fig. 8.35 **Fibrinolytic system.**

(a) Conversion of plasminogen to plasmin

(b) Plasmin α₂-antiplasmin complex

Fig. 8.36 **Fibrinolysis.**
(a) The conversion of plasminogen to plasmin by plasminogen activator (t-PA) occurs most efficiently on the surface of fibrin, which has binding sites for both plasminogen and t-PA.
(b) Free plasmin in the blood is rapidly inactivated by α₂-antiplasmin. Plasmin generated on the fibrin surface is partially protected from inactivation. The lysine-binding sites on plasminogen are necessary for the interaction between plasmin(ogen) and fibrin and between plasmin and α₂-antiplasmin.

multimeric forms of vWF are the most effective in promoting platelet function (see p. 467 and Fig. 8.37).

Limitation of coagulation

Antithrombin. Antithrombin (AT), a member of the serine protease inhibitor (serpin) superfamily, is a potent inhibitor of coagulation. It inactivates the serine proteases by forming stable complexes with them, and its action is greatly potentiated by heparin.

Activated protein C. This is generated from its vitamin K-dependent precursor by the action of thrombin; thrombin activation of protein C is enhanced when thrombin is bound to thrombomodulin, which is an endothelial cell receptor (Fig. 8.34). Activated protein C destroys factor V and factor VIII, reducing further thrombin generation.

Protein S. This is a cofactor for protein C which acts by enhancing binding of activated protein C to the phospholipid surface. It circulates bound to C4b binding protein but some 30–40% remains unbound and active (free protein S).

Other inhibitors. Other natural inhibitors of coagulation include α₂-macroglobulin, α₁-antitrypsin and α₂-antiplasmin.

Fibrinolysis

Fibrinolysis, which helps to restore vessel patency, also occurs in response to vascular damage. In this system (Fig. 8.35), an inactive plasma protein – plasminogen – is converted to plasmin by plasminogen activators derived from the plasma or blood cells (intrinsic activation) or the tissues (extrinsic activation).

Plasmin is a serine protease which breaks down fibrinogen and fibrin into fragments X, Y, D and E, collectively known as fibrin (and fibrinogen) degradation products (FDPs). D-dimer is produced when cross-linked fibrin is degraded. Its presence in the plasma indicates that the coagulation mechanism has been activated (see p. 467). Plasmin is also capable of breaking down coagulation factors such as factors V and VIII.

The fibrinolytic system is activated by the presence of fibrin. Plasminogen is specifically adsorbed to fibrin and

fibrinogen by lysine-binding sites. However, little plasminogen activation occurs in the absence of fibrin, as fibrin also has a specific binding site for plasminogen activators, whereas fibrinogen does not (Fig. 8.36).

The major plasminogen activator is tissue-type plasminogen activator (t-PA); vascular endothelium is the major source of t-PA in plasma. Its release is stimulated by a number of mediators, including thrombin. Another plasminogen activator is urokinase, synthesized in the kidney and released into the urogenital tract. Intrinsic plasminogen activators such as factor XII and pre-kallikrein are of minor physiological importance.

t-PA is inactivated by plasminogen activator inhibitor-1 (PAI-1). Activated protein C inactivates PAI-1 and therefore induces fibrinolysis (Fig. 8.34). Inactivators of plasmin such as α₂-antiplasmin (Fig. 8.36) and thrombinactivatable fibrinolysis inhibitor (TAFI) also contribute to the regulation of fibrinolysis.

Investigation of bleeding disorders

Although the precise diagnosis of a bleeding disorder may depend on laboratory tests, much information may be obtained from the history and physical examination:

- **Is there a generalized haemostatic defect?** Supportive evidence for this includes bleeding from multiple sites, spontaneous bleeding, and excessive bleeding after injury.
- **Is the defect inherited or acquired?** A family history of a bleeding disorder should be sought. Severe inherited defects usually become apparent in infancy, while mild inherited defects may only come to attention later in life, for example with excessive bleeding after surgery, childbirth, dental extractions or trauma. Some defects are revealed by routine coagulation screens which are performed before surgical procedures.
- **Is the bleeding suggestive of a vascular/platelet defect or a coagulation defect?**

Vascular/platelet bleeding is characterized by easy bruising and spontaneous bleeding from small vessels. There is often bleeding into the skin. The term purpura includes both petechiae, which are small skin haemorrhages varying from pinpoint size to a few millimetres in diameter and which do not blanch on pressure, and ecchymoses, which are larger areas of bleeding into the skin. Bleeding also occurs from mucous membranes especially the nose and mouth.

Coagulation disorders are typically associated with haemarthroses and muscle haematomas, and bleeding after injury or surgery. There is often a short delay between the precipitating event and overt haemorrhage or haematoma formation.

Laboratory investigations

- **Blood count and film** show the number and morphology of platelets and any blood disorder such as leukaemia or lymphoma. The normal range for the platelet count is $150–400 \times 10^9/L$.
- **Bleeding time** measures platelet plug formation in vivo. It is determined by applying a sphygmomanometer cuff to the arm and inflating it to 40 mmHg. Two 1 mm deep, 1 cm long incisions are made in the forearm with a template. Each wound is blotted every 30 s and the time taken for bleeding to stop is recorded, normally between 3 and 10 minutes. Prolonged bleeding times are found in patients with platelet function defects, and there is a progressive prolongation with platelet counts less than $80 \times 10^9/L$. The bleeding time should not be performed at low platelet counts.
- **Coagulation tests** are performed using blood collected into citrate, which neutralizes calcium ions and prevents clotting.

The *prothrombin time* (PT) (also see p. 480) is measured by adding tissue thromboplastin in the form of animal brain extract, or a recombinant equivalent, and calcium to the patient's plasma ('extrinsic' system). The normal PT is 16–18 s, and it is prolonged with abnormalities of factors VII, X, V, II or I, liver disease, or if the patient is on warfarin.

The *activated partial thromboplastin time* (APTT) is also sometimes known as the PTT with kaolin (PTTK). It is performed by adding a surface activator (such as kaolin), phospholipid (as platelet substitute) and calcium to the patient's plasma ('intrinsic' system). The normal APTT is 30–50 s depending on the exact methodology, and it is prolonged with deficiencies or inhibitors of one or more of the following factors: XII, XI, IX, VIII, X, V, II or I (but not factor VII) (see Fig. 8.33).

The *thrombin time* (TT) is performed by adding thrombin to the patient's plasma. The normal TT is about 12 s, and it is prolonged with fibrinogen deficiency, dysfibrinogenaemia (normal level of fibrinogen but abnormal function) or inhibitors such as heparin or FDPs.

Correction tests can be used to differentiate prolonged times in the PT, APTT and TT due to various coagulation factor deficiencies and inhibitors of coagulation. Prolonged PT, APTT or TT because of coagulation factor deficiencies are corrected by addition of normal plasma to the patient's plasma; no correction of an abnormal result after the addition of normal plasma is suggestive of the presence of an inhibitor of coagulation.

Factor assays are used to confirm coagulation defects, especially where a single inherited disorder is suspected.

Special tests of coagulation will often be required to confirm the precise haemostatic defect. Such tests include estimation of fibrinogen and FDPs, platelet function tests such as platelet aggregation and tests of the fibrinolytic pathway which include the euglobulin clot lysis time (ELT) and assays of plasminogen, t-PA and PAI-1. The ELT involves precipitation by acidification of the euglobulin fraction of plasma, which contains fibrinogen, plasminogen and plasminogen activators but excluding α_2-antiplasmin. The euglobulin fraction is clotted with thrombin and the time taken for lysis of the fibrin clot is a measure of fibrinolytic activity; the normal range is 60–270 minutes. Factor XIII can be estimated by a clot stability screening test or by direct assay.

VASCULAR DISORDERS

The vascular disorders (Table 8.23) are characterized by easy bruising and bleeding into the skin. Bleeding from mucous membranes sometimes occurs but the bleeding is rarely severe. Laboratory investigations including the bleeding time are normal. The vascular disorders include the following.

Hereditary haemorrhagic telangiectasia is a rare disorder with autosomal dominant inheritance. Dilatation of capillaries and small arterioles produces characteristic small red spots that blanch on pressure in the skin and mucous membranes, particularly the nose and gastrointestinal tract. Recurrent epistaxis and chronic gastrointestinal bleeding are the major problems and may cause chronic iron deficiency anaemia.

Table 8.23	Vascular disorders
Congenital	**Allergic**
Hereditary haemorrhagic telangiectasia (Osler–Weber–Rendu disease)	Henoch–Schönlein purpura
	Drugs
	Steroids
Connective tissue disorders (Ehlers–Danlos syndrome, osteogenesis imperfecta, pseudoxanthoma elasticum, Marfan's syndrome)	Sulphonamides
	Others
	Senile purpura
	Easy bruising syndrome
	Scurvy
Acquired	Factitious purpura
Severe infections: septicaemia meningococcal infections measles typhoid	

Table 8.24 Clinical effects caused by different levels of platelet count

Platelet count ($\times 10^9$/L)	Clinical defect
> 500	Haemorrhage or thrombosis
500–100	No clinical effect
100–50	Moderate haemorrhage after injury
50–20	Purpura may occur
	Haemorrhage after injury
< 20	Purpura common
	Spontaneous haemorrhage from mucous membranes
	Intracranial haemorrhage (rare)

By permission of Colvin BT (2004) *Medicine* 32(5): 27–33

Table 8.25 Causes of thrombocytopenia

Impaired production	Excessive destruction
Bone marrow failure	Immune
Megaloblastic anaemia	ITP
Leukaemia	Secondary immune (SLE, CLL, viruses, drugs, e.g. heparin)
Myeloma	
Myelofibrosis	
Solid tumour infiltration	Alloimmune neonatal thrombocytopenia
Aplastic anaemia:	Post-transfusion purpura
drugs	
chemicals	**Sequestration**
viruses	Hypersplenism
paroxysmal nocturnal haemoglobinuria	**Dilutional**
	Massive transfusion
	Other
	Disseminated intravascular coagulation
	Thrombotic thrombocytopenic purpura

Easy bruising syndrome is a common benign disorder occurring in otherwise healthy women. It is characterized by bruises on the arms, legs and trunk with minor trauma, possibly because of skin vessel fragility. It may give rise to the suspicion of a serious bleeding disorder.

Senile purpura and purpura due to steroids are both due to atrophy of the vascular supporting tissue.

Purpura due to infections is mainly caused by damage to the vascular endothelium. The rash of meningococcal septicaemia is particularly characteristic (p. 75).

Henoch–Schönlein purpura (p. 629) occurs mainly in children. It is a type III hypersensitivity reaction that is often preceded by an acute upper respiratory tract infection. Purpura is mainly seen on the legs and buttocks. Abdominal pain, arthritis, haematuria and glomerulonephritis also occur. Recovery is usually spontaneous, but some patients develop renal failure.

Episodes of inexplicable bleeding or bruising may represent abuse, either self-inflicted or caused by others. These various forms of artificial or factitious purpura are expressions of severe emotional or psychiatric disturbances.

PLATELET DISORDERS

Bleeding due to thrombocytopenia or abnormal platelet function is characterized by purpura and bleeding from mucous membranes. Bleeding is uncommon with platelet counts above 50×10^9/L, and severe spontaneous bleeding is unusual with platelet counts above 20×10^9/L (Table 8.24).

Thrombocytopenia

This is caused by reduced platelet production in the bone marrow or excessive peripheral destruction of platelets (Table 8.25). The underlying cause may be revealed by history and examination but a bone marrow examination will show whether the numbers of megakaryocytes are reduced, normal or increased, and will provide essential information on morphology. Specific laboratory tests may be useful to confirm the presence of such conditions as paroxysmal nocturnal haemoglobinuria (PNH) or systemic lupus erythematosus (SLE).

In patients with thrombocytopenia due to failure of production, no specific treatment may be necessary but the underlying condition should be treated if possible. Where the platelet count is very low or the risk of bleeding is very high, then platelet concentrate administration is indicated.

Idiopathic thrombocytopenic purpura (ITP)

Thrombocytopenia is due to immune destruction of platelets. The antibody-coated platelets are removed following binding to Fc receptors on macrophages.

ITP in children

The condition is usually acute but self-limiting and may follow a viral infection or immunization. Bone marrow examination is not usually performed unless treatment becomes necessary on clinical grounds.

ITP in adults

The presentation is usually less acute than in children. Adult ITP is characteristically seen in women and may be associated with other autoimmune disorders such as SLE, thyroid disease and autoimmune haemolytic anaemia (Evans' syndrome), in patients with chronic lymphocytic leukaemia and solid tumours, and after infections with viruses such as HIV. Platelet autoantibodies are detected in about 60–70% of patients, and are presumed to be present, although not detectable, in the remaining patients; the antibodies often have specificity for platelet membrane glycoproteins IIb/IIIa and/or Ib.

Clinical features

Major haemorrhage is rare and is seen only in patients with severe thrombocytopenia. Easy bruising, purpura, epistaxis and menorrhagia are common. Physical examination is normal except for evidence of bleeding. Splenomegaly is rare.

Investigation

The only blood count abnormality is thrombocytopenia. Normal or increased numbers of megakaryocytes are found in the bone marrow (if examination is performed), which is otherwise normal. The detection of platelet auto-antibodies is not essential for confirmation of the diagnosis, which often depends on exclusion of other causes of excessive destruction of platelets.

Treatment

Children

Children do not usually require treatment. Where this is necessary on clinical grounds, high-dose prednisolone is effective, given for a very short course. Intravenous immunoglobulin (i.v. IgG) should be reserved for very serious bleeding or urgent surgery. Chronic ITP is rare and requires specialist management, avoiding cytotoxic agents.

Adults

Patients with platelet counts greater than $30 \times 10^9/L$ require no treatment unless they are about to undergo a surgical procedure.

First-line therapy consists of oral corticosteroids 1 mg/kg body weight but i.v. IgG is useful where a rapid rise in platelet count is desired, especially before surgery. There are also advocates for high-dose corticosteroids as initial therapy.

Second-line therapy involves splenectomy, to which the majority of patients respond, but a wide range of treatments is available in chronic ITP. These include high-dose corticosteroids, high-dose i.v. IgG, intravenous anti-D, vinca alkaloids, danazol, immunosuppressive agents such as azathioprine, ciclosporine and dapsone. There is also interest in the use of specific monoclonal antibodies such as rituximab, as well as recombinant thrombopoietin.

Platelet transfusions are reserved for intracranial or other extreme haemorrhage, where emergency splenectomy may be justified.

Other immune thrombocytopenias

Drugs cause immune thrombocytopenia by the same mechanisms as described for drug-induced immune haemolytic anaemia (p. 450). The same drugs can be responsible for immune haemolytic anaemia, thrombocytopenia or neutropenia in different patients.

Heparin-induced thrombocytopenia. See page 480.

Neonatal alloimmune thrombocytopenia is due to feto-maternal incompatibility for platelet-specific antigens, usually for HPA-1a (human platelet alloantigen) and is the platelet equivalent of haemolytic disease of the newborn (HDN). The mother is HPA-1a-negative and produces antibodies which destroy the HPA-1a-positive fetal platelets.

Thrombocytopenia is self-limiting after delivery, but platelet transfusions may be required initially to prevent or treat bleeding associated with severe thrombo-cytopenia; platelets are prepared from HPA-1a-negative volunteers or the mother herself. Severe bleeding such as intracranial haemorrhage may also occur in utero. Antenatal treatment of the mother – with platelet trans-fusions given directly to the fetus by ultrasound-guided needling of the umbilical vessels – has been effective in preventing haemorrhage in severely affected cases.

Post-transfusion purpura (PTP) is rare, occurring 2–12 days after a blood transfusion. PTP is associated with a platelet-specific alloantibody, usually anti-HPA-1a in an HPA-1a-negative individual. PTP almost invariably occurs in females who have been previously immunized by pregnancy or blood transfusion. The cause of the destruction of the patient's own platelets is not well understood, but they may be destroyed as 'bystanders' during the acute immune response to HPA-1a. PTP is self-limiting, but high-dose intravenous immunoglobulin may limit the period of thrombocytopenia.

Thrombotic thrombocytopenic purpura (TTP)
(p. 636)

TTP is a rare, but very serious condition, in which platelet destruction leads to profound thrombocytopenia. There is a characteristic symptom complex of florid purpura, fever, fluctuating cerebral dysfunction and haemolytic anaemia with red cell fragmentation, often accompanied by renal failure. The coagulation screen is usually normal but lactic dehydrogenase (LDH) levels are markedly raised as a result of haemolysis.

The underlying cause is not fully understood but TTP seems to be due to endothelial damage associated with the presence in the circulation of very-high-molecular-weight multimers of von Willebrand factor (vWF) which accumulate owing to the absence of a protease which is normally responsible for vWF degradation. This absence is due to mutations in the *ADAMTS 13* gene. In some cases there is a true deficiency of the protease, while in others an immune response appears to reduce protease activity temporarily. TTP is associated with pregnancy, oral contraceptives, systemic lupus erythematosus, infection and drug treatment, including the use of ticlopidine and clopidogrel, but many cases have no obvious cause.

Treatment consists of plasma exchange, using cryoprecipitate-depleted FFP (cryo-poor supernatant) or solvent detergent-treated FFP, both of which contain reduced amounts of high-molecular-weight vWF multi-mers. It is also thought that FFP supplies the missing protease. Most patients are also treated with prednisone 1 mg/kg daily and low-dose aspirin 75 mg daily is often given as the platelet count rises above $50 \times 10^9/L$. Disease activity is monitored by measuring the platelet count and serum LDH. Platelet concentrates are contraindicated.

The untreated condition has a mortality of up to 90% but modern management has reduced this figure to about 10%. Recurrent and relapsing TTP occurs, often associated with a persistent lack of vWF protease.

Platelet function disorders

These are usually associated with excessive bruising and bleeding and, in some of the acquired forms, with thrombosis. The platelet count is normal or increased and the bleeding time is prolonged. The rare inherited defects of platelet function require more detailed investigations such as platelet aggregation studies and factor VIII:C and vWF assays, if von Willebrand's disease is suspected.

Inherited types of platelet dysfunction
- *Glanzmann's thrombasthenia* – lack of the platelet membrane glycoprotein IIb/IIIa complex resulting in defective fibrinogen binding and failure of platelet aggregation.
- *Bernard–Soulier syndrome* – lack of platelet membrane glycoprotein Ib, the binding site for factor vWF. This causes a failure of platelet adhesion and moderate thrombocytopenia.
- *Storage pool disease* – lack of the storage pool of platelet dense bodies, causing poor platelet function.

Acquired types of platelet dysfunction
- Myeloproliferative disorders
- Renal and liver disease
- Paraproteinaemias
- Drug-induced, such as by aspirin or other platelet inhibitory drugs.

If there is serious bleeding or if the patient is about to undergo surgery, drugs with antiplatelet activity should be withdrawn and any underlying condition should be corrected if possible. In patients with renal failure, the haematocrit should be increased to greater than 0.30 and the use of desmopressin may be helpful. Platelet transfusions may be required if these measures are unsuccessful or if the risk of bleeding is high.

Thrombocytosis

The platelet count may rise above $400 \times 10^9/L$ as a result of:

- splenectomy
- Hodgkin's lymphoma and other malignancies
- inflammatory disorders such as rheumatoid arthritis, ulcerative colitis and Crohn's disease
- major surgery.

Thus thrombocytosis is part of the acute-phase reaction, although following splenectomy platelet numbers are also elevated because of the loss of a major site of platelet destruction.

Essential thrombocythaemia, a myeloproliferative disorder which is described on page 455, and other myeloproliferative conditions such as polycythaemia vera (PV) and chronic myeloid leukaemia (CML) may also be associated with a high platelet count.

A persistently elevated platelet count can lead to arterial or venous thrombosis. It is usual to treat the underlying cause of the thrombocytosis but a small dose of aspirin (75 mg) is also sometimes given. In myeloproliferative disease there is also a paradoxical risk of abnormal bleeding and specific action to reduce the platelet count, usually with hydroxycarbamide (hydroxyurea) is often taken.

INHERITED COAGULATION DISORDERS

Coagulation disorders may be inherited or acquired. The inherited disorders are uncommon and usually involve deficiency of one factor only. The acquired disorders occur more frequently and almost always involve several coagulation factors; they are considered in the next subsection.

In inherited coagulation disorders, deficiencies of all factors have been described. Those leading to abnormal bleeding are rare, apart from haemophilia A (factor VIII deficiency), haemophilia B (factor IX deficiency) and von Willebrand's disease.

Haemophilia A

In haemophilia A, the level of factor VIII:C is reduced but the level of factor vWF is normal (see Fig. 8.37). The prevalence of haemophilia A is about 1 in 5000 of the male population. It is inherited as an X-linked disorder. If a female carrier has a son, he has a 50% chance of having haemophilia, and a daughter has a 50% chance of being a carrier. All daughters of men with haemophilia are carriers and the sons are normal.

The human factor VIII gene is enormous, constituting about 0.1% of the X chromosome, encompassing 186 kilobases of DNA. Various genetic defects have been found, including deletions, duplications, frameshift mutations and insertions. In approximately 50% of families with severe disease, the defect is an inversion. There is a high mutation rate, with one-third of cases being apparently sporadic with no family history of haemophilia.

Clinical and laboratory features
The clinical features depend on the level of factor VIII:C.

- *Levels of less than 1%* are associated with frequent spontaneous bleeding from early life. Haemarthroses are common and may lead to joint deformity and crippling if adequate treatment is not given. Bleeding into muscles is also common, and intramuscular injections should be avoided.

Fig. 8.37 (a) Normal factor VIII synthesis. (b) Haemophilia A showing defective synthesis of factor VIIIc. (c) von Willebrand's disease showing reduced synthesis of vWF.

- *Levels of 1–5%* are associated with severe bleeding following injury and occasional apparently spontaneous episodes.
- *Levels above 5%* produce mild disease, usually with bleeding only after injury or surgery. It should be noted that patients with mild haemophilia can still bleed badly once haemostasis has failed. Diagnosis in this group is often delayed until quite late in life.

The most common causes of death in people with haemophilia are cancer and heart disease, as for the general population. Cerebral haemorrhage is much more frequent however, and in recent years, HIV infection and liver disease (due to hepatitis C) have become a more common cause of death.

The main laboratory features of haemophilia A are shown in Table 8.26. The abnormal findings are a prolonged APTT and a reduced level of factor VIII:C. The PT, bleeding time and vWF level are normal.

Treatment

Bleeding is treated by administration of factor VIII concentrate by intravenous infusion.

- *Minor bleeding*: the factor VIII:C level should be raised to 20–30%.

- *Severe bleeding*: the factor VIII:C should be raised to at least 50%.
- *Major surgery*: the factor VIII:C should be raised to 100% preoperatively and maintained above 50% until healing has occurred.

Factor VIII has a half-life of 12 hours and therefore must be administered at least twice daily to maintain the required therapeutic level. Continuous infusion is sometimes used to cover surgery. Factor VIII concentrate is freeze-dried and may be stored in domestic refrigerators at 4°C. This allows it to be administered by the patient immediately after bleeding has started, reducing the likelihood of chronic damage to joints and the need for inpatient care.

Recombinant factor VIII concentrate is well established as the treatment of choice for people with haemophilia, but economic constraints and limited production capacity for recombinant factors have resulted in many previously treated patients still being offered treatment with plasma-derived concentrates, particularly in developing countries.

The majority of severely affected patients are given prophylaxis three times per week from early childhood in an attempt to prevent permanent joint damage.

Synthetic vasopressin (Desmopressin – an anologue of vasopressin) – intravenous, subcutaneous or intranasal – produces a rise in factor VIII:C proportional to the initial level of factor VIII. It avoids the complications associated with blood products and is useful for treating bleeding episodes in mild haemophilia and as prophylaxis before minor surgery. It is ineffective in severe haemophilia.

People with haemophilia should be registered at comprehensive care centres (CCC), which take responsibility for their full medical care, including social and psychological support. Each person with haemophilia carries a special medical card giving details of the disorder and its treatment.

Table 8.26 Blood changes in haemophilia A, von Willebrand's disease and vitamin K deficiency

	Haemophilia A	von Willebrand's disease	Vitamin K deficiency
Bleeding time	Normal	↑	Normal
PT	Normal	Normal	↑
APTT	↑+	↑±	↑
VIII:C	↓++	↓	Normal
vWF	Normal	↓	Normal

Complications

Up to 30% of people with severe haemophilia will develop antibodies to factor VIII:C during their lifetime, usually after the first few treatment doses of factor VIII. The prevalence of antibodies in the UK haemophilia population is 5–10% because they uncommonly develop in more mildly affected patients and often disappear spontaneously or with continued treatment.

Management of such patients may be very difficult, and even extremely high doses of factor VIII may not produce a rise in the plasma level of factor VIII:C. Purified porcine factor VIII may not cross-react with the patient's antibody. Some factor IX concentrates contain activated factors, which may 'bypass' the inhibitor and stop the bleeding. Recombinant factor VIIa also has this bypassing potential and shows great promise as an agent for treating patients with inhibitors. There is a growing interest in immune tolerance induction, especially in the management of recently developed inhibitors in young people. Similar strategies, including immunosuppression and immunoabsorption, have been described.

The risk of viral transmission has been virtually eliminated in developed countries by excluding high-risk blood donors, testing all donations for HBsAg, HCV and HIV antibodies, and by including steps to inactivate viruses during the preparation of plasma-derived concentrate.

Hepatitis A and B vaccination is offered routinely to all patients with haemophilia and von Willebrand's disease. The clinical consequences of haemophilia patients infected with HIV are similar to other HIV-infected patients (see p. 132), except that Kaposi's sarcoma does not occur. A number of patients with hepatitis C will progress to develop chronic liver disease and cirrhosis (see p. 372).

The use of recombinant factor VIII eliminates any residual risk of transfusion-transmitted infection, and it is safe and effective; but there is a similar incidence of inhibitor development as with plasma-derived factor VIII.

Carrier detection and antenatal diagnosis

Determination of carrier status in females begins with a family history and coagulation factor assays. Female carriers usually have a factor VIII level of about 50% of normal, but the exact value is very variable, partly because of lyonization. Owing to this process early in embryonic life (that is, random inactivation of one chromosome; see p. 172), some carriers have very low levels of factor VIII while others will have normal levels. Carriers could be diagnosed with reasonable confidence if the level of factor VIII:C was 50% or less of that expected from the level of factor vWF measured at the same time, but often no clear-cut answer was provided by this method. Carrier detection can be carried out using molecular genetic testing, either by direct detection of mutations within the factor VIII gene or by tracking of the abnormal gene using DNA polymorphisms as markers.

Antenatal diagnosis may be carried out by molecular analysis of fetal tissue obtained by chorionic villus biopsy at 11–12 weeks' gestation.

Haemophilia B (Christmas disease)

Haemophilia B is caused by a deficiency of factor IX. The inheritance and clinical features are identical to haemophilia A, but the incidence is only about 1 in 30 000 males. The gene is smaller at 34 kilobases and the half-life of the factor is longer at 18 hours. Haemophilia B is treated with factor IX concentrates, recombinant factor IX now being available, and prophylactic doses are given twice a week. Desmopressin is ineffective.

Von Willebrand's disease (vWD)

In vWD, there is defective platelet function as well as factor VIII:C deficiency, and both are due to a deficiency or abnormality of vWF (see Fig. 8.37). vWF plays a role in platelet adhesion to damaged subendothelium as well as stabilizing factor VIII:C in plasma (see p. 467).

The vWF gene is located on chromosome 12 and numerous mutations of the gene have been identified. vWD has been classified into three types:

- *Type 1* is characterized by a mild reduction in vWF and is usually inherited as an autosomal dominant.
- *Type 2* is due to a decrease in the proportion of high-molecular-weight multimers, and it too is usually inherited as an autosomal dominant.
- *Type 3* is recessively inherited and patients have barely detectable levels of factor vWF (and therefore also of factor VIII:C). Their parents are often phenotypically normal.

Many subtypes have also been described, such as type 2B where increased vWF avidity for platelets causes mild thrombocytopenia, and type 2N where there is an abnormal vWF binding site for VIII:C.

Clinical features. These are variable. Type 1 and type 2 patients usually have mild clinical features. Bleeding follows minor trauma or surgery, and epistaxis and menorrhagia often occur. Haemarthroses are rare. Type 3 patients have more severe bleeding but rarely experience the joint and muscle bleeds seen in haemophilia A.

Characteristic laboratory findings are shown in Table 8.26. These also include defective platelet aggregation with ristocetin.

Treatment depends on the severity of the condition and may be similar to that of mild haemophilia, including the use of Desmopressin where possible. Intermediate purity factor VIII or von Willebrand factor concentrates should be used to treat bleeding or to cover surgery in patients who require replacement therapy, especially in type 3 (severe) disease. Cryoprecipitate should be avoided because of the greater risk of transfusion-transmitted infection, since cryoprecipitate is not a virally inactivated product.

ACQUIRED COAGULATION DISORDERS

Vitamin K deficiency (see also p. 242)

Vitamin K is necessary for the γ-carboxylation of glutamic acid residues on coagulation factors II, VII, IX and X and on proteins C and S. Without it, these factors cannot bind calcium.

Deficiency of vitamin K may be due to:

- *inadequate stores*, as in haemorrhagic disease of the newborn and severe malnutrition (especially when combined with antibiotic treatment) (see p. 352)
- *malabsorption of vitamin K*, a fat-soluble vitamin, which occurs in cholestatic jaundice owing to the lack of intraluminal bile salts
- *oral anticoagulant drugs*, which are vitamin K antagonists.

The PT and APTT are prolonged (see Table 8.26) and there may be bruising, haematuria and gastrointestinal or cerebral bleeding. Minor bleeding is treated with phytomenadione (vitamin K$_1$) 10 mg intravenously. Some correction of the PT is usual within 6 hours but it may not return to normal for 2 days.

Newborn babies have low levels of vitamin K, and this may cause minor bleeding in the first week of life (*classical haemorrhagic disease of the newborn*). Vitamin K deficiency may also cause *late haemorrhagic disease of the newborn*, which occurs 2–26 weeks after birth and may result in severe bleeding such as intracranial haemorrhage. Most infants with these syndromes have been exclusively breast-fed, and both conditions may be prevented by administering 1 mg i.m. vitamin K to all neonates (p. 242). Concerns about the safety of this are unfounded.

Liver disease

Liver disease may result in a number of defects in haemostasis:

- *Vitamin K deficiency*. This occurs owing to intrahepatic or extrahepatic cholestasis.
- *Reduced synthesis*. Reduced synthesis of coagulation factors may be the result of severe hepatocellular damage. The use of vitamin K does not improve the results of abnormal coagulation tests, but it is generally given to ensure that a treatable cause of failure of haemostasis has not been missed.
- *Thrombocytopenia*. This results from hypersplenism due to splenomegaly associated with portal hypertension or from folic acid deficiency.
- *Functional abnormalities*. Functional abnormalities of platelets and fibrinogen are found in many patients with liver failure.
- *Disseminated intravascular coagulation*. DIC (see below) may occur in acute liver failure.

Disseminated intravascular coagulation (DIC)

There is widespread generation of fibrin within blood vessels, owing to activation of coagulation by release of

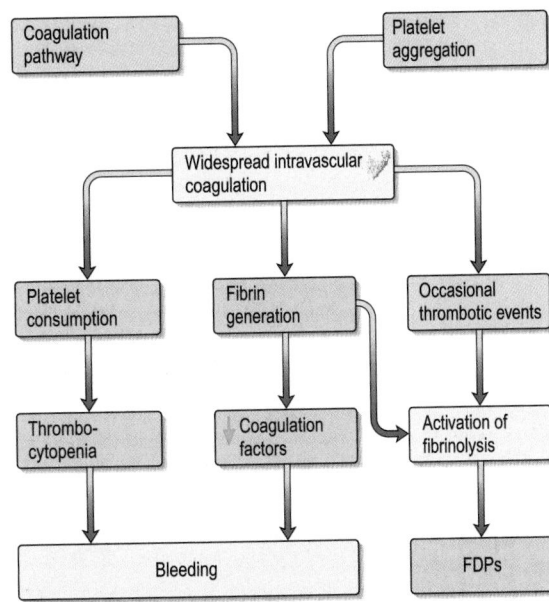

Fig. 8.38 Disseminated intravascular coagulation. FDP, fibrin degradation products.

procoagulant material, and by diffuse endothelial damage or generalized platelet aggregation. Activation of leucocytes, particularly monocytes causing expression of tissue factor and the release of cytokines, may play a role in the development of DIC.

There is consumption of platelets and coagulation factors and secondary activation of fibrinolysis leading to production of fibrin degradation products (FDPs), which may contribute to the coagulation defect by inhibiting fibrin polymerization (Fig. 8.38). The consequences of these changes are a mixture of initial thrombosis followed by a bleeding tendency due to consumption of coagulation factors and fibrinolytic activation.

Causes of DIC

These include:

- malignant disease
- septicaemia (e.g. Gram-negative and meningococcal)
- haemolytic transfusion reactions
- obstetric causes (e.g. abruptio placentae, amniotic fluid embolism)
- trauma, burns, surgery
- other infections (e.g. falciparum malaria)
- liver disease
- snake bite.

Clinical features

The underlying disorder is usually obvious. The patient is often acutely ill and shocked. The clinical presentation of DIC varies from no bleeding at all to profound haemostatic failure with widespread haemorrhage. Bleeding may occur from the mouth, nose and venepuncture sites and there may be widespread ecchymoses.

Thrombotic events may occur as a result of vessel occlusion by fibrin and platelets. Any organ may be involved, but the skin, brain and kidneys are most often affected.

Investigations

The diagnosis is often suggested by the underlying condition of the patient.

Severe cases with haemorrhage
- The PT, APTT and TT are usually very prolonged and the fibrinogen level markedly reduced.
- High levels of FDPs, including D-dimer are found owing to the intense fibrinolytic activity stimulated by the presence of fibrin in the circulation.
- There is severe thrombocytopenia.
- The blood film may show fragmented red blood cells.

Mild cases without bleeding
- Increased synthesis of coagulation factors and platelets
- Normal PT, APTT, TT and platelet counts
- FDPs are raised.

Treatment

The underlying condition is treated and this may be all that is necessary in patients who are not bleeding. Maintenance of blood volume and tissue perfusion is essential. Transfusions of platelet concentrates, FFP, cryoprecipitate and red cell concentrates is indicated in patients who are bleeding. The use of heparin to prevent intravascular coagulation is rarely indicated. Inhibitors of fibrinolysis such as tranexamic acid should not be used in DIC as dangerous fibrin deposition may result. Antithrombin and/or activated protein C concentrates have been used in selected cases.

Excessive fibrinolysis

Excessive fibrinolysis may occur during surgery involving tumours of the prostate, breast, pancreas and uterus owing to release of tissue plasminogen activators.

Primary hyperfibrinolysis is very rare but activation of fibrinolysis occurs in DIC as a secondary event in response to intravascular deposition of fibrin.

The clinical picture is similar to DIC with widespread bleeding. Laboratory investigations are also similar with a prolonged PT, APTT and TT, a low fibrinogen level, and increased FDPs, although fragmented red cells and thrombocytopenia are not seen, since disseminated coagulation is not present.

If the diagnosis is certain, fibrinolytic inhibitors such as e-aminocaproic acid (EACA) or tranexamic acid should be considered. If DIC cannot be excluded, it is safer to treat as for DIC.

Massive transfusion

Few platelets and reduced levels of factors V and VIII are found in stored blood, although there are adequate amounts of the other coagulation factors. During massive transfusion (defined as transfusion of a volume of blood equal to the patient's own blood volume within 24 hours,

e.g. approximately 10 units in an adult), the platelet count and PT and APTT should be checked at intervals. Transfusion of platelet concentrates and FFP should be given if thrombocytopenia or defective coagulation are thought to be contributing to continued blood loss. Other problems of massive transfusion are described on page 974.

Inhibitors of coagulation

In addition to the factor VIII:C alloantibodies that are found in 5–10% of people with severe haemophilia A, factor VIII:C autoantibodies arise occasionally in patients with autoimmune disorders such as SLE, in elderly patients, and sometimes after childbirth. There can be severe bleeding. The antibodies sometimes disappear spontaneously, but treatment with plasma exchange, high-dose intravenous immunoglobulin and immunosuppressive drugs may be required in addition to any replacement therapy with factor concentrates (see above).

Lupus anticoagulant antibodies (p. 534) are autoantibodies directed against phospholipids (antiphospholipid antibodies). They are found in about 10% of patients with SLE and also occur in otherwise healthy individuals. They lead to prolongation of phospholipid-dependent coagulation tests, particularly the APTT, but do not inhibit coagulation factor activity. Bleeding does not occur unless there is coexistent severe immune thrombocytopenia. The main clinical problems are thrombosis and recurrent miscarriages (p. 577).

FURTHER READING

Bolton-Maggs PHB, Pasi KJ (2003) Haemophilias A and B. *Lancet* **361**: 1801–1809.

Levi M, ten Cate H (1999) Disseminated intravascular coagulation. *New England Journal of Medicine* **341**: 586–592.

Moake JL (2002) Thrombotic microangiopathies. *New England Journal of Medicine* **347**: 589–600.

Schafer AI (2004) Thrombocytosis. *New England Journal of Medicine* **350**: 1211–1219.

THROMBOSIS

A thrombus is defined as a solid mass formed in the circulation from the constituents of the blood during life. Fragments of thrombi (emboli) may break off and block vessels downstream. Thromboembolic disease is much more common than abnormal bleeding; nearly half of adult deaths in England and Wales are due to coronary artery thrombosis, cerebral artery thrombosis or pulmonary embolism.

A thrombus results from a complex series of events involving coagulation factors, platelets, red blood cells and the vessel wall.

Arterial thrombosis

This usually occurs in association with atheroma, which tends to form at areas of turbulent blood flow such as the bifurcation of arteries. Platelets adhere to the damaged vascular endothelium and aggregate in response to ADP and TXA_2 to form a 'white thrombus'. The growth of the platelet thrombus is limited at its margins by PGI_2 and NO. Plaque rupture leads to the exposure of blood containing factor VIIa to tissue factor within the plaque which may trigger blood coagulation and lead to thrombus formation. This results in complete occlusion of the vessel or embolization that produces distal obstruction. The risk factors for arterial thrombosis are related to the development of atherosclerosis (see p. 799).

Arterial thrombi may also form in the heart, as mural thrombi in the left ventricle after myocardial infarction, in the left atrium in mitral valve disease, or on the surfaces of prosthetic valves.

Venous thrombosis

Unlike arterial thrombosis, venous thrombosis often occurs in normal vessels. Major causes are stasis and hypercoagulability. The majority of venous thrombi occur in the deep veins of the leg, originating around the valves as 'red thrombi' consisting mainly of red cells and fibrin. The propagating thrombus is formed of fibrin and platelets and is particularly liable to embolize. Chronic venous obstruction following thrombosis in the deep veins of the leg frequently results in a permanently swollen limb and may lead to ulceration (post-phlebitic syndrome).

Risk factors for venous thrombosis are shown in Table 8.27. Venous thrombosis may occur with changes in blood cells such as polycythaemia and thrombocythaemia, and with coagulation abnormalities (thrombophilia; see below).

Table 8.27 Risk factors of venous thromboembolism

Patient factors	Disease or surgical procedure
Age	Trauma or surgery, especially
Obesity	of pelvis, hip or lower limb
Varicose veins	Malignancy
Long air travel	Cardiac failure
Immobility (bed rest	Recent myocardial infarction
> 4 days)	Infection
Pregnancy and puerperium	Inflammatory bowel disease
Previous deep vein	Nephrotic syndrome
thrombosis or	Polycythaemia
pulmonary embolism	Thrombocythaemia
Thrombophilia	Paroxysmal nocturnal
Antithrombin deficiency	haemoglobinuria
Protein C or S deficiency	Sickle cell anaemia
Resistance to activated	
protein C (caused by	
factor V Leiden variant)	
Prothrombin gene variant	
Homocysteinaemia	
Antiphospholipid	
antibody/lupus	
anticoagulant	
Oestrogen therapy	
including HRT	

The clinical features and diagnosis of venous thrombosis are discussed on page 870.

Thrombophilia

Thrombophilia is a term describing inherited or acquired defects of haemostasis leading to a predisposition to venous or arterial thrombosis. It should be considered in patients with:

- recurrent venous thrombosis
- venous thrombosis for the first time under age 40 years
- an unusual venous thrombosis such as mesenteric or cerebral vein thrombosis
- unexplained neonatal thrombosis
- recurrent miscarriages
- arterial thrombosis in the absence of arterial disease.

Coagulation abnormalities
Factor V Leiden

Factor V Leiden is formed by a single nucleotide substitution (Arg506gln) in the factor V gene (factor V Leiden mutation). This makes factor V less likely to be cleaved by activated protein C. Factor V is a cofactor for thrombin generation (see Fig. 8.33) and the failure of activated protein C to inactivate factor V (see Fig. 8.34) results in a tendency to thrombosis. Factor V Leiden is found in 3–5% of healthy individuals in the western world and in about 20% of patients with venous thrombosis.

The risk of venous thrombosis is increased in women with factor V Leiden who are pregnant or taking oral contraceptives. Screening for the defect before prescribing oral contraceptives or during pregnancy would be costly and might deny oral contraception to a substantial number of women who would then be at an increased risk of pregnancy, and therefore thrombosis. In addition, the use of oral anticoagulants in pregnancy carries a risk of fatal maternal bleeding, which may equal the risk of death due to postpartum thrombosis, and the fetus is also at risk of complications from the use of oral anticoagulants (see p. 481).

Prothrombin variant

A mutation in the 3' untranslated region of the prothrombin gene has been described (G20210A). This variant is associated with elevated levels of prothrombin and a two- to threefold increase in the risk of venous thrombosis. There is an interaction with factor V Leiden and contraceptive pill use or pregnancy. The prevalence is 2% in Caucasian populations, 6% in unselected patients with thrombosis and about 18% in families with unexplained thrombophilia.

Antithrombin (AT) deficiency

This deficiency can be inherited as an autosomal dominant. Many variations have been described that lead to a conformational change in the protein. It can also be acquired following trauma, with major surgery and with the contraceptive pill. Low levels are also seen in severe proteinuria (e.g. the nephrotic syndrome). Recurrent thrombotic episodes occur starting at a young age in the inherited variety. Patients are relatively resistant to heparin as antithrombin is required for its action. Anti-thrombin III concentrates are available.

Protein C and S deficiency

These autosomal dominant conditions result in an increased risk of venous thrombosis, often before the age of 40 years. Homozygous protein C or S deficiency causes neonatal purpura fulminans, which is fatal without immediate replacement therapy. Protein C concentrate and a recombinant activated protein C are available.

Antiphospholipid antibody

See pages 534 and 577.

Investigations

Haemostatic screening tests

- **Full blood count** including platelet count
- **Coagulation screen** including a fibrinogen level.

These tests will detect erythrocytosis, thrombocytosis, and dysfibrinogenaemia and the possible presence of a lupus anticoagulant.

Testing for specific causes of thrombophilia

- **Assays** for naturally occurring anticoagulants such as AT, protein C and protein S
- **Assay** for activated protein C resistance and molecular testing for factor V Leiden and the prothrombin variant
- **Screen for a coagulation factor** inhibitor including a lupus anticoagulant (and anticardiolipin antibodies) (see p. 534)
- **Fibrinolytic pathway tests** (see p. 469).

Prevention and treatment of arterial thrombosis

Attempts to prevent or reduce arterial thrombosis are directed mainly at minimizing factors predisposing to atherosclerosis. Treatment of established arterial thrombosis includes the use of antiplatelet drugs and thrombolytic therapy.

Antiplatelet drugs

Platelet activation at the site of vascular damage is crucial to the development of arterial thrombosis, and this can be altered by the following drugs (Table 8.28):

- *Aspirin* irreversibly inhibits the enzyme cyclo-oxygenase (COX), resulting in reduced platelet production of TXA_2 (see Fig. 8.32). At the low doses used in cardiovascular disease prevention or treatment, there is selective inhibition of the isoform COX-1 found within platelets. This inhibition cannot be repaired and is effective for the life of the circulating platelet, which is about 1 week.
- *Dipyridamole* – which inhibits platelet phosphodiesterase, causing an increase in cyclic AMP with potentiation of the action of PGI_2 – has been used widely as an anti-thrombotic agent, but there is little evidence that it is effective.

Table 8.28 Drugs used in the treatment of thrombotic disorders

Antiplatelet	Anticoagulant
Aspirin	Heparin:
Dipyridamole	unfractionated (or standard)
Clopidogrel	low molecular weight
Gp, IIb/IIIa inhibitors, e.g. abciximab, eptifibatide, tirofiban	Hirudins, e.g. lepirudin
	Fondaparinux
Epoprostenol	Warfarin
	Ximelagatran

Thrombolytic
Streptokinase
Tissue-type plasminogen activator (t-PA or alteplase)
Reteplase (r-PA)
Tenecteplase (TNK-tPA)

- *Clopidogrel* – affects the ADP-dependent activation of the glycoprotein IIb/IIIa complex. It is similar to ticlopidine but has fewer side-effects. Trials support its use in acute coronary syndromes (p. 808), particularly if aspirin is contraindicated.
- *Glycoprotein IIb/IIIa receptor antagonists* block a receptor on the platelet for fibrinogen and von Willebrand factor (Fig. 8.39). Three classes have been described:
  (a) murine–human chimeric antibodies (e.g. abciximab)
  (b) synthetic peptides (e.g. eptifibatide)
  (c) synthetic non-peptides (e.g. tirofiban).
  They have been used as an adjunct in invasive coronary intervention and as primary medical therapy in coronary heart disease. Excessive bleeding has been a problem.
- *Epoprostenol* is a prostacyclin which is used to inhibit platelet aggregation during renal dialysis (with or without heparin) and is also used in primary pulmonary hypertension.

The indications for and results of antiplatelet therapy are discussed in the appropriate sections (pp. 806 and 1215).

Thrombolytic therapy
Streptokinase

Streptokinase is a purified fraction of the filtrate obtained from cultures of haemolytic streptococci. It forms a complex with plasminogen, resulting in a conformational change which activates other plasminogen molecules to form plasmin.

Streptokinase is antigenic and the development of streptococcal antibodies precludes repeated use. Activation of plasminogen is indiscriminate so that both fibrin in clots and free fibrinogen are lysed, leading to low fibrinogen levels and the risk of haemorrhage.

Plasminogen activators (PA)

Tissue-type plasminogen activators (alteplase (t-PA), tenecteplase (TNK-PA)) are produced by recombinant technology. Reteplase (r-PA) is also a recombinant plasminogen activator. They are not antigenic and do not give allergic reactions. They have a slightly higher risk of intracerebral haemorrhage (see also p. 813).

Fig. 8.39 **The role of glycoprotein IIb/IIIa in platelet aggregation and the inhibition of platelet aggregation by inhibitors of glycoprotein IIb/IIIa receptors.** Modified from Lefkovits J, Plow EF, Topol EJ (1995) *New England Journal of Medicine* **332**: 1554, with permission.

Indications

The use of thrombolytic therapy in myocardial infarction is discussed on page 813. The combination of aspirin with thrombolytic therapy produces better results than thrombolytic therapy alone. The extent of the benefit depends on how quickly treatment is given. They are also used in cerebral infarction (p. 1214) and occasionally in massive pulmonary embolism.

The main risk of thrombolytic therapy is bleeding. Treatment should not be given to patients who have had recent bleeding, uncontrolled hypertension or a haemorrhagic stroke, or surgery or other invasive procedures within the previous 10 days.

Prevention and treatment of venous thromboembolism

Venous thromboembolism is a common problem after surgery, particularly in high-risk patients such as the elderly, those with malignant disease and those with a history of previous thrombosis (Table 8.29). The incidence is also high in patients confined to bed following trauma, myocardial infarction or other illnesses. The prevention and treatment of venous thrombosis includes the use of anticoagulants.

Anticoagulants

Heparin (standard or unfractionated)

Heparin is not a single substance but a mixture of polysaccharides. Commercially available unfractionated heparin consists of components with molecular weights varying from 5000 to 35 000 with an average of about 13 000. It was initially extracted from liver (hence its name) but it is now prepared from porcine gastric mucosa.

Heparin has an immediate effect on coagulation by potentiation of the formation of irreversible complexes between antithrombin and activated serine protease coagulation factors (thrombin, XIIa, XIa, Xa, IXa and VIIa).

Table 8.29 **Classification of risk of deep vein thrombosis and pulmonary embolism for hospital patients**

Low risk (proximal vein thrombosis 0.4%; fatal pulmonary embolism < 0.2%)
Patients < 40 years undergoing major surgery (> 30 minutes) with no other risk factors
Patients undergoing minor surgery (< 30 minutes) with no other risk factors
Patients with minor trauma or illness with no thrombophilia but history of deep vein thrombosis or previous pulmonary embolism

Medium risk (proximal vein thrombosis 2–4%; fatal pulmonary embolism 0.2–0.5%)
Major general, urological, gynaecological, cardiothoracic, vascular or neurological surgery in patients > 40 years or with one or more other risk factor(s)
Major acute medical illness such as myocardial infarction, heart failure, chest infection, cancer or inflammatory bowel disease
Major trauma
Minor surgery, trauma or illness in patients with previous deep vein thrombosis, pulmonary embolism or thrombophilia
Plastercast immobilization of the leg in patients with minor injury

High risk (proximal vein thrombosis 10–20%; fatal pulmonary embolism 1–5%)
Fracture or major orthopaedic surgery of pelvis, hip or leg
Major pelvic or abdominal surgery for cancer
Major surgery, trauma or illness in patients with previous deep vein thrombosis, pulmonary embolism or thrombophilia
Leg paralysis
Critical leg ischaemia or major leg amputation

Verstraete M (1997) Fortnightly review: prophylaxis of venous embolism. *BMJ* **314**:124, with permission of the BMJ.

Low-molecular-weight heparins (LMW heparins)

These are produced by enzymatic or chemical degradation of standard heparin, producing fractions with molecular weights in the range of 2000–8000. Potentiation of thrombin inhibition (anti-IIa activity) requires a minimum length of the heparin molecule with an approximate molecular weight of 5400, whereas the inhibition of factor Xa requires only a smaller heparin molecule with a molecular weight of about 1700.

LMW heparins have the following properties:

- Bioavailability is better than that of unfractionated heparin.
- They have greater activity against factor Xa than against factor IIa, suggesting that they may produce an equivalent anticoagulant effect to standard heparin but have a lower risk of bleeding, although this has not generally been confirmed. In addition, LMW heparins cause less inhibition of platelet function.
- They have a longer half-life than standard heparin and so can be given as a once-daily subcutaneous injection instead of every 8–12 hours.
- They produce little effect on tests of overall coagulation, such as the APTT at doses recommended for prophylaxis. They are not fully neutralized by protamine.

LMW heparins are widely used for antithrombotic prophylaxis, e.g. high-risk surgical patients and for the treatment of established thrombosis (see p. 870).

The main complication of all heparin treatment is bleeding. This is managed by stopping heparin. Very occasionally it is necessary to neutralize unfractionated heparin with protamine. Other complications include osteoporosis with prolonged therapy and thrombocytopenia.

Heparin-induced thrombocytopenia (HIT). HIT is an uncommon complication of heparin therapy and usually occurs 5–14 days after first heparin exposure. It is due to an immune response directed against heparin/platelet factor 4 complexes. All forms of heparin have been implicated but the problem occurs less often with LMW heparins. A separate and unimportant immediate thrombocytopenia has also been described.

HIT is paradoxically associated with severe thrombosis and when diagnosed all forms of heparin must be discontinued, including heparin flush. Unfortunately the diagnosis can be difficult to make because patients on heparin are often very sick and may be thrombocytopenic for many other reasons. Laboratory tests based on bioassay or immunoassay are available but are neither sensitive nor specific and management decisions often have to be made before results are available.

It is usually necessary to continue some form of anticoagulation in patients with HIT and the choice lies between the heparinoid danaparoid and the antithrombin hirudin. The introduction of warfarin should be covered by one of these agents, as warfarin alone may be ineffective or even exacerbate thrombosis as protein C levels fall.

Fondaparinux

This is a new synthetic pentasaccharide which inhibits activated factor X, similar to the LMW heparins. It will now be necessary to establish comparative efficacy (prevention or treatment of thrombosis) against risk of side-effects (bleeding) before the position of fondaparinux becomes clear.

Hirudin

A recombinant form of hirudin, lepirudin, is available. Lepirudin is used for anticoagulation in patients with HIT. Hirudins act directly on thrombin and can be monitored by the use of the APTT. They are excreted by the kidney and must be used with caution in renal failure.

Oral anticoagulants

These act by interfering with vitamin K metabolism. There are two types of oral anticoagulants, the coumarins and indanediones. The coumarin warfarin is most commonly used because it has a low incidence of side-effects other than bleeding.

The dosage is controlled by PT tests. Thromboplastin reagents for PT testing are derived from a variety of sources and give different PT results for the same plasma. It is standard practice to compare each thromboplastin with an international reference preparation so that it can be assigned an international sensitivity index (ISI). The international normalized ratio (INR) is the ratio of the patient's PT to a normal control when using the international reference preparation. Therapeutic ranges using the INR for oral anticoagulation in various conditions are shown in Box 8.2.

Each laboratory can use a chart adapted to the ISI of their thromboplastin to convert the patient's PT to the INR. Suitably selected control plasmas can also be used to achieve the same objective. The use of this system means that PT tests on a given plasma sample using different thromboplastins result in the same INR and that anticoagulant control is comparable in different hospitals across the world.

 Box 8.2   Indications for oral anticoagulation and target INR (British Society for Haematology 1998)

Target INR

2.5	Pulmonary embolism, proximal and calf deep vein thrombosis, recurrence of venous thromboembolism when no longer on warfarin therapy, symptomatic inherited thrombophilia, atrial fibrillation, cardioversion, mural thrombus, cardiomyopathy.
3.5	Recurrence of venous thromboembolism while on warfarin therapy, antiphospholipid syndrome, mechanical prosthetic heart valve, coronary artery graft thrombosis.

Contraindications to the use of oral anticoagulants are seldom absolute and include:

- severe uncontrolled hypertension
- non-thromboembolic strokes
- peptic ulceration (unless cured by *Helicobacter pylori* eradication)
- severe liver and renal disease
- pre-existing haemostatic defects
- non-compliance.

Oral anticoagulants should be avoided in pregnancy because they are teratogenic in the first trimester and may be associated with fetal haemorrhage later in pregnancy. When anticoagulation is considered essential in pregnancy, specialist advice should be sought. Self-administered subcutaneous heparin should be used as an alternative, although this may not be as effective for women with prosthetic cardiac valves.

Many drugs interact with warfarin (see Ch. 16). More frequent PT testing should accompany changes in medication, which should occur with the full knowledge of the anticoagulant clinic.

An increased anticoagulant effect due to warfarin (Emergency box 8.1) is usually produced by one of the following mechanisms:

- drugs causing a reduction in the metabolism of warfarin, including tricyclic antidepressants, cimetidine, sulphonamides, phenothiazines and amiodarone
- drugs such as clofibrate and quinidine which increase the sensitivity of hepatic receptors to warfarin

- drugs interfering with vitamin K absorption (such as broad-spectrum antibiotics and colestyramine) which also potentiate the action of warfarin
- displacement of warfarin from its binding site on serum albumin by drugs such as sulphonamides (this is not usually responsible for clinically important interactions)
- drugs that inhibit platelet function (such as aspirin) which increase the risk of bleeding
- alcohol excess, cardiac failure, liver or renal disease, hyperthyroidism and febrile illnesses which result in potentiation of the effect of warfarin.

A decreased anticoagulant effect due to warfarin. This is usually produced by drugs that increase the clearance of warfarin by induction of hepatic enzymes that metabolize warfarin, such as rifampicin and barbiturates.

Ximelagatran

This oral direct thrombin inhibitor is a potential alternative to warfarin and has already been evaluated in patients with venous thromboembolism, atrial fibrillation and myocardial infarction. It has a rapid onset of action and can be administered in a fixed dose without the need for monitoring. Drug interactions are also less than for warfarin but elimination is primarily renal and abnormalities of liver function have been described during its use.

Prophylaxis to prevent venous thromboembolism

Prophylactic measures to prevent venous thrombosis during surgery are aimed at procedures for preventing stasis, such as early mobilization, elevation of the legs, compression stockings, and possibly calf-muscle stimulation and passive calf-muscle exercises during surgery, and methods for preventing hypercoagulability, usually using heparin.

Low-risk patients (Table 8.29) require no specific measures other than early mobilization.

Moderate-risk patients should receive a standard dose of LMW heparin e.g. enoxaparin 20 mg (2000 i.u.) subcutaneously daily until the patient is ambulatory.

In *high-risk patients*, such as patients undergoing total hip replacement, LMW heparin once daily, such as enoxaparin 40 mg (4000 i.u.), has been shown to be more effective than standard low-dose heparin in preventing thrombosis. There is evidence to suggest that it is most effective when administered for a total of 1 month postoperatively rather than merely during the admission for surgery.

LMW heparin has replaced standard low-dose heparin for all surgical prophylaxis and is increasingly used for medical prophylaxis.

Treatment of established venous thromboembolism

The aim of anticoagulant treatment is to prevent further thrombosis and pulmonary embolization while resolution

---

> **!** **Emergency Box 8.1**
> **Management of bleeding and excessive oral anticoagulation (modified from British Society for Haematology 1998)**

INR > 3.0 < 6.0 (target INR 2.5) INR > 4.0 < 6.0 (target INR 3.5)	(1) reduce warfarin dose or stop (2) restart warfarin when INR < 5.0
INR > 6.0 < 8.0 no bleeding or minor bleeding	(1) stop warfarin (2) restart when INR < 5.0
INR > 8.0, no bleeding or minor bleeding	(1) stop warfarin (2) restart warfarin when INR < 5.0 (3) if other risk factors for bleeding give 0.5–2.5 mg of vitamin K (oral)
Major bleeding	(1) stop warfarin (2) give prothrombin complex concentrate 50 units/kg or FFP 15 mL/kg (3) give 5 mg of vitamin K (oral or i.v.)

If unexpected bleeding occurs investigate the possibility of a local anatomical cause.

of venous thrombi occurs by natural fibrinolytic activity. Anticoagulation is started with heparin as it produces an immediate anticoagulant effect. There is no evidence that it is necessary to use heparin for any longer than it takes for simultaneously administered warfarin to produce an anticoagulant effect (INR 2.5) usually about 3–4 days.

LMW heparin (e.g. tinzaparin 175 units/kg daily) is equally effective and as safe as unfractionated heparin in the immediate treatment of deep vein thrombosis and pulmonary embolism. This creates the opportunity for treatment of venous thromboembolism without admission to hospital, in compliant patients without coexisting risk factors for haemorrhage.

Anticoagulation (with warfarin approximately 3–9 mg daily for 6 weeks) is sufficient for patients after their first thrombosis provided there are no persisting risk factors. There is much interest in the use of longer-term anticoagulation in patients with previous thrombosis. It has

been suggested that a lower INR might be safer and equally effective but the current view is that the target INR should be 2.0 to 3.0 where oral anticoagulation is used. Secondary prophylaxis should be offered to patients with unprovoked venous thromboembolism, for a period of 6–12 months. Very long-term treatment should be reserved for those with repeated episodes or continuing risk factors. Outpatient anticoagulation is best supervised in anticoagulant clinics. Patients are issued with national booklets for recording INR results and anticoagulant doses.

The role of thrombolytic therapy in the treatment of venous thrombosis is not established. It is sometimes used in patients with massive pulmonary embolism and in patients with extensive deep venous thrombi.

Thrombolytic therapy should be followed by anticoagulation with heparin for a few days and then by oral anticoagulants for a few months to prevent rethrombosis.

FURTHER READING

British Society for Haematology guidelines documents:
(1998) Guidelines on oral anticoagulation, 3rd edition. *British Journal of Haematology* **101**: 374–387
(2000) Guidelines on the investigation and management of the antiphospholipid syndrome. *British Journal of Haematology* **109**: 704–715
(2001) Investigation and management of heritable thrombophilia. *British Journal of Haematology* **114**: 512–528
(2003) Guideline on the diagnosis and management of the thrombotic microangiopathic haemolytic anaemias. *British Journal of Haematology* **120**: 556–573
(2003) Guidelines for the investigation and management of idiopathic thrombocytopenic purpura in adults, children and in pregnancy. *British Journal of Haematology* **120**: 574–596
(2004) The diagnosis for deep vein thrombosis in symptomatic outpatients and the potential for clinical assessment and D-dimer assays to reduce the need for diagnostic imaging. *British Journal of Haematology* **124**: 15–25.

Online. Available: http://www.bcshguidelines.com; http://www.bcsh.org.uk; http://www.transfusionguidelines-org.uk.
Buller, HR, Prins MH (2003) Secondary prophylaxis with warfarin for venous thromboembolism. *New England Journal of Medicine* **349**: 702–704.
Dahlback B (2000) Blood coagulation. *Lancet* **355**: 1627–1632.
George JN (2000) Platelets. *Lancet* **355**: 1531–1539.
Gerhardt A et al. (2000) Prothrombin and factor V mutations in women with a history of thrombosis during pregnancy and the puerperium. *New England Journal of Medicine* **342**: 374–380.
Lowe GDO, Sanderock PAG, Rosedaal FR (2003) Prevention of venous thromboembolism after major orthopaedic surgery: is fondaparinux an advance? *Lancet* **362**: 504–505.
Shapiro SS (2003) Treating thrombosis in the 21st century. *New England Journal of Medicine* **349**: 1762–1764.
Topol EJ, Byzova TV, Plow EF (1999) Platelet GP IIb-IIIa blockers. *Lancet* **353**: 227–231.

CHAPTER BIBLIOGRAPHY

Beutler E, Lichtman MA, Coller BS, Kipps TJ, Seligsohn U (2001) *Williams Hematology*, 6th edn. New York: McGraw-Hill.
Hoffbrand AV, Pettit J (2000). *Atlas of Clinical Haematology*, 3rd edn, Edinburgh: Churchill Livingstone.

Hoffbrand AV, Pettit J, Moss P (2001) *Essential Haematology*, 4th edn. Oxford: Blackwell Science.
Murphy MF, Pamphilon D (2001) *Practical Transfusion Medicine*. Oxford: Blackwell Science.
Provan D, Gribben J (2000) *Molecular Haematology*. Oxford: Blackwell Science.
Weatherall D, Clegg J (2001) *The Thalassaemia Syndromes*, 4th edn. Oxford: Blackwell Science.

SIGNIFICANT WEBSITES

http://www.bloodline.net
General website on haematology
http://www.transfusion.org
Journal of the American Association of Blood Banks
http://www.shotuk.org
Serious Hazards of Transfusion (SHOT) scheme, covering UK and Ireland NHS and private hospitals, affiliated to the Royal College of Pathologists (based Manchester Blood Transfusion Centre)
http://www.blood.co.uk
UK National Blood Service

http://www.doh.gov.uk/bbt2
UK CMO's Better Blood Transfusion Conference
http://www.bcshguidelines.com
British Society for Haematology guidelines
http://www.wfh.org
World Federation of Hemophilia
http://www.hemophilia.org
US National Hemophilia Foundation
http://www.med.unc.edu/isth/
International Society on Thrombosis and Haemostasis (ISTH)

Malignant disease

The term 'malignant disease' encompasses a wide range of illnesses, including common ones such as lung, breast and colorectal cancer (Table 9.1), as well as rare ones, like the acute leukaemias. Malignant disease is widely prevalent and, in the West, almost a third of the population will develop cancer at some time during their life. It is second only to cardiovascular disease as the cause of death. Although the mortality of cancer is high, many advances have been made, both in terms of treatment, and in understanding the biology of the disease at the molecular level.

Treatment is given with curative or palliative intent, depending upon the evidence from continuing clinical trials. For many people, the word 'cancer' implies certain death, although this is clearly not always the case. Physicians have an obligation to be honest with their patients, combining realism about the prognosis with compassion and understanding so that patients can take an informed part in treatment decisions.

AETIOLOGY AND EPIDEMIOLOGY

In most patients the cause of their cancer remains unknown and is probably multifactorial. Several environmental factors have, however, been identified as being associated with the development of malignancy (Table 9.2).

Tobacco

The incidence of lung cancer in both men and women has increased dramatically in the last 25 years. The association of smoking with lung cancer is indisputable and causative mechanisms have been identified: cigarette tobacco is responsible for one-third of all deaths from cancer in the UK. Smoking not only causes lung cancer, it is also associated with cancer of the mouth, larynx, oesophagus and bladder. Smoking is discussed on page 893.

Alcohol

Alcohol is associated with cancers of the upper respiratory and gastrointestinal tracts (Table 9.2), and it also interacts

Table 9.1 Epidemiology of cancer by site of origin in England and Wales

Type	% of all cancers (1998)	% of cancer deaths	M : F
Oral cavity/pharynx	1	1.2	2.3 : 1
Oesophagus	2.3	4.4	2 : 1
Stomach	3.7	4.7	2.4 : 1
Colorectal	11.1	11.0	1.4 : 1
Pancreas	2.3	4.3	1.5 : 1
Lung	13.6	22.2	1.6 : 1
Melanoma	1.8	1.0	0.6 : 1
Other skin	14.1	0.3	1.5 : 1
Breast	12.2	8.6	0.01 : 1
Cervix	1.2	1.1	
Uterus	1.5	0.7	
Ovary	2.0	2.9	
Prostate	7.4	6.3	
Bladder	4.5	3.5	3.6 : 1
Kidney	1.8	2.0	2.1 : 1
Brain	1.3	2.1	1.4 : 1
Non-Hodgkin's lymphoma	2.8	2.9	1.5 : 1
Myeloma	1.1	1.6	1.5 : 1
Leukaemias	2.1	2.6	1.5 : 1

Cancers < 1% have been excluded
Derived from Doll R, Peto R (2003) In: *Oxford Textbook of Medicine*. 4th edn. Oxford: Oxford University Press

Table 9.2   Some causative factors associated with the development of cancer at various sites

Smoking	Mouth, pharynx, oesophagus, larynx, lung, bladder, lip
Alcohol	Mouth, pharynx, larynx, oesophagus, colorectal
Iatrogenic:	
Alkylating agents	Bladder, bone marrow
Oestrogens	Endometrium, vagina, breast
Androgens	Prostate
Radiotherapy	e.g. mantle radiotherapy – carcinoma of breast and bronchus
Diet:	
High-fat diet	Colorectal cancer
Environmental/ occupation:	
Vinyl chloride	Liver (angiosarcoma)
Polycyclic hydrocarbons	Skin, lung, bladder, myeloid leukaemia
Aromatic amines	Bladder
Asbestos	Lung, mesothelium
Ultraviolet light	Skin, lip
Radiation	e.g. leukaemia, thyroid cancer
Aflatoxin	Liver
Biological agents:	
Hepatitis B virus	Liver (hepatocellular carcinoma)
Hepatitis C virus	Liver (hepatocellular carcinoma)
Human T cell leukaemia virus	Leukaemia/lymphoma
Epstein–Barr virus	Burkitt's lymphoma Hodgkin's lymphoma
Schistosoma japonicum	Bladder
Helicobacter pylori	Stomach

with tobacco in the aetiology of these tumours. It may be associated with an increased risk of breast cancer.

Diet

Dietary factors have been attributed to account for a third of cancer deaths, although it is often difficult to differentiate these from other epidemiological factors. For example, the incidence of stomach cancer is particularly high in the Far East, while breast and colon cancers are more common in the western, economically more developed countries. Many associations have been observed without a causative mechanism being identified between the incidence of cancer and the consumption of dietary fibre, red meat, saturated fats, salted fish, vitamin E, vitamin A and many others. Food and its role in the causation of gastrointestinal cancer is discussed in Chapter 5.

Environmental/occupational

Ultraviolet light is known to increase the risk of skin cancer (basal cell, squamous cell and melanoma). The incidence of melanoma is therefore particularly high in the white Anglo-Celtic population of Australia, New Zealand and South Africa, where exposure to UV light is combined with a genetically predisposed population.

Occupational factors. In 1775, Percival Pott described the association between carcinogenic hydrocarbons in soot and the development of scrotal epitheliomas in chimney sweeps.

The principal causes now are asbestos (lung and mesothelial cancer) and combustion of fossil fuels releasing polycyclic hydrocarbons (skin, lung, bladder cancers). Organic chemicals such as benzene may cause molecular abnormalities associated with the development of myeloid leukaemia.

Infectious agents

The geographical distribution of a rare malignancy may suggest that it might be caused by, or associated with, an infective agent. For example, a specific type of T-cell leukaemia, seen almost exclusively in residents of the southern island of Japan and in the West Indies, is caused by infection with the retrovirus, HTLV-1 (human T-cell leukaemia virus) which is endemic in these areas.

Hepatocellular carcinoma occurs in patients with hepatitis B and C virus infections, and Burkitt's lymphoma and nasopharyngeal carcinoma are associated with the Epstein–Barr virus. EBV is also linked with Hodgkin's lymphoma (p. 508). Patients with HIV infection or immunosuppression from organ transplantation have an increased incidence of EBV-related lymphoma and herpesvirus-8-associated Kaposi's sarcoma. The incidence of cervical cancer is increasing amongst younger women in association with human papillomavirus infection. Early sexual activity and multiple sexual partners have both been found to be associated with increased risk.

Bacterial infection with *Helicobacter pylori* predisposes to the development of gastric cancer and gastric lymphoma, while *Schistosoma japonicum* infection predisposes to the development of squamous carcinomas in the bladder.

Iatrogenic

Drugs. Oestrogens have been implicated in the development of vaginal, endometrial and breast carcinoma. Alkylating agents and radiotherapy given, for example, for Hodgkin's lymphoma (see later) are themselves associated with an increased incidence of secondary acute myelogenous leukaemia (AML), bladder and lung cancer. The epipodophyllotoxin drug, etoposide, has also been shown to be associated with the development of secondary AML.

Radiation. The nuclear disasters of Hiroshima, Nagasaki and Chernobyl led to an increased incidence of leukaemia after 5–10 years in the exposed population. Increased incidences of thyroid and breast cancer have also been reported. Radiotherapy used, for example, in ankylosing spondylitis and Hodgkin's lymphoma, has led to increased incidences of cancer.

Geographical distribution

The incidence of specific tumours varies with geographical location but the cause varies; for example England, Scotland and Wales have the highest death rate from malignant disease in the world, mainly because of the very high incidence of lung cancer due to smoking. India also has the highest incidence of cancers of the gall bladder, mouth and lower pharynx. Breast, colon and prostatic cancer have a relatively low incidence in Asian countries. Liver cancer occurs world-wide but is rare in Europe and North America where the HBV carrier rate is low. Stomach cancer is particularly prevalent in Japan and is thought to be due to dietary factors.

Environmental factors have been clearly implicated. For example, subsequent generations of people moving from countries with a low incidence to those with a high incidence of breast or colon cancer acquire the cancer incidence of the country to which they have moved. This suggests that for these specific cancers, environmental factors are more significant than genetic ones.

THE BIOLOGY OF CANCER

Most human neoplasms are monoclonal in origin, i.e. they arise from genetic mutations within a single affected cell. However, over subsequent cell divisions heterogeneity develops with the accumulation of further abnormalities. The genes most commonly affected can be characterized as those controlling cell cycle check points, DNA repair and DNA damage recognition, apoptosis, differentiation, and growth signalling. Proliferation may continue at the expense of differentiation, which together with the failure of apoptosis leads to tumour formation with the accumulation of abnormal cells varying in size, shape and nuclear morphology as viewed down the light microscope.

The *kinetics* of cancer cell growth are exponential; however, the doubling times of human tumours are enormously variable. Mutations are common in the genes controlling a series of intracellular proteins, such as the cyclins and cyclin-dependent kinases (p. 157), and oncogene products such as c-*myc*, and the *ras* proteins (see Cancer genetics, p. 188) that regulate proliferation. Proliferation may also be abnormal due to defects in the nuclear enzyme telomerase, contact with other cells, nutrient supply or cytokine signalling. Telomerase is an enzyme that prevents the normal shortening of DNA with each cell division that leads to senescence. Persistent telomerase activity helps to maintain the neoplastic state in cancer cells.

Epithelial growth factor (EGF) and its receptors are overexpressed in many human epithelial tumours, constitutively switching on unrestrained growth of these tumours. Transforming growth factor-β (TGF-β), a cytokine which has effects on extracellular matrix proteins, angiogenesis (see below) and immune effector cells, is also often overexpressed in tumour cells, and defects in TGF-β signalling are often found in cancer cells. This signalling pathway is activated by cytoplasmic proteins, e.g. MADH4. Defects in tumour suppressor genes such as *MADH4* (*SMAD4* or *DPC4*) and *p53* (see p. 189) have a major part to play and occur, for example, in most pancreatic cancers.

Apoptosis and growth

Tumour cell death may also be dysregulated. Normal cells usually die by an active and tightly regulated process known as apoptosis, or 'programmed cell death' (p. 162). Apoptosis can occur in response to a number of physiological or pathological stimuli (tumour necrosis factor, Fas ligand, and DNA-damaging cytotoxic drugs) and is mediated within the cell by a family of proteins known as caspases. Caspase activity is, in turn, regulated by intracellular inhibitors such as the Bcl-2 family of proteins and the inhibitor of apoptosis proteins (IAPs). Disturbances in the normal balance of these various proteins have been identified which favour survival of tumour cells over their normal counterparts. An example is the upregulation of the bcl-2 protein in follicular non–Hodgkin's lymphoma.

Tumour immunology

Tumour cells are usually not recognized and killed by the immune system. There are two main causes. The first is failure to express molecules such as HLA and costimulatory B7 molecules which are required for activation of cytotoxic, or 'killer', T lymphocytes, since expression of these 'costimulatory' molecules following gene transfection may augment an immune response. Secondly, tumours may also actively secrete immunosuppressive cytokines and cause a generalized immunosuppression, leading for example to the reactivation of latent herpes zoster in shingles associated with malignancy.

Angiogenesis

For many tumours, there is a progressive slowing of the rate of growth as the tumours become larger. This occurs for many reasons, but outgrowing the blood supply is paramount. Tumours need to establish a new blood supply. This new vessel formation (angiogenesis) is stimulated by a variety of peptides produced both by tumour cells and by host inflammatory cells, such as basic fibroblast growth factor (bFGF), angiopoietin 2 and vascular endothelial growth factors (VEGFs), which are stimulated by hypoxia. Inhibition of angiogenesis is a potentially novel method of cancer therapy, as new vessel formation within and around tumours not only provides the cancer with nutrients and oxygen, but permits haematogenous spread, or metastasis.

Invasion and metastasis

Cancers spread by both local invasion and by metastasis in vessels of the blood or lymphatic systems. Infiltration into surrounding tissues is associated with loss of cell–cell cohesion. Cohesion is mediated by active homotypic cell adhesion molecules (CAMs). The cadherin molecules are transmembrane glycoproteins able to mediate cellular attachment. Epithelial cadherin (E-cadherin) is expressed by many carcinomas, e.g. gastric carcinoma (p. 289), and loss of E-cadherin expression is associated with an increase in invasion of the tumour.

Invasion is partly determined by the balance of activators to inhibitors of proteolysis. Secretion of proteolytic enzymes, including the matrix metalloproteinases (particularly the collagenases), occurs from adjacent fibroblasts owing to failure of production of tissue inhibitors. The balance between the expression and activity of the matrix metalloproteinases (MMPs) and their tissue inhibitors (TIMPs) is involved in tumour growth, invasion, metastasis and angiogenesis. Some TIMPs may regulate cell proliferation and survival of cancer cells independently of MMP activity.

Dissemination of tumour cells occurs when they enter the vascular and lymphatic vessels. Here they must survive host-defence mechanisms so as to spread throughout the body. The disseminated cancer cells lodge in distant sites, partly by chance, but also because of specific interactions between receptors/ligands found on endothelial cells and on tumour cells. This may account for the specific pattern of metastases with certain tumours; for example, breast tumours frequently metastasize to long bones (see below).

The attachment of tumour cells to the endothelial cells is partly through adhesion molecules. Integrins are transmembrane heterodimeric glycoproteins formed by non-covalent association of α and β chains. These molecules are normally responsible for cell-substrate adhesion. Patterns of integrin expression in tumours are complex but, nevertheless, certain tumours demonstrate upregulation of specific integrins, such as the alpha v family, during tumour progression, and this may allow migration of tumour cells through the extracellular matrix substrate and invasion through the basement membrane and formation of a metastatic deposit. Integrins also act as receptors for signals regulating gene expression and apoptosis.

Bone metastases. These occur in 75% of patients with advanced breast and prostate cancer and in 25% of patients with other solid tumours, e.g. lung, GI tract, thyroid, bladder or kidney.

Metastases are either osteolytic or osteoblastic with some patients having both.

Prostate cancer is predominantly osteoblastic while most patients with breast cancer have osteolytic lesions.

In multiple myeloma (p. 517) the lesions are purely osteolytic.

Bone is a frequent site of metastases due to:

- high blood flow
- tumour cell production of adhesins which bind them to marrow stromal cells
- growth factors in bone, including TGFβ, insulin-like growth factor (ILG)-1 and 2, platelet-derived growth factor and fibroblastic growth factors.

Osteolytic metastases (Fig. 9.1). The destruction of bone is mediated by osteoclasts and not the tumour cells. Tumour cells produce parathyroid hormone-related peptide, IL-6, prostaglandin E$_2$, TNF and macrophage

Fig. 9.1 Mechanisms of osteolytic metastases. Tumour cells secrete hormones as shown. These increase various factors, e.g. RANKL, and lead to increased osteoclastic activity. Bone destruction (resorption) in turn produces factors which increase tumour growth. Osteoprotegerin (see p. 592) has an inhibitory effect on RANKL. BMPs, bone morphogenic proteins; FGF, fibroblast growth factor; IGF, insulin-like growth factor; IL-6, interleukin 6; JNK, jun N-terminal kinase; M-CSF, macrophage colony-stimulating factor; NFκB, nuclear factor kappa B; PDGF, platelet-derived growth factor; PGE2, prostaglandin E2; PTH-RP, parathyroid hormone-related peptide; RANKL, receptor activator of NFκB ligand; TGF, transforming growth factor; TNF, tumour necrosis factor.

colony-stimulating factor (M-CSF) which increase the expression of receptor activity of nuclear factor κB ligand (RANKL) which directly induces formation of osteoclasts and bone resorption. Bone destruction increases calcium levels, which promotes both tumour growth and the production of PTH-related peptide, which is a major factor in osteolytic bone destruction in many tumours. In multiple myeloma there is, additionally, inhibition of osteoblast activity (p. 517).

Osteoblastic metastases. The mechanism for this is less clear. It has been suggested that osteoclastic activity precedes osteoblastic activity and bone formation. It is also possible that the vicious circle (as in osteoclastic activity) may be in action, whereby the tumour induces osteoblastic activity and the release of growth factors for osteoblasts, which then increases the growth of tumours. Endothelin 1 has been shown to stimulate bone formation and its levels are increased in, for example, prostate and breast cancers.

Cancer genetics

The development of cancer is associated with a fundamental genetic change within the cell. Evidence for the genetic origin of cancer is based on the following:

- Some cancers show a familial predisposition.
- Most known carcinogens act through induced mutations.

- Susceptibility to some carcinogens depends on the ability of cellular enzymes to convert them to a mutagenic form.
- Genetically determined traits associated with a deficiency in the enzymes required for DNA repair are associated with an increased risk of cancer.
- Some cancers are associated with chromosome 'instability' because of deficiencies in mismatch repair genes.
- Many malignant tumours represent clonal proliferations of neoplastic cells.
- Many tumours contain well-described cytogenetic abnormalities, which involve mutated or abnormally regulated oncogenes and tumour suppressor genes with transforming activity in cell lines.

Mutations may occur in the germline and therefore be present in every cell in the body, or they may occur by somatic mutation in response, for example, to carcinogens, and therefore be present only in the cells of the tumour.

Expression of the mutation and hence carcinogenesis will depend upon the penetrance (due to level of expression and presence of other genetic events) of the gene and whether the mutated allele has a dominant or recessive effect. There are a small group of autosomal dominant inherited mutations such as *RB* (in retinoblastoma) and a small group of recessive mutations (Table 9.3). Carriers of the recessive mutations are at risk of developing cancer if the second allele becomes mutated, leading to 'loss of heterozygosity' within the tumour, although this is seldom sufficient as carcinogenesis is a multistep process.

Malignant transformation may result from a gain in function as cellular proto-oncogenes become mutated, (e.g. *ras*), amplified (e.g. *HER2*), or translocated (e.g. *BCR-ABL*). However, these mutations are insufficient to cause malignant transformation by themselves. Alternatively, there may be a loss of function of tumour suppressor genes that normally suppress growth and differentiation. A third mechanism involves alterations in the genes controlling the transcription of the oncogenes or tumour suppressor genes (e.g. p. 189) (Tables 9.3 and 9.4).

DNA repair

Autosomal recessive

Some relatively rare autosomal *recessive* diseases associated with abnormalities of DNA repair predispose to the development of cancer (Table 9.3).

- *Xeroderma pigmentosum.* There is an inability to repair DNA damage caused by ultraviolet light and by some chemicals, leading to a high incidence of skin cancer.
- *Ataxia telangiectasia.* Mutation results in an increased sensitivity to ionizing radiation and an increased incidence of lymphoid tumours.
- *Bloom's syndrome and Fanconi's anaemia.* An increased susceptibility to lymphoid malignancy is seen.

It is not known why these chromosome-break syndromes predispose to tumours of lymphatic tissue.

Autosomal dominant

The following are examples of cancer syndromes that exhibit *dominant* inheritance (Table 9.3):

- *Retinoblastoma*, an eye tumour found in young children. It occurs in both hereditary (40%) and non-hereditary (60%) forms. The 40% of patients with the hereditary form have a germline mutation on the long arm of chromosome 13 that predisposes to retinoblastoma. In addition to the latter, children inheriting this mutation

Table 9.3 Familial cancer syndromes

	Gene	Neoplasms
Autosomal dominant		
Retinoblastoma	RB1	Eye
Wilms' tumour	WT1	Kidney
Li–Fraumeni	p53	Sarcoma/ brain/ leukaemia
Neurofibromatosis type 1	NF1	Neurofibromas
Familial adenomatous polyposis (FAP)	APC	Colon
Hereditary non-polyposis colon cancer (HNPCC)	MLH1 and MSH2	Colon, endometrium
Breast ovary families	BRCA1 and BRCA2	Breast/ovary
Melanoma	p16	Skin
Von Hippel–Lindau	VHL	Renal cell carcinoma and haemangio-blastoma
Multiple endocrine neoplasia Type 1	MEN1	Pituitary, pancreas, parathyroid
Multiple endocrine neoplasia Type 2	RET	Thyroid, adrenal medulla
Autosomal recessive		
Xeroderma pigmentosa	XP	Skin
Ataxia telangiectasia	AT	Leukaemia, lymphoma
Fanconi's anaemia	FA	Leukaemia, lymphoma
Bloom's syndrome	BS	Leukaemia, lymphoma

Table 9.4 Examples of acquired/somatic mutations and proto-oncogenes

Point mutation	
K-ras	Pancreatic cancer
DNA amplification	
myc	Neuroblastoma
HER2-neu	Breast cancer
Chromosome translocation	
BCR-ABL	CML, ALL
PML-RAR	APML
Bcl-2/IgH	Follicular lymphoma
c-myc and Ig	Burkitt's lymphoma

CML, chronic myeloid leukaemia; ALL, acute lymphoblastic leukaemia; APML, acute promyelocytic leukaemia at the so-called *RB1* locus are at risk for developing other tumours, particularly osteosarcoma.

- *Breast and ovarian cancer.* Two genes have been identified – *BRCA1* and *BRCA2*. A strong family history along with germline mutation of these genes accounts for most cases of familial breast cancer and over half of ovarian cancers. BRCA1 and 2 proteins bind to the DNA repair enzyme Rad51 to make it functional in repairing DNA breaks. Mutations in the *BRCA* genes will lead to accumulation of unrepaired mutations in tumour-suppressor genes and crucial oncogenes.

- *Neurofibromatosis.* Inactivation of the *NF1* gene will lead to constitutive activation of *ras* proteins.

- *Multiple-endocrine-adenomatosis syndromes* (p. 1099). Multiple endocrine neoplasia type 1 is associated with the *MEN1* gene and type 2 (MEN2) is associated with mutations in the *RET* proto-oncogene on chromosome 10 and as such are the exception to all the other syndromes which involve tumour suppressor genes.

FURTHER READING

Murphy RM (2001) Chemokines and the molecular basis of cancer metastases. *New England Journal of Medicine* **345**: 833–835.

Pedersen-Bjergaard J (2001) Molecular cytogenetics in cancer. *Lancet* **357**: 491–492.

Roodman GD (2004) Mechanisms of bone metastases. *New England Journal of Medicine* **350**: 1655–1664.

Stewart AK, Schuh AC (2000) White cells 2: Impact of understanding the molecular basis of haematological malignant disorders on clinical practice. *Lancet* **355**: 1447–1453.

Wyllie AH, Bellamy CO, Bubb VJ et al. (1999) Apoptosis and carcinogenesis. *British Journal of Cancer* **80** (Suppl. 1): 34–37.

THE DIAGNOSIS OF MALIGNANCY

Most common cancers (but not the haematological cancers) start as focal microscopic clones of transformed cells, and diagnosis only becomes likely once sufficient tumour bulk has accumulated to cause symptoms or signs. In order to try to make an earlier diagnosis and increase the curative possibilities, an increasing number of screening programmes are being investigated which target the asymptomatic or preinvasive stages of the cancer.

Screening

Genetic screening is used to target screening to those people at most risk of developing cancer. The aim is to improve individual and/or population survival. This strategy is dependent upon finding tests that are sufficiently sensitive and specific, using detection methods that identify cancer before it has spread, and having curative treatments that are practical and consistent with maintenance of a normal lifestyle and quality of life.

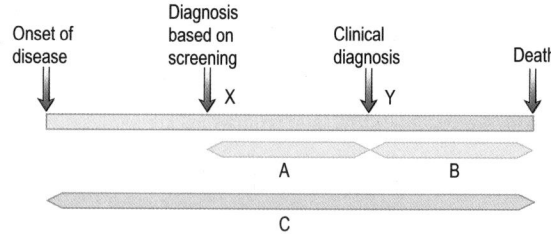

Fig. 9.2 Lead time bias. Earlier diagnosis, at X, made by screening tests before the clinical diagnosis, at Y, suggests an increased survival time of A + B. The actual survival time (C) remains unchanged.

The ability to detect cancer at its very early stages when the patient is asymptomatic is the goal of every healthcare system.

Screening is provided to populations, e.g. for breast and cervical cancer in the UK, and also to individuals via annual check-ups, or opportunistic when patients see their doctor for other reasons.

Unfortunately, earlier diagnosis does not necessarily mean longer survival. The patient is merely treated at an earlier date and hence the survival appears longer, death still occurs at the same time from the point of genesis of the cancer. This is called lead time bias (Fig. 9.2). With length time bias, a greater number of slowly growing tumours are detected when screening asymptomatic individuals.

An effective screening procedure should:

- be affordable to the healthcare system
- be acceptable to all social groups so that they attend the screening session
- have a good discriminatory index between benign and malignant lesions
- show a reduction in mortality from the cancer.

Cervical cancer

This test is cheap and safe but cervical smears require a well-trained cytologist to identify the early changes (dyskaryosis and cervical intraepithelial neoplasia (CIN)). This test reduces the incidence and mortality from cervical cancer.

Breast cancer

The UK NHS Breast Screening Programme (i.e. mammography) for women aged 50–64 years has been shown to reduce mortality from breast cancer, and randomized control studies from other countries have also shown reductions in mortality. The test is acceptable to most women with 75% of women attending for screening.

The cost is estimated to be between £250 000 and £1.3 million per life saved, money which according to critics of screening, could be used more appropriately in better treatment.

Other population-based screening programmes that are being used or are in trials are:

Prostate cancer

There is an easy, cheap, effective test – serum prostate-specific antigen (PSA) for the detection of this cancer, which is on the increase. The problems are that no easy acceptable treatment is available (p. 686) and the natural history of the disease is unclear (many men over 70 have evidence of prostate cancer at post-mortem with no symptoms of the disease) and no survival advantage has yet been shown.

Colorectal cancer (CRC)

Faecal occult blood is an acceptable and cheap test for the detection of CRC. The false-positive rates are high, meaning many unnecessary colonoscopies (p. 330). Screening with flexible sigmoidoscopy is discussed on p. 331. No clear benefit on survival has yet been shown.

Symptoms of cancer

Patients present with tumour site-specific symptoms, e.g. pain, and physical signs, e.g. a mass, which readily identify the primary site of the cancer. On the other hand, many seek medical attention when more systemic and non-specific symptoms occur such as weight loss, fatigue, and anorexia. These usually indicate a more advanced stage of the disease except in some paraneoplastic and ectopic endocrine syndromes (see below). Other patients are only diagnosed upon the discovery of established metastases such as the back pain of metastatic prostatic cancer or the liver enlargement of metastatic gastro-intestinal cancer.

Other indirect effects of the cancer manifest as paraneoplastic syndromes (Box 9.1) that are often associated with specific types of cancer and are reversible with treatment of the cancer. The effects and mechanisms can be very variable. For example in the Lambert–Eaton syndrome (p. 1269) there is cross-reactivity between tumour antigens and the normal tissues, e.g. the acetylcholine release at neuromuscular junctions.

The *coagulopathy of cancer* may present with thrombophlebitis, deep venous thrombosis and pulmonary emboli, particularly in association with cancers of pancreas, stomach and breast.

Other symptoms are related to peptide or hormone release, e.g. carcinoid or Cushing's syndrome.

Cachexia of advanced cancer is due to release of chemokines such as tumour necrosis factor (TNF), as well as the fact that patients have a loss of appetite.

Cancer-associated immunosuppression can lead to reactivation of latent infections such as herpes zoster.

Physical examination

A general examination should be performed to include:

- main symptomatic areas, e.g. site, size of mass and associated lymphadenopathy
- precursor lesions, e.g. solar keratosis, dysplastic naevi
- general signs, e.g. jaundice, clubbing
- functional capacity (see Table 9.6).

Box 9.1 Paraneoplastic syndromes

Syndrome	Tumour
Neurological	
Lambert–Eaton syndrome	Lung (small cell)
Peripheral sensory neuropathy	Lung (small cell), breast and ovary
Cerebellar degeneration	Lung (particularly small cell)
Endocrine/metabolic	
SIADH	Lung (small cell)
Ectopic ACTH secretion	Lung (small cell)
Hypercalcaemia	Renal, breast
Musculoskeletal	
Hypertrophic pulmonary osteoarthropathy	Lung (non-small cell)
Clubbing	Lung
Skin	
Dermatomyositis/polymyositis	Lung and upper GI
Acanthosis nigricans	Mainly gastric
Hyperpigmentation	Lung (small cell)
Pemphigus	
Haematological	
Erythrocytosis	Renal cell carcinoma, hepatocellular carcinoma, cerebellar haemangioblastoma
Migratory thrombophlebitis	Pancreatic adenocarcinoma
DIC	Adenocarcinoma

SIADH, syndrome of inappropriate antidiuretic hormone secretion; ACTH, adrenocorticotrophic hormone; DIC, disseminated intravascular coagulation

Histology

The diagnosis of cancer may be suspected by both patient and doctor but advice about treatment can usually only be given on the basis of a tissue diagnosis. This may be obtained by surgical biopsy or on the basis of cytology (e.g. lung cancer diagnosed by sputum cytology or cervix cancer diagnosed on the basis of a cervical smear). Malignant lesions can be distinguished morphologically from benign by the pleomorphic nature of the cells, increased numbers of mitoses, nuclear abnormalities in size, chromatin pattern and nucleolar organization, and evidence of invasion into surrounding tissues.

The degree of differentiation (or conversely of anaplasia) of the tumour has prognostic significance: generally speaking, more differentiated tumours have a better prognosis than poorly differentiated ones. Immunocytochemistry, using monoclonal antibodies against tumour antigens, is very helpful in differentiating between lymphoid and epithelial tumours and between some subsets of these, for example T and B cell lymphomas, germ cell tumours, prostatic tumours, neuroendocrine tumours, melanomas, and sarcomas. However, many adenocarcinomas and squamous carcinomas do not bear any distinctive immunohistochemical markers that are diagnostic of their primary site of origin.

There are several tests for genetic markers in tissue sections. For example, fluorescent in situ hybridization (FISH, p. 177) can be used to look for characteristic chromosomal translocations, deletions or duplications (see genetic basis of cancer, p. 486). Tissue microarrays can identify genomic imbalances, e.g. in breast cell cancer lines and lymphoma (see p. 170).

Staging

Before a decision about treatment can be made, not only the type of tumour but also its extent and distribution need to be established. Various 'staging investigations' are therefore performed before a treatment decision is made. To be useful clinically the staging system must subdivide the patients into groups of different prognosis which can guide treatment selection.

The staging systems vary according to the type of tumour and may be site specific (see Hodgkin's lymphoma, p. 510), or the TNM (tumour, node, metastases) classification shown in Table 9.5 which can be applied to most common cancers.

Performance status

In addition to anatomical staging, the person's age and general state of health need to be taken into account when planning treatment. The latter has been called 'performance status' and is of great prognostic significance for all tumour types (Table 9.6). Performance status reflects the effects of the cancer on the patient's functional capacity. An alternative performance rating scale is by Karnowsky.

Tumour markers (Table 9.7)

Tumour markers are intracellular proteins or cell surface glycoproteins released into the circulation and detected by immunoassays. Alpha-fetoprotein, β-human chorionic gonadotrophin and prostate-specific antigen are useful in the diagnosis of cancer but the remainder in Table 9.7 should be used with great care in diagnosis because of low specificity. They can be useful in the serial monitoring of response to treatment, as they can be quite sensitive to changes in the tumour burden.

CANCER TREATMENT

Aims of treatment

Cancer treatment requires the cooperation of a multidisciplinary team to coordinate the delivery of the appropriate treatment (surgery, chemotherapy, radiotherapy and biological/endocrine therapy), supportive and symptomatic care, and psychosocial support. While all members will have the patient's care as their central concern, someone, often the oncologist, has to take responsibility for the coordination of the many professionals involved. Central to this endeavour is the

---

Table 9.5   TNM classification as used for lung cancer

T = extent of primary tumour; N = extent of regional lymph node involvement; M = presence of distant metastases

Tx	Positive cytology only
T1	< 3 cm diameter
T2	> 3 cm/extends to hilar region/invades visceral pleura/partial atelectasis
T3	Involvement of chest wall, diaphragm, pericardium, mediastinum, pleura, total atelectasis
T4	Involvement of heart, great vessels, trachea, oesophagus, malignant effusion
N1	Peribronchial, ipsilateral hilar lymph node involvement
N2	Ipsilateral mediastinal
N3	Contralateral mediastinal, scalene or supraclavicular
M0	No distant metastases
M1	Metastases present

Table 9.6   Eastern Cooperative Oncology Group (ECOG) performance status scale

Status	Description
0	Asymptomatic, fully active and able to carry out all predisease performance without restrictions
1	Symptomatic, fully ambulatory but restricted in physically strenuous activity and able to carry out performance of a light or sedentary nature, e.g. light housework, office work
2	Symptomatic, ambulatory and capable of all self-care but unable to carry out any work activities. Up and about more than 50% of waking hours: in bed less than 50% of day
3	Symptomatic, capable of only limited self-care, confined to bed or chair more than 50% of waking hours, but not bedridden
4	Completely disabled. Cannot carry out any self-care. Totally bedridden

Table 9.7 Serum tumour markers	
α-Fetoprotein	Hepatocellular carcinoma, and non-seminomatous germ cell tumours of the gonads
β-Human chorionic gonadotrophin (β-HCG)	Choriocarcinomas, germ cell tumours and lung cancers
Prostate-specific antigen (PSA)	Carcinoma of prostate
Carcinoma embryonic antigen (CEA)	Gastrointestinal cancers
CA-125	Ovarian cancer
CA-19-9	Gastrointestinal cancers particularly pancreatic cancer
CA-15-3	Breast cancer

involvement of the patient, through education as to the nature of their disease and the treatment options available. An informed choice can then be made, even if in the end it is simply to abide by the decisions made by the professionals. Good communication embodies a humane approach which preserves hope at an appropriate level through empathy and understanding of the patient's position.

Curing cancer

For most solid tumours local control is possible but not sufficient for cure because of the presence of systemic (microscopic) disease, while haematological cancers are usually disseminated from the outset. Improvement in the rate of cure of most cancers is thus dependent upon earlier detection and effective systemic treatment. The likelihood of cure of the systemic disease depends upon the type of cancer, its chemo-/hormonal sensitivity, and tumour bulk (microscopic or clinically detectable). A few rare cancers are so chemosensitive that even bulky metastases can be cured, e.g. leukaemia, lymphoma, gonadal germ cell tumours, and choriocarcinoma. For most common solid tumours such as breast and colorectal cancer, there is no current cure of bulky (clinically detectable) metastases, but micrometastatic disease treated by adjuvant chemotherapy (see below) after surgery can be cured in 10–20% of patients.

Palliation

When cure is no longer possible, palliation, i.e. relief of tumour symptoms and prolongation of life, is possible in many cancers in proportion to their chemo- and radiosensitivity. There is on average a 2–18 months prolongation in median life expectancy with treatments for solid tumours and up to 5–8 years for some leukaemias and lymphomas, with those with the most responsive tumours experiencing the greatest benefit. The development of more effective chemotherapeutic drugs and better supportive care such as antiemetics has done much to reduce the side-effects of chemotherapy and to improve the cost/benefit ratio for the patient receiving palliative treatment. In addition, through early assessment during treatment, it is possible to stop if there is no evidence of benefit within 6–8 weeks of starting, so as to minimize exposure to toxic and unsuccessful treatment.

Measuring response to treatment

A measurable response to treatment can serve as a useful early surrogate marker when assessing whether to continue a given treatment for an individual patient.

Response to treatment can be subjective or objective. A *subjective response* is one perceived by the patient in terms of, for example, relief of pain and dyspnoea, or improvement in appetite, weight gain or energy. Such subjective response is a major aim of most palliative treatments. Quantitative measurements of these subjective symptoms form a part of the assessment of response to chemotherapy, especially in those situations where cure is not possible and where the aim of treatment is to provide prolongation of good-quality life. In these circumstances, measures of quality of life enable an estimate of the balance of benefit and side-effects to be made.

Objective response to treatment is measured either as a complete response, which is a complete disappearance of all detectable disease clinically and radiologically or partial response, which is conventionally defined as more than a 50% reduction in the size of the tumour. The terms used to evaluate the responses of tumours are given in Box 9.2. The term 'remission' is often used synonymously with 'response' which if complete means an absence of detectable disease without necessarily implying a cure of the cancer.

Oncological emergencies

- *Superior vena caval obstruction* can arise from any upper mediastinal mass but is most commonly associated with lung cancer and lymphoma. The patient presents with difficulty breathing and/or swallowing, with stridor, swollen, oedematous facies and venous congestion. *Treatment* is with immediate steroids, vascular stents, anticoagulation and mediastinal radiotherapy or chemotherapy. Some tumours, e.g. lymphomas and germ cell tumours, are so sensitive to chemotherapy that this is preferred to radiotherapy, as the masses are likely to be both large and associated with more disseminated disease elsewhere. An early decision is necessary on the patient's likely prognosis, as ventilatory support may be required until treatment has had time to relieve the obstruction.

i **Box 9.2** Definitions of response

Complete response	Complete disappearance of all detectable disease
Partial response	More than 50% reduction in the product of the bidimensional diameters of the tumour
Stable disease	No change, or < 50% reduction and < 25% increase
Progressive disease	Increase in size of tumour by at least 25% at any site

- *Spinal cord compression* (p. 1250) needs to be rapidly diagnosed and urgent treatment arranged to salvage as much functional capacity as possible. Early neurological clinical features may be incomplete, more subjective than objective and gradual in onset. MR scanning is the investigation of choice. *Treatment* should begin with high-dose steroids followed by surgical decompression and radiotherapy to the affected vertebrae to achieve the best disease control and palliation.
- *Neutropenic sepsis* (p. 495).
- *Acute lysis syndrome.* This occurs if treatment produces a massive breakdown of tumour cells, leading to increased serum levels of urate, potassium and phosphate. Urate deposition in the renal tubules can cause renal failure (hyperuricaemic nephropathy) requiring dialysis. The xanthene oxidase inhibitor (allopurinol) is given before treatment is started. Intravenous rasburicase, a recombinant urate oxidase, is occasionally used for prophylaxis and treatment but is very expensive.
- *Acute hypercalcaemia* presents with vomiting, confusion, constipation and oliguria Treatment is by resuscitation with intravenous fluids until a saline diuresis is established, followed by i.v. pamidronate (Emergency box 18.2).
- *Raised intracranial pressure* due to intracerebral metastases presents classically with headache, nausea and vomiting. However, for many there is a slower onset with non-specific symptoms such as drowsiness or mental deterioration. *Treatment* is by high-dose steroids and investigation by MRI as to whether surgery is appropriate or chemotherapy and radiotherapy are required.
- *Hyperviscosity* affects those with a very high haematocrit (> 50), white cell count (> 100×10^9/L) or platelet cell count (> 1000×10^9/L) from untreated acute leukaemia, or polycythaemia. *Treatment* is by leucopheresis and plasmapheresis followed by chemotherapy treatment for the underlying malignancy.

Adjuvant therapy for solid tumours

This is defined as treatment given in the absence of macroscopic evidence of metastases, to patients at risk of recurrence from micrometastases, after treatment of the primary lesion has been given. 'Neoadjuvant' therapy is given before primary therapy, which may shrink the tumour size and treat any micrometastases as soon as possible.

Micrometastatic spread by lymphatic or haematological dissemination often occurs early in the development of the primary tumour, and can be demonstrated by molecular biological methods capable of detecting the small numbers (1 in 10^6) of circulating cells. Studies correlating prognosis with histological features of the primary cancer, e.g. differentiation or presence of early metastatic invasion of blood vessels or regional lymph nodes, have led to an increasing ability to predict which patients are at high risk of local or distant recurrence from micrometastatic disease.

Trials of treatment with local radiotherapy or endocrine, biological or chemotherapy treatments have shown a significant improvement in survival in common adult cancers such as breast, bowel, prostate, head and neck, cervical cancer, choriocarcinoma and gonadal germ cell cancers. Central to these studies has been the careful selection of patients according to defined risk criteria, and the reduction of treatment toxicity to reach a balanced risk/benefit ratio. Absolute improvements in survival of 5–10% and relative risk reductions in the order of 12–25% (dependent upon the pre-existing risk) have been achieved in common epithelial cancers such as bowel, breast and prostate, with greater absolute improvements of 25% in the more sensitive germ cell tumours.

While these improvements currently translate into many lives saved from common diseases at a public health level, the majority who receive such treatment do not benefit because they were already cured, or because the cancer is resistant to the treatment. Better tests in the future will identify those with the micrometastases who really need treatment. On an individual patient basis the decision on whether adjuvant treatment will be worthwhile must include consideration of other factors such as the patient's life expectancy, concurrent medical conditions, and lifestyle priorities.

Treatment of malignancy in sanctuary sites

A 'sanctuary site' is the term used to indicate that metastatic disease has involved a site that is not accessible to conventional drug therapy. An example of this is leukaemic infiltration of the meninges in children with acute lymphoblastic leukaemia. Because of the blood–brain barrier, agents such as vincristine and prednisolone do not enter the subarachnoid space in sufficient quantity to eliminate all the leukaemic cells, and are therefore ineffective in preventing the development of meningeal infiltration. In order to treat these cells, intrathecal chemotherapy and/or cranial irradiation are required for patients at risk (p. 505).

PRINCIPLES OF CHEMOTHERAPY

Chemotherapy employs systemically administered drugs that directly damage cellular DNA (and RNA). It kills cells by promoting apoptosis and sometimes frank necrosis. There is a narrow therapeutic window between effective treatment of the cancer and normal tissue toxicity, because the drugs are not cancer specific (unlike some of the biological agents), and the increased proliferation in cancers is not much greater than in normal tissues (see tumour growth and failure of apoptosis, p. 162). The dose and schedule of the chemotherapy is limited by the normal tissue tolerance, especially in those more proliferative tissues of the bone marrow and gastrointestinal tract mucosa. All tissues can be affected, however, depending upon the pharmacokinetics of the drug and affinity for particular tissues (e.g. heavy metal compounds for kidneys and nerves).

The therapeutic effect on the cancer is achieved by a variety of mechanisms which seek to exploit differences between normal and transformed cells. While most of the drugs have been derived in the past by empirical testing of many different compounds, e.g. alkylating agents, the new molecular biology is leading to targeting of particular genetic defects in the cancer (see tyrosine kinase inhibitors for CML, p. 506).

Toxicity to normal tissue can be limited in some instances by supplying growth factors such as granulocyte colony-stimulating factor (G-CSF) or by the infusion of stem cell preparations to diminish myelotoxicity. The use of more specific biological agents with relatively weak pro-apoptotic effects in combination with the general cytotoxics will also improve the therapeutic ratio (see trastuzumab and breast cancer, p. 521).

Most tumours rapidly develop resistance to single agents given on their own. For this reason the principle of intermittent combination chemotherapy was developed. Several drugs are combined together, chosen on the basis of differing mechanisms of action and non-overlapping toxicities. These drugs are given over a period of a few days followed by a rest of a few weeks, during which time the normal tissues have the opportunity for regrowth. If the normal tissues are more proficient at DNA repair than the cancer cells, it may be possible to deplete the tumour while allowing the restoration of normal tissues between chemotherapy cycles (Fig. 9.3).

In many experimental tumours it has been shown that there is a log–linear relationship between drug dose and number of cancer cells killed and that the maximum effective dose is very close to the maximum tolerated dose at which dose-limiting toxicity is reached. With a chemosensitive tumour, relatively small increases in dose may have a large effect on tumour cell kill. It is therefore apparent that where cure is a realistic option the dose administered is critical and may need to be maintained despite toxicity. In situations where cure is not a realistic possibility and palliation is the aim, a sufficient dose to exceed the therapeutic threshold, but not cause undue toxicity, is required as the short-term quality of life becomes a major consideration.

Classification of cytotoxic drugs (Table 9.8)

DNA damaging
Alkylating agents
Alkylating agents act by covalently binding alkyl groups, and their major effect is to cross-link DNA strands, interfering with DNA synthesis and causing strand breaks. Despite being among the earliest cytotoxic drugs developed, they maintain a central position in the treatment of cancer. Melphalan is one of the original nitrogen mustards and is used in multiple myeloma. Chlorambucil is used in Hodgkin's lymphoma and chronic lymphocytic leukaemia. Other common alkylating agents include cyclophosphamide and ifosfamide, as well as the nitrosoureas, carmustine (BCNU) lomustine (CCNU) and busulfan used in chronic myeloid leukaemia. Tetrazines also alkylate DNA; dacarbazine is used in malignant melanoma and temozolomide in malignant gliomas.

Platinum compounds
Cisplatin, carboplatin and oxaliplatin cause interstrand cross-links of DNA and are often regarded as non-classical alkylating agents. They have transformed the treatment of testicular cancer and have a major role against many other tumours, including lung, ovarian and head and neck cancer. Toxicity, as for other heavy metals, includes renal and peripheral nerve damage.

Antimetabolites
Antimetabolites are usually structural analogues of naturally occurring metabolites that interfere with normal synthesis of nucleic acids by falsely substituting purines and pyrimidines in metabolic pathways. Antimetabolites can be divided into:

Fig. 9.3 Effects of multiple courses of cytotoxic chemotherapy.

Table 9.8 Chemotherapy: some cytotoxic drugs
DNA damaging
Free radicals – alkylators, e.g. cyclophosphamide
DNA cross-linking – platinum, e.g. cisplatin, carboplatin, oxaliplatin
Antimetabolites
Thymidine synthesis, e.g. 5-fluorouracil, methotrexate, cytarabine and mercaptopurine
DNA repair inhibitors
Topoisomerase inhibitors – epipodophyllotoxins, e.g. etoposide; campothecins, e.g. irinotecan
DNA intercalation – anthracyclines, e.g. doxorubicin
Antitubulin
Tubulin binding – alkaloids, e.g. vincristine, vinorelbine
Taxanes – e.g. paclitaxel, docetaxel

■ *Folic acid antagonist*, e.g. methotrexate. This is structurally very similar to folic acid and binds preferentially to dihydrofolate reductase, the enzyme responsible for the conversion of folic acid to folinic acid. It is used widely in the treatment of solid tumours and haematological malignancies. Folinic acid is often given to 'rescue' normal tissues from the effects of methotrexate.

■ *Pyrimidine antagonists*. 5-Fluorouracil (5-FU) consists of a uracil molecule with a substituted fluorine atom. It acts by blocking the enzyme thymidylate synthase, which is essential for pyrimidine synthesis. 5-Fluorouracil has a major role in the treatment of solid tumours, particularly gastrointestinal cancers. Capecitabine is metabolized to 5-FU, and is useful in colorectal cancer. Tegafur with uracil is used with calcium folinate in metastatic colorectal cancer.

■ *Arabinosides* inhibit DNA synthesis by inhibiting DNA polymerase. Cytosine arabinoside (cytarabine) is used almost exclusively in the treatment of acute myeloid leukaemia where it remains the backbone of therapy, while its analogue gemcitabine is proving useful in a number of solid cancers such as lung and ovary. Fludarabine is used in the treatment of B cell chronic lymphocytic leukaemia; it is also used in reduced intensity stem cell transplantation (p. 496) because of its immunosuppressive effect.

■ *Purine antagonists*, e.g. 6-mercaptopurine and 6-tioguanine, which are both used almost exclusively in the treatment of acute leukaemia.

DNA repair inhibitors
Epipodophyllotoxins
These are semisynthetic derivatives of podophyllotoxin, which is an extract from the mandrake plant. Etoposide is a drug used in a wide range of cancers and works by maintaining DNA strand breaks by acting on the enzyme topoisomerase II. Topoisomerase I inhibitors such as irinotecan and topotecan have also proved active against a variety of solid tumours. Both these enzymes allow unwinding and uncoiling of supercoiled DNA.

Cytotoxic antibiotics
These drugs such as doxorubicin and bleomycin act by intercalating adjoining nucleotide pairs on the same strand of DNA and by inhibiting DNA repair. They have a wide spectrum of activity in haematological and solid tumours. Doxorubicin is one of the most widely used of all cytotoxic drugs but has cumulative toxicity to the myocardium, while bleomycin has particular toxicity for the lungs. Pegylated liposomal doxorubicin is used as second-line treatment for advanced ovarian cancer with reduction of cardiotoxicity, but infusion reactions occur.

Antitubulin agents
Vinca alkaloids
Drugs such as vincristine, vinblastine and vinorelbine act by binding to tubulin and inhibiting microtubule formation (see p. 158). They are used in the treatment of haematological and non-haematological cancers. They are associated with neurotoxicity due to their anti-microtubule effect and must never be given intrathecally.

Taxanes
Paclitaxel is isolated from the bark of the western yew. Docetaxel is a semisynthetic taxane. They bind to tubulin dimers and prevent their assembly into microtubules. They are active drugs against many cancers such as ovarian, breast and lung cancer. Taxanes can cause neurotoxicity and hypersensitivity reactions and patients should be premedicated with steroids, H_1 and H_2 histamine antagonists prior to treatment.

Side-effects of chemotherapy

Chemotherapy carries many potentially serious side-effects and should be used only by trained practitioners. The four most common side-effects are vomiting, hair loss, tiredness and myelosuppression (Table 9.9). Side-effects are much more directly dose related than anti-cancer effects and it has been the practice to give drugs at doses close to their maximum tolerated dose, although this is not always necessary to achieve their maximum anticancer effect. Common combination chemotherapeutic regimens are shown in Table 9.10.

Nausea and vomiting
The severity of this common side-effect varies with the cytotoxic and it can be eliminated in 75% of patients by using modern antiemetics. Nausea and vomiting are particular problems with platinum analogues and with doxorubicin. A stepped policy with antiemetics such as metoclopramide and domperidone or $5-HT_3$ serotonin antagonists (e.g. ondansetron, granisetron) combined with dexamethasone should be used to match the emetogenic potential of the chemotherapy. Aprepitant, a neurokinin receptor antagonist is helpful in preventing acute and delayed nausea and vomiting associated with cisplatin-based chemotherapy. It is used with dexamethasone and a $5-HT_3$ antagonist.

Table 9.9 Side-effects of chemotherapy

Common
Nausea and vomiting
Hair loss
Myelosuppression
Mucositis
Fatigue

Drug-specific
Cardiotoxicity, e.g. anthracyclines
Pulmonary toxicity, e.g. bleomycin
Neurotoxicity, e.g. cisplatinum, vinca alkaloids, taxanes
Nephrotoxicity, e.g. cisplatinum
Skin plantar–palmar dermatitis, e.g. 5-fluorouracil
Sterility, e.g. alkylating agents
Secondary malignancy, e.g. alkylating agents, epipodophyllotoxins

Table 9.10 **Some chemotherapy regimens**

Hodgkin's lymphoma	ABVD	Doxorubicin, bleomycin, vinblastine, dacarbazine
	BEACOPP	Bleomycin, etoposide, doxorubicin, cyclophosphamide, vincristine, procarbazine, prednisolone
Non-Hodgkin's lymphoma	CHOP	Cyclophosphamide, hydroxy-doxorubicin, vincristine, prednisolone
Breast	CMF	Cyclophosphamide, methotrexate, 5-fluorouracil
	AC	Doxorubicin, cyclophosphamide
	MM	Mitoxantrone, methotrexate
Lung	PE	Cisplatin, etoposide
	MIC	Mitomycin, ifosfamide, cisplatin
Stomach	ECF	Epirubicin, cisplatin, 5-fluorouracil

Box 9.3 Febrile neutropenia treatment

Resuscitation with intravenous fluids to restore circulatory function, e.g. urine output, followed by cultures of blood, urine, sputum and stool and empirical antibiotics:

- Commonly used antibiotics should include activity against pseudomonas, e.g. ceftazidime or ticarcillin with gentamicin
- May require antibiotics against *Staph. aureus* especially with indwelling venous access lines, e.g. flucloxacillin or vancomycin.

If the patient deteriorates clinically and/or temperature still elevated after 48 hours, change antibiotics according to culture results or empirically increase Gram-negative and Gram-positive cover.

- Consider adding treatment for opportunistic infections if fever not responding to broad-spectrum antibiotics, e.g. amphotericin B
liposomal amphotericin B or voriconazole (latter two are very expensive) or caspofungin – fungus
high-dose co-trimoxazole – pneumocystis
clarithromycin – mycoplasma.

Hair loss

Many but not all cytotoxic drugs are capable of causing hair loss. Scalp cooling can sometimes be used to reduce hair loss but in general this side-effect can only be avoided by selection of drugs where this is possible. Hair always regrows on completion of chemotherapy.

Bone marrow suppression and immunosuppression

Suppression of the production of red blood cells, white blood cells and platelets occurs with most cytotoxic drugs and is a dose-related phenomenon. Severely myelosuppressive chemotherapy may be required if treatment is to be given with curative intent despite the potential for rare but fatal infection or bleeding. Anaemia and thrombocytopenia are managed by erythropoetin or red cell or platelet transfusions.

Neutropenic patients are at high risk of bacterial and fungal infection, often from enteric bowel flora. Those with a fever > 37°C and less than 0.5×10^9 neutrophils/L are managed by the immediate introduction of broad-spectrum antibiotics intravenously for the treatment of infection (Box 9.3). Initial empirical therapy should be reviewed following microbiological results. Haemopoietic growth factors and peripheral blood stem cells can reduce the duration of neutropenia significantly, benefiting patients at high risk of infectious complications.

Mucositis

This common side-effect of chemotherapy reflects the sensitivity of the mucosa to antimitotic agents. It causes severe pain and problems with swallowing. Treatment is with antiseptic and anticandidal mouthwash and, if severe, fluid and antibiotic support, as the mouth is a portal for entry of enteric organisms. A recent study has shown a keratinocyte growth factor to be helpful (palifermin).

Cardiotoxicity

This is a rare side-effect of chemotherapy, usually associated with anthracyclines such as doxorubicin. It is dose-related and can largely be prevented by restricting the cumulative total dose of anthracyclines within the safe range (equivalent to 450 mg/m^2 body surface area cumulative doxorubicin dose).

Neurotoxicity

This occurs predominantly with the plant alkaloids, vinca, taxanes and platinum analogues (but not carboplatin). It is dose-related and cumulative. Chemotherapy is usually stopped before the development of a significant polyneuropathy, which once established is only partially reversible. Vincristine must *never* be given intrathecally as the neurological damage is progressive and fatal.

Nephrotoxicity

Cisplatin (but not oxaliplatin or carboplatin), methotrexate and ifosfamide can potentially cause renal damage. This can usually be prevented by maintaining an adequate diuresis during treatment.

Sterility

Some anticancer drugs, particularly alkylating agents, may cause sterility, which may be irreversible. In males the storage of sperm prior to chemotherapy should be offered to the patient when chemotherapy is given with curative intent. In females it may be possible to collect oocytes to be fertilized in vitro and cryopreserved as embryos. Cryopreservation of ovarian tissue and retrieval of viable oocytes for subsequent fertilization is still experimental.

Secondary malignancies

Anticancer drugs have mutagenic potential and the development of secondary malignancies, predominantly acute leukaemia, is an uncommon but particularly unwelcome long-term side-effect in patients otherwise cured of their primary malignancies. The alkylating agents and epipodophyllotoxins are particularly implicated in this complication.

Drug resistance

Drug resistance is one of the major obstacles to curing cancer with chemotherapy. Some tumours have an inherently low level of resistance to currently available treatment and are often cured. These include gonadal germ cell tumours, Hodgkin's lymphoma and childhood acute leukaemia. Solid tumours such as small-cell lung cancer initially appear to be chemosensitive, with the majority of patients responding, but most patients eventually relapse with resistant disease. In other tumours such as melanoma the disease is largely chemoresistant from the start.

Most resistance occurs as a result of genetic mutation and becomes more likely as the number of tumour cells increases. It has also been shown that anticancer drugs can themselves increase the rate of mutation to resistance. Resistance to cytotoxic drugs is often multiple and is then known as multidrug resistance (MDR), e.g. resistance to doxorubicin is often associated with resistance to vinca alkaloids and epipodophyllotoxins, and is mediated through increased expression of P-glycoprotein (a 170 kDa membrane phosphoglycoprotein), which mediates the efflux of cytotoxic drugs out of the cells. Many other mechanisms may also be involved in resistance to chemotherapy, such as the upregulation of anti-apoptotic proteins Bcl-2 and Bax.

High-dose therapy

Most anticancer drugs have a sigmoid dose–response relationship which suggests that, up to a point, a higher dose of a cytotoxic drug will induce a greater response. However, increasing cytotoxic drug doses is often not possible, owing to toxicity. For many chemotherapeutic agents the toxicity which limits the dose is bone marrow failure, and infusion of stem cells is necessary to restore the lymphohaemopoietic system.

Haemopoietic stem cell transplantation

Bone marrow and transplanted cells may be:

- autologous – from self or identical twin
- syngeneic – from identical twin
- allogeneic – from non-identical donor (matched or sometimes mismatched)
- from umbilical cord blood. This is increasingly being used for adult and childhood leukaemia.

It usually takes 2–3 weeks for engraftment to take and during this time patients need supportive care with nursing in isolated cubicles with air filtration.

Principles of autologous stem cell transplantation

Autologous stem cells are used as rescue from myeloablative chemotherapy. Haemopoietic stem cells are collected from the patients' bone marrow, or more commonly by leucopheresis from peripheral blood following administration of the growth factor granulocyte colony-stimulating factor (G-CSF) prior to chemotherapy. They are stored by cryopreservation. These cells are then re-infused intravenously after an intensive, myeloablative chemotherapy regimen. This approach has been particularly effective in relapsed leukaemias, lymphomas and in myeloma. There is no risk of graft rejection or graft-versus-host disease (GVHD) but the graft-versus-tumour effect is lost (see below).

Principles of allogeneic stem cell transplantation

Historically, the transplantation of donor haemopoietic cells has been combined with myeloablative chemotherapy ± radiotherapy. This has the dual effects of treating the malignancy as well as immunosuppression that allows the graft 'to take'. Anti-T cell antibodies are often given to reduce graft-versus-host disease and immune-related infection. It is thought that the engraftment of the donor immune system, with antitumour activity (graft versus tumour), is primarily responsible for the increased effectiveness of this approach. In general, ideal donors are fully matched at the major HLA antigens. Thus siblings are more likely to be found to be potential donors than unrelated volunteers. Some degree of HLA antigen mismatch may be tolerated in children, but is problematic in adults. Allogeneic transplantation has been successfully used in acute and chronic leukaemias, and myeloma.

Complications include 'graft-versus-host disease', an immune reaction of the donor cells against normal host organs, which can affect 30–50% of transplant recipients and is potentially fatal in some cases. Immunosuppression, both from conditioning therapy and from the immunosuppressive drugs (ciclosporin or tacrolimus) given to prevent graft-versus-host disease, results in a high incidence of opportunistic infections. All patients receive prophylactic antibacterial, antifungal and antiviral drugs but infections still occur. Mortality therefore from conventional allogeneic stem cell transplantation is a major problem, with 20–40% at risk of dying from the procedure, depending on the age and status of the recipient, and the degree of HLA compatibility of the donor (see also Immunotherapy, p. 498).

Non-myeloablative allogenoic stem cell transplantation

In this procedure, also known as 'reduced intensity' transplantation, conditioning therapy is non-myeloablative without radiation therapy but it is immunosuppressant. The principle is that the anticancer effect of the stem cell transplantation will still be present without the complications of conventional allogeneic stem cell transplantation. Mortality (mainly GVHD) is lower, and the technique is being used more widely, particularly in the elderly.

PRINCIPLES OF ENDOCRINE THERAPY

Oestrogens are capable of stimulating the growth of breast and endometrial cancers, and androgens the growth of prostate cancer. Removal of these growth factors by manipulation of the hormonal environment may result in apoptosis and regression of the cancer. Endocrine therapy can be curative in a proportion of patients treated for micrometastatic disease in the adjuvant setting for breast and prostate cancer and provides a minimally toxic non-curative (palliative) treatment in advanced/metastatic disease. The presence of detectable cellular receptors for the hormone markedly increases the likelihood that the therapy will be effective. Figure 9.4 shows the binding of the hormone to the receptor.

Oestrogens and progestogens
Breast cancer (see Table 9.21)
About one-third of patients have receptors for oestrogens and progesterones. Hormonal manipulation includes the use of tamoxifen, which blocks oestrogen receptors, and the reduction of endogenous oestrogen by oophorectomy or 'medical oophorectomy' via pituitary downregulation using a gonadotrophin-releasing hormone (GnRH) analogue such as goserelin.

Tamoxifen is used as an adjuvant therapy to surgery and in advanced metastatic breast disease (see p. 519).

Progestogens have a direct effect on breast tumour cells through progesterone receptors, as well as effects on

the pituitary/ovarian (premenopausal) and adrenal/pituitary axis (postmenopausal) and can be as effective as tamoxifen.

In postmenopausal women, androgens are synthesized by the adrenal glands and converted in subcutaneous fat to estrone by the enzyme aromatase. Aromatase inhibitors, for example anastrozole, letrozole and exemestane, reduce circulating oestrogen levels and oestrogen synthesis in tumour cells and have shown greater efficacy than tamoxifen in the treatment of metastatic breast cancer and equivalence in the adjuvant setting in the postmenopausal woman.

Endometrial cancers
Endometrial cancers have receptors for both oestrogens and progestogens. Approximately 20% of receptor-positive metastases will regress for a median 20 months with synthetic progestogens such as medroxyprogesterone acetate but paradoxically tamoxifen has little effect. Trials to date with adjuvant progestogens have not been successful in increasing survival.

Androgens
In advanced prostate cancer, androgen deprivation induces regression in 70% of cases for a median duration of 24 months. GnRH agonists, e.g. goserelin, and orchidectomy, are equally effective; however, androgen receptor blockers such as flutamide are less so. Combinations of goserelin and flutamide may be used in the initial phase of treatment to avoid a disease flare from the initial agonist action of GnRH analogues, but prolonged combination therapy has been no more effective than goserelin alone. In the adjuvant setting, the addition of androgen deprivation to prostatic radiotherapy or surgery has improved survival.

PRINCIPLES OF BIOLOGICAL THERAPY

The group includes a range of protein molecules, from small peptide chemokines, larger cytokines, to complex antibody molecules, made available by genetic engineering.

Interferons
Interferons (p. 202) are naturally occurring cytokines that mediate the cellular immune response. They have many actions in treatment of malignant disease with both antiproliferative activity and stimulation of humoral and cell-mediated immune responses to the tumour that can result in an antitumour effect if the host effector mechanisms are present and fully competent.

Alpha-interferon (IFN-α) has been used against several malignancies to treat established disease such as melanoma, renal cell carcinoma and chronic myeloid leukaemia. In the latter, it results in a reduction in the number of Philadelphia (Ph) chromosome-positive cells in at least 50% of patients, with total elimination in 10%.

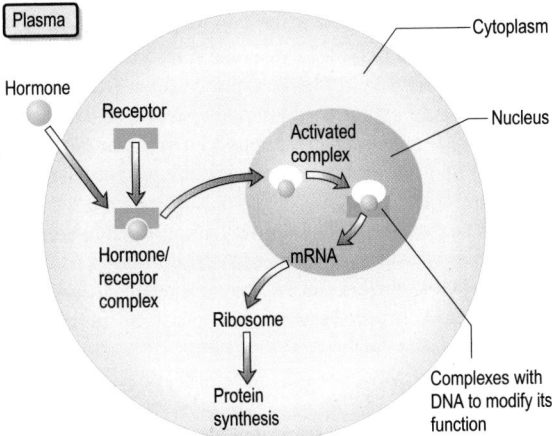

Fig. 9.4 Mechanism of the interaction between a steroid hormone and its receptor. This interaction modifies DNA activity and hence cell growth and replication.

It has been replaced by imatinib first-line treatment (p. 506). Interferon has also been used to maintain remission after cytotoxic treatment by suppressing microscopic residual disease, e.g. myeloma. In renal cell carcinoma alpha-interferon has a low (10–15%) but significant anticancer effect and prolongation of survival.

Treatment with IFN has side-effects (p. 371), most commonly flu-like symptoms which tend to diminish with time, and fatigue which generally does not and can be treatment limiting. IFN was given as a daily subcutaneous injection, but conjugation with polyethylene glycol (PEG interferon) has led to a reduction in frequency of injection and severity of side-effects.

Interleukins

Originally described for their activity in modulating leucocyte activation, these cytokines have widespread activity in coordinating cellular activity in many organs. Interleukin-2, a recombinant protein, is used to activate T cell responses, often in conjunction with interferon-stimulated B cell activation. Antitumour activity has been observed in renal cell carcinoma and melanoma with responses in 10–20% of patients, occasionally for prolonged periods. Toxicity is common; acutely this includes the capillary leak syndrome with hypotension, whilst pulmonary oedema, autoimmune thyroiditis and vitiligo occur later.

Haemopoietic growth factors

Erythropoietin for anaemia and granulocyte (G-CSF) or granulocyte–macrophage colony-stimulating factor (GM-CSF) are used:

- to reduce the duration of neutropenia following chemotherapy
- with or without chemotherapy, to stimulate the proliferation of haemopoietic progenitor cells in the marrow so that they enter the circulation and can be collected from the peripheral blood to support high-dose chemotherapy treatment, particularly in myeloma (p. 518).

Monoclonal antibodies (Table 9.11)

Monoclonal antibodies directed against tumour cell surface antigens are 'humanized' by being genetically engineered as a chimera comprising a human constant region with the murine heavy and light chains of the antigen-combining site, to reduce formation of blocking human anti-mouse antibodies when used in patients. Uses include:

- *In vitro,* in conjunction with complement, they are used to deplete autologous bone marrow of tumour cells in patients with leukaemia and lymphoma receiving high-dose treatment with autologous haemopoietic progenitor cell support.
- *In vitro* in immunoadsorption columns to select the CD34-positive (stem cell) fraction from peripheral blood progenitor cell or autologous bone marrow collections, to support high-dose treatment in haematological and other malignancies.

Table 9.11	Biological therapies	
Drug	**Function**	**Malignancy**
Imatinib	Tyrosine kinase inhibitor	Stromal cell tumour Chronic myeloid leukaemia
Gefitinib	Tyrosine kinase inhibitor	Non-small-cell lung cancer
Cetuximab	Anti-EGF receptor	Colorectal cancer
Bevacizumab	Anti-VEGF	Colorectal cancer
Rituximab	Anti-CD20 on B cells	Lymphoma
Dallizumab	Anti-CD25	Leukaemia/lymphoma
Alemtuzumab	Anti-CD52	Chronic lymphocytic leukaemia
Trastuzumab	Anti-HER-2 protein	Breast cancer
Bortezomib	Proteosome inhibitor	Leukaemia Myeloma

- As direct treatment for B cell non-Hodgkin's lymphoma (e.g. Rituximab anti-CD20 surface antigen). Tumour cell lysis occurs by both complement- and antibody-dependent cellular cytotoxicity.
- *As a carrier molecule* to target toxins or radioisotopes to the tumour cells, e.g. anti-CD20 conjugated to radioactive iodine is being used as treatment for non-Hodgkin's lymphoma.
- As anti-growth factor agents added to chemotherapy, e.g. trastuzumab against the Her2/ Neu or c-erbB2 antigen, a member of the epidermal growth factor receptor family, to increase the apoptotic response to cytotoxics with improved survival in metastatic breast cancer or with bevacizumab in colorectal cancer.

Immunotherapy

Activation of the immune system using bacille Calmette–Guérin (BCG) for bladder cancer or interleukin-2 for renal cancer induces responses in 60% and 10% of patients respectively. Certain antigens that are specific to cancer cells, such as sequences of tumour immunoglobulin from B cell lymphomas or melanoma antigens have been used as tumour vaccines. Antigen-presenting cells (dendritic cells) from the patient can be genetically engineered to present both antigen and cytokines such as interleukin-2 or granulocyte–macrophage colony-stimulating factor, and clinical responses have been observed. Another approach has used dendritic cells to further improve the vaccination strategy by engineering them to display the full range of HLA and B7 costimulatory molecules.

The use of non-myeloablative haemopoietic stem cell and donor lymphocyte infusions, while losing some of the specificity, has produced the strongest evidence for the efficacy of immunotherapy at the risk of the greatest toxicity.

Gene therapy

Antisense oligonucleotides are short sequences of DNA bases which specifically inhibit complementary sequences of either DNA or RNA. As a result, they can be generated against genetic sequences which are specific for tumour cells. Their clinical development has been hampered by poor uptake by tumour cells and rapid degradation by natural endonucleases. However, one antisense sequence directed against the *Bcl-2* oncogene has been shown to have an antitumour effect in patients with non-Hodgkin's lymphoma. Creation of reliable vectors for the transfection of tumour cells in vivo still forms a major barrier to the greater application of this modality.

Intracellular signal inhibitors

The recognition that many cancer cells are transformed by the activity of the protein products of oncogenes has led to the search for peptides or other compounds which inhibit these proteins, or their intracellular signal pathways. An example is the tyrosine kinase inhibitor imatinib, which specifically inhibits the fusion oncoprotein BCR-ABL. This compound is an extremely effective treatment for chronic myeloid leukaemia, a disease characterized by the presence of the BCR-ABL fusion protein. Many other similar molecules, inhibiting enzymes involved in cell cycling or cytokine signalling, are in preclinical or early clinical development. Examples include farnesyl transferase inhibitors, which inhibit ras proteins, inhibitors of the platelet-derived growth factor receptor, and drugs which inhibit matrix metalloproteinases.

PRINCIPLES OF RADIATION THERAPY

Radiation delivers energy to tissues, causing ionization and excitation of atoms and molecules. The biological effect is exerted through the generation of single- and double-strand DNA breaks, inducing apoptosis of cells as they progress through the cell cycle, and through the generation of short-lived free radicles, particularly from oxygen, which damage proteins and membranes.

The most commonly used form of radiotherapy is *external beam* or *teletherapy* from a linear accelerator source which provides X-rays, the energy of which is transmitted as photons. Cobalt-60 generators can also provide gamma rays and high-energy photons.

Brachytherapy is the use of radiation sources in close contact with the tissue to provide intense exposure over a short distance to a restricted volume.

Systemic radionuclides, e.g. iodine-131, or radioisotope-labelled monoclonal antibodies and hormones can be administered by intravenous or intracavitary routes to provide radiation targeted to particular tissue uptake via surface antigens or receptors.

The radiation dose is measured in grays (Gy), where 1 gray = 1 joule absorbed per kilogram of absorbing tissue and 1 centigray = 1 rad. The biological effect is dependent upon the dose rate, duration, volume irradiated, and the tissue sensitivity. Sensitivity to photon damage is greatest during the G_2–M phase of the cell cycle and is also dependent upon the DNA repair capacity of the cell. Fractionation is the delivery of the radiation dose in increments separated by at least 4–6 hours to try to exploit any advantage in DNA repair between normal and malignant cells. Radiation dose is thus described by three factors:

- total dose in cGy
- number of fractions
- time for completion.

Most treatments are delivered in 150–200 cGy fractions daily for 5 days per week, although a regimen of two fractions daily (hyperfractionation) had improved survival benefit in a lung cancer trial.

The radiation effect will also depend upon the intensity of the radiation source, measured as the linear energy transfer or frequency of ionizing events per unit of path, which is subject to the inverse square law as the energy diminishes with the distance from the source.

The generation of free radicles depends upon the degree of oxygenation/hypoxia in the target tissues. This can affect the biological effect by up to threefold and is the subject of continuing research for hypoxic cell sensitizers.

The depth of penetration of biological tissues by the photons depends upon the energy of the beam. Low-energy photons from an 85 kV source are suitable for superficial treatments, while high-energy 35 MeV sources produce a beam with deeper penetration, less scatter both at the initial skin boundary (skin sparing) and at the margins of the beam, and less absorption by bone. Superficial radiation may be also delivered by electron beams from a linear accelerator that has had the target electrode that generates the X-rays removed.

Radiotherapy treatment planning involves both detailed physics of the applied dose and knowledge of the biology of the cancer and whether the intention is to treat the tumour site alone, or include the likely loco-regional patterns of spread. Normal tissue tolerance will determine the extent of the side-effects, and a balanced decision is made according to the curative or palliative intent of the treatment and the likely early or late side-effects.

The cancers for which radiotherapy is usually employed as primary curative when the tumour is anatomically localized are listed in Table 9.12 along with those in which radiotherapy has curative potential when used in addition to surgery (adjuvant radiotherapy). Palliative treatments are frequently used to provide relief of symptoms to improve quality if not duration of survival (Box 9.4).

Side-effects of radiotherapy

Radiotherapy side-effects may occur early within days to weeks of treatment when they are usually self-limiting but associated with general systemic disturbance (Table 9.13). The side-effects will depend upon tissue sensitivity, fraction size and treatment volume and are managed with supportive measures until normal tissue repair occurs. The toxicity may also be enhanced by exposure to other radiation-sensitizing agents, especially some cytotoxics, e.g. bleomycin, actinomycin, anthracyclines, cisplatin and 5-fluorouracil.

Table 9.12 Curative radiotherapy treatment

Primary modality
Retina
CNS
Skin
Oropharynx and larynx
Cervix and vagina
Prostate
Lymphoma

Adjuvant to primary surgery
Lung
Breast
Uterus
Bladder
Rectum
Testis-seminoma
Sarcoma

Table 9.13 Side-effects of radiotherapy

Acute side-effects
Anorexia, nausea, malaise
Mucositis, oesophagitis, diarrhoea
Alopecia
Myelosuppression

Late side-effects

Skin	Ischaemia, ulceration
Bone	Necrosis, fracture, sarcoma
Mouth	Xerostomia, sialitis, ulceration
Bowel	Stenosis, fistula, diarrhoea
Bladder	Cystitis
Vagina	Dyspareunia, stenosis
Lung	Fibrosis
Heart	Pericardial fibrosis, cardiomyopathy
CNS	Myelopathy
Gonads	Infertility, menopause
Second malignancies,	e.g. Leukaemia Cancer, e.g. thyroid

Box 9.4 Palliative benefits of radiotherapy

- Pain relief, e.g. bone metastases
- Reduction of headache and vomiting in raised intracranial pressure from CNS metastases
- Relief of obstruction of bronchus, oesophagus, ureter, and lymphatics
- Preservation of skeletal integrity from metastases in weight-bearing bones
- Reversal of neurological impairment from spinal cord or optic nerve compression by metastases

Later side-effects occur from months to years later, unrelated to the severity of the acute effects because of their different mechanism. Late effects reflect both the loss of slowly proliferating cells and a local endarteritis which produces ischaemia and proliferative fibrosis.

Growth may be arrested if bony epiphyses are not yet fused and are irradiated, leading to distorted skeletal growth in later life.

Secondary malignancies following radiotherapy typically appear 10–20 years after the cure of the primary cancer. Haematological malignancies tend to occur sooner than solid tumours from the irradiated tissues. The latter are very dependent upon the status of the tissue at the time of treatment, e.g. the pubertal breast is up to 300 times more sensitive to malignant transformation than the breast tissues of a woman in her thirties. Patients who smoke are more liable to develop lung cancer. Treatment of these secondary cancers can be successful providing there is normal bone marrow to reconstitute the haemopoietic system or the whole tissue at risk (e.g. thyroid after mantle radiotherapy for lymphoma) can be resected.

FURTHER READING
Gregor A (2000) How to improve effects of radiation and control its toxicity. *Annals of Oncology* **11** (Suppl. 3): 231–234.

HAEMATOLOGICAL MALIGNANCIES

The leukaemias, the lymphomas and multiple myeloma are an interrelated spectrum of malignancies of the myeloid and lymphoid systems. They are uncommon but not rare, the lymphomas alone being the seventh commonest cancer in the UK. The aetiology of these diseases is unknown, although viruses, irradiation, cytotoxic poisons and immune suppression have been implicated in a small proportion of cases (p. 501). The pathogenesis involves at least one or usually more molecular abnormalities, and non-random chromosomal abnormalities have been detected in several leukaemias and lymphomas. Classification has become increasingly complex, with the universally applied WHO scheme demanding morphological, cytogenetic and sometimes molecular criteria to be fulfilled. Treatment options are multiple. Patients need to be supported through treatment involving prolonged myelosuppression and immunosuppression. These are potentially life-threatening but can also be curative. This has given rise to the need for highly skilled staff and specialist facilities, and patients should be referred to these centres for treatment.

Large multicentre Phase III trials have validated single centre data and show that curative therapy can be delivered in the community.

In the management of these diseases it is critical that patients are appraised of the natural history, its potential modification by treatment and the risks of both severe morbidity and mortality. It must be made clear from the outset whether a curative or palliative strategy is most appropriate and why. If cure is to be pursued, the patient must be appraised of the approximate probability of success and its potential price. The possibility of failure needs to be addressed at the outset and not at the last minute.

THE LEUKAEMIAS

These are relatively rare diseases with an incidence of about 10 per 100 000 per year. They are classified as being acute (short natural history) or chronic (long natural history), and of myeloid or lymphoid origin. More than half of the leukaemias present acutely (ALL, AML) with the remainder being chronic types (CLL, CML). The type of leukaemia varies with age; acute lymphoblastic leukaemia (ALL) is mainly seen in childhood and chronic lymphocytic leukaemia is a disease of the elderly. The myelodysplastic syndromes are considered pre-leukaemic and are discussed on page 453. Leukaemia can be diagnosed by examination of a stained slide of peripheral blood and bone marrow, with immune phenotyping, cytogenetics and molecular genetics being essential for complete subclassification and prognostication.

General classification

The characteristics of leukaemic cells can be assessed by light microscopy, expression of cytosolic enzymes and expression of surface antigens. These will reflect the lineage and degree of maturity of the leukaemic clone. Thus, leukaemia can be divided on the basis of the speed of evolution of the disease into acute or chronic. Each of these is then further subdivided into myeloid or lymphoid, according to the cell type involved.

- acute myeloid leukaemia (AML)
- acute lymphoblastic leukaemia (ALL)
- chronic myeloid leukaemia (CML)
- chronic lymphocytic leukaemia (CLL).

Aetiology

This is unknown but several factors have been associated:

- *Radiation*. This can induce genetic damage to haemopoietic precursors and ALL, AML and CML have been seen in increased incidences in survivors of Hiroshima and Nagasaki and in patients treated with ionizing radiation.
- *Chemical and drugs*. Exposure to benzene used in industry, may lead to marrow damage. AML occurs after treatment with alkylating agents, e.g. melphalan.
- *Genetic*. The incidence of leukaemia is increased in identical twins and in syndromes of somatic cell chromosomal aneuploidy, e.g. Down's syndrome, Klinefelter's syndrome.
- *Viruses*. Leukaemias are associated with human T cell lymphotropic virus type 1 (HTLV-1), which is found particularly in Japan and the Caribbean.

Genetic abnormalities in leukaemia

Leukaemic cells often have a somatically acquired cytogenetic abnormality, which may be of prognostic, as well as diagnostic, importance.

These genetic alterations change the normal cell regulating process by interfering with the control of normal proliferation, blocking differentiation, maintaining an unlimited capacity for self-renewal and lastly, promoting resistance to death signals, i.e. decreased apoptosis.

The first non-random chromosomal abnormality to be described was the Philadelphia (Ph) chromosome, which is associated with chronic myeloid leukaemia (CML) in 97% of cases. The Ph chromosome is also found in ALL, the incidence in the latter illness increasing with age. The translocation is shown schematically in Figure 9.5. The Ph chromosome is an abnormal chromosome 22, resulting from a reciprocal translocation between part of the long arm of chromosome 22 and chromosome 9. The resulting karyotype is described as t(9;22)(q34;q11). The molecular consequences of the translocation are that part of the Abelson proto-oncogene (c-*ABL*) normally present on chromosome 9 is translocated to chromosome 22, where it comes into juxtaposition with a region of chromosome 22 named the 'breakpoint cluster region' (BCR). The translocation creates a hybrid transcription unit consisting of the 5' end of the *BCR* gene and the c-*ABL* proto-oncogene.

The new 'fusion' gene *BCR-ABL* is capable of being expressed as a chimeric messenger RNA which has been identified in cells from patients with CML. When translated, this produces a fusion protein that has tyrosine kinase activity and enhanced phosphorylating activity compared with the normal protein, resulting in altered cell growth, stromal attachment and apoptosis. The breakpoint differs in CML and Ph-positive ALL, leading to the production of two different tyrosine kinase proteins with molecular weights of 210 kDa and 190 kDa respectively. It is unclear whether the presence of *BCR-ABL* is sufficient for the development of the disease. It has recently been shown that normal subjects can carry low levels of the *BCR-ABL* fusion gene in their blood without developing leukaemia.

Almost all patients with acute promyelocytic leukaemia (APML), a subtype of acute myelogenous leukaemia,

Fig. 9.5 The Philadelphia chromosome (Ph). The long arm (q) of chromosome 22 has been shortened by the reciprocal translocation with chromosome 9.

have the t(15;17) reciprocal translocation, which occurs at the q25 band on chromosome 15 and the q22 band on chromosome 17. The breakpoint on chromosome 17 occurs in the gene encoding the retinoic acid receptor, fusing it with part of the *PML* gene. This is to some extent the explanation for the responsiveness of patients with APML to all-*trans*-retinoic acid (ATRA, see p. 504). Other genetic and cytogenetic abnormalities are often seen in leukaemic cells (see Table 9.14).

Cell surface markers

These can be used to classify acute leukaemias. Immature myeloid cells have cell surface markers, e.g. CD13, CD14, CD33, CD34, which can be identified using monoclonal antibodies. The majority of patients with ALL (60%), for example, show the common ALL antigen (CALLA – CD10).

ACUTE LEUKAEMIAS

The acute leukaemias are predominantly diseases of adulthood, increasing in incidence with advancing age. Acute myeloid (myeloblastic, myelogenous) leukaemia (AML) has a median age at presentation of 65 years and may arise 'de novo' or against a background of myelodysplasia, either of unknown aetiology or related to cytotoxic chemotherapy. Acute lymphoid (lymphoblastic) leukaemia (ALL) has a substantially lower median age at presentation and in addition is the commonest malignancy in childhood. The WHO classification is shown in Table 9.14.

Clinical features

The majority of patients with acute leukaemia, regardless of subtype present with symptoms arising from:

- anaemia – shortness of breath on effort; excessive tiredness, weakness
- leucopoenia – recurrent infections
- thrombocytopenia – bleeding and bruising (particularly acute promyelocytic leukaemia)
- marrow infiltration – bone pain.

Examination may be unremarkable, but features include:

- pallor
- fever (due to infection, not the disease itself)
- petechiae, purpura, bruises, fundal haemorrhage (particularly acute promyelocytic leukaemia)
- lymphadenopathy, hepatosplenomegaly (more notable in lymphoblastic leukaemia)
- violacious skin lesions (acute myelomonocytic leukaemia)
- testicular enlargement (acute lymphoblastic leukaemia)
- cranial nerve palsies occasionally found (acute lymphoblastic leukaemia).

Investigations
Confirmation of diagnosis (Fig. 9.6)

- **Blood count**. Hb low, WBC raised usually (sometimes low), platelets low.

Table 9.14 WHO classification of acute leukaemia

(a) Acute myeloid leukaemia
AML with recurrent genetic abnormalities
AML with t(8;21)(q22;q22), (AML1/ETO)
AML with abnormal bone marrow eosinophils and
    inv(16)(p13;q22) or t(16;16)(p13;q22), (CBFβ/MYH1 1)
Acute promyelocytic leukaemia with t(15;17)(q22;q12),
    PML/RAR-alpha and variants
AML with 11q23 (MLL) abnormalities

AML with multilineage dysplasia
Following MDS or MDS/MDP
Without antecedent MDS or MDS/MDP, but with dysplasia
    in at least 50% of cells in two or more myeloid lineages

AML and myelodysplastic syndromes, therapy related
Alkylating agent/radiation-related type
Topoisomerase II inhibitor-related type
Other

AML, not otherwise categorized*
AML, minimally differentiated
AML without maturation
AML with maturation
Acute myelomonocytic leukaemia
Acute monoblastic/acute monocytic leukaemia
Acute erythroid leukaemia (erythroid/myeloid and pure
    erythroleukaemia variants)
Acute megakaryoblastic leukaemia
Acute basophilic leukaemia
Acute panmyelosis with myelofibrosis
Myeloid sarcoma

(b) Acute lymphoid leukaemia
Precursor B cell acute lymphoblastic leukaemia
    t(9;22)(q34;q11); BCR/ABC fusion gene
    t(4;11)(q21;q23); MLL-AF4 fusion gene
    t(1;19)(q23;p13.3); E2A/PBX1 fusion gene
    t(12;21)(p13;q22); TEL/AMLI
Precursor T cell acute lymphoblastic leukaemia
Burkitt-cell leukaemia

* The entities included in this group are defined almost identically to the corresponding entity in the French–American–British (FAB) classification
MDS, myelodysplastic syndromes; MPD, myeloproliferative diseases
Modified from Jaffe ES, Harris NL, Stein H, Vardiman JW (eds) (2001) *World Health Organization Classification of Tumours. Pathology and Genetics of Tumours of Haematopoietic and Lymphoid Tissues.* Lyon: IARC Press, with permission

- **Blood film**. Blast cells almost invariably seen, (Fig. 9.6a), lineage identified morphologically, confirmed with immunophenotyping.
- **Bone marrow aspirate**. Increased cellularity, reduced erythropoiesis, reduced megakaryocytes, sometimes trilineage dysplasia. Blast cells > 20% (often approaching 100%) (Fig. 9.6b). Lineage confirmation by immunophenotyping (FISH), cytogenetic and molecular genetics.
- **Chest X-ray**. Mediastinal widening often present in T lymphoblastic leukaemia.

Blast cell →

(a)

(b)

Fig. 9.6 **(a) Peripheral blood film showing characteristic blast cells**. The arrow points to the abnormal blast cell. **(b) Bone marrow aspirate** showing particle with increased cellularity. Courtesy of Dr Manzoor Mangi.

For planning therapy

- Biochemistry, serum urate, renal and liver biochemistry.
- Cardiac function; ECG and direct tests of left ventricular function, e.g. echocardiogram or MUGA scan (p. 756).

Principles of management

Untreated acute leukaemia is invariably fatal, most often within months, though with judicious palliative care it may be extended to perhaps a year. Treatment with curative intent may be successful, or may fail, either because the leukaemia cannot be eradicated or because the patient cannot sustain the therapy, death occurring as early as if treatment had not been initiated.

At initial presentation, acute leukaemias range from being probably curable (most favourable risk – childhood acute lymphoblastic leukaemia) through possibly curable (de novo low-risk AML) to probably incurable (AML with adverse cytogenetic features in the elderly, secondary AML, recurrent acute leukaemia). Since curative treatment even for 'low-risk' acute leukaemia carries considerable morbidity and potential mortality and that for 'high-risk' acute leukaemia even more, it is essential that the 'risk/benefit' ratio is clearly understood by physician and patient alike.

In AML, patients with t(15;17) t(8;17) or inv(16) (or its variant t16;16), i.e. low risk, do not benefit from allogeneic stem cell transplantation during their first complete remission because the risks outweigh benefits. Patients with adverse factors (high risk) – (5/del5q), -7, abnormal 3q, t(9;22) or a complex karyotype – should have transplantation because they respond poorly to conventional chemotherapy. Other poor prognostic factors (high risk) include developing the disease over 60 years of age, leukaemia following myelodysplastic syndrome (MDS), relapsed disease, secondary leukaemia and extramedullary disease.

Palliative therapy

The patient must understand that the decision to manage palliatively does not mean 'no therapy', or abandonment, but rather the recognition of a different goal from prolongation of life, though this may also be achieved to some degree. Every attempt should be made to ensure that the patients are at home as much as possible, whilst making available the full range of supportive care. Palliation may well include both chemotherapy and irradiation in addition to blood product support. 'Moral' support is invaluable.

Curative therapy

The decision to treat with curative intent, particularly if successful, implies severe disruption of normality for the patient and family for at least 6 months and often up to a year, and, regardless of success, life is never quite the same again. In the short term, it may demand transfer to another hospital, as acute leukaemia should only be treated in units seeing at least 10 such cases per year. It is highly likely to involve admission to hospital for up to a month in the first instance, with further, partly predictable, subsequent admissions of several days' to weeks' duration, requiring discussions and decisions about work or education.

The decision to treat with curative intent implies that cure is possible, and that the chance of cure justifies the risks of the therapy. It does not imply that cure is guaranteed or even expected. The failure rate may be high, and the patient must know that he or she will be told if cure becomes an unrealistic goal. Treating with curative intent may well involve rapid decisions about resuscitation with transfer to the intensive care unit, the possibility of which is discussed in advance.

Active therapy

Supportive care

This forms the basis of treatment whether for cure or palliation:

- Avoidance of symptoms of anaemia (haemoglobin > 10 g/dL) – repeated transfusion of packed red cells (sometimes irradiation of cells is required).
- Prevention or control of bleeding (platelet count < 10 × 10^9/L in the uninfected, and 20 × 10^9/L in the infected patient).
- Treatment of infection:
  (a) *Prophylactically.* Education of patients, relatives and staff about hand washing and isolation facilities. The use of selected antibiotics and antifungals.

(b) *Therapeutically.* Management of fever with protocol/ algorithm of antibiotic and antifungal combinations.

- Control of hyperuricaemia with hydration, prophylactic allopurinol and very occasionally rasburicase (p. 492).

Specific treatment

The initial requirement of therapy is to return the peripheral blood and bone marrow to normal (complete remission; CR) with 'induction chemotherapy' tailored to the particular leukaemia and the individual patient's risk factors. Since this treatment is not leukaemia specific but also impairs normal bone marrow function, it leads to a major risk of life-threatening infection, which increases the risk of early death in the short term. Since infection is the major problem, it is necessary to conduct the early therapy in hospital, the patient sleeping in a single room with en-suite lavatory and washing facilities ('some' isolation).

Successful remission induction is always followed by further treatment (consolidation), the details being determined by the type of leukaemia and the patient's risk factors (and the patient's tolerance of treatment). Recurrence is almost invariable if 'consolidation' therapy is not given. This reflects the lack of sensitivity of the definition of 'complete remission', which has until very recently been solely morphological. Cytogenetics and molecular genetic techniques can identify residual leukaemic cells not detected morphologically, and they are highly predictive of recurrence. Recommendations have recently been made to modify the definition of remission to reflect this. Failure to achieve morphological CR with two cycles of therapy carries almost as bad a prognosis as the leukaemia untreated. If CR can be achieved, e.g. by new experimental approaches, cure may still be possible with stem cell transplantation (p. 496).

Fig. 9.7 **Acute myeloid leukaemia: overall survival with or without myeloablative therapy.** BXIII = treatment group. (from Rohatiner AZS et al. (2000) *Annals of Oncology* **11**: 1007–1015 with permission).

'high risk AML' is commoner with increasing age, but is only curable with allogeneic transplantation, and the toxicity of this treatment increases dramatically with age.

Complete remission will be achieved in about three-quarters of patients under the age of 60, failure being due to either resistant leukaemia or death due to infection or (rarely) bleeding. It may be expected that approximately 50% of those entering complete remission will be cured. (i.e. approximately 30% overall) (Fig. 9.7). The management of recurrence is undertaken on an individual basis, since the overall prognosis is very poor despite the fact that second remissions may be achieved. Long survival following recurrence is rarely achieved without allogeneic transplantation. Experimental therapy should be considered.

Acute myeloid leukaemia (AML; excluding APML, p. 504)

Treatment with curative intent is undertaken in the majority of adults below the age of 60 years, provided there is no significant co-morbidity. Risk of failure is based on the cytogenetic pattern (p. 503). Those at 'low risk' are treated with moderately intensive combination chemotherapy always including an anthracycline antibiotic such as daunorubicin and cytosine arabinoside (cytarabine) and consolidation with a minimum of four cycles of treatment given at 3- to 4-week intervals. Those at 'high risk' may only be treated with curative intent if an HLA-identified sibling is available for stem cell transplantation.

Those at ' intermediate risk' are a heterogeneous group but when possible they should be given consolidating chemotherapy to induce remission followed by sibling matched allogeneic transplantation, despite its attendant risks.

The initial treatment of the older patient is much more contentious. Intuitively, biological age should determine the management of the individual patient. Unfortunately

Acute promyelocytic leukaemia (APML)

This is an uncommon variant of AML characterized by the translocation t(15;17) (p. 501). There is an almost invariable coagulopathy, which was a major cause of death. The empirical discovery that all-*trans*-retinoic acid (ATRA) causes differentiation of promyelocytes and rapid reversal of the bleeding tendency was a major breakthrough. It is now conventional to treat APML with ATRA combined with chemotherapy and to follow successful remission induction with maintenance ATRA. Allogeneic transplantation may be necessary either if the leukaemia is not eliminated at the molecular level, or following a second remission after recurrence. Arsenic trioxide, which induces apoptosis via activation of the caspase cascade (p. 162) is also effective.

Complete remission and molecular remission occur in at least 80% of younger adults with APML (it is uncommon in the elderly). At least 60% will expect to be cured. In contrast to the other subtypes of AML, the prognosis after recurrence is quite favourable with prolonged second remissions being possible with further blocks of ATRA and chemotherapy even if allogeneic transplant is not performed, though it is the treatment of choice.

Acute lymphoblastic leukaemia (ALL)

The overall strategy for the treatment of ALL differs in detail from that for AML (Fig. 9.8). Remission induction is undertaken with combination chemotherapy including vincristine, prednisolone, asparaginase (crisantaspase) and usually an anthracycline antibiotic, e.g. doxorubicin. Once remission is achieved, the details of consolidation will be determined by the anticipated risk of failure.

Allogeneic transplantation is only recommended for those at highest risk, i.e. those with t(9;22) since this is otherwise incurable with conventional therapy. It is unclear yet what the role of imatinib (see below) will be in this setting. Patients with certain subtypes receive maintenance therapy for 2 years.

The other major difference between therapy for ALL and AML is the need for central nervous system directed therapy. Prophylaxis should be given with intrathecal chemotherapy under platelet cover if necessary, as soon as blasts are cleared from the blood. Depending upon risk this may be continued for up to 2 years, and complemented by high doses of systemic cytosine arabinoside (cytarabine) or methotrexate. Cranial irradiation previously given to all patients is reserved for those at very high risk and those who are symptomatic (Fig. 9.8).

Prognosis

The prognosis of ALL in childhood is now excellent: complete remission is achieved in almost all, with up to 80% being alive without recurrence at 5 years. Failure occurs most frequently in those with high blast count and t(9;22) translocation.

The situation is far less satisfactory for adults, the prognosis getting worse with advancing years. Co-morbidity and t(9;22) translocation increases in frequency with age. Overall the complete remission rate is 70–80%, failure being due partly to resistant leukaemia and partly to failure of supportive care. Failure to achieve complete remission with first-line therapy carries a very poor prognosis. If CR can be achieved with new therapies, it should be consolidated with sibling or possibly even unrelated donor transplantation despite the high risk of graft-versus-host disease. Thirty to 40% of patients continue in durable first remissions, resulting in approximately 25–30% overall patient cure.

As with AML, most recurrences occur within the first 3 years and the outcome is extremely poor. Second remissions, though usually achieved, are rarely durable except following allogeneic transplantation. Isolated extramedullary recurrences, however, may be cured.

CHRONIC LEUKAEMIAS

Chronic myeloid leukaemia (CML)

Chronic myeloid leukaemia (CML) accounts for about 14% of all leukaemias, is almost exclusively a disease of adults with the peak of presentation being at 40–60 years and is characterized by the presence of the Philadelphia chromosome (Fig. 9.9). Unlike the acute leukaemias which are either rapidly reversed or rapidly fatal, CML has a more slowly progressive course which if not initially cured will be followed eventually by blast crisis (90% myeloid, 20% lymphoid) or myelofibrosis and death after 3–4 years.

Clinical features

CML usually presents in the chronic phase and some patients have no symptoms. Symptoms include:

- shortness of breath due to anaemia
- abdominal discomfort due to splenomegaly
- weight loss
- fever, sweats, NOT due to infection

Fig. 9.8 **Treatment regimen for acute lymphoblastic leukaemia.**

Fig. 9.9 **Philadelphia chromosome.** This is formed by a reciprocal translocation of part of the long arm (q) of chromosome 22 to chromosome 9. It is seen in 90–95% of patients with chronic myeloid leukaemia. The karyotype is expressed as 46XX, (9;22)(q34;q11).

- headache (occasionally) due to hyperleucocytosis
- bruising, bleeding (uncommon).

Signs
- Pallor
- Splenomegaly, often massive
- Lymphadenopathy, at times of blast crisis
- Retinal haemorrhage due to leucostasis.

Investigations

- **Blood count.** Hb low or normal, WBC raised, platelets low, normal or raised.
- **Blood film.** Neutrophilia with the whole spectrum of myeloid precursors including occasional blasts.
- **Bone marrow aspirate.** Increased cellularity, increased myeloid precursors. Cytogenetics reveals t(9;22) translocation (the Philadelphia chromosome) (Fig. 9.9)
- **Fluorescein-in-situ hybridization** (FISH), reverse transcriptase polymerase chain reaction (RT-PCR) or microarray expression may be needed to demonstrate the cytogenetic/molecular abnormality.
- **LAP is usually reduced.**

Management

Imatinib, a *tyrosine kinase inhibitor* that specifically blocks the enzymatic action of the BCR-ABL fusion protein is first-line treatment *for the chronic phase*. It has replaced alpha-interferon. Imatinib produces a complete haematological response in over 95% of patient, and 70–80% of these have no detectable BCR-ABL transcripts in the blood. Event-free, and overall, survival appear to be better than for other treatments. Imatinib can be continued indefinitely.

In the acute phase (blast transformation) most patients have only a short-lived response to imatinib, and other treatments (see below) will be necessary.

Side-effects of imatinib, which usually are well tolerated, include nausea, headaches, rashes and cytopenia. Resistance to imatinib as a single agent has developed and further clinical studies are necessary.

Stem cell transplantation (SCT)

Allogeneic haemopoietic stem cell transplantation can cure approximately 70% of chronic phase CML patients but with a risk of complications and death due to graft-versus-host disease (GVHD) and opportunistic infections.

Factors making complications more likely include:

- increasing age
- SCT in acute phase
- degree of histocompatibility between donor and recipient.

Graft-versus-leukaemia effect plays a role in the increased survival following SCT so that reduced-intensity transplantation is being more frequently used.

The exact role of SCT in the imatinib era is unclear but failure to respond to that agent is an indication. Monitoring of patients following either SCT or imatinib is by measuring BCR-ABL transcripts using the reverse transcriptase PCR.

Chronic lymphocytic leukaemia (CLL)

This is the commonest leukaemia, occurring predominantly in later life and increasing in frequency with advancing years. It is almost invariably B lymphocytic in origin. In many patients it is a chance finding with no symptoms, while others present with the features of marrow failure or immunosuppression. The median survival may be 10 years, and may be found to correlate with various presentation features (Table 9.15). It is becoming increasingly recognized that cytogenic and molecular abnormalities carry prognostic significance (see below).

Clinical features

Common symptoms are:

- recurrent infection because of (functional) leucopenia and immune failure (reduced immunoglobulins)
- anaemia due to haemolysis or marrow infiltration
- painless lymphadenopathy
- splenic discomfort.

The commonest findings on examination are:

- anaemia
- fever (due to infection)
- generalized lymphadenopathy
- hepatosplenomegaly, sometimes massive.

However, none of these may be present.

Investigations

- **Blood count.** Hb normal or low; WBC raised, and may be very high; platelets normal or low.
- **Blood film.** Lymphocytes increased above $5 \times 10^9/L$.
- **Bone marrow.** Reflects peripheral blood, often very heavily infiltrated with lymphocytes.
- **Immunophenotyping** shows mainly CD19/20 + CD5$^+$ B cells. They may weakly express surface immunoglobulin.
- **Cytogenetics** can help assess prognosis. Abnormalities include deletions at trisomy 12 (40%) 13q14 (60%), long arms of 6, 11 and 13 and abnormalities in the *p53* gene. There are mutations of IgVH (on B cells) which help in assessing prognosis. IgVH is difficult to measure. However, intracellular ZAP-70 (zeta-associated protein) which correlates closely with the IgVH mutated status can be measured by flow cytometry in a general laboratory.
- **Coombs' test.** May be positive if there is haemolysis.
- **Immunoglobulins.** Low or normal.

Management

In CLL, the major consideration is when to treat. Treatment depends on the 'stage' (Table 9.15) of the disease, although the cytogenic markers are being increasingly used. In particular, low levels of ZAP-70 indicate a good prognosis with no treatment necessary. Conversely unmutated IgVH (high levels of ZAP-70) indicate a poor prognosis.

Early-stage disease is usually managed expectantly, advanced-stage disease is always treated immediately

Table 9.15   The Rai and Binet staging systems for chronic lymphocytic leukaemia*

System and stage	Risk	Manifestations	Percent of patients	Median survival	Recommended treatment
Rai staging system					
0	Low	Lymphocytosis	31	> 10	Watch and wait
I	Intermediate	Lymphadenopathy	35	9	Treat only with progression[†]
II	Intermediate	Splenomegaly, lymphadenopathy, or both	26	7	Treat only with progression[†]
III	High	Anaemia, organomegaly,	6	5	Treatment indicated in most cases
IV	High	One or more of the following: anaemia, thrombocytopenia and organomegaly	2	5	Treatment indicated in most cases
Binet staging system					
A	Low	Lymphocytosis, < 3 lymphoid areas enlarged[‡]	63§	> 10	Watch and wait
B	Intermediate	≥ 3 Lymphoid areas enlarged[‡]	30	7	Treatment indicated in most cases
C	High	Anaemia, thrombocytopenia or both	7	5	Treatment indicated in most cases

* Lymphocytosis is present in all stages of the disease
[†] Progression is defined by weight loss, fatigue, fever, massive organomegaly and a rapidly increasing lymphocyte count
[‡] Enlarged lymphoid areas may include the cervical, axillary and inguinal lymph nodes; the spleen or liver may be enlarged
§ Stage A includes all patients with Rai stage 0 disease, two-thirds of patients with Rai stage I disease and one-third of those with Rai stage II
From Dighiero G, Binet JL (2000) *New England Journal of Medicine* **343**: 1800

and the approach to the intermediate stage is variable. The absolute indication for treatments are:

- anaemia (especially due to haemolysis)
- recurrent infection
- splenic discomfort
- progressive disease manifest by doubling of the lymphocyte count in 6 months.

General/supportive treatment

Anaemia due to haemolysis is treated with steroids. If it is refractory or recurrent, or if splenic discomfort is a problem, a splenectomy is performed. Anaemia due to marrow infiltration is treated with chemotherapy and, when necessary, blood transfusion. Erythropoietin (p. 422) may avoid the need for transfusions, particularly in patients receiving chemotherapy.

Infection is treated with antibiotics, with prophylactic therapy being given during periods of chemotherapy. Immunoglobulin replacement may be helpful.

Allopurinol is given to prevent hyperuricaemia.

Specific treatment

Chlorambucil, given in modest doses, usually reduces the blood count and decreases lymphadenopathy and splenomegaly, and successfully palliates the disease. The bone marrow rarely returns to normal. Treatment is usually limited to a few months' duration and then withheld until progression.

Since the introduction of the purine analogues, fludarabine alone or in combination with cyclophosphamide or mitoxantrone (with or without steroids), treatment has had a much greater impact on the bone marrow and can induce complete or molecular complete remission. More recently, the addition of rituximab (relatively ineffective alone) in combination therapy has been reported to result in a dramatic improvement in the response rate. Myeloablative chemotherapy with autologous stem cell rescue and allogeneic stem cell transplantation with myeloablative or non-myeloablative condition regimens are currently undergoing trials.

Outcome

Survival correlates closely with cytogenetic findings and Rai or Binet stage at any time. The median survival from diagnosis is very variable with normal life expectancy in some groups and rapid progression in others. Poor prognostic factors include a high Rai and Binet stage, a short lymphocyte doubling time (< 12 months), diffuse bone marrow infiltration, cytogenetic abnormalities involving *p53* dysfunction, *Ilq23*, trisomy 12 and CD38/ZAP-70 positivity, male gender and developing the disease over 60 years of age. Intervention, when indicated, usually causes improvement in symptoms and in the blood count. The effect on survival is unclear. More aggressive treatments, particularly combinations of cytotoxic chemotherapy with antibody therapy, result in better quality remission of longer duration. These improvements may translate into a survival advantage, to accompany the improvement in quality of life afforded by good supportive care.

Hairy cell leukaemia (HCL)

HCL is a clonal proliferation of abnormal B (or very rarely T) cells which, as in CLL, accumulate in the bone marrow and spleen. It is a rare disease, median age at presentation is 52 years old and the male to female ratio is 4 : 1. The bizarre name relates to the appearance of the cells on a blood film and in the bone marrow – they have an irregular outline owing to the presence of filament-like cytoplasmic projections. They show a strong acid phosphatase reaction that is resistant to tartaric acid. The cells express many cellular differentiation markers including CD19, 20 and 103 but not CD21 or 5.

Clinical features include anaemia, fever and weight loss. Splenomegaly occurs in 80%, lymphadenopathy is uncommon. Anaemia, neutropenia, thrombocytopenia and low monocyte counts are found.

Treatment

The purine analogues 2-chloroadenosine acetate (2-CDA) (cladribine) and pentostatin have specific activity in this condition; complete remission is achieved in 90% with just one cycle of treatment. The remissions sometimes last for several years and patients can be retreated. Rituximab is used in cases who do not respond to the above drugs.

Prolymphocytic leukaemia

Prolymphocytic leukaemia is another rare disorder, often mistaken for CLL. It may be of B or of T cell lineage. It is characterized by bone marrow failure (anaemia, neutropenia and thrombocytopenia) and – as in HCL –

FURTHER READING

Chiorazzi N, Rai KR, Ferrarini M (2005) Chronic lymphocytic leukaemia. *New England Journal of Medicine* **352**: 804–815.

Goldman JM, Melo JV (2003) Chronic myeloid leukaemia – advances in biology and new approaches to treatment. *New England Journal of Medicine* **349**: 1451–1464.

Hamblin TJ (2004) Predicting progression – ZAP-70 in CLL. *New England Journal of Medicine* **351**: 856–857.

Henderson ES, Lister TA, Greaves MF (eds) (2002) *Leukemia*, 7th edn. Philadelphia: Saunders.

Jaffe ES, Harris NL, Stein H, Vardiman JW (eds) (2001) *World Health Organization Classification of Tumours. Pathology and Genetics of Tumours of Haematopoietic and Lymphoid Tissues.* Lyon: IARC Press.

Lister TA, Rohatiner A (guest eds) (2002) Non-Hodgkin's lymphoma. *Best Practice and Research, Clinical Haematology* **15**: 3

National Institute for Clinical Excellence (2003) *Guidance on Cancer Services: Improving Outcomes in Haematological Cancers. The Manual.* London: NICE.

Oscier D, Fegan C, Hillmen P et al.; Guidelines Working Group of the UK CLL Forum. British Committee for Standards in Haematology (2004) Guidelines on the diagnosis and management of chronic lymphocytic leukaemia. *British Journal of Haematology* **125**: 294–317.

Pui CH, Relling MV, Downing JR (2004) Mechanisms of disease: acute lymphoblastic leukemia. *New England Journal of Medicine* **350**: 1535–1548.

splenomegaly. Treatment generally comprises chlorambucil as for CLL, although splenectomy may be indicated and fludarabine can be useful.

THE LYMPHOMAS

The lymphomas are commoner than the leukaemias and are increasing in incidence for reasons which are unclear. They arise as the result of abnormal proliferation of the lymphoid system, and hence occur at any site where lymphoid tissue is found. Most commonly they are manifest by the development of lymphadenopathy at single or multiple sites, although primary extranodal presentations account for up to 20% of non-Hodgkin's lymphoma. The prognosis is determined by the specific subtype of lymphoma and the anatomical extent of disease and its bulk, the clinical course ranging from months to years.

The guiding principles of management are broadly the same as for the leukaemias. The precise diagnosis is established, appropriate further investigation is conducted to allow a management plan to be formulated, both for the short and long term, and the situation is clearly explained to the patient.

Lymphomas are currently classified on the basis of histological appearance into:

- Hodgkin's lymphoma
- non-Hodgkin's lymphoma.

The distinction between lymphoid leukaemia and lymphoma is not always clear.

HODGKIN'S LYMPHOMA (HL)

This is a rare disease involving primarily the lymph nodes. The incidence in the UK is approximately 2.5/100 000 with a male to female ratio of 1.3 : 1. Its peak incidence is in the third decade. The incidence is stable.

Aetiology

There is epidemiological evidence linking previous infective mononucleosis with HL and up to 40% of patients with HL have increased EBV antibody titres at the time of diagnosis and several years prior to the clinical development of HL. EBV DNA has been demonstrated in tissue from patients with HL. These data suggest a role for EBV in pathogenesis. Other viruses have not been detected. Other environmental and occupational exposure to pathogens have been postulated.

Pathology

The hallmark of HL is the Reed–Sternberg cell (Fig. 9.10) which is usually derived from germinal centre B cells or, rarely, peripheral T cells. CD30 and CD25 are almost always expressed in the majority of cases of classical HL.

The WHO classification of HL is shown in Table 9.16. Classical HL can be divided into:

Table 9.16 Pathological classification of Hodgkin's lymphoma

Nodular lymphocyte-predominant Hodgkin's lymphoma
Classical Hodgkin's lymphoma
   Nodular sclerosis HL
   Lymphocyte-rich HL
   Mixed cellularity HL
   Lymphocyte-depleted HL

From Harris NL et al. (1999) *Journal of Clinical Oncology*
17: 3835–3849

Fig. 9.10 Histological appearance of Hodgkin's lymphoma. There is a background rich in benign small lymphocytes and histiocytes together with scattered mononuclear Hodgkin's cells and a classical malignant binucleate Reed–Sternberg cell (arrow) to the right of centre. Courtesy of Dr AJ Norton.

- *Nodular sclerosing HL* (70% of cases) where many fibrotic bands are present. This type is typically seen in young females, involving particularly lymph nodes in the mediastinum and neck.
- *Lymphocyte-rich HL* appears in 5% and is characterized by an infiltrate of many small lymphocytes and Reed–Sternberg cells. It often occurs in peripheral lymph nodes. It is often an indolent disease.
- *Mixed cellularity HL*. Approximately 25% of cases have mixed cellularity with lymphocytes, eosinophils, neutrophils and histiocytes. Reed–Sternberg cells are present but no fibrotic bands. It is more common in men and is associated with B symptoms.
- *Lymphocyte-depleted HL* is rare and there is lack of cellular infiltrate with numerous Reed–Sternberg cells. It is seen in HL associated with HIV.

In addition to classical HL, *nodular lymphocyte-predominant HL* (5% of cases) contains malignant L and H cells (lymphocytic and/or histiocytic Reed–Sternberg cell variants, also called 'popcorn' cells) which are positive for CD20, CD45, BCL6, CD79a without expressing CD15 or CD30.

Pathogenesis

This remains unclear but several factors have been identified in classical HL:

B cells. There is a lack of expression of surface immunoglobulin (or BCR) in the Hodgkin and Reed–Sternberg cell. This may be due to destructive mutations or non-functional rearrangements in the immunoglobulin genes, and/or a lack of immunoglobulin-specific transcription factors.

Resistance to apoptosis. The malignant lymphoma cell may have acquired a Fas-resistant phenotype that prevents its death in the germinal centre. Destruction mutations have been found in the Fas gene inactivating the Fas pathway.

Development of non-regulatory growth signals. It has been suggested that the transforming Reed–Sternberg cell may acquire self-sufficiency in growth signals and develop non-regulated, permanent transcription activity by NFκB. Mutations have been reported in the $I\kappa\beta\alpha$ gene

Environmental. A delayed exposure to ubiquitous infections in childhood may suggest that HL is a late infection with a common virus. See EBV above.

Genetic factors. Monozygotic twins have a 100 times greater risk of concordantly developing HL. No increase has been seen in dizygotic twins.

It is clear that several pathways may lead to HL but the central issue must be that lymphocytes of the B-cell lineage not expressing immunoglobulins somehow escape apoptosis.

Clinical features

- Lymph node enlargement, most often of the cervical nodes (other causes are shown in Table 9.17); these are usually painless and with a rubbery consistency.
- Enlargement of the spleen/liver.
- 'B' symptoms: fever, (25%) drenching night sweats, weight loss of > 10% bodyweight (see Table 9.18).
- Other constitutional symptoms, such as pruritus, fatigue, anorexia and, occasionally, alcohol-induced pain at the site of enlarged lymph nodes.
- Symptoms due to involvement of other organs (e.g. lung – cough and breathlessness).

Investigations

- **Blood count** may be normal, or there can be a normochromic, normocytic anaemia. Lymphopenia and occasionally eosinophilia are present.
- **Erythrocyte sedimentation rate** (ESR) is usually raised and is an indicator of disease activity.
- **Liver biochemistry** is often abnormal, with or without liver involvement.
- **Serum lactate dehydrogenase**; raised level is adverse prognostic factor.
- **Uric acid** is normal or raised.
- **Chest X-ray** may show mediastinal widening, with or without lung involvement.
- **CT scans** show involvement of intrathoracic nodes in 70% of cases. Abdominal or pelvic lymph nodes are also found. It is the investigation of choice for staging

Table 9.17 Differential diagnosis of cervical lymph node enlargement

Infections	Primary lymph node
Acute	**malignancies**
Pyogenic infections	Hodgkin's lymphoma
Infective mononucleosis	Non-Hodgkin's lymphoma
Toxoplasmosis	Chronic lymphocytic
Cytomegalovirus infection	leukaemia
Infected eczema	Acute lymphoblastic
Cat scratch fever	leukaemia
Acute childhood exanthema	
	Secondary malignancies
Chronic	Nasopharyngeal
Tuberculosis	Thyroid
Syphilis	Laryngeal
Sarcoidosis	Lung
HIV infection	Breast
	Stomach
Connective tissue disorders	
Rheumatoid arthritis	**Miscellaneous**
	Kawasaki's syndrome
Drug reactions	
Phenytoin	

Table 9.18 Cotswolds modification of Ann Arbor staging classification

Stage	Description
Stage I	Involvement of a single lymph-node region or lymphoid structure (e.g. spleen, thymus, Waldeyer's ring) or involvement of a single extralymphatic site
Stage II	Involvement of two or more lymph-node regions on the same side of the diaphragm (hilar nodes, when involved on both sides, constitute stage II disease); localized contiguous involvement of only one extranodal organ or site and lymph-node region(s) on the same side of the diaphragm (IIE). The number of anatomic regions involved should be indicated by a subscript (e.g. II$_3$)
Stage III	Involvement of lymph-node regions on both sides of the diaphragm (III), which may also be accompanied by involvement of the spleen (IIIS) or by localized involvement of only one extranodal organ site (IIIE) or both (IIISE)
III1	With or without involvement of splenic, hilar, coeliac, or portal nodes
III2	With involvement of para-aortic, iliac, and mesenteric nodes
Stage IV	Diffuse or disseminated involvement of one or more extranodal organs or tissues, with or without associated lymph-node involvement

Designations applicable to any disease state	
A	No symptoms
B	Fever (temperature > 38°C), drenching night sweats, unexplained loss of more than 10% of body weight within the previous 6 months
X	Bulky disease (a widening of the mediastinum by more than one-third of the presence of a nodal mass with a maximal dimension greater than 10 cm)
E	Involvement of a singe extranodal site that is contiguous or proximal to the known nodal site

From Diehl V et al. (2004) Hodgkin's lymphoma – diagnosis and treatment. Reprinted with permission from Elsevier (*Lancet Oncology* **5**: 19–26).

(Table 9.18), although PET scanning is increasingly being used.

- **Bone marrow aspirate and trephine biopsy** are seldom done but show involvement in patients with advanced disease. This is unusual at initial presentation.
- **Lymph node biopsy** is required for a definitive diagnosis (Fig. 9.10).

A typical chest X-ray and CT scan in one patient are shown in Figure 9.11.

Management

Treatment is almost always recommended and under-taken with curative intent and considerable expectation of success (Figs 9.12 and 9.13). Expectant management may be reasonable in some cases of lymphocyte-predominant Hodgkin's lymphoma, although the rationale for this must be made clear to the patient and there needs to be close early surveillance.

Specific treatment is based otherwise on the anatomical distribution of disease, its 'bulk' and the presence or absence of 'B' symptoms. ('stage': Table 9.18).

'Early stage' (I^A, II^A no bulk)

The treatment of choice now is brief chemotherapy followed by involved field irradiation. Extended field megavoltage irradiation was used with 70% of patients being cured, and probably half of those in whom it failed were 'salvageable' with combination chemotherapy. Large field irradiation has come under recent criticism because of a significantly increased incidence of breast cancer in young women, lung cancer in smokers and cardiac disease following supradiaphragmatic 'mantle' field irradiation. 'Moderate' chemotherapy ABVD (Table 9.10), 2–4 cycles (i.e. non sterilizing and low secondary cancer risk) followed by involved field irradiation (20–30 Gy) has become standard care. Current trials are evaluating the role of PET scanning to see if patients who become 'PET' negative can be spared irradiation altogether.

Advanced disease

This is also curable for a significant proportion of patients, the median survival exceeding 5 years. Cyclical combination chemotherapy with or without irradiation to sites of 'bulk' disease is the treatment of choice for all these patients. The 'gold standard' combination is ABVD (Table 9.10) given to a total of 6–8 cycles each month, the blood count permitting. All patients with mediastinal bulk receive irradiation whether or not the CT scan returns to normal. It may well be that in the future PET scanning, as for those with early disease, may reduce the need for irradiation. This approach will be curative for approximately 50–60% of those with advanced disease, the major potential toxicity in the short term being

Fig. 9.11 (a) **Chest X-ray of a large mediastinal mass that is due to Hodgkin's lymphoma. (b) CT scan of the same patient.** The mass is indicated here by crossed lines.

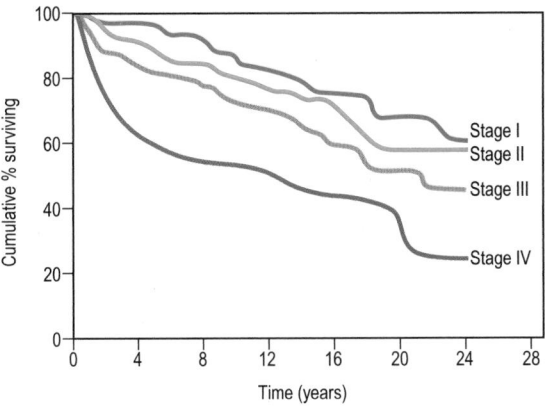

Fig. 9.12 **Survival in Hodgkin's lymphoma related to Ann Arbor stage at presentation.**

Fig. 9.13 **Survival of patients with Hodgkin's lymphoma.** From Oza AM et al. (1993) Patterns of survival in patients with Hodgkin's disease: long follow-up in a single centre. From Oza AM et al. (1993) *Annals of Oncology* **4**: 385–392, with permission.

myelosuppression with a mortality of ~ 1%. In the long term the risks are to the heart and lungs. Infertility and second malignancy are much less common than following the previous gold standard therapy MOPP (or MVPP). The 15-year survival of this group of patients is approximately 65%.

Twenty-five per cent of patients fail to achieve remission of advanced Hodgkin's lymphoma with the initial ABVD chemotherapy. 'Intensification' of treatment by increasing the number of drugs, alternating combinations, or hybrids may have reduced this proportion in resistant patients. Recently two schedules, one given cyclically with many drugs, some in high doses, and the other as a continuous 12-week programme of chemotherapy (both complemented with significant amounts of irradiation) have been reported to reduce the failure rate substantially in the short term. Confirmation of these results with longer follow-up is awaited. Clearly, the development of a prognostic index to identify these resistant patients prospectively would be a major step forward, although the highest-risk group is very small. The alternative to the strategy of overtreating some for the benefit of the few, is to undertreat the few to the advantage of the many, and then 'salvage' the failures. Limited success with myeloablative chemotherapy with haemopoietic stem cell rescue has been reported in those with 'refractory disease'.

Recurrent Hodgkin's lymphoma, certainly after 'conventional'-dose chemotherapy is potentially very serious though not necessarily fatal. The median survival from the first recurrence is more than 10 years; it may be influenced by the duration of first remission: it may not be so good if failure occurs after more intensive initial therapy. Second, and third remissions are achieved more often than not with 'appropriate' re-induction chemotherapy. It is conventional to consolidate remission in this group when possible, with high-dose therapy and peripheral blood cell progenitor rescue (PBPCR). Registry data suggest that this may be curative in up to 50%, although follow-up does not extend beyond 15 years.

Experimental approaches for recurrent and refractory disease include new cytotoxic drugs, monoclonal antibodies and reduced-intensity allogeneic transplantation.

FURTHER READING

Diehl V et al. (2004) Hodgkin's lymphoma – diagnosis and treatment. *Lancet Oncology* **5**: 19–26.

Thomas RK et al. (2004) Hodgkin's lymphoma – molecular biology of Hodgkin and Reed–Sternberg cells. *Lancet Oncology* **5**: 11–18.

NON-HODGKIN'S LYMPHOMA (NHL)

These are malignant tumours of the lymphoid system classified separately from Hodgkin's lymphoma. Most (70%) are of B cell origin although T cell tumours are increasingly being recognized.

The incidence of these tumours is approximately 15/100 000 per year in developed countries, an incidence which has increased over the last 20–30 years. There is a slight male predominance. The median age of presentation is 55–75 years.

Aetiology

The cause is unknown. There is wide geographical variation which probably reflects different environmental factors. NHL is associated with the EBV virus (Burkitt's lymphoma) and the human T cell lymphotropic virus which is prevalent in Japan, Africa, South America and the Caribbean. Herpesvirus 8 is associated with primary effusion lymphomas and Castleman's disease; there is an increase in lymphoma in patients with AIDS. *Helicobacter pylori* is an aetiological factor in gastric MALT lymphoma.

Lymphomas also occur in congenital immunodeficiency, post-transplantation and in autosomal family cancer syndromes (Table 9.3). Other causes, e.g. occupation, dietary and exposure to chemicals, have been linked to the increasing incidence but the evidence is unconfirmed.

Pathogenesis

There is a malignant clonal expansion of lymphocytes which might occur at a different stage of lymphocyte development. In general, neoplasms of non-dividing mature lymphocytes are indolent whereas those of proliferating cells (e.g. lymphoblasts, immunoblasts) are much more aggressive. This malignant transformation is usually due to errors in gene rearrangements which occur during the class switch, or gene recombinations for immunoglobulins and T cell receptors. Thus, many of the errors occur within immunoglobulin loci or T cell receptor loci. For example, an abnormal gene translocation may lead to the activation of a proto-oncogene next to a promoter sequence for the immunoglobulin heavy chains (Ig-H).

Cytogenetic features (Table 9.19)

Burkitt's lymphoma was the first tumour in which a cytogenetic change was shown to involve the translocation of a specific gene. The most frequent change is a translocation between chromosomes 8 and 14 in which the *myc* oncogene moves from chromosome 8 to a position near the constant region of the immunoglobulin heavy chain gene on chromosome 14, resulting in upregulation of *myc*. Similar rearrangements involving the light chain loci are seen in the alternative Burkitt's lymphoma translocations between chromosome 8 and either chromosome 2 or 22. Other somatic cytogenetic abnormalities associated with human lymphoma are the t(14;18) in follicular lymphoma, involving upregulation of the *Bcl-2* gene, or the upregulation of *Bcl-1* (also called cyclin D1) as a result of t(11;14) in mantle cell lymphoma.

Immunophenotypes

All NHL B cells express CD20 and surface immunoglobulin. Individual lymphomas vary in their expression, e.g. follicular lymphomas express CD10, mantle cell CD43, while the diffuse large B cell lymphoma expresses both CD10 and CD43. They can be used in the classification. T cell lymphomas do not express CD20 but variably express CD3, 4, 8 and 30.

Classification

The WHO classification (2001) which is based on the Revised European American Lymphoma (REAL) system is shown in Table 9.20. Previous classifications have divided lymphomas into indolent (or low grade) and aggressive (or high grade), and the WHO classification has been modified to include aggressive or highly aggressive lymphomas.

Clinical features

- *Peripheral lymphadenopathy.* Most patients present with painless, superficial lymph node enlargement.
- *Systemic symptoms (B symptoms).* Fever, sweats, anorexia and weight loss.
- *Extranodal presentation.* This is more common than in HL and may involve the gastrointestinal tract, lung,

Table 9.19	Chromosome translocations in non-Hodgkin's lymphoma		
Type	**Translocation**	**Genes**	**Function**
Follicular	t(14;18)	Bcl-2/IgH	Suppresses apoptosis
Lymphoplasmacytic	t(9;14)	PAX5	Transcription factor
Mantle cell	t(11;14)	Bcl-1 (cyclin D1)	Cell cycle regulator
Diffuse large B cell	t(3;4)	Bcl-6	Cell cycle regulator
Burkitt's	t(8;14) t(2;8)	c-myc and Ig	Transcription factor
Anaplastic	t(2;5)	NPM1/ALK	Tyrosine kinase
MALT	t(11;18)	BIRC3/MALT1 fusion protein	Suppresses apoptosis

MALT, mucosal associated lymphoid tissue

Table 9.20 Modified WHO classification of lymphoid neoplasms other than ALL (2001)

B cell lymphomas

Precursor B cell lymphoma	Precursor B lymphoblastic lymphoma/leukaemia (*highly aggressive*)
Mature B cell lymphoma	Chronic lymphocytic leukaemia/small lymphocytic lymphoma
	Lymphoplasmacytic lymphoma
	Splenic marginal zone lymphoma
	Extranodal marginal zone B cell lymphoma of mucosa-associated lymphoid tissue (MALT-lymphoma)
	Nodal marginal zone B cell lymphoma
	Follicular lymphoma (*aggressive*)
	Mantle cell lymphoma
	Diffuse large B cell lymphoma (*aggressive*)
	Mediastinal (thymic) large B cell lymphoma
	Intravascular large B cell lymphoma
	Primary effusion lymphoma
	Burkitt's lymphoma/leukaemia (*highly aggressive*)

T/NK cell lymphomas

Precursor T cell lymphoma	Precursor T cell lymphoblastic leukaemia/lymphoma (*highly aggressive*)
	Blastic NK cell lymphoma
Mature T/NK cell lymphoma	Adult T cell leukaemia/lymphoma (*very aggressive*)
	Extranodal NK/T cell lymphoma, nasal type
	Enteropathy-type T cell lymphoma
	Hepatosplenic T cell lymphoma
	Subcutaneous panniculitis-like T cell lymphoma
	Mycosis fungoides
	Sézary syndrome
	Primary cutaneous anaplastic large cell lymphoma
	Peripheral T cell lymphoma, unspecified (*aggressive*)
	Angioimmunoblastic T cell lymphoma
	Anaplastic large cell lymphoma (*aggressive*)

NK, natural killer

Modified from Jaffe ES, Harris NL, Stein H, Vardiman JW (eds) (2001) *World Health Organization Classification of Tumours. Pathology and Genetics of Tumours of Haematopoietic and Lymphoid Tissues.* Lyon: IARC Press

brain, testes, thyroid and skin. Abdominal involvement may reveal hepatosplenomegaly. Skin involvement (T cell lymphomas) presents as mycosis fungoides (p. 1352) and Sézary syndrome (p. 1353).

- *Oropharyngeal involvement* occurs rarely.
- HIV predisposes to NHL.

Investigations

- **Full blood count**. Normochromic, normocytic anaemia, an elevated white cell count or neutropenia and thrombocytopenia are suggestive of bone marrow infiltration.
- **ESR** may be elevated.
- **Urea and electrolytes**. Patients may have renal impairment as a consequence of ureteric obstruction secondary to intra-abdominal or pelvic lymph node enlargement.
- **Serum uric acid level** may be raised.
- **Liver biochemistry**. This may be abnormal if there is hepatic involvement.
- **Serum lactate dehydrogenase and β_2-microglobulin** are prognostic indicators.
- **Serum immunoglobulins** – decreased levels may occur with paraproteinaemia.
- **Chest X-ray, CT scans** of chest, abdomen and pelvis. **PET and gallium scans** help in staging.
- **Bone marrow aspirate** and trephine biopsy are always performed.
- **Lymph node biopsy** (or Trucut needle biopsy, often under radiological guidance, in the case of surgically inaccessible nodes). Immunophenotyping and cytogenetic/molecular analysis (DNA micro-array analysis), to distinguish type of NHL.

Follicular lymphoma

These comprise 20% of all B cell lymphomas. Most patients with follicular lymphoma present feeling well but with painless lymphadenopathy. Investigation usually reveals multiple sites of disease: involvement of the bone marrow is common. Managed conservatively it is a remitting and recurring disease with a clinical course running over a median of 10 (1–20 years) years during which there will be about three 'episodes' of relapse. Death occurs because of resistant disease, transformation to diffuse large B cell lymphoma (LBCL) or the effects of therapy.

The 'well' patient should be managed with no specific therapy until progression is documented. Repeat biopsy should be performed at this time in case there has been histological transformation to LBCL as this has specific implications for therapy.

The indications for the initiation of therapy are:

- *Stage I presentation (10–15%)*. This is treated with 'involved' field irradiation, which almost invariably induces 'complete remission'. The median time to progression is 10–15 years. Some patients may be cured. There is no evidence that mortality is affected by treatment, but the therapy has a low morbidity and mortality.
- *Advanced disease* with:
  - constitutional 'B' symptoms
  - 'organ impairment', i.e. bone marrow failure
  - 'bulky' disease, i.e. lymph node mass > 10 cm
  - progressive disease after expectant management, documented if necessary on two scans 3 months apart

– histological transformation.

■ *Philosophy of patient and physician*.

A specific follicular lymphoma international prognostic index (FLIPI) has been formulated, defining 'low', 'intermediate' and 'high' risk groups. This may provide a more objective basis for the decision to begin therapy, and with what.

A recent study showed that survival can be predicted by the different genes expressed on accompanying T cells and dendritic cells (not tumour cells) identified by DNA micro-array analysis of tumour tissue.

Treatment options

Standard initial treatment in the UK is with an alkylating agent, e.g. chlorambucil, or a combination containing an alkylating agent, e.g. COP (cyclophosphamide, vincristine and prednisolone), given usually over 3–6 months. The overall response rate is high (~ 80%), but the proportion of complete remissions is low. It may be possible to push those patients for whom the first treatment fails into remission with a second therapy. Progression is the rule after a median of 2–3 years: there is no evidence of cure. Provided transformation has not occurred, further remissions (an average of three) can be achieved with the same or other single agents or combination of drugs. The remission becomes significantly shorter after the third, and death supervenes. Quality of life, except during treatment (and often during treatment), is normal until the disease becomes refractory.

Thus, managed conventionally, follicular lymphoma is a paradigm for the 'indolent' but incurable malignancy. Whilst this overall approach is acceptable for the elderly it is manifestly unsatisfactory for the younger patient.

Other therapies

■ Aggressive combination chemotherapy gives high complete remission rates and molecular remission.
■ High-dose chemotherapy with PBPCR. Open Phase II trials, comparing outcome with historical controls and now Phase III trials suggest an advantage over conventional therapy in first or second remission (molecular remission also occurs).
■ Antibody therapy. The monoclonal antibody rituximab induces remission (partial) in 30–70% of patients, almost without toxicity. Molecular remissions are observed. Complications include the cytokine release syndrome, with fever, vomiting and allergic reactions (angio-oedema, bronchospasm and dyspnoea).
■ Rituximab/chemotherapy combination. These have now been reported to improve the complete remission rate (with disappearance of Bcl-2 positive cells from the bone marrow in 100% of patients), freedom from progression and event-free survival, even though there is (as yet) no effect on overall survival. This may become the standard therapy for CD20 positive lymphoma.
■ Antibody-targeted irradiation. This short-term therapy using anti-CD20 to deliver either ^{131}I or ^{90}Y yields 'durable' complete remission.

In addition, two major additional biological therapies are under evaluation:

■ vaccine therapy
■ reduced intensity allogeneic transplantation.

The median survival of follicular lymphoma appears to have been extended from 5 years to 10 years following the introduction of alkylating agent chemotherapy. There are grounds for optimism that the new approaches outlined above will improve it further or even result in cure. The challenge, beyond giving the best current advice to the patient today is to devise the initial strategy which will convert follicular lymphoma from a treatable to a curable disease. If the strategy brings greater potential toxicity, the risks have to be weighed carefully against *potential* long-term benefits. The same strategy will not be right for all patients.

Lymphoplasmacytic lymphoma

This is an uncommon B cell lymphoma often presenting with heavy bone marrow infiltration, and is almost the only lymphoma to be diagnosed on bone marrow biopsy alone. There is frequently splenomegaly and anaemia, and in some an associated paraprotein IgM with associated immune paresis (Waldenström's macroglobulinaemia; WM) occurs. Patients in this group are usually older and commonly present with the symptoms of bone marrow failure or hyperviscosity. It may be a chance diagnosis.

Management may be expectant, the indications for treatment being:

■ symptomatic anaemia
■ recurrent infection
■ symptoms of hyperviscosity, e.g. headache, visual disturbance
■ progression.

Treatment is supportive in the first instance. Transfusion and/or erythropoietin is given for the anaemia, particularly if chemotherapy is being given. Plasmapheresis is an excellent means of controlling the paraproteinaemia both in the short and longer term.

Chlorambucil is the conventional treatment, the 'response criteria' for WM being different from those of the rest of the lymphomas. The paraprotein will be reduced by 50% (response) in 50–70% of cases in the short term. Progression is the rule and as with follicular lymphoma there may be further response. The purine analogue fludarabine is also 'effective'.

It is not clear how much the use of chemotherapy has actually influenced overall survival, and quality of life is poorly recorded. The median survival is several years.

A heightened awareness of this relatively uncommon but symptomatic lymphoma has led to more enthusiastic exploration of the new therapies being tested on the other B cell lymphomas (see above).

Mantle cell lymphoma

This is an uncommon lymphoma (6% of non-Hodgkin's

lymphoma) with a median survival of 3–4 years. It occurs predominantly in the elderly and is almost always widely disseminated at presentation, with lymphadenopathy and frequent involvement of the bone marrow and gastrointestinal tract. Treatment is often compromised by co-morbidity.

Combination chemotherapy is the most usual first-line therapy, if possible: the response rate may be above 50% but the complete remission rate is low. The addition of rituximab has been reported to improve this. Intensifying chemotherapy appears to improve the results, but recurrence is almost invariable. New approaches are greatly needed.

Large B cell lymphoma (DLBCL)

This is the commonest lymphoma and is almost invariably fatal without therapy within months, and was previously classified as aggressive or high-grade lymphoma. Now > 50% of young patients are cured. The only indications for a palliative approach at the initial presentation are extreme co-morbidity and the will of the patient. Expectant management is inappropriate. Patients present with rapidly progressive lymphadenopathy and progressive infiltration of many organs, e.g. spinal cord, gastrointestinal tract.

Treatment

Treatment decisions are based on the stage and may be tailored by the International Prognostic Index (Box 9.5).

In the absence of relevant co-morbidity all patients should receive cyclical combination chemo-immuno-therapy, the gold standard being cyclophosphamide, hydroxydaunorubicin, vincristine, prednisolone and rituximab (CHOP + R). Sixty to seventy percent of those with early stage disease (I, II$_A$ without bulk) may expect to be cured either with 6 cycles or 3 cycles followed by involved field irradiation. Those with more extensive disease conventionally receive 6–8 cycles. There has been a suggestion that decreasing the interval between cycles may be feasible (with growth factor support), and this may improve the results. There are conflicting reports about the advantages of increasing the intensity of initial treatment for those perceived to be at 'high risk'. There is also controversy about the indications for central nervous system prophylaxis and which form it should take.

For those with advanced disease the cure fraction, which was about 30%, has been increased with the incorporation of rituximab as standard therapy, by 15%.

Progression during therapy or failure of the initial treatment to achieve complete remission has a very poor prognosis. Second-line therapy e.g. platinum or gemcitabine should be initiated with a view, if possible, to high-dose therapy and PBPCR if further response is achieved. This is not usually possible and long-term success is rare. Proper consideration should be given to palliation or experimental therapy. In contrast, recurrence after a disease-free interval is potentially still curable. The complete remission rate after a second treatment is 40–50%: it is conventional to consolidate such remissions with high-dose therapy which will cure perhaps half (i.e. 25% 'cure' overall of the selected younger patients in whom curative therapy is attempted).

Burkitt's lymphoma

This is an uncommon lymphoma in the western world. It is endemic to Africa in the mosquito belt: there is a close association with the Epstein–Barr virus and it is a disease with a very high proliferative index which is very rapidly fatal without therapy.

The clinical presentation worldwide is usually that of lymphadenopathy, often with an abdominal mass and frequently with bone marrow infiltration (and 'leukaemia'). Central nervous system involvement is common, up to 30% having meningitis at the time of presentation. In Africa, by far the two commonest presentations are the abdominal mass or a large tumour involving the jaw (Fig. 9.14); the bone marrow and central nervous system are also frequently involved.

Treatment

Treatment, whilst undoubtedly toxic with both morbidity and mortality, is much less dangerous than the disease. It relieves symptoms and is potentially curable in a high proportion of cases.

Supportive care is with hydration and prevention of hyperuricaemia with allopurinol associated with rapid tumour lysis. Rasburicase is a major advance.

> ### Box 9.5 Prognostic factors in non-Hodgkin's lymphoma
>
> Adverse factors:
> - Age > 60 years
> - Stage III or IV, i.e. advanced disease
> - High serum lactate dehydrogenase level
> - Performance status (ECOG 2 or more)
> - More than one extranodal site involved
>
> ECOG, Eastern Cooperative Oncology Group

Fig. 9.14 A child with Burkitt's lymphoma.

Drug therapy

The management of the newly diagnosed case in Europe is straightforward but in Africa it may be very difficult.

Cyclical combination chemotherapy, incorporating at least high doses of cyclophosphamide and methotrexate as well as vincristine and doxorubicin, is followed by further cycles including high-dose cytarabine depending on the extent of disease at presentation. Up to six cycles must be given at about monthly intervals. While both the high-dose systemic methotrexate and cytarabine cross the blood–brain barrier in tumoricidal doses, many prefer to supplement them with intrathecal chemotherapy also. The role of cranial irradiation is unclear. In Africa, treatment can be difficult to coordinate but is based on the same principles.

This treatment will be tolerated quite well by the majority of patients, who tend to be young. The reported complete remission rate is very high, 70–90% depending on age (and excluding those with concurrent HIV infection), with very few recurrences occurring after 1 year. Hence 60–70% may be cured. Demonstrating improvements on this will be difficult but rituximab may have a role.

The management of progression despite treatment is difficult and rarely successful. Remission induction with alternative therapy, possibly including cisplatin, is the first line of attack. If achieved, it is consolidated with high-dose therapy or allogeneic transplantation.

T Cell lymphomas

These are much less common than the B cell counterparts. In the main, the overall treatment strategies are the same, but success is much more limited.

Primary extranodal lymphoma

The WHO classification does not distinguish between primarily nodal or extranodal at the time of presentation if the histological picture is the same.

Primary cerebral lymphoma

This is a very aggressive disease with survival untreated measured in months. It is particularly dangerous within the setting of HIV infection. Irradiation plus corticosteroids has, until recently, been the treatment of first choice. It is rarely curative, and may be associated with severe cerebral toxicity when given in high enough doses to eliminate lymphoma, particularly in the elderly. Even following irradiation, the median time to progression is less than a year. Subsequent management is palliative.

Recent data suggest that a very aggressive approach, involving sequential very high doses of methotrexate followed by cytarabine may obviate the need for irradiation and be curative in a proportion of cases. Followed by irradiation this treatment may eliminate lymphoma in an even higher proportion of cases, but the potential central nervous system toxicity is considered by most to be unacceptable.

Primary gastric lymphoma

In a high proportion of cases, particularly in Northern Italy, lymphoma is associated with *Helicobacter pylori* infection (p. 283). Biopsy of the gastric lesion usually shows lymphoma ('low-grade' B cell pathologically, of extranodal marginal zone type) and *H. pylori* is usually detected. Treatment to eradicate *H. pylori* is with antibiotics (and a proton pump inhibitor) for 2 weeks. Symptomatic relief is usually rapid. Provided there is no evidence of disease outside the stomach, further treatment is not given but surveillance endoscopy is performed, first at 3 months then 6-monthly. Partial or complete remission is the rule, but may take many months to achieve. Treatment of progression (always confirmed by biopsy) is with more antibiotics initially. Both irradiation and alkylating agent therapy are effective. Rituximab is being investigated. There is no role for surgery in the management of gastric lymphoma.

Primary cutaneous lymphoma (see p. 1352)

This is much commoner than generally perceived. It must be carefully distinguished from cutaneous infiltration with lymphocytes in a patient with nodal disease. It is usually of T cell origin (Sézary syndrome, mycosis fungoides). It is often multifocal and responds well to local therapy even when it appears histologically aggressive. Survival may be very long without chemotherapy, and in many cases treatment may only serve to disrupt the quality of life.

FURTHER READING

Dave SS, Wright G, Tan B et al. (2004) Prediction of survival in follicular lymphoma based on molecular features of tumour-infiltrating immune cells. *New England Journal of Medicine* **351**: 2159–2169.

Hennessy BT et al. (2004) Non-Hodgkin lymphoma: an update. *Lancet Oncology* **5**: 341–353.

Mauch PM, Armitage JO, Coiffier B et al. (2003) *Non-Hodgkin's Lymphomas*. Philadelphia: Lippincott Williams & Wilkins.

MYELOMA

Myeloma is a malignant disease of the plasma cells of bone marrow, accounting for 1% of all malignant disease. There is a clonal expansion of abnormal, proliferating plasma cells producing a monoclonal paraprotein, mainly IgG (55%) or IgA (20%) and rarely IgD. The paraproteinaemia may be associated with excretion of light chains in the urine (Bence Jones protein), which are either kappa or lambda. In approximately 20% there is no paraproteinaemia, only light chains in the urine.

Clinicopathological features

Myeloma is a disease of the elderly, the median age at presentation being over 60 years. It is rare under 40 years of age. The annual incidence is 4 per 100 000 and it is commoner in males and in black Africans but less common in Asians. There is:

■ *Bone destruction*, often causing fractures of long bones or vertebral collapse (which can cause spinal cord compression) and hypercalcaemia

■ *Bone marrow infiltration* with plasma cells, resulting in anaemia, neutropenia, thrombocytopenia, together with production of the paraprotein which may (rarely) result in symptoms of hyperviscosity

■ *Renal impairment* (p. 637) owing to a combination of factors – deposition of light chains in the renal tubules, hypercalcaemia, hyperuricaemia, use of NSAIDs and (rarely) in patients who have had the disease for some time, deposition of amyloid.

In addition there is a reduction in the normal immunoglobulin levels (immune paresis), contributing to the tendency for patients with myeloma to have recurrent infections, particularly of the respiratory tract.

Cytogenetics

Abnormalities of chromosomes were found in only 50% of patients with old techniques. However, with fluorescent in situ hybridization and microarray techniques abnormalities are found in most. Abnormalities of chromosome 13 and hypodiploidy have been shown to be associated with poor survival, as have t(4;14), t(14;16) and p53 deletions.

Bone metastases

There is dysregulation of bone remodelling which leads to the typical lytic lesions, e.g. spine, skull. In myeloma there is increased osteoclastic activity with no increased osteoblast formation of bone. Bisphosphonates that inhibit osteoclast activity are useful in myeloma but surprisingly there is no increase in bone deposition (see below).

Adhesion of stromal cells to myeloma cells stimulates the production of RANKL, IL-6, and also VEGF (which plays a role in angiogenesis). RANKL also stimulates osteoclast formation and the lytic lesions (see Fig. 9.1). Myeloma cells also produce dickkopf-1 (DKK1) which *inhibits* osteoblast activity and therefore production of new bone. This occurs because DKK1 binds to the Wnt co-receptor, lipoprotein receptor-related protein 5 (LRP5), inhibiting Wnt signalling and osteoblast differentiation.

Symptoms

■ Bone pain – most commonly backache owing to vertebral involvement (60%)
■ Symptoms of anaemia
■ Recurrent infections
■ Symptoms of renal failure (20–30%)
■ Symptoms of hypercalcaemia
■ Rarely, symptoms of hyperviscosity and bleeding due to thrombocytopenia.

Patients can be asymptomatic, the diagnosis being suspected by 'routine' abnormal blood tests. Life-threatening complications are shown in Box 9.6.

> ### Box 9.6 Life-threatening complications of myeloma
>
> ■ Renal impairment – often a consequence of hypercalcaemia – requires urgent attention and patients may need to be considered for long-term peritoneal or haemodialysis.
> ■ Hypercalcaemia should be treated by rehydration and use of bisphosphonates such as pamidronate.
> ■ Spinal cord compression due to myeloma is treated with dexamethasone, followed by radiotherapy to the lesion delineated by a magnetic resonance imaging (MRI) scan.
> ■ Hyperviscosity due to high circulating levels of paraprotein may be corrected by plasmapheresis.

Investigations

■ **Full blood count**. Hb is normal or low. WCC is normal or low. The platelet count is normal or low.
■ **ESR**. This is almost always high.
■ **C-reactive protein** is always raised.
■ **Blood film**. There may be rouleaux formation as a consequence of the paraprotein.
■ **Urea and electrolytes**. There may be evidence of renal failure (see above)
■ **Serum β_2-microglobulin** > 2.5 mg/L ⎫ useful in
■ **Serum lactate dehydrogenase (LDH)** ⎭ prognosis.
■ **Serum calcium** is normal or raised.
■ **Serum alkaline phosphatase** is usually normal.
■ **Total protein** is normal or raised.
■ **Serum albumin** is normal or low.
■ **Serum protein electrophoresis or immunofixation** characteristically shows a monoclonal band.
■ **Uric acid** is normal or raised.
■ **Skeletal survey**. This may show characteristic lytic lesions, most easily seen in the skull (Fig. 9.15). CT,

Fig. 9.15 Myeloma affecting the skull. Note the rounded lytic translucencies produced by infiltration of the skull with myeloma cells.

Fig. 9.16 **Multiple myeloma**. Histology shows replacement of the medullary cavity by abnormal plasma cells with some binucleate forms. A residual bony trabeculum is present towards the right. Courtesy of Dr AJ Norton.

MRI and PET are used in plasmacytomas (bone lesions without plasma cells in the blood).

- **DXA scanning** is valuable for follow-up of treatment.
- **24-hour urine immunofixation** is used for assessment of light-chain excretion.
- **Bone marrow aspirate** or trephine shows characteristic infiltration by plasma cells (Fig. 9.16). Amyloid may be found.

Diagnosis

Two out of three diagnostic features should be present:

- paraproteinaemia or Bence Jones protein
- radiological evidence of lytic bone lesions
- an increase in bone marrow plasma cells.

An international prognostic index which would help in staging the disease is being developed; the Durie–Salmon criteria are no longer used.

Monoclonal gammopathy of unknown significance (MGUS). MGUS describes an isolated finding of a monoclonal paraprotein in the serum, usually in the elderly; 20–30% go on to develop multiple myeloma.

Treatment

With good supportive care and chemotherapy with autologous or allogeneic stem cell transplantation, median survival is now 5 years with some patients surviving to 10 years. Young patients receiving more intensive therapy may live longer.

Supportive therapy

- Anaemia should be corrected; blood transfusion may be required. Erythropoietin often helps.
- Infection should be treated promptly with antibiotics. Give yearly flu vaccinations.
- Bone pain can be helped most quickly by radiotherapy. NSAIDs are also useful (beware of use in renal involvement).
- Pathological fractures may also be prevented by prompt orthopaedic surgery (kyphoplasty) with pinning of lytic bone lesions seen on the skeletal survey.

Specific therapy

Conventional treatment, incorporating first-class supportive care including long-term bisphosphonates, e.g. zoledronate or clodronate, which inhibit osteoclast activity, reduces progression of bone disease. Initial chemotherapy with melphalan and prednisolone has a response rate of approximately 50%. Complete remission is never attained and all patients will relapse without further treatment. High-dose melphalan therapy and peripheral blood stem cell rescue (autotransplantation) has undoubtedly improved the duration of remission and overall survival of younger patients, even if cure has not been attained. 'Reduced-intensity' allogeneic stem cell transplants are also used, with a reduction of mortality over normal-intensity allogeneic transplants, but still with graft-versus-myeloma effect.

'New' approaches are showing considerable promise and may lead to greater improvements:

- *Thalidomide.* This anti-angiogenesis agent has been shown, outside the context of pregnancy, to reduce the paraprotein in heavily pretreated patients with myeloma. Phase III trials in combination with chemotherapy are in progress and new analogues are becoming available.
- *Bortazemab.* This proteosome inhibitor has now been licensed in the USA on the basis of single agent data. As with thalidomide, Phase II trials with chemotherapy have been most encouraging and Phase III trials are underway.

> **FURTHER READING**
> Bruno B (2004) New drugs for treatment of multiple myeloma. *Lancet Oncology* **5**: 430–442.
> Sirohi B, Powles R (2004) Multiple myeloma. *Lancet* **363**: 875–887.

COMMON SOLID TUMOUR TREATMENT

Common solid cancer mortality is listed in Table 9.1; the improvements over the past 10 years have come from advances in the prevention, diagnosis, and treatment. The presentation, diagnosis, and natural history of the common cancers are described in the relevant organ system chapters. In this section the systemic therapy of the common cancers is described, and in addition the treatment of germ cell tumours illustrates what can be achieved when chemotherapy resistance is overcome. The decision to treat and the aim of that treatment whether for palliation or cure, require knowledge of the disease, prognostic factors, the patient's performance status, and the potential efficacy of treatment. Management should be carried out by multidisciplinary teams, usually led by an oncologist.

Lung cancer (p. 947)

Prognostic factors

Presentation, diagnosis and surgery are discussed on p. 948.

Lung cancer histology is divided into two main types; small-cell (neuroendocrine) lung cancers (SCLC) and non-small-cell lung cancers (NSCLC). In addition, tumour stage and patient performance status are used in selecting treatment and predicting response and prognosis. While overall 5-year survival has remained approximately 15%, treatment is beginning to have an impact in selected groups and the multidisciplinary team can greatly aid in the appropriate application of treatment and the avoidance of nihilism.

Non-small-cell lung cancer
Prognostic factors

The staging is classified according to the TNM system (Table 9.5), by which the disease can be divided into local, locally advanced, and advanced stages with 5-year survival varying from 55–67%, to 23–40%, to 1–3% respectively. The addition of CT and PET scanning has increased the accuracy of staging and improved the selection of patients for surgery and adjuvant therapy.

Treatment

In *operable disease* stages T1N0 to T3N2 (stage I to IIIa) adjuvant radiotherapy and chemotherapy are still of uncertain benefit, although recently the international adjuvant lung cancer trial showed that cisplatin-based combination chemotherapy produced an improvement in 5-year survival of 4% from 40.4% to 44.5%. Uracil and tegafur given for 2 years after complete resection can improve survival in stage I adenocarcinoma.

For *unresectable disease,* the combination of concurrent cisplatin with radiotherapy when compared with radiotherapy alone has increased the resection rate and 3-year survival from 11% to 23% at the expense of greater oesophageal toxicity.

In *advanced disease* cisplatin or carboplatin in combination with one other drug such as paclitaxel or gemcitabine for 12 weeks produces a symptomatic improvement in 40%, and increases median survival from 6 to 10 months compared with best supportive care, with 10–20% alive at 1 year.

Small-cell lung cancer
Prognostic factors

The staging of small-cell lung cancer is divided into limited and extensive disease according to whether or not it is confined to a single anatomical area or radiation field.

Treatment

Limited disease is present in approximately 30% of patients and is best treated with concurrent chemo- and radiotherapy using a combination of cisplatin and etoposide or irinotecan, which increases the survival at 5 years from 15% to 25% compared with radiotherapy alone. A similar degree of improvement can also be achieved with hyperfractionated radiotherapy. Prophylactic whole-brain radiation to prevent cerebral metastases can reduce symptomatic CNS disease and improve overall survival by 5%.

Extensive disease can be palliated with the combination of carboplatin and etoposide or irinotecan, which when compared with best supportive care can increase median survival from 6 months to 9–13 months and 2-year survival to 20%.

Breast cancer

Breast cancer is the most common cancer in women who do not smoke. The screening programme in the UK, with mammography every 3 years in women aged 50–64 and improvements in multimodality treatment have improved overall survival and rates of cure, while breast-conserving surgery has greatly ameliorated the psychosexual impact of the disease.

Symptoms and signs

Most women present with a painless increasing mass which may also be associated with nipple discharge, skin tethering, ulceration and, in inflammatory cancers, oedema and erythema. In developing countries, 80% present with advanced disease.

Investigations

The triple assessment of any symptomatic breast mass by palpation, radiology (mammography, ultrasound and MRI scan) and fine-needle aspiration cytology is the most reliable way to differentiate breast cancer from the 15 times more common benign breast masses. Assessment should be carried out in a dedicated one-stop clinic able to provide the appropriate support and referral accordingly. Staging is both surgical with respect to tumour size and axillary lymph node status and, in advanced disease, by investigation of common sites of metastasis by chest X-ray, bone and liver scan. At present, only 20% of patients are diagnosed with no evidence of microscopic nodal metastases.

Prognostic factors

The size of the primary tumour, the histological subtype (most are infiltrating ductal carcinoma), histological grade/differentiation, oestrogen and progesterone receptor status, patient age and menopausal status are all significant independent predictors of risk of recurrence. Expression of c-*erbB2* is linked to the above and a predictor of treatment response.

Early breast cancer
The prognosis (10-year survival) can be predicted from the independent prognostic factors in Box 9.7. Survival

> **Box 9.7 Poor prognostic factors for breast cancer**
>
> - Young age
> - Premenopausal
> - Large tumour size
> - High tumour grade
> - Oestrogen and progesterone receptor negative
> - Positive nodes

will vary from 90% for small (< 1 cm) low-grade node-negative tumours to 20% for large high-grade tumours with more than three axillary nodes involved and no adjuvant therapy.

Local treatment

Surgery with wide local excision and breast conservation, or mastectomy with or without reconstruction, is dictated by the location and extent of the breast mass, and patient preferences. Surgery of the axilla may require full dissection or sentinel lymph node guided sampling in order to gain local control and provide prognostic information to guide adjuvant treatment if there are clinically involved nodes. The greater the amount of axillary surgery the more the risk of post-operative lymph-oedema. Radiotherapy is given to the conserved breast after wide local excision to reduce local recurrence, and after mastectomy if there are risk factors such as proximity to surgical margins or lymph node metastases, to complete the local control measures. Adjuvant radiotherapy reduces the risk of local recurrence by 25% and improves 10-year survival by 3%. Recent data suggest that women over 70 years with oestrogen receptor positive cancers up to 2 cm may be offered surgery and tamoxifen alone without radiotherapy, without compromising outcome.

Adjuvant systemic treatment

Tamoxifen (p. 497) adjuvant therapy immediately following surgery for oestrogen and/or progesterone receptor-positive disease has reduced the 10-year relative risk of women dying from breast cancer by about 25% and the absolute 10-year death rate by 12%. A meta-analysis of all randomized trials of adjuvant therapy in breast cancer has shown that for *premenopausal women* with axillary lymph node metastases or other high-risk features (Box 9.7), adjuvant chemotherapy with CMF (cyclophosphamide, 5-fluorouracil plus methotrexate) or more effective regimens with epirubicin, or ataxane (Epi-CMF or FEC) for 6 months, reduces the absolute 10-year death rate by about 10% and the relative risk of death by 20%. Ovarian ablation is equally effective as CMF chemotherapy. The effects of tamoxifen and chemotherapy are additive and most effective given serially, not concurrently.

For *postmenopausal women* with oestrogen and/or progesterone receptor-positive disease, adjuvant tamoxifen or aromatase inhibitors given for 5 years reduces the risk of death from breast cancer by a similar 25%. Aromatase inhibitors avoid the adverse effects of tamoxifen on the uterus and venous thromboembolism but add risks of osteoporosis. Menopausal status does not affect the relative efficacy of tamoxifen or chemotherapy; however, since the risk of recurrence is lower after the menopause, the absolute improvement in survival is less. Toxicity may also be higher in this age group so that treatment decisions may need to be more individualized in discussion between the patient and her doctors. The combined effect of radiotherapy, chemotherapy and tamoxifen or aromatase inhibitor halves the risk of dying of breast cancer for appropriately selected patients.

Advanced breast cancer

Patients with established metastatic disease may require endocrine therapy, chemotherapy or radiotherapy. The treatment is not curative but may be of great palliative benefit and consistent often with many years of good-quality life. Little additional benefit has been gained by adding endocrine and chemotherapy together, although the addition of anti-HER2 (antibodies) to chemotherapy has produced a modest survival advantage. In general, therefore, the serial use of intermittent courses of the different hormonal and chemotherapies seems most consistent with maintaining a good quality of life for as long as possible.

Endocrine therapy (p. 497)

Women who have high levels of oestrogen receptors and progesterone receptors in their tumour have a greater chance of responding to endocrine treatments. In addition, certain clinical features can predict the likelihood of responding to hormonal manipulations (Box 9.8).

Endocrine therapy is usually tried first in those patients who have characteristics suggesting they are likely to respond and who do not have immediately life-threatening disease. Remission lasts on average 2 years and is consistent with an excellent quality of life. When relapse occurs, further treatment with alternative agents may produce another remission. A range of hormonal manipulations is available (Table 9.21).

Chemotherapy (p. 492)

Chemotherapy is considered for patients who are unlikely to respond to hormonal treatment or who fail to respond to endocrine therapy or who require a rapid response if at risk of, for example, liver or respiratory failure. If chosen carefully, chemotherapy can provide

---

> **Box 9.8 Clinical features that increase the likelihood of response to endocrine treatment for metastatic disease**
>
> ■ Oestrogen or progesterone receptor positive (60% vs 10% response in oestrogen receptor (ER) negative disease)
> ■ Long interval (more than 2 years) from initial surgery to time of relapse

---

Table 9.21 Endocrine therapy of metastatic breast cancer

For premenopausal patients
(a) Suppression of ovarian function by means of oophorectomy, radiation-induced ovarian ablation or a GnRH analogue, e.g. goserelin
(b) Oestrogen receptor antagonist, tamoxifen, fulvestrant
(c) Progesterone

For postmenopausal patients
(a) Oestrogen receptor antagonists, tamoxifen, fulvestrant
(b) Progesterone
(c) Aromatase inhibitors (e.g. anastrozole, letrozole and exemestane)

good-quality palliation and prolongation of life. The most common regimens used include:

- CMF (cyclophosphamide, methotrexate, 5-fluorouracil)
- MM (mitoxantrone (mitozantrone) and methotrexate)
- doxorubicin and cyclophosphamide
- paclitaxel or docetaxel used as single agents or in combination with an anthracycline or capecitabine
- vinorelbine
- capecitabine.

There is very little difference in efficacy between the different regimens for metastatic disease, with response rates varying from 40% to 60% for median duration of 8 months. More recently, the addition of trastuzumab (p. 498) monoclonal antibody to the cytotoxic drugs has significantly improved survival for those women whose tumour over-expresses the c-erbB2/Her2 oncogene. The addition of capecitabine to docetaxel or trastuzumab, has also improved survival in metastatic breast cancer. The regimens do differ in toxicity with MM being one of the least toxic. The multiple regimens provide the possibility of avoiding drug resistance over several episodes of treatment interspersed with treatment-free periods so that the disease can be palliated, often for several years.

Gastrointestinal cancer

Presentation, diagnosis and local treatments are described in Chapter 6.

Oesophageal cancer

Histology, stage, age and performance status are critical to treatment decisions, which should be made by a multi-disciplinary team in designated units. The prognosis for the majority of symptomatic patients is poor, 50% have distant metastases at the time of diagnosis and the majority of the remainder will have loco-regional spread into mediastinal structures.

Treatment

Neoadjuvant therapy for potentially resectable squamous carcinomas with cisplatin, 5-fluorouracil and concurrent radiotherapy achieves complete remission in 20–40% with 25–35% of patients alive 5-years after surgery. There is an increased perioperative mortality. Postoperative chemotherapy for adenocarcinomas has failed to improve overall survival.

Locally advanced or metastatic disease can be palliated with 5-fluorouracil chemotherapy in approximately 30%, increasing to 45–55% with the addition of oxaliplatin or irinotecan for a median duration of 6–8 months.

Gastric cancer

Presentation and diagnosis are described on page 288.

Prognostic factors

The histological grade and staging with respect to the presence of serosal involvement (T3) and nodal involvement (N1–2) are the main factors in prognosis. For the majority of patients with node-positive disease the 5-year survival is only 20% following surgery alone.

Treatment

A recent study of combined chemo-radiotherapy with cisplatin and 5-fluorouracil compared with surgery alone showed significantly increased median survival from 28 to 35 months and 3-year survival from 41% to 50%. This was achieved mainly through improvement in loco-regional control but is suitable only for good performance status patients.

Advanced disease may be palliated with chemotherapy such as epirubicin, cisplatin, and infusional 5-fluorouracil in 40–50% of patients for a median of 8–10 months but is suitable only for the younger fitter patient.

Colorectal cancer

Presentation and diagnosis are described on page 329.

The site of the disease, above or below the pelvic peritoneal reflection, and TNM stage are the main prognostic factors (see Table 6.17).

Treatment

Local therapy is discussed on page 330.

Adjuvant chemotherapy with 5-fluorouracil and folinic acid for rectal and colonic adenocarcinoma significantly increases 5-year survival for node-positive disease stage III (Dukes' C) by 5% from 40% to 45%. A further 6% improvement in a recent trial was achieved by the addition of oxaliplatin, and trials are examining the addition of monoclonal antibody to the EGF receptor (cetuximab) or VEGF (bevacizumab).

Advanced colorectal cancer is successfully palliated with little toxicity by 5-fluorouracil and folinic acid regimens in approximately 30% of patients for a median of 12–14 months. The addition of irinotecan or oxaliplatin increases the proportion who benefit to 55% but with increased toxicity. The monoclonal antibody bevacizumab (and possibly cetuximab) increases the response rate to chemotherapy and in one trial the median survival from 14 to 21 months.

Epithelial ovarian cancer

Epithelial ovarian cancer comprises 80% of all ovarian cancers, the remainder being of germ cell or stromal origin.

Symptoms and signs

Ovarian cancer typically causes few specific symptoms, sometimes there is a sensation of a pelvic mass, which may become (acutely) painful, often there is only vague abdominal distension and epigastric discomfort.

Investigation

Pelvic examination should be complemented by a trans-vaginal ultrasound and serum CA125. Magnetic resonance imaging is the definitive imaging technique for the pelvis.

Prognostic factors

Histological subtype, grade/differentiation stage, and extent of residual disease following surgery are all significant independent prognostic factors for survival.

Treatment

Surgery (with total abdominal hysterectomy, bilateral salpingo-oophorectomy and omentectomy) has a major role in the treatment of ovarian cancer. For patients in whom the disease is confined to the ovary, the surgery can be curative in 80–90% if the histology is well to moderately differentiated. For patients with poorly differentiated or more advanced disease, with spread throughout the peritoneal cavity, surgery still has a major role in staging the patient and improving survival when it is possible to debulk optimally to < 1 cm residual. Primary chemotherapy and delayed surgery is an alternative approach currently under investigation.

Drugs used to treat ovarian cancer are cisplatin and its analogue carboplatin, which is associated with fewer side-effects. Response is achieved in approximately two-thirds of patients. Paclitaxel has been shown to improve the survival of many patients when added to a platinum-based treatment.

Adjuvant treatment with carboplatin and paclitaxel for stage I high-risk disease increases the absolute 5-year survival by 9% from 70% to 79%. In advanced disease 75% of patients will respond to combination chemotherapy and the median survival is approximately 3 years. Up to 30% of those with metastatic disease may be alive after 5 years, although this falls to 5–10% if the cancer is not able to be debulked at operation or has spread outside the peritoneal cavity.

Prostate cancer

Early prostate cancer

Presentation and diagnosis are described on page 685.

Prognostic factors

The histological appearances are graded and accorded a Gleason Score which together with the height of the serum PSA plus accurate staging of the local extent of disease with pelvic MRI and transrectal ultrasound can identify prognostic groups. This allows the selection of patients with good prognosis who may reasonably choose to be kept under surveillance with no active treatment and, like 75% of men over the age of 80, die with, but not because of, their prostate cancer.

Treatment

Curative surgery (radical prostatectomy) and either external beam radiotherapy or brachytherapy can achieve equivalent survival rates but differ in the spectrum of unwanted side-effects with respect to incontinence and sexual dysfunction. In appropriately selected series of patients a 5-year survival of 85% can be achieved. Discussion between patient and clinician is vital before treatment is started.

Adjuvant androgen deprivation treatment such as monthly depot goserelin has not improved the survival from surgery but when given before and during radiotherapy can improve the overall survival at 3 years from 62% to 78%.

Advanced prostate cancer

Treatment

Metastatic prostate cancer with either local or skeletal spread is rapidly and effectively palliated in 70% of patients by androgen deprivation. The median duration of response is 2 years and, on the development of hormone resistance, mitoxantrone or docetaxel possibly with estramustine, chemotherapy can be guided by PSA response to provide some further months' palliation when compared with best supportive care. Radiotherapy provides a very effective palliation of painful skeletal metastases and can be delivered systemically by intravenous bone-seeking strontium-labelled bisphosphonate for patients with multiple affected sites.

Testicular and ovarian germ cell tumours

Germ cell tumours are the most common cancers in men aged 15–35 years but comprise only 1–2% of all cancers. They are much less common in women. There are two main histological types, seminoma (dysgerminoma in women) and teratoma. Teratomas may comprise varying proportions of mature and immature elements. Germ cell tumours may rarely occur in extragonadal sites in the midline from pituitary, mediastinum or retroperitoneum but should be treated in a similar manner.

Symptoms and signs

Most men present with a testicular mass which is often painful, some with symptoms of metastases to the para-aortic lymph nodes with back pain. In women the mass presents with vague pelvic symptoms but at a younger age than the more common epithelial ovarian cancers.

Investigations

Ultrasound scanning of the testicle or ovary is required, with assay of serum tumour markers, α-fetoprotein (AFP) and β-human chorionic gonadotrophin (β-HCG), and lactic dehydrogenase (LDH), followed by CT or MRI scan for distant metastases. Surgery for men is by the inguinal approach to avoid spillage of highly metastatic tumour in the scrotum. Surgery for diagnosis and staging should be conservative in women with preservation of fertility because of the efficacy of chemotherapy.

Treatment

Seminomas

Seminomas are the least common of these tumours and are very radiosensitive and chemosensitive. Seminomas are associated with a raised serum LDH but only rarely a mildly raised HCG and never a raised AFP. Stage I disease limited to the gonad is associated with a 30% risk of recurrence with surgery alone. Adjuvant therapy with either chemo- or radiotherapy leads to greater than 95% cure in early-stage disease but chemotherapy with single-agent cisplatin or carboplatin does not have the long-term risks of secondary malignancy associated with radiotherapy. Combination chemotherapy (e.g. cisplatin, etoposide and bleomycin) will cure 90% of those with metastatic disease.

Teratomas

The risk of relapse with stage I disease varies from 5% to 40% depending upon the histological differentiation and extent of local invasion. Adjuvant chemotherapy for those at moderate to high risk (e.g. cisplatin, etoposide and bleomycin) leads to a 95% cure rate. Metastatic disease commonly involves para-aortic lymph nodes and lungs but may spread rapidly, especially if there are trophoblastic (HCG-producing) elements present. HCG can be associated with gynaecomastia and can be tested for in any young male with a urinary pregnancy test to enable rapid institution of potentially life-saving treatment. About 80% of teratomas will express either HCG or AFP and almost all metastatic disease will be associated with an elevation of the less-specific serum marker lactate dehydrogenase (LDH). Chemotherapy cure for metastatic teratoma varies from over 90% for those with small-volume to 40% for those with large-volume metastases and associated rises of AFP > 10 000 and β-HCG > 100 000 IU/L.

Although approximately 20% of men will be infertile due to azoospermia at the time of diagnosis, the majority of the remainder will retain their fertility after chemotherapy and be able to father normal children. Similarly, most women retain their fertility, although less is known about the association with infertility at presentation owing to the much lower frequency of germ cell tumours in women.

Cancer with unknown primary

Patients presenting with symptoms of their metastases without a clinically obvious primary after investigation represent a common clinical problem and comprise 5–10% of patients in a specialist oncological centre. As a result of several systematic studies, some with postmortem follow-up, the following guidance should aid the choice of appropriate investigation and treatment.

Diagnosis

Diagnosis requires histology first and foremost, as it will lead to the identification of several distinct groups.

1. *Squamous cancers* – mostly presenting in the lymph nodes of the cervical region, 80% will be associated with an occult head and neck primary, the remainder arising from the lung. Inguinal nodes point usually to a primary of the genital tract or anal canal. Treatment with radiotherapy and chemotherapy may have curative potential.
2. *Poorly differentiated or anaplastic cancers* – this group will contain the majority of the curable cancers such as

 Box 9.9 Adenocarcinoma with unknown primary: primary sites with major treatment benefits

- Breast, e.g. isolated axillary lymphadenopathy
- Ovary, e.g. peritoneal carcinomatosis
- Prostate, e.g. pelvic lymphadenopathy

high-grade lymphomas and germ cell tumours identifiable by their immunocytochemistry and tumour markers. Treatment and prognosis is as outlined in the respective primary sites.
3. *Adenocarcinomas* form the majority, and their investigation should be guided by the desire to identify the most treatable options and the knowledge that the largest proportion will have arisen from the lung or pancreas, with relatively poor treatment prospects (Box 9.9). Investigations should therefore comprise a chest X-ray and abdominal CT scan with, in men, serum PSA and rectal ultrasound to identify prostate cancers, and in women, mammography to identify occult breast cancer, and pelvic CT or MRI to identify ovarian cancer. Tumour markers for other solid cancers, although highly sensitive, are too non-specific to be useful as diagnostic aids in this situation.

Further investigation may require MRI for breast and ovarian masses, PET for head and neck, lung and possibly other primaries, and radioisotope scans for thyroid and carcinoid tumours.

For good prognosis patients wishing to have palliative chemotherapy, investigations such as endoscopy to identify lung, colon or stomach primaries are indicated to guide the choice of chemotherapy agents.

Prognosis

The histological type and extent of the disease, and performance status of the patient are the key factors. Most large series report an overall median survival of 12 weeks but considerably better survival amongst the special subgroups below.

Patients presenting with isolated nodal metastases do have a significantly better prognosis than the majority with visceral and/or bone metastases and may warrant more extensive investigation.

Treatment

In women, an isolated axillary lymph node metastasis should be treated as for lymph-node-positive breast cancer. Malignant ascites in women should have a trial of chemotherapy as for epithelial ovarian cancer. The prognosis for those responding to the therapeutic trial is similar to the disease of known primary origin. For men, the occasional occult prostatic cancer found from a raised serum PSA offers some palliative treatment prospects. An increasing choice of chemotherapy agents for gastrointestinal cancers has potential to improve the palliation of patients with liver metastases. If after all efforts, no primary has been identified, palliative chemotherapy treatment can achieve responses in 20–40% in highly selected series, with median survivals of 9–10 months and 5–10% surviving to 5 years.

FURTHER READING

Bosl GJ, Motzer RJ (1997) Testicular germ cell cancer. *New England Journal of Medicine* **337**: 242–253.

Cannistra SA (2004) Cancer of the ovary. *New England Journal of Medicine* **351**: 2519–2529.

Smith I (2003) Cancer of the breast – treatment. *New England Journal of Medicine* **348**: 2431–2438.

Veronesi U et al (2005) Breast cancer. *Lancet* **365**: 1727–1741.

PALLIATIVE MEDICINE AND SYMPTOM CONTROL

Palliative care may be defined as the active, total care of patients whose disease is no longer responsive to curative treatment. The goal of this care is to achieve the best possible quality of life for patients and their families by controlling physical symptoms as well as recognizing psychological, social and spiritual problems. Death is accepted as a normal process, which should neither be hastened nor postponed and the need to provide a support system for the family in bereavement is also recognized.

Many symptoms suffered in incurable illness have a complex aetiology in which the physical component may be overlaid by psychosocial issues. For such patients considerable input from a multidisciplinary team of specialist palliative care professionals may be needed to resolve the symptoms. There is good evidence that integration of palliative care and antitumour management early in the course of disease will reduce long-term distress and difficulty in symptom management. This view moves away from the traditional concentration on the provision of palliative care at the end of life.

The most appropriate first step in providing care in complex situations is often to deal with physical symptoms.

Pain

The symptom most feared by cancer patients is pain, although only two-thirds suffer significant pain throughout the course of their disease. Those patients who suffer pain may present with several pains of differing aetiology, with cancer being directly responsible for about 70%. Pain may be related to associated problems such as rapid weight loss or pressure sores, or may have a separate, non-malignant cause, such as arthritis. The principles of pain relief are careful assessment and diagnosis of the cause of pain, use of analgesics according to the analgesic ladder, and regular review of the effectiveness of the prescribed drugs (Fig. 9.17).

The analgesic ladder

The cancer pain relief programme of the World Health Organization groups drugs into three main classes:

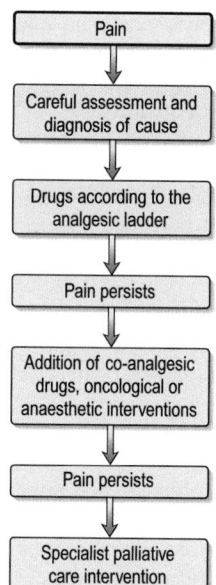

Fig. 9.17 **Management of cancer pain.**

1. non-opioid drugs, such as paracetamol or aspirin and other non-steroidal anti-inflammatory medications
2. weak opioid drugs, such as codeine, dextropropoxyphene and combinations of codeine with paracetamol
3. strong opioid drugs, such as morphine and diamorphine.

The analgesic ladder states that, if optimal use of a drug from the non-opioid class (e.g. 1000 mg of paracetamol 6-hourly) does not result in satisfactory pain relief, the prescription should be increased up one step to a weak opioid. If the equivalent of codeine 60 mg 4-hourly is not sufficient to control pain, the patient will require a strong opioid. Adjuvant, co-analgesic drugs may be added to each step of the ladder.

Strong opioid drugs

Morphine is the drug of choice and in most circumstances should be given regularly by mouth. The dose can be tailored to the individual patient's needs by the addition of 'as required' doses; morphine has no ceiling analgesic effect. A suitable starting dose of morphine is 10 mg 4-hourly, or 5 mg if the patient is elderly or frail. Patients with renal failure will have impaired excretion of morphine metabolites; they should receive a single dose of morphine and be carefully observed for the return of pain in order to determine the approximate rate of excretion of the metabolites.

If a 10 mg dose of morphine relieves the pain but the relief does not last for 4 hours, a 50% increase in the dose should be made (i.e. 10, 15, 20, 30, 45, 60, 90, 120, 180 mg) until satisfactory pain control is achieved.

When the patient's 24-hour morphine requirement has been established, the prescription may be converted to a *controlled-release preparation*. There are both 12-hour and 24-hour release preparations available. The appropriate dose may be calculated by simple addition. For example:

> 20 mg morphine elixir 4-hourly
> = 120 mg morphine per day
> = 60 mg twice-daily of a 12-hour preparation
>   or 120 mg daily of a 24-hour preparation.

If the patient is unable to take oral medication because of nausea or vomiting, gastrointestinal obstruction or altering levels of consciousness, the opioid should be given rectally or parentally. For cancer patients who need long-term analgesia, continuous subcutaneous infusion is the preferred route. Diamorphine is used in this situation because of its greater solubility. By subcutaneous or intramuscular injection, diamorphine is approximately twice as potent as morphine orally. Hence the conversion from oral morphine may be calculated as follows:

> 30 mg oral morphine 4-hourly
> = 180 mg morphine per day
> = 90 mg diamorphine subcutaneously over 24 hours.

Side-effects. *Constipation* caused by analgesic drugs is almost universal. The prescription of a stimulant laxative such as dantron 1–3 capsules at night should be mandatory at the same time as morphine is started. No tolerance develops to this side-effect and laxative medication must be continued as long as analgesics are prescribed.

Nausea or vomiting may occur in 30–60% of patients first started on morphine. However, for those who have worked up the analgesic ladder and who have no other cause for vomiting, the prescription of an 'as required' centrally acting antiemetic is usually sufficient. Tolerance will develop to this side-effect, usually within 4–5 days.

Confusion, nightmares and hallucinations occur in a small percentage of patients. Tolerance to these side-effects does not develop and a change of opiate drug is usually required.

Pain not responsive to opioids

Not all cancer pains are relieved by opioids. In some situations the addition of co-analgesic drugs will result in improved pain control. An increasing number of different classes of drugs have been used in this setting. Some of the most common include the following.

Non-steroidal anti-inflammatory drugs used in addition to a weak or strong opioid for bone pain. Published studies have most frequently used naproxen (500 mg twice-daily) but there is no clear evidence of any one drug being superior in effect. It may be that idiosyncratic side-effects require a trial of a different NSAID.

Pains of nerve destruction called dysaesthetic or deafferentation pain are generally only marginally improved by strong opiates. Several classes of drug, including steroids, have been found to be helpful in reducing the symptoms. In cases of constant burning dysaesthesia, the tricyclic antidepressants are helpful. Amitriptyline 10 mg at night increasing incrementally to 75–100 mg is usually sufficient (compare with the doses required for mood elevation) and the response, if achieved, can be expected in about a week. Anticonvulsant drugs are useful in the management of lancinating, neuropathic pains. Carbamazepine starting at a dose of 100 mg twice-daily is most commonly used, but sodium valproate 300 mg twice-daily may cause fewer adverse side-effects. Gabapentin and pregabalin are of benefit in some forms of neuropathic pain.

In addition to drugs, many other techniques such as radiotherapy, anaesthetic and neurosurgical intervention are employed for the treatment of specific pains.

Regular review of the patient is necessary to achieve optimal pain control. Pain is a complex experience unique to each individual and its perception is modulated by the psychosocial and spiritual situation of the patient. If pain is proving difficult to control, it will be necessary to pay further attention to these other significant factors.

Gastrointestinal symptoms

Anorexia, malaise and weakness are among the most frequently troublesome symptoms in advanced cancer. Endogenously produced cytokines (e.g. tumour necrosis factor and interleukins) are mediators of the anorexia/cachexia syndrome. There is at present no specific therapy, but the approach to treatment depends on adequate management of associated symptoms. Care should be given to addressing the psychological distress caused by a change in body image, with attention to nutrition including dietary advice and the judicious use of steroids.

Nausea and vomiting occur in up to two-thirds of cancer patients in the last 6 weeks of life. The approach to treatment should be similar to that required for pain, involving careful assessment and diagnosis of the cause. It may, however, be more difficult to reach a diagnosis and a somewhat empirical approach to treatment is often adopted. In order to ensure adequate absorption of the antiemetic, parenteral administration, preferably by the subcutaneous route, may be helpful for the first 24–48 hours.

Antiemetics are classified according to their affinities for neurotransmitter receptor sites. A gastrokinetic dopamine antagonist such as metoclopramide 10 mg every 6–8 hours would be helpful in vomiting related to upper gastrointestinal tract stasis or to liver metastases. Metoclopramide should be avoided in cases of intestinal obstruction as it increases peristalsis in the upper bowel. Centrally acting antiemetics such as the phenothiazines, e.g. prochlorperazine 10 mg 8-hourly, cyclizine 50 mg 8-hourly, or the dopamine antagonist butyrophenone, haloperidol 1.5 mg 8-hourly are the drugs of choice in vomiting caused by drugs or metabolic disturbance. As with the prescription of analgesics, antiemetics will be most effective if prescribed on a regular rather than 'as-required' basis.

Bowel obstruction

Bowel obstruction may present acutely or in a more chronic manner and the cause is often multifactorial.

A small number of patients may benefit from surgical intervention, so consideration must be given to this modality of treatment in every case. Most patients will not be suitable for surgery and can be managed medically. The active medical management of malignant bowel obstruction includes:

- the relief of intestinal colic using an antispasmodic such as hyoscine butylbromide 60–80 mg daily; loperamide is sometimes helpful
- treating continuous pain with adequate analgesia such as diamorphine
- treating vomiting if nausea is a problem with a centrally acting antiemetic such as cyclizine 150 mg daily or haloperidol 5–10 mg daily.

It will be necessary to administer all of these medicines parenterally and the subcutaneous route is most appropriate.

Evidence suggests that the use of corticosteroids or the somatostatin analogue octreotide may shorten the length of episodes of obstruction. Octreotide also reduces the volume of fluids secreted into the bowel, thus reducing the volume of nasogastric aspirate or vomit.

Patients may be allowed to drink and eat low-residue diets which are mostly absorbed in the proximal gastro-intestinal tract. It is usually possible, with adequate mouth care, to prevent a sensation of thirst, and routine parenteral fluids are not required. A few patients with intractable vomiting due to a high intestinal block may benefit from continuous nasogastric aspiration or gastrostomy drainage.

Respiratory symptoms

Respiratory symptoms, in particular breathlessness, cause great distress to patients and their carers. Management is based on an accurate diagnosis of the cause and active treatment of all potentially reversible situations. Infections should be treated, pleural and pericardial effusions drained and symptomatic anaemic patients transfused. Radiotherapy, cytotoxic agents and local laser therapy or stent insertions may relieve specific areas of bronchial tree obstruction. The place of oxygen in managing breathlessness is not clear, but it may be helpful in patients with correctable hypoxia.

The sensation of breathlessness and a cycle of respiratory panic may be partially relieved by the prescription of regular benzodiazepines. Regular doses of short-acting opioids 5–20 mg 4-hourly are also helpful, as they are postulated to have a local as well as a central effect. Nebulization of a morphine solution may reduce the sensation of breathlessness in a proportion of patients.

Persistent unproductive cough is a very troublesome symptom. Opiates, codeine, methadone or morphine elixir are helpful as antitussive agents. Antitumour therapy may be required to alleviate pressure on a large airway. Nebulized local anaesthetic may also be helpful in the prevention of cough.

Other physical symptoms

Patients with cancer may develop a large number of physical symptoms. These may be related directly to the presence of the tumour (e.g. vaginal blood loss from a cervix carcinoma) or to the treatment received (e.g. lymphoedema of the arm following breast surgery and radiotherapy). Management of these symptoms will be specific and may require the intervention of other specialists.

Patients may also develop symptoms as a reflection of their debility, such as pressure sores, urinary incontinence, jaundice or recurrent infections. These symptoms may be managed according to the overall expectations and requirements of the patient and their family. These situations of multiple symptomatology in frail patients put considerable demands on the expertise and creativity of clinicians as they present a great challenge for the maintenance of the best possible quality of life.

Psychological symptoms

Effective communication with all patients and their families is a fundamental tenet of clinical practice but is particularly necessary in the stressful situations which surround fatal disease. Basic communication skills include allowing time for the patient to talk, using language which is appropriate to the circumstances, being prepared to repeat information, and being aware that both the patient and the family may receive bad news by blocking or denying it. Remember that it is not always necessary to have an answer or a solution to every problem that is presented, but that considerable support may be given by sympathetic listening.

Care of cancer patients should be designed to allow them to spend as much time as possible in their own homes. Effective liaison between the cancer centre, the palliative care team and the primary healthcare team is essential to ensure total care. You must avoid misinterpretation of any information that may be given regarding treatment and prognosis.

Approximately 60% of cancer patients will die in general hospital wards under the care of the physician or surgeon who first diagnosed their tumour, although many are transferred to hospice care. Every clinician should develop some basic skills in symptom control and the ability to recognize those patients who require more specialist intervention. Caring for this group of patients demands detailed attention to alleviating physical symptoms and the establishment of a secure environment for the patient and family to obtain information and support.

The practice of specialist palliative medicine has traditionally been confined to patients with cancer, although most services cover HIV and AIDS and some of the rapidly fatal neurological diseases. These are all conditions in which the clinical situation is changing rapidly and where difficult symptoms exist. There are undoubtedly patients with non-malignant disease such as end-stage renal or cardiac failure who benefit from a similar multidisciplinary approach to their care. Expansion of specialist palliative medicine into non-malignant situations is being actively pursued. The patient-orientated principles of palliative medicine can, however, be usefully applied throughout all medical practice.

FURTHER READING

Hardy J (2000) Sedation in terminally ill patients. *Lancet* **356**: 1866–1867.

Morrison RS, Meier DE (2004) Palliative care. *New England Journal of Medicine* **350**: 2582–2590.

SIGNIFICANT WEBSITES

http://www.cancerbacup.org.uk
  UK patient organization
http://www.cancerresearchuk.org/
  UK charity (formed from merged Imperial Cancer Research Fund and Cancer Research Campaign).

http://www.cancer.org
  US cancer organisation
http://www.palliativemedjournal.com
  Journal of Palliative Medicine

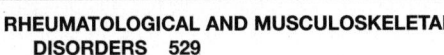

Rheumatology and bone disease

RHEUMATOLOGICAL AND MUSCULOSKELETAL DISORDERS

Many common locomotor problems are short-lived and self-limiting or settle with a course of simple analgesia and/or physical treatment; for example, physiotherapy or osteopathy. Nonetheless, they represent 20–30% of the workload of the primary care physician. Recognition and appropriate early treatment of many painful rheumatic conditions may help reduce the incidence of chronic pain disorders. Early recognition and subsequent treatment of inflammatory arthritis by specialist multidisciplinary teams leads to better symptom control and prevents long-term joint damage and disability. A wide selection of pamphlets offer helpful advice for patients, and their use should be encouraged. Most of the musculoskeletal diseases are seen world-wide, although the prevalence of individual conditions varies.

Fig. 10.1 **The synovial joint.**

THE NORMAL JOINT

There are two types of joints – synovial and fibrocartilaginous.

Synovial joints (Fig. 10.1)
These include the ball-and-socket joints (e.g. hip) and the hinge joints (e.g. interphalangeal).

They possess a cavity and permit the opposed cartilaginous articular surfaces to move painlessly over each other. Movement is restricted to a required range, and stability is maintained during use. The load is distributed across the surface, thus preventing damage by overloading or disuse.

Synovium and synovial fluid
Normal synovium is a few cells thick and vascular. Its surface is smooth and non-adherent and is permeable to proteins and crystalloids. As there are no macroscopic gaps, it is able to retain normal joint fluid even under pressure. The surface layer comprises macrophages and

fibroblast-like cells. The fibroblasts release hyaluronan into the joint space, which helps to retain fluid in the joint. Synovial fluid is a highly viscous fluid secreted by the synovial cells and has a similar consistency to plasma. Glycoproteins ensure a low coefficient of friction between the cartilaginous surfaces. Tendon sheaths and bursa are also lined by synovium.

Fibrocartilaginous joints

These include the intervertebral discs, the sacroiliac joints, the pubic symphysis and the costochondral joints.

Juxta-articular bone

The bone which abuts a joint (epiphyseal bone) differs structurally from the shaft (metaphysis). It is highly vascular and comprises a light framework of mineralized collagen enclosed in a thin coating of tougher, cortical bone. The ability of this structure to withstand pressure is low and it collapses and fractures when the normal intra-articular covering of hyaline cartilage is worn away – as, for example, in osteoarthritis (OA). Loss of surface cartilage also leads to the abnormalities of bone growth and remodelling typical of OA (see p. 551).

Hyaline cartilage

This forms the articular surface and is avascular. It relies on diffusion from synovial fluid for its nutrition. It is rich in type II collagen that forms a meshwork enclosing giant macromolecular aggregates of proteoglycan. These heterogeneous macromolecules comprise protein chains (aggrecans) to which are attached side-chains of the carbohydrates keratan and chondroitin sulphate. These molecules retain water in the structure by producing a dynamic tension between the retaining force of the collagen matrix and the expansive effect of osmotic pressure. Intermittent pressure from 'loading' of the joint is essential to normal cartilage function and encourages movement of water, minerals and nutrients between cartilage and synovial fluid. Chondrocytes secrete collagen and proteoglycans and are embedded in the cartilage. They migrate towards the joint surface along with the matrix they produce.

Ligaments and tendons

These structures stabilize joints. Ligaments are variably elastic and this contributes to the degree of stiffness or laxity of joints (see p. 587). Tendons are inelastic and transmit muscle power to bones. The joint capsule is formed by intermeshing tendons and ligaments. The point where a tendon or ligament joins a bone is called an *enthesis* and may be the site of inflammation.

Components of extracellular matrix

All connective tissues contain an extracellular matrix of macromolecules – collagens, elastins, non-collagenous glycoproteins and proteoglycans – in addition to cells, e.g. fibroblasts. There are several different types of cell surface receptors that bind extracellular matrix proteins including the integrins, CD44 and the proeoglycan-family of receptors e.g. syndecans.

Collagens

Collagens consist of three polypeptide chains (alpha chains) wound into a triple helix These alpha chains contain repeating sequences of *Gly–x–y* triplets, where *x* and *y* are often prolyl and hydroxyprolyl residues. Collagen fibres show considerable genetic heterogeneity, with genes on at least 12 chromosomes. The majority of collagen in the body is type I – the major component of bone, tendon, ligament, skin, sclera, cornea, blood vessels and the hollow organs. Types III, V and VI are also present in most tissues although little collagen type III is found in bone or cartilage. Other types of collagen are tissue specific, i.e. types II, IX, X and XI are found in hyaline cartilage, type IV in basement membrane and type VII in anchoring structures at junctions between epithelium and mesenchyme. There are several classes of collagen genes, based on their protein structures, and abnormalities of these may lead to specific diseases (see p. 602).

Elastin

Elastin is an insoluble protein polymer and is the main component of elastic fibres. Tropoelastin, its precursor, is synthesized by vascular smooth muscle cells and skin fibroblasts. Cross-linkages with desmosine and iso-desmosine are specific to elastin fibres.

Glycoproteins

Fibronectin is the major non-collagenous glycoprotein in the extracellular matrix. Its molecule contains a number of functional domains, or cell recognition sites that bind ligands and are involved in cellular adhesion. A peptide sequence (*Arg–Gly–Asp*), which mimics some of the functions of fibronectin, is also found in other adhesion proteins (e.g. vitronectin, laminin and collagen type VI). Fibronectin plays a major role in tissue remodelling. Its production is stimulated by interferon-gamma and by transforming growth factor-beta and inhibited by tumour necrosis factor and interleukin-1.

Proteoglycans

These proteins contain glycosaminoglycan (GAG) side-chains and are of variable form and size. Many have been identified at different sites in connective tissue, e.g. aggrecan, biglycan, fibromodulin, decorin (in extracellular matrix), syndecan, CD44, fibroglycan (on cell surfaces), cerebroglycan (in brain), serglycan (in intracellular tissues) and perglycan (in basement membranes). Their function is to bind extracellular matrix together, retain soluble molecules in the matrix and assist with cell binding. Abnormalities of any of these structures may lead to periarticular or articular symptoms and/or predispose to the development of arthritis.

Joint sensation

The ligaments, periosteum, synovial tissue and capsule of the joint are richly supplied by blood vessels and nerves. Pain usually derives from inflammation of these sites because the synovial membrane is relatively insensitive.

CLINICAL APPROACH TO THE PATIENT

TAKING A MUSCULOSKELETAL HISTORY

The following questions are helpful in assessing the problem and making a diagnosis. A history, taken carefully, can often lead to a diagnosis. Pattern recognition is the key to accurate diagnosis in rheumatic diseases.

Pain

- *Where is it? Is it localized or generalized?* The pattern of joint involvement is a useful clue to the diagnosis (e.g. distal interphalangeal joints in osteoarthritis).
- *Is it arising from joints, the spine, muscles or bone?* Soft tissue lesions and inflamed joints are locally tender.
- *Could it be referred from another site?* Joint pain is localized but may radiate distally – shoulder to upper arm; hip to thigh and knee.
- *Is it constant, intermittent or episodic? How severe is it – aching or agonizing?* For example, the pain of gout, or of septic arthritis in a previously fit, non-immuno-compromised patient is agonizing. Joint pain lasting a day or so may indicate palindromic rheumatism, whilst longer bouts of a few days are typical of untreated gout or pseudogout. Constant pain, especially pain at night, may be due to an underlying malignancy.
- *Are there aggravating or precipitating factors?* For example:
  - Mechanical problems are made worse by activity and eased by rest.
  - Inflammatory joint and spine pain are worse after rest and improve with activity.
  - Trauma is a common cause of musculoskeletal pain.
- *Are there any associated neurological features?* Numbness, pins and needles and/or loss of power suggest 'nerve' pain. Consider carpal tunnel syndrome (see p. 539), a spinal problem such as disc prolapse (p. 542) or spondylosis (p. 541), or neurological disease. Nerve root pain, such as that due to a disc prolapse, reflects the anatomical distribution of the affected root.

Stiffness

- *Is it generalized or localized?* Spine or joint stiffness is common after injury.
- *Does it affect the limb girdles or periphery?*
- *Is it worse in the morning and relieved by activity?* Joints that are stiff for more than 15 minutes each morning are usually inflamed – think of rheumatoid arthritis (RA) (see p. 555) or another cause of inflammatory arthritis. Spinal stiffness and pain which is much worse in the morning may indicate ankylosing spondylitis (p. 564), especially in patients in their twenties or thirties. Shoulder and pelvic girdle stiffness and pain, which are worse in the morning in a patient over 55 years, may be polymyalgia rheumatica (p. 582).

Swelling

- *Is it of one joint, or of several?* Look for symmetry or asymmetry, and/or a peripheral or proximal pattern; these are important clues to the type of arthritis. Rheumatoid arthritis is typically polyarticular. An acute monarthritis may be due to trauma, gout (in a middle-aged male) or sepsis (fever or immunosuppression).
- *Is it constant or episodic?*
- *Are episodes of swelling short-lived, or longer?*
- *Is there associated inflammation (redness and warmth)?*

Gender

Gout (see p. 568), reactive arthritis (p. 566) and ankylosing spondylitis (p. 564) are more common in men. Rheumatoid arthritis and other autoimmune connective tissue diseases are more common in women.

Age

- *Is the person young, middle-aged or older?* Injury is common in young people but can occur at any age.
- *How old was the patient when the problem first started?* Osteoarthritis (see p. 550) and polymyalgia rheumatica (p. 582) rarely affect the under-fifties. Rheumatoid arthritis starts most commonly in women aged 20–50 years.

General health

- *Is there any associated ill-health or other worrying feature, such as weight loss or fever?* Systemic illness is a common feature of many rheumatic diseases. If there is weight loss and/or fever, think of autoimmune rheumatic disease, sepsis (joint infection may be due to septicaemia and is a medical emergency) or malignancy.
- *Are there other associated medical conditions that may be relevant?* Psoriasis (see p. 1331) or inflammatory bowel disease is associated with asymmetrical arthritis. Charcot's joints (p. 589) are seen in diabetics.

Medication

Could a drug be a cause? Diuretics may precipitate gout in men and older women. Hormone replacement therapy or the oral contraceptive pill may precipitate systemic lupus erythematosus (SLE) (p. 574). Steroids can cause avascular necrosis. Some drugs cause a lupus-like syndrome (p. 576).

Race

Is this relevant? Sickle cell disease causes joint pain in young black Africans, but osteoporosis (see p. 594) is uncommon in older black Africans.

Past history

Have there been any similar episodes or is this the first? Are there any clues from previous medical conditions? Gout is recurrent; the episodes settle without treatment in about 10 days. Acute episodes of palindromic rheumatism may predate the onset of rheumatoid arthritis (see p. 557).

Family history

Does anyone in the family have a similar problem or another related disorder? Osteoarthritis may be familial. Seronegative spondyloarthropathies (see p. 564) is seen in families with a history of arthritis, psoriasis, ankylosing spondylitis, iritis or inflammatory bowel disease. Autoimmunity has a familial tendency.

Occupational history

What job does the patient do? This can be a factor in soft tissue problems and osteoarthritis (e.g. in heavy labourers and dancers). Work-related problems are becoming more common and are complained of more.

Psychosocial history

■ *Has there been an injury for which a legal case for compensation is pending?*
■ *Has there been any recent major stress in family or working life? Could this be relevant?* Stress rarely causes rheumatic disease but may precipitate a flare-up of inflammatory arthritis. Stress also tends to reduce a person's ability to cope with pain or disability. Remember that the diagnosis of a chronic arthritis has a major influence on the lifestyle of patients and their families. The extent of disability should be noted.

Extent of disability

The World Health Organization describes the impact of disease on an individual in terms of:

■ *Impairment:* any loss or abnormality of psychological or anatomical structure or function
■ *Disability* (activity limitation): any restriction or lack of ability to perform an activity in the manner or within the range considered normal for a human being
■ *Handicap* (participation restriction): a disadvantage for an individual resulting from an impairment or disability that limits or prevents the fulfilment of a role that is normal for that individual.

The patient's own perception of limitation must be taken into account during assessment, as well as the impact of physical causes due to disease. Subjective and objective assessments must be made. Quality of life (QoL) involves physical and psychosocial factors. The aim of treatment is to reduce or cure physical and/or psychological disease and to reduce the impact of any impairment or disability on the individual. A variety of different standard questionnaires can be used to assess pain, disease impact and outcome (e.g. Health Assessment Questionnaire (HAQ), Arthritis Impact Measurement Scale (AIMS)).

EXAMINATION OF THE JOINTS

Always observe a patient, looking for disabilities, as he or she walks into the room and sits down. General and neurological examinations are often necessary. Guidelines for rapid examinations of the limbs and spine are shown in Practical box 10.1.

Examining an individual joint involves three stages – looking, feeling and moving:

■ *Appearance.* Look at it for swelling, rash or erythema, muscle wasting, deformity such as a distal bone

---

 Practical Box 10.1
Rapid examinations of the limb and spine

Rapid examination of the upper limbs
■ *Raise arms sideways to the ears (abduction). Reach behind neck and back.* Difficulties with these movements indicate a shoulder or rotator cuff problem.
■ *Hold the arms forward, with elbows straight and fingers apart, palm up and palm down.* Fixed flexion at the elbow indicates an elbow problem. Examine the hands for swelling, wasting and deformity.
■ *Place the hands in the 'prayer' position with the elbows apart.* Flexion deformities of the fingers may be due to arthritis, flexor tenosynovitis or skin disease. Painful restriction of the wrist limits the person's ability to move the elbows out with the hands held together.
■ *Make a tight fist.* Difficulty with this indicates a loss of flexion or grip. Grip strength can be measured.

Rapid examination of the lower limbs
■ *Ask the patient to walk* a short distance away from and towards you, and to stand still. Look for abnormal posture or stance.
■ *Ask the patient to stand on each leg.* Severe hip disease causes the pelvis on the non-weight-bearing side to sag (positive Trendelenburg test).
■ *Watch the patient stand and sit,* looking for hip and/or knee problems.
■ *Ask the patient to straighten and flex each knee.*
■ *Ask the patient to place each foot in turn on the opposite knee with the hip externally rotated.* This tests for painful restriction of hip or knee. Abnormal hips or knees must be examined lying.
■ *Move each ankle up and down.* Examine the ankle joint and tendons, medial arch and toes whilst standing.

Rapid examination of the spine
Stand behind the patient.

■ *Ask the patient to (a) bend forwards to touch the toes with straight knees, (b) extend backwards, (c) flex sideways, and (d) look over each shoulder, flexing and extending and side-flexing the neck.* Observe abnormal spinal curves – scoliosis (lateral curve), kyphosis (forward bending) or lordosis (backward bending). A cervical and lumbar lordosis and a thoracic kyphosis are normal. Muscle spasm is worse whilst standing and bending. Leg length inequality leads to a scoliosis which decreases on sitting or lying (the lengths are measured lying).
■ *Ask the patient to lie supine.* Examine any restriction of straight-leg raising (see disc prolapse, p. 542).
■ *Ask the patient to lie prone.* Examine for anterior thigh pain during a femoral stretch test (flexing knee whilst prone), which indicates a high lumbar disc problem.
■ *Palpate* the spine and buttocks for tender areas.

---

displaced laterally as in knock knees (genu valgus) or bowed legs (genu varus), fixed flexion or hyperextension, loss of normal range and lack of fluidity of movement, and any pain caused by movement.
■ *Feel* it for tenderness, warmth (indicates inflammation) and swelling which may be due to fluid, soft tissue or

bone. Common descriptors are 'fluctuant' (fluid), 'firm' or 'boggy' (swelling of the synovium), and 'hard' (bony).

- *Movement.* Move it to assess the passive range of movement (e.g. flexion, extension, abduction, adduction and rotation), any instability, or the production of pain and crepitus (grating) seen with cartilage damage. The normal range varies between individuals. Comparing right with left and asking the patient about any change in range help to assess whether the endpoints are normal or not. A screening examination of the loco-motor system, known by the acronym GALS (global assessment of the locomotor system) has been devised.

X-ray of the joint often forms an integral part of the examination.

INVESTIGATIONS

Investigations are unnecessary in many of the common regional musculoskeletal problems and osteoarthritis (OA); the diagnosis is clear from the history and examination findings. Tests help to exclude another condition and to reassure the patient or their primary care physician.

Useful blood screening tests

- **Full blood count**
  Haemoglobin. Normochromic, normocytic anaemia occurs in chronic inflammatory and autoimmune diseases. Hypochromic, microcytic anaemia indicates iron deficiency, often due to non-steroidal anti-inflammatory drug (NSAID) induced gastrointestinal bleeding.
  White cell count. Neutrophilia is seen in bacterial infection (e.g. septic arthritis). It also occurs with corticosteroid treatment. Lymphopenia occurs with viral illnesses or active systemic lupus erythematosus (SLE). Neutropenia may reflect drug-induced bone marrow suppression. Eosinophilia is seen in the Churg–Strauss syndrome (p. 938).
  Platelets. Thrombocythaemia occurs with chronic inflammation. Thrombocytopenia is seen in drug-induced bone marrow suppression.
- **Erythrocyte sedimentation rate (ESR) and C-reactive protein (CRP).** An increase reflects inflammation. Plasma viscosity is also raised in inflammatory disease and measured in some laboratories in place of the sedimentation rate.
- **Bone and liver biochemistry.** A raised serum alkaline phosphatase may indicate liver or bone disease. A rise in liver enzymes is seen with drug-induced toxicity. For other investigations of bone, see page 593.

Other blood and urine tests

- *Protein electrophoretic strip and urinary Bence Jones protein* – to exclude myeloma as a cause of a raised ESR.
- *Serum uric acid* – for gout.
- *Antistreptolysin-O titre* – in rheumatic fever.

Serum autoantibody studies

Rheumatoid factors (RFs)

IgM rheumatoid factors are detected by agglutination tests using IgG-coated latex particles (the Rose–Waaler test) or sensitized sheep red cells (sheep cell agglutination test or SCAT). They are antibodies (usually IgM, but occasionally IgG or IgA) against the Fc portion of IgG and are detected in 70% of patients with rheumatoid arthritis (RA), but are not diagnostic. A high titre in early RA indicates a poor prognosis. Positive titres occasionally predate the onset of RA. Titres may fluctuate. RFs are detected in many autoimmune rheumatic disorders (e.g. SLE), in chronic infections, and in asymptomatic older people (Table 10.1).

Citrullinated cyclic peptide (CCP) antibodies

These are measured by an ELISA technique and have a high specificity for RA (90% with a sensitivity of 60%). They are helpful in early disease to distinguish it from acute transient synovitis (see Box 10.7, p. 557).

Antinuclear antibodies (ANAs)

These are detected by indirect immunofluorescent staining of fresh-frozen sections of rat liver or kidney or Hep-2 cell lines. Different patterns reflect a variety of antigenic specificities that occur with different clinical pictures (for example, anti-DNA/histone (homogeneous) antibodies suggest active SLE; anticentromere antibodies suggest systemic sclerosis) and are detected in many autoimmune diseases. ANA is used as a screening test for SLE, but low titres occur in RA and chronic infections and in normal individuals, especially the elderly (Table 10.2). Hep-2 staining patterns are a guide to likely antigenic specificity, and some such as anticentromere are un-equivocal. Antinucleolar staining patterns are associated with several hallmarks of systemic sclerosis reactivities (see below).

Table 10.1 Conditions in which rheumatoid factor is found in the serum

Autoimmune rheumatic diseases	RF (IgM) %
Rheumatoid arthritis	70
Systemic lupus erythematosus	25
Sjögren's syndrome	90
Systemic sclerosis	30
Polymyositis/dermatomyositis	50
Juvenile idiopathic arthritis	Variable

Viral infections	Hyperglobinaemias
Hepatitis	Chronic liver disease
Infectious mononucleosis	Sarcoidosis
	Cryoglobulinaemia

Chronic infections	Normal population
Tuberculosis	Elderly
Leprosy	Relatives of patients
Infective endocarditis	with RA
Syphilis	

Table 10.2 Conditions in which serum antinuclear antibodies (%) are found	
Systemic lupus erythematosus	95
Systemic sclerosis	70
Sjögren's syndrome	80
Polymyositis and dermatomyositis	40
Rheumatoid arthritis	30
Juvenile idiopathic arthritis	Variable
Other diseases	
Autoimmune hepatitis	100
Drug-induced lupus	> 95
Myasthenia gravis	50
Fibrosing alveolitis	30
Diabetes mellitus	25
Infectious mononucleosis	5–10
Normal population	8

Anti-double-stranded-DNA (dsDNA) antibodies

These are usually detected by a precipitation test (Farr assay), by ELISA, or by an immunofluorescent test using *Crithidia luciliae* (which contains double-stranded DNA). They are diagnostic of active SLE but may be negative in mild or inactive disease. High titres of IgG anti-dsDNA indicate a poor prognosis and are specific to SLE. Anti-single-stranded DNA antibodies are non-specific.

Anti-extractable nuclear antigen (ENA) antibodies

These produce a speckled ANA fluorescent pattern and can be distinguished by ELISA:

- anti-Ro (SS-A) – SLE + Sjögren's syndrome
- anti-La (SS-B) – Sjögren's syndrome
- anti-Sm – SLE
- anti-U1-RNP – a range of diseases, including SLE, overlap syndrome.

Anti Jo-1 antibodies

These antibodies to the enzyme histidyl tRNA synthase block its amino-acylation and are found in polymyositis and dermatomyositis.

Anti-topoisomerase 1 (ScL-70) antibodies

These are seen in systemic sclerosis.

Anti-neutrophil cytoplasmic antibodies (ANCAs) (see p. 634)

These are detected on fixed human neutrophils. Two major ANCA patterns are recognized:

- proteinase 3 (PR3-ANCA), formerly called cytoplasmic or cANCA
- myeloperoxidase (MPO-ANCA), formerly called perinuclear or pANCA.

PR3-ANCA is present in up to 90% of serum from patients with Wegener's granulomatosis. MPO-ANCA is found in up to 60% of other vasculitides, such as microscopic polyarteritis (polyangiitis) and Churg–Strauss syndrome. An MPO-ANCA is found in inflam-matory bowel disease and rheumatic disease, which is not associated with vasculitis.

Antiphospholipid antibodies

These are detected in the antiphospholipid syndrome and SLE (p. 577).

The principal autoantigen is β_2-glycoprotein 1 (apolipoprotein H), which binds to cardiolipin and other anionic phospholipids. Anticardiolipin antibody and β_2-glycoprotein are measured by ELISA. The lupus anticoagulants are antibodies against β_2-glycoprotein 1 as well as prothrombin and annexin. They are detected by coagulation tests, such as prolongation of the activated partial thromboplastin time (APTT), as some of these antibodies interfere with phospholipid-dependent clotting systems in vitro.

Anti-RNA polymerase antibodies I, II and III

I and III are present in systemic sclerosis (see p. 579).

Immune complexes

Immune complexes are infrequently measured, largely because of variability between assays and difficulty in interpreting their meaning. Assays based on the poly-ethylene glycol precipitation method (PEG) or C1q binding are available commercially.

Complement

Low complement levels indicate consumption and suggest an active disease process in SLE.

Joint aspiration (Practical box 10.2)

Examination of joint (or bursa) fluid is used mainly to diagnose septic, reactive or crystal arthritis. The nature of the fluid is an indicator of the level of inflammation. Clear

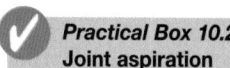
Practical Box 10.2
Joint aspiration

This is a sterile procedure which should be carried out in a clean environment
Explain the procedure to the patient; obtain consent

1. Decide on the site to insert the needle and mark it.
2. Clean the skin and your hands scrupulously; remove rings and wristwatch. Gloves are not obligatory, but many prefer to use them.
3. Draw up local anaesthetic (and corticosteroid if it is being used) and then use a new needle.
4. Warn the patient, insert the needle, injecting local anaesthetic as it advances and, if a joint effusion is suspected, attempt to aspirate as you advance it.
5. If fluid is obtained, change syringes and aspirate fully.
6. Examine the fluid in the syringe and decide whether or not to proceed with a corticosteroid injection.
7. Cover the injection site and advise the patient to rest the affected area for a few days. Warn the patient that the pain may increase initially but to report urgently if this persists beyond a few days, if the swelling worsens, or if they become febrile, since this might indicate an infected joint.

fluid indicates little inflammation in the joint, whereas translucent or opaque fluid indicates increasing cellularity and underlying inflammation. Purulent fluid is seen in septic arthritis, but crystal arthritis and reactive arthritis may also produce a highly cellular effusion. The procedure is often undertaken in combination with injection of a corticosteroid. Aspiration alone is therapeutic in crystal arthritis.

Diagnostic imaging and visualization

- **X-rays** can be diagnostic in certain conditions (e.g. rheumatoid arthritis), but remember the following points:
  - **(a)** In acute low back pain, X-rays are indicated only if the pain is persistent, recurrent, associated with neurological symptoms or signs, or worse at night. They should also be performed if the pain is associated with such symptoms as fever or weight loss, which might indicate a more sinister underlying pathology.
  - **(b)** Radiological changes are common in older people and may not indicate symptomatic osteoarthritis or spondylosis.
  - **(c)** X-rays are of little diagnostic value in early inflammatory arthritis but are useful as a baseline from which to judge later change.
- **Ultrasound (US)** is particularly useful for periarticular structures, soft tissue swellings and tendons. It is increasingly used to examine the shoulder and other structures during movement. This visualizes shoulder impingement syndrome (see p. 538). US can be used to guide local injections. Quantitative ultrasound of the heel may prove a convenient and portable means of assessing bone density.
- **Magnetic resonance imaging (MRI)** shows bone changes and intra-articular structures in striking detail. It is more sensitive than X-rays in the early detection of articular disease. It is the investigation of choice for most spinal disorders but is inappropriate in uncomplicated mechanical low back pain. Gadolinium injection enhances inflamed tissue. MRI can also detect muscle changes, e.g. myositis.
- **Computerized axial tomography (CT)** is useful for detecting changes in calcified structures.
- **Bone scintigraphy** utilizes radionuclides, usually ^{99m}Tc, and detects abnormal bone turnover and blood circulation and, although non-specific, helps in detecting areas of inflammation, infection or malignancy. It is best used in combination with other anatomical imaging techniques.
- **DXA scanning** uses very low doses of X-irradiation to measure bone density and is used in the screening and monitoring of osteoporosis.
- **Positron emission tomography (PET)** scanning uses radionuclides which decay by emission of positrons. Fluorine-18 in deoxyglucose indicates areas of increased glucose metabolism, locates tumours, demonstrates large vessel vasculitis, e.g. Takayasu's arteritis (see p. 869). PET scans are combined with CT or MRI to improve anatomical details.

- **Arthroscopy** is a direct means of visualizing a joint, particularly the knee or shoulder. Biopsies can be taken, surgery performed in certain conditions (e.g. repair or trimming of meniscal tears), and loose bodies removed.

Examination of synovial fluid

This is described in Box 10.1.

FURTHER READING

Bellamy N (2003) Principles of outcome assessment. In: Hochberg MC, Silman AJ, Smolen JS et al. (eds) *Rheumatology*, 3rd edn. London: Mosby, Vol. 1, Section 1, Ch. 4.

Doherty M, Dacre J, Dieppe P, Snaith M (1992) The 'GALS' locomotor screen. *Annals of the Rheumatic Diseases* **51**: 1165–1169.

Isenberg D, Renton, P (2003) *Imaging in Rheumatology*. Oxford University Press.

Morrow J, Nelson L, Watts R, Isenberg D (1999) *Autoimmune Rheumatic Diseases*, 2nd edn. Oxford: Oxford Medical Publications.

COMMON REGIONAL MUSCULOSKELETAL PROBLEMS (Fig.10.2)

Analgesic and anti-inflammatory drugs used for treatment of musculoskeletal problems are discussed on page 549.

ⓘ Box 10.1 Examination of synovial fluid

The fluid can be examined directly in a clear syringe or sterile pot. The characteristics of synovial fluid show a trend from clear to purulent which indicates roughly the type of arthritis.

Colour	Diagnosis	WCC per mm³
Clear, yellow and viscous	OA	< 3000
Translucent and thin	RA	
Very cloudy	Seronegative arthritis Reiter's disease Crystal arthritis	3000–40 000
Purulent	Sepsis	750 000

Polarized light microscopy with a red filter needs to be undertaken by an expert:

- Gout – negatively birefringent, needle-shaped crystals of sodium urate
- Pyrophosphate arthropathy (pseudogout) – rhomboidal, weakly positively birefringent crystals of calcium pyrophosphate.

Gram staining is essential if septic arthritis is suspected and may identify the organism immediately. Joint fluid should be cultured and antibiotic sensitivities requested.

RA, rheumatoid arthritis; OA, osteoarthritis

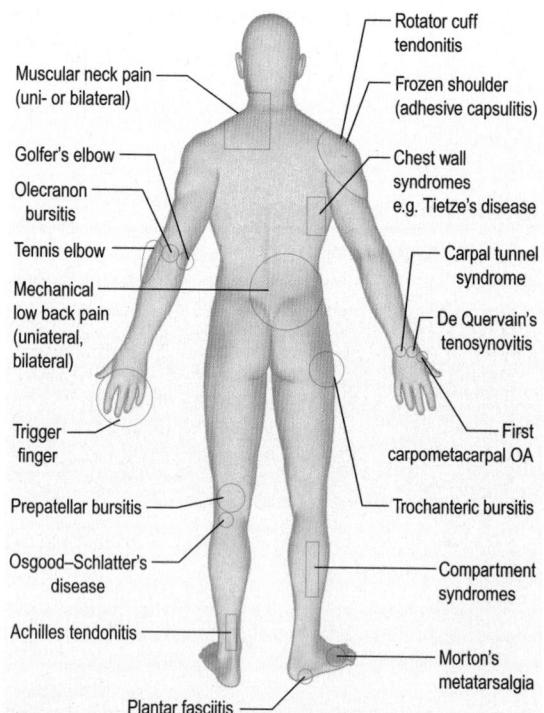

Muscular neck pain (uni- or bilateral)

Golfer's elbow

Olecranon bursitis

Tennis elbow

Mechanical low back pain (uniateral, bilateral)

Trigger finger

Prepatellar bursitis

Osgood–Schlatter's disease

Achilles tendonitis

Plantar fasciitis

Rotator cuff tendonitis

Frozen shoulder (adhesive capsulitis)

Chest wall syndromes e.g. Tietze's disease

Carpal tunnel syndrome

De Quervain's tenosynovitis

First carpometacarpal OA

Trochanteric bursitis

Compartment syndromes

Morton's metatarsalgia

Fig. 10.2 Common regional musculoskeletal problems.

Table 10.3 Pain in the neck and shoulder

Trauma (for example, a fall)
Mechanical or muscular neck pain
Whiplash injury
Disc prolapse – nerve root entrapment (p. 1265)
Ankylosing spondylitis
Shoulder lesions:
    Rotator cuff tendonitis
    Calcific tendonitis or bursitis
    Impingement syndrome or rotator cuff tear
    Adhesive capsulitis (true 'frozen' shoulder)
    Inflammatory arthritis or osteoarthritis
Polymyalgia rheumatica
Fibromyalgia
Chronic (work-related) upper limb pain syndrome
Tumour

musculature (shoulder girdle pain). Pain often radiates upwards to the occiput but rarely laterally to the tip of the shoulder. It is commonly associated with unilateral or bilateral tension headaches; pain radiating over the head to the temple and eye, described as like a pressure or tight band. These features are also seen in fibromyalgia (see p. 547).

Treatment

Patients are given short courses of analgesic therapy along with reassurance and explanation. Physiotherapists can help to relieve spasm and pain, teach exercises and relaxation techniques, and improve posture. An occupational therapist can advise about the ergonomics of the workplace if the problem is work-related (see p. 548).

PAIN IN THE NECK AND SHOULDER
(Table 10.3)

Mechanical or muscular neck pain (shoulder girdle pain)

Unilateral or bilateral muscular-pattern neck pain is common and usually self-limiting. It can follow injury, falling asleep in an awkward position, or prolonged keyboard working. Chronic burning neck pain occurs because of muscle tension from anxiety and stress.

Spondylosis (see p. 1264) seen on X-ray increases after the age of 40 years, but it is not always causal. Spondylosis can, however, cause stiffness and increases the risk of mechanical or muscular neck pain. Muscle spasm can be palpable, is tender and may lead to abnormal neck posture (e.g. acute torticollis). Muscular-pattern neck pain is not localized but affects the trapezius muscle, the C7 spinous process and the paracervical

Nerve root entrapment

This is caused by an acute cervical disc prolapse or pressure on the root from spondylotic osteophytes narrowing the root canal.

Acute cervical disc prolapse presents with unilateral pain in the neck, radiating to the interscapular and shoulder regions. This diffuse, aching dural pain is followed by sharp, electric shock-like pain down the arm, in a nerve root distribution, often with pins and needles, numbness, weakness and loss of reflexes (see Table 10.4).

Cervical spondylosis occurs in the older patient with posterior osteophytes compressing the nerve root and causing root pain (see Fig. 21.42, p. 1265), commonly at

Table 10.4 Cervical nerve root entrapment – symptoms and signs

Nerve root	Sensory changes	Reflex loss	Weakness
C5	Lateral arm	Biceps	Shoulder abduction
			Elbow flexion
C6	Lateral forearm	Biceps	Elbow flexion
	Thumb and index finger	Supinator	Wrist extension
C7	Middle finger	Triceps	Elbow extension
C8	Medial forearm	None	Finger flexion
	Little and ring fingers		
T1	Medial upper arm	None	Finger ab- and adduction

Fig. 10.3 **MRI of cervical spine**, showing a large central disc prolapse impinging on the spinal cord (arrow) at the C6/7 level.

C5/C6 or C6/C7; it is seen on oblique radiographs of the neck. An MRI scan shows facet joint OA and any associated disc prolapse clearly.

Treatment

A support collar, rest, analgesia and sedation are used as necessary. Patients should be advised not to carry heavy items. It usually recovers in 6–12 weeks. MRI is the investigation of choice if surgery is being considered or the diagnosis is uncertain (Fig. 10.3). A cervical root block administered under direct vision by an experienced pain specialist may relieve pain while the disc recovers. Neurosurgical referral is essential if the pain persists or if the neurological signs of weakness or numbness are severe or bilateral. Bilateral root pain is a neurosurgical emergency because a central disc prolapse may compress the cervical spinal cord.

Whiplash injury

Whiplash injury results from acceleration–deceleration forces applied to the neck, usually in a road traffic accident when the car of a person wearing a seat belt is struck from behind. Delayed recovery depends in part upon the severity of the initial injury. A simple decision plan based on clinical criteria helps to distinguish those most at risk and who warrant radiography. There is a low probability of serious bony injury if there is no midline cervical tenderness, no focal neurological deficit, normal alertness, no intoxication and no painful distracting injury. CT scans are reserved for those with bony injury. MRI scans occasionally show severe soft tissue injury. Whiplash injuries commonly lead to litigation.

Whiplash injury is a common cause of chronic neck pain, although most people recover within a few weeks or months. The pattern of chronic neck pain is often complex, involving pain in the neck, shoulder and arm. Headache, dizziness, and loss of memory and poor concentration sometimes accompany this. The subjective nature of these symptoms has led to controversy about their cause. The problem is more commonly seen in industrialized countries. It has often been suggested that the syndrome is caused in part by the prospect of financial compensation. This may not be wholly conscious and may be contributed to in part by the conflictive nature of the compensation process. There appears to be a direct relationship between poor prognosis and potential for compensation – elimination of compensation for pain and suffering due to this type of injury may lead to an improved prognosis.

Treatment is with reassurance (as the patient may be very anxious), analgesia, a short-term collar and physiotherapy. Pain may take a few weeks or months to settle and the patient should be warned of this.

FURTHER READING

Malleson A (2002) *Whiplash and Other Useful Illnesses.* Montreal: McGill–Queens University Press.

Steill IG, Clement CM, McKnight RD et al. (2003). The Canadian C-spine Risk versus the NEXUS Low-Risk Criteria in patients with trauma. *New England Journal of Medicine* **349**: 2510–2518.

PAIN IN THE SHOULDER

The shoulder is a shallow joint with a large range of movement. The humeral head is held in place by the rotator cuff (Fig. 10.4) which is part of the joint capsule. It comprises the tendons of infraspinatus and teres minor posteriorly, supraspinatus superiorly and teres major and subscapularis anteriorly. The rotator cuff (particularly

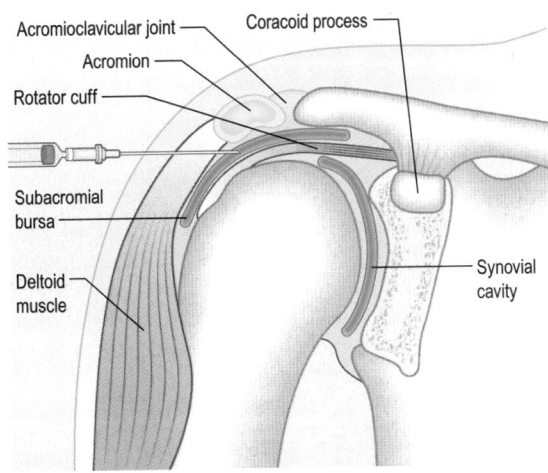

Fig. 10.4 **The shoulder region**, showing site of injection and subacromial space.

> ⓘ **Box 10.2** Differential diagnosis of 'shoulder' pain
>
> - Rotator cuff tendonitis pain is worse at night and radiates to the upper arm.
> - Painful shoulders produce secondary muscular neck pain.
> - Muscular neck pain (also known as shoulder girdle pain) does not radiate to the upper arm.
> - Cervical nerve root pain is usually associated with pins and needles or neurological signs in the arm.

supraspinatus) prevents the humeral head blocking against the acromion during abduction; the deltoid pulls up and the supraspinatus pulls in to produce a turning moment. This permits the greater tuberosity to glide under the acromion without impingement.

Pain in the shoulder can sometimes be due to problems in the neck. The differential diagnosis of this is shown in Box 10.2. Although the term 'frozen shoulder' is commonly used for any painful stiff shoulder, true frozen shoulder (adhesive capsulitis) is uncommon – see below. A painful, stiff shoulder can result from rotator cuff lesions and is also seen following hemiplegia, chest or breast surgery or myocardial infarction. Painful shoulders may also be the initial presentation of RA, less commonly a seronegative spondyloarthropathy, and of polymyalgia rheumatica in the elderly.

Rotator cuff (supraspinatus) tendonitis

This is a common cause of painful restriction of the shoulder at all ages. It follows trauma in 30% of cases and is bilateral in under 5%. The pain radiates to the upper arm and is made worse by arm abduction and elevation, which are often limited. The pain is often worse during the middle of the range of abduction, reducing as the arm is raised fully and the painful part of the tendon rotates through to the proximal side of the acromion – a so-called painful arc syndrome. When examined from behind, the scapula rotates earlier during elevation. Passive elevation reduces impingement and is less painful. Severe pain virtually immobilizes the joint, although some rotation is retained (cf. adhesive capsulitis). There is also painful spasm of the trapezius. X-rays are necessary only when rotator cuff tendonitis is persistent or the diagnosis is uncertain.

Treatment

Analgesics or NSAIDs may suffice, but severe pain responds to an injection of corticosteroid (Fig. 10.4). Patients should be warned that 10% will develop worse pain for 24–48 hours after injection. Seventy per cent improve over 5–20 days and mobilize the joint themselves. Physiotherapy helps persistent stiffness but further injections may be needed.

Calcific tendonitis and bursitis

Calcium pyrophosphate deposits in the tendon are visible on X-ray, but they are not always symptomatic. The pathogenesis is unclear, although the part of the tendon affected is likely to be affected by relative ischaemia. The deposit is usually just proximal to the greater tuberosity. It may lead to acute or chronic recurrent shoulder pain and restriction of movement. A local corticosteroid injection may relieve the pain. The calcification may persist or resolve. Aspiration of the deposit under X-ray or ultrasound control may be required for persistent pain. Rarely, arthroscopic removal is necessary.

Shedding of crystals into the subacromial bursa causes severe pain and shoulder restriction. The shoulder feels hot and is swollen, and an X-ray will show a diffuse opacity in the bursa. The differential diagnosis of calcific bursitis is gout, pseudogout or septic arthritis.

Aspiration and injection with corticosteroid can help.

Torn rotator cuff

This is caused by trauma in the young but also occurs spontaneously in the elderly and in rheumatoid arthritis (RA). It prevents active abduction of the arm, but patients learn to initiate elevation using the unaffected arm. Once elevated, the arm can be held in place by the deltoid muscle. In younger people, the tear is repaired surgically but this is rarely possible in the elderly or in RA. Repeated trauma of the cuff between humerus and acromion/acromioclavicular joint causes osteophyte and cyst formation.

Shoulder impingement syndrome causes pain and crepitus on abduction and rotation. Some patients require arthroscopic surgery.

Adhesive capsulitis (true 'frozen' shoulder)

This is uncommon. Severe shoulder pain is associated with complete loss of all shoulder movements, including rotation. High doses of NSAIDs and intra-articular injections of corticosteroids are helpful. Once the pain settles, a manipulation under anaesthetic is advisable. When untreated, it recovers in 1–2 years.

Ultrasound examination can distinguish the above shoulder problems accurately and allows a guided corticosteroid injection.

FURTHER READING
Smidt N, Green S (2003) Is the diagnosis important for the treatment of patients with shoulder pain? *Lancet* **362**: 1867–1868.

PAIN IN THE ELBOW

Pain in the elbow can be due to epicondylitis, inflammatory arthritis or occasionally osteoarthritis.

Epicondylitis

Two common sites where the insertions of tendons into bone become inflamed (*enthesitis*) are the insertions of the

Fig. 10.5 Injection for tennis elbow.

wrist extensor tendon into the lateral epicondyle ('tennis elbow') and the wrist flexor tendon into the medial epicondyle ('golfer's elbow'). Both are usually unrelated to either sporting activity.

There is local tenderness. Pain radiates into the forearm on using the affected muscles – typically, holding a heavy bag in tennis elbow or carrying a tray in golfer's elbow. Pain at rest also occurs.

Treatment

Advise rest and arrange review by a physiotherapist. A local injection of corticosteroid at the point of maximum tenderness is helpful when the pain is severe (Fig. 10.5). Avoid the ulnar nerve when injecting golfer's elbow. Both conditions settle spontaneously eventually, but occasionally become disabling.

PAIN IN THE HAND AND WRIST (Table 10.5)

Hand pain is commonly caused by injury or repetitive work-related use. When associated with pins and needles or numbness it suggests a neurological cause arising at the wrist, elbow or neck. Pain and stiffness that are worse in the morning are due to tenosynovitis or inflammatory arthritis. The distribution of hand pain often indicates the diagnosis.

Table 10.5 Pain in the hand and wrist – causes

All ages	Older patients
Trauma/fractures	Nodal OA:
Tenosynovitis:	DIPs (Heberden's nodes)
Flexor with/without	PIPs (Bouchard's nodes)
triggering	First carpometacarpal
Dorsal	joint
De Quervain's	Trauma – scaphoid fracture
Carpal tunnel syndrome	Pseudogout
Ganglion	Gout:
Inflammatory arthritis	Acute
Raynaud's syndrome (p. 869)	Tophaceous
Chronic regional pain	
syndrome type I (p. 548)	

DIPs, PIPs, distal and proximal interphalangeal joints

Tenosynovitis

The finger flexor tendons run through a series of synovial sheaths and under loops which hold them in place. Inflammation occurs with repeated or unaccustomed use, or in inflammatory arthritis when the thickened sheaths are often palpable.

Flexor tenosynovitis causes finger pain when gripping and stiffness of the fingers in the morning. Occasionally a tendon causes a trigger finger, when the finger remains flexed after gripping and has to be pulled straight. A tendon nodule is palpable, usually in the distal palm.

Dorsal tenosynovitis is less common except in rheumatoid arthritis. The swelling is on the back of the hand and wrist.

De Quervain's tenosynovitis causes pain and swelling around the radial styloid where the abductor pollicis longus tendon is held in place by a retaining band. There is local tenderness, and the pain at the styloid is worsened by flexing the thumb into the palm.

Treatment

Therapeutic ultrasound helps some people. Usually corticosteroid is injected alongside the tendon under low pressure (not into the tendon itself). Occasionally surgery is needed.

Other conditions causing pain

Carpal tunnel syndrome

This is due to thickened tendons or synovitis in the carpal tunnel and the causes are discussed on page 1260. The history is usually typical and diagnostic with the patient waking with numbness, tingling and pain in a median nerve distribution. The pain radiates to the forearm. The fingers feel swollen but usually are not. Wasting of the abductor pollicis brevis develops with sensory loss in the palm and radial three and a half fingers. Tinel's sign may be positive, i.e. reproduction of the pain on tapping the nerve in the carpal tunnel.

Treatment is with a splint to hold the wrist in dorsiflexion overnight. This relieves the symptoms and is diagnostic; used nightly for several weeks it may produce full recovery. If it does not, a corticosteroid injection into the carpal tunnel helps in about 70% of cases, although it may recur. Persistent symptoms or nerve damage requires nerve conduction studies and surgical decompression of the carpal tunnel.

Inflammatory arthritis

This may present with pain, swelling and stiffness of the hands. In RA the wrists, proximal interphalangeal (PIP) joints and metacarpophalangeal (MCP) joints are affected symmetrically. In psoriatic arthritis and Reiter's disease a finger may be swollen (dactylitis) or the distal interphalangeal (DIP) joints are affected asymmetrically.

Nodal osteoarthritis

This affects the DIP and less commonly PIP joints, which are initially swollen and red. The inflammation and pain settle but bony swellings remain. There is often a strong family history and it rarely presents before 50 years of age. Reassurance and local treatment are all that is needed.

First carpometacarpal osteoarthritis

This causes pain at the base of the thumb when gripping, or painless stiffness at the base of the thumb.

Scaphoid fractures

These cause pain in the anatomical snuffbox. They may not be seen immediately on X-ray. Untreated scaphoid fractures eventually cause pain because of failed union.

Ganglion

A ganglion is a jelly-filled, often painless swelling caused by a partial tear of the joint capsule. The wrist is a common site. Treatment is not essential as many resolve or cause little trouble. They rarely respond to injection, and surgical excision is possibly the best option.

Dupuytren's contracture

This is a painless, palpable fibrosis of the palmar aponeurosis, with fibroblasts invading the dermis. It causes puckering of the skin and gradual flexion of the affected fingers, usually the ring and little fingers. It is more common in males, Caucasians, in diabetes mellitus and in those who abuse alcohol. It is associated with Peyronie's disease of the penis – a painful inflammatory disorder of the corpora cavernosa, leading eventually to painless fibrosis and angulation of the penis during erection. Plastic surgical release of the contracture is restricted to those with severe deformity of the fingers.

PAIN IN THE LOWER BACK

Low back pain is a common symptom. It is often traumatic and work-related, although lifting apparatus and other mechanical devices are used to avoid it. Episodes are generally short-lived and self-limiting, and patients attend a physiotherapist or osteopath more often than a doctor. Chronic back pain is the cause of 14% of long-term disability in the UK. The causes are listed in Table 10.6, and the management of back pain is summarized in Box 10.3.

Investigations

- **Spinal X-rays** are required only if the pain is associated with certain 'red flag' symptoms or signs, which indicate a high risk of more serious underlying problems:
  - (a) starts before the age of 20 or after 50 years
  - (b) is persistent and a serious cause is suspected
  - (c) is worse at night or in the morning, when an inflammatory arthritis (e.g. ankylosing spondylitis), infection or a spinal tumour may be the cause
  - (d) is associated with a systemic illness, fever or weight loss
  - (e) is associated with neurological symptoms or signs.

Table 10.6 **Pain in the back (lumbar region) – causes**

Mechanical
Trauma
Muscular and ligamentous pain
Fibrositic nodulosis
Postural back pain (sway back)
Lumbar spondylosis
Facet joint syndrome
Lumbar disc prolapse
Spinal and root canal stenosis
Spondylolisthesis
Disseminated idiopathic skeletal hyperostosis (DISH)
Fibromyalgia (see p. 547)

Inflammatory
Infective lesions of the spine
Ankylosing spondylitis/sacroiliitis (see p. 564)

Metabolic
Osteoporotic spinal fractures (see p. 595)
Osteomalacia (see p. 600)
Paget's disease (see p. 599)

Neoplastic (see p. 588)
Metastases
Multiple myeloma
Primary tumours of bone
Referred pain

> ### *i* Box 10.3 Management of back pain
>
> - Most back pain presenting to a primary care physician needs no investigation.
> - Pain between ages 20 and 55 years is likely to be mechanical and is managed with analgesia, brief rest and physiotherapy.
> - Patients should stay active within the limits of their pain.
> - Early treatment of the acute episode, advice and exercise programmes reduce long-term problems and prevent chronic pain syndromes.
> - Physical manipulation of uncomplicated back pain produces short-term relief and enjoys high patient satisfaction ratings.
> - Psychological and social factors may influence the time of presentation.
> - Appropriate early management reduces long-term disability.

- **MRI** is preferable to **CT** scanning when neurological signs and symptoms are present.
- **Bone scans** are useful in infective and malignant lesions but are also positive in degenerative lesions.
- **Full blood count, ESR and biochemical tests** are required only when the pain is likely to be due to malignancy, infection or a metabolic cause.

Mechanical low back pain

Mechanical low back pain starts suddenly, may be recurrent and is helped by rest. Mechanical back pain is often precipitated by an injury and may be unilateral or bilateral. It is usually short-lived.

Examination

The back is stiff and a scoliosis may be present when the patient is standing. Muscular spasm is visible and palpable and causes local pain and tenderness. It lessens when sitting or lying. Patients with spondylosis on X-ray probably have an increased risk of developing mechanical back pain but changes are often absent in the young and may be coincidental in the elderly. Pain relief and physiotherapy are helpful. The patient needs to be re-educated in lifting and shown exercises to prevent recurrent attacks of chronic pain. Once a patient has presented to a general practitioner with low back pain, although the episode itself is usually self-limiting, there is a significantly increased risk of further back pain episodes. Risk factors for recurrent back pain include female sex, increasing age, pre-existing chronic wide-spread pain (fibromyalgia) and such psychosocial factors as high levels of psychological distress, poor self-rated health and dissatisfaction with employment. Chronic low back pain is a major cause of disability and time off work and is reduced by appropriate early management.

Spinal movement occurs at the disc and the posterior facet joints, and stability is normally achieved by a complex mechanism of spinal ligaments and muscles. Any of these structures may be a source of pain. An exact anatomical diagnosis is difficult, but some typical syndromes are recognized (see below). They are often associated with radiological spondylosis (see p. 1265).

Postural back pain develops in individuals who sit in poorly designed, unsupportive chairs.

Fibrositic nodulosis

This causes unilateral or bilateral low back pain, radiating to the buttock and upper posterior thigh. There are tender nodules in the upper buttock and along the iliac crest. Such nodules are relevant only if they are tender and associated with pain. They are probably traumatic. Local, intralesional corticosteroid injections help.

Postural back pain and sway back of pregnancy

Low back pain is common in pregnancy and reflects altered spinal posture and increased ligamentous laxity. There is usually a hyperlordosis on examining the patient standing. Weight control and pre- and postnatal exercises are helpful, and the pain usually settles after delivery. Analgesics and NSAIDs are best avoided during pregnancy and breast-feeding. Epidurals during delivery are not associated with an increased incidence of subsequent back pain. Poor posture causes a similar syndrome in the non-pregnant, owing to obesity or muscular weakness. Poor sitting posture at work is a frequent cause of chronic low back pain.

Lumbar spondylosis

The fundamental lesion in spondylosis is in an inter-vertebral disc, a fibrous joint whose tough capsule inserts into the rim of the adjacent vertebrae. This capsule encloses a fibrous outer zone and a gel-like inner zone. The disc allows rotation and bending.

Changes in the discs may start in teenage years or early twenties and increase with age. The gel changes chemically, breaks up, shrinks and loses its compliance. The surrounding fibrous zones develop circumferential or radial fissures. In the majority this is initially asymptomatic but visible on MRI as decreased hydration. Later the discs become thinner and less compliant. These changes cause circumferential bulging of the intervertebral ligaments.

Reactive changes develop in adjacent vertebrae; the bone becomes sclerotic and osteophytes form around the rim of the vertebra (Fig. 10.6). The most common sites of lumbar spondylosis are L5/S1 and L4/L5. Disc prolapse through an adjacent vertebral endplate to produce a Schmorl's node on X-ray is painless but may accelerate disc degeneration.

Spondylosis may be symptomless, but it can cause:

- episodic mechanical spinal pain
- progressive spinal stiffening
- facet joint pain
- acute disc prolapse, with or without nerve root irritation
- spinal stenosis
- spondylolisthesis.

Fig. 10.6 **MRI of lumbar spine**, showing a central disc prolapse at the L4/L5 level (arrow). The signal from the L4/L5 and L5/S1 discs indicates dehydration, while the L3/L4 signal appearance is normal.

Facet joint syndrome

Lumbar spondylosis also causes secondary osteoarthritis of the facet joints. Pain is typically worse on bending backwards and when straightening from flexion. It is lumbar in site, unilateral or bilateral and radiates to the buttock. The facet joints are well seen on MRI and may show osteoarthritis, an effusion or a ganglion. Diagnostic local anaesthetic injections into the joints (under X-ray vision) can be followed by a corticosteroid injection. The long-term value of this is unclear but many patients find the procedure helpful. Physiotherapy to reduce hyperlordosis and reducing weight are helpful.

Treatment of mechanical back pain

Adequate analgesia to allow normal mobility and avoid bed rest is best, combined with physical treatments. The evidence base for physiotherapy, back muscle training regimens and manipulation is not good. Manipulation produces more rapid pain relief in some patients. A positive approach probably reduces the development of chronic pain. A comfortable sleeping position should be adopted using a mattress of medium (not hard) firmness.

Acute lumbar disc prolapse

The central disc gel may extrude into a fissure in the surrounding fibrous zone and cause acute pain and muscle spasm, which in turn leads to a forwards and sideways tilt when standing. These events are often self-limiting. A disc prolapse occurs when the extrusion extends beyond the limits of the fibrous zone (Fig. 10.6). The weakest point is posterolateral, where the disc may impinge on emerging spinal nerve roots in the root canal.

The episode starts dramatically during lifting, twisting or bending and produces a typical combination of low back pain and muscle spasm, and severe, lancinating pains, paraesthesia, numbness and neurological signs in one leg (rarely both). The back pain is diffuse, usually unilateral and radiates into the buttock. The muscle spasm leads to a scoliosis that reduces when lying down. The nerve root pain develops with, or soon after, the onset. The site of the pain and other symptoms is determined by the root affected (Table 10.7). A central high lumbar disc prolapse may cause spinal cord compression and long tract signs (i.e. upper motor neurone). Below L2/L3 it produces lower motor neurone lesions.

On examination, the back often shows a marked scoliosis and muscle spasm. The lying, straight-leg-raising test is positive in a lower lumbar disc prolapse – raising the straight leg beyond 30 degrees produces pain in the leg; slight limitation or pain in the back limiting the movement is not significant. Pain in the affected leg produced by a straight raise of the other leg suggests a large or central disc prolapse. Look for perianal sensory loss, which might indicate a cauda equina lesion – a neurosurgical emergency. An upper lumbar disc prolapse produces a positive femoral stretch test – pain in the anterior thigh when the knee is flexed in the prone position.

Treatment

Advise a short period (2–3 days) of bed rest – lying flat for a lower disc but semi-reclining for a high lumbar disc – and prescribe analgesia and muscle relaxants. Once the pain is tolerable, encourage the patient to mobilize and refer to a physiotherapist for exercises and preventative advice. An X-ray-guided epidural or nerve root canal injection by a pain specialist reduces pain, although the evidence that it speeds resolution or prevents surgery is unclear. Caudal epidural injections are less effective than lumbar ones. Resuscitation equipment must be available for these procedures. Referral to a surgeon for possible microdiscectomy or hemilaminectomy is necessary if the neurological signs are severe, if the pain persists and is severe for more than 6–10 weeks, or if the disc is central. If bladder or anal sphincter tone is affected it becomes a neurosurgical emergency.

Spinal and root canal stenosis

Progressive loss of disc height, OA of the facet joints, posterolateral osteophytes and hypertrophy of the ligamentum flavum all contribute to root canal stenosis. This causes nerve root pain or spinal root claudication – pain and paraesthesiae in a root distribution brought on by walking and relieved slowly by rest. The associated sensory symptoms, slow recovery when the patient rests and presence of normal foot pulses distinguish this from peripheral arterial claudication.

Spinal canal stenosis at more than one level is often associated with a congenitally narrow spinal canal. It causes buttock and bilateral leg pain, paraesthesiae and numbness when walking. Rest helps, as does bending forwards, a manoeuvre that opens the spinal canal. Specialist surgical advice is necessary.

Table 10.7	Lumbar nerve root entrapment – symptoms and signs			
Nerve root	**Sensory changes**	**Reflex loss**	**Weakness**	**Usual disc prolapse**
L2	Front of thigh	None	Hip flexion/ adduction	L2/3
L3	Inner thigh and knee	Knee	Knee extension	L2/3
L4	Inner calf	Knee	Knee extension	L3/4
L5	Outer calf Upper, inner foot	None	Inversion of foot Dorsiflexion of toes	L4/5
S1	Posterior calf Lateral border of foot	Ankle	Plantar flexion of foot	L5/S1

Spondylolisthesis

This occurs in adolescents and young adults when bilateral congenital pars interarticularis defects cause instability and permit the vertebra to slip, with or without preceding injury. Rarely a cauda equina syndrome with loss of bladder and anal sphincter control and saddle-distribution anaesthesia develops (p. 1265). It is diagnosed radiologically. Low back pain in adolescents warrants investigation, and spondylolisthesis requires orthopaedic assessment. It needs careful monitoring during the growth spurt.

A degenerative spondylolisthesis may also develop in older people with lumbar spondylosis.

Diffuse idiopathic skeletal hyperostosis (DISH)

DISH (Forrestier's disease) affects the spine and extra-spinal locations. It causes bony overgrowths and ligamentous ossification and is characterized by flowing calcification over the anterolateral aspects of the vertebrae. The spine is stiff but not always painful, despite the dramatic X-ray changes. Ossification at muscle insertions around the pelvis produces radiological 'whiskering'. Similar changes occur at the patella and in the feet.

Treatment is with analgesics or NSAIDs for pain, and exercise to retain movement and muscle strength.

Osteoporotic crush fracture of the spine

Osteoporosis is asymptomatic but leads to an increased risk of fracture of peripheral bones, particularly neck of femur and wrist, and thoracic or lumbar vertebral crush fractures. Such vertebral fractures develop without trauma, after minimal trauma, or as part of a major accident. They may develop painlessly or cause agonizing localized pain that radiates around the ribs and abdomen. Multiple fractures lead to an increased thoracic kyphosis ('widow's stoop'). The diagnosis is confirmed by X-rays, showing loss of anterior vertebral body height and wedging, with sparing of the vertebral end-plates and pedicles (see Fig. 10.37, p. 595).

Treatment

Advise bed rest and analgesia until the severe pain subsides over a few weeks, then gradual mobilization. It may warrant hospitalization. There may be some residual pain. Bone density measurement and preventative treatment of osteoporosis are essential (see p. 596).

Ankylosing spondylitis (see also p. 564)

Buttock pain and low-back stiffness in a young adult suggests ankylosing spondylitis, especially if it is worse at night and in the morning.

FURTHER READING
McConnell J (2003) Mattresses for a pain in the back. *Lancet* **362**; 1594–1595.

Table 10.8 Pain in the hip – causes

Hip region problems	Main sites of pain
Osteoarthritis of hip	Groin, buttock, front of thigh to knee
Trochanteric bursitis (or gluteus medius tendonopathy)	Lateral thigh to knee
Meralgia paraesthetica	Anterolateral thigh to knee
Referred from back	Buttock
Facet joint pain	Buttock and posterior thigh
Fracture of neck of femur	Groin and buttock
Inflammatory arthritis	Groin, buttock, front of thigh to knee
Sacroiliitis (AS)	Buttock(s)
Avascular necrosis	Lumbar spine and buttocks
Polymyalgia rheumatica	Lumbar spine, buttocks and thighs

AS, ankylosing spondylitis

PAIN IN THE HIP (Table 10.8)

'Hip' refers to a wide area between the upper buttock, trochanter and groin. It is useful to ask the patient to point to the site of pain and its field of radiation. Pain arising from the hip joint itself is felt in the groin, lower buttock and anterior thigh, and may radiate to the knee. Occasionally and inexplicably, hip arthritis causes pain only in the knee.

Osteoarthritis (OA) (see also p. 552)

OA is the most common cause of hip joint pain in a person over the age of 50 years. It causes pain in the buttock and groin on standing and walking. Stiff hip movements cause difficulty in putting on a sock and may produce a limp.

Trochanteric bursitis and gluteus medius tendinopathy

This may be due to trauma or unaccustomed exercise, but sometimes has an unknown cause. It also occurs in inflammatory arthritis. The pain over the trochanter is worse going up stairs and when abducting the hip, and the trochanter is tender to lie on. A local corticosteroid injection onto the surface of the trochanter is helpful. A tear of the gluteus medius tendon at its insertion into the trochanter causes a syndrome that is similar but does not respond to injection. MRI scans have demonstrated this new syndrome. Its best management is unclear.

Meralgia paraesthetica (see also p. 1260)

This causes numbness and burning dysaesthesia (increased sensitivity to light touch) over the anterolateral thigh and may be precipitated by a sudden increase in weight, an injury or during pelvic surgery. It is usually self-limiting but can be helped by amitriptyline 10 mg at night or gabapentin starting with 300 mg.

Fracture of the femoral neck

This usually occurs after a fall, occasionally spontaneously. There is pain in the groin and thigh, weight-bearing is painful or impossible, and the leg is shortened and externally rotated. Occasionally a fracture is not displaced and remains undetected. X-rays are diagnostic. Anyone with a hip fracture, especially after minimal trauma, should be reviewed for osteoporosis (see p. 595).

Avascular necrosis (osteonecrosis) of the femoral head

This is uncommon but occurs at any age. There is severe hip pain. X-rays are diagnostic after a few weeks, when a well-demarcated area of increased bone density is visible. In the femur this lies at the upper pole of the femoral head. The affected bone may collapse. Early, the X-ray is normal but bone scintigraphy or MRI demonstrate the lesion. Risk factors include treatment with corticosteroids or heparin, exposure to high barometric pressures (divers and tunnellers), excessive alcohol consumption, and sickle cell disease.

Inflammatory arthritis of the hip

This produces pain in the groin and stiffness, which are worse in the morning. Rheumatoid arthritis (RA) rarely presents with hip pain, although the hip is involved eventually in severe RA. Ankylosing spondylitis and other seronegative spondyloarthropathies cause inflammatory hip arthritis in younger people.

Polymyalgia rheumatica (see also p. 582)

Bilateral hip, buttock and thigh pain and stiffness that are worse in the morning in an elderly patient may be attributable to polymyalgia rheumatica.

PAIN IN THE KNEE (Table 10.9)

The knee depends on ligaments and quadriceps muscle strength for stability. It is frequently injured, particularly during sports. Trauma or overuse of the knee leads to a

---

Table 10.9   Pain in the knee

Trauma and overuse:
  Periarticular problems:
    Anterior knee pain or medial knee pain
    Internal derangements – meniscal tears or cruciate
      ligament tears

Osteoarthritis

Inflammatory arthritis:
  Acute monarthritis:
    Gout, pseudogout, Reiter's disease or septic arthritis
  Pauciarticular (< 4 joints):
    Seronegative spondyloarthropathy or atypical
      rheumatoid arthritis
  Polyarticular:
    Rheumatoid arthritis

Popliteal (Baker's) cyst/ruptured cyst

Osteochondritis dissecans

Hypermobility syndrome

Referred from hip joint

---

variety of peri- and intra-articular problems. Some are self-limiting, others require physiotherapy, local corticosteroid injections or surgery.

The knee is also a common site of inflammatory arthritis and osteoarthritis. Minor radiographic changes of osteoarthritis (see Fig. 10.9, p. 551) are common in the over-fifties and often coincidental, the cause of the pain being periarticular. Knee pain should not be attributed to osteoarthritis until other causes have been excluded. Symptomatic osteoarthritis of the knee correlates poorly with the severity of the radiological changes.

Common periarticular knee lesions

Medial knee pain

There may be medial or lateral ligament strain, but the medial ligament is more commonly affected. There is pain at the ligament's insertion into the upper medial tibia, which is worsened by standing or stressing the affected ligament.

Anserine bursitis causes pain and localized tenderness 2–3 cm below the posteromedial joint line in the upper part of the tibia at the site of the bursa. It occurs in obese women, often with valgus deformities, and in breaststroke swimmers.

Treatment is with physiotherapy and a local corticosteroid injection.

Anterior knee pain

Anterior knee pain is common in adolescence. In many cases no specific cause is found despite careful investigation. This is called 'anterior knee pain syndrome' and settles with time. Isometric quadriceps exercises and avoidance of high heels both help the condition. Patient and parents often need firm reassurance. Abnormal patellar tracking may be a cause and need surgical treatment.

Pre- and infrapatellar bursitis are caused by unaccustomed kneeling ('housemaid's knee'). There is local pain, tenderness and fluctuant swelling. Avoidance of kneeling and a local corticosteroid injection are helpful. Septic bursitis can occur.

Chondromalacia patellae is diagnosed arthroscopically. The retropatellar cartilage is fibrillated. In most cases the pain settles eventually. When there is patellar misalignment it may need surgery, as does recurrent patellar dislocation in adolescent girls.

Osgood–Schlatter's disease causes pain and swelling over the tibial tubercle. It is a traction apophysitis of the patellar tendon and occurs in enthusiastic teenage sports players.

Hypermobility of joints causes joint pain (see also p. 587).

Common intra-articular traumatic lesions of the knee

Torn meniscus

The menisci are partially attached fibrocartilages that stabilize the rounded femoral condyles on the flat tibial plateaux. In the young they are resilient but this decreases exercises. Loose fragments can be fixed arthroscopically or removed. A similar lesion affecting the lateral femoral condyle occurs in older people.

Knee joint effusions

An effusion of the knee causes swelling, stiffness and pain. The pain is more severe with an acute onset and with increasing inflammation, because of stretching of the capsule that contains the pain receptors. A full clinical history and examination must include a past medical, family and drug history.

Inflammatory arthritis affects the knees and causes warmth and swelling. An acute inflammatory monarthritis of the knee is a common presentation of a seronegative spondyloarthropathy and occasionally is the first sign of RA.

Monarthritis of the knee, associated with severe pain and marked redness, may be due to septic arthritis, or gout in the middle-aged male, or to gout or pseudogout in an older male or female. A cool, clear, viscous effusion is seen in elderly patients with moderate or severe symptomatic OA.

Examination

A large and tense effusion is easily seen and felt on each side of the patella and in the suprapatellar pouch, and is fluctuant. The effusion delays the patella tapping against the femur when it is pressed firmly and quickly (the 'patellar tap' sign). Small effusions also demonstrate the 'bulge' sign when the patient is lying with the quadriceps relaxed. For this, apply a gentle sweeping pressure, first to the medial side of the joint and then, watching the medial dimple, to the lateral side. Slightly delayed bulging of the medial dimple indicates fluid in the joint.

Investigations

These are (a) blood biochemistry, and (b) aspiration and examination of the knee effusion. The basic technique of aspiration is described in Practical box 10.2 on page 534.

If there is a flexion deformity, externally rotate the leg or support the knee. Stand on the side opposite the joint and insert the needle between the patella, just proximal to its mid point, and the medial femoral condyle. Angle the needle slightly backwards and inject small volumes of local anaesthetic, advancing until aspiration detects fluid. Then change the syringe for a larger one and aspirate as much fluid as possible. Examine the fluid (see Box 10.1, p. 535) and decide whether to inject corticosteroid or arrange microbiological tests.

Haemarthrosis of the knee

This is caused by:

- trauma – meniscal, cruciate or synovial lining tear
- clotting or bleeding disorders, such as haemophilia, sickle cell disease or von Willebrand's disease.

Popliteal cyst (Baker's cyst)

In approximately 5% of patients with a knee effusion, a swollen, painful popliteal cyst develops. This is usually

Fig. 10.7 **MRI of a knee**, showing a complete tear of the posterior horn of the medial meniscus, extending to its lower surface (arrow).

with age. They can be torn by a twisting injury, commonly in sports that involve twisting and bending. The history is usually diagnostic. There is immediate medial or lateral knee pain and dramatic swelling within a few hours. The affected side is tender. If the tear is large the knee may lock flexed. The immediate treatment is to apply ice. MRI demonstrates the tear (Fig. 10.7). In most circumstances, especially in active sportsmen, early arthroscopic repair or trimming of the torn meniscus is essential. Surgical intervention reduces recurrent pain, swelling and locking but not the risk of secondary osteoarthritis. The long-term benefit of repairing tears is not yet known. Post-surgical quadriceps exercises aid a return to sport.

Torn cruciate ligaments

Torn cruciate ligaments account for around 70% of knee haemarthroses in young people. They often coexist with a meniscal tear. Partial cruciate tears are difficult to diagnose clinically. On flexing the knee to 90 degrees, a torn anterior cruciate allows the tibia to be pulled forwards on the femur. MRI is the investigation of choice. Such injuries need urgent orthopaedic referral. There is a significant incidence of secondary OA.

Osteochondritis dissecans

This occasionally causes knee pain and swelling in adolescents and young adults, more commonly males. It is probably traumatic, possibly with hereditary predisposing factors. A fragment of bone and its attached cartilage detach by shearing, most commonly from the lateral aspect of the medial femoral condyle.

There is aching pain after activity and, if the fragment becomes loose, locking or 'giving way' occurs. The lesion is seen on a tunnel-view X-ray, but MRI is more sensitive, especially if the fragment is undisplaced. Undisplaced lesions are treated with rest, then isometric quadriceps due to a bursa (usually the semimembranosus bursa), which in some individuals has a valve-like connection to the knee. This allows the effusion to flow into the bursa but not back. Occasionally there is a synovial herniation through the posterior joint capsule. The cyst is best seen and felt in the popliteal fossa with the patient standing.

Ruptured popliteal cyst

A popliteal cyst may rupture if the patient is mobile, particularly on standing up quickly or climbing stairs. Fluid escapes into the soft tissue of the popliteal fossa and upper calf, causing sudden and severe pain, swelling and tenderness of the upper calf. Dependent oedema of the ankle develops and the knee effusion reduces dramatically in size and may be undetectable.

A history of previous knee problems and the sudden onset of pain and tenderness high in the calf suggest a ruptured cyst rather than a deep vein thrombosis (DVT). However, the diagnosis is often missed and treated inappropriately with anticoagulants. A diagnostic ultrasound examination distinguishes a ruptured cyst from a DVT (see p. 870). Analgesics or NSAIDs, rest with the leg elevated, and aspiration and injection with corticosteroids into the knee joint are required.

PAIN IN THE FOOT AND HEEL (Table 10.10)

The feet are subjected to extreme pressures by weight-bearing and inappropriate shoes. They are commonly painful. Broad, deep, thick-soled shoes are essential for sporting activities, prolonged walking or standing, and in people with congenitally flat or arthritic feet.

There are two common types of foot deformity:

- flat feet stress the ankle and throw the hindfoot into a valgus (everted) position – a flat foot is rigid and inflexible
- high-arched feet place pressure on the lateral border and ball of the foot.

The foot is affected by a variety of inflammatory arthritic conditions. After the hand, the foot joints are the most

Table 10.10 Pain in the foot and heel – causes

Structural (flat (pronated) or high arched (supinated))
Hallux valgus/rigidus (± OA)
Metatarsalgia
Morton's neuroma
Stress fracture
Inflammatory arthritis
Acute, monarticular – gout
Chronic, polyarticular – RA
Chronic, pauciarticular – seronegative spondyloarthropathy
Tarsal tunnel syndrome
Heel pain
  Plantar fasciitis   Below heel
  Plantar spur   Below heel
  Achilles tendonitis/bursitis   Behind heel
  Sever's disease   Behind heel
Arthritis of ankle/subtaloid joints

commonly affected by rheumatoid arthritis. The diagnosis depends upon careful assessment of the distribution of the joints affected, the pattern of other joint problems, or by finding the associated condition (e.g. psoriasis, see p. 1331).

Hallux valgus

The great toe migrates laterally. In the congenital form the first metatarsal is displaced medially (metatarsus primus varus). The shape of modern shoes causes later onset of hallux valgus. It is a common complication of RA.

Hallux rigidus

Osteoarthritis of the first MTP joint in a normally aligned or valgus joint causes hallux rigidus – a stiff, dorsiflexed and painful great toe. Careful choice of footwear and the help of a podiatrist suffice for most cases, but some require surgery.

Metatarsalgia

This is common, especially in women who wear high heels, after trauma and in those with hammer toes. The ball of the foot is painful to walk and stand on. Callosities and pressure-induced bursae develop under the metatarsal heads. Rheumatoid arthritis causes misalignment of the metatarsal bones and severe metatarsalgia.

Treatment is with podiatry and the wearing of appropriate shoes. Surgery is occasionally needed, particularly in the rheumatoid forefoot.

Morton's metatarsalgia is due to a neuroma, usually between the third and fourth toes. It causes pain, burning and numbness in the adjacent surfaces of the affected toes when walking. It is helped by wearing wider, cushioned-soled shoes. Occasionally a steroid injection is necessary.

Stress (march) fractures

These cause sudden, severe weight-bearing pain in the distal shaft of the fractured metatarsal bone. They occur after unaccustomed walking or with new shoes. There is local tenderness and swelling, but initially X-rays are normal and diagnosis delayed. A radioisotope bone scan reveals the fracture earlier than X-rays. Reduced weight-bearing for a few weeks usually suffices.

Tarsal tunnel syndrome

This is an entrapment neuropathy of the posterior tibial nerve as it rounds the medial malleolus. It produces burning, tingling and numbness of the toes, sole and medial arch. The nerve is tender below the malleolus and, when tapped, produces a shock-like pain (Tinel's sign). A local steroid injection under the retinaculum, between the medial malleolus and calcaneum, is helpful.

Pain under the heel

Plantar fasciitis is an enthesitis at the insertion of the tendon into the calcaneum. It produces localized pain when standing and walking, and tenderness in the midline. It occurs alone or in seronegative spondyloarthropathy.

Plantar spurs are traction lesions at the insertion of the plantar fascia in older people and are usually asymptomatic. They become painful after trauma.

Calcaneal bursitis is a pressure-induced (adventitious) bursa that produces diffuse pain and tenderness under the heel. Compression of the heel pad from the sides is painful, which distinguishes it from plantar fascia pain.

Whatever the cause, the pain is always worse in the morning as soon as weight is placed on the foot.

All of these lesions are treated with heel pads, and reduced walking; they are often self-limiting. A splint at night to hold the foot dorsiflexed and to stretch the plantar fascia is preferable to a local corticosteroid injection in plantar fasciitis. When an injection is necessary, a medial approach is used, rather than through the heel pad, under a posterior tibial nerve block.

Pain behind the heel and leg

Sever's disease is a traction apophysitis of the Achilles tendon in young people (cf. Osgood–Schlatter's disease p. 588).

Achilles tendonitis is an *enthesitis* at the insertion of the tendon into the calcaneum. This is traumatic or it can complicate seronegative spondyloarthropathy. Raising the shoe heel reduces pain. Occasionally a low-pressure corticosteroid injection near the enthesis is necessary.

Achilles tendonosis causes a painful, tender swelling a few centimetres above the tendon's insertion. Advise against walking barefoot and jumping. Therapeutic ultrasound is helpful. (Caution – a local injection may cause the tendon to rupture.)

Achilles' bursitis lies clearly anterior to the tendon and can be safely injected with corticosteroid.

Compartment syndromes

The muscles of the lower leg are enclosed in fascial compartments, with little room for expansion to occur. Compartment syndromes can be acute and severe, such as following exercise.

In the *anterior tibial syndrome* there is severe pain in the front of the shin, occasionally with foot drop. Immediate surgical decompression to prevent muscle necrosis is sometimes required.

Chronic compartment syndrome produces pain in the lower leg that is aggravated by exercise and may therefore be mistaken for a vascular or neurological disorder.

PAIN IN THE CHEST

Musculoskeletal conditions are sometimes a cause of chest pain. An example is Tietze's disease. In this condition, pain arises from the costosternal junctions. It is usually unilateral and affects one, two or three ribs. There is local tenderness, which helps to make the diagnosis. The condition is benign and self-limiting. It often responds well to anti-inflammatory drugs. Other causes of chest wall pain include rib fractures due to trauma or osteoporosis or a malignant deposit. Costochondral pain occurs in ankylosing spondylitis (see p. 565).

CHRONIC PAIN SYNDROMES
(see also p. 1282)

Chronic pain syndromes are difficult to manage. Psychological factors are at least as important as inflammation or damage in determining a patient's perception of pain. It is essential to be objective and non-judgmental when dealing with them, discussing physical, psychological and social factors without assuming which is primary. Chronic pain syndromes are difficult to explain scientifically and it is all too easy for a doctor to 'blame' the patient for this lack of explanation. Some chronic pain states may be caused partly by the process of litigation that may follow an injury.

Any chronic painful condition can change the way a person copes. Some people with chronic diseases or chronic pain cope well, but others adopt coping strategies and patterns of behaviour which make things worse. They become anxious, depressed or socially isolated, and their quality of life is reduced. In chronic pain syndromes patients need help to lead a more normal life despite their pain, and are best referred to a specialist, multidisciplinary pain service.

Psychological states such as depression and anxiety produce physical symptoms, of which one is pain, while people with frank physical diseases are often understandably anxious and depressed.

Fibromyalgia (fibrositis syndrome)

'Fibromyalgia' (p. 1282) is a useful diagnosis of exclusion although it is not universally accepted as a diagnosis. Patients value a name to explain symptoms previously dismissed or attributed simply to psychological or social problems. A typical feature of fibromyalgia is tender trigger points. The tenderness is not 'all over', a point which distinguishes it from anxiety states. The patient is usually a middle-aged woman who struggles on with her work and/or housework despite the pain. Such individuals are difficult to live with and there is often family discord. Many patients have sleep disturbances, so they awake unrefreshed and have poor concentration. It can occur at any age and is increasingly recognized in teenagers.

The pain is a widespread, unremitting, aching discomfort. There are often other health problems, such as chronic fatigue syndrome (see below), irritable bowel syndrome, premenstrual syndrome, tension headache, anxiety and depression; doctors sometimes inappropriately label them 'heart sink' patients. The patient's frustration is compounded by the fact that most tests are normal, and they fear doctors believe it is 'all in their mind'.

Treatment

A sympathetic approach is appropriate, with reassurance for the patient that fibromyalgia often improves and is not inevitably disabling. A graded aerobic exercise regimen over 3 months is safe and effective. When depression is present, it should be treated, but potentially addictive anxiolytic agents are best avoided. A behavioural psychologist may persuade the person to pace their life more effectively and to cope better, although patients often resist referral for psychological help.

Drugs

Analgesics or NSAIDs help in some cases but are best used intermittently.

Low doses of sedative antidepressant drugs, such as amitriptyline or dosulepin, help when taken a few hours before bedtime. They act by increasing the levels of serotonin in the CNS. It should be explained that these doses are analgesic and not antidepressant, and their side-effects should be outlined.

Trigger-point injections with local anaesthetic, corticosteroids or acupuncture are sometimes helpful.

Oral corticosteroids are not helpful.

Chronic fatigue syndrome

Diffuse muscular pain and stiffness is common in this condition, which is described on page 1281.

Chronic (work-related) upper-limb pain syndrome

This name is preferred to 'repetitive strain injury' (RSI). The predominant symptoms are pain in all or part of one or both arms. A specific lesion, such as tennis elbow or carpal tunnel syndrome, or muscular-pattern neck pain often develops first, and early recognition and treatment may prevent chronicity. After a variable period, the pain becomes more diffuse and no longer simply work-related, and there is often severe distress. It is seen in keyboard workers and others who perform the same task without breaks for prolonged periods, and in musicians. When it arises at work, it is often at a time of changing work practices, shortage of staff or disharmony. Middle managers find it difficult to deal with and this compounds the stress.

It is seen throughout the developed world. It peaked in incidence in Australia in the 1970s and 1980s but has largely disappeared there, apparently because of changes in work practices, improvements in early medical management, changes in workers' compensation legislation, and reduced media discussion of the problem.

Treatment

If possible there should be a brief period off work and a gradual return to activity once the pain has settled. Cautious use of analgesia and NSAIDs, with physiotherapy, is helpful during the initial phase to prevent a vicious circle developing.

A review of working practices and the positioning of screen, keyboard and chair are essential, as is support of the patient by their manager. Musicians are helped by expert advice on playing technique and should reduce playing times temporarily, but not stop completely.

Temporomandibular pain dysfunction syndrome

This is a disorder of the temporomandibular joint associated with nocturnal tooth grinding or abnormalities of bite. It particularly occurs in anxious people. It gives rise to pain in one or both temporomandibular joints.

Dental correction of the bite helps a few but when no dental cause is found, low-dose tricyclic antidepressant therapy is used. Many patients are exposed to much unnecessary dental treatment.

Chronic regional pain syndrome type 1 (previously called reflex sympathetic dystrophy or Sudek's atrophy)

This is defined as 'a complex disorder or group of disorders that may develop as a consequence of trauma affecting the limbs, with or without obvious nerve lesions'. It may also develop after central nervous system lesions (e.g. strokes) or without cause. It occurred in 1.5% of soldiers injured in Vietnam. Its features are pain and other sensory abnormalities, including hyperaesthesia, autonomic vasomotor dysfunction, leading to abnormal blood flow and sweating, and motor system abnormalities. This leads to structural changes of superficial and deep tissues (trophic changes). Not all components need be present. The sensory, motor and sympathetic nerve changes are not restricted to the distribution of a single nerve and may be remote from the site of injury. The early phase – with pain, swelling and increased skin temperature – is difficult to diagnose but potentially reversible.

After a period of weeks or months, a second, still painful, dystrophic phase develops, characterized by articular stiffness, cold skin and trophic changes, often with localized osteoporosis.

A late phase involves continued pain, skin and muscle atrophy, and muscle contractures, and is extremely disabling.

Diagnosis is initially clinical – a high index of suspicion and recognizing the unusual distribution of the pain. A three-phase bone scan shows diffuse or patchy increase in uptake in the affected limb in all three phases: early (a few seconds – arterial); middle (a few minutes – soft tissue); and late (several hours – mineral). The bone phase abnormalities appear early and well before demineralization is seen on X-ray. There is never loss of joint space, which distinguishes the appearances from the periarticular osteoporosis of inflammatory joint disease.

Treatment

Management is difficult and the problem often very disabling. The evidence base to treatment is poor, as in many rare disorders. Early diagnosis, effective pain relief and general care of the patient are essential. NSAIDs and corticosteroids are used in the early phase, together with active exercise of the limb. Calcitonin or intravenous disodium pamidronate may also help at this stage. If pain persists despite initial treatment, a phentolamine test is used to test for evidence of sympathetically maintained pain (i.v. infusion of up to 40 mg with careful cardiac monitoring). If this is positive, a stellate ganglion block is used for upper limb and a sympathetic chain block for lower limb involvement. Guanethidine (an alpha-blocking agent) or lidocaine administered to the limb under tourniquet is also useful. Referral to a pain management clinic is advisable.

Chronic regional pain syndrome type II is discussed on page 1198.

FURTHER READING

Clauw DJ, Simon LS (2003) Chronic generalized musculoskeletal pain. *Clinical Rheumatology* **17**(4)
Jayson MIV (ed) (1993) *The Lumbar Spine and Back Pain*, 4th edn. London: Churchill Livingstone.
Yassi A (1997) Repetitive strain injuries. *Lancet* **349**: 943–947.

ANALGESIC AND ANTI-INFLAMMATORY DRUGS FOR MUSCULOSKELETAL PROBLEMS

The key to using drugs, particularly in chronic disorders and the elderly, is to balance risk and benefit and constantly to review their appropriateness. Box 10.4 shows the main drugs available.

Simple and compound analgesic agents

Simple agents such as paracetamol, aspirin, or codeine compounds (or combination preparations), used when necessary or regularly, relieve pain and improve function. Paracetamol with dextropropoxyphene (co-proximal) should not be prescribed and is being withdrawn. Sleep may also be improved. Side-effects are relatively infrequent, although drowsiness and constipation occur with codeine preparations, especially in the elderly.

Stronger analgesics, such as dihydrocodeine or morphine derivatives, should be used only with severe pain.

Non-steroidal anti-inflammatory drugs (NSAIDs)

NSAIDs have anti-inflammatory and centrally acting analgesic properties. They inhibit cyclo-oxygenase (COX), a key enzyme in the formation of prostaglandins, prostacyclins and thromboxanes (see Fig. 14.32). There are three specific cyclo-oxygenase enzymes: COX-1, the constitutive form; COX-2, the form mainly induced by inflammation; and COX-3 found in the brain. Most of the older NSAIDs block all three enzymes but with variable specificity; their therapeutic effect depends on blocking COX-2 and their side-effects mainly on blocking COX-1.

COX-1 is a constitutive enzyme present in many normal tissues. Inhibition of the enzyme by NSAIDs produces side-effects caused, for example, by the loss of gastric mucosal protection and a decrease in renal blood flow.

COX-2 is induced in response to pro-inflammatory cytokines and is not found in most normal tissues. It is associated with oedema and the nociceptive and pyretic effects of inflammation. COX-2 appears to be constitutive in the kidney. COX-2 specific NSAIDs are available, but see page 550.

COX-3 is present in the brain and is responsible for pain and hyperpyrexia. It is blocked weakly by paracetamol and by COX non-specific drugs. COX-2 specific drugs appear not to block COX-3, an observation which may explain their weaker analgesic action.

Uses

- *Short courses* of NSAIDs are used occasionally in osteoarthritis and spondylosis, even when there is minimal inflammation. They are commonly used in musculoskeletal pain but simple analgesia is often more appropriate.
- *In crystal synovitis*, NSAIDs have a true anti-inflammatory effect (see p. 570).
- *In chronic inflammatory synovitis*, NSAIDs do not alter the chronic inflammatory process, nor decrease the risk of joint damage, but they do reduce pain and stiffness.

 Box 10.4 Analgesics and NSAIDs

Analgesics (in order of potency)
Advise that they be taken *only* if needed. Maximum doses are indicated here.

Paracetamol	500–1000 mg	6-hourly
Paracetamol with codeine	1–2 tablets	6-hourly
Paracetamol with dihydrocodeine	1–2 tablets	Every 6–8 hours
Dihydrocodeine	30–60 mg	Every 6–8 hours

Non-steroidal anti-inflammatory drugs (NSAIDs)
Always to be taken with food. Use slow-release preparations in inflammatory conditions or if more regular pain control is needed. Examples:

Ibuprofen	200–400 mg	Every 6–8 hours
Ibuprofen slow release	600–800 mg	Every 1–3 days
Diclofenac	25–50 mg	8-hourly
Diclofenac slow release	75–100 mg	× 1–2 daily
Celecoxib*	100–200 mg	× 2 daily

*COX-2-specific NSAID

- Slow-release preparations are useful for *inflammatory arthritis* and when more constant pain control is needed.
- NSAID gels have some value in chronic arthritis.

Side-effects

The most common with COX non-specific NSAIDs are indigestion or skin rashes. Gastric erosions and peptic ulceration with perforation and bleeding also occur. Proton-pump inhibitors are probably the best drugs to protect those at high risk from serious gastrointestinal events. H_2 blockers also help as gastroprotective agents. The value of prostaglandin E_2 analogues is limited by their tendency to cause nausea and diarrhoea. In the elderly, NSAIDs may cause gastric mucosal damage and gastrointestinal bleeding without warning symptoms, thereby causing significant morbidity and mortality. They may also reduce renal function, especially in the elderly. They should only be prescribed with a proton pump inhibitor in this group.

COX-2 specific NSAIDs produce fewer gastrointestinal side-effects (6% compared to 16% in one trial) but renal complications and fluid retention still occur. Rofecoxib has been withdrawn because of an increase in cardiovascular events with prolonged use. Celecoxib has also been implicated suggesting that this may be a 'class' phenomenon. Cox-2 specific NSAID should therefore only be used in patients with a high risk of gastro-intestinal disease and with no cardiovascular risk.

FURTHER READING

Fitzgerald GA, Patrono C (2004) Coxibs and cardiovascular disease. *New England Journal of Medicine* **351**: 1709–1711.

Graham DY (2002) NSAIDs, *Helicobacter pylori* and Pandora's box. *New England Journal of Medicine* **347**: 2162–2163.

Schwab JM, Schluesener HJ, Lante S (2003). COX 3. *Lancet* **361**: 981–982.

OSTEOARTHRITIS (OA)

Osteoarthritis is a disease of synovial joints characterized by cartilage loss with an accompanying periarticular bone response. There is no simple definition of OA as it requires consideration of three overlapping areas – pathological changes, radiological features and clinical consequences. Pathologically, there is an alteration in cartilage structure, radiologically there are osteophytes and joint space narrowing, and clinically some patients complain of pain and disability.

Epidemiology

Osteoarthritis is the most common type of arthritis. The prevalence increases with age, and most people over 60 years will have some radiological evidence of it. It occurs world-wide, although OA of the hip is less common in black Africans and Chinese populations than

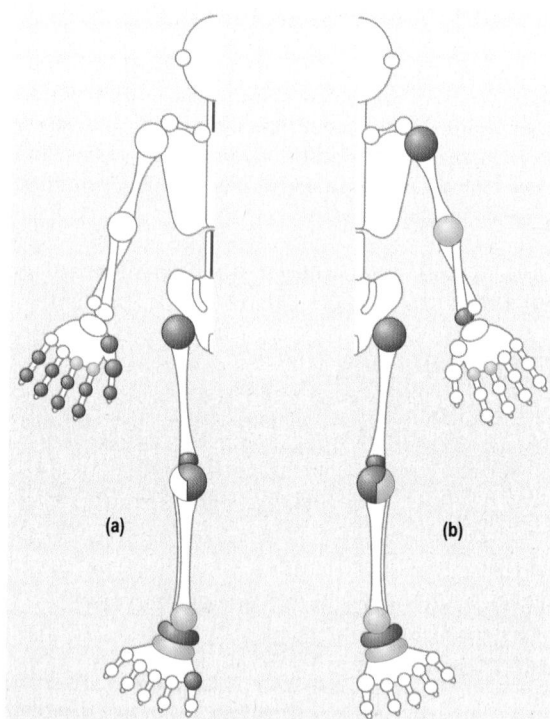

Fig. 10.8 Typical distribution of affected joints in (a) primary generalized OA and (b) pyrophosphate arthropathy. ●, more commonly affected; ◐, less commonly affected.

in Caucasians. Most epidemiological studies have been based on radiological evidence, which is much more frequent than symptomatic OA. Women over 55 years are affected more commonly than are men of a similar age. There is a familial pattern of inheritance with distal interphalangeal joint involvement as the hallmark (nodal OA) and also with primary generalized OA. OA has a variable distribution (Fig. 10.8). The resulting disabilities have major socio-economic resource implications, particularly in the developed world.

Aetiology

Genes that encode collagen type II have been proposed as candidate genes for familial OA. Osteoarthritis is the result of active, sometimes inflammatory but potentially reparative processes rather than the inevitable result of trauma and ageing. Focal destruction of the articular cartilage is the common pathological feature. The spectrum of OA ranges from atrophic disease in which cartilage destruction occurs without any subchondral bone response, to hypertrophic disease in which there is massive new bone formation at the joint margins.

Cartilage is a matrix of collagen fibres (mainly type II, see p. 530), enclosing a mixture of proteoglycans and water. Proteoglycans are present mainly as large molecular aggrecans, which consist of a protein core with attached chondroitin sulphate and keratan sulphate chains. The gene for human aggrecan has been cloned, and polymorphisms of the gene have been correlated with OA of the hand in older men.

Cartilage is smooth-surfaced and shock-absorbing. Under normal circumstances there is a dynamic balance between cartilage degradation by wear and its production by chondrocytes. Early in the development of OA this balance is lost and, despite increased synthesis of extracellular matrix, the cartilage becomes oedematous. Focal erosion of cartilage develops. Chondrocytes die and, although repair is attempted from adjacent cartilage, the process is disordered. Eventually the synthesis of extracellular matrix fails and the surface becomes fibrillated and fissured. Cartilage ulceration exposes underlying bone to increased stress, producing micro-fractures and cysts. The bone attempts repair but produces abnormal sclerotic subchondral bone and overgrowths at the joint margins, called *osteophytes* (Fig. 10.9). There is some secondary inflammation.

Pathogenesis

Several mechanisms have been suggested for the pathogenesis:

- Matrix loss is caused by the action of matrix metalloproteinases such as collagenase (MMP-1), gelatinase (MMP-2) and stromelysin (MMP-3). These are secreted by chrondrocytes in an inactive form. Extracellular activation then leads to the degradation of collagen and proteoglycans.
- Tissue inhibitors of metalloproteinases (TIMPs) regulate the MMPs. Disturbance of this regulation may lead to increased cartilage degradation and contribute to the development of OA.
- There is synovial inflammation in OA, producing interleukin-1 (IL-1) and tumour necrosis factor (TNF-α). These cytokines stimulate metalloproteinase production and IL-1 inhibits type II collagen production.
- Growth factors, including insulin-like growth factor (IGF-1) and transforming growth factor (TGF-β), are involved in collagen synthesis, and their deficiency may play a role in impairing matrix repair.
- Vascular endothelial growth factor from macrophages is a potent stimulator of angiogenesis and may contribute to inflammation and neovascularization in OA.
- Mutations in the gene for type II collagen (COL2A1) have been associated with early polyarticular OA.
- Twin studies suggest a strong hereditary element underlying OA, and further studies may reveal genetic markers for the disease. The influence of genetic factors is estimated at 35–65%.
- In the Caucasian population there is an inverse relationship between the risk of developing OA and osteoporosis.
- A large population study has suggested that a high intake of vitamin C and other antioxidants may reduce the risk of OA. The lack of antioxidants is thought to contribute to many ageing processes.
- In women, weight-bearing sports produce a two- to threefold increase in risk of OA of the hip and knee.

Fig. 10.9 Diagram and X-ray of a knee, showing early osteoarthritis. There is a medial compartment narrowing owing to cartilage thinning with subarticular sclerosis and marginal osteophyte formation (arrows).

- In men, there is an association between hip OA and certain occupations – farming and labouring.
- Obesity is a risk factor for developing OA in later life.

The term primary OA is sometimes used when there is no obvious known predisposing factor.

Box 10.5 shows some of the predisposing factors for the development of OA, whilst Table 10.11 shows other conditions that sometimes cause secondary arthritis.

Clinical features

Osteoarthritis affects many joints, with diverse clinical patterns. Hip and knee OA is the major cause of disability. Early OA is rarely symptomatic unless accompanied by a joint effusion, whilst advanced radiological and patho-logical OA is not always symptomatic.

Some flare-ups are due to inflammation but are not associated with an increased ESR or CRP. Focal synovitis

Box 10.5 Factors predisposing to osteoarthritis

- *Obesity* – Predicts later risk of radiological and symptomatic OA in population studies.
- *Heredity* – Familial tendency to develop nodal and generalized OA.
- *Gender* – Polyarticular OA is more common in women; a higher prevalence after the menopause suggests a role for sex hormones.
- *Hypermobility* (see p. 587) – Increased range of joint motion and reduced stability lead to OA.
- *Osteoporosis* – There is reduced risk of OA.
- Other diseases – See Table 10.11.
- *Trauma* – A fracture through any joint. Meniscal and cruciate ligament tears cause OA of the knee.
- *Congenital joint dysplasia* – Alters joint biomechanics and leads to OA. Mild acetabular dysplasia is common and leads to earlier onset of hip OA.
- *Joint congruity* – Congenital dislocation of the hip or a slipped femoral epiphysis or Perthes' disease; osteonecrosis of the femoral head (see p. 588) in children and adolescents causes early-onset OA.
- *Occupation* – Miners develop OA of the hip, knee and shoulder, cotton workers OA of the hand, and farmers OA of the hip.
- *Sport* – Repetitive use and injury in some sports causes a high incidence of lower-limb OA.

Table 10.11 **Causes of osteoarthritis**

Primary OA	No known cause
Secondary OA	Pre-existing joint damage:
	Rheumatoid arthritis
	Gout
	Seronegative spondyloarthropathy
	Septic arthritis
	Paget's disease
	Avascular necrosis, e.g.
	corticosteroid therapy
	Metabolic disease:
	Chondrocalcinosis
	Hereditary haemochromatosis
	Acromegaly
	Systemic diseases:
	Haemophilia – recurrent haemarthrosis
	Haemoglobinopathies, e.g. sickle cell
	disease
	Neuropathies

is caused by fragments of shed bone or cartilage. Radiological OA is usually, but not inevitably, progressive. This progression may be stepwise or continual. Radiological improvement is uncommon but has been observed, suggesting that repair is possible. This may be the basis for effective drug treatments in the future.

Symptoms
- Joint pain
- Joint gelling (stiffening and pain after immobility)
- Joint instability
- Loss of function.

Table 10.12 **Features of nodal OA**

Familial
Has a higher incidence in women
Typical pattern of polyarticular involvement of the hand joints
Develops in late middle age
Has a generally good long-term functional outcome
Associated with OA of the knee, hip and spine

Signs
- Joint tenderness
- Crepitus on movement
- Limitation of range of movement
- Joint instability
- Joint effusion and variable levels of inflammation
- Bony swelling
- Wasting of muscles.

Clinical subsets

Localized OA
Nodal OA (Table 10.12)
Joints of the hand are usually affected one at a time over several years, with the distal interphalangeal joints (DIPs) being more often involved than the proximal interphalangeal joints (PIPs). The onset may be painful and associated with tenderness, swelling and inflammation and impairment of hand function. The inflammation often occurs around the female menopause. PIP-predominant nodal OA has a superficial similarity to early rheumatoid arthritis. Even if a weakly positive rheumatoid factor is found, it is of no significance. The inflammatory phase settles after some months or years, leaving painless bony swellings posterolaterally – Heberden's nodes (DIPs) and Bouchard's nodes (PIPs), along with stiffness and deformity (Fig. 10.10). Functional impairment is slight for most, although PIP osteoarthritis restricts gripping more than DIP involvement. On X-ray, the nodes are marginal osteophytes and there is joint space loss.

Carpometacarpal and metacarpophalangeal OA of the thumb coexist with nodal OA and cause pain, which decreases as the joint stiffens. The 'squared' hand in OA is caused by bony swelling of the carpometacarpal joint and fixed adduction of the thumb. Function is rarely severely compromised.

Polyarticular hand OA is associated with a slightly increased frequency of OA at other sites.

Hip OA
Hip OA affects 7–25% of white adult Caucasians but is significantly less common in black African populations. There are two major subgroups defined by the radiological appearance. The most common is *superior-pole hip OA*, where joint space narrowing and sclerosis predominantly affect the weight-bearing upper surface of the femoral head and adjacent acetabulum. This is most common in men and unilateral at presentation, although both hips may become involved because the disease is progressive. Early onset of hip OA is associated with acetabular dysplasia. Less commonly, *medial cartilage loss*

compartment is most commonly affected and leads to a varus (bow-legged) deformity. There is often also retropatellar OA. Previous trauma, meniscal and cruciate ligament tears are risk factors for developing knee OA.

Primary generalized OA

This is less common than nodal OA of the hands but is usually seen in combination. It is also called 'nodal generalized OA' (NGOA). The other joints affected are the knees, first MTP, hip, and intervertebral (spondylosis). There is a female preponderance and a strong familial tendency. NGOA is associated with immune complex deposition and may have an autoimmune cause. Its onset is often sudden and severe.

Erosive OA

This is rare. The DIPs and PIPs are inflamed and equally affected. In contrast to nodal OA, the functional outcome is poor. Radiologically, there are marked subchondral cysts. Erosive OA may develop into RA and may not be a true subset of OA.

Crystal-associated OA

This is most commonly seen with calcium pyrophosphate deposition in the cartilage (chondrocalcinosis). *Chondrocalcinosis* increases in frequency with age, but is usually asymptomatic. The joints most commonly affected are the knees (hyaline cartilage and fibrocartilage) and wrists (triangular fibrocartilage). There is patchy linear calcification on X-ray (Fig. 10.11).

A chronic arthropathy (pseudo-OA) occurs, predominantly in elderly women with severe chondrocalcinosis. There is a florid inflammatory component and marked osteophyte and cyst formation visible on X-rays. The joints affected differ from NGOA – being predominantly the knees, then wrists and shoulders, but also elbows, ankles and hips. Chondrocalcinosis is associated with pseudogout, an acute crystal-induced arthritis (see p. 571).

Fig. 10.10 Severe nodal osteoarthritis. The DIP joints demonstrate Heberden's nodes. The middle finger DIP joint is deformed and unstable. The thumb is adducted and the bony swelling of the first carpometacarpal joint is clearly shown – 'the squared hand of nodal OA'.

occurs. This is most common in women and associated with hand involvement (nodal generalized OA – NGOA), and is usually bilateral. It is more rapidly disabling.

Knee OA

The prevalence of knee OA is 40% in individuals aged over 75 years. It is commoner in women than in men. There is a strong relationship with obesity. The disease is generally bilateral and strongly associated with *polyarticular OA of the hand* in elderly women. The medial

Fig. 10.11 Chondrocalcinosis of the knee. Note the linear calcification in the hyaline cartilage and calcification of the lateral meniscus (plus mild secondary OA).

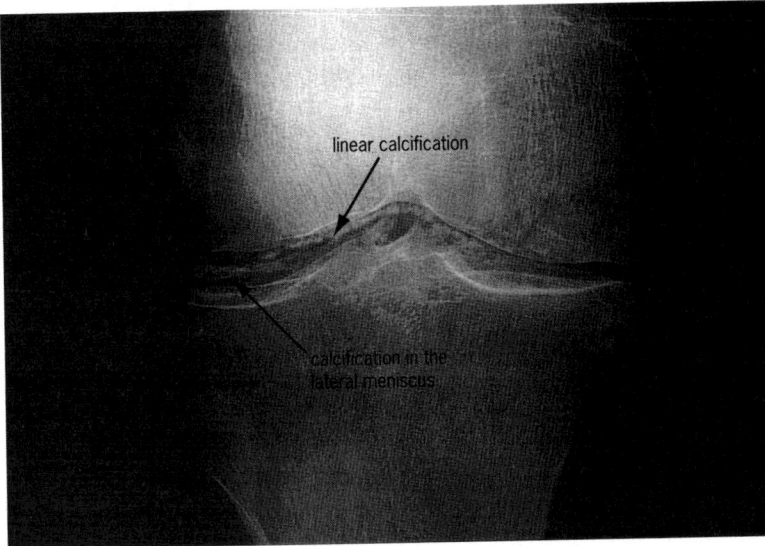

linear calcification

calcification in the lateral meniscus

A rare, rapidly destructive arthritis in elderly women, affecting shoulders, hips and knees, is associated with finding crystals of calcium apatite in a bloody joint effusion. The outlook is poor and joints require early surgical replacement.

Investigations in OA

- **Blood tests**. There is no specific test; the ESR and CRP are normal. Rheumatoid factor and antinuclear antibodies are negative.
- **X-rays** are abnormal only when the damage is advanced.
- **MRI** demonstrates early cartilage and subchondral bone changes.
- **Arthroscopy** reveals early fissuring and surface erosion of the cartilage.

Treatment

The guiding principle is to treat the symptoms and disability, not the radiological appearances; depression and poor quadriceps strength are better predictors of pain than is radiological severity in OA of the knee. Education of the individual about the disease and its effects reduces pain, distress and disability and increases compliance with treatment. Psychological or social factors alter the impact of the disease.

Physical measures

Weight loss and exercises for strength and stability are useful. Hydrotherapy helps, especially in lower-limb OA. Local heat, ice packs, massage and rubifacients or local NSAID gels are all used, although the value of NSAID gels is probably marginal.

Complementary medicine is commonly used and, despite lack of scientific evidence, little is lost in trying it since a number of patients do seem to be helped.

Medication

Balance the potential benefit against potential side-effects. Drugs usually should be used only in severe disease. Patients should be prescribed short courses of simple analgesics before NSAIDs (see Box 10.4). NSAIDs should be used intermittently. It has been suggested that some NSAIDs may increase the cartilage damage, while others are 'chondroprotective', but these claims remain unproven.

Intra-articular corticosteroid injections produce short-term improvement when there is a painful joint effusion. Frequent injections into the same joint should be avoided.

The role of chondroitin sulphate and glycosaminoglycan (sold as food supplements) is still under investigation and unproven. They appear to do no harm and some patients benefit.

Surgery

Total replacement arthroplasty has transformed the management of severe OA. The safety of hip and knee replacements is now equal, with a complication rate of about 1%; loosening, and late blood-borne infection are the most serious. Unicompartmental knee replacement is a less major procedure and appropriate for some patients.

These slight but definite risks make it essential that the patient is certain that surgery is wanted, when all else has been tried. For the vast majority, a total hip or knee replacement reduces pain and stiffness and greatly increases function.

Other surgical procedures include realignment osteotomy of the knee or hip, excision arthroplasty of the first MTP and base of the thumb, and fusion of a first MTP joint.

FURTHER READING
Brandt KD, Doherty M, Lohmander LS (eds) (1998) *Osteoarthritis.* Oxford: Oxford University Press.
Cicuttini F, Spector TD (1998) Osteoarthritis. *Medicine* **26**(6): 68–71.
Doherty M (2001) Risk factors for progression of knee osteoarthritis. *Lancet* **358**: 775–776.

INFLAMMATORY ARTHRITIS

Inflammatory arthritis includes a large number of arthritic conditions in which the predominant feature is synovial inflammation. This disparate group includes postviral arthritis, rheumatoid arthritis, seronegative spondyloarthropathy, crystal arthritis and Lyme arthritis. The diagnosis of these conditions is helped by the pattern of joint involvement (Table 10.13), along with any nonarticular disease; a past and family history may be helpful. The distribution of the affected joints (symmetrical or asymmetrical; large or small) as well as the periodicity of the arthritis (single acute, relapsing, chronic and progressive) may also help in the diagnosis.

Certain nonarticular diseases – for example, psoriasis, iritis, inflammatory bowel disease, non-specific urethritis or recent dysentery – may suggest a seronegative spondyloarthropathy. There may be evidence of recent viral illness (rubella, hepatitis B or parvovirus), of rheumatic fever, or of a tick bite and skin rash (Lyme

Table 10.13   Pattern of joint involvement in inflammatory arthritis

Diseases presenting as an inflammatory monarthritis
Crystal arthritis, e.g. gout, pseudogout
Septic arthritis
Palindromic rheumatism
Traumatic ± haemarthrosis
Arthritis due to juxta-articular bone tumour
Occasionally, psoriatic, reactive, rheumatoid may present as monarthritis

Diseases presenting as an inflammatory polyarthritis
Rheumatoid arthritis
Reactive arthritis
Seronegative arthritis associated with psoriasis or ankylosing spondyloarthropathy
Postviral arthritis
Lyme arthritis
Enteropathic arthritis
Arthritis associated with erythema nodosum

disease). In early arthritis it may not be possible to make a specific diagnosis until the disease has evolved.

There is a distinct genetic separation of rheumatoid-pattern synovitis and the seronegative group; RA (see below) is associated with a genetic marker in the class II major histocompatibility genes, whilst seronegative spondyloarthropathy shares certain alleles in the B locus of class I MHC genes, usually B27 (see p. 564).

In general the pain and stiffness of inflammatory arthritis are worse in the morning and after rest. This early-morning exacerbation may last several hours, in contrast to the much shorter post-rest gelling of OA. Inflammatory markers (ESR and CRP) are often raised in inflammatory arthritis, and there is often a normochromic, normocytic anaemia. Specific types of arthritis are discussed below.

RHEUMATOID ARTHRITIS (RA)

Rheumatoid arthritis is a chronic symmetrical poly-arthritis of unexplained cause. It is a systemic disorder characterized by chronic inflammatory synovitis of mainly peripheral joints. Its course is extremely variable and it is associated with nonarticular features.

Aetiology and pathogenesis

- *Geographical.* RA has a world-wide distribution and affects 0.5–3% (depending on the definition) of the population. It is a significant cause of disability and mortality and carries a high socio-economic cost.
- *Age.* RA presents from early childhood (when it is rare) to late old age. The most common age of onset is between 30 and 50 years.
- *Gender.* Women before the menopause are affected three times more often than men. After the menopause the frequency of onset is similar between the sexes, suggesting an aetiological role for sex hormones. The use of oral contraceptives may delay the onset of RA but does not reduce the risk of developing it.
- *Familial.* The disease is familial but sporadic. In occasional families it affects several generations. It is estimated to account for 50% of disease susceptibility.
- *HLA types.* There is a strong association between susceptibility to RA and certain HLA haplotypes. HLA-DR4, which occurs in 50–75% of patients, correlates with a poor prognosis, as does HLA-DRβ1* 0404/0401. The possession of a specific pentapeptide (QK/RAA) in the third allelic hypervariable region of HLA-DRβ1 increases susceptibility. Combined with a positive rheumatoid factor it identifies individuals with a 13 times greater risk for developing bone erosions in early disease.
- *Anti-CCP (anti-citrullinated cyclic peptide) antibodies* react with proteins where arginine has been replaced by citrulline. They predate the clinical disease by several years. They help distinguish early RA from transient polyarthritis.

Immunology

The chronic synovial inflammation may be caused by ongoing *T cell activation*. Alternatively it may be maintained by the local production of rheumatoid factors and *continuous stimulation of macrophages* via IgG Fc receptors. Considering the extent of synovial inflammation and lymphocytic infiltration, there are only minimal amounts of factors normally produced by T cells (interferon and interleukin-2 and -4). Conversely, the cytokines (IL-1, IL-8, TNF-α, granulocyte–macrophage colony-stimulating factor) and chemokines produced by macrophages (macrophage inflammatory protein (MIP) and monocyte chemoattractant protein (MCP)) and fibroblasts (producing IL-6) are abundant. Activated mast cells which release histamine and TNF-α may also play a role.

CD4-specific antibodies, when used therapeutically, produce a specific helper T-cell lymphopenia but do not significantly alter the disease, raising the possibility that T cells play a lesser role.

Temporary B cell ablation (a technique used for treating B cell lymphomas) induces remission, reinforcing the central place of rheumatoid factor production in maintaining the chronic inflammation of RA.

Antibodies to TNF-α, IL-1 or specific blocking agents produce marked short-term improvement in synovitis, indicating the pivotal role of these cytokines in the chronic synovitis (see p. 562). They also reduce the malaise felt in active RA.

Synovial fibroblasts have high levels of the *adhesion molecule*, vascular cell adhesion molecule (VCAM-1), a molecule which supports B lymphocyte survival and differentiation, and of decay accelerating factor (DAF), a factor that prevents complement-induced cell lysis. These molecules may facilitate the formation of ectopic lymphoid tissue in synovium. High-affinity antibodies are not a feature of RA, unlike other autoimmune diseases.

The triggering antigen remains unclear, although it is suggested that the glycosylation pattern of immuno-globulins may be abnormal in RA and lead to their becoming potentially antigenic. There is little evidence that collagen type II is the triggering antigen, although it is a cause of arthritis in animal models of RA.

Bacterial or slow virus infections have been implicated but are unproven. It has been suggested that an immune response to any pathogen is to produce autoantibodies by B cell clonal expansion. In susceptible individuals such clones may persist.

Pathology

Rheumatoid arthritis is typified by widespread persisting synovitis (inflammation of the synovial lining of joints, tendon sheaths or bursae). The cause of this is unclear, but the production of rheumatoid factors (RFs, see below) by plasma cells in the synovium and the local formation of immune complexes play a part. In RA, the normal synovium becomes greatly thickened to the extent that it is palpable as a 'boggy' swelling around the joints and tendons. There is proliferation of the synovium into folds and fronds, and it is infiltrated by a variety of inflammatory cells, including polymorphs, which transit through the tissue into the joint fluid, and lymphocytes and plasma cells. There are disorganized lymphoid follicles that are responsive to exogenous antigens. The normally sparse surface layer of lining cells becomes hyperplastic and thickened (Fig. 10.12). There is marked vascular proliferation. Increased permeability of blood vessels and the synovial lining layer leads to joint effusions that contain lymphocytes and dying polymorphs.

The hyperplastic synovium spreads from the joint margins on to the cartilage surface. This 'pannus' of inflamed synovium damages the underlying cartilage by blocking its normal route for nutrition and by the direct effects of cytokines on the chondrocytes. The cartilage becomes thinned and the underlying bone exposed. Local cytokine production and joint disuse combine to cause juxta-articular osteoporosis during active synovitis.

Fibroblasts from the proliferating synovium also grow along the course of blood vessels between the synovial margins and the epiphyseal bone cavity and damage the bone. This is shown by MRI to occur in the first 3–6 months following onset of the arthritis, and before the

Fig. 10.13 **X-ray of early RA**, showing typical erosions at the thumb and middle MCP joints and at the ulnar styloid.

diagnostic, ill-defined juxta-articular bony 'erosions' appear on X-ray (Fig. 10.13). This early damage justifies the use of DMARDs (see p. 561) within 3–6 months of onset of the arthritis. Low-dose steroids delay and anti-TNF-α agents halt or even reverse erosion formation. Erosions lead to a variety of deformities and contribute to long-term disability.

Rheumatoid factors (RFs)

These are circulating autoantibodies, which have the Fc portion of IgG as their antigen. The nature of the antigen means that they self-aggregate into immune complexes and thus activate complement and stimulate inflammation, causing chronic synovitis. Transient production of RFs is an essential part of the body's normal mechanism for removing immune complexes, but in RA they show a much higher affinity and their production is persistent and occurs in the joints. They may be of any immunoglobulin class (IgM, IgG or IgA), but the most common tests employed clinically detect IgM rheumatoid factor. Around 70% of patients with polyarticular RA have IgM rheumatoid factor in the serum.

The term seronegative RA is used for patients in whom the standard tests for IgM rheumatoid factor are persistently negative. They tend to have a more limited pattern of synovitis.

IgM rheumatoid factor is not diagnostic of RA, nor does its absence rule the disease out; but it is a useful predictor of prognosis. A persistently high titre in early disease implies more persistently active synovitis, more joint damage and greater disability eventually, and justifies earlier use of DMARDs.

(a)

(b)

Fig. 10.12 **Histological appearance of RA synovium.**
(a) Normal synovium. (b) Synovial appearances in established RA, showing marked hypertrophy of the tissues with infiltration by lymphocytes and plasma cells. From Shipley M (1993) *Colour Atlas of Rheumatology*, 3rd edn. Wolfe Mosby, with permission.

RF and the antibody to CCP (see p. 533) together are more specific, and anti-CCP indicates a worse prognosis.

CLINICAL FEATURES OF RA

Typical presentation

The most typical presentation of rheumatoid arthritis (approximately 70% of cases) begins as a slowly progressive, symmetrical, peripheral polyarthritis, evolving over a period of a few weeks or months. Women are affected three times more often than are men. The patient is usually in her thirties to fifties, but the disease can occur at any age. Less commonly (15%) a rapid onset can occur over a few days (or explosively overnight) with a severe symmetrical polyarticular involvement. These patients often have a better prognosis. A worse than average prognosis (with a predictive accuracy of about 80%) is indicated by being female, a gradual onset over a few months, and a positive IgM rheumatoid factor, and/or anaemia within 3 months of onset. The differential diagnosis of early RA is shown in Box 10.6.

Symptoms and signs

The majority of patients complain of pain and stiffness of the small joints of the hands (metacarpophalangeal, MCP), proximal and distal interphalangeal (PIP, DIP) and feet (metatarsophalangeal, MTP). The wrists, elbows, shoulders, knees and ankles are also affected. In most cases many joints are involved, but 10% present with a monarthritis of the knee or shoulder or with a carpal tunnel syndrome. The hips are rarely affected early in the disease.

The patient feels tired and unwell and the pain and stiffness are significantly worse in the morning and may improve with gentle activity. Sleep is disturbed.

The joints are usually warm and tender with some joint swelling. There is limitation of movement and muscle wasting. Deformities develop as the disease progresses. Nonarticular features develop (see below).

Other presentations

The presentation and progression of RA is variable. Presentations are shown in Box 10.7. Relapses and remissions occur either spontaneously or in response to drug therapy. In some patients the disease remains active, producing progressive joint damage. Rarely the process may cease ('burnt-out RA').

A *seronegative, limited synovitis* initially affects the wrists more often than the fingers and has a less symmetrical joint involvement. It has a better long-term prognosis, but some cases progress to severe disability. This form can be confused with psoriatic arthropathy, which

> ### Box 10.6 Differential diagnosis of early rheumatoid arthritis
>
> - Postviral arthritis – rubella, hepatitis B or parvovirus
> - Seronegative spondyloarthropathies
> - Polymyalgia rheumatica
> - Acute nodal osteoarthritis (PIPs and DIPs involved)

> ### Box 10.7 Typical presentations of rheumatoid arthritis
>
> - **Palindromic** – Monarticular attacks lasting 24–48 hours; 50% progress to other types of RA.
> - **Transient** – A self-limiting disease, lasting less than 12 months and leaving no permanent joint damage. Usually seronegative for IgM rheumatoid factor. Some of these may be undetected postviral arthritis.
> - **Remitting** – There is a period of several years during which the arthritis is active but then remits, leaving minimal damage.
> - **Chronic, persistent** – The most typical form, it may be seropositive or seronegative for IgM rheumatoid factor. The disease follows a relapsing and remitting course over many years. Seropositive patients tend to develop greater joint damage and long-term disability. They warrant earlier and more aggressive treatment with disease-modifying agents.
> - **Rapidly progressive** – The disease progresses remorselessly over a few years and leads rapidly to severe joint damage and disability. It is usually seropositive, has a high incidence of systemic complications and is difficult to treat.

has a similar distribution. There may be a family history of psoriasis or the patient may develop psoriasis later.

Palindromic rheumatism is unusual (5%) and consists of short-lived (24–72 h) episodes of acute monarthritis. The joint becomes acutely painful, swollen and red, but resolves completely. Further attacks occur in the same or other joints. About 50% go on to develop typical chronic rheumatoid synovitis after a delay of months or years. The rest remit or continue to have acute episodic arthritis. The detection of IgM rheumatoid factor predicts conversion to chronic, destructive synovitis.

Complications (Table 10.14)

Septic arthritis

This is a serious complication with significant morbidity and mortality. The joint (or joints) may be hot and inflamed with accompanying fever and a neutrophil leucocytosis in the blood. However, these signs are often absent, and any effusion, particularly of sudden onset, should be aspirated. *Staphylococcus aureus* is the most common organism. Treatment is with systemic antibiotics (see p. 571) and drainage.

Table 10.14 Complications of rheumatoid arthritis
Complications of the condition
Ruptured tendons
Ruptured joints (Baker's cysts)
Joint infection
Spinal cord compression (atlantoaxial or upper cervical spine)
Amyloidosis (rare)
Side-effects of therapy
See Table 10.15

Amyloidosis (see p. 1142)

Amyloidosis is found in a very small number of people with severe rheumatoid arthritis. RA is the most common cause of secondary amyloidosis. Primary amyloidosis causes a polyarthritis that resembles RA in distribution and is also often associated with carpal tunnel syndrome and subcutaneous nodules.

Joint involvement in RA

Hands and wrists

The impact of RA on the hands is severe. In early disease the fingers are swollen, painful and stiff. Inflamed flexor tendon sheaths increase functional impairment and may cause carpal tunnel syndrome. Joint damage causes a variety of typical deformities. Most typical is a combination of ulnar drift and palmar subluxation of the MCPs (Fig. 10.14). This leads to unsightly deformity, but function may be remarkably good once the patient has learned to adapt, and pain is controlled. Fixed flexion (buttonhole or boutonnière deformity) or fixed hyperextension (swan-neck deformity) of the PIP joints impairs hand function.

Swelling and dorsal subluxation of the ulnar styloid leads to wrist pain and may cause rupture of the finger

(a)

(b)

Fig. 10.14 **(a) Characteristic hand deformities in RA. (b) Early rheumatoid arthritis** – dorsal tenosynovitis of the right wrist and small joints of both hands with spindling of the fingers.

extensor tendons, leading in turn to a sudden onset of finger drop of the little and ring fingers predominantly, which needs urgent surgical repair.

Shoulders

RA commonly affects the shoulders. Initially the symptoms mimic rotator cuff tendonitis (see p. 538) with a painful arc syndrome and pain in the upper arms at night. As the joints become more damaged, global stiffening occurs. Late in the disease rotator cuff tears are common (see p. 538) and interfere with dressing, feeding and personal toilet.

Elbows

Synovitis of the elbows causes swelling and a painful fixed flexion deformity. In late disease flexion may be lost and severe difficulties with feeding result, especially combined with shoulder, hand and wrist deformities.

Feet

One of the earliest manifestations of RA is painful swelling of the MTP joints. The foot becomes broader and a hammer-toe deformity develops. Exposure of the metatarsal heads to pressure by the forwards migration of the protective fibrofatty pad (Fig. 10.15) causes pain. Ulcers or callouses may develop over the metatarsal heads and the dorsum of the toes. Mid- and hindfoot RA causes a flat medial arch and loss of flexibility of the foot. The ankle often assumes a valgus position. Appropriate broad, deep shoes are essential but rarely wholly adequate, and walking is often painful and limited. Podiatry helps and surgery may be required.

Knees

Massive synovitis and knee effusions occur, but respond well to aspiration and steroid injection (see p. 534). A

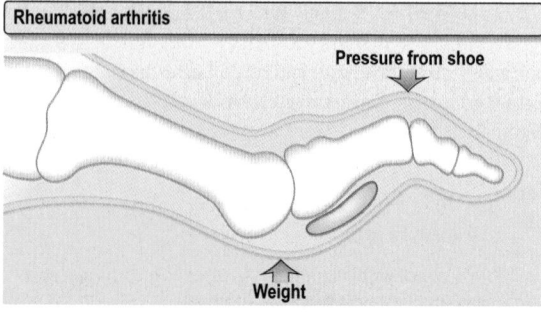

Fig. 10.15 **The toes in RA**, showing exposure of the metatarsal heads with forward migration of the soft tissue pad.

persistent effusion increases the risk of popliteal cyst formation and rupture (see p. 546). In later disease, erosion of cartilage and bone causes loss of joint space on X-ray and damage to the medial and/or lateral and/or retropatellar compartments of the knees. Depending on the pattern of involvement, the knees may develop a varus or valgus deformity. Secondary OA follows. Total knee replacement is often the only way to restore mobility and relieve pain.

Hips

The hips are rarely affected in early RA and are less commonly affected than the knees at all stages of the disease. Pain and stiffness are accompanied by radiological loss of joint space and juxta-articular osteoporosis. The latter may permit medial migration of the acetabulum (protrusio acetabulae). Later, secondary OA develops. Hip replacement is usually necessary.

Cervical spine

Painful stiffness of the neck in RA is often muscular, but it may be due to rheumatoid synovitis affecting the synovial joints of the upper cervical spine and the bursae which separate the odontoid peg from the anterior arch of the atlas and from its retaining ligaments. This synovitis leads to bone destruction, damages the ligaments and causes atlantoaxial or upper cervical instability. Subluxation and local synovial swelling may damage the spinal cord, producing pyramidal and sensory signs. MRI is the best way of visualizing this, but lateral flexed and extended neck X-rays can demonstrate instability. In late RA, difficulty walking which cannot be explained by articular disease, weakness of the legs or loss of control of bowel or bladder may be due to spinal cord compression and is a neurosurgical emergency. Image the cervical spine in flexion and extension in patients with RA before surgery or upper gastrointestinal endoscopy to check for instability and reduce the risk of cord injury during intubation.

Other joints

The temporomandibular, acromioclavicular, sternoclavicular, cricoarytenoid and any other synovial joint can be affected.

Nonarticular manifestations (Fig. 10.16)

Soft tissue surrounding joints

Subcutaneous nodules are firm, intradermal and generally occur over pressure points, typically the elbows, the finger joints and the Achilles tendon. They may ulcerate and become infected, but usually resolve when the disease comes under control. The nodules can be removed surgically or injected with corticosteroids if causing a problem. They tend to recur. Histologically there is a necrotic centre surrounded by rows of activated macrophages. This resembles synovitis without a synovial space.

The olecranon and other bursae may be swollen (*bursitis*).

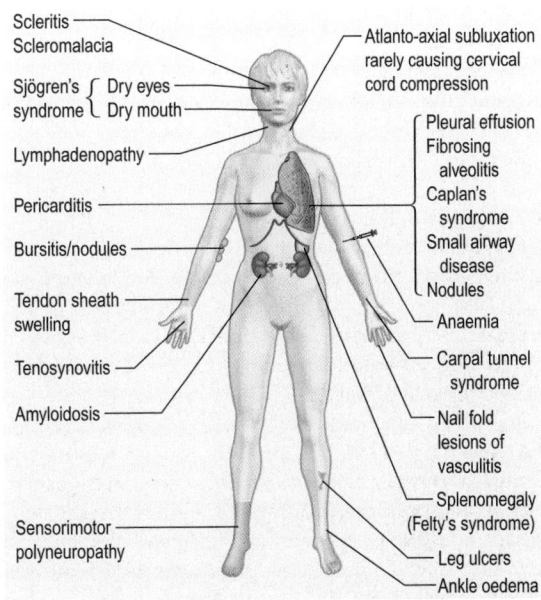

Fig. 10.16 **Nonarticular manifestations of RA.**

Tenosynovitis of affected flexor tendons in the hand can cause a trigger finger. Swelling of the extensor tendon sheath over the dorsum of the wrist is common.

Muscle wasting around joints is common. Muscle enzyme concentrations are normal; myositis is extremely rare. Corticosteroid-induced myopathy may occur.

Lungs (see also p. 937)

Peripheral, intrapulmonary nodules are usually asymptomatic but may cavitate. When pneumoconiosis is present (Caplan's syndrome), large cavitating lung nodules develop.

Other manifestations are:

- serositis causing pleural effusion
- pleural nodules
- fibrosing alveolitis
- obstructive bronchiolitis.

Vasculitis

Vasculitis (see p. 581) is caused by immune complex deposition in arterial walls. It is uncommon. Smoking is a risk factor. Other manifestations are:

- nail-fold infarcts due to cutaneous vasculitis
- widespread cutaneous vasculitis with necrosis of the skin (seen in patients with very active, strongly seropositive disease)
- mononeuritis multiplex (p. 1260)
- bowel infarction due to necrotizing arteritis of the mesenteric vessels (this may be indistinguishable from polyarteritis nodosa).

The heart and peripheral vessels

Clinical pericarditis is rare. In strongly seropositive RA, echocardiogram or post-mortem studies, however, show that 30–40% of patients have pericardial involvement.

Endocarditis and myocardial disease are rarely seen clinically, although found at post-mortem in approximately 20% of cases. These are secondary to vasculitis.

Raynaud's syndrome may occur (see p. 869).

The nervous system

Neuropathies, either mononeuritis multiplex or a sensory loss in a glove and stocking pattern, are due to vasculitis of the vasa nervorum. Compression neuropathies such as carpal or tarsal tunnel syndrome are due to local synovial hypertrophy. Atlantoaxial subluxation can cause serious neurological abnormalities.

The eyes

Scleritis and episcleritis occur in severe, seropositive disease and produce painful red lesions in the eye. Scleritis may lead to perforation of the eye (scleromalacia perforans) and requires active treatment with local and systemic corticosteroids.

Sicca syndrome causes dry mouth and eyes (see Sjögren's syndrome, p. 581).

The kidneys

Amyloidosis causes the nephrotic syndrome and renal failure. Presentation is with proteinuria. It occurs rarely in severe, long-standing rheumatoid disease and is due to the deposition of highly stable serum amyloid A protein (SAP) in the intercellular matrix of a variety of organs. SAP is an acute-phase reactant, produced normally in the liver. It is rare, and proteinuria in RA is more commonly due to DMARDs.

The spleen, lymph nodes and blood

Felty's syndrome is splenomegaly and neutropenia in a patient with RA. Leg ulcers or sepsis are complications. HLA-DR4 is found in 95% of patients, compared with 50–75% of patients with RA alone.

The lymph nodes may be palpable, usually in the distribution of affected joints. There may be peripheral lymphoedema of the arm or leg.

Anaemia is almost universal and is usually the normochromic, normocytic anaemia of chronic disease. It may be iron-deficient owing to gastrointestinal blood loss from NSAID ingestion, or rarely haemolytic (Coombs' positive). There may be a pancytopenia due to hypersplenism in Felty's syndrome or as a complication of DMARD treatment. A high platelet count occurs with active disease.

DIAGNOSIS AND INVESTIGATIONS

The diagnosis relies on the clinical features described above. The American College of Rheumatology (ACR) criteria are shown in Box 10.8 and are useful for epidemiological and investigative studies but are unhelpful in early disease.

Initial investigations include:

- **Blood count**. Anaemia may be present. The ESR and/ or CRP are raised in proportion to the activity of the

Box 10.8 Criteria for the diagnosis of rheumatoid arthritis (American College of Rheumatology, 1987 revision)

- Morning stiffness > 1 hour ⎫
- Arthritis of three or more joints ⎬ For 6 weeks or
- Arthritis of hand joints and wrists ⎭ more
- Symmetrical arthritis
- Subcutaneous nodules
- A positive serum rheumatoid factor
- Typical radiological changes (erosions and/or periarticular osteopenia)

Four or more criteria are necessary for diagnosis.

inflammatory process and are useful in monitoring treatment.
- **Serology**. Rheumatoid factor is present in approximately 70% of cases and ANA at low titre in 30%.
- **X-rays** of the affected joint(s) to establish a baseline. Only soft tissue swelling is seen in early disease. MRI demonstrates early erosions but is rarely warranted.
- **Aspiration of the joint** if an effusion is present. The aspirate looks cloudy owing to white cells. In a suddenly painful joint septic arthritis should be suspected (see p. 571).

Other investigations will depend on the clinical picture as outlined above. In severe disease extensive imaging of joints may be required. MRI is the technique of choice, especially for the knee and cervical spine.

MANAGEMENT OF RA (Box 10.9)

The diagnosis of RA inevitably causes concern and fear in the patient and requires a lot of explanation and reassurance. The doctor and therapist should retain a positive approach and remind the patient that with the help of drugs most will continue to lead a more or less normal life despite their arthritis; 25% will recover completely. The earliest years are often the most difficult and people should try to stay at work during this phase.

Box 10.9 Management of rheumatoid arthritis

- Establish the diagnosis clinically.
- Use NSAIDs and analgesics to control symptoms.
- Try to induce remission with i.m. depot methylprednisolone 80–120 mg if synovitis persists beyond 6 weeks.
- If synovitis recurs, refer to a rheumatologist to start sulfasalazine or methotrexate. Give a second dose of i.m. depot methylprednisolone.
- Refer for physiotherapy and general advice through a specialist team.
- If there is no significant improvement in 6–12 weeks as measured by less pain, less morning stiffness and reduced acute-phase response, use a combination of methotrexate and sulfasalazine.
- If no better, use an alternative agent, such as gold, d-penicillamine, leflunamide or anti-TNF-α therapy

Uncertainty about when the disease will remit and flare, when and if drugs will work, and whether they may produce side-effects, makes planning from day to day difficult. People learn to adjust remarkably but this takes time and support. A rheumatology unit will have a team, including doctors, specialist nurses and physiotherapists, to help the patient learn to cope. Leaflets give helpful advice, as do local patient groups. Patients from socially deprived backgrounds and smokers have a worse prognosis. Statins have been shown to be of benefit in reducing cardiovascular risk and possibly inflammation whatever the cholesterol level; more studies are required.

Drug therapy

There is no curative agent available for RA. Symptoms are controlled with analgesia and NSAIDs. Recent data support the use of DMARDs early in the disease to prevent the long-term irreversible damaging effects of inflammation of the joints, and TNF-α blocking drugs are revolutionizing the management of RA.

Non-steroidal anti-inflammatory drugs (NSAIDs)

Most patients with RA are unable to cope without an NSAID to relieve night pain and morning stiffness. NSAIDs do not reduce the underlying inflammatory process. They all act on the cyclo-oxygenase (COX) pathway (see Fig. 14.32). The individual response to NSAIDs varies greatly. It is desirable therefore to try several different drugs for a particular patient in order to find the best (see Box 10.4). Each compound should be given for at least a week. Start with an inexpensive NSAID with few side-effects and with which you are familiar. Regular doses are needed to be effective. The major side-effects of NSAIDs are discussed on page 549. If gastrointestinal side-effects are prominent, or the patient is over 65 years, add a proton pump inhibitor. Slow-release preparations (e.g. slow-release diclofenac, 75 mg, taken after supper), or a suppository at bedtime, usually work well and can be given in addition to daytime therapy if necessary. For additional relief a simple analgesic is taken as required (e.g. paracetamol or a combination of dihydrocodeine and paracetamol). Many patients need night sedation.

Disease-modifying anti-rheumatic drugs

(Table 10.15)

DMARDs, which mainly act through cytokine inhibition, reduce inflammation, as reflected by a reduction of joint swelling, a fall in the plasma acute-phase reactants and slowing of the development of joint erosions and irreversible damage. Their beneficial effect is not immediate (hence 'slow-acting agents') and may be partial or transient. The problem with many DMARDs is that their effect is often only partial, achieving between 20–50% improvement by ACR criteria for disease remission. Drugs which achieve 70% improvement are required and TNF-α blocking agents are close to achieving this goal in around 20% of patients. There is good evidence that

DMARDs control symptoms and signs of joint inflammation and that their withdrawal leads to a flare. Methotrexate, sulfasalazine, leflunamide, TNF-α blockers and ciclosporin have all been shown to reduce the rate of progressive joint damage in early and late disease.

Generally DMARDs are used after symptomatic treatment. However, in patients positive for RF and anti-CCP with a poor prognosis they should be used early, and certainly before the appearance of erosions on X-rays of hands and feet. The early use of depot injections of a corticosteroid at 6–12 weeks may induce remission. Studies of early RA suggest that intervention with DMARDs at 6 weeks to 6 months improves the outcome. The use of combinations of three or four drugs (steroids, methotrexate, sulfasalazine and hydroxychloroquine) in early RA (the inverted pyramid approach), reducing the number of agents once remission has been achieved, is more controversial and its long-term efficacy is yet to be proven. Toxicity appears to be reduced with such combinations, possibly because inflammation is controlled effectively. You must not overtreat people who are not going to develop erosions. Most prognostic assessments in early disease are only 80% accurate for risk of erosion and subsequent disability, and clinical judgement retains a central place in managing RA. DMARDs are usually prescribed by a rheumatologist (Table 10.15).

Sulfasalazine

This is a combination of sulfapyridine and 5-aminosalicylic acid. Sulfapyridine is probably the active component. It is well tolerated and for many is the first-choice DMARD, especially in younger patients. It produces a response in about half the patients in the first 3–6 months. Serious side-effects are rare, being mainly leucopenia and thrombocytopenia.

Methotrexate

This is considered by many to be the drug of choice. It should not be used in pregnancy. Conception should be delayed for at least 3 months off the drug for either partner. It is given at an initial weekly dose of 2.5–7.5 mg orally, increased up to 15–25 mg if necessary. It is well tolerated and this therapy can be introduced early in the disease. Nausea or poor absorption may limit its efficacy. It can be self-administered by subcutaneous injection. Oral folic acid should be given in addition to reduce side-effects, although it may marginally reduce efficacy. Full blood counts and liver biochemistry should be monitored carefully. It usually works within 1–2 months. More patients remain on this agent than on most other DMARDs, indicating that it is effective and has relatively few side-effects.

Leflunamide

This DMARD exerts an immunomodulatory effect by preventing pyrimidine production in proliferating lymphocytes through blockade of the enzyme dihydroorotate dehydrogenase. Most cells are able to bypass this blockade but T cells cannot – thus it has a specific effect to

Table 10.15	Disease-modifying anti-rheumatic drugs (DMARDs)		
Drug	**Dose**	**Side-effects**	**Monitoring**
Sulfasalazine (enteric coated)	500 mg daily after food, increasing to 2–3 g daily	Nausea	
		Skin rashes and mouth ulcers	
		Neutropenia and/or thrombocytopenia	Initial, fortnightly, then 4-monthly
		Abnormal liver biochemistry	Initial, monthly, then 4-monthly
Methotrexate	2.5 mg increasing to 25 mg weekly, orally or s.c.	Nausea, mouth ulcers and diarrhoea	
		Abnormal liver biochemistry	Initial, fortnightly, then monthly
		Neutropenia and/or thrombocytopenia	Initial, weekly, then monthly
		Renal impairment	Initial, then every 3–6 months
		Pulmonary fibrosis (rare)	Baseline chest X-ray
Leflunamide	100 mg daily for 1–3 days, then 20 (or 10) mg daily or 10–20 mg daily	Diarrhoea	
		Neutropenia and/or thrombocytopenia	Initial, then fortnightly; monthly at 6 months
		Abnormal liver biochemistry	Initial, then fortnightly; monthly at 6 months
		Alopecia	
		Hypertension	
TNF-α blockade Etanercept. Infliximab and adalimumab (used with methotrexate)	For use in specialist centre – central registry of patients	Infections including tuberculosis, septicaemia	See British Society of Rheumatology guideline
		Hypersensitivity reactions	Stop if no response after 3 months
Less commonly used			
Sodium aurothiomalate	10 mg test dose i.m., then 20–50 mg weekly Monthly with improvement	Skin rashes and mouth ulcers	
		Neutropenia and/or thrombocytopenia	Initial and with each injection
		Renal impairment	Test urine for blood/protein weekly
Hydroxychloroquine	200–400 mg daily, reduce to 5 days/week	Skin rashes	
		Corneal deposits	Test visual fields at 6 months and fundoscopy if abnormal
		Retinal damage (very rare before 6 years' therapy)	
D-penicillamine	125 mg, increasing slowly to 500–1000 mg daily before food	Nausea or loss of taste	
		Skin rashes and mouth ulcers	
		Neutropenia and/or thrombocytopenia	Initial, fortnightly, then monthly
		Renal impairment	Test urine for blood/protein weekly
		Lupus-like syndrome	
Azathioprine	25 mg, increasing to 150 mg daily (max 2.5 mg/kg/day)	Nausea	
		Neutropenia and/or thrombocytopenia	Initial, then weekly, then monthly
		Abnormal liver biochemistry	Initial, then monthly
Ciclosporin	2.5 mg/kg/day for 6 weeks, then 4 mg/kg/day. Reduce if creatinine doubles or BP rises	Renal impairment	Initial, then fortnightly, then monthly
		Hypertension	Initial, then fortnightly, then monthly
Anakinra	100 mg × 1 daily sc	Headache, infections, neutropenia	Initial, then monthly

block clonal expansion of T cells by slowing progression through the maturation phases G to S1. It is 80% absorbed by mouth and there is no significant interaction with food. It has a long half-life of 4–28 days. The loading dose is 100 mg daily for 1–3 days, then 20 mg daily (10 mg if diarrhoea is a problem). The main side-effects are diarrhoea, nausea, alopecia and rash. Diarrhoea diminishes with time. Blood monitoring is obligatory. Its onset of action is 4 weeks compared with 6 weeks for methotrexate. The initial response is similar to sulfasalazine but improvement continues and is better sustained at 2 years.

Leflunamide works in some patients who have failed to respond to methotrexate, or it can be administered with methotrexate to enhance the response. It is probably more effective when given without folate supplements. It needs a 'washout' of 2 years before conception (3 months in men) so is best avoided in premenopausal women.

Tumour necrosis factor (TNF-α), IL-1 blockers and new therapies
The availability of agents that block TNF-α has significantly changed the traditional use of DMARDs. They are

used after at least two DMARDs (usually sulfasalazine and methotrexate) have been tried (NICE guidelines).

- *Etanercept* is a fully humanized p75 TNF-α receptor IgG1 fusion protein given by subcutaneous injection. Around 65% of patients respond well. Some develop an injection reaction.
- *Infliximab* is a monoclonal antibody against TNF-α, given intravenously and co-prescribed with methotrexate to prevent loss of efficacy because of antibody formation.
- *Adalimumab* is a fully human monoclonal antibody against TNF-α given along with methotrexate.

These products slow or halt erosion formation in up to 70% of patients with RA and produce healing in a few. Patients often comment that their malaise and tiredness improve in a manner that is not seen with other DMARDs. They represent a major therapeutic advance in the treatment of RA and juvenile idiopathic arthritis. There is no evidence to date of increased tumour development. Some people become ANA positive and develop a reversible lupus-like syndrome. Reactivation of old TB may occur. These agents are extremely expensive when compared with traditional DMARDs and will cause funding problems for most healthcare systems even if they save costs in the longer term by reducing disability and the need for hospitalization. Their use should be restricted to specialist centres, and patients should be included in long-term cohort studies to unequivocally prove efficiency and to search for potential serious late-onset side-effects.

Anakinra is a human recombinant IL-1 receptor antagonist which, in combination with methotrexate, is licensed for use in RA.

Anti-citrullinated peptide has been shown to slow the development of RA erosions. Cytotoxic T-lymphocyte-associated antigen-4 (CTLA-4) is promising in trials.

Rituximab (p. 498), which causes lysis of B cells, has been shown to produce significant short-term improvement when used alone or in combination with cyclophosphamide or methotrexate.

Corticosteroids

The use of oral corticosteroids has a number of problems (Box 10.10). They are powerful disease-controlling drugs, but are avoided in the long term because side-effects are inevitable. Early intensive short-term regimens are used in some centres. Others use doses of 5–7.5 mg as maintenance therapy. There is some evidence that increased physical activity because of better symptom control reduces the risk of osteoporosis. Corticosteroids are also invaluable to patients with severe disease with extra-articular manifestations such as vasculitis.

Intra-articular injections with semicrystalline steroid preparations have a powerful but sometimes only short-lived effect.

Intramuscular depot injections (40–120 mg depot methylprednisolone) help to control severe disease flares, or can be used before a holiday or other life event, but should be used with caution and also infrequently.

> **i** **Box 10.10 Problems associated with the use of corticosteroids**
>
> - Patients are increasingly anxious about the use of corticosteroids because of adverse publicity about their potential side-effects. This must be discussed frankly and the risks of not using corticosteroids in treatment should be described and balanced against the risks of the drugs themselves.
> - Patients must be warned to avoid sugars and saturated fats and to eat less because of the risk of weight gain.
> - The skin becomes thin and easily damaged.
> - Monitor for diabetes and hypertension.
> - Cataract formation may be accelerated.
> - Osteoporosis develops within 6 months on doses above 7.5 mg daily, monitor with DXA scan and treat with calcium and vitamin D and bisphosphonate (see p. 597).

Drugs used less commonly

Gold (sodium aurothiomalate) is given by deep intramuscular injection. A test dose of 10 mg is followed by weekly doses of 50 mg until response occurs, usually in about 3 months. If there is no remission after a total dose of 1 g, treatment should be stopped. If a response is obtained, the interval between injections is increased to 4 weeks, continued for up to 5 years. Side-effects occur in a third of patients on i.m. gold. Rare side-effects include pulmonary fibrosis, colitis, polyneuropathy and cholestatic jaundice. Gold-induced glomerulonephritis can occur, particularly in patients who are HLA-DR3 positive, and routine urinalysis for proteinuria is performed.

The antimalarial, hydroxychloroquine is well tolerated. It is used alone in mild disease or as an adjunct to other DMARDs. Retinopathy is the most serious side-effect, but this is rare before 6 years of treatment. Patients should have 6-monthly checks of macular function with an Amsler chart, as retinopathy is irreversible.

D-penicillamine is given *before food* and for at least 3 months before improvement occurs. Penicillamine should not be continued if there is no improvement within 1 year. If proteinuria exceeds 2 g/24 h the drug must be stopped. Loss of taste is reversible. Other rare side-effects include a lupus erythematosus-like syndrome and a myasthenia gravis-like syndrome.

Azathioprine at a maximum dose of 2.5 mg/kg and cyclophosphamide 1–2 mg/kg have been used, usually when other DMARDs have been ineffective. They are often used when extra-articular features are severe, particularly with vasculitis. They are also used in patients who have been treated with corticosteroids and who have developed the severe side-effects of those agents.

Ciclosporin 2.5–4 mg/kg is used for active rheumatoid arthritis when conventional therapy has been ineffective. Side-effects include a rise in creatinine level and hypertension.

Physical measures

Patients with RA need constant advice and support from

physiotherapists and nurse specialists, especially while they are learning to adjust. A combination of rest for active arthritis and exercises to maintain joint range and muscle power is essential. Exercise in a hydrotherapy pool is popular and effective. Advice about managing activities of daily living despite the arthritis, and about gadgets, seating or structural changes in the home or at work are helpful.

Surgery

Surgery has a useful role in the long-term approach to patient management. Its main objectives are prophylactic, to prevent joint destruction and deformity, and reconstructive, to restore function.

Single-joint disease can be treated by surgical synovectomy to reduce the bulk of inflamed tissue and prevent damage. Excision arthroplasty of the ulnar styloid reduces pain and the risk of extensor tendon damage. Excision arthroplasties of the metatarsal heads reduce metatarsal pain and relieve pressure points. The major surgical advance has been the development of total replacement arthroplasty of the hip, knee, finger joints, elbows and shoulders. Such procedures need careful planning and preparation, and the expected outcomes and risks should be explained to the patient.

FURTHER READING

Buckley CD (2003) Why does chronic inflammatory joint disease persist? *Clinical Medicine* **3**: 361–366.

Choi HK, Hernán MA, Saegar JD, Robins JM, Wolfe F (2002) Methotrexate and mortality in patients with RA. *Lancet* **359**: 1173–1177.

Lee DM, Weinblatt ME (2001) Rheumatoid arthritis. *Lancet* **358**: 903–911.

O'Dell JR (2004) Therapeutic strategies for rheumatoid arthritis. *New England Journal of Medicine* **350**: 2951–2602.

Olsen NJ, Stein CM (2004) New drugs for rheumatoid arthritis. *New England Journal of Medicine* **350**: 2167–2179.

SERONEGATIVE SPONDYLOARTHROPATHIES

This awkward title describes a group of conditions affecting the spine and peripheral joints, which cluster in families and are linked to certain type 1 HLA antigens (Table 10.16).

The joint involvement is more limited than that seen in RA and its distribution is different. There are associated extra-articular and genetic features. These diseases occasionally present in childhood.

Histologically the synovitis itself is difficult to distinguish from that of RA, but there is no production of rheumatoid factors – hence 'seronegative'. Inflammation of the enthesis (junction of ligament or tendon and bone) and joint ankylosis develop more commonly than in RA.

Table 10.16 Seronegative spondyloarthropathies

Ankylosing spondylitis (AS)
Psoriatic arthritis
Reactive arthritis
Sexually acquired (Reiter's disease)
Post-dysenteric reactive arthritis
Enteropathic arthritis (ulcerative colitis/Crohn's disease)

All are associated with an increased frequency of sacroiliitis and an increased frequency of HLA-B27.

Aetiology

The common aetiological thread of these disorders is their striking association with HLA-B27, particularly ankylosing spondylitis (AS). This was the first demonstrated disease association of any HLA type (B27 is present in > 90% of Caucasians with AS but only 8% of controls). Its aetiological relevance remains unclear. The role of class I HLA antigens in pathogenesis is supported by the fact that HLA-B27 transgenic mice spontaneously develop arthritis, skin, gut and genitourinary lesions.

There are clues that infections play a role, possibly by molecular mimicry, with parts of the organism which are structurally similar to the HLA molecule triggering cross-reactive antibody formation. This is unproven. AIDS is increasing the prevalence of reactive arthritis and spondylitis in sub-Saharan Africa even in the absence of HLA-B27. The explanation for this changing epidemiology is unclear.

The types of arthritis that follow a precipitating infection are called reactive arthritis (p. 566).

The specialized immune systems of the gut and genitourinary mucous membranes may also play a causal role, perhaps reacting to local infections or to antigens which cross the damaged mucosa.

ANKYLOSING SPONDYLITIS (AS)

This is an inflammatory disorder of the spine affecting mainly young adults. The frequency of AS in different populations is roughly paralleled by the incidence of HLA-B27; Africans and Japanese have a low incidence of both HLA-B27 and ankylosing spondylitis, while the North American Haida Indians have a high incidence of both. There are at least 11 subtypes of HLA-B27 (B*2701–B*2711). Some appear to increase risk; others have a protective role. Twin studies indicate a much higher disease concordance in HLA-B27-positive monozygotic twins than in dizygotic twins. Other genetic loci appear to be involved. The disease occurs in men and women (2.5 : 1). It is milder in women, so men are more likely to present with symptoms of the disease (in a ratio of 4 : 1). There is lymphocyte and plasma cell infiltration and local erosion of bone at the attachments of the intervertebral and other ligaments (enthesitis). This heals with new bone (syndesmophyte) formation.

Box 10.11 Nonarticular problems in seronegative spondyloarthropathies

- Uveitis, in all types
- Cutaneous lesions in reactive arthritis (keratoderma blenorrhagica), histologically identical to pustular psoriasis
- Nail dystrophy, in psoriasis and reactive arthritis
- Aortitis, occasionally in AS and reactive arthritis

Clinical features

Episodic inflammation of the sacroiliac joints in the late teenage years or early twenties is the first manifestation of AS. Pain in one or both buttocks and low back pain and stiffness are typically worse in the morning and relieved by exercise. Initially the diagnosis is often missed because the patient is asymptomatic between episodes and radiological abnormalities are absent. Retention of the lumbar lordosis during spinal flexion is an early sign. Later, paraspinal muscle wasting develops. Spinal stiffness can be measured by Schoeber's test – a tape measure is placed in the midline 10 cm above the dimples of Venus. Any movement of a marker at 15 cm during flexion is recorded. A reading of less than 5 cm implies spinal stiffness. Individuals may be able to touch the floor with a stiff back if they have good hip movements but serial movement of the finger tip to floor distance highlights any change. Non-spinal complications (uveitis or costochondritis) suggest the diagnosis (Box 10.11). Costochondral junction inflammation causes anterior chest pain. Measurable reduction of chest expansion is due to costovertebral joint involvement.

Peripheral joint involvement is asymmetrical and affects a few, predominantly large joints. Hip involvement leads to fixed flexion deformities of the hips and further deterioration of the posture. Young teenage boys occasionally present with a lower-limb monarthritis (see p. 587).

Acute anterior uveitis is strongly associated with HLA-B27 in AS and related diseases and is occasionally the presenting complaint. Severe eye pain, photophobia and blurred vision are an emergency (see p. 1169). Overall clinical assessment is based on pain, tenderness, stiffness and fatigue using, for example, the Bath Ankylosing Spondylitis Disease Activity Index.

Investigations

- **Blood**. The ESR and CRP are usually raised.
- **HLA testing** is rarely of value because of the high frequency of HLA-B27 in the population, but may give supporting evidence in a difficult case.
- **X-rays**. The medial and lateral cortical margins of both sacroiliac joints lose definition owing to erosions and eventually become sclerotic (Fig. 10.17). The earliest radiological appearances in the spine are blurring of the upper or lower vertebral rims at the thoracolumbar junction (best seen on a lateral X-ray) caused by an enthesitis at the insertion of the intervertebral ligaments. These changes may eventually affect the whole spine. Persistent inflammatory enthesitis causes bony

Fig. 10.17 X-ray of ankylosing spondylitis. The sacroiliac joints are eroded and show marginal sclerosis (white arrows). There is bridging syndesmophyte formation at the thoracolumbar junction (black arrows).

spurs (syndesmophytes). Syndesmophytes are more vertically oriented than the beak-like osteophytes of spondylosis and the disc is preserved, unlike in spondylosis (see p. 541). Syndesmophytes cause bony ankylosis and permanent stiffening. The sacroiliac joints eventually fuse, as may the costovertebral joints, reducing chest expansion. Calcification of the intervertebral ligaments and fusion of the spinal facet joints and syndesmophytes leads to what is often called a 'bamboo' spine (Fig. 10.18).

Treatment

The key to effective management of AS is early diagnosis so that a regimen of preventative exercises is started before syndesmophytes have formed. Morning exercises aim to maintain spinal mobility, posture and chest expansion. Failure to control pain and to encourage regular spinal and chest exercises leads to an irreversible dorsal kyphosis and wasted paraspinal muscles. This, along with stiffening of the cervical spine, makes forward vision difficult.

When the inflammation is active, the morning pain and stiffness are too severe to permit effective exercise. An evening dose of a long-acting or slow-release NSAID or an NSAID suppository improves sleep, pain control and exercise compliance. Peripheral arthritis and

Fig. 10.18 **X-ray of bamboo spine in ankylosing spondylitis.** In advanced disease there is calcification of the interspinous ligaments and fusion of the facet joints as well as syndesmophytes at all levels. The sacroiliac joints fuse.

enthesitis are managed with NSAIDs or local steroid injections. Sulfasalazine or methotrexate may help the peripheral arthritis but there is little evidence that they control spinal disease.

TNF-α blocking drugs are effective in severe disease and help both spinal and peripheral joint inflammation in the short term. Relapse occurs on stopping therapy.

Prognosis

With exercise and pain relief, the prognosis is excellent and over 80% of patients are fully employed. The back may be stiff, but disability is minimal unless the hips are involved.

Most patients with AS are HLA-B27 positive and they should be made aware that they risk passing the gene to 50% of their children. HLA-B27 positive offspring then have a 30% risk of developing AS.

PSORIATIC ARTHRITIS (see also p. 1331)

The term 'psoriatic arthritis' describes a variety of different patterns of arthritis and enthesitis seen in people with psoriasis or with a family history of psoriasis. Five to eight per cent of individuals with psoriasis develop one of several different patterns of arthritis for which there is no serological marker. Activated CD4+ T lymphocytes appear to cause the lesions. Different subtypes of activated lymphocyte migrate to skin or joint, accounting for the skin and joint disease flaring at different times. There is compelling evidence that this is a reaction to organisms, such as group A streptococci, producing an autoimmune response in psoriatic skin plaques. These activated T lymphocytes release cytokines (interleukin 1, TNF-β and interferon).

Clinical features

The arthritis is typically more limited in distribution and less severe than in RA. The skin disease can be mild and may develop after the arthritis.

The most typical pattern of joint involvement in psoriasis is distal interphalangeal arthritis. It is unsightly, but rarely disabling, and there is often adjacent nail dystrophy. Cutaneous lesions, interphalangeal joint synovitis and tenosynovitis causing a 'sausage' finger or toe (dactylitis) are seen in pauciarticular psoriatic arthritis (and in reactive arthritis).

A seronegative symmetrical polyarthritis similar to rheumatoid arthritis also occurs.

Radiologically, psoriatic arthritis is erosive but the erosions are central in the joint, not juxta-articular, and produce a 'pencil in cup' appearance (Fig. 10.19).

Arthritis mutilans affects about 5% of patients with psoriatic arthritis and causes marked periarticular osteolysis and bone shortening ('telescopic' fingers) (Fig. 10.20), in which, despite the deformity, pain may be mild and function often surprisingly good.

Individuals with psoriasis may develop unilateral or bilateral sacroiliitis and typical AS, but with early involvement of the neck; only 50% are HLA-B27 positive.

Treatment and prognosis

NSAIDs and/or analgesics help the pain but they can occasionally worsen the skin lesions. Local synovitis responds to intra-articular corticosteroid injections.

In milder, polyarticular cases, sulfasalazine slows the development of joint damage.

When the disease is severe, methotrexate or ciclosporin is given because they control both the skin lesions and the arthritis. Anti-TNF-α agents, e.g. etanercept (see p. 563), are highly effective and safe for severe skin and joint disease. Corticosteroids orally may destabilize the skin disease and are best avoided.

The prognosis for the joint involvement is generally better than in RA.

REACTIVE ARTHRITIS

Reactive arthritis is a sterile synovitis, which occurs following an infection (see also post-streptococcal arthritis, p. 587).

Seronegative spondyloarthropathy develops in 1–2% of patients after an acute attack of dysentery, or a sexually acquired infection – non-specific urethritis (NSU) in the male, non-specific cervicitis in the female. In male patients who are HLA-B27 positive the relative risk is 30–50. Being HLA-B27 positive is not obligatory, however. Women are less commonly affected.

Aetiology

A variety of organisms can be the trigger, including some strains of *Salmonella* or *Shigella* spp. in bacillary dysentery. *Yersinia enterocolitica* causes diarrhoea and a reactive arthritis. In NSU the organisms are *Chlamydia trachomatis* or *Ureaplasma urealyticum*.

Fig. 10.19 **X-ray of psoriatic arthritis.** There is osteolysis of the metatarsal heads and central erosion of the proximal phalanges to produce the 'pencil in cup' appearance (circle). All the lesser toes are subluxed.

Fig. 10.20 **Hand showing psoriatic arthritis mutilans.** All the fingers are shortened and the joints unstable, owing to underlying osteolysis.

Bacterial antigens or bacterial DNA have been found in the inflamed synovium of affected joints, suggesting that this persistent antigenic material is driving the inflammatory process. Other environmental factors may explain why even in susceptible individuals, repeated infections do not necessarily produce a reactive arthritis. The methods by which HLA-B27 increases susceptibility to reactive arthritis may include:

- T cell receptor repertoire selection
- molecular mimicry causing autoimmunity against HLA-B27 and/or other self antigens
- mode of presentation of bacteria-derived peptides to T lymphocytes.

These are not mutually exclusive.

There are other organisms that also trigger reactive arthritis but have a different genetic basis; see post-streptococcal arthritis (p. 587), gonococcal arthritis (p. 572) and brucellosis (p. 572). In these, the borderline between reactive arthritis and septic arthritis is more indistinct and they can cause both.

Clinical features (Fig. 10.21)

The arthritis is typically an acute, asymmetrical, lower-limb arthritis, occurring a few days to a couple of weeks

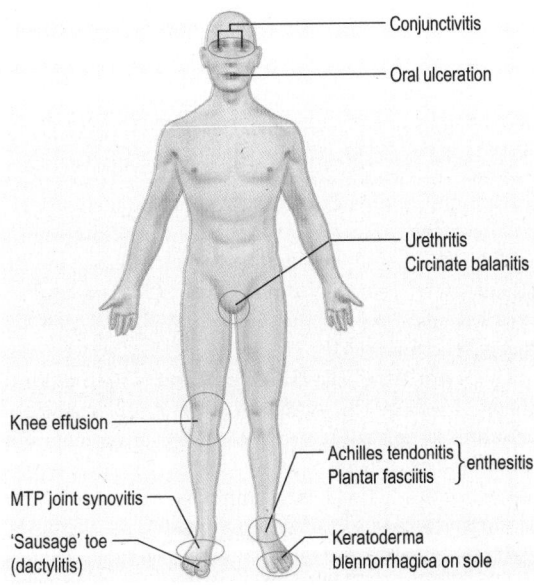

Fig. 10.21 **Clinical features of reactive arthritis.**

- Conjunctivitis
- Oral ulceration
- Urethritis / Circinate balanitis
- Knee effusion
- Achilles tendonitis / Plantar fasciitis } enthesitis
- MTP joint synovitis
- 'Sausage' toe (dactylitis)
- Keratoderma blennorrhagica on sole

after the infection. The arthritis may be the presenting complaint if the infection is mild or asymptomatic. Enthesitis is common, causing plantar fasciitis or Achilles tendonitis (see p. 546). Seventy per cent recover fully within 6 months but many have a relapse.

In susceptible individuals with reactive arthritis, sacroiliitis and spondylitis may also develop. Acute anterior uveitis may complicate more severe or relapsing disease but is not synchronous with the arthritis.

The skin lesions resemble psoriasis:

- *Circinate balanitis* in the uncircumcised male causes painless superficial ulceration of the glans penis. In the circumcised male the lesion is raised, red and scaly. Both heal without scarring.
- *Keratoderma blenorrhagica* – the skin of the feet and hands develops painless, red and often confluent raised plaques and pustules histologically similar to pustular psoriasis.
- *Nail dystrophy* may occur.

Other features

These include:

- bilateral conjunctivitis occurs in 30%
- the classically described triad of Reiter's disease – urethritis, arthritis and conjunctivitis.

Treatment

There is some evidence that treating persisting infection with antibiotics will alter the course of the arthritis, once it has developed. Cultures should be taken and any infection treated. Sexual partners may require specialist advice about, and treatment for, sexually acquired diseases.

Pain responds well to NSAIDs and local corticosteroid injections. The majority of individuals with reactive arthritis have a single attack which settles, but a few develop a disabling relapsing and remitting arthritis. Relapsing cases are sometimes treated with sulfasalazine or methotrexate (see Table 10.15). There is a likely but unproven role for TNF-α blocking agents in severe disease.

ENTEROPATHIC ARTHRITIS ASSOCIATED WITH INFLAMMATORY BOWEL DISEASE

Enteropathic synovitis occurs in approximately 10–15% of patients with ulcerative colitis and Crohn's disease (see p. 312). The link between the bowel disease and the inflammatory arthritis is not clear. Selective mucosal leakiness may expose the individual to antigens that trigger synovitis.

The arthritis is asymmetrical and predominantly affects lower-limb joints. An HLA-B27-associated sacroiliitis or spondylitis is seen in 5% of patients with inflammatory bowel disease and is independent of disease activity. The joint symptoms may predate the development of bowel disease and lead to its diagnosis.

Remission of ulcerative colitis or total colectomy usually leads to remission of the joint disease, but arthritis may persist even in well-controlled Crohn's disease.

Treatment

The inflammatory bowel disease should be treated (see p. 314). In all cases of enteropathic arthritis, the joint disease should be managed symptomatically with NSAIDs, although they may make diarrhoea worse. A monoarthritis is best treated by intra-articular corticosteroids. Sulfasalazine is frequently prescribed as this may help both bowel and joint disease. TNF-α blocking drugs are effective in inducing remission in Crohn's disease but not in ulcerative colitis.

FURTHER READING

Lebwohl M (2003) Psoriasis. *Lancet* **361**: 1197–1204.
Nuki G (1998) Ankylosing spondylitis, HLA B27, and beyond. *Lancet* **351**: 767–769.

CRYSTAL ARTHRITIS

Aetiology

Two main types of crystal account for the majority of crystal-induced arthritis. They are sodium urate and calcium pyrophosphate and are distinguished by their different shapes and refringence properties under polarized light with a red filter (Fig. 10.22). Rarely, crystals of calcium apatite (see p. 554) or cholesterol cause acute synovitis.

Neutrophils ingest the crystals and release pro-inflammatory enzymes from their phagosomes into the joint, thus triggering complement activation and attracting more neutrophils. Crystals may be found in asymptomatic joints. Why they initiate an attack is unclear. In pseudogout (p. 571), crystal shedding from the cartilage causes an attack.

GOUT AND HYPERURICAEMIA

Gout is an inflammatory arthritis associated with hyperuricaemia.

Epidemiology

The prevalence of gout in Europe and the USA is approximately 0.2%, although hyperuricaemia in this population occurs in about 5%. The prevalence of gout is increasing and is mainly seen in developed countries. Gout develops in men more than women (10 : 1) and rarely occurs before young adulthood (when it suggests a specific enzyme defect), and seldom in premenopausal females. The prevalence in older females is increasing with increased diuretic use. Hyperuricaemia is common in certain ethnic groups (e.g. Maoris).

Uric acid levels start to rise after puberty and are higher in men than in women until the female menopause. There is a normal distribution of serum uric acid in the population with a skewed distribution at the upper end of the range. Hyperuricaemia is defined as a serum uric acid level greater than two standard deviations from the mean (420 µmol/L in males, 360 µmol/L in females). This is close to the limit of urate solubility.

Fig. 10.22 **(a) Needle-shaped urate crystals**, viewed under polarized light with a red filter. **(b) A small intracellular pyrophosphate crystal**, viewed under polarized light with a red filter.

Most people with hyperuricaemia are asymptomatic. The range for gouty individuals is higher than for normals, but the curves overlap (Fig. 10.23). Serum uric acid levels increase with age, obesity, a high-protein diet, a high alcohol consumption (particularly beer drinkers), combined hyperlipidaemia, diabetes mellitus, ischaemic heart disease and hypertension. There is often a family history of gout.

Pathogenesis

Causes of hyperuricaemia are shown in Table 10.17. In many patients with gout there is no obvious cause. Hyperuricaemia is the major determinant for developing gout.

Uric acid levels in the blood depend on the balance between purine synthesis and the ingestion of dietary purines, and the elimination of urate by the kidney and

Table 10.17 Causes of hyperuricaemia

Impaired excretion of uric acid
Chronic renal disease (clinical gout unusual)
Drug therapy, e.g. thiazide diuretics, low-dose aspirin
Hypertension
Lead toxicity
Primary hyperparathyroidism
Hypothyroidism
Increased lactic acid production from alcohol, exercise, starvation
Glucose-6-phosphatase deficiency (interferes with renal excretion)

Increased production of uric acid
Increased purine synthesis de novo due to:
  Hypoxanthine-guanine-phosphoribosyl transferase (HGPRT) reduction (an X-linked inborn error causing the Lesch–Nyhan syndrome)
  Phosphoribosyl-pyrophosphate synthase overactivity
  Glucose-6-phosphatase deficiency with glycogen storage disease type 1 (patients who survive develop hyperuricaemia due to increased production as well as decreased excretion)
Increased turnover of purines due to:
  Myeloproliferative disorders, e.g. polycythaemia vera
  Lymphoproliferative disorders, e.g. leukaemia
  Others, e.g. carcinoma, severe psoriasis

Fig. 10.23 **Serum uric acid levels in normals and in patients with gout.** 7.9 mg/dL is equivalent to 474 μmol/L, 5.1 mg/dL is equivalent to 306 μmol/L. From Snaith ML, Scott JT (1977) *Annals of Rheumatic Disease*, with permission.

intestine. The body pool is about 1000 mg and 60% is turned over daily.

Uric acid synthesis. Uric acid is the last step in the breakdown pathway of purines. The last two steps, the conversion of hypoxanthine to xanthine and of xanthine to uric acid, are catalysed by the enzyme xanthine oxidase. Humans lack the enzyme uricase.

Uric acid excretion (Fig. 10.24). Uric acid is completely filtered by the glomerulus; 98–100% is then reabsorbed in the proximal tubule and 50% is secreted by the distal tubule. Some post-secretory reabsorption also takes place. Low-dose aspirin blocks urate secretion. High-dose aspirin also blocks its reabsorption, leading to increased

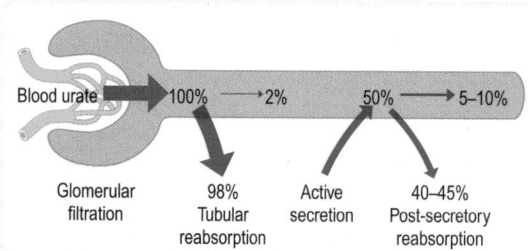

Fig. 10.24 Urate renal transport. The net result is that about 5–10% of the glomerular load is excreted in the urine under normal circumstances.

net excretion. Insulin resistance enhances urate resorption. Ninety per cent of patients with gout have impaired excretion of urate, 10% have increased production also and in less than 1% an inborn error of metabolism leads to purine overproduction. One-third of uric acid is eliminated in the faeces.

Clinical features

Hyperuricaemia causes four clinical syndromes:

- acute urate synovitis – gout
- chronic polyarticular gout
- chronic tophaceous gout
- urate renal stone formation (p. 649).

Acute gout presents typically in a middle-aged male with sudden onset of agonizing pain, swelling and redness of the first MTP joint. The attack occurs at any time, but may be precipitated by too much food or alcohol, by dehydration or by starting a diuretic. Untreated attacks last about 7 days. Recovery is typically associated with desquamation of the overlying skin. In 25% of attacks, a joint other than the great toe is affected.

In severe attacks, overlying crystal cellulitis makes gout difficult to distinguish clinically from infective cellulitis. A family or personal history of gout and the finding of a raised serum urate suggest the diagnosis but, if in doubt, blood and other cultures should be taken.

Chronic polyarticular gout is unusual, except in elderly people on long-standing diuretic treatment, in renal failure, or occasionally in men who have been started on treatment with allopurinol too soon after an acute attack.

Chronic tophaceous gout (see below).

Investigations

The clinical picture is often diagnostic, as is the rapid response to NSAIDs.

- **Joint fluid microscopy** is the most specific and diagnostic test but is technically difficult.
- **Serum urate** is usually raised (> 600 μmol/L). If it is not, recheck it several weeks after the attack, as the level falls immediately after an acute attack. Acute gout never occurs with a serum uric acid in the lower half of the normal range.
- **Serum urea and creatinine** are monitored for signs of renal impairment.

Treatment

The use of NSAIDs in high doses rapidly reduces the pain and swelling. Initial doses, taken with food, are:

- naproxen: 750 mg immediately, then 500 mg every 8–12 hours
- diclofenac: 75–100 mg immediately, then 50 mg every 6–8 hours
- indometacin: 75 mg immediately, then 50 mg every 6–8 hours.

After 24–48 hours, reduced doses are given for a further week. *Caution*: NSAIDs may cause renal impairment. In individuals with renal impairment or a history of peptic ulceration, alternative treatments include:

- colchicine: 1000 μg immediately, then 500 μg every 6–12 hours, but this causes diarrhoea
- corticosteroids: intramuscular or intra-articular depot methylprednisolone.

Dietary advice

The first attacks may be separated by many months or years and are managed symptomatically. Individuals should be advised to reduce their alcohol intake, especially beer, which is high in purines. A diet which reduces total calorie and cholesterol intake and avoids such foods as offal, some fish and shellfish and spinach, all of which are rich sources of purines, is advised. This can reduce serum urate by 15% and delay the need for drugs that reduce serum urate levels.

Treatment with agents that reduce serum urate levels

Only when the attacks are frequent and severe, despite dietary changes, or associated with renal impairment or tophi, or when the patient finds NSAIDs or colchicine difficult to tolerate should allopurinol be used. It should never be started within a month of an acute attack and always be started under cover of a course of NSAID or colchicine for the first 2–4 weeks before and 4 weeks after starting allopurinol.

Allopurinol (300–600 mg) blocks the enzyme xanthine oxidase, which converts xanthine into urate (see Fig. 15.11). It reduces serum urate levels rapidly and is relatively non-toxic but should be used at low doses (50–100 mg) in renal impairment. Skin rashes are the most common side-effect. Bone marrow suppression is very rare. Allopurinol may induce acute gout when it is first introduced.

Uricosuric agents are no longer routinely available. The angiotensin I-receptor antagonist, losartan, is uricosuric in hypertensive patients on diuretics.

Chronic tophaceous gout

Individuals with very high levels of urate can present with different clinical pictures. In chronic tophaceous gout, sodium urate forms smooth white deposits (tophi) in skin and around joints. They may occur on the ear, the fingers or the Achilles tendon. Large deposits are unsightly and ulcerate. There is chronic joint pain and sometimes superimposed acute gouty attacks.

Periarticular deposits lead to a halo of radio-opacity and clearly defined ('punched out') bone cysts on X-ray.

Tophaceous gout is often associated with renal impairment and/or the long-term use of diuretics. There may be acute or chronic urate nephropathy or renal stone formation. Whenever possible, stop the diuretics or change to less urate-retaining ones, such as bumetamide.

FURTHER READING
Terkeltaub RA (2003) Gout. *New England Journal of Medicine* **349**: 1647–1655.

PSEUDOGOUT (PYROPHOSPHATE ARTHROPATHY)

Calcium pyrophosphate deposits in hyaline and fibro-cartilage produce the radiological appearance of chondrocalcinosis (see p. 553). Shedding of crystals into a joint precipitates acute synovitis which resembles gout, except that it is more common in elderly women and usually affects the knee or wrist. The attacks are often very painful. In young people it may be associated with haemochromatosis, hyperparathyroidism, Wilson's disease or alkaptonuria.

Diagnosis

The diagnosis is made by detecting rhomboidal, weakly positively birefringent crystals in joint fluid, or deduced from the presence of chondrocalcinosis on X-ray. The joint fluid looks purulent. Septic arthritis must be excluded and joint fluid should be sent for culture.

The attacks may be associated with fever and a raised white blood cell count.

Treatment

Aspiration of the joint reduces the pain dramatically but it is usually necessary to use an NSAID or colchicine, as for gout. If infection can be excluded, an intra-articular injection of a corticosteroid helps.

INFECTIONS OF JOINTS AND BONES

Joints may become infected by direct injury or by blood-borne infection from an infected skin lesion or other site.

Chronically inflamed joints (e.g. in rheumatoid arthritis) are more prone to infection than are normal joints. Individuals who are immunosuppressed, by AIDS or by immunosuppressive agents, are particularly at risk, as are infants, the elderly and those who abuse alcohol. Artificial joints are also potential sites for infection.

SEPTIC ARTHRITIS

The organism that most commonly causes septic arthritis is *Staphylococcus aureus*. Other organisms include streptococci, other species of staphylococcus, *Neisseria gonorrhoeae*, *Haemophilus influenzae* in children, and these and other Gram-negative organisms in the elderly or complicating RA.

Clinical features

Suspected septic arthritis is a medical emergency. In young and previously fit people, the joint is hot, red, swollen, and agonizingly painful and held immobile by muscle spasm. In the elderly and immunosuppressed and in RA the clinical picture is less dramatic, so a high index of suspicion is needed to avoid missing treatable but potentially severely destructive septic arthritis. In 20% the sepsis affects more than one joint.

Investigations

- **Aspirate** the joint and send the fluid for urgent Gram staining and culture. The fluid is usually frankly purulent. The culture techniques should include those for gonococci and anaerobes.
- **Blood cultures** are often positive.
- **Leucocytosis** is usual, unless the person is severely immunosuppressed.
- **X-rays** are of no value in diagnosis.
- **Skin wound swabs, sputum and throat swab or urine** may be positive and indicate the source of infection.

Treatment

This should be started immediately on diagnosis because joint destruction occurs in days. The joint should be immobilized initially and then physiotherapy started early to prevent stiffness and muscle wasting. Intravenous antibiotics should be given for 1–2 weeks. It is usual to give two antibiotics to which the organism is sensitive for 6 weeks, then one for a further 6 weeks orally. Monitor clinically and with the ESR and CRP.

Empirical treatment in septic arthritis

This is started before the results of culture are obtained. Discuss the case with a microbiologist. Intravenous flucloxacillin 1–2 g is given 6-hourly, plus fusidic acid 500 mg orally 8-hourly. If the patient is allergic to penicillin, replace flucloxacillin with erythromycin 1 g i.v. 6-hourly or clindamycin 600 mg i.v. 8-hourly. In immuno-suppressed patients, flucloxacillin 1–2 g i.v. 6-hourly plus gentamicin (to cover Gram-negative organisms) should be used. Change the antibiotics if the organism is not sensitive. Drainage of the joint and arthroscopic joint washouts are helpful in relieving pain.

Management of infected prostheses

If chronically infected, the prosthesis is removed and the joint space filled with an antibiotic-impregnated spacer for 3–6 weeks before a new prosthesis is inserted. The whole process is covered by antibiotics.

Prognosis

Surgical drainage may be required if there is joint destruction and osteomyelitis. Patients can start weight-bearing as soon as the inflammation subsides. Resolution of the septic arthritis with complete recovery can occur in a few days or weeks. It may lead to secondary osteoarthritis (see p. 552).

SPECIFIC TYPES OF BACTERIAL ARTHRITIS

Gonococcal arthritis

This is the most common cause of a septic arthritis in previously fit young adults, more commonly affecting women and homosexual men.

Initially the patient becomes febrile and develops characteristic pustules on the distal limbs. Polyarthralgia and tenosynovitis are common at this stage and about 40% have a gonococcaemia. This phase settles and blood cultures usually become negative. Later, large-joint mon- or pauciarticular arthritis may follow. Culture is usually positive from the genital tract, although the joint fluid may be sterile. It is not clear whether this is simply a septic arthritis – although it responds rapidly to antibiotics – or whether there is also a reactive element to bacterial lipopolysaccharide.

Treatment consists of oral penicillin, ciprofloxacin or doxycycline for 2 weeks, and joint rest.

Tuberculous arthritis

Around 1% of patients with tuberculosis develop joint and/or bone involvement. It occurs as the primary disease in children. In adults, it is usually due to haematogenous spread from secondary pulmonary or renal lesions. The onset is insidious and diagnosis often delayed.

The organism invades the synovium or intervertebral disc. There are caseating granulomas and rapid destruction of cartilage and adjacent bone. Some patients develop a reactive polyarthritis (Poncet's disease).

A hip or knee (30%) is quite commonly affected, but around 50% develop spinal disease. The patient is febrile, has night sweats, is anorexic and loses weight. The usual risk factors for tuberculosis apply – debility, alcohol abuse or immunosuppression. HIV-positive/AIDS patients are at particular risk.

Investigations should include culture of fluid, and culture and biopsy of the synovium. *M. tuberculosis* is the usual organism, but atypical mycobacteria are occasionally implicated. A chest X-ray should be performed. Initially joint or spinal X-rays may be normal but joint-space reduction and bone destruction develop rapidly if treatment is delayed. MRI shows the abnormality earlier in the spine and MRI-guided biopsy from the affected disc is necessary to obtain cultures.

Treatment is as for tuberculosis (see p. 932). The joint should be rested and the spine immobilized in the acute phase.

Meningococcal arthritis

This may complicate a meningococcal septicaemia and presents as a migratory polyarthritis. Organisms can only rarely be cultured from the joint and most cases are due to immune complex deposition. Treatment is with penicillin.

Infective endocarditis

This may present with arthralgia, polymyalgia rheumatica-like symptoms or an infective arthritis. It is discussed on page 828.

Lyme arthritis

A person with Lyme disease (see p. 79) develops a fever and headache, and an expanding, erythematous rash called erythema chronicum migrans. About 25% of cases develop an acute pauciarticular arthritis. This usually resolves but 20% of untreated cases go on to develop a chronic arthritis. It is unclear whether this and other late manifestations are due to chronic infection or are antibody-induced.

Diagnosis is by the detection of IgM antibodies against the spirochaete *Borrelia burgdorferi*.

Treatment with antibiotics (amoxicillin or doxycycline) is highly effective in early disease. The response of chronic arthritis to antibiotic treatment may be delayed for months.

Brucellosis

Brucellosis (see p. 77) has a world-wide distribution. The most common cause of chronic brucellosis and of arthritis is *Brucella melitensis*. There is usually a peripheral mon- or oligoarticular arthritis, which may be septic or reactive. Arthritis is more common in chronic infections of more than 6 months.

Syphilitic arthritis

Congenital syphilis (see p. 123) can cause an acute painful epiphysitis or osteochondritis sometimes associated with para-articular swelling in the first few weeks of life. Later, at age 8–16 years, painless effusion of the knees may occur (Clutton's joints).

In acquired syphilis, arthralgia and arthritis occur in the secondary stage. Charcot's (neuropathic) joints usually involve the knees in tabes dorsalis (see p. 589).

Actinomycetes infection

Actinomycetes (see p. 90) can affect the mandible or vertebrae.

ARTHRITIS IN VIRAL DISEASE

A transient polyarthritis or arthralgia can occur before, during or after many viral illnesses. These include infectious mononucleosis, chickenpox, mumps, adenovirus, rubella, parvovirus B19, hepatitis B and C, arboviral infections and HIV. In most of these it is due to a direct toxic effect or immune complex deposition.

In *rubella* (see p. 52) the virus can occasionally be isolated from the joint. This arthritis occurs most commonly in up to 50% of young adult females a few days after rubella infection (6% of men). It is a symmetrical polyarthritis involving the MCP or PIP joints most commonly, but many joints can be affected. It closely resembles rheumatoid arthritis. IgM rubella antibodies are present. It resolves within a few weeks in most cases. A mild arthritis occurs rarely 2–4 weeks after rubella vaccination.

Parvovirus B19 (p. 48) causes an acute, self-limiting arthritis and is associated with erythema infectiosum ('slapped cheek disease').

In *hepatitis B infection* (see p. 366) a sudden symmetrical polyarticular arthritis of the small joints of the hands occurs in approximately one-third of patients, often in the prodromal phase and mostly resolving before the onset of jaundice. *Hepatitis C* causes type II mixed cryoglobulinaemia (see p. 628).

Arbovirus infections (see p. 52) which are endemic in many parts of the world give rise to an arthralgia and/or arthritis. For example, the Ross River virus has caused an epidemic polyarthritis in Australia and the South Pacific; it involves the small joints of the hands and clears in 2–4 weeks. Other viral infections causing epidemic arthritis include chikungunya (p. 53) and O'nyong-nyong (p. 52).

Musculoskeletal aspects of infection with human immunodeficiency virus (HIV) and acquired immunodeficiency syndrome (AIDS)

The clinical features seen in these patients are due to a number of causes such as opportunistic infections and drug therapy and are not usually caused directly by HIV. Infective arthritis seen in these immunosuppressed patients often has minimal symptoms and signs. Some of the antiviral agents cause an acute arthritis, possibly because of crystallization in the joint.

Arthralgia is common in AIDS. There is a seronegative, predominantly lower-limb arthritis, similar to psoriasis or Reiter's disease. Spondylitis also occurs but is not HLA-B27 associated. Avascular necrosis, possibly associated with corticosteroids or alcohol, is seen.

Nonarticular diseases such as Sjögren's- and lupus-like syndromes, systemic vasculitis of the necrotizing and hypersensitivity types and myositis also occur.

FUNGAL INFECTION

Fungal infections of joints occur rarely. Bone abscesses may be seen. Destructive joint lesions can also occur with blastomycosis. A benign polyarthritis accompanied by erythema nodosum occasionally occurs in coccidioidomycosis and histoplasmosis. Culture of purulent synovial fluid and skin tests for fungi may help the diagnosis.

BONE INFECTIONS

Acute and chronic osteomyelitis

Osteomyelitis can be due either to metastatic haematogenous spread (e.g. from a boil) or to local infection. Malnutrition, debilitating disease and decreased immunity may play a part in the pathogenesis.

Staphylococcus is the organism responsible for 90% of cases of acute osteomyelitis. Other organisms include *Haemophilus influenzae* and salmonella; infection with the latter may occur as a complication of sickle cell anaemia. The classic presentation is with fever and localized pain with overlying erythema. Diagnosis and treatment within a few days carries a good prognosis. Delayed treatment leads to chronic osteomyelitis. In chronic osteomyelitis sinus formation is usual. Subacute osteomyelitis is associated with a chronic abscess within the bone (Brodie's abscess). Symptoms may be limited to local pain.

Treatment of osteomyelitis is with immobilization and antibiotic therapy with flucloxacillin and fusidic acid. Surgical drainage and removal of dead bone (sequestrum) may be possible but recurrence is common.

Tuberculous osteomyelitis

This is usually due to haematogenous spread from a reactivated primary focus in the lungs or gastrointestinal tract. The disease starts in intra-articular bone. The spine is commonly involved (Pott's disease), with damage to the bodies of two neighbouring vertebrae leading to vertebral collapse and acute angulation of the spine (gibbus). Later an abscess forms ('cold abscess'). Pus can track along tissue planes and discharge at a point far from the affected vertebrae. Symptoms consist of local pain and later swelling if pus has collected. Systemic symptoms of malaise, fever and night sweats occur.

Treatment is as for pulmonary tuberculosis (see p. 932) together with initial immobilization.

FURTHER READING

Berendt T, Byren I (2004) Bone and joint infection. *Clinical Medicine* 4: 510–518.

Espinoza LR (ed.) (2003) Infections and rheumatic diseases. *Rheumatic Diseases Clinics of North America* 29(1).

Goldenberg DL (1998) Septic arthritis. *Lancet* 351: 197–202.

AUTOIMMUNE DISEASES (CONNECTIVE TISSUE DISORDERS)

Autoimmune diseases are conditions in which the immune system damages specific organs or causes systemic ill-health. Organ-specific autoimmune diseases include Graves' disease, Hashimoto's thyroiditis, pernicious anaemia and insulin-dependent diabetes mellitus. In most of the autoimmune rheumatic diseases it is thought that self-antigens provide the drive, although the trigger may yet prove to be exogenous. They are clinically diverse but are unified by the detection of non-organ-specific autoantibodies in the serum and various tissues. Rheumatoid arthritis (RA, see p. 555) is the most common autoimmune rheumatic disease.

Some of the diseases in this section, e.g. systemic lupus erythematosus (SLE), polymyositis and dermatomyositis and systemic sclerosis, are discussed because of their similar pathophysiology. They are sometimes referred to as connective tissue disorders.

SYSTEMIC LUPUS ERYTHEMATOSUS (SLE) AND LUPUS-LIKE DISEASES

SLE is an inflammatory, multisystem disorder with arthralgia and rashes as the most common clinical features, and cerebral and renal disease as the most serious problems.

Epidemiology

SLE occurs world-wide but the prevalence varies from country to country, with the most common prevalence of 1:250 being in African American women. In other populations the prevalence varies between 1:1000 and 1:10 000. It is about nine times as common in women as in men, with a peak age of onset between 20–40 years.

Aetiology

The cause is unknown but there are several predisposing factors:

- *Heredity*. There is a higher concordance rate in monozygotic twins (up to 25%) compared to dizygotic twins (3%). First-degree relatives have a 3% chance of developing the disease, but approximately 20% have autoantibodies.
- *Genetics*. There is an increased frequency of HLA-B8 and DR3 in Caucasians. There is a stronger association with HLA-DR2 in Japanese lupus patients.
- *Complement*. There is an inherited deficiency of C2 and C4 (which are in linkage disequilibrium with HLA-DR3 and DR2) in some patients. A functional deficiency of C_1q has been suggested.
- *Sex hormone status*. Premenopausal women are most frequently affected. In addition, SLE has been seen in males with Klinefelter's syndrome (XXY) (see p. 1064). In New Zealand mice, a lupus-like disease is ameliorated by oophorectomy or treatment with male hormones.

Immunological factors

Loss of 'self'-tolerance has several consequences:

- *B cell activation* results in increased autoantibody (mainly IgG) production to a variety (up to 2000) of antigens (nuclear, cytoplasmic and plasma membrane), e.g. ANA, anti-dsDNA.
- Development of and failure to remove *immune complexes* from the circulation leads to deposition of complexes in the tissue, causing vasculitis and disease (e.g. glomerulonephritis). Immune complexes also form in situ and this may play a role in glomerulonephritis, skin disease and possible cerebral involvement. Both renal and cerebral lupus are associated with high titre of anti-dsDNA.
- There is impaired *T cell regulation* of the immune response.

- There is *abnormal cytokine production* (IL-1 and IL-2), although its exact role in the pathogenesis is unknown. IL-6 and IL-10 levels are often raised.
- *TNF-α promoter polymorphisms* have also been linked to SLE and appear to be independent of susceptibility alleles.

Environmental triggers

Drugs such as hydralazine, methyldopa, isoniazid, D-penicillamine and minocycline can induce lupus not associated with anti-dsDNA (see below). Flare-ups can be induced by the contraceptive pill and hormone replacement therapy (HRT). Ultraviolet light is another well-recognized trigger, probably via increased apoptosis (see below). Viral aetiology has also been proposed. Increased cell turnover or immunological activation due to environmental agents may be a unifying mechanism.

Pathogenesis

Although much interest has been focused on immunological abnormalities in relation to lupus, there seems to be little wrong with the process itself but rather there is a failure to clear apoptotic material efficiently. Nuclear constituents, e.g. DNA and histones, are released from cells and their inefficient removal may lead to their being present in excess and possibly in some altered form. The nuclear material is then taken up by antigen-presenting cells and presented to T cells which in turn stimulate B cells to produce antibodies directed against nuclear antigens, e.g. Ro, La. The formation of some of these autoantibodies is due to proteases such as granzyme B which are active during apoptosis. Different subsets of autoantibodies may be related to the different clinical patterns.

Pathology

SLE is characterized by a widespread vasculitis affecting capillaries, arterioles and venules. Fibrinoid (an eosinophilic amorphous material) is found along blood vessels and tissue fibres. The synovium of joints may be oedematous and also contain fibrinoid deposits, which contain immune complexes. Haematoxylin bodies (rounded blue homogeneous haematoxylin-stained deposits) are seen in inflammatory infiltrates and are thought to result from the interaction of antinuclear antibodies and cell nuclei.

The pathology of lesions in other organs is described in the appropriate chapters.

Clinical features

SLE is extremely variable in its manifestations and most of the clinical features are due to the consequences of vasculitis. Mild cases may present only with arthralgia and fatigue, and can be difficult to diagnose (Fig. 10.25).

General features

Fever is common in exacerbations, occurring in up to 50% of cases. Patients complain of marked malaise and tiredness and these symptoms do not correlate with disease activity or severity of organ-based complications.

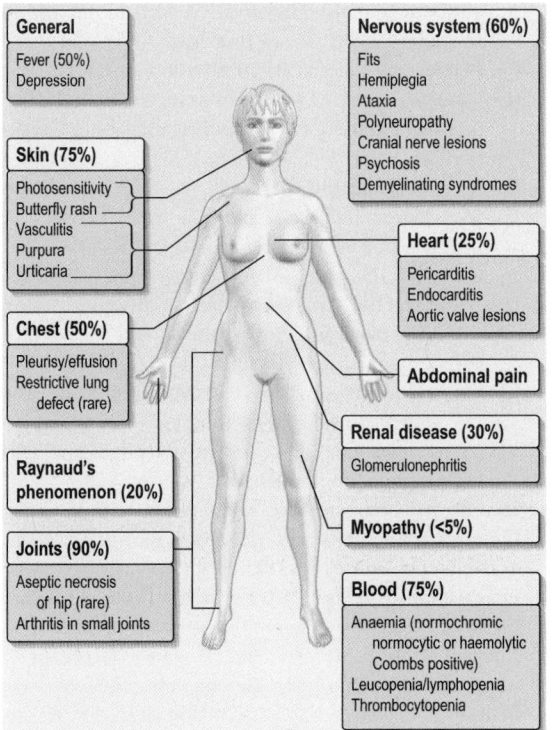

General	
Fever (50%) Depression	

Skin (75%)	
Photosensitivity Butterfly rash Vasculitis Purpura Urticaria	

Chest (50%)	
Pleurisy/effusion Restrictive lung defect (rare)	

Raynaud's phenomenon (20%)	

Joints (90%)	
Aseptic necrosis of hip (rare) Arthritis in small joints	

Nervous system (60%)	
Fits Hemiplegia Ataxia Polyneuropathy Cranial nerve lesions Psychosis Demyelinating syndromes	

Heart (25%)	
Pericarditis Endocarditis Aortic valve lesions	

Abdominal pain	

Renal disease (30%)	
Glomerulonephritis	

Myopathy (<5%)	

Blood (75%)	
Anaemia (normochromic normocytic or haemolytic Coombs positive) Leucopenia/lymphopenia Thrombocytopenia	

Fig. 10.25 Clinical features of systemic lupus erythematosus (SLE).

The joints and muscles

Joint involvement is the most common clinical feature (≥ 90%). Patients often present with symptoms resembling RA with symmetrical small joint arthralgia. Joints are painful but characteristically appear clinically normal, although sometimes there is slight soft-tissue swelling surrounding the joint. Deformity because of joint capsule and tendon contraction is rare, as are bony erosions. Rarely, major joint deformity resembling RA (known as Jaccoud's arthropathy) may be seen. Aseptic necrosis affecting the hip or knee is a rare complication of the disease.

Myalgia is present in up to 50% of patients but a true myositis is seen only in < 5%. Overlap connective tissue disease (p. 581) is likely if myositis is prominent.

The skin (see p. 1341)

This is affected in 75% of cases. Erythema, in a 'butterfly' distribution on the cheeks of the face and across the bridge of the nose (see Fig. 23.26) is characteristic. Vasculitic lesions on the finger tips and around the nail folds, purpura and urticaria occur. In one-third of cases there is photosensitivity, and prolonged exposure to sunlight can lead to exacerbations of the disease. Livedo reticularis, palmar and plantar rashes, pigmentation and alopecia may be seen. Raynaud's phenomenon (see p. 869) is common and may precede the development of arthralgia and other clinical problems by years.

Immunofluorescence of 'normal' non-sun-exposed skin, obtained on biopsy (for example from the buttock), will show immunoglobulin and complement deposition at the dermoepidermal junction (known as the positive lupus band test).

Discoid lupus is described on page 1343.

The lungs (see p. 938)

Up to 50% of patients will have lung involvement sometime during the course of the disease. Recurrent pleurisy and pleural effusions (exudates) are the most common manifestations and are often bilateral. Pneumonitis and atelectasis may be seen; eventually a restrictive lung defect develops with loss of lung volumes and raised hemidiaphragms. This 'shrinking lung syndrome' is poorly understood but may have a neuromuscular basis. Rarely, pulmonary fibrosis occurs, more commonly in overlap syndromes. Intrapulmonary haemorrhage associated with vasculitis is a rare but potentially life-threatening complication.

The heart and cardiovascular system

The heart is involved in 25% of cases. Pericarditis, with small pericardial effusions detected by echocardiography, is common. A mild myocarditis also occurs, giving rise to arrhythmias. Aortic valve lesions and a cardiomyopathy can rarely be present. A non-infective endocarditis involving the mitral valve (Libman–Sacks syndrome) is very rare. Raynaud's, vasculitis, arterial and venous thromboses can occur, especially in association with the antiphospholipid syndrome. There is an increased frequency of atherosclerotic disease in SLE. This partly reflects treatment with corticosteroids but it is likely that SLE itself, perhaps due to effects on endothelial cell activation or sustained elevation in inflammatory proteins, is an independent risk factor for macrovascular disease. Homozygosity for mannan-binding lectin variant (p. 201) is associated with an increased risk of arterial thrombosis in SLE. Trials to assess the benefit of intensive treatment of cardiovascular risk factors in SLE are underway. The benefit of statin therapy in the absence of significant hypercholesterolaemia remains to be proven.

The kidneys

The WHO classification of types of nephritis is on page 627. Autopsy studies suggest that histological changes are very frequent, but clinical renal involvement occurs in only approximately 30% of cases. All patients should have regular screening of urine for blood and protein. Proteinuria should be quantified and haematuria should prompt examination for urinary casts or fragmented red cells that suggest glomerulonephritis. Renal vein thrombosis can occur in nephrotic syndrome or associated with procoagulant antiphospholipid antibodies.

The nervous system

Involvement of the nervous system occurs in up to 60% of cases and symptoms may fluctuate. There may be a mild depression but occasionally more severe psychiatric disturbances occur. Epilepsy, migraines, cerebellar ataxia, aseptic meningitis, cranial nerve lesions, cerebrovascular disease or a polyneuropathy may be seen. The pathogenic mechanism for cerebral lupus is complex. Lesions may be due to vasculitis or immune-complex deposition, thrombosis or non-inflammatory microvasculopathy. The commonest finding on MRI scan is of increased white matter signal abnormality. In patients with cerebral lupus, infection should be excluded or treated in parallel with administration of corticosteroids and immuno-suppression.

The eyes

Retinal vasculitis can cause infarcts (cytoid bodies) which appear as hard exudates, and haemorrhages. There may be episcleritis, conjunctivitis or optic neuritis, but blindness is uncommon. Secondary Sjögren's syndrome may be seen in about 15% of cases.

The gastrointestinal system

SLE causes gastrointestinal symptoms, of which mouth ulcers are the commonest and may be a presenting feature. These may be painless or become secondarily infected and painful. Mesenteric vasculitis can produce inflammatory lesions involving the small bowel (infarction or perforation). Liver involvement is unusual, although lupoid antibodies are described in autoimmune hepatitis. Pancreatitis is uncommon.

Lupus variants

Chronic discoid lupus is a benign variant of the disease, in which skin involvement is often the only feature, although systemic abnormalities may occur with time. The rash is characteristic and appears on the face as well-defined erythematous plaques that progress to scarring and pigmentation (see p. 1343). Subacute cutaneous lupus erythematosus, a rare variant, is described on page 1344.

Drug-induced SLE is usually characterized by arthralgia and mild systemic features, rashes and pericarditis, but seldom renal or cerebral disease. It usually disappears when the drug causing it is stopped. Hydralazine and procainamide are the most likely causes, but other drugs have occasionally been implicated. Anti-histone antibodies are associated.

Overlap syndrome is discussed on page 581.

Antiphospholipid syndrome (see below) was originally described in SLE and the presence of antiphospholipid antibodies partially accounts for the increased tendency to thrombosis.

Investigations

- **Blood**:
  - (a) *A full blood count* usually shows a leucopenia, lymphopenia and/or thrombocytopenia. An autoimmune haemolytic anaemia occurs. The ESR is raised in proportion to the disease activity. In contrast, the CRP is normal.
  - (b) *Serum antinuclear antibodies* (ANA) are positive in almost all cases. Double-stranded DNA (dsDNA) binding is specific for SLE, although it is only present in 50% of cases, particularly those with severe systemic involvement (e.g. renal disease). Antinucleosome antibodies predate anti-dsDNA antibodies. Antibodies to RNA (ss and ds) anti-Ro and anti-La can also be detected.
  - (c) *Rheumatoid factor* is positive in 25% of the patients.
  - (d) *Serum complement levels* are reduced during active disease. Isolated C4 deficiency may be a genetic variant.
  - (e) *Anti-phospholipid antibodies*:
    - (i) *Anticardiolipin antibodies* are present in 35–45% of the patients.
    - (ii) *Anti β2-glycoprotein 1 antibodies* are also detected in vitro with pathogenic anti-phospholipid antibodies.
    - (iii) *Lupus anticoagulant tests* are often positive in association with anticardiolipin and other antiphospholipid antibodies.
  - (f) *Immunoglobulins* are raised (usually IgG and IgM) with a polyclonal pattern.
- **Histology**. Characteristic histological and immuno-fluorescent abnormalities are seen in biopsies from, for example, the kidney and skin.
- **Diagnostic imaging**. CT scans of the brain sometimes show infarcts or haemorrhage with evidence of cerebral atrophy. MR can detect lesions in white matter which are not seen on CT. However, it can be very difficult to distinguish true vasculitis from small thrombi.

Management

The disease and its management should be discussed, pointing out that the prognosis is much improved, though patients are advised to avoid excessive exposure to sunlight and should reduce cardiovascular risk factors.

Drug therapy should be used for active disease. There is no evidence that treatment in remission alters the progression of the disease.

- Arthralgia, arthritis, fever and serositis all respond well to standard doses of NSAIDs. Antimalarial drugs (chloroquine or hydroxychloroquine) (see Table 10.15) help mild skin disease, fatigue and arthralgias that cannot be controlled with NSAIDs. They have been shown to reduce the frequency of flares in SLE and are recommended in all but the mildest cases unless contraindicated. Patients should be warned about visual side-effects but self-monitoring of vision is sufficient for hyroxychloroquine unless there is other ocular pathology.
- Corticosteroids orally or as intravenous boluses are helpful, with dose determined by clinical severity. Immunosuppressive drugs such as azathioprine, cyclophosphamide or mycophenolate mofetil are essential for more severe disease (glomerulonephritis, vasculitis, cerebral disease or blood dyscrasias) and when the symptoms are poorly controlled.
- Newer therapies include anti-CD20 monoclonal antibodies, which are undergoing clinical trials. They deplete subpopulations of B lymphocytes.

Course and prognosis

An episodic course is characteristic, with exacerbations and complete remissions that may last for long periods.

These remissions often occur even in patients with severe organ-based disease. However, SLE can also be a chronic persistent condition. Earlier estimates of the mortality in SLE were exaggerated; 10-year survival rate is about 90%, although much lower if major organ-based complications are present. In most cases the pattern of the disease becomes established in the first 10 years; if serious problems have not developed in this time, they are unlikely to do so. The arthritis is usually intermittent but arthralgia and fatigue are often more persistent. Chronic progressive destruction of joints as seen in RA and OA occurs rarely, but a few patients develop deformities such as ulnar deviation. Increased frequency of macrovascular disease appears to be a significant problem for late-stage SLE.

Pregnancy and SLE

Fertility is usually normal except in severe disease and there is no major contraindication to pregnancy. Barrier methods of contraception rather than the pill are advisable. Recurrent miscarriages occur and these may be associated with antiphospholipid antibodies. Remission and exacerbations can occur during pregnancy with frequent exacerbations of the disease postpartum. The patient's usual treatment should be continued during pregnancy. Hypertension must be controlled. With severe renal disease and high antiphospholipid antibodies, fetal mortality is high (> 25%).

ANTIPHOSPHOLIPID SYNDROME

The antiphospholipid syndrome is associated with autoantibodies which have specificity for negatively charged phospholipids (see p. 534). A small proportion of these patients have SLE. Recurrent arterial and venous thromboses and miscarriages are the hallmark of the syndrome. The paradoxical association between a prothrombotic state and the presence of autoantibodies with in-vitro anticoagulant effects is not fully understood. However, β_2-glycoprotein (β_2GP1) (apolipoprotein H) undergoes a conformational change in the protein, exposing an antigenic epitope which has been identified as the target for both anticardiolipin antibodies and lupus anticoagulant. It is also associated with pathogenic antiphospholipid antibodies.

Clinical features

Arterial and venous thromboses

Approximately 20% of strokes occurring under the age of 45 years are thought to be due to the antiphospholipid syndrome. Thromboses of different types occur and cause other features of the disease, including the Budd–Chiari syndrome and Addison's disease.

Abortions

Twenty-seven per cent of women who have had more than two spontaneous abortions have the anticardiolipin syndrome. Antiphospholipid antibodies reduce the levels of annexin V, a protein with potent anticoagulant activity found in the placenta and vascular endothelium.

Other features

These include:

- thrombocytopenia
- chorea, migraine and epilepsy
- valvular heart disease
- cutaneous manifestations (e.g. livedo reticularis)
- positive Coombs' test.

The syndrome may also be involved in the development of accelerated atheroma.

Investigations

Anticardiolipin antibodies (detected by ELISA) are diagnostic. Lupus anticoagulant antibodies are found in coagulation assays (p. 534). The ESR is usually normal and antinuclear antibodies are usually negative.

Treatment

Current guidelines recommend aggressive anticoagulation for patients who have suffered thrombosis. High levels of antibody – especially IgG, and particularly if lupus anticoagulant or anti-β_2GP1 is positive – may warrant treatment even in the absence of thrombosis. Aspirin is most often prescribed, although clopidogel or warfarin is also used in some cases. Heparin and aspirin are given in early pregnancy, because warfarin is toxic to the fetus and because of the adverse effects of high-titre antibodies in pregnancy.

SYSTEMIC SCLEROSIS (SCLERODERMA)
(see p. 1343)

Systemic sclerosis (SSc) is a multisystem disease of unknown cause. It falls within the scleroderma spectrum of diseases but is distinct from the localized scleroderma syndromes that do not involve internal organ disease and are rarely associated with vasospasm (Raynaud's phenomenon). SSc has the highest case-specific mortality of any of the autoimmune rheumatic diseases. SSc occurs world-wide but there may be racial or ethnic differences in clinical features. For example, renal involvement is less frequent in Japanese cases.

The incidence of SSc is 10/million population per year with a 3:1 female to male ratio. The peak incidence is between 30 and 50 years of age. It is rare in children.

Environmental risk factors for scleroderma-like disorders include exposure to vinyl chloride, silica dust, adulterated rapeseed oil and trichlorethylene. Drugs such as bleomycin may also produce a similar picture. Although unusual, familial cases are reported and twin cohorts suggest higher concordance in monozygotic pairs, consistent with genetic determinants of aetiology.

Pathology and pathogenesis

Figure 10.26 shows the pathogenic interaction and mechanisms in systemic sclerosis.

Vascular features

An early lesion is widespread vascular damage involving small arteries, arterioles and capillaries. There is initial

Fig. 10.26 **Pathogenic mechanisms in systemic sclerosis.** EC, endothelial cell.

endothelial cell damage with release of cytokines including endothelin-1, the latter causing vasoconstriction. There is continued intimal damage with increasing vascular permeability, leading to cellular activation, activation of adhesion molecules (E-selectin, VCAM, ICAM-1) (Table 4.2, p. 198), with migration of cells into the extracellular matrix. Migrating lymphocytes are IL-2-producing cells, expressing surface antigens such as CD3, CD4 and CD5 (Table 4.7, p. 209). All these factors cause release of other mediators (e.g. interleukin-1, -4, -6 and -8, TGF-β and PDGF) (Table 4.5, p. 203) with activation of fibroblasts.

The damage to small blood vessels also produces widespread obliterative arterial lesions and subsequent chronic ischaemia.

Fibrotic features

Fibroblasts synthesize increased quantities of collagen types I and III, as well as fibronectin and glycosaminoglycans, producing fibrosis in the lower dermis of the skin as well as the internal organs.

Humoral immunity

Humoral immunity is also involved because at least 90% of patients have antinuclear antibodies (see below).

Clinical features

Raynaud's phenomenon

Raynaud's phenomenon is seen in almost 100% of cases and can precede the onset of the full-blown disease by many years, especially for limited cutaneous disease (see below).

Limited cutaneous scleroderma (LcSSc) – 70% of cases

This usually starts with Raynaud's phenomenon many years (up to 15) before any skin changes. The skin involvement is limited to the hands, face, feet and forearms. The skin is tight over the fingers and often produces flexion deformities of the fingers. Involvement of the skin of the face produces a characteristic 'beak'-like nose and a small mouth (microstomia). Painful digital ulcers and telangiectasia with dilated nail-fold capillary loops are seen. Digital ischaemia may lead to gangrene. Gastrointestinal tract involvement is common in this group. Pulmonary hypertension develops in 10–15% of this group and pulmonary interstitial disease may occur.

The CREST syndrome (Calcinosis, Raynaud's phenomenon, Esophageal involvement, Sclerodactyly and skin changes in the fingers, Telangiectasia) was the term previously used to describe this syndrome.

Diffuse cutaneous scleroderma (DcSSc) – 30% of cases

Initially oedematous in onset, skin sclerosis rapidly follows. Raynaud's phenomenon usually starts just before or concomitant with the oedema.

Diffuse swelling and stiffness of the fingers is rapidly followed by more extensive sclerosis which can involve most of the body in the severest cases. Later the skin becomes atrophic. Early involvement of other organs occurs with general symptoms of lethargy, anorexia and weight loss.

- Heartburn, reflux or dysphagia due to oesophageal involvement are almost invariable and anal incontinence occurs in many patients. Malabsorption from bacterial overgrowth due to dilatation and atony of the small bowel is not infrequent, and more rarely dilatation and atony of the colon occurs. Pseudo-obstruction is a known complication.
- Renal involvement may be acute or chronic. Acute hypertensive renal crisis used to be the most common cause of death in systemic sclerosis. ACE inhibitors and better care along with dialysis and renal transplantation have changed this.

- Lung disease, both fibrosis and pulmonary hypertension (PHT), contribute significantly to mortality in SSc. PHT can be isolated or secondary to fibrosis, and high plasma levels of endothelin-1 are seen.
- Myocardial fibrosis leads to arrhythmias and conduction defects. Pericarditis is found occasionally.

Sometimes these systemic features occur without skin involvement (*scleroderma sine scleroderma*). Overlap syndromes with additional features of SLE, RA or inflammatory muscle disorder occur.

Investigations

- **Full blood count**. A normochromic, normocytic anaemia may occur and a microangiopathic haemolytic anaemia is seen in some patients with renal disease.
- **Urea and electrolytes**.
- **Autoantibodies**:
  (a) *In LcSSc*: speckled, nucleolar or anticentromere antibodies (ACAs) occur in 70–80% of cases.
  (b) *In DcSSc*: there are antitopoisomerase-1 antibodies in 30% of cases, and anti-RNA polymerase (I, II and III) antibodies in 20–25%.
  (c) *Rheumatoid factor* is positive in 30%.
  (d) *ANA* is positive in 70%.
- **Urine**. Microscopy and, if there is proteinuria, a 24-hour urine collection for protein and creatinine clearance.
- **Imaging**:
  (a) CXR – used to exclude other pathology, changes in cardiac size and established lung disease.
  (b) Hands – deposits of calcium around fingers (in severe cases, erosion and absorption of the tufts of the distal phalanges – termed acrosteolysis).
  (c) Barium swallow generally confirms impaired oesophageal motility. Scintigraphy, manometry and upper GI endoscopy are also valuable.
  (d) High-resolution CT – to demonstrate fibrotic lung involvement. This should be performed prone to exclude dependent fluid changes mimicking very early bibasal fibrosis.
- Other investigations of gastrointestinal tract (e.g. see Fig. 6.4, p. 274), lung, renal and cardiac as appropriate.

Management

Treatment should be organ-based in order to try to control the disease. Currently there is no cure.

- Education, counselling and family support are essential.
- Regular exercises and skin lubricants may limit contractures.
- Raynaud's may be improved by hand warmers, oral vasodilators (calcium-channel blockers, ACE inhibitors) and parenteral vasodilators (prostacyclin analogues and calcitonin gene-related peptide). Lumbar sympathectomy can help foot symptoms. Radical microarteriolysis (digital sympathectomy) is indicated in severe digital ischaemia.
- Oesophageal symptoms can almost always be improved by proton-pump inhibitors, and prokinetic drugs are also helpful.
- Symptomatic malabsorption requires nutritional supplements and rotational antibiotics (see p. 304) to treat small intestinal bacterial overgrowth.
- Renal involvement requires intensive control of hypertension. First drug of choice is an ACE inhibitor. Vigilance for hypertensive scleroderma renal crisis (SRC) is critical, especially in early-stage dcSSc with rapidly progressive skin and tendon friction rubs. High-dose corticosteroids (above 10 mg prednisolone daily) may increase the risk of SRC.
- Intermittent or short-term continuous intravenous prostacyclin may be helpful for severe Raynaud's, digital ulceration, critical digital ischaemia.
- Pulmonary hypertension is treated with oral vasodilators, oxygen, warfarin. Advanced cases should receive prostacyclin therapy (inhaled, subcutaneous or intravenous) or the oral endothelin-receptor antagonist bosentan. Right heart failure is treated conventionally and transplantation (heart–lung or single lung) should be considered in eligible cases.
- Pulmonary fibrosis is currently treated with immunosuppression, most often with cyclophosphamide or azathioprine combined with low-dose oral prednisolone.
- No effective anti-fibrotic therapies are yet of proven efficacy.

Prognosis

In limited cutaneous scleroderma the disease is often milder, with much less severe internal organ involvement and a 70% 10-year survival. Pulmonary hypertension is a significant later cause of death. Lung fibrosis and severe gut involvement also determine mortality. In diffuse disease, where organ involvement is often severe at an earlier stage, many patients die of pulmonary, cardiac or renal involvement. Overall, pulmonary involvement (vascular or interstitial) accounts for around 50% of scleroderma-related deaths.

Localized forms of scleroderma occur either in patches (morphoea, p. 1343) or linear forms. These are more commonly seen in children and adolescents and do not convert into systemic forms, although ANA may occur in localized scleroderma and very occasionally there is coexistence of localized and systemic forms.

POLYMYOSITIS (PM) AND DERMATOMYOSITIS (DM)

Polymyositis is a rare disorder of unknown cause, in which the clinical picture is dominated by inflammation of striated muscle, causing proximal muscle weakness. When the skin is involved it is called 'dermatomyositis'. These are rare disorders (incidence 2–10/million population per annum) and occur in all races and at all ages. The aetiology is unknown, although viruses (e.g. Coxsackie, rubella, influenza) have been implicated and persons with HLA-B8/DR3 appear to be genetically predisposed.

Clinical features

The clinical subsets are:

- adult polymyositis
- adult dermatomyositis
- adult polymyositis, dermatomyositis with malignancies
- PM/DM in association with other connective tissue diseases
- childhood DM.

Adult polymyositis

Women are affected three times more commonly than men.

The onset can be insidious, over months, but can be acute. General malaise, weight loss and fever can develop during the acute phase.

The major feature of polymyositis is proximal muscle weakness which is progressive. There is wasting of the shoulder and pelvic girdle muscles with weakness. Pain and tenderness are uncommon features. Involvement of pharyngeal, laryngeal and respiratory muscles can lead to dysphagia, dysphonia and respiratory failure. The changes can occur at a frightening speed but are often less rapid. Patients have difficulty squatting, going up stairs, rising from a chair, raising their hands above the head and holding their head up.

Respiratory muscles are affected in severe disease and this compounds the effects of interstitial fibrosis (especially in those with anti-Jo-1 antibodies) and patients may require ventilation. Dysphagia is seen in about 50% owing to oesophageal muscle involvement. Arthralgia is seen in about 25% but is mild and Raynaud's phenomenon occurs in some patients. Antibodies to Jo-1 and other t-RNA synthetases are associated and may predict worse outcome. Hardening and fissuring of skin over the pulp surface of the fingers (mechanic's hands) is typical.

Adult dermatomyositis

This also is more common in women.

Cutaneous features include a heliotrope (purple) discoloration of the eyelids and periorbital oedema. Scaly, purple-red raised vasculitic patches occur over the extensor surfaces of joints and fingers (collodion patches). Ulcerative vasculitis and calcinosis of the subcutaneous tissue occurs in 25% of cases. Muscle weakness is common. Myalgia, polyarthritis and Raynaud's phenomenon occur in this group. In the long term, muscle fibrosis and contractures of joints occur.

Associated with other connective tissue diseases

There is an association with other autoimmune rheumatic diseases (e.g. SLE, RA and systemic sclerosis) with their associated clinical features such as deforming arthritis, malar rash and skin sclerosis.

Association with malignancies

The relative risk of cancer is 2.4 for male and 3.4 for female patients, and a wide variety of cancers have been reported. The onset and clinical picture does not differ from that of typical DM/PM. The associated cancer may not become apparent for 2–3 years, and recurrent or refractory dermatomyositis should prompt a search for occult malignancy.

There is also an association with malignancy (e.g. lung, ovary, breast, stomach), which can predate the onset of myositis. This occurs particularly in males with dermatomyositis.

Childhood dermatomyositis

This most commonly affects children between the ages of 4 and 10 years. The typical rash of dermatomyositis is usually accompanied by muscle weakness. Muscle atrophy, subcutaneous calcification and contractures may be widespread and severe. Ulcerative skin vasculitis is common and recurrent abdominal pain due to vasculitis is also a feature.

Investigations

- **Serum creatine kinase (CK)**, aminotransferases and aldolase are usually raised and are useful guides to the muscle damage but may not reflect activity.
- **The ESR** is raised in about 5% of cases.
- **Serum autoantibody studies**. Antinuclear antibody testing is commonly positive in patients with dermatomyositis. Rheumatoid factor is present in up to 50% and many myositis-specific antibodies (MSAs) have been recognized and correlate with certain subsets. Antibodies to Jo-1 (antibodies to histidyl tRNA synthase) are predictive of pulmonary fibrosis but are rarely seen in patients with dermatomyositis.
- **Electromyography** (EMG) shows a typical triad of changes with myositis: spontaneous fibrillation potentials at rest; polyphasic or short-duration potentials on voluntary contraction; and salvos of repetitive potentials on mechanical stimulation of the nerve.
- **MRI** can be used to detect abnormal muscle.
- **Needle muscle biopsy** shows fibre necrosis and regeneration in association with an inflammatory cell infiltrate with lymphocytes around the blood vessels and between muscle fibres. Open biopsy allows more thorough assessment.
- **Screening for malignancy** is usually limited to relatively non-invasive investigation such as CXR mammography, pelvic/abnormal ultrasound, urine microscopy and a search for circulating tumour markers.

Treatment

Bed rest is usually helpful but must be combined with an exercise programme. Prednisolone is the mainstay of treatment; 0.5–1.0 mg/kg bodyweight as initial therapy given for at least 1 month after myositis has become clinically and enzymatically inactive. Tapering of steroids must be slow. Early intervention with steroid-sparing agents such as methotrexate, azathioprine, ciclosporin, cyclophosphamide and mycophenolate mofetil is common. Intravenous immunoglobulin therapy (IVIG) is helpful in some recalcitrant cases.

SJÖGREN'S SYNDROME AND KERATOCONJUNCTIVITIS SICCA

The syndrome of dry eyes (keratoconjunctivitis sicca) in the absence of rheumatoid arthritis or any of the auto-immune diseases is known as 'primary Sjögren's syndrome'. There is an association with HLA-B8/DR3. Dryness of the mouth, skin or vagina may also be a problem. Salivary and parotid gland enlargement is seen.

Associated systemic features include:

- arthralgia and occasional non-progressive polyarthritis, like that seen in SLE (but much less common)
- Raynaud's phenomenon
- dysphagia and abnormal oesophageal motility as seen in systemic sclerosis (but less common)
- other organ-specific autoimmune disease, including thyroid disease, myasthenia gravis, primary biliary cirrhosis and autoimmune hepatitis
- renal tubular defects (uncommon) causing nephrogenic diabetes insipidus and renal tubular acidosis
- pulmonary diffusion defects and fibrosis
- polyneuropathy, fits and depression
- vasculitis
- increased incidence of non-Hodgkin's B cell lymphoma.

Pathology and investigations

Biopsies of the salivary gland or of the lip show a focal infiltration of lymphocytes and plasma cells.

- **Schirmer tear test**. This is a standard strip of filter paper placed on the inside of the lower eyelid; wetting of < 10 mm in 5 minutes indicates defective tear production.
- **Rose Bengal staining** of the eyes shows punctate or filamentary keratitis.
- **Laboratory abnormalities**. These include raised immunoglobulin levels, circulating immune complexes and many autoantibodies. Rheumatoid factor is usually positive. Antinuclear antibodies are found in 60–70% of cases and antimitochondrial antibodies in 10%. Anti-Ro (SSA) antibodies are found in 70%, compared with 10% of cases of RA and secondary Sjögren's syndrome. This antibody is of particular interest because it can cross the placenta and cause congenital heart block.

Treatment is with artificial tears and saliva-replacement solutions.

'OVERLAP' SYNDROME AND UNDIFFERENTIATED CONNECTIVE TISSUE DISEASE

Patients may present with varied clinical and serologic features not within the accepted boundaries of a single disease entity but sufficiently differentiated to fit more than one diagnosis. Those that have unequivocal evidence for a connective tissue disease but demonstrate features that cross classification criteria for two or more conditions such as SLE, PM, RA or SSc are described as overlap syndromes. Many cases that were previously labelled mixed connective tissue disease (MCTD) are probably better termed overlap connective tissue disease. Some patients demonstrate clinical features suggesting a connective tissue disease such as Raynaud's phenomenon, arthralgia, rash or serological abnormalities including positive ANA. However, they may fail to fulfil classification criteria for a connective tissue disease. These individuals may be operationally labelled as having undifferentiated connective tissue disorder (UCTD). They should be followed up as many develop defined diseases over time.

SYSTEMIC INFLAMMATORY VASCULITIS

Vasculitis is an inflammation of the vessel wall. The classification remains controversial, but is usually based on the type of artery affected (Fig. 10.27 and Table 10.18). There is some overlap and some cases are difficult to classify, partly because in many conditions there is always some vasculitis histologically. Table 10.19 shows other infective and non-infective conditions in which a vasculitis is seen.

The disorders are characterized by inflammation in or through a blood vessel wall, with fibrinoid necrosis with or without granuloma formation. Histologically there are several different patterns: necrotizing vasculitis; giant cell arteritis; and granulomatous angiitis. The clinical

Table 10.18 Types of systemic vasculitis

Non-infective

Large	Giant cell arteritis
	Takayasu's arteritis
Medium	Classical polyarteritis nodosum (PAN)
	Kawasaki's disease
Small	Microscopic polyangiitis ⎫
	Wegener's granulomatosis ⎬ ANCA associated
	Churg–Strauss syndrome ⎭
	Henoch–Schönlein purpura
	Cutaneous leucocytoclastic vasculitis
	Essential cryoglobulinaemia

Table 10.19 Other conditions associated with vasculitis (see also Table 10.18)

Infective	e.g. Subacute infective endocarditis
Non-infective	Vasculitis with rheumatoid arthritis
	Systemic lupus erythematosus
	Scleroderma
	Polymyositis/dermatomyositis
	Drug-induced Behçet's disease
	Goodpasture's syndrome
	Hypocomplementaemia
	Serum sickness
	Paraneoplastic syndromes
	Inflammatory bowel disease

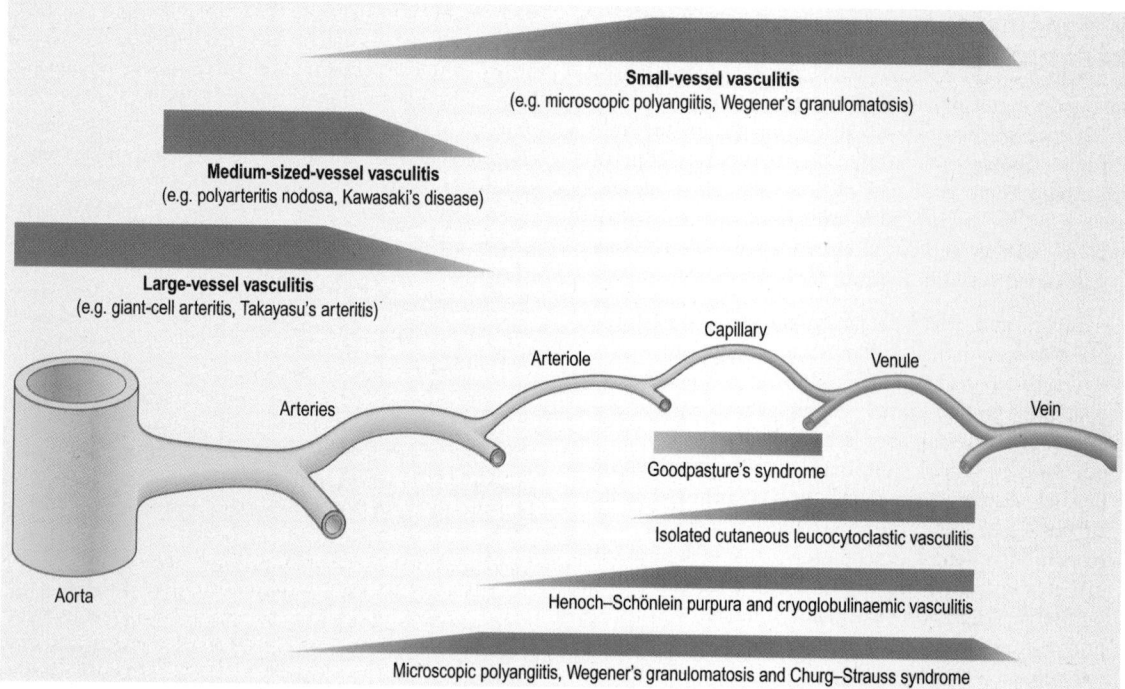

Fig. 10.27 **Sites of vascular involvement by vasculitides.** From Jeanette JC and Falk RJ (1997) *New England Journal of Medicine* **337**: 1512–1523. Copyright © 1997 Massachusetts Medical Society. All rights reserved.

manifestations are due to ischaemic necrosis and vary with the size and type of blood vessel affected. The vasculitides are systemic diseases which affect the skin and musculo-skeletal, renal and gastrointestinal systems. Skin lesions are palpable and commonly urticarial. Many types of systemic non-autoimmune vasculitis are associated with antineutrophilic cytoplasmic antibody (ANCA, see p. 633).

- *Large vessel* refers to the aorta and its major tributaries.
- *Medium vessel* refers to medium and small-sized arteries and arterioles.
- *Small vessel* refers to small arteries (ANCA-associated disease only), arterioles, venules and capillaries.

LARGE VESSEL VASCULITIS

Polymyalgia rheumatica (PMR) and giant cell (temporal) arteritis are systemic illnesses of the elderly. Both are associated with the finding of a giant cell arteritis on temporal artery biopsy.

Polymyalgia rheumatica (PMR)

PMR causes a sudden onset of severe pain and stiffness of the shoulders and neck, and of the hips and lumbar spine; a limb girdle pattern. These symptoms are worse in the morning, lasting from 30 minutes to several hours. The clinical history is usually diagnostic and the patient is always over 50 years.

Patients develop systemic features of tiredness, fever, weight loss, depression and occasionally nocturnal

 Box 10.12 Symptom patterns in some muscle disorders

- **Polymyositis** – proximal muscle ache and weakness
- **Polymyalgia rheumatica** – proximal morning stiffness and pain
- **Myopathy** – weakness, but no pain or stiffness

sweats if it is not diagnosed and treated early. A differential diagnosis is shown in Box 10.12.

Investigation of PMR

- **A raised ESR and/or CRP** is a hallmark of this condition. It is rare to see PMR without an acute-phase response. If it is absent, the diagnosis should be questioned and the tests repeated a few weeks later before treatment is started.
- **Serum alkaline phosphatase and γ-glutamyl-transpeptidase** may be raised as markers of the acute phase.
- **Anaemia** (mild normochromic, normocytic) is often present.
- **Temporal artery biopsy** shows giant cell arteritis in 10–30% of cases, but is not usually performed.

Giant cell arteritis (GCA)

GCA is inflammatory granulomatous arteritis of large arteries which occurs in association with PMR. The patient may have current PMR, a history of recent PMR, or be on treatment for PMR. It is extremely rare under 50 years of age. It may present with the symptoms of GCA with severe headaches, tenderness of the scalp (combing the hair may be painful) or of the temple, claudication of the jaw when eating, tenderness and swelling of one or more temporal or occipital arteries, and can cause sudden painless temporary or permanent visual loss (see p. 1249). Systemic manifestations of severe malaise, tiredness and fever occur.

Investigation of GCA

- **Normochromic, normocytic anaemia**.
- **ESR** is usually raised (in the region of 50–120 mm/h) and the CRP very high.
- **Liver biochemistry**. Abnormalities occur, as in PMR. The albumin may be low.
- **A temporal artery biopsy** from the affected side is the definitive diagnostic test. This should be taken before, or within 7 days of starting, high doses of corticosteroids. Start the drug first if the patient is very ill, in severe pain or has experienced visual loss or stroke. The lesions are patchy and the whole length of the biopsy (> 1 cm long) must be examined.

The histological features of GCA are:

- intimal hypertrophy
- inflammation of the intima and sub-intima
- breaking up of the internal elastic lamina
- giant cells, lymphocytes and plasma cells in the internal elastic lamina.

Treatment of PMR or GCA

Corticosteroids produce a dramatic reduction of symptoms within 24–48 hours of starting treatment, provided the dose is adequate. This should reduce the risk of patients with PMR developing GCA. NSAIDs are less effective and should not be used.

In GCA, corticosteroids are obligatory because they significantly reduce the risk of irreversible visual loss and other focal ischaemic lesions, but much higher doses are needed. Both diseases settle after 12–36 months of treatment in about 75% of patients, but the remaining 25% continue to require low doses of corticosteroids for years. Starting doses of prednisolone are:

- **PMR**: 10–15 mg prednisolone as a single dose in the morning
- **GCA**: 60–100 mg prednisolone, usually in divided doses.

With GCA it is best to start at the higher dose, as the response is more dramatic and diagnostic. The dose should then be reduced gradually in weekly or monthly steps. While the dose is above 20 mg, the step reductions are 5 mg, reducing the evening doses first. Between 20 mg and 10 mg the reduction can be in 2.5 mg steps, but below 10 mg the rate should be slower and the steps each of 1 mg. Steroid-sparing immunosuppressive agents are used in refractory cases.

Dose reduction (and increases when necessary) are titrated against the response or recurrence of symptoms and a fall or rise in the ESR or CRP.

Calcium and vitamin D supplements and bisphosphonates are necessary to prevent osteoporosis whilst steroids are being used.

Takayasu's arteritis

This is a granulomatous inflammation of the aorta and its major branches and is discussed on page 869.

MEDIUM-SIZED VESSEL VASCULITIS

Polyarteritis nodosa (PAN)

Classical PAN is a rare condition which, unlike other vasculitic diseases, usually occurs in middle-aged men. It is accompanied by severe systemic manifestations, and its occasional association with hepatitis B antigenaemia suggests a vasculitis secondary to the deposition of immune complexes. Pathologically, there is fibrinoid necrosis of vessel walls with microaneurysm formation, thrombosis and infarction.

Clinical features

These include fever, malaise, weight loss and myalgia. These initial symptoms are followed by dramatic acute features that are due to organ infarction.

- *Neurological* – mononeuritis multiplex is due to arteritis of the vasa nervorum.
- *Abdominal* – pain due to arterial involvement of the abdominal viscera, mimicking acute cholecystitis, pancreatitis or appendicitis. Gastrointestinal haemorrhage occurs because of mucosal ulceration.
- *Renal* – presents with haematuria and proteinuria. Hypertension and acute/chronic renal failure occur.
- *Cardiac* – coronary arteritis causes myocardial infarction and heart failure. Pericarditis may occur.
- *Skin* – subcutaneous haemorrhage and gangrene occur. A persistent livedo reticularis is seen in chronic cases. Cutaneous and subcutaneous palpable nodules occur, but are uncommon.
- *Lung* – involvement is rare.

Investigations and treatment

- **Blood count**. Anaemia, leucocytosis and a raised ESR occur.
- **Biopsy** material from an affected organ shows features listed above.
- **Angiography**. Demonstration of microaneurysms in hepatic, intestinal or renal vessels if necessary.
- **Other investigations** as appropriate (e.g. ECG and abdominal ultrasound), depending on the clinical problem. ANCA is positive only rarely in classic PAN.

Treatment is with corticosteroids, usually in combination with immunosuppressive drugs such as azathioprine.

Kawasaki's disease

This is an acute systemic vasculitis involving medium-sized vessels, affecting mainly children under 5 years of age. It is very frequent in Japan, and an infective trigger is suspected. It occurs world-wide and is also seen in adults.

Clinical features and treatment

The clinical features are:

- fever lasting 5 days or more
- bilateral conjunctival congestion 2–4 days after onset
- dryness and redness of the lips and oral cavity 3 days after onset
- acute cervical lymphadenopathy accompanying the fever
- polymorphic rash involving any part of the body
- redness and oedema of the palms and soles 2–5 days after onset.

Five of these six features should be present to make the diagnosis, or four of six if coronary aneurysms can be seen on two-dimensional echocardiography or angiography.

Cardiovascular changes in the acute stage include pancarditis and coronary arteritis leading to aneurysms or dilatation. Other features include diarrhoea, albuminuria, aseptic meningitis and arthralgia and, in most, there is a leucocytosis, thrombocytosis and a raised CRP. Anti-endothelial cell autoantibodies are often detectable.

Treatment is with high-dose intravenous immuno-globulin, which prevents the coronary artery disease, followed after the acute phase by aspirin 200–300 mg daily.

SMALL VESSEL VASCULITIS

This can be separated into those that are positive or negative for antineutrophilic cytoplasmic antibody (ANCA) (see p. 633).

The clinical features and diagnosis of small vessel vasculitis are shown in Table 10.20.

ANCA-positive vasculitis

- Wegener's granulomatosis – see page 938.
- Churg–Strauss granulomatosis – see page 938.
- Microscopic polyangiitis – see page 938.

ANCA-negative small-vessel vasculitis

This includes Henoch–Schönlein purpura – see pages 587 and 629.

Cutaneous leucocytoclastic vasculitis

This is the characteristic acute purpuric lesion which histologically involves the dermal post-capillary venules. This lesion affects only the skin and should be differentiated from similar lesions produced in systemic vasculitis. The purpura may be accompanied by arthralgia and glomerulonephritis. Hepatitis C infection is common and may be an aetiological agent. The condition can also be caused by drugs such as sulphonamides and penicillin.

Treatment of small cell vasculitis

Small vessel vasculitis may be self-limiting and requires little treatment. Aggressive therapy with corticosteroids and immunosuppressive agents is required for severe disease.

BEHÇET'S DISEASE

Behçet's disease is an inflammatory disorder of unknown cause. There is a striking geographical distribution, it being most common in Turkey, Iran and Japan. The prevalence per 100 000 is 10–15 in Japan and 80–300 in

Table 10.20   Diagnosis and clinical features of small vessel vasculitis

	Wegener's granulomatosis	Churg-Strauss syndrome	Microscopic polyangiitis	Henoch–Schönlein purpura	Cryoglobulinaemic vasculitis
Features					
ANCA (in blood) PR3	90%	+	+	–	–
MPO	–	60%	60%		
Necrotizing granulomas	+	+	–	–	–
Cryoglobulins (in blood and vessels)	–	–	–	–	–
IgA immune deposits (mainly)	–	–	–	+	–
Asthma and eosinophilia	–	+	–	–	–
Organs involved					
Skin	40	60	40	90	90
Kidneys	80	45	90	50	55
Lungs	90	70	50	< 5	< 5
ENT	90	50	35	< 5	< 5
Musculoskeletal	60	50	60	75	70
Neurological	20	70	30	10	40
Gastrointestinal	50	50	50	60	30

Modified from Jeanette JC, Falk RJ (1997) Small vessel vasculitis. *New England Journal of Medicine* **337**: 1512–1523

Turkey. There is a link to the HLA-B51 allele (a split antigen of B5), with a relative risk of 5–10; this association is not seen in patients in the USA and Europe.

Clinical features

The cardinal clinical feature is recurrent oral ulceration. The international criteria for diagnosis require oral ulceration and any two of the following: genital ulcers, defined eye lesions, defined skin lesions, or a positive skin pathergy test (see below). Oral ulcers can be aphthous or herpetiform. The eye lesions include an anterior or posterior uveitis or retinal vascular lesions. Cutaneous lesions consist of erythema nodosum, pseudofolliculitis and papulopustular lesions.

Other manifestations include a self-limiting peripheral mon- or oligoarthritis affecting knees, ankles, wrists and elbows; gastrointestinal symptoms of diarrhoea, abdominal pain and anorexia; pulmonary and renal lesions; a brainstem syndrome, organic confusional states and a meningoencephalitis. All the common manifestations are self-limiting except for the ocular attacks. Repeated attacks of uveitis can cause blindness.

The pathergy reaction is highly specific to Behçet's disease. Skin injury, by a needle prick for example, leads to papule or pustule formation within 24–48 hours. An intradermal injection of urate crystals is also used.

Treatment

Corticosteroids, immunosuppressant agents and ciclosporin-A are used for chronic uveitis and the rare neurological complications. Colchicine helps erythema nodosum and joint pain. Thalidomide may be useful in some cases although side-effects of drowsiness and peripheral neuropathy are common. It should not be used in pregnant women because of phocomelia (limb abnormalities).

DIFFERENTIAL DIAGNOSIS OF RHEUMATIC COMPLAINTS IN THE ELDERLY (Fig.10.28)

Musculoskeletal problems

These are common at all ages. In the elderly, pain arises from a combination of age-related changes and injury.

Back and neck pain (see pp. 540 and 536)

These are commonly associated with spondylosis on X-ray. Complications include spinal stenosis or nerve root claudication. Look for locally tender areas, which might be injected. Mechanical back pain may be worse in the morning, especially when spondylosis is severe or there is marked deformity; there is a normal ESR and CRP, which distinguishes this from polymyalgia rheumatica. Rarely, elderly women present with previously undiagnosed ankylosing spondylitis.

Osteoporotic fractures

Osteoporotic fractures of the spine cause acute pain or deformity and subsequent postural back pain. The acute pain may warrant a period of bed rest (see p. 596). The management of such problems in the elderly is the same as for younger people but a response to treatment is less predictable. Advice about posture, exercise, general fitness and about medication to reduce the risk of further fractures is necessary but must be tempered by the patient's general health.

Symptomatic osteoarthritis (see p. 552)

This increases with increasing age and is uncommon below the age of 50 years. It is necessary to look for possible reversible causes of pain and disability, such as periarticular lesions or a joint effusion. Caution about drug treatment is necessary because of the increased risk of side-effects in older patients. Joint replacement surgery

FURTHER READING

Black CM (1997) Systemic sclerosis. In: Klippel JH, Dieppe PA (eds) *Management in Rheumatology*, 2nd edn. London: Mosby, Section 7, Ch. 11: 1–10.

Callen JP (2000) Dermatomyositis. *Lancet* **355**: 53–57.

CME Section (2001) Rheumatological and immunological disorders. *Clinical Medicine* **1**(1): 7–20.

Denton CP, Black CM (2000) Scleroderma and related disorders: therapeutic aspects. *Baillière's Clinical Rheumatology* **14**(1): 17–35.

Pickering MC, Haskard DP (2000) Behçet's syndrome. *Journal of the Royal College of Physicians London* **24**: 169–177.

Sakane T, Takeno M, Suzuki N, Inaba G (1999) Behçet's disease. *New England Journal of Medicine* **341**: 1284–1291.

Scott DGI, Watts RA (2000) Systemic vasculitis: epidemiology, classification and environmental factors. *Annals of Rheumatology* **59**: 161–163.

Fig. 10.28 **The differential diagnosis of arthritis in the elderly.**

has transformed the outlook for many older people with OA by offering pain control and increased mobility and independence.

Rheumatoid arthritis (see p. 555)

RA may present in the elderly as a dramatic onset of symmetrical polyarthritis. This has a reasonable prognosis and responds well to low doses of prednisolone and other drug therapy. RA in the older patient may mimic polymyalgia rheumatica; the synovitis becomes apparent as the corticosteroid dose is reduced. Treat with DMARDs as for RA in order to reduce the corticosteroid dose.

Polymyalgia rheumatica and giant cell arteritis (see p. 582)

These must be recognized and treated. Failure to respond to adequate doses of prednisolone should trigger a search for an alternative disease, such as RA, vasculitis, infection or malignancy.

Chondrocalcinosis

This increases with increasing age and is seen on over 40% of knee X-rays in the over-80s. It may produce a variety of arthritic conditions (see p. 553).

Pseudogout (see p. 571)

This causes acute monarthritis of the wrist or knee in older people. It responds well to aspiration and intra-articular corticosteroids or oral NSAIDs.

Gout

Gout causes acute monarthritis in the elderly but may also present as a polyarticular inflammatory arthritis, especially in elderly women on long-term diuretic treatment, or as tophaceous gout (p. 570).

Septic arthritis (see p. 571)

Septic arthritis in the elderly and frail produces articular symptoms, and signs that may be muted. The patient usually has septicaemia and the best way to ensure its recognition is to retain it in the differential diagnosis of all musculoskeletal presentations in unwell, elderly people.

Treatment

In all cases the management is similar to that described in the main part of the chapter, but special care should be taken to reduce doses of medication where possible and to think about possible adverse drug effects or interactions.

ARTHRITIS IN CHILDREN

Joint and limb pains are common in children but arthritis is fortunately rare. Babies and young children may present with immobility of a joint or a limp, but the diagnosis can be extremely difficult. Figure 10.29 summarizes the differential diagnosis.

For chronic conditions, the child and family often need a great deal of support from physiotherapists, occupational therapists, psychologists, teachers, social workers and

Juvenile idiopathic arthritis	Other conditions
Systemic arthritis Oligoarthritis (persistent) Oligoarthritis (extended) Polyarticular arthritis (rheumatoid factor-positive) Polyarticular arthritis (rheumatoid factor-negative) Juvenile spondyloarthropathy Psoriatic arthritis Unclassified	Henoch–Schönlein purpura Infections, e.g. tuberculosis, septic arthritis, viral arthritis Rheumatic fever Hypermobility syndrome Leukaemia Sickle cell disease SLE and other autoimmune connective tissue disease Transient synovitis of the hip

Fig. 10.29 The differential diagnosis of arthritis in children.

orthopaedic surgeons. These are best obtained in specialist paediatric centres.

JUVENILE IDIOPATHIC ARTHRITIS (JIA)

Systemic arthritis

Still's disease (which accounts for 10% of cases of JIA) affects boys and girls equally up to 5 years of age; then girls are more commonly affected. Adult-onset Still's disease is extremely rare.

Clinical features include a high, swinging, early-evening pyrexia, an evanescent pink maculopapular rash with arthralgia and arthritis, myalgia and generalized lymphadenopathy. Hepatosplenomegaly and pericarditis and pleurisy occur. The differential diagnoses include malignancy, in particular leukaemia and neuroblastoma, and infection. Laboratory tests show a high ESR and CRP, neutrophilia and thrombocytosis. Autoantibodies are negative.

Oligoarthritis (persistent)

This is the most common form of JIA (50–60%) but is still a relatively uncommon condition. It affects, by definition, four or fewer joints – especially knees, ankles and wrists – often in an asymmetrical pattern. It affects mainly girls, with a peak age of 3 years. The prognosis is generally good with most going into remission. Uveitis (often with a positive ANA) occurs and requires regular screening by a 3-monthly slit-lamp examination. Blindness can occur if it is untreated. Prognosis is generally good, with remission occurring eventually in most patients.

Oligoarthritis (extended)

In approximately 25% of patients, oligoarthritis extends to affect many more joints after around 6 months. This form of arthritis can be very destructive.

Polyarticular JIA

The rheumatoid factor-positive form occurs in older girls, usually over 8 years. It is a systemic disease; the arthritis commonly involves the small joints of the hands, wrists, ankles and feet initially, and eventually larger joints. It can be a very destructive arthritis and needs aggressive treatment.

The rheumatoid factor-negative form is commoner. It usually affects girls under 12 years but can occur at any age. They may be ANA positive, with a risk of chronic uveitis. The arthritis is often asymmetrical, with a distribution similar to that seen in the RF-positive form. It may also affect the cervical spine, temporomandibular joints and elbows.

Enthesitis-related arthritis (juvenile spondyloarthropathy)

This affects teenage and younger boys mainly, producing an asymmetrical arthritis of lower-limb joints and enthesitis. It is associated with HLA-B27 and a risk of acute anterior uveitis. It is the childhood equivalent of adult ankylosing spondylitis but spinal involvement is rare in childhood. Approximately one in three develops spinal disease in adulthood.

Psoriatic arthritis

This may occur in children and is similar in pattern to the adult form. The arthritis may be very destructive. Psoriasis may develop long after the arthritis but is found commonly in a first-degree relative.

Treatment of JIA

JIA should always be referred to a specialist paediatric rheumatology unit with facilities to assess and design treatment plans which aim to prevent long-term disability. These units also need facilities for rehabilitation, education and surgical intervention. NSAIDs reduce pain and stiffness but disease-modifying agents such as methotrexate are used to control moderate and severe disease. Corticosteroids are often required in systemic disease: intravenous pulsed methylprednisolone is used, followed by methotrexate ($10-15\,\text{mg/m}^2$) weekly to control disease and prevent growth suppression. Anti-TNF agents (see Table 10.15) are used if methotrexate fails, and are highly effective in all types except systemic-onset disease where the results are variable. Sulfasalazine is used only in enthesitis-related JIA. Aspirin may be a cause of Reye's syndrome and should not be used under the age of 12 years.

Prognosis

Up to 50% of children develop long-term disability; 25% may continue to have active arthritis into adult years. Death may be due to infection or systemic disease with pericarditis or amyloidosis.

OTHER TYPES

Henoch–Schönlein purpura (see also p. 629)

This is the commonest systemic vasculitis seen in children. IgA immune complexes deposit in the small vessels. It often occurs after upper respiratory tract infections. Other manifestations include lower limb purpura, a transient non-migratory polyarthritis, and abdominal pain. Fifty per cent of these patients will have haematuria and proteinuria, due to a glomerulonephritis; treatment of this is discussed on page 629. The prognosis is excellent, although 1% develop chronic renal damage.

Rheumatic fever

Rheumatic fever still occurs occasionally in developed countries but is more common in developing countries. It is described on page 76.

The arthritis affects large joints and migrates between joints, each being affected for a few days at a time. This is unlike Still's disease, where arthritis is usually much more persistent in each affected joint. The fever is persistent but rarely as high as in Still's disease (see above) and the temperature often remains above normal. A child may not volunteer a history of sore throat and the carditis may be silent. Isolated arthritis is the presenting symptom in 14–42%. The disease is easily missed if not included in the differential diagnosis of acute childhood arthritis.

Treatment is described on page 77.

Hypermobility syndrome

Five to ten per cent of children are hypermobile. A proportion of them will develop various musculoskeletal complaints in early childhood, such as late walking, flat feet, or nocturnal leg pains, possibly due to hypermobile ankles and knees suffering recurrent sprains and strains after exercise. Joint effusions, subluxation, dislocation and ligamentous injuries may occur throughout childhood. Low back pain may develop in affected adolescents. There may be some risk of the early development of osteoarthritis in adulthood. More severe hypermobility is also seen in Ehlers–Danlos and Marfan's syndromes (see pp. 602 and 1356).

Treatment is with exercise directed at improving the strength of muscles that cross affected joints, as well as overall fitness and endurance. It may be necessary to reduce or change sporting and other activities.

Miscellaneous conditions

Some children develop *idiopathic musculoskeletal pain* that can become chronic. Management of these children requires exclusion of the causes shown in Figure 10.29, but without performing unnecessary laboratory investigations. *Nocturnal musculoskeletal pains* are episodic and may be associated with hypermobility. They may be called 'growing pains'. They often last 15–30 minutes and awaken the child from sleep, and may require physiotherapy and analgesics, together with advice and support to the parents.

Low back pain in children may reflect psychosocial problems at home or school as much as any obvious musculoskeletal pathology.

Osteochondritis can affect the ossification centre of the ends of bones. A typical condition is *Osgood–Schlatter disease*, which is characterized by localized pain and swelling over the tibial tubercle or at the patellar tendon insertion. It is usually seen in athletic teenagers and responds to local treatment and changes of sporting activities. *Sever's disease* is an osteochondritis of the insertion of the Achilles tendon into the calcaneum.

Perthes' disease is an idiopathic, possibly avascular, necrosis of the proximal femoral epiphysis, of unknown aetiology. It presents as a painless limp, usually in boys aged 3–12 years, and is occasionally bilateral. If severe it may require surgical correction.

Transient synovitis of the hip (irritable hip) causes painful limitation of movement, usually of one hip, after an upper respiratory infection in young children (usually boys). Symptoms usually resolve within a few weeks (2–3% develop Perthes' disease) but other more serious causes of hip pain should be excluded. Treatment is with rest and analgesia until the pain resolves.

> **FURTHER READING**
> Cassidy JT, Petty RS (2001) *Textbook of Paediatric Rheumatology,* 4th edn. Philadelphia: Saunders.
> Woo P, Wedderburn LR (1998) Juvenile chronic arthritis. *Lancet* **351**: 969–973.

RHEUMATOLOGICAL PROBLEMS SEEN IN OTHER DISEASES

Gastrointestinal and liver disease

- *Enteropathic synovitis* – see page 568.
- *Autoimmune hepatitis* (see p. 373) may be accompanied by an arthralgia similar to that seen in systemic lupus erythematosus. Joint pain occurs in a bilateral, symmetrical distribution, with the small joints of the hands being prominently affected. Joints usually look normal but sometimes there is a slight soft-tissue swelling. These patients often have positive tests for antinuclear antibodies.
- *Primary biliary cirrhosis* patients occasionally have a symmetrical arthropathy.
- *Hereditary haemochromatosis* is associated with arthritis in 50% of cases; this is often the first sign of the disease and chondrocalcinosis is common.
- *Whipple's disease* (see p. 305) is accompanied by fever and arthralgia.

Malignant disease

It is not uncommon for malignant diseases to present with musculoskeletal symptoms. Bone pain may be due to multiple myeloma, lymphoma, a primary tumour of bone or secondary deposits. The pain is typically unremitting, worse at night and there are other clinical clues such as weight loss or ill-health. Secondary gout occurs in conditions such as chronic myeloid leukaemia.

Table 10.21   Malignant neoplasms of bone

Metastases (osteolytic)
Bronchus
Breast
Prostate (often osteosclerotic as well)
Thyroid
Kidney

Multiple myeloma

Primary bone tumours (rare; seen in the young) e.g.
Osteosarcomas
Fibrosarcomas
Chondromas
Ewing's tumour

Neoplastic disease of bone

Malignant tumours of bone are shown in Table 10.21. The most common tumours are metastases from the bronchus, breast and prostate. Metastases from kidney and thyroid are less common. Primary bone tumours are rare and usually seen only in children and young adults.

Symptoms are usually related to the anatomical position of the tumour, with local bone pain. Systemic symptoms (e.g. malaise and pyrexia) and aches and pains occur and are occasionally related to hypercalcaemia (see p. 1092). The diagnosis of metastases can often be made from the history and examination, particularly if the primary tumour has already been diagnosed. Symptoms from bony metastases may, however, be the first presenting feature.

Investigations

Skeletal isotope scans show bony metastases as 'hot' areas before radiological changes occur.

- **X-rays** may show metastases as osteolytic areas with bony destruction. Osteosclerotic metastases are characteristic of prostatic carcinoma.
- **Serum alkaline phosphatase** (from bone) is usually raised.
- **Hypercalcaemia** is seen in 10–20% of patients with malignancies. It is associated chiefly with metastases, but can also result from ectopic parathormone or parathyroid hormone-related protein secretion.
- **Prostate-specific antigen** (PSA) and serum acid phosphate are raised in the presence of prostatic metastases.

Treatment

Treatment is usually with analgesics and anti-inflammatory drugs. Local radiotherapy to bone metastases relieves pain and reduces the risk of pathological fracture. Some tumours respond to chemotherapy; others are hormone-dependent and respond to hormonal therapy. Occasionally pathological fractures require internal fixation.

Hypertrophic pulmonary osteoarthropathy

Hypertrophic osteoarthropathy is most often associated with carcinoma of the bronchus. It is a non-metastatic complication and may be the presenting feature of the disease. It occurs only rarely with other conditions that also cause clubbing. It is seen most often in middle-aged men, who present with pain and swelling of the wrists and ankles. Other joints are involved occasionally.

The diagnosis is made on the presence of clubbing of the fingers, which is usually gross, and periosteal new bone formation along the shafts of the distal ends of the radius, ulna, tibia and fibula on X-ray. A chest X-ray usually shows the malignancy.

Treatment should be directed at the underlying carcinoma; if this can be removed, the arthropathy disappears. NSAIDs relieve the symptoms.

Paraneoplastic polyarthritis

This is seen with carcinoma of the breast in women and of the lung in men, and also with renal cell carcinoma. The neoplasm may be occult at onset and the diagnosis is then difficult to make.

Skin disease

Psoriatic arthritis

This is discussed on page 566.

Erythema nodosum (p. 1341)

This is accompanied by arthritis in over 50% of cases. The knees and ankles are particularly affected, being swollen, red and tender. The arthritis subsides, along with the skin lesions, within a few months. Treatment is with NSAIDs or occasionally steroids.

Neurological disease

Neuropathic joints (Charcot's joints) are joints damaged by trauma as a result of the loss of the protective pain sensation. They were first described by Charcot in relation to tabes dorsalis. They are also seen in syringomyelia, diabetes mellitus and leprosy. The site of the neuropathic joint depends upon the localization of the pain loss:

- in tabes dorsalis, the knees and ankles are most often affected
- in diabetes mellitus, the joints of the tarsus are involved
- in syringomyelia, the shoulder is involved.

Neuropathic joints are not painful, although there may be painful episodes associated with crystal deposition. Presentation is usually with swelling and instability. Eventually severe deformities develop.

The characteristic finding is a swollen joint with abnormal but painless movement. This is associated with neurological findings that depend upon the underlying disease (e.g. dissociated sensory loss in syringomyelia or polyneuropathy in diabetes). X-ray changes are characteristic, with gross joint disorganization and bony distortion.

Treatment is symptomatic. Surgery may be required in advanced cases.

Blood disease

Arthritis due to haemarthrosis is a common presenting feature of *haemophilia* (see p. 472). Attacks begin in early childhood in most cases and are recurrent. The knee is the most commonly affected joint but the elbows and ankles are sometimes involved. The arthritis can lead to bone destruction and disorganization of joints. Apart from replacement of factor VIII, affected joints require initial immobilization followed by physiotherapy to restore movement and measures to prevent and correct deformities.

Sickle cell crises (p. 443) are often accompanied by joint pain that particularly affects the hands and feet in a bilateral, symmetrical distribution. Affected joints usually look normal but are occasionally swollen. This condition may also be complicated by avascular necrosis (see p. 544) and by osteomyelitis.

Arthritis can also occur in *acute leukaemia*; it may be the presenting feature in childhood. The knee is particularly affected and is very painful, warm and swollen. Treatment is directed at the underlying leukaemia. Arthritis may also occur in *chronic leukaemia*, with leukaemic deposits in and around the joints.

Individuals with *thalassaemia major* (see p. 441) are living longer and are presenting with back pain due to premature disc degeneration, secondary spondylosis and crush fractures due to osteoporosis. There is marked discal calcification.

Endocrine and metabolic disorders

Hypothyroid patients may complain of pain and stiffness of proximal muscles, resembling polymyalgia rheumatica. They may also have carpal tunnel syndrome. Less often, there is an arthritis accompanied by joint effusions, particularly in the knees, wrist and small joints of the hands and feet. These problems respond rapidly to thyroxine.

Hyperparathyroidism may be complicated by chondrocalcinosis and acute pseudogout.

In *acromegaly*, arthralgia occurs in about 50% of patients. It particularly affects the small joints of the hands and knees. There may be carpal tunnel syndrome.

In *Cushing's disease*, back pain is common.

Joint disorders related to diabetes mellitus are described on page 1131.

Familial hypercholesterolaemia is associated with oligo- or polyarthritis usually with tendon xanthomata. Arthritis also occurs in combined hyperlipidaemia.

MISCELLANEOUS ARTHROPATHIES

Familial Mediterranean fever (FMF)

FMF is inherited as an autosomal recessive condition and occurs in certain ethnic groups, particularly Arabs, Turks, Armenians and Sephardic Jews. The gene, called *MEFV*, has been localized to chromosome 16. It encodes for pyrin or marenostrin, which activate the biosynthesis of a chemotactic-factor inactivator in neutrophils. Failure to produce this leads to FMF attacks.

These are characterized by recurrent attacks of fever, arthritis and serositis. Abdominal or chest pain due to peritonitis or pleurisy occurs. The arthritis is usually monarticular and attacks last up to 1 week. The condition may be mistaken for palindromic rheumatism, but such attacks are not usually accompanied by fever.

The diagnosis can be made by PCR, if available, but usually it is based on the clinical picture and exclusion of other conditions.

Treatment regularly with colchicine 1000–1500 µg daily can usually prevent the attacks. In general the disorder is benign but in 25% of cases renal amyloidosis develops.

Sarcoidosis (see also p. 935)

The most common type of arthritis is that associated with erythema nodosum, which occurs in 20% of cases of sarcoidosis at or soon after the onset of the disease. The most useful diagnostic test is a chest X-ray, which shows hilar lymphadenopathy in 80% of cases.

Other patterns of arthritis occur later in the disease. These include a transient rheumatoid-like polyarthritis and an acute monarthritis that can be mistaken for gout.

Treatment is with NSAIDs, but if these fail to control the symptoms, corticosteroids are usually very effective.

Osteochondromatosis

In this condition, foci of cartilage form within the synovial membrane. These foci become calcified and then ossified (osteochondromas). They may give rise to loose bodies within the joint. The condition occurs in a single joint of a young adult and X-rays are usually diagnostic.

Treatment involves removal of loose bodies and synovectomy.

Pigmented villonodular synovitis

This is characterized by exuberant synovial proliferation that occurs either in joints or in tendon sheaths. The main manifestation in joints is recurrent haemarthrosis. It may produce progressive local bone destruction but a malignant form is seen occasionally.

Treatment is synovectomy or radiotherapy. In tendon sheaths, the condition gives rise to a nodular mass that requires excision.

Relapsing polychondritis

Relapsing polychondritis is a rare inflammatory condition of cartilage. It occurs equally in males and females, usually the elderly. Tenderness, inflammation and eventual destruction of cartilage occur, mainly in the ear, nose, larynx or trachea. A seronegative polyarthritis occurs, as well as episcleritis and evidence of a vasculitis (e.g. glomerulonephritis). The diagnosis is clinical with laboratory evidence of acute inflammation.

Treatment involves corticosteroids and immunosuppressive agents.

DISEASES OF BONE

Bone is a specialized connective tissue, serving three major functions:

- *mechanical* – providing structure and muscular attachment for movement
- *metabolic* – as a reserve of calcium and phosphate
- *protective* – enclosing bone marrow and vital organs.

STRUCTURE AND PHYSIOLOGY

Long bones (e.g. femur, tibia, humerus) and flat bones (e.g. skull, scapula, mandible) have different embryological templates, with cortical and trabecular bone in varying proportions (Fig. 10.30).

- *Cortical* (*compact or lamellar*) *bone* forms the shaft (diaphysis) of long bones and the outer shell of flat bones. It has mainly mechanical and protective functions.
- *Trabecular* (*cancellous*) *bone* is found at the end of long bones (epiphysis) and inside the cortex of flat bones, consisting of a network of interconnecting trabecular plates and rods. It is the major site of bone remodelling and mineral homeostasis.
- *Woven bone* lacks this organized structure and is characterized by random orientation of collagen fibres. It is formed in the first few years of life, in fracture repair, and in high-turnover bone diseases, e.g. Paget's disease.

Bone comprises cells and a matrix of organic (mainly protein) and inorganic (mineral) elements.

Matrix components

Type I collagen is the main component of bone matrix, forming parallel lamellae in a highly organized structure. In cortical bone, concentric lamellae form around blood vessels in Haversian canals, which communicate via transverse (Volkmann's) canals. Non-collagenous proteins include osteocalcin, osteopontin and fibronectin. Bone mineral consists mainly of calcium hydroxyapatite, which gives bone its resistance to compressive forces.

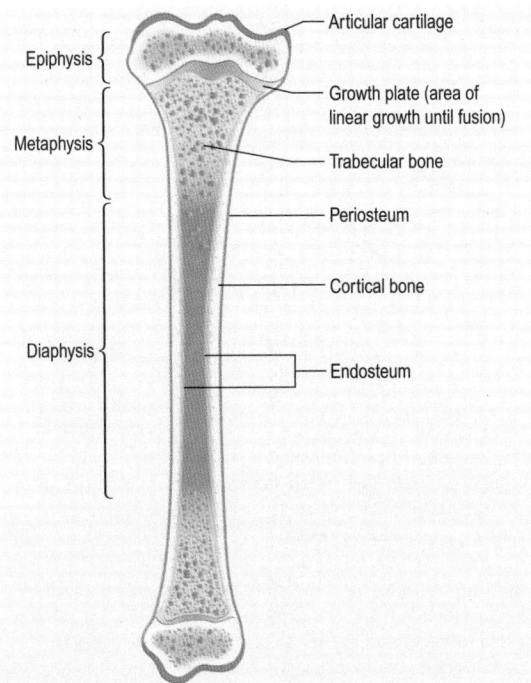

Fig. 10.30 Diagram of a longitudinal section of a growing long bone.

Bone cells

Osteocytes

These small cells are embedded within bone and act as transducers of mechanical stress, their cytoplasmic processes communicating with other osteocytes and osteoblastic cells on the bone surface.

Osteoblasts

Derived from local mesenchymal stem cells, osteoblasts are present on the bone surface and synthesize bone matrix (osteoid) and regulate its mineralization, after which a large proportion of the redundant osteoblasts are removed by apoptosis. Some remain as lining cells on the surface or become embedded in newly mineralized bone as osteocytes. Osteoblasts are also critical in the regulation of osteoclast generation and function through production of the stimulatory factor RANK-L (the *ligand* for *receptor activator* of *nuclear* factor *kappa*-B) and the inhibitory factor osteoprotegerin (OPG). Osteoblasts are rich in alkaline phosphatase and express many receptors, including those for glucocorticoids, parathyroid hormone (PTH), 1,25-dihydroxyvitamin D_3 (1,25-$(OH)_2D_3$), oestrogen, prostaglandins, interleukins, tumour necrosis factor alpha (TNF-α) and transforming growth factor (TGF)-β.

Osteoclasts

Osteoclasts develop from haemopoietic stem cells of the macrophage/monocyte lineage. They express receptors for colony-stimulating factor-1 (M-CSF), RANK-L and calcitonin, but not for PTH. They attach to bone, forming a ruffled border to create a series of extracellular lysosomal

compartments. Hydrogen ions are secreted into this space, the acid environment dissolving the crystals and exposing the matrix, which is then degraded by cysteine protease enzymes (e.g. cathepsin K) functioning at their optimal pH.

Bone growth and remodelling

Longitudinal growth occurs at the epiphyseal growth plate (between the epiphysis and metaphysis). Cartilage is produced by chondrocytes and ossified until skeletal maturity at 18–21 years of age, when the epiphysis and metaphysis fuse.

In adults, bone is remodelled in basic multicellular units (Fig. 10.31). Osteocytes communicate mechanical strain to osteoblasts on the bone surface via cytoplasmic projections. The osteoblast responds to this or to other signals (PTH, 1,25-$(OH)_2D_3$, cytokines and growth factors) by increasing production of RANK-L and M-CSF and reducing OPG production. This promotes osteoclast formation from circulating monocyte precursors and directs osteoclasts to the area of bone to be resorbed. Unknown inhibitory signals (see p. 486) limit osteoclast recruitment and activity. Macrophages remove apoptotic osteoclasts and prepare the resorbed surface (the cement line). Growth factors drive osteoblast formation from local stem cells (coupling of resorption and formation), producing osteoid which is mineralized to form new bone. The cycle is completed in about 120 days. Remodelling is balanced if there has been no net change in the amount of bone, i.e. the amount formed is the same as the amount resorbed.

The control of bone remodelling is complex and results from the interaction of mechanical stresses, systemic hormones and locally produced cytokines, growth factors, prostaglandins and other factors such as nitric oxide. Genetic factors are also involved. Oestrogen is a major regulator of bone remodelling both in females and males and acts mainly by inhibiting osteoclastogenesis and increasing osteoclast apoptosis.

FURTHER READING

Bland R (2000) Steroid hormone receptor expression and action in bone. *Clinical Science* **98**: 217–240.
Compston JE (2001) Sex steroids and bone. *Physiological Reviews* **81**: 419–447.
Suda T et al. (1999) Modulation of osteoclast differentiation and function by the new members of the tumor necrosis factor receptor and ligand families. *Endocrinology Reviews* **20**: 345–357.

CALCIUM HOMEOSTASIS AND ITS REGULATION

Calcium homeostasis is regulated by the effects of PTH and 1,25-$(OH)_2D_3$ on gut, kidney and bone. Calcium-sensing receptors are present in the parathyroid gland, kidney, brain and other organs.

Fig. 10.31 **A diagram of bone remodelling, representing a cross-section of a groove in a flat area of bone at a single time-point.** (Resorption and formation in fact occur simultaneously at different points along the groove or tunnel.) On the left, the multinucleate osteoclast is resorbing bone at the groove's apex, in response to increased RANK-L and M-CSF (and reduced osteoprotegerin) from adjacent osteoblasts which have been activated by hormones, cytokines or by osteocytes under mechanical strain. Macrophages appear in the osteoclasts' wake, clearing apoptotic cells (reversal) and preparing the resorbed bone surface as a 'cement line'. Growth factors released from the bone stimulate differentiation of local stem cells to osteoblasts that form new bone, completing the cycle. TNF, tumour necrosis factor; IL, interleukin.

CALCIUM ABSORPTION AND DISTRIBUTION
(Fig. 10.32)

Daily calcium consumption, primarily from dairy foods, should ideally be around 20–25 mmol (800–1000 mg). Dietary calcium deficiency is rarely a significant cause of bone disease. Intestinal absorption of calcium is reduced by vitamin D deficiency and in malabsorptive states.

Vitamin D metabolism (Fig. 10.33)

The primary source of vitamin D in humans is photoactivation (in the skin) of 7-dehydrocholesterol to cholecalciferol, which is then converted in the liver to

25-hydroxycholecalciferol $(25\text{-}(OH)D_3)$ and further converted by renal 1α-hydroxylase to the active metabolite 1,25-dihydroxycholecalciferol $(1,25\text{-}(OH)_2D_3)$. (This step can occur in lymphomatous and sarcoid tissue, resulting in the hypercalcaemia that may complicate these diseases.) A less active metabolite, $24,25\text{-}(OH)_2D_3$, is formed if vitamin D supplies are adequate. Regulation of this enzyme is by PTH, phosphate and by feedback inhibition by $1,25\text{-}(OH)_2D_3$.

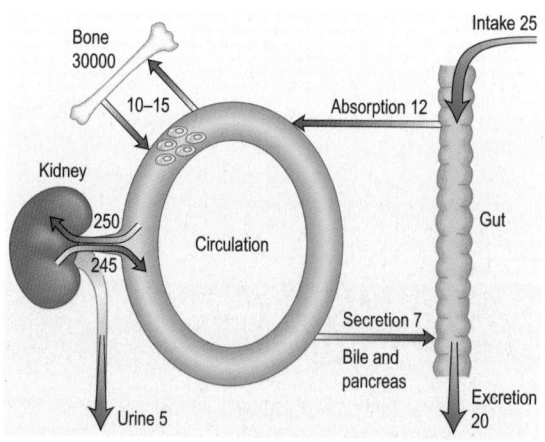

Fig. 10.32 **Calcium exchange in the normal human.** The amounts are shown in mmol per day.

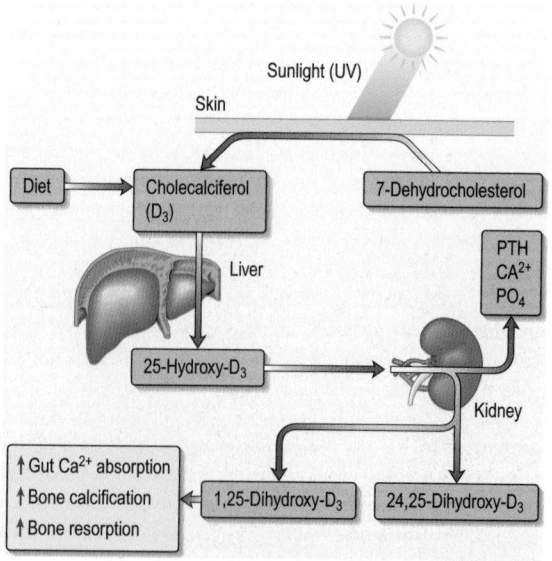

Fig. 10.33 **The metabolism and actions of vitamin D.**

Parathyroid hormone (PTH)

PTH, an 84-amino-acid hormone, is secreted from the chief cells of the parathyroid glands (normally situated posterior to the thyroid, but occasionally in the neck or mediastinum). PTH increases renal phosphate excretion, and increases plasma calcium by:

- increasing osteoclastic resorption of bone (occurring rapidly)
- increasing intestinal absorption of calcium (a slower response)
- increasing synthesis of 1,25-$(OH)_2D_3$
- increasing renal tubular reabsorption of calcium.

Hypomagnesaemia can suppress the normal PTH response to hypocalcaemia.

Calcitonin

Calcitonin is produced by thyroid C cells. Calcitonin inhibits osteoclastic bone resorption and increases the renal excretion of calcium and phosphate. However, neither total thyroidectomy (absent calcitonin) or medullary carcinoma of the thyroid (excess calcitonin) has significant skeletal effects in humans.

INVESTIGATION OF BONE AND CALCIUM DISORDERS (Fig.10.34)

Total plasma calcium

(reference range 2.2–2.6 mmol/L)
About 40% is ionized and physiologically active; the remainder is complexed or protein-bound, particularly to albumin. Ionized calcium is difficult to measure and not routinely assessed. Total plasma calcium is corrected for protein binding by adding or subtracting 0.02 mmol/L for every gram per litre of a simultaneous albumin level below or above 40 g/L. For critical measurements, samples should be taken in the fasting state and without a tourniquet (the latter may increase local plasma protein concentration).

Plasma phosphate (reference range 0.8–1.4 mmol/L)

Phosphate is essential to most biological systems. Primary hyperparathyroidism is associated with low levels of plasma phosphate. High levels are found in renal failure or in hypoparathyroidism.

PTH measurements (reference range 10–65 ng/L)

The PTH assay measures the intact PTH molecule. Raised levels are found in primary, secondary and tertiary hyperparathyroidism and in familial hypocalciuric hypercalcaemia. Lithium toxicity may also be associated with raised PTH levels. In hypercalcaemia due to other causes, PTH levels are suppressed.

25-hydroxyvitamin D (reference range depends on season of year, but generally levels ≥20 ng/mL [50 nmol/L] are considered normal)

Serum 25-OHD levels provide an assessment of vitamin D status. Vitamin D deficiency or insufficiency is often associated with increased serum PTH levels. Measurements of 1,25-$(OH)_2D_3$ are seldom helpful clinically.

Urinary calcium (normal range 2.5–7.5 mmol/24 h)

This is increased where renal tubular reabsorption of calcium is decreased, or in hypercalcaemia. An exception to the latter is familial hypocalciuric hypercalcaemia, where urinary calcium excretion is inappropriately low in the presence of hypercalcaemia (p. 1094). The main role of urinary calcium assay is in the investigation of renal calculi.

Markers of bone formation

- *Alkaline phosphatase* is derived from liver, bone, pancreas, kidney and placenta. Bone-specific alkaline phosphatase is synthesized by osteoblasts; serum levels are raised in the growing child and in bone diseases in which bone turnover is increased (Fig. 10.34).
- *Osteocalcin* is produced by osteoblasts. Serum levels are often elevated in high-turnover bone disease and are reduced by glucocorticoids.
- *Type I collagen propeptides* are by-products of collagen synthesis. Carboxyterminal propeptide of collagen I (P1CP) and the aminoterminal propeptide (P1NP) can both be measured in serum.

Markers of bone resorption

- *Pyridinoline or deoxypyridinoline cross-links of collagen* are produced by collagen degradation, and excreted in urine. Deoxypyridinoline is bone-specific, and both are more sensitive than urinary hydroxyproline.
- *N-terminal and C-terminal cross-linked telopeptides* also reflect bone resorption and may alter more rapidly in

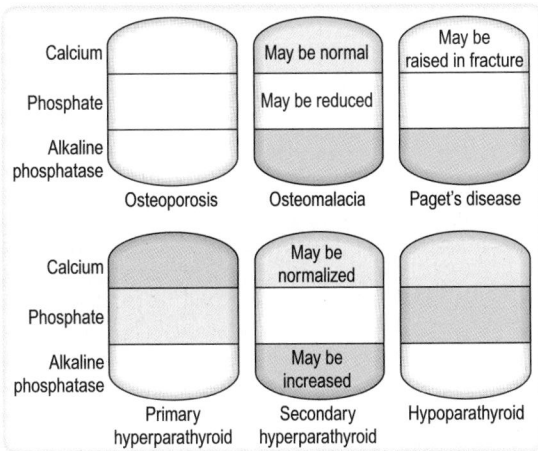

Fig. 10.34 **Changes in serum calcium, phosphate and alkaline phosphatase in main bone disorders.** Shading represents increased (red), reduced (blue) or normal (white) levels.

response to disease or treatment. They can be assessed in urine or serum.

Diagnostic imaging

- *Plain radiographs* identify fracture, tumours and infections. Features characteristic of specific metabolic bone diseases may be seen (see separate sections).
- *Radionuclide scans.* Technetium-99m-labelled methylene bisphosphonate uptake is predominantly dependent on blood flow and osteoblastic activity, detecting increased bone activity in cases of fracture, infection, metastases or in metabolic bone disease with greater sensitivity than X-rays.
- *Magnetic resonance imaging* allows detailed assessment of subchondral and other bone areas. Variations in technique (T1, T2, STIR (which suppresses the high signal from fat in bone marrow)) offer specific diagnostic or prognostic information, for example in suspected avascular necrosis.

Bone density measurements (see p. 596)

Bone biopsy

A core of bone is removed (from cortex to cortex of the iliac crest) with a trephine, and the non-decalcified specimen is examined for indices of bone turnover and remodelling. A fluorochrome (usually oral tetracycline), given for 2 days on two occasions 10 days apart before the biopsy, enables measurement of actively forming surfaces of bone. In clinical practice, bone biopsy is most useful in the diagnosis of osteomalacia and renal osteodystrophy.

OSTEOPOROSIS

Definition and incidence

Osteoporosis is defined as 'a disease characterized by low bone mass and micro-architectural deterioration of bone tissue, leading to enhanced bone fragility and an increase in fracture risk'. Bone is normally mineralized but is deficient in quantity, quality and structural integrity (Fig. 10.35).

The World Health Organization (WHO) defines osteoporosis as a bone density more than 2.5 standard deviations (SDs) below the young adult mean value (T-score < −2.5). Values between 1 and 2.5 SDs below the young adult mean are termed 'osteopenia'.

As the risk of fracture increases exponentially with age, changing population demographics will increase the burden of disease (currently costing almost £1.75 billion annually in the UK). The remaining lifetime risk of hip fracture for a white woman at age 50 is around 15%, 5% for men, with equal risks around 11–13% for Colles' or vertebral fractures. Of those surviving to 80 years of age, 30% of women and 15% of men will suffer a hip fracture. Caucasian and Asian races are particularly at risk.

Fig. 10.35 **The microarchitecture of (a) normal and (b) osteoporotic bone.** There is thinning and a loss of trabecular plates in **(b)**.

Pathogenesis

The changes in bone mass with age are shown in Figure 10.36. Peak bone mass is attained between 20–30 years of age. From around the age of 40 years, age-related bone loss occurs in both men and women and persists thereafter throughout life. In women there is an acceleration of bone loss around the time of the menopause which probably lasts between 5 and 10 years.

Oestrogen deficiency is a major factor in the pathogenesis of postmenopausal osteoporosis and also in osteoporosis in men. In the elderly, vitamin D insufficiency and consequent secondary hyperparathyroidism are pathogenetic factors.

Bone mass therefore depends on the peak mass attained and on the rate of loss later in life. Genetic factors are the single most significant influence on peak bone mass but multiple genes are involved, including the collagen type IA1, vitamin D receptor and oestrogen receptor genes. Nutritional factors, sex hormone status and physical activity also affect the peak mass attained.

Risk factors associated with increased bone loss may be considered as endogenous or exogenous.

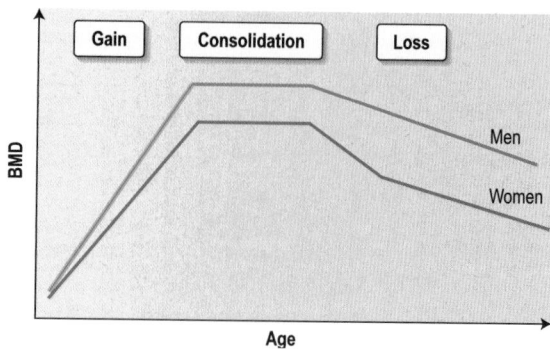

Fig. 10.36 Schematic representation of lifetime changes in bone mineral density (BMD).

- Endogenous factors include ethnicity, female gender, advancing age, family history of fracture.
- Exogenous factors include hypogonadism (male or female), glucocorticoid treatment, low body mass index, previous fracture, smoking, immobilization, and excess alcohol. Vitamin D insufficiency is particularly relevant in the elderly

Hyperparathyroidism, hyperthyroidism, coeliac disease, inflammatory bowel or joint diseases, chronic liver or renal disease increase the risk of osteoporosis. Recently raised serum homocysteine levels have been shown to be predictive for hip fractures in older people.

Falls contribute significantly to fracture risk, particularly in the elderly. Environment (e.g. poor lighting, uneven floor surface), neuromuscular and cardiovascular disease and commonly prescribed drugs (diuretics, sedatives, anxiolytics) are often overlooked causes of falls in the elderly. Some of these risk factors exert their effect through bone mineral density (BMD) whilst others are independent (Table 10.22).

Not all causes of osteoporosis affect bone remodelling and architecture in the same way. An early consequence of oestrogen deficiency (possibly transient) is reduced osteoclast apoptosis. Increased numbers of basic multicellular units (BMUs) appear, with increased resorption depth exceeding the synthetic capacity of osteoblasts, causing a loss of resistance to fracture not entirely reflected by measured BMD. Hyperparathyroidism and hyperthyroidism are also associated with increased turnover. In older individuals, reduced formation is more significant than increased resorption. Glucocorticoid-induced osteoporosis is initially associated with a high turnover state,

though chronic glucocorticoid use is associated with reduced bone formation and low turnover.

Clinical features

Fracture is the only cause of symptoms in osteoporosis. Sudden onset of severe pain in the spine, localized at the affected level and often radiating around to the front, suggests vertebral crush fracture. However, only about one in three vertebral fractures is symptomatic. Pain from mechanical derangement, increasing kyphosis, height loss and abdominal protuberance follow crushed vertebrae. Colles' fractures typically follow a fall on an outstretched arm. Fractures of the neck of the femur usually occur in older individuals falling on their side or back. Other causes of low-trauma fractures must not be overlooked, including metastatic disease and myeloma.

Investigations

If fracture suspected

Plain radiographs usually show a fracture and may reveal previous asymptomatic vertebral deformities (Fig. 10.37). Where plain films are normal, fractures (especially of pelvis) may be detected by bone scintigraphy.

(a)

Table 10.22 Risk factors for osteoporosis	
BMD-dependent	**BMD-independent**
Female sex	Increasing age
Caucasian/Asian	Previous fragility fracture
Hypogonadism	Low body mass index
Immobilization	Smoking
Alcohol abuse	Glucocorticoid therapy
Low dietary calcium intake	High bone turnover
Vitamin D insufficiency	Increased risk of falling
Drugs:	
Heparin	
Ciclosporin	
Anticonvulsants	
Endocrine disease:	
Cushing's syndrome	
Hyperthyroidism	
Hyperparathyroidism	
Other diseases:	
Chronic renal disease	
Chronic hepatic disease	
Malabsorption	
Inflammatory bowel disease	
Rheumatoid arthritis	
Mastocytosis	
Multiple myeloma	
Osteogenesis imperfecta	

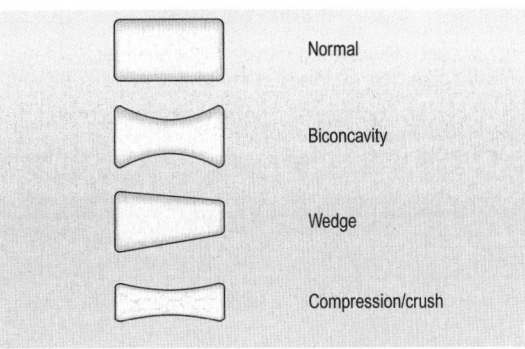

(b)

Fig. 10.37 (a) Lateral X-ray of the thoracic spine showing a compression fracture (arrowed). (b) Types of vertebral deformity in osteoporosis.

Bone density

■ *Conventional radiographs* are relatively insensitive for detecting osteopenia.

■ *Dual energy X-ray absorptiometry* (DXA) measures areal bone density (mineral per surface area rather than a true volumetric density), usually of the lumbar spine and proximal femur. It is precise, accurate, uses low doses of radiation and is the gold standard in osteoporosis diagnosis (Fig. 10.38). Because of osteophytes, spinal deformity and vertebral fractures, spinal values should be interpreted with caution in the elderly. Indications for DXA scanning are listed in Table 10.23.

■ *Quantitative CT scanning* allows true volumetric assessment, and distinction between trabecular and cortical bone. However, it is more expensive, requires higher radiation than other techniques, and to date offers no clinical advantage.

■ *Quantitative ultrasound* of the calcaneum. This does not require ionizing radiation and is cheaper than other methods. It has been shown to predict fracture risk in men and women.

Associated disease and risk factors

Investigations to exclude other diseases or identify contributory factors associated with osteoporosis should be performed and are particularly necessary in men, in whom secondary causes are more common (Table 10.22).

Selection of individuals for treatment: risk assessment

At present, population screening for osteoporosis is not recommended and a case-finding strategy is used to select individuals for bone density measurement, based on risk factors. In general, a BMD T score below −2.5 is used as a starting point for decisions about intervention; however, other independent risk factors for fracture should also be taken into account (see Fig. 10.39 and Table 10.22). Algorithms using this approach are currently being developed to assess fracture probability over a time period of 5–10 years, which provides a more appropriate interventional threshold.

Prevention and treatment (Box 10.13)

New vertebral fractures may require bed rest for 1–2 weeks with strong analgesia (e.g. meptazinol) and transcutaneous electrical nerve stimulation (TENS) may be helpful. Muscle relaxants (e.g. diazepam 2 mg three times daily), subcutaneous calcitonin (50–100 IU daily) or a single intravenous infusion of pamidronate (60–90 mg) are useful for pain relief, and physiotherapy helps restore confident mobilization. Non-spinal fractures should be treated by conventional orthopaedic means.

Predisposing lifestyle factors should be addressed, and those at significant risk can be identified for DXA.

■ *Diet* should include 700–1000 mg of calcium daily (ideally 1500 mg postmenopausally) and 400–800 IU of vitamin D in individuals not receiving adequate exposure to sunlight.

Fig. 10.38 Dual energy X-ray absorptiometry of the lumbar spine. The AP image of the lumbar spine is shown on the left and on the right, the patient's value is expressed in relation to the reference range.

Table 10.23 Indications for DXA scan
Radiographic osteopenia
Loss of height or thoracic kyphosis
Hypogonadism
Previous fragility fracture
Glucocorticoid therapy
Body mass index < 19 (kg/m²)
Maternal history of hip fracture
Diseases associated with osteoporosis (Table 10.22)

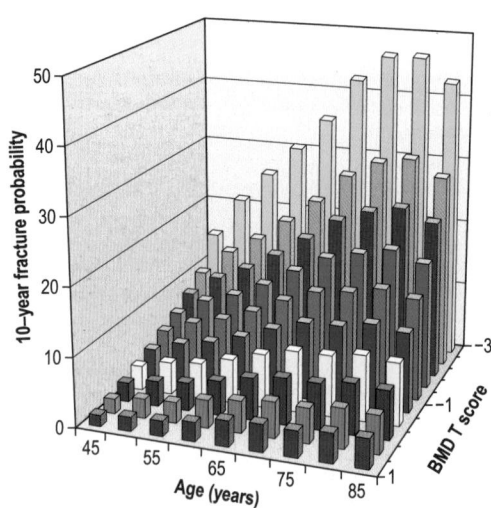

Fig. 10.39 A graph illustrating the combined effects of age (x-axis) and reduced bone mass (expressed as T scores on the z-axis) on the 10-year probability of fracture (y-axis) in a population of women. Reduced bone mass osteopenia, T scores between −1 and −2.5. Osteoporotic bone (T scores less than −2.5) is shown in pale green. Note that the risk of fracture may be greater in an older woman with osteopenia than in a young woman with osteoporosis. Data from Kanis JA (2002) Diagnosis of osteoporosis and assessment of fracture risk. *Lancet* **359**: 1929–1936.

Box 10.13 Management of osteoporosis

In all individuals
- Assess risk factors
- If present, proceed to DXA (may not be necessary in all patients with fragility fractures)
- Exclude secondary causes in patients with osteoporosis

In patients with previous fragility fracture and those aged over 65 years with BMD T score ≤ –2.5 measured by DXA
- Offer lifestyle advice (e.g. exercise, diet, smoking cessation)
- Offer treatment:
  First-line option alendronate or risedronate
  Also – raloxifene in women with vertebral osteoporosis
       – teriparatide in women with very severe osteoporosis, or if intolerant to other therapies
  Give calcium and vitamin D supplements where appropriate

In younger patients with BMD T score ≤ –2.5 (measured by DXA, hip ± spine)
- Assess need for treatment based on age and other independent risk factors
- Offer lifestyle advice
- Offer treatment as above, if appropriate

In frail older individuals
- Offer lifestyle advice
- Fall risk assessment and advice where appropriate
- Give calcium and vitamin D supplements
- Hip protectors for individuals in nursing homes

See also Royal College of Physicians' Guidelines (in list for further reading)

Box 10.14 Medication to reduce risk of fractures

- Efficacy against vertebral, non-vertebral and hip fractures:
  Bisphosphonates (alendronate, risedronate)
  Strontium ranelate
- Established efficacy against vertebral fractures:
  Raloxifene
- Established efficacy against non-vertebral and hip fractures:
  Combined calcium and vitamin D
- Established efficacy against vertebral and non-vertebral fractures:
  Teriparatide
- Conflicting evidence for efficacy:
  Calcitonin
  Calcitriol

- *Exercise.* Thirty minutes of weight-bearing exercise three times a week may increase BMD, though this has not been a universal finding in all studies. Gentle exercise in the elderly may reduce the risk of falls and improve the protective responses to falling.
- *Smoking cessation.* Smoking is associated with lower BMD and increased fracture risk. Alcohol abuse should be avoided.
- *Reduce falls.* Physiotherapy and assessment of home safety may be required. Hip protectors for elderly patients in residential care may reduce fracture risk.

Pharmacological intervention

Most interventions used act by inhibiting bone resorption (anti-resorptives) although teriparatide stimulates bone formation and strontium ranelate (a new drug) does both. In clinical trials all interventions have been assessed against a background of calcium and vitamin D repletion, and in clinical practice supplements should therefore be given if there is any evidence or risk of deficiency.

The evidence base for anti-fracture efficacy of interventions varies. Adequately powered randomized controlled trials, with fracture as end-point, exist for alendronate, risedronate, raloxifene, hormone replacement therapy, teriparatide (recombinant human PTH peptide 1-34) and combined calcium/vitamin D (the latter in frail older individuals only). Some interventions have been shown to reduce fracture at vertebral and non-vertebral sites, including the hip, whereas others have not been demonstrated to be effective at all sites (Box 10.14). Since a fracture at one site increases the risk of subsequent fracture at any site, treatments with efficacy at all major fracture sites (particularly spine and hip) are preferable. Hence the bisphosphonates or strontium ranelate are generally regarded as the first-line options in the majority of women with osteoporosis.

- *Bisphosphonates,* synthetic analogues of bone pyrophosphate (Fig. 10.40) adhere to hydroxyapatite and inhibit osteoclasts. *Alendronate* and *risedronate* increase bone mass at the hip and spine, and reduce the incidence of fractures at vertebral, hip and other sites, particularly in women who have already sustained a vertebral fracture. These can be given as daily (10 mg and 5 mg respectively) or once-weekly doses; (70 mg and 35 mg respectively) are preferred by the vast majority of patients. Etidronate is given cyclically, alternating 2 weeks of the drug with 76 days of calcium supplement. It has been shown to reduce vertebral fractures and, in observational studies, a

Fig. 10.40 The chemical structures of the aminophosphonates alendronate and risedronate are compared with the structure of pyrophosphate.

reduction in non-vertebral fractures has also been shown. The optimal duration of bisphosphonate therapy is unknown; prolonged suppression of bone turnover may have adverse effects, and it is currently advised to reassess treatment after 5–10 years. Nitrogen-containing bisphosphonates (e.g. alendronate, risedronate) may cause upper gastro-intestinal side-effects, and adherence to a strict dosing regimen is necessary. The tablets should be taken in the fasting state with a large drink of water, while the patient is standing or sitting upright. The patient should subsequently remain upright and avoid food and drink for at least 30 minutes. Bisphosphonates should be used with caution in patients with renal impairment.

■ *Raloxifene* is a selective oestrogen-receptor modulator (SERM). It has no stimulatory effect on the endometrium but activates oestrogen receptors in bone. It prevents BMD loss at the spine and hip in post-menopausal women, though fracture rates were only reduced in the spine. It also reduces the incidence of oestrogen-receptor-positive breast carcinoma in women treated for up to 4 years. Leg cramps and flushing may occur and the risk of thromboembolic complications is also increased to a degree similar to that seen with HRT. It is given as a daily oral dose (60 mg).

■ *Recombinant human parathyroid hormone peptide 1-34* (*teriparatide*) is an anabolic agent that stimulates bone formation. It has been shown to reduce vertebral and non-vertebral fractures in postmenopausal women with established osteoporosis, although data on hip fracture are not available. It is given by daily subcutaneous injection in a dose of 20 µg. Its use is mainly indicated in very severe cases of osteoporosis or in women who are intolerant of or fail to respond to other therapies. Teriparatide causes only mild transient hypercalcaemia and routine monitoring is not required. Nausea and headache may occur.

■ *Strontium ranelate* is a new dual action bone agent that has anti-resorptive and anabolic effects. It reduces the risk of vertebral and non-vertebral fractures, including hip fractures in post-menopausal women with osteoporosis. The dose is 2 g daily (granules are dissolved in water at night). Nausea, diarrhoea and headache are infrequent side effects and there is a small increase in the risk of venous thromboembolic disease.

■ *Combination therapy of calcium with vitamin D* has been shown to reduce non-vertebral fractures, including hip fractures, in elderly women living in residential care The recommended dose is 800 IU of vitamin D and 1 g calcium daily.

Strategies used less commonly
These include:

■ *Hormone replacement therapy* (HRT) prevents bone loss and reduces vertebral and non-vertebral fractures. However, because of adverse effects on breast cancer and cardiovascular disease risk it is now not used except in perimenopausal women with osteoporosis

who also have menopausal symptoms and in women who are intolerant of other therapies (for a suggested maximum of 5 years).

■ *Combination therapies*, either with two anti-resorptive agents or an anti-resorptive and an anabolic agent often produce larger increases in BMD than mono-therapy but have not been shown to result in greater fracture reduction than with monotherapy.

■ *Calcitriol* (1,25-(OH)$_2$D$_3$) may reduce vertebral fracture rate, although the data are inconsistent. Hypercalcaemia and hypercalciuria may occur and monitoring is necessary.

■ *Calcitonin*. Nasal or subcutaneous calcitonin may be used; vertebral fracture rates may be reduced, although this has not been a universal finding.

Glucocorticoid-induced osteoporosis
Individuals requiring oral glucocorticoid therapy for 3 months or more (at any dose) should be assessed for coexisting risk factors (age, previous fracture, hormone status). Primary prevention is recommended in men and women aged over 65 years and in individuals who have sustained a fragility fracture aged 40 years or more. DXA results guide treatment for other patients. Bisphosphonates (etidronate, alendronate and risedronate) are the only approved agents for this indication. Calcium and vitamin D supplementation should also be given.

Osteoporosis in men
Alendronate (10 mg daily) has been shown to increase BMD and to reduce vertebral fractures in men with osteoporosis and is approved for this indication. In men with osteoporosis who have clinical and biochemical evidence of hypogonadism, testosterone replacement can be used.

FURTHER READING
Beral V, Banks E, Reeves G (2002) Evidence from randomized trials on the long-term effects of hormone replacement therapy. *Lancet* **360**: 942–944.

Bone and Tooth Society, National Osteoporosis Society and Royal College of Physicians (2002) *Glucocorticoid-induced Osteoporosis. Guidelines for Prevention and Treatment*. Royal College of Physicians, London

Bone HG et al. (2004) Ten year's experience with alendronate for osteoporosis in post-menopausal women. *New England Journal of Medicine* **350**: 1189–1199.

Cummings SR, Melton LJ (2002) Epidemiology and outcomes of osteoporotic fractures. *Lancet* **359**: 1761–1767.

Delmas PD (2002) Treatment of postmenopausal osteoporosis. *Lancet* **359**: 2018–2026.

Kanis JA (2002) Diagnosis of osteoporosis and assessment of fracture risk. *Lancet* **359**: 1929–1936.

Riggs BL, Hartmann LC (2003) Selective estrogen receptor modulators – mechanisms of action and application to clinical practice. *New England Journal of Medicine* **348**: 618–629.

Royal College of Physicians (2000) *Osteoporosis: Clinical Guidelines for Prevention and Treatment. Update on Pharmacological Interventions and an Algorithm for Management.* London: Royal College of Physicians.
Seeman E (2002) Pathogenesis of bone fragility in women and men. *Lancet* **359**: 1841–1850.

PAGET'S DISEASE

Osteitis deformans or Paget's disease is a focal disorder of bone remodelling. The initial event of excessive resorption is followed by a compensatory increase in new bone formation, increased local bone blood flow and fibrous tissue in adjacent bone marrow. Ultimately, formation exceeds resorption but the new bone is structurally abnormal.

Epidemiological studies are difficult because most patients are asymptomatic. Most often seen in Europe and particularly in northern England, it affects men and women (2 : 3) over age 40 years. Incidence approximately doubles per decade thereafter, with up to 10% radiologically affected by the age of 90. A positive family history is noted in about 14%.

Aetiology and pathogenesis

A number of genes have been implicated in Paget's disease, including sequestsome p62, nuclear factor kappa B (NFkB), osteoprotegerin and *bcl2*. Intracellular inclusions in the osteoclasts in a pagetic lesion are believed to be paramyxovirus nucleocapsid (e.g. canine distemper virus, measles or respiratory syncytial virus). However, similar microfilaments are seen in other bone disorders, and theories of a viral aetiology in Paget's remain contentious. Altered expression of c-*fos* (an oncogene) is one suggested mechanism linking viral infection with the pathogenic changes in osteoclasts, which are more numerous, and contain an increased number of nuclei (up to 100). Increased osteoclastic bone resorption is followed by formation of woven bone; which is softer and may lead to deformity and increased fracture risk. Unaffected bone remains normal throughout life (i.e. Paget's disease does not spread, but can become symptomatic at previously silent sites).

Clinical features (Fig. 10.41)

Most (60–80%) patients with radiologically identified Paget's disease are asymptomatic. Diagnosis often follows the finding of an asymptomatic elevation of serum alkaline phosphatase, or a plain X-ray performed for other indications. The disease may involve one bone (monostotic, in 15%) or many (polyostotic). The most common sites in order of frequency are pelvis, lumbar spine, femur, thoracic spine, sacrum, skull, tibia.

Symptoms can include:

- bone pain, most often in the spine or the pelvis
- joint pain when an involved bone is close to a joint, leading to cartilage damage and osteoarthritis
- deformities, in particular bowed tibia and skull changes
- complications from:
  (a) nerve compression (deafness from VIIIth cranial nerve involvement; also cranial nerves II, V, VII may be involved; spinal stenosis, hydrocephalus)
  (b) increased bone blood flow (myocardial hypertrophy and high-output cardiac failure)
  (c) pathological fractures
- osteogenic sarcoma in pagetic bone (fewer than 1% of cases, but a 30-fold increased risk compared with non-pagetic patients).

Investigations

- **X-ray** features vary from predominantly lytic lesions (osteoporosis circumscripta in the skull is characteristic), through a mixed phase, to a mainly sclerotic phase of bone expansion, thickening of trabeculae and loss of distinction between cortex and trabeculae (de-differentiation).
- **Bone scans** show the extent of skeletal involvement, but are unable to distinguish between Paget's disease and sclerotic metastatic carcinoma (especially breast and prostate).
- **Increased serum alkaline phosphatase** with normal serum calcium and phosphate, reflects increased bone turnover. Levels may be normal with limited or monostotic Paget's. Levels are reduced with treatment and are a marker of relapse. Mild hypercalcaemia follows immobilization only when there is very extensive disease. Urinary hydroxyproline excretion is also increased and, together with serum alkaline phosphatase levels, may be used as a marker of disease activity.

Treatment

Bisphosphonates are the mainstay of treatment. New bone formed after treatment is lamellar, not woven (reflecting normalization of bone turnover rather than a direct effect on osteoblasts). In addition to treating symptomatic patients (the minority), studies to date indicate that treatment of asymptomatic lesions is appropriate if there is a significant risk of potential complications, e.g. fracture in weight-bearing long bones or the spine, nerve entrapment or deafness with skull involvement, and treatment before orthopaedic procedures in involved bone (to reduce vascularity).

Intravenous bisphosphonates

Intravenous pamidronate is highly efficacious. Regimens vary widely but up to 360 mg is given in divided doses over 6 weeks and then repeated as required after 6 months or longer. Pamidronate can be associated with a first-dose reaction characterized by 'flu-like' symptoms including a transient pyrexia over 24–48 hours.

Oral bisphosphonates

Tiludronate is indicated for the treatment of Paget's disease in a dose of 400 mg daily for 12 weeks, repeated as necessary after 6 weeks or longer. Ibandronate, 30 mg daily for 2 months, repeated if necessary after at least 2 months, is also approved for this indication. Risedronate,

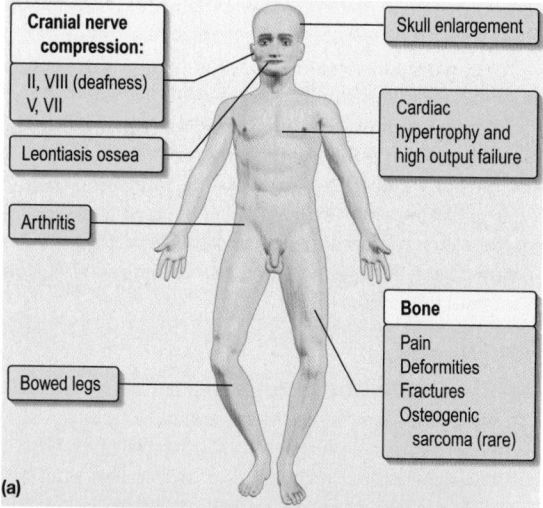

(a)

Cranial nerve compression:
II, VIII (deafness)
V, VII

Leontiasis ossea

Arthritis

Bowed legs

Skull enlargement

Cardiac hypertrophy and high output failure

Bone
Pain
Deformities
Fractures
Osteogenic sarcoma (rare)

(b)

(c)

Fig. 10.41 **Paget's disease. (a)** Clinical features. **(b)** Picture of the legs showing bowing of the tibia, caused by increased bone growth. Note the erythema ab igne on the medial aspect of the thigh. **(c)** X-ray appearance of the pelvis, showing osteolytic and osteosclerotic lesions.

30 mg/day for 2 months, repeated as necessary after at least 2 months, may also be used. Etidronate is also approved but is less often used because of its lower potency.

Treatment is monitored by regular measurement of serum alkaline phosphatase levels ± urinary hydroxyproline excretion.

Surgery

Joint replacement or osteotomy is sometimes necessary to correct deformity or pain due to (secondary) degenerative joint disease. Intra-articular injection of lidocaine can be useful to differentiate joint or bone disease. Neurosurgery may be required where there is spinal disease. Osteosarcoma usually requires amputation, though wide excision and limb-salvage can be successful at distal sites.

FURTHER READING

Lyles KW et al. (2001) A clinical approach to diagnosis and management of Paget's disease of bone. *Journal of Bone and Mineral Research* **16**: 1379–1387.

RICKETS AND OSTEOMALACIA

Rickets (in children) and osteomalacia (in adults) result from inadequate mineralization of bone matrix (osteoid). They are usually caused by a defect in vitamin D availability or metabolism.

Pathology

In children, the growth plate is elongated with distortion of the arrangement of chondrocytes. Calcification is delayed and vascularization impaired. In adults, osteomalacia is characterized by increased osteoid width (> 15 μm) and increased mineralization lag time.

Double tetracycline labelling shows lack of uptake of tetracycline in osteoid seams. Changes of secondary hyperparathyroidism are often present, except in hypophosphataemic osteomalacia.

Aetiology (Table 10.24)

Vitamin D deficiency is usually due to inadequate sunlight

Table 10.24 Causes of rickets and osteomalacia

Vitamin D deficiency
Inadequate synthesis in skin
Low dietary intake
Malabsorption:
   Coeliac disease
   Intestinal resection
   Chronic cholestasis, e.g. primary biliary cirrhosis

Renal disease
Chronic renal failure
Bone disease due to dialysis
Tubular disorders, e.g. renal tubular acidosis, Fanconi's
   syndrome

Miscellaneous
Vitamin-D-dependent rickets types I and II
Dent's disease (X-linked hypophosphataemia – vitamin-D-
   resistant rickets)
Tumour-induced hypophosphataemic rickets and
   osteomalacia

exposure and/or dietary insufficiency (Fig. 10.33). Asian women and elderly individuals, especially those who are housebound, are particularly at risk. Anticonvulsant therapy (especially phenytoin and phenobarbital) affects vitamin D metabolism and predisposes to vitamin D deficiency. Malabsorption of vitamin D occurs in some gastrointestinal diseases, particularly coeliac disease and small intestinal Crohn's disease.

Chronic renal failure results in reduced 1α-hydroxylation of 25-(OH)D$_3$. Mutations in the P450$_{c1}$ α gene (chromosome 12) cause 1α-hydroxylase deficiency, also known as *vitamin D-dependent rickets type I*, an autosomal recessive disease (see p. 711). In *type II vitamin D-dependent rickets* there is a defect in the intracellular 1,25-(OH)$_2$D$_3$ receptor. X-linked hypophosphataemic rickets, resulting in lower-limb deformities and stunted growth rate in affected males, is caused by mutations in the *PHEX* gene (see p. 711). In the Fanconi syndrome and in renal tubular acidosis, osteomalacia can develop, mainly because of the continuous phosphaturia.

Hypophosphataemic osteomalacia has been associated with mesenchymal tumours which are believed to produce humoral factors ('phosphatonins') including fibroblast growth factor 23 (FGF23), which increases phosphate excretion. Treatment of the tumour results in remineralization.

Clinical features

Adult osteomalacia may produce vague symptoms of bone or muscle pain and tenderness. Pathological fractures may occur. Occasionally a marked proximal myopathy leads to a characteristic 'waddling' gait. Deformity is uncommon. In modern practice many cases are detected biochemically in high-risk patients, especially those with gastrointestinal disease or surgery, before clear symptoms are present. Occasionally, tetany or other hypocalcaemic features may occur.

At birth, neonatal rickets may present as craniotabes (thin deformed skull). In the first few years of life there may be widened epiphyses at the wrists and beading at the costochondral junctions, producing the 'rickety rosary', or a groove in the rib cage (Harrison's sulcus). In older children, lower limb deformities are seen. A myopathy may also occur. Hypocalcaemic tetany may occur in severe cases.

Investigations

- **Increased serum alkaline phosphatase**, indicating increased osteoblast activity, is the most common abnormality (note: alkaline phosphatase is elevated during skeletal growth).
- **Plasma calcium** is usually normal, in association with secondary hyperparathyroidism and a raised PTH., but may be low in severe cases.
- **Serum phosphate** may be low, owing to increased PTH-dependent phosphaturia, though this is variable.
- **Serum 25-hydroxyvitamin D$_3$** is usually low (exceptions being vitamin-D-resistant rickets).
- **X-rays** are often normal in adults, but may show defective mineralization, especially in the pelvis, long bones and ribs, with 'Looser's zones' – linear areas of low density surrounded by sclerotic borders.
- **Iliac crest biopsy** with double tetracycline labelling (see above) is occasionally necessary if biochemical tests are equivocal.

Treatment

Treatment should be directed towards correction of the cause where possible, with increase in vitamin D intake and sunlight exposure.

Multiple formulations of vitamin D and its metabolites are available. When deficiency is nutritional, 'replacement' doses of the native vitamin are needed (400–800 IU daily). Higher 'pharmacological' doses, sometimes administered parenterally, may be needed in some patients with gastrectomy, malabsorption or liver disease, although many respond to more conventional doses. Treatment with calcitriol or alfacalcidol is indicated where there is defective 1α-hydroxylation, e.g. chronic renal disease, vitamin D resistance and hypophosphataemic rickets and osteomalacia.

FURTHER READING
Wharton B, Bishop N (2003) Rickets. *Lancet* **362**: 1389–1400.

SKELETAL DYSPLASIAS

These include a large group of heterogeneous disorders of bone and connective tissue.

Collagen defects

Collagen is responsible for many of the structural, tensile and load-bearing properties in the various tissues where it is found. The structure of collagen is discussed on page 530. Twenty-eight dispersed genes encode for more than 16 different types of collagen:

- The fibrillar collagens, e.g. types I, II, III, V and XI, are encoded by *COL1A1–2, COL2A1, COL3, COL5, COL11.* Mutations of these genes produce osteogenesis imperfecta and Ehlers–Danlos syndrome.
- Basement membrane collagen, type IV, is encoded by *COL4A1–5.* Mutations lead to Alport's disease (see p. 631).
- Fibril-associated collagens with interrupted triple helices (FACIT), e.g. types IX, XII and XIV, are encoded by *COL9, COL12.*
- Filament producing collagen type VI is encoded by *COL6A1, 2, 3.*
- Network-forming collagens types VIII and X are encoded by *COL8A1, COL10A1.*
- Anchoring fibril collagen, e.g. type VII, is encoded by *COL7A1.* Mutations of this gene produce epidermolysis bullosa (p. 1348).

Ehlers–Danlos syndrome

This is a heterogeneous group of disorders of collagen. Ten different types have been recognized with varying degrees of skin fragility, skin hyperextensibility and joint hypermobility. Types I, II and III are inherited in an autosomal dominant fashion; the biochemical basis is unknown. No abnormalities in *COL1A1, COL1A2* and *COL2A1* genes have been found.

Type IV is also autosomal dominant and involves arteries, the bowel and uterus, as well as the skin. Mutations in *COL3A1* gene produce abnormalities in structure, synthesis or secretion of type III collagen.

Type VI is a recessively inherited disorder and results from a mutation in the gene that encodes lysyl hydroxylase.

Type VII is an autosomal dominant disorder where there is a defect in the conversion of procollagen to collagen; *COL1A1* and *COL1A2* mutations delete the *N*-proteinase cleavage sites.

Other forms of Ehlers–Danlos are very rare and their defects have not been elucidated. The clinical features are described on page 1356.

Osteogenesis imperfecta (fragilitas ossium, brittle bone syndrome)

This is a heterogeneous group of mainly autosomally dominant inherited disorders. In the majority there are mutations in the genes encoding the chains in type I collagen, i.e. *COL1A1, COL1A2.* There are four main types with very variable clinical pictures ranging from death in the perinatal period (type II), severe bone deformity (type III), to a normal lifespan (types I and IV). Recently three separate clinical subtypes have been identified (V, VI and VII).

The major clinical feature is very fragile and brittle bones but other collagen-containing tissues are also involved, such as tendons, the skin and the eyes. Osteogenesis imperfecta tarda (type I) has mild bony deformities, blue sclerae, defective dentine, early-onset deafness, hypermobility of joints, and heart valve disorders. More severe forms present with multiple fractures and gross deformities. Treatment is with bisphosphonates, which enhances bone cortical thickness. Prognosis is variable, depending on the severity of the disease.

Osteochondrodysplasia

There are over 150 variants, some, but not all, due to mutations in the *COL2A1* gene that encodes type II collagen. Many types have not been clearly identified. All show abnormalities of the vitreous humour of the eye and abnormalities of articular cartilage, both of which have abundant type II collagen.

Miscellaneous defects

Osteopetrosis (marble bone disease)

This condition may be inherited in either an autosomal dominant or an autosomal recessive manner; the recessive type is severe and the dominant type is mild. In addition, another recessive form associated with renal tubular acidosis is due to carbonic anhydrase II deficiency.

In the severe form, bone density is increased throughout the skeleton but bones tend to fracture easily. Involvement of the bone marrow leads to a leucoerythroblastic anaemia. There is mental retardation and early death.

In the mild form there may be only X-ray changes, but fractures and infection can occur. The acid phosphate level is raised.

Marfan's syndrome

This is described on page 1356.

Fibroblast growth factor receptor defect

Achondroplasia ('dwarfism') is diagnosed in the first years of life. The disease is inherited in an autosomal dominant manner and is caused by a defect in the fibroblast growth factor receptor-3 gene. The trunk is of normal length but the limbs are very short and broad. The vault of the skull is enlarged, the face is small and the nose bridge is flat. Intelligence is normal.

FURTHER READING

Rauch F, Glorieux FH (2004) Osteogenesis imperfecta. *Lancet* **363**: 1377–1385.
Tolar J, Teitelbaum SL, Orchard PJ (2004) Osteopetrosis. *New England Journal of Medicine* **351**: 2839–2849.

CHAPTER BIBLIOGRAPHY

Favus MJ (ed.) (2000) *Primer on the Metabolic Bone Diseases and Disorders of Mineral Metabolism*, 4th edn. Philadelphia: Lippincott Raven, American Society for Bone and Mineral Research.

Scriver CR, Beaudet AL, Sly WS, Valle D (2000) *The Metabolic Basis of Inherited Disease*, 8th edn. New York: McGraw-Hill.

SIGNIFICANT WEBSITES

http://www.rheumatology.org
  American College of Rheumatology
http://www.arc.org.uk
  UK Arthritis Research Campaign
http://www.rheumatology.org.uk/
  British Society of Rheumatology – useful, patient-oriented information
http://www.nos.org.uk/
  UK National Osteoporosis Society – useful information and reviews of ongoing research

http://www.osteo.org/
  US National Institute of Health's bone-diseases page, with useful links from there for osteoporosis, Paget's and osteomalacia
http://www.cbcu.cam.ac.uk/calreviews
  Cambridge University site – links to quizzes, pathology images, etc.
http://www.rcplondon.ac.uk
  Royal College of Physicians Guidelines
http://www.catchword.com
  Clinical Medicine journal

Renal disease 11

FUNCTIONAL ANATOMY

The kidneys are paired organs, 11–14 cm in length in adults, 5–6 cm in width and 3–4 cm in depth. The kidneys lie retroperitoneally on either side of the vertebral column at the level of T12 to L3. The renal parenchyma comprises an outer cortex and an inner medulla. The functional unit of the kidney is the nephron of which each contains approximately one million. *Each nephron* is made up of a glomerulus, proximal tubule, loop of Henle, distal tubule and collecting duct. The renal capsule and ureters are innervated via T10–12 and L1 nerve roots, and renal pain is felt over the corresponding dermatomes.

Arterial blood is supplied to the kidneys via the renal arteries, which branch off the abdominal aorta, and venous blood is conveyed to the inferior vena cava via the renal veins. Approximately 25% of humans possess dual or multiple renal arteries on one or both sides. The left renal vein is longer than the right and for this reason the left kidney, where possible, is usually chosen for live donor transplant nephrectomy.

The *renal artery* undergoes a series of divisions within the kidney (Fig. 11.1) forming successively the *interlobar arteries*, which run radially to the corticomedullary junction, *arcuate arteries*, which run circumferentially along the corticomedullary junction, and *interlobular arteries* which run radially through the renal cortex towards the surface of the kidney. *Afferent glomerular arterioles* arise from the interlobular arteries to supply the glomerular capillary bed, which drains into *efferent glomerular arterioles*. Efferent arterioles from the outer cortical glomeruli drain into a peritubular capillary network within the renal cortex and thence into increasingly large and more proximal branches of the renal vein. By contrast, blood from the juxtamedullary glomeruli passes via the vasa recta in the medulla and then turns back towards the area of the cortex from which the vasa recta originated. *Vasa recta* possess fenestrated walls, which facilitates movement of diffusible substances. The collecting ducts merge in the inner medulla to form the ducts of Bellini, which empty at the apices of the papillae into the calyces. The calyces, in common with the renal pelvis, ureter and bladder are lined with transitional cell epithelium.

The *glomerulus* comprises four main cell types: (1) endothelial cells which are fenestrated with 500–1000 Å pores; (2) visceral epithelial cells (podocytes) which support the delicate glomerular basement membrane by means of an extensive trabecular network (foot processes); (3) parietal epithelial cells which cover the Bowman's capsule; (4) mesangial cells (see Fig. 11.11). Mesangial cells are believed to be related to macrophages of the reticuloendothelial

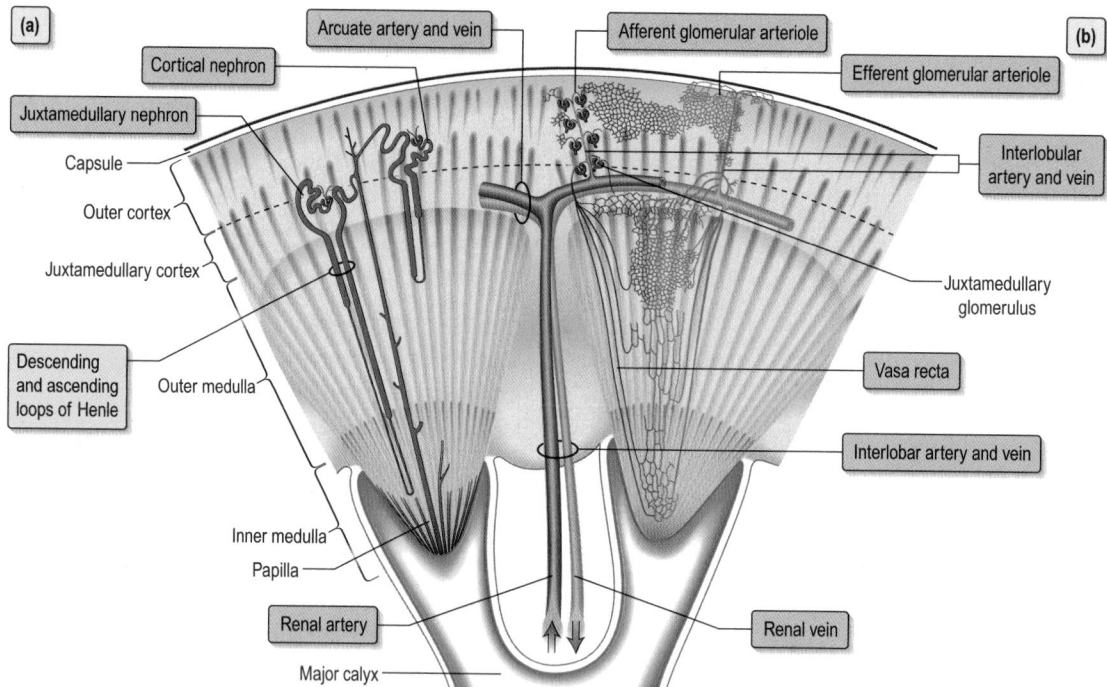

Fig. 11.1 **Functional anatomy of the kidney. (a)** The nephrons. **(b)** Arterial and venous supply. After Williams PL (ed) (1995) *Gray's Anatomy*, 38th edn. Edinburgh: Churchill Livingstone, with permission from Elsevier.

system and have a phagocytic function and contractile capabilities that can control blood flow and filtration surface area along the glomerular capillaries in response to a host of mediators. They also secrete the mesangial matrix, which provides skeletal framework for the entire glomerular capillaries. The glomerular capillary basement membrane lies between the endothelial and the visceral epithelial cells. The latter put out multiple long foot processes which interdigitate with those of adjacent epithelial cells. Together the endothelial cells, basement membrane and epithelial cells form the filtration barrier or sieve.

The *renal tubules* are lined by epithelial cells, which are cuboidal except in the thin limb of the loop of Henle where they are flat. Proximal tubular cells differ from other cells of the system as they have a luminal brush border. The cortical portion of the collecting ducts contains two cell types with different functions, namely principal cells and intercalated cells (see p. 694). Fibroblast-like cells in the renal cortical interstitium have been identified and shown to produce erythropoietin in response to hypoxia (p. 611).

The *juxtaglomerular apparatus* comprises the macula densa, the extraglomerular mesangium and the terminal portion of the afferent glomerular arteriole (which contains renin-producing granular cells) together with the proximal portion of the efferent arteriole. The macula densa is a plaque of cells containing large, tightly packed cell nuclei (hence the name macula densa) within the thick ascending limb of the loop of Henle. This anatomical arrangement is such as to allow changes in the renal tubule to influence behaviour of the adjacent glomerulus (tubulo-glomerular feedback).

RENAL FUNCTION

PHYSIOLOGY

A conventional diagrammatic representation of the nephron is shown in Figure 11.2a and a physiological version in Figure 11.2b.

An essential feature of renal function is that a large volume of blood – 25% of cardiac output or approximately 1300 mL per minute – passes through the two million glomeruli.

A hydrostatic pressure gradient of approximately 10 mmHg (a capillary pressure of 45 mmHg minus 10 mmHg of pressure within Bowman's space and 25 mmHg of plasma oncotic pressure) provides the driving force for ultrafiltration of virtually protein-free and fat-free fluid across the glomerular capillary wall into Bowman's space and so into the renal tubule (Fig. 11.3).

The *ultrafiltration rate* (glomerular filtration rate; GFR) varies with age and sex but is approximately 120–130 mL/min per 1.73 m^2 surface area in adults. This means that, each day, ultrafiltration of 170–180 L of water and unbound small-molecular-weight constituents of blood occurs. If these large volumes of ultrafiltrate were excreted unchanged as urine, it would be necessary to ingest huge amounts of water and electrolytes to stay in balance. This is avoided by the selective reabsorption of water, essential electrolytes and other blood constituents, such as glucose and amino acids, from the filtrate in transit along the nephron. Thus, 60–80% of filtered water and sodium are reabsorbed in the proximal tubule along with virtually all the potassium, bicarbonate, glucose and

Fig. 11.2 (a) Principal parts of the nephron. The point where the distal tubule is in close proximity to its own glomerulus is called the juxtaglomerular apparatus. This contains the macula densa.
(b) Diagrammatic representation of the counter-current system.
(i) Vasa recta: these vessels descend from the cortex into the medulla and then turn back towards the cortex. *(ii) Cortical nephron*: these have short descending limbs extending into the outer medulla. *(iii) Juxtamedullary nephron*: the descending limb dips deeply into the hypertonic inner medulla. Numbers indicate approximate osmolalities.

Fig. 11.3 Pressures controlling glomerular filtration.
1, capillary hydrostatic pressure (45 mmHg); **2**, hydrostatic pressure in Bowman's space (10 mmHg); **3**, plasma protein oncotic pressure (25 mmHg). Arrows (1, 2, 3) indicate the direction of a pressure gradient.

amino acids (Fig. 11.2b). Additional water and sodium chloride are reabsorbed more distally, and fine tuning of salt and water balance is achieved in the distal tubules and collecting ducts under the influence of aldosterone and antidiuretic hormone (ADH). The final urine volume is thus 1–2 L daily. Calcium, phosphate and magnesium are also selectively reabsorbed in proportion to the need to maintain a normal electrolyte composition of body fluids.

The urinary excretion of some compounds is more complicated. For example, potassium is freely filtered at the glomerulus, almost completely reabsorbed in the proximal tubule, and secreted in the distal tubule and collecting ducts. A clinical consequence of this is that the ability to eliminate unwanted potassium is less dependent on GFR than is the elimination of urea or creatinine. Other compounds filtered and reabsorbed or secreted to a variable extent include urate and many organic acids, including many drugs or their metabolic breakdown products. The more tubular secretion of a compound that occurs, the less dependent elimination is on the GFR; penicillin and cefradine are examples of compounds secreted by the tubules.

Urine concentration and the countercurrent system

Urine is concentrated by a complex interaction between the loops of Henle, the medullary interstitium, medullary blood vessels (vasa recta) and the collecting ducts (see p. 691). The proposed mechanism of urine concentration is termed 'the countercurrent mechanism'. The countercurrent hypothesis states that: 'a small difference in osmotic concentration at any point between fluid flowing in opposite directions in two parallel tubes connected in a hairpin manner is multiplied many times along the length of the tubes'. Tubular fluid moves from the renal cortex towards the papillary tip of the medulla via the proximal straight tubule and the thin descending limb of the loop of Henle, which is permeable to water and impermeable to sodium. The tubule then loops back towards the cortex so that the direction of the fluid movement is reversed in the ascending limb, which is impermeable to water but permeable to sodium. This results in a large osmolar concentration difference between the corticomedullary junction and the hairpin loop at the tip of the papilla, and hence countercurrent multiplication. There is an analogy with heat exchangers.

Since the urine that emerges from the proximal tubule is iso-osmotic, the first nephron segment actually involved in urinary concentration is the descending limb of Henle's loop. There are two types of descending limbs (Fig. 11.2b). The short loops originate in superficial and midcortical glomeruli, which turn in the outer medulla. The long loops, which originate in the deep cortical and juxtamedullary glomeruli, penetrate the outer medulla up to the tip of the papilla. Approximately 15% of nephrons have long loops and the remaining 85% have short loops. Both the ascending limb in the outer and inner medulla and the first part of the distal tubule are impermeable to water and urea. Through the $Na^+/K^+/2Cl$ cotransporter, the thick ascending limb actively transports sodium chloride, increasing the interstitial tonicity, resulting in tubular dilution with no net movement of water and urea on account of low permeability. The hypotonic fluid under ADH action undergoes osmotic equilibration with the interstitium in the late distal and the cortical and outer medullary collecting duct, resulting in water removal. Urea concentration in the tubular fluid rises on account of low urea permeability. At the inner medullary collecting duct, which is highly permeable to urea and water, especially in response to ADH, the urea enters the interstitium down its concentration gradient, preserving interstitial hypertonicity and generating high urea concentration in the interstitium.

The hypertonic interstitium causes abstraction of water from the descending limb of the loop of Henle, which is relatively impermeable to NaCl and urea, making the tubular fluid hypertonic with high NaCl concentration as it arrives at the bend of the loop of Henle. Urea plays a key role in the generation of medullary interstitial hypertonicity. The urea that is reabsorbed into the inner medullary stripe from the terminal inner medullary collecting duct is carried out of this region by ascending vasa recta, which deposits urea into the adjacent descending limb of both short and long loops of Henle, thus recycling the urea to the inner medullary collecting tubule. This process is facilitated by the close anatomical relationship that the hairpin loop of Henle and the vasa recta share.

Acid–base balance

Tubular function is also critical to the control of acid–base balance. Thus, filtered bicarbonate is largely reabsorbed and hydrogen ions are excreted mainly buffered by phosphate (see p. 713).

Glomerular filtration rate (GFR)

In health, the GFR remains remarkably constant owing to intrarenal regulatory mechanisms. In disease, with a reduction in intrarenal blood flow, damage to or loss of glomeruli, or obstruction to the free flow of ultrafiltrate along the tubule, the GFR will fall and the ability to eliminate waste material and to regulate the volume and composition of body fluid will decline. This will be manifest as a rise in the plasma urea or creatinine and in a reduction in measured GFR.

The concentration of urea or creatinine in plasma represents the dynamic equilibrium between production and elimination. In healthy subjects there is an enormous reserve of renal excretory function, and serum urea and creatinine do not rise above the normal range until there is a reduction of 50–60% in the GFR. Thereafter, the level

Table 11.1 Factors influencing serum urea levels

Production	Elimination
Increased by	**Increased by**
High-protein diet	Elevated GFR, e.g. pregnancy
Increased catabolism	
Surgery	**Decreased by**
Infection	Glomerular disease
Trauma	Reduced renal blood flow
Corticosteroid therapy	Hypotension
Tetracyclines	Dehydration
Gastrointestinal bleeding	Urinary obstruction
Cancer	Tubulointerstitial nephritis
Decreased by	
Low-protein diet	
Reduced catabolism,	
e.g. old age	
Liver failure	

GFR, glomerular filtration rate

of urea depends both on the GFR and its production rate (Table 11.1). The latter is heavily influenced by protein intake and tissue catabolism. The level of creatinine is much less dependent on diet but is more related to age, sex and muscle mass. Once it is elevated, serum creatinine is a better guide to GFR than urea and, in general, measurement of serum creatinine is a good way to monitor further deterioration in the GFR.

It must be re-emphasized that a normal serum urea or creatinine is not synonymous with a normal GFR.

Measurement of the glomerular filtration rate

Measurement of the GFR is necessary to define the exact level of renal function. It is essential when the serum (plasma) urea or creatinine is within the normal range.

Inulin clearance – the gold standard of physiologists – is not practical or necessary in clinical practice. The most widely used measurement is the creatinine clearance (Fig. 11.4).

Creatinine clearance is dependent on the fact that daily production of creatinine (principally from muscle cells) is remarkably constant and little affected by protein intake. Serum creatinine and urinary output thus vary very little throughout the day. This permits the use of 24-hour urine collections, which reduce collection errors, and the measurement of a single serum creatinine value during the 24 hours.

Creatinine excretion is, however, by both glomerular filtration and tubular secretion, although at normal serum levels the latter is relatively small. As most laboratory methods for measurement of serum creatinine give slight overestimates, the calculation of clearance fortuitously gives a value close to that of inulin.

With progressive renal failure, creatinine clearance may overestimate GFR but, in clinical practice, this is seldom significant. Certain drugs – for example cimetidine, trimethoprim, spironolactone and amiloride – reduce tubular secretion of creatinine, leading to a rise in serum creatinine and a fall in measured clearance.

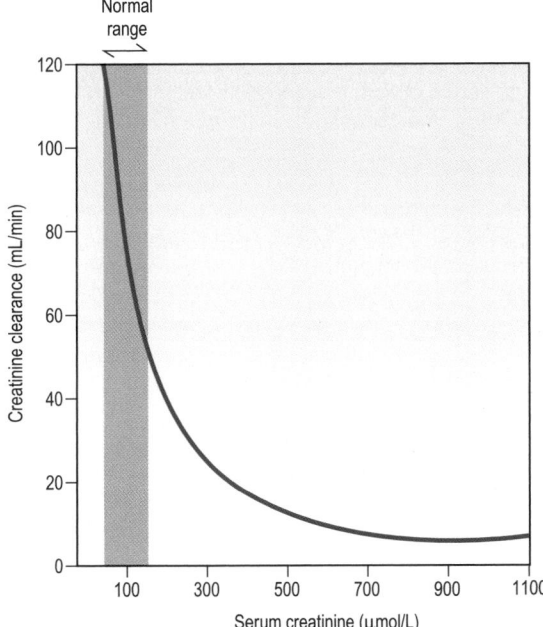

Fig. 11.4 Creatinine clearance versus serum creatinine. Note that the serum creatinine does not rise above the normal range until there is a reduction of 50–60% in the glomerular filtration rate (creatinine clearance).

Given these observations, creatinine clearance, nevertheless, is a reasonably accurate measure of GFR in those situations in which it is most required – normal or near normal renal function. Urine is collected over 24 hours for measurement of urinary creatinine. A plasma level of creatinine is measured sometime during the 24-hour period. Creatinine clearance is obtained from the formula:

$$U \times V/P$$

where U = urine concentration of creatinine; V = rate or urine flow in mL/min; P = plasma concentration of creatinine. Normal ranges: men 90–140 mL/min; women 80–125 mL/min.

Where urine collections are difficult (e.g. with ileal conduits) or deemed inaccurate, the GFR may be measured by the single injection of compounds such as [51Cr]EDTA (ethylenediaminetetraacetic acid), [99mTc]DTPA (diethylenetriaminepentaacetic acid) or [125I]iothalamate, their excretion being primarily by glomerular filtration. Following intravenous injection of the compound, three blood samples are obtained at 2, 3 and 4 hours (or rather longer intervals if the patient is oedematous or if renal failure is suspected). The GFR may then be calculated from the slope of the exponential fall in blood level of the compound. Increasingly, iohexol (a low-osmolality, non-ionic contrast medium) is being used, particularly in study settings. It is non-radioactive and can be measured reliably by a routine biochemical HPLC (high-pressure liquid chromatography) technique. Iohexol clearance correlates with radioisotopic techniques and can be assessed from finger-prick blood samples.

Cystatin C is an endogenous cysteine protease inhibitor. It is a low-molecular-weight protein filtered freely by the glomerulus and is produced at a constant rate. It is not secreted by tubules and therefore correlates with GFR. The cystatin C level is unaffected by gender, and correction for surface area is not needed. Studies suggest that cystatin C levels correlate better with radioisotope estimation of GFR than do creatinine levels and are more sensitive to mild renal impairment, particularly when the creatinine level is still normal. However, there is a lack of prospective studies and the plasma normal range can be affected by malignancy and steroid therapy.

Calculated GFR. Measurement of true GFR is cumbersome, time consuming and may be inaccurate if 24-hour urine collections are incomplete. Therefore, several formulae have been developed that allow a prediction of creatinine clearance or GFR from serum creatinine and demographics. The Cockroft–Gault formula is used most frequently and takes into account the patient's age, gender, weight and plasma creatinine (Box 11.1). Recently, a new prediction equation has been developed based on the data derived from the Modification of Diet in Renal Disease (MDRD) study in patients with chronic renal failure (Box 11.1). This equation is based on, age, sex, serum urea, creatinine and albumin. In addition, unlike Cockroft–Gault it also considers racial background of the patient, which makes it more reliable in ethnically diverse

---

 Box 11.1 Calculation of creatinine clearance

Cockroft–Gault equation

Men

$$\text{Creatinine clearance} = \frac{1.23 \times (140 - \text{Age}) \times (\text{Weight in kg})}{\text{Serum creatinine } (\mu\text{mol/L})}$$

Women
Use the same equation but multiply by 1.04 instead of 1.23.

Modification of diet in renal disease (MDRD)
$$\text{GFR} = 170 \times (\text{S creatinine (mg/dL)}^{-0.999}) \times (\text{Age}^{-0.176})$$
$$\times \text{S urea mg/dL}^{-0.70}) \times (\text{S albumin g/dL}^{+0.318})$$
$$(\times 0.762 \text{ if female}: \times 1.180 \text{ if black})$$
S = serum.

To convert creatinine values in µmol/L to mg/dL multiply by 0.0113.
To convert serum urea in mmol/L to mL/dL multiply by 2.8.

See http://www.nephron.com for MDRD calculator.

National Kidney Foundation – clinical practice guidelines formula

$$\text{GFR} = 186 \times \left(\frac{S_{Cr}}{88}\right)^{-1.154} \times \text{Age}^{-0.203}$$

S_{Cr} = serum creatinine (µmol/L)

For woman – multiply by 0.742.
If black African – multiply by 1.212.

TUBULAR FUNCTION

The major function of the tubule is the selective reabsorption or excretion of water and various cations and anions to keep the volume and electrolyte composition of body fluid normal (see Ch. 12).

The active reabsorption from the glomerular filtrate of compounds such as glucose and amino acids also takes place. Within the normal range of blood concentrations these substances are completely reabsorbed by the proximal tubule. However, if blood levels are elevated above the normal range, the amount filtered (filtered load = GFR × plasma concentration) may exceed the maximal absorptive capacity of the tubule and the compound 'spills over' into the urine. Examples of this occur with hyperglycaemia in diabetes mellitus or elevated plasma phenylalanine in phenylketonuria.

Conversely, inherited or acquired defects in tubular function may lead to incomplete absorption of a normal filtered load, with loss of the compound in the urine (a lowered 'renal threshold'). This is seen in renal glycosuria, in which there is a genetically determined defect in tubular reabsorption of glucose. It is diagnosed by demonstrating glycosuria in the presence of normal blood glucose levels. Inherited or acquired defects in the tubular reabsorption of amino acids, phosphate, sodium, potassium and calcium also occur, either singly or in combination. Examples include cystinuria and the Fanconi syndrome (see p. 1144 and Ch. 12). Tubular defects in the reabsorption of water result in nephrogenic diabetes insipidus (p. 1091). Under normal circumstances, antidiuretic hormone induces an increase in the permeability of water in the collecting ducts by attachment to receptors with subsequent activation of adenyl cyclase. This then activates a protein kinase, which induces preformed cytoplasmic vesicles containing water channels (termed 'aquaporins') to move to and insert into the tubular luminal membrane. This allows water entry into tubular cells down a favourable osmotic gradient. Water then crosses the basolateral membrane and enters the bloodstream. When the effect of ADH wears off, water channels return to the cell cytoplasm (Fig. 12.5).

Investigation of tubular function in clinical practice

Various tubular mechanisms could theoretically be investigated, but, in clinical practice, tests of tubular function are required less often than glomerular function. *Twenty-four-hour sodium output* may be helpful in determining whether a patient is complying with a low-salt diet and in the management of salt-losing nephropathy. *Tests of proximal tubular function* may be required in the diagnosis of Fanconi's syndrome or isolated proximal tubular defects (e.g. urate clearance). Bicarbonate, glucose, phosphate and amino acid are all reabsorbed in the proximal tubule. Their presence in the urine is abnormal, and though formal methods of measuring maximal reabsorption are available, they are seldom necessary. *Retinal-binding protein* and *β_2-microglobulin* are normally reabsorbed by the proximal tubule, and their urinary excretion is non-specifically increased by diseases of the proximal tubule.

Two tests of distal tubular function are commonly applied in clinical practice: measurement of urinary concentrating capacity in response to water deprivation, and measurement of urinary acidification. These tests are dealt with on pages 1090 and 718.

ENDOCRINE FUNCTION

Renin–angiotensin system (see also p. 1096)

The juxtaglomerular apparatus is made up of specialized arteriolar smooth muscle cells that are sited on the afferent glomerular arteriole as it enters the glomerulus. These cells synthesize prorenin, which is cleaved into the active proteolytic enzyme renin. Active renin is then stored in and released from secretary granules. Prorenin is also released in the circulation and comprises 50–90% of circulating renin, but its physiological role remains unclear as it cannot be converted into active renin in the systemic circulation. Renin converts angiotensinogen in blood to angiotensin I. Angiotensin-converting enzyme (ACE), which is located in the lung, luminal border of endothelial cells, glomeruli and other organs, converts angiotensin I (decapeptide) to angiotensin II (octapeptide). Renin release is controlled by:

- pressure changes in the afferent arteriole
- sympathetic tone
- chloride and osmotic concentration in the distal tubule via the macula densa (Fig. 11.2a)
- local prostaglandin and nitric oxide release.

Angiotensin II has two major systemic effects: systemic vasoconstriction and sodium and water retention. Both of these actions will tend to reverse the hypovolaemia or hypotension that is usually responsible for the stimulation of renin release. Angiotensin II promotes renal NaCl and water absorption by direct stimulation of Na^+ reabsorption in the early proximal tubule and by increased adrenal aldosterone secretion which enhances Na^+ transport in the collecting duct. In addition to influencing systemic haemodynamics, angiotensin II also regulates GFR. Although it constricts both afferent and efferent arterioles, vasoconstriction of efferent arterioles is three times greater than that of afferent, resulting in increase of glomerular capillary pressure and maintenance of GFR. In addition, angiotensin II constricts mesangial cells, reducing the filtration surface area, and sensitizes the afferent arteriole to the constricting signal of tubuloglomerular feedback (see p. 606). The net result is that angiotensin II has opposing effects on the regulation of GFR: (a) an increase in glomerular pressure and consequent rise in GFR; (b) reduction in renal blood

groups of individuals. It is very popular in large population-based epidemiological studies where weight of the patient is usually not available. A clinical practice guideline formula produced by the National Kidney Foundation is also shown in Box 11.1.

flow and mesangial cell contraction, reducing filtration. In renal artery stenosis with resultant low perfusion pressure, angiotensin II maintains GFR. However, in cardiac failure and hypertension, GFR may be reduced by angiotensin II.

Erythropoietin (see also p. 422)

Erythropoietin is the major stimulus for erythropoiesis. It is a glycoprotein produced principally by fibroblast-like cells in the renal interstitium. Under hypoxic conditions both the alpha and beta subunits of hypoxia inducible factor 1 (HIF-1) are expressed, leading to subsequent erythropoietin gene transcription via the combined effects of hepatic nuclear factor 4 (HNF-4), p300, and HIF-1-alpha and -beta. Erythropoietin, once formed, binds to its receptors on erythroid precursor cells. Under normal oxygen conditions, only the HIF-1-beta subunit is expressed. The alpha subunit undergoes proline hydroxylation in the presence of iron and oxygen by prolyl hydoxylase. The hydroxylated HIF-1-alpha subunit binds to von Hippel–Lindau protein and a ubiquitin ligase complex is activated. This leads to ubiquitination and subsequent degradation of HIF-1-alpha via proteosomes so that no erythropoietin is transcribed.

Loss of renal substance, with decreased erythropoietin production, results in a normochromic, normocytic anaemia. Conversely, erythropoietin secretion may be increased, with resultant polycythaemia, in patients with polycystic renal disease, benign renal cysts or renal cell carcinoma. Recombinant human erythropoietin has been biosynthesized and is available for clinical use, particularly in patients with renal failure (see p. 673).

Vitamin D metabolism (see also p. 592)

Naturally occurring vitamin D (cholecalciferol) requires hydroxylation in the liver at position 25 and again by a 1α-hydroxylase enzyme (mitochondrial cytochrome P450) mainly in the distal convoluted tubule, the cortical and inner medullary part of the collecting ducts and the papillary epithelia of the kidney to produce the powerfully metabolically active 1,25-dihydroxycholecalciferol (1,25-$(OH)_2D_3$). The 1α-hydroxylase activity is increased by high plasma levels of parathyroid hormone (PTH), low phosphate and low 1,25-$(OH)_2D_3$. 1,25-Dihydroxycholecalciferol and 25-hydroxycholecalciferol are degraded in part by being hydroxylated at position 24 by 24-hydroxylase. The activity of this enzyme is reduced by PTH and increased by 1,25-$(OH)_2D_3$ (which therefore promotes its own inactivation).

Reduced 1α-hydroxylase activity in diseased kidneys results in relative deficiency of 1,25-$(OH)_2D_3$. As a result, gastrointestinal calcium and to a lesser extent phosphate absorption is reduced and bone mineralization impaired. Receptors for 1,25-$(OH)_2D_3$ exist in the parathyroid glands, and reduced occupancy of the receptors by the vitamin alters the set-point for release of PTH in response to a given decrement in plasma calcium concentration. Gut calcium malabsorption, which induces a tendency to hypocalcaemia, and relative lack of 1,25-$(OH)_2D_3$, contri-

bute therefore to the hyperparathyroidism seen regularly in patients with renal impairment, even of modest degree.

Autocrine function

Endothelins

The endothelins ET-1, ET-2 and ET-3 are a family of similar potent vasoactive peptides that also influence cell proliferation and epithelial solute transport. They do not circulate but act locally. ETs are produced by most types of cells in the kidney. The vascular actions are mediated by two receptors, with ET_A (specific for ET-1) mediating vasoconstriction and ET_B (responsive to all ETs) causing vasodilatation. Endothelins inhibit sodium and water absorption by suppressing Na^+/K^+-ATPase and Na^+/H^+ antiporter activity in the proximal tubule and antagonizing the action of ADH and aldosterone in the collecting duct. Tubular transport actions are mediated by ET_B. Endothelins, through vasoconstriction by ET_A and salt and water retention via ET_B receptors, cause hypertension. Endothelins, mainly through ET_A receptors, can also alter cell proliferation and matrix accumulation by increasing tissue inhibitor of metalloproteinase, cytokines, fibronectin and collagen. These peptides also stimulate the proliferation of a variety of renal cell types.

Prostaglandins

Prostaglandins are unsaturated, oxygenated fatty acids, derived from the enzymatic metabolism of arachidonic acid, mainly by constitutively expressed cyclo-oxygenase-1 (COX-1) or inducible COX-2 (see Fig. 14.32). COX-1 is highly expressed in the collecting duct, while COX-2 expression is restricted to the macula densa. Both COX isoforms convert arachidonic acid to the same product, the bioactive but unstable prostanoid precursor, prostaglandin H_2 (PGH_2). PGH_2 is converted to:

- PGE_2 (formed by PDE_2 synthase in the collecting duct, responsible for natriuretic and diuretic effects)
- PGD_2 (undetermined significance, produced in proximal tubule)
- prostacyclin (PGI_2) (mainly synthesized in the interstitial and vascular compartment)
- thromboxane A_2 (vasoconstrictor, mainly synthesized in glomerulus).

They all act through G-coupled transmembrane receptors.

Prostaglandins maintain renal blood flow and glomerular filtration rate in the face of reductions induced by vasoconstrictor stimuli such as angiotensin II, catecholamines and α-adrenergic stimulation. In the presence of renal underperfusion, inhibition of prostaglandin synthesis by non-steroidal anti-inflammatory drugs results in a further reduction in GFR, which is sometimes sufficiently severe as to cause acute renal failure. Renal prostaglandins also have a natriuretic renal tubular effect and antagonize the action of antidiuretic hormone. Renal prostaglandins do not regulate salt and water excretion in normal subjects, but in some circumstances, such as chronic renal failure, prostaglandin-induced vasodilatation is involved in maintaining renal blood flow. Patients with chronic renal failure are thus vulnerable to further deterioration in renal function on exposure to non-steroidal anti-inflammatory drugs, as are elderly patients in many of whom renal function is compromised by renal vascular disease and/or the effects of ageing upon the kidney. Moreover, in conditions such as volume depletion, which are associated with high renin release (facilitated by prostaglandins), inhibition of prostaglandin synthesis may lead to hyperkalaemia due to hyporeninaemic hypoaldosteronism (since angiotensin II is the main stimulus for aldosterone).

Urodilatin: renal natriuretic peptide
(see also p. 1096)
A 32-amino-acid atrial natriuretic-like peptide (ANP-like peptide), putatively synthesized by connecting and collecting ducts in the kidney, has been isolated from human urine. Its natriuretic potency equals or exceeds that of atrial ANP by increasing cGMP production in the collecting duct. It is postulated that cardiac ANP is primarily a regulator of the cardiovascular system through its vascular effects and that renal natriuretic peptide participates in the intrarenal regulation of sodium and chloride transport.

Nitric oxide and the kidney
Nitric oxide (Fig. 15.10), a molecular gas, is formed by the action of three isoforms of nitric oxide synthase (NOS). All three enzymes, neuronal (nNOS or NOS1), inducible (iNOS or NOS2) and endothelial (eNOS or NOS3), which are cytochrome P450-like proteins, facilitate the addition of the guanidine nitrogen of the amino acid arginine to molecular oxygen, producing nitric oxide and water. In general nNOS and eNOS are constitutively active, producing low levels of nitric oxide dependent upon intracellular calcium elevation. In contrast, the transcriptional regulation of iNOS can be markedly induced, particularly by inflammatory cytokines, resulting in extremely large amounts of nitric oxide. The most recognized cellular target of nitric oxide is soluble guanylate cyclase. The stimulation of this enzyme enhances the synthesis of cyclic GMP from GTP. All three isoforms, are expressed in the kidney with eNOS in the vascular compartment, nNOS mainly in the macula densa and inner medullary collecting duct and iNOS in several tubule segments. Nitric oxide mediates the following physiological actions in the kidney:

- regulation of renal haemodynamics
- natriuresis by inhibiting Na^+/K^+-ATPase and Na^+/H^+ antiporter and antagonizing ADH
- modulation of tubuloglomerular feedback so that the composition of tubular fluid delivered to the macula densa changes the filtration rate of the associated glomerulus.

Protein and polypeptide metabolism
The kidney is a major site for the catabolism of many small-molecular-weight proteins and polypeptides, including many hormones such as insulin, PTH and calcitonin by endocytosis carried out by megalin–cubilin complex in the brush border of proximal tubular cells. In renal failure the metabolic clearance of these substances is reduced and their half-life is prolonged. This accounts, for example, for the reduced insulin requirements of diabetic patients as their renal function declines.

FURTHER READING
Breyer MD (2002) Beyond cyclooxygenase. *Kidney International* **62**: 1898–1889.
Hendry BM, James AF (1997) Endothelin antagonists in renal disease. *Lancet* **350**: 381–382.
Kone BC, Baylis C (1997). Biosynthesis and homeostatic roles of nitric oxide in the normal kidney. *American Journal of Physiology* **272**: F561–F566.

INVESTIGATIONS

EXAMINATION OF THE URINE
Appearance

This is of little value in the differential diagnosis of renal disease except in the diagnosis of haematuria. Overt 'bloody' urine is usually unmistakable but should be checked using dipsticks (Stix testing). Very concentrated urine may also appear dark or smoky. Other causes of discoloration of urine include cholestatic jaundice, haemoglobinuria, drugs such as rifampicin, use of fluorescein or methylthioninium chloride (methylene blue), and ingestion of beetroot. Discoloration of urine after standing for some time occurs in porphyria, alkaptonuria and in patients ingesting the drug L-dopa.

Volume

In health, the volume of urine passed is primarily determined by diet and fluid intake. In temperate climates it lies within the range 800–2500 mL per 24 hours. The minimum amount passed to stay in fluid balance is determined by the amount of solute – mainly urea and electrolytes – being excreted and the maximum concentrating power of the kidneys. On a normal diet, some 800 mOsm of solute are passed daily. Since the maximum urine concentration is approximately 1200 mOsm/kg, the minimum volume of urine obligated by excretion of 800 mOsm of solute would thus be approximately 650 mL. A diet rich in carbohydrate and fat and low in protein and salt results in a lower solute excretion and as little as 300 mL of urine per day may be required. Conversely, a high-salt, high-protein intake obligates a larger urine flow and, via the thirst mechanism, a higher fluid intake. The appropriateness of a given daily urine output must therefore be related to factors such as diet, body size and fluid intake.

In diseases such as chronic renal failure or diabetes insipidus, impairment of concentrating ability requires increased volumes of urine to be passed, given the same daily solute output. An increased solute output, such as in glycosuria or increased protein catabolism following surgery or associated with sepsis, also demands increased urine volumes.

The maximum urine output depends on the ability to produce dilute urine. Intakes of 10 or even 20 L daily can be tolerated by normal humans but, given a daily solute output of 800 mOsm, require the ability to dilute to 80 and 40 mOsm/kg, respectively. Where diluting ability is impaired such as inappropriate secretion of ADH, the ability to excrete large volumes of ingested water is also impaired.

Oliguria

Oliguria, usually defined as the excretion of less than 300 mL of urine per day, may be 'physiological', as in patients with hypotension and hypovolaemia, where urine is maximally concentrated in an attempt to conserve water. More often, it is due to intrinsic renal disease or obstructive nephropathy (see p. 654).

Anuria (no urine) suggests urinary tract obstruction until proved otherwise; bladder outflow obstruction must always be considered first.

Polyuria

Polyuria is a persistent, large increase in urine output, usually associated with nocturia. It must be distinguished from frequency of micturition with the passage of small volumes of urine. Documentation of fluid intake and output may be necessary. Polyuria is the result of an excessive (hysterical) intake of water, an increased excretion of solute (as in hyperglycaemia and glycosuria), or a defective renal concentrating ability or failure of production of ADH.

Specific gravity and osmolality

Urine specific gravity is a measure of the weight of dissolved particles in urine, whereas urine osmolality reflects the number of such particles. Usually the relationship between the two is close. An exception exists when a relatively small number of relatively large particles are present in urine, such as in multiple myeloma. Measurement of urine specific gravity or osmolality is required only in limited circumstances, such as the differential diagnosis of oliguric renal failure or the investigation of polyuria or inappropriate ADH secretion. Specific gravity is usually fixed at 1.010 in chronic failure or acute tubular necrosis as compared to prerenal acute renal failure where specific gravity is very high close to 1.025.

Urinary pH

Measurement of urinary pH is unnecessary except in the investigation and treatment of renal tubular acidosis (see p. 716).

Chemical (Stix) testing

Routine Stix testing of urine for blood, protein and sugar is obligatory in all patients suspected of having renal disease.

Blood

Haematuria may be overt, with bloody urine, or microscopic and found only on chemical testing. Currently used Stix tests for blood are very sensitive, being positive if two or more red cells are visible under the high-power field of a light microscope. Indeed, the test is too sensitive, sometimes giving positive results in normal individuals. A further disadvantage is that Stix testing cannot distinguish between blood and free haemoglobin. A positive Stix test must always be followed by microscopy of fresh urine to confirm the presence of red cells and so exclude the relatively rare conditions of haemoglobinuria or myoglobinuria. In females with a positive Stix test result for blood, it is essential to enquire whether the patient is menstruating. Bleeding may come from any site within the urinary tract (Fig. 11.5):

- *Overt bleeding from the urethra* is suggested when blood is seen at the start of voiding and then the urine becomes clear.
- *Blood diffusely present* throughout the urine comes from the bladder or above.
- *Blood only at the end of micturition* suggests bleeding from the prostate or bladder base.

Careful urine microscopy is mandatory as the presence of red-cell casts is diagnostic of bleeding from the kidney itself, most often due to glomerulonephritis. In the absence of red-cell casts, further investigations, such as urine cytology, renal imaging and cystoscopy, are required to define the site of bleeding. Renal biopsy may be required (see p. 618).

Protein

Proteinuria is one of the most common signs of renal disease. Detection is primarily by Stix testing. Most

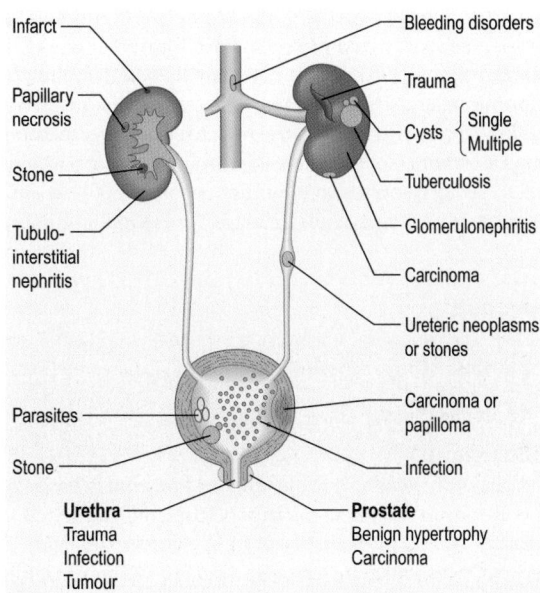

Fig. 11.5 **Sites and causes of bleeding from the urinary tract.**

reagent strips can detect a concentration of 100–200 mg/L or more in urine. They react primarily with albumin and are relatively insensitive to globulin and Bence Jones proteins.

If proteinuria is confirmed on repeated Stix testing, protein excretion in 24-hour urine collections should be measured (but see below). Healthy adults excrete up to 30 mg daily of albumin. Pyrexia, exercise and adoption of the upright posture all increase urinary protein output. Proteinuria, while occasionally benign, always requires further investigation. In some glomerular disease the protein leak is selective (e.g. minimal change) and urine electrophoresis can demonstrate the relative leaks, e.g. IgA or albumin.

Postural proteinuria. This term is used to refer to proteinuria present on dipstick testing which becomes undetectable after a period of hours lying flat. Typically, a negative dipstick result is obtained on the first urine passed on rising in the morning, whereas subsequent specimens give a positive result. This is regarded even for insurance purposes as a benign condition.

Microalbuminuria

The term microalbuminuria is an unfortunate one since the albumin referred to is of normal molecular size and weight. Normal individuals excrete less than 20 µg of albumin per minute (30 mg in 24 hours). Dipsticks, however, detect albumin only in a concentration above 200 mg/L (300 mg per 24 hours if urine volume is normal). An increase in albumin excretion between these two levels – so-called microalbuminuria – is now known to be an early indicator of diabetic glomerular disease. It is widely used as a predictor of the development of nephropathy in diabetics and may be extended to other conditions.

Timed 24-hour urinary excretion rates provide the most precise measure of microalbuminuria. However, in clinical practice it is more convenient to test for microalbuminuria using random urine samples in which albumin concentration is related to urinary creatinine concentration. Generally an albumin : creatinine ratio of 2.5 to 20 corresponds to albuminuria of 30–300 mg daily respectively. Kits are available to test for microalbuminuria.

Glucose

Renal glycosuria is uncommon, so that a positive test for glucose always requires exclusion of diabetes mellitus.

Bacteriuria

Dipsticks are available for testing for bacteriuria based on the detection of nitrite produced from the reduction of urinary nitrate by bacteria and also for the detection of leucocyte esterase, an enzyme specific for neutrophils. Although each test on its own has limitations, a positive reaction with both tests has a high predictive value for urinary tract infection (p. 640).

Microscopy

Urine microscopy should be carried out in all patients suspected of having renal disease. Care must be taken to obtain a 'clean' sample of mid-stream urine. The presence of numerous skin squames suggests a contaminated, poorly collected sample that cannot be properly interpreted.

If a clean sample of urine cannot be obtained, suprapubic aspiration is required in suspected urinary tract infections, particularly in children.

White cells

The presence of 10 or more white blood cells (WBCs) per cubic millimetre in fresh unspun mid-stream urine samples is abnormal and indicates an inflammatory reaction within the urinary tract. Most commonly it is due to urinary tract infection (UTI), but it may also be found in sterile urine in patients during antibiotic treatment of urinary infection or within 14 days of treatment. Sterile pyuria also occurs in patients with stones, tubulointerstitial nephritis, papillary necrosis, tuberculosis, and interstitial cystitis.

Red cells

The presence of one or more red cells per cubic millimetre in unspun urine samples results in a positive Stix test for blood and is abnormal. It is claimed that red cells of glomerular origin can be identified by their dysmorphic appearance, especially on phase-contrast microscopy, but the method is subject to observer error and has not gained wide acceptance.

Casts (see Fig. 11.6)

These cylindrical bodies, which are moulded ('cast') in the shape of the distal tubular lumen, may be hyaline, granular or cellular. Hyaline casts and fine granular casts represent precipitated protein and may be seen in normal urine, particularly after exercise. More coarsely granular casts occur with pathological proteinuria in glomerular and tubular disease. Red-cell casts – even one – always indicate renal disease. If red cells degenerate, a rusty coloured 'haemoglobin' granular cast is seen. White cell casts may be seen in acute pyelonephritis. They may be confused with the tubular cell casts that occur in patients with acute tubular necrosis.

Bacteria

The demonstration of bacteria on Gram staining of the centrifuged deposit of a clean-catch mid-stream urine sample is highly suggestive of urinary infection and can be of value in the immediate differential diagnosis of UTI. If accompanied by pyuria it may be accepted as evidence of UTI in the ill and febrile patient and treatment should be initiated.

Urine for quantitative culture (see p. 640) must always be obtained prior to starting antibiotic treatment in order to confirm the diagnosis and to allow definition of bacterial antibiotic sensitivities.

Stix testing for blood or protein is of no value in the diagnosis of UTI, as both may be absent from the urine of many patients with bacteriuria.

Fig. 11.6 **Red-cell cast**. Note aggregation of red cells as a 'cast' of the tubule.

BLOOD AND QUANTITATIVE TESTS

The use of serum urea, creatinine and GFR as measures of renal function is discussed on page 608. Other quantitative tests of disturbed renal function are described under the relevant disorders.

IMAGING TECHNIQUES

Plain X-ray

A plain radiograph of the abdomen is always taken prior to urography. Its main value is to identify renal calcification or radiodense calculi in the kidney, renal pelvis, line of the ureters or bladder (Fig. 11.7).

Excretion urography

Excretion urography, also known as intravenous urography (IVU) or intravenous pyelography (IVP), still plays a role in renal diagnosis, especially in patients with haematuria and stone disease, but has in part been replaced by ultrasonography and CT scanning. An organic iodine-containing contrast medium is given intravenously. A small proportion of patients will have an 'allergic' reaction to contrast medium. With low-osmolality contrast media the risk is relatively low (e.g. 1% develop bronchospasm or urticaria, less than 0.003% develop more severe complications such as cardiac arrhythmias and convulsions and the mortality is of the order 1 in 200 000). Patients who have had a previous contrast medium reaction, who have asthma or a history of allergy requiring medical treatment should receive steroid prophylaxis before contrast medium (e.g. prednisolone 30 mg 12 hours and 2 hours before contrast medium). Contrast media do not cause renal damage in normovolaemic patients with normal renal function, but may be nephrotoxic in patients with impaired renal function, especially when this results from diabetic nephropathy or multiple myeloma. The IVU series should be inspected

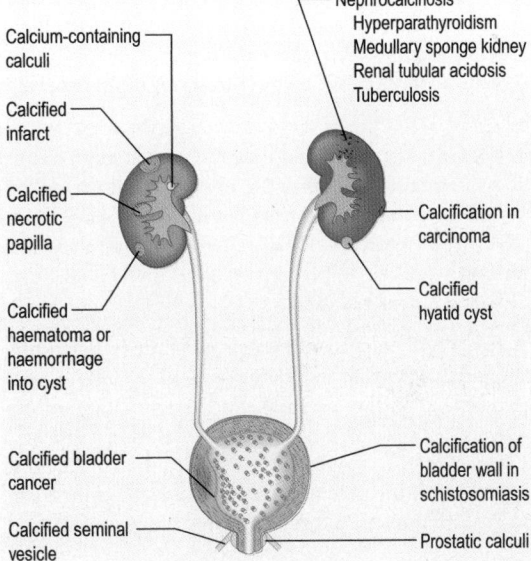

Fig. 11.7 **Calcification in the renal tract**. Calculi can occur at any site.

for renal size and position (kidneys span over three lumbar vertebrae and the left is higher than the right). Any distortion of the smooth renal outline, calyceal dilatation (e.g. due to obstruction), filling defects in renal pelves (e.g. stones, tumour), ureteric obstruction and displacement (e.g. retroperitoneal fibrosis) should be noted. The bladder should be examined both pre- and postmicturition for abnormalities of contour and residual volume.

Ultrasonography

Ultrasonography of the kidneys and bladder has the advantage over X-ray techniques of avoiding ionizing radiation and intravascular contrast medium. In renal diagnosis it is the method of choice for:

- renal measurement and for renal biopsy or other interventional procedures
- checking for pelvicalyceal dilatation as an indication of renal obstruction when chronic renal obstruction is suspected; in suspected acute ureteric obstruction either intravenous urography or unenhanced spiral CT are the methods of choice
- characterizing renal masses as cystic or solid
- diagnosing polycystic kidney disease
- detecting intrarenal and/or perinephric fluid (e.g. pus, blood)
- demonstrating renal arterial perfusion or detecting renal vein thrombosis using Doppler technique.

Doppler ultrasonography is based on the principle that, when incident sound waves are reflected from a moving structure, their frequency is shifted by an amount proportional to the velocity of the reflector (e.g. an RBC); this shift can be quantified and displayed as a spectral Doppler scan or colour overlay (colour Doppler).

Ultrasonography of the distended bladder is used to measure bladder wall thickness and to check for bladder tumours and stones. A scan obtained after voiding allows bladder emptying to be assessed.

The disadvantages of using ultrasonography to assess the urinary tract are:

- It does not show detailed pelvicalyceal anatomy.
- It does not fully visualize the normal adult ureter.
- It may miss small renal calculi and does not detect the majority of ureteric calculi. CT may be required (see below).
- It is operator-dependent.

In patients with suspected benign prostatic hypertrophy, examination of the bladder before and after voiding, with measurement of the prostate, and examination of the kidneys to check for pelvicalyceal dilatation suffice. If prostate cancer is suspected, more detailed ultrasound examination of the prostate with a transrectal transducer, usually with transrectal prostate biopsy, is necessary.

Computed tomography (CT)

Computed tomography is used mainly as a second-line imaging method in the urinary tract, but increasingly as a first-line investigation in cases of suspected ureteric colic. Spiral CT has both improved image resolution and allows reconstruction of the imaging data in a variety of planes. CT is used:

- to characterize renal masses which are indeterminate at ultrasonography
- to stage renal tumours
- to detect 'lucent' calculi; low-density calculi which are lucent on plain films (e.g. uric acid stones) are well seen on CT
- to evaluate the retroperitoneum for tumours, retroperitoneal fibrosis (periaortitis) and other causes of ureteric obstruction
- to assess severe renal trauma

- to visualize the renal arteries and veins by helical or spiral CT
- to stage bladder and prostate tumours; MRI is, however, increasingly used to stage prostate cancer.

The use of spiral unenhanced CT in suspected ureteric colic permits diagnosis of causes of pain other than calculi more readily than does urography.

Magnetic resonance imaging (MRI)

MRI is used:

- to characterize renal masses as an alternative to CT
- to stage renal, prostate and bladder cancer
- to demonstrate the renal arteries by *magnetic resonance angiography* with gadolinium as contrast medium. In experienced hands its sensitivity and specificity approaches renal angiography.

Magnetic resonance urography is preferred over IVU in patients with chronic urolithiasis or intrinsic or extrinsic ureteric tumour, and in paediatric uroradiology. It is analogous to IVU. Gadolinium is used as contrast medium, which is regarded as less nephrotoxic than iodine-containing agents used in IVU.

Antegrade pyelography (Fig. 11.8)

Antegrade pyelography involves percutaneous puncture of a pelvicalyceal system with a needle and the injection of contrast medium to outline the pelvicalyceal system and ureter to the level of obstruction. It is used when ultrasonography has shown a dilated pelvicalyceal system in a patient with suspected obstruction. Antegrade pyelography is the preliminary to percutaneous placing of a drainage catheter or ureteric stent in the obstructed pelvicalyceal system (percutaneous nephrostomy).

Retrograde pyelography

Following cystoscopy, preferably under screening control, a catheter is either impacted in the ureteral orifice or passed a short distance up the ureter, and contrast medium is injected. Retrograde pyelography is mainly used to investigate lesions of the ureter and to define the lower level of ureteral obstruction shown on excretion urography or ultrasound plus antegrade studies. It is invasive, commonly requires a general anaesthetic, and may result in the introduction of infection.

Micturating cystourethrography (MCU)

This involves catheterization and the instillation of contrast medium into the bladder. The catheter is then removed and the patient screened during voiding to check for vesicoureteric reflux and to study the urethra and bladder emptying. It is used primarily in children with recurrent infection (see p. 639).

MCU is not an appropriate investigation in adults because vesicoureteric reflux and urinary tract infection

Fig. 11.8 Antegrade pyelography via percutaneous catheter (small arrow) of obstructed system. Percutaneous drainage catheter (large arrow) has been inserted.

cause renal scarring and calyceal distortion in early life, but reflux tends to disappear by the time adulthood is reached. If reflux is detected in an adult with normal renal anatomy, it is thought not to induce kidney damage later. The absence of reflux in an adult does not therefore exclude the diagnosis of reflux nephropathy. Therefore, whatever the finding on micturating cystourethrography, management is not altered.

The presence or absence of vesicoureteric reflux may also be investigated by scintigraphy (see below).

Aortography or renal arteriography

Conventional or digital subtraction angiography (DSA) is used. The latter allows the use of smaller doses of contrast medium which can be injected via a central venous catheter (venous DSA) or via a fine transfemoral arterial catheter (arterial DSA). Angiography is mainly used to define extrarenal or intrarenal arterial disease. Arteriography is still the 'gold standard' method of renal artery imaging but magnetic resonance angiography and spiral CT angiography are being used increasingly (Fig. 11.9). Complications include cholesterol embolizations (p. 648) and contrast-induced kidney damage.

Venography is only used occasionally to exclude renal vein thrombosis. In most instances this can be done less invasively with Doppler ultrasonography, CT or MRI.

Fig. 11.9 Magnetic resonance angiogram of normal renal arteries.

Renal scintigraphy

Renal scintigraphy using a gamma camera is divided into:

- dynamic studies in which the function of the kidney is examined serially over a period of time, most often using a radiopharmaceutical excreted by glomerular filtration
- static studies involving imaging of tracer that is taken up and retained by the renal tubule.

Dynamic scintigraphy

The radiopharmaceutical technetium-labelled diethyl-enetriaminepentaacetic acid, [^{99m}Tc]DTPA is excreted by glomerular filtration. ^{123}I-labelled ortho-iodohippuric acid (Hippuran) is both filtered and secreted by the tubules and mercaptoacetyltriglycine (MAG3) labelled with technetium (^{99m}Tc) is excreted by renal tubular secretion. Following venous injection of a bolus of tracer, emissions from the kidney can be recorded by gamma camera. This information allows examination of blood perfusion of the kidney, uptake of tracer as a result of glomerular filtration, transit of tracer through the kidney, and the outflow of tracer-containing urine from the collecting system.

Renal blood flow

Dynamic studies can be used to investigate patients in whom renal artery stenosis is suspected as a cause for hypertension and in patients with severe oliguria (post-traumatic, post-aortic surgery, or after a kidney transplant) to establish whether, and to what extent, there is renal perfusion. In patients with unilateral renal artery stenosis there is, typically, a slowed and reduced uptake of tracer with delay in reaching a peak. Studies carried out before and after administration of an ACE inhibitor may demonstrate a fall in uptake that is suggestive of functional arterial stenosis. Both false-positive and false-negative results occur, particularly in patients with renal impairment, and renal arteriography remains the 'gold standard' in the diagnosis of main renal artery stenosis. In patients with total renal artery occlusion, no kidney uptake of tracers is observed.

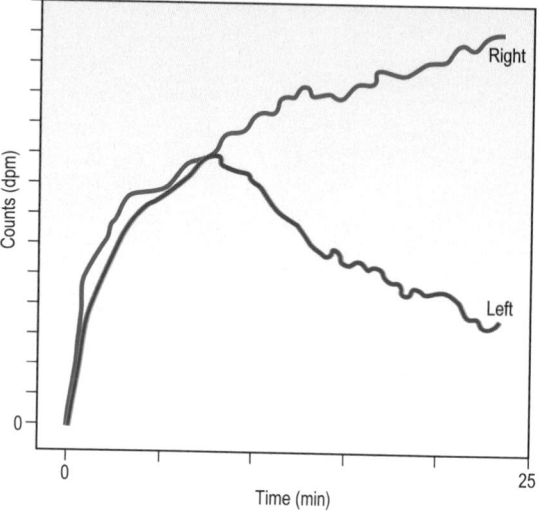

Fig. 11.10 Dynamic scintigram. Note the progressive rise of the right kidney curve to a plateau (in contrast to the normal left kidney curve) owing to urinary tract obstruction on the right side.

Investigation of obstruction

Renal scintigraphy provides functional evidence of obstruction. After injection usually of (^{99m}Tc)MAG3 a rise in resistance to flow in the pelvis or ureter prolongs the parenchymal transit of tracer and there is usually a delay in emptying the pelvis. On whole-kidney renograms, the time–activity curve fails to fall after an initial peak, or continues to rise (Fig. 11.10).

When the possibility of obstruction is suspected, a dynamic renal scintigram is performed with diuresis. Furosemide (frusemide) (0.5 mg/kg, adult dose 40 mg) is given intravenously about 18–20 minutes into the study. Time–activity curves show an immediate fall after the injection of furosemide in the normal and in the absence of obstruction. In the presence of obstruction, the retention of activity in the pelvis persists, the activity–time curve fails to fall or falls to a lesser extent than the previous rate of rise of the activity–time curve.

A decision as to whether conservative surgery or nephrectomy should be carried out in unilateral obstruction is facilitated by renographic assessment of the contribution of each kidney.

Bladder emptying

At the end of dynamic studies, bladder emptying may be investigated and any postmicturition residual urine measured. Vesicoureteric reflux may be observed, although the sensitivity for detection of this is low. Increased sensitivity can be obtained by direct isotope cystography when a dilute isotope solution is instilled into the bladder by catheter.

Glomerular filtration rate

This is discussed on page 608.

Static scintigraphy

This is usually performed using [^{99m}Tc]DMSA (dimercaptosuccinic acid), which is taken up by tubular cells. Uptake is proportional to renal function.

Relative renal function

Function is normally evenly divided between the kidneys, with a range of 45–55%. Static studies are particularly useful in unilateral renal disease, where the relative uptake of the two kidneys can be calculated.

Kidney visualization

Normal kidneys show a uniform uptake with a smooth renal outline. Scars can be identified as photon-deficient 'bites'. Static scintigraphy is of considerable value in identifying ectopic kidneys or 'pseudotumours' of the kidneys (i.e. normally functioning renal tissue abnormally placed within the kidney).

Localization of infection

The use of citrate labelled with gallium-67 or isotopically labelled leucocytes that are taken up by inflammatory tissue may be of value in defining localized infection, such as renal abscesses or infection within a renal cyst.

TRANSCUTANEOUS RENAL BIOPSY
(Practical box 11.1)

The renal biopsy is carried out under ultrasound control in specialized centres and requires interpretation by an experienced pathologist. The pathologist should provide information that helps clinical management. Renal biopsy is helpful in the investigation of the nephritic and nephrotic syndromes, acute and chronic renal failure, haematuria after urological investigations and renal graft dysfunction. Native renal biopsy material must be

 Practical Box 11.1
Transcutaneous renal biopsy

Before biopsy
1. A coagulation screen is performed. It must be normal.
2. The serum is grouped and saved for crossmatching.
3. The patient is given a full explanation of what is involved and consent obtained.

During biopsy
1. The patient lies prone with a hard pillow under the abdomen.
2. The kidney is localized by ultrasound.
3. Local anaesthetic is injected along the biopsy track.
4. The patient holds a breath when the biopsy is performed.

After biopsy
1. A pressure dressing is applied to the biopsy site and the patient rests in bed for 24 hours.
2. The fluid intake is maximized to prevent clot colic.
3. The pulse and blood pressure are checked regularly.
4. The patient is advised to avoid heavy lifting or gardening for 2 weeks.

Table 11.2 Complications of transcutaneous renal biopsy

Macroscopic haematuria – about 20%
Pain in the flank, sometimes referred to shoulder tip
Perirenal haematoma
Arteriovenous aneurysm formation – about 20%, almost
    always of no clinical significance
Profuse haematuria demanding blood transfusion – 1–3%
Profuse haematuria demanding occlusion of bleeding
    vessel at angiography or nephrectomy – approximately
    1 in 400
Introduction of infection
The mortality rate is about 0.1%

Fig. 11.11 **Diagram showing a normal (left) and proteinuric (right) glomerulus**. A capillary loop showing normal glomerular morphology on the left with an epithelial cell with pseudopodia (foot processes). In the proteinuric diagram (right) there is fusion of the foot processes characteristic of many diseases. BM, basement membrane; MC, mesangial cell; MM, mesangial matrix. After Marsh FP (1985) *Postgraduate Nephrology*. Butterworth Heinemann.

examined by conventional histochemical staining, by electron microscopy, and by immunoperoxidase or immunofluorescence. Techniques like in situ hybridization and polymerase chain reaction analysis are also widely used in renal biopsy specimens.

The complications of transcutaneous renal biopsy are shown in Table 11.2.

GLOMERULAR DISEASES

A glomerulus consists of a collection of capillaries which come from the afferent arteriole and are confined within the urinary space (Bowman's capsule); this is continuous with the proximal tubule. The capillaries are partially attached to mesangium, a continuation of the arteriolar wall consisting of mesangial cells and the matrix. The free wall of glomerular capillaries (across which filtration takes place) consists of basement membrane covered by visceral epithelial cells with individual foot processes and lined by endothelial cells (Fig. 11.11). The normal thickness of the basement membrane equals about 250–300 nm. The spaces between foot processes, with diameters of 20–60 nm, are called filtration pores. It is believed they are the pores by which filtered fluid reaches the urinary space. The endothelial cells on the luminal aspect of the basement membrane are fenestrated (diameter 70–100 nm). The basement membrane is arranged in three zones – lamina rara externa, lamina rara densa and lamina rara interna – and is composed of type IV collagen and negatively charged proteoglycans (heparan sulphate).

Glomerular disease includes glomerulonephritis, i.e. inflammation of the glomeruli and glomerulopathies when there is no evidence of inflammation. There is an overlap between these terms.

GLOMERULOPATHIES

Glomerulopathies are the third most common cause of end-stage renal disease (after diabetes and hypertension) in Europe and the USA, accounting for some 10–15% of such patients.

Glomerulopathy (GN) is a general term for a group of disorders in which:

- there is primarily an immunologically mediated injury to glomeruli, although renal interstitial damage is a regular accompaniment
- kidneys are involved symmetrically
- secondary mechanisms of glomerular injury come into play following an initial immune insult such as fibrin deposition, platelet aggregation, neutrophil infiltration and free radical-induced damage.
- renal lesion may be part of a generalized disease (e.g. systemic lupus erythematosus, SLE).

Pathogenesis

GN is considered to be an immunologically mediated disorder with involvement of cellular immunity (T lymphocytes, macrophages/dendritic cells), humoral immunity (antibodies, immune complexes, complement), and other inflammatory mediators (including cytokines, chemokines and the coagulation cascade). The immune response can be directed against known target antigens, particularly when GN complicates infections, neoplasia or drugs. More frequently the underlying antigenic target is unknown. Primary GN may occur in genetically susceptible individuals following an environmental insult. The genetic susceptibility is usually determined by major histocompatibilty complex (HLA) genes (e.g. HLA-A1, B8, DR2, DR3). The environmental factors may be drugs (e.g. hydralazine), chemicals (e.g. gold, silica, hydrocarbons) or infectious agents. The known predisposing factors are discussed in more detail below. The physical evidence of immune reactions is indicated by the presence of circulating autoantibodies and/or abnormalities in serum complement and glomerular deposition of antibodies, immune complexes, complement and fibrin.

Pathological terms in glomerular disease

The most commonly used terms are:

- *Focal*: some but not all the glomeruli contain the lesion
- *Diffuse* (global): most of the glomeruli (> 75%) contain the lesion
- *Segmental*: only a part of the glomerulus is affected (most focal lesions are also segmental, e.g. focal segmental glomerulosclerosis)
- *Proliferative*: an increase in cell number due to hyperplasia of one or more of the resident glomerular cells with or without inflammation
- *Membrane alterations*: capillary wall thickening due to deposition of immune deposits or alterations in basement membrane
- *Crescent formation*: epithelial cell proliferation with mononuclear cell infiltration in Bowman's space.

Classification of glomerulopathies

There is no complete correlation between the histopathological types of GN and the clinical features of disease. Glomerular diseases have been classified in numerous ways. Here they are organized and discussed as they relate to four major glomerular syndromes:

- *Nephrotic syndrome* – massive proteinuria (> 3.5 g/day), hypoalbuminaemia, oedema, lipiduria and hyperlipidaemia.
- *Acute glomerulonephritis* (*acute nephritic syndrome*) – abrupt onset of glomerular haematuria (RBC casts or dysmorphic RBC), non-nephrotic range proteinuria, oedema, hypertension and transient renal impairment.
- *Rapidly progressive glomerulonephritis* – features of acute nephritis, focal necrosis with or without crescents and rapidly progressive renal failure over weeks.
- *Asymptomatic haematuria, proteinuria or both.*

Certain types of GN, particularly those that are a part of a systemic disease, can present as more than one syndrome, e.g. lupus nephritis, cryoglobulinaemia, and Henoch–Schönlein purpura, but more typically they are associated with the nephrotic syndrome and will be discussed below. Investigation of glomerular diseases are shown in Table 11.3.

NEPHROTIC SYNDROME

Pathophysiology

Hypoalbuminaemia.
Urinary protein loss of the order 3.5 g daily or more in an adult is required to cause hypoalbuminaemia. In children, proportionately less proteinuria results in hypoalbuminaemia. The normal dietary protein intake in the UK is of the order 70 g daily and the normal liver can synthesize albumin at a rate of 10–12 g daily. How then does a urinary protein loss of the order of 3.5 g daily result in hypoalbuminaemia? This can be partly explained

Table 11.3 Investigation of glomerular diseases

Investigations	Positive findings
Urine microscopy	Red cells, red-cell casts
Urinary protein	Nephrotic or sub-nephrotic range proteinuria
Serum urea	May be elevated
Serum creatinine	May be elevated
Culture (throat swab, discharge from ear, swab from inflamed skin)	Nephritogenic organism (not always)
Antistreptolysin-O titre	Elevated in post-streptococcal nephritis
C3 and C4 levels	May be reduced
Antinuclear antibody	Present in significant titre in systemic lupus erythematosus
ANCA	Positive in vasculitis
Anti-GBM	Positive in Goodpasture's syndrome
Cryoglobulins	Increased in cryoglobulinaemia
Creatinine clearance	Normal or reduced
Chest X-ray	Cardiomegaly, pulmonary oedema (not always)
Renal imaging	Usually normal
Renal biopsy	Any glomerulopathy

by increased catabolism of reabsorbed albumin in the proximal tubules during the nephrotic syndrome even though actual albumin synthesis rate is increased. However, in addition, dietary intake of protein increases albuminuria, so that the plasma albumin concentration tends to decrease during consumption of a high-protein diet. If the increase in urinary albumin excretion that follows dietary augmentation is prevented by administration of ACE inhibitors (ACEI), a high-protein diet causes an increase in plasma albumin concentration in the nephrotic syndrome. Therefore, to maximize serum albumin concentration in nephrotic patients, a reduction in urinary albumin excretion with an ACEI is always necessary.

Proteinuria. The mechanism of the proteinuria is complex. It occurs partly because structural damage to the glomerular basement membrane leads to an increase in the size and number of pores, allowing passage of more and larger molecules. Electrical charge is also involved in glomerular permeability. Fixed negatively charged components are present in the glomerular capillary wall, which repel negatively charged protein molecules. Reduction of this fixed charge occurs in glomerular disease and appears to be a key factor in the genesis of heavy proteinuria.

Hyperlipidaemia. The characteristic disorder is an increase in the low-density lipoprotein (LDL), very-low-density lipoprotein (VLDL), and/or intermediate-density lipoprotein (IDL) fractions, but no change or decrease in HDL. This results in an increase in the LDL/HDL cholesterol ratio. Hyperlipidaemia is the consequence of increased synthesis of lipoproteins (such as apolipoprotein B, C-III, Lp(a) lipoprotein), as a direct consequence of a low plasma albumin. There is also a reduced clearance of the principal triglycerides bearing lipoprotein (chylomicrons and VLDL) in direct response to albuminuria.

Oedema in hypoalbuminaemia.   See Chapter 12 (p. 696).

Management

General measures

- Initial treatment should be with dietary sodium restriction and a thiazide diuretic (e.g. bendroflumethiazide). Unresponsive patients require furosemide 40–120 mg daily with the addition of amiloride (5 mg daily), but the serum potassium concentration should be monitored carefully. Nephrotic patients may malabsorb diuretics (as well as other drugs) owing to gut mucosal oedema. Resistance to oral diuretic treatment may demand parenteral administration for a time. Patients are sometimes hypovolaemic, and moderate oedema may have to be accepted in order to avoid postural hypotension.
- A high-protein diet (approximately 80–90 g protein daily) increases proteinuria and can be harmful in the long term. Normal protein intake is advisable.

    Infusion of albumin produces only a transient effect. It is normally only employed in diuretic-resistant patients and those with oliguria and uraemia in the absence of severe glomerular damage, e.g. in minimal-change nephropathy. Albumin infusion is combined with diuretic therapy. Diuresis, when once initiated in this way, often continues with diuretic treatment alone.

- Hypercoagulable states predispose to venous thrombosis. The hypercoagulable state is due to loss of clotting factors (e.g. antithrombin) in the urine and an increase in hepatic production of fibrinogen. Prolonged bed rest should therefore be avoided as thromboembolism is very common in the nephrotic syndrome. In the absence of any contraindication, long-term prophylactic anticoagulation is desirable. Once renal vein thrombosis has occurred, permanent anticoagulation is required.
- Sepsis is a major cause of death in nephrotic patients. The increased susceptibility to infection is partly due to loss of immunoglobulin in the urine. Pneumococcal infections are particularly common and pneumococcal vaccine should be given. Early detection and aggressive treatment of infections, rather than long-term antibiotic prophylaxis, is the best approach.
- Lipid abnormalities are responsible for an increase in the risk of myocardial infarction or peripheral vascular disease in patients with proteinuria. Treatment of hypercholesterolaemia is best with an HMG-CoA reductase inhibitor, with fibrates if necessary (p. 1141).
- ACE inhibitors and/or angiotensin II receptor antagonists (AIIRA) are increasingly used for their antiproteinuric properties in all types of GN. These groups of drugs reduce proteinuria by lowering

---

Table 11.4   Glomerulopathies associated with the nephrotic syndrome

Nephrotic syndrome with 'bland' urine sediments
Primary glomerular disease
    Minimal-change glomerular lesion
    Congenital nephrotic syndrome
    Focal segmental glomerular sclerosis
    Membranous nephropathy

Secondary glomerular disease
    Amyloidosis
    Diabetic nephropathy

Nephrotic syndrome with 'active' urine sediments (mixed nephrotic/nephritic)
Primary glomerular disease
    Mesangiocapillary glomerulonephritis
    Mesangial proliferative glomerulonephritis

Secondary glomerular disease
    Systemic lupus erythematosus
    Cryoglobulinaemic disease
    Henoch–Schönlein syndrome
    Idiopathic fibrillary glomerulopathy
    Immunotactoid glomerulopathy

---

glomerular capillary filtration pressure; the blood pressure and renal function should be monitored regularly.

Specific measures

The aim is to reverse the abnormal urinary protein leak. These are discussed in detail below.

Table 11.4 shows the glomerular lesions commonly associated with the nephrotic syndrome. These are divided into diseases with or without RBC casts (bland or active urine sediments). Each of these entities may occur as a primary renal lesion or as a secondary component of a systemic disease.

Nephrotic syndrome with 'bland' urine sediments

Minimal-change glomerular lesion (minimal-change nephropathy)

In this condition the glomeruli appear normal on light microscopy (Fig. 11.12). The only abnormality seen on electron microscopy is fusion of the foot processes of epithelial cells (podocytes) (Fig. 11.11). This is a non-specific finding and is seen in many conditions associated with proteinuria. Neither immune complexes nor anti-GBM antibody can be demonstrated by immunofluorescence. However, the immunological pathogenesis of this condition is suggested by three factors:

- its response to steroids and immunosuppressive drugs
- its occurrence in Hodgkin's lymphoma, with remission following successful treatment
- patients with the condition and their family members have a high incidence of asthma and eczema; remission of the nephrotic syndrome following desensitization or antigen avoidance has been described.

Fig. 11.12 Normal glomerulus on light microscopy in minimal change disease.

A suggested explanation for the proteinuria is the production by T lymphocytes of a factor that increases glomerular permeability to protein.

Clinical features

Minimal-change nephropathy is most common in children, particularly males, accounting for the large majority of cases of nephrotic syndrome (proteinuria is usually highly selective) in childhood. Oedema is present and in children this may be facial. The condition accounts for 20–25% of cases of adult nephrotic syndrome. It is often regarded as a condition that does not lead to chronic renal failure (but see focal sclerosis below).

Management

High-dose corticosteroid therapy with prednisolone 60 mg/m^2 daily (up to a maximum of 80 mg/day) for a maximum of 4–6 weeks followed by 40 mg/m^2 every other day for a further 4–6 weeks corrects the urinary protein leak in more than 95% of children. Response rates in adults are significantly lower and response may occur only after many months (12 weeks with daily steroid therapy and 12 weeks of maintenance with alternate-day therapy). Spontaneous remission also occurs and steroid therapy should, in general, be withheld if urinary protein loss is insufficient to cause hypoalbuminaemia or oedema.

In children, one-third subsequently do not relapse, but further courses of corticosteroids are indicated in the remainder. One-third of these patients relapse regularly on steroid withdrawal, and remission is once more induced with steroid therapy; a course of cyclophosphamide 1.5–2.0 mg/kg daily is given for 8–12 weeks with concomitant prednisolone 7.5–15 mg/day. This increases the likelihood of long-term remission. Steroid unresponsive patients may also respond to cyclophosphamide. No more than two courses of cyclophosphamide should be prescribed in children because of the risk of side-effects, which include azoospermia.

In both children and adults, if remission lasts for 4 years after steroid therapy, further relapse is very rare.

An alternative to cyclophosphamide is ciclosporin 3–5 mg/kg/day, which is effective but must be continued long term to prevent relapse on stopping treatment. Excretory function and ciclosporin blood levels (recommended trough levels 80–150 ng/mL) must be monitored carefully, as ciclosporin is potentially nephrotoxic. In corticosteroid-dependent children, the anthelminthic agent levamisole 2.5 mg/kg to a maximum of 150 mg on alternate days is useful in maintenance of remission but its mode of action is unexplained. Most of the controlled studies have been conducted in the paediatric age group, making recommendations on treatment in adults difficult.

Congenital nephrotic syndrome

Congenital nephrotic syndrome (Finnish type) is an autosomal recessively inherited disorder due to mutations in the gene coding for a transmembrane protein, nephrin, that occurs with a frequency of 1 per 8200 live births in Finland. Nephrin was the first slit-diaphragm protein identified. Its loss of function results in massive proteinuria shortly after birth; these patients usually have an enlarged placenta. This disorder can be diagnosed in utero; increased alpha-fetoprotein in amniotic fluid is a common feature. The microscopic features of the kidney are varied. Some glomeruli are small and infantile, whereas others are enlarged, more mature and have diffuse mesangial hypercellularity. Because of the massive proteinuria, some tubules develop microcysts and are dilated. On electron microscopy, complete effacement of the foot processes of visceral epithelial cells is observed. This condition is characterized by relentless progression to end-stage renal failure. Other inherited nephrotic syndromes involve mutations in other genes that encode podocyte proteins such as podocin, alpha-actinin-4 and Wilms' tumour suppressor gene.

Focal segmental glomerulosclerosis (FSGS)

This is a disease of unknown aetiology. It usually presents as massive proteinuria (usually non-selective), haematuria, hypertension and renal impairment. Patients with nephrotic syndrome are often resistant to steroid therapy. All age groups are affected. It usually recurs in transplanted kidneys, sometimes within days of transplantation, particularly in patients with aggressive native renal disease.

Aetiology

It is generally believed that a circulating permeability factor (with serine protease activity) causes the increased protein leak because plasma from patients increases membrane permeability in isolated glomeruli. Kidneys transplanted into murine models of FSGS develop the lesion, but kidneys from FSGS-prone mice transplanted to a normal strain are protected. Removal of this factor by plasmapheresis results in transient amelioration of proteinuria. Upregulation of CD80 in podocytes has a major role in the co-stimulatory immune response pathway. Anti-CD80 antibodies, used in renal transplantation, are likely to be used in FSGS in the future.

Pathology

This glomerulopathy is defined primarily by its appearance on light microscopy. Segmental glomerulosclerosis is seen, which later progresses to global sclerosis. The deep glomeruli at the corticomedullary junction are affected first. These may be missed on transcutaneous biopsy, leading to a mistaken diagnosis of a minimal-change glomerular lesion. A pathogenetic link may exist between minimal-change nephropathy and focal glomerulosclerosis, as a proportion of cases classified as having the former condition develop progressive renal impairment. Immunofluorescence may show deposits of C3 and IgM in affected portions of the glomerulus. The other glomeruli are usually enlarged but may be of normal size. In some patients mesangial hypercellularity is a feature. Focal tubular atrophy and interstitial fibrosis are invariably present. Electron microscopic findings mirror light microscopic features with capillary obliteration by hyaline deposits (mesangial matrix and basement membrane material) and lipids. The other glomeruli exhibit primarily foot process effacement, occasionally in patchy distribution.

Two histological variants of FSGS exist. In *classic FSGS* (Fig. 11.13a) the involved glomeruli show sclerotic segments in any location of the glomerulus. The *glomerular tip lesion* is characterized by segmental sclerosis at an early evolution, at the tubular pole of all the affected glomeruli (tip FSGS) (Fig. 11.13b). Capillaries contain foam cells, and overlying visceral epithelial cells are enlarged and adherent to the most proximal portion of proximal tubules. These patients have a more favourable response to steroids and run a more benign course. In the other variant, known as *collapsing FSGS* (Fig. 11.13c) the visceral cells are usually enlarged and coarsely vacuolated with wrinkled and collapsed capillary walls. These features indicate a severe lesion, with a corresponding progressive clinical course of the disease. Collapsing FSGS is commonly seen in young blacks with human immunodeficiency virus (HIV) infection or disease and is known as HIV-associated nephropathy (HIVAN) (see p. 134).

Similar glomerular changes are seen as a secondary phenomenon when the number of functioning nephrons is reduced for any reasons (e.g. nephrectomy, hypertension, gross obesity, ischaemia, sickle nephropathy, reflux nephropathy, heroin abuse, chronic allograft nephropathy, IgA nephropathy and scarring following renal vasculitis), leading to the hypothesis that FSGS results from overloading (glomerular hyperfiltration) of the remaining nephrons.

Treatment

Prednisolone 0.5–2 mg/kg/day is used in most patients and continued for 6 months before declaring the patient resistant to therapy; this is common. The use of ciclosporin at doses to maintain serum trough levels at

(a) Classic FSGS showing sclerotic segments (arrow) in glomerulus.

(b) Glomerular tip lesions showing segmental sclerosis (arrow) at pole of glomerulus.

(c) Collapsing FSGS (arrow).

Fig. 11.13 **Focal segmental glomerulosclerosis (FSGS).**

150–300 ng/mL may be effective in reducing or stopping urinary protein excretion. Relapse after reducing or stopping ciclosporin is very common. Long-term use may be required to maintain remission. Cyclophosphamide, chlorambucil or azathioprine is used for second-line therapy in adults. In FSGS patients with mesangial hypercellularity and tip lesion, use of cyclophosphamide 1–1.5 mg/kg/day with 60 mg of prednisolone for 3–6 months followed by prednisolone and azathioprine as maintenance therapy has found some success. About 50% of patients progress to end-stage renal failure within 10 years of diagnosis, particularly those who are resistant to therapy.

Membranous glomerulopathy

This condition occurs mainly in adults, predominantly in males. Patients present with asymptomatic proteinuria or frank nephrotic syndrome. Microscopic haematuria, hypertension and/or renal impairment may accompany the nephrotic syndrome. Like all nephritides, hypertension and the degree of renal impairment are poor prognostic signs. The clinical evolution of membranous GN over time has shown that almost half of patients undergo spontaneous or therapy-related remission. However, eventually about 40% develop chronic renal failure, usually in association with persistent nephrotic range proteinuria. Younger patients, females and those with asymptomatic proteinuria of modest degree at the time of presentation do best.

Aetiopathogenesis

An identical glomerular histological picture is seen in the primary or idiopathic form (which comprises 75% of the cases) and also when membranous GN is secondary to drugs (e.g. penicillamine, gold, NSAIDs, probenecid, mercury, captopril), autoimmune disease (e.g. SLE, thyroiditis), infectious disease (e.g. hepatitis B, hepatitis C, schistosomiasis, *Plasmodium malariae*), neoplasia (e.g. carcinoma of lung, colon, stomach, breast and lymphoma) and other causes (e.g. sarcoidosis, kidney transplantation, sickle cell disease). The changes seen by light and electron microscopy mirror one another quite well and represent morphological progression that is dependent on the duration of the disease. At all stages, immunofluorescence shows the presence of uniform granular capillary wall deposits of IgG and complement C3. In the early stage the deposits are small and can be missed on light microscopy. Electron microscopy reveals small electron-dense deposits in the subepithelial aspects of the capillary walls. In the intermediate stage the deposits are encircled by basement membrane, which gives an appearance of spikes of basement membrane perpendicular to the basement membrane on silver staining. Late in the disease the deposits are completely surrounded by basement membrane and are undergoing resorption, which appears as uniform thickening of the capillary basement membrane on light microscopy (Fig. 11.14a, b and c).

An animal model (Heymann nephritis) in which the morphological appearances closely resemble the human

(a)

(b)

(c)

Fig. 11.14 **Membranous glomerulopathy. (a)** Schematic representation of membranous nephropathy showing the early, middle and late stages. D, subepithelial deposits; MC, mesangial cell; MM, mesangial matrix; S, spikes. (After Marsh FP (1985) *Postgraduate Nephrology*. Butterworth Heinemann.) **(b)** Light microscopy of membranous nephropathy showing thickened basement membrane (arrow). **(c)** Silver stain showing spikes (arrow) in membranous nephropathy.

condition can be induced in susceptible rats by immunization with renal autoantigens such as the brush border component of proximal tubular cells, megalin (gp330). However, the target autoantigen is unknown in humans, as megalin is absent from human podocytes. Several neutral endopeptidases located in the brush border and glomeruli are potential target autoantigens. Immune complexes are formed in situ after reacting with autoantibodies directed against these renal autoantigens.

Treatment

Oral high-dose corticosteroids are ineffective in producing either a sustained remission of nephrotic syndrome or preserving renal function in patients with membranous GN. The use of azathioprine is not associated with any significant benefits. The alkylating agents, cyclophosphamide and chlorambucil, are both effective in the management of membranous GN. Because of growing concern about long-term toxicity, these drugs should be reserved for patients who exhibit clinical features, such as severe or prolonged nephrosis (i.e. proteinuria > 6 g/day for > 6 months), renal insufficiency and hypertension, that predict a high likelihood of progression to end-stage renal failure. Chlorambucil (0.2 mg/kg/day in months 2, 4 and 6 alternating with oral prednisolone 0.4 mg/kg/day in months 1, 3 and 5) and cyclophosphamide (1.5–2.5 mg/kg/day for 6–12 months with 1 mg/kg/day of oral prednisolone on alternate days for the first 2 months) are equally effective. Ciclosporin and mycophenolate with oral steroids may become the agents of choice for membranous GN. As membranous GN is caused by circulating autoantibodies, anti-B lymphocyte therapy would seem more logical than broad-spectrum immunosuppressive agents, which are more effective against T lymphocytes. Anti-CD20 antibodies (rituximab, which ablates B lymphocytes), has been shown to improve renal function, reduce proteinuria and increase the serum albumin; no significant adverse affects have been shown in the short term.

(a)

(b)

Fig. 11.15 **Amyloid.** **(a)** Light microscopy of eosinophilic amyloid deposits (arrow). **(b)** Congo red stain under polarized light showing apple green refringence.

Amyloidosis (p. 1147)

Amyloidosis is an acquired or inherited disorder of protein folding, in which normally soluble proteins or fragments are deposited extracellularly as abnormal insoluble fibrils.

Pathology

On light microscopy, eosinophilic deposits are seen in the mesangium, capillary loops and arteriolar walls. Staining with Congo red renders these deposits pink and they show green birefringence under polarized light (Fig. 11.15). Immunofluorescence is unhelpful, but on electron microscopy the characteristic fibrils of amyloid can be seen. Amyloid consisting of immunoglobulin light chains (AL amyloid) can be identified by immunohistochemistry in only 40% of the cases as compared to almost 100% of patients with protein found in secondary amyloid (amyloid protein A, AA amyloid).

Diagnosis and treatment (see p. 1148)

The *diagnosis* can often be made clinically when features of amyloidosis are present elsewhere. On imaging, the kidneys are often large. Scintigraphy with radiolabelled serum amyloid P (SAP), a technique for quantitatively imaging amyloid deposits in vivo, is desirable because of its ability to detect the rate of regression or progression of amyloidsis over a period of time (p. 1148). Renal biopsy is necessary in all suspected cases of renal involvement.

Treatment of the underlying cause should be undertaken. Renoprotective measures should be started (p. 672). The success of dialysis and kidney transplantation is dependent upon the extent of amyloid deposition in extrarenal sites, especially the heart.

Diabetic nephropathy

Diabetic renal disease is the leading cause of end-stage renal failure in the western world. Type 1 and type 2

Fig. 11.16 Diabetes mellitus. Advanced diabetic glomerulopathy and arteriolar sclerosis (arrow).

diabetic patients (see p. 1126) have equivalent rates of proteinuria, azotaemia, and ultimately end-stage renal failure. Both types of diabetes show strong similarities in their rate of renal functional deterioration, and onset of co-morbid complications.

Pathology

The kidneys enlarge initially and there is glomerular hyperfiltration (GFR > 150 mL/min). The major early histological lesions seen are glomerular basement membrane thickening and mesangial expansion. Later, glomerulosclerosis develops with nodules (Kimmelstiel–Wilson lesion) and hyaline deposits in the glomerular arterioles (see Fig. 11.16). These later changes are associated with heavy proteinuria. The lesions seen in type 1 are also seen in type 2. The pathophysiology is discussed on page 1126.

Treatment

The timing of renoprotection therapy in diabetes is a subject of current investigation. Lifestyle changes (cessation of smoking and increase in exercise), hypertension, poor metabolic regulation, and hyperlidaemia should be addressed in every diabetic. Microalbuminuria is a reason to start treatment with ACE inhibitors or an angiotensin II receptor antagonist (AIIRA) in either type of diabetes, regardless of blood pressure elevation. Like other kidney diseases, however, nearly the entire course of renal injury in diabetes is clinically silent. Medical intervention during this silent phase (Box 11.3) is renoprotective, as judged by slowed loss of glomerular filtration. Despite intensified metabolic control and antihypertension treatment in diabetic patients, a substantial number still go on to develop end-stage renal failure.

Nephrotic syndrome with 'active' urine sediments (mixed nephrotic/nephritic)

Mesangiocapillary (membranoproliferative) glomerulonephritis (MCGN)

This uncommon lesion has three subtypes with similar clinical presentations: the nephrotic syndrome, haematuria, hypertension and renal impairment. They also have similar microscopic findings although the pathogenesis may be different. Electron microscopy defines:

- Type 1 MCGN. There is mesangial cell proliferation, with mainly subendothelial immune deposition and apparent splitting of the capillary basement membrane, giving a 'tram-line' effect. It can be associated with persistently reduced plasma levels of C3 and normal levels of C4 due to activation of the complement cascade by the classical pathway. It may be idiopathic or may occur with chronic infection (abscesses, infective endocarditis, infected ventriculoperitoneal shunt) or cryoglobulinaemia secondary to hepatitis C infections (Fig. 11.17a).
- Type 2 MCGN. There is mesangial cell proliferation with electron-dense, linear intramembranous deposits that usually stain for C3 only (Fig. 11.17b). This type may be idiopathic or be associated with partial lipodystrophy (loss of subcutaneous fat on face and upper trunk). MCGN affects young adults. These patients have low C3 levels like in type 1 but this is due to the activation of the alternative pathway of the complement cascade; they also have autoantibodies to C3 convertase enzyme.
- Type 3 MCGN has features of both types 1 and 2. Complement activation appears to be via the final common pathway of the cascade.

Most patients eventually go on to develop renal failure over several years. Type 2 MCGN recurs in virtually 100% of renal transplant patients but recurrence is less common in type 1 (25%). However, recurrence does not interfere with long-term graft function.

Management

For all age groups, for idiopathic MCGN with normal renal function, non-nephrotic range proteinuria, no specific therapy is required. Close follow-up every four months, with specific attention to blood pressure control is recommended.

In children with the nephritic syndrome and/or impaired renal function, a trial of steroids is warranted (alternate-day prednisolone 40 mg/m² for a period of 6–12 months). If no benefit is seen, this treatment is discontinued. Regular follow-up with control of blood pressure, use of agents to reduce proteinuria and correction of lipid abnormalities is necessary.

In adults with the nephritic syndrome and/or renal impairment, aspirin (325 mg) or dipyridamole (75–100 mg) or a combination of the two, should be given for 6–12 months. Again if no benefits are seen, the treatment should be stopped. Treatment to slow the rate of progression of renal failure is instituted (p. 672).

Fig. 11.17 **Mesangiocapillary glomerulonephritis (MCGN). (a) Type I MCGN** showing expanded mesangial matrix and mesangial cells, thickened capillary wall, large subendothelial deposits and formation of a new layer of basement membrane (tram-line effect). **(b) Type II MCGN.** This shows a variable glomerular appearance, very electron-dense material has replaced the Bowman's capsule and tubular basement membrane and part of the capillary. There is some proliferation of mesangial cells. (After Marsh FP (1985) *Postgraduate Nephrology.* Butterworth Heinemann.)

Mesangial proliferative GN (IgM nephropathy, C1q nephropathy)

In addition to minimal-change disease, there are two other disorders that usually present with heavy proteinuria with only minor changes on light microscopy.

IgM nephropathy is characterized by increased mesangial cellularity in most of the glomeruli, associated with granular immune deposits (IgM and complement) in the mesangial regions. Patients present with episodic or persistent haematuria with the nephrotic syndrome. Unlike minimal-change disease, the prognosis is not uniformly good, as steroid response is only 50% compared to 90% in minimal-change disease. Between 10% and 30% develop progressive renal insufficiency with signs of secondary FSGS on repeat biopsy. A trial of cyclophosamide with prednisolone is used with persistent nephrotic syndrome, particularly with a rising plasma creatinine concentration.

C1q nephropathy is very similar to IgM nephropathy in presenting features and microscopic appearance with the exception of C1q deposits in the mesangium. Sometimes it is misdiagnosed as lupus nephritis, particularly in patients with negative serology (so-called seronegative lupus.) The distinguishing features are intense C1q staining and absence of tubuloreticular inclusions (attributable to high circulating alpha-interferon) on electron microscopy. Only some patients are steroid dependent. Progression to renal failure is, as in most glomerular diseases, most likely to occur in patients with heavy proteinuria and renal insufficiency.

Systemic lupus erythematosus (lupus glomerulonephritis) (see also p. 575)

Overt renal disease occurs in at least one-third of SLE patients and, of these, 25% reach end-stage renal failure within 10 years. Histologically almost all patients will have changes which are classified by the World Health Organization (modified with added clinical manifestations) as:

- Type I – Mesangial immune deposits (normal glomeruli on light microscopy). Asymptomatic.
- Type II – Mesangial immune deposits with mesangial cell hypercellularity and matrix expansion. Clinically there is mild renal disease.
- Type III – Focal proliferative glomerulonephritis (involving < 50% of the total number of glomeruli on renal biopsy) with subdivisions for active or sclerotic lesions. Haematuria and proteinuria are seen in almost all.
- Type IV – Diffuse proliferative glomerulonephritis (involving > 50% of total number of glomeruli on renal biopsy) either with segmental (class IV-S) or global (class IV-G) involvement, and also with subdivisions for active or sclerotic lesions (Fig. 11.18). Clinically, as in type III, but the nephrotic syndrome, hypertension and renal insufficiency are often seen.
- Type V – Membranous GN. Heavy proteinuria is seen, with signs of the nephrotic syndrome, haematuria and hypertension.
- Type VI – Advanced sclerosing lesions (> 90% glomeruli are sclerosed). Progressive renal failure is seen.

Serial renal biopsies show that in approximately 25% of patients, histological appearances alter from one histological classification to another during the interbiopsy interval. The prognosis is better in patients with types I, II and V. Immune deposits in the glomeruli and mesangium are characteristic of SLE and stain positive for IgG, IgM, IgA and the complement components C3, C1q and C4 on immunofluorescence.

Pathophysiology

SLE is now known to be an autoantigen-driven, T-cell-dependent and B-cell-mediated autoimmune disease (p. 574). Lupus nephritis typically has circulating auto-

Fig. 11.18 **Lupus nephritis type IV – a diffuse proliferative nephritis.** There is proliferation of endothelial and mesangial cells.

antibodies to cellular antigens (particularly anti-dsDNA, anti-Ro) and complement activation which leads to reduced levels of C3, C4, and particularly C1q. C1q is the first component of the classical pathway of the complement cascade (see p. 201) and is involved in the activation of complement and clearance of self-antigens generated during apoptosis. Anti-C1q antibodies may help in distinguishing a renal from a non-renal relapse. However, not all autoantibodies are pathogenic to the kidney. These nephritogenic antibodies have specific physicochemical characteristics and correlate well with the pattern of renal injury. DNA was thought to be the inciting autoantigen, but now nucleosomes (structures comprising DNA and histone, generated during apoptosis) are the most likely autoantigen. Nucleosome-specific T cells, antinucleosome antibodies and nephritogenic immune complexes are generated. Positively charged histone components of the nucleosome bind to the negatively charged heparan sulphate (within the glomerular basement membrane) inciting an inflammatory reaction and resulting in mesangial cell proliferation, mesangial matrix expansion and inflammatory leucocytes. Other pathogenic mechanisms include infarction of glomerular segments, thrombotic microangiopathy, vasculitis and glomerular sclerosis.

The extraglomerular features of lupus nephritis include tubulointerstitial nephritis (75% of patients), renal vein thrombosis and renal artery stenosis. Thrombotic manifestations are associated with autoantibodies to phospholipids (anticardiolipin or lupus anticoagulant).

Management

Initial treatment depends on the clinical presentation but hypertension and oedema should be treated. A definite histopathological diagnosis is required. Type I requires no treatment. Type II usually runs a benign course but some are treated with steroids.

There have been a number of clinical trials with immunosuppressive agents in types III, IV and V. At present, steroids and cyclophosphamide are usually used for induction, with azathioprine and mycophenolate mofetil for maintenance therapy.

B cell depletion with rituximab (anti-CD20) has been shown to be effective in a small study.

Prognosis

Treatment leading to the normalization of proteinuria, hypertension and renal dysfunction indicates a good prognosis. Glomerulosclerosis (type VI) usually predicts end-stage renal disease (p. 665).

Cryoglobulinaemic renal disease

Cryoglobulins (CG) are immunoglobulins and complement components, which precipitate reversibly in the cold. Three types are recognized:

In *type I*, the cryoprecipitable immunoglobulin is a single monoclonal type, as is found in multiple myeloma and lymphoproliferative disorders.

Types II and *III* cryoglobulinaemias are mixed types. In each, a polyclonal IgG antigen is bound to an antiglobulin. In type II, the antiglobulin component, which is usually of the IgM or IgA class with rheumatoid factor activity, is monoclonal, while in type III it is polyclonal. Type II CGs account for 40–60% cases, whilst 40–50% of all CG cases are of type III.

Glomerular disease is more common in type II than in type III cryoglobulinaemia. In approximately 30% of these 'mixed' cryoglobulinaemias, no underlying or associated disease is found (essential cryoglobulinaemia). Recognized associations include viral infections (hepatitis B and C, HIV, cytomegalovirus, Epstein–Barr infection), fungal and spirochaetal infections, malaria and infective endocarditis and autoimmune diseases (SLE, rheumatoid arthritis and Sjögren's syndrome). Glomerular pathological changes resemble MCGN (Fig. 11.17).

Presentation is usually in the fourth or fifth decades of life, and women are more frequently affected than men. Systemic features include purpura, arthralgia, leg ulcers, Raynaud's phenomenon, evidence of systemic vasculitis, a polyneuropathy, and hepatic involvement. The glomerular disease presents typically as asymptomatic proteinuria, microscopic haematuria or both, but presentation with an acute nephritic and nephrotic syndrome (commonest presentation) or features of renal impairment also occurs.

Serological investigation reveals a reduction in concentration of early complement components with an elevation of later components, detection of CGs, monoclonal gammopathy, rheumatoid factor, autoantibodies and antiviral antibodies or mRNA of hepatitis C, depending on the associated disorder.

Spontaneous remission occurs in about one-third of cases and approximately one-third pursue an indolent course. Corticosteroid and/or immunosuppressive therapy with cyclophosphamide may be of benefit, but evaluation of treatment is difficult owing to the rarity of the disease and the occurrence of spontaneous remissions. Intensive plasma exchange or cryofiltration has been used in selected cases. Interferon reduces the viraemia in hepatitis C but does not influence the cryoglobulinaemia.

Henoch–Schönlein syndrome

This clinical syndrome comprises a characteristic skin rash, abdominal colic, joint pain and glomerulonephritis. Approximately 30–70% have clinical evidence of renal disease with haematuria and/or proteinuria. The renal disease is usually mild but the nephrotic syndrome and acute renal failure can occur. The renal lesion is a focal segmental proliferative glomerulonephritis, sometimes with mesangial hypercellularity. In the more severe cases, epithelial crescents may be present. Immunoglobulin deposition, mainly of IgA, is seen in the glomerular mesangium, similar to IgA nephropathy. There is no treatment of proven benefit. Treatment is usually supportive but with crescentic GN aggressive immunosuppression has been tried with variable outcome.

Idiopathic fibrillary glomerulopathy

In this rare condition, characteristic microfibrillary structures are seen in the mesangium and glomerular capillary wall on electron microscopy that are clearly different from those seen in amyloidosis; the fibrils are larger than those in amyloidosis (20–30 versus 10 nm diameter) and do not stain with Congo red. The median age at presentation is approximately 45 years (range 10–80 years). Patients present with proteinuria, mostly in the nephrotic range (60%), and microscopic haematuria (70%), hypertension and renal impairment (50%) that may progress rapidly: 40–50% of patients develop end-stage renal failure within 2–6 years.

No treatment is known to be of benefit, although isolated instances of an apparent response to corticosteroid and immunosuppressive therapy have been reported.

Immunotactoid glomerulopathy

In this disorder, microtubules which are much larger (30–40 nm diameter) than the fibrils in fibrillary glomerulopathy are seen on electron microscopy. The majority of patients have circulating paraprotein or monoclonal immunoglobulin deposition is seen in the glomeruli on immunofluorescence microscopy. A lymphoproliferative disease is the underlying cause in over 50% of cases. The clinical presentation and course are similar to fibrillary glomerulopathy, although therapy can be effective in patients with lymphoproliferative disease and/or paraproteinaemia. Complete or partial remission of the nephrotic syndrome can be achieved by various chemotherapeutic agents in over 80% of patients.

ACUTE GLOMERULONEPHRITIS (ACUTE NEPHRITIC SYNDROME) (Table 11.5)

This comprises:

- haematuria (macroscopic or microscopic) – red-cell casts are typically seen on urine microscopy

Table 11.5 Diseases commonly associated with the acute nephritic syndrome

Post-streptococcal glomerulonephritis
Non-streptococcal post-infectious glomerulonephritis, e.g. *Staphylococcus*, pneumococcus, *Legionella*, syphilis, mumps, varicella, hepatitis B and C, echovirus, Epstein–Barr virus, toxoplasmosis, malaria, schistosomiasis, trichinosis
Infective endocarditis
Shunt nephritis
Visceral abscess
Systemic lupus erythematosus (see p. 575)
Henoch–Schönlein syndrome (see p. 587)
Cryoglobulinaemia (see p. 628)

- proteinuria
- hypertension
- oedema (periorbital, leg or sacral)
- temporarily oliguria and uraemia.

The histological pattern is characterized by cellular proliferation (mesangial and endothelial) and inflammatory cell infiltration (neutrophils, macrophages).

Post-streptococcal glomerulonephritis (PSGN)

The patient, usually a child, suffers a streptococcal infection 1–3 weeks before the onset of the acute nephritic syndrome. Streptococcal throat infection, otitis media or cellulitis may all be responsible. The infecting organism is a Lancefield group A β-haemolytic streptococcus of a nephritogenic type. The latent interval between the infection and development of symptoms and signs of renal involvement reflects the time taken for immune complex formation and deposition and glomerular injury to occur. PSGN is now rare in developed countries. Renal biopsy shows diffuse, florid, acute inflammation in the glomerulus (without necrosis but occasionally cellular crescents), with neutrophils and deposition of immunoglobulin (IgG) and complement (Fig. 11.19a, b). Ultrastructural findings are those of electron-dense deposits, characteristically but not solely in the subepithelial aspects of the capillary walls. Endothelial cells often are swollen. Similar biopsy findings may be seen in *non-streptococcal post-infectious glomerulonephritis* – shown in Table 11.5.

Management

The acute phase should be treated with antihypertensives, diuretics, salt restriction and dialysis as necessary. If recovery is slow, corticosteroids may be helpful. The prognosis is usually good in children. A small number of adults develop hypertension and/or renal impairment later in life. Therefore in older patients, an annual blood pressure check, and an estimation of serum creatinine, is a reasonable precaution, even after apparent complete recovery. Evidence in support of long-term penicillin prophylaxis after the development of glomerulonephritis is lacking. In non-streptococcal post-infectious glomerulonephritis, prognosis is equally good if the underlying infection is eradicated.

(a)

(b)

Fig. 11.19 **Post-streptococcal glomerulonephritis.**
(a) Diagram showing large aggregates of immune material (humps) in the extracapillary area. There is an increase in mesangial matrix and mesangial cells with occlusion of the capillary lumen by endothelial cell cytoplasm, leucocytes and mesangial cell cytoplasm. After Marsh FP (1985) *Postgraduate Nephrology.* Butterworth Heinemann, with permission.
(b) Light microscopy showing acute inflammation of the glomerulus with neutrophils.

Glomerulonephritis with infective endocarditis

GN occurs rarely in patients with infective endocarditis (usually i.v. drug abusers). It usually manifests itself as acute nephritic syndrome. A similar presentation is in patients with infected ventriculoperitoneal shunt (*shunt nephritis*). Microscopic appearances resemble post-infectious GN, but lesions are usually focal and segmental. Crescentic GN with acute renal failure has been described, particularly with *Staphylococcus aureus* infection. Appropriate antibiotic therapy or surgical eradication of infection in fulminant cases (embolic infarct of the kidney) usually results in a return of normal renal function.

Glomerulonephritis associated with visceral abscesses (mainly pulmonary)

Clinical and microscopic features are indistinguishable from post-infectious GN, but usually complement levels are normal and immune deposits are absent on biopsy.

Antibiotic therapy and surgical drainage of the abscess results in complete recovery of renal function in approximately 50% of patients.

Asymptomatic urinary abnormalities

A variety of renal lesions may present as either isolated proteinuria or haematuria, alone or with proteinuria. *Isolated proteinuria* without haematuria in asymptomatic patients is usually an incidental finding. It is usually in the sub-nephrotic range without an active urine sediment and there is normal renal function. Over 50% of these patients have postural proteinuria. The outcome of isolated proteinuria (postural or non-postural) is excellent in the majority of patients, with a gradual decline in proteinuria. Occasionally, it may be an early sign of a serious glomerular lesion such as membranous GN, IgA nephropathy, FSGS, diabetic nephropathy or amyloidosis. Moreover, mild proteinuria may accompany a febrile illness, congestive heart failure or infectious diseases with no clinical renal significance.

Haematuria with or without sub-nephrotic range proteinuria in an asymptomatic patient may lead to early discovery of potentially serious glomerular disease such as SLE, Henoch–Schönlein purpura, post-infectious GN or idiopathic hypercalciuria in children. Asymptomatic haematuria is also the primary presenting manifestation of a number of specific glomerular diseases discussed below.

IgA nephropathy (Fig. 11.20a, b)

This disease has replaced post-streptococcal glomerulo-nephritis as the commonest form of glomerulonephritis world-wide. There is a focal and segmental proliferative glomerulonephritis with mesangial deposits of polymeric IgA_1. In some cases IgG, IgM and C3 may also be seen in the glomerular mesangium. The disease may be a result of an exaggerated bone marrow and tonsillar IgA_1 immune response to viral or other antigens and is associated with an abnormality in O-linked galactosylation in the hinge region of the IgA_1 molecule. Quantitative and structural changes of IgA_1 play a key role in the development of disease due to functional abnormalities of two IgA receptors: CD89 expressed on blood myeloid cells and the transferring receptor (CD71) on mesangial cells. Abnormal IgA_1 induces the release of soluble CD89, which is responsible for the formation of circulating IgA complexes. These complexes may then be trapped by CD71, which is overexpressed on mesangial cells in IgA nephropathy patients, allowing IgA complex formation in the mesangium. Up to 50% of patients exhibit elevated serum IgA (polyclonal) concentration. Superimposed crescent formation is frequent, particularly following macroscopic haematuria due to upper respiratory tract infection. Several diseases may be associated with IgA deposits, including Henoch–Schönlein purpura, chronic liver disease, malignancies (especially carcinoma of bronchus), seronegative spondyloarthrides, coeliac disease, mycosis fungoides and psoriasis.

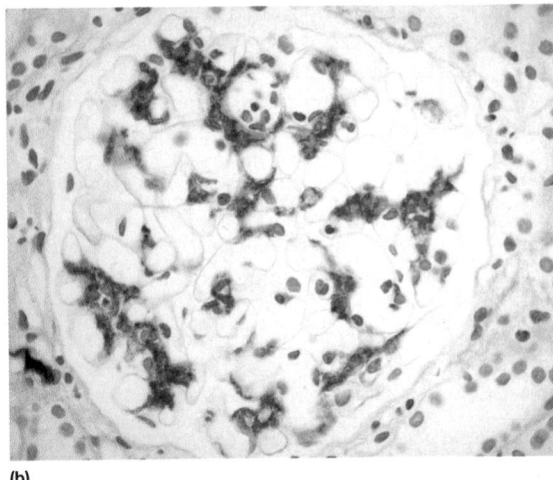

Fig. 11.20 **IgA nephropathy. (a)** Light microscopy. Showing mesangial cell proliferation (arrow) and increased matrix. **(b)** IgA deposits on immunoperoxidase staining.

Clinical presentation

IgA nephropathy tends to occur in children and young males. They present with asymptomatic microscopic haematuria or recurrent macroscopic haematuria sometimes following an upper respiratory or gastrointestinal viral infection. Proteinuria occurs and 5% can be nephrotic. The prognosis is usually good, especially in those with normal blood pressure, normal renal function and absence of proteinuria at presentation. Surprisingly, recurrent macroscopic haematuria is a good prognostic sign, although this may be due to 'lead-time bias' (p. 488), as patients with overt haematuria come to medical attention at an earlier stage of their illness. The risk of eventual development of end-stage renal failure is about 25% in those with proteinuria of more than 1 g per day, elevated serum creatinine, hypertension, ACE gene polymorphism (DD isoform) and tubulointerstitial fibrosis on renal biopsy.

Management

Patients with proteinuria over 1–3 g/day, mild glomerular changes only and preserved renal function should be treated with steroids. Steroids reduce proteinuria and stabilize renal function. The combination of cyclophosphamide, dipyridamole and warfarin should not be used, nor should ciclosporin. In patients with progressive disease (creatinine clearance less than 70 mL/min), fish oil or prednisolone with cyclophosphamide for 3 months followed by maintenance with prednisolone and azathioprine may be tried. A tonsillectomy can reduce proteinuria and haematuria in those patients with recurrent tonsillitis. All patients, with or without hypertension and proteinuria, should receive a combination of ACE inhibitor and angiotensin II receptor antagonist rather than each agent alone because reduction of proteinuria and preservation of renal function are better with combination therapy despite similar blood pressure control. Mesangial IgA deposits are commonly found in

the allografts of transplanted patients but loss of graft function as a result is uncommon.

Alport's syndrome

Alport's syndrome is a rare condition characterized by an hereditary nephritis with haematuria, proteinuria (less than 1–2 g/day) progressive renal failure and high-frequency nerve deafness. Approximately 15% of cases may have ocular abnormalities such as bilateral anterior lenticonus and macular and perimacular retinal flecks. In about 85% of patients with Alport's syndrome there is X-linked inheritance of a mutation in the *COLIVα5* gene encoding the COLIVα5 collagen chain. In female carriers, penetrance is variable and depends on the type of mutation or degree of mosaicism following hybridization of the X chromosome. Patients with autosomal recessive or dominant modes of inheritance have also been described with mutations in *COLIVα3* or *COLIVα4* genes. In families with stromal cell tumours there is an additional mutation in the *COLIVα6* gene.

Mutations present in Alport's syndrome that produce post-translational defects in α3, α4 and α5 chains result in incorrect assembly or folding of monomers; such defective monomers are rapidly degraded. These mutations arrest the normal developmental switch and cause the persistence of embryonic α1,α1 and α2 networks in glomerular basement membrane. The α1,α1 and α2 network is more susceptible to endoproteolysis and oxidative stress than the α3, α4 and α5 network. Over time, patients with Alport's syndrome probably become more sensitive to selective basement membrane proteolysis, which may explain why their glomerular membranes thicken unevenly, split and ultimately deteriorate.

The primary glomerular filtration barrier of the glomerular capillary consists of the basement membrane and the outer slit diaphragm formed between adjacent podocytes. Loss of slit function causes massive proteinuria (congenital nephrotic syndrome, p. 622) but deterioration of glomerular basement produces only mild proteinuria. Proteinuria in Alport's syndrome is the result of glomerular sclerosis, rather than primary loss of slit pores. In pedigrees with a history of renal failure, disease progresses from concomitant interstitial fibrosis, macrophage and lymphocyte infiltration secondary to tubular basement disruption and trans-differentiation of epithelial mesenchymal cells to fibroblasts. This fibrogenic response destroys renal architecture. The renal histology characteristically shows split basement membrane. In some patients with Alport's syndrome and carriers, thin basement membrane, as seen in benign familial haematuria, is the only abnormality detected on histology. For this reason, the boundary between Alport's and benign familial haematuria has become increasingly vague.

Management

The disease is progressive and accounts for some 5% of cases of end-stage renal failure in childhood or adolescence. Patients with early renal failure can be treated with ACE inhibitors to attenuate proteinuria and slow the rate of progression. Anti-GBM antibody does not adhere normally to the glomerular basement membrane of affected individuals but development of crescentic glomerulonephritis in the transplanted kidney due to anti-GBM alloantibody is a well-recognized complication.

Thin glomerular basement membrane disease

The condition is inherited as an autosomal dominant and typically presents with persistent microscopic glomerular haematuria (RBC casts or dysmorphic RBCs). The diagnosis is made by renal biopsy, which shows thinning of the glomerular capillary basement membrane on electron microscopy. The condition was underdiagnosed and is much commoner than previously believed. The prognosis for renal function is usually very good but some patients develop renal insufficiency over decades. The cause of renal impairment in this condition is not known but may be due to secondary FSGS or concomitant IgA nephropathy. Misdiagnosis occurs with Alport's syndrome which shares similar histological features. No treatment is of known benefit.

RAPIDLY PROGRESSIVE GLOMERULONEPHRITIS (RPGN)

RPGN is a syndrome with glomerular haematuria (RBC casts or dysmorphic RBCs), rapidly developing acute renal failure over weeks to months and focal glomerular necrosis (Fig. 11.21) with or without glomerular crescent development on renal biopsy. The 'crescent' is an aggregate of macrophages and epithelial cells in Bowman's space (Fig. 11.21). RPGN can develop with immune deposits (anti-GBM or immune complex type) or without immune deposits (pauci-immune). It can also develop as an idiopathic primary glomerular disease or can be superimposed on other glomerular diseases, primary or secondary. The classification used here is based on the immunofluorescence information obtained from renal histology (Table 11.6).

Anti-GBM glomerulonephritis (Fig. 11.22a)

Anti-GBM glomerulonephritis, characterized by linear capillary loop staining with IgG and C3 and extensive crescent formation, accounts for 15–20% of all cases of RPGN, although overall it accounts for less than 5% of all forms of glomerulonephritis. This condition is rare, with an incidence of 1 per 2 million in the general population. About two-thirds of these patients have Goodpasture's syndrome with associated lung haemorrhage (p. 940). The remainder have a renal restricted anti-GBM RPGN, which is seen in people above 50 years and affects both genders equally.

(a)

(b)

Fig. 11.21 **Rapidly progressive glomerulonephritis (RPGN).** Arrows show 'crescents' with aggregates of macrophages and epithelial cells in Bowman's space. **(a)** Focal necrotizing glomerulonephritis. **(b)** Crescentic glomerulonephritis.

Fig. 11.22 **Immunofluorescence. (a)** Showing antiglomerular basement membrane antibody (anti-GBM) deposition in a linear pattern typical of Goodpasture's syndrome. **(b)** Showing immune complex deposition in a diffuse granular pattern.

Anti-GBM antibodies (detected by ELISA) are present in serum and are directed against the non-collagenous (NCl) component of $\alpha3$ (IV) collagen of basement membrane. This target antigen must be present as a component of the native $\alpha3$, $\alpha4$, $\alpha5$ (IV) network of selected basement membrane in order for pulmonary and renal disease to develop. Consequently, there are no known cases of anti-GBM glomerulonephritis in patients with Alport's syndrome (p. 631). Anti-GBM RPGN is restricted by the major histocompatibilty complex; HLA-DRB1*1501 and HLA-DRB1*1502 alleles increase susceptibility, whereas HLA-DR7 and HLA-DR1 are protective. The thymus expresses $\alpha3$ (IV) NCl peptides that can eliminate autoreactive CD4$^+$ helper T cells, but a few such cells escape deletion and are kept in check by circulating regulatory cells. Breakdown of this peripheral tolerance (the mechanism of which is unknown) results in these autoreactive CD4$^+$ cells producing anti-GBM antibodies. These antibodies are very specific as shown by the fact that antibodies against $\alpha1,\alpha1$ and $\alpha2$ NCl

domains do not cause RPGN. Since the $\alpha3$ (IV) NCl epitope is hidden within the $\alpha3$, $\alpha4$ and $\alpha5$ (IV) promoter, it is presumed that an environmental factor, such as exposure to hydrocarbons or tobacco smoke, is required in order to reveal cryptic epitopes to the immune system.

The mechanism of renal injury is complex. When anti-GBM antibody binds basement membrane it activates complement and proteases and results in disruption of the filtration barrier and Bowman's capsule, causing proteinuria and the formation of crescents. Crescent formation is facilitated by interleukin-12 and gamma-interferon which are produced by resident and infiltrating inflammatory cells.

Management

This is based on counteracting the factors involved in the pathogenesis. Thus plasma exchange is used to remove circulating antibodies, steroids to suppress inflammation from antibody already deposited in the tissue and cyclophosphamide to suppress further antibody synthesis. The prognosis is directly related to the extent of glomerular damage (measured by percentage of crescents, serum creatinine and need for dialysis) at the initiation of treatment. When oliguria occurs or serum creatinine rises above 600–700 µmol/L, renal failure is usually irreversible. Once the active disease is treated, this condition, unlike other autoimmune diseases, does not follow a remitting/relapsing course. Furthermore, if left untreated, autoantibodies diminish spontaneously within 3 years and autoreactive T cells cannot be detected in the convalescent patients. This is suggestive of re-establishment of peripheral tolerance which coincides with re-emergence of regulatory CD25$^+$ cells in the peripheral blood; these play a key role in inhibiting the autoimmune response. The emergence and persistence of these regulatory cells may underlie the 'single hit' nature of this condition.

ANCA-positive vasculitides (see also p. 584)

Inflammation and necrosis of the blood vessel wall occurs in many primary vasculitic disorders. Wegener's granulomatosis, microscopic polyangiitis and Churg–Strauss syndrome are described as small vessel vasculitides and

---

Table 11.6 Types of rapidly progressive glomerulonephritis (RPGN)

Linear immunofluorescent pattern (Fig. 11.22a)
Idiopathic anti-GBM antibody-mediated RPGN
Goodpasture's syndrome

Granular immunofluorescent pattern (immune complex-mediated RPGN) (Fig. 11.22b)
Idiopathic immune complex-mediated RPGN
Associated with other primary GN
   Mesangiocapillary GN (type II > type I)
   IgA nephropathy
   Membranous glomerulopathy
Associated with secondary GN
   Post-infectious GN
   Systemic lupus erythematosus
   Henoch–Schönlein syndrome
   Cryoglobulinaemia

Negative immunofluorescent pattern (pauci-immune RPGN)
ANCA-associated systemic vasculitides

Fig. 11.23 **Vasculitic rash.**

are commonly associated with antineutrophil cytoplasm antibodies (ANCA). These diseases share common pathology with focal necrotizing lesions, which affect many different vessels and organs; in the lungs, a capillaritis may cause lung haemorrhage; within the glomerulus of the kidney, crescentic GN and/or focal necrotizing lesions may cause acute renal failure (Fig. 11.21a, b); in the dermis, a purpuric rash (Fig. 11.23) or vasculitic ulceration. Wegener's and Churg–Strauss syndrome may have additional granulomatous lesions.

Autoantibodies directed against constituents of the cytoplasm of normal human granulocytes and monocytes are useful in the understanding of the above disorders. Two forms of antineutrophil cytoplasmic antibodies (ANCA) can be demonstrated; proteinase-3 (PR3)-ANCA and myeloperoxidase (MPO)-ANCA. Binding of PR3-ANCA to neutrophils in indirect immunofluorescence assays produces a granular cytoplasmic stain – hence the use of the old term 'cytoplasmic (c)-ANCA'. MPO-ANCA produces a perinuclear stain – hence the old term 'perinuclear (p)-ANCA'. If ELISA and indirect immunofluorescence techniques are combined, diagnostic specificity is 99%.

PR3-ANCA positivity is found in the large majority of patients with active Wegener's granulomatosis and in up to 50% of patients with microscopic polyangiitis. Anti-MPO positivity is present in the majority of patients with idiopathic crescentic glomerulonephritis and in a variable number of cases of microscopic polyangiitis. Churg–Strauss syndrome may have either anti-MPO- or anti-PR3-ANCA. Testing for antineutrophil cytoplasmic antibodies should be accompanied by appropriate tests of autoantibodies directed against DNA and the glomerular basement membrane antigen. The simultaneous occurrence of ANCA and anti-GMB antibody is well documented; such patients tend to follow the natural history of Goodpasture's disease. Variations in the ANCA titres have been used in the assessment of disease activity. Several drugs (e.g. propylthiouracil, hydralazine, minocycline, penicillamine) may induce vasculitides associated with ANCA. Most patients reported with drug-induced ANCA-associated vasculitis have MPO-ANCA, often in very high titres. In addition to MPO-ANCA, most also have antibodies to elastase or to lactoferrin. A relatively small number have PR3-ANCA. Many cases of drug-induced ANCA-associated vasculitis present with constitutional symptoms, arthralgias/arthritis, and cutaneous vasculitis. However, the full range of clinical features associated with ANCA, including crescentic GN and lung haemorrhage, can also occur.

It remains unclear how and why autoimmunity with formation of ANCA antibodies occurs. However, a recent study, using material from patients with anti-PR3 suggests that such patients also have autoantibodies to a peptide translated from the antisense DNA strand of PR-3 (complementary PR-3; cPR-3) or to a mimetic of this peptide. This suggests that autoimmunity can be initiated through an immune response against a peptide that is antisense or complementary to the autoantigen, which then induces anti-idiotypic antibodies (autoantibodies) that cross-react with the autoantigen.

There is some evidence to suggest that ANCA are pathogenic and not just markers of disease; for example, development of drug-induced ANCA and associated vasculitic lesions in humans. Studies in MPO knockout mice further highlight the pathogenic significance of ANCA.

ANCA do not act alone. There may be multiple factors that contribute to the initiation of an ANCA autoimmune response and the induction of injury by ANCA, such as genetic predisposition (α_1-antitrypsin deficiency; Pi-Z allele) and environmental factors (e.g. silica exposure, viral infection, *Staph. aureus* infection) can result in high local or systemic pro-inflammatory cytokines such as tumour necrosis factor (TNF).

Treatment

The sooner treatment is instituted the more chance there is of recovery of renal function. Corticosteroids and cyclophosphamide are of benefit: high-dose oral prednisolone (maximum 80 mg/day reducing over time to 15 mg/day by 3 months) and cyclophosphamide (2 mg/kg/day, adjusted for age, renal function and prevailing WBC count). Intravenous pulse, rather than daily oral, cyclophosphamide is associated with an equivalent response with better side-effect profile but is associated with higher relapse rate. The best indicators of prognosis are pulmonary haemorrhage and severity of renal failure at presentation. Patients who present with fulminant disease need intensification of immunosuppression with adjuvant plasma exchanges (7 × 3–4 L over 14 days) or intravenous pulse methyl prednisolone (1 g/day for 3 consecutive days). In a recent randomized control study of patients with severe renal failure at presentation (creatinine > 500 µmol/day) plasma exchange appeared to have better outcome than pulse methyl prednisolone.

Once remission has been achieved, azathioprine should be substituted for cyclophosphamide. In cases of intolerance to azathioprine or cyclophosphamide, mycophenolate has been tried with some success. Colonization of the upper respiratory tract with *Staph. aureus* increases the risk of relapse, and treatment with sulphamethoxazole/trimethoprim reduces the relapse rate. Relapse after complete cessation of immunosuppressive therapy has been observed relatively frequently, and therefore long-term, albeit relatively low-dose, immunosuppression is necessary. Long-term follow-up of patients is mandatory. Intravenous immunoglobulin (ATG directed against activated T lymphocytes causes lymphopenia) and anti-TNF therapy show promise in the treatment of severe and drug-resistant cases.

OTHER GLOMERULAR DISORDERS

HIV-associated nephropathy (HIVAN) (p. 134)

A number of renal lesions have been described in association with HIV infection. These include glomerulonephritis of various histological types and the haemolytic uraemic syndrome. The most common (80–90%) histological abnormality is a focal glomerulosclerosis (FGS).

HIV-associated FGS

A characteristic 'collapsed' appearance of glomeruli is often seen on light microscopy similar to that seen in other causes of focal segmental glomerulosclerosis (see Fig. 11.13c). In HIVAN many visceral epithelial cells (podocytes) are enlarged, hyperplastic, coarsely vacuolated, contain protein absorption droplets and overlie capillaries with varying degrees of wrinkling and collapse of the walls. It is associated with loss of podocyte-specific markers such as Wilms' tumour factor and synaptopodin. There is now clear evidence that HIV-1 infects podocytes of patients with HIVAN. HIVAN has striking predilection; over 90% of patients are black. Clinically HIVAN presents with proteinuria in the nephrotic range, oedema and a 'bland' urine. Hypertension is unusual. If untreated, patients go on to renal failure which can be rapid in progression.

IgA may be an integral feature of HIV-1 infection, as is IgA nephropathy. In this setting, HIV antigen may be a part of the glomerular immune complexes and circulating immune complexes.

Highly active antiretroviral therapy (HAART) may result in stabilization of renal function and prevention of progression to end-stage renal failure (efficacy 23%) and HIV-associated mortality in patients with end-stage renal failure. A cyclin-dependent kinase inhibitor, roscovitine, has been successfully used in the treatment of experimental HIVAN.

Fabry's disease

This is the result of deficiency of the enzyme alpha-galactosidase with accumulation of sphingolipids in many cells. In the kidney, accumulations of sphingolipids especially affects podocytes, which on light microscopy appear enlarged and vacuolated. Ultrastructurally, these inclusion bodies appear as zebra or myeloid bodies representing sphingolipids. These structures can also be found in endothelial, mesangial, and arterial and arteriolar smooth muscle cells. The most common renal manifestation is proteinuria and progressive renal failure.

Treatment (p. 1147).

Sickle nephropathy

Sickle disease or trait is complicated relatively commonly by papillary sclerosis or necrosis, nephrogenic diabetes insipidus and incomplete renal tubular acidosis. Glomerular lesions are rare and can sometimes be traced to hepatitis B or C infection acquired through repeated blood transfusions. Occasionally, proteinuria or nephrotic syndrome with progressive renal insufficiency is seen without prior infection. The rare glomerular lesion is that of membranous GN or mesioproliferative GN with IgG deposits. No form of effective therapy is known.

Glomerulopathy associated with pre-eclampsia

The glomerular lesion of pre-eclampsia is characterized by marked endothelial swelling and obliteration of capillary lumina. Fibrinogen–fibrin deposits may be found in the mesangium. The renal lesion may not be reversible as 30% of patients have changes for 6 months or longer. Patients who have had pre-eclampsia are more likely to develop hypertension in subsequent pregnancies. Severe proteinuria may occur during the course of pre-eclampsia and from time to time produce features of nephrotic syndrome. Ordinarily, proteinuria disappears after delivery.

In severe cases, associated with cortical necrosis, there may be microangiopathic haemolytic anaemia. Vascular endothelial growth factor (VEGF) and placental growth factor (PLGF) play a key role in the development of the placenta. Relative deficiency of either factor can theoretically cause implantation abnormalities normally seen in pre-eclampsia. A soluble fms-like tyrosine kinase (sFlt1) receptor, which is an antagonist of PLGF and specifically of VEGF, is upregulated in the placenta of patients with pre-eclampsia. Excessive free radical generation in the placenta of pre-eclamptic patients is due to upregulation of NADPH oxidase activity caused by generation of an angiotensin II receptor agonist antibody.

RENAL INVOLVEMENT IN OTHER DISEASES

Polyarteritis nodosa (PAN) (see also p. 583)

Classical PAN is a multisystem disorder. Aneurysmal dilatation of medium-sized arteries may be seen on renal arteriography. The condition is more common in men and in the elderly and, typically, the patient is ANCA-negative. Hypertension, polyneuropathy, and features indicating ischaemic infarction of various organs including the kidney are presenting features. It may be associated with drug abuse and hepatitis B infection. This form of polyangiitis is associated with slowly progressive renal failure, often accompanied by severe hypertension. Rapidly progressive renal failure is rare. Treatment with immunosuppression is less effective than it is for microscopic polyangiitis.

Haemolytic uraemic syndrome (HUS)

HUS is characterized by intravascular haemolysis with red cell fragmentation (microangiopathic haemolysis), thrombocytopenia and acute renal failure due to thrombosis in small arteries and arteriole (Fig. 11.24). These features are also seen in disseminated intravascular coagulation, but coagulation tests are typically normal in HUS. The syndrome often follows a febrile illness, particularly gastroenteritis (also known as diarrhoea-associated HUS – D+HUS) often associated with *Escherichia coli*, notably strain O157. This strain of *E. coli* produces verocytotoxin (shiga toxin), which has an A unit and five B units. The A unit is pathogenic by inhibiting protein synthesis and initiating endothelial damage. The role of B units is to facilitate the entry of the A unit into the endothelial cells by binding to a receptor (Gb3) on the endothelial cell. The toxins are transported to endothelial cells from the gut on neutrophils. Most patients with D+HUS recover renal function, but supportive care including maintenance of fluid and electrolyte balance, antihypertensive medication, nutritional support and dialysis is commonly required. Plasmapheresis is not beneficial but is usually tried as last resort. About 5% die during the acute episode, 5% develop chronic renal failure and 30% exhibit evidence of long-term damage with persistent proteinuria. Antibiotic and antimotility agents for the diarrhoea increase the risk of the HUS and its complications.

Recurrent episodes of HUS have been described in the same individual, and familial forms of the disease (with both recessive and dominant inheritance) exist. It is sug-

gested that the non-diarrhoeal-induced form of HUS (D–HUS) may be a complement-driven illness related to deficiency of complement factor H. Factor H is a soluble protein produced by the liver, which regulates the activity of the alternative complement activation pathway; in particular, it protects host cell surfaces from complement-mediated damage. In some families with D–HUS, a mutation has been traced to another complement regulatory protein known as membrane cofactor protein (MCP). This protein is highly expressed in the kidney and normally prevents glomerular C3 activation. A loss of function mutation in MCP may result in unopposed complement activation and development of HUS. Treatment is often very difficult because of severe hypertension and the possibility of frequent recurrences. The course of the disease is often indolent and progressive. *Post-renal transplant* recurrences are frequent. Plasmapheresis or plasma infusion, although unproven, is still recommended. Liver transplantation is potentially the only curative treatment.

Sporadic cases of D–HUS can be associated with pregnancy, SLE, scleroderma, malignant hypertension, metastatic cancer, HIV infection and various drugs including oral contraceptives, ciclosporin, tacrolimus, chemotherapeutic agents (e.g. cisplatin, mitomycin C, bleomycin) and heparin. Treatment is supportive with removal of the offending agent or specific treatment of the underlying cause. There is no evidence in favour of plasma infusion or plasmapheresis in these sporadic cases but it is tried, usually as last resort.

Pneumococcus-associated HUS: This rare complication of *Streptococcus pneumoniae* infection was previously associated with a high morbidity and mortality. This organism produces an enzyme (possibly neuroaminidase) which can expose an antigen (Thomsen antigen) present on RBCs, platelets and glomeruli. Antibodies to the Thomsen antigen result in an antigen–antibody reaction and can lead to HUS and anaemia. The improved outcome is due to increasing awareness of this complication, judicious use of blood products (washed blood products) and avoiding plasma infusion or plasmapheresis.

Thrombotic thrombocytopenic purpura (TTP) (p. 471)

TTP is characterized by microangiopathic haemolysis, renal failure and evidence of neurological disturbance. Young adults are most commonly affected.

Antiphospholipid syndrome (APS) (p. 577)

The central feature of APS is recurrent thrombosis (both venous and arterial) and fetal loss in the presence of antiphospholipid antibodies. Such antibodies may be primary or secondary to infections (HIV, hepatitis C) or autoimmune disease (SLE). There are many types of antibodies but one, which binds to β_2-glycoprotein, changes the endothelial cell profile to being procoagulant and proinflammatory: 50% have renal involvement with proteinuria. Thrombotic microangiopathy is a rare but

Fig. 11.24 **Typical haemolytic uraemic syndrome (HUS) renal lesion** – light microscopy. Arrow shows microthrombi.

well-recognized presentation. In some cases a lupus nephritis-like (usually membranous GN) lesion is seen. The only proven treatment for APS is warfarin with an INR of 3–4. Use of steroids or plasmapheresis is reserved for patients with APS and life-threatening renal involvement with thrombotic microangiopathy. Treatment is variably successful (30–70%).

Multiple myeloma

Acute renal failure is relatively common in myeloma, occurring in 20–30% of affected individuals at the time of diagnosis, and is mainly due to the nephrotoxic effects of the abnormal immunoglobulins. The following types of renal lesions are associated with myeloma.

1. Light chain cast nephropathy – intratubular deposition of light chains, particularly kappa chains facilitated by Tamm–Horsfall glycoprotein, which characteristically appear on renal histology as fractured casts with giant cell reaction (Fig. 11.25).
2. AL amyloidosis – deposition of amyloid fibrils of light chains (Congo red positive)
3. Light chain deposition disease – nodular glomerulo-sclerosis with granular deposits of usually lambda light chains (Congo red negative)
4. Plasma cell infiltration – often incidental finding at autopsy
5. Fanconi's syndrome – tubular toxicity due to light chains
6. Hypercalcaemic nephropathy – bone resorption causing hypercalcaemia
7. Hyperuricaemic nephropathy – tumour lysis causing tubular crystallization of uric acid.
8. Radiocontrast nephropathy – interaction between light chains and radiocontrast.

Acute renal failure due to cast nephropathy is usually irreversible. Treatment of underlying myeloma is indicated (p. 518).

Fig. 11.25 **Cast nephropathy in a patient with multiple myeloma**. Light microscopy picture showing characteristic fractured cast and giant cell reaction (arrows).

FURTHER READING

Cattran DC (guest editor) (1999) Management of glomerulonephritis. *Kidney International. Supplement* **70**: whole issue.

Cohen RA, Brown RS (2003) Microscopic haematuria. *New England Journal of Medicine* **348**: 2330–2338.

Davin JC, Ten Berge IK, Weening JJ (2001) What is the difference between IgA nephropathy and Henoch–Schonlein purpura nephritis? *Kidney International* **59**: 823–834.

Eddy AA, Symons JM (2003) Nephrotic syndrome in childhood. *Lancet* **362**: 629–639.

Flanc RS, Roberts MA, Stripoli GF et al. (2004) Treatment of diffuse proliferative lupus nephritis: A meta-analysis of randomized trials. *American Journal of Kidney Diseases* **43**: 197–208.

Hudson BG, Tryggvason K, Sundaramoorthy M, Neilson EG (2003) Alport's syndrome, Goodpasture's syndrome and type IV collagen. *New England Journal of Medicine* **348**: 2543–2556.

Luft FC (2003) Pieces of the preeclampsia puzzle. *Nephrology, Dialysis, Transplantation* **18**: 2209–2210.

Madaio SW (2003) Recent advances in the pathogenesis of lupus nephritis: autoantibodies and B cells. *Seminars in Nephrology* **23**: 564–568.

Pendergraft WF, Preston GA, Shah RR et al. (2004) Autoimmunity is triggered by cPR-3, a protein complementary to human auto-antigen proteinase-3. *Nature Medicine* **10**: 72–79.

Peniket AJ, Littlewood TJ, Winearls CG (2003) The radical treatment of paraprotein disorders affecting the kidney. *Nephrology, Dialysis, Transplantation* **18**: 431–434.

Tarr PL, Gordon CA, Chandler WL (2005) Shiga-toxin-producing E. coli and haemolytic uraemic syndrome. *Lancet* **365**: 1073–1086.

Tsai HM (2003) Advances in the pathogenesis, diagnosis and the treatment of thrombotic thrombocytopenic purpura. *Journal of the American Society of Nephrology* **14**: 1072–1081.

URINARY TRACT INFECTION

Urinary tract infection (UTI) is common in women, in whom it usually occurs in an anatomically normal urinary tract. Conversely, it is uncommon in men and children, and the urinary tract is often abnormal and requires investigation. The incidence of UTI is 50 000 per million persons per year and accounts for 1–2% of patients in primary care. Recurrent infection causes considerable morbidity; if complicated, it can cause severe renal disease including end-stage renal failure. It is also a common source of life-threatening Gram-negative septicaemia.

Aetiology and pathogenesis

Infection is most often due to bacteria from the patient's own bowel flora (Table 11.7). Transfer to the urinary tract may be via the bloodstream, the lymphatics or by direct extension (e.g. from a vesicolic fistula), but is most often via the ascending transurethral route (Fig. 11.26).

Symptomatic infection is related to the virulence of the organisms, which competes with the innate host defence system, However, inflammation and injury are determined by the host response and not by the bacterium.

Virulence.   Ability to adhere to epithelial cells determines the degree of virulence of the organism. For *E. coli*, these factors include flagellae (for motility), aerobactin (for iron acquisition in the iron-poor environment of the urinary tract), haemolysin (for pore forming) and above all, the presence of adhesins on the bacterial fimbriae and on the cell surface. There are two types of *E. coli*: those with *type 1 fimbriae* (with adhesin known as FimH) associated with cystitis; and those with *type P fimbriae* (with adhesin known as PapG) commonly responsible for pyelonephritis. Bacterial adhesins are necessary for attachment of bacteria to the mucous membranes of the perineum and urothelium. There are several molecular forms of adhesins. The most studied is the PapG adhesin, which is located on the tip of P fimbriae. This lectin (one of the P blood group antigens) structure recognizes binding sites consisting of oligosaccharide sequences present on the mucosal surface.

Innate host defence.   The following hosts defence mechanisms are necessary to prevent UTI:

Table 11.7 Organisms causing urinary tract infection in domiciliary practice

Organism	Approximate frequency (%)
Escherichia coli and other 'coliforms'	68+
Proteus mirabilis	12
*Klebsiella aerogenes**	4
*Enterococcus faecalis**	6
Staphylococcus saprophyticus or *epidermidis*[†]	10

* More common in hospital practice
[†] More common in young women (20–30%)

- *Neutrophils* – adhesins activate receptors, e.g. Toll 4, on the mucosal surface, resulting in IL-8 production and expression of its receptor CXCR1 on neutrophil surfaces. Activation of neutrophils is essential for bacterial killing. Defective IL-8 production or reduced expression of CXCR1 results in impaired function of neutrophils predisposing an individual to severe UTI.
- *Urine osmolality and pH* – urinary osmolality > 800 mOsm/kg and low or high pH reduce bacterial survival.
- *Complement* – complement activation with IgA production by uroepithelium (acquired immunity) also plays a major role in defence against UTI.
- *Commensal organisms* – such as lactobacilli, coryne-bacteria, streptococci and bacteroides are part of the normal host defence. Eradication of these commensal organisms by spermicidal jelly or disruption by certain antibiotics results in overgrowth of *E. coli*.
- *Urine flow* – urine flow and normal micturition wash out bacteria. Urine stasis promotes UTI.
- *Uroepithelium* – mannosylated proteins such as Tamm–Horsfall proteins (THP), which are present in the mucus and glycocalyx covering uroepithelium, have antibacterial properties. These proteins interfere with bacterial binding to uroepithelium. Disruption of this uroepithelium by trauma (e.g. sexual intercourse or catheterization) predisposes to UTI. Cranberry juice (blueberry juice) contains a large-molecular-weight factor (proanthrocyanidins) that prevents binding of *E. coli* to the uroepithelium (see p. 641).
- *Blood group antigens* – women who are non-secretors of ABH blood group antigens are three to four times more likely to have recurrent UTIs.

Natural history

UTI is commonly an isolated, rather than a repeated, event (Fig. 11.27).

Complicated versus uncomplicated infection
(Fig. 11.28)

It is necessary to distinguish between UTI occurring in patients with functionally normal urinary tracts and in those with abnormal tracts.

Functionally normal urinary tracts (with normal renal imaging).   Here, persistent or recurrent infection seldom results in serious kidney damage (uncomplicated UTI).

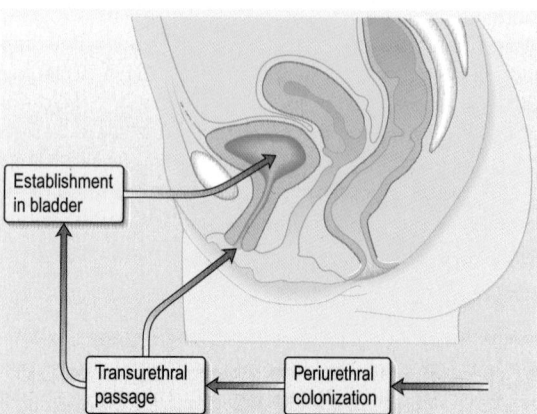

Fig. 11.26 Ascending infection of the urinary tract.

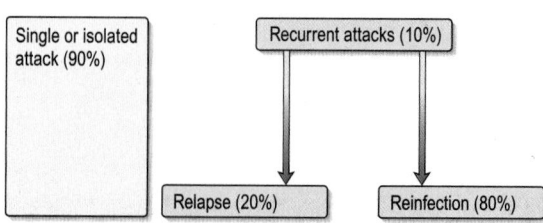

Fig. 11.27 The natural history of urinary tract infection.

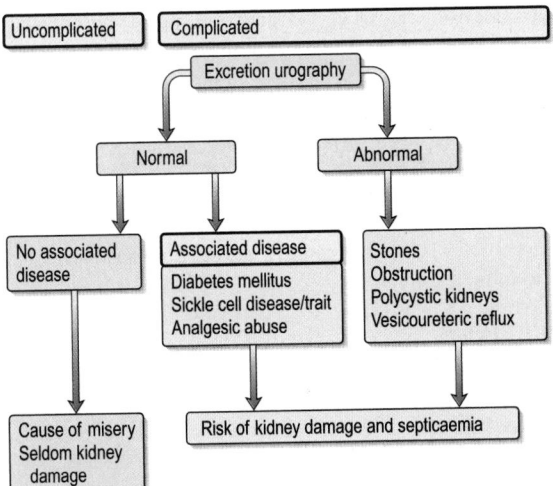

Fig. 11.28 **Complicated versus uncomplicated urinary tract infection.**

Fig. 11.29 **CT scan showing a wedge-shaped area of renal cortical loss (arrow) following acute pyelonephritis.**

Abnormal urinary tracts. Tracts with stones, or associated diseases such as diabetes mellitus which themselves cause kidney damage, may be made worse with infection (complicated UTI). UTI, particularly with *Proteus*, may predispose to stone formation. The combination of infection and obstruction results in severe, sometimes rapid, kidney damage (obstructive pyonephrosis) and is a major cause of Gram-negative septicaemia.

Acute pyelonephritis

The combination of fever, loin pain with tenderness and significant bacteriuria usually implies infection of the kidney (acute pyelonephritis). Small renal cortical abscesses and streaks of pus in the renal medulla are often present. Histologically there is focal infiltration by polymorphonuclear leucocytes and many polymorphs in tubular lumina.

Although, with antibiotics, significant permanent kidney damage in adults with normal urinary tracts is rare, CT scanning can show wedge-shaped areas of inflammation in the renal cortex (Fig. 11.29) and hence damage to renal function.

Reflux nephropathy

This was called chronic pyelonephritis or atrophic pyelonephritis, and it results from a combination of:

- vesicoureteric reflux, and
- infection acquired in infancy or early childhood.

Normally the vesicoureteric junction acts as a one-way valve (Fig. 11.30), urine entering the bladder from above; the ureter is shut off during bladder contraction, thus preventing reflux of urine. In some infants and children – possibly even in utero – this valve mechanism is incompetent, bladder voiding being associated with variable reflux of a jet of urine up the ureter. A secondary consequence is incomplete bladder emptying, as refluxed urine returns to the bladder after voiding. This latter

Fig. 11.30 **Findings in reflux nephropathy compared with normal.**

event predisposes to infection, and the reflux of infected urine leads to kidney damage.

Typically there is papillary damage, tubulointerstitial nephritis and cortical scarring in areas adjacent to 'clubbed calyces'.

Diagnosis is based on CT scan of the kidneys, which shows irregular renal outlines, clubbed calyces and a variable reduction in renal size. The condition may be unilateral or bilateral and affect all or part of the kidney.

Reflux usually ceases around puberty with growth of the bladder base. Damage already done persists and progressive renal fibrosis and further loss of function occur in severe cases even though there is no further infection.

Reflux nephropathy cannot occur in the absence of reflux and therefore does not begin in adult life. Consequently, adult females with bacteriuria and a normal urogram can be reassured that kidney damage will not develop.

Chronic reflux nephropathy acquired in infancy predisposes to hypertension in later life and, if severe, is a relatively common cause of end-stage renal failure in childhood or adult life. Meticulous early detection and control of infection, with or without ureteral reimplantation to create a competent valve, can prevent further scarring and allow normal growth of the kidneys. No proof exists, however, that reimplantation surgery confers long-term benefit.

Reinfection versus relapsing infection

When UTI is recurrent it is necessary to distinguish between relapse and reinfection.

Relapse is diagnosed by recurrence of bacteriuria with the same organism within 7 days of completion of antibacterial treatment and implies failure to eradicate infection (Fig. 11.31) usually in conditions such as stones, scarred kidneys, polycystic disease or bacterial prostatitis.

Reinfection is when bacteriuria is absent after treatment for at least 14 days, usually longer, followed by recurrence of infection with the same or different organisms. This is not due to failure to eradicate infection, but is the result of reinvasion of a susceptible tract with new organisms. Approximately 80% of recurrent infections are due to reinfection.

Symptoms and signs of UTI

The most typical symptoms of UTI are:

- frequency of micturition by day and night
- painful voiding (dysuria)
- suprapubic pain and tenderness
- haematuria
- smelly urine.

These symptoms relate to bladder and urethral inflammation, commonly called 'cystitis', and suggest lower urinary tract infection. Loin pain and tenderness, with fever and systemic upset, suggest extension of the infection to the pelvis and kidney, known as pyelitis or pyelonephritis. However, localization of the site of infection on the basis of symptoms alone is unreliable.

UTI may also be present with minimal or no symptoms or may be associated with atypical symptoms such as abdominal pain, fever or haematuria in the absence of frequency or dysuria.

In small children, who cannot complain of dysuria, symptoms are often 'atypical'. The possibility of UTI must always be considered in the fretful, febrile sick child who fails to thrive.

Diagnosis

This is based on quantitative culture of a clean-catch midstream specimen of urine and the presence or absence of pyuria. The criteria for the diagnosis of UTI, particularly in symptomatic women, are shown in Table 11.8. A diagnosis based on rigid adherence to a bacterial count of at least 10^5 organisms per millilitre of urine in symptomatic women is incorrect. Diagnosis of 'low count bacteriuria' ($\geq 10^2$ organisms) demands additionally the presence of pyuria.

Dipstick tests can be used to detect nitrites in urine. Most Gram-negative organisms reduce nitrates to nitrites and produce a red colour in the reagent square. False-negative results are common. Dipsticks that detect significant pyuria depend on the release of esterases from leucocytes. Dipstick tests positive for both nitrite and leucocyte esterase are highly predictive of acute infection (sensitivity of 75% and specificity of 82%).

Abacteriuric frequency or dysuria ('urethral syndrome')

Causes of truly abacteriuric frequency/dysuria include postcoital bladder trauma, vaginitis, atrophic vaginitis or urethritis in the elderly, and interstitial cystitis (Hunner's ulcer). In symptomatic young women with 'sterile pyuria', *Chlamydia* infection and tuberculosis must be excluded.

Interstitial cystitis is an uncommon but distressing complaint, most often affecting women over the age of 40 years. It presents with frequency, dysuria and often severe suprapubic pain. Urine cultures are sterile. Cysto-

Fig. 11.31 A comparison of reinfection, relapse and treatment failure in urinary tract infection.

Table 11.8   Criteria for diagnosis of bacteriuria
Symptomatic young women
$\geq 10^2$ coliform organisms/mL urine plus pyuria (> 10 WCC/mm^3)
OR
$\geq 10^5$ any pathogenic organism/mL urine
OR
any growth of pathogenic organisms in urine by suprapubic aspiration
Symptomatic men
$\geq 10^3$ pathogenic organisms/mL urine
Asymptomatic patients
$\geq 10^5$ pathogenic organisms/mL urine on two occasions

scopy shows typical inflammatory changes with ulceration of the bladder base. It is commonly thought to be an autoimmune disorder. Various treatments are advocated with variable success. These include oral prednisolone therapy, bladder instillation of sodium cromoglicate or dimethyl sulphoxide and bladder stretching under anaesthesia.

Predominant frequency and passage of small volumes of urine ('irritable bladder') is possibly consequent on previous UTI or conditioned by psychosexual factors. Such patients must be distinguished from those with frequency due to polyuria. Repeated courses of antibiotics in patients with genuine abacteriuric frequency or dysuria are quite inappropriate and detract from identifying the true nature of the problem.

Special investigations

Uncomplicated UTI usually does not require radiological evaluation unless it is recurrent or affecting males and children or there are unusually severe symptoms. Patients with predisposing conditions such as diabetes mellitus or immunocompromised states may also benefit from early imaging. If pyonephrosis is suspected, early imaging and possible drainage is warranted. Intravenous urography and ultrasound are used in the assessment of these patients, allowing the detection of calculi, obstruction, and incomplete emptying, but only in the adult. CT is a more sensitive modality for diagnosis and follow-up of complicated renal tract infection. Contrast-enhanced CT allows different phases of excretion to be studied and can define the extent of disease and identify significant complications or obstruction. Nuclear medicine has a limited role in the evaluation of UTI in adults. Its main role is in the assessment of renal function, often prior to surgery. MRI is particularly useful in those with iodinated contrast allergies, offering an ionizing radiation-free alternative in the diagnosis of both medical and surgical diseases of the kidney.

Treatment

Single isolated attack

Pretreatment urine culture is desirable but not mandatory. In primary care, a positive dipstick test for nitrite and leucocyte esterase is sufficient. Treatment is over 3–5 days with amoxicillin (250 mg three times daily), nitrofurantoin (50 mg three times daily), trimethoprim (200 mg twice daily) or an oral cephalosporin. The treatment regimen is modified in light of the result of urine culture and sensitivity testing, and/or the clinical response. For resistant organisms the alternative drugs are co-amoxiclav or ciprofloxacin.

A high (2 L daily) fluid intake should be encouraged during treatment and for some subsequent weeks. Urinalysis, microscopy and culture should be repeated 5 days after treatment. 'Single-shot' treatment with 3 g of amoxicillin or 1.92 g of co-trimoxazole can be used for patients with bladder symptoms of less than 36 hours' duration who have no previous history of UTI.

If the patient is acutely ill with high fever, loin pain and tenderness (acute pyelonephritis), a broad-spectrum antibiotic is given intravenously, such as aztreonam, cefuroxime, ciprofloxacin or gentamicin (2–5 mg/kg daily in divided doses) switching to a further 7 days' treatment with oral therapy as symptoms improve. Intravenous fluids may be required to achieve a good urine output.

In patients presenting for the first time with high fever, loin pain and tenderness, urgent renal ultrasound examination is required to exclude an obstructed pyonephrosis. If this is present it should be drained by percutaneous nephrostomy (p. 616).

Recurrent infection

Pretreatment and post-treatment urine cultures are mandatory to confirm the diagnosis and identify whether recurrent infection is due to relapse or reinfection.

In *relapse*, a search should be made for a cause (e.g. stones or scarred kidneys), and this should be eradicated if possible, for example by the removal of stones. Intense or prolonged treatment – intravenous or intramuscular aminoglycoside for 7 days or oral antibiotics for 4–6 weeks – is required. If this fails, long-term antibiotics are required.

Reinfection implies that the patient has a predisposition to periurethral colonization or poor bladder defence mechanisms. Contraceptive practice should be reviewed and the use of a diaphragm and spermicidal jelly discouraged. Atrophic vaginitis should be identified in postmenopausal women, who should be treated (see below). All patients must undertake prophylactic measures:

- a 2 L daily fluid intake
- voiding at 2- to 3-hour intervals with double micturition if reflux is present
- voiding before bedtime and after intercourse
- avoidance of spermicidal jellies and bubble baths and other chemicals in bathwater
- avoidance of constipation, which may impair bladder emptying.

Evidence of impaired bladder emptying on excretion urography/ultrasound requires urological assessment. If UTI continues to recur, treatment for 6–12 months with low-dose prophylaxis (trimethoprim 100 mg, co-trimoxazole 480 mg, cefalexin 125 mg at night, or macrocrystalline nitrofurantoin) is required; it should be taken last thing at night when urine flow is low. An alternative for infrequent attacks is immediate self-treatment with a conventional antibiotic for 3–5 days. When infection is clearly related to coitus, a single dose of macrocrystalline nitrofurantoin following intercourse may reduce the total drug usage for prophylaxis. Intravaginal oestrogen therapy has been shown to produce a reduction in the number of episodes of UTI in postmenopausal women. Cranberry juice is said to reduce the risk of symptoms and reinfection by 12–20% but studies are limited.

Urinary infections in the presence of an indwelling catheter

Colonization of the bladder by a urinary pathogen is common after a urinary catheter has been present for more than a few days, partly due to organisms forming biofilms. So long as the bladder catheter is in situ, antibiotic treatment is likely to be ineffective and will encourage the development of resistant organisms. Treatment with antibiotics is indicated only if the patient has symptoms or evidence of infection, and should be accompanied by replacement of the catheter. Prevention of infection with sterile insertion and closed drainage systems plays a major role. Catheters should not be used unnecessarily. Bladder stones may form in patients with long-term indwelling catheters, further complicating the situation.

Infection by *Candida* is a frequent complication of prolonged bladder catheterization. Treatment should be reserved for patients with evidence of invasive infection or those who are immunosuppressed, and should consist of removal or replacement of the catheter and in severe infections intravesical amphotericin.

Bacteriuria in pregnancy

The urine of pregnant women must always be cultured as 2–6% have asymptomatic bacteriuria. Whilst asymptomatic bacteriuria in the non-pregnant female seldom leads to acute pyelonephritis and often does not require treatment, acute pyelonephritis frequently occurs in pregnancy under these circumstances. Failure to treat may thus result in severe symptomatic pyelonephritis later in pregnancy, with the possibility of premature labour. Asymptomatic bacteriuria, in the presence of previous renal disease, may predispose to pre-eclamptic toxaemia, anaemia of pregnancy, and small or premature babies. Therefore bacteriuria must always be treated and be shown to be eradicated. Reinfection may require prophylactic therapy. Tetracycline, trimethoprim, sulphonamides and 4-quinolones must be avoided in pregnancy. Amoxicillin and ampicillin, nitrofurantoin and oral cephalosporins may safely be used in pregnancy.

Bacterial prostatitis

Bacterial prostatitis is a relapsing infection which is difficult to treat. It presents as perineal pain, recurrent epididymo-orchitis and prostatic tenderness, with pus in expressed prostatic secretion. Treatment is for 4–6 weeks with drugs that penetrate into the prostate, such as trimethoprim or ciprofloxacin. Long-term low-dose treatment may be required. Prostadynia (prostatic pain in the absence of active infection) may be a very persistent sequel to bacterial prostatitis. Amitriptyline and carbamazepine may alleviate the symptoms.

Renal carbuncle

Renal carbuncle is an abscess in the renal cortex caused by a blood-borne *Staphylococcus*, usually from a boil or carbuncle of the skin. It presents with a high swinging fever, loin pain and tenderness, and fullness in the loin. The urine shows no abnormality as the abscess does not communicate with the renal pelvis, more often extending into the perirenal tissue. Staphylococcal septicaemia is common. Diagnosis is by ultrasound or CT scanning. Treatment involves antibacterial therapy with flucloxacillin and surgical drainage.

Tuberculosis of the urinary tract

Tuberculous infection is on the increase world-wide, partly due to the reservoir of infection in susceptible HIV-infected individuals and by the emergence of drug-resistant strains. Tuberculosis of the urinary tract presents with frequency, dysuria or haematuria. In the UK it is mainly seen in the Asian immigrant population. Cortical lesions result from haematogenous spread in the primary phase of infection. Most heal, but in some, infection persists and spreads to the papillae, with the formation of cavitating lesions and the discharge of mycobacteria into the urine. Infection of the ureters and bladder commonly follows, with the potential for the development of ureteral stricture and a contracted bladder. Rarely, cold abscesses may form in the loin. In males the disease may present with testicular or epididymal discomfort and thickening.

Diagnosis depends on constant awareness, especially in patients with sterile pyuria. Excretion urography may show cavitating lesions in the renal papillary areas, commonly with calcification. There may also be evidence of ureteral obstruction with hydronephrosis. Diagnosis of active infection depends on culture of mycobacteria from early-morning urine samples. The urogram may be normal in diffuse interstitial renal tuberculosis when diagnosis is made by renal biopsy. Some patients present with small unobstructed kidneys, when the diagnosis is easy to miss.

Treatment. The treatment is as for pulmonary tuberculosis (see p. 932). Renal ultrasonography or excretion urography should be carried out 2–3 months after initiation of treatment as ureteric strictures may first develop in the healing phase.

Xanthogranulomatous pyelonephritis

This is an uncommon chronic interstitial infection of the kidney, most often due to *Proteus*, in which there is fever, weight loss, loin pain and a palpable enlarged kidney. It is usually unilateral and associated with staghorn calculi. CT scanning shows up intrarenal abscesses as lucent areas within the kidney. Nephrectomy is the treatment of choice; antibacterial treatment rarely, if ever, eradicates the infection.

Malakoplakia

This is a rare condition in which plaques of abnormal inflammatory tissue grow within the urinary tract in the presence of urinary infection. The histological appearances are characteristic. It is thought that the condition is caused by an acquired inability of macrophages to kill phagocytosed bacteria. Muscarinic agonists and ascorbic acid may improve macrophage function; ciprofloxacin penetrates the macrophage well and is the antibiotic of choice. Prolonged treatment is often needed.

FURTHER READING
Fihn SD (2003) Acute uncomplicated urinary tract infection in women. *New England Journal of Medicine* **349**: 259–266.
Urinary tract infection (symposium) (2001) *Journal of Infectious Diseases* **183** (Suppl. 1).

TUBULOINTERSTITIAL NEPHRITIS (TIN)

Diseases of the kidney primarily affect the glomeruli, vasculature, or the remainder of the renal parenchyma that consists of the tubules and interstitium. Although the tubules and the interstitium are distinct functional entities, they are intimately related. Injury involving one of them invariably results in damage to the other.

Acute tubulointerstitial nephritis (TIN)

In approximately 70% of the cases, acute TIN is due to a hypersensitivity reaction to drugs (Table 11.9), most commonly drugs of the penicillin family and non-steroidal anti-inflammatory drugs (NSAIDs). Fifteen per cent are infection related, 8% are idiopathic and 5% are cases of tubulointerstitial nephritis with uveitis (TINU) syndrome.

Drug induced acute TIN. Patients present with fever, arthralgia, skin rashes and acute oliguric or non-oliguric renal failure. Many have eosinophilia and eosinophiluria. Renal histology shows an intense interstitial cellular infil-

Table 11.9 Common causes of acute tubulointerstitial nephritis

Drugs (70%)
Penicillins	Rifampicin
Sulphonamides	Diuretics:
Non-steroidal anti-	furosemide
inflammatory drugs	thiazides
Phenindione	Cimetidine
Allopurinol	Phenytoin
Cephalosporins	

Infection (15%)
Viruses, e.g. hantavirus
Bacteria, e.g. streptococci

Idiopathic (8%)

Tubulointerstitial nephritis with uveitis (TINU) (5%)

Systemic inflammatory disorders, e.g. systemic lupus erythematosus (SLE)

trate, often including eosinophils, with variable tubular necrosis. Rarely, NSAIDs can cause a glomerular minimal-change lesion in addition to TIN and present as the nephrotic syndrome. *Treatment* involves withdrawal of offending drugs. High-dose steroid therapy (prednisolone 60 mg daily) is commonly given but its efficacy has not been proven. Patients may require dialysis for management of the acute renal failure. Most patients make a good recovery in kidney function, but some may be left with significant interstitial fibrosis and a persistent high serum creatinine.

Infection causing acute TIN. Acute pyelonephritis leads to inflammation of the tubules, producing a neutrophilic cellular infiltrate. TIN can complicate systemic infections with viruses (hantavirus, Epstein–Barr virus, HIV, measles, adenovirus), bacteria (*Legionella, Leptospira*, streptococci, *Mycoplasma, Brucella, Chlamydia*) and others (*Leishmania, Toxoplasma*). Hantavirus causes haemorrhagic fever with TIN and can be fatal. Epstein–Barr virus DNA has been found in renal biopsy tissue of cases of idiopathic TIN; if confirmed, this could potentially become a relatively common cause of acute TIN. In immunocompromised patients such as post-renal transplantation, CMV, polyoma, and herpes simplex virus can cause acute TIN in the renal graft. *Treatment* involves eradication of infection by appropriate antibiotics or antiviral agents.

Acute TIN as part of multisystem inflammatory diseases. Several non-infectious inflammatory disorders such as Sjögren's syndrome, SLE and Wegener's granulomatosis can cause acute or chronic TIN rather than glomerulonephritis. Sjögren's syndrome may additionally present as renal tubular acidosis. Sarcoidosis presents as granulomatous TIN in up to 20% of patients. Associated hypercalcaemia causes acute renal failure. These heterogeneous conditions with TIN generally respond to steroids.

TINU syndrome. In this syndrome, uveitis generally coincides with acute TIN. It is common in childhood, but has been reported in adulthood. Among adults it is more common in females, but its cause remains unknown. Patients present with weight loss, anaemia and raised ESR. A prolonged course of steroids leads to improvement in both renal function and uveitis.

Chronic tubulointerstitial nephritis

The major causes of chronic tubulointerstitial nephritis are given in Table 11.10. In many cases no cause is found. Chronic TIN changes evolve in progressive primary glomerular or vascular disease of the kidney, where its severity is a better predictor of long-term renal survival than the primary site of insult.

The patient usually either presents with polyuria and nocturia, or is found to have proteinuria or uraemia. Proteinuria is usually slight (less than 1 g daily). Papillary necrosis with ischaemic damage to the papillae occurs in

Table 11.10 Causes of chronic tubulointerstitial nephritis

Common	Uncommon
Reflux nephropathy	Alport's syndrome
Non-steroidal anti-inflammatory drugs	Balkan nephropathy and herbal nephropathy
Diabetes mellitus	Irradiation
Sickle cell disease or trait	Sjögren's syndrome
Cadmium or lead intoxication	Hyperuricaemic nephropathy

a number of tubulointerstitial nephritides, for example in analgesic abuse, diabetes mellitus, sickle cell disease or trait. The papillae can separate and be passed in the urine. Microscopic or overt haematuria or sterile pyuria also occurs, and occasionally a sloughed papilla may cause ureteric colic or produce acute ureteric obstruction. The radiological appearances must be distinguished from those of reflux nephropathy (Fig. 11.32).

Tubular damage to the medullary area of the kidney leads to defects in urine concentration and sodium conservation with polyuria and salt wasting. Fibrosis progressing into the cortex leads to loss of excretory function and uraemia.

Analgesic nephropathy

The chronic consumption of large amounts of analgesics (especially those containing phenacetin) and NSAIDs leads to chronic tubulointerstitial nephritis and papillary necrosis. Analgesic nephropathy is twice as common in women as in men and presents typically in middle-age. Patients are often depressed or neurotic. Presentation may be with anaemia, chronic renal failure, UTIs, haematuria, or urinary tract obstruction (owing to sloughing of a renal papilla). Salt and water-wasting renal disease may occur. Chronic analgesic abuse also predisposes to the development of uroepithelial tumours.

The consumption of the above analgesics should be discouraged. If necessary, dihydrocodeine or paracetamol is a reasonable alternative. This may result in the arrest of the disease and even in improvement in function. UTI, hypertension (if present) and saline depletion will require appropriate management. The development of flank pain or an unexpectedly rapid deterioration in renal function should prompt ultrasonography to screen for urinary tract obstruction due to a sloughed papilla.

Balkan nephropathy

This is a chronic TIN endemic in areas along the tributaries of the River Danube. Inhabitants of the low-lying plains, which are subjected to frequent flooding and where the water supply comes from shallow wells, are affected, whereas the disease does not occur in hillside villages where surface water provides the water supply. Its cause is unknown. The disease is insidious in onset, with mild proteinuria progressing to renal failure in 3 months to 10 years. Patients exhibit a high incidence of uroepithelial tumours. There is no treatment.

Chinese herb nephropathy

Chinese herbal medicines have been increasingly used in the West, e.g. for slimming, and have caused a nephropathy. The renal histology is similar to Balkan nephropathy but the clinical course is very aggressive. The causal agent has been identified as aristolochic acid produced as a result of fungal contamination of the herbal medicine. It is characterized by relentless progression to end-stage renal failure. There is a high incidence of uroepithelial tumours.

Other forms of chronic tubulointerstitial nephritis

These are rare (see Table 11.10). Diagnosis of all forms depends on a history of drug ingestion or industrial exposure to nephrotoxins. In patients with unexplained renal impairment with normal-sized kidneys, renal biopsy must always be undertaken to exclude a treatable tubulointerstitial nephritis such as granulomatous TIN due to renal sarcoidosis, which may be the first presentation of sarcoidosis (see p. 935). Renal sarcoidosis generally responds rapidly to steroids.

Hyperuricaemic nephropathy (see p. 570)

Acute hyperuricaemic nephropathy is a well-recognized cause of acute renal failure in patients with marked hyperuricaemia that is usually due to lympho-proliferative or myeloproliferative disorders. It may

Papillary necrosis

Always bilateral

Spurs

Hooks

Ring sign (sloughed papilla)

No loss of cortex

Clubbed calyces (sloughed papilla)

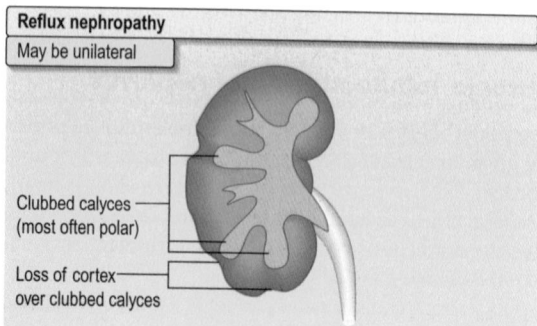

Reflux nephropathy

May be unilateral

Clubbed calyces (most often polar)

Loss of cortex over clubbed calyces

Fig. 11.32 A comparison of radiological appearances of papillary necrosis and reflux nephropathy.

occur prior to treatment but most often follows commencement of treatment, when there is rapid lysis of malignant cells, release of large amounts of nucleoprotein and increased uric acid production. Renal failure is due to intrarenal and extrarenal obstruction caused by deposition of uric acid crystals in the collecting ducts, pelvis and ureters. The condition is manifest as oliguria or anuria with increasing uraemia. There may be flank pain or colic. Plasma urate levels are above 0.75 mmol/L and may be as high as 4.5 mmol/L. Diagnosis is based on the hyperuricaemia and the clinical setting. Ultrasound may demonstrate extrarenal obstruction due to stones, but a negative scan does not exclude this where there is coexistent intrarenal obstruction.

Allopurinol 100–200 mg three times daily for 5 days is given prior to and throughout treatment with radiotherapy or cytotoxic drugs. A high rate of urine flow must be maintained by oral or parenteral fluid and the urine kept alkaline by the administration of sodium bicarbonate 600 mg four times daily and acetazolamide 250 mg three times daily, since uric acid is more soluble in an alkaline than in an acid medium. Rasburicase (p. 492) is occasionally used. In severely oliguric or anuric patients, dialysis is required to lower the plasma urate.

There is no convincing evidence for *chronic hyperuricaemia nephropathy*.

FURTHER READING

Baker RJ, Pusey CD (2004) The changing profile of acute tubulointerstitial nephritis. *Nephrology, Dialysis, Transplantation* 19: 8–11.
Gobel U, Kettritz R, Schneider W et al. (2001) The protean face of renal sarcoidosis. *Journal of the American Society of Nephrology* **12**: 616–623.

HYPERTENSION AND THE KIDNEY

Hypertension can be the cause or the result of renal disease. It is often difficult to differentiate between the two on clinical grounds. Routine tests as described on page 860 should be performed on all hypertensive patients, but renal imaging is usually unnecessary. A guide to how patients should be fully investigated is given on page 1095.

The mechanisms responsible for the normal regulation of arterial blood pressure and the development of essential primary hypertension are unclear (p. 858). One basic concept is that the long-term regulation of arterial pressure is closely linked to the ability of the kidneys to excrete sufficient salt to maintain normal sodium balance, extracellular fluid volume, and normal blood volume at normotensive arterial pressures. Several studies point to the kidney as involved in the genesis of essential primary hypertension. Cross-transplantation experiments suggest that hypertension travels with the kidney, in that hypertension will develop in a normotensive recipient of a kidney genetically programmed for hypertension. Likewise patients with end-stage renal failure due to hypertension become normotensive after receiving a renal allograft from normotensive donors, provided the new kidney works.

One of many renal factors involved in the genesis of hypertension is the total number of nephrons in the kidney. There is now circumstantial as well direct evidence to suggest that patients with hypertension and normal renal function have a significantly reduced number of nephrons in each kidney alongside enlargement of the remaining glomeruli due to glomerular hyperfiltration. Moreover, certain races (blacks, Hispanics) with predilection for hypertension have increased glomerular volume, a surrogate marker for a reduced number of nephrons.

Whether the reduced number of nephrons is caused by genetic or environmental factors is unclear. Changes in the intrauterine environment may lead to retarded renal growth before birth, low birthweight and hypertension during adult life. In humans, an association has been found between low birthweight and reduced renal volume, possibly indicating reduced numbers of nephrons.

ESSENTIAL HYPERTENSION

Pathophysiology

In benign essential hypertension, arteriosclerosis of major renal arteries and changes in the intrarenal vasculature (nephrosclerosis) occur as follows:

- In small vessels and arterioles, intimal thickening with reduplication of the internal elastic lamina occurs and the vessel wall becomes hyalinized.
- In large vessels, concentric reduplication of the internal elastic lamina and endothelial proliferation produce an 'onion skin' appearance.
- Reduction in size of both kidneys may occur; this may be asymmetrical if one major renal artery is more affected than the other.
- The proportion of sclerotic glomeruli is increased compared with age-matched controls.

Deterioration in excretory function accompanies these changes, but severe renal failure is unusual in whites (1 in 10 000). In black Africans, by contrast, hypertension much more often results in the development of renal failure with a fourfold higher incidence of end-stage renal failure in blacks compared to whites. This racial difference in incidence of hypertensive renal disease may be due to overestimation of diagnosis on clinical grounds, poor compliance with medication, higher incidence of hypertension, which is usually a salt-sensitive type, and reduced number of nephrons.

In accelerated, or malignant-phase hypertension:

- Arteriolar fibrinoid necrosis occurs, probably as a result of plasma entering the media of the vessel through splits in the intima. It is prominent in afferent glomerular arterioles.
- Fibrin deposition within small vessels is often associated with thrombocytopenia and red-cell fragmentation

seen in the peripheral blood film (microangiopathic haemolytic anaemia).

Microscopic haematuria, proteinuria, usually of modest degree (1–3 g daily), and progressive uraemia occur. If untreated, fewer than 10% of patients survive 2 years.

Management

The management of benign essential and malignant hypertension is described on page 861.

If treatment is begun before renal impairment has occurred, the prognosis for renal function is good. Stabilization or improvement in renal function with healing of intrarenal arteriolar lesions and resolution of microangiopathic haemolysis occur with effective treatment of malignant-phase hypertension. Lifelong follow-up of the patient is mandatory. In blacks with hypertensive nephrosclerosis and renal impairment, a blood pressure target of < 140/85 mmHg should be achieved. ACE inhibitors appear to be more effective than beta-blockers, and, if possible, calcium-channel blockers of the dihydropyridine group (e.g. amlodipine) should be avoided.

RENAL HYPERTENSION

Hypertension commonly complicates bilateral renal disease such as chronic glomerulonephritis, bilateral reflux nephropathy (chronic atrophic pyelonephritis of childhood), polycystic disease and analgesic nephropathy. Two main mechanisms are responsible:

- activation of the renin–angiotensin–aldosterone system
- retention of salt and water owing to impairment in excretory function, leading to an increase in blood volume and hence blood pressure.

The second of these assumes greater significance as renal function deteriorates.

Hypertension occurs earlier, is more common and tends to be more severe in patients with renal cortical disorders, such as glomerulonephritis, than in those with disorders affecting primarily the renal interstitium, such as reflux or analgesic nephropathy.

Management is described on page 861. Meticulous control of the blood pressure is necessary to prevent further deterioration of renal function secondary to vascular changes produced by the hypertension itself. There is good evidence that ACE-inhibitor drug treatment confers an additional renoprotective effect for a given degree of blood pressure control than other hypotensive drugs.

Renovascular disease

Narrowing of the renal arteries (renal artery stenosis) usually is caused by one of two pathological entities: fibromuscular disease or atherosclerotic renovascular disease (ARVD). The epidemiology and the natural history of these two conditions differ and they are considered separately.

Mechanism of hypertension

Renal ischaemia results in a reduction in the pressure in afferent glomerular arterioles. This leads to an increase in the production and release of renin from the juxtaglomerular apparatus (see p. 606) with a consequent increase in angiotensin II, a very potent vasoconstrictor. Angiotensin II also causes hypertension by upregulating NADPH oxidase enzyme with excessive superoxide generation. Superoxide chelates nitric oxide (a potent vasodilator) resulting in reduced vasodilator activity and also hypertension.

Physiological changes in renal artery stenosis

In renal artery stenosis, renal perfusion pressure is reduced and nephron transit time is prolonged on the side of the stenosis; salt and water reabsorption is therefore increased. As a result, urine from the ischaemic kidney is more concentrated and has a lower sodium concentration than urine from the contralateral kidney. Inulin, creatinine and *p*-aminohippuric acid (PAH) clearances are decreased on the ischaemic side.

Fibromuscular disease of the renal arteries

Fibromuscular disease accounts for 20–40% of renal vascular disease and encompasses four distinct types: (1) medial fibroplasia (65–85%); (2) perimedial fibroplasia (10–15%); (3) intimal fibroplasia (5–10%); and (4) medial hyperplasia (5%). Medial fibroplasia usually follows a benign course and never follows a progressive course after the age of 40 years. The other two types of fibroplasia follow a progressive course and may lead to total occlusion. Medial hyperplasia is a distinct but rare entity, which accounts for only 1% of renovascular disease. It commonly affects young females, who exhibit elevated blood pressures but with well-preserved renal function. Angiography reveals a characteristic string of beads appearance. Angioplasty (occasionally stent insertion) is usually successful in improving or even curing hypertension in affected individuals, and overall prognosis is very good.

Atherosclerotic renovascular disease (ARVD)

This is a common cause of hypertension and chronic renal failure due ischaemic nephropathy. Its incidence increases with age, rising from 5% under 60 years to 16% in those over 60 years old. In most patients the atherosclerotic lesion is ostial (within 1 cm of the origin of the renal artery) and usually associated with symptomatic atherosclerotic vascular disease elsewhere. Patients with peripheral vascular disease (39%), coronary artery disease (10–29%), congestive cardiac failure (34%) and aortic aneurysm (38%) are at high risk of developing significant renal artery stenosis.

Many patients are asymptomatic and are discovered incidentally during investigation for other conditions. Aortography experience from the USA shows 11% of asymptomatic patients have significant unilateral stenosis and 4% have bilateral disease. The renal consequences of ARVD are functional, such as hypertension (present in 50%), sodium retention (ankle and flash pulmonary oedema), proteinuria (usually sub-nephrotic range) and decreased GFR. The morphological features of the affected kidneys include vascular sclerosis, tubular atrophy, interstitial fibrosis with inflammatory cellular infiltrate, atubular glomeruli, cholesterol emboli, and secondary FSGS changes. Baseline renal function is related to the extent of renal parenchymal injury rather than to the degree of stenosis, as is the response (improvement in hypertension and renal function) to revascularization.

Renovascular disease is easy to miss and should be considered in patients with hypertension and/or chronic renal failure. Other clues to the diagnosis include: abdominal audible bruits, as well as over carotid arteries suggestive of generalized arterial disease; ultrasonography showing > 1.5 cm renal asymmetry; recurrent flash pulmonary oedema without cardiopulmonary disease; progressive chronic renal failure in patients with evidence of generalized atherosclerosis.

Screening for renovascular disease

Radionuclide studies (see p. 617). These can demonstrate decreased renal perfusion on the affected side. In unilateral renal artery stenosis, a disproportionate fall in uptake of isotope on the affected side following administration of captopril or aspirin is suggestive of the presence of significant renal artery stenosis. A completely normal result renders the diagnosis unlikely.

Doppler ultrasound. This method is very sensitive but highly operator-dependent and time-consuming. It generates data about intrarenal vascular resistance, which can be valuable in predicting the success of revascularization procedures. A resistive index of ≥ 80 is a predictor of poor response following intervention.

Magnetic resonance angiography. MRA can be used to visualize the renal arteries and there is a good – though not perfect – correlation between MRA findings and those of renal arteriography.

Helical ('spiral') CT scanning. This permits noninvasive imaging of the renal arteries. It is much less expensive than MRI but does expose the patient to ionizing radiation and to contrast injection and is less reliable than MRI.

Renal arteriography (see p. 617) remains the 'gold standard' investigation in the diagnosis of renal arterial disease.

Treatment

The aim of treatment is to correct hypertension and improve renal perfusion and excretory function. Renal artery stenosis can progress to occlusion, particularly in patients with stenosis > 75% as shown by serial angiography, necessitating revascularization in ARVD. The options in renal artery stenosis include transluminal angioplasty to dilate the stenotic region, insertion of stents across the stenosis (sometimes the only endoscopic option when the stenosis occurs close to the origin of the renal artery from the aorta, rendering angioplasty technically difficult or impossible), reconstructive vascular surgery and nephrectomy. Revascularization is indicated in vessels with stenosis > 75% and recurrent flash pulmonary oedema, drug resistant severe hypertension, ARVD affecting solitary functioning kidney, patients with cardiac failure needing ACE inhibitors, unexplained progressive renal failure and dialysis-dependent renal failure. With good selection of patients, hypertension is cured or improved by intervention in more than 50%. Occasional dramatic improvements in renal function ensue but results are generally disappointing. All patients with ARVD should be treated with a combination of aspirin, statins and optimal control of blood pressure as prophylaxis against progression of atherosclerosis.

Mortality is high because of other associated co-morbidities, and ARVD patients have generalized endothelial dysfunction. ARVD patients with end-stage renal failure have higher rates than those with good renal function. Five-year survival is only 18% in patients with end-stage renal failure due to ARVD.

Systemic sclerosis (see also p. 577)

Interlobular renal arteries are affected with intimal thickening, and fibrinoid changes occur in afferent glomerular arterioles similar to renal changes in malignant hypertension. Glomerular changes are non-specific. The pathogenesis is unknown and neither steroid nor immunosuppressive therapy is of value. Serum ANCA is not present. Treatment with ACE-inhibitor drugs is of immense benefit, reducing proteinuria and often halting or even partially reversing decline in renal function. 'Scleroderma renal crisis' is a term applied to rapid loss of renal function owing to rapid progression of renal microvascular disease in this condition. Early ACE inhibitor treatment may be of benefit, as may continuous intravenous infusion of prostacyclin.

FURTHER READING

Higashi Y, Sasaki S, Nakagama K et al. (2002) Endothelial function and oxidative stress in renovascular hypertension. *New England Journal of Medicine* **346**: 1954–1962.

Keller G, Zimmer G, Mall G et al. (2003) Nephron number in patients with primary hypertension. *New England Journal of Medicine* **348**: 101–108.

Radermacher J, Chavan A, Bleck J et al. (2001) Use of Doppler ultrasonography to predict the outcome of therapy for renal-artery stenosis. *New England Journal of Medicine* **344**: 410–417.

Safian RD, Textor SC (2001) Medical progress: renal artery stenosis. *New England Journal of Medicine* **343**: 431–442.

OTHER VASCULAR DISORDERS OF THE KIDNEY

Renal artery occlusion

This occurs from thrombosis in situ usually in a severely damaged atherosclerotic vessel or more commonly from embolization. Both lead to renal infarction, resulting in a wide spectrum of clinical manifestations depending on the size of the artery involved. Occlusion of a small branch artery may produce no effect, but occlusion of larger vessels results in dull flank pain and varying degrees of renal failure.

Embolization may occur from the heart (e.g. in atrial fibrillation). Intra-arterial thrombolytic therapy has been tried with mixed results.

Cholesterol embolization

Showers of cholesterol-rich atheromatous material from ulcerated plaques may reach the kidney from the aorta and/or renal arteries, particularly after catheterization of the abdominal aorta or attempts at renal artery angioplasty. Anticoagulants and thrombolytic agents may also precipitate cholesterol embolization. Renal failure from cholesterol emboli may be acute or slowly progressive. Clinical features include fever, eosinophilia, back and abdominal pain, and evidence of embolization elsewhere, for example to the retina or digits. The diagnosis can be confirmed by renal biopsy. No treatment is of proven benefit.

Renal vein thrombosis

This is usually of insidious onset, occurring in the nephrotic syndrome, with a renal cell carcinoma, and in conditions associated with an increased risk of venous thrombosis (e.g. antithrombin deficiency or the presence of anticardiolipin antibodies). Anticoagulation is indicated.

CALCULI AND NEPHROCALCINOSIS

Renal and vesical calculi

In the UK, approximately 2% of people have a urinary tract stone at any given time. Prevalence of stone disease is much higher in the Middle East. Most stones occur in the upper urinary tract; the incidence of bladder stones has declined in the UK, but in some developing countries they are still common.

Most stones are composed of calcium oxalate and phosphate; these are more common in men (Table 11.11). Mixed infective stones, which account for about 15% of all calculi, are twice as common in women as in men. The overall male to female ratio of stone disease is 2 : 1.

Stone disease is frequently a recurrent problem. More than 50% of patients with a history of nephrolithiasis will

Table 11.11 Type and frequency of renal stones in the UK

Type of renal stone	Approximate frequency (%)
Calcium oxalate usually with calcium phosphate	65
Calcium phosphate alone	15
Magnesium ammonium phosphate (struvite)	10–15
Uric acid	3–5
Cystine	1–2

develop a recurrence within 10 years. The risk of recurrence increases if a metabolic or other abnormality predisposing to stone formation is present and is not modified by treatment.

Aetiology

Inhibitors of crystal formation are present in normal urine preventing the formation of stones, as the concentrations of stone-forming substances exceed their maximum solubility in water. Many stone-formers have no detectable metabolic defect, although microscopy of warm, freshly passed urine reveals both more and larger calcium oxalate crystals than are found in normal subjects. Factors predisposing to stone formation in these so-called 'idiopathic stone-formers' are:

- chemical composition of urine that favours stone crystallization
- production of a concentrated urine as a consequence of dehydration associated with life in a hot climate or work in a hot environment
- impairment of inhibitors that prevent crystallization in normal urine. Postulated inhibitors include inorganic magnesium, pyrophosphate and citrate. Organic inhibitors include glycosaminoglycans and nephrocalcin (an acidic protein of tubular origin). Tamm–Horsfall protein may have a dual role in both inhibiting and promoting stone formation.

Recognized causes of stone formation are listed in Table 11.12.

Hypercalcaemia

If the GFR is normal, hypercalcaemia almost invariably leads to hypercalciuria. The common causes of hypercalcaemia leading to stone formation are:

- primary hyperparathyroidism
- vitamin D ingestion
- sarcoidosis.

Table 11.12 Causes of urinary tract stone formation

Dehydration	Infection
Hypercalcaemia	Cystinuria
Hypercalciuria	Renal tubular acidosis
Hyperoxaluria	Primary renal disease
Hyperuricaemia and hyperuricosurea	(polycystic kidneys, medullary sponge kidneys)
	Drugs

Of these, primary hyperparathyroidism (see p. 901) is the most common cause of stones.

Hypercalciuria

This is by far the most common metabolic abnormality detected in calcium stone-formers.

Approximately 8% of men excrete in excess of 7.5 mmol of calcium in 24 hours. Calcium stone formation is more common in this group, but as the majority of even these individuals do not form stones the definition of 'pathological' hypercalciuria is arbitrary. A reasonable definition is 24-hour calcium excretion of more than 7.5 mmol in male stone-formers and more than 6.25 mmol in female stone-formers.

The kidney is the major site for plasma calcium regulation. Approximately 90% of the ionized calcium filtered by the kidney is reabsorbed. Renal tubular reabsorption is controlled largely by parathyroid hormone (PTH).

Approximately 65% of the filtered calcium is absorbed in the proximal convoluted tubule, 20% by the thick ascending limb of the loop of Henle, and 15% by the distal convoluted tubule and collecting ducts.

Causes of hypercalciuria are:

- hypercalcaemia
- an excessive dietary intake of calcium
- excessive resorption of calcium from the skeleton, such as occurs with prolonged immobilization or weightlessness
- idiopathic hypercalciuria.

Idiopathic hypercalciuria is a common risk factor for the formation of stones, and uncontrolled hypercalciuria is a cause of recurrences. The majority of patients with idiopathic hypercalciuria have increased absorption of calcium from the gut. Moreover, studies have shown that animal protein and salt also have a considerable influence on calcium excretion.

Hyperoxaluria

There are two inborn errors of glyoxalate metabolism that cause increased endogenous oxalate biosynthesis, and are inherited in an autosomal recessive manner. In both types, calcium oxalate stone formation occurs.

The prognosis is poor owing to widespread calcium oxalate crystal deposition in the kidneys. Renal failure typically develops in the late teens or early twenties. Successful liver transplantation has been shown to cure the metabolic defect.

Much more common causes of mild hyperoxaluria are:

- excess ingestion of foodstuffs high in oxalate, such as spinach, rhubarb and tea
- dietary calcium restriction, with compensatory increased absorption of oxalate
- gastrointestinal disease (e.g. Crohn's), usually with an intestinal resection, associated with increased absorption of oxalate from the colon.
- Dehydration secondary to fluid loss from the gut also plays a part in stone formation.

Hyperuricaemia and hyperuricosuria

Uric acid stones account for 3–5% of all stones in the UK, but in Israel the proportion is as high as 40%. Uric acid is the end-point of purine metabolism. Hyperuricaemia (see p. 569) can occur as a primary defect in idiopathic gout, and as a secondary consequence of increased cell turnover, for example in myeloproliferative disorders. Increased uric acid excretion occurs in these conditions, and stones will develop in some patients. Some uric acid stone-formers have hyperuricosuria (> 4 mmol per 24 hours on a low-purine diet) without hyperuricaemia.

Dehydration alone may also cause uric acid stones to form. Patients with ileostomies are at particular risk both from dehydration and from the fact that loss of bicarbonate from gastrointestinal secretions results in the production of an acid urine (uric acid is more soluble in an alkaline than in an acid medium).

Some patients with calcium stones also have hyperuricaemia and/or hyperuricosuria; it is believed the calcium salts precipitate upon an initial nidus of uric acid in such patients.

Urinary tract infection

Mixed infective stones are composed of magnesium ammonium phosphate together with variable amounts of calcium. Such struvite stones are often large, forming a cast of the collecting system (staghorn calculus). These stones are usually due to UTI with organisms such as *Proteus mirabilis* that hydrolyse urea, with formation of the strong base ammonium hydroxide. The availability of ammonium ions and the alkalinity of the urine favour stone formation. An increased production of mucoprotein from infection also creates an organic matrix on which stone formation can occur.

Cystinuria (see also p. 1146)

Cystinuria results in the formation of cystine stones. About 1–2% of all stones are composed of cystine.

Primary renal diseases

There is a high prevalence of stone disease in patients with polycystic renal disease (see p. 681).

Medullary sponge kidney is also associated with stones. There is dilatation of the collecting ducts with associated stasis and calcification (Fig. 11.33). Approximately 20% of these patients have hypercalciuria and a similar proportion have a renal tubular acidification defect.

Renal tubular acidoses, both inherited and acquired, are associated with nephrocalcinosis and stone formation, owing, in part, to the production of a persistently alkaline urine and reduced urinary citrate excretion.

Drugs

Some drugs promote calcium stone formation (e.g. loop diuretics, antacids, glucocorticoids, theophylline, vitamins D and C, acetazolamide); some promote uric acid stones (e.g. thiazides, salicylates,); and some precipitate into stones (e.g. indinavir, triamterene).

(a)

(b)

Fig. 11.33 **Medullary sponge kidney. (a)** Plain film showing 'spotty' calcification in the renal areas (arrow). **(b)** After injection of contrast, the calcification is shown to be small calculi in the papillary zones.

Aetiology of bladder stones

Bladder stones are endemic in some developing countries. The cause of this is unknown but dietary factors probably play a role. Bladder stones may be the result of:

- bladder outflow obstruction (e.g. urethral stricture, neuropathic bladder, prostatic obstruction)
- the presence of a foreign body (e.g. catheters, non-absorbable sutures).

Significant bacteriuria is usually found in patients with bladder stones. Some stones found in the bladder have been passed down from the upper urinary tract.

Pathology

Stones may be single or multiple and vary enormously in size from minute, sand-like particles to staghorn calculi or large stone concretions in the bladder. They may be located within the renal parenchyma or within the collecting system. Pressure necrosis from a large calculus may cause direct damage to the renal parenchyma, and stones regularly cause obstruction, leading to hydronephrosis. They may ulcerate through the wall of the collecting system, including the ureter. A combination of obstruction and infection accelerates damage to the kidney.

Clinical features

Most people with urinary tract calculi are asymptomatic. Pain is the most common symptom and may be sharp or dull, constant, intermittent or colicky (Table 11.13).

When urinary tract obstruction is present, measures that increase urine volume, such as copious fluid intake or diuretics, including alcohol, make the pain worse.

Table 11.13 Clinical features of urinary tract stones
Asymptomatic
Pain: renal colic
Haematuria
Urinary tract infection
Urinary tract obstruction

Physical exertion may cause mobile calculi to move, precipitating pain and, occasionally, haematuria. Ureteric colic occurs when a stone enters the ureter and either obstructs it or causes spasm during its passage down the ureter. This is one of the most severe pains known. Radiation from the flank to the iliac fossa and testis or labium in the distribution of the first lumbar nerve root is common. Pallor, sweating and vomiting often occur and the patient is restless, tending to assume a variety of positions in an unsuccessful attempt to obtain relief from the pain. Haematuria often occurs. Untreated, the pain of ureteric colic typically subsides after a few hours.

When urinary tract obstruction and infection are present, the features of acute pyelonephritis or of a Gram-negative septicaemia may dominate the clinical picture.

Vesical calculi associated with bladder bacteriuria may present with frequency, dysuria and haematuria; severe introital or perineal pain may occur if trigonitis is present. A calculus at the bladder neck or an obstruction in the urethra may cause bladder outflow obstruction, resulting in anuria and painful bladder distension.

A history of possible aetiological factors should be obtained, including:

- occupation and residence in hot countries likely to be associated with dehydration
- a history of vitamin D consumption
- gouty arthritis.

Calcified papillae may mimic ordinary calculi, so that causes of papillary necrosis such as analgesic abuse should be considered.

Physical examination should include a search for corneal or conjunctival calcification, gouty tophi and arthritis and features of sarcoidosis.

Investigations

These should include a mid-stream specimen of urine for culture and measurement of serum urea, electrolyte, creatinine and calcium levels.

Fig. 11.34 **X-rays showing calculus. (a)** The calculus (arrow) is overlying bone on the left (easily missed). **(b)** The same patient 1 week later: the calculus has descended and is easily seen in the pelvis of the left side (arrow).

Plain abdominal X-ray and excretion urography are still used widely for diagnosis, although unenhanced helical (spiral) CT is the best diagnostic test available. Ureteric stones can be missed by ultrasound.

Pure uric acid stones are radiolucent. Mixed infective stones in which organic matrix predominates are barely radiopaque. Calcium-containing and cystine stones are radiopaque. Calculi overlying bone are easily missed (Fig. 11.34). Staghorn calculi may be missed if the plain abdominal X-ray carried out before contrast injection during urography is not inspected (Fig. 11.35). Uric acid stones may present as a filling defect after injection of contrast medium (Fig. 11.36). Such stones are readily seen on CT scanning (Fig. 11.37).

Excretion urography is carried out during the episode of pain; a normal urogram excludes the diagnosis of pain due to calculous disease. The urographic appearances in a patient with acute left ureteric obstruction are shown in Figure 11.38. The urine of the patient should be passed through a sieve to trap any calculi for chemical analysis.

Management

Adequate analgesia should be given. An NSAID, e.g. diclofenac 75 mg by i.v. infusion, compares favourably with pethidine and does not cause nausea. Stones less than 0.5 cm diameter usually pass spontaneously. Stones greater than 1 cm diameter usually require urological or radiological intervention. Extracorporeal shock wave lithotripsy (ESWL) will fragment most stones, which then pass spontaneously. Ureteroscopy with a Yag laser can be

Fig. 11.35 **Staghorn calculus**. X-ray appearances before and after contrast on the right side are identical owing to a staghorn calculus in a non-functioning right kidney. A plain film may be confused with those taken after contrast injection.

Fig. 11.36 **Excretion urogram, showing a lucent filling defect (uric acid stone; arrow) in the left renal pelvis.** The differential diagnosis includes a sloughed papilla and a transitional cell tumour.

Fig. 11.37 CT scan, showing a uric acid stone, which appears as a bright lesion in the left kidney (arrow).

used for larger stones. Percutaneous nephrolithotomy is also used. Open surgery is rarely needed.

Investigating the cause of stone formation

In an elderly patient who has had a single episode with one stone, only limited investigation is required. Younger patients and those with recurrent stone formation require detailed investigation.

- **Renal imaging** is necessary to define the presence of a primary renal disease predisposing to stone formation.
- **Significant bacteriuria** may indicate mixed infective stone formation, but relapsing bacteriuria may be a consequence of stone formation rather than the original cause.
- **Chemical analysis** of any stone passed may be of great value and all that is required in the diagnosis of cystinuria or uric acid stone formation.
- **Serum calcium concentration** should be estimated and corrected for serum albumin concentration (see p. 593). Hypercalcaemia, if present, should be investigated further (see p. 1093).

- **Serum urate concentration** is often, but not invariably, elevated in uric acid stone-formers.
- **A screening test for cystinuria** should be carried out by adding sodium nitroprusside to a random unacidified urine sample; a purple colour indicates that cystinuria may be present. Urine chromatography is required to define the diagnosis precisely.
- **Urinary calcium, oxalate and uric acid output** should be measured in two consecutive carefully collected 24-hour urine samples. After withdrawing aliquots for estimation of uric acid, it is necessary to add acid to the urine in order to prevent crystallization of calcium salts upon the walls of the collection vessel, which would give falsely low results for urinary calcium and oxalate.
- **Plasma bicarbonate** is low in renal tubular acidosis. The finding of a urine pH that does not fall below 5.5 in the face of metabolic acidosis is diagnostic of this condition (see p. 716).

Prophylaxis

The age of the patient and the severity of the problem affect both the need for and the type of prophylaxis.

Idiopathic stone-formers

Where no metabolic abnormality is present, the mainstay of prevention is maintenance of a high intake of fluid throughout the day and night. The aim should be to ensure a daily urine volume of 2–2.5 L, which requires a fluid intake in excess of this, substantially so in the case of those who live in hot countries or work in a hot environment.

Idiopathic hypercalciuria

Severe dietary calcium restriction is inappropriate (see p. 649). Patients should be encouraged to consume a normal-calcium (30 mmol/day) diet. Dietary calcium restriction results in hyperabsorption of oxalate, and so foods containing large amounts of oxalate should also be limited. A high fluid intake should be advised as for

Fig. 11.38 X-ray, showing acute left ureteric obstruction. Note the increased density of the nephrogram and the absence of a pyelogram on the left side 15 minutes after contrast injection. From Cox TM, Firth D, Benz J et al (eds) (2003) *Oxford Textbook of Medicine*, 3rd edn, by permission of Oxford University Press.

idiopathic stone-formers. Patients who live in a hard-water area may benefit from drinking softened water.

If hypercalciuria persists and stone formation continues, a thiazide is used (e.g. bendroflumethiazide 2.5 or 5 mg each morning). Thiazides reduce urinary calcium excretion by a direct effect on the renal tubule. They may precipitate diabetes mellitus or gout and worsen hypercholesterolaemia. Reduction of animal proteins to 50 g/day and sodium intake to 50 mmol/day is also advisable, as a randomized controlled trial has found that a diet restricted in animal protein and salt but with normal calcium was more effective in the prevention of calcium and particularly oxalate stones than a diet restricted in calcium.

Mixed infective stones

Recurrent stones should be prevented by maintenance of a high fluid intake and meticulous control of bacteriuria. This will require long-term follow-up and often the use of long-term low-dose prophylactic antibacterial agents.

Uric acid stones

Dietary measures are probably of little value and are difficult to implement. Effective prevention can be achieved by the long-term use of allopurinol to maintain the serum urate and urinary uric acid excretion in the normal range. A high fluid intake should also be maintained. Uric acid is more soluble at alkaline pH, and long-term sodium bicarbonate supplementation to maintain an alkaline urine is an alternative approach in those few patients unable to take allopurinol. However, alkalinization of the urine facilitates precipitation of calcium oxalate and phosphate.

Cystine stones

These can be prevented and indeed will dissolve slowly with a high fluid intake. Five litres of water is drunk each 24 hours, and the patient must wake twice during the night to ingest 500 mL or more of water. Many patients cannot tolerate this regimen. An alternative, though potentially more troublesome, option is the long-term use of the chelating agent penicillamine; this causes cystine to be converted to the more soluble penicillamine–cysteine complex. Side-effects include drug rashes, blood dyscrasias and immune complex-mediated glomerulonephritis. However, it is especially effective in promoting dissolution of cystine stones already present.

Mild hyperoxaluria with calcium oxalate stones

A high fluid intake and dietary oxalate restriction are required. Dietary advice as in hypercalciuria is also advisable.

Nephrocalcinosis

The term 'nephrocalcinosis' means diffuse renal parenchymal calcification that is detectable radiologically (Fig. 11.39). The condition is typically painless. Hypertension and renal impairment commonly occur. The main causes of nephrocalcinosis are listed in Table 11.14.

Fig. 11.39 X-ray of nephrocalcinosis.

Table 11.14 Causes of nephrocalcinosis

Mainly cortical (rare)
Renal cortical necrosis (tram-line calcification)

Mainly medullary
Hypercalcaemia (primary hyperparathyroidism, hypervitaminosis D, sarcoidosis)
Renal tubular acidosis (inherited and acquired)
Primary hyperoxaluria
Medullary sponge kidney
Tuberculosis

Dystrophic calcification occurs following renal cortical necrosis. In hypercalcaemia and hyperoxaluria, deposition of calcium oxalate results from the high concentration of calcium and oxalate within the kidney.

In renal tubular acidosis (see p. 716) failure of urinary acidification and a reduction in urinary citrate excretion both favour calcium phosphate and oxalate precipitation, since precipitation occurs more readily in an alkaline medium and the calcium-chelating action of urinary citrate is reduced.

Treatment and prevention of nephrocalcinosis consist of treatment of the cause.

FURTHER READING
Bihl G, Meyers A (2001) Recurrent renal stone disease – advances in pathogenesis and management. *Lancet* **358**: 651–656.
Borghi L et al. (2002) Comparison of two diets for the prevention of recurrent stones in idiopathic hypercalciuria. *New England Journal of Medicine* **346**: 77–84.
Teichman JMH (2004) Acute renal colic from ureteral calculus. *New England Journal of Medicine* **350**: 684–693.

URINARY TRACT OBSTRUCTION

The urinary tract may be obstructed at any point between the kidney and the urethral meatus. This results in dilatation of the tract above the obstruction. Dilatation of the renal pelvis is known as hydronephrosis.

Aetiology

Obstructing lesions may lie within the lumen, or in the wall of the urinary tract, or outside the wall, causing obstruction by external pressure. The major causes of obstruction are shown in Table 11.15. Overall, the frequency is the same in men and women. However, in the elderly, urinary tract obstruction is more common in men owing to the frequency of bladder outflow obstruction.

Pathophysiology

Obstruction with continuing urine formation results in:

- progressive rise in intraluminal pressure
- dilatation proximal to the site of obstruction
- compression and thinning of the renal parenchyma, eventually reducing it to a thin rim and resulting in a decrease in the size of the kidney.

Acute obstruction is followed by transient renal arterial vasodilatation succeeded by vasoconstriction, probably

Table 11.15 Causes of urinary tract obstruction

Within the lumen	Pressure from outside
Calculus	Pelviureteric compression
Blood clot	(bands; aberrant vessels)
Sloughed papilla	Tumours (e.g. retroperitoneal
(diabetes; analgesia	tumour or glands;
abuse; sickle cell	carcinoma of colon;
disease or trait)	tumours in pelvis, e.g.
Tumour of renal pelvis	carcinoma of cervix)
or ureter	Diverticulitis
Bladder tumour	Aortic aneurysm
	Retroperitoneal fibrosis
Within the wall	(periaortitis)
Pelviureteric neuromuscular	Accidental ligation of ureter
dysfunction (congenital,	Retrocaval ureter (right-sided
10% bilateral)	obstruction)
Ureteric stricture	Prostatic obstruction
(tuberculosis, especially	Phimosis
after treatment; calculus;	
after surgery)	
Ureterovesical stricture	
(congenital; ureterocele;	
calculus; schistosomiasis)	
Congenital megaureter	
Congenital bladder neck	
obstruction	
Neuropathic bladder	
Urethral stricture	
(calculus; gonococcal;	
after instrumentation)	
Congenital urethral valve	
Pin-hole meatus	

mediated mainly by angiotensin II and thromboxane A_2. Ischaemic interstitial damage mediated by free oxygen radicals and inflammatory cytokines compounds the damage induced by compression of the renal substance.

Clinical features

Symptoms of upper tract obstruction

Loin pain occurs which can be dull or sharp, constant or intermittent. It may be provoked by measures that increase urine volume and hence distension of the collecting system, such as a high fluid intake or diuretics, including alcohol. Complete anuria is strongly suggestive of complete bilateral obstruction or complete obstruction of a single kidney.

Conversely, polyuria may occur in partial obstruction owing to impairment of renal tubular concentrating capacity. Intermittent anuria and polyuria indicates intermittent complete obstruction.

Infection complicating the obstruction may give rise to malaise, fever and septicaemia.

Symptoms of bladder outflow obstruction

Symptoms may be minimal. Hesitancy, narrowing and diminished force of the urinary stream, terminal dribbling and a sense of incomplete bladder emptying are typical features. The frequent passage of small volumes of urine occurs if a large volume of residual urine remains in the bladder after urination. Incontinence of such small volumes of urine is known as 'overflow incontinence' or 'retention with overflow'.

Infection commonly occurs, causing increased frequency, urgency, urge incontinence, dysuria and the passage of cloudy smelly urine. It may precipitate acute retention.

Signs

Loin tenderness may be present. An enlarged hydronephrotic kidney is often palpable. In acute or chronic retention the enlarged bladder can be felt or percussed. Examination of the genitalia, rectum and vagina is essential, since prostatic obstruction and pelvic malignancy are common causes of urinary tract obstruction. However, the apparent size of the prostate on digital examination is a poor guide to the presence of prostatic obstruction.

Investigations

Routine blood and biochemical investigations may be abnormal; for example, there may be a raised serum urea or creatinine, hyperkalaemia, anaemia of chronic disease or blood in the urine. Nevertheless, the diagnosis of obstruction cannot be made on these tests alone and further investigations must be performed.

Ultrasonography (see p. 615)
This is a reliable means of ruling out upper urinary tract dilatation. Ultrasound cannot distinguish a baggy, low-pressure unobstructed system from a tense, high-pressure obstructed one, so that false-positive scans are seen. However, in the hands of an experienced observer, a normal

scan does rule out urinary tract obstruction, except in very rare circumstances such as, for example, encasement of the kidney by fibrous or malignant tissue.

Radionuclide studies (see p. 617)

These have no place in the initial investigation of acute obstruction. Their main role is in possible long-standing obstruction to differentiate true obstructive nephropathy from retention of tracer in a baggy, low-pressure, unobstructed pelvicalyceal system.

Excretion urography

A plain film is necessary to detect calcification. However, calculi overlying bone are easily missed.

In recent unilateral obstruction, the affected kidney is enlarged and smooth in outline. The nephrogram is delayed owing to a reduction in the GFR. The calyces and pelvis fill with contrast medium later than on the normal side.

In time, the nephrogram on the affected side becomes denser than normal, owing to the prolonged nephron transit time, which allows greater than normal concentration of contrast medium within the tubules. Later, the site of obstruction may be seen, with dilatation of the system proximal to the level of the block (Fig. 11.40).

A full-length film should be taken after an attempt at bladder emptying by the patient. Complete emptying indicates either that no obstruction to bladder outflow exists or that intravesical pressure can be raised sufficiently to overcome it. Apparent bladder outflow impairment may be the result of nervousness or embarrassment on the part of the patient, or failure to carry out the X-ray before the bladder has refilled with contrast medium from above, or it may be due to an atonic but non-obstructed bladder. Vesicoureteric reflux can result in contrast medium returning to the bladder from above, giving the appearance of a partially full bladder.

Helical (spiral) CT scanning

This is used to outline in detail the cause of the obstruction.

Antegrade pyelography and ureterography
(see p. 616)

This defines the site and cause of obstruction. It can be combined with drainage of the collecting system by percutaneous needle nephrostomy.

Retrograde ureterography (see p. 616)

This is indicated if antegrade examination cannot be carried out or if there is the possibility of dealing with ureteric obstruction from below at the time of examination. The technique carries the risk of introducing infection into an obstructed urinary tract.

In obstruction due to neuromuscular dysfunction at the pelviureteric junction or retroperitoneal fibrosis, the collecting system may fill normally from below.

Cystoscopy, urethroscopy and urethrography

Obstructing lesions within the bladder and urethra can be seen directly by endoscopic examination.

Urethrography involves introducing contrast medium into the bladder by catheterization or suprapubic bladder puncture, and taking X-ray films during voiding to show obstructing lesions in the urethra. It is of particular value in the diagnosis of urethral valves and strictures.

Treatment

Aims

Treatment involves:

- relieving the obstruction
- treating the underlying cause
- preventing and treating infection.

The ultimate aim of treatment is to relieve symptoms and to preserve renal function.

Temporary external drainage of urine by nephrostomy may be valuable, as this allows time for further investigation when the site and nature of the obstructing lesion are uncertain, doubt exists as to the viability of the obstructed kidney, or when immediate definitive surgery would be hazardous.

Recent, complete upper urinary tract obstruction demands urgent relief to preserve kidney function, particularly if infection is present.

In contrast, with partial urinary tract obstruction, particularly if spontaneous relief is expected – such as by passage of a calculus – there is no immediate urgency.

Fig. 11.40 **X-ray taken 24 hours after injection of contrast, showing a delayed nephrogram and pyelogram on the left side and dilatation of the system to the level of the block.** By this time contrast medium has disappeared from the normal right side.

Surgical management

This depends on the cause of the obstruction and local expertise. Dialysis may be required in the ill patient prior to surgery.

Diuresis usually follows relief of obstruction at any site in the urinary tract. Massive diuresis may occur following relief of bilateral obstruction owing to previous sodium and water overload and the osmotic effect of retained solutes combined with a defective renal tubular reabsorptive capacity (as in the diuretic phase of recovering acute tubular necrosis). This diuresis is associated with increased blood volume and high levels of atrial natriuretic peptide (ANP). Defective renal tubular reabsorptive capacity cannot be the sole mechanism of severe diuresis since this phenomenon is not observed following relief of unilateral obstruction. The diuresis is usually self-limiting, but a minority of patients will develop severe sodium, water and potassium depletion requiring appropriate intravenous replacement. In milder cases, oral salt and potassium supplements together with a high water intake are sufficient.

Specific causes of obstruction

Calculi

These are discussed on page 617.

Pelviureteric junction obstruction (Fig. 11.41)

This results from a functional disturbance in peristalsis of the collecting system in the absence of mechanical obstruction. Surgical attempts at correction of the obstruction by open or percutaneous pyeloplasty are indicated in patients with recurrent loin pain and those in whom serial excretion urography, or measurements of GFR indicate progressive kidney damage. Nephrectomy to remove the risk of developing pyonephrosis and septicaemia is indicated if long-standing obstruction has destroyed kidney function.

Obstructive megaureter

This childhood condition may become evident only in adult life. It results from the presence of a region of defective peristalsis at the lower end of the ureter adjacent to the ureterovesical junction. The condition is more common in males. It presents with UTI, flank pain or haematuria. The diagnosis is made on excretion urography or, if necessary, ascending ureterography.

Excision of the abnormal portion of ureter with reimplantation into the bladder is always indicated in children, and in adults when the condition is associated with evidence of progressive deterioration in renal function, bacteriuria that cannot be controlled by medical means, or recurrent stone formation.

Retroperitoneal fibrosis (chronic periaortitis)

In this condition the ureters become embedded in dense retroperitoneal fibrous tissue with resultant unilateral or bilateral obstruction. The condition may extend from the level of the second lumbar vertebra to the pelvic brim. The incidence of the condition in men is three times that

Fig. 11.41 X-ray, showing left pelviureteric junction obstruction (arrow).

in women. An autoallergic response to leakage of material, probably ceroid, derived from atheromatous plaques is considered to be the underlying cause of the condition. Recognized associations are with abdominal aortic aneurysm and prolonged exposure to the drug methysergide and ergot-derived dopamine receptor agonists, e.g. cabergoline, and asbestos. The differential diagnosis includes retroperitoneal lymphoma or cancer.

Malaise, back pain, normochromic anaemia, uraemia and a raised erythrocyte sedimentation rate (ESR) are typical features. Excretion urography shows bilateral or unilateral ureteric obstruction commencing at the level of the pelvic brim. A periaortic mass may be seen on a CT scan (Fig. 11.42).

Obstruction is relieved surgically by ureterolysis. Biopsy should be performed to determine whether there is an underlying lymphoma or carcinoma. Corticosteroids are of benefit, and in bilateral obstruction in frail patients it may be best to free only one ureter and to rely upon steroid therapy to induce regression of fibrous tissue on the contralateral side, since bilateral ureterolysis is a major operation. In some patients, surgery alone or steroid therapy alone may suffice, but in the majority both surgery and subsequent corticosteroid therapy appear to be necessary. An alternative approach is placement of a

Fig. 11.42 Retroperitoneal fibrosis (periaortitis). Note the large mass surrounding the abdominal aorta on this CT scan (arrow).

ureteric stent or stents and corticosteroid therapy. A disadvantage is that an adequate biopsy of the mass – readily obtainable on open operation – is not easily obtained, and regular (usually 6-monthly) changes of the stent or stents is required if the periaortic mass does not regress.

Response to treatment and disease activity are assessed by serial measurements of ESR and GFR supplemented by isotopic and imaging techniques including CT scanning. Relapse after withdrawal of steroid therapy may occur and treatment may need to be continued for years. Mycophenolate or tamoxifen are also effective. Long-term follow-up is mandatory.

Benign prostatic hypertrophy

Benign prostatic hypertrophy is a common cause of urinary tract obstruction. It is described on page 685.

Prognosis of urinary tract obstruction

The prognosis depends upon the cause and the stage at which obstruction is relieved. In obstruction, four factors influence the rate at which kidney damage occurs, its extent and the degree and rapidity of recovery of renal function after relief of obstruction. These are:

- whether obstruction is partial or complete
- the duration of obstruction
- whether or not infection occurs
- the site of obstruction.

Complete obstruction for several weeks will lead to irreversible or only partially reversible kidney damage. If the duration of complete obstruction is several months, total irreversible destruction of the affected kidney will result. Partial obstruction carries a better prognosis, depending upon its severity. Bacterial infection coincident with obstruction rapidly increases kidney damage. Obstruction at or below the bladder neck may induce hypertrophy and trabeculation of the bladder without a rise in pressure within the upper urinary tract, in which case the kidneys are protected from the effects of backpressure.

FURTHER READING
Yaqoob M, Junaid I (2003) Urinary tract obstruction. In: Warrell DA, Cox TM, Firth JD (eds) *Oxford Textbook of Medicine*. Oxford: Oxford University Press

DRUGS AND THE KIDNEY

Drug-induced impairment of renal function

Prerenal

Impaired perfusion of the kidneys can result from drugs that cause:

- hypovolaemia – for example:
  (a) potent loop diuretics such as furosemide, especially in elderly patients
  (b) renal salt and water loss, such as from hypercalcaemia induced by vitamin D therapy (since hypercalcaemia adversely affects renal tubular salt and water conservation)
- decrease in cardiac output, which impairs renal perfusion (e.g. beta-blockers)
- decreased renal blood flow (e.g. ACE inhibitors particularly in the presence of renovascular disease).

Renal

Several mechanisms of drug-induced renal damage exist and may coexist.

- *Acute tubular necrosis produced by direct nephrotoxicity.* Examples include prolonged or excessive treatment with aminoglycosides (e.g. gentamicin, streptomycin), amphotericin B, heavy metals or carbon tetrachloride. The combination of aminoglycosides with furosemide is particularly nephrotoxic.
- *Acute tubulointerstitial nephritis* (see p. 643) with interstitial oedema and inflammatory cell infiltration. This cell-mediated hypersensitivity nephritis occurs with many drugs, including penicillins, sulphonamides and NSAIDs.
- *Chronic tubulointerstitial nephritis* due to drugs. See page 643.
- *Immune complex-mediated glomerulonephritis.* Examples include penicillamine.

Postrenal

Retroperitoneal fibrosis with urinary tract obstruction may result from the use of drugs (p. 656).

Use of drugs in patients with impaired renal function (Box 11.2)

Many aspects of drug handling are altered in patients with renal impairment.

Absorption

This may be unpredictable in uraemia as nausea and vomiting are frequently present.

Box 11.2 Safe prescribing in renal disease

Safe prescribing in renal failure demands knowledge of the clinical pharmacology of the drug and its metabolites in normal individuals and in uraemia. The clinician should ask the following questions when prescribing:

1 Is treatment mandatory? Unless it is, it should be withheld.
2 Can the drug reach its site of action? For example, there is little point in prescribing the urinary antiseptic, nitrofurantoin, in renal failure since bacteriostatic concentrations will not be attained in the urine.
3 Is the drug's metabolism altered in uraemia?
4 Will accumulation of the drug or metabolites occur? Even if accumulation is a potential problem owing to the drug or its metabolites being excreted by the kidneys, it is not necessarily an indication to change the drug given. The size of the loading dose will depend upon the size of the patient and is unrelated to renal function.
    Avoidance of toxic levels of drug in blood and tissues subsequently requires the administration of normal doses of the drug at longer time intervals than usual or smaller doses at the usual time intervals.
5 Is the drug toxic?
6 Are the effective concentrations of the drug in biological tissues similar to the toxic concentrations? Should blood levels of the drug be measured?
7 Will the drug worsen the uraemic state by means other than nephrotoxicity, e.g. steroids tetracycline?
8 Is the drug a sodium or potassium salt? These are potentially hazardous in uraemia.

Not surprisingly, adverse drug reactions are more than twice as common in renal failure as in normal individuals. Elderly patients, in whom unsuspected renal impairment is common, are particularly at risk. Careful attention to the above and careful titration of the dose of drugs employed should reduce the problem.
    The dose may be titrated by:

▪ observation of its clinical effect, e.g. hypotensive agents
▪ early detection of toxic effects
▪ measurement of drug levels in the blood, e.g. gentamicin levels.

Metabolism

Oxidative metabolism of drugs by the liver may be altered in uraemia. This is rarely of clinical significance.
    The rate of drug metabolism by the kidney is reduced as a result of two factors:

▪ *Reduced drug catabolism.* Insulin, for example, is in part catabolized by the normal kidney. In renal disease, insulin catabolism is reduced. The insulin requirements of diabetics decline as renal function deteriorates, for this reason.
▪ *Reduced conversion of a precursor to a more active metabolite,* such as the conversion of 25-hydroxycholecalciferol to the more active 1,25-$(OH)_2D_3$. The 1α-hydroxylase enzyme responsible for this conversion is located in the kidney. In renal disease, production of the enzyme declines and deficiency of 1,25-$(OH)_2D_3$ results.

Protein binding

Reduced protein binding of a drug potentiates its activity and increases the potential for toxic side-effects. Measurement of the total plasma concentration of such a drug can give misleading results. For example, the serum concentration of phenytoin required to produce an antiepileptic effect is much higher in normal individuals than in those with renal failure, since in the latter proportionately more drug is present in the free form.

    Some patients with renal disease are hypoproteinaemic and reduced drug-binding to protein results. This is not the sole mechanism of reduced drug-binding in such patients. For example, hydrogen ions, which are retained in renal failure, bind to receptors for acidic drugs such as sulphonamides, penicillin and salicylates, thus enhancing their potential for causing toxicity.

Volume of distribution

Salt and water overload or depletion may occur in patients with renal disease. This affects the concentration of drug obtained from a given dose.

End-organ sensitivity

The renal response to drug treatment may be reduced in renal disease. For example, mild thiazide diuretics have little diuretic effect in patients with severe renal impairment.

Renal elimination

The major problem in the use of drugs in renal failure concerns the reduced elimination of many drugs normally excreted by the kidneys.

    Water-soluble drugs such as gentamicin that are poorly absorbed from the gut, typically given by injection and are not metabolized by the liver, give rise to far more problems than lipid-soluble drugs such as propranolol, which are well absorbed and principally metabolized by the liver. Metabolites of lipid-soluble drugs, however, may themselves be water-soluble and potentially toxic.

Drugs causing uraemia by effects upon protein anabolism and catabolism

Tetracyclines, with the exception of doxycycline, have a catabolic effect and as a result the concentration of nitrogenous waste products is increased. They may also cause impairment of GFR by a direct effect. Corticosteroids have a catabolic effect and so also increase the production of nitrogenous wastes. A patient with moderate impairment of renal function may therefore become severely uraemic if given tetracyclines or corticosteroid therapy.

    Drugs and toxic agents causing specific renal tubular syndromes include mercury, lead, cadmium and vitamin D.

Problem patients

Particular problems are presented by patients in whom renal function is altering rapidly, such as those with recovering acute tubular necrosis. In addition, drugs may be removed by dialysis and haemofiltration, which will affect the dosage required.

FURTHER READING
British Medical Association and Royal Pharmaceutical Society of Great Britain (2005) Renal impairment. In: British National Formulary, 50th edn. Bath: Bath Press.

ACUTE RENAL FAILURE (ARF)

The term 'renal failure' means failure of renal excretory function due to depression of the glomerular filtration rate. This is accompanied to a variable extent by failure of erythropoietin production (see p. 611), vitamin D hydroxylation (p. 611), regulation of acid–base balance (p. 714) and regulation of salt and water balance and blood pressure (p. 610).

Definition

Acute renal failure means abrupt deterioration in parenchymal renal function, which is usually, but not invariably, reversible over a period of days or weeks. In clinical practice, such deterioration in renal function is sufficiently severe to result in uraemia. Oliguria is usually, but not invariably, a feature. Acute renal failure may cause sudden, life-threatening biochemical disturbances and is a medical emergency. The distinction between acute and chronic renal failure may not be readily apparent in a patient presenting with uraemia. Patients with chronic renal impairment are not immune from the development of a superimposed acute-on-chronic renal failure under appropriate circumstances.

Epidemiology

The observed incidence and outcomes of ARF are highly dependent upon the populations studied and the definition of ARF employed. The incidence of hospital-acquired ARF has increased from 4.9% in the 1970s to 7% in the 1990s. However, the incidence of community-acquired ARF on admission to hospital is approximately 1% with ARF superimposed on chronic renal failure accounting for 50% of these patients. The incidence of severe ARF (creatinine > 500 μmol/L) is about 130–140/million population and in patients with creatinine levels of up to 177 μmol/L or a 50% rise from baseline (less severe) it is about 200/million/year. Uncomplicated ARF can usually be managed outside the intensive care unit (ITU) setting and carries a good prognosis, with mortality rates less than 5–10%. In contrast, ARF complicating non-renal organ system failure (in the ITU setting) is associated with mortality rates of 50–70%, which have not changed for several decades. Moreover, sepsis-related ARF has a significantly worse prognosis than ARF in the absence of sepsis.

Classification

Renal failure results in reduced excretion of nitrogenous

Table 11.16 Causes of altered serum urea and creatinine concentration other than altered renal function

	Decreased concentration	Increased concentration
Urea	Low protein intake Liver failure Sodium valproate treatment	Corticosteroid treatment Tetracycline treatment Gastrointestinal bleeding
Creatinine	Low muscle mass	High muscle mass Red meat ingestion Muscle damage (rhabdomyolysis) Decreased tubular secretion (e.g. cimetidine, trimethoprim therapy)

waste products of which urea is the most commonly measured. A raised serum urea concentration (uraemia) is classified as: (i) prerenal, (ii) renal or (iii) postrenal. More than one category may be present in an individual patient. Other causes of altered serum urea and creatinine concentration are shown in Table 11.16.

Prerenal uraemia

In prerenal uraemia, there is impaired perfusion of the kidneys with blood. This results either from hypovolaemia, hypotension, impaired cardiac pump efficiency or vascular disease limiting renal blood flow, or combinations of these factors. Usually the kidney is able to maintain glomerular filtration close to normal despite wide variations in renal perfusion pressure and volume status – so-called 'autoregulation'. Further depression of renal perfusion leads to a drop in glomerular filtration and development of prerenal uraemia. Drugs which impair renal autoregulation, such as ACE inhibitors and NSAIDs, increase the tendency to develop prerenal uraemia. All causes of prerenal uraemia may lead to established parenchymal kidney damage and the development of acute renal failure. By definition, excretory function in prerenal uraemia improves once normal renal perfusion has been restored.

A number of criteria have been proposed to differentiate between prerenal and intrinsic renal causes of uraemia (Table 11.17).

Table 11.17 Criteria for distinction between prerenal and intrinsic causes of renal dysfunction

	Prerenal	Intrinsic
Urine specific gravity	> 1.020	< 1.010
Urine osmolality (mOsm/kg)	> 500	< 350
Urine sodium (mmol/L)	< 20	> 40
$FE_{Na} = \dfrac{U_{Na}}{P_{Na}} \div \dfrac{U_{Cr}}{P_{Cr}} \times 100$	< 1%	> 1%

FE, fractional excretion; P, plasma; U, urine; Cr, creatinine; Na, sodium

- *Urine specific gravity and urine osmolality* are easily obtained measures of concentrating ability but are unreliable in the presence of glycosuria or other osmotically active substances in the urine.
- *Urine sodium* is low if there is avid tubular reabsorption, but may be increased by diuretics or dopamine.
- *Fractional excretion of sodium* (FE_{Na}), the ratio of sodium clearance to creatinine clearance, increases the reliability of this index but may remain low in some 'intrinsic' renal diseases, including contrast nephropathy and myoglobinuria.

Laboratory tests, however, are no substitute for clinical assessment. A history of blood or fluid loss, sepsis potentially leading to vasodilatation, or of cardiac disease may be helpful. Hypotension (especially postural), a weak rapid pulse and a low jugular venous pressure will suggest that the uraemia is prerenal. In doubtful cases, measurement of central venous pressure is often invaluable, particularly with fluid challenge (see p. 969).

Management

If the prerenal uraemia is a result of hypovolaemia and hypotension, prompt replacement with appropriate fluid is essential to correct the problem and prevent development of ischaemic renal injury and acute renal failure (p. 974). Since prerenal and renal uraemia may coexist, and fluid challenge in the latter situation may lead to volume overload with pulmonary oedema, careful clinical monitoring is vital. Blood pressure should be checked regularly and signs of elevated jugular venous pressure and of pulmonary oedema sought frequently. Central venous pressure monitoring is usually advisable (see p. 968). If the problem relates to cardiac pump insufficiency or occlusion of the renal vasculature, appropriate measures – albeit often unsuccessful – need to be taken.

Postrenal uraemia

Here, uraemia results from obstruction of the urinary tract at any point from the calyces to the external urethral orifice. The causes and presentation of urinary tract obstruction are dealt with on page 654. Screening for urinary tract obstruction is by renal ultrasonography. Urinary tract obstruction may present in an acute fashion (if obstruction of a single functioning kidney by, for example, a calculus occurs) but typically is of insidious onset.

Acute uraemia due to renal parenchymal disease

Causes

This is most commonly due to acute renal tubular necrosis (Table 11.18). Other causes include disease affecting the intrarenal arteries and arterioles as well as glomerular capillaries, such as a vasculitis (p. 581), accelerated hypertension, cholesterol embolism, haemolytic uraemic syndrome, thrombotic thrombocytopenic purpura

Table 11.18   Some causes of acute tubular necrosis

Haemorrhage	Haemoglobinaemia (due to
Burns	haemolysis, e.g. in
Diarrhoea and vomiting,	falciparum malaria,
fluid loss from fistulae	'blackwater fever')
Pancreatitis	Hepatorenal syndrome
Diuretics	Radiological contrast agents
Myocardial infarction	Drugs, e.g. aminoglycosides,
Congestive cardiac failure	NSAIDs, ACE inhibitors,
Endotoxic shock	platinum derivatives
Snake bite	Abruptio placentae
Myoglobinaemia	Pre-eclampsia and eclampsia

(TTP), pre-eclampsia and crescentic glomerulonephritis. Acute tubulointerstitial nephritis (p. 643) may also cause acute renal failure. This also occurs when renal tubules are acutely obstructed by crystals, for example following sulphonamide therapy in a dehydrated patient (sulphonamide crystalluria) or after rapid lysis of certain malignant tumours following chemotherapy (acute hyperuricaemic nephropathy). Acute bilateral suppurative pyelonephritis or pyelonephritis of a single kidney can cause acute uraemia.

Acute tubular necrosis
Causes

Acute tubular necrosis (ATN) is common, particularly in hospital practice. It results most often from renal ischaemia but can also be caused by direct renal toxins including drugs such as the aminoglycosides, lithium and platinum derivatives (Table 11.18).

Kidneys appear to be particularly vulnerable to ischaemic injury when cholestatic jaundice is present, and more than one ischaemic factor appears to be present in some situations. For example, disseminated intravascular coagulation complicating Gram-negative septicaemia and complications of pregnancy such as placental rupture, pre-eclampsia and eclampsia, may result in occlusion or partial occlusion of intrarenal vessels, exacerbating the ischaemic insult resulting from hypotension associated with the underlying condition.

Myoglobinaemia and haemoglobinaemia consequent upon muscle injury (rhabdomyolysis) complicating trauma, pressure necrosis or heroin use predispose to ATN, perhaps in part owing to occlusion of renal tubules by myoglobin and haemoglobin casts. In liver failure, acute renal failure appears to result from rapidly reversible vasomotor abnormalities within the kidney. A kidney removed from a patient with hepatic cirrhosis and liver failure dying with oliguric renal failure may function normally immediately after transplantation into a normal individual. Efferent glomerular arteriolar dilatation resulting from ACE-inhibitor drug therapy, with consequent lowering of glomerular filtration pressure, may cause acute deterioration in excretory function if renal arterial disease is also present. The effect is compounded by concomitant use of non-steroidal anti-inflammatory agents which reduce prostaglandin production, opposing this effect.

Pathogenesis

Factors postulated to be involved in the development of ATN include:

- *Intrarenal microvascular vasoconstriction:*
  (a) Vasoconstriction is increased in response to endothelin, adenosine, thromboxane A_2, leukotrienes and sympathetic nerve activity. However, endothelin antagonists failed to show any beneficial effect in the clinical setting.
  (b) Vasodilatation is reduced in response to: (i) nitric oxide, prostaglandins (PGE_2), acetylcholine and bradykinin; (ii) increased endothelial and vascular smooth muscle cell structural damage; (iii) increased leucocyte–endothelial adhesion, vascular congestion and obstruction, leucocyte activation and inflammation. After success in the prevention of ARF in animal models, anti-ICAM (intercellular adhesion molecule) in the clinical setting failed to live up to its initial promise.

- *Tubular cell injury.* Ischaemic injury results in rapid depletion of intracellular ATP stores resulting in cell death either by necrosis or apoptosis, due to the following: (i) entry of calcium into cells with an increase in cytosolic cell calcium concentration; (ii) induction by hypoxia of inducible nitric oxide synthases with increased production of nitric oxide causing cell death; (iii) increased production of intracellular proteases such as calpain, which cause proteolysis of cytoskeletal proteins and cell wall collapse; (iv) activation of phospholipase A_2 with increased production of free fatty acids, particularly arachidonic acid, due to its action on the lipid layer of cell membranes; (v) cell injury resulting from reperfusion with blood after initial ischaemia causing excessive free radical generation; (vi) tubular obstruction by desquamated viable or necrotic cells and casts; (vii) loss of cell polarity, i.e. integrins located on the basolateral side of the cell are translocated to the apical surface, which when combined with other desquamated cells forms casts, with tubular obstruction and back leak of tubular fluid.

Tubular cellular recovery. Tubular cells have the capacity to regenerate rapidly and to reform the disrupted tubular basement membrane, which explains the reversibility of ATN. Multiple growth factors, including insulin like growth factor 1, epidermal growth factor and hepatocyte growth factor and their receptors are upregulated during the regenerative process after injury. Clinical utility of growth factors in the treatment of ARF is unproven.

In established ATN renal blood flow is much reduced, particularly blood flow to the renal cortex. Ischaemic tubular damage contributes to a reduction in glomerular filtration by a number of interrelated mechanisms:

- *Glomerular contraction* reducing the surface area available for filtration, due to reflex afferent arteriolar spasm mediated by increased solute delivery to the macula densa. Increased solute delivery is due to impaired sodium absorption in the proximal tubular cells because of loss of cell polarity with mislocalization of the Na^+/K^+-ATPase and impaired tight junction integrity, resulting in decreased apical-to-basal transcellular sodium absorption.
- *'Back leak' of filtrate* in the proximal tubule owing to loss of function of the tubular cells.
- *Obstruction of the tubule* by debris shed from ischaemic tubular cells.

Course

The clinical course of acute renal failure associated with ATN is variable depending on the severity and duration of the renal insult. Oliguria is common in the early stages: non-oliguric renal failure is usually a result of a less severe renal insult. Recovery of renal function typically occurs after 7–21 days, although recovery is delayed by continuing sepsis. In the recovery phase, GFR may remain low while urine output increases, sometimes to many litres a day owing to defective tubular reabsorption of filtrate. The clinical course is variable and ATN may last for up to 6 weeks, even after a relatively short-lived initial insult. Eventually renal function usually returns almost to normal or to normal, although exceptions exist (e.g. in renal cortical necrosis – see below).

No treatment is, as yet, known which will reduce the duration of acute renal tubular necrosis once it has occurred. The use of intravenous mannitol, furosemide or 'renal-dose' dopamine is not supported by controlled trial evidence, and none of these treatments is without risk. The synthetic analogue of atrial natriuretic factor, anaritide, did not reduce the duration of or mortality from ATN. However, oliguric patients did appear to do better whilst non-oliguric ones did worse when treated with this agent in a large clinical trial. Moreover, use of exogenous IGF-1 failed to show any beneficial effect in clinical ARF.

Whether a state of 'incipient' ATN exists in some patients with prerenal uraemia, and whether ATN can be prevented by administration of mannitol, furosemide or dopamine, also remain uncertain. Many nephrologists will administer one or more of these agents if correction of prerenal factors does not initiate a diuresis, but proof of benefit is lacking.

Clinical and biochemical features

These are the features of the causal condition together with features of rapidly progressive uraemia. The rate at which serum urea and creatinine concentrations increase is dependent upon the rate of tissue breakdown in the individual patient. This is increased in the presence of trauma, sepsis and following surgery. *Hyperkalaemia* is common, particularly following trauma to muscle and in haemolytic states. *Metabolic acidosis* is usual unless hydrogen ion loss by vomiting or aspiration of gastric contents is a feature. *Hyponatraemia* may be present owing to water overload if patients have continued to drink in the face of oliguria, or if overenthusiastic fluid replacement with 5% dextrose has been carried out. *Pulmonary* oedema owing to salt and water retention is not uncommon, particularly after inappropriate attempts to initiate a diuresis by infusion of normal 0.9% saline without adequate monitoring of the patient's volume status. *Hypocalcaemia* due to reduced renal production of 1,25-dihydroxycholecalciferol and *hyperphosphataemia* due to phosphate retention are common.

Symptoms of uraemia such as anorexia, nausea, vomiting and pruritus develop, followed by intellectual clouding, drowsiness, fits, coma and haemorrhagic episodes. Epistaxes and gastrointestinal haemorrhage are relatively common. Severe infection may have initiated the acute renal failure or have complicated it owing to the impaired immune defences of the uraemic patient or ill-considered management, such as the insertion and retention of an unnecessary bladder catheter with complicating urinary tract infection and bacteraemia.

Investigation of the uraemic emergency

Investigations are aimed at defining whether the patient has acute or chronic uraemia, whether uraemia results from prerenal, renal or postrenal factors, and establishing the cause.

Acute or chronic uraemia?

The distinction between acute and chronic uraemia depends in part on the history, duration of symptoms and previous urinalysis or measurements of renal function.

A rapid rate of change of serum urea and creatinine with time suggests an acute process. A normochromic, normocytic anaemia suggests chronic disease, but anaemia may complicate many of the diseases that cause acute renal failure, owing to a combination of haemolysis, haemorrhage and deficient erythropoietin production.

Ultrasound assessment of renal echogenicity and size is helpful. Small kidneys of increased echogenicity are diagnostic of a chronic process, although the reverse is not true; the kidney may remain normal in size in diabetes and amyloidosis, for instance.

Evidence of renal osteodystrophy (for example, digital subperiosteal erosions due to hyperparathyroid bone disease) is indicative of chronic disease.

Measurement of carbamylated haemoglobin (a product of non-enzymatic reaction between urea and haemoglobin, cf. glycosylated haemoglobin) is not widely employed.

Prerenal, renal or postrenal uraemia?

Bladder outflow obstruction is ruled out by insertion of a urethral catheter or flushing of an existing catheter, which should then be removed unless a large volume of urine is obtained. Absence of upper tract dilatation on renal ultrasonography will, with very rare exceptions, rule out urinary tract obstruction.

The distinction between prerenal and renal uraemia may be difficult (see p. 659). Assessment of the patient's volume status is essential and central venous pressure measurement may be extremely helpful. If volume status is low, appropriate corrective measures are indicated. If no diuresis ensues, acute intrinsic renal failure is present.

Use of low-dose dopamine, mannitol or furosemide (frusemide) is unhelpful and they should not be given.

Other investigations

These include urinalysis, urine microscopy, particularly for red cells and red-cell casts (indicative of glomerulonephritis), and urine culture. Blood tests include measurement of serum urea, electrolytes, creatinine, calcium, phosphate, albumin, alkaline phosphatase and urate concentrations, as well as full blood count and examination of the peripheral blood film where necessary. Coagulation studies, blood cultures and measurements of nephrotoxic drug blood levels should be carried out. Urine should be tested for free haemoglobin and myoglobin, where appropriate.

Management

The aim of management of acute renal tubular necrosis is to keep the patient alive until spontaneous recovery of renal function occurs. Ideally patients should be managed by a nephrologist or intensivist with access to facilities for blood purification and fluid removal (see p. 663). Early specialist referral is advisable. Poor initial management and late referral result in the arrival in the specialist centre of a patient who is severely uraemic, acidotic and hyperkalaemic, with pulmonary oedema following over-enthusiastic intravenous fluid administration and with a Gram-negative septicaemia complicating the presence of an unnecessary indwelling bladder catheter.

General measures

Good nursing and physiotherapy are vital. Regular oral toilet, chest physiotherapy and consistent documentation of fluid intake and output, and where possible measurement of daily bodyweight to assess fluid balance changes, all have a role. The patient should be confined to bed only if essential.

Emergency measures
Hyperkalaemia

This is a life-threatening complication owing to the risk of cardiac dysrhythmias, particularly ventricular fibrillation. Treatment is outlined in Emergency box 12.1. Correction of acidosis with intravenous sodium bicarbonate will also reduce serum potassium concentration, but administration of sodium may be inappropriate if the patient is salt and water overloaded. Rapid correction of acidosis in a hypocalcaemic patient may also trigger tetany, since hydrogen ions displace calcium from albumin-binding sites, thus increasing the physiologically active calcium concentration in blood. Ion exchange resins are used to prevent subsequent hyperkalaemia rather than to deal with the acute emergency. In many patients, hyperkalaemia will be controlled only by dialysis or haemofiltration.

Pulmonary oedema

Unless a diuresis can be induced with intravenous furosemide (frusemide), dialysis or haemofiltration will be required.

Sepsis

Infections, when detected, should be treated promptly, bearing in mind the need to avoid nephrotoxic drugs and to use drugs with appropriate monitoring and drug levels (e.g. gentamicin, vancomycin). Prophylactic antibiotics or barrier nursing is not recommended in all cases.

Use of drugs

Great care must be exercised in the use of drugs (see p. 657).

Fluid and electrolyte balance

Twice-daily clinical assessment is needed. In general, once the patient is euvolaemic, daily fluid intake should equal urine output plus losses from fistulae and from vomiting, plus an allowance of 500 mL daily for insensible loss. Febrile patients will require an additional allowance. Sodium and potassium intake should be minimized. If abnormal losses of fluid occur, for example in diarrhoea, additional fluid and electrolytes will be required. The development of signs of salt and water overload (peripheral oedema, basal crackles, elevation of jugular venous pressure) or of hypovolaemia should prompt reappraisal of fluid intake. Large changes in daily weight reflecting change in fluid balance status should also prompt a reappraisal of the situation.

Diet

With rare exceptions, sodium and potassium restriction are appropriate. The place of dietary protein restriction is controversial. If it is hoped to avoid dialysis or haemo-filtration, protein intake is sometimes restricted to approximately 40 g daily. This poses the risk of a negative nitrogen balance despite attempts to reduce endogenous protein catabolism by maintenance of a high energy intake in the form of carbohydrate and fat. Patients treated by blood purification techniques are more appropriately managed by providing 70 g protein daily or more. Hyper-catabolic patients will require an even higher nitrogen intake to prevent negative nitrogen balance.

Routes of intake are, in preferred order, enteral by mouth, enteral by nasogastric tube, and parenteral. The last of these is, however, only necessary if vomiting or bowel dysfunction render the enteral route inappropriate.

Vitamin supplements are usually supplied. Vitamin D analogue therapy and pharmacological doses of erythro-poietin are not employed routinely.

Dialysis and haemofiltration

The main indications for blood purification and/or excess fluid removal by these techniques are:

- symptoms of uraemia
- complications of uraemia, such as pericarditis
- severe biochemical derangement in the absence of symptoms (especially if a rising trend is observed in an oliguric patient and in hypercatabolic patients)
- hyperkalaemia not controlled by conservative measures
- pulmonary oedema

- severe acidosis
- for removal of drugs causing the acute renal failure, e.g. gentamicin, lithium, severe aspirin overdose.

The main options are peritoneal dialysis, intermittent haemodialysis (HD) combined with ultrafiltration, if necessary, intermittent haemofiltration, continuous arteriovenous or venovenous haemofiltration, and haemodiafiltration. For reasons that are incompletely understood, adverse cardiovascular effects are much less during haemofiltration than during haemodialysis. Continuous treatments are superior to intermittent ones in this respect.

Continuous renal replacement treatments (CRRT)

Blood flow is achieved either by using the patient's own blood pressure to generate arterial blood flow through a filter or by the use of a blood pump to draw blood from the lumen of a dual-lumen catheter placed in the jugular, subclavian or femoral vein.

Continuous arteriovenous or venovenous haemofiltration (CAVH, CVVH) refers to the continuous removal of ultrafiltrate from the patient, usually at rates of up to 1000 mL/h, combined with simultaneous infusion of replacement solution. For instance, in a fluid-overloaded patient one might remove filtrate at 1000 mL/h and replace at a rate of 900 mL/h, achieving a net fluid removal of 100 mL/h.

Continuous haemodiafiltration (CAVHDF, CVVHDF) is a combination of haemofiltration and haemodialysis, involving both the net removal of ultrafiltrate from the blood and its replacement with a replacement solution, together with the countercurrent passage of dialysate (which may be identical to the replacement solution). Both the ultrafiltrate and the spent dialysate appear as 'waste'.

Comparisons of dialysis modalities

Peritoneal dialysis (PD) is used infrequently in the management of ARF, with decreasing utilization over the past 5–10 years. Drawbacks to the use of PD in ARF are: (i) low efficiency in fluid and solute removal compared to CRRT or intermittent HD; (ii) ARF complicating intra-abdominal pathology is unsuitable for PD; (iii) increasing intra-abdominal pressure can compromise lung function; (iv) use of dialysis fluids with a high dextrose content may produce hyperglycaemia and other metabolic derangements. Data suggest that PD is significantly less effective than CRRT in the management of ARF and should be reserved for situations where other modalities of therapy are not available.

A meta-analysis of 13 studies comparing intermittent HD to CRRT in ARF failed to demonstrate any difference in mortality between the two modalities. There are thus insufficient data to favour either HD or CRRT as a superior mode of therapy in ARF. However, there is consensus that in haemodynamically unstable patients, CRRT is better tolerated.

Membrane biocompatibility

The concept of membrane 'biocompatibility' relates to the activation of cellular (neutrophils, platelets) and humoral (complement system and coagulation cascade) components upon contact between blood and dialysis membranes. As a general rule, unsubstituted cellulosic membranes (cuprophan) are the least biocompatible, with biocompatibility improving with substitution of free hydroxyl groups by tertiary amino groups (hemophan), acetate (cellulose acetate, diacetate, triacetate) or the use of synthetic polymers (e.g. polysulphone, polyamide, polyacrilonitrile and polymethylmethacrylate).

In a recent meta-analysis, synthetic membranes appeared to confer a significant survival advantage over unsubstituted cellulose (cuprophan)-based membranes but no benefit on recovery of renal function was observed.

Acute renal failure in the intensive care unit

In the UK, increasing numbers of patients with acute renal failure are managed in the setting of an intensive care unit. Many such patients have multiorgan failure, sepsis or both, with associated cardiovascular instability. Continuous methods of blood purification and control of fluid balance, such as venovenous haemofiltration, are preferable to intermittent haemodialysis or peritoneal dialysis in such patients. Advantages include:

- much less disturbance of cardiovascular stability
- the ability to generate as much 'space' for fluid administration as is required, which can be adjusted flexibly to the needs of the patient (many patients require large volumes of fluid to be administered for nutritional and other reasons)
- the removal of potentially harmful substances such as inflammatory cytokines via the more porous membrane employed in haemofiltration.

Acute respiratory distress syndrome (ARDS) is not uncommon in patients with multiorgan failure, including acute renal failure, requiring intensive therapy. In such patients the wish to remove as much fluid from the patient as possible to reduce pulmonary congestion must be balanced against the need of organs, including the kidneys, for an adequate blood flow, if recovery is to occur.

Management of the recovery phase

Usually, after 1–3 weeks, renal function improves, as evidenced by an increase in urine volume and improvement in serum biochemistry. Dialysis or haemofiltration, if they have been required, can be discontinued. A careful watch on clinical state, salt and water balance, and serum chemistry is required at this stage, particularly if a major diuretic phase develops owing to recovery of glomerular filtration at a time when renal tubular reabsorptive capacity for sodium, potassium and water remains impaired. Intravenous fluid replacement is sometimes required together with supplements of sodium chloride and potassium. Typically, the diuretic phase lasts for only a few days.

Acute cortical necrosis

Renal hypoperfusion results in diversion of blood flow from the cortex to the medulla, with a drop in GFR. Medullary ischaemic damage is largely reversible owing to the capacity of the tubular cells for regeneration. In contrast, glomerular ischaemic injury does not heal with regeneration but with scarring – glomerulosclerosis. Prolonged cortical ischaemia may lead to irreversible loss of renal function termed 'cortical necrosis'. This may be patchy or complete. Any cause of acute tubular necrosis, if sufficiently severe or prolonged, may lead to cortical necrosis. This outcome is particularly common if acute renal failure has been accompanied by derangements of the vascular endothelial system or coagulation system, such as occurs in haemolytic uraemic syndrome and complications of pregnancy.

Contrast nephropathy

In patients with impaired renal function, iodinated radiological contrast media may be nephrotoxic, possibly by causing renal vasoconstriction and by a direct toxic effect upon renal tubules. The effect is dose-dependent and therefore more commonly seen in procedures that require large amounts of contrast media, such as angiography with or without angioplasty. In many patients the effect is mild, transient, fully reversible and of no clinical significance. The risk and severity of contrast nephropathy is amplified by the presence of hypovolaemia and renal impairment, especially if due to diabetic nephropathy. Diabetes per se is not a risk factor.

Prevention involves minimization as far as possible of the dose of contrast employed and use of a low-osmolality contrast medium. Pre-hydration with intravenous saline is of proven benefit. A popular regimen involves infusion of 1 L of saline during the 12 hours before and 12 hours after contrast exposure. Care must be taken to avoid volume overload in susceptible patients.

N-acetylcysteine (NAC; a potent antioxidant) given 48 hours prior to radiological intervention may be of benefit in preventing worsening of pre-existing renal impairment following intravenous contrast, but the effect on morbidity and mortality is unknown. Routine use of dopamine, theophylline (adenosine antagonist) and prophylactic haemodialysis (removing contrast agent from circulation) are of no benefit. In patients with advanced CRF who are undergoing coronary angiography, periprocedural haemofiltration given in an ITU setting appears to be effective in preventing the deterioration of renal function due to contrast agent-induced nephropathy and is associated with improved in-hospital and long-term outcomes.

When deterioration in renal function occurs after intra-arterial injection of contrast (for example, after coronary angiography) it may be difficult to differentiate the effects of contrast-induced damage from those of atheromatous embolization (see p. 648). The latter carries a worse prognosis.

Hepatorenal syndrome (HRS)

The renal failure observed in HRS results from profound renal vasoconstriction with histologically normal kidneys (p. 384). Although many of the features of HRS resemble prerenal ARF, the defining feature is a lack of improvement in renal function with volume expansion. Renal recovery is usually observed after restoration of hepatic function after successful liver transplantation.

FURTHER READING

Bonventre JV, Weinberg JM (2003) Recent advances in the pathophysiology of ischaemic renal failure. *Journal of the American Society of Nephrology* **13**: 2199–2210.

Lameire N, Van Biesen W, Vanholder R (2005) Acute renal failure. *Lancet* **365**: 417–430.

Phu NH, Hein TT, Mai NT et al. (2002) Haemofiltration and peritoneal dialysis in infection associated acute renal failure in Vietnam. *New England Journal of Medicine* **347**: 97–104.

CHRONIC RENAL FAILURE (CRF)

Chronic renal failure implies long-standing, and usually progressive, impairment in renal function. In many instances, no effective means are available to reverse the primary disease process. Exceptions include correction of urinary tract obstruction, immunosuppressive therapy for systemic vasculitis and Goodpasture's syndrome, treatment of accelerated hypertension, and correction of critical narrowing of renal arteries causing renal impairment. The rate of deterioration in renal function can, however, be slowed (see p. 672). A list of causes of CRF is given in Table 11.19.

Wide geographical variations in the incidence of disorders causing CRF exist. The most common cause of glomerulonephritis in sub-Saharan Africa is malaria. Schistosomiasis is a common cause of renal failure due to urinary tract obstruction in parts of the Middle East, including southern Iraq. The incidence of end-stage renal failure varies between racial groups, as does the relative importance of different causes of chronic renal failure. End-stage renal failure is three to four times as common in black Africans in the UK and USA as it is in whites, and hypertensive nephropathy is a much more frequent cause of end-stage renal failure in this group. The prevalence of diabetes mellitus and hence of diabetic nephropathy is higher in some Asian groups than in whites. The age is of relevance; CRF due to atherosclerotic renal vascular disease is much more common in the elderly than in the young.

Table 11.19 Causes of chronic renal failure

Congenital and inherited disease
Polycystic kidney disease (adult and infantile forms)
Medullary cystic disease
Tuberose sclerosis
Oxalosis
Cystinosis
Congenital obstructive uropathy

Glomerular disease
Primary glomerulonephritides including focal glomerulosclerosis
Secondary glomerular disease (systemic lupus, polyangiitis, Wegener's granulomatosis, amyloidosis, diabetic glomerulosclerosis, accelerated hypertension, haemolytic uraemic syndrome, thrombotic thrombocytopenic purpura, systemic sclerosis, sickle cell disease)

Vascular disease
Hypertensive nephrosclerosis (common in black Africans)
Reno-vascular disease
Small and medium-sized vessel vasculitis

Tubulointerstitial disease
Tubulointerstitial nephritis – idiopathic, due to drugs (especially nephrotoxic analgesics), immunologically mediated
Reflux nephropathy
Tuberculosis
Schistosomiasis
Nephrocalcinosis
Multiple myeloma (myeloma kidney)
Balkan nephropathy
Renal papillary necrosis (diabetes, sickle cell disease and trait, analgesic nephropathy)
Chinese herb nephropathy

Urinary tract obstruction
Calculus disease
Prostatic disease
Pelvic tumours
Retroperitoneal fibrosis
Schistosomiasis

Clinical approach to the patient with CRF or any other form of renal disease

History

Particular attention should be paid to:

- *duration of symptoms*
- *drug ingestion*, including non-steroidal anti-inflammatory agents, analgesic and other medications, and unorthodox treatments such as herbal remedies
- *previous medical and surgical history*, e.g. previous chemotherapy, multisystem diseases such as SLE
- *previous occasions* on which urinalysis or measurement of urea and creatinine might have been performed, e.g. pre-employment or insurance medical examinations, new patient checks
- *family history* of renal disease.

Symptoms

The early stages of renal failure are often completely asymptomatic, despite the accumulation of numerous metabolites. Serum urea and creatinine concentrations are measured in renal failure since methods for their determination are available and a rough correlation exists between urea and creatinine concentrations and symptoms. These substances are, however, in themselves not particularly toxic. The nature of the metabolites that are involved in the genesis of symptoms is unclear. Such metabolites must be products of protein catabolism (since dietary protein restriction may reverse symptoms associated with renal failure) and many of them must be of relatively small molecular size (since haemodialysis employing membranes which allow through only relatively small molecules improves symptoms). Little else is known with certainty.

Symptoms are common when the serum urea concentration exceeds 40 mmol/L, but many patients develop uraemic symptoms at lower levels of serum urea. Symptoms include:

- malaise, loss of energy
- loss of appetite
- insomnia
- nocturia and polyuria due to impaired concentrating ability
- itching
- nausea, vomiting and diarrhoea
- paraesthesiae due to polyneuropathy
- 'restless legs' syndrome (overwhelming need to frequently alter position of lower limbs) (p. 1287)
- bone pain due to metabolic bone disease
- paraesthesiae and tetany due to hypocalcaemia
- symptoms due to salt and water retention – peripheral or pulmonary oedema
- symptoms due to anaemia (see p. 424)
- amenorrhoea in women; erectile dysfunction in men.

In more advanced uraemia (serum urea > 50–60 mmol/L), these symptoms become more severe, and CNS symptoms are common:

- mental slowing, clouding of consciousness, and seizures
- myoclonic twitching.

Severe depression of glomerular filtration can result in oliguria. This can occur with either acute renal failure or in the terminal stages of chronic renal failure. However, even if the GFR is profoundly depressed, failure of tubular reabsorption may lead to very high urine volumes; the urine output is therefore not a useful guide to renal function.

Examination

There are few physical signs of uraemia per se. Findings include:

- *short stature* – in patients who have had chronic renal failure in childhood
- *pallor* – due to anaemia
- *increased photosensitive pigmentation* – which may make the patient look misleadingly healthy
- *brown discoloration of the nails*
- *scratch marks* due to uraemic pruritus
- *signs of fluid overload* (p. 695)
- *pericardial friction rub*

- *flow murmurs* – mitral regurgitation due to mitral annular calcification; aortic and pulmonary regurgitant murmurs due to volume overload
- *glove and stocking peripheral sensory loss* (rare).

The kidneys themselves are usually impalpable unless grossly enlarged as a result of polycystic disease, obstruction or tumour. Rectal and vaginal examination may disclose evidence of an underlying cause of renal failure, particularly urinary obstruction, and should always be performed.

In addition to these findings, there may be physical signs of any underlying disease which may have caused the renal failure, for instance:

- cutaneous vasculitic lesions in systemic vasculitides
- retinopathy in diabetes
- evidence of peripheral vascular disease
- evidence of spina bifida or other causes of neurogenic bladder.

An assessment of the central venous pressure, skin turgor, blood pressure both lying and standing and peripheral circulation should also be made. The major symptoms and signs of chronic renal failure are shown in Figure 11.43.

Investigations

The following investigations are common for all renal patients. This includes patients with glomerular or non-

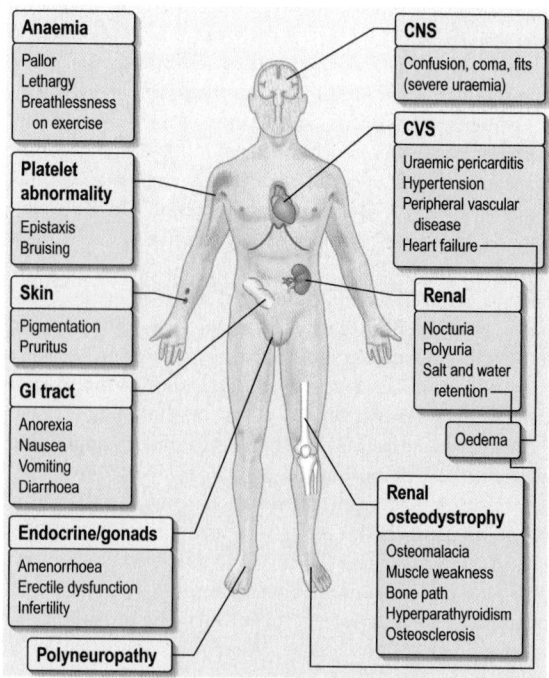

Fig. 11.43 Symptoms and signs of chronic renal failure. Oedema may be due to a combination of primary renal salt and water retention and heart failure.

glomerular disease, renal involvement in systemic diseases, ARF and CRF, as renal symptoms and signs are non-specific.

Urinalysis

- *Haematuria* may indicate glomerulonephritis, but other sources must be excluded. Haematuria should not be assumed to be due to the presence of an indwelling catheter.
- *Proteinuria*, if heavy, is strongly suggestive of glomerular disease. Urinary infection may also cause proteinuria.
- *Glycosuria* with normal blood glucose is common in CRF.

Urine microscopy (see p. 614)

- *White cells* in the urine usually indicate active bacterial urinary infection, but this is an uncommon cause of renal failure; sterile pyuria suggests papillary necrosis or renal tuberculosis.
- *Eosinophiluria* is strongly suggestive of allergic tubulointerstitial nephritis or cholesterol embolization.
- *Granular casts* are formed from abnormal cells within the tubular lumen, and indicate active renal disease.
- *Red-cell casts* are highly suggestive of glomerulonephritis.
- *Red cells in the urine* may be from anywhere between the glomerulus and the urethral meatus (Fig. 11.5).

Urine biochemistry

- *24-hour creatinine clearance* is useful in assessing the severity of renal failure.
- *Measurements of urinary electrolytes* are unhelpful in chronic renal failure. The use of urinary sodium concentration in the distinction between prerenal and intrinsic renal disease is discussed on page 659.
- *Urine osmolality* is a measure of concentrating ability. A low urine osmolality is normal in the presence of a high fluid intake but indicates renal disease when the kidney should be concentrating urine, such as in hypovolaemia or hypotension.
- *Urine electrophoresis and immunofixation* is necessary for the detection of light chains, which can be present without a detectable serum paraprotein.

Serum biochemistry

- *Urea and creatinine.*
- *Electrophoresis and immunofixation* should be performed for myeloma.
- *Extreme elevations of creatine kinase* and a disproportionate elevation in serum creatinine and potassium compared to urea suggest rhabdomyolysis.

Haematology

- *Eosinophilia* suggests vasculitis, allergic tubulointerstitial nephritis, or cholesterol embolism.
- *Markedly raised viscosity or ESR* suggests myeloma or vasculitis.
- *Fragmented red cells and/or thombocytopenia* suggests intravascular haemolysis due to accelerated hypertension, haemolytic uraemic syndrome or thrombotic thrombocytopenic purpura.

- *Tests for sickle cell disease* should be performed when relevant.

Immunology

- *Complement components* may be low in active renal disease due to SLE, mesangiocapillary glomerulonephritis, post-streptococcal glomerulonephritis, and cryoglobulinaemia.
- *Autoantibody screening* is useful in detection of SLE (p. 576), scleroderma (p. 579), Wegener's granulomatosis and microscopic polyangiitis (p. 938), and Goodpasture's syndrome (p. 632).
- *Cryoglobulins* should be sought in patients with unexplained glomerular disease, particularly mesangiocapillary glomerulonephritis.
- *Urine culture* should always be performed.
- *Early-morning urine samples* should be cultured if tuberculosis is possible.
- *Antibodies to streptococcal antigens* (ASOT, anti-DNase B) should be sought if post-streptococcal glomerulonephritis is possible.
- *Antibodies to hepatitis B and C* may point to polyarteritis or membranous nephropathy (hepatitis B) or to cryoglobulinaemic renal disease (hepatitis C).
- *Antibodies to HIV* raise the possibility of HIV-associated renal disease.
- *Malaria* is a major cause of glomerular disease in the tropics.

Radiological investigation

- *Ultrasound.* Every patient should undergo ultrasonography (for renal size and to exclude hydronephrosis), and plain abdominal radiography and CT (without contrast) to exclude low-density renal stones or nephrocalcinosis, which may be missed on ultrasound.
- *Intravenous urography* is seldom necessary in advanced renal disease.
- *CT* is also useful for the diagnosis of retroperitoneal fibrosis and some other causes of urinary obstruction, and may also demonstrate cortical scarring.
- *MRI.* Magnetic resonance angiography in renovascular disease.

Renal biopsy (see p. 618)

This should be performed in every patient with unexplained renal failure and normal-sized kidneys, unless there are strong contraindications. If rapidly progressive glomerulonephritis is possible, this investigation must be performed within 24 hours of presentation if at all possible, to guide immunosuppressive treatment.

COMPLICATIONS OF CHRONIC RENAL FAILURE

Anaemia

Several factors have been implicated:

- *erythropoietin deficiency* (the most significant)
- *bone marrow toxins* retained in renal failure

- *bone marrow fibrosis* secondary to hyperparathyroidism
- *haematinic deficiency* – iron, vitamin B_{12}, folate
- *increased red cell destruction*
- *abnormal red cell membranes* causing increased osmotic fragility
- *increased blood loss* – occult gastrointestinal bleeding, blood sampling, blood loss during haemodialysis or because of platelet dysfunction
- *ACE inhibitors* (may cause anaemia in chronic renal failure, probably by interfering with the control of endogenous erythropoietin release).

Red cell survival is reduced in renal failure. Increased red cell destruction may occur during haemodialysis owing to mechanical, oxidant and thermal damage.

Bone disease: renal osteodystrophy

The term 'renal osteodystrophy' embraces the various forms of bone disease that may develop alone or in combination in chronic renal failure – hyperparathyroid bone disease, osteomalacia, osteoporosis, osteosclerosis and adynamic bone disease (Fig. 11.44). Most patients with chronic renal failure are found, histologically, to have mixed bone disease. Covert renal osteodystrophy is present in many patients with moderate renal impairment and in almost all of those with end-stage renal failure.

Pathogenesis of bone disease

Decreased renal production of the 1α-hydroxylase enzyme results in reduced conversion of 25-$(OH)_2D_3$ to the more metabolically active $1,25$-$(OH)_2D_3$.

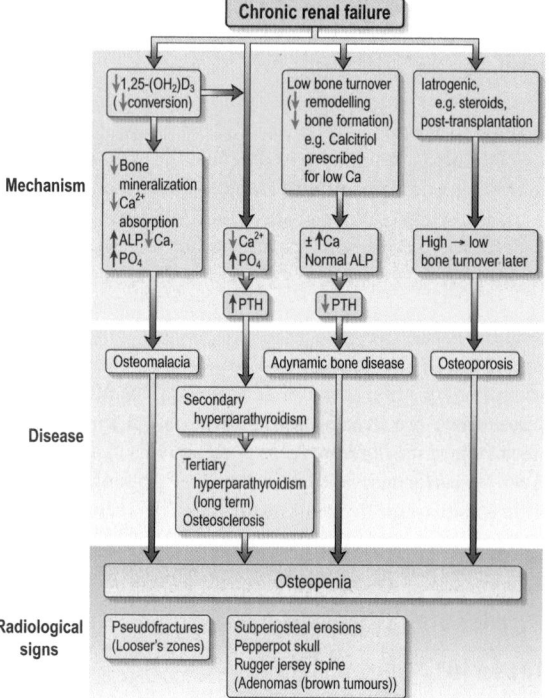

Fig. 11.44 Renal osteodystrophy: Pathogenesis and radiological features of renal bone disease. ALP, alkaline phosphatase.

- Reduced activation of vitamin D receptors in the parathyroid glands leads to increased release of parathyroid hormone.
- 1,25-Dihydroxycholecalciferol deficiency also results in gut calcium malabsorption.
- Phosphate retention owing to reduced excretion by the kidneys, also indirectly by lowering ionized calcium (and probably directly via a putative but unrecognized phosphate receptor), results in an increase in PTH synthesis and release.
- PTH promotes reabsorption of calcium from bone and increased proximal renal tubular reabsorption of calcium, and this opposes the tendency to develop hypocalcaemia induced by $1,25$-$(OH)_2D_3$ deficiency and phosphate retention. This '*secondary*' hyperparathyroidism leads to increased osteoclastic activity, cyst formation and bone marrow fibrosis (osteitis fibrosa cystica).

Radiologically, digital subperiosteal erosions and 'pepperpot skull' are seen. Long-standing secondary hyperparathyroidism ultimately leads to hyperplasia of the glands with *autonomous* or '*tertiary*' *hyperparathyroidism* in which hypercalcaemia is present. Serum alkaline phosphatase concentration is raised in both secondary and tertiary hyperparathyroidism. Long-standing parathyroid hormone excess is also thought to cause increased bone density (osteosclerosis) seen particularly in the spine where alternating bands of sclerotic and porotic bone give rise to a characteristic 'rugger jersey' appearance on X-ray.

$1,25$-$(OH)_2D_3$ deficiency and hypocalcaemia result in impaired mineralization of osteoid (*osteomalacia*). Such impaired mineralization also occurs when osteoblasts are inhibited by, for example, aluminium given as gut phosphorus binders, or accumulated in bone as a result of exposure to aluminium in source water used to make up dialysate for haemodialysis. In this situation, serum alkaline phosphatase concentration tends to be low or normal.

The condition of 'adynamic bone disease' in which both bone formation and resorption are depressed (in the absence of aluminium bone disease or overtreatment with vitamin D) is also seen. The pathogenesis of this condition is unclear and it is not known whether it leads to an increased risk of fractures or other complications. There may be hypercalcaemia; the serum alkaline phosphatase is normal, the PTH is low. X-rays and DEXA scan show osteopenia. No treatment is of proven benefit.

Osteoporosis is commonly found in CRF, often after transplantation and the use of corticosteroids. Monitoring is with yearly DEXA scan.

Management is discussed on page 596.

Skin disease

Pruritus (itching) is common in severe renal failure and is usually attributed in the main to retention of nitrogenous waste products of protein catabolism. Certainly, marked improvement often follows the institution of dialysis. Other causes of pruritus include:

- hypercalcaemia
- hyperphosphataemia
- elevated calcium × phosphate product
- hyperparathyroidism (even if calcium and phosphate levels are normal)
- iron deficiency.

In dialysis patients, inadequate dialysis is a cause of pruritus. Nevertheless, a significant number of dialysis patients who are well dialysed and in whom other causes of pruritus can be excluded suffer persistent itching. The cause is unknown and no effective treatment exists.

Many patients with renal failure suffer from dry skin for which simple aqueous creams are helpful. Eczematous lesions, particularly in relation to the region of an arteriovenous fistula, are relatively common. Chronic renal failure may also cause porphyria cutanea tarda (PCT), a blistering photosensitive skin rash. This results from a decrease in hepatic uroporphyrinogen decarboxylase combined with a decreased clearance of porphyrins in the urine or by dialysis. Pseudoporphyria a condition similar to PCT but without enzyme deficiency is also seen in CRF with increased frequency.

Gastrointestinal complications
These include:

- decreased gastric emptying and increased risk of reflux oesophagitis
- increased risk of peptic ulceration
- increased risk of acute pancreatitis
- constipation – particularly in patients on continuous ambulatory peritoneal dialysis (CAPD).

Elevations of *serum amylase* of up to three times normal may be found in chronic renal failure without any evidence of pancreatic disease, owing to retention of high-molecular-weight forms of amylase normally excreted in the urine.

Metabolic abnormalities
Gout. Urate retention is a common feature of chronic renal failure. Treatment of clinical gout is complicated by the nephrotoxic potential of NSAIDs. Colchicine is useful in treatment of the acute attack, and allopurinol should be introduced later under colchicine cover to prevent further attacks. The dose of allopurinol should be reduced in renal impairment.

Insulin. Insulin is catabolized by and to some extent excreted via the kidneys. For this reason, insulin requirements in diabetic patients decrease as renal failure progresses. By contrast, end-organ resistance to insulin is a feature of advanced renal impairment resulting in modestly impaired glucose tolerance when a standard glucose tolerance test is carried out. Insulin resistance may contribute to hypertension and lipid abnormalities.

Lipid metabolism abnormalities. These are common in renal failure, and include:

- impaired clearance of triglyceride-rich particles
- hypercholesterolaemia (particularly in advanced renal failure).

The situation is further complicated in end-stage renal disease, when regular heparinization (in haemodialysis), excessive glucose absorption (in CAPD) and immunosuppressive drugs (in transplantation) may all contribute to lipid abnormalities. Correction of lipid abnormalities by, for example, HMG-CoA reductase inhibitor therapy (statins) is used in renal failure patients, although without formal proof of benefit derived from prospective controlled trials.

Endocrine abnormalities
These include:

- hyperprolactinaemia, which may present with galactorrhoea in men as well as women
- increased luteinizing hormone (LH) levels in both sexes, and abnormal pulsatility of LH release
- decreased serum testosterone levels (only seldom below the normal level); sexual dysfunction and decreased spermatogenesis are common
- absence of normal cyclical changes in female sex hormones, resulting in oligomenorrhoea or amenorrhoea
- complex abnormalities of growth hormone secretion and action, resulting in impaired growth in uraemic children (pharmacological treatment with recombinant growth hormone and insulin-like growth factor is used)
- abnormal thyroid hormone levels, partly because of altered protein binding.

Measurement of thyroid-stimulating hormone (TSH) is the best way to assess thyroid function. True hypothyroidism occurs with increased frequency in renal failure. Posterior pituitary gland function is normal in renal failure.

Muscle dysfunction
Uraemia appears to interfere with muscle energy metabolism, but the mechanism is uncertain. Decreased physical fitness (cardiovascular deconditioning) also contributes.

Nervous system
Central nervous system
Severe uraemia causes an unusual combination of depressed cerebral function and decreased seizure threshold. However, convulsions in a uraemic patient are much more commonly due to other causes such as accelerated hypertension, thrombotic thrombocytopenic purpura, or drug accumulation. Asterixis, tremor and myoclonus are also features of severe uraemia.

Rapid correction of severe uraemia by haemodialysis leads to 'dialysis disequilibrium' owing to osmotic cerebral swelling. This can be avoided by correcting uraemia gradually by short, repeated haemodialysis treatments or by the use of peritoneal dialysis.

'Dialysis dementia' is a syndrome of progressive intellectual deterioration, speech disturbance, myoclonus and fits, which is due to aluminium intoxication; it may be accompanied by aluminium bone disease and by microcytic anaemia. Low-grade aluminium exposure may also cause more subtle, subclinical deterioration in intellectual function. Prevention involves removal of aluminium from source water used to manufacture dialysis fluid, and restriction or avoidance of aluminium-containing gut-phosphorus binders. Treatment is with the chelating agent desferrioxamine.

Autonomic nervous system
Autonomic dysfunction is common in renal impairment. Findings include:

- increased circulating catecholamine levels associated with down-regulation of α-receptors
- impaired baroreceptor sensitivity
- impaired efferent vagal function.

Overactivity of the sympathetic nervous system in chronic renal failure is believed to play a part in the genesis of hypertension in this condition. All of these abnormalities improve to some extent after institution of regular dialysis and resolve after successful renal transplantation.

Peripheral nervous system
Median nerve compression in the carpal tunnel is common, usually due to β_2-microglobulin-related amyloidosis. 'Restless legs' syndrome (p. 666) is common in uraemia. The syndrome is difficult to treat. Iron deficiency should be treated if present. Attention should be paid to adequacy of dialysis. Symptoms may improve with the correction of anaemia by erythropoietin. Clonazepam is sometimes useful. Renal transplantation cures the problem. A polyneuropathy occurs in patients who are inadequately dialysed.

Psychiatric problems are common. Patients can have anxiety, depression, phobias and psychoses.

Cardiovascular disease
Life expectancy remains severely reduced compared with the normal population owing to a greatly increased (16-fold) incidence of cardiovascular disease, particularly myocardial infarction, cardiac failure, sudden cardiac death and stroke.

Risk factors
Hypertension is a frequent complication of renal failure. Diabetes mellitus is the commonest cause of end-stage renal failure. Dyslipidaemia is universal in uraemic patients. Furthermore, smoking is as common as in the general population and male gender is over-represented in patients with CRF. Cardiac hypertrophy is common, as is systolic and diastolic dysfunction. Diastolic dysfunction is largely attributable to left ventricular hypertrophy and contributes to hypotension during fluid removal on haemodialysis. Systolic dysfunction may be due to:

- myocardial fibrosis
- abnormal myocyte function owing to uraemia

- calcium overload and hyperparathyroidism
- carnitine and selenium deficiency.

Left ventricular hypertrophy is a risk factor for early death in renal failure, as in the general population. Systolic dysfunction is also a marker for early death in renal failure.

Coronary artery calcification. Traditional risk factors (e.g. smoking, diabetes) can only in part explain the risk differential between the general population and the population of patients with chronic nephropathies. Coronary artery calcification is more common in patients with end-stage renal failure than in normal individuals and it is highly likely that this contributes significantly to cardiovascular mortality. Vascular calcification is frequent in all sizes of vessel in renal failure. In addition to the classical risk factors for atherosclerosis, a raised calcium × phosphate product causes medial calcification. Hyperparathyroidism may also contribute independently to the pathogenesis by increasing intracellular calcium. It is now believed that vascular calcification in uraemia is an active process whereby vascular smooth muscle cells acquire osteoblast-like characteristics, possibly in response to elevated phosphate or calcium × phosphate product. Recently, inflammation has emerged as a potent mediator of vascular calcification by inhibition of fetuin (a glycoprotein synthesized by liver, which is a potent inhibitor of vascular calcification). The impact of vascular calcification is the reduction of vascular compliance, which manifests by increased pulse pressure and pulse wave velocity, and increased afterload contributing further to left ventricular hypertrophy. In addition to myocardial abnormalities, vascular calcification with its associated biomechanical vessel wall alterations is a strong predictor of all-cause and cardiovascular morbidity and mortality in patients with CRF. Diffuse calcification of the myocardium is also common; the causes are similar.

Other cardiovascular risk factors. These include hyperhomocysteinaemia, *Chlamydia pneumoniae* infection, oxidative stress and elevated endogenous inhibitor of nitric oxide synthase and asymmetric dimethyl arginine (ADMA) levels. High ADMA levels in uraemia are in part caused by oxidative stress and can possibly explain the 52% increase in the risk of death and 34% increase in the risk of cardiovascular events in uraemic patients. The use of antioxidants, vitamin E or *N*-acetylcysteine has been associated with a significant reduction in all-cause and cardiovascular mortality.

Pericarditis
This is common and occurs in two clinical settings:

- Uraemic pericarditis is a feature of severe, pre-terminal uraemia or of underdialysis. Haemorrhagic pericardial effusion and atrial arrhythmias are often associated. There is a danger of pericardial tamponade, and anticoagulants should be used with caution. Pericarditis usually resolves with intensive dialysis.

- Dialysis pericarditis occurs as a result of an intercurrent illness or surgery in a patient receiving apparently adequate dialysis.

Malignancy

The incidence of malignancy is raised in patients with CRF and with dialysis. Malignant change can occur in multicystic kidney disease. Lymphomas, primary liver cancer and thyroid cancers also occur.

Management

Successful renal transplantation improves some, but not all, of the complications of CRF, therefore, attempts should be made to prevent these complications by careful monitoring with ECG, echocardiography, angiography (if necessary) and nuclear imaging. CT (electron beam tomography, spiral CT) and/or MRI are useful in the assessment of arterial calcification. Treatment is with the control of risk factors (p. 670) as well as the treatment of hypercalcaemia and hyperparathyroidism (p. 670).

PROGRESSION OF CHRONIC RENAL IMPAIRMENT

Once established, and whatever the initial cause, chronic renal impairment tends to progress inexorably to end-stage renal failure, although the rate of progression may depend upon the underlying nephropathy. Patients with chronic glomerular diseases tend to deteriorate more quickly than those with chronic tubulointerstitial nephropathies. Hypertension and heavy proteinuria are bad prognostic indicators in this context. A non-specific renal scarring process common to renal disorders of different aetiologies may be responsible for progression.

In 1982, the hypothesis of 'glomerular hyperfiltration' in response to nephron loss was postulated as a common pathway of progression of renal failure. A rise in intraglomerular capillary pressure and adaptive glomerular hypertrophy due to reduced arteriolar resistance and increased glomerular blood flow under conditions of reduced nephron mass have been postulated as causes of glomerular scarring and proteinuria. Since the afferent arteriolar tone decreases more than efferent arteriolar tone, intraglomerular pressure and the amount of filtrate formed by a single nephron rises. Angiotensin II produced locally modulates intraglomerular capillary pressure and GFR. Angiotensin II predominantly causes vasoconstriction of postglomerular arterioles, thereby increasing the glomerular hydraulic pressure and filtration fraction (Fig. 11.45). In addition, by its effect on mesangial cells and podocytes, it increases the pore sizes and impairs the size-selective function of basement membrane for macromolecules. Angiotensin II also modulates cell growth directly and indirectly by upregulating TGF-β, a potent fibrogenic cytokine, increases collagen synthesis and also causes epithelial cell transdifferentiation to myofibroblasts which contribute to excessive matrix formation. Furthermore, angiotensin II by upregulating plasminogen activator inhibitor-1 (PAI-1) inhibits matrix proteolysis by plasmin, resulting in accumulation of excessive matrix and scarring both in the glomeruli and interstitium.

Renal interstitial scarring is also a factor. The prognosis for renal function in chronic glomerular disorders is judged more accurately by interstitial histological appearances than by glomerular morphology. The cause of this progressive interstitial damage and fibrosis is mutifactorial. In addition to non-haemodynamic effects of angiotensin II, proteinuria per se by exposing tubular cells to albumin and its bound fatty acids and cytokines promotes secretion of pro-inflammatory mediators, which by promoting interstitial inflammatory cell infiltrate further augments fibrosis and progression of renal failure. Therapeutic manoeuvres aimed at inhibiting angiotensin II and reducing proteinuria mainly by ACEI and angiotensin-receptor antagonists have beneficial effects in slowing the rate of progression of renal failure in both diabetic and non-diabetic renal diseases in humans.

Fig. 11.45 **Glomerular dynamics**: Effect of the renin–angiotensin system. AI, angiotensin I; AII, angiotensin II.

MANAGEMENT OF CHRONIC RENAL FAILURE

The underlying cause of renal disease should be treated aggressively wherever possible.

Renoprotection

The multidrug approach to chronic nephropathies has been formalized in an international protocol (Box 11.3).

Correction of complications

Hyperkalaemia

Hyperkalaemia often responds to dietary restriction of potassium intake. Drugs which cause potassium retention (see p. 708) should be stopped. Occasionally it may be necessary to prescribe ion-exchange resins to remove potassium in the gastrointestinal tract. Emergency treatment of severe hyperkalaemia is described on page 709.

Acidosis

Correction of acidosis helps to correct hyperkalaemia in chronic renal failure, and may also decrease muscle catabolism. Sodium bicarbonate supplements are often effective (4.8 g (57 mmol) of Na^+ and HCO_3^- daily), but may cause oedema and hypertension owing to extracellular fluid expansion. Calcium carbonate, also used as a calcium supplement and phosphate binder, has a beneficial effect on acidosis.

Calcium and phosphate control and suppression of PTH

Hypocalcaemia and hyperphosphataemia should be treated aggressively, preferably with regular (e.g. 3-monthly) measurements of serum PTH to assess how effectively hyperparathyroidism is being suppressed.

Box 11.3 Renoprotection

Goals of treatment
BP < 120/80
Proteinuria < 0.3 g/24 hours

Treatment
Patients with chronic renal failure and proteinuria
> 1 g/24 hours:
■ ACE inhibitor increasing to maximum dose
■ Add angiotensin receptor antagonist if goals are not achieved*
■ Add diuretic to prevent hyperkalaemia and help to control BP
■ Add calcium-channel blocker (verapamil or diltiazem) if goals not achieved

Additional measures
■ Statins to lower cholesterol to < 4.5 mmol/L
■ Stop smoking (threefold higher rate of deterioration in CRF)
■ Treat diabetes (HbA_{1c} < 7%)
■ Normal protein diet (0.8–1 g/kg bodyweight)

*In type 2 diabetes start with angiotensin receptor antagonist

Suppression of PTH levels to below two or three times the upper limit of 'normal' carries a high risk of development of adynamic bone disease.

Dietary restriction of phosphate is seldom effective alone, because so many foods contain it. Oral calcium carbonate or acetate reduces absorption of dietary phosphate but is contraindicated where there is hypercalcaemia or hypercalciuria. Aluminium-containing gut phosphate binders are very effective but absorption of aluminium poses the risk of aluminium bone disease and development of cognitive impairment. Regular monitoring of plasma aluminium should be carried out, and signs of aluminium toxicity mandate chelation with desferrioxamine. The polymer sevelamer is also used as a gut phosphate binder. It reduces the calcium load and attenuates vascular calcification and also lowers cholesterol levels by 10%. Lanthanum carbonate is a new non-calcium, non-aluminium phosphate binder that is effective and has a good safety profile. It is currently undergoing approval in Europe and the USA for clinical use. An alternative to phosphate binders is nicotinamide, which blocks the intestinal sodium/inorganic phosphate (Na/Pi) cotransporter. Preliminary results are very promising in that it reduced phosphate levels and PTH levels in dialysis patients alongside improvement in the lipid profile. This approach may become a useful alternative for the suppression of hyperparathyroidism and reduction of phosphate levels without inducing hypercalcaemia.

Treatment with calcitriol or a vitamin D analogue such as alfacalcidol in early renal impairment has no deleterious effect upon renal function provided hypercalcaemia is avoided. New vitamin D metabolites (22-oxacalcitriol, paricalcitol, doxercalciferol) are less calcaemic. However, with the exception of paricalcitol (19-nor-1,25 dihydroxyvitamin D_2, which may have survival advantage), their usefulness over conventional but less expensive calcitriol or alphacalcidol remains to be established. Treatment with vitamin D analogues should be started only if serum PTH level is three times or more above the upper limit of normal, in order to prevent the development of adynamic bone disease (see p. 668). Vitamin D therapy has the disadvantage that it increases not only calcium but also phosphate absorption and may therefore exacerbate hyperphosphataemia and ectopic calcification including calciphylaxis (calcification of small vessels). Calcimimetic agents (e.g. cinacalcet – calcium-sensing receptor agonist) have also been tried in established secondary hyperparathyroidism with successful suppression of PTH levels and lowering of calcium × phosphate product. Long-term safety and efficacy of these agents remains to be established.

Drug therapy

This should be minimized in patients with chronic renal impairment. Tetracyclines (with the possible exception of doxycycline) should be avoided in view of their anti-anabolic effect and tendency to worsen uraemia. Drugs excreted by the kidneys, such as gentamicin, should be prescribed with caution and drug levels monitored if feasible. Non-steroidal anti-inflammatory drugs should be avoided. Potassium-sparing agents, such as spironolactone and amiloride, pose particular dangers, as do artificial salt substitutes, all of which contain potassium.

Anaemia

The anaemia of erythropoietin (EPO) deficiency can be treated with synthetic (recombinant) human EPO (erythropoietin-alpha or -beta, or the longer-acting darbopoietin-alpha). Subcutaneous administration of erythropoietin-alpha is contraindicated (see below) in CRF and the intravenous route is used, initially 50 U/kg of epoietin-alpha over 1–5 min three times weekly. Blood pressure, haemoglobin concentration and reticulocyte count are measured every 2 weeks and the dose adjusted to maintain a target haemoglobin of 10–12 g/dL.

Failure to respond to 300 U/kg weekly, or a fall in haemoglobin after a satisfactory response, may be due to iron deficiency, bleeding, malignancy, infection or formation of anti-EPO neutralizing antibodies. The demand for iron by the bone marrow is enormous when erythropoietin is commenced. Patients on EPO therapy are regularly monitored for iron status and considered iron deficient if plasma ferritin is < 100 μg/L, hypochromic RBCs > 5%, transferin saturation < 20%. Intravenous (rather than oral) iron supplements optimize response to EPO treatment by repletion of iron stores.

Correction of anaemia with EPO improves quality of life, exercise tolerance, sexual and cognitive function in dialysis patients, and leads to regression of left ventricular hypertrophy. Avoidance of blood transfusion also lessens the chance of sensitization to HLA antigens, which may otherwise be a barrier to successful renal transplantation.

The disadvantages of erythropoietin therapy are that it is expensive and causes a rise in blood pressure in up to 30% of patients, particularly in the first 6 months. Peripheral resistance rises in all patients, owing to loss of hypoxic vasodilatation and to increased blood viscosity. A rare complication is encephalopathy with fits, transient cortical blindness and hypertension. Recently, several reports of anti-EPO antibody-mediated pure red cell aplasia in patients receiving subcutaneous EPO therapy (particularly EPO alpha) have been described. The exact cause is unknown but interventions such as using the intravenous route and changes in manufacture have reduced the number of cases by 80%. Other causes of anaemia should be looked for and treated appropriately (see p. 423).

Male erectile dysfunction

Testosterone deficiency should be corrected. The oral phosphodiesterase inhibitors, e.g. sildenafil, tadalafil and vardenafil, are effective in end-stage renal failure and are the first line of therapy. The use of nitrates is a contraindication to this treatment. Other treatments are discussed on page 1055.

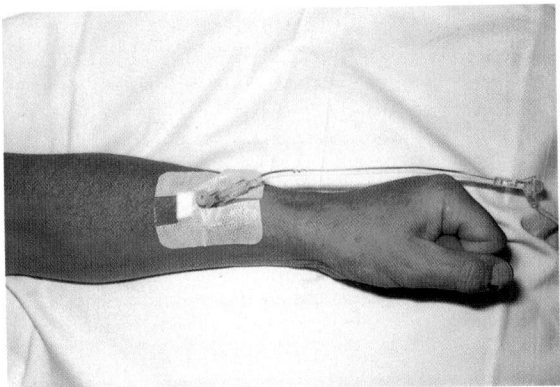

Fig. 11.46 **Intravenous cannula in exactly the wrong place**, in a right-handed patient with chronic renal impairment who will in future need a left (non-dominant arm) radiocephalic fistula.

EARLY REFERRAL OF PATIENTS WITH CHRONIC RENAL FAILURE

Patients with chronic renal impairment should be referred to a nephrologist with access to facilities for renal replacement therapy at an early stage since late referral has been shown to be associated with increased mortality and morbidity when such patients commence renal replacement therapy. Old age is no bar to referral in the reasonably fit elderly patient.

Patients need time to adjust to the demands of chronic renal failure and its treatment, and to absorb information. Veins required in the future for fashioning of an arteriovenous fistula should not be rendered useless by cannulation (Fig. 11.46).

If the patient opts for regular haemodialysis, fashioning of an arteriovenous fistula should be carried out well in advance of the need for dialysis, when serum creatinine is of the order 400–500 mmol/L in non-diabetics and at an even earlier stage in diabetics with poorer vasculature. Such fistulae require several weeks to mature and become usable for vascular access.

RENAL REPLACEMENT THERAPY

Approximately 100 white individuals per million population commence renal replacement therapy in the UK each year. The corresponding figure in black Africans and Asians in the UK is three to four times higher, largely owing to diabetic and hypertensive nephropathy. The aim of all renal replacement techniques is to mimic the excretory functions of the normal kidney, including excretion of nitrogenous wastes, maintenance of normal electrolyte concentrations, and maintenance of a normal extracellular volume.

Haemodialysis

Basic principles

In haemodialysis, blood from the patient is pumped through an array of semipermeable membranes (the

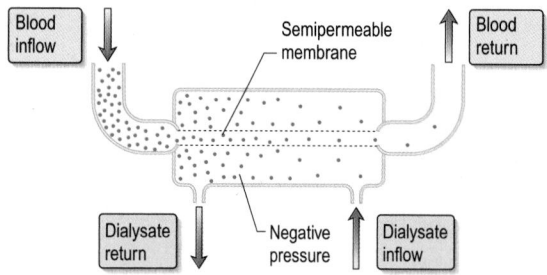

Fig. 11.47 Changes across a semipermeable dialysis membrane.

Table 11.20 Range of concentrations (mmol/L) in routinely available final dialysates used for haemodialysis	
Sodium	130–145
Potassium	0.0–4.0
Calcium	1.0–1.6
Magnesium	0.25–0.85
Chloride	99–108
Bicarbonate	35–40
OR	
Acetate	35–40
Glucose	0–10

dialyser, often called an 'artificial kidney') which bring the blood into close contact with dialysate, flowing countercurrent to the blood. The plasma biochemistry changes towards that of the dialysate owing to diffusion of molecules down their concentration gradients (Fig. 11.47).

The dialysis machine comprises a series of blood pumps, with pressure monitors and bubble detectors and a proportionating unit, also with pressure monitors and blood leak detectors. Blood flow during dialysis is usually 200–300 mL per minute and the dialysate flow usually 500 mL per minute. The efficiency of dialysis in achieving biochemical change depends on blood and dialysate flow and the surface area of the dialysis membrane.

Dialysate is prepared by a proportionating unit, which mixes specially purified water with concentrate, resulting in fluid with the composition described in Table 11.20. Highly permeable synthetic membranes allow more rapid haemodialysis than with cellulose-based membranes (high-flux haemodialysis).

Access for haemodialysis

Adequate dialysis requires a blood flow of at least 200 mL per minute. The most reliable long-term way of achieving this is surgical construction of an arteriovenous fistula (Fig. 11.48a, b), using the radial or brachial artery and the cephalic vein. This results in distension of the vein and thickening ('arterialization') of its wall, so that after 6–8 weeks, large-bore needles may be inserted to take blood to and from the dialysis machine. In patients with poor-quality veins or arterial disease (e.g. diabetes mellitus) arteriovenous polytetrafluoroethylene (PTFE)

(a)

(b)

Fig. 11.48 Arteriovenous (radiocephalic) fistula. **(a)** In the left forearm. **(b)** One way of reminding the anaesthetic, nursing and surgical team about the presence of an existing arteriovenous fistula in a haemodialysis patient about to undergo surgery. In particular, the fistula should not be compressed during surgery to avoid thrombosis within it.

grafts are used for access. However, these grafts have a very high incidence of thrombosis and 2-year graft patency is only 50–60%. Dipyridamole or fish oils improve graft patency but warfarin, aspirin and clopidogrel do not and are associated with a high incidence of complications.

If dialysis is needed immediately, a large-bore double-lumen cannula may be inserted into a central vein – usually the subclavian, jugular or femoral. *Semipermanent dual-lumen venous catheters* can also be used, usually inserted via a skin tunnel to lessen the risk of infection. Nevertheless, local and systemic sepsis is high, with increased morbidity and mortality. Stenosis of the subclavian vein is also common, and the jugular route is preferred.

Dialysis prescription

Dialysis must be tailored to an individual patient to obtain optimal results.

Dry weight

This is the weight at which a patient is neither fluid overloaded nor depleted. Patients are weighed at the start of each dialysis session and the transmembrane pressure adjusted to achieve fluid removal equal to the amount by which they exceed their dry weight.

The dialysate buffer

The dialysate buffer is usually acetate or bicarbonate. The sodium and calcium concentrations of the dialysate buffer are carefully monitored. A high dialysate sodium causes thirst and hypertension. A high dialysate calcium causes hypercalcaemia, whilst a low-calcium dialysate combined with poor compliance of medication with oral calcium carbonate and vitamin D may result in hyperparathyroidism.

Frequency and duration

Frequency and duration of dialysis are adjusted to achieve adequate removal of uraemic metabolites and to avoid excessive fluid overload between dialysis sessions. An adult of average size usually receives 4–5 hours' treatment three times a week. Twice-weekly dialysis is adequate only if the patient has considerable residual renal function.

Short-duration dialysis using very biocompatible high-flux membranes is commonly employed. Advantages include shorter duration of treatment and hence increased patient convenience. Disadvantages include higher cost of the membranes employed and, in all probability, higher prevalence of hypertension in such patients, requiring hypotensive medication. It should not be forgotten that normal kidneys work for 24 hours a day, 7 days a week, and that dialysis is a poor substitute for the natural state.

Adequate/optimal dialysis should be adjusted to individual patient's needs. All patients are anticoagulated (usually with heparin) during treatment as contact with foreign surfaces activates the clotting cascade. In the UK, a small number of patients manage self-supervised home haemodialysis.

Complications

Hypotension during dialysis is the major complication. Contributing factors include: an excessive removal of extracellular fluid, inadequate 'refilling' of the blood compartment from the interstitial compartment during fluid removal, abnormalities of venous tone, autonomic neuropathy, acetate intolerance (acetate acts as a vasodilator) and left ventricular hypertrophy.

Very rarely patients may develop anaphylactic reactions to ethylene oxide, which is used to sterilize most dialysers. Patients receiving ACE inhibitors are at risk of anaphylaxis if polyacrylonitrile dialysers are used.

Other potential, rare, complications include the hard-water syndrome (caused by failure to soften water resulting in a high calcium concentration prior to mixing with dialysate concentrate), haemolytic reactions and air embolism.

Adequacy of dialysis

Dialysis treatment is empirical since the size, number and nature of 'uraemic toxins' is unclear. The only true measure of adequacy is patient mortality and morbidity. Adequate nutrition of the patient as well as adequate dialysis is necessary to reduce morbidity and mortality.

Symptoms of underdialysis are non-specific and include insomnia, itching, fatigue despite adequate correction of anaemia, restless legs and a peripheral sensory neuropathy.

Adequacy of dialysis may be assessed by computerized calculation of urea kinetics, requiring measurement of the residual renal urea clearance, the rate of rise of urea concentration between dialysis sessions, and the reduction in urea concentration during dialysis. The dialysis dose is normally defined in terms of urea reduction ratio (URR) and/or equilibrated urea clearance, eKt/V (where K is the dialyser clearance, t is the duration of dialysis in minutes, and V is the urea distribution volume estimated as total body water). Kt/V of 1.0–1.2 and/or URR of 65% per dialysis session is the minimum threshold required for well-nourished dialysis patients dialysed three times per week. It is unclear whether a higher eKt/V is associated with a better outcome, although no additional benefits of high (1.53) compared to standard (1.16) eKt/V were seen over 5 years follow-up. It is likely that duration of haemodialysis session is a factor in itself in addition to the efficiency with which small molecules such as urea are cleared. The best haemodialysis outcome data are seen in renal units where long hours (8 hours per session) of dialysis are routinely practiced.

Haemodialysis is the most efficient way of achieving rapid biochemical improvement, for instance in the treatment of acute renal failure or severe hyperkalaemia. This advantage is offset by disadvantages such as haemodynamic instability, especially in acutely ill patients with multiorgan disease, and over-rapid correction of uraemia can lead to 'dialysis disequilibrium'. This is characterized by nausea and vomiting, restlessness, headache, hypertension, myoclonic jerking, and in severe instances seizures and coma owing to rapid changes in plasma osmolality leading to cerebral oedema.

These problems have led to the increasing adoption of gentler continuous methods for the treatment of acute renal failure (see below).

Haemofiltration

This involves removal of plasma water and its dissolved constituents (e.g. K^+, Na^+, urea, phosphate) by convective flow across a high-flux semipermeable membrane, and replacing it with a solution of the desired biochemical composition (Fig. 11.49). Lactate is used as buffer in the replacement solution because rapid infusion of acetate causes vasodilatation and bicarbonate may cause precipitation of calcium carbonate.

Haemofiltration can be used for both acute and chronic renal failure. High volumes need to be exchanged in order to achieve adequate small molecule removal; typically a 22 L exchange three times a week for maintenance treatment and 1 L per hour in acute renal failure. Financial costs of disposable items (such as filters and replacement fluid) are high and only a tiny minority of

Fig. 11.49 **Principles of haemofiltration.**

Table 11.21 Range of concentrations (mmol/L) in routinely available CAPD dialysate*	
Sodium	130–134
Potassium	0
Calcium	1.0–1.75
Magnesium	0.25–0.75
Chloride	95–104
Lactate	35–40
Glucose	77–236
Total osmolality	356–511 mOsm/kg

* Glucose content is often expressed as g/dL of anhydrous glucose (e.g. 1.36% = 77 mmol/L). An even more hypertonic dialysate (6.36%) is available for acute (intermittent) peritoneal dialysis

patients with end-stage renal failure are managed in this way. However, nursing costs are reduced when acute renal failure is managed in an intensive care unit setting since haemofiltration can be managed by ITU nursing staff rather than renal unit nurses.

Peritoneal dialysis

Peritoneal dialysis utilizes the peritoneal membrane as a semipermeable membrane, avoiding the need for extracorporeal circulation of blood. This is a very simple, low-technology treatment compared to haemodialysis. The principles are simple (Fig. 11.50).

- A tube is placed into the peritoneal cavity through the anterior abdominal wall.
- Dialysate is run into the peritoneal cavity, usually under gravity.
- Urea, creatinine, phosphate, and other uraemic toxins pass into the dialysate down their concentration gradients.
- Water (with solutes) is attracted into the peritoneal cavity by osmosis, depending on the osmolarity of the dialysate. This is determined by the glucose or polymer (icodextrin) content of the dialysate (Table 11.21).
- The fluid is changed regularly to repeat the process.

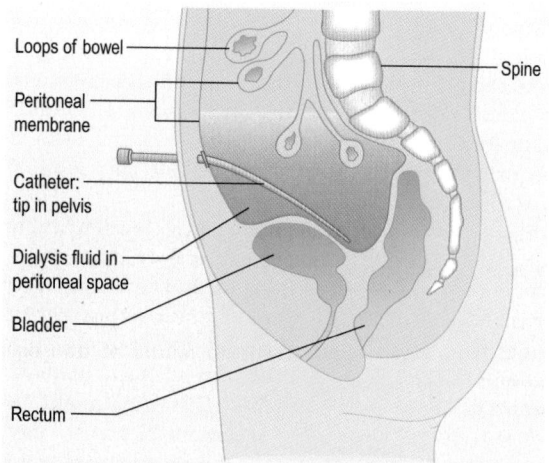

Fig. 11.51 **The siting of a Tenckhoff peritoneal dialysis catheter.**

Chronic peritoneal dialysis requires insertion of a soft catheter, with its tip in the pelvis, exiting the peritoneal cavity in the midline and lying in a skin tunnel with an exit site in the lateral abdominal wall (Fig. 11.51).

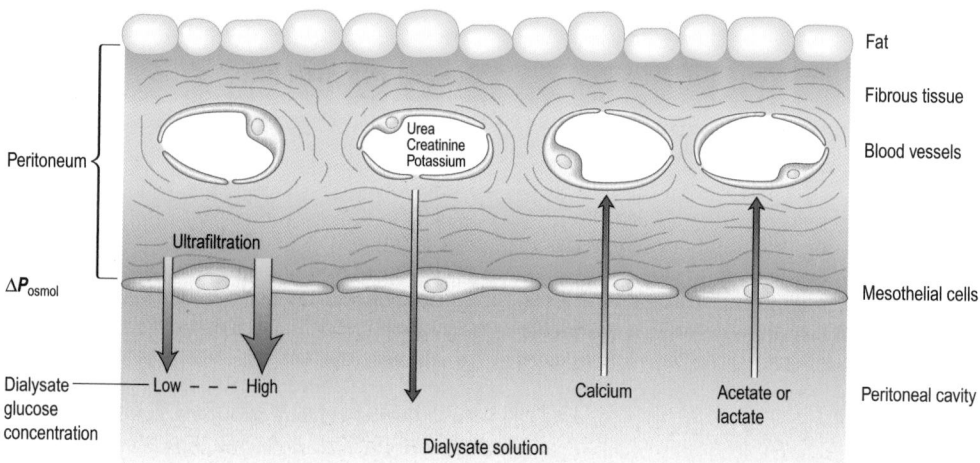

Fig. 11.50 **Principles of peritoneal dialysis.** Water is attracted into the peritoneal cavity depending on the osmolarity of the dialysate.

This form of dialysis can be adapted in several ways.

- **Continuous ambulatory peritoneal dialysis (CAPD).** Dialysate is present within the peritoneal cavity continuously, except when dialysate is being exchanged. Dialysate exchanges are performed three to five times a day, using a sterile no-touch technique to connect 1.5–3 L bags of dialysate to the peritoneal catheter; each exchange takes 20–40 minutes. This is the technique most often used for maintenance peritoneal dialysis in patients with end-stage renal failure.
- **Nightly intermittent peritoneal dialysis (NIPD).** An automated device is used to perform exchanges each night while the patient is asleep. Sometimes dialysate is left in the peritoneal cavity during the day in addition, to increase the time during which biochemical exchange is occurring.
- **Tidal dialysis.** A residual volume is left within the peritoneal cavity with continuous cycling of smaller volumes in and out.

Osmotic removal of excess plasma water and solutes is achieved using hypertonic dialysate, which exerts an osmotic 'drag'. Depending on the patient's fluid intake and residual urine output, it may be necessary to use one or more hypertonic dialysate bags daily to achieve fluid balance in CAPD. Fluid overload is a relatively common problem in CAPD, and is due to failure of transport across the peritoneal membrane.

Complications

Peritonitis

Bacterial peritonitis is the most common serious complication of CAPD and other forms of peritoneal dialysis. Clinical presentations include abdominal pain of varying severity (guarding and rebound tenderness are unusual), and a cloudy peritoneal effluent – without which, the diagnosis cannot be made. Microscopy reveals a neutrophil count of above 100 cells per mL. Nausea, vomiting, fever and paralytic ileus may be seen if peritonitis is severe. The incidence of CAPD-associated peritonitis has been much reduced (to about one episode every two patient years) by use of a Y-disconnect system in preference to previous methods.

CAPD peritonitis must be investigated with culture of peritoneal effluent. Empirical antibiotic treatment is started, with a spectrum which covers both Gram-negative and Gram-positive organisms. Antibiotics may be given by the oral, intravenous or intraperitoneal route; most centres rely on intraperitoneal antibiotics. Common causative organisms are listed in Table 11.22.

Staph. aureus peritonitis should lead to a search for nasal carriage of this organism, and *Staph. epidermidis* peritonitis may indicate contamination from the patient's (or helper's) skin. Relapsing *Staph. epidermidis* peritonitis with an organism with the same antibiotic sensitivity pattern on each occasion may indicate that the Tenckhoff catheter has become colonized: often this is difficult to eradicate without replacement of the catheter under antibiotic cover.

Table 11.22 Some causes of CAPD peritonitis*

	Approximate percentage of cases
Staphylococcus epidermidis	40–50
Escherichia coli, Pseudomonas and other Gram-negative organisms	25
Staphylococcus aureus	15
Mycobacterium tuberculosis	2
Candida and other fungal species	2

* In approximately 20%, no bacteria are found

Gram-negative peritonitis may complicate septicaemia from urinary or bowel infection. A mixed growth of Gram-negative and anaerobic organisms strongly suggests bowel perforation, and is an indication for laparotomy.

Fungal peritonitis often follows antibacterial treatment but may occur de novo. Clinical presentation is very variable. It is rare to be able to cure fungal peritonitis without catheter removal as well as antifungal treatment. Intraperitoneal amphotericin has been associated with the formation of peritoneal adhesions.

Infection around the catheter site

Infection where the catheter exits through the skin is relatively common. It should be treated aggressively (with systemic and/or local antibiotics) to prevent spread of the infection into the subcutaneous tunnel and the peritoneum. The most common causative organisms are staphylococci.

Other complications

CAPD is often associated with constipation, which in turn may impair flow of dialysate in and out of the pelvis. Occasionally dialysate may leak through a diaphragmatic defect into the thoracic cavity, causing a massive pleural 'effusion'. The glucose content of the effusion is usually diagnostic, or the diagnosis may be made by instillation of methylthioninium chloride (methylene blue) with dialysate and the demonstration of a blue colour on pleural tap. Dialysate may also leak into the scrotum down a patent processus vaginalis.

Failure of peritoneal membrane function is a predictable complication of long-term CAPD, resulting in worsening biochemical exchange and decreased ultrafiltration with hypertonic dialysate. It is thought that this problem may be accelerated by excessive reliance on hypertonic dialysate to remove fluid.

Sclerosing peritonitis is a potentially fatal complication of CAPD. The cause is often unclear, but recurrent peritonitis, and exposure of the peritoneum to unphysiological high glucose concentrations, is responsible in most cases. Progressive thickening of the peritoneal membrane occurs in association with adhesions and strictures, turning the small bowel into a mass of matted loops and causing repeated episodes of small bowel obstruction. CAPD should be abandoned. Improvement may follow renal transplantation or treatment with prednisolone or azathioprine.

Contraindications

There are few absolute contraindications apart from unwillingness or inability on the patient's part to learn the technique.

Previous peritonitis causing peritoneal adhesions may make peritoneal dialysis impossible: but the extent of adhesions is difficult to predict, and it may be worth an attempted surgical placement of a dialysis catheter.

The presence of a stoma (colostomy, ileostomy, ileal urinary conduit) makes successful placement of a dialysis catheter extremely unlikely.

Active intra-abdominal sepsis, for instance due to diverticular abscesses, is an absolute contraindication to peritoneal dialysis although diverticular disease per se is not.

Abdominal hernias may often expand during CAPD as a result of increased intra-abdominal pressure, and should ideally be repaired before or at the time of CAPD catheter insertion.

Visual impairment may make it difficult for a patient to perform dialysate exchanges, but completely blind patients can be trained in the technique if adequately motivated.

Severe arthritis makes it difficult to perform the exchanges, but a large number of mechanical aids are available. Sterilization of connections by heat or ultraviolet light reduces the risk of peritonitis.

Recent studies suggest that end-stage renal failure patients with coronary artery disease or congestive heart failure have significantly higher morbidity and mortality on CAPD compared to HD. Moreover, elderly patients do worse on CAPD than younger patients. It is advisable to consider HD as the first-choice dialysis modality in these patients where it is possible.

Adequacy of peritoneal dialysis

No consensus yet exists on how the adequacy of peritoneal dialysis should be measured and the optimum degree of removal of urea and other waste products to be obtained in unit time. Urea kinetic modelling may be employed, as with haemodialysis. Based on observational studies, weekly Kt/V of 2.0 coupled with a creatinine clearance target of 60 L per week has been recommended. However, in a recent randomized prospective study (ADEMEX), standard daily exchanges of 8 L in total (creatinine clearance 40 L per week) compared to a creatinine clearance of 60 L per week yielded similar patient and technique survival. Peritoneal dialysis inadequacy becomes common when residual renal function declines to zero. With increasing time on treatment, adequacy may become impaired owing to alterations in the efficiency of the peritoneal membrane in transporting waste products, fluid and electrolytes.

Complications of long-term dialysis

Cardiovascular disease (see p. 670) and sepsis are the leading causes of death in long-term dialysis patients.

Causes of fatal sepsis include peritonitis complicating peritoneal dialysis and *Staph. aureus* infection (including endocarditis) complicating the use of indwelling access devices for haemodialysis.

Dialysis amyloidosis

This is the accumulation of amyloid protein (p. 1147) as a result of failure of clearance of β_2-microglobulin, a molecule of 11.8 kDa. This protein is the light chain of the class I HLA antigens and is normally freely filtered at the glomerulus but is not removed by cellulose-based haemodialysis membranes. The protein polymerizes, possibly after modification by non-enzymic glycosylation, to form amyloid deposits, which may cause median nerve compression in the carpal tunnel or a dialysis arthropathy – a clinical syndrome of pain and disabling stiffness in the shoulders, hips, hands, wrists and knees. β_2-microglobulin-related amyloid may be demonstrated in the synovium. Amyloid deposits can also cause pathological bone cysts and fractures, pseudotumours and gastrointestinal bleeding caused by amyloid deposition around submucosal blood vessels. The extent of amyloid deposition is best assessed by nuclear imaging, either using [^{99m}Tc]DMSA, or, more specifically, by the use of radiolabelled serum amyloid P component.

Rapid improvement after renal transplantation is probably due to steroid therapy as low-dose prednisolone alone can also cause an improvement. A change to a biocompatible synthetic membrane has also been reported to be of benefit: again, the mechanism for this improvement is not clear.

Transplantation

Successful renal transplantation offers the potential for almost complete rehabilitation in end-stage renal failure. This mode of renal replacement therapy has significant survival advantage compared to dialysis patients on transplant waiting lists. It allows freedom from dietary and fluid restriction; anaemia and infertility are corrected; and the need for parathyroidectomy is reduced. It is the treatment of choice for most patients with end-stage renal failure. The supply of donor organs (in the UK, 30/million/year) is greatly exceeded by demand (48/million/year), and donor organs are therefore scarce and a valuable resource that must be used optimally.

The technique involves the anastomosis of an explanted human kidney, usually either from a cadaveric donor or from a living close relative, on to the iliac vessels of the recipient (Fig. 11.52). The donor ureter is placed into the recipient's bladder. Unless the donor is genetically identical (i.e. an identical twin), immunosuppressive treatment is needed, for as long as the transplant remains in place, to prevent rejection. Refinements in patient selection and assessment of donor–recipient compatibility, improvements in surgical techniques and the development of more efficient immunosuppressive regimens have increased patient and graft survival. Eighty per cent of grafts now survive for 5–10 years in the best centres, and 50% for 10–30 years.

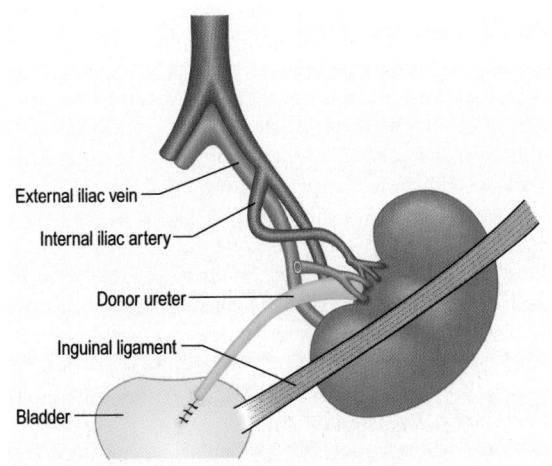

External iliac vein

Internal iliac artery

Donor ureter

Inguinal ligament

Bladder

Fig. 11.52 **Anatomy of a renal transplant operation.**

Factors affecting success

ABO (blood group) compatibility between donor and recipient is required. However, in some centres, particularly in Japan where a cadaveric organ-donation programme is not well established, ABO-incompatible renal transplants are increasingly performed after desensitizing with immunoadsorption to remove pre-formed antibodies, splenectomy, anti-CD20 antibodies to remove B lymphocytes, and intravenous pooled immunoglobulins for immunomodulation or anti-idiotypic antibodies. In experienced hands, results are acceptable.

Matching donor and recipient for HLA type

Matching for HLA-DR antigens appears to have the most impact on graft survival. Studies have shown that matching at the HLA-B locus has only a minor effect on graft outcomes. Complete compatibility at A, B and DR offers the best chance of success, followed by a single HLA mismatch (i.e. antigen possessed by the donor and not possessed by the recipient). The effect of further degrees of mismatching upon graft survival in first transplants is of modest degree. Nationwide matching schemes for kidneys retrieved from cadaver donors are in existence. However, with availability of more efficient immunosuppressive agents, the value of HLA matching in the overall transplant outcome is, if any, only modest. Transplantation with completely mismatched kidneys, particularly when the donor is the patient's partner, is routinely practiced and results are as good as, if not better than, beneficially matched cadaveric kidneys.

Adequate immunosuppressive treatment

See below.

The donor kidney

Cadaveric donation

Most countries allow the removal of kidneys and other organs from patients who have suffered irretrievable brain damage ('brainstem death') while their hearts are still beating (see p. 989).

Living related donation

A close relative may volunteer as a potential donor. A sibling donor may be HLA identical or share one or no haplotypes with the potential recipient. In the UK, donor age must be 18 years or more.

Potential living related donors are subjected to an intensive preoperative evaluation, including clinical examination and measurement of renal function, tests for carriage of hepatitis B, C, HIV and cytomegalovirus, and detailed imaging of renal anatomy, to be sure that transplantation will be technically feasible.

Unrelated living donors may be accepted provided no inducement (financial or otherwise) is involved. Paid live non-related donor transplantation is illegal in the UK.

Immunosuppression for transplantation

Long-term drug treatment for the prevention of rejection is employed in all cases apart from living related donation from an identical twin. Some degree of immunological tolerance does develop, and the risk of rejection is highest in the first 3 months after transplantation. In the early months rejection episodes occur in less than 30% of cadaver kidney recipients. Most are reversible. A combination of immunosuppressive drugs is usually used.

Corticosteroids. Corticosteroids have a non-specific anti-inflammatory (inhibition of phospholipase A_2 and arachidonic acid cascade) and immunosuppressive action (inhibition of gamma-interferon-dependent adhesion molecules and thereby dendritic cell and T lymphocyte interaction). High-dose methylprednisolone is used as the primary treatment for acute rejection.

Azathioprine. Azathioprine prevents cell-mediated rejection by blocking purine synthesis and replication of lymphocytes. A recent study suggests that azathioprine and its metabolite 6-mercaptopurine can convert a CD28-dependent costimulatory Rac1 signal (proliferation and differentiation) upon dendritic cell and T-lymphocyte interaction into an apoptotic response by their ability to form 6-thio-GTP. 6-Thio-GTP competes with GTP for Rac1, preventing its anti-apoptotic action. Adverse effects include suppression of red cell and platelet production, an increased incidence of infections (particularly viral), and hepatotoxicity. It also interacts with allopurinol, which increases levels of the active metabolites of azathioprine (6-mercaptopurinol), resulting in toxicity.

Mycophenolate mofetil is metabolized to mycophenolic acid and blocks inosine monophosphate dehydrogenase (IMPD) an enzyme in the de-novo synthetic pathway of purine synthesis. It may be more specific for lymphocytes because unlike in other cells an alternative purine synthetic salvage pathway is absent from lymphocytes. It is more potent than azathioprine, as trials have shown a reduction in rejection episodes. Gastrointestinal symptoms such as nausea, vomiting and diarrhoea are more than with azathioprine but the drug can be used with allopurinol.

Ciclosporin (CSA). Ciclosporin, a calcineurin inhibitor, prevents the activation of T lymphocytes in response to new antigens and is highly effective in preventing rejection, while leaving the functioning of the rest of the immune system largely intact. Intracellularly, CSA forms complexes with cyclophilin (isomerase) and inhibits calmodulin–calcineurin-induced phosphorylation of NF-AT transcription factor for IL-2 and possibly other T cell activation genes. Its introduction has revolutionized organ transplantation. Disadvantages include high cost and nephrotoxicity. Even with careful adjustment of the dose in response to trough blood levels, renal function may be adversely affected.

Tacrolimus, also a calcineurin inhibitor, blocks T-cell activation by a mechanism very similar to that of ciclosporin with the exception that tacrolimus forms a complex with immunophilin FK binding protein-12 (FKBP-12) instead of cyclophilin. The downstream actions are the same as with CSA. It is more potent than CSA and is therefore used both as a rescue agent for treating rejection and as a maintenance agent. Its side-effects are broadly similar to those of CSA except it is more diabetogenic.

Sirolimus and the structural analogue everolimus are newer immunosuppressants that are synergistic with CSA but lack nephrotoxicity. Sirolimus, like tacrolimus, binds to FKBP (particularly the -25 rather than the -12 isoform) but instead of calcineurin inhibition, acts on targets of rapamycin signalling (target of rapamycin – TOR) and prevents cell entry into G1 phase of the cell cycle. It may lead to poor wound healing and delay the recovery of proximal tubular cell injury sustained during transplantation. Its main side-effects are thombocytopenia and hyperlipidaemia. Its role in renal transplantation is being explored.

Antibodies. Both polyclonal anti-thymocytic globulin (ATG) and anti-lymphocytic globulin (ALG) and monoclonal (OKT3) antibodies are potent immunosuppressive agents. Antibodies may be derived from mouse, rabbit, horse, or 'humanized', and directed against any of a number of lymphocycte surface marker proteins, enabling neutralization or killing of lymphocytes with certain functions (e.g. T cells, activated T cells, cells expressing adhesion molecules). They are mainly used for the treatment of steroid-resistant rejections and as an induction therapy for high immunological risk patients (previously sensitized with circulating anti-HLA antibodies). Basiliximab (chimeric) and dacluzimab (humanized) anti-CD25 monoclonal antibodies bind to IL-2 receptors on activated T lymphocytes only (therefore having few side-effects), inhibiting IL-2-driven proliferative responses. They have largely replaced ATG and ALG in transplant induction protocols.

Complications

Acute tubular necrosis (ATN)

ATN is the commonest cause of cadaveric graft dysfunction (up to 40–50%), particularly after asystolic donation and prolonged cold ischaemia time (> 24 hours).

Kidneys from elderly (> 55 years) donors and those with a history of hypertension are liable to develop ATN. Delayed graft function due to ATN is associated with worse long-term outcome and also predisposes the graft to rejection. It is usual practice to use induction with antibodies and use 50% of the starting dose of calcineurin inhibitors in recipient of grafts at high risk for ATN.

Technical failures

There may be occlusion or stenosis of the arterial anastomosis, occlusion of the venous anastomosis, and urinary leaks owing to damage to the lower ureter, or defects in the anastomosis between ureter and recipient bladder. If urine output drops, these diagnoses should be considered using Doppler ultrasonography, DTPA scanning and/or renal angiography. Surgical re-implantation may be required.

Acute rejection (AR)

AR is seen in up to 30% of transplant recipients and usually presents with declining renal function within the first 3 months. Renal biopsy confirms the diagnosis and also assesses the severity. Therapy in cellular rejection is high-dose pulse steroid; in acute vascular rejection, ATG, ALG or OKT3 is used. More than one rejection within the first 3 months, delayed rejection and failure of serum creatinine to return to baseline are associated with worse long-term outcome.

Infections

In the first month post-transplantation, infections tend to be from bacterial sources seen typically in the surgical population. Cytomegalovirus (CMV) infections develop weeks or months after transplantation in 70% of CMV-seronegative recipients receiving grafts from a sero-positive donor and in patients receiving biological agents (antibodies) as induction or therapy for rejection, unless prophylaxis with valganciclovir or valaciclovir is given. Prophylaxis is also routinely given against *Pneumocystis carinii* (co-trimoxazole) and oral candidiasis (nystatin or amphotericin lozenges). Polyomavirus infections (BK nephropathy) result in graft dysfunction and eventual loss due to mainly tubulointerstitial nephritis. There is no known specific treatment with the exception of tapering immunosuppression.

Post-transplantation lymphoproliferative disorders

Epstein–Barr virus-associated malignancies are common in patients who received biological agents and in children. Cautious tapering of ciclosporin or tacrolimus and monitoring for the reappearance of cytotoxic lymphocytes has improved the outcome.

Chronic allograft nephropathy (CAN)

CAN remains the most common cause of late graft failure. The process is mediated by immunological and non-immunological factors and results in a progressive irreversible decline in graft function with mild to modest proteinuria (< 3 g/day). Unfortunately there is no established therapy of proven efficiency.

Malignancy

Immunosuppressive therapy increases the risk of skin tumours, including basal and squamous cell carcinoma. In white recipients, exposure to ultraviolet light should be minimized and sun-block creams employed. Other common cancers are renal, cervical and vaginal. In female recipients, regular yearly cervical smears should be carried out.

Cardiovascular disease

Cardiovascular disease is the cause of death post-transplantation in 50% of cases. This is due to increased incidence of hypertension, obesity, diabetes and insulin resistance lipid disorders. Use of a statin (fluvastatin) was associated with reduction in cardiac end-points (myocardial infarction or revascularization) post-transplantation but overall mortality remained unchanged in a randomized prospective study.

Post-transplant osteoporosis

This is common following transplantation owing to treatment with steroids. Maximum bone loss occurs within the first 3 months and regular DXA scans are necessary. Bisphosphonates (alendronate, palmidronate), and alphacalcidol with or without calcium carbonate have proven to be effective in control studies.

Recurrent disease

Recurrence of renal disease is surprisingly common. Primary FSGS often recurs and causes early graft loss. Mesangiocapillary GN, diabetic nephropathy and IgA nephropathy also commonly recur but seldom cause renal insufficiency.

FURTHER READING

Amann K, Ritz C, Adamczak M, Ritz E (2003) Why is coronary heart disease of uraemic patients so frequent and so devastating? *Nephrology, Dialysis, Transplantation* **18**: 631–640.

Meguid EL, Nahas A, Bello AK (2005) Chronic kidney disease: the global challenge. *Lancet* **365**: 331–340.

Eknoyan G, Beck GJ, Cheung KA (2002) Effect of dialysis dose and membrane flux in maintenance haemodialysis. *New England Journal of Medicine* **347**: 2010–2019.

Halloran PF (2004) Immunosuppressive drugs for kidney transplantation. *New England Journal of Medicine* **351**: 2715–2729.

Liu Y (2004) Epithelial to mesenchymal transition in renal fibrogenesis: pathologic significance, molecular mechanism and therapeutic intervention. *Journal of the American Society of Nephrology* **15**: 1–14.

Murphy B (2003) Transplantation. *Nephrology Self-Assessment Program (NephSAP)* **2**(4): 121–198.

Schieppati A, Remuzzi G (2003) The future of renoprotection: frustration and promises. *Kidney International* **64**: 1947–1955.

CYSTIC RENAL DISEASE

Solitary or multiple renal cysts are common, especially with advancing age: 50% of those aged 50 years or more have one or more such cysts. They have no special significance except in the differential diagnosis of renal tumours (see p. 684). Such cysts are often asymptomatic and are found on excretion urography or ultrasound examination performed for some other reason. Occasionally they may cause pain and/or haematuria owing to their large size, or bleeding may occur into the cyst. Cystic degeneration (the formation of multiple cysts which enlarge with time) occurs regularly in the kidneys of patients with end-stage renal failure treated by dialysis and/or transplantation. Malignant tumour formation seems to be more common in such kidneys than in the general population.

Autosomal-dominant polycystic kidney disease

Autosomal-dominant polycystic kidney disease (ADPKD) is an inherited disorder usually presenting in adult life. It is characterized by the development of multiple renal cysts, variably associated with extrarenal (mainly hepatic and cardiovascular) abnormalities. ADPKD is by far the most common inherited nephropathy, with a prevalence rate ranging from 1 : 400 to 1 : 1000 in white populations. It accounts for 3–10% of all patients commencing regular dialysis in the West.

In about 85% of cases, the gene responsible (*PKD1*) has been located on chromosome 16. A second gene, *PKD2*, which has been mapped on chromosome 4, accounts for the vast majority of other cases. These genetic abnormalities are distinct from the autosomal recessive form of polycystic disease (due to mutations in the *PKHD1* gene on chromosome 6p21.1–p12), which is often lethal in early life. The protein corresponding to the *PKD1* gene, polycystin 1, appears to be an integral membrane glycoprotein involved in cell-to-cell and/or cell-to-matrix interaction and functions as a mechanosensor. The protein corresponding to the *PKD2* gene appears to function as a calcium ion channel, regulating calcium influx and/or release from intracellular stores. Polycystin-1 acts as the regulator of PKD2 channel activity by its co-localization on cilia of collecting tubular cells. Disruption of the polycystin pathway results in reduced cytoplasmic calcium, which in principal cells of the collecting duct causes increase in cAMP via stimulation of calcium-inhibitable adenyl cyclase and inhibition of cAMP phosphodiesterases.

Clinical features

Clinical presentation may be at any age from the second decade. Presenting symptoms include:

■ acute loin pain and/or haematuria owing to haemorrhage into a cyst, cyst infection or urinary tract stone formation

- loin or abdominal discomfort owing to the increasing size of the kidneys
- subarachnoid haemorrhage associated with berry aneurysm rupture
- complications of hypertension
- complications of associated liver cysts
- symptoms of uraemia and/or anaemia associated with chronic renal failure.

Erythraemia is a rare complication and presentation of ADPKD.

The natural history of the disease is one of progressive renal impairment, sometimes punctuated by acute episodes of loin pain and haematuria, and commonly associated with the development of hypertension. The rate of progression to renal failure is variable. The determinants of progression are both genetic and non-genetic. In the PKD2 form, renal cysts develop more slowly and end-stage renal failure (ESRF) occurs 10–15 years later than in the PKD1 form. Gender affects renal prognosis. Males with ADPKD reach end-stage renal failure 5–6 years earlier than females. There is a large variability in the age at ESRF within families, even between affected monozygotic twins.

Complications and associations

Pain

A minority of patients suffer chronic renal pain resistant to common analgesics, presumably owing to the pressure effect of large cysts. Surgical decompression of such cysts appears to be of benefit in about two-thirds of patients. Laparoscopic cyst decortication is a minimally invasive alternative technique.

Cyst infection

The response to standard antibacterial therapy is often poor owing to poor penetration of conventional antibiotics across the cyst wall. Lipophilic antibiotics active against Gram-negative bacteria, such as co-trimoxazole and fluoroquinolones, penetrate into the cysts better and their use has greatly improved the treatment of this complication.

Renal calculi

These are diagnosed in about 10–20% of patients with ADPKD. Frequently they are composed of uric acid and hence radiolucent. Obstructing or painful stones are treated no differently than are stones in patients with normal urinary tracts. Percutaneous stone removal and extracorporeal lithotripsy may safely be employed.

Hypertension

Hypertension is an early and very common feature of ADPKD. Elevation of blood pressure, still within the normal range, is detectable in young affected individuals and is associated with an increase in left ventricular mass. It appears that left ventricular hypertrophy occurs to a greater degree for a given rise in blood pressure in ADPKD compared with other renal disorders and with essential hypertension. Intrarenal activation of the renin–angiotensin system is involved in pathogenesis, and ACE inhibitors are logical first-line agents in treatment. Early control of blood pressure is essential as cardiovascular complications are a major cause of death in ADPKD.

Progressive renal failure

This is the most serious complication of ADPKD. At glomerular filtration rates below 50 mL/min, the rate of decline in GFR averages 5 mL/min each year, which is more rapid than in other primary renal disorders. The probability of being alive without requiring dialysis or transplantation by the age of 70 years is of the order of 30%. Survival rates on regular haemodialysis and after renal transplantation in ADPKD are similar to those of patients with other primary renal diseases.

Hepatic cysts

Approximately 30% of patients have hepatic cysts and in a minority of patients massive enlargement of the polycystic liver is seen. Pain, infection of cysts and, more rarely, compression of the bile duct, portal vein or hepatic venous outflow occur. Rarely, percutaneous drainage of painful cysts, laparoscopic fenestration or even partial hepatectomy may be necessary. Infected cysts may require drainage.

Intracranial aneurysm formation

About 10% of ADPKD patients have an asymptomatic intracranial aneurysm and the prevalence is twice as high in the subgroup of patients with a family history of such aneurysms or of subarachnoid haemorrhage. Such haemorrhage is preceded in from 20% to 40% of cases by premonitory headaches from a few hours up to 2 weeks before the onset of subarachnoid bleeding. Headache of sudden onset or unusual character or severity in a patient with ADPKD should prompt investigation. Contrast-enhanced spiral CT or MR angiography are the best investigations. Screening for intracranial aneurysm in ADPKD is currently recommended for patients aged 18–40 years who have a positive family history.

Mitral valve prolapse

This is found in 20% of individuals with ADPKD.

Diagnosis

Physical examination commonly reveals large, irregular kidneys and possibly hepatomegaly. Definitive diagnosis is established by ultrasound examination (Fig. 11.53). However, such renal imaging techniques may be equivocal, especially in subjects under the age of 20 years.

Screening

The children and siblings of patients with established ADPKD should, in general, be offered screening. Affected individuals should have regular blood pressure checks and should be offered genetic counselling. Screening by ultrasonography should not be carried out before the age of 20 years, as excluding the condition may be difficult and hypertension is unusual before this age. Even at age 20, renal ultrasonography may give a false-negative

Fig. 11.53 Ultrasound scan of a polycystic kidney, showing an enlarged kidney with many cysts of varying size.

result. Gene linkage analysis can be utilized in many families.

Therapy

No therapy is yet available but potential agents include *vasopressin receptor antagonists*, which have been studied in animal models of polycystic kidney disease, which is closely related to human ADPKD, where they have halted cyst progression or caused disease regression. ADPKD kidneys may be particularly vulnerable to *adenylyl cyclase agonists* or *cAMP phosphodiesterase inhibitors*. Caffeine at clinically relevant concentrations has been found to enhance the effect of desmopressin to stimulate chloride secretion in cultured epithelial cells from ADPKD cysts.

Medullary cystic disease ('juvenile nephronophthisis')

Juvenile nephronophthisis that develops early in childhood is commonly inherited in an autosomal recessive manner. Mutations in the genes *NPHP1–4* have recently been found. The proteins mutated, nephrocystin and inversin, are co-localized in the cilia of the renal tubules. A similar condition developing later in childhood (medullary cystic disease) is inherited as an autosomal dominant trait, but sporadic cases occur in both conditions. Despite its name, the dominant histological finding is interstitial inflammation and tubular atrophy, with later development of medullary cysts. Progressive glomerular failure is a secondary consequence.

The dominant features are polyuria, polydipsia and growth retardation. Diagnosis is based on the family history and renal biopsy, the cysts rarely being visualized by imaging techniques.

Medullary sponge kidney

Medullary sponge kidney is an uncommon but not rare condition that usually presents with renal colic or haematuria. Although it is most often sporadic, a few affected families have been reported. The condition is characterized by dilatation of the collecting ducts in the papillae, sometimes with cystic change. In severe cases the medullary area has a sponge-like appearance. The condition may affect one or both kidneys or only part of one kidney. Cyst formation is commonly associated with the development of small calculi within the cyst. In about 20% of patients there is associated hypercalciuria or renal tubular acidosis (see p. 716). Hemihypertrophy of the skeleton has been described in this condition.

The diagnosis is made by excretion urography, which shows small calculi in the papillary zones with an increase in radiodensity around these following injection of contrast medium as the dilated or cystic collecting ducts are filled with contrast (see Fig. 11.33).

The natural history is one of intermittent colic with passage of small stones or haematuria. Renal function is usually well maintained and renal failure is unusual, except where obstructive nephropathy develops owing to the presence of stones in the pelvis or ureters.

FURTHER READING

Gattone VH II, Wang W, Harris PC, Torres VE (2003) Inhibition of renal cystic disease development and progression by a vasopressin V2 receptor antagonist. *Nature Medicine* **9**: 1323–1326.

Joly D, Hummel A, Ruello A, Knebelmann B (2003) Ciliary function of polycystins: a new model for cystogenesis. *Nephrology, Dialysis, Transplantation* **18**: 1689–1692.

TUMOURS OF THE KIDNEY AND GENITOURINARY TRACT

MALIGNANT RENAL TUMOURS

These comprise 1–2% of all malignant tumours, and the male to female ratio is 2 : 1.

Renal cell carcinoma

Renal cell carcinomas (RCC) arise from proximal tubular epithelium. They are the most common renal tumour in adults. They rarely present before the age of 40 years, the average age of presentation being 55 years.

In von Hippel–Lindau disease, an autosomal dominant disorder, bilateral renal cell carcinomas are common and haemangioblastomas, phaeochromocytomas and renal cysts are also found. Polymorphic probes from chromosome 3p, the region implicated in renal cell carcinoma, have demonstrated genetic linkage between them and von Hippel–Lindau disease. It seems likely, therefore, that mutation of the same tumour suppressor gene may be responsible for both renal cell carcinoma and von Hippel–Lindau disease. Deletion of the short arm of chromosome 3 is the most consistent cytogenetic finding in sporadic tumours. Renal cell carcinomas are highly vascular tumours. Microscopically most tumours are composed of large cells containing clear cytoplasm.

Clinical features

Patients present with haematuria, loin pain and a mass in the flank. Malaise, anorexia and weight loss (30%) may occur, and 5% of patients have polycythaemia (see p. 454).

Thirty per cent of patients have hypertension due to secretion of renin by the tumour with anaemia due to depression of erythropoietin in approximately the same number. Pyrexia is present in about one-fifth of patients and approximately one-quarter present with metastases. Rarely, a left-sided varicocele may be associated with left-sided tumours that have invaded the renal vein and caused obstruction to drainage of the left testicular vein.

Diagnosis

Excretion urography will reveal a space-occupying lesion in the kidney; 10% of these show calcification. Ultrasonography is used to demonstrate the solid lesion and to examine the patency of the renal vein and inferior vena cava. A small (< 3 cm) renal cell carcinoma may be missed on excretion urography and ultrasonography. CT scanning can also be used to identify the renal lesion and involvement of the renal vein or inferior vena cava. MRI is better than CT for tumour staging. Renal arteriography will reveal the tumour's circulation but is now seldom employed. Urine cytology for malignant cells is of no value. The ESR is usually raised. Liver biochemistry may be abnormal, returning to normal after surgery.

Treatment

Treatment is by nephrectomy unless bilateral tumours are present or the contralateral kidney functions poorly, in which case conservative surgery such as partial nephrectomy may be indicated. If metastases are present, nephrectomy may still be warranted since regression of metastases has been reported after removal of the main tumour mass. Medroxyprogesterone acetate is of some value in controlling metastatic disease. Treatment with interleukin-2 and beta-interferon produces a remission in about 20% of cases. A striking regression of metastases has been reported after non-myeloablative chemotherapy followed by allogeneic (sibling) peripheral blood stem-cell transplantation. Given the frequency of mutation in tumour suppression gene *VHL* and oversecretion of vascular endothelial growth factor (VEGF) in RCC, a trial with neutralizing antibody to VEGF (bevacizumab) caused significant slowing in the rate of progression of metastatic renal cell carcinoma but did not prolong the overall patient survival. Similarly in a recent study, adjuvant autologous renal tumour cell vaccine given intradermally every 4 weeks for 6 months at the time of radical nephrectomy for non-metastatic RCC was associated with an increase in 5-year disease progression-free survival – 77% compared to 68% in the placebo group. These exciting new studies may help to improve the prognosis of RCC.

Prognosis

The prognosis depends upon the degree of differentiation of the tumour and whether or not metastases are present. The 5-year survival rate is 60–70% with tumours confined to the renal parenchyma, 15–35%, with lymph node involvement, and only approximately 5% in those who have distant metastases.

Nephroblastoma (Wilms' tumour)

This tumour is seen mainly within the first 3 years of life and may be bilateral. It presents as an abdominal mass, rarely with haematuria. Diagnosis is established by excretion urography followed by arteriography. A combination of nephrectomy, radiotherapy and chemotherapy has much improved survival rates, even in children, with metastatic disease. Overall, 5-year survival rate in UK children diagnosed between 1971 and 1985 was 79%.

UROTHELIAL TUMOURS

The calyces, renal pelvis, ureter, bladder and urethra are lined by transitional cell epithelium. Transitional cell tumours account for about 3% of deaths from all forms of malignancy. Such tumours are uncommon below the age of 40 years, and the male to female ratio is 4 : 1. Bladder tumours are about 50 times as common as those of the ureter or renal pelvis.

Predisposing factors include:

- cigarette smoking
- exposure to industrial carcinogens such as β-naphthylamine and benzidine (workers in the chemical, cable and rubber industries are at particular risk) or ingestion of aristolochic acid found in some herbal weight-loss preparations
- exposure to drugs (e.g. phenacetin, cyclophosphamide)
- chronic inflammation (e.g. schistosomiasis, usually associated with squamous carcinoma).

Presentation

Painless haematuria is the most common presenting symptom of bladder malignancy, although pain may occur owing to clot retention. Symptoms suggestive of UTI may develop in the absence of significant bacteriuria. In patients with bladder cancer, pain may also result from local nerve involvement. Presenting symptoms may result from local metastases.

Transitional cell carcinomas in the kidney and ureter may present with haematuria. They may also give rise to flank pain, particularly if urinary tract obstruction is present.

Investigations

Cytological examination of urine for malignant cells and renal imaging (ultrasonography and CT) should be performed in all patients. Cystoscopy is necessary unless pathology is found in the upper urinary tract. It may be omitted in men under 20 and women under 30 years if significant bacteriuria accompanies the haematuria and ceases following control of the infection, provided urine cytology and renal imaging are normal. With these exceptions, haematuria should always be investigated. In cases where the tumour is not clearly outlined on ultrasonography or CT, retrograde ureterography may be helpful.

Treatment

Pelvic and ureteric tumours. These are treated by nephroureterectomy. Radiotherapy and chemotherapy appear to be of little or no value. Subsequently, cystoscopy should be regularly carried out, since about half the patients will develop bladder tumours.

Bladder tumours. Treatment depends upon the stage of the tumour (in particular whether it has penetrated the bladder muscle) and its degree of differentiation.

Superficial bladder tumours are treated by transurethral resection or local diathermy with follow-up check cystoscopies and cytological examination of the urine. Bladder instillation of doxorubicin, mitomycin and thiotepa is used for recurrent tumours, as is instillation of BCG (bacille Calmette–Guérin).

Invasive bladder tumours are treated with radical cystectomy in patients under 70 years and radical radiotherapy in those over 70 years with salvage cystectomy for recurrences. Cystectomy requires a new bladder to be made out of small bowel, joining this to the urethra if possible or making an ileal conduit.

Prognosis

The prognosis ranges from a 5-year survival rate of 80–90% for lesions not involving bladder muscle to 5% for those presenting with metastases.

Testicular tumours are discussed on page 522.

DISEASES OF THE PROSTATE GLAND

Benign enlargement of the prostate gland

Benign prostatic enlargement occurs most often in men over the age of 60 years. Such enlargement is much less common in Asian individuals. It is unknown in eunuchs. The aetiology of the condition is unknown. Microscopically, hyperplasia affects the glandular and connective tissue elements of the prostate. Enlargement of the gland stretches and distorts the urethra, obstructing bladder outflow.

Clinical features

Frequency of urination, usually first noted as nocturia, is a common early symptom. Difficulty or delay in initiating urination, with variability and reduced forcefulness of the urinary stream and post-void dribbling, are often present. Acute retention of urine (see below) or retention with overflow incontinence may occur. Occasionally, severe haematuria results from rupture of prostatic veins or as a consequence of bacteriuria or stone disease. Occasional patients present with severe renal failure.

Abdominal examination for bladder enlargement together with examination of the rectum are essential. A benign prostate feels smooth. An accurate impression of prostatic size cannot be obtained on rectal examination.

Management and prognosis

Patients with mild-to-moderate symptoms should be managed by 'watchful waiting', because symptoms following therapy are sometimes greater than those with no therapy at all.

Patients with moderate prostatic symptoms can be treated medically. A number of drugs have been employed, including alpha-blockers such as tamsulosin. Finasteride is a competitive inhibitor of 5α-reductase, which is the enzyme involved in the conversion of testosterone to dihydrotestosterone. This is the androgen primarily responsible for prostatic growth and enlargement. Finasteride decreases prostatic volume with an increase in urine flow. Deterioration in renal function or the development of upper tract dilatation requires surgery.

In acute retention or retention with overflow, the first priorities are to relieve pain and to establish urethral catheter drainage. If urethral catheterization is impossible, suprapubic catheter drainage should be carried out. The choice of further management is then between immediate prostatectomy, a period of catheter drainage followed by prostatectomy, or the acceptance of a permanent indwelling suprapubic or urethral catheter.

Prostatic carcinoma

Prostatic carcinoma accounts for 7% of all cancers in men and is the fourth most common cause of death from malignant disease in men in England and Wales. Malignant change within the prostate becomes increasingly common with advancing age. By the age of 80 years, 80% of men have malignant foci within the gland, but most of these appear to lie dormant. Histologically, the tumour is an adenocarcinoma. Hormonal factors are thought to play a role in the aetiology.

Clinical features

Presentation may be with symptoms of lower urinary tract obstruction or of metastatic spread, particularly to bone. The diagnosis may be made by the incidental finding of a hard irregular gland on rectal examination, or as an unexpected histological result after prostatectomy for what was believed to be benign prostatic hypertrophy. In developed countries, patients now present as a result of screening for prostate cancer by measurement of prostate-specific antigen (PSA). However, on the evidence available, national programmes of screening are not justified. Treatment of well people carries a high morbidity of urinary incontinence and sexual dysfunction with no evidence as yet of increased survival. In future, screening of 'at-risk' groups may be useful.

Investigations

These include transrectal ultrasound of the prostate and prostatic biopsy. A histological diagnosis is essential before treatment. The Gleason scoring system is based on the histological appearances. If metastases are present, serum prostate-specific antigen levels are usually markedly elevated (> 16 μg/L); it is a myth that elevated levels occur as a result of rectal examination.

Ultrasonography and transrectal ultrasonography are also of value in defining the size of the gland and staging any tumour present. The upper renal tracts can be examined by ultrasonography for evidence of dilatation. Bone metastases may appear as osteosclerotic lesions on X-ray and are detected by isotopic bone scans.

Treatment (see also p. 685)

Prophylactic finasteride therapy can prevent or delay the appearance of prostatic carcinoma in men above the age of 55 years but usually at the expense of sexual side-effects and increased risk of high-grade prostatic cancer. Microscopic, impalpable tumours can sometimes be managed expectantly. Treatment for disease confined to the gland is radical prostatectomy (provided the patient is fit for the procedure) or radiotherapy. A randomized trial comparing radical prostatectomy with watching and waiting in early prostate cancer revealed radical prostatectomy significantly reduced disease-specific mortality, but there was no significant difference between surgery and watching and waiting in terms of overall survival. Locally extensive disease is managed with radiotherapy with or without androgen ablation therapy. Metastatic disease can be treated with orchidectomy, but many men refuse. Luteinizing hormone-releasing hormone (LHRH) analogues such as buserelin or goserelin are equally effective and preferred by many. Non-hormonal chemotherapy is usually unhelpful. The duration of survival depends on the age of the patient and the degree of differentiation and extent of the tumour.

RENAL DISEASE IN THE ELDERLY

Renal failure in the elderly more often results from renal vascular disease or urinary tract obstruction than in younger age groups. In males, obstruction is most often due to benign or malignant prostatic enlargement, while in females it results from pelvic cancer.

Progressive sclerosis of glomeruli occurs with ageing and this, together with the development of atheromatous renal vascular disease, accounts for the progressive reduction in GFR seen with advancing years. A GFR of 50–60 mL/min (about half the normal value for a young adult) may be regarded as 'normal' in patients in their eighties. The reduction in muscle mass often seen with ageing may mask this deterioration in renal function in that the serum creatinine concentration may be less than 0.12 mmol/L in an elderly patient whose GFR is 50 mL/min or lower. The use of serum creatinine as a measure of renal function in the elderly must take this into account. This is especially so in the elderly when prescribing drugs whose excretion is in whole or in part by the kidney.

Urinary tract infections

UTIs are common in the elderly, in whom impaired bladder emptying due to prostatic disease in males and neuropathic bladder – especially common in females – is frequently found. Symptoms may be atypical, the major complaints being incontinence, nocturia, smelly urine or vague change in well-being with little in the way of dysuria. Demonstration of significant bacteriuria in the presence of such symptoms requires treatment.

Urinary incontinence

This is defined as involuntary passage of urine sufficient to be a health or social problem. It is common in the elderly with 25% of women and 15% of men over 65 having a problem.

- *Urge incontinence* is usually due to detrusor over-activity with leakage of urine because the bladder is perceived to be full. This is common in the elderly; it occurs as an isolated event or secondary to local factors, e.g. bladder infection or stones, or to central factors, e.g. stroke, dementia or Parkinson's disease.
- *Stress incontinence* occurs when the intra-abdominal pressure is increased, e.g. after a cough or sneeze and there is a weak pelvic floor or urethral sphincter. It is common in women after childbirth.
- *Overflow incontinence* occurs with leakage of urine from a full distended bladder. It occurs commonly in men with prostatic obstruction, following spinal cord injury or in women with cystoceles or after gynae-cological surgery.
- *Functional incontinence*. Passage of urine occurs owing to inability to get to a toilet because of disability, e.g. stroke, trauma, the unavailability of toilet facilities or dementia.

Management

- Physical examination for local problems, e.g. prostatic enlargement in men, gynaecological disorders in women, and for central problems, e.g. neurological disorders or dementia.
- Urine analysis, e.g. glycosuria and culture for UTI.
- Treatment of contributing causes, e.g. constipation, drug therapy, other co-existing disease.
- Urge incontinence – bladder training, antimuscarinics, e.g. oxybutynin and tolterodine.
- Stress incontinence – pelvic floor exercises.
- Overflow – removal of obstruction.
- Functional – improve facilities, regular urine voiding, absorbent padding.

Further evaluation with urodynamics is necessary in patients who do not respond and have a potentially curable problem. An expert and committed incontinence advisory and treatment service combining nursing and medical skills is invaluable for elderly patients with this distressing problem. Home visits to ensure the availability of commodes and toilets is essential. For established incontinence, catheterization may be necessary but should be avoided if at all possible. Incontinence and its treatment are matters of major importance and are by no means confined solely to the elderly.

FURTHER READING

Joachim D, Richter A, Hoffman L et al. (2004) Adjuvant autologous renal tumour cell vaccine and risk of tumour progression in patients with renal cell carcinoma after radical nephrectomy: phase III randomized controlled trial. *Lancet* **363**: 594–599.

Motzer RJ, Bander NH, Nanus DM (1996) Medical progress: renal cell carcinoma. *New England Journal of Medicine* **335**: 865–875.

Nelson WG, de Marzo A, Isaacs WB (2003) Prostate cancer. *New England Journal of Medicine* **349**: 366–381.

Prostate cancer series (2003) *Lancet* **361**: 859–864; 955–964; 1045–1053; 1122–1128.

Slavin S (2000) Cancer immunotherapy with alloreactive lymphocytes. *New England Journal of Medicine* **343**: 802–803.

Thompson IM, Goodman PJ, Tangen CM et al. (2003) The influence of finasteride on the development of prostate cancer. *New England Journal of Medicine* **349**: 215–224.

Yang JC, Howarth L, Sherry RM et al. (2003) A randomized trial of bevacizumab as anti-vascular endothelial growth factor antibody, for metastatic renal cancer. *New England Journal of Medicine* **349**: 427–434.

CHAPTER BIBLIOGRAPHY

Cameron JS, Davison AM, Grunfeld JP et al. (eds) (2004) *Oxford Textbook of Clinical Nephrology.* Oxford: Oxford University Press.

Parsons M, Cardozo L (2004) *Female Urinary Incontinence in Practice.* London: Royal Society of Medicine.

Schrier RW (ed) (1997) *Renal Electrolyte Disorders*, 5th edn. Philadelphia: Lippincott Raven.

Current Opinion in Nephrology and Hypertension is a monthly journal with review articles, each issue devoted to one or two topics.

Journal of the American Society of Nephrology is the highest impact journal in nephrology with bimonthly self-assessment programme (SAP) supplements.

Kidney International is the major journal associated with the International Society of Nephrology – monthly with original and review articles.

Nephrology, Dialysis, Transplantation is the major European journal devoted to the subject, with review articles, editorial comments and original papers.

SIGNIFICANT WEBSITES

http://www.tinkershop.net/nephro.htm
  Nephrology calculator
http://www.nephronline.org
  For healthcare professionals involved in the management of patients with kidney disease
http://www.renalnet.org
  Kidney information clearing house database
http://www.kidney.org.uk/
  UK charity run by and for patients

Water, electrolytes and acid–base balance

In health, the volume and biochemical composition of both extracellular and intracellular fluid compartments in the body remains remarkably constant. Many different disease states result in changes of control, either of extracellular fluid volume or of the electrolyte composition of extracellular fluid. An understanding of these abnormalities is therefore essential for the management of a wide range of clinical disorders.

DISTRIBUTION AND COMPOSITION OF BODY WATER

In normal persons, the total body water constitutes 50–60% of lean bodyweight in men and 45–50% in women. In a healthy 70 kg male, total body water is approximately 42 L. This is contained in three major compartments:

- the intracellular fluid (28 L, about 35% of lean bodyweight)
- the interstitial fluid that bathes the cells (9.4 L, about 12%)
- plasma (4.6 L, about 4–5%).

In addition, small amounts of water are contained in bone, dense connective tissue, and epithelial secretions, such as the digestive secretions and cerebrospinal fluid.

The intracellular and interstitial fluids are separated by the cell membrane; the interstitial fluid and plasma are separated by the capillary wall (Fig. 12.1). In the absence of solute, water molecules move randomly and in equal numbers in either direction across a permeable membrane. However, if solutes are added to one side of the membrane, the intermolecular cohesive forces reduce the activity of the water molecules. As a result, water tends to stay in the solute-containing compartment because there

Fig. 12.1   Distribution of water between the vascular and extravascular (interstitial) spaces. This is determined by the equilibrium between hydrostatic pressure, which tends to force fluid out of the capillaries, and oncotic pressure, which acts to retain fluid within the vessel. The net flow of fluid outwards is balanced by 'suction' of fluid into the lymphatics, which returns it to the bloodstream. Similar principles govern the volume of the peritoneal and pleural spaces.

is less free diffusion across the membrane. This ability to hold water in the compartment can be measured as the osmotic pressure.

Osmotic pressure

Osmotic pressure is the primary determinant of the distribution of water among the three major compartments. The concentrations of the major solutes in these fluids differ, and each compartment has one solute that is primarily limited to that compartment and therefore determines its osmotic pressure: K^+ salts in the intra-

Table 12.1 Electrolyte composition of intracellular and extracellular fluids

	Plasma (mmol/L)	Interstitial fluid (mmol/L)	Intracellular fluid (mmol/L)
Na^+	142	144	10
K^+	4	4	160
Ca^{2+}	2.5	2.5	1.5
Mg^{2+}	1.0	0.5	13
Cl^-	102	114	2
HCO_3^-	26	30	8
PO_4^{2-}	1.0	1.0	57
SO_4^{2-}	0.5	0.5	10
Organic acid	3	4	3
Protein	16	0	55

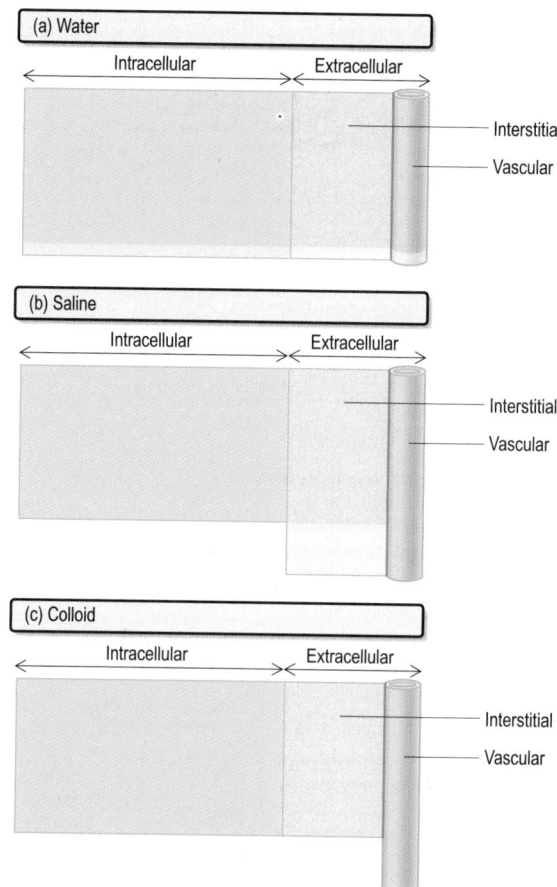

Fig. 12.2 Relative effects of the addition of 1 L of (a) water, (b) saline 0.9%, and (c) a colloid solution.

cellular fluid (most of the cell Mg^{2+} is bound and osmotically inactive), Na^+ salts in the interstitial fluid, and proteins in the plasma. Regulation of the plasma volume is somewhat more complicated because of the tendency of the plasma proteins to hold water in the vascular space by an oncotic effect which is in part counterbalanced by the hydrostatic pressure in the capillary that is generated by cardiac contraction (Fig. 12.1). The composition of intracellular and extracellular fluids is shown in Table 12.1.

A characteristic of an osmotically active solute is that it cannot freely leave its compartment. The capillary wall, for example, is relatively impermeable to plasma proteins, and the cell membrane is 'impermeable' to Na^+ and K^+ because the Na^+/K^+-ATPase pump largely restricts Na^+ to the extracellular fluid and K^+ to the intracellular fluid. By contrast, Na^+ freely crosses the capillary wall and achieves similar concentrations in the interstitium and plasma; as a result, it does not contribute to fluid distribution between these compartments. Similarly, urea crosses both the capillary wall and the cell membrane and is osmotically inactive. Thus, the retention of urea in renal failure does not alter the distribution of the total body water.

A conclusion from these observations is that body Na^+ stores are the primary determinant of the extracellular fluid volume. Thus the extracellular volume – and therefore tissue perfusion – are maintained by appropriate alterations in Na^+ excretion. For example, if Na^+ intake is increased, the extra Na^+ will initially be added to the extracellular fluid. The associated increase in extracellular osmolality will cause water to move out of the cells, leading to extracellular volume expansion. Balance is restored by excretion of the excess Na^+ in the urine.

Distribution of different types of replacement fluids

Figure 12.2 shows the relative effects on the compartments of the addition of identical volumes of water, saline and colloid solutions. Thus, 1 L of water given intravenously as 5% dextrose is distributed equally into all compartments, whereas the same amount of 0.9% saline remains in the extracellular compartment. The latter is thus the correct treatment for extracellular water

depletion – sodium keeping the water in this compartment. The addition of 1 L of colloid with its high oncotic pressure stays in the vascular compartment and is the treatment for hypovolaemia.

Regulation of extracellular volume (Fig. 12.3)

The extracellular volume is determined by the sodium concentration. The regulation of extracellular volume is dependent upon a tight control of sodium balance, which is exerted by normal kidneys. Renal Na^+ excretion varies directly with the effective circulating volume. In a 70 kg man, plasma fluid constitutes one-third of extracellular volume (4.6 L), of which 85% (3.9 L) lies in the venous side and only 15% (0.7 L) resides in the arterial circulation. The unifying hypothesis of extracellular volume regulation in health and disease proposed by Schrier states that the fullness of the arterial vascular compartment – or the so-called effective arterial blood volume (EABV) – is the primary determinant of renal sodium and water excretion. Thus effective arterial blood volume constitutes effective circulatory volume for the purposes of body fluid homeostasis. The fullness of the arterial compartment depends upon a normal ratio between cardiac output and peripheral arterial resistance.

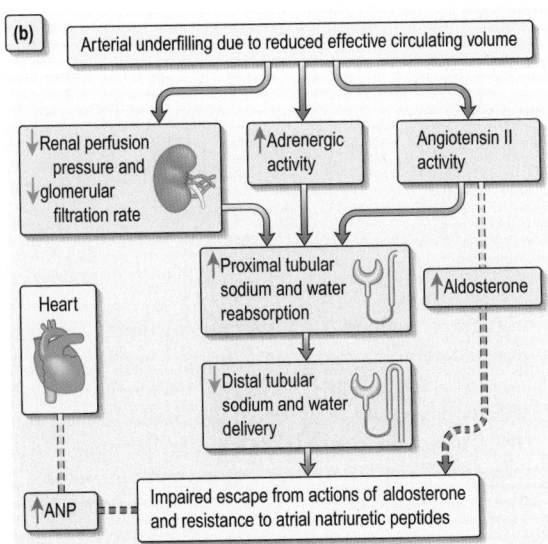

Fig. 12.3 (a) Sequence of events in which a decrease in cardiac output or peripheral arterial dilatation initiates renal sodium and water retention.
(b) Mechanism of impaired escape from the actions of aldosterone and resistance to atrial natriuretic peptides (ANP). Modified from Schrier RW (1997) *Renal and Electrolyte Disorders*, 5th edn.

Thus, diminished EABV is initiated by a fall in cardiac output or a fall in peripheral arterial resistance (an increase in the holding capacity of the arterial vascular tree). When the EABV is expanded, the urinary Na$^+$ excretion is increased and can exceed 100 mmol/L. In contrast, the urine can be rendered virtually free of Na$^+$ in the presence of EABV depletion and normal renal function.

These changes in Na$^+$ excretion can result from alterations both in the filtered load, determined primarily by the glomerular filtration rate (GFR), and in tubular reabsorption, which is affected by multiple factors. In general, it is changes in tubular reabsorption that constitute the main adaptive response to fluctuations in the effective circulating volume. How this occurs can be appreciated from Table 12.2 and Figure 12.4, which depicts the sites and determinants of segmental Na$^+$ reabsorption. Although the loop of Henle and distal tubule make a major overall contribution to net Na$^+$ handling, transport in these segments primarily varies with the amount of Na$^+$ delivered; that is, reabsorption is flow-dependent. In comparison, the neurohumoral regulation of Na$^+$ reabsorption according to body needs occurs primarily in the proximal and collecting tubules.

Table 12.2   Mechanisms of sodium transport in the various nephron segments

Tubule segment	Filtered Na⁺ reabsorbed (%)	Major mechanism of luminal Na⁺ entry	Major factors regulating transport
Proximal tubule	60–70	$Na^+ - H^+$ exchange and cotransport of Na^+ with glucose, phosphate and other organic solutes	Angiotensin II Norepinephrine (noradrenaline)
Loop of Henle	20–25	$Na^+ - K^+ - 2Cl^-$ cotransport	Flow dependent Pressure natriuresis mediated by nitric oxide
Distal tubule	5	$Na^+ - Cl^-$ cotransport	Flow dependent
Collecting ducts	4	Na^+ channels	Aldosterone Atrial natriuretic peptide

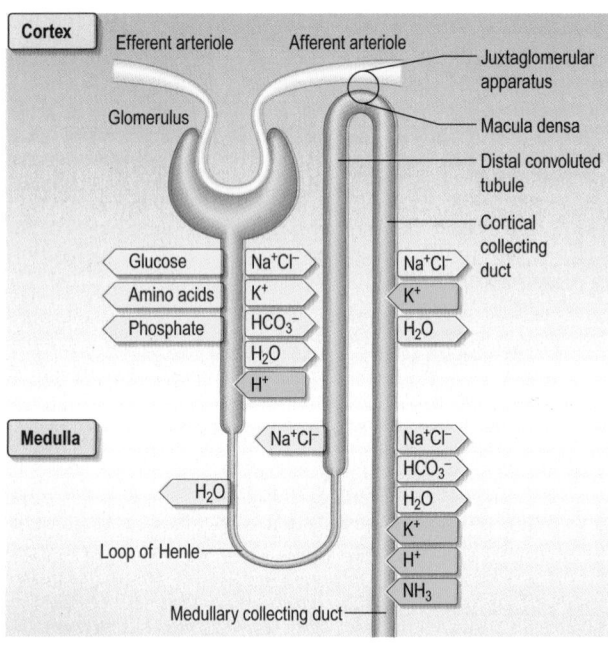

Fig 12.4   The nephron – sites of removal or addition of electrolytes from or into tubular fluid.

Neurohumoral regulation of extracellular volume

This is mediated by volume receptors that sense changes in the EABV rather than alterations in the sodium concentration. These receptors are distributed in both the renal and cardiovascular tissues.

■ *Intrarenal receptors.* Receptors in the walls of the afferent glomerular arterioles respond, via the juxta-glomerular apparatus, to changes in renal perfusion, and control the activity of the renin–angiotensin–aldosterone system (p. 1096). In addition, sodium concentration in the distal tubule and sympathetic nerve activity alter renin release from the juxtaglomerular cells. Prostaglandins I_2 and E_2 are also generated within the kidney in response to angiotensin II, acting to maintain glomerular filtration rate and sodium and water excretion, modulating the sodium-retaining effect of this hormone.

■ *Extrarenal receptors.* These are located in the vascular tree in the left atrium and major thoracic veins, and in the carotid sinus body and aortic arch. These volume receptors respond to a slight reduction in effective circulating volume and result in increased sympathetic nerve activity and a rise in catecholamines. In addition, volume receptors in the cardiac atria control the release of a powerful natriuretic hormone – atrial natriuretic peptide (ANP) – from granules located in the atrial walls (p. 1096).

High-pressure arterial receptors (carotid, aortic arch, juxtaglomerular apparatus) predominate over low-pressure volume receptors in volume control in mammals. The low-pressure volume receptors are distributed in thoracic tissues (cardiac atria, right ventricle, thoracic veins, pulmonary vessels) and their role in the volume regulatory system is marginal.

Aldosterone and possibly atrial natriuretic peptide (ANP) are responsible for day-to-day variations in Na⁺ excretion, by their respective ability to augment and diminish Na⁺ reabsorption in the collecting ducts.

■ A *salt load*, for example, leads to an increase in the effective circulatory and extracellular volume, raising both renal perfusion pressure, and atrial and arterial filling pressure. The increase in the renal perfusion pressure reduces the secretion of renin, and subsequently that of angiotensin II and aldosterone (Fig. 18.27), whereas the rise in atrial and arterial filling pressure increases the release of ANP. These factors combine to reduce Na⁺ reabsorption in the collecting duct, thereby promoting excretion of excess Na⁺.

- In contrast, in patients on *low Na⁺ intake* or in those who become volume-depleted as a result of vomiting and diarrhoea, the ensuing decrease in effective volume enhances the activity of the renin–angiotensin–aldosterone system and reduces the secretion of ANP. The net effect is enhanced Na⁺ reabsorption in the collecting ducts, which accounts for the appropriate fall in Na⁺ excretion in this setting. It tends to increase the extracellular volume towards normal.

With more marked hypovolaemia, a decrease in GFR leads to an increase in proximal and thin ascending limb Na⁺ reabsorption which contributes to Na⁺ retention. This is brought about by enhanced sympathetic activity acting directly on kidneys and indirectly by stimulating the secretion of renin/angiotensin II (see Fig. 12.3b) and nonosmotic release of antidiuretic hormone (ADH). The pressure natriuresis phenomenon may be the final defence against changes in the effective circulating volume. Marked persistent hypovolaemia leads to systemic hypotension and increased salt and water absorption in the proximal tubules and ascending limb of Henle. This process may be mediated by changes in renal interstitial hydrostatic pressure and local prostaglandin and nitric oxide production.

Volume regulation in oedematous conditions
Sodium and water are retained despite increased extracellular volume in oedematous conditions such as cardiac failure, hepatic cirrhosis and hypoalbuminaemia. Here the principal mediator of salt and water retention is the concept of arterial underfilling due either to reduced cardiac output or diminished peripheral arterial resistance. Arterial underfilling in these settings leads to reduction of pressure or stretch (i.e. 'unloading' of arterial volume receptors) which results in activation of the sympathetic nervous system, activation of the renin–angiotensin–aldosterone system and nonosmotic release of antidiuretic hormone (ADH). These neurohumoral mediators promote salt and water retention in the face of increased extracellular volume. The common nature of the degree of arterial fullness and neurohumoral pathway in the regulation of extracellular volume in health and disease states forms the basis of Schrier's unifying hypothesis of volume homeostasis (Fig. 12.3a).

Mechanism of impaired escape from actions of aldosterone and resistance to ANP
Not only is the activity of the renin–angiotensin–aldosterone system increased in oedematous conditions such as cardiac failure, hepatic cirrhosis and hypo-

albuminaemia, but also the action of aldosterone is more persistent than in normal subjects and patients with Conn's syndrome, who have increased aldosterone secretion (p. 1097). In normal subjects, high doses of mineralocorticoids initially increase renal sodium retention so that the extracellular volume is increased by 1.5–2 litres. However, renal sodium retention then ceases, sodium balance is re-established, and there is no detectable oedema. This escape from mineralocorticoid-mediated sodium retention explains why oedema is not a characteristic feature of primary hyperaldosteronism (Conn's syndrome). The escape is dependent on an increase in delivery of sodium to the site of action of aldosterone in the collecting ducts. The increased distal sodium delivery is achieved by high extracellular volume-mediated arterial overfilling. This suppresses sympathetic activity and angiotensin II generation, and increases cardiac release of ANP with resultant increase in renal perfusion pressure and GFR. The net result of these events is reduced sodium absorption in the proximal tubules and increased distal sodium delivery which overwhelms the sodium-retaining actions of aldosterone.

In patients with oedematous conditions such as cardiac failure, hepatic cirrhosis and hypoalbuminaemia escape from the sodium-retaining actions of aldosterone does not occur and therefore they continue to retain sodium in response to aldosterone. Accordingly they have substantial natriuresis when given spironolactone, which blocks mineralocorticoid receptors. Alpha-adrenergic stimulation and elevated angiotensin II increase sodium transport in the proximal tubule, and reduced renal hypoperfusion and GFR further increase sodium absorption from the proximal tubules by presenting less sodium and water in the tubular fluid. Sodium delivery to the distal portion of the nephron, and thus the collecting duct, is reduced. Similarly, increased cardiac ANP release in these conditions requires optimum sodium concentration at the site of its action in the collecting duct for its desired natriuretic effects. Decreased sodium delivery to the collecting duct is therefore the most likely explanation for the persistent aldosterone-mediated sodium retention, absence of escape phenomenon and resistance to natriuretic peptides in these patients (Fig. 12.3b).

Regulation of water excretion
Body water homeostasis is effected by thirst and the urine concentrating and diluting functions of the kidney. These in turn are controlled by intracellular osmoreceptors, principally in the hypothalamus, to some extent by volume receptors in capacitance vessels close to the heart, and via the renin–angiotensin system. Of these, the major and best-understood control is via osmoreceptors. Changes in the plasma Na⁺ concentration and osmolality are sensed by osmoreceptors that influence both thirst and the release of ADH (also called vasopressin) from the supraoptic and paraventricular nuclei.

ADH plays a central role in urinary concentration by increasing the water permeability of the normally impermeable cortical and medullary collecting ducts. The ability of ADH to increase the urine osmolality is related indirectly to transport in the ascending limb of the loop of Henle, which reabsorbs NaCl without water. This process, which is the primary step in the countercurrent mechanism, has two effects: it makes the tubular fluid dilute and the medullary interstitium concentrated. In the absence of ADH, little water is reabsorbed in the collecting ducts, and a dilute urine is excreted. In contrast, the presence of ADH promotes water reabsorption in the collecting ducts down the favourable osmotic gradient between the tubular fluid and the more concentrated interstitium. As a result, there is an increase in urine osmolality and a decrease in urine volume.

The cortical collecting duct has two cell types (see also p. 714) with very different functions:

- *Principal cells* (about 65%) have sodium and potassium channels in the apical membrane and, as in all sodium-reabsorbing cells, Na^+/K^+-ATPase pumps in the basolateral membrane.
- *Intercalated cells*, in comparison, do not transport NaCl (since they have a lower level of Na^+/K^+-ATPase activity) but play a role in hydrogen and bicarbonate handling and in potassium reabsorption in states of potassium depletion.

The ADH-induced increase in collecting duct water permeability occurs primarily in the principal cells. ADH acts on V2 (vasopressin) receptors located on the basolateral surface of principal cells, resulting in the activation of adenyl cyclase. This leads to protein kinase activation and to preformed cytoplasmic vesicles that contain unique water channels (called aquaporins) moving to and then being inserted into the luminal membrane. The water channels span the luminal membrane and permit water movement into the cells down a favourable osmotic gradient (Fig. 12.5). This water is then rapidly returned to the systemic circulation across the basolateral membrane. When the ADH effect has worn off, the water channels aggregate within clathrin-coated pits, from which they are removed from the luminal membrane by endocytosis and returned to the cytoplasm. A defect in any step in this pathway, such as in attachment of ADH to its receptor or the function of the water channel, can cause resistance to the action of ADH and an increase in urine output. This disorder is called *nephrogenic diabetes insipidus*.

Plasma osmolality

In addition to influencing the rate of water excretion, ADH plays a central role in osmoregulation because its release is directly affected by the plasma osmolality. At a plasma osmolality of less than 275 mOsm/kg, which usually represents a plasma Na^+ concentration of less than 135–137 mmol/L, there is essentially no circulating ADH. As the plasma osmolality rises above this threshold, however, the secretion of ADH increases progressively.

Two simple examples will illustrate the basic mechanisms of osmoregulation, which is so efficient that the plasma Na^+ concentration is normally maintained within 1–2% of its baseline value.

Ingestion of a water load leads to an initial reduction in the plasma osmolality, thereby diminishing the release of

Fig. 12.5 **Aquaporin-mediated water transport in the renal collecting duct.** Stimulation of the vasopressin 2 receptor causes cAMP-mediated insertion of the aquaporin into the apical membrane, allowing water transport down the osmotic gradient. Adapted from Connolly DL, Shanahan CM, Weissberg PL (1996) *Lancet* **347**: 211.

ADH. The ensuing reduction in water reabsorption in the collecting ducts allows the excess water to be excreted in a dilute urine.

Water loss resulting from sweating is followed by, in sequence, a rise in both plasma osmolality and ADH secretion, enhanced water reabsorption, and the appropriate excretion of a small volume of concentrated urine. This renal effect of ADH minimizes further water loss but does not replace the existing water deficit. Thus, optimal osmoregulation requires an increase in water intake, which is mediated by a concurrent stimulation of thirst. The importance of thirst can also be illustrated by studies in patients with central diabetes insipidus, who are deficient in ADH. These patients often complain of marked polyuria, which is caused by the decline in water reabsorption in the collecting ducts. However, they do not typically become hypernatraemic, because urinary water loss is offset by the thirst mechanism.

Osmoregulation versus volume regulation

A common misconception is that regulation of the plasma Na^+ concentration is closely correlated with the regulation of Na^+ excretion. However, it is related to volume regulation, which has different sensors and effectors (volume receptors) from those involved in water balance and osmoregulation (osmoreceptors).

The roles of these two pathways should be considered separately when evaluating patients.

- *A water load* is rapidly excreted (in 4–6 hours) by inhibition of ADH release. This process is normally so efficient that volume regulation is not affected and there is no change in ANP release or in the activity of the renin–angiotensin–aldosterone system. Thus, a dilute urine is excreted, and there is little alteration in the excretion of Na^+.

- *Isotonic saline* administration, in contrast, causes an increase in volume but no change in plasma osmolality. In this setting, ANP secretion is increased, aldosterone secretion is reduced, and ADH secretion does not change. The net effect is the appropriate excretion of the excess Na^+ in a relatively iso-osmotic urine.

In some cases, both volume and osmolality are altered and both pathways are activated. For example, if a person with normal renal function eats salted potato chips and peanuts without drinking any water, the excess Na^+ will increase the plasma osmolality, leading to osmotic water movement out of the cells and increased extracellular volume. The rise in osmolality will stimulate both ADH release and thirst (the main reason why many restaurants and bars supply free salted foods), whereas the hypervolaemia will enhance the secretion of ANP and suppress that of aldosterone. The net effect is increased excretion of Na^+ without water.

This principle of separate volume and osmoregulatory pathways is also evident in the syndrome of inappropriate ADH secretion (SIADH). Patients with SIADH (p. 1091) have impaired water excretion and hyponatraemia caused by the persistent presence of ADH. However, the release of ANP and aldosterone is not impaired and, thus, Na^+ handling remains intact. These findings have implications for the correction of the hyponatraemia in this setting and require restriction of water intake.

ADH is also secreted by nonosmotic stimuli such as stress (e.g. surgery, trauma), markedly reduced effective circulatory volume (cardiac failure, hepatic cirrhosis), psychiatric disturbance, and nausea, irrespective of plasma osmolality. This is mediated by the effects of sympathetic overactivity on supraoptic and paraventricular nuclei. In addition to water retention, ADH release in these conditions promotes vasoconstriction owing to the activation of V1 (vasopressin) receptors distributed in the vascular tissue.

Regulation of cell volume

Maintenance of a constant volume in the face of extracellular and intracellular osmotic alterations is a critical problem faced by all cells. Most cells respond to swelling or shrinkage by activating specific metabolic or membrane-transport processes that return cell volume to its normal resting state. Within minutes after exposure to hypotonic solutions and resulting cell swelling, a common feature of many cells is the increase in plasma membrane potassium and chloride conductance. Although extrusion of intracellular potassium certainly contributes to a regulatory volume decrease, the role of chloride efflux itself is modest, given the relatively low intracellular chloride concentration. Indeed other intracellular osmolytes, such as taurine and other amino acids, are transported out of the cell to achieve a regulatory volume decrease. In contrast, these regulatory mechanisms are operative in reverse to protect cell volume under hyper-

tonic conditions, as is the case in the renal medulla. The tubular cells at the tip of renal papillae, which are constantly exposed to a hypertonic extracellular milieu, maintain their cell volume on a long-term basis by actively taking up smaller molecules, such as betaine, taurine and myoinositol, and by synthesizing more sorbitol and glycerophosphocholine.

Increased extracellular volume

Increased extracellular volume occurs in numerous disease states. The physical signs depend on the distribution of excess volume and on whether the increase is local or systemic. According to Starling principles, distribution depends on:

- venous tone, which determines the capacitance of the blood compartment and thus hydrostatic pressure
- capillary permeability
- oncotic pressure – mainly dependent on serum albumin
- lymphatic drainage.

Depending on these factors, fluid accumulation may result in expansion of interstitial volume, blood volume, or both.

Clinical features

Peripheral oedema is caused by expansion of the extracellular volume by at least 2 L (15%). The ankles are normally the first part of the body to be affected, although they may be spared in patients with lipodermatosclerosis (where the skin is tethered and cannot expand to accommodate the oedema). Oedema may be noted in the face, particularly in the morning. In a patient in bed, oedema may accumulate in the sacral area. Expansion of the interstitial volume also causes pulmonary oedema, pleural effusion, pericardial effusion and ascites. Expansion of the blood volume (overload) causes a raised jugular venous pressure, cardiomegaly, added heart sounds, basal crackles as well as a raised arterial blood pressure in certain circumstances.

Causes

Extracellular volume expansion is due to sodium chloride retention. Increased salt intake does not normally cause volume expansion because of rapid homeostatic mechanisms which increase salt excretion. However, a rapid intravenous infusion of a large volume of saline will cause volume expansion. Thus, most causes of extracellular volume expansion are associated with renal sodium chloride retention.

Heart failure

Reduction in cardiac output and the consequent fall in effective circulatory volume and arterial filling lead to activation of the renin–angiotensin–aldosterone system, nonosmotic release of ADH, and increased activity of the renal sympathetic nerves via volume receptors and baroreceptors (Fig. 12.3a). Sympathetic overdrive also indirectly augments ADH and renin–angiotensin–aldosterone response in these conditions. The cumulative effect of these mediators results in increased peripheral and renal arteriolar resistance and water and sodium retention. These factors result in extracellular volume expansion and increased venous pressure, causing oedema formation.

Hepatic cirrhosis

The mechanism is again complex, but involves peripheral vasodilatation (possibly owing to increased nitric oxide generation) resulting in reduced effective arterial blood volume (EABV) and arterial filling. This leads to an activation of a chain of events common to cardiac failure and other conditions with marked peripheral vaso-dilatation (Fig. 12.3a and b). The cumulative effect results in increased peripheral and renal resistance, water and sodium retention, and oedema formation.

Nephrotic syndrome

Interstitial oedema is a common clinical expression of hypoalbuminaemia and particularly nephrotic syndrome. Expansion of the interstitial compartment is secondary to the accumulation of sodium in the extracellular compart-ment. This is due to an imbalance between oral (or parenteral) sodium intake and urinary sodium output, as well as alterations of fluid transfer across capillary walls. The intrarenal site of sodium retention is the cortical collecting duct (CCD) where Na^+/K^+-ATPase expression and activity are increased threefold along the basolateral surface (Fig. 12.4). In addition, amiloride-sensitive epi-thelial sodium channel activity is also increased in the CCD. The renal sodium retention should normally be counterbalanced by increased secretion of sodium in the inner medullary collecting duct, brought about by the release of ANP. This regulatory pathway is curtailed in patients with nephrotic syndrome by enhanced catabolism of cyclic GMP (the second messenger for ANP) following phosphodiesterase activation.

Oedema generation was classically attributed to the decrease in the plasma oncotic pressure and the sub-sequent increase in transcapillary oncotic gradient. However, the oncotic pressure and transcapillary oncotic gradient remain unchanged and the transcapillary hydrostatic pressure gradient is not altered. Conversely, capillary hydraulic conductivity (a measure of per-meability) is increased. This is determined by intercellular macromolecular complexes between the endothelial cells consisting of tight junctions (made of occludins, claudins and ZO proteins) and adherens junctions (made of cadherin, catenins and actin cytoskeleton). It seems that elevated TNF-α levels in nephrotic syndrome activate protein kinase C, which changes phosphorylation of occludin and capillary permeability. In addition, increased circulating ANP can increase capillary hydraulic conductivity by altering the permeability of intercellular junctional complexes. Furthermore, reduction in effective circulatory volume and the consequent fall in cardiac output and arterial filling can lead to a chain of events as in cardiac failure and cirrhosis (see above and Fig. 12.3). These factors result in extracellular volume expansion and oedema formation.

Sodium retention

A decreased GFR decreases the renal capacity to excrete sodium. This may be acute, as in the acute nephritic syndrome (p. 629), or may occur as part of the presen-tation of chronic renal failure. In end-stage renal failure, extracellular volume is controlled by the balance between salt intake and its removal by dialysis.

Numerous drugs may cause renal sodium retention, particularly in patients whose renal function is already impaired:

- *Oestrogens* cause mild sodium retention, which has a weak aldosterone-like effect. This is the cause of weight gain in the premenstrual phase.
- *Mineralocorticoids and liquorice* (the latter potentiates the sodium-retaining action of cortisol) have aldosterone-like actions.
- *NSAIDs* cause sodium retention in the presence of activation of the renin–angiotensin–aldosterone system by heart failure, cirrhosis and in renal artery stenosis.

Substantial amounts of sodium and water may accumu-late in the body without clinically obvious oedema or evidence of raised venous pressure. In particular, several litres may accumulate in the pleural space or as ascites; these spaces are then referred to as 'third spaces'. Bone may also act as a 'sink' for sodium and water.

Other causes of oedema

- Initiation of insulin treatment for type 1 diabetes and refeeding after malnutrition are both associated with the development of transient oedema. The mechanism is complex.
- Oedema may result from increased capillary pressure owing to relaxation of precapillary arterioles. The best example is the peripheral oedema caused by dihydropyridine calcium-channel blockers such as nifedipine.
- Oedema may be caused by increased interstitial oncotic pressure as a result of increased capillary permeability to proteins. This can occur as part of a rare complement-deficiency syndrome; with thera-peutic use of interleukin-2 in cancer chemotherapy; or in ovarian hyperstimulation syndrome (p. 1061).

Idiopathic oedema of women

This, by definition, occurs in women without heart failure, hypoalbuminaemia, renal or endocrine disease. Oedema is intermittent and often worse in the premenstrual phase. The condition remits after the menopause. Patients complain of swelling of the face, hands, breasts and thighs, and a feeling of being bloated. Sodium retention during the day and increased sodium excretion during recumbency are characteristic; an abnormal fall in plasma volume on standing caused by increased capillary permeability to proteins may be the cause of this. The oedema may respond to diuretics, but returns when they are stopped. A similar syndrome of diuretic-dependent sodium retention can be caused by abuse of diuretics, for instance as part of an attempt to lose weight; but not all women with idiopathic oedema admit to having taken diuretics, and the syndrome was described before diuretics were introduced for clinical use.

Local increase in oedema

This does not reflect disturbances of extracellular volume control per se, but can cause clinical confusion. Examples are ankle oedema due to venous damage following thrombosis or surgery, ankle or leg oedema due to immobility, oedema of the arm due to subclavian thrombosis, and facial oedema due to superior vena caval obstruction. Local loss of oncotic pressure may result from increased capillary permeability to proteins, caused by inflammatory mediators such as histamine and interleukins (e.g. a bee sting). Lastly, local loss of lymphatic drainage causes lymphoedema (see p. 1356).

Treatment

The underlying cause should be treated where possible. Heart failure, for example, should be treated, and offending drugs such as NSAIDs withdrawn.

Sodium restriction has only a limited role, but is useful in patients who are resistant to diuretics. Sodium intake can easily be reduced to approximately 100 mmol daily; reductions below this are often difficult to achieve without affecting the palatability of food.

Manoeuvres that increase venous return stimulate salt and water excretion by effects on cardiac output and ANP release. This is the rationale for strict bed rest in congestive cardiac failure. Water immersion also causes redistribution of blood towards the central veins, but is seldom of practical use. Venous compression stockings or bandages may help to mobilize oedema in heart failure.

The mainstay of treatment is the use of diuretic agents, which increase sodium, chloride and water excretion in the kidney (Table 12.3). These agents act by interfering with membrane ion pumps which are present on numerous cell types; they mostly achieve specificity for the kidney by being secreted into the proximal tubule, resulting in much higher concentrations in the tubular fluid than in other parts of the body.

Clinical use of diuretics

Loop diuretics (see Fig. 12.6, p. 705)

These potent diuretics are useful in the treatment of any cause of systemic extracellular volume overload. They stimulate excretion of both sodium chloride and water by blocking the sodium–potassium–2-chloride channel in the thick ascending limb of Henle and are useful in stimulating water excretion in states of relative water overload. They also act by causing increased venous capacitance, resulting in rapid clinical improvement in patients with left ventricular failure, preceding the diuresis. Unwanted effects include:

- urate retention causing gout
- hypokalaemia
- hypomagnesaemia
- decreased glucose tolerance
- allergic tubulo-interstitial nephritis and other allergic reactions
- myalgia – especially with bumetanide
- ototoxicity (due to an action on sodium pump activity in the inner ear) – particularly with furosemide (frusemide)

Table 12.3 Types and clinical uses of diuretics				
Class	**Major action**	**Examples**	**Clinical uses**	**Potency**
Loop diuretics	↓ Na^+–Cl^-–K^+ cotransport in thick ascending limb of loop of Henle	Furosemide Bumetanide Torasemide	Volume overload (CCF, nephrotic syndrome, CRF) ?Acute renal failure SIADH	+++
Thiazide and related diuretics	↓ Na^+–Cl^- cotransport in early distal convoluted tubule	Bendroflumethiazide Chlortalidone Metolazone Indapamide	Hypertension Volume overload (CCF) Hypercalciuria	++
Potassium sparing	↓ Na^+ reabsorption (in exchange for K^+) in collecting duct (principal cells)	Aldosterone antagonist, e.g. spironolactone, eperenone	Hyperaldosteronism (primary and secondary) Bartter's syndrome Heart failure Cirrhosis with fluid overload	+
		Others: amiloride triamterene	Prevention of K^+ deficiency in combination with loop or thiazide	
Carbonic anhydrase inhibitors	↓ Na^+ HCO_3^- reabsorption in proximal collecting duct ↓ Aqueous humour formation	Acetazolamide	Metabolic alkalosis Glaucoma	+

CCF, congestive cardiac failure; CRF, chronic renal failure; SIADH, syndrome of inappropriate antidiuretic hormone secretion

■ interference with excretion of lithium, resulting in toxicity.

In most situations there is little to choose between the drugs in this class. Bumetanide has a better oral bioavailability than furosemide, particularly in patients with severe peripheral oedema, and has more beneficial effects than furosemide on venous capacitance in left ventricular failure. It can cause severe muscle cramps when used in high doses.

Thiazide diuretics (see Fig. 12.7, p. 706)
These are less potent than loop diuretics. They act by blocking a sodium chloride channel in the distal convoluted tubule. They cause relatively more urate retention, glucose intolerance and hypokalaemia than loop diuretics. They interfere with water excretion and may cause hyponatraemia, particularly if combined with amiloride or triamterene. This effect is clinically useful in diabetes insipidus. Thiazides reduce peripheral vascular resistance by mechanisms that are not completely understood but do not appear to depend on their diuretic action, and are widely used in the treatment of essential hypertension. They are also used extensively in mild to moderate cardiac failure. Thiazides reduce calcium excretion. This effect is useful in patients with idiopathic hypercalciuria, but may cause hypercalcaemia. Numerous agents are available, with varying half-lives but little else to choose between them. Metolazone is not dependent for its action on glomerular filtration, and therefore retains its potency in renal impairment.

Potassium-sparing diuretics (see Fig. 12.8)
These are relatively weak and are most often used in combination with thiazides or loop diuretics to prevent potassium depletion. They are of two types.

■ *Aldosterone antagonists*, which compete with aldosterone in the collecting ducts and reduce sodium absorption, e.g. spironolactone and eplerenone (which has a shorter half-life). Spironolactone is used in patients with heart failure because it significantly reduces the mortality in these patients by antagonizing the fibrotic effect of aldosterone on the heart. Eplerenone, which is devoid of antiandrogenic or antiprogesterone properties, is likely to be used as the first-line aldosterone antagonist in the future.
■ *Amiloride and triamterene* inhibit sodium uptake by blocking epithelial sodium channels in the collecting duct and reduce renal potassium excretion by reducing lumen-negative transepithelial voltage. They are mainly used as potassium sparing agents with thiazide or loop diuretics.

Carbonic anhydrase inhibitors
These are relatively weak diuretics and are seldom used except in the treatment of glaucoma. They may cause metabolic acidosis and hypokalaemia.

Aquaretics (vasopressin or ADH receptor blockers)
Vasopressin V2 receptor antagonists may become very useful agents in the treatment of conditions associated with elevated levels of vasopressin, such as heart failure, cirrhosis and SIADH (see p. 1091). Non-peptide vasopressin V2 receptor antagonists are efficacious in producing free water diuresis in humans. Studies in patients with heart failure and cirrhosis suggest that such agents will allow normalization of serum osmolality with less water restriction. Additional benefits of combined V1 and V2 receptor antagonism in heart failure are possible but remain unproven in patients. Safe use of these agents will require avoidance in hypovolaemic patients and caution with regard to rate of correction of dilutional hyponatraemia commonly present in heart failure and cirrhosis.

Resistance to diuretics
Resistance may occur as a result of:

■ poor bioavailability
■ reduced GFR, which may be due to decreased circulating volume despite oedema (e.g. nephrotic syndrome, local causes of oedema) or intrinsic renal disease
■ activation of sodium-retaining mechanisms, particularly aldosterone.

Management. Intravenous administration may establish a diuresis. High doses of loop diuretics may be required to achieve adequate concentrations in the tubule if GFR is depressed. However, the daily dose of furosemide (frusemide) must be limited to a maximum of 2 g for an adult, because of ototoxicity. *Intravenous albumin* solutions restore plasma oncotic pressure temporarily in the nephrotic syndrome and may allow mobilization of oedema but fail to potentiate the natriuretic effect of loop diuretics.

Combinations of various classes of diuretics are extremely helpful in patients with resistant oedema. A loop diuretic plus a thiazide inhibit two major sites of sodium reabsorption; this effect may be further potentiated by addition of a potassium-sparing agent. Metolazone in combination with a loop diuretic is particularly useful in refractory congestive cardiac failure, because its action is less dependent on glomerular filtration. However, this potent combination can cause severe electrolyte imbalance. Both aminophylline and dopamine increase renal blood flow and may be useful in refractory cardiogenic sodium retention. In addition, theophyllines, by inhibiting phosphodiesterase activity in the inner medullary collecting duct, prolong the action of cyclic GMP (a second messenger of ANP).

Effects on renal function
All diuretics may increase plasma urea concentrations by increasing urea reabsorption in the medulla. Thiazides may also promote protein breakdown. In certain situations diuretics may also decrease GFR:

■ Excessive diuresis may cause volume depletion and prerenal failure.
■ Diuretics may cause allergic tubulo-interstitial nephritis.

- Thiazides may directly cause a drop in GFR; the mechanism is complex and not fully understood.

Decreased extracellular volume

Deficiency of sodium and water causes shrinkage both of the interstitial space and of the blood volume and may have profound effects on organ function.

Clinical features

Symptoms are variable. Thirst, muscle cramps, nausea and vomiting, and postural dizziness may occur. Severe depletion of circulating volume causes hypotension and impairs cerebral perfusion, causing confusion and eventual coma.

Signs can be divided into those due to loss of interstitial fluid and those due to loss of circulating volume.

- *Loss of interstitial fluid* leads to loss of skin elasticity ('turgor') – the rapidity with which the skin recoils to normal after being pinched. Skin turgor decreases with age, particularly at the peripheries. The turgor over the anterior triangle of the neck or on the forehead is a very useful sign in all ages.
- *Loss of circulating volume* leads to decreased pressure in the venous and (if severe) arterial compartments. Loss of up to 1 L of extracellular fluid in an adult may be compensated for by venoconstriction and may cause no physical signs. Loss of more than this causes the following:

Postural hypotension

Normally the blood pressure rises if a subject stands up, as a result of increased venous return due to venoconstriction (this maintains cerebral perfusion). Loss of extracellular fluid (underfill) prevents this and causes a fall in blood pressure. This is one of the earliest and most reliable signs of volume depletion, as long as the other causes of postural hypotension are excluded (Table 12.4).

Low jugular venous pressure

In hypovolaemic patients, the jugular venous pulsation can be seen only with the patient lying completely flat, or even head down, because the left atrial pressure is lower than 5 cmH$_2$O.

Peripheral venoconstriction

This causes cold skin with empty peripheral veins, which are difficult to cannulate just when the patient needs intravenous therapy the most! This sign is often absent in sepsis, where peripheral vasodilatation contributes to effective hypovolaemia.

Tachycardia

This is not always a reliable sign. Beta-blockers and other antiarrhythmics may prevent tachycardia, and hypovolaemia may activate vagal mechanisms and actually cause bradycardia.

Causes

Salt and water may be lost from the kidneys, from the gastrointestinal tract, or from the skin. Examples are given in Table 12.5.

In addition, there are a number of situations where signs of volume depletion occur despite a normal or increased body content of sodium and water.

- Septicaemia causes vasodilatation of both arterioles and veins, resulting in greatly increased capacitance of the vascular space. In addition, increased capillary permeability to plasma proteins leads to loss of fluid from the vascular space to the interstitium.
- Diuretic treatment of heart failure or nephrotic syndrome may lead to rapid reduction in plasma volume. Mobilization of oedema may take much longer.
- There may be inappropriate diuretic treatment of oedema (e.g. when the cause is local rather than systemic).

Investigations

Blood tests are in general not helpful in the assessment of extracellular volume. Plasma urea may be raised owing to increased urea reabsorption and, later, to prerenal failure (when the creatinine rises as well), but this is very nonspecific. Urinary sodium is low if the kidneys are functioning normally, but is misleading if the cause of the volume depletion involves the kidneys (e.g. diuretics, intrinsic renal disease). Urine osmolality is high in

---

Table 12.4 Postural hypotension: some causes of a fall in blood pressure from lying to standing

Decreased circulating volume (hypovolaemia)	**Interference with peripheral vasoconstriction by drugs**
	Nitrates
Autonomic failure	Calcium-channel blockers
Diabetes mellitus	α-Adrenoreceptor blocking
Systemic amyloidosis	drugs
Shy–Drager syndrome	
	Prolonged bed rest
Interference with autonomic function by drugs	**(cardiovascular deconditioning)**
Ganglion blockers	
Tricyclic antidepressants	

Table 12.5 Causes of extracellular volume depletion

Haemorrhage	**Renal losses**
External	Diuretic use
Concealed, e.g. leaking	Impaired tubular sodium
aortic aneurysm	conservation
	Reflux nephropathy
Burns	Papillary necrosis
	Analgesic nephropathy
Gastrointestinal losses	Diabetes mellitus
Vomiting	Sickle cell disease
Diarrhoea	
Ileostomy losses	
Ileus	

volume depletion (owing to increased water reabsorption), but may also often mislead.

Treatment

The overriding principle is to aim to replace what is missing.

Haemorrhage

This involves the loss of blood. The rational treatment of acute haemorrhage is therefore the infusion of a combination of red cells and a plasma substitute or (if unavailable) whole blood. (Chronic anaemia causes salt and water retention rather than volume depletion by a mechanism common to conditions with peripheral vasodilatation.)

Loss of plasma

Loss of plasma, as occurs in burns or severe peritonitis, should be treated with human plasma or a plasma substitute (see p. 463).

Loss of water and electrolytes

Loss of water and electrolytes, as occurs with vomiting, diarrhoea, or excessive renal losses, should be treated by replacement of the loss. If possible, this should be done with oral water and sodium salts. These are available as slow sodium (600 mg, approximately 10 mmol of each Na^+ and Cl^- per tablet), the usual dose of which is 6–12 tablets per day with 2–3 L of water. It is used in mild or chronic salt and water depletion, such as that associated with renal salt wasting.

Sodium bicarbonate (500 mg, 6 mmol each of Na^+ and HCO_3^- per tablet) is used in doses of 6–12 tablets per day

with 2–3 L of water. This is used in milder chronic sodium depletion with acidosis (e.g. chronic renal failure, post-obstructive renal failure, renal tubular acidosis). Sodium bicarbonate is less effective than sodium chloride in causing positive sodium balance.

Oral rehydration solutions are described in Box 2.9 (see p. 71). Intravenous fluids may sometimes be required (Table 12.6). Rapid infusion (e.g. 1000 mL per hour or even faster) is necessary if there is hypotension and evidence of impaired organ perfusion (e.g. oliguria, confusion); in these situations, plasma expanders (colloids) are often used in the first instance to restore an adequate circulating volume (see p. 974). Repeated clinical assessments are vital in this situation, usually complemented by frequent measurements of central venous pressure (see Ch. 15, p. 968, for the management of shock). Severe hypovolaemia induces venoconstriction, which maintains venous return; over-rapid correction does not give time for this to reverse, resulting in signs of circulatory overload (e.g. pulmonary oedema) even if a total body ECF deficit remains. In less severe ECF depletion (such as in a patient with postural hypotension complicating acute tubular necrosis), the fluid should be replaced at a rate of 1000 mL every 4–6 hours, again with repeated clinical assessment. If all that is required is avoidance of fluid depletion during surgery, 1–2 L may be given over 24 hours, remembering that surgery is a stimulus to sodium and water retention and that over-replacement may be as dangerous as under-replacement. Regular monitoring by fluid balance charts, bodyweight and plasma biochemistry is mandatory.

Loss of water alone

This causes extracellular volume depletion only in severe cases, because the loss is spread evenly among all the compartments of body water. In the rare situations where there is a true deficiency of water alone, as in diabetes insipidus or in a patient who is unable to drink (after surgery, for instance), the correct treatment is to give water.

If intravenous treatment is required, water is given as 5% dextrose, because pure water would lead to osmotic lysis of blood cells.

Table 12.6 Intravenous fluids in general use for fluid and electrolyte disturbances					
	Na^+ (mmol/L)	K^+ (mmol/L)	HCO_3^- (mmol/L)	Cl^- (mmol/L)	Indication (see footnote)
Normal plasma values	142	4.5	26	103	
Sodium chloride 0.9%	150	–	–	150	1
Sodium chloride 0.18% + glucose 4%	30	–	–	30	2
Glucose 5% + potassium chloride 0.3%	–	40	–	40	3
Sodium bicarbonate 1.26%	150	–	150	–	4

1. Volume expansion in hypovolaemic patients. Rarely to maintain fluid balance when there are large losses of sodium. The sodium (150 mmol/L) is higher than in plasma and hypernatraemia can result. It is often necessary to add KCl 20–40 mmol/L.
2. Maintenance of fluid balance in normovolaemic, normonatraemic patients.
3. To replace *water*. Can be given with or without potassium chloride. May be alternated with 0.9% saline as an alternative to (2).
4. For volume expansion in hypovolaemic, acidotic patients alternating with (1). Occasionally for maintenance of fluid balance combined with (2) in salt-wasting, acidotic patients.

FURTHER READING

Allison S (2004) Fluid, electrolytes and nutritition. *Clinical Medicine* 4(6).

Lee CR, Watkins MI, Patterson JH et al. (2003) Vasopressin: a new target for the treatment of heart failure. *American Heart Journal* 146(1): 9–18.

Marples D (2000) Water channels: who needs them? Editorial. *Lancet* 355: 1571–1572.

Mortimer PS, Levick JR (2004) Chronic peripheral oedema. *Clinical Medicine* 4: 448–453.

Plant L (2003) Clinical use of diuretics. *Clinical Medicine* 3: 517–520.

Schrier RW (1992) A unifying hypothesis of body fluid regulation. *Journal of the Royal College of Physicians, London* 26: 295–299.

Sterns RH (2003) Fluid, electrolyte, and acid base disturbances. *Nephrology Self-Assessment Program* 2(1): 1–40.

DISORDERS OF SODIUM CONCENTRATION

These are best thought of as disorders of body water content. As discussed above, sodium content is regulated by volume receptors; water content is adjusted to maintain, in health, a normal osmolality and (in the absence of abnormal osmotically active solutes) a normal sodium concentration. Disturbances of sodium concentration are caused by disturbances of water balance.

HYPONATRAEMIA

Hyponatraemia (Na < 135 mmol/L) is one of the most common abnormalities detected in biochemistry laboratories. It may be associated with normal extracellular volume and total body sodium content (Table 12.7). The differential diagnosis of hyponatraemia depends on an assessment of extracellular volume.

Rarely, hyponatraemia may be a 'pseudo-hyponatraemia'. This occurs in hyperlipidaemia (either high cholesterol or high triglyceride) or hyperproteinaemia where there is a spuriously low measured sodium concentration, the sodium being confined to the aqueous phase but having its concentration expressed in terms of the total volume of plasma. In this situation, plasma osmolality is normal and therefore treatment of 'hyponatraemia' is unnecessary. Artefactual 'hyponatraemia' caused by taking blood from the limb into which fluid of low sodium concentration is being infused should be excluded!

Salt-deficient hyponatraemia

This is due to salt loss in excess of water; the causes are listed in Table 12.8. In this situation, ADH secretion is initially suppressed (via the hypothalamic osmoreceptors); but as fluid volume is lost, volume receptors override the osmoreceptors and stimulate both thirst and the release of ADH. This is an attempt by the body to defend circulating volume at the expense of osmolality.

Table 12.7   Causes of hyponatraemia with normal extracellular volume

Abnormal ADH release	**Increased sensitivity to ADH**
Vagal neuropathy (failure of inhibition of ADH release)	Chlorpropamide
Deficiency of adrenocorticotrophic hormone (ACTH) or glucocorticoids (Addison's disease)	Tolbutamide
	ADH-like substances
	Oxytocin
	Desmopressin
Hypothyroidism	
Severe potassium depletion	**Unmeasured osmotically active substances stimulating osmotic ADH release**
Syndrome of inappropriate antidiuretic hormone (see Table 18.36)	Glucose
	Chronic alcohol abuse
	Mannitol
Major psychiatric illness	Sick-cell syndrome (leakage of intracellular ions)
'Psychogenic polydipsia' Nonosmotic ADH release? Antidepressant therapy	

Table 12.8   Causes of hyponatraemia with decreased extracellular volume

Gut	Kidney
Vomiting	Osmotic diuresis (e.g. hyperglycaemia, severe uraemia)
Diarrhoea	Excessive use of diuretics
Haemorrhage	Adrenocortical insufficiency
	Tubulo-interstitial renal disease
	Unilateral renal artery stenosis
	Recovery phase of acute tubular necrosis

With extrarenal losses and normal kidneys, the urinary excretion of sodium falls in response to the volume depletion, as does water excretion, leading to concentrated urine containing less than 10 mmol/L of sodium. However, in salt-wasting kidney disease, renal compensation cannot occur and the only physiological protection is increased water intake in response to thirst.

Clinical features

With sodium depletion the clinical picture is usually dominated by features of volume depletion (see p. 699). The diagnosis is usually obvious where there is a history of gut losses, diabetes mellitus or diuretic abuse.

Table 12.9 shows the potential daily losses of water and electrolytes from the gut. Losses due to renal or adrenocortical disease may be less easily identified and are suggested by a urinary sodium concentration of more than 20 mmol/L in the presence of clinically evident volume depletion.

Treatment

This is directed at the primary cause whenever possible. *In a healthy patient:*

- give oral electrolyte–glucose mixtures (p. 71)
- increase salt intake with slow sodium 60–80 mmol/day.

Table 12.9 Average concentrations and potential daily losses of water and electrolytes from the gut

	Na⁺ (mmol/L)	K⁺ (mmol/L)	Cl₃⁻ (mmol/L)	Volume (mL in 24 hours)
Stomach	50	10	110	2500
Small intestine				
Recent ileostomy	120	5	110	1500
Adapted ileostomy	50	4	25	500
Bile	140	5	105	500
Pancreatic juice	140	5	60	2000
Diarrhoea	130	10–30	95	1000–2000+

In a patient with vomiting or severe volume depletion:

- give intravenous 0.9% saline with potassium supplements
- correction of acid–base abnormalities is usually not required.

Hyponatraemia due to water excess (dilutional hyponatraemia)

This results from an intake of water in excess of the kidney's ability to excrete it. With normal kidney function, dilution hyponatraemia is uncommon even if a patient drinks approximately 1 L per hour. The most common iatrogenic cause is overgenerous infusion of 5% glucose into postoperative patients; in this situation it is exacerbated by an increased ADH secretion in response to stress. Postoperative hyponatraemia is a common clinical problem (almost 1% of patients) with symptomatic hyponatraemia occurring in 20% of these patients. Marathon runners drinking excess water and 'sports drinks' can become hyponatraemic. Premenopausal females are at most risk for developing hyponatraemic encephalopathy postoperatively, with postoperative ADH values in young females being 40 times higher than in young males. To prevent hyponatraemia, avoid using hypotonic fluids postoperatively and administer isotonic saline unless otherwise clinically contraindicated. The serum sodium should be measured daily in any patient receiving continuous parenteral fluid.

Some degree of hyponatraemia is usual in acute oliguric renal failure, while in chronic renal failure it is most often due to ill-given advice to 'push' fluids. The most common presentation of hyponatraemia due to water excess is in patients with severe cardiac failure, hepatic cirrhosis or the nephrotic syndrome in which there is evidence of volume overload (Table 12.10). In all these conditions there is usually an element of reduced glomerular filtration rate with avid reabsorption of sodium and chloride in the proximal tubule. This leads to reduced delivery of chloride to the 'diluting' ascending

Table 12.10 Causes of hyponatraemia with increased extracellular volume

Heart failure
Liver failure
Oliguric renal failure
Hypoalbuminaemia

limb of Henle's loop and a reduced ability to generate 'free water', with a consequent inability to excrete dilute urine. This is commonly compounded by the administration of diuretics that block chloride reabsorption and interfere with the dilution of filtrate either in Henle's loop (loop diuretics) or distally (thiazides).

Clinical features

Dilutional hyponatraemia symptoms are common when this develops acutely. Symptoms rarely occur until the serum sodium is less than 120 mmol/L and are more usually associated with values around 110 mmol/L or lower. They are principally neurological and are due to the movement of water into brain cells in response to the fall in extracellular osmolality.

Hyponatraemic encephalopathy symptoms and signs are non-specific and include headache, confusion, and restlessness leading to drowsiness, myoclonic jerks, generalized convulsions, and eventually coma. Other features depend on the cause, such as signs of congestive cardiac failure or liver disease.

Risk factors for developing hyponatraemic encephalopathy. The brain's adaptation to hyponatraemia initially involves extrusion of blood and CSF, as well as sodium, potassium and organic osmolytes, in order to decrease brain osmolality. Various factors can interfere with successful adaptation. These factors rather than the absolute change in serum sodium predict whether a patient will suffer hyponatraemic encephalopathy. *Children* under 16 years are at increased risk due to their relatively larger brain-to-intracranial volume ratio compared to adults. *Premenopausal women* are more likely to develop encephalopathy than postmenopausal females and males because of inhibitory effects of sex hormones and the effects of vasopressin on cerebral circulation resulting in vasoconstriction and hypoperfusion of brain. *Hypoxaemia* is a major risk factor for hyponatraemic encephalopathy. Patients with hyponatraemia can develop hypoxia due to either non-cardiac pulmonary oedema or hypercapnic respiratory failure. Respiratory failure in symptomatic hyponatraemia can be of very sudden onset. Recent data have shown that hypoxia is the strongest predictor of mortality in patients with symptomatic hyponatraemia.

Investigations

No further investigation of hyponatraemia is usually necessary if it is associated with clinically detectable extracellular volume excess. The cause of hyponatraemia with apparently normal extracellular volume is usually less obvious, and this category requires careful investigations to:

- exclude Addison's disease
- exclude hypothyroidism
- consider 'syndrome of inappropriate ADH secretion' (SIADH) and drug-induced water retention.

Remember, potassium and magnesium depletion potentiate ADH release and are causes of diuretic-associated hyponatraemia.

The syndrome of inappropriate ADH secretion is often over-diagnosed. Some causes are associated with a lower set-point for ADH release, rather than completely autonomous ADH release; an example is chronic alcohol abuse.

Treatment

The underlying cause should be corrected where possible. Most cases are simply managed by restriction of water intake (to 1000 or even 500 mL per day) with review of diuretic therapy. Magnesium and potassium deficiency must be corrected. In mild sodium deficiency, 0.9% saline given slowly is sufficient. Hypertonic saline (3%, 513 mmol/L) should be used with extreme care and restricted only for patients with acute water retention in whom there are severe neurological signs, such as fits or coma. It should be given very slowly (not more than 70 mmol per hour), the aim being to increase the serum sodium by 8–10 mmol/L in the first 4 hours, but the absolute change should not exceed 15–20 mmol/L over 48 hours. In general, the plasma sodium should not be corrected to greater than 125–130 mmol/L. Assuming that total body water comprises 50% of total bodyweight, 1 mL/kg of 3% sodium chloride will raise the plasma sodium by 1 mmol/L. In some cases furosemide can be used to prevent pulmonary congestion and to increase the rate of sodium correction. Hypertonic saline must *not* be given to patients who are already fluid overloaded because of the risk of acute heart failure; in this situation, 100 mL of 20% mannitol may be infused in an attempt to increase renal water excretion (see below).

If hyponatraemia has developed slowly, as it does in the majority of patients, the brain will have adapted by decreasing intracellular osmolality. A rapid rise in extracellular osmolality, particularly if there is an 'overshoot' to high serum sodium and osmolality, will result in severe shrinking of brain cells and in the syndrome of 'central pontine myelinolysis', which may be fatal. However, recent evidence suggests that the development of demyelination lesions is not associated with the rate of correction of sodium in hyponatraemic states. The factors associated with demyelination are pre-existing hypoxaemia, liver disease and CNS radiation. A new approach which holds promise in aiding the treatment of hyponatraemic encephalopathy is the use of vasopressin V2 receptor antagonists (see p. 691) which produce a free water diuresis. V2 antagonists are currently available for research purposes only.

Syndrome of inappropriate ADH secretion

This is described in Chapter 18.

HYPERNATRAEMIA

This is much rarer than hyponatraemia and nearly always indicates a water deficit. This may be due to (Table 12.11):

- impaired thirst or impaired conscious state
- pituitary diabetes insipidus (see p. 1090) (failure of ADH secretion)
- nephrogenic diabetes insipidus (failure of response to ADH)
- osmotic diuresis, e.g. diabetic ketoacidosis
- excessive loss of water through the skin or lungs.

Excessive administration of hypertonic sodium may also contribute, for example:

- excessive reliance on 0.9% (150 mmol/L) saline for volume replacement
- administration of drugs with a high sodium content (e.g. piperacillin)
- use of 8.4% sodium bicarbonate after cardiac arrest.

Hypernatraemia is always associated with increased plasma osmolality, which is a potent stimulus to thirst. None of the above cause hypernatraemia unless thirst sensation is abnormal or access to water limited. For instance, a patient with diabetes insipidus will maintain a normal serum sodium concentration by maintaining a high water intake until an intercurrent illness prevents this. Thirst is frequently deficient in elderly people, making them more prone to water depletion. Hypernatraemia may occur in the presence of normal, reduced or expanded extracellular volume, and does not necessarily imply that total body sodium is increased.

Clinical features

Symptoms of hypernatraemia are non-specific. Nausea, vomiting, fever and confusion may occur. A history of long-standing polyuria, polydipsia and thirst suggests diabetes insipidus. There may be clues to a pituitary cause. A drug history may reveal ingestion of nephrotoxic drugs. Assessment of extracellular volume status guides

Table 12.11 Causes of hypernatraemia	
ADH deficiency Diabetes insipidus	**Osmotic diuresis** Total parenteral nutrition Hyperosmolar diabetic coma
Iatrogenic Administration of hypertonic sodium solutions	
	PLUS Deficient water intake
Insensitivity to ADH (nephrogenic diabetes insipidus) Lithium Tetracyclines Amphotericin B Acute tubular necrosis	

resuscitation. Mental state should be assessed. Convulsions occur in severe hypernatraemia.

Investigations

Simultaneous urine and plasma osmolality and sodium should be measured. Plasma osmolality is high in hypernatraemia. Passage of urine with an osmolality lower than that of plasma in this situation is clearly abnormal and indicates diabetes insipidus. In pituitary diabetes insipidus, urine osmolality will increase after administration of desmopressin; the drug (a vasopressin analogue) has no effect in nephrogenic diabetes insipidus. If urine osmolality is high this suggests either an osmotic diuresis due to an unmeasured solute (e.g. in parenteral feeding) or excessive extrarenal loss of water (e.g. heat stroke).

Treatment

Treatment is that of the underlying cause, for example:

- in ADH deficiency, replace ADH in the form of desmopressin, a stable non-pressor analogue of ADH
- remember to withdraw nephrogenic drugs where possible and replace water either orally or, if necessary, intravenously.

In severe (> 170 mmol/L) hypernatraemia, 0.9% saline (150 mmol/L) should be used initially. Avoid too rapid a drop in serum sodium concentration; the aim is correction over 48 hours, as over-rapid correction may lead to cerebral oedema.

In less severe (e.g. > 150 mmol/L) hypernatraemia, the treatment is 5% dextrose or 0.45% saline; the latter is obviously preferable in hyperosmolar diabetic coma. Very large volumes – 5 L a day or more – may need to be given in diabetes insipidus.

If there is clinical evidence of volume depletion (see p. 699, this implies that there is a sodium deficit as well as a water deficit. Treatment of this is discussed on page 700.

FURTHER READING

Adrogue HJ, Madias NE (2000) Hypernatremia. *New England Journal of Medicine* **342**: 1493–1499.

Adrogue HJ, Madias NE (2000) Hyponatremia. *New England Journal of Medicine* **342**: 1581–1589.

Cadnapaphornchai MA, Schrier RW (2000) Pathogenesis and management of hyponatremia. *American Journal of Medicine* **109**: 688–692.

Moritz ML, Carlos Ayus J (2003). The pathophysiolgy and treatment of hyponatraemic encephalopathy: an update. *Nephrology, Dialysis, Transplantation* **18**: 2486–2491.

DISORDERS OF POTASSIUM CONTENT AND CONCENTRATION

Regulation of serum potassium concentration

The usual dietary intake varies between 80 and 150 mmol daily, depending upon fruit and vegetable intake. Most of the body's potassium (3500 mmol in an adult man) is intracellular. Serum potassium levels are controlled by:

- uptake of K^+ into cells
- renal excretion
- extrarenal losses (e.g. gastrointestinal).

Uptake of potassium into cells is governed by the activity of the Na^+/K^+-ATPase in the cell membrane and by H^+ concentration.

Uptake is *stimulated* by:

- insulin
- β-adrenergic stimulation
- theophyllines.

Uptake is *decreased* by:

- α-adrenergic stimulation
- acidosis – K^+ exchanged for H^+ across cell membrane
- cell damage or cell death – resulting in massive K^+ release.

Renal excretion of potassium is increased by aldosterone, which stimulates K^+ and H^+ secretion in exchange for Na^+ in the collecting duct (see Fig. 12.8). Because H^+ and K^+ are interchangeable in the exchange mechanism, acidosis decreases and alkalosis increases the secretion of K^+. Aldosterone secretion is stimulated by hyperkalaemia and increased angiotensin II levels, as well as by some drugs, and this acts to protect the body against hyperkalaemia and against extracellular volume depletion. The body adapts to dietary deficiency of potassium by reducing aldosterone secretion. However, because aldosterone is also influenced by volume status, conservation of potassium is relatively inefficient, and significant potassium depletion may therefore result from prolonged dietary deficiency.

A number of drugs affect K^+ homeostasis by affecting aldosterone release (e.g. heparin, NSAIDs) or by directly affecting renal potassium handling (e.g. diuretics).

Normally only about 10% of daily potassium intake is excreted in the gastrointestinal tract. Vomit contains around 5–10 mmol/L of K^+, but prolonged vomiting may cause hypokalaemia by inducing sodium depletion, stimulating aldosterone, which increases renal potassium excretion. Potassium is secreted by the colon, and diarrhoea contains 10–30 mmol/L of K^+; profuse diarrhoea can therefore induce marked hypokalaemia. Colorectal villous adenomas may rarely produce profuse diarrhoea and K^+ loss.

HYPOKALAEMIA

Causes

The most common causes of chronic hypokalaemia are diuretic treatment (particularly thiazides) and hyperaldosteronism. Acute hypokalaemia is often caused by intravenous fluids without potassium and redistribution into cells. The common causes are shown in Table 12.12.

Rare causes
Bartter's syndrome

This consists of metabolic hypokalaemia, alkalosis,

Table 12.12 Causes of hypokalaemia

Increased renal excretion	Reduced intake
Diuretics:	Intravenous fluids without K^+
thiazides	Dietary deficiency
loop diuretics	
	Redistribution into cells
Increased aldosterone	β-Adrenergic stimulation
secretion	Acute myocardial infarction
Liver failure	Beta-agonists: e.g. fenoterol,
Heart failure	salbutamol
Nephrotic syndrome	Insulin treatment, e.g.
Cushing's syndrome	treatment of diabetic
Conn's syndrome	ketoacidosis
ACTH-producing tumours	Correction of megaloblastic
	anaemia, e.g. B_{12} deficiency
Exogenous	Alkalosis
mineralocorticoid	Hypokalaemic periodic
Corticosteroids	paralysis
Carbenoxolone	
Liquorice (potentiates renal	**Gastrointestinal losses**
actions of cortisol)	Vomiting
	Severe diarrhoea
Renal disease	Purgative abuse
Renal tubular acidosis	Villous adenoma
types 1 and 2	Ileostomy or
Renal tubular damage	uterosigmoidostomy
(diuretic phase)	Fistulae
Acute leukaemia	Ileus/intestinal obstruction
Cytotoxic treatment	
Nephrotoxicity	
Amphotericin	
Aminoglycosides	
Release of urinary tract	
obstruction	
Bartter's syndrome	
Liddle's syndrome	
Gitelman's syndrome	

Fig. 12.6 Transport mechanisms in the thick ascending limb of the loop of Henle. Sodium chloride is reabsorbed in the thick ascending limb by the bumetanide-sensitive sodium–potassium–2-chloride cotransporter (NKCC2). The electroneutral transporter is driven by the low intracellular sodium and chloride concentrations generated by the Na^+/K^+-ATPase and the kidney-specific basolateral chloride channel (ClC-Kb). The availability of luminal potassium is rate-limiting for NKCC2, and recycling of potassium through the ATP-regulated potassium channel (ROMK – rat outer medulla K^+ channel) ensures the efficient functioning of the NKCC2 and generates a lumen-positive transepithelial potential.

Genetic studies have identified putative loss-of-function mutations in the genes encoding NKCC2 ☐1, ROMK ☐2, ClC-Kb ☐3, and barttin ☐4 in subgroups of patients with **Bartter's syndrome**. In contrast to the normal condition, loss of function of NKCC2 ☐1 impairs reabsorption of sodium and potassium. Inactivation of the basolateral ClC-Kb ☐3 and barttin ☐4 reduces transcellular reabsorption of chloride. Loss of function of any of these will reduce the transepithelial potential and thus decrease the driving force for the paracellular reabsorption of cations (K^+, Mg^{2+}, Ca^{2+} and Na_4^+). Paracellin-1 is necessary for the paracellular transport of Ca^{2+} and Mg^{2+}. In most patients with Bartter's syndrome, urinary calcium excretion is increased. Hypercalcaemia or increased activation of calcium-sensing receptor inactivates ROMK and causes Bartter's syndrome. Ka and Kb, kidney-specific basolateral chloride channel. ROMK, renal outer medullary potassium channel.

hypercalciuria, normal blood pressure, and an elevated plasma renin and aldosterone. The primary defect in this disorder is an impairment in sodium and chloride reabsorption in the thick ascending limb of the loop of Henle (Fig. 12.6). Mutation in the genes encoding either the sodium–potassium–2-chloride cotransporter (NKCC2), the ATP-regulated renal outer medullary potassium channel (ROMK) or kidney-specific basolateral chloride channels (ClC-Kb) – Bartter's types I, II and III respectively – causes loss of function of these channels, with consequent impairment of sodium and chloride reabsorption. There is also an increased intrarenal production of prostaglandin E_2 which is secondary to sodium and volume depletion, hypokalaemia and the consequent neurohumoral response rather than a primary defect. PE_2 causes vasodilatation and may explain why the blood pressure remains normal.

A recent molecular finding was the identification of barttin, a beta-subunit for ClC-Ka and ClC-Kb chloride channels. Barttin is a protein encoded by the *BSND* (Barter's syndrome with sensori-neural deafness) gene; a loss of function mutation causes type IV Bartter's syndome associated with sensorineural deafness and renal failure. Barttin co-localizes with a subunit of the chloride channel in basolateral membranes of the renal tubule and inner ear epithelium. It appears to mediate chloride exit in the thick ascending limb (TAL) of the loop of Henle and chloride recycling in potassium-secreting strial marginal cells in the inner ear. A very rare variant of type IV is a disorder with an impairment of both chloride channels (ClC-Ka and ClC-Kb) produces the same phenotypic defects.

A gain of function mutation of the calcium sensing receptor (CaSR) which leads to autosomal dominant hypocalcaemia has also been recognized in Bartter's syndrome. In the kidney, the CaSR is expressed mainly in the basolateral membrane of cortical TAL. Activation of CaSR by high calcium or magnesium or by gain-of-function mutation triggers intracellular signalling, including release of arachidonic acid and inhibition of adenylate cyclase. Both actions result in inhibition of ROMK activity, which in turn leads to reduction in the lumen-positive electrical potential and transcellular absorption of calcium. This effect of CaSR explains why patients with mutations in this receptor may present with both hypocalcaemia, hypercalciuria and renal wasting of NaCl, resulting in a Bartter-like syndrome.

In summary, these defects in sodium chloride transport are thought to initiate the following sequence, which is almost identical to that seen with chronic ingestion of a loop diuretic. The initial salt loss leads to mild volume depletion, resulting in activation of the renin–angiotensin–aldosterone system. The combination of hyperaldosteronism and increased distal flow (owing to the reabsorptive defect) enhances potassium and hydrogen secretion at the secretory sites in the collecting tubules, leading to hypokalaemia and metabolic alkalosis.

Diagnostic pointers include high urinary potassium and chloride despite low serum values as well as increased plasma renin (NB: in primary aldosteronism, renin levels are low). Hyperplasia of the juxtaglomerular apparatus is seen on renal biopsy (careful exclusion of diuretic abuse is necessary). Hypercalciuria is a common feature but magnesium wasting, though rare, may also occur. *Treatment* is with combinations of potassium supplements, amiloride and indometacin.

Gitelman's syndrome

Gitelman's syndrome is a phenotype variant of Bartter's syndrome characterized by hypokalaemia, metabolic alkalosis, hypocalciuria, hypomagnesaemia, normal blood pressure, and elevated plasma renin and aldosterone. There are striking similarities between the Gitelman syndrome and the biochemical abnormalities induced by chronic thiazide diuretic administration. Thiazides act in the distal convoluted tubule to inhibit the function of the apical sodium–chloride cotransporter (NCCT) (Fig. 12.7). Analysis of the gene encoding the NCCT has identified loss of function mutations in Gitelman's syndrome.

Like Bartter's syndrome, defective NCCT function leads to increased solute delivery to the collecting duct, with resultant solute wasting, volume contraction and an aldosterone-mediated increase in potassium and hydrogen secretion. Unlike Bartter's syndrome, the degree of volume depletion and hypokalaemia is not sufficient to stimulate prostaglandin E_2 production. Impaired function of NCCT is predicted to cause hypocalciuria, as does thiazide administration. Impaired sodium reabsorption across the apical membrane coupled with continued intracellular chloride efflux across the basolateral membrane, causes the cell to become hyperpolarized. This in turn stimulates calcium reabsorption via apical, voltage-activated calcium channels. Decreased intracellular sodium also facilitates calcium efflux via the basolateral sodium–calcium exchanger. The mechanism for urinary magnesium losses is not known. *Treatment* consists of potassium and magnesium supplementation ($MgCl_2$) and a potassium-sparing diuretic. Volume resuscitation is usually not necessary, because patients are not dehydrated. Elevated

Fig. 12.7 **Transport mechanisms in the distal convoluted tubule.** Under normal conditions, sodium chloride is reabsorbed by the apical thiazide-sensitive sodium–chloride cotransporter (NCCT) in the distal convoluted tubule. The electroneutral transporter is driven by the low intracellular sodium and chloride concentrations generated by the Na^+/K^+-ATPase and an, as yet, undefined basolateral chloride channel. In this nephron segment, there is an apical calcium channel and a basolateral sodium-coupled exchanger. Physiological evidence indicates that the mechanisms for the transport of magnesium are similar to those for calcium.

In **Gitelman's syndrome**, putative loss-of-function mutations in the sodium–chloride cotransporter (*NCCT* (**X**)) lead to decreased reabsorption of sodium chloride and increased reabsorption of calcium. Functional overactivity of NCCT leads to **Gordon's syndrome** by a new mechanism (see text).

prostaglandin E_2 does not occur (see above) and, therefore, NSAIDs are not indicated in this disorder.

Liddle's syndrome

This is characterized by potassium wasting, hypo-kalaemia and alkalosis, but is associated with low renin and aldosterone production, and high blood pressure. There is a mutation in the gene encoding for the amiloride-sensitive epithelial sodium channel in the distal tubule/collecting duct. This leads to constitutive activation of the epithelial sodium channel, resulting in excessive sodium reabsorption with coupled potassium and hydrogen secretion. Unregulated sodium reabsorption across the collecting tubule results in volume expansion, inhibition of renin and aldosterone secretion and development of low renin hypertension (Fig. 12.8).

Therapy consists of sodium restriction along with amiloride or triamterene administration, both potassium-sparing diuretics which directly close the sodium channels. The mineralocorticoid antagonist spironolactone is ineffective, since the increase in sodium-channel activity is not mediated by aldosterone.

Hypokalaemic periodic paralysis (p. 1271)

This condition may be precipitated by carbohydrate intake, suggesting that insulin-mediated potassium

LUMEN · CELL · INTERSTITIAL FLUID/BLOOD

Aldosterone

Epithelial sodium channel

Mineralcorticoid receptor

Fig. 12.8 Aldosterone-regulated transport in the cortical collecting ducts. Under normal conditions, the epithelial sodium channel is the rate-limiting barrier for the normal entry of sodium from the lumen into the cell. The resulting lumen-negative transepithelial voltage (indicated by the minus sign) drives potassium secretion from the principal cells and proton secretion from the α-intercalated cells (see Fig. 12.12).

In **Liddle's syndrome**, a mutation in the gene encoding the epithelial sodium channel results in persistent unregulated reabsorption of sodium and increased secretion of potassium (not shown).

In **pseudo-hypoaldosteronism type I autosomal recessive**, loss-of-function mutations (**X**) in this gene inactivate the channel.

In the **autosomal dominant variety**, the mutation is in the gene encoding the mineralocorticoid regulation of the activity of the epithelial sodium channel. Either mechanism reduces the activity of the epithelial sodium channel, thus causing salt wasting and decreasing the secretion of potassium and protons.

influx into cells may be responsible. This syndrome also occurs in association with hyperthyroidism in Chinese patients.

Clinical features

Hypokalaemia is usually asymptomatic, but severe hypokalaemia (< 2.5 mmol) may cause muscle weakness. Potassium depletion may also cause symptomatic hyponatraemia (see p. 701).

Hypokalaemia is associated with an increased frequency of atrial and ventricular ectopic beats. This association may not always be causal, because adrenergic activation (for instance after myocardial infarction) causes both hypokalaemia and increased cardiac irritability. Hypokalaemia in patients without cardiac disease is unlikely to lead to serious arrhythmias.

Hypokalaemia seriously increases the risk of digoxin toxicity by increasing binding of digoxin to cardiac cells, potentiating its action, and decreasing its clearance.

Chronic hypokalaemia is associated with interstitial renal disease, but the pathogenesis is not completely understood.

Table 12.13 Treatment of hypokalaemia

Cause	Treatment
Dietary deficiency	Increase intake of fresh fruit/ vegetables or oral potassium supplements (20–40 mmol daily) (Potassium supplements can cause gastrointestinal irritation)
Hyperaldosteronism, e.g. cirrhosis, thiazide therapy	Spironolactone
	Co-prescription of a potassium-sparing diuretic with a similar onset and duration of action
Intravenous fluid replacement	Add 20 mmol/L of K+ with monitoring

Treatment

The underlying cause should be identified and treated where possible. Table 12.13 shows some examples.

Acute hypokalaemia may correct spontaneously. In most cases, withdrawal of oral diuretics or purgatives, accompanied by the oral administration of potassium supplements in the form of slow-release potassium or effervescent potassium, is all that is required. Intravenous potassium replacement is required only in conditions such as cardiac arrhythmias, muscle weakness or severe diabetic ketoacidosis. When using intravenous therapy in the presence of poor renal function, replacement rates > 20 mmol per hour should be used only, with hourly monitoring of serum potassium and ECG changes. Ampoules of potassium should be thoroughly mixed in 0.9% saline; do not use glucose solution as this would make hypokalaemia worse.

The treatment of adrenal disorders is described on page 1086.

Failure to correct hypokalaemia may be due to concurrent hypomagnesaemia. Serum magnesium should be measured and any deficiency corrected.

HYPERKALAEMIA

Causes

Acute self-limiting hyperkalaemia occurs normally after vigorous exercise and is of no pathological significance. Hyperkalaemia in all other situations is due either to increased release from cells or to failure of excretion (Table 12.14). The most common causes are renal impairment and drug interference with potassium excretion. The combination of ACE inhibitors with potassium-sparing diuretics or NSAIDs is particularly dangerous.

Rare causes

Hyporeninaemic hypoaldosteronism

This is also known as type 4 renal tubular acidosis (see p. 717). Hyperkalaemia occurs because of acidosis and hypoaldosteronism.

Table 12.14 Causes of hyperkalaemia

Decreased excretion	Increased extraneous load
Renal failure*	Potassium chloride
Drug:* direct effect on potassium handling	Salt substitutes
Amiloride	Transfusion of stored blood*
Triamterene	**Spurious**
Spironolactone	*Increased in vitro release from abnormal cells*
Aldosterone deficiency	Leukaemia
Hyporeninaemic hypoaldosteronism (RTA type 4)	Infectious mononucleosis
Addison's disease	Thrombocytosis
ACE inhibitors*	Familial
NSAIDs	pseudohyperkalaemia
Ciclosporin treatment	haemolysis in syringe
Heparin treatment	*Increased release from muscles*
Acidosis*	Vigorous fist clenching
Gordon's syndrome	during phlebotomy

Increased release from cells (decreased Na$^+$/K$^+$-ATPase activity)
Acidosis
Diabetic ketoacidosis
Rhabdomyolysis/tissue damage
Tumour lysis
Succinylcholine (amplified by muscle denervation)
Digoxin poisoning
Vigorous exercise (α-adrenergic; transient)

*Common causes

Pseudo-hypoaldosteronism type 1 (autosomal recessive and dominant types)

This is a disease of infancy, apparently due to resistance to the action of aldosterone. It is characterized by hyperkalaemia and evidence of sodium wasting (hyponatraemia, extracellular volume depletion). Autosomal recessive forms result from loss of function because of mutations in the gene for epithelial sodium channel activity (opposite to Liddle's syndrome). This disorder involves multiple organ systems and is especially marked in the neonatal period. With aggressive salt replacement and control of hyperkalaemia, these children can survive and the disorder appears to become less severe with age. The autosomal dominant type is due to mutations affecting the mineralocorticoid receptor (Fig. 12.8). These patients present with salt wasting and hyperkalaemia but do not have other organ-system involvement.

Hyperkalaemic periodic paralysis (see p. 1271)

This is precipitated by exercise, and is caused by an autosomal dominant mutation of the skeletal muscle sodium channel gene.

Gordon's syndrome (familial hyperkalaemic hypertension, pseudohypoaldosteronism type 2)

This appears to be a mirror image of Gitelman's syndrome (see p. 706), in which primary renal retention of sodium causes hypertension, volume expansion, low renin/aldosterone, hyperkalaemia and metabolic acidosis. There is also an increased sensitivity of sodium reabsorption to thiazide diuretics, suggesting that the thiazide-sensitive sodium–chloride cotransporter (NCCT) is involved. Genetic analyses, however, have excluded abnormalities in NCCT. The involvement of two loci on chromosomes 1 and 12 and a further genetic heterogeneity has also been found. These genes do not correspond to ionic transporters but to unexpected proteins, WNK (*W*ith *N*o lysine *K*inase) 1 and WNK 4, which are two closely related members of a novel serine – threonine kinase family. WNK 4 normally inhibits NCCT by preventing its membrane translocation from the cytoplasm. Loss of function mutation in WNK 4 results in escape of NCCT from normal inhibition and its overactivity as seen from the patient's phenotype. WNK 1 is an inhibitor of WNK 4 and in some patients with Gordon's syndrome, gain of function mutation in WNK 1 results in functional deficiency of WNK 4 and overactivity of NCCT.

Suxamethonium and other depolarizing muscle relaxants

These cause release of potassium from cells. Induction of muscle paralysis during general anaesthesia may result in a rise of plasma potassium of up to 1 mmol/L. This is not usually a problem unless there is pre-existing hyperkalaemia.

Clinical features

Serum potassium of greater than 7.0 mmol/L is a medical emergency and is associated with ECG changes (Fig. 12.9). Severe hyperkalaemia may be asymptomatic and may predispose to sudden death from asystolic cardiac arrest. Muscle weakness is often the only symptom, unless (as is commonly the case) the hyperkalaemia is associated with metabolic acidosis, causing Kussmaul respiration. Hyperkalaemia causes depolarization of cell membranes, leading to decreased cardiac excitability, hypotension, bradycardia, and eventual asystole.

Treatment

Treatments for severe hyperkalaemia require both urgent measures to save lives and maintenance therapy to keep potassium down, as summarized in Emergency box 12.1. The cause of the hyperkalaemia should be found and treated.

High potassium levels are cardiotoxic as they inactivate sodium channels. Divalent cations, e.g. calcium, restore the voltage dependability of the channels.

Calcium ions protect the cell membranes from the effects of hyperkalaemia but do not alter the potassium concentration. Supraphysiological *insulin* (20 units) drives potassium into the cell and lowers plasma potassium by 1 mmol in 60 minutes, but must be accompanied by glucose to avoid hypoglycaemia. Regular measurements of blood glucose for at least 6 hours after use of insulin should be performed and extra glucose must be available for immediate use. The use of glucose alone in non-diabetic patients, to stimulate endogenous

Emergency Box 12.1
Correction of severe hyperkalaemia

IMMEDIATE
Attach ECG monitor and IV access

Protect myocardium
10 mL of 10% calcium gluconate IV over 5 mins
Effect is temporary but dose can be repeated after
    15 mins

Drive K⁺ into cells
Insulin 10 units + 50 mL of 50% glucose IV over
    10–15 mins followed by regular checks of blood
    glucose and plasma K⁺
Repeat as necessary

and/or correction of severe acidosis (pH < 6.9) – infuse
    $NaHCO_3$ (1.26%)

and/or salbutamol 0.5 mg in 100 mL of 5% glucose over
    15 min (rarely used)

LATER

Deplete body K⁺ (to decrease plasma K⁺ over next 24 h)
Polystyrene sulphonate resins:
    15 g orally up to three times daily with laxatives
    30 g rectally followed 3–6 hours later by an enema
Haemodialysis or peritoneal dialysis if the above fails

(a) Normal

(c) Reduced P wave with increased QRS complex

(b) Tented T wave

(d) 'Sine wave' pattern (pre-cardiac arrest)

Fig. 12.9 **Progressive ECG changes with increasing hyperkalaemia.**

insulin release does not produce the high levels of insulin required and therefore is not recommended.

Intravenous or nebulized salbutamol (10–20 mg) has not yet found widespread acceptance and may cause disturbing muscle tremor at the doses required.

Correction of acidosis with hypertonic (8.4%) sodium bicarbonate causes volume expansion and should not be used; 1.26% is used with severe acidosis (pH < 6.9) (p. 719). *Gastric aspiration* will remove potassium and leads to alkalosis.

Ion-exchange resins (polystyrene sulphonate resins) are used as maintenance therapy to keep potassium down

after emergency treatment. They make use of the ion fluxes which occur in the gut to remove potassium from the body, and are the only way short of dialysis of removing potassium from the body. They may cause fluid overload (resonium contains Na⁺) or hypercalcaemia (calcium resonium). Recent evidence suggests that resins do not significantly enhance the excretion of potassium beyond the effect of diarrhoea induced by osmotic or secretory cathartics.

In general, all of these measures are simply ways of buying time either to correct the underlying disorder or to arrange removal of potassium by dialysis, which is the definitive treatment for hyperkalaemia.

FURTHER READING
Amerlate I, Dawson KP (2000) Bartter's syndrome; an overview. *Quarterly Journal of Medicine* **93**: 207–215.
Halperin ML, Kamel KS (1998) Electrolyte quintet. Potassium. *Lancet* **352**: 135–140.
Yang CL, Angell J, Mitchell R, Ellison DH (2003) WNK kinases regulate thiazide sensitive Na–Cl cotransport. *Journal of Clinical Investigation* **111**: 1039–1045.
Watanabe S, Fukumoto S, Chang H (2002) Association between activating mutation of CaSR and Bartter's syndrome. *Lancet* **360**: 692–694.

DISORDERS OF MAGNESIUM CONCENTRATION

Plasma magnesium levels are normally maintained within the range 0.7–1.1 mmol/L. Magnesium balance is a function of intake and excretion. The average daily magnesium intake is 15 mmol. One-third of this magnesium is absorbed, principally in the small bowel. In the healthy adult, there is no net gain or loss of magnesium from bone, so that balance is achieved by the urinary excretion of the net magnesium absorbed.

Primary disturbance of magnesium balance is uncommon; hypo- or hypermagnesaemia usually developing on a background of more obvious fluid and electrolyte disturbances. Disturbance in magnesium balance should always be suspected in association with other fluid and electrolyte disturbances when the patient develops unexpected neurological signs or symptoms.

Renal handling of magnesium

Magnesium transport differs from that of most other ions in that the proximal tubule is not the major site of reabsorption. Only 15–25% of the filtered magnesium is reabsorbed passively in the proximal tubule and 5–10% in the distal tubule. The major site of magnesium transport is the cortical thick ascending limb (cTAL) of the loop of Henle, where 60–70% of the filtered load is reabsorbed (Fig. 12.6). It was demonstrated that this transport is passive and paracellular, driven by the lumen positive electrochemical gradient, characteristic of this segment. Conversely, magnesium reabsorption in the distal convoluted tubule (DCT) is of transcellular and active nature (Fig 12.7). The reabsorption rate in the DCT (5–15%) is much lower than in the cTAL, but it defines the final urinary excretion, as there is no significant reabsorption in the collecting duct. Three to five per cent of filtered magnesium is finally excreted in the urine. TAL magnesium reabsorption varies with changes in the plasma magnesium concentration, which is the main physiological regulator of urinary magnesium excretion. Hypermagnesaemia inhibits loop transport, while hypomagnesaemia stimulates magnesium transport. Hypercalcaemia inhibits magnesium loop transport by an unknown mechanism.

Another factor that can influence loop magnesium transport is the rate of sodium chloride reabsorption. This effect is relatively unimportant in normal subjects, but decreased reabsorption and magnesium wasting can be induced by the administration of a loop diuretic (Fig. 12.6).

HYPOMAGNESAEMIA

This most often develops as a result of deficient intake, defective gut absorption, or excessive gut or urinary loss (Table 12.15). It can also occur with acute pancreatitis, possibly owing to the formation of magnesium soaps in the areas of fat necrosis. Calcium deficiency usually develops with hypomagnesaemia. The serum magnesium is usually < 0.7 mmol/L.

Isolated dominant hypomagnesaemia (IDH)

IDH follows an autosomal dominant mode of inheritance, presenting as hypomagnesaemia and hypocalciuria. It has similarities with Gitelman's syndrome but lacks hypokalaemia and metabolic alkalosis. The *FXYD2* gene,

Table 12.15 Causes of hypomagnesaemia

Decreased magnesium absorption	Gut losses
Malabsorption (severe)	Prolonged nasogastric suction
Malnutrition	Excessive purgation
Alcohol excess	Gastrointestinal/biliary fistulae
	Severe diarrhoea
Increased renal excretion	**Miscellaneous**
Drugs:	Acute pancreatitis
loop diuretics	Inherited tubular wasting
thiazide diuretics	Isolated dominant
digoxin	hypomagnesaemia
Diabetic ketoacidosis	Familial hypomagnesaemia,
Gitelman's syndrome (p. 706)	hypercalciuria and
Hyperaldosteronism	nephrocalcinosis
SIADH	
Alcohol excess	
Hypercalciuria	
1,25-(OH)-vitamin D_3	
deficiency	
Drug toxicity:	
amphotericin	
aminoglycosides	
cisplatin	
ciclosporin	

SIADH, syndrome of inappropriate antidiuretic hormone secretion

encoding the gamma-subunit of Na^+/K^+-ATPase which is mainly expressed in TAL and DCT, is mutated, resulting in the inhibition of Na^+/K^+-ATPase activity and limiting the amount of potassium entry into the cell. Closing of potassium-sensitive apical magnesium channels cause reduced magnesium absorption and hypomagnesaemia in patients with IDH.

Familial hypomagnesaemia, hypercalciuria and nephrocalcinosis (FHHNC)

This disorder is characterized by excessive renal magnesium and calcium wasting. In addition, affected individuals develop bilateral nephrocalcinosis and progressive renal failure. Patients also have elevated PTH levels, which precedes any reduction in GFR. A substantial proportion of patients show incomplete distal renal tubular acidosis, hypocitraturia and hyperuricaemia. Extrarenal involvement such as myopia, nystagmus, chorioretinitis has been reported. Based on clinical observation and clearance studies, the main defect in magnesium and calcium reabsorption lies in cTAL. Ten different mutations have been identified in a novel gene (*CLND16*) which encodes for paracellin-1 (claudin 16), a member of the claudin family of tight junction proteins.

Clinical features

Symptoms and signs include irritability, tremor, ataxia, carpopedal spasm, hyperreflexia, confusional and hallucinatory states, and epileptiform convulsions. An ECG may show a prolonged QT interval, broad flattened T waves, and occasional shortening of the ST segment.

Treatment

This involves the withdrawal of precipitating agents such as diuretics or purgatives and the parenteral infusion of 50 mmol of magnesium chloride in 1 L of 5% dextrose or other isotonic fluid over 12–24 hours. This should be repeated daily until the plasma magnesium level is normal.

HYPERMAGNESAEMIA

This primarily occurs in patients with acute or chronic renal failure given magnesium-containing laxatives or antacids. It can also be induced by magnesium-containing enemas. Mild hypermagnesaemia may occur in patients with adrenal insufficiency. Causes are given in Table 12.16.

Clinical features

Symptoms and signs relate to neurological and cardiovascular depression, and include weakness with hyporeflexia proceeding to narcosis, respiratory paralysis and cardiac conduction defects. Symptoms usually develop when the plasma magnesium level exceeds 2 mmol/L.

Treatment

Treatment requires withdrawal of any magnesium

Table 12.16   Causes of hypermagnesaemia

Impaired renal excretion
Chronic renal failure
Acute renal failure

Increased magnesium intake
Purgatives, e.g. magnesium sulphate
Antacids, e.g. magnesium trisilicate

Haemodialysis with high [Mg^{2+}] dialysate

Table 12.17   Causes of hypophosphataemia

Redistribution	**Decreased intake/absorption**
Respiratory alkalosis	Dietary
Treatment of diabetic ketoacidosis (insulin drives phosphate into cells)	Malabsorption
	Vomiting
	Gut phosphate binders, e.g. aluminium hydroxide
Carbohydrate refeeding after fasting	Vitamin D deficiency
After parathyroidectomy (hungry bone disease)	Alcohol withdrawal

Renal losses
Hyperparathyroidism
Renal tubular defects
Dent's disease
Tumour-induced osteomalacia
X-linked ⎫
Autosomal ⎬ dominant hypophosphataemic rickets
Diuretics ⎭

therapy. An intravenous injection of 10 mL of calcium gluconate 10% (2.25 mmol calcium) is given to antagonize the effects of hypermagnesaemia, along with dextrose and insulin (as for hyperkalaemia) to lower the plasma magnesium level. Dialysis may be required in patients with severe renal failure.

DISORDERS OF PHOSPHATE CONCENTRATION

Phosphate forms an essential part of most biochemical systems, from nucleic acids downwards. About 80% of all body phosphorus is within bone, plasma phosphate normally ranging from 0.80 to 1.40 mmol/L. Phosphate reabsorption from the kidney (85% from the proximal tubule) is decreased by parathyroid hormone (PTH) mediated by a cyclic AMP-dependent mechanism; thus hyperparathyroidism is associated with low plasma levels of phosphate. Other factors that are known to control phosphate reabsorption in the proximal tubule are 1,25-dihydroxyvitamin D_3, sodium delivery to the proximal tubule, serum concentrations of calcium, bicarbonate, carbon dioxide tension, glucose, alanine, serotonin, dopamine and sympathetic activity. The regulation of plasma phosphate level is closely linked to calcium.

HYPOPHOSPHATAEMIA

Significant hypophosphataemia (< 0.4 mmol/L) occurs in a number of clinical situations, owing to redistribution into cells, to renal losses, or to decreased intake (Table 12.17). It may cause:

- muscle weakness, e.g. diaphragmatic weakness, decreased cardiac contractility, skeletal muscle rhabdomyolysis
- a left-shift in the oxyhaemoglobin dissociation curve (reduced 2,3-bisphosphoglycerate (2,3-BPG)) and rarely haemolysis
- confusion, hallucinations and convulsions.

Mild hypophosphataemia often resolves without specific treatment. However, diaphragmatic weakness may be severe in acute hypophosphataemia, and may impede weaning a patient from a ventilator. Interestingly, chronic hypophosphataemia (in X-linked hypophosphataemia) is associated with normal muscle power.

Diseases associated with altered serum phosphate concentrations

Decreased reabsorption of phosphate occurs in patients with tumour-induced osteomalacia (TIO), X-linked dominant hypophosphataemic rickets (XLR) and autosomal-dominant hypophosphataemic rickets (ADHR). These syndromes have similar biochemical and osseous phenotypes. Patients have osteomalacia or rickets, reduced tubular phosphate reabsorption, hypophosphataemia, normal or low serum calcium, normal PTH and PTH-related protein concentrations and normal or low 1,25-dihydroxyvitamin D_3. Urinary cyclic AMP levels are generally in the normal range.

In TIO, there is excessive production of phosphatonins, e.g. fibroblast growth factor 23 (FGF-23), matrix extracellular phosphoglycoprotein (MEPG) and frizzled related protein 4 (FRP-4). These cannot be degraded by normal concentrations of PHEX (phosphate regulating gene with homologies to endopeptidases on the X chromosome). This results in net excess of inhibitors of the sodium–phosphate cotransporter in the proximal tubule, and phosphaturia.

In ADHR, FGF-23 is mutated so that it is resistant to PHEX proteolysis. *In XLR*, mutations in PHEX prevent binding to FGF-23 and FRP-4, resulting in a net relative excess of phosphatonins.

Normal adaptive increases in 1,25-dihydroxyvitamin D_3 synthesis in response to low phosphate levels do not occur in TIO, ADHR and XLR, aggravating phosphaturia (Fig. 12.10).

Dent's disease is now the generally accepted name for a group of hereditary tubular disorders including X-linked recessive nephrolithiasis with renal failure, X-linked recessive hypophosphataemic rickets and idiopathic low-molecular-weight proteinuria. Dent's disease is characterized by low-molecular-weight proteinuria, hypercalciuria, hyperphosphaturia, nephrocalcinosis, kidney stones and eventual renal failure, with some patients developing rickets or osteomalacia. It is caused by loss of

LUMEN   CELL   INTERSTITIAL FLUID/BLOOD

Fig. 12.10   PHEX regulation of phosphate transport and vitamin D metabolism in the proximal tubule. The hormone, phosphatonin is an inhibitor of sodium–phosphate cotransporter (NPT2). When bound to PHEX (phosphate-regulating gene with homologies to endopeptidase on the X chromosome) it is bioinactive and is thought to stimulate phosphate reabsorption via the sodium–phosphate cotransporter (NPT2) and to retard the degradation of 1,25-dihydroxyvitamin D by downregulating 24-hydroxylase activity. Over-production of phosphatonins occurs in tumour-induced osteomalacia, gain of function mutation as in autosomal dominant hypophosphataemic rickets and loss of function mutation in PHEX as X-linked hypophosphataemia. This causes renal phosphate wasting, as well as increased 1,25-dihydroxyvitamin D degradation. Modified from Rowe PSN (1998).

function mutation of a proximal tubular endosomal chloride channel, ClC5. This chloride channel, along with the proton pump is essential for acidification of proximal tubular endosomes. The process is linked with normal endocytosis, degradation and recycling of absorbed proteins, vitamins and hormones. Defective endosomal acidification (owing to the mutated *CLCN5* gene) results in impaired endosomal degradation and recycling of endocytosed hormones such as PTH. High PTH concentration activates apical receptors, increases endocytosis of the sodium–phosphate cotransporter and produces increased phosphaturia. It also results in increased 1α-hydoxylase activity, causing excess production of 1,25-$(OH)_2$ D_3, hypercalciuria, renal stones and nephrocalcinosis. Moreover, the receptors (megalin and cubilin) for reabsorption of low-molecular-weight proteins and albumin in the proximal tubules are decreased in Dent's disease. This is secondary to the defective acidification of endosomes, which can explain low-molecular-weight proteinuria and excessive urinary leaks of cytokines, hormones and chemokines. This urinary profile is associated with progressive renal fibrosis and more rapid decline in renal function.

Treatment includes combined therapy with phosphate supplementation and calcitriol (1,25-dihydroxyvitamin D) administration.

Treatment of acute hypophosphataemia, if warranted, is with intravenous phosphate at a maximum rate of 9 mmol every 12 hours, with repeated measurements of calcium and phosphate, as over-rapid administration of phosphate may lead to severe hypocalcaemia, particularly in the presence of alkalosis. Chronic hypophosphataemia can be corrected, if warranted, with oral effervescent sodium phosphate.

HYPERPHOSPHATAEMIA

Hyperphosphataemia is common in patients with chronic renal failure (see p. 668 and Table 12.18). Hyperphosphataemia is usually asymptomatic but may result in precipitation of calcium phosphate, particularly in the presence of a normal or raised calcium or of alkalosis. Uraemic itching may be caused by a raised calcium × phosphate product. Prolonged hyperphosphataemia causes hyperparathyroidism, and periarticular and vascular calcification.

Usually no treatment is required for acute hyperphosphataemia, as the causes are self-limiting. Treatment of chronic hyperphosphataemia is with gut phosphate binders and dialysis (see p. 672).

FURTHER READING
Calverie Martin F, Gonzalez Acosta H, Flores C et al. (2003) De novo insertion of an Alu sequence in the coding region of the CLCN5 gene results in Dent's disease. *Human Genetics* **113**(6): 480–485.
Konrad M, Weber S (2003) Recent advances in molecular genetics of hereditary magnesium losing disorders. *Journal of the American Society of Nephrology* **14**: 249–260.
Schiavi SC, Kumar R (2004) The phosphatonin pathway: new insights in phosphate homeostasis. *Kidney International* **65**: 1–14.
Weiseinger JR, Bellorin-Fort E (1998) Electrolyte quintet. Magnesium and phosphate. *Lancet* **352**: 391–396.

Table 12.18   Causes of hyperphosphataemia
Chronic renal failure
Phosphate-containing enemas
Tumour lysis
Myeloma-abnormal phosphate-binding protein
Rhabdomyolysis

ACID–BASE DISORDERS

The concentration of hydrogen ions in both extracellular and intracellular compartments is extremely tightly controlled, and very small changes may lead to major cell dysfunction. The blood pH is tightly regulated and is normally maintained at between 7.38 and 7.42. Any deviation from this range indicates a change in the hydrogen ion concentration $[H^+]$ because blood pH is the negative logarithm of $[H^+]$ (Table 12.19). The $[H^+]$ at a physiological blood pH of 7.40 is 40 nmol/L. An increase

Table 12.19	Relationship between [H⁺] and pH
pH	[H⁺] (nmol/L)
6.9	126
7.0	100
7.1	79
7.2	63
7.3	50
7.4	40
7.5	32
7.6	25

in the [H⁺] – a fall in pH – is termed acidaemia. A decrease in [H⁺] – a rise in the blood pH – is termed alkalaemia. The disorders that cause these changes in the blood pH are acidosis and alkalosis, respectively.

Normal acid–base physiology

The normal adult diet contains 70–100 mmol of acid. Throughout the body, there are buffers that minimize any changes in blood pH that these ingested hydrogen ions might cause. Such buffers include intracellular proteins (e.g. haemoglobin) and tissue components (e.g. the calcium carbonate and calcium phosphate in bone) as well as the bicarbonate–carbonic acid buffer pair generated by the hydration of carbon dioxide. This buffer pair is clinically most relevant, in part because its contribution can be measured and because alterations in this buffer pair reveal changes in all other buffer systems. Bicarbonate ions [HCO_3^-] and carbonic acid (H_2CO_3) exist in equilibrium; and in the presence of carbonic anhydrase, carbonic acid dissociates to carbon dioxide and water, as expressed in the following equation:

$$H^+ + HCO_3^- \rightleftharpoons H_2CO_3 \overset{\text{carbonic anhydrase}}{\rightleftharpoons} CO_2 + H_2O.$$

The addition of hydrogen ions drives the reaction to the right, decreasing the plasma bicarbonate concentration [HCO_3^-] and increasing the arterial carbon dioxide pressure (P_aCO_2). As shown in the following Henderson–Hasselbalch equation, a fall in the plasma [HCO_3^-] increases [H^+] and thus lowers blood pH:

$$[H^+] = 181 \times P_aCO_2 \, [HCO_3^-]$$

where [H^+] is expressed in nmol per litre, P_aCO_2 in kilopascals, [HCO_3^-] in mmol per litre, and 181 is the dissociation coefficient of carbonic acid. Alternatively the equation can be expressed as:

$$pH = pK + \log \, [HCO_3^-]/[H_2CO_3]$$

where pK = 6.1. Thus, the bicarbonate used in the buffering process must be regenerated to maintain normal acid–base balance.

Although the acidaemia stimulates an increase in ventilation, which blunts this change in pH, increased ventilation does not regenerate the bicarbonate used in the buffering process. Consequently, the kidney must excrete hydrogen ions to return the plasma [HCO_3^-] to normal. Maintenance of a normal plasma [HCO_3^-] under physiological conditions depends not only on daily regeneration of bicarbonate but also on reabsorption of all bicarbonate filtered across the glomerular capillaries.

Renal reabsorption of bicarbonate

The plasma [HCO_3^-] is normally maintained at approximately 25 mmol/L. In individuals with a normal glomerular filtration rate (120 mL/min), about 4500 mmol of bicarbonate is filtered each day. If this filtered bicarbonate were not reabsorbed, the plasma [HCO_3^-] would fall, along with blood pH. Thus, maintenance of a normal plasma [HCO_3^-] requires that essentially all of the bicarbonate in the glomerular filtrate be reabsorbed (Fig. 12.11).

The proximal convoluted tubule reclaims 85–90% of filtered bicarbonate; in contrast, the distal nephron reclaims very little. This difference is caused by the greater quantity of luminal carbonic anhydrase in the proximal tubule than in the distal nephron. As a result of these quantitative differences, bicarbonate that escapes reabsorption in the proximal tubule is excreted in the urine.

Proximal tubular bicarbonate reabsorption is catalysed by the Na⁺/K⁺-ATPase pump located in the basolateral cell membrane. By exchanging peritubular potassium ions for intracellular sodium ions, the pump keeps the intracellular sodium concentration low, allowing sodium ions to enter the cell by moving down the sodium concentration gradient from the tubule lumen to the cell interior. Hydrogen ions are transported in the opposite

Fig. 12.11 Resorption of sodium bicarbonate in the renal (mainly proximal) tubule. Bicarbonate is reclaimed by the secretion of H⁺ into the tubule in exchange for Na⁺. This results in the formation of H_2CO_3, which is then broken down to CO_2. This is reabsorbed and converted back to H_2CO_3, which now dissociates into H⁺ and HCO_3^-. The net result is reabsorption of Na⁺ and HCO_3^-. This process is dependent on carbonic anhydrase within the cells and on the luminal surface of the tubular cell.

direction (at the Na^+–H^+ antiporter), thereby maintaining electroneutrality. Before bicarbonate enters the proximal tubule, it combines with secreted hydrogen ions, forming carbonic acid. In the presence of luminal carbonic anhydrase (CA-IV) carbonic acid rapidly dissociates into carbon dioxide and water, which can then rapidly enter the proximal tubular cell. In the cell, carbon dioxide is hydrated by cytosolic carbonic anhydrase (CA-II), ultimately forming bicarbonate, which is then transported down an electrical gradient from the cell interior, across the membrane into the peritubular fluid, and into the blood. In this process, each hydrogen ion secreted into the proximal tubule lumen is reabsorbed and can be resecreted; there is no net loss of hydrogen ions or net gain of bicarbonate ions.

Renal excretion of [H^+] (Fig. 12.12)
More acid is secreted into the proximal tubule (up to 4500 nmol of hydrogen ions each day) than into any other nephron segment. However, the hydrogen ions secreted into the proximal tubule are almost completely reabsorbed with bicarbonate; consequently, proximal tubular hydrogen ion secretion does not contribute significantly to hydrogen ion elimination from the body. The excretion of the daily acid load requires hydrogen ion secretion in more distal nephron segments.

Most dietary hydrogen ions come from sulphur-containing amino acids that are metabolized to sulphuric acid (H_2SO_4), which then reacts with sodium bicarbonate as follows:

$$H_2SO_4 + 2NaHCO_3 \rightarrow Na_2SO_4 + 2CO_2 + 2H_2O.$$

Excess sulphate is excreted in the urine, whereas excess hydrogen ions are buffered by bicarbonate and lower the plasma [HCO_3^-]. This fall in plasma [HCO_3^-] leads to a slight decrease in the blood pH, although a smaller decrease in the blood pH than would have occurred if buffer were unavailable. The subsequent excretion of hydrogen ions takes place primarily in the collecting duct and results in the regeneration of 1 mmol of bicarbonate for every mmol of hydrogen ions excreted in the urine.

The collecting duct has two types of cell:

- *The principal cell* with an aldosterone-sensitive Na^+ absorption site. These cells reabsorb Na^+ and H_2O and secrete K^+ under the influence of aldosterone.
- *The α-intercalated cell*, which possesses the proton pump for the active secretion of hydrogen ions in exchange for reabsorption of K^+ ions. Aldosterone increases H^+ ion secretion.

Secretion of hydrogen ions from the cortical collecting duct is indirectly linked to sodium reabsorption. Aldosterone has several facilitating effects on hydrogen ion secretion. Aldosterone opens sodium channels in the luminal membrane of the principal cell and increases Na^+/K^+-ATPase activity. The subsequent movement of cationic sodium into the principal cell creates a negative charge within the tubule lumen. Potassium ions from the principal cells and hydrogen ions from the α-intercalated cells move out from the cells down the electrochemical gradient and into the lumen. Aldosterone also stimulates directly the H^+-ATPase in the α-intercalated cell, further enhancing hydrogen ion secretion.

When hydrogen ions are secreted into the lumen of the collecting tubule, a tiny, but physiologically critical, fraction of these excess hydrogen ions remains in solution. Here, they increase the urinary [H^+] and lower urinary pH below 4.0. Nevertheless, below this urine pH, inhibition of proton-secreting pumps such as H^+-ATPase severely restricts kidney secretion of more hydrogen ions. Consequently, secretion of hydrogen ions depends on the presence of buffers in the urine that maintain the urine pH at a level higher than 4.0.

Fig. 12.12 **Renal excretion of H^+.** Secretion of H^+ from the cortical collecting ducts is indirectly linked to Na^+ reabsorption. Intracellular potassium is exchanged for sodium in the principal cell. Aldosterone stimulates H^+ secretion by entering the principal cell, where it opens Na^+ channels in the luminal membrane and increases Na^+/K^+-ATPase activity. The movement of cationic Na^+ into the principal cells then creates a negative charge within the tubule lumen. K^+ moves from the electrochemical gradient and into the lumen.

Aldosterone apparently also stimulates the H^+-ATPase directly in the intercalated cell, further enhancing H^+ secretion. When the urinary pH falls to 4.0–4.5, further H^+ secretion by the α-intercalated cells ceases. The filtration of titratable acids (e.g. phosphoric acid) raises the intraluminal pH and permits this process to continue. Secreted H^+ binds to the conjugate anion of a titratable acid (HPO_4^{2-} in this case) and is excreted in the urine. The H^+ to be secreted arises from the reassociation of H_2O and CO_2 in the presence of carbonic anhydrase; thus, a bicarbonate molecule is regenerated each time an H^+ is eliminated in the urine.

Buffer systems in acid excretion
Two buffer systems are involved in acid excretion: the titratable acids such as phosphate, and the ammonia system. Each system is responsible for excreting about half of the daily acid load of 50–100 mmol under physiological conditions (Fig. 12.12).

Titratable acid

A titratable acid is a filtered buffer substance having a conjugate anion that can be titrated within the pH range occurring physiologically in the urine. Phosphoric acid (pK_a 6.8) is the usual titratable urinary buffer. Hydrogen ions bind to the conjugate anions of the titratable acids and are excreted in the urine. For each hydrogen ion excreted in this form, a bicarbonate ion is regenerated within the cell and returned to the blood (Fig. 12.12).

Ammonium (NH_4^+)

In the setting of metabolic acidosis, titratable acids cannot increase significantly because the availability of titratable acid is fixed by the plasma concentration of the buffer and by the GFR. The ammonia buffer system, in contrast, can increase several 100-fold when necessary. Consequently, impaired renal excretion of hydrogen ions is always associated with a defect in ammonium excretion (Fig. 12.13).

All ammonia used to buffer urinary hydrogen ions in the collecting tubule is synthesized in the proximal convoluted tubule. Glutamine is the primary source of ammonia. It undergoes deamination catalysed by glutaminase, resulting in α-ketoglutaric acid (see Fig. 12.13) and ammonia. Once formed, ammonia can diffuse into the proximal tubule lumen and become acidified, forming ammonium. Once in the proximal tubule lumen, ammonium flows along the tubule to the thick ascending limb of Henle's loop. Here, it is transported out of the tubule into the medullary interstitium. Ammonium then dissociates to ammonia, leading to a high interstitial ammonia concentration. Ammonia diffuses down its concentration gradient into the lumen of the collecting

Fig. 12.13 **The ammonia buffering system in the kidney.** All ammonia used to buffer H^+ in the collecting duct is synthesized in the proximal convoluted tubule, and glutamine is the main source of this ammonia. As glutamine is metabolized, α-ketoglutarate (α-KG) is formed, which ultimately breaks down to bicarbonate that is then secreted into the peritubular fluid at an Na^+–HCO_3^- cotransporter.

tubule. Here, it reacts with the hydrogen ions secreted by the collecting tubular cells to form ammonium. Because ammonium (NH_4) is not lipid-soluble, it is trapped in the lumen and excreted in the urine as ammonium chloride. Two conditions predominantly promote ammonia synthesis by the proximal tubular cell: systemic acidosis and hypokalaemia.

Controversy still exists about whether glutamine metabolism and ureagenesis in the liver play a role in acid–base homeostasis. Ureagenesis in the liver consumes up to 1000 mmol of bicarbonate/day in humans as a result of $2NH_4 + 2HCO_3$ = urea + CO_2 + H_2O. The liver is believed to contribute to regulation of acid–base balance by controlling the rate of ureagenesis and therefore bicarbonate consumption in response to changes in plasma acidity. Recent studies in human volunteers have shown that metabolic acidosis increases ureagenesis and potentially makes it worse by consuming more bicarbonate. Similarly, metabolic alkalosis decreases ureagenesis, whereby less bicarbonate is consumed, resulting in an increase of alkali load in the face of alkalosis. In the light of these new human data it is concluded that ureagenesis is a maladaptive process for acid–base regulation and that ureagenesis has no discernible homeostatic effect on acid–base equilibrium in humans.

Causes of acid–base disturbance

Acid–base disturbance may be caused by:

- abnormal CO_2 removal in the lungs ('respiratory' acidosis and alkalosis)
- abnormalities in the regulation of bicarbonate and other buffers in the blood ('metabolic' acidosis and alkalosis).

Both may, and usually do, coexist. For instance, metabolic acidosis causes hyperventilation (via medullary chemoreceptors, see p. 877), leading to increased removal of CO_2 in the lungs and partial compensation for the acidosis. Conversely, respiratory acidosis is accompanied by renal bicarbonate retention, which could be mistaken for primary metabolic alkalosis. The situation is even more complex if a patient has both respiratory disease and a metabolic disturbance.

Diagnosis

Clinical history and examination usually point to the correct diagnosis. Table 12.20 shows the typical changes, but in complicated patients the acid–base nomogram (Fig. 12.14) is invaluable. The $[H^+]$ and P_aCO_2 are measured in arterial blood (for precautions see p. 713) as well as the bicarbonate. If the values from a patient lie in one of the bands in the diagram, it is likely that only one abnormality is present. If the $[H^+]$ is high (pH low) but the P_aCO_2 is normal, the intercept lies between two bands: the patient has respiratory dysfunction, leading to failure of CO_2 elimination, but this is partly compensated for by metabolic acidosis, stimulating respiration and CO_2 removal (this is the most common 'combined' abnormality in practice).

Table 12.20	Changes in arterial blood gases		
	pH	P_aco_2	HCO_3^-
Respiratory acidosis	N or ↓	↑↑	↑ (compensated)
Respiratory alkalosis	N or ↑	↓↓	↓ (slight)
Metabolic acidosis	N or ↓	↓	↓↓
Metabolic alkalosis	N or ↑	↑ (slight)	↑↑

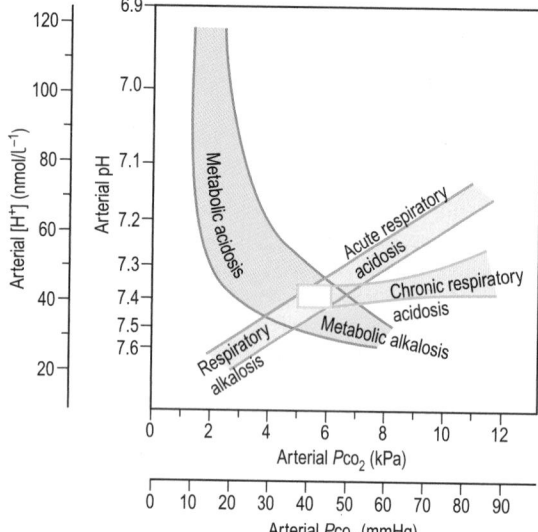

Fig. 12.14   **The Flenley acid–base nomogram.** This was derived from a large number of observations in patients with 'pure' respiratory or metabolic disturbances. The bands show the 95% confidence limits representing the individual varieties of acid–base disturbance. The central white box shows the approximate limits of arterial pH and $P\text{co}_2$ in normal individuals.

RESPIRATORY ACIDOSIS AND ALKALOSIS

Respiratory acidosis
This is caused by retention of CO_2. The P_aco_2 and $[H^+]$ rise. Renal retention of bicarbonate may partly compensate, returning the $[H^+]$ towards normal (see p. 713).

Respiratory alkalosis
Increased removal of CO_2 is caused by hyperventilation, so there is a fall in P_aco_2 and $[H^+]$ (see p. 877).

METABOLIC ACIDOSIS

This is due to the accumulation of any acid other than carbonic acid, and there is a primary decrease in the plasma $[HCO_3^-]$. Several disorders can lead to metabolic acidosis: acid administration, acid generation (e.g. lactic acidosis during shock or cardiac arrest), impaired acid excretion by the kidneys, or bicarbonate losses from the gastrointestinal tract or kidneys. From a diagnostic viewpoint, calculation of the plasma anion gap is extremely useful in narrowing this differential diagnosis.

The anion gap
The first step is to identify whether the acidosis is due to retention of H^+Cl^- or to another acid. This is achieved by calculation of the anion gap. The principles underlying this calculation are straightforward:

- The normal cations present in plasma are Na^+, K^+, Ca^{2+}, Mg^{2+}.
- The normal anions present in plasma are Cl^-, HCO_3^-, negative charges present on albumin, phosphate, sulphate, lactate, and other organic acids.
- The sums of the positive and negative charges are equal.
- Measurement of plasma $[Na^+]$, $[K^+]$, $[Cl^-]$ and $[HCO_3^-]$ is usually easily available.

$$\text{ANION GAP} = \{[Na^+] + [K^+]\} - \{[HCO_3^-] + [Cl^-]\}$$

Because there are more unmeasured anions than cations, the normal anion gap is 10–18 mmol/L, although calculations with more sensitive methods place this at 6–12 mmol/L. Albumin normally makes up the largest portion of these unmeasured anions. As a result, a fall in the plasma albumin concentration from the normal value of about 40 g/L to 20 g/L may reduce the anion gap by as much as 6 mmol/L, because each 1 g/L of albumin has a negative charge of 0.2–0.28 mmol/L.

Metabolic acidosis with a normal anion gap

If the anion gap is normal in the presence of acidosis, this suggests that H^+Cl^- is being retained or that $Na^+HCO_3^-$ is being lost. Causes of a normal-anion-gap acidosis are given in Table 12.21. In these conditions, plasma bicarbonate decreases and is replaced by chloride to maintain electroneutrality. Consequently, these disorders are sometimes referred to collectively as hyperchloraemic acidoses.

Renal tubular acidosis (RTA)
This term refers to systemic acidosis caused by impairment of the ability of the renal tubules to maintain

Table 12.21 Causes of metabolic acidosis with a normal anion gap	
Increased gastrointestinal bicarbonate loss	**Decreased renal hydrogen ion excretion**
Diarrhoea	Distal (type 1) renal tubular
Ileostomy	acidosis
Ureterosigmoidostomy	Type 4 renal tubular acidosis
	(aldosterone deficiency)
Increased renal	
bicarbonate loss	**Increased HCl production**
Acetazolamide	Ammonium chloride ingestion
Proximal (type 2) renal	Increased catabolism of lysine,
tubular acidosis	arginine
Hyperparathyroidism	
Tubular damage,	
e.g. drugs, heavy metals,	
paraproteins	

acid–base balance. This group of disorders is uncommon and only rarely a cause of significant clinical disease. Renal tubular acidosis may be secondary to immunological, drug-induced or structural damage to the tubular cells, an inherited abnormality, or an isolated ('primary') abnormality. As with most disorders that are not well understood, the nomenclature is confusing.

Type 4 renal tubular acidosis

Also called 'hyporeninaemic hypoaldosteronism', this is probably the most common of these disorders. The cardinal features are hyperkalaemia and acidosis occurring in a patient with mild chronic renal insufficiency, usually caused by tubulo-interstitial disease (e.g. reflux nephropathy) or diabetes (Gordon's syndrome shares biochemical abnormalities but differs in having normal GFR and hypertension). Plasma renin and aldosterone are found to be low, even after measures which would normally stimulate their secretion (Table 12.22). An identical syndrome may be caused by chronic ingestion of NSAIDs, which impair renin and aldosterone secretion. In the presence of acidosis, urine pH may be low. Treatment is with fludrocortisone, sodium bicarbonate, diuretics, or ion exchange resins to remove potassium, or some combination of these. Dietary potassium restriction alone is ineffective.

Type 3 renal tubular acidosis (RTA)

This condition is vanishingly rare, and represents a combination of type 1 and type 2. Inherited type 3 RTA is caused by mutations resulting in carbonic anhydrase type II deficiency, which is characterized by osteopetrosis, RTA of mixed type, cerebral calcification and mental retardation. Typical radiographic features of osteopetrosis are present and histopathological study of the iliac crest reveals unreabsorbed calcified primary spongia.

Type 2 ('proximal') renal tubular acidosis

This is very rare in adult practice (Table 12.23). It is caused by failure of sodium bicarbonate reabsorption in the proximal tubule. The cardinal features are acidosis, hypokalaemia, an inability to lower the urine pH below

Table 12.23 Causes of proximal renal tubular acidosis (type 2 RTA)

Cystinosis	Vitamin D deficiency/ hyperparathyroidism
Tyrosinaemia	
Wilson's disease	**Toxins and drugs**
Glycogen storage disease, type I	Carbonic anhydrase inhibitors
	Lead
Pyruvate carboxylase deficiency	Cadmium
	Mercury
	Uranium
Multiple myeloma	Copper
	Outdated tetracycline ingestion

5.5 despite systemic acidosis, and the appearance of bicarbonate in the urine despite a subnormal plasma bicarbonate. This disorder normally occurs as part of a generalized tubular defect, together with other features such as glycosuria and amino-aciduria. Inherited forms of isolated type 2 RTA are described as both autosomal dominant and recessive patterns of inheritance, where putative mutations are in the Na^+–H^+ antiporter in the apical membrane and Na^+–HCO_3^- cotransporter in the basolateral membrane of proximal tubular cells respectively (Fig. 12.11) Treatment is with sodium bicarbonate: massive doses may be required to overcome the renal 'leak'.

Type 1 ('distal') renal tubular acidosis

This is due to a failure of H^+ excretion in the distal tubule (Table 12.24). It consists of:

- acidosis
- hypokalaemia (few exceptions)
- inability to lower the urine pH below 5.3 despite systemic acidosis
- low urinary ammonium production.

Table 12.22 Diagnosis of hyporeninaemic hypoaldosteronism (type 4 renal tubular acidosis)

Hyperkalaemia
(In the absence of drugs known to cause hyperkalaemia)

Low plasma bicarbonate and hyperchloraemia

Normal ACTH stimulation test

Low basal 24-hour urinary aldosterone

Subnormal response of plasma renin and plasma aldosterone to stimulation
Samples taken over 2 hours supine and again after 40 mg furosemide (80 mg if creatinine > 120 µmol/L) and 4 hours upright posture

Correction of hyperkalaemia by fludrocortisone 0.1 mg daily

Table 12.24 Causes of distal renal tubular acidosis (type 1 RTA)

Primary	**Drugs and toxins**
Idiopathic	Amphotericin B
	Lithium carbonate
Genetic	NSAIDs
Familial	Lead
Marfan's syndrome	
Ehlers–Danlos syndrome	**Autoimmune diseases**
Sickle cell anaemia	Sjögren's syndrome*
	Thyroiditis
Nephrocalcinosis	Autoimmune hepatitis
Chronic hypercalcaemia	Primary biliary cirrhosis
Medullary sponge kidney	Systemic lupus erythematosus
Hypergammaglobulinaemic states	
Amyloidosis*	**Renal transplant rejection***
Cryoglobulinaemia	
Chronic liver disease	

*May also cause proximal renal tubular acidosis

Practical Box 12.1
Diagnosis of renal tubular acidosis

Plasma HCO_3^- < 21 mmol/L, urine pH > 5.3 = renal tubular acidosis

To differentiate between proximal (very rare) and distal (rare) requires bicarbonate infusion test

Plasma HCO_3^- > 21 mmol/L but suspicion of partial renal tubular acidosis (e.g. nephrocalcinosis-associated diseases): **acid load test** required as follows:

Give 100 mg/kg ammonium chloride by mouth

Check urine pH hourly and plasma HCO_3^- at 3 hours

Plasma HCO_3^- should drop below 21 mmol/L unless the patient vomits (in which case the test should be repeated with an antiemetic)

If urine pH remains > 5.3 despite a plasma HCO_3^- of 21 mmol/L, the diagnosis is confirmed

These features may be present only in the face of increased acid production; hence the need for an acid load test in diagnosis (Practical box 12.1). Other features include:

- low urinary citrate (owing to increased citrate absorption in the proximal tubule where it can be converted to bicarbonate)
- hypercalciuria.

These abnormalities result in osteomalacia, renal stone formation and recurrent urinary infections. Osteomalacia is caused by buffering of H^+ by Ca^{2+} in bone, resulting in depletion of calcium from bone. Renal stone formation is caused by hypercalciuria, hypocitraturia (citrate inhibits calcium phosphate precipitation), and alkaline urine (which favours precipitation of calcium phosphate). Recurrent urinary infections are caused by renal stones. Both autosomal dominant and recessive inheritance patterns have been reported in primary distal RTA. Patients in South East Asia with an autosomal dominant type have a milder phenotype and may have an associated ovalocytosis. In this form the $Cl^--HCO_3^-$ exchanger in the basolateral surface of intercalated cells is mutated. However, in the autosomal recessive distal RTA, a substantial proportion of patients have sensorineural deafness, and this is associated with a loss of function mutation in the H^+-ATPase at the apical surface of intercalated cells.

Treatment is with sodium bicarbonate, potassium supplements and citrate. Thiazide diuretics are useful by causing volume contraction and increased proximal sodium bicarbonate reabsorption.

Urinary anion gap

Another useful tool in the evaluation of metabolic acidosis with a normal anion gap is the urinary anion gap:

URINARY ANION GAP =
{urinary $[Na^+]$ + urinary $[K^+]$} – urinary $[Cl^-]$.

This calculation can be used to distinguish the normal-anion-gap acidosis caused by diarrhoea (or other gastro-intestinal alkali loss) from that caused by distal renal tubular acidosis. In both disorders, the plasma $[K^+]$ is characteristically low. In patients with renal tubular acidosis, urinary pH is always greater than 5.3.

Although excretion of urinary hydrogen ions in the patient with diarrhoea should acidify the urine, hypokalaemia leads to enhanced ammonia synthesis by the proximal tubular cells. Despite acidaemia, the excess urinary buffer increases the urine pH to a value above 5.3 in some patients with diarrhoea.

Whenever urinary acid is excreted as ammonium chloride, the increase in urinary chloride excretion decreases the urinary anion gap. Thus, the urinary anion gap should be negative in the patient with diarrhoea, regardless of the urine pH. On the other hand, although hypokalaemia may result in enhanced proximal tubular ammonia synthesis in distal renal tubular acidosis, the inability to secrete hydrogen ions into the collecting duct in this condition limits ammonium chloride formation and excretion; thus, the urinary anion gap is positive in distal renal tubular acidosis.

Metabolic acidosis with a high anion gap

If the anion gap is increased, one may conclude that an unmeasured anion is present in increased quantities. This may be either one of the acids normally present in small, but unmeasured quantities, such as lactate, or an exogenous acid. Causes of a high-anion-gap acidosis are given in Table 12.25.

Table 12.25 Causes of metabolic acidosis with an increased anion gap

Renal failure (sulphate, phosphate)

Accumulation of organic acids

Lactic acidosis
L-lactic
   Type A – anaerobic metabolism in tissues
      Hypotension/cardiac arrest
      Sepsis
   Poisoning – e.g. ethylene glycol, methanol
   Type B – decreased hepatic lactate metabolism
      Insulin deficiency (decreased pyruvate dehydrogenase activity)
      Metformin accumulation (chronic renal failure)
      Haematological malignancies
      Rare inherited enzyme defects
D-lactic (fermentation of glucose in bowel by abnormal bowel flora, complicating abnormal small bowel anatomy, e.g. blind loops)

Ketoacidosis
Insulin deficiency
Alcohol excess
Starvation

Exogenous acids
Salicylate

Lactic acidosis

Increased lactic acid production occurs when cellular respiration is abnormal, because of either a lack of oxygen in the tissues ('type A') or a metabolic abnormality, such as drug-induced ('type B') (Table 12.25). The most common cause in clinical practice is type A lactic acidosis, occurring in septic or cardiogenic shock. Significant acidosis can occur despite a normal blood pressure and P_aCO_2, owing to splanchnic and peripheral vasoconstriction. Acidosis worsens cardiac function and vasoconstriction further, contributing to a downward spiral and fulminant production of lactic acid.

Diabetic ketoacidosis (see p. 1119)

This is a high-anion-gap acidosis resulting from the accumulation of organic acids, acetoacetic acid and hydroxybutyric acid, owing to increased production and some reduced peripheral utilization.

Uraemic acidosis

Kidney disease may cause acidosis in several ways. Reduction in the number of functioning nephrons decreases the capacity to excrete ammonia and H^+ in the urine. In addition, tubular disease may cause bicarbonate wasting. Acidosis is a particular feature of those types of chronic renal failure in which the tubules are particularly affected, such as reflux nephropathy and chronic obstructive uropathy.

Chronic acidosis is most often caused by chronic renal failure, where there is a failure to excrete fixed acid. Up to 40 mmol of hydrogen ions may accumulate daily. These are buffered by bone, in exchange for calcium. Chronic acidosis is therefore a major risk factor for renal osteodystrophy and hypercalciuria.

Chronic acidosis has also been shown to be a risk factor for muscle wasting in renal failure, and may also contribute to the inexorable progression of some types of renal disease.

Uraemic acidosis should be corrected because of the effects of chronic acidosis on growth, muscle turnover and bones. Oral sodium bicarbonate 2–3 mmol/kg daily is usually enough to maintain serum bicarbonate above 20 mmol/L, but may contribute to sodium overload. Calcium carbonate improves acidosis and also acts as a phosphate binder and calcium supplement, and is commonly used. Acidosis in end-stage renal failure is usually fully corrected by adequate dialysis.

Mixed metabolic acidosis

Both types of acidosis may coexist. For instance, cholera would be expected to cause a normal-anion-gap acidosis owing to massive gastrointestinal losses of bicarbonate, but the anion gap is often increased owing to renal failure and lactic acidosis as a result of hypovolaemia.

Clinical features

Clinically the most obvious effect is stimulation of respiration, leading to the clinical sign of 'air hunger', or Kussmaul respiration. Interestingly, patients with pro-found hyperventilation may not complain of breathlessness, although in others it may be a presenting complaint.

Acidosis increases delivery of oxygen to the tissues by shifting the oxyhaemoglobin dissociation curve to the right, but it also leads to inhibition of 2,3-BPG production, which returns the curve towards normal (see p. 960). Cardiovascular dysfunction is common in acidotic patients, although it is often difficult to dissociate the numerous possible causes of this. There is no doubt that acidosis is negatively inotropic. Severe acidosis also causes venoconstriction, resulting in redistribution of blood from the peripheries to the central circulation, and increased systemic venous pressure, which may worsen pulmonary oedema caused by myocardial depression. Arteriolar vasodilatation also occurs, further contributing to hypotension.

Cerebral dysfunction is variable. Severe acidosis is often associated with confusion and fits, but numerous other possible causes are usually present.

As mentioned earlier, acidosis stimulates potassium loss from cells, which may lead to potassium deficiency if renal function is normal, or to hyperkalaemia if renal potassium excretion is impaired.

General treatment of acidosis

Treatment should be aimed at correcting the primary cause. In lactic acidosis caused by poor tissue perfusion ('type A'), treatment should be aimed at maximizing oxygen delivery to the tissues by protecting the airway, improving breathing and circulation. This usually requires inotropic agents, mechanical ventilation and invasive monitoring. In 'type B' lactic acidosis, treatment is that of the underlying disorder; e.g.

- insulin in diabetic ketoacidosis
- treatment of methanol and ethylene glycol poisoning with ethanol
- removal of salicylate by dialysis.

The question of whether severe acidosis should be treated with bicarbonate is extremely controversial. Severe acidosis ($[H^+] > 100$ nmol/L, pH < 7.0) is associated with a very high mortality, which makes many doctors keen to correct it. Since acidosis is known to impair cardiac contractility, it would seem sensible to correct acidosis with bicarbonate in a sick patient. However:

- Rapid correction of acidosis may result in tetany and fits owing to a rapid decrease in ionized calcium.
- Administration of sodium bicarbonate (8.4%) provides 1 mmol/mL of sodium, which may lead to extracellular volume expansion, exacerbating pulmonary oedema.
- Bicarbonate therapy increases CO_2 production and will therefore correct acidosis only if ventilation can be increased to remove the added CO_2 load.
- The increased amounts of CO_2 generated may diffuse more readily into cells than bicarbonate, worsening intracellular acidosis.

Administration of sodium bicarbonate (50 mmol, as 50 mL of 8.4% sodium bicarbonate intravenously) is still occasionally given during cardiac arrest and is often necessary before arrhythmias can be corrected. Correction of hyperkalaemia associated with acidosis is also of undoubted benefit. In other situations there is no clinical evidence to show that correction of acidosis improves outcome, but it is standard practice to administer sodium bicarbonate when [H⁺] is above 126 nmol/L (pH < 6.9), using intravenous 1.26% (150 mmol/L) bicarbonate. Intravenous sodium lactate should never be given.

METABOLIC ALKALOSIS

Metabolic alkalosis is common, comprising half of all the acid–base disorders in hospitalized patients. This observation should not be surprising since vomiting, the use of diuretics, and nasogastric suction are common among hospitalized patients. The mortality associated with metabolic alkalosis is substantial; the mortality rate is 45% in patients with an arterial pH of 7.55 and 80% when the pH is greater than 7.65. Although this relationship is not necessarily causal, severe alkalosis should be viewed with concern.

Classification and definitions

Metabolic alkalosis has been classified on the basis of underlying pathophysiology (Table 12.26).

The most common group is due to chloride depletion which can be corrected without potassium repletion. The other major grouping is that due to potassium depletion, usually with mineralocorticoid excess. Metabolic alkalosis due to both potassium and chloride depletion also occurs.

Table 12.26   Causes of metabolic alkalosis

Chloride depletion
Gastric losses: vomiting, mechanical drainage, bulimia
Chloruretic diuretics: e.g. bumetanide, furosemide chlorothiazide, metolazone
Diarrhoeal states: villous adenoma, congenital chloridorrhoea
Cystic fibrosis (high sweat chloride)

Potassium depletion/mineralocorticoid excess
Primary aldosteronism
Secondary aldosteronism
Apparent mineralocorticoid excess
   Primary deoxycorticosterone excess: 11α- and 17α-hydroxylase deficiencies
   Drugs: liquorice (glycyrrhizic acid) as a confection or flavouring, carbenoxolone
   Liddle's syndrome
Bartter's and Gitelman's syndromes and their variants
Laxative abuse, clay ingestion

Hypercalcaemia states
Hypercalcaemia of malignancy
Acute or chronic milk–alkali syndrome

Others
Ampicillin, penicillin therapy
Bicarbonate ingestion: massive or with renal insufficiency
Recovery from starvation
Hypoalbuminaemia

Chloride may be lost from the gut, kidney or skin. The loss of gastric fluid rich in acid results in alkalosis because bicarbonate generated during the production of gastric acid returns to the circulation. In Zollinger–Ellison syndrome (p. 416) or gastric outflow obstruction these losses can be massive. Although sodium and potassium loss in the gastric juice is variable, the obligate urinary loss of these cations is intensified by bicarbonaturia, which occurs during disequilibrium.

Chloruretic agents all directly produce loss of chloride, sodium and fluid in the urine. These losses in turn promote metabolic alkalosis by several mechanisms:

- diuretic-induced increases in sodium delivery to the distal nephron enhance potassium and hydrogen ion secretion
- extracellular volume contraction stimulates renin and aldosterone secretion, which blunts sodium losses but accelerates potassium and hydrogen ion secretion
- potassium depletion augments bicarbonate reabsorption in the proximal tubule, and
- stimulates ammonia production which in turn will increase urinary net acid excretion.

Urinary losses of chloride exceed those for sodium and are associated with alkalosis even when potassium depletion is prevented. The cessation of events that generate alkalosis is not necessarily accompanied by resolution of the alkalosis. A widely accepted hypothesis for the maintenance of alkalosis is chloride depletion rather than volume depletion. Although normal functioning of the proximal tubule is essential for bicarbonate absorption, the collecting duct appears to be the major nephron site for altered electrolyte and proton transport in both maintenance and recovery from metabolic alkalosis. During maintenance, the α-intercalated cells in the cortical collecting duct do not secrete bicarbonate because insufficient chloride is available for bicarbonate exchange. When chloride is administered and luminal or cellular chloride concentration increases, bicarbonate is promptly excreted and alkalosis is corrected.

Metabolic alkalosis in hypokalaemia is generated primarily by an increased intracellular shift of hydrogen ion causing intracellular acidosis. Potassium depletion is also associated with enhanced ammonia production with increased obligate net acid excretion. However, the role of intracellular acidosis is supported by the correction of the alkalosis by infusion of potassium without any suppression of renal net excretion. The correction is assumed to occur by the movement of potassium into and of hydrogen ion out of the cell, which titrates extracellular fluid bicarbonate.

Milk–alkali syndrome in which both bicarbonate and calcium are ingested produces alkalosis by vomiting, calcium-induced bicarbonate absorption and reduced GFR. Cationic antibiotics in high doses can cause alkalosis by obligatory bicarbonate loss in the urine.

Clinical features

The symptoms of metabolic alkalosis per se are difficult to separate from those of chloride, volume, or potassium depletion. Tetany (see p. 1095), apathy, confusion, drowsiness, cardiac arrhythmias and neuromuscular irritability are common when alkalosis is severe. The oxyhaemoglobin dissociation curve is shifted to the left. Respiration may be depressed.

Treatment

Chloride-responsive metabolic alkalosis. Although replacement of the chloride deficit is essential in chloride depletion states, selection of the accompanying cation – sodium, potassium or proton – is dependent on the assessment of extracellular fluid volume status (p. 699), the presence or absence of associated potassium depletion, and the degree and reversibility of any depression of GFR. If kidney function is normal, bicarbonate and base equivalents will be excreted with sodium or potassium, and metabolic alkalosis will be rapidly corrected as chloride is made available.

If chloride and extracellular depletion coexist then isotonic saline solution is appropriate therapy.

In the clinical settings of fluid overload, saline is contraindicated. In such situations, intravenous use of hydrochloride acid or ammonium chloride can be given. If GFR is adequate, acetazolamide, which causes bicarbonate diuresis by inhibiting carbonic anhydrase, can also be used. When the kidney is incapable of responding to chloride repletion, dialysis is necessary.

Chloride-resistant metabolic alkalosis. Metabolic alkalosis due to potassium depletion is managed by the correction of the underlying cause (see hypokalaemia). Mild to moderate alkalosis requires oral potassium chloride administration. However, the presence of cardiac arrhythmia or generalized weakness requires intravenous potassium chloride.

FURTHER READING

Adrogue HJ, Madias NE (1998) Management of life-threatening acid–base disorders. *New England Journal of Medicine* **338**: 26–34 and 107–111.

Borthwick KJ, Karet F (2002) Inherited disorders of the H$^+$-ATPase. *Current Opinion in Nephrology and Hypertension* **11**(5): 563–568.

Karet F (2002) Inherited distal renal tubular acidosis. *Journal of the American Society of Nephrology* **13**: 2178–2184.

Schrier RW (eds) (1997) In: *Renal and Electrolyte Disorders*. New York: Lippincott–Raven, pp. 1–240.

CASE STUDIES

Case 12.1
A 44-year-old patient with known chronic liver disease secondary to hepatitis B presented with marked exertional dyspnoea. Examination revealed: blood pressure 130/80, elevated JVP at 8 cm, bilateral pleural effusions, ascites and marked pitting pedal oedema. Investigations revealed: plasma sodium 136 mmol/L, potassium 3.6 mmol/L, bicarbonate 32 mmol/L, chloride 96 mmol/L, urinary sodium <10 mmol/day, urinary potassium 60 mmol/day.

Question
(a) Explain the persistent retention of sodium in the face of salt and water overload?

Answer
(a) In crisis, arterial vasodilatation due to nitric oxide overactivity leads to arterial underfilling. This is perceived by the pressure and volume receptors as hypovolaemia, with consequent activation of the sympathetic system, nonosmotic release of ADH and activation of the renin–angiotensin–aldosterone system. These mediators lead to salt and water reduction (see Fig. 12.3a, p. 691).

Case 12.2
A 32-year-old patient was referred for investigation of refractory hypertension. His blood pressure was elevated at 210/110 with grade 3 hypertensive retinopathy despite taking beta-blockers, a calcium antagonist and an ACE inhibitor. The rest of the examination was normal. Investigations revealed: sodium 148 mmol/L, potassium 3 mmol/L, bicarbonate 32 mmol/L, urea 4 mmol/L, glucose 4 mmol/L, urine dipstick negative for proteins.

Questions
(a) What is the likely diagnosis?
(b) What is the cause of absence of oedema in this patient?

Answers
(a) Conn's syndrome (p. 1097).
(b) This is due to the escape from the action of aldosterone. The escape is dependent on an increase in delivery of sodium to the site of aldosterone in the collecting duct. The increase in sodium delivery is achieved by high extracellular volume-mediated arterial overfilling. This suppresses sympathetic activity and angiotensin II generation, and increases cardiac release of ANP with resultant increase in renal perfusion pressure and GFR. The net result of these events is reduced sodium absorption in the proximal

tubules and increased sodium delivery, which over-whelms the sodium-retaining actions of aldosterone (see Fig. 12.3b, p. 691).

Case 12.3

A 62-year-old woman is found lying on the floor of her house. On examination she is bradycardic and peripherally shut down. ECG confirms sinus bradycardia with changes consistent with inferior myocardial infarction. Emergency electrolyte measurements revealed: sodium 136 mmol/L, potassium 4 mmol/L, bicarbonate 10 mmol/L, chloride 102 mmol/L, urea 7.5 mmol/L.

Question

(a) Comment on the biochemistry and how you will confirm your diagnosis?

Answer

(a) The biochemical picture is one of high-anionic-gap metabolic acidosis. In the presence of myocardial infarction and hypotension, the likely cause would be lactic acidosis. Measurement of plasma lactate (normally < 2 mmol/L) would confirm the diagnosis. Correction of the underlying cause will correct the acidosis by itself.

Case 12.4

The plasma biochemistry of a patient who presented with severe loin pain is as follows: sodium 138 mmol/L, potassium 2.5 mmol/L, urea 3.8 mmol/L, chloride 114 mmol/L, bicarbonate 14.5 mmol/L, urinary pH 6.5.

Questions

(a) What is the cause of this metabolic abnormality?
(b) What is the cause of the loin pain?

Answers

(a) Distal renal tubular acidosis (see the section on renal tubular acidosis).
(b) Nephrocalcinosis and renal colic due to renal stones are characteristic features of renal tubular acidosis.

Case 12.5

An 18-year-old boy was referred for the investigation of chronic fatigue syndrome. His mother comments that he is easily tired by sport and is not doing well at school. He is normotensive. Investigations revealed: sodium 145 mmol/L, potassium 2.8 mmol/L, bicarbonate 35 mmol/L, chloride 80 mmol/L, magnesium 0.6 mmol/L (normal range > 0.8 mmol/L), urea 5 mmol/L, glucose 5.2 mmol/L, urinary sodium excretion of 60 mmol and potassium excretion of 60 mmol/day.

Question

(a) What is the likely diagnosis?

Answer

(a) This patient has classic Gitelman's syndrome. It is similar to Bartter's but hypomagnesaemia favours Gitelman's syndrome.

Case 12.6

A 36-year-old woman with a past medical history of peptic ulceration presented with a history of 3 days of vomiting. She looked unwell and investigations revealed: haemoglobin 16.3 mmol/L, sodium 138 mmol/L, potassium 2.8 mmol/L, urea 14.3 mmol/L, pH 7.52, bicarbonate 36 mmol/L, chloride 75 mmol/L.

Questions

(a) What is the likely metabolic abnormality?
(b) What is the likely diagnosis?
(c) What is the pH of the patient's urine?

Answers

(a) This patient suffers from hypochloraemic metabolic alkalosis.
(b) The underlying cause is pyloric stenosis.
(c) The patient's urine is paradoxically acid, despite alkalosis.

Case 12.7

A 72-year-old man was admitted with a 3-week history of feeling unwell, poor appetite and diarrhoea. On examination, he was clearly dehydrated and had acidotic breathing. His blood pressure was 90/70; the postural drop to 60/30. He was frail. The rest of the general and system examination was unremarkable. The initial biochemistry revealed: sodium 121 mmol/L, potassium 1.9 mmol/L, chloride 83 mmol/L, bicarbonate 4 mmol/L, urea 90 mmol/L, creatinine 960 μmol/L, pH 7.1, P_{O_2} 15.7 kPa, P_{CO_2} 2.2 kPa, serum osmolality 334 mOsm/kg, urine osmolality 404 mOsm/kg, urinary sodium 2 mmol/L and potassium 28 mmol/L. He continued to pass between 50–80 mL of urine per hour.

Questions

(a) How would you describe the metabolic abnormality?
(b) What was the likely cause?
(c) Why did this patient remain polyuric in the face of severe dehydration?

Answers

(a) This patient suffers from volume depletion syndrome characterized by dehydration, hypokalaemia, and hypochloraemic metabolic acidosis with high ionic gap. He has severe acute prerenal failure with normal urine output and dilute urine.

(b) The only single diagnosis which can explain this abnormality is secretory villous adenoma.

(c) His polyuria in the face of severe dehydration is due to nephrogenic diabetes insipidus secondary to chronic hypokalaemia. Hypokalaemia downregulates aquaporin II, which is essential for ADH-dependent water absorption from the collecting duct.

Cardiovascular disease 13

ESSENTIAL ANATOMY, PHYSIOLOGY AND EMBRYOLOGY OF THE HEART

Introduction

Myocardial cells constitute 75% of the heart mass but only about 25% of the cell number. They are designed to perform two fundamental functions: initiation and conduction of electrical impulses and contraction. Although most myocardial cells are able to perform both these functions, the vast majority are predominantly contractile cells (myocytes) and a small number are specifically designed as electrical cells. The latter, collectively known as the conducting system of the heart, are not nervous tissue but modified myocytes lacking in myofibril components. They have the ability to generate electrical impulses which are then conducted to the myocytes, leading to contraction by a process known as excitation–contraction coupling. The rate of electrical impulse generation and the force of myocardial contraction are modified by numerous factors including autonomic input and stretch.

Three epicardial coronary arteries supply blood to the myocardium, and a more complex network of veins is responsible for drainage. In the face of continuous arterial pressure fluctuations, blood vessels, especially in the cerebral circulation, maintain constant tissue perfusion by a process known as '*autoregulation*'; blood vessel control is, however, complex involving additional local and central mechanisms.

The conduction system of the heart

The sinus node

The sinus node is a complex spindle-shaped structure that lies in the lateral and epicardial aspects of the junction between the superior vena cava and the right atrium (Fig. 13.1). Physiologically, it generates impulses automatically by spontaneous depolarization of its membrane at a rate quicker than any other cardiac cell type. It is therefore the natural pacemaker of the heart.

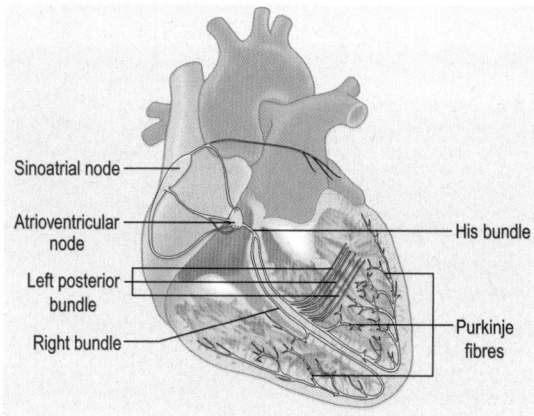

Fig. 13.1 **The conducting system of the heart.**

Sinoatrial node

Atrioventricular node

Left posterior bundle

Right bundle

His bundle

Purkinje fibres

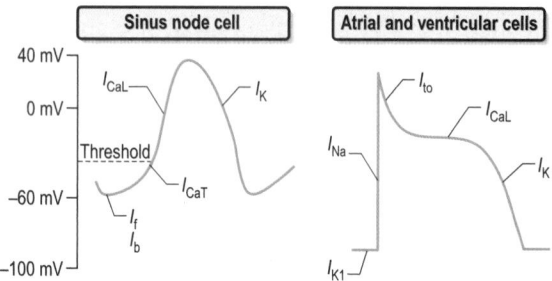

Sinus node cell

Atrial and ventricular cells

Fig. 13.2 **Myocardial action potentials.** I_b, background inward sodium current; I_f, 'funny' current; I_{CaT}, transient (or 'T' type) and I_{CaL}, long-lasting (or 'L' type) calcium channels; I_{Na}, inward sodium current; I_{to}, transient outward potassium current; I_{K1}, inwards rectifier current; I_K delayed rectifier potassium current.

A number of factors are responsible for the spontaneous decay of the sinus node cell membrane potential ('the pacemaker potential'), the most significant of which is a small influx of sodium ions into the cells. This small sodium current has two components: the background inward current (I_b) and the 'funny' (I_f) current (or pacemaker current) (Fig. 13.2). The term 'funny' current denotes ionic flow through channels activated in *hyperpolarized* cells (–60 mV or greater), unlike other time- and voltage-dependent channels activated by *depolarization*. The rate of depolarization of the sinus node membrane potential is modulated by autonomic tone (i.e. sympathetic and parasympathetic input), stretch, temperature, hypoxia, blood pH and in response to other hormonal influences (e.g. triiodothyronine and serotonin).

Atrial and ventricular myocyte action potentials

Action potentials in the sinus node trigger depolarization of the atrial and subsequently the ventricular myocytes. These cells have a different action potential from that of sinus node cells. Their resting membrane potential is a consequence of a small flow of potassium ions into the cells through open 'inward rectifier' channels; at this stage sodium and calcium channels are closed. The arrival of adjacent action potentials triggers the opening of voltage-

gated, fast, self-inactivating sodium channels, resulting in a sharp depolarization spike. This is followed by a partial repolarization of the membrane due to activation of 'transient outward' potassium channels.

The plateau phase which follows is unique to myocytes and results from a small, but sustained inward calcium current through L-type calcium channels lasting 200–400 ms. This calcium influx is caused by a combined increase in permeability of the cell and especially the sarcolemmal membranes to calcium (Fig. 13.3). This plateau (or refractory) phase in myocyte action potential prevents early reactivation of the myocytes and directly determines the strength of contraction. The gradual inactivation of the calcium channels activates delayed rectifier potassium channels repolarizing the membrane. Atrial tissue is activated like a 'forest fire', but the activation peters out when the insulating layer between the atrium and the ventricle – the annulus fibrosus – is reached. Controversy still exists about whether impulses from the sinoatrial (SA) node travel over specialized conducting 'pathways' or over ordinary atrial myocardium.

The AV node, His bundle and Purkinje fibres

The depolarization continues to conduct slowly through the atrioventricular (AV) node. This is a small, bean-shaped structure that lies beneath the right atrial endocardium within the lower inter-atrial septum. The AV node continues as the His bundle, which penetrates the annulus fibrosus and conducts the cardiac impulse rapidly towards the ventricle. The His bundle reaches the crest of the interventricular septum and divides into the right bundle branch and the main left bundle branch.

The right bundle branch continues down the right side of the interventricular septum to the apex, from where it radiates and divides to form the Purkinje network, which spreads throughout the subendocardial surface of the right ventricle. *The main left bundle branch* is a short structure, which fans out into many strands on the left side of the interventricular septum. These strands can be grouped into an anterior superior division (the anterior hemi-bundle) and a posterior inferior division (the posterior hemi-bundle). The anterior hemi-bundle supplies the subendocardial Purkinje network of the anterior and superior surfaces of the left ventricle, and the inferior hemi-bundle supplies the inferior and posterior surfaces. Impulse conduction through the AV node is slow and depends on action potentials largely produced by slow transmembrane calcium flux. In the atria, ventricles and His–Purkinje system, conduction is rapid and is due to action potentials generated by rapid transmembrane sodium diffusion.

The cellular basis of myocardial contraction – excitation contraction coupling

Each myocyte, approximately 100 μm long, branches and interdigitates with adjacent cells. An intercalated disc permits electrical conduction to adjacent cells. Myocytes contain bundles of parallel myofibrils. Each myofibril is made up of a series of sarcomeres (Fig. 13.4). A sarcomere (which is the basic unit of contraction) is bound by two

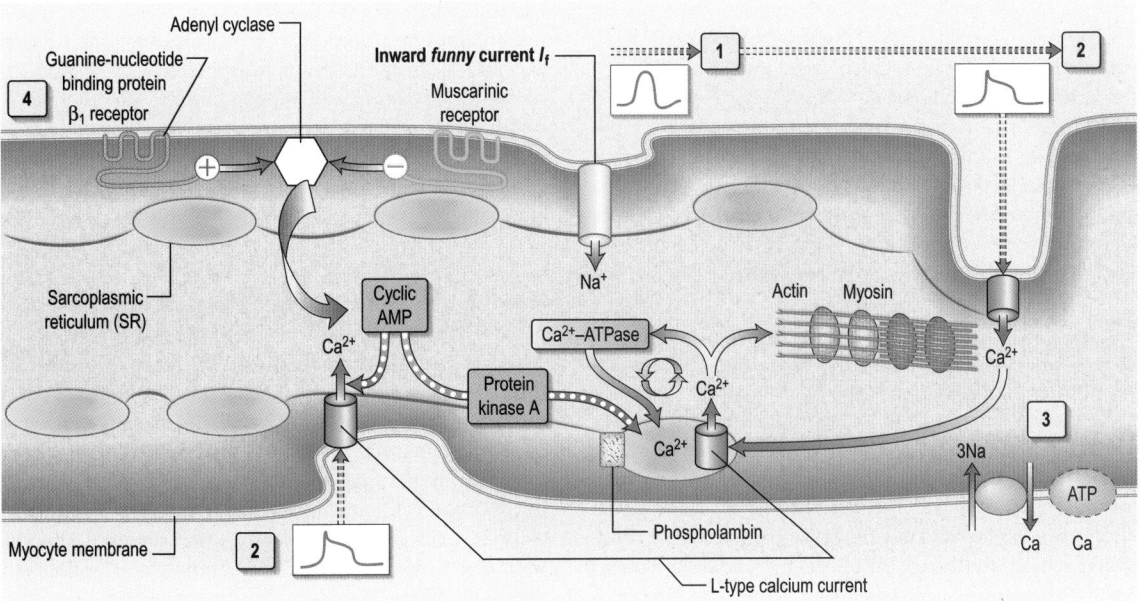

Fig. 13.3 **The 'complete' cardiac cell.**

1. Spontaneous depolarization in sinus node cells due to sodium (Na) influx through the 'funny' current generates the 'pacemaker' potential.
2. This activates other atrial and ventricular myocytes, triggering action potentials and activating L-type calcium (Ca) channels in the surface and transverse tubule membranes (at top and bottom of figure).
3. The resulting Ca influx acts on Ca-induced Ca release channels (RyR2) on the sarcoplasmic reticulum (SR), resulting in release of stored Ca and acts together on actin and myosin fibrils, resulting in contraction. Ca reuptake pumps in the SR, regulated by phospholambin replenish the stores; various exchange pumps also expel Ca from the cell.
4. Autonomic input has either a positive chronotropic/inotropic effect (β₁ receptors) or a negative chronotropic/inotropic effect (muscarinic receptors).

Fig. 13.4 **Schematic diagram showing the structure of a myofibril within a myocyte.** The myofibrils are made up of a series of sarcomeres joined at the Z line.

transverse Z lines, to each of which is attached a perpendicular filament of the protein actin. The actin filaments from each of the two Z bands overlap with thicker parallel protein filaments known as myosin. Actin and myosin filaments are attached to each other by crossbridges that contain ATPase, which breaks down adenosine triphosphate (ATP) to provide the energy for contraction.

Two chains of actin molecules form a helical structure, with another molecule, tropomyosin, in the grooves of the actin helix, and a further molecule, troponin, is attached to every seven actin molecules. During cardiac contraction the length of the actin and myosin monofilaments does not change. Rather, the actin filaments slide between the myosin filaments when ATPase splits a high-energy bond of ATP. To supply the ATP, the myocyte (which cannot stop for a rest) has a very high mitochondrial density (35% of the cell volume). As calcium ions bind to troponin C, the activity of troponin I is inhibited, which induces a conformational change in tropomyosin. This event unlocks the active site between actin and myosin, enabling contraction to proceed.

Calcium is made available during the plateau phase of the action potential by calcium ions entering the cell and by being mobilized from the sarcoplasmic reticulum through the ryanodine receptor (RyR2) calcium-release channel. RyR2 activity is regulated by the protein calstabin 2 (see p. 852) and nitric oxide. The force of cardiac muscle contraction ('inotropic state') is thus regulated by the influx of calcium ions into the cell through calcium channels (Fig. 13.3). T (transient) calcium channels open when the muscle is more depolarized, whereas L (long-lasting) calcium channels require less depolarization. The extent to which the sarcomere can shorten determines the stroke volume of the ventricle. It is maximally shortened in response to powerful inotropic drugs or severe exercise.

Starling's law of the heart

The contractile function of an isolated strip of cardiac tissue can be described by the relationship between the velocity of muscle contraction, the load that may be moved by the contracting muscle, and the extent to which the muscle is stretched before contracting. As with all other types of muscle, the velocity of contraction of myocardial tissue is reduced by increasing the load against which the tissue must contract. However, in the non-failing heart, pre-stretching of cardiac muscle improves the relationship between the force and velocity of contraction (Fig. 13.5).

This phenomenon was described in the intact heart as an increase of stroke volume (ventricular performance) with an enlargement of the diastolic volume (preload), and is known as 'Starling's law of the heart' or the 'Frank–Starling relationship'. It has been transcribed into more clinically relevant indices. Thus, stroke work (aortic pressure × stroke volume) is increased as ventricular end-diastolic volume is raised. Alternatively, within certain limits, cardiac output rises as pulmonary capillary wedge pressure increases. This clinical relationship is described by the ventricular function curve (Fig. 13.5), which also shows the effect of sympathetic stimulation.

Nerve supply of the myocardium

Adrenergic nerves supply atrial and ventricular muscle fibres as well as the conduction system. β_1-Receptors predominate in the heart with both epinephrine (adrenaline) and norepinephrine (noradrenaline) having positive inotropic and chronotropic effects. Cholinergic nerves from the vagus supply mainly the SA and AV nodes via M_2 muscarinic receptors. The ventricular myocardium is sparsely innervated by the vagus. Under basal conditions, vagal inhibitory effects predominate over the sympathetic excitatory effects, resulting in a slow heart rate.

Adrenergic stimulation and cellular signalling

β_1-Adrenergic stimulation enhances Ca^{2+} flux in the myocyte and thereby strengthens the force of contraction (Fig. 13.3). Binding of catecholamines, e.g. norepinephrine (noradrenaline), to the myocyte β_1-adrenergic receptor stimulates membrane-bound adenylate kinases. These enzymes enhance production of cyclic AMP that activates intracellular protein kinases, which in turn phosphorylate cellular proteins, including L-type calcium channels within the cell membrane. β_1-Adrenergic stimulation of the myocyte also enhances myocyte relaxation.

The return of calcium from the cytosol to the sarcoplasmic reticulum (SR) is regulated by phospholamban (PL), a low-molecular-weight protein in the SR membrane. In its dephosphorylated state, PL inhibits Ca^{2+} uptake by the SR ATPase pump (Fig. 13.3). However, β_1-adrenergic activation of protein kinase phosphorylates PL, and blunts its inhibitory effect. The subsequently greater uptake of calcium ions by the SR hastens Ca^{2+} removal from the cytosol and promotes myocyte relaxation.

The increased cAMP activity also results in phosphorylation of troponin I, an action that inhibits actin–myosin interaction, and further enhances myocyte relaxation.

The cardiac cycle

The cardiac cycle (Fig. 13.6) consists of precisely timed rhythmic electrical and mechanical events that propel

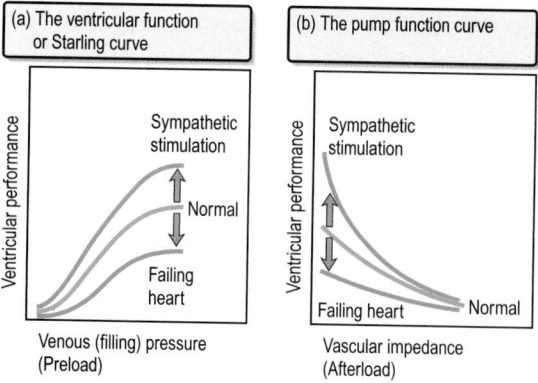

Fig. 13.5 The Frank–Starling mechanism, showing the effect on ventricular contraction of alteration in filling pressures and outflow impedance in the normal, failing and sympathetically stimulated ventricle.

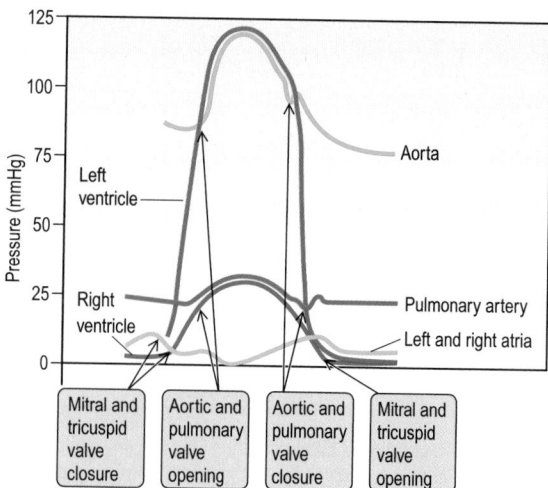

Fig. 13.6 The cardiac cycle.

blood into the systemic and pulmonary circulations. The first event in the cardiac cycle is atrial depolarization (a P wave on the surface ECG) followed by right atrial and then left atrial contraction. Ventricular activation (the QRS complex on the ECG) follows after a short interval (the PR interval). Left ventricular contraction starts and shortly thereafter right ventricular contraction begins. The increased ventricular pressures exceed the atrial pressures, and close first the mitral and then the tricuspid valves.

Until the aortic and pulmonary valves open, the ventricles contract with no change of volume (isovolumetric contraction). When ventricular pressures rise above the aortic and pulmonary artery pressures, the pulmonary valve and then the aortic valve open and ventricular ejection occurs. As the ventricles begin to relax, their pressures fall below the aortic and pulmonary arterial pressures, and aortic valve closure is followed by pulmonary valve closure. Isovolumetric relaxation then occurs. After the ventricular pressures have fallen below the right atrial and left atrial pressures, the tricuspid and mitral valves open. The cardiac cycle can be graphically depicted as the relationship between the pressure and volume of the ventricle. This is shown in Figure 13.7, which illustrates the changing pressure–volume relationships in response to increased contractility and to exercise.

The coronary circulation

The coronary arterial system (Fig. 13.8) consists of the right and left coronary arteries. These arteries branch from the aorta, arising immediately above two cusps of the aortic valve. These arteries are unique in that they fill during diastole, when not occluded by valve cusps and

(a)

(b)

Fig. 13.7 **Pressure–volume loop.** AB, diastole – ventricular filling; BC systole – isovolumetric ventricular contraction; CD, systole – ventricular emptying; DA, diastole – isovolumetric ventricular relaxation.

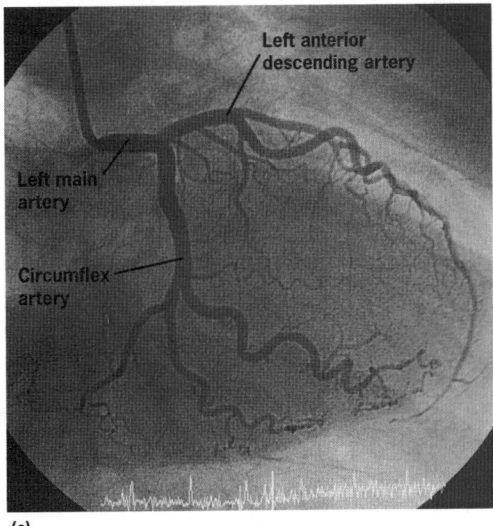

(c)

Fig. 13.8 (a) **Diagram of the normal coronary arterial anatomy. (b) Angiogram of non-dominant right coronary system. (c) Angiogram of dominant left coronary system from the same patient.** Right anterior oblique projection.

when not squeezed by myocardial contraction. The right coronary artery arises from the right coronary sinus and courses through the right side of the atrioventricular groove, giving off vessels that supply the right atrium and the right ventricle. The vessel usually continues as the posterior descending coronary artery, which runs in the posterior interventricular groove and supplies the posterior part of the interventricular septum and the posterior left ventricular wall.

Within 2.5 cm of its origin from the left coronary sinus, the left main coronary divides into the left anterior descending artery and the circumflex artery. The left anterior descending artery runs in the anterior inter-ventricular groove and supplies the anterior septum and the anterior left ventricular wall. The left circumflex artery travels along the left atrioventricular groove and gives off branches to the left atrium and the left ventricle (marginal branches).

The sinus node and the AV node are supplied by the right coronary artery in about 60% and 90% of people, respectively. Therefore, disease in this artery may cause sinus bradycardia and AV nodal block. The majority of the left ventricle is supplied by the left coronary artery, so that stenosis in the left main artery is extremely dangerous; total obstruction of this vessel is rarely compatible with life.

Some blood from the capillary beds in the wall of the heart drains directly into the cavities of the heart by tiny veins, but the majority returns by veins which accompany the arteries, to empty into the right atrium via the coronary sinus. An extensive lymphatic system drains into vessels that travel along the coronary vessels and then into the thoracic duct.

Blood vessel control and functions of the vascular endothelium

In functional terms, the tunica intima with the vascular endothelium and the smooth-muscle-cell-containing tunica media are the main constituents of blood vessels. These two structures are closely interlinked by a variety of mechanisms to regulate vascular tone. The central control of blood vessels is achieved via the neuro-endocrine system. Sympathetic vasoconstrictor and parasympathetic vasodilator nerves regulate vascular tone in response to daily activity. Where neural control is impaired, or in various pathological states, e.g. haemor-rhage, endocrine control of blood vessels mediated through epinephrine (adrenaline), angiotensin and vaso-pressin takes over.

At a local level, tissue perfusion is maintained automatically and by the effect of various factors synthesized and/or released in the immediate vicinity. In the face of fluctuating arterial pressures, blood vessels vasoconstrict independently of nervous input when blood pressure drops and vice versa. This process of *auto-regulation* is a consequence of:

- the *Bayliss myogenic* response – the ability of blood vessels to constrict when distended

- the *vasodilator washout* effect – the vasoconstriction triggered by a decrease in the concentration of tissue metabolites.

The vascular endothelium is a cardiovascular endocrine organ, which occupies a strategic interface between blood and other tissues. It produces various compounds (e.g. nitrous oxide (NO), prostacyclin (PGI_2), endothelin, endothelial derived hyperpolarizing factor (ERHF), adhesion molecules, vascular endothelial growth factor (VEGF)) and has enzymes located on the surface control-ling the levels of circulating compounds such as angiotensin, bradykinin and serotonin. It has many regulatory roles:

Vasomotor control

NO is a diffusible gas with a very short half-life, pro-duced in endothelial cells from the amino acid L-arginine via the action of the enzyme NO synthase (NOS), which is controlled by cytoplasmic calcium/calmodulin (Fig. 13.9). It is produced in response to various stimuli (Table. 13.1), triggering vascular smooth muscle relax-ation through activation of guanylate cyclase, leading to an increase in the intracellular levels of cyclic 3,5-guanine monophosphate (cGMP). Its cardiovascular effects protect against atherosclerosis, high blood pressure, heart failure and thrombosis. NO is also the neurotransmitter in various 'nitrergic' nerves in the central and peripheral

Fig. 13.9 **Nitric oxide: the stimulus for production and function of nitric oxide (NO).** Various stimuli lead to the production of nitric oxide via cytoplasmic calcium/calmodulin. NO triggers smooth muscle relaxation via the activation of guanylyl cyclase. ROC, receptor-operated Ca^{2+} channel; SAC, stretch-activated Ca^{2+} channel; IP3, inositol triphosphate; ER, endoplasmic reticulum; GTP, guanine triphosphate; cGMP, cyclic guanine monophosphate.

Table 13.1 Some of the products and functions of the vascular endothelium

Endothelial product	Function(s)	Stimulus

Nitrous oxide (NO)	Vasodilatation
	Inhibits platelet aggregation
	Inhibits transcription of adhesion molecules
	Inhibits vascular smooth muscle proliferation
		Shear stress, e.g. induced by exercise
		Agonists: thrombin, acetylcholine,
		  endothelin, bradykinin, serotonin, substance P
		  Inflammation/endotoxin shock

Prostacyclin (PGI$_2$)	Vasodilatation Inhibits platelet aggregation	Agonist: thrombin Inflammation
Prostanoids	Vasoconstriction	Hypoxia
Endothelin	Vasoconstriction	Thrombin, angiotensin II, vasopressin Hypoxia *NB:* Inhibited by shear stress
Endothelial-derived hyperpolarizing factor	Vasodilatation	Agonists: bradykinin, acetylcholine
Angiotensin-converting enzyme	Vasoconstriction	Expressed naturally
Von Willebrand factor	Promotes platelet aggregation Stabilizes factor VIII	Agonists: thrombin, epinephrine (adrenaline)

Adhesion molecules
  P, L, E selectins
	Margination of white blood cells (WBC)	Inflammatory mediators: histamine, thrombin,
		  TNF, IL-6

ICAM, VCAM, PECAM	Binding and diapedesis of WBC into vessel wall	
Vascular endothelial growth factor (VEGF)	Angiogenesis Vasodilatation Increased vascular permeability	Pregnancy Hypoxia Inflammation: rheumatoid arthritis, trauma, tumours

ICAM, intracellular adhesion molecule; VCAM, vascular cell adhesion molecule; PECAM, platelet/endothelial cell adhesion molecule; TNF, tumour necrosis factor; IL, interleukin

nervous systems and may play a role in the central regulation of vascular tone. The new class of drugs used to treat erectile dysfunction, the phosphodiesterase (PDE$_5$) inhibitors, prevent the breakdown of cGMP and promote vasodilatation.

PGI$_2$ is synergistic to NO and also plays a role in the local regulation of vasomotor tone. *Endothelin* is a 21-amino-acid peptide that counteracts the effects of NO. Its production is inhibited by shear stress, i.e. the stress exerted on the vessel wall by the flowing blood, and it causes profound vasoconstriction and vascular smooth muscle hypertrophy. It is thought to play a role in the genesis of hypertension and atheroma. *Angiotensin-converting enzyme* located on the endothelial cell membrane converts circulating angiotensin I (synthesized by the action of renin on angiotensinogen) to angiotensin II which has vasoconstrictor properties and leads to aldosterone release (Fig. 18.27). Aldosterone promotes sodium absorption from the kidney and together with the angiotensin-induced vasoconstriction provides haemodynamic stability. Other factors which influence vasomotor tone include histamine (released by mast cells), bradykinin (synthesized from kininogen by the action of coagulation factor XIIa) and serotonin released by platelets.

Anti- and prothrombotic mechanisms

PGI$_2$, produced from arachidonic acid in the endothelial cell membrane by the action of the enzyme cyclo-oxygenase (Fig. 14.32), inhibits platelet aggregation. Low-dose aspirin prevents activation of the cyclo-oxygenase pathway in platelets but only to a degree that does not affect PGI$_2$ synthesis, unlike higher doses. Other antithrombotic agents such as clopidogrel (ADP receptor antagonist) and glycoprotein IIb/IIIa inhibitors achieve their effects by acting directly on platelet receptors. The antithrombotic effect of PGI$_2$ is aided by NO, affecting platelets via activation of guanylate cyclase. The endothelial cell membrane also produces other anticoagulant molecules such as thrombomodulin, heparin sulphate and various fibrinolytic factors. Clinically used, fast-acting, heparin preparations are identical to this naturally occurring molecule; slower-acting warfarin inhibits the synthesis of various coagulation factors from vitamin K in the liver; ximelagatran is a direct thrombin inhibitor.

In addition to their ability to prevent clotting, endothelial cells also aid thrombosis. They are responsible for the production of von Willebrand factor through a unique organelle called the Weibal–Palade body, which not only acts as a carrier for factor VIII but also promotes platelet adhesion by binding to exposed collagen (p. 479).

Modulation of immune responses

In response to various inflammatory mediators, the vascular endothelium expresses various so-called 'adhesion molecules' which promote leucocyte attraction, adhesion and infiltration into the blood vessel wall (p. 149).

Regulation of vascular cell growth

The endothelial cells are also responsible for the development of new blood vessels ('angiogenesis') in the placenta, wound healing, tissue repair and tumour growth. This process is facilitated by the vascular endothelial growth factor (VEGF).

Fetal circulation

In utero, the pulmonary circulation is largely unnecessary because fetal blood is oxygenated by placental blood flow, a parallel and integral element in the systemic circulation. In the fetus, systemic venous blood returning to the right atrium is partly deflected through the foramen ovale to the left atrium. Blood that passes through the right ventricle is diverted from the pulmonary artery to the aorta through the ductus arteriosus. Thus, the systemic venous return, which is a mixture of oxygenated and deoxygenated blood, is mostly returned to the systemic arterial system.

At birth, inspiration dilates the pulmonary arterioles, resulting in a dramatic reduction of pulmonary vascular resistance. Blood therefore flows through the pulmonary circulation. The increased oxygen tension and reduced levels of prostaglandins trigger closure of the ductus arteriosus, and the reduced right atrial pressure and increasing left atrial pressure tend to close the foramen ovale. Thus, the circulation is divided into two separate circuits connected in series.

In the fetus the left and right heart both propel blood from the systemic veins to the systemic arteries; thus, severe abnormalities of the heart may not compromise fetal blood flow.

FURTHER READING

Chong AY, Blann AD, Lip GY (2003) Assessment of endothelial damage and dysfunction: observations in relation to heart failure. *Quarterly Journal of Medicine* 96(4): 253–267.

Hambrecht R et al. (2000) Effect of exercise on coronary endothelial function in patients with coronary artery disease. *New England Journal of Medicine* **342**: 454–460.

Levick JR (2003) *An Introduction to Cardiovascular Physiology,* 4th edn. London: Arnold.

Nabel EG (2003) Cardiovascular disease. *New England Journal of Medicine* **349**: 60–72.

Rich S, McLaughlin VV (2003) Endothelin receptor blockers in cardiovascular disease. *Circulation* **108**: 2184–2190.

SYMPTOMS OF HEART DISEASE

Eliciting a good history is invaluable in diagnosing, and managing heart disease. There is overlap between symptoms arising from cardiovascular disease and those originating from other pathology. The following symptoms occur with heart disease:

- chest pain
- dyspnoea
- palpitations
- syncope
- fatigue
- peripheral oedema

The severity of anginal pain, dyspnoea, palpitations or fatigue may be classified according to the New York Heart Association grading of 'cardiac status' (Table 13.2).

Chest pain

This is the symptom most commonly associated with heart disease.

The pain of angina pectoris and myocardial infarction is due to myocardial hypoxia. Classically, it is felt as crushing, gripping or heavy pain behind the sternum in the centre of the chest, radiating to the neck, shoulder or jaw, or more rarely to the teeth, back or abdomen. It may be associated with pain, paraesthesia or heaviness in one (commonly the left) or both arms. Typically, the pain of angina pectoris is provoked by exercise and promptly relieved by rest or short-acting nitrates. Angina occurring on lying flat is termed decubitus angina. The level of exertion required to provoke pain – for example, after walking on the flat for 200 yards – should be elicited.

Angina that is becoming more frequent or unpredictable, or occurs at rest is classified as unstable, a component of the 'acute coronary syndrome' (p. 808). Even quite significant ischaemia/infarction may not be associated with chest pain but rather with dyspnoea, nausea and sweating. This is 'silent' ischaemia due to loss of pain-sensing fibres within the heart, and is more common in the diabetic and elderly. Ischaemia may also present with atypical (e.g. dyspeptic) pain.

Central chest pain *radiating to the back* may be due to cardiac ischaemia but a dissecting or enlarging thoracic aortic aneurysm also produces a similar pain and sometimes ECG changes.

Pericarditis pain is also felt at the centre of the chest. However, its character is similar to pleuritic pain, i.e. sharp, exacerbated by movement, respiration and cough-

Table 13.2 The New York Heart Association grading of 'cardiac status' (modified)

Grade 1	Uncompromised (no breathlessness)
Grade 2	Slightly compromised (on severe exertion)
Grade 3	Moderately compromised (on mild exertion)
Grade 4	Severely compromised (breathless at rest)

Table 13.3   Differential diagnosis of chest pain

Central	Lateral/peripheral
Cardiac	**Pulmonary**
Ischaemic heart disease (infarction or angina)	Infarction
Coronary artery spasm	Pneumonia
Pericarditis/myocarditis	Pneumothorax
Mitral valve prolapse	Lung cancer
Aortic aneurysm/dissection	Mesiothelioma
	Non-pulmonary
Non-cardiac	Bornholm disease (epidemic myalgia)
Pulmonary embolism	Herpes zoster
Oesophageal disease	Trauma (ribs/muscular)
Mediastinitis	
Costochondritis (Tietze's disease)	
Trauma (soft tissue, rib)	
Functional	

ing. Unlike pleuritic pain, however, some relief may be afforded by sitting forwards.

Left submammary stabbing pain, so-called 'precordial catch', is usually associated with anxiety (called effort syndrome or Da Costa's syndrome), although cardiac conditions such as mitral valve prolapse may produce a similar sensation. Oesophageal disease may also produce central (retrosternal) chest pain, which can be difficult to differentiate from cardiac pain (see Box 6.4). The differential diagnosis of chest pain is listed in Table 13.3.

Dyspnoea

Dyspnoea is an abnormal awareness of breathlessness. Pain, particularly within the chest and abdomen, may also lead to dyspnoea. However, the main causes are cardiac and pulmonary pathologies; in the cardiovascular system, this is most commonly due to left ventricular failure (LVF).

Left ventricular failure causes dyspnoea due to oedema of the pulmonary interstitium and alveoli. This makes the lungs stiff (less compliant), thus increasing the respiratory effort required to ventilate the lungs. Tachypnoea (increased respiratory rate) is usually also present owing to stimulation of pulmonary stretch receptors.

It is clinically valuable to grade dyspnoea in a similar manner to chest pain (see above), by the level of exertion required to provoke its onset and by the patient's cardiac status (Table 13.2) as this is an indication of severity. As LVF worsens, other forms of breathlessness such as orthopnoea and paroxysmal nocturnal dyspnoea occur.

Orthopnoea refers to breathlessness on lying flat. Blood is redistributed from the legs into the torso leading to an increase in central and pulmonary blood volume, worsening pulmonary oedema. Furthermore, whilst recumbent, the abdominal contents push up against the diaphragm, restricting its movement (splinting). Orthopnoea is usually overcome by the patient using an increasing number of pillows to sleep. The number of pillows required indicates the severity.

Paroxysmal nocturnal dyspnoea (PND) occurs when a patient is woken from sleep fighting for breath, a dramatic and frightening experience. The patient sits up, stands or opens the window for fresh air. PND is in essence a variation of orthopnoea, in that it is due to the same mechanisms. However, as sensory awareness is reduced whilst asleep, the pulmonary oedema can become quite severe before the patient is awoken.

Some symptoms of LVF may mimic *respiratory pathology* leading to diagnostic difficulty. Most notoriously, oedema of the bronchial endothelium can cause a 'cardiac wheeze' leading to the misdiagnosis of airways disease. Pulmonary oedema may also produce a cough, productive of a frothy blood-tinged sputum. Conversely, PND-like episodes with coughing may occur in asthma, but conventionally the term PND is reserved for cardiac problems.

In severe heart failure, alternate episodes of hyperventilation and apnoea may occur (*Cheyne–Stokes respiration*). If hypopnoea occurs rather than apnoea, the phenomenon is termed 'periodic breathing', but the two variations are known together as *central sleep apnoea syndrome* (*CSAS*). This occurs due to malfunctioning of the respiratory centre in the brain, caused by poor cardiac output with concurrent cerebrovascular disease.

The symptoms of CSAS, such as daytime somnolence and fatigue, are similar to those of obstructive sleep apnoea syndrome (OSAS, p. 907) and there is considerable overlap with the symptoms of heart failure. CSAS is believed to lead to myocardial hypertrophy and fibrosis, deterioration in cardiac function and complex arrhythmias including non-sustained ventricular tachycardia, hypertension and stroke. Studies conducted on patients with heart failure show that patients with CSAS have a worse prognosis compared to similar patients without CSAS.

Palpitations

Palpitations represent an increased awareness of the normal heartbeat or the sensation of slow, rapid or irregular heart rhythms.

The normal heartbeat may be sensed because of anxiety, excitement, exercise or recumbency on the left side. Therefore, a careful history may help to rule out a pathological cause for palpitations. The most common arrhythmias felt as palpitations are premature ectopic beats and paroxysmal tachycardias. A useful trick is to ask patients to tap out the rate and rhythm of their palpitations, as the different arrhythmias have different characteristics.

Premature beats are felt by the patient as a pause followed by a forceful beat. This is because premature beats are usually followed by a pause before the next normal beat, as the heart resets itself. The next beat is more forceful as the heart has had a longer diastolic period and therefore filled with more blood before this beat. These premature beats may occur in clusters and may lead to great anxiety although they are usually benign.

Paroxysmal tachycardias start abruptly and may be felt as a sudden racing heartbeat. They may terminate as suddenly, but often tend to slow down first, therefore leading to the sensation of the palpitations fading away. Paroxysmal atrial fibrillation is irregular in rhythm whereas other supraventricular or ventricular tachycardias are regular. Paroxysmal tachycardias, especially when prolonged, may lead to other symptoms such as syncope, presyncope, dyspnoea or chest pain. Supraventricular arrhythmias, especially atrial fibrillation and AV nodal re-entry, may also produce polyuria after the palpitations owing to the release of atrial natriuretic peptide (ANP), which leads to sodium and water loss from the kidneys.

Some patients experience *tachycardia on standing*, associated with a mild drop in blood pressure and symptoms of dizziness or near syncope. This is due to a form of autonomic dysfunction termed the postural orthostatic tachycardia syndrome (POTS) and is due to sinus tachycardia (p. 766).

Bradycardias may be appreciated as slow, regular, heavy or forceful beats. Most often, however, they are simply not sensed. All palpitations may be graded by the NYHA cardiac status (Table 13.2).

Syncope

Transient loss of consciousness due to inadequate cerebral blood flow is termed syncope, and may be due to a variety of causes. The cardiovascular causes, which may be grouped as vascular, obstructive or arrhythmic, are listed in Table 13.4.

Vascular. The most common cause of syncope is the *vasovagal attack*, also known as neurocardiogenic or situational syncope (p. 1226), or more commonly as a simple faint. It may be triggered by prolonged orthostatic (standing upright) stress or strong emotion. The

Table 13.4 Cardiovascular causes of syncope
Vascular
Neurocardiogenic (vasovagal)
Postural hypotension
Postprandial hypotension
Micturition syncope
Carotid sinus syncope
Obstructive
Aortic stenosis
Hypertrophic obstructive cardiomyopathy
Pulmonary stenosis
Tetralogy of Fallot
Pulmonary hypertension/embolism
Atrial myxoma/thrombus
Defective prosthetic valve
Arrhythmias
Rapid tachycardias
Profound bradycardias (Stokes–Adams)
Significant pauses (in rhythm)
Artificial pacemaker failure

mechanism begins with peripheral vasodilatation and venous pooling of blood leading to a reduction in the amount of blood returned to the heart. The near-empty heart responds by contracting vigorously, which in turn stimulates mechanoreceptors (stretch receptors) in the inferoposterior wall of the left ventricle. These in turn trigger reflexes via the central nervous system, which act to reduce ventricular stretch (i.e. further vasodilatation and sometimes profound bradycardia), but this causes a drop in blood pressure and therefore syncope. These episodes are usually associated with a prodrome of dizziness, nausea, sweating, tinnitus, yawning and a sinking feeling. Recovery occurs within a few seconds, especially if the patient lies down.

A drop in systolic blood pressure of 20 mmHg or more on standing from a sitting or lying position is termed *postural (orthostatic) hypotension*. This occurs as blood pools in the legs because of gravity. Usually, reflex vasoconstriction prevents a drop in pressure but if this is absent or the patient is fluid-depleted, postural hypotension can occur. This condition is more prevalent in the elderly because of age-related autonomic dysfunction, but also may be related to *vasodilating* or *diuretic drugs*.

Postprandial hypotension is commonly defined as a drop in systolic blood pressure of 20 mmHg or more within 2 hours of the start of a meal. It is also said to occur if the systolic blood pressure drops from above 100 mmHg to under 90 mmHg in the same time period. It is thought to occur very commonly, even more so than postural hypotension, especially in the elderly and hypertensive populations. The mechanism has not been firmly established but it is believed to commence with pooling of blood in the splanchnic vessels. In normal subjects, this elicits a homeostatic response via activation of baroreceptors and the sympathetic system, peripheral vasoconstriction and an increase in cardiac output. Abnormalities in these mechanisms are believed to cause postprandial hypotension.

Micturition syncope refers to loss of consciousness whilst micturating. Some cases occur due to orthostatic hypotension. Bladder evacuation may produce parasympathetic overactivity, resulting in bradycardia and vasodilatation.

Carotid sinus syncope occurs when there is an exaggerated vagal response to carotid sinus stimulation, again leading to bradycardia and vasodilatation. It may be so severe as to provoke syncope by wearing a tight collar, looking upwards or turning the head.

Obstructive. *Obstructive cardiac causes* listed in Table 13.4 all lead to syncope due to restriction of blood flow from the heart into the rest of the circulation, or between the different chambers of the heart.

Arrhythmias. *Stokes–Adams attacks* have been defined as sudden loss of consciousness unrelated to posture. It is usually due to intermittent high-grade atrioventricular block, profound bradycardia or ventricular standstill. Without warning, the patient falls to the ground, pale and deeply unconscious. The pulse is usually very slow or absent. After a few seconds the patient flushes brightly and recovers consciousness as the pulse quickens. Often there are no sequelae, but patients may injure themselves during falls.

Occasionally a generalized convulsion may occur if the period of cerebral hypoxia is prolonged, leading to a misdiagnosis of epilepsy.

Fatigue

Fatigue may be a symptom of inadequate systemic perfusion in heart failure. However, other factors may be responsible:

- poor sleep due to paroxysmal nocturnal dyspnoea, orthopnoea, decubitus angina, nocturia (due to diuretic therapy) or nightmares (due to amiodarone therapy)
- direct side-effect of medication, particularly beta-blockers
- electrolyte imbalance due to diuretic therapy
- as a systemic manifestation of infection such as endocarditis.

Peripheral oedema

Heart failure results in salt and water retention due to renal underperfusion and consequent activation of the renin–angiotensin–aldosterone system (p. 1096). This leads to dependent pitting oedema.

EXAMINATION OF THE CARDIOVASCULAR SYSTEM

GENERAL EXAMINATION

General features of the patient's well-being should be noted as well as the presence of conjunctival pallor, obesity, jaundice and cachexia.

Clubbing (p. 884)

The most common cardiac cause of clubbing is congenital cyanotic heart disease, particularly Fallot's tetralogy. Clubbing is seen in 10% of patients with subacute infective endocarditis. Clubbing takes months to develop and is not seen in acute endocarditis or in neonates or infants with cyanotic heart disease. Clubbing in cor pulmonale is due to the underlying pulmonary disease (e.g. bronchiectasis or fibrosing alveolitis).

Splinter haemorrhages

These small, subungual linear haemorrhages are frequently due to trauma, but are also seen in infective endocarditis.

Cyanosis

This is a dusky blue discoloration of the skin (particularly at the extremities) or of the mucous membranes when the capillary oxygen saturation is less than 85%.

Central cyanosis is seen in the tongue and lips, and is due to desaturation of central arterial blood. This occurs in cardiac and respiratory disorders associated with shunting of deoxygenated venous blood into the systemic circulation, as in the presence of a right-to-left heart shunt.

Peripheral cyanosis is seen in the hands and feet, which are cold. A patient who is centrally cyanosed will also be peripherally cyanosed but isolated peripheral cyanosis occurs in conditions associated with peripheral vasoconstriction and stasis of blood in the extremities leading to increased peripheral oxygen extraction. Such conditions include congestive heart failure, circulatory shock, exposure to cold temperatures and abnormalities of the peripheral circulation.

THE ARTERIAL PULSE

A pulse is felt by compressing an artery against a bone. The first pulse to be examined is the right radial pulse. The timings of the left radial and femoral pulses are then compared with that of the right radial pulse. Delayed femoral pulsation occurs because of a proximal stenosis, particularly of the aorta (coarctation).

Pulse rate

The pulse rate should be between 60 and 80 beats per minute (b.p.m.) when an adult patient is lying quietly in bed. Young children may have higher pulse rates, and athletes and elderly adults may have slower rates. The exact rate is often less valuable than the changes in heart rate observed over time (seen on a pulse chart). When the pulse is irregular, not all ventricular systolic beats may be detected by palpation of the radial pulse. Such apex–radial pulse deficits may be appreciated by counting the radial pulse whilst simultaneously listening to the heartbeat with a stethoscope, and are commonly associated with atrial fibrillation and ventricular ectopy.

Rhythm

In normal subjects the pulse is regular except for a slight quickening in early inspiration and a slowing in expiration (sinus arrhythmia). Irregularities of the pulse rhythm are usually due to premature beats, intermittent heart block or atrial fibrillation.

Premature beats occur as occasional or repeated irregularities superimposed on a regular pulse rhythm. Similarly, intermittent heart block is revealed by occasional beats dropped from an otherwise regular rhythm. A more irregular pattern (irregularly irregular) of heartbeats in which no pattern is recognizable occurs in atrial fibrillation. This irregular pattern persists when the pulse quickens in response to exercise, in contrast to pulse irregularity due to ectopic beats, which usually disappears on exercise. However, this is not a reliable way to distinguish ectopic beats from other causes of pulse irregularity.

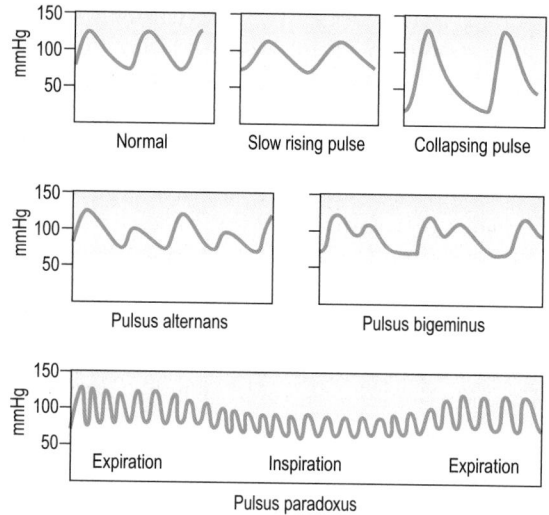

Fig. 13.10 Arterial waveforms.

Carotid pulse

Carotid pulsations are not normally apparent on inspection of the neck but may be visible (Corrigan's sign) in conditions associated with a large-volume pulse, including high output states (such as thyrotoxicosis, anaemia or fever) and in aortic regurgitation. The carotid pulse may also be visible when the carotid artery is aneurysmal or kinked. The amplitude and shape of the carotid pulse is normally examined by palpation of the right carotid artery. Light palpation should be used to detect the presence of a thrill.

A large-volume pulse may also be associated with the large stroke volume that is necessary if bradycardia is present. A 'collapsing' or 'water hammer' pulse is a large-volume pulse characterized by a short duration with a brisk rise and fall. This is best appreciated by palpating the radial artery with the palmer aspect of four fingers whilst elevating the patient's arm above the level of the heart. A collapsing pulse is characteristic of aortic valvular regurgitation or a persistent ductus arteriosus.

A small-volume pulse is seen in cardiac failure, shock and obstructive valvular or vascular disease. It may also be present during tachyarrhythmias. The pulse of aortic stenosis is not only small in volume but is slow in rising to a peak (*plateau pulse*) and is often associated with a notch on the upstroke (anacrotic pulse) or a systolic shudder or thrill (Fig. 13.10).

Paradoxical pulse

Paradoxical pulse is a misnomer, as it is actually an exaggeration of the normal pattern (Fig. 13.10). In normal subjects, the systolic pressure and the pulse pressure (the difference between the systolic and diastolic blood pressures) fall during inspiration. The normal fall of systolic pressure is less than 10 mmHg, and this can be measured using a sphygmomanometer. It is due to increased pulmonary intravascular volume during

inspiration. In severe airflow limitation (especially severe asthma) there is an increased negative intrathoracic pressure on inspiration which enhances the normal fall in blood pressure. In patients with cardiac tamponade, the fluid in the pericardium increases the intrapericardial pressure, thereby impeding diastolic filling of the heart. The normal inspiratory increase in venous return to the right ventricle is at the expense of the left ventricle, as both ventricles are confined by the accumulated pericardial fluid within the pericardial space. Paradox can occur through a similar mechanism in constrictive pericarditis but is less common.

Alternating pulse (pulsus alternans)

This is characterized by regular alternate beats that are weak and strong. It is a feature of severe myocardial failure and is due to the prolonged recovery time of damaged myocardium; it indicates a very poor prognosis. It is easily noticed when taking the blood pressure because the systolic pressure may vary from beat to beat by as much as 50 mmHg. Pulsus alternans may also occur when there is rapid, abnormal tachycardia. In this case it acts as a compensatory mechanism and does not indicate a poor prognosis. Pulsus alternans should be distinguished from a bigeminal pulse (see below).

Bigeminal pulse (pulsus bigeminus)

This is due to a premature ectopic beat following every sinus beat. The rhythm is not regular (Fig. 13.10) because every weak pulse is premature.

Pulsus bisferiens

This is a pulse that is found in hypertrophic obstructive cardiomyopathy and in mixed aortic valve disease (regurgitation combined with stenosis). The first systolic wave is the 'percussion' wave produced by the transmission of the left ventricular pressure in early systole. The second peak is the 'tidal' wave caused by recoil of the vascular bed. This normally happens in diastole (the dicrotic wave), but when the left ventricle empties slowly or is obstructed from emptying completely, the tidal wave occurs in late systole. The result is a palpable double pulse.

THE BLOOD PRESSURE

The peak systemic arterial blood pressure is produced by transmission of left ventricular systolic pressure. Vascular tone and an intact aortic valve maintain the diastolic blood pressure. The normal blood pressure is discussed on page 737. How to take the blood pressure is outlined in Practical box 13.1.

Variations in blood pressure

The systolic blood pressure varies by up to 10 mmHg between the right and left brachial arteries. Standing

Practical Box 13.1
Taking the blood pressure

1. The blood pressure is taken in the (right) arm with the patient relaxed and comfortable.
2. The sphygmomanometer cuff is wrapped around the upper arm with the inflation bag placed over the brachial artery.
3. The cuff is inflated until the pressure exceeds the arterial pressure – when the radial pulse is no longer palpable.
4. The diaphragm of the stethoscope is positioned over the brachial artery just below the cuff.
5. The cuff pressure is slowly reduced until sounds (Korotkoff sounds) can be heard (phase 1). This is the **systolic pressure**.
6. The pressure is allowed to fall further until the Korotkoff sounds become suddenly muffled (phase 4).
7. The pressure is allowed to fall still further until they disappear (phase 5).

The **diastolic pressure** is usually taken as phase 5 because this phase is more reproducible and nearer to the intravascular diastolic pressure. The Korotkoff sounds may disappear (phase 2) and reappear (phase 3) between the systolic and diastolic pressures. Do not mistake phase 2 for the diastolic pressure or phase 3 for the systolic pressure.

usually causes a slight reduction of the systolic pressure (< 20 mmHg) and an increase in the diastolic pressure (< 10 mmHg). In postural (orthostatic) hypotension, a large postural fall of both the systolic and diastolic pressures is associated with dizziness. When an irregular heart rhythm such as atrial fibrillation is present, the blood pressure is variable. Because the blood pressure is normally liable to variation, it must be estimated on several occasions before it can be declared elevated.

JUGULAR VENOUS PRESSURE

There are no valves between the internal jugular vein and the right atrium. Observation of the column of blood in the internal jugular system is therefore a good measure of right atrial pressure. The external jugular cannot be relied upon because of its valves and because it may be obstructed by the fascial and muscular layers through which it passes; it can only be used if typical venous pulsation is seen, indicating no obstruction to flow.

Measurement of jugular venous pressure (JVP)
(Practical box 13.2)
Hepatojugular reflux can be seen when the abdomen is compressed causing a temporary increase in central and hence jugular venous pressure. It is a simple way of confirming the venous nature of a pulsation in the neck.

An abnormally low jugular venous pressure cannot be measured clinically. Causes include haemorrhage and other forms of hypovolaemia.

Elevation of the jugular venous pressure occurs in heart failure. It is also produced by:

 Practical Box 13.2
Measurement of jugular venous pressure

The patient is positioned at about 45° to the horizontal (between 30° and 60°), wherever the top of the venous pulsation can be seen in a good light.

The jugular venous pressure is measured as the vertical distance between the manubriosternal angle and the top of the venous column.

The normal jugular venous pressure is usually less than 3 cm H_2O, which is equivalent to a right atrial pressure of 8 cm H_2O when measured with reference to a point midway between the anterior and posterior surfaces of the chest. The venous pulsations are not usually palpable (except for the forceful venous distension associated with tricuspid regurgitation).

- constrictive pericarditis
- cardiac tamponade
- renal disease with salt and water retention
- overtransfusion or excessive infusion of fluids
- superior vena caval obstruction (but in this case pulsation is absent).

In constrictive pericarditis or cardiac tamponade, ventricular filling is reduced during inspiration because the ventricles are squeezed by the pericardial fluid or non-compliant pericardium, which tightens as the diaphragm descends. Thus, the level of venous pressure increases during inspiration (Kussmaul's sign). Other causes of an increased jugular pressure also distort the shape of the pressure wave and are considered below.

The jugular venous pressure wave

This consists of three peaks and two troughs (Fig. 13.11). The peaks are described as *a*, *c* and *v* waves and the troughs are known as *x* and *y* descents:

- The *a* **wave** is produced by atrial systole.
- The *x* **descent** occurs when the atrial contraction finishes.
- As the pressure falls there is a small transient increase that produces a positive deflection called the *c* **wave**. This is caused by transmission of the rapidly increasing right ventricular pressure before the tricuspid valve closes.
- The *v* **wave** develops as the venous return fills the right atrium during continued ventricular systole.
- The *y* **descent** follows the *v* wave when the tricuspid valve opens.

The *a* wave can be distinguished from the *v* wave by observing the venous pulse while palpating the carotid artery. The *a* wave occurs immediately before carotid pulsation and the *v* wave occurs simultaneously with carotid pulsation.

The main abnormalities of the shape of the jugular venous pressure wave are elevations of the *a* and *v* waves and steepness of the *y* descent (Fig. 13.11).

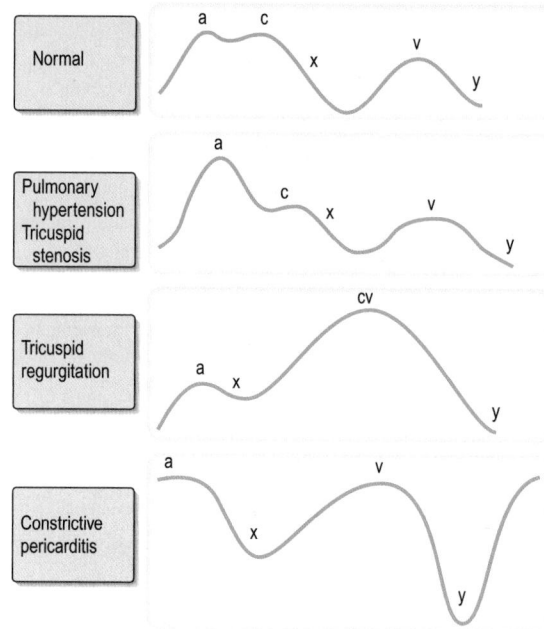

Fig. 13.11 **Jugular venous waveforms.**

Large *a* waves

These are caused by increased resistance to ventricular filling, as seen with right ventricular hypertrophy due to pulmonary hypertension or pulmonary stenosis. They may also be caused by tricuspid stenosis, but this is unusual because patients with tricuspid stenosis are usually in atrial fibrillation and therefore do not have *a* waves.

A very large *a* wave occurs when the atrium contracts against a closed tricuspid valve; this is known as a 'cannon wave'. Cannon waves occur irregularly in complete heart block and in ventricular tachycardia. In both these situations there is atrioventricular dissociation, and by random chance there is occasional simultaneous atrial and ventricular contraction. In junctional rhythms the atria and ventricles usually contract simultaneously and rapid, regular cannon waves are produced.

Large *v* waves

Tricuspid regurgitation results in giant *v* waves (systolic waves) because the right ventricular pressure is transmitted directly to the right atrium and the great veins.

Steep *y* descent

Diastolic collapse of elevated venous pressure can occur in right ventricular failure but is more dramatic in constrictive pericarditis and tricuspid regurgitation. At the end of ventricular systole the elevated atrial pressure suddenly falls when the tricuspid valve opens. However, the ventricles are stiff and cannot be distended and therefore, the venous pressure rapidly rises again. This rapid fall and rise of the jugular venous pulse is known as Friedreich's sign.

EXAMINATION OF THE PRECORDIUM

Inspection

Look for deformities like pectus excavatum and kyphoscoliosis, which can give rise to an ejection systolic murmur arising from compression of the large vessels. Place the patient at 45° and look tangentially for any precordial bulge of cardiac enlargement. Note the position of the apex beat and any other cardiac pulsations; a left ventricular aneurysm may produce eccentric pulsations separate from the apex beat, while a heave may be seen over the left parasternal region due to right ventricular hypertrophy or from an enlarged left atrium.

Palpation

Localize the apex beat, which is the most outward and downward point of cardiac impulse. It can be classified into several abnormal forms:

- **Tapping** apex is a palpable first sound and is felt as a sudden but brief cardiac impulse. It is typically present in early mitral stenosis (when valve leaflets are still pliable), but can also be felt in tachycardic states, e.g. following exercise, especially in thin-built persons.
- **Forceful** apex is vigorous in volume overload conditions, e.g. mitral or aortic regurgitation, or sustained (heaving) in pressure overload situations arising from left ventricular hypertrophy, e.g. aortic stenosis, systemic hypertension and hypertrophic cardiomyopathy.
- The apex beat is **impalpable** in emphysema, obesity and pericardial or pleural effusions.
- **Double pulsation** – two apical impulses with each heartbeat – may be felt in hypertrophic cardiomyopathy, the first pulsation being from atrial contraction. A double impulse can also be due to an outward movement of the myocardium in late systole in a ventricular aneurysm.

A sustained left parasternal impulse or heave is felt with right ventricular hypertrophy or left atrial enlargement. A left atrial impulse can be distinguished from that due to right ventricular hypertrophy as it occurs just before the apex beat or carotid pulsation.

Pulsations from a dilated pulmonary artery may be felt in the second left interspace as a palpable second sound in severe pulmonary hypertension. Similarly, in systemic hypertension, the aortic component of the second sound may be palpable.

Thrills are palpable murmurs and imply a definite abnormality, e.g. systolic thrill of aortic stenosis or mitral regurgitation and diastolic thrill of mitral stenosis.

Auscultation

Use the bell of the stethoscope to hear low-pitched sounds, i.e. heart sounds and the mid-diastolic murmur of mitral stenosis. High-pitched systolic murmurs, early diastolic murmurs, ejection clicks and opening snaps are best appreciated with the help of the diaphragm.

Fig. 13.12 **Normal and additional heart sounds.** S1, first heart sound; S2, second heart sound; A2, aortic component of the second sound; P2, pulmonary component of the second sound; EC, ejection systolic click; OS, opening snap; S3, third heart sound; S4, fourth heart sound.

Fig. 13.13 Variations of the second sound. S1, first heart sound; A2, aortic component and P2, pulmonary component of the second sound; ASD, atrial septal defect; RBBB, right bundle branch block; LBBB, left bundle branch block; RVH, right ventricular hypertrophy; LVH, left ventricular hypertrophy.

Analyse each sound and murmur separately and time them with the carotid pulse. Follow a routine and examine the mitral, tricuspid, pulmonary and aortic areas in turn.

Characteristics of heart sounds (Fig. 13.12)

First heart sound (S1). This is best heard at the apex. It is usually single or narrowly split.

Loud S1 is heard in thin-built persons and hyperdynamic circulation (exercise, fever, anaemia, and thyrotoxicosis). It is also loud if valve leaflets are still widely open when ventricular systole begins, e.g. tachycardia, mild or moderate mitral stenosis and conditions with short PR interval (Wolff–Parkinson–White syndrome).

Soft S1 is heard in obesity, emphysema, pericardial effusion, severe calcific mitral stenosis (immobile leaflets), mitral or tricuspid regurgitation, heart failure and cardiogenic shock. It is also soft when the leaflets are already partly closed due to prolonged diastolic filling before ventricular systole begins, e.g. bradycardia and conditions where the PR interval is prolonged (first-degree heart block).

Variable intensity of S1 is heard when the relationship between atrial and ventricular systole is not constant (e.g. ventricular tachycardia, complete heart block).

Second heart sound (S2). The pulmonary component of S2 (P2) closely follows the aortic component (A2), as right heart emptying usually finishes after the stronger left heart has emptied. Normal or physiological splitting of S2 during inspiration is commonly heard in children or young adults (Fig. 13.13).

For additional sounds see Figure 13.12 and Figure 3.13.

Heart murmurs (Fig. 13.14)

Murmurs are caused by turbulent blood flow, which can occur because of high blood flow through a normal valve or normal flow through an abnormal valve (or into a dilated chamber). The intensity or loudness of a murmur depends upon the flow volume, flow velocity and the distance of the source of murmur from the stethoscope. Thus, systolic murmurs can be graded between 1 and 6, and diastolic between 1 and 4 according to their increasing loudness.

Murmurs due to high-velocity blood flow, e.g. mitral or aortic regurgitation, are often described as 'blowing' or high-pitched in quality and are best heard with the diaphragm of the stethoscope.

Low-velocity murmurs, e.g. mitral stenosis, are 'rumbling' and low-pitched in quality and are best heard with the bell of the stethoscope. Right-sided murmurs become louder on inspiration, since inspiration increases venous return to the right heart. Innocent or flow murmurs are soft, early systolic, short and non-radiating in nature. These are best heard with the diaphragm near the left sternal edge and originate from either the left or right ventricular outflow tracts. They arise in normal hearts and are commonly heard in children and young adults. Flow murmurs are accentuated by physiological manoeuvres that increase the cardiac output, such as exercise, and are also present in other high cardiac output states, e.g. fever, chronic anxiety, anaemia, thyrotoxicosis, beriberi and pregnancy. Skeletal abnormalities like kyphoscoliosis or funnel chest can also produce similar murmurs.

Murmur	Timing and duration	Characteristics	Conditions
Ejection systolic		Crescendo–decrescendo intensity pattern with peaking in mid-systole S1 and S2 clearly audible May follow aortic or pulmonary ejection clicks Best heard over left sternal border and base Radiates to carotids and suprasternal notch	Aortic stenosis Pulmonary stenosis Aortic or pulmonary flow murmurs (e.g. atrial septal defect) Left (e.g. hypertrophic cardiomyopathy) or right (Fallot's tetralogy) outflow tract obstruction
Pansystolic		Loud and 'blowing' in nature Maintains a constant intensity Extends from S1 throughout systole, up to and beyond S2 Best heard at apex (MR) or lower left sternal edge (TR; VSD) Radiates to axilla (MR), base (TR; MR) or whole precordium (VSD)	Mitral regurgitation (MR) Tricuspid regurgitation (TR) Ventricular septal defects (VSD) (harsh murmur and usually a thrill palpable)
Late systolic		Unusual and occurs when prolapsed valve leaflets become incompetent in mid–late systole	Mitral valve prolapse (may be associated with a mid-systolic click) Hypertrophic cardiomyopathy with dynamic outflow tract obstruction
Early diastolic		High-pitched murmurs Decrescendo pattern Best heard with the diaphragm at upper and mid left sternal edge with patient sitting forwards and breath held in expiration	Aortic regurgitation (AR) Pulmonary regurgitation (Graham Steell murmur due to severe pulmonary hypertension secondary to mitral stenosis)
Mid-diastolic		Low-pitched rumbling murmurs Due to increased or turbulent flow across mitral or tricuspid valves Best heard with bell of stethoscope at apex with the patient turned in left lateral position (mitral stenosis), or lower left sternal edge (tricuspid stenosis)	Mitral stenosis (MS) Austin Flint murmur (in severe AR, the regurgitant jet impinges on the anterior mitral leaflet causing partial obstruction of mitral valve) Tricuspid stenosis (TS) Increased flow across mitral or tricuspid valve as in severe MR and TR; left-to-right shunts, e.g. large atrial septal defect
Continuous murmurs		Occur due to combination of systolic and diastolic flow owing to a connection between arterial and venous system or due to high rates of venous flow (e.g. venous hums)	Patent ductus arteriosus Arteriovenous fistulae (congenital, iatrogenic and those associated with increased collateral circulation, as in coarctation of aorta) 'Mammary souffle' due to high mammary blood flow in pregnancy or lactation Venous hum in the neck due to high venous flow in young children or severe anaemia

Fig. 13.14 **Types of cardiac murmurs.** MR, mitral regurgitation; TR, tricuspid regurgitation; ASD, atrial septal defect; VSD, ventricular septal defect.

Murmurs should be assessed by careful systematic auscultation. While examining, the timing of the murmur, its behaviour during respiration, the point and position where murmur is best heard, the direction of selective propagation (radiation) and the character of murmur must be noted. The presence or absence of any valvular or structural cardiac abnormality should be confirmed by echocardiography.

Extracardiac sounds

Bruits are high-pitched, blowing murmurs that arise from stenosis of a peripheral artery, including the distal aorta.

Pericardial friction rub is a high-pitched, scratching or crunching noise caused by the movement of the inflamed pericardium. It is best heard over the left lower sternal edge in systole, but can also be heard in early diastole or synchronously with atrial contraction.

CARDIAC INVESTIGATIONS

Chest X-ray

Ideally, this is taken in the postero-anterior (PA) direction at maximum inspiration with the heart close to the X-ray film to minimize magnification with respect to the thorax. A lateral may give additional information if the PA is abnormal. The cardiac structures and great vessels that can be seen on these X-rays are indicated in Figure 13.15. An antero-posterior (AP) view is only taken in an emergency.

Heart size

Heart size can be reliably assessed only from the PA chest film. The maximum transverse diameter of the heart is compared with the maximum transverse diameter of the thorax measured from the inside of the ribs (the cardio-thoracic ratio).

The cardiothoracic ratio (CTR) is usually less than 50%, except in neonates, infants, athletes and patients with skeletal abnormalities such as scoliosis and funnel chest. A transverse cardiac diameter of more than 15.5 cm is abnormal. Pericardial effusion or cardiac dilatation causes an increase in the ratio.

A *pericardial effusion* produces a globular, sharp-edged shadow (Fig. 13.113, p. 855). This enlargement may occur quite suddenly and, unlike in heart failure, there is no associated change in the pulmonary vasculature. The echocardiogram is more specific than the chest X-ray for the diagnosis of pericardial effusion, partly because at least 250 mL of fluid must accumulate before X-ray changes are apparent.

Certain patterns of specific chamber enlargement may be seen on the chest X-ray:

Left atrial dilatation. This results in prominence of the left atrial appendage and a straightening or convex bulging of the upper left heart border, a double atrial shadow to the right of the sternum, and splaying of the carina because a large left atrium elevates the left main bronchus (Fig. 13.16). On a lateral chest X-ray an enlarged left atrium bulges backwards, impinging on the oesophagus.

Left ventricular enlargement. This results in an increase in the CTR and a smooth elongation and increased convexity of the left heart border. A left ventricular aneurysm may produce a distinct bulge or distortion of the left heart border (see Fig. 13.17, p. 743).

Right atrial enlargement. This results in the right border of the heart projecting into the right lower lung field.

Right ventricular enlargement. This can be due to congenital heart disease. It results in an increase of the CTR and an upward displacement of the apex of the heart because the enlarging right ventricle pushes the left ventricle leftwards, upwards and eventually backwards. Differentiation of left from right ventricular enlargement may be difficult from the shape of the left heart border alone, but the lateral view shows enlargement anteriorly for the right ventricle and posteriorly for the left ventricle.

Ascending aortic dilatation or enlargement. This is seen as a prominence of the aortic shadow to the right of the mediastinum between the right atrium and superior vena cava.

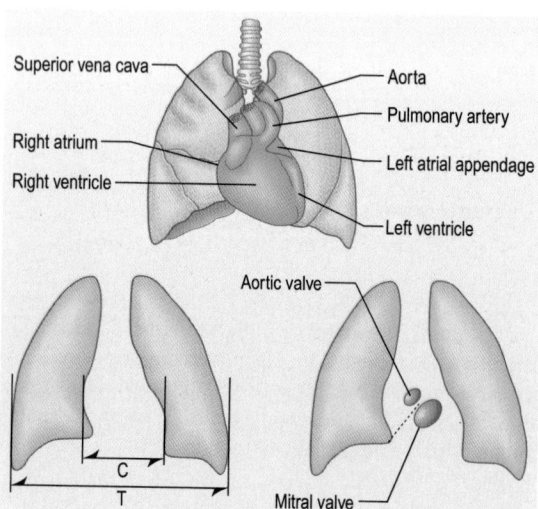

Fig. 13.15 Diagrams to show the heart silhouette on the chest X-ray, measurements of the cardiothoracic ratio (CTR) and the location of the cardiac valves. The dotted line is an arbitrary line from the left hilum to the right cardiophrenic angle: a calcified aortic valve is seen above this line. CTR = (C/T) × 100%; normal CTR < 50%.

Fig. 13.16 Plain PA chest X-ray of a patient with mixed mitral valve disease. The left atrium is markedly enlarged **(a)**. Note the large bulge on the left heart border (left atrium) and the 'double shadow' (border of the right and left atria) **(b)** on the right side of the heart. There is cardiac (left ventricular) enlargement due to mitral regurgitation.

Dissection of the ascending aorta. This is seen as a widening of the mediastinum, although it is often difficult to assess on an AP chest X-ray. A left-sided pleural effusion may be evident if the aneurysm is leaking or there may be blood around the apex of the lung ('capping').

Enlargement of the pulmonary artery. Enlargement of the pulmonary artery in pulmonary hypertension, pulmonary artery stenosis and left-to-right shunts produces a prominent bulge on the left-hand border of the mediastinum below the aortic knuckle.

Calcification

Calcification in the cardiovascular system occurs because of tissue degeneration. Calcification is visible on a lateral or a penetrated PA film, but is best studied by fluoroscopy or CT scanning. Various types of calcification can occur.

Pericardial calcification. This is seen as plaque-like opacities over the surface of the heart, but particularly concentrated in the atrioventricular groove. Such calcification often results from tuberculous pericarditis and may be associated with pericardial constriction (see Fig. 13.114, p. 856).

Valvular calcification. This results from long-standing rheumatic or bicuspid aortic valve disease. On a frontal view a calcified aortic valve is seen above a line joining the left hilum to the right cardiophrenic angle (Fig. 13.15, p. 742). On the lateral film, a calcified aortic valve is seen on or above a line joining the carina to the sternophrenic angle. Mitral valvular calcification is seen below and behind this line.

Myocardial calcification. This occurs after myocardial infarction, especially in association with a left ventricular aneurysm (Fig. 13.17).

Calcification of the aorta. Calcification of the aorta is a common, normal finding in patients over the age of 40 years and appears as a curvilinear opacity around the circumference of the aortic knuckle. Calcification in the ascending aorta usually denotes syphilitic aortitis, whereas in the descending aorta it is due to atheroma or, in the younger patient, to non-specific aortitis.

Coronary arterial calcification. Coronary arterial calcification, especially of the proximal left coronary artery, is associated with coronary atheroma but does not necessarily correspond to the site of maximal stenosis. Electron beam computed tomography is a technique which is now often used to grade coronary calcification. A high score (corrected for age and gender) predicts coronary atherosclerosis.

Lung fields

Pulmonary plethora results from left-to-right shunts (e.g. atrial or ventricular septal defects). It is seen as a general increase in the vascularity of the lung fields and as an

Fig. 13.17 **Left ventricular aneurysm: plain PA chest X-ray demonstrating a cardiac silhouette with a 'bulge' (arrow) on the left lateral border.** This bulge is due to aneurysm formation of many years following a myocardial infarction. A thin line of calcification can be seen along the edge of this bulge.

increase in the size of hilar vessels (e.g. in the right lower lobe artery), which normally should not exceed 16 mm diameter.

Pulmonary oligaemia is a paucity of vascular markings and a reduction in the width of the arteries. It occurs in situations where there is reduced pulmonary blood flow, such as pulmonary embolism, severe pulmonary stenosis and Fallot's tetralogy.

Pulmonary arterial hypertension may result from pulmonary embolism, chronic lung disease or chronic left heart disease, such as shunts due to a ventricular septal defect or mitral valve stenosis. In addition to X-ray features of these conditions, the pulmonary arteries are prominent close to the hila but are reduced in size (pruned) in the peripheral lung fields. This pattern is usually symmetrical.

Pulmonary venous hypertension occurs in left ventricular failure or mitral valve disease. Normal pulmonary venous pressure is 5–14 mmHg at rest. Mild pulmonary venous hypertension (15–20 mmHg) produces isolated dilatation of the upper zone vessels. Interstitial oedema occurs when the pressure is between 21 and 30 mmHg. This manifests as fluid collections in the interlobar fissures, interlobular septa (Kerley B lines) and pleural spaces. This gives rise to indistinctness of the hilar regions and haziness of the lung fields. Alveolar oedema occurs when the pressure exceeds 30 mmHg, appearing as areas of consolidation and mottling of the lung fields (Fig. 13.18) and pleural effusions. Patients with long-standing elevation of the pulmonary venous pressure have reactive

(a)

(b)

Fig. 13.18 **Acute pulmonary oedema.** This pair of chest X-rays were taken from a patient before **(a)** and after **(b)** treatment of acute pulmonary oedema. The X-ray taken when the oedema was present demonstrates hilar haziness, Kerley B lines, upper lobe venous engorgement and fluid in the right horizontal interlobar fissure. These abnormalities are resolved on the film taken after successful treatment.

thickening of the pulmonary arteriolar intima, which protects the alveoli from pulmonary oedema. Thus, in these patients the pulmonary venous pressure may increase to well above 30 mmHg before frank pulmonary oedema develops.

Fluoroscopy

Fluoroscopy is an X-ray procedure used to observe the form and motion of deep structures of the body. It has been largely superseded by echocardiography. However, it is still essential for the insertion of cardiac catheters and pacemaker electrodes, and sometimes used to assess mechanical prosthetic valves.

Electrocardiography

The electrocardiogram (ECG) is a recording of the electrical activity of the heart. It is the vector sum of the depolarization and repolarization potentials of all myocardial cells (Fig. 13.2). At the body surface these generate potential differences of about 1 mV, and the fluctuations of these potentials create the familiar P-QRS-T pattern. At rest the intracellular voltage of the myocardium is polarized at −90 mV compared with that of the extracellular space. This diastolic voltage difference occurs because of the high intracellular potassium concentration, which is maintained by the sodium–

potassium pump despite the free membrane permeability to potassium. Depolarization of cardiac cells occurs when there is a sudden increase in the permeability of the membrane to sodium. Sodium rushes into the cell and the negative resting voltage is lost (phase 0 in Fig. 13.39, p. 765). The depolarization of a myocardial cell causes the depolarization of adjacent cells and, in the healthy heart, the entire myocardium is depolarized in a coordinated fashion. During repolarization, cellular electrolyte balance is slowly restored (phases 1, 2 and 3). Slow diastolic depolarization (phase 4) follows until the threshold potential is reached. Another action potential then follows.

The ECG is recorded from two or more simultaneous points of skin contact (electrodes). When cardiac activation proceeds towards the positive contact, an upward deflection is produced on the ECG. Correct representation of a three-dimensional spatial vector requires recordings from three mutually perpendicular (orthogonal) axes. The shape of the human torso does not make this easy, so the practical ECG records 12 projections of the vector, called 'leads' (Fig. 13.19 and Practical box 13.3).

Six of the leads are obtained by recording voltages from the limbs (I, II, III, AVR, AVL and AVF). The other six leads record potentials between points on the chest surface and an average of the three limbs: RA, LA and LL. These are designated V_1–V_6 and aim to select activity

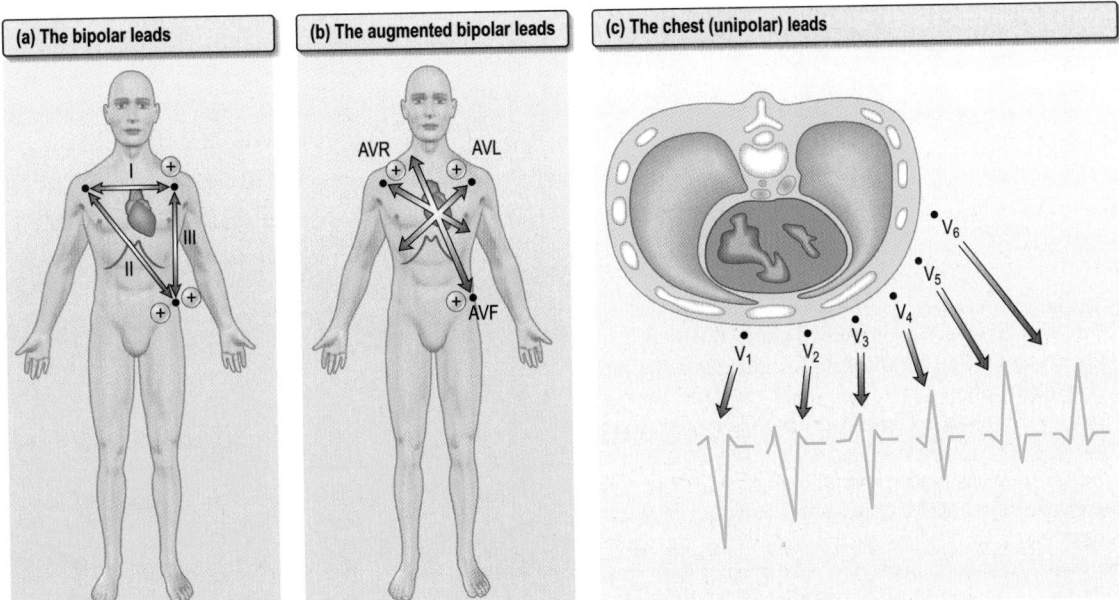

(a) The bipolar leads

(b) The augmented bipolar leads

(c) The chest (unipolar) leads

Fig. 13.19 The connections or directions that comprise the 12–lead electrocardiogram.

from the right ventricle (V_1–V_2), interventricular septum (V_3–V_4) and left ventricle (V_5–V_6). Note that leads AVR and V_1 are oriented towards the cavity of the heart, leads II, III and AVF face the inferior surface, and leads I, AVL and V_6 face the lateral wall of the left ventricle. A V_4 on the right side of the chest (V_4R) is occasionally useful (e.g. for the diagnosis of right ventricular infarction).

Most ECG machines are simultaneous three-channel recorders with output either as a continuous strip or with automatic channel switching. Many ECG machines also analyse the recordings and print the analysis on the record. Usually the machine interpretation is correct, but many arrhythmias still defy automatic analysis.

The ECG waveform

The shape of the normal ECG waveform (Fig. 13.20) has similarities, whatever the orientation. The first deflection is caused by atrial depolarization, and it is a low-amplitude slow deflection called a *P wave*. The *QRS complex* reflects ventricular activation or depolarization and is sharper and larger in amplitude than the P wave. An initial downward deflection is called the *Q wave*. An initial upward deflection is called an *R wave*. The *S wave* is the last part of ventricular activation. The *T wave* is another slow and low-amplitude deflection that results from ventricular repolarization.

Practical Box 13.3
ECG leads

Standard leads (bipolar):
Lead I   Right arm (–ve) to left arm (+ve)
Lead II   Right arm (–ve) to left leg (+ve)
Lead III   Left arm (–ve) to left leg (+ve)

Augmented leads (augmented bipolar):
AVR   Right arm (+ve) to left arm and left leg (–ve)
AVL   Left arm (+ve) to left leg and right arm (–ve)
AVF   Left leg (+ve) to left arm and right arm (–ve)

Chest leads (unipolar) are derived by connecting the V lead against the three extremity leads – the exploring electrodes are placed as follows:
V_1 4th intercostal space just to the right of the sternum
V_2 4th intercostal space just to the left of the sternum
V_3 Halfway between V_2 and V_4
V_4 5th intercostal space in the left mid-clavicular line
V_5 On same horizontal as V_4 in anterior axillary line
V_6 On same horizontal as V_4 in mid-axillary line

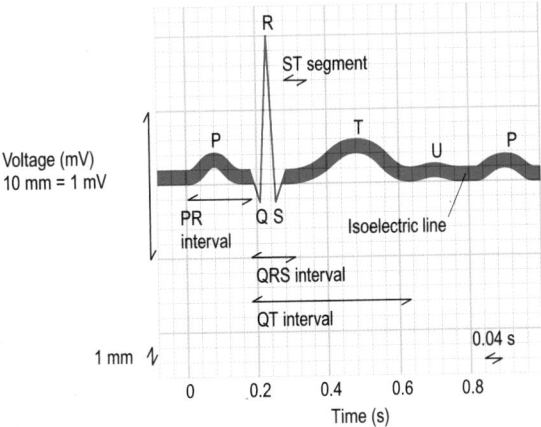

Fig. 13.20 The waves and elaboration of the normal electrocardiogram. From Goldman MJ (1976) *Principles of Clinical Electrocardiography*, 9th edn. Los Altos: Lange.

Table 13.5	Normal ECG intervals
P wave duration	≤ 0.12 s
PR interval	0.12–0.22 s
QRS complex duration	≤ 0.10 s
Corrected QT (QT$_c$)	≤ 0.44 s in males
	≤ 0.46 s in female
$QT_{cB} = QT/(R - R)\sqrt{2}$	Bazett's square root formula
$QT_{cF} = QT/(R - R)\sqrt{3}$	Fridericia's cube root formula

Fig. 13.21 **A normal 12-lead electrocardiogram.**

The PR interval is the length of time from the start of the P wave to the start of the QRS complex. It is the time taken for activation to pass from the sinus node, through the atrium, AV node and the His–Purkinje system to the ventricle.

The QT interval extends from the start of the QRS complex to the end of the T wave. This interval represents the time taken to depolarize and repolarize the ventricular myocardium. QT interval varies greatly with heart rate and is often represented as a corrected QT interval (or QTc) for a given heart rate. There are a number of formulae that exist for derivation of QTc, but the most widely accepted are Bazett's formula and Fridericia's correction (Table 13.5).

Abnormally prolonged QTc can predispose to a risk of dangerous ventricular arrhythmias. Prolongation of QT interval may be congenital or can occur in many acquired conditions (see Table 13.14, p. 777).

The *ST segment* is the period between the end of the QRS complex and the start of the T wave. In the normal heart, all cells are depolarized by this phase of the ECG, i.e. the ST segment represents ventricular repolarization.

A normal ECG is shown in Fig. 13.21, and the normal values for the electrocardiographic intervals are indicated in Table 13.5. Leads that face the lateral wall of the left ventricle have predominantly positive deflections, and leads looking into the ventricular cavity are usually negative. Detailed patterns depend on the size, shape and rhythm of the heart and the characteristics of the torso.

Cardiac vectors

At any point in time during depolarization and repolarization, electrical potentials are being propagated in different directions. Most of these cancel each other out and only the net force is recorded. This net force in the frontal plane is known as the cardiac vector.

The mean QRS vector can be calculated from the six standard leads (Fig. 13.22):

- normal between −30° and +90°
- left axis deviation between −30° and −90°
- right axis deviation between +90° and +150°.

Calculation of this vector is useful in the diagnosis of some cardiac disorders.

Exercise electrocardiography

This is a technique used to assess the cardiac response to exercise. The ECG is recorded whilst the patient walks or runs on a motorized treadmill. The test is based upon the principle that exercise increases myocardial demand on coronary blood supply which may be inadequate during exercise, and at peak stress can result in relative myocardial ischaemia. Most exercise tests are performed according to a standardized method, e.g. the Bruce protocol. Recording an ECG after exercise is not an adequate form of stress test. Normally there is little change in the T wave or ST segment during exercise.

The patient's exercise capacity (the total time achieved) will depend on many factors; however, patients who can only exercise for less than 6 minutes generally have a poorer prognosis.

Myocardial ischaemia provoked by exertion results in ST segment depression (> 1 mm) in leads facing the affected area. The form of ST segment depression provoked by ischaemia is characteristic: it is either planar or shows down-sloping depression (Fig. 13.23). Up-sloping depression is a non-specific finding. The degree of ST segment depression is positively correlated to the degree of myocardial ischaemia.

ST segment elevation during an exercise test is induced much less frequently than ST depression. When it occurs, it reflects transmural ischaemia caused by coronary spasm or critical stenosis.

Although most abnormalities are detected in leads V$_5$ (anterior and lateral ischaemia) or AVF (inferior ischaemia), it is best to record a full 12-lead ECG. During an exercise test the blood pressure and rhythm responses to exercise are also assessed. Exercise normally causes an increase in heart rate and blood pressure. A sustained fall in blood

Fig. 13.22 Cardiac vectors. (a) The hexaxial reference system, illustrating the six leads in the frontal plane, e.g. lead I is 0°, lead II is +60°, lead III is +120°. **(b) Calculating the direction of the cardiac vector.** In the first column the QRS complex with zero net amplitude (i.e. when the positive and negative deflections are equal) is seen in lead III. The mean QRS vector is therefore perpendicular to lead III and is either −150° or +30°. Lead I is positive, so the axis must be +30°, which is normal. In left axis deviation (second column) the main deflection is positive (R wave) in lead I and negative (S wave) in lead III. In right axis deviation (third column) the main deflection is negative (S wave) in lead I and positive (R wave) in lead III. The frontal plane QRS axis is normal only if the QRS complexes in leads I and II are predominantly positive.

pressure usually indicates severe coronary artery disease. A slow recovery of the heart rate to basal levels has also been reported to be a predictor of mortality.

Frequent premature ventricular depolarizations during the test are associated with a long-term increase in the risk of death from cardiovascular causes and further testing is required in these patients. Use of the exercise test in angina is described on page 805.

24-Hour ambulatory taped electrocardiography
This is a technique for recording transient changes such as a brief paroxysm of tachycardia, an occasional pause in

Fig. 13.23 Electrocardiographic changes during exercise test. Upper trace – significant horizontal ST segment depression during exercise. Lower trace – ST elevation during exercise.

the rhythm, or intermittent ST segment shifts (Fig. 13.24). A conventional 12-lead ECG is recorded in less than a minute and usually samples less than 20 complexes. In a 24-hour period over 100 000 complexes are recorded. Such a large amount of data must be analysed by automatic or semi-automatic methods. This technique is called 'Holter' electrocardiography after its inventor.

Event recording is another technique that is used to record less frequent arrhythmias. The patient is provided with a pocket-sized device that can record and store a short segment of the ECG. The device may be kept for several days or weeks until the arrhythmia is recorded. Most units of this kind will also allow transtelephonic ECG transmission so that the physician can determine the need for treatment or the continued need for monitoring.

A very small event recorder, known as an implantable loop recorder (ILR), can also be implanted subcutaneously, triggered by events or a magnet, and interrogated by the physician.

Other tests
Non-invasive methods that make use of digitalized Holter recordings to identify increased risk of ventricular arrhythmias include assessment of heart rate variability, signal averaged ECG (SAECG), and T-wave alternans.

Heart rate variability (HRV) can be assessed from a 24-hour ECG. HRV is decreased in some patients following myocardial infarction and represents an abnormality of autonomic tone or cardiac responsiveness. Low HRV is a major risk factor for sudden death and ventricular arrhythmias in patients discharged following myocardial infarction.

Signal-averaged ECG (SAECG) is a technique that requires amplification and averaging of abnormal low-amplitude signals which occur beyond the end of the QRS complex and extend well into the ST segment. These signals are therefore also known as late potentials and are too small to be detected on a surface ECG. They arise in

(a)

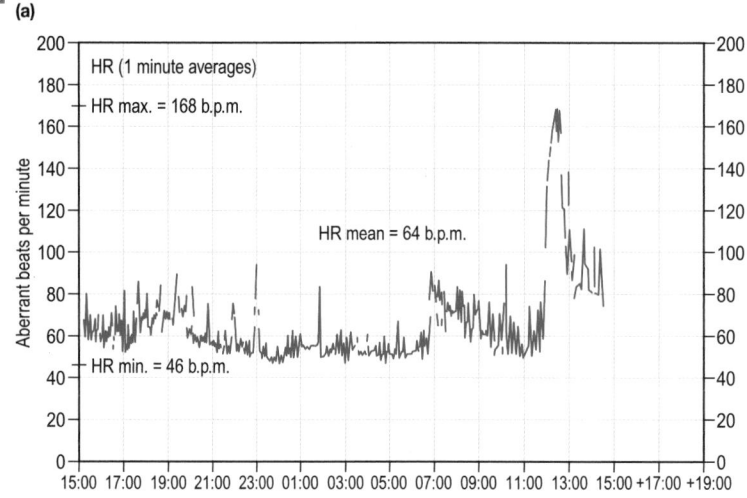

Fig. 13.24 **Examples of Holter recordings. (a)** Tachograph showing sudden increase in heart rate between 1100 and 1300 hours.

(b)

(b) Ambulatory ECG record of the same patient, revealing supraventricular tachycardia.

(c)

(c) Ambulatory ECG showing ST depression in a patient with silent myocardial ischaemia.

areas of slow conduction in the myocardium, such as the border zone of an infarct, where re-entrant ventricular arrhythmias can originate.

T-wave alternans (TWA) is a valuable technique used as a non-invasive marker of susceptibility to ventricular arrhythmias and sudden cardiac death. TWA represents microvolt level changes in the morphology of the T waves in every other beat and can be detected during acute myocardial ischaemia using amplification techniques.

Visible TWA on an ordinary surface ECG is quite a rare phenomenon, except in patients with long QT syndromes, particularly during emotion or exercise.

Tilt testing

Patients with suspected neurocardiogenic (vasovagal) syncope should be investigated by upright tilt testing. The patient is secured to a table which is tilted to + 60° to the vertical for 45 minutes or more. The ECG and blood

Fig. 13.25 **Tilt test**. The ECG (top trace) and arterial blood pressure recorded during a tilt test. After 1 minute of tilt, hypotension, bradycardia and syncope occur.

pressure are monitored throughout. If neither symptoms nor signs develop, isoprenaline may be slowly infused or glyceryl trinitrate inhaled and the tilt repeated. A positive test results in hypotension, sometimes bradycardia (Fig. 13.25) and presyncope/syncope, and supports the diagnosis of neurocardiogenic syncope. If symptoms and signs appear, placing the patient flat can quickly reverse them. The effect of treatment can be evaluated by repeating the tilt test, but it is not always reproducible.

Carotid sinus massage

Carotid sinus massage (p. 772, Practical box 13.4) may lead to asystole (> 3 s) and/or a fall of blood pressure (> 50 mmHg). This hypersensitive response occurs in many of the normal (especially elderly) population, but may also be responsible for loss of consciousness in some patients with carotid sinus syndrome (p. 766). In one-third of cases carotid sinus massage is only positive when the patient is standing. Atherosclerosis can cause narrowing and stenosis of carotid arteries. Carotid sinus massage should thus be avoided in patients with carotid bruits.

FURTHER READING
Benditt DG et al. (1996) Tilt table testing for assessing syncope. American College of Cardiology. *Journal of the American College of Cardiology* **28**(1): 263–275.
Gibbons RJ et al. (2002) ACC/AHA 2002 guideline update for exercise testing. A report of the American College of Cardiology/American Heart Association Task Force on Practice Guidelines. *Journal of the American College of Cardiology* **40**(8): 1531–1540.
Gold MR et al. (2000) A comparison of T-wave alternans, signal averaged ECG and programmed ventricular stimulation for arrhythmia risk stratification. *Journal of the American College of Cardiology* **36**(7): 2247–2253.
Kadish, AH et al. (2001) ACC/AHA clinical competence statement on electrocardiography and ambulatory electrocardiograph: a report of the ACC/AHA/ACP-ASIM task force on clinical competence (ACC/AHA Committee to develop a clinical competence statement on electrocardiography and ambulatory electrocardiography) endorsed by the International Society for Holter and noninvasive electrocardiology. *Circulation* 104(25): 3169–3178.
Malik M (ed) (2001) *Risk of Arrhythmia and Sudden Death*. London: BMJ Books.

Echocardiography

Echocardiography is a non-invasive diagnostic technique that is widely used in clinical cardiology. It involves the use of ultrasound (either alone or with contrast agent) to assess cardiac structure and function.

Physics

Echocardiography uses transmitted ultrasound wavelengths of 1 mm or less, which correspond to frequencies of approximately 2 MHz (2 million cycles per second) or more. At such high frequencies, the ultrasound waves can be focused into a 'beam' and aimed at a particular region of the heart. The waves are generated in very short bursts or pulses a few microseconds long by a crystal transducer, which also detects returning echoes and converts them into electrical signals.

When the handheld crystal transducer is placed on the body surface the emitted ultrasound pulses encounter interfaces between various body tissues as they pass through the body. In crossing each interface, some of the wave energy is reflected, and if the beam path is approximately at right angles to the plane of the interface, the reflected waves return to the transducer as an echo. Since the velocity of sound in body tissues is almost constant (1550 m/s), the time delay for the echo to return measures the distance of the reflecting interface. Thus, if a single ultrasound pulse is transmitted, a series of echoes return, the first of which is from the closest interface.

Echocardiographic modalities
M mode
M mode echocardiography is a technique that details the changing motion of structures along the ultrasound beam with time. Thus the motion of the interventricular septum during the cardiac cycle (either towards or away from the transducer placed on the chest wall) can be assessed and quantified. Stationary structures thus generate horizontal straight lines, the distances of which from the top of the screen indicate their depths, and movements, such as those of heart valves, are indicated by zigzag lines (Fig. 13.26c).

Two-dimensional echocardiography
Alternatively, a series of views from different positions can be obtained in the form of a two-dimensional image (cross-sectional 2-D echocardiography) (Fig. 13.26a, b, d).

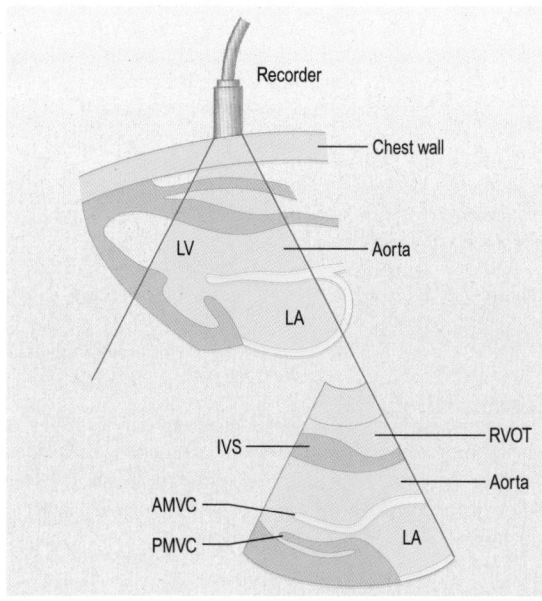

(a)

Fig. 13.26 **Echocardiograms**.

(a) Diagram showing the anatomy of the area scanned and a diagrammatic representation of the echocardiogram.

(b)–(e) Echocardiograms from a normal subject:

(b) *Two-dimensional long-axis view.*
(c) *M-mode recording* with the ultrasound beam directed across the left ventricle, just below the mitral valve.
(d) *Two-dimensional short-axis view* at the level of the tips of the papillary muscles.
(e) *Apical four-chamber view*. Note that the convention that shows the position of the transducer (the apex of the sector image) at the top of the paper causes the heart to appear 'upside down' in these views. AMVC, anterior mitral valve cusp; Ao, aorta; IVS, interventricular septum; LA, left atrium; LV, left ventricle; LV(d), LV(s), left ventricular end-diastolic and end-systolic dimensions; MV, mitral valve; PM, papillary muscle; PMVC, posterior mitral valve cusp; PVW, posterior ventricular wall; RA, right atrium; RV, right ventricle; RVOT, right ventricular outflow tract.

(b)

(c)

(d)

(e)

This method is useful for delineating anatomical structures and for quantifying volumes of cardiac chambers. It is conventional for different imaging planes to be used to create standard 2-D views. Ultrasound machines are commercially available that create moving three-dimensional images of the heart in real time. The clinical use of 3-D is evolving and is likely to involve better assessment of valve morphology.

Doppler echocardiography

Echocardiography imaging utilizes echoes from tissue interfaces. Using high amplification, it is also possible to detect weak echoes scattered by small targets, including those from red blood cells. Blood velocity in the heart chambers is typically much more rapid (> 1 m/s) than the movement of myocardial tissue. If the blood is moving in the same direction as the direction of the ultrasound beam, the frequency of the returning echoes will be changed according to the Doppler phenomenon. The Doppler shift frequency is directly proportional to the blood velocity. Blood velocity data can be acquired and displayed in several ways.

Pulsed-wave (PW) Doppler extracts velocity data from the pulse echoes used to form a two-dimensional image and gives useful qualitative information. PW echoes can be specified from locations within an image identified by a sample volume cursor placed on the screen. Such information from the left ventricular outflow tract (LVOT) and right ventricular outflow tract provides the stroke distance, and is used to estimate cardiac output (CO) and also to quantify intracardiac shunts.

Cardiac output can then be derived using the formula: CO = stroke volume × heart rate. Stroke volume is the stroke distance multiplied by the area of the LVOT, which can also be measured echocardiographically. PW Doppler of the flow across the mitral valve and into the left atrium through the pulmonary veins can be used as part of the estimation of left ventricular filling pressure.

Colour flow Doppler. Doppler colour flow imaging uses one colour for blood flowing towards the transducer and another colour for blood flowing away. This technique allows the direction, velocity and timing of the flow to be measured with a simultaneous view of cardiac structure and function. Colour flow Doppler is used to help assess valvular regurgitation (Fig. 13.27) and may be useful in the assessment of coronary blood flow.

Continuous-wave (CW) Doppler collects all the velocity data from the path of the beam and analyses it to generate a spectral display. This is unlike PW Doppler, which provides information from a particular sample volume at one location along a line. Thus, CW Doppler does not provide any depth information.

The outline of the envelope of the spectral display is used to estimate the value of peak velocity throughout the cardiac cycle. CW Doppler is used typically to assess valvular obstruction, which then causes increased velocities. For example, normal velocities are of the order

Fig. 13.27 Colour Doppler shows blood flowing away from the echocardiography probe as a blue signal and towards the probe as a red signal. In this patient with tricuspid regurgitation, blood leaks from the right ventrical to the right atrium during cardiac systole.

of 1 m/s across the normal aortic valve, but if there is a severe obstructive lesion, such as a severely stenotic aortic valve, velocities of 4 m/s or more can occur (Fig. 13.28a, b). These velocities are generated by the pressure gradient that exists across the lesion.

According to the Bernoulli equation, the pressure difference between two chambers is calculated as: 4 multiplied by the square of the CW Doppler velocity between chambers. Thus a velocity of 5 m/s across the aortic valve suggests a peak gradient of 4 × 5 × 5 = 100 mmHg between the ascending aorta and the left ventricle. This equation has been validated in a wide variety of clinical situations, including valve stenoses, ventricular septal defects and intraventricular obstruction (as in hypertrophic cardiomyopathy). It is often clinically unnecessary to resort to invasive methods such as cardiac catheterization to measure intracardiac pressure gradients.

Similarly, pulmonary artery (PA) systolic pressure and right ventricular diastolic pressure can be calculated using the Bernoulli equation. In this case, CW Doppler tracing of the tricuspid regurgitant jet is used to estimate the pressure gradient between the right ventricle and the right atrium. The PA systolic pressure is then calculated by adding the estimated right atrial pressure to the pressure gradient between the right ventricle and the right atrium.

Tissue Doppler. Tissue Doppler is similar to PW Doppler. It measures myocardial tissue velocities within a particular sample volume placed on the image. Such velocities are of the order of 1 cm/s. Currently, tissue Doppler of the mitral annulus is used as part of the estimation of left ventricular filling pressure.

(a)

(b)

Fig. 13.28 **(a) Two-dimensional echocardiogram (long-axis view)** in a patient with **calcific aortic stenosis**. The calcium in the valve generates abnormally intense echoes. There is some evidence of the associated left ventricular hypertrophy.
(b) Continuous-wave (CW) Doppler signals obtained from the right upper parasternal edge, where the high-velocity jet from the stenotic valve is coming towards the transducer. AV, aortic valve; LA, left atrium; MV, mitral valve; LV, left ventricle; IVS, interventricular septum; PVW, posterior ventricular wall.

Other ultrasound modalities. Harmonic power Doppler, pulse inversion Doppler and ultraharmonics are used to detect and amplify microsphere-specific signals as part of the echocardiographic assessment of myocardial perfusion.

The echocardiographic examination

Transthoracic echocardiography is a 'non-invasive' procedure that causes the patient no discomfort and is harmless. A physician or technician performs the studies and a comprehensive examination takes 15–45 minutes. The ultrasound machines are either mobile on wheels, or are handheld.

The technical issue associated with echocardiography is that the lungs and rib cage obstruct the passage of ultrasound to the heart in the adult subject. Small 'windows' can usually be found in the third and fourth left intercostal spaces (termed left parasternal); just below the xiphoid process of the sternum (subcostal); and, with the subject turned to the left and exhaling, from the point where the apical beat is palpated (apical). By positioning the transducer successively over these sites and angling and rotating it to line up with the scan plane, a series of standard sectional views is obtained. In children, and some adults, the aortic arch can be visualized from a supra-sternal position.

The standard nomenclature for two-dimensional echocardiographic images is shown in Figure 13.26a. The parasternal position of the transducer gives access to the long-axis and short-axis planes. The apical approach gives a second view of the long-axis plane, but with the apex in the foreground, and also shows the four-chamber plane (Fig. 13.26e). A three-chamber apical view is sometimes also obtained. The convention adopted in most adult cardiology units of showing the transducer position at the top of the image results in the apical views being 'upside-down' compared to the anatomic position of the heart. M-mode recordings are obtained from the para-sternal position to document motion patterns of the aorta, aortic valve and left atrium, the mitral valve, and the left and right ventricles (Fig. 13.26c).

Quantification in echocardiography

Quantification is helpful because of the relative inaccuracy of *subjective* assessment of chamber size and cardiac function. M mode is used to assess lengths in a single plane. The 1 cm calibration markers on M-mode recordings permit measurement of cardiac dimensions at any point in the cardiac cycle with a typical accuracy of ± 2–3 mm. M mode can be used to estimate LV systolic function by comparing end-diastolic and end-systolic dimensions. For example, the percentage reduction in the left ventricular cavity size ('shortening fraction' – SF) is given by:

$$SF = \frac{LVDD - LVSD}{LVDD} \times 100\%$$

where LVDD is left ventricular diastolic diameter and LVSD is left ventricular systolic diameter, at the base of the heart. The normal range is 30–45%.

This method is easy to perform, but is an inaccurate measure of ejection fraction (EF) because it does not take account of reduced regional function of the mid or apical myocardium, due to infarction for example. For this reason, estimation of EF based upon the difference in LV volumes from systole to diastole, derived from planimetered measurements of LV area in at least two planes, is more accurate. A normal EF is > 55%. This method is helpful in assessing the response of the patient with heart failure to therapy. This method also permits estimation of LV mass.

Transoesophageal echocardiography (TOE)

This involves placing the transducer mounted on a flexible tube into the oesophagus. This involves the use of local anaesthesia and sometimes intravenous sedation. High-resolution images can be obtained because of the close proximity of the heart to the transducer in the oesophagus, and also because of the higher frequencies that are used relative to transthoracic imaging.

TOE is most commonly used in the assessment of valve structure and function (to assess for reparability of mitral valve prolapse), for features and complications of infective endocarditis, to assess the aorta for aortic dissection, and to assess for cardiac source of embolus.

Wall motion stress echocardiography

Echocardiography can be used clinically to evaluate the patient for the presence of myocardial scars and for the presence of reversible ischaemia. Since ultrasound cannot directly detect red blood cells in capillaries, myocardial wall motion is used as a surrogate for perfusion. Myocardial segments that demonstrate a change in function (defined as a change or reduction in thickening) from rest to stress can be assumed to be supplied by a flow-limiting stenosis in the epicardial artery or graft.

Stress for this indication needs to be inotropic to induce true ischaemia. Physiological stress includes treadmill exercise, which is complicated by the difficulty in obtaining reliable images rapidly as the patient comes off the treadmill, before heart rate reduces back to sub-maximal levels. Alternatively, pharmacological stress can be induced with dobutamine at graded doses. This is relatively safe but complications such as ventricular arrhythmia have been reported.

This technique can also be used to assess for viability of the myocardium and for hibernating or stunned myocardium.

Myocardial perfusion echocardiography

In order to assess myocardial perfusion by echocardiography (MPE), microspheres of similar size to red blood cells are used as an intravenous contrast agent. Microsphere-specific ultrasound modes such as harmonic power Doppler can be used for detection. MPE involves the use of intravenous infusion of contrast to fill the myocardium. A pulse of ultrasound destroys microspheres within the capillaries (and not the LV cavity), and the time taken to replenish the capillaries is a measure of myocardial blood flow. The time taken to fill should be significantly shorter at stress than at rest.

Clinical use of echocardiography

The echocardiographic findings in particular conditions are discussed in relevant sections, but a brief overview is given below.

Valve stenosis

Congenitally abnormal aortic or pulmonary valves show a characteristic 'dome' shape in systole because the cusps cannot separate fully and a bicuspid configuration may be demonstrated. The presence of calcium in a valve gives rise to intense echoes that generate multiple, parallel lines on M-mode recordings. CW Doppler (p. 751) directed from the apex measures velocity of the jet crossing the diseased valve, from which the pressure gradient can be calculated (Fig. 13.28b).

Mitral stenosis

The M-mode shows restriction and reversal of direction of the posterior leaflet motion (Fig. 13.29c). A short-axis view shows the shape of the mitral orifice in diastole, and its area can be measured directly from the image. Peak, mean and end-diastolic pressure gradients can be obtained from CW Doppler. Additional imaging views indicate the size of the left atrium, and may show the presence of left atrial thrombus.

Valve regurgitation

Doppler is extremely sensitive for detecting valve regurgitation and care must be taken not to overestimate severity of regurgitation. Transthoracic echocardiography is as accurate as angiography in the evaluation of valvular regurgitation, provided appropriate algorithms for interpretation are used. Echocardiography can determine the underlying cause such as rheumatic disease or mitral valve prolapse.

Aortic aneurysms and dissections

Dilatation of the aortic root can be measured accurately and the presence of a reflecting structure within the lumen of the aorta is strongly suggestive of an intimal flap associated with dissection. Transoesophageal views are particularly suitable for detecting pathology in the ascending and descending aorta. In some hospitals this is the investigation of first choice when aortic dissection is suspected although MRI is increasingly used.

Prosthetic heart valves

Each type of mechanical heart valve prosthesis has characteristic echocardiographic features. Irregularity or restriction of movement can be shown. Bioprostheses can also be assessed echocardiographically. The presence of stenosis or regurgitation may be documented by colour flow and continuous wave Doppler. Prosthetic valves imaged transthoracically cast acoustic shadows that obscure the area behind the valve. For this reason a transoesophageal approach is often used to inspect a prosthetic mitral valve for evidence of endocarditis or thrombosis.

Infective endocarditis

Vegetations > 2 mm can be detected (Fig. 13.87a, p. 831). Complications of endocarditis such as valvar regurgitation and abscess can be identified.

Cardiac failure

Left ventricular function and response to treatment is

Fig. 13.29 Echocardiograms in rheumatic mitral valve disease. (a) *Two-dimensional long-axis view* showing enlarged left atrium and 'hooked' appearance of the mitral valve leaflets resulting from commissural fusion.
(b) *Magnified short-axis view* showing the mitral valve orifice as seen from the direction of the arrow in (a). The orifice area can be planimetered to assess the severity; in this case it is 1.5 cm², indicating moderately severe disease.
(c) *M-mode recording* of the mitral valve showing restricted motion of the thickened leaflets.
(d) *Continuous-wave (CW) Doppler recording* showing slow rate of decay of flow velocity from the left atrium to the left ventricle during diastole. It is also possible to derive the valve orifice area from the velocity decay rate. LA, left atrium; LV, left ventricle; AMVL, PMVL, anterior and posterior mitral valve leaflets.

readily assessed and should be performed in all patients with known or suspected heart failure. Left- and right-sided heart cardiac output and filling pressures can also be estimated.

Cardiomyopathies

Dilated cardiomyopathy is characterized by an enlarged, globular shaped, thin-walled left ventricle with poor function and low stroke output shown by reduced movements of the valves (Fig. 13.107, p. 850).

Hypertrophic cardiomyopathy (HCM) (Fig. 13.109, p. 851) shows that the left ventricle is typically small and hypertrophied, with a thickened, interventricular septum (asymmetric septal hypertrophy – ASH). There is a characteristic, displacement of the mitral valve apparatus towards the septum in systole (systolic anterior motion – SAM). Some patients have outflow tract or other LV

obstruction and others have regional hypertrophy of other segments.

Restrictive cardiomyopathy shows the typical appearances of conditions such as amyloid, and LV diastolic function can be evaluated.

Pericardial effusion

Fluid in the pericardial cavity shows as an echo-free region between the myocardium and the intense echo of the parietal pericardium (Fig. 13.30). The most severe manifestation of pericardial effusion is tamponade, which is a clinical and not an echocardiographic diagnosis. The size of a pericardial effusion alone does not indicate tamponade. Echocardiographic features of haemo-dynamically significant effusions include marked (> 25%) respiratory variation of tricuspid, aortic or mitral Doppler tracings. If the inferior vena cava is small and collapses

Fig. 13.30 Two-dimensional echocardiogram (short-axis view) from a patient with a large **pericardial effusion** associated with pulmonary tuberculosis. The exudate is seen between the visceral and parietal layers of the pericardium and would give a false impression of cardiomegaly on a chest X-ray. Note the multiple fibrous strands within the effusion, showing that it is consolidating and will probably lead to constriction of cardiac function. LV, left ventricle; RV, right ventricle; EFF, effusion.

with respiration it is unlikely that the patient is in tamponade.

Masses within the heart

Echocardiography is a sensitive method for detecting masses within the heart (Fig. 13.103, p. 847), and their haemodynamic significance.

Ischaemic disease

Coronary arteries cannot be imaged adequately using echo techniques, but images may be useful for the diagnosis of complications related to myocardial infarction, such as mitral papillary muscle rupture, tamponade or ventricular septal rupture. The use of stress echocardiography to identify chronic coronary artery disease is discussed above (p. 753).

In the post-infarction period, echocardiography and Doppler are used to diagnose left ventricular aneurysm, left ventricular thrombus, mitral regurgitation and pericardial effusion as well as to assess left ventricular function (ejection fraction).

Congenital heart disease

Echocardiography has largely replaced cardiac catheterization and angiography. The aim of the examination is first to establish the sequence of blood flow through the heart, and to define anatomical abnormalities as well to evaluate the postoperative status of the operated congenital heart patients.

Contrast echo for LV opacification

Intravenous contrast agents are available that permit opacification of the left ventricle and definition of the endocardial border. Their clinical utility has reduced with the advent of harmonic imaging, which has improved image quality in previously difficult to image patients. It is likely that the use of ultrasound contrast agents in echocardiography will increase when there is approval for perfusion imaging.

Intravascular (coronary) ultrasound

Intravascular (coronary) ultrasound probes can be used to image proximal coronary arteries as part of a percutaneous transluminal coronary angioplasty (PTCA) procedure, for example to assess for adequacy of deployment of intracoronary stents.

Nuclear imaging

Nuclear imaging may be used to detect myocardial infarction or to measure myocardial function, perfusion or viability, depending on the radiopharmaceutical used and the technique of imaging. These data are particularly valuable when used in combination.

Image type

Gamma cameras produce a planar image in which structures are superimposed as in a standard radiograph. Single-photon-emission computed tomography (SPECT) imaging uses similar raw data to construct tomographic images, just as a CT image is reconstructed from X-rays. This gives finer anatomical resolution, but is technically demanding. These methods may be used with any of the radiopharmaceuticals.

Myocardial perfusion and viability

Thallium-201 is rapidly taken up by the myocardium, so an image taken immediately after injection reflects the distribution of blood flow to the myocardium. Areas of ischaemia or infarction receive less ^{201}Tl and appear dark. Between 2 and 24 hours after injection, ^{201}Tl is redistributed so that all cardiac myocytes contain a comparable concentration. Images at this time show dark areas where the myocardium has infarcted, but normal density in ischaemic areas. Comparison of the early and late images is one method of predicting whether an ischaemic area of myocardium contains enough viable tissue to justify coronary bypass or angioplasty.

Technetium-99-labelled tetrofosmin (Fig. 13.31) is also taken up rapidly by cardiac myocytes, but does not undergo redistribution. When this substance is injected during exercise, its distribution in the myocardium reflects the distribution of blood at the time of the exercise, even if the image is taken several hours later. This is a sensitive method of detecting myocardial viability. Images produced following injection of ^{99m}Tc-tetrofosmin during exercise can be compared to images produced following injection at rest to decide which areas of ischaemia are reversible (p. 795). In patients unable to exercise, the heart can be stressed with drugs, e.g. dipyridamole or dobutamine.

Fig. 13.31 Myocardial SPECT study acquired with ^{99}Tc tetrofosmin tracer. Left panel – three short axis slices, a horizontal and a vertical axis plane of the left ventricle after stress and following a resting re-injection of tracer. The rest images demonstrate normal tracer uptake (orange signal) in the whole of the left ventricle. The stress images demonstrate reduced tracer uptake (purple-blue signal) in the anterior and septal walls consistent with a significant stenosis in the left anterior descending artery. Middle panel – polar maps of the whole myocardium can localize the ischaemic territory. Right panel – quantitative analysis can help define the extent and reversibility of the ischaemia.

Infarct imaging

Perfusion images produced using compounds labelled with ^{201}Tl or ^{99m}Tc-sestamibi show a myocardial infarction as a perfusion defect or 'cold spot'. These methods are sensitive for detecting and localizing the infarct, but give no information about its age. ^{99m}Tc pyrophosphate is preferentially taken up by myocardium which has undergone infarction within the previous few days. Images are difficult to interpret because the isotope is also concentrated by bone and cartilage.

Radionuclide angiography

Two methods are used to obtain blood pool images:

- A MUGA (multigated acquisition) or equilibrium image is obtained by intravenous injection of ^{99m}Tc, which attaches to the patient's own red cells in vivo and which is therefore retained in the vascular space. Over 200 heartbeats are imaged. Comparison of the study with the ECG allows systolic and diastolic points of the cycle to be identified.
- A first-pass study images the heart as a bolus of isotope makes a single pass through the circulation.

These techniques are complementary, but both outline the cardiac chambers, particularly the left ventricle, by imaging the isotope within the central circulation during systole and diastole. The percentage of the left ventricular volume ejected with each systole (the ejection fraction) can be measured accurately, and any section of the left ventricular wall that contracts abnormally (a wall motion defect) can be visualized (Fig. 13.32).

Positron emission tomography (PET)

This is a technique based on detection of high-energy emissions caused by annihilation of positrons released from unstable isotopes. There are several advantages of PET over other techniques, e.g. improved spatial resolution, accurate quantification, the use of biological isotopes of carbon, nitrogen, and oxygen. However, PET is expensive and requires a cyclotron to produce the short-lived tracers. PET has become a useful investigation in the detection of viable myocardium in patients who are suitable for revascularization.

Myocardial perfusion and ischaemia can be determined with ^{13}N-ammonia or oxygen-15 with greater sensitivity

(a) Before sublingual nitrate
End-diastolic   **End-systolic**

(b) After sublingual nitrate

Fig. 13.32 **MUGA scan of patient with left ventricular aneurysm**. End-diastolic and end-systolic images were recorded **(a)** before administration of sublingual nitrate and **(b)** again after administration. The apical aneurysm is not altered by administration of nitrate, although the remainder of the left ventricle shows a reduced end-systolic size (arrows).

than SPECT. Myocardial metabolism and viability can be detected with the use of ^{18}F-fluorodeoxyglucose (FDG), which the cardiac myocyte utilizes for energy production in the presence of reduced oxygen supply and blood flow. There may be reduced perfusion to infarcted or fibrotic myocardium, but also reduced FDG uptake. In hibernating myocardium, with viable but dysfunctional myocardium, PET can demonstrate reduced myocardial perfusion but with preserved or increased FDG uptake.

Cardiac catheterization

Cardiac catheterization is the introduction of a thin radio-opaque tube (catheter) into the circulation. The right heart is catheterized by introducing the catheter into a peripheral vein (usually the right femoral or internal jugular vein) and advancing it through the right atrium and ventricle into the pulmonary artery. The pressures in the right heart chambers, and pulmonary artery can be measured directly. An indirect measure of left atrial pressure can be obtained by 'wedging' a catheter into the distal pulmonary artery (p. 971). In this position the pressure from the right ventricle is obstructed by the catheter and only the pulmonary venous and left atrial pressures are recorded.

Left heart catheterization is usually performed via the right femoral artery, although the brachial and radial arteries are sometimes used in patients with significant peripheral vascular disease. A pigtail catheter is advanced up the aorta and manipulated through the aortic valve into the left ventricle. Pressure tracings are taken from the left ventricular cavity. The end-diastolic pressure is invariably elevated in patients with left ventricular dysfunction. A power injection of radio-opaque contrast material is used to opacify the left ventricular cavity (left ventriculography) and thereby assesses left ventricular systolic function. Figure 13.33 presents a normal angiogram showing normal left ventricular function. The catheter is then withdrawn across the aortic valve into the aorta and the 'pullback' gradient across the valve is measured.

Aortography (a power injection into the aortic root) can be performed to assess the aortic root and the presence and severity of aortic regurgitation.

Specially designed catheters are then used to selectively engage the left and right coronary arteries, and contrast cine-angiograms are taken in order to define the coronary circulation and identify the presence and severity of any coronary artery disease. Coronary angiography is described further on page 805.

During cardiac catheterization, blood samples may be withdrawn to measure the concentration of ischaemic metabolites (e.g. lactate) and the oxygen content. These estimations are used to gauge ischaemia, quantify intracardiac shunts, and measure cardiac output.

Digital subtraction angiography
This technique permits the injection of small volumes of radio-contrast agents during cardiac catheterization with the production of computer-analysed high-quality angiograms.

Unfortunately, peripheral injection of contrast does not give adequate visualization of the coronary arteries, but aortic lesions can be visualized.

Fig. 13.33 **Normal angiogram**. Diastolic (left) and systolic (right) frames recorded after X-ray contrast was injected into the left ventricle (contrast left ventriculogram). Normal left ventricular function is demonstrated.

(a)   (b)

CT scanning

CT scanning is limited because an image must be obtained in approximately 50 ms to eliminate cardiac motion. Both conventional and spiral CT are used to image the thoracic aorta and mediastinum. CT involves ionizing radiation, requires intravascular contrast media and has been largely superseded by MRI. Electron-beam CT, which produces a faster beam image, has been developed, but is expensive.

Cardiovascular magnetic resonance (CMR)

Cardiovascular magnetic resonance (a non-invasive imaging technique that does not involve harmful radiation) is a rapidly developing investigation in cardiology. CMR scanners employ cardiac and respiratory gating to effectively suspend cardio-respiratory motion. The use of different CMR sequences can provide black-blood or white-blood images, still or moving images, anatomical and functional information. Synchronization with the ECG allows cardiac images in systole and diastole to be obtained (Fig. 13.34). Intravenous gadolinium can be used with a myocardial perfusion study, contrast-enhanced angiography or for myocardial infarct imaging. The major contraindications are permanent pacemaker or defibrillator, intracerebral clips, significant claustrophobia. Patients with coronary stents and prosthetic valves can be safely scanned. The current indications for CMR are provided in Table 13.6.

FURTHER READING
Ashley EA, Myers J, Froelicher U (2000) Exercise testing in clinical medicine. *Lancet* **356**: 1592–1597.
Cheitlin MD et al. (2003) ACC/AHA/ASE 2003 Guidline update for the clinical application of echocardiography: summary article. A report of the American College of Cardiology/American Heart Association Task Force on Practice Guidelines (ACC/AHA/ASE Committee to Update the 1997 Guidelines for the Clinical Application of Echocardiography). *Journal of the American Society of Echocardiography* **16**(10): 1091–1100.
Constantine G (2004) Role of MRI in clinical cardiology. *Lancet* **363**: 2162–2171.
Orro CM (2002) *The Practice of Clinical Echocardiography*. Philadelphia: WB Saunders
Pennell DJ, Prvulovich E (1995) *Nuclear Cardiology*. London: BPC Wheatons, British Nuclear Society.
Peterson KL, Nicol P (1996) *Cardiac Catheterization. Methods, Diagnosis and Therapy*. Philadelphia: WB Saunders.

Table 13.6 Cardiovascular magnetic resonance (CMR)

Indications
1. Congenital heart disease: (CHD)
   - anatomical assessment following echocardiography, particularly in patients with complex CHD or following surgical intervention
   - follow-up/surveillance studies
   - anomalous pulmonary or systemic venous return
   - assessment of right or left ventricular function/dilatation
2. Cardiomyopathies/cardiac infiltration/pericardial disease
3. Disease of the aorta, including aortic dissection, aneurysm, coarctation
4. Valvular heart disease:
   - quantification of stenosis and regurgitation
   - accurate ventricular dimensions/function
   - planimetry of valvular stenosis
5. Coronary artery disease:
   - left and right ventricular function
   - wall motion assessment during dobutamine stress
   - myocardial perfusion during adenosine stress
   - coronary artery and coronary artery bypass graft imaging
   - myocardial infarct imaging and viability assessment with dobutamine CMR or delayed enhancement
6. Pulmonary vessels

(a)

(b)

Fig. 13.34 **Magnetic resonance image (MRI),** showing a pair of axial images taken through the mid-thorax at the level of the mitral valve. **(a)** A view of end-systole. **(b)** Taken at end-diastole. Note the clear differentiation between the atria and ventricles. This is a normal study. LA, left atrium; LV, left ventricle; MV, mitral valve; RA, right atrium; RV, right ventricle.

THERAPEUTIC PROCEDURES

Cardiac resuscitation

When cardiac arrest occurs, basic life support must be started immediately. The longer the period of respiratory and circulatory arrest, the lower is the chance of restoring healthy life. After 3 minutes, irreversible anoxic cerebral damage occurs.

All healthcare professionals should be familiar with basic procedures. Organization and teamwork are essential to a successful outcome. In hospitals the prior identification of patients who should be resuscitated ensures that treatment is appropriately focused. Medical emergency teams and critical care outreach teams have increasing roles to play in the prevention of cardiac arrests.

Basic life support (BLS)

The first step is to ensure the safety of the victim and rescuer. The next is to ascertain that the victim is unresponsive by shaking him/her and shouting into one ear. If no response is obtained, help should be sought immediately prior to commencement of basic life support. If the likely cause of the unconsciousness is due to a breathing problem (e.g. trauma, drowning, choking, drug/alcohol intoxication or if the victim is an infant or child) then the rescuer should perform resuscitation for about 1 minute before going for help. Basic life support is easily remembered as A (airway), B (breathing) and C (circulation) (Emergency box 13.1).

Airway

Debris (e.g. blood and mucus) in the mouth and pharynx should be removed. Loose or ill-fitting dentures should be removed. The airway should be opened gently by flexing the neck and extending the head ('sniffing the morning air' position). This manoeuvre is not recommended if a cervical spine injury is suspected. Any obstruction deep in the oral cavity or upper respiratory tract may require abdominal and or chest thrusts (Heimlich manoeuvre, p. 899).

Emergency Box 13.1
Basic life support

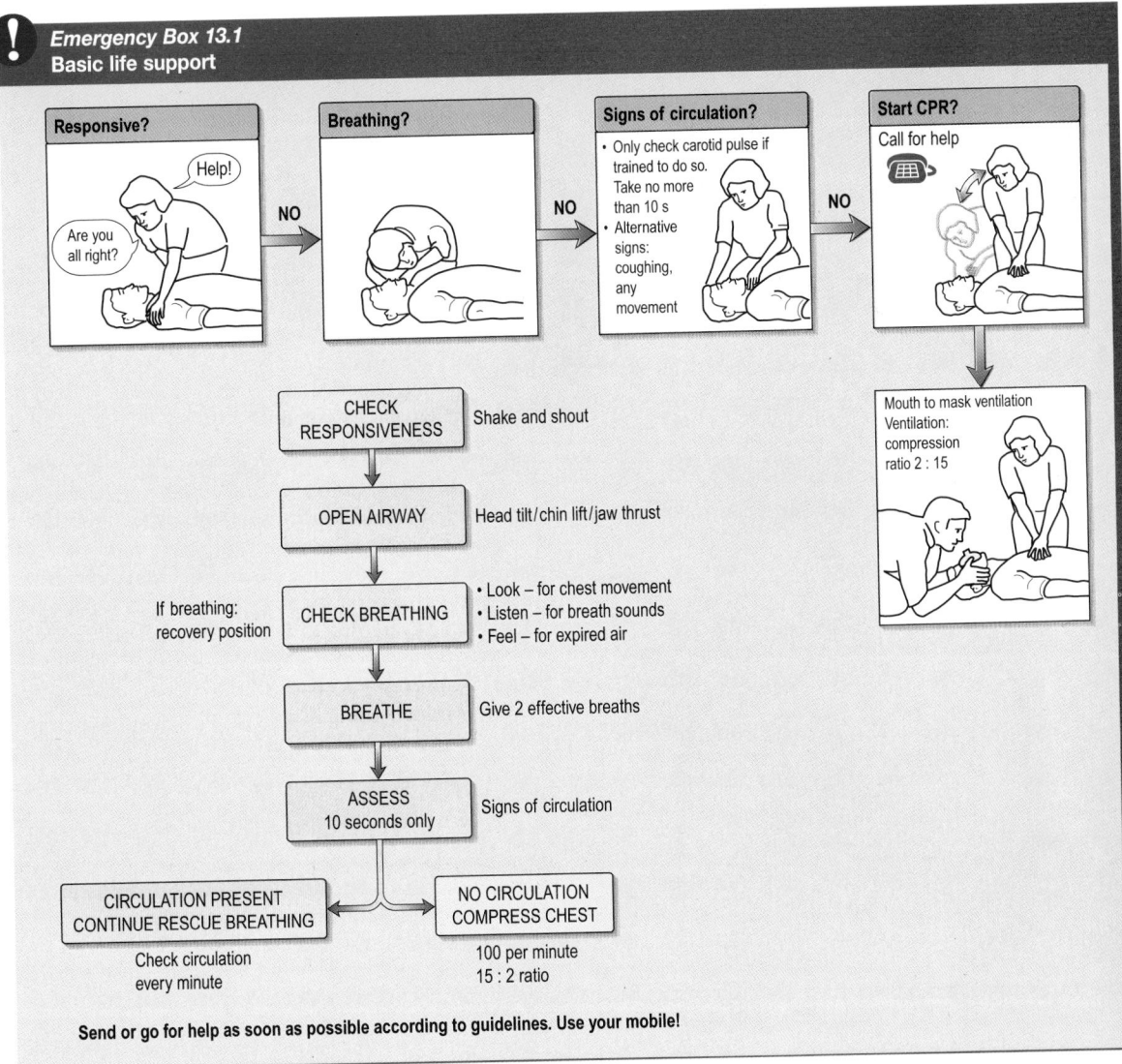

Send or go for help as soon as possible according to guidelines. Use your mobile!

Breathing

Once a clear airway has been established the victim's breathing should be assessed by the 'look, listen and feel' method. By placing a cheek close to the victim's mouth, breath sounds can be felt and heard and the rise and fall of the chest and abdomen observed. If there is no evidence of breathing, expired air ventilation should be commenced.

With the head of the victim tilted backwards (*head tilt*), the chin pulled forward (*chin lift*) or *jaw thrust* and the nostrils pinched firmly, the rescuer takes a deep breath and seals his/her lips around the mouth of the victim. Two effective breaths are given over 2 seconds each. Expired air respiration is the only method of artificial respiration that successfully ventilates the patient. If resistance to these puffs is experienced, the airway needs to be reassessed and/or the head tilt and jaw lift corrected.

If the rescuer feels reluctant to give mouth-to-mouth resuscitation because of safety concerns (e.g. potentially infective material such as blood or vomitus in the oropharynx) it is acceptable to perform chest compressions alone.

Circulation

Cardiac arrest is accompanied by circulatory collapse. Absence of the carotid pulse confirms this and should be assessed for at least 10 seconds by someone trained to do so. The carotid pulse lies lateral and posterior to the thyroid cartilage and medial to the medial border of sternocleidomastoid: it can sometimes be difficult to palpate.

If absent, the circulation is best re-established by external chest compression. The heel of one hand is placed over the lower half of the victim's sternum and the heel of the second hand is placed over the first with the fingers interlocked. The arms are kept straight and the sternum is rhythmically depressed by 2–5 cm at a rate of approximately 100 per minute. Chest compressions do not massage the heart. The thorax acts as a pump and the heart provides a system of one-way valves to ensure forward circulation. Respiratory and circulatory support is continued by providing two effective breaths for every 15 cardiac compressions (15 : 2 for one or two persons).

It is better to give compressions without interruption. This maintains adequate cerebral and coronary perfusion pressures. There is evidence to suggest that if the person performing compressions tires, the quality of resuscitation deteriorates.

Advanced cardiac life support

By the time effective life support has been established, more help should have arrived and advanced cardiac life support can begin. This consists of ECG monitoring, endotracheal intubation and setting up an intravenous infusion in a large peripheral vein or a central vein. Immediate therapy includes defibrillation, oxygen and cardioactive drugs. It is not possible to recommend an exact sequence of management because it will depend on the arrival of skilled personnel and equipment and the nature of the cardiac arrest.

As soon as possible the cardiac rhythm should be established. At first this is easily achieved by monitoring the ECG through the paddles of a defibrillator. Later, ECG monitoring can be set up. If the ECG shows ventricular fibrillation or if there is any doubt as to the nature of the rhythm (e.g. 'fine' VF may be confused with asystole), no time should be lost before defibrillating the patient. If initial defibrillation attempts are unsuccessful, time can then be spent intubating the patient and setting up an intravenous infusion whilst the circulation is supported by external chest compression.

If there is any difficulty in intubating the patient, ventilation should be continued by means of an airway, a ventilating bag and oxygen. Intravenous epinephrine (adrenaline) results in vasoconstriction and increases the proportion of the cardiac output delivered to the brain.

Causes of unexpected cardiac arrest

Each year in the UK there are approximately 100 000 unexpected deaths occurring within 24 hours of the development of cardiac symptoms. About half of these deaths are almost instantaneous. There are several causes (see Table 13.7).

Most deaths are due to ventricular fibrillation or rapid ventricular tachycardia, and a small proportion are due to severe bradyarrhythmias. Coronary artery disease accounts for approximately 80% of the sudden cardiac death in western society. Transient ischaemia is suspected as the major trigger factor; however, only a small proportion of survivors have clinical evidence of acute myocardial infarction.

There are two mechanisms of sudden unexpected cardiac arrest:

- ventricular fibrillation or pulseless ventricular tachycardia (VF/VT)
- non-VF/VT (asystole and pulseless electrical activity also known as electromechanical dissociation).

The principal difference in the management of these two groups of arrhythmias is the need for attempted defibrillation in those patients with VF/VT (Fig. 13.35).

Three-quarters of arrests are due to ventricular fibrillation or rapid ventricular tachycardia. Only a very small proportion are due to pulseless electrical activity. The remainder are due to asystole. An agonal rhythm is characterized by an inexorable slowing and widening of the QRS complexes associated with falling blood pressure and cardiac output. This type of arrhythmia is very difficult to reverse and usually no attempt should be made because it is the result rather than the cause of death.

Table 13.7 Causes of unexpected cardiac arrest

Cardiac arrhythmias (e.g. ventricular fibrillation)
Sudden pump failure (e.g. acute myocardial infarction)
Acute circulatory obstruction (e.g. pulmonary embolism)
Cardiovascular rupture (e.g. aortic dissection, myocardial rupture)
Vasomotor collapse (e.g. in pulmonary hypertension)

Fig. 13.35 **Universal advanced life-support algorithm**. Reproduced by permission of the European Resuscitation Council and Laerdal Medical Ltd. CPR, cardiopulmonary resuscitation; EMD, electromechanical dissociation; VF/VT, ventricular fibrillation/ventricular tachycardia.

Arrests are treated in the following ways:

- Ventricular fibrillation or pulseless ventricular tachycardia is readily treated with IMMEDIATE defibrillation, CPR and drugs. Intravenous amiodarone is the first-line drug in refractory VF/pulseless VT.
- Asystole is more difficult to treat but the heart may respond to atropine or epinephrine (adrenaline). Recently vasopressin has been shown to be successful. If there is any sign of slow electromechanical activity (e.g. bradycardia with a weak pulse), emergency pacing should be used.
- Pulseless electrical activity: several potentially reversible causes are listed in the universal algorithm. It carries a

very poor prognosis. Effective treatment involves addressing the underlying cause.

Figure 13.35 shows the treatments recommended by the European Resuscitation Council and the Resuscitation Council UK.

Defibrillation

This technique is used to convert ventricular fibrillation to sinus rhythm. When the defibrillator is discharged, a high-voltage field envelopes the heart which depolarizes the myocardium and allows an organized heart rhythm to emerge. Electrical energy is discharged through two paddles placed on the chest wall. Initially 200 J is used for defibrillation.

The paddles are placed in one of two positions:

- One paddle is placed to the right of the upper sternum and the other over the cardiac apex.
- One paddle is placed under the tip of the left scapula and the other is placed over the anterior wall of the left chest.

Electrode jelly or electrolyte gel pads should be used to ensure good contact between the electrode paddles and the skin. Jelly smeared carelessly across the chest may cause short-circuits and arcing of the charge. All personnel should stand clear of the patient. The person performing defibrillation has the responsibility for ensuring the safety of the patient and other people present.

Conventional defibrillators employ a damped monophasic waveform. Biphasic defibrillators which require less energy are becoming increasingly common. Automated external defibrillators (AEDs) which recognize ventricular fibrillation automatically deliver a shock if indicated. These are available in some public places. It is the responsibility of all healthcare practitioners to be familiar with the range of defibrillators they may be called on to use in their workplace.

DC-cardioversion (DCC)

Tachyarrhythmias that do not respond to medical treatment or that are associated with haemodynamic compromise (e.g. hypotension, worsening heart failure) may be converted to sinus rhythm by the use of a transthoracic electric shock. A short-acting general anaesthetic is used. Muscle relaxants are not usually given.

When the arrhythmia has definite QRS complexes, the delivery of the shock should be timed to occur with the downstroke of the QRS complex (synchronization) (Fig. 13.36). The machine being used to perform the cardioversion will do this automatically if the appropriate button is pressed. There is a crucial difference between defibrillation and cardioversion: a non-synchronized shock is used to defibrillate. Accidental defibrillation of a patient who does not require it may itself precipitate ventricular fibrillation.

Typical indications for DCC include:

- atrial fibrillation
- atrial flutter

Tachycardia | Sinus rhythm

Synchronized DC shock

Fig. 13.36 DC-cardioversion of a supraventricular tachycardia to sinus rhythm. The direct current shock is delivered synchronously with the QRS complex.

- sustained ventricular tachycardia
- junctional tachyarrhythmias.

If atrial fibrillation or flutter has been present for more than a few days, it is necessary to anticoagulate the patient adequately for 4 weeks before elective cardioversion to reduce the risk of embolization. The duration of anticoagulation after successful cardioversion for atrial fibrillation is a complex issue and depends on a number of factors: it should be at least for 6 weeks after the procedure and may well be for much longer.

Digoxin toxicity may lead to ventricular arrhythmias or asystole following cardioversion. Therapeutic digitalization does not increase the risks of cardioversion, but it is conventional to omit digoxin several days prior to elective cardioversion in order to be sure that toxicity is not present.

Cardiac enzyme levels may rise after a cardioversion.

Temporary pacing

Therapeutic cardiac pacing is employed in any patient with sustained symptomatic or haemodynamically compromising bradycardia. Bradycardias may be due to either a slow intrinsic heart rate (e.g. sinus node dysfunction) or atrioventricular block. Prophylactic cardiac pacing is employed in asymptomatic patients with either bradycardia or conduction abnormalities in whom the risk of progression to symptomatic bradycardia justifies such a strategy.

Transvenous pacing is the preferred method in patients with symptomatic bradycardias. In summary a thin (French gauge 5 or 6), bipolar pacing electrode wire is inserted via an internal jugular vein, a femoral vein or a subclavian vein and is positioned at the right ventricular apex using cardiac fluoroscopy. The energy needed for successful pacing (the pacing threshold) is assessed by reducing the energy until the pacemaker fails to stimulate the tissue (loss of capture). The output energy is then set at three times the threshold value to prevent inadvertent loss of capture. If the threshold increases above 5 V, the pacemaker wire should be resited. A temporary pacemaker unit (Fig. 13.37a) is almost always set to work 'on demand' – to fire only when a spontaneous beat has not occurred. The rate of temporary pacing is usually 60–80 per minute.

Transcutaneous pacing is the preferred method in selected patients with asymptomatic bradycardia or conduction abnormalities and may be life-saving for patients in whom a cardiac arrest is precipitated by bradycardia. In this method the myocardium is depolarized by current flow between two large adhesive electrodes positioned anteriorly and posteriorly on the chest wall. Transcutaneous pacing is uncomfortable for the conscious patient. However, it can usually be tolerated until a temporary transvenous pacemaker is inserted.

Permanent pacing

Permanent pacemakers are fully implanted in the body and connected to the heart by one or two electrode leads (Fig. 13.37b). The pacemaker is powered by solid-state lithium batteries, which usually last 5–10 years. Pacemakers are 'programmable' in that their operating characteristics (e.g. the pacing rate) can be changed by a programmer that transmits specific electromagnetic signals through the skin. The pacemaker leads are passed transvenously to the right heart chambers.

Pacemakers are designed to both pace and sense either the ventricles or the atria or more commonly both chambers. A single chamber ventricular pacemaker is described as a 'VVI' unit because it paces the ventricle (V), senses the ventricle (V) and is inhibited (I) by a spontaneous ventricular signal. Occasionally (e.g. in symptomatic sinus bradycardia), an atrial pacemaker (AAI) may be implanted. Pacemakers that are connected to both the right atrium and ventricle ('dual chamber' pacemakers) are used to simulate the natural pacemaker and activation sequence of the heart. This form of pacemaker is called DDD because it paces the two (dual) chambers, senses both (D) and reacts in two (D) ways – pacing in the same chamber is inhibited by spontaneous atrial and ventricular signals, and ventricular pacing is triggered by spontaneous atrial events (Fig. 13.37c).

In addition, pacemakers may be 'rate responsive' (R). A rate-responsive pacemaker detects motion (level of vibration or acceleration), respiration, or changes in QT interval, and by employing one or more biosensors, changes its rate of pacing so that it is appropriate to the level of exertion.

The choice of pacemaker mostly depends on the underlying rhythm abnormality and the general condition of the patient. For example, complete heart block in patients with sinus rhythm should be treated with a dual-chamber device in order to maintain AV synchrony,

(a)

(b)

(c)

N   N   N   N

V

(c)

Fig. 13.37 **Pacemakers.** (**a**) A temporary pacemaker unit.
(**b**) A permanent pacemaker with atrial (placed in the right
atrium, usually in its high lateral wall) and ventricular (placed in
the right ventricular apex) leads.
(**c**) An electrocardiogram showing dual (atrial and ventricular)
chamber pacing. A wide QRS complex results from abnormal
activation of the ventricles from the right ventricular apex.

whereas inactive or infirm patients may not benefit from
the most sophisticated units. Specialized biventricular
pacemakers have been introduced for the treatment of
severe heart failure.

Permanent pacemakers are inserted under local
anaesthetic using fluoroscopy to guide the insertion of the
electrode leads via the cephalic or subclavian veins.

Perioperative prophylactic antibiotics are routinely
prescribed. The pacemaker is usually positioned subcutaneously in front of the pectoral muscle. Following
surgery, which usually takes 60–90 minutes, the patient
rests in bed for 6–12 hours before being discharged.
Patients may not drive for at least 1 week after implantation, and must inform the licensing authorities and their
motor insurers.

Complications are few but can prove to be very
difficult to manage, and patients should be referred to the
pacemaker clinic. They include the following:

- infection
- erosion
- pocket haematoma
- lead displacement
- electromagnetic interference.

Pericardiocentesis

A pericardial effusion is an accumulation of fluid between
the parietal and visceral layers of pericardium. Fluid is
removed to relieve symptoms that are due to haemodynamic embarrassment or for diagnostic purposes. This
can be a technically difficult procedure, particularly in the
acute setting. In an emergency it can be performed at the
bedside.

Pericardial aspiration or pericardiocentesis is performed
by inserting a needle into the pericardial space, usually
via a subxiphisternal route under ultrasound guidance.
Certain effusions, particularly posterior ones, require
surgical drainage under a general anaesthetic. If a large
volume of fluid is to be removed, a wide-bore needle and
cannula are inserted. The needle may be removed and the
cannula left in situ to drain the fluid. Fluid that is removed
is sent for chemical analysis, microscopy, including
cytology, Gram-stain, and culture. If a reaccumulation of
pericardial fluid is anticipated, the cannula may be left in
place for several days or an operation can be performed
to cut a window in the parietal pericardium (fenestration)
or to remove a large section of the pericardium.

Right-heart bedside catheterization
(Fig. 15.19)

Bedside catheterization of the pulmonary artery with a
pulmonary artery balloon flotation catheter (Swann–
Ganz catheter) is performed in patients with:

- cardiac failure
- cardiogenic shock
- doubtful fluid status.

Intra-aortic balloon pumping

This is a technique used to assist temporarily the failing
left ventricle. A catheter with a long sausage-shaped
balloon at its tip is introduced percutaneously into the
femoral artery and manipulated under X-ray control so
that the balloon lies in the descending aorta just below the

aortic arch. The balloon is rhythmically deflated and inflated with carbon dioxide gas. Using the ECG or intra-aortic pressure changes, the inflation is timed to occur during ventricular diastole to increase diastolic aortic pressure and consequently to improve coronary and cerebral blood flow. During systole the balloon is deflated, resulting in a reduction in the resistance to left ventricular emptying. Intra-aortic balloon pumping is used for circulatory support in the following acute situations:

- *Cardiogenic shock.* Balloon pumping is used to improve cardiac output when there is a transient or reversible depression of left ventricular function, such as in a patient with severe mitral valve regurgitation who is awaiting surgical replacement of the mitral valve, or in a patient with a ventricular septal defect that is due to septal infarction. It may also be used to support patients awaiting heart transplantation.
- *Unstable angina pect*oris. Balloon pumping is used to treat unstable angina pectoris by improving coronary flow and decreasing myocardial oxygen consumption by reducing the 'afterload'. This technique may be successful, even when medical therapy has failed. It is followed by early angiography and appropriate definitive therapy such as surgery or coronary angioplasty.

Balloon pumping should not be used when there is no remediable cause of cardiac dysfunction. It is also unsuitable in patients with severe aortic regurgitation, aortic dissection and severe peripheral vascular disease.

Complications of balloon pumping occur in about 20% of patients and include aortic dissection, leg ischaemia, emboli from the balloon, and balloon rupture. Embolic complications are reduced by anticoagulation with heparin.

FURTHER READING

British Medical Association, Resuscitation Council (UK) and Royal College of Nursing (2001) *Decisions Relating to Cardiopulmonary Resuscitation.* A joint statement from the British Medical Association, Resuscitation Council (UK) and the Royal College of Nursing. London: BMA.

De Latorre F et al. (2001) European Resuscitation Council Guidelines. *Resuscitation* 48: 211–221.

Eisenberg MS, Mengert TJ (2001) Cardiac resuscitation. *New England Journal of Medicine* **344**: 1304–1313.

Lockey AS, Nolan JP (2001) Cardiopulmonary resuscitation in adults. *British Medical Journal* **323**: 819–820.

Resuscitation Council (UK) (2001) *Resuscitation Guidelines 2000.* London: Resuscitation Council (UK).

Email: enquiries[commat]resus.org.uk (website: www.resus.org.uk).

CARDIAC ARRHYTHMIAS

An abnormality of the cardiac rhythm is called a cardiac arrhythmia. Arrhythmias may cause sudden death, syncope, heart failure, dizziness, palpitations or no symptoms at all. There are two main types of arrhythmia:

- bradycardia: the heart rate is slow (< 60 b.p.m.)
- tachycardia: the heart rate is fast (> 100 b.p.m.).

Tachycardias are more symptomatic when the arrhythmia is fast and sustained. Tachycardias are subdivided into supraventricular tachycardias, which arise from the atrium or the atrioventricular junction, and ventricular tachycardias, which arise from the ventricles.

Some arrhythmias occur in patients with apparently normal hearts, and in others arrhythmias originate from scar tissue as a result of underlying structural heart disease. When myocardial function is poor, arrhythmias are more symptomatic and are potentially life-threatening.

SINUS NODE FUNCTION

The normal cardiac pacemaker is the sinus node (p. 725) and, like most cardiac tissue, it depolarizes spontaneously.

The rate of sinus node discharge is modulated by the autonomic nervous system. Normally the parasympathetic system predominates, resulting in slowing of the spontaneous discharge rate from approximately 100 to 70 b.p.m. A reduction of parasympathetic tone or an increase in sympathetic stimulation leads to tachycardia; conversely, increased parasympathetic tone and decreased sympathetic stimulation produces bradycardia. The sinus rate in women is slightly faster than in men. Normal sinus rhythm is characterized by P waves that are upright in leads I, and II of the ECG (Fig. 13.21, p. 746), but inverted in the cavity leads AVR and V1 (Fig. 13.38a).

Sinus arrhythmia

Fluctuations of autonomic tone result in phasic changes of the sinus discharge rate. During inspiration, parasympathetic tone falls and the heart rate quickens, and on expiration the heart rate falls. This variation is normal, particularly in children and young adults. Typically sinus arrhythmia results in a regularly irregular pulse.

Sinus bradycardia

A sinus rate of less than 60 b.p.m. during the day or less than 50 b.p.m. at night is known as sinus bradycardia.

It is usually asymptomatic unless the rate is very slow. It is normal in athletes owing to increased vagal tone. Other causes may be divided into systemic or cardiac and are discussed under Bradycardias and heart block (p. 766).

Sinus tachycardia

Sinus rate acceleration to more than 100 b.p.m. is known as sinus tachycardia. Again, causes may be divided into systemic or cardiac and are discussed under Supraventricular tachycardias (p. 770).

Fig. 13.38 **(a) An ECG showing normal sinus rhythm** (PR interval < 0.2 s). P wave preceding each QRS complex.
(b) A patient with sick sinus syndrome. This shows sinus arrest (only occasional sinus P waves) and junctional escape beats (J). P waves are inverted in the cavity leads that are shown here.

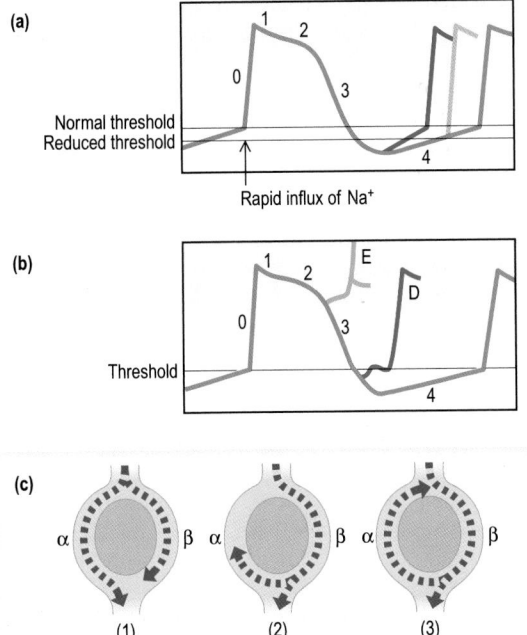

Fig. 13.39 **Mechanisms of arrhythmogenesis.(a) and (b)**
Action potentials (i.e. the potential difference between intracellular and extracellular fluid) of ventricular myocardium after stimulation.
(a) Increased (accelerated) automaticity due to reduced threshold potential or an increased slope of phase 4 depolarization (see p. 744).
(b) Triggered activity due to early (E) or delayed (D) 'after depolarizations' reaching threshold potential.
(c) Mechanism of circus movement or re-entry. In panel (1) the impulse passes down both limbs of the potential tachycardia circuit. In panel (2) the impulse is blocked in one pathway (a) but proceeds slowly down pathway β, returning along pathway α until it collides with refractory tissue. In panel (3) the impulse travels so slowly along pathway β that it can return along pathway α and complete the re-entry circuit, producing a circus movement tachycardia.

Mechanisms of arrhythmia production

Abnormalities of automaticity, which could arise from a single cell, and abnormalities of conduction, which require abnormal interaction between cells, account for both bradycardia and tachycardia. Sinus bradycardia is a result of abnormally slow automaticity while bradycardia due to AV block is caused by abnormal conduction within the AV node or the distal AV conduction system. The mechanisms generating tachycardia are shown in Figure 13.39.

Accelerated automaticity (Fig. 13.39a)

The normal mechanism of spontaneous cardiac rhythmicity is slow depolarization of the transmembrane voltage during diastole until the threshold potential is reached and the action potential of the pacemaker cells takes off. This mechanism may be accelerated by increasing the rate of diastolic depolarization or changing the threshold potential. For example, sympathetic stimulation releases epinephrine (adrenaline), which enhances automaticity. Abnormal automaticity can occur in virtually all cardiac tissues and may initiate arrhythmias. Such changes are thought to produce sinus tachycardia, escape rhythms and accelerated AV nodal (junctional) rhythms.

Triggered activity (Fig. 13.39b)

Myocardial damage can result in oscillations of the transmembrane potential at the end of the action potential. These oscillations, which are called 'after depolarizations', may reach threshold potential and produce an arrhythmia. If they occur before the transmembrane potential reaches its threshold (at the end of phase 3 of the action potential), they are called 'early afterdepolarizations' (E in Fig. 13.39b). When they develop after the transmembrane potential is completed, they are called 'delayed afterdepolarizations' (D in the figure).

The abnormal oscillations can be exaggerated by pacing, catecholamines, electrolyte disturbances, and some medications, which may then trigger arrhythmia. The atrial tachycardias produced by digoxin toxicity are due to triggered activity. The initiation of ventricular arrhythmia in the long QT syndrome (p. 777) may be caused by this mechanism.

Re-entry (or circus movements) (Fig. 13.39c)

The mechanism of re-entry occurs when a 'ring' of cardiac tissue surrounds an inexcitable core (e.g. in a region of scarred myocardium). Tachycardia is initiated if an ectopic beat finds one limb refractory (α) resulting in unidirectional block and the other limb excitable. Provided conduction through the excitable limb (β) is slow enough, the other limb (α) will have recovered and will allow retrograde activation to complete the re-entry loop. If the time to conduct around the ring is longer than the recovery times (refractory periods) of the tissue within the ring, circus movement will be maintained, producing a run of tachycardia. The majority of regular paroxysmal tachycardias are produced by this mechanism.

BRADYCARDIAS AND HEART BLOCK

Bradycardias may be due to failure of impulse formation (sinus bradycardia) or failure of impulse conduction from the atria to the ventricles (atrioventricular block).

Bradycardia

Sinus bradycardia

Sinus bradycardia is due to extrinsic factors influencing a relatively normal sinus node or due to intrinsic sinus node disease. The mechanism can be acute and reversible or chronic and degenerative. Common causes of sinus bradycardia include:

Extrinsic causes

- Hypothermia, hypothyroidism, cholestatic jaundice and raised intracranial pressure.
- Drug therapy with beta-blockers, digitalis and other antiarrhythmic drugs.
- Neurally mediated syndromes (see below).

Intrinsic causes

- Acute ischaemia and infarction of the sinus node (as a complication of acute myocardial infarction).
- Chronic degenerative changes such as fibrosis of the atrium and sinus node (sick sinus syndrome).

Sick sinus syndrome or *sinoatrial disease* is usually caused by idiopathic fibrosis of the sinus node. Other causes of fibrosis such as ischaemic heart disease, cardiomyopathy or myocarditis can also cause the syndrome. Patients develop episodes of sinus bradycardia or sinus arrest (Fig. 13.38b) and commonly, owing to diffuse atrial disease, experience paroxysmal atrial tachyarrhythmias (tachy–brady syndrome).

Neurally mediated syndromes

Neurally mediated syndromes are due to a reflex (called Bezold–Jarisch) that may result in both bradycardia (sinus bradycardia, sinus arrest and AV block) and reflex peripheral vasodilatation. These syndromes usually present as syncope or presyncope (dizzy spells).

Carotid sinus syndrome occurs in the elderly and mainly results in bradycardia. Syncope occurs (see p. 734).

Neurocardiogenic (vasovagal) syncope (syndrome) usually presents in young adults but may present for the first time in elderly patients. It results from a variety of situations (physical and emotional) that affect the autonomic nervous system. The efferent output may be predominantly bradycardic, predominantly vasodilatory or mixed.

Postural orthostatic tachycardia syndrome (POTS) is a sudden and significant increase in heart rate associated with normal or mildly reduced blood pressure produced by standing. The underlying mechanism is a failure of the peripheral vasculature to appropriately constrict in response to orthostatic stress, which is compensated by an excessive increase in heart rate.

Many medications, such as antihypertensives, tricyclic antidepressants, and neuroleptics can be the cause of syncope, particularly in the elderly. Careful dose titration and avoidance of combining two agents with potential to cause syncope help to prevent iatrogenic syncope.

Treatment

The management of sinus bradycardia is first to identify and if possible remove any extrinsic causes. Temporary pacing may be employed in patients with reversible causes until a normal sinus rate is restored and in patients with chronic degenerative conditions until a permanent pacemaker is implanted.

Chronic symptomatic sick sinus syndrome requires permanent pacing (AAI), with additional antiarrhythmic drugs (or ablation therapy) to manage any tachycardia element. Thromboembolism is common in tachy–brady syndrome and patients should be anticoagulated unless there is a contraindication.

Patients with carotid sinus hypersensitivity (asystole > 3 s), especially if symptoms are reproduced by carotid sinus massage, and in whom life-threatening causes of syncope have been excluded, benefit from pacemaker implantation.

Treatment options in neurocardiogenic syndrome include avoidance, if possible, of situations known to cause syncope in a particular patient. Increased salt intake, compression of the lower legs with hose, and drugs such as beta-blockers, alpha-agonists or myocardial negative inotropes (such as disopyramide) may be helpful. In selected patients with 'malignant' neurocardiogenic syncope (syncope associated with injuries) permanent pacemaker therapy is helpful. These patients benefit from dual chamber pacemakers with a feature called 'rate drop response' which, once activated, paces the heart at a fast rate for a set period of time in order to prevent syncope.

Fig. 13.40 An ECG showing first-degree atrioventricular block with a prolonged PR interval. In this trace coincidental ST depression is also present.

Heart block

Heart block or conduction block may occur at any level in the conducting system. Block in either the AV node or the His bundle results in atrioventricular (AV) block, whereas block lower in the conduction system produces bundle branch block.

Atrioventricular block

There are three forms:

First-degree AV block

This is simple prolongation of the PR interval to more than 0.22 s. Every atrial depolarization is followed by conduction to the ventricles but with delay (Fig. 13.40).

Second-degree AV block

This occurs when some P waves conduct and others do not. There are several forms (Fig. 13.41):

- *Mobitz I block* (Wenckebach block phenomenon) is progressive PR interval prolongation until a P wave fails to conduct. The PR interval before the blocked P wave is much longer than the PR interval after the blocked P wave.
- *Mobitz II block* occurs when a dropped QRS complex is not preceded by progressive PR interval prolongation.
- *2 : 1 or 3 : 1 (advanced) block* occurs when every second or third P wave conducts to the ventricles. This form of second-degree block is neither Mobitz I nor II.

Wenckebach AV block in general is due to block in the AV node, whereas Mobitz II block signifies block at an infra-nodal level such as the His bundle. The risk of progression to complete heart block is greater and the reliability of the resultant escape rhythm is less with Mobitz II block. Therefore pacing is usually indicated in Mobitz II block, whereas patients with Wenckebach AV block are usually monitored.

Acute myocardial infarction may produce *second-degree heart block.* In inferior myocardial infarction, close monitoring and transcutaneous temporary back-up pacing are all that is required. In anterior myocardial infarction, second-degree heart block is associated with a high risk of progression to complete heart block, and temporary pacing followed by permanent pacemaker implantation is usually indicated. 2 : 1 Heart block may either be due to block in the AV node or at an infra-nodal level. Management depends on the clinical setting in which it occurs.

(a)

(b)

(c)

Fig. 13.41 Three varieties of second-degree atrioventricular (AV) block.
(a) *Wenckebach (Mobitz type I) AV block.* The PR interval gradually prolongs until the P wave does not conduct to the ventricles (arrow).
(b) *Mobitz type II AV block.* The P waves that do not conduct to the ventricles (arrows) are not preceded by gradual PR interval prolongation.
(c) *Two P waves to each QRS complex.* The PR interval prior to the dropped P wave is always the same. It is not possible to define this type of AV block as type I or type II Mobitz block and it is, therefore, a third variety of second-degree AV block (arrows show P waves).

(a)

(b)

Fig. 13.42 **Two examples of complete heart block.**
(a) Congenital complete heart block. The QRS complex is narrow (0.08 s) and the QRS rate is relatively rapid (52 b.p.m.).
(b) Acquired complete heart block. The QRS complex is broad (0.13 s) and the QRS rate is relatively slow (38 b.p.m.).

Third-degree (complete) AV block

Complete heart block occurs when all atrial activity fails to conduct to the ventricles (Fig. 13.42). In patients with complete heart block the aetiology needs to be established (Table 13.8). In this situation life is maintained by a spontaneous escape rhythm.

Narrow complex escape rhythm (< 0.125 QRS complex), implies that it originates in the His bundle and therefore that the region of block lies more proximally in the AV node. The escape rhythm occurs with an adequate rate (50–60 b.p.m.) and is relatively reliable.

Treatment depends on the aetiology. Recent-onset narrow-complex AV block due to transient causes may respond to intravenous atropine, but temporary pacing facilities should be available for the management of these patients. Chronic narrow-complex AV block requires permanent pacing (dual chamber, p. 762) if it is symptomatic or associated with heart disease. Pacing is also advocated for isolated, congenital AV block, even if asymptomatic.

Broad complex escape rhythm (> 0.125) implies that the escape rhythm originates below the His bundle and therefore that the region of block lies more distally in the His–Purkinje system.

The resulting rhythm is slow (15–40 b.p.m.) and relatively unreliable. Dizziness and blackouts (Stokes–Adams attacks) often occur. In the elderly, it is usually caused by degenerative fibrosis and calcification of the distal conduction system (Lev's disease). In younger individuals, a proximal progressive cardiac conduction disease due to the inflammatory process is known as Lenegre's syndrome. Sodium channel abnormalities have recently been identified in both syndromes. Broad-complex AV block may also be caused by ischaemic heart disease, myocarditis or cardiomyopathy. Temporary pacing followed by permanent pacemaker implantation (p. 762) is indicated, as pacing considerably reduces the mortality. Because ventricular arrhythmias are not uncommon, an implantable cardioverter–defibrillator (ICD) may be indicated.

Bundle branch block

The His bundle gives rise to the right and left bundle branches. The left bundle subdivides into the anterior and posterior divisions of the left bundle. Various conduction disturbances can occur.

Bundle branch conduction delay. This produces trivial widening of the QRS complex (up to 0.11 s). It is known as incomplete bundle branch block.

Table 13.8 Aetiology of complete heart block	
Congenital Autoimmune (e.g. maternal SLE) Structural heart disease (e.g. transposition of the great vessels)	**Cardiac surgery** e.g. following aortic valve replacement, CABS, VSD repair
Idiopathic fibrosis Lev's disease (progressive fibrosis of distal His–Purkinje system in elderly patients) Lenegre's disease (proximal His–Purkinje fibrosis in younger patients)	**Iatrogenic** Radiofrequency AV node ablation and pacemaker implantation **Drug-induced** e.g. digoxin, amiodarone
Ischaemic heart disease Acute myocardial infarct Ischaemic cardiomyopathy	**Infections** Endocarditis Lyme disease Chagas' disease **Connective tissue diseases** e.g. SLE, rheumatoid arthritis
Non-ischaemic heart disease Calcific aortic stenosis Idiopathic dilated cardiomyopathy Infiltrations (e.g. amyloidosis, sarcoidosis, neoplasia)	**Neuromuscular diseases** e.g. Duchenne muscular dystrophy

SLE, systemic lupus erythematosus; CABS, coronary artery bypass surgery; VSD, ventricular septal defect; AV, atrioventricular

Fig. 13.43 **Right bundle branch block versus bifascicular block. (a)** A 12-lead ECG showing right bundle branch block. Note an rsR pattern with the tall R in lead V_1–V_2 and the broad S waves in leads I and V_5–V_6. **(b)** Compare with an ECG showing bifascicular block. In addition to right bundle branch block, note left axis deviation and deep S waves in leads III and AVF typical for left anterior hemiblock.

Complete block of a bundle branch. This is associated with a wider QRS complex (0.12 s or more). The shape of the QRS depends on whether the right or the left bundle is blocked.

Right bundle branch block (Fig. 13.43a) produces late activation of the right ventricle. This is seen as deep S waves in leads I and V_6 and as a tall late R wave in lead V_1 (late activation moving towards right- and away from left-sided leads).

Left bundle branch block (Fig. 13.44) produces the opposite – a deep S wave in lead V_1 and a tall late R wave in leads I and V_6. Because left bundle branch conduction is normally responsible for the initial ventricular activation, left bundle branch block also produces abnormal Q waves.

Hemiblock. Delay or block in the divisions of the left bundle branch produces a swing in the direction of depolarization (electrical axis) of the heart. When the anterior division is blocked (left anterior hemiblock), the left ventricle is activated from inferior to superior. This produces a superior and leftwards movement of the axis (left axis deviation). Delay or block in the postero-inferior division swings the QRS axis inferiorly to the right (right axis deviation).

Bifascicular block (Fig. 13.43b). This is a combination of a block of any two of the following: the right bundle branch, the left antero-superior division and the left postero-inferior division. Block of the remaining fascicle will result in complete AV block.

Clinical features

Bundle branch blocks are usually asymptomatic. Right bundle branch block causes wide but physiological splitting of the second heart sound. Left bundle branch block may cause reverse splitting of the second sound. Patients with intraventricular conduction disturbances may complain of syncope. This is due to intermittent complete heart block or to ventricular tachyarrhythmias. ECG monitoring and electrophysiological studies are needed to determine the cause of syncope in these patients.

Causes

Right bundle branch block occurs as an isolated congenital anomaly or is associated with cardiac or pulmonary conditions (Table 13.9). Right bundle branch block alone does not alter the electrical axis of the heart.

Fig. 13.44 **A 12-lead ECG showing left bundle branch block.** The QRS duration is greater than 0.12 s. Note the broad notched R waves with ST depression in leads I, AVL, and V_6, and the broad QS waves in V_1–V_3.

Table 13.9 Causes of right bundle branch block

It is also a normal finding in 1% of young adults and 5% of elderly adults

Congenital heart disease	Myocardial disease
Atrial septal defect	Acute myocardial infarction
Fallot's tetralogy	Cardiomyopathy
Pulmonary stenosis	Conduction system fibrosis
Ventricular septal defect	

Pulmonary disease
Cor pulmonale
Recurrent pulmonary embolism
Acute pulmonary embolism (transient)

Table 13.10 Causes of left bundle branch block

Left ventricular outflow obstruction	Coronary artery disease
Aortic stenosis	Acute myocardial infarction
Hypertension	Severe coronary disease (two- to three-vessel disease)

Axis deviations signify right ventricular hypertrophy (RV overload) or coexistent fascicular block. The combination of right bundle branch block with left axis deviation is associated with ostium primum atrial septal defects. Complete left bundle branch block is often associated with extensive left ventricular disease. The most common causes are listed in Table 13.10 and are similar to those of complete heart block.

SUPRAVENTRICULAR TACHYCARDIAS

Supraventricular tachycardias (SVTs) arise from the atrium or the atrioventricular junction. Conduction is via the His–Purkinje system; therefore the QRS shape during tachycardia is usually similar to that seen in the same patient during baseline rhythm. A classification of supraventricular tachycardia is listed in Table 13.11. Some of these are discussed in more detail below.

Inappropriate sinus tachycardia

Inappropriate sinus tachycardia is a persistent increase in resting heart rate unrelated to or out of proportion with the level of physical or emotional stress. It is found predominantly in women and is not uncommon in health professionals. Sinus tachycardia due to intrinsic sinus node abnormalities such as enhanced automaticity, or abnormal autonomic regulation of the heart with excess sympathetic and reduced parasympathetic input, is extremely rare.

In general, sinus tachycardia is a secondary phenomenon and the underlying causes need to be actively investigated. Depending on the clinical setting, acute causes include exercise, emotion, pain, fever, infection, acute heart failure, acute pulmonary embolism and hypovolaemia. Chronic causes include pregnancy, anaemia, hyperthyroidism and catecholamine excess. The underlying cause should be found and treated, rather than treating the compensatory physiological response. If necessary, beta-blockers may be used to slow the sinus rate, e.g. in hyperthyroidism (p. 1073).

Atrioventricular junctional tachycardias

AV nodal re-entry and AV re-entry tachycardias are usually referred to as paroxysmal SVTs and are often seen in young patients with no or little structural heart disease, although congenital heart abnormalities (e.g. Ebstein's anomaly, atrial septal defect, Fallot's tetralogy) can coexist in a small proportion of patients with these arrhythmias. The first presentation is common between ages 12 and 30, and the prevalence is approximately 2.5 per 1000.

In these tachycardias the AV node is an essential component of the re-entry circuit.

Atrioventricular nodal re-entry tachycardia (AVNRT)

This tachycardia is twice as common in women. Clinically, the tachycardia often strikes suddenly without

Table 13.11 Causes of supraventricular tachycardia (SVT)

Tachycardia	ECG features	Comment
Sinus tachycardia	P wave morphology similar to sinus rhythm	Need to determine underlying cause
AV nodal re-entry tachycardia (AVNRT)	No visible P wave, or inverted P wave immediately before or after QRS complex	Commonest cause of palpitations in patients with normal hearts
AV reciprocating tachycardia (AVRT)	P wave visible between QRS and T wave complexes	Due to an accessory pathway. If pathway conducts in both directions, ECG during sinus rhythm may be pre-excited
Atrial fibrillation	Irregularly irregular RR intervals and absence of organized atrial activity	Commonest tachycardia in patients over 65 years
Atrial flutter	Visible flutter waves at 300/min (saw-tooth appearance) usually with 2 : 1 AV conduction	Suspect in any patient with regular SVT at 150/min
Atrial tachycardia	Organized atrial activity with P wave morphology different from sinus rhythm	Usually occurs in patients with structural heart disease
Multifocal atrial tachycardia	Multiple P wave morphologies ($\geq$ 3) and irregular RR intervals	Rare arrhythmia; most commonly associated with significant chronic lung disease
Accelerated junctional tachycardia	ECG similar to AVNRT	Rare in adults

obvious provocation, but exertion, coffee, tea and alcohol may aggravate or induce the arrhythmia. An attack may stop spontaneously or may continue indefinitely until medical intervention.

In AVNRT, there are two functionally and anatomically different pathways within the AV node: one is characterized by a short effective refractory period and slow conduction, and the other has a longer effective refractory period and conducts faster. In sinus rhythm, the atrial impulse that depolarizes the ventricles usually conducts through the fast pathway. If the atrial impulse (e.g. an atrial premature beat) occurs early when the fast pathway is still refractory, the slow pathway takes over in propagating the atrial impulse to the ventricles. It then travels back through the fast pathway which has already recovered its excitability, thus initiating the most common 'slow–fast', or typical, AVNRT.

The rhythm is recognized on ECG by normal regular QRS complexes, usually at a rate of 140–240 per minute (Fig. 13.45a). Sometimes the QRS complexes will show typical bundle branch block. P waves are either not visible or are seen immediately before or after the QRS complex because of simultaneous atrial and ventricular activation. Less commonly observed (5–10%) is tachycardia when the atrial impulse conducts anterogradely through the fast pathway and returns through the slow pathway, producing a long RP' interval ('fast–slow', or long RP' tachycardia).

Atrioventricular reciprocating tachycardia (AVRT)

In AVRT there is a large circuit comprising the AV node, the His bundle, the ventricle and an abnormal connection from the ventricle back to the atrium. This abnormal connection consists of myocardial fibres that span the atrioventricular groove; it is called an accessory pathway or bypass tract. Bypass tracts result from incomplete separation of the atria and the ventricles during fetal development.

In contrast to AVNRT, this tachycardia is due to a macro-reentry circuit and each part of the circuit is activated sequentially. As a result atrial activation occurs after ventricular activation and the P wave is usually clearly seen between the QRS and T complexes (Fig. 13.45b).

Accessory pathways are most commonly situated on the left but may occur anywhere around the AV groove. The most common accessory pathways known as *Kent bundles* are in the free wall or septum. In about 10% of cases multiple pathways occur. *Mahaim fibres* are atrio-fascicular or nodo-fascicular fibres entering the ventricular myocardium in the region of the right bundle branch. Accessory pathways that conduct from the ventricles to the atria only are not visible on the surface ECG during sinus rhythm and are therefore 'concealed'. Accessory pathways that conduct bidirectionally usually are manifest on the surface ECG. If the accessory pathway conducts from the atrium to the ventricle during sinus rhythm, the electrical impulse can conduct quickly over this abnormal connection to depolarize part of the

Fig. 13.45 **Atrioventricular junctional tachycardia.**
(a) Atrioventricular *nodal re-entry* tachycardia. The QRS complexes are narrow and the P waves cannot be seen.
(b) *Atrioventricular re-entry* tachycardia (Wolff–Parkinson–White syndrome). The tachycardia P waves are clearly seen after narrow QRS complexes.
(c) An electrocardiogram taken in a patient with Wolff–Parkinson–White syndrome during sinus rhythm. Note the short PR interval and the δ wave (arrow).
(d) Atrial fibrillation in the Wolff–Parkinson–White syndrome. Note tachycardia with broad QRS complexes with fast and irregular ventricular rate.

ventricles abnormally (pre-excitation). A pre-excited ECG is characterized by a short PR interval and a wide QRS complex that begins as a slurred part known as the δ wave (Fig. 13.45c). Patients with a history of palpitations and a pre-excited ECG have a syndrome known as Wolff–Parkinson–White (WPW) syndrome.

During AVRT the AV node and ventricles are activated normally (orthodromically), resulting usually in a narrow QRS complex. Less commonly, the tachycardia circuit can be reversed, with activation of the ventricles via the accessory pathway and atrial activation via retrograde conduction through the AV node (antidromic AVRT). This results in a broad complex tachycardia. These patients are also prone to atrial fibrillation.

During atrial fibrillation, the ventricles may be depolarized by impulses travelling over both the abnormal and the normal pathways. This results in pre-excited atrial fibrillation, a characteristic tachycardia that is characterized by irregularly irregular broad QRS complexes (Fig. 13.45d). If an accessory pathway has a short antegrade effective refractory period (< 250 ms), it may conduct to the ventricles at an extremely high rate and may cause ventricular fibrillation. The incidence of sudden death is 0.15–0.39% per patient-year and it may be a first manifestation of the disease in younger individuals. Verapamil and digoxin may allow a higher rate of conduction over the abnormal pathway and precipitate ventricular fibrillation. Therefore, neither verapamil nor digoxin should be used to treat atrial fibrillation associated with the WPW syndrome.

Symptoms

The leading symptom of most SVTs, in particular AV node re-entry and AV re-entry tachycardias, is rapid regular palpitations, usually with abrupt onset, which can occur spontaneously or be precipitated by simple movements. A common feature is termination by Valsalva manoeuvres. In younger individuals with no structural heart disease, the rapid heart rate can be the main pathological finding.

Irregular palpitations may be due to atrial premature beats, atrial flutter with varying AV conduction block, atrial fibrillation or multifocal atrial tachycardia. In patients with depressed ventricular function, uncontrolled atrial fibrillation can reduce cardiac output and cause hypotension and congestive heart failure.

Other symptoms may include anxiety, dizziness, dyspnoea, neck pulsation, central chest pain, and weakness. Polyuria may occur because of release of atrial natriuretic peptide in response to increased atrial pressures during the tachycardia. Prominent jugular venous pulsations due to atrial contractions against closed atrioventricular valves may be observed during AVNRT or AVRT.

Syncope has been reported in 10–15% patients, usually just after initiation of the arrhythmia or in association with a prolonged pause following its termination. However, in older patients with concomitant heart disease, such as aortic stenosis, hypertrophic cardiomyopathy, and cerebrovascular disease, significant hypotension and syncope may result from moderately fast ventricular rates.

Acute management

In emergency, distinguishing between AVNRT and AVRT may be difficult, but it is usually not critical as both tachycardias respond to the same treatment. Patients presenting with SVTs and haemodynamic instability (e.g. hypotension, pulmonary oedema) require emergency cardioversion. If the patient is haemodynamically stable, vagal manoeuvres, including right carotid massage (Practical box 13.4), Valsalva manoeuvre (Practical box 13.5) and facial immersion in cold water can be successfully employed.

Practical Box 13.4
Carotid sinus massage

- Ensure there is no significant carotid artery disease (carotid bruits).
- Provide continuous electrocardiographic monitoring.
- Patient is in supine position with the head slightly extended.
- Start with right carotid sinus massage.
- Apply firm rotary pressure to the carotid artery at the level of the third cervical vertebra for 5 seconds.
- Alternatively, steady pressure can be applied. If no response, massage left carotid sinus.
- Generally, right carotid sinus massage decreases the sinus node discharge, and left carotid sinus massage slows atrioventricular conduction.
- Do not massage both carotid sinuses at the same time.
- Single application of carotid sinus pressure may be effective in about 20–30% of patients with paroxysmal supraventricular tachycardias; multiple applications can terminate tachycardia in about 50% of patients.
- Asystole is a potential but rare complication.

Practical Box 13.5
Valsalva manoeuvre

- Valsalva manoeuvre is an abrupt voluntary increase in intrathoracic and intra-abdominal pressures by straining.
- Provide continuous electrocardiographic monitoring.
- Patient is in supine position.
- Patient should not take deep inspiration before straining.
- Ideally, the patient blows into the mouthpiece of a manometer against a pressure of 30–40 mmHg for 15 seconds.
- Alternatively, the patient strains for 15 seconds while breath-holding.
- Transient acceleration of tachycardia usually occurs during the strain phase as a result of sympathetic excess.
- On release of strain, the rate of tachycardia slows because of the compensatory increase in vagal tone (baroreceptor reflex) and it may be terminated in about 50% of patients.
- Termination of tachycardia may be followed by pauses and transient ventricular ectopics.

Of these techniques, the Valsalva manoeuvre is the best and often easier for the patient to perform successfully. It should be undertaken when the patient is resting in the supine position (thus avoiding elevated background sympathetic tone). Several seconds after the release of strain, the resulting intense vagal effect may terminate AVNRT or AVRT or may produce sufficient AV block to reveal an underlying atrial tachyarrhythmia.

If physical manoeuvres have not been successful, intravenous adenosine (up to 0.25 mg/kg) should be tried. This is a very short-acting (half-life < 10 s) naturally occurring purine nucleoside that causes complete heart block for a fraction of a second following i.v. administration. It is highly effective at terminating AVNRT and AVRT or unmasking underlying atrial activity. It rarely affects ventricular tachycardia. The side-effects of adenosine are very brief but include:

- bronchospasm
- flushing
- chest pain
- heaviness of the limbs.

It is contraindicated in patients with a history of asthma. In some patients, adenosine can induce atrial fibrillation.

An alternative treatment is verapamil 5–10 mg i.v. over 5–10 minutes, i.v. diltiazem, or beta-blockers (esmolol, propranolol, metoprolol). Verapamil (or diltiazem) must not be given after beta-blockers *or* if the tachycardia presents with broad (> 0.12 s) QRS complexes.

Long-term management

Patients with suspected cardiac arrhythmias should always be referred to the cardiologist for electro-physiological evaluation and long-term management, as both pharmacological and non-pharmacological alter-natives, including ablation of an accessory pathway, are readily available. Verapamil, diltiazem, and beta-blockers have proven effective in 60–80% of patients. Sodium-channel blockers (flecainide and propafenone), potassium repolarization current blockers (sotalol, dofetilide, azimilide), and the multichannel blocker amiodarone may also prevent the occurrence of tachycardia.

Refinement of catheter ablation techniques has rendered many AV junctional tachycardias entirely curable. Modification of the slow pathway is successful in 96% of patients with AVNRT, although a 1% risk of AV block is present. In AVRT, the target for catheter ablation is the accessory pathway(s). The success rate for ablation of a single accessory pathway is approximately 95%, with a recurrence rate of 5%, requiring a repeat procedure.

Atrial tachyarrhythmias

Atrial tachyarrhythmias including atrial fibrillation, atrial flutter, atrial tachycardia and atrial ectopic beats all arise from the atrial myocardium. They share common aetiologies, which are listed in Table 13.12.

Atrial fibrillation

This is a common arrhythmia, occurring in 5–10% of patients over 65 years of age. It also occurs, particularly in a paroxysmal form, in younger patients. Any condition resulting in raised atrial pressure, increased atrial muscle mass, atrial fibrosis, or inflammation and infiltration of the atrium, may cause atrial fibrillation. There are also many systemic causes of atrial fibrillation (Table 13.12).

Hypertension and heart failure are most often associ-ated with non-rheumatic atrial fibrillation. Hyper-thyroidism may provoke atrial fibrillation, sometimes as virtually the only feature of the disease, and thyroid function tests are mandatory in any patient with unaccounted atrial fibrillation. Atrial fibrillation occurs in one-third of patients after coronary bypass surgery and in

Table 13.12 Causes of atrial tachyarrhythmias

Cardiac	Non-cardiac
Hypertension	Thyrotoxicosis
Congestive heart failure	Phaeochromocytoma
Coronary artery disease and myocardial infarction	Acute and chronic pulmonary disease (pneumonia, chronic obstructive pulmonary disease)
Valvular heart disease	
Cardiomyopathy: dilated, hypertrophic	Pulmonary vascular disease (pulmonary embolism)
Myocarditis and pericarditis	
Wolff–Parkinson–White syndrome	Electrolyte disturbances (hypokalaemia)
Sick sinus syndrome	Increased sympathetic tone (exercise, adrenergically mediated arrhythmia)
Cardiac tumours	
Cardiac surgery	
Familial tachyarrhythmia (e.g. lone atrial fibrillation)	Increased parasympathetic tone (vagally induced and postprandial arrhythmia)
	Alcohol abuse ('holiday heart' and long-term use)
	Caffeine, smoking, recreational drug use

more than half of those undergoing valvular surgery. It usually manifests during the first 4 days and is associated with increased morbidity and mortality, largely due to stroke and circulatory failure, and longer hospital stay.

In some patients no cause can be found, and this group are labelled as 'lone' atrial fibrillation. The pathogenesis of 'lone', or 'idiopathic', atrial fibrillation is unknown but genetic predisposition or even specific genetically pre-determined forms of the arrhythmia have been proposed. Recently, a gene defect linked to chromosome 10q22–q24 has been identified in three Catalonian families, half the members of which presented with atrial fibrillation at a relatively young age. The mutated genes responsible for atrial fibrillation have been mapped to other chromosomes but have not yet been identified.

Atrial fibrillation is maintained by continuous, rapid (300–600 per minute) activation of the atria by multiple meandering re-entry wavelets, often driven by rapidly depolarizing automatic foci. The atria respond electrically at this rate but there is no coordinated mechanical action and only a proportion of the impulses are conducted to the ventricles. The ventricular response depends on the rate and regularity of atrial activity, particularly at the entry to the AV node, the refractory properties of the AV node itself, and the balance between sympathetic and parasympathetic tone.

Symptoms and signs

Symptoms attributable to atrial fibrillation are highly variable. In some patients (about 30%) it is an incidental finding, whilst others attend hospital as an emergency following the onset of atrial fibrillation. Most patients experience some deterioration of exercise capacity or well-being, but this may only be appreciated once sinus rhythm is restored. When caused by rheumatic mitral stenosis, the onset of atrial fibrillation results in con-siderable worsening of cardiac failure.

The patient has a very irregular pulse, as opposed to a basically regular pulse with an occasional irregularity (e.g. extrasystoles) or recurring irregular patterns (e.g. Wenckebach block). The irregular nature of the pulse in atrial fibrillation is maintained during exercise.

The ECG shows fine oscillations of the baseline (so-called fibrillation or f waves) and no clear P waves. The QRS rhythm is rapid and irregular. Untreated, the ventricular rate is usually 120–180 per minute, but it slows with treatment.

The clinical classification of atrial fibrillation includes first detected, paroxysmal, persistent, and permanent forms of the arrhythmia and is essential for the decision-making between rhythm restoration and rate control. For example, atrial fibrillation may be asymptomatic and the 'first detected episode' should not be regarded as necessarily the true onset.

Management

When atrial fibrillation is due to an acute precipitating event such as alcohol toxicity, chest infection or hyperthyroidism, the provoking cause should be treated. Strategies for the acute management of AF are ventricular rate control or cardioversion (± anticoagulation). Ventricular rate control is achieved by drugs which block the AV node (see below), while the cardioversion is achieved electrically by DC shock (p. 761) or medically either by intravenous infusion of an anti-arrhythmic drug such as a class Ic or a class III agent or by taking an oral agent previously tested in hospital and found to be safe in a particular patient ('pill-in-pocket' approach).

The choice depends upon:

- how well the arrhythmia is tolerated (is cardioversion urgent?)
- whether anticoagulation is required before considering elective cardioversion
- whether spontaneous cardioversion is likely (previous history? reversible cause?).

Conversion to sinus rhythm can be achieved by electrical DC cardioversion 200 J, then 2 × 360 J (p. 761) in about 80% of patients. Biphasic waveform defibrillation is more effective than conventional (monophasic) defibrillation, and biphasic defibrillators are becoming available. In some cases, internal transvenous low-energy (4 J) cardioversion is capable of restoring sinus rhythm where conventional transthoracic cardioversion has failed. Patients are anticoagulated with warfarin for 4 weeks before cardioversion. Anticoagulants are used to minimize the risk of thromboembolism associated with cardioversion unless atrial fibrillation is of less than 1–2 days' duration. Transoesophageal echocardiography is being used to document the presence or absence of atrial thrombus as a guide to the necessity for long-term anticoagulation.

Two strategies are available for the long-term management of atrial fibrillation:

- 'rhythm control' (antiarrhythmic drugs plus DC cardioversion *plus warfarin*)
- 'rate control' (AV nodal slowing agents *plus warfarin*).

(a)

(b)

(c)

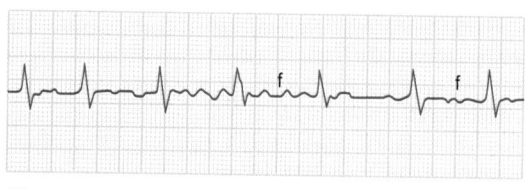

(d)

Fig. 13.46 ECGs of a variety of atrial arrhythmias.
(a) Atrial premature beats (arrows). The premature P wave is different from the sinus P wave and conducts to the ventricle with a slightly prolonged PR interval.
(b) Atrial tachycardia with second-degree atrioventricular block. Note the fast atrial (P wave) rate of 150/min and the slower ventricular (R wave) rate of 75/min.
(c) Atrial flutter. Some flutter waves are marked with an F. In this case the flutter frequency is 240/min. Every fourth flutter wave is transmitted to the ventricles and the ventricular rate is therefore 60/min.
(d) Atrial fibrillation. Note absolute rhythm irregularity and baseline undulations (f waves).

Which strategy to adopt needs to be assessed for each individual patient. Factors to consider include the likelihood of maintaining sinus rhythm and the safety/tolerability of antiarrhythmic drugs in a particular patient. Recurrent paroxysms may be prevented by oral medication. In general, class Ic agents are employed in patients with no significant heart disease and class III agents are preferred in patients with significant structural heart disease.

Rate control as a primary strategy may be appropriate in patients who:

- have the permanent form of the arrhythmia associated with mild symptoms which can be further improved by slowing heart rate

- are older than 65 years with recurrent atrial tachyarrhythmias (primary 'accepted' atrial fibrillation)
- have persistent tachyarrhythmias and have failed cardioversion(s) and serial prophylactic antiarrhythmic drug therapy and in whom the risk/benefit ratio from using specific antiarrhythmic agents is shifted towards increased risk
- do not have heart failure or left ventricular dysfunction that can be improved by restoring sinus rhythm.

Rate control is usually achieved by a combination of *digoxin, beta-blockers* or *calcium-channel blockers* (*verapamil* or *diltiazem*). The ventricular rate response is generally considered controlled if the heart rate is between 60 and 80 beats per minute at rest and 90 and 115 beats per minute during moderate exercise. To assess the adequacy of rate control, an ECG rhythm strip may be sufficient in an elderly patient but ambulatory 24-hour Holter monitoring and an exercise stress test (treadmill) are needed in younger individuals. Patients with poor rate control despite optimal medical therapy should be considered for AV node ablation and pacemaker implantation (*'ablate and pace' strategy*). These patients usually experience a marked symptomatic improvement but because of the ongoing risk of thromboembolism require life-long *anticoagulation*.

Anticoagulation (target INR 2.0–3.0)

This is indicated in patients with atrial fibrillation and one of the following major or two of the moderate risk factors:

Major risk factors

- Prosthetic heart valve
- Rheumatic mitral valve disease
- Prior history of CVA/TIA
- Age > 75 years
- Hypertension
- Coronary artery disease with poor LV function.

Moderate risk factors

- Age 65–75 years
- Coronary artery disease but normal LV function
- Diabetes mellitus.

In addition, other features, e.g. left atrial enlargement, LV dysfunction of any cause, evidence of atrial thrombus or a reduced atrial appendage emptying velocity, also encourage anticoagulation with warfarin.

In most other patients, aspirin is prescribed. Young patients (< 65 years) with no heart disease (lone atrial fibrillation) usually require no thromboembolic prophylaxis but should be treated with *aspirin* 300 mg. A new oral anticoagulant, ximelagatran, which is effective and easier to use, is currently under trials.

Younger patients with lone paroxysmal atrial fibrillation should be carefully assessed to rule out a single atrial ectopic focus triggering atrial fibrillation. Such foci are usually located in the pulmonary veins. This form of atrial fibrillation can be effectively cured by catheter ablation (*pulmonary vein isolation*).

Atrial flutter

Atrial flutter is often associated with atrial fibrillation and often shares clinical presentation requiring a similar initial therapeutic approach. Atrial flutter is usually an organized atrial rhythm with an atrial rate typically between 250 and 350 beats per minute. Typical, or isthmus-dependent, atrial flutter involves a macro re-entrant right atrial circuit around the tricuspid annulus. The wavefront circulates down the lateral wall of the right atrium, through the Eustachian ridge between the tricuspid annulus and the inferior vena cava, and up the inter-atrial septum, giving rise to the most frequent pattern, referred to as counterclockwise flutter. Re-entry can also occur in the opposite direction (clockwise or reverse flutter).

The ECG shows regular sawtooth-like atrial flutter waves (F waves) between QRS complexes (Fig. 13.46c). In typical counterclockwise atrial flutter, the F waves are negative in the inferior leads and positive in leads V_1 and V_2. In clockwise atrial flutter, the deflection of the F waves is the opposite. If F waves are not clearly visible, it is worth accentuating them by slowing AV conduction by carotid sinus massage or by the administration of AV nodal blocking drugs such as adenosine or verapamil.

Symptoms are largely related to the degree of AV block. Most often, every second flutter beat conducts, giving a ventricular rate of 150 b.p.m.. Occasionally, every beat conducts, producing a heart rate of 300 b.p.m. More often, especially when patients are receiving treatment, AV conduction block reduces the heart rate to approximately 75 b.p.m.

Management

Treatment of a symptomatic acute paroxysm is electrical *cardioversion*. Patients who have been in atrial flutter more than 1–2 days should be treated in a similar manner to patients with atrial fibrillation and *anticoagulated* for 4 weeks prior to cardioversion.

Recurrent paroxysms may be prevented by oral medication. In general, *class Ic* agents are employed in patients with no significant heart disease and *class III* agents are preferred in patients with significant structural heart disease. *AV nodal blocking agents* may be used to control the ventricular rate if the arrhythmia persists. However, the treatment of choice for patients with recurrent atrial flutter is radiofrequency catheter *ablation* (p. 782). This technique offers patients whose only arrhythmia is typical atrial flutter an almost certain chance of a cure.

Atrial tachycardia

This is an uncommon arrhythmia. Its prevalence is believed to be less than 1% in patients with arrhythmias It is usually associated with structural heart disease but in many cases it is referred to as idiopathic. Macro re-entrant tachycardia often occurs after surgery for congenital heart disease Atrial tachycardia with block is often a result of digitalis poisoning.

The mechanisms of atrial tachycardia are attributed to enhanced automaticity, triggered activity or intra-atrial re-entry. Atrial re-entry tachycardia is usually relatively slow (125–150 b.p.m.) and can be initiated and terminated by atrial premature beats. The P'P' intervals are regular. The PR interval depends on the rate of tachycardia and is longer than in sinus rhythm at the same rate.

Automatic tachycardia usually presents with higher rates (125–250 b.p.m.) and is often characterized by a progressive increase in the atrial rate with onset of the tachycardia ('warm-up') and progressive decrease prior to termination ('cool-down'). Atrial tachycardia is typically caused by a focus which is frequently located along the crista terminalis in the right atrium, adjacent to a pulmonary vein in the left atrium, or around one of the atrial appendages. Automatic atrial tachycardia may also present as an incessant variety leading to tachycardia-induced cardiomyopathy.

Figure 13.46b demonstrates an atrial tachycardia at an atrial rate of 150 per minute. The P waves are abnormally shaped and occur in front of the QRS complexes. Carotid sinus massage may increase AV block during tachycardia, thereby facilitating the diagnosis, but does not usually terminate the arrhythmia. Treatment options include *cardioversion, antiarrhythmic drug therapy* to maintain sinus rhythm, *AV nodal slowing agents* to control rate and, in selected cases, radiofrequency catheter *ablation*.

Atrial ectopic beats

These often cause no symptoms, although they may be sensed as an irregularity or heaviness of the heartbeat. On the ECG they appear as early and abnormal P waves, and are usually, but not always, followed by normal QRS complexes (Fig. 13.46a). Treatment is not normally required unless the ectopic beats provoke more significant arrhythmias, when *beta-blockers* may be effective.

VENTRICULAR TACHYARRHYTHMIAS

Ventricular tachyarrhythmias can be considered under the following headings:

- life-threatening ventricular tachyarrhythmias
- torsades de pointes
- normal heart ventricular tachycardia
- non-sustained ventricular tachycardia
- ventricular premature beats

Life-threatening ventricular tachyarrhythmias

Sustained ventricular tachycardia and ventricular fibrillation with haemodynamic instability (e.g. syncope, hypotension) are life-threatening ventricular tachyarrhythmias.

Sustained ventricular tachycardia

Sustained ventricular tachycardia (> 30 s) often results in *presyncope* (dizziness), *syncope, hypotension* and *cardiac arrest*, although it may be remarkably well tolerated in some patients. Examination reveals a pulse rate typically between 120 and 220 b.p.m. Usually there are clinical signs of atrioventricular dissociation (i.e. intermittent cannon 'a' waves in the neck, p. 738) and variable intensity of the first heart sound).

Table 13.13 ECG distinction between supraventricular tachycardia (SVT) with bundle branch block and ventricular tachycardia (VT)

VT is more likely than SVT with bundle branch block where there is:

- a very broad QRS (> 0.14 s)
- atrioventricular dissociation
- a bifid, upright QRS with a taller first peak in V_1
- a deep S wave in V_6
- a concordant (same polarity) QRS direction in all chest leads (V_1–V_6)

The ECG shows a rapid ventricular rhythm with broad (often 0.14 s or more), abnormal QRS complexes. AV dissociation may result in visible P waves which appear to march through the tachycardia, capture beats (intermittent narrow QRS complex owing to normal ventricular activation via the AV node and conducting system) and fusion beats (intermediate between ventricular tachycardia beat and capture beat).

Supraventricular tachycardia with bundle branch block may resemble ventricular tachycardia on the ECG. However, if a broad complex tachycardia is due to SVT with either right or left bundle branch block, then the QRS morphology should resemble a typical RBBB or LBBB pattern (Figs 13.43 and 13.44). Other ECG criteria to differentiate VT from SVT with aberrancy are indicated in Table 13.13. Eighty per cent of all broad complex tachycardias are due to ventricular tachycardia, and the proportion is even higher in patients with structural heart disease. Therefore, in all cases of doubt, ventricular tachycardia should be diagnosed.

Treatment may be urgent, depending on the haemodynamic situation. If the patient is haemodynamically compromised (e.g. hypotensive or pulmonary oedema) emergency DC cardioversion may be required. On the other hand, if the blood pressure and cardiac output are well maintained, intravenous therapy with class I drugs or amiodarone is usually used. First-line drug treatment consists of lidocaine (50–100 mg i.v. over 5 minutes) followed by a lidocaine infusion (2–4 mg i.v. per minute). DC cardioversion is necessary if medical therapy is unsuccessful.

Ventricular fibrillation

This is very rapid and irregular ventricular activation with no mechanical effect. The patient is pulseless and becomes rapidly unconscious, and respiration ceases (cardiac arrest). The ECG shows shapeless, rapid oscillations and there is no hint of organized complexes (Fig. 13.47). It is usually provoked by a ventricular ectopic beat. Ventricular fibrillation rarely reverses spontaneously. The only effective treatment is electrical defibrillation. Basic and advanced cardiac life support is needed (p. 759).

If the attack of ventricular fibrillation occurs during the first day or two of an acute myocardial infarction, it is

Fig. 13.47 **Ventricular fibrillation.** Four beats of sinus rhythm followed by a ventricular ectopic beat that initiates ventricular fibrillation. The ST segment during sinus rhythm is elevated owing to acute myocardial infarction in this case.

probable that prophylactic therapy will be unnecessary. If the ventricular fibrillation was not related to an acute infarction, the long-term risk of recurrent cardiac arrest and sudden death is high.

Survivors of these ventricular tachyarrhythmias are, in the absence of an identifiable reversible cause (e.g. acute myocardial infarction, severe metabolic disturbance), at high risk of sudden death. Implantable cardioverter–defibrillators (ICDs) are first-line therapy in the management of these patients (p. 782).

The Brugada syndrome

This inheritable condition accounts for part of a group of patients with idiopathic ventricular fibrillation who have no evidence of causative structural cardiac disease. It is more common in young male adults and in South East Asia. The diagnosis is made by identifying the classic ECG changes that may be present spontaneously or provoked by the administration of a class I anti-arrhythmic (flecainide or ajmaline): right bundle branch block with coved ST elevation in leads V_1–V_3 (Fig. 13.48).

In 20% of cases it is a monogenic inheritable condition associated with cardiac sodium channel (*SCN5A*) mutations. It can present with sudden death during sleep, resuscitated cardiac arrest and syncope, or the patient may be asymptomatic and diagnosed incidentally or during familial assessment. There is a high risk of sudden death, particularly in the symptomatic patient or those with spontaneous ECG changes. The only successful treatment is an ICD. Beta-blockade is not helpful and may be harmful in this syndrome.

Torsades de pointes

Torsades de pointes arises when ventricular repolarization (QT interval) is greatly prolonged (long QT syndrome). The causes of long QT syndrome and torsades de pointes are listed in Table 13.14.

Congenital long QT syndrome may (Jervell–Lange-Nielsen syndrome) or may not (Romano–Ward syndrome) be associated with congenital deafness. QT prolongation and torsades de pointes can be precipitated by increased adrenergic drive (exertion or emotion), sudden arousal (e.g. being woken from sleep by an alarm) or it can occur even when asleep. In acquired long QT syndrome, QT prolongation and torsades de pointes are usually provoked by bradycardia.

Torsades de pointes causes palpitations and syncope but usually terminates spontaneously. It may, however,

Fig. 13.48 **The Brugada ECG.** ST elevation in V_1–V_3 with right bundle branch block.

Table 13.14 Causes of long QT syndrome and torsades de pointes tachycardia

Congenital syndromes
Jervell–Lange-Nielsen (autosomal recessive)
Romano–Ward (autosomal dominant)

Electrolyte abnormalities
Hypokalaemia
Hypomagnesaemia
Hypocalcaemia

Drugs
Quinidine, disopyramide
Sotalol, amiodarone
Amitriptyline (and other tricyclic antidepressants)
Chlorpromazine (and other phenothiazine drugs)
Erythromycin, other macrolides and fluoroquinolones

Poisons
Organophosphate insecticides

Miscellaneous
Bradycardia
Mitral valve prolapse
Acute myocardial infarction
Prolonged fasting and liquid protein diets (long term)
Central nervous system diseases, e.g. dystrophia myotonica

degenerate to ventricular fibrillation resulting in sudden death. It is characterized on the ECG by rapid, irregular, sharp complexes that continuously change from an upright to an inverted position (Fig. 13.49a).

Between spells of tachycardia or immediately preceding the onset of tachycardia the ECG shows a prolonged QT interval; the corrected QT (Table 13.5, p. 746) is equal to or greater than 0.44 s. Figure 13.49b shows examples of three forms of long QT interval prolongation. Acute management is as follows:

- Any electrolyte disturbance is corrected.
- Causative drugs are stopped.
- The heart rate is maintained with atrial or ventricular pacing.
- Magnesium sulphate 8 mmol (mg^{2+}) over 10–15 min for acquired long QT.

- Intravenous isoprenaline may be effective when QT prolongation is acquired (isoprenaline is contraindicated for congenital long QT syndrome).

Long-term management of acquired long QT syndrome involves avoidance of all drugs known to prolong the QT interval. Congenital long QT syndrome is generally treated by beta-blockade, left cardiac sympathetic denervation, and pacemaker therapy. Patients who remain symptomatic despite conventional therapy and those with a strong family history of sudden death usually need ICD therapy.

The molecular biology of the congenital long QT syndromes has been shown to be heterogeneous. It is usually a monogenic disorder and has been associated with mutations in cardiac potassium and sodium channel genes (Table 13.15). The different genes involved appear to correlate with different phenotypes (Fig. 13.49b) that

(a)

Fig. 13.49 Prolonged QT. (a) An ECG demonstrating a supraventricular rhythm with a long QT (LQT) interval giving way to atypical ventricular tachycardia (torsades de pointes). The tachycardia is short-lived and is followed by a brief period of idioventricular rhythm.

(b) Further examples of a prolonged QT interval corresponding to three different types of LQT.

(b)

Table 13.15 Single gene mutations responsible for congenital long QT syndrome

Subtype	Chromosome	Product	Channel
LQT1	11	KCNQ1	I_{ks} α subunit
LQT2	7	HERG	I_{kr} α subunit
LQT3	3	SCN5A	I_{Na} α subunit
LQT4	4	Ankyrin B	Unknown
LQT5	21	KCNE1	I_{ks} β subunit
LQT6	21	KCNE2	I_{kr} β subunit

can exhibit such variable penetrance that carriers may have completely normal ECGs. It is likely that identification of the mutation involved will not only improve diagnostic accuracy but also guide future therapy for the congenital long QT syndrome.

Normal heart ventricular tachycardia

Monomorphic ventricular tachycardia in patients with structurally normal hearts (idiopathic VT) is usually a benign condition with an excellent long-term prognosis. Occasionally, it is incessant (so called Galavardin's tachycardia) and if untreated may lead to cardiomyopathy.

Normal heart VT either arises from a focus in the right ventricular outflow tract or in the left ventricular septum. Treatment of symptoms is usually with beta-blockers. There is a special form of verapamil-sensitive tachycardia that responds well to non-dihydropyridine calcium antagonists. In symptomatic patients, radiofrequency catheter ablation is highly effective, resulting in a cure in > 90% cases.

Non-sustained ventricular tachycardia

Non-sustained ventricular tachycardia (NSVT) is defined as ventricular tachycardia that is ≥ 5 consecutive beats but lasts < 30 s (Fig. 13.50d). NSVT can be found in 6% of patients with normal hearts and usually does not require treatment. NSVT is documented in up to 60–80% of patients with heart disease. There is insufficient evidence on prognosis, but an ICD has been shown to improve survival of patients with particularly poor left ventricular function (ejection fraction 30% or less) by preventing arrhythmic death. Antiarrhythmic suppression of NSVT is not usually advocated but beta-blockers may improve quality of life in symptomatic individuals.

Ventricular premature beats

These may be uncomfortable, especially when frequent. The patient complains of extra beats, missed beats or heavy beats because it may be the premature beat, the post-ectopic pause or the next sinus beat that is noticed by the patient. The pulse is irregular owing to the premature beats. Some early beats may not be felt at the wrist. When a premature beat occurs regularly after every normal beat, 'pulsus bigeminus' may occur.

These premature beats (Fig. 13.50a–c) have a broad (> 0.12 s) and bizarre QRS complex because they arise from an abnormal (ectopic) site in the ventricular myocardium. Following a premature beat there is usually a complete compensatory pause because the AV node or

(a)

(b)

(c)

(d)

Fig. 13.50 **Varieties of ventricular ectopic activity.**
(a) Two ventricular ectopic beats of different morphology (multimorphological).
(b) Two ventricular premature beats (VPBs) occurring one after the other (a pair or couplet of VPBs).
(c) Frequently repetitive ventricular ectopic activity of a single morphology.
(d) Brief run of ventricular tachycardia (non-sustained ventricular tachycardia) that follows previous ectopic activity.

ventricle is refractory to the next sinus impulse. Early 'R-on-T' ventricular premature beats (occurring simultaneously with the upstroke or peak of the T wave of the previous beat) may induce ventricular fibrillation in patients with heart disease, particularly in patients following myocardial infarction.

Ventricular premature beats are usually treated only if symptomatic. Usually simple measures such as reassurance and beta-blocker therapy are all that is required.

LONG-TERM MANAGEMENT OF CARDIAC TACHYARRHYTHMIAS

Options for the long-term management of cardiac tachyarrhythmias include:

- antiarrhythmic drug therapy
- ablation therapy
- device therapy.

To determine the optimal strategy for a given patient the following questions must be addressed:

- Is the principal aim of treatment symptom relief or prevention of sudden death?
- Is maintaining sinus rhythm or controlling ventricular rates the treatment goal?

Commonly employed treatment strategies for the management of specific tachyarrhythmias are outlined in Table 13.16.

Antiarrhythmic drugs

Drugs that modify the rhythm and conduction of the heart are used to treat cardiac arrhythmias. Antiarrhythmic drugs may aggravate or produce arrhythmias (proarrhythmia) and they may also depress ventricular contractility and must therefore be used with caution. They are classified according to their effect on the action potential (Vaughan Williams' classification; Table 13.17 and Fig. 13.51).

Class I drugs

These are membrane-depressant drugs that reduce the rate of entry of sodium into the cell (sodium-channel

Table 13.16 Long-term management of tachyarrhythmias

Tachycardia	Management aims	Management strategies
AV node re-entry tachycardia (AVNRT)	Relieve symptoms	AV-node-blocking agents Class Ic or class III Catheter ablation
AV reciprocating tachycardia (AVRT)	Relieve symptoms	AV-node-blocking agents Class Ic or class III Catheter ablation
Wolff–Parkinson–White (WPW) syndrome	Relieve symptoms Prevent sudden death (esp. if documented pre-excited atrial fibrillation)	Class Ic or class III Catheter ablation

Atrial fibrillation	Relieve symptoms
	Prevent worsening heart failure due to poor rate control
	Prevent thromboembolic complications
		Maintenance of sinus rhythm:
		    class Ic or class III ± cardioversion
		    catheter ablation of ectopic focus
		Rate control:
		    AV-node-slowing agents
		    AV node ablation plus pacemaker
		Anticoagulation

Atrial flutter	Relieve symptoms Prevent worsening heart failure due to poor rate control Prevent thromboembolic complications	Class Ic or class III Catheter ablation AV-node-blocking agents Anticoagulation
Atrial tachycardia	Relieve symptoms Prevent worsening heart failure due to poor rate control Prevent thromboembolic complications	Class Ic or class III Catheter ablation AV-node-blocking agents Anticoagulation
Life-threatening ventricular tachyarrhythmias	Prevent sudden death	Implantable cardioverter–defibrillator (ICD) Beta-blockers
Congenital long QT	Prevent sudden death	Beta-blockers ± pacemaker ICD Correct bradycardia Correct electrolytes
Acquired long QT Normal heart ventricular tachycardias	Prevent sudden death Relieve symptoms	Avoidance of all QT-prolonging drugs Beta-blockers, calcium-channel blockers Catheter ablation
Non-sustained VT (NSVT)	Relieve symptoms Prevent sudden death in certain situations	Beta-blockers Class Ic or class III ICD in clearly defined subgroups

Table 13.17 Vaughan Williams' classification of antiarrhythmic drugs

Class I	Membrane-depressant drugs (sodium-channel blockers)
Ia	Disopyramide, procainamide, quinidine
Ib	Lidocaine (lignocaine), mexiletine
Ic	Flecainide, propafenone
Class II	β-Adrenoceptor blocking drugs, e.g. atenolol, propranolol, esmolol
Class III	Prolong action potential, e.g. amiodarone, sotalol
Class IV	Calcium-channel blockers, e.g. verapamil, diltiazem
(Other	Adenosine, digoxin)

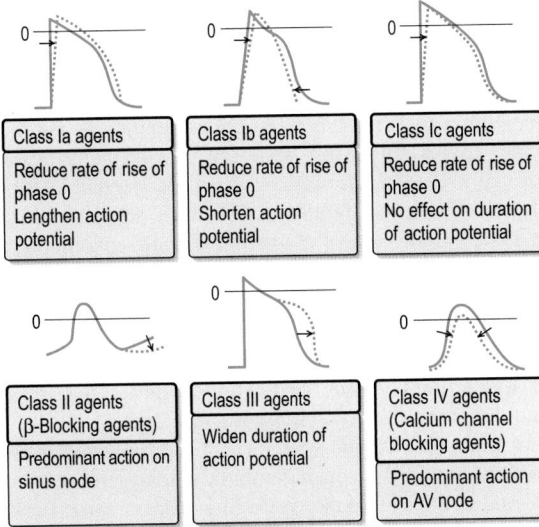

Fig. 13.51 Vaughan Williams' classification of antiarrhythmic drugs based on their effect on cardiac action potentials. 0, 0 mV. The dotted curves indicate the effects of the drugs.

blockers). They may slow conduction, delay recovery or reduce the spontaneous discharge rate of myocardial cells. Class Ia drugs (e.g. disopyramide) lengthen the action potential, class Ib drugs (e.g. lidocaine) shorten the action potential, and class Ic (flecainide, propafenone) do not affect the duration of the action potential. Class I agents have been found to increase mortality compared to placebo in post-myocardial infarction patients with ventricular ectopy (Cardiac Arrhythmia Suppression Trial (CAST) trials – class Ic agents) and in patients treated for atrial fibrillation (class Ia agent, quinidine). In view of this, class Ic agents such as flecainide and indeed all other class I drugs should be reserved for patients who do not have significant coronary artery disease, left ventricular dysfunction, or other forms of significant structural hearts disease.

Class II drugs (see Table 13.49)

These antisympathetic drugs prevent the effects of catecholamines on the action potential. Most are β-adrenoceptor antagonists. Cardioselective beta-blockers (β_1) include metoprolol, atenolol and acebutalol. Beta-blockers suppress AV node conduction, which may be effective in preventing attacks of junctional tachycardia, and may help to control ventricular rates during paroxysms of other forms of SVT (e.g. atrial fibrillation). In general beta-blockers are anti-ischaemic, and anti-adrenergic and have proven beneficial effects in patients post-myocardial infarction (by preventing ventricular fibrillation) and in patients with congestive heart failure. It is therefore advisable to consider beta-blocker therapy either alone or in combination with other antiarrhythmic drugs in patients with symptomatic tachyarrhythmias, particularly in patients with coronary artery disease.

Class III drugs

These prolong the action potential and do not affect sodium transport through the membrane. The drugs in this class are amiodarone and sotalol. Sotalol is also a beta-blocker.

Some drugs, such as ibutilide and dofetilide, are only available in some countries. Sotalol may result in acquired long QT syndrome and torsades de pointes. The risk of torsades is increased in the setting of hypokalaemia, and particular care should be taken in patients taking diuretic therapy. Amiodarone therapy in contrast to most other antiarrhythmic drugs carries a low risk of pro-arrhythmia in patients with significant structural heart disease. Because it has many toxic and potentially serious side-effects, patients need to be counselled prior to commencing amiodarone and monitored carefully at regular follow-up intervals. Dofetilide has been used to treat atrial fibrillation and flutter in patients with recent myocardial infarction and poor LV function.

Class IV drugs (see also Table 13.28)

The non-dihydropyridine calcium antagonists that reduce the plateau phase of the action potential are particularly effective at slowing conduction in nodal tissue. Verapamil and diltiazem are two drugs in this group. These drugs can prevent attacks of junctional tachycardia (AVNRT and AVRT) and may help to control ventricular rates during paroxysms of other forms of SVT (e.g. atrial fibrillation).

Drug therapy is commonly used for symptomatic relief in patients who do not have life-threatening tachy-arrhythmias. Patient safety is the main factor determining the choice of antiarrhythmic therapy and proarrhythmic risks need to be carefully assessed prior to initiating therapy. As a generalization, class Ic agents are employed in patients with structurally normal hearts and class III agents are used in patients with structural heart disease.

In order to administer antiarrhythmic agents as safely as possible it is helpful to be familiar with the different proarrhythmia mechanisms and their main predisposing risk factors (Table 13.18).

Patients with structurally normal hearts and normal QT intervals, or with implantable defibrillators, are either at very low risk of proarrhythmia or are protected from any life-threatening consequences, and in these patients it

Table 13.18 Proarrhythmia mechanisms and the predisposing risk factors

Prearrhythmia mechanism	Drug	Predisposing risk factors
Torsades de pointes	Class Ia (disopyramide, procainamide, quinidine) Sotalol 'Pure' class III (ibutilide)	Baseline QT prolongation Female gender Hypokalaemia/diuretic use Clinical heart failure Advanced structural heart disease Conversion of AF to sinus rhythm
Atrial flutter with 1 : 1 AV conduction and wide QRS complexes	Class I_a (disopyramide, quinidine) Class I_c (flecainide, propafenone)	Risk reduced by adding an AV-nodal-slowing agent
'Late' sudden death (arrhythmic mechanism not clearly defined)	Class I_c (flecainide) Quinidine	Myocardial ischaemia

is possible to persevere with drug therapy until an efficacious, well-tolerated agent is identified.

Catheter ablation

Radiofrequency catheter ablation is frequently employed in the management of symptomatic tachyarrhythmias. Ablations are performed by placing three or four electrode catheters into the heart chambers in order to record and pace from various sites. Pacing the atria or the ventricles is used to trigger the tachycardia and to study the tachycardia mechanism. Successful ablation depends on accurate identification of either the site of origin of a focal tachycardia or of a critical component of a macro-reentry tachycardia. The following tachyarrhythmias can be readily ablated:

- AV node re-entry tachycardia (AVNRT)
- AV re-entry tachycardia (AVRT) with an accessory pathway, including WPW syndrome
- normal heart VT
- atrial flutter
- atrial tachycardia.

Symptomatic patients with a pre-excited ECG because of accessory pathway conduction (WPW syndrome) are advised to undergo catheter ablation as first-line therapy, owing to the risk of sudden death associated with this condition. This is especially the case in patients with pre-excited atrial fibrillation. Patients with accessory pathways that only conduct retrogradely from the ventricles to the atrium are not at increased risk of sudden death but experience symptoms due to AVRT. These patients are commonly offered an ablation procedure if simple measures such as AV nodal slowing agents fail to suppress tachycardia. The main risk associated with accessory pathway ablation is thromboembolism in patients with left-sided accessory pathways. The success rate for catheter ablation of AVNRT and accessory pathways is greater than 95%.

Patients with normal hearts and documented ventricular tachycardia should be referred for specialist evaluation. Unlike VT in patients with structural heart disease, normal heart VT is not associated with increased risk of sudden death and is easily cured by catheter ablation.

Catheter ablation is recommended in patients with atrial flutter that is not easily managed medically. Ablation of typical flutter is effective in 90–95% cases. In the direct comparison of catheter ablation and anti-arrhythmic therapy, the rate of recurrence was significantly lower following ablation. Atrial tachycardia, especially in patients with structurally normal hearts, may also be cured by catheter ablation. In atrial fibrillation, adequate control of ventricular rates is sometimes not possible despite optimal medical therapy. These patients experience a marked symptomatic improvement following AV node ablation and pacemaker implantation. Unlike other forms of catheter ablation this does not cure the arrhythmia; atrial fibrillation continues and anti-coagulation is still required following ablation.

In younger patients with structurally normal hearts, atrial ectopic beats, which commonly arise from a focus situated in the pulmonary veins, may trigger atrial fibrillation. Catheter ablation of this ectopic focus includes the application of radiofrequency energy in or around the pulmonary veins in order to abolish the connection between the sleeves of arrhythmogenic atrial myocardium surrounding or extending into the veins from the remaining atrium (pulmonary vein isolation). The trigger is therefore eliminated and the arrhythmia does not recur. The complications of the procedure involve pulmonary vein stenosis, thrombosis and stroke. The complication rate is small and the success rate is 60–80% in patients with paroxysmal atrial fibrillation and 20–40% in those with a persistent form of the arrhythmia.

Implantable cardioverter–defibrillator (ICD)

Life-threatening ventricular arrhythmias (ventricular fibrillation or rapid ventricular tachycardia with hypotension) result in death in up to 40% within 1 year of diagnosis. Large multicentre prospective trials such as the Antiarrhythmics (amiodarone) Versus Implantable Defibrillator (AVID) trial have proven that implantable defibrillators improve overall survival in patients who have experienced an episode of life-threatening ventricular tachyarrhythmia (Fig. 13.52).

The ICD recognizes ventricular tachycardia or fibrillation and automatically delivers pacing or a shock to the

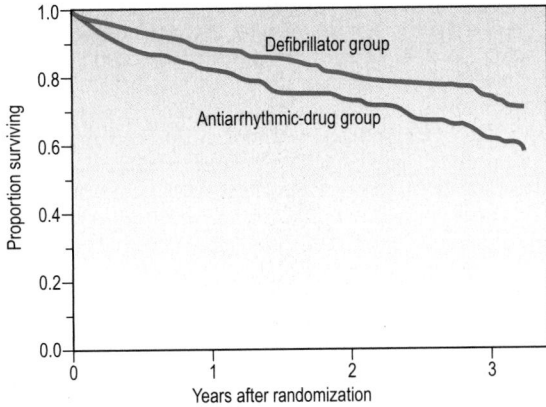

Fig. 13.52 Survival curves of the Multicentre Automatic Defibrillator Implantation Trial (MADIT) following myocardial infarction. Patients with left ventricular ejection fractions of ≤ 0.35 and documented asymptomatic non-sustained ventricular tachycardia and inducible ventricular tachycardia were randomized to receive an ICD or conventional therapy.

heart to cause cardioversion to sinus rhythm. Modern ICDs are only a little larger than a pacemaker and are implanted in a pectoral position (Fig. 13.53). The device may have leads to sense and pace both the right atrium and ventricle, and the lithium batteries employed are able to provide energy for over 100 shocks each of around 30 J. ICD discharges are painful if the patient is conscious. However, ventricular tachycardia may often be terminated by overdrive pacing the heart, which is painless. The ICD is superior to all other treatment options at preventing sudden cardiac death. The use of this device has cut the sudden death rate in patients with a history of serious ventricular arrhythmias to approximately 2% per year. However, the majority of these patients have significant structural heart disease and overall cardiac mortality due to progressive heart failure remains high. As a result ICDs are now first-line therapy in the secondary prevention of sudden death.

Implantable cardioverter–defibrillators are also employed in the primary prevention of sudden cardiac death. The chances of surviving an out of hospital cardiac arrest are as low as 10%. Therefore selected patients who have never experienced a spontaneous episode of life-

(a)

(b)

(c)

Fig. 13.53 Implantable cardioverter–defibrillator. **(a) X-ray of a 'dual-chamber' ICD** in a left pectoral position with atrial and ventricular leads. **(b) An implantable dual-chamber cardioverter–defibrillator** (GEM III DR). **(c) Termination of ventricular fibrillation** by the direct current shock at 20 J. Electrogram recorded internally from the ventricular lead of an ICD reveals chaotic ventricular activity consistent with ventricular fibrillation. This is confirmed by an electrocardiogram (lead V_2). The marker channel demonstrates that the device detects ventricular fibrillation correctly (FS, fibrillation sensing, lower line) and delivers an appropriate shock (CD) that terminates the arrhythmia and restores normal sinus rhythm (VS, ventricular sensing, lower line). Incidentally, atrial fibrillation is also detected before shock delivery (upper line on the marker channel).

threatening ventricular tachyarrhythmia but who are assessed to be at high risk of sudden death are advised to undergo ICD implantation. In two large primary prevention ICD trials, Multicenter Automated Defibrillator Implantation Trial (MADIT II) and Sudden Cardiac Death in Heart Failure Trial (SCD-HeFT), therapy with an ICD reduced mortality by 23–31% on top of conventional treatment, which included revascularization, beta-blockers, and angiotensin-converting enzyme inhibitors.

The following groups of patients may merit prophylactic ICD placement:

- patients with coronary artery disease; significant impairment of left ventricular function (LVEF ≤ 35–40%), spontaneous non-sustained ventricular tachycardia in whom sustained ventricular tachycardia was induced by pacing the heart during an electrophysiological study
- patients with very poor LV function post-MI (LVEF ≤ 30%); however a recent study has shown no overall reduction in mortality
- patients with dilated and particularly hypertrophic cardiomyopathy, long QT syndrome and Brugada syndrome who have a strong family history of sudden cardiac death.

FURTHER READING

Albers GW, Dalen JE, Laupacis A et al. (2001) Antithrombotic therapy in atrial fibrillation. *Chest* **119** (1 Suppl.): 194S–206S.

Blomstrom-Lundqvist C et al.; European Society of Cardiology Committee, NASPE–Heart Rhythm Society (2003) ACC/AHA/ESC guidelines for the management of patients with supraventricular arrhythmias – executive summary. A report of the American College Of Cardiology/American Heart Association task force on practice guidelines and the European SOCiety of Cardiology committee for practice guidelines (writing committee to develop guidelines for the management of patients with supraventricular arrhythmias) developed in collaboration with NASPE–Heart Rhythm Society. *Journal of the American College of Cardiology* 2003 **42**(8): 1493–1531.

Fuster V et al.; American College of Cardiology/American Heart Association Task Force on Practice Guidelines; European Society of Cardiology Committee for Practice Guidelines and Policy Conferences (Committee to Develop Guidelines for the Management of Patients With Atrial Fibrillation); North American Society of Pacing and Electrophysiology (2001) ACC/AHA/ESC Guidelines for the Management of Patients With Atrial Fibrillation: Executive Summary A Report of the American College of Cardiology/American Heart Association Task Force on Practice Guidelines and the European Society of Cardiology Committee for Practice Guidelines and Policy Conferences (Committee to Develop Guidelines for the Management of Patients With Atrial Fibrillation) Developed in Collaboration With the North American Society of Pacing and Electrophysiology. *Circulation* **104**(17): 2118–2150.

Gregoratos G, Abrams J, Epstein AE et al.; American College of Cardiology/American Heart Association Task Force on Practice Guidelines American College of Cardiology/American Heart Association/North American Society for Pacing and Electrophysiology Committee (2002) ACC/AHA/NASPE 2002 guideline update for implantation of cardiac pacemakers and antiarrhythmia devices: summary article. A report of the American College of Cardiology/American Heart Association Task Force on Practice Guidelines (ACC/AHA/NASPE Committee to Update the 1998 Pacemaker Guidelines). *Journal of Cardiovascular Electrophysiology* **13**(11): 1183–1199.

HEART FAILURE

Heart failure is a complex syndrome that can result from any structural or functional cardiac disorder that impairs the ability of the heart to function as a pump to support a physiological circulation.

The incidence of heart failure increases with advancing age. The average annual incidence is 2–4% between 35 and 64 years, and 10% in patients over 65 years. The prognosis of heart failure has improved over the past 10 years, but the mortality rate is still high with approximately 50% of patients dead at 5 years. Heart failure accounts for 5% of admissions to hospital medical wards. The cost of managing heart failure in the UK exceeds £1 billion per year. Coronary artery disease is the commonest cause of heart failure in western countries.

The causes of heart failure are shown in Table 13.19.

Factors aggravating or precipitating heart failure

Any factor that increases myocardial work may aggravate existing heart failure or initiate failure. The most common are arrhythmias, anaemia, thyrotoxicosis, pregnancy, obesity, infective endocarditis, pulmonary infection, change of heart failure therapy including poor compliance. Readmission rates range from 29% and 47% within 3–6 months of hospital discharge.

PATHOPHYSIOLOGY

When the heart fails, considerable changes occur to the heart and peripheral vascular system in response to the haemodynamic changes associated with heart failure (Table 13.20). These physiological changes are compensatory and maintain cardiac output and peripheral perfusion. However, as heart failure progresses, these mechanisms are overwhelmed and become pathophysiological. The development of pathological peripheral vasoconstriction and sodium retention in heart failure by activation of the renin–angiotensin–aldosterone system, is a loss of beneficial compensatory mechanisms and

Table 13.19 Causes of heart failure

Main causes
Ischaemic heart disease (35–40%)
Cardiomyopathy (dilated) (30–34%)
Hypertension (15–20%)

Other causes
Cardiomyopathy (undilated): hypertrophic/obstructive, restrictive (amyloidosis, sarcoidosis)
Valvular heart disease (mitral, aortic, tricuspid)
Congenital heart disease (ASD, VSD)
Alcohol and drugs (chemotherapy)
Hyperdynamic circulation (anaemia, thyrotoxicosis, haemochromatosis, Paget's disease)
Right heart failure (RV infarct, pulmonary hypertension, pulmonary embolism, cor pulmonale (COPD))
Tricuspid incompetence
Arrhythmias (atrial fibrillation, bradycardia (complete heart block, the sick sinus syndrome))
Pericardial disease (constrictive pericarditis, pericardial effusion)

Table 13.20 Pathophysiological changes in heart failure

Ventricular dilatation
Myocyte hypertrophy
Increased collagen synthesis
Altered myosin gene expression
Altered sarcoplasmic Ca^{2+}-ATPase density
Increased ANP secretion
Salt and water retention
Sympathetic stimulation
Peripheral vasoconstriction

represents cardiac decompensation. Factors involved are venous return, outflow resistance, contractility of the myocardium, and salt and water retention.

Venous return (preload)

In the intact heart, myocardial failure leads to a reduction of the volume of blood ejected with each heartbeat and an increase in the volume of blood remaining after systole. This increased diastolic volume stretches the myocardial fibres and, as Starling's law of the heart would suggest, myocardial contraction is restored. However, the failing myocardium results in depression of the ventricular function curve (cardiac output plotted against the ventricular diastolic volume) (Fig. 13.5, p. 728).

Mild myocardial depression is not associated with a reduction in cardiac output because it is maintained by an increase in venous pressure (and hence diastolic volume). However, the proportion of blood ejected with each heartbeat (ejection fraction) is reduced early in heart failure. Sinus tachycardia also ensures that any reduction of stroke volume is compensated for by the increase in heart rate; cardiac output (stroke volume × heart rate) is therefore maintained.

When there is more severe myocardial dysfunction, cardiac output can be maintained only by a large increase

in venous pressure and/or marked sinus tachycardia. The increased venous pressure contributes to the development of dyspnoea, owing to the accumulation of interstitial and alveolar fluid, and to the occurrence of hepatic enlargement, ascites and dependent oedema, due to increased systemic venous pressure. However, the cardiac output at rest may not be much depressed, but myocardial and haemodynamic reserve is so compromised that a normal increase in cardiac output cannot be produced by exercise.

In very severe heart failure the cardiac output at rest is depressed, despite high venous pressures. The inadequate cardiac output is redistributed to maintain perfusion of vital organs, such as the heart, brain and kidneys, at the expense of the skin and muscle.

Outflow resistance (afterload) (see Figs 15.3 and 15.4)

This is the load or resistance against which the ventricle contracts. It is formed by:

- pulmonary and systemic resistance
- physical characteristics of the vessel walls
- the volume of blood that is ejected.

An increase in afterload decreases the cardiac output. This results in a further increase of end-diastolic volume and dilatation of the ventricle itself, which further exacerbates the problem of afterload. This is expressed by Laplace's law: the tension of the myocardium (T) is proportional to the intraventricular pressure (P) multiplied by the radius of the ventricular chamber (R): i.e. $T \propto PR$.

Myocardial contractility (inotropic state)

The state of the myocardium also influences performance. The sympathetic nervous system is activated in heart failure via baroreceptors as an early compensatory mechanism, which provides inotropic support and maintains cardiac output. Chronic sympathetic activation, however, has deleterious effects by further increasing neurohormonal activation and myocyte apoptosis. This is compensated by a downregulation of β-receptors. Increased contractility (positive inotropism) can result from increased sympathetic drive, and this is a normal part of the Frank–Starling relationship (Fig. 13.5, p. 728). Conversely, myocardial depressants (e.g. hypoxia) decrease myocardial contractility (negative inotropism).

Neurohormonal and sympathetic system activation: salt and water retention

The increase in venous pressure that occurs when the ventricles fail leads to retention of salt and water and their accumulation in the interstitium, producing many of the physical signs of heart failure. Reduced cardiac output also leads to diminished renal perfusion, activating the renin–angiotensin system and enhancing salt and water retention (Fig. 12.3, p. 691), which further increases venous pressure (Fig. 13.54). The retention of sodium is in part compensated by the action of circulating atrial natriuretic peptides and antidiuretic hormone (see p. 691 and below).

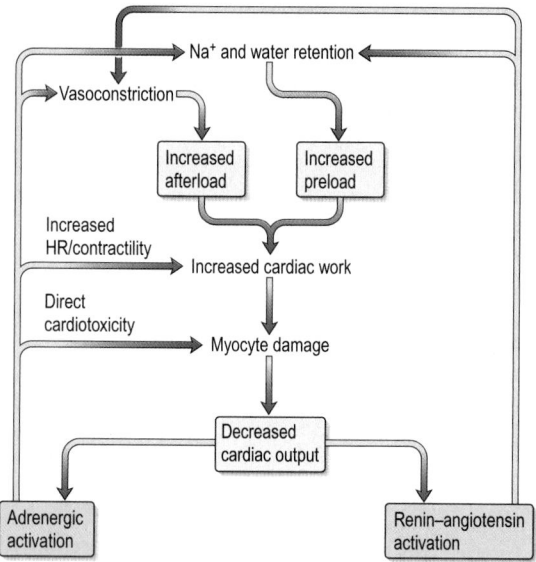

Fig. 13.54 The compensatory physiological response to heart failure. Chronic activation of the renin–angiotensin and adrenergic systems results in a 'vicious cycle' of cardiac deterioration that further exacerbates the physiological response.

The interaction of haemodynamic and neurohumoral factors in the progression of heart failure remains unclear. Increased ventricular wall stress promotes ventricular dilatation and further worsens contractile efficiency. In addition, prolonged activation of the sympathetic nervous and renin–angiotensin–aldosterone systems exerts direct toxic effects on myocardial cells.

Myocardial remodelling in heart failure

Left ventricular remodelling is a process of progressive alteration of ventricular size, shape, and function owing to the influence of mechanical, neurohormonal, and possibly genetic factors in several clinical conditions, including myocardial infarction, cardiomyopathy, hypertension, and valvular heart disease. Its hallmarks include hypertrophy, loss of myocytes, and increased interstitial fibrosis. Remodelling continues for months after the initial insult, and the eventual change in the shape of the ventricle becomes responsible for significant impairment of overall function of the heart as a pump (Fig. 13.55a). In cardiomyopathy, the process of progressive ventricular dilatation or hypertrophy occurs without ischaemic myocardial injury or infarction (Fig. 13.55b).

Changes in myocardial gene expression

Haemodynamic overload of the ventricle stimulates changes in cardiac contractile protein gene expression. The overall effect is to increase protein synthesis, but many proteins also switch to fetal and neonatal isoforms. Human myosin is composed of a pair of heavy chains and two pairs of light chains. Myosin heavy chains (MHC) exist in two isoforms, α and β, that have different contractile properties and ATPase activity. $\alpha\alpha$-MHC predominates in the atria and $\beta\beta$-MHC in the ventricles. In animal models, pressure overload results in a shift from $\alpha\alpha$- to $\beta\beta$-MHC in the atria, in parallel with atrial size. This results in reduction in atrial contractility but reduced energy demands. This shift is less significant in the human ventricle, as the $\beta\beta$-MHC isoform already predominates. Other genes affected in heart failure include those encoding Na^+/K^+-ATPase, Ca^{2+}-ATPase and β_1-adrenoceptors.

Abnormal calcium homeostasis

Calcium ion flux within myocytes plays a pivotal role in the regulation of contractile function. Excitation of the myocyte cell membrane causes the rapid entry of calcium

Fig. 13.55 Ventricular remodelling in (a) ischaemic (MI) and (b) non-ischaemic heart failure, e.g. in cardiomyopathy.
From Jessop M, Brozana S (2003) *New England Journal of Medicine* **348**: 2011, with permission. Copyright © 2003 Massachusetts Medical Society. All rights reserved.

into myocytes from the extracellular space via calcium channels. This triggers the release of intracellular calcium from the sarcoplasmic reticulum and initiates contraction (see Fig. 13.3). Relaxation results from the uptake and storage of calcium by the sarcoplasmic reticulum (see Fig. 13.9) controlled by changes in nitric oxide. In heart failure, there is a prolongation of the calcium current in association with prolongation of contraction and relaxation.

Apoptosis (see also p. 162)

Apoptosis (or 'programmed cell death') of myocytes has been demonstrated in animal models of ischaemic reperfusion, rapid ventricular pacing, mechanical stretch, and pressure overload. Apoptosis is associated with irreversible congestive heart failure, and the spiral of ventricular dysfunction, characteristic of heart failure, results from the initiation of apoptosis by cytokines, free radicals and other triggers.

Natriuretic peptides (ANP, BNP and C-type)

Atrial natriuretic peptide (ANP) is released from atrial myocytes in response to stretch. ANP induces diuresis, natriuresis, vasodilatation and suppression of the renin–angiotensin system. Levels of circulating ANP are increased in congestive cardiac failure and correlate with functional class, prognosis and haemodynamic state. The renal response to ANP is attenuated in heart failure, probably secondarily to reduced renal perfusion, receptor downregulation, increased peptide breakdown, renal sympathetic activation, and excessive renin–angiotensin activity. *Brain natriuretic peptide* (*BNP*) (so called because it was first discovered in brain) is predominantly secreted by the ventricles and has an action similar to that of ANP but it has greater diagnostic and prognostic value (p. 789). *C-type peptide*, which is limited to vascular endothelium and the central nervous system, has similar effects to those of ANP and BNP. The therapeutic benefits of the natriuretic peptides have been investigated by administration of ANP and by the inhibition of the enzyme responsible for breakdown of the peptides (neutral endopeptidase – NEP).

Endothelial function in heart failure

The endothelium has a central role in the regulation of vasomotor tone. In patients with heart failure, endothelium-dependent vasodilatation in peripheral blood vessels is impaired and may be one mechanism of exercise limitation. The cause of abnormal endothelial responsiveness relates to abnormal release of both nitric oxide and vasoconstrictor substances, such as endothelin (ET). The activity of nitric oxide, a potent vasodilator, is blunted in heart failure. ET secretion from a variety of tissues is stimulated by many factors, including hypoxia, catecholamines and angiotensin II. The plasma concentration of ET is elevated in patients with heart failure, and levels correlate with the severity of haemodynamic disturbance. The major source of circulating ET in heart failure is the pulmonary vascular bed.

ET has many actions that potentially contribute to the pathophysiology of heart failure: vasoconstriction, sympathetic stimulation, renin–angiotensin system activation and left ventricular hypertrophy. Acute intravenous administration of endothelin antagonists improves haemodynamic abnormalities in patients with congestive cardiac failure, and oral endothelin antagonists are being developed. Plasma concentrations of some cytokines, in particular TNF, are increased in patients with heart failure.

Antidiuretic hormone (vasopressin)

Antidiuretic hormone (ADH) is raised in severe chronic heart failure, particularly in patients on diuretic treatment. High ADH concentration precipitates hyponatraemia which is an ominous prognostic indicator.

CLINICAL SYNDROMES OF HEART FAILURE

Various terms are used in clinical practice to mean 'heart failure' without following any guideline definition of heart failure or diagnostic criteria.

The terms 'biventricular' or 'congestive' heart failure are used variously but are best restricted to cases where right heart failure results from pre-existing left heart failure.

Biventricular cardiac failure is the most common manifestation of heart failure. It is clinically useful to divide heart failure into the syndromes of left and right cardiac failure, but it is rare for any part of the heart to fail in isolation.

Chronic heart failure can be 'compensated' or 'decompensated'. In *compensated heart failure*, symptoms are stable and overt features of fluid retention are absent. *Decompensated heart failure* refers to an acute or continuing deterioration. Causes, such as ischaemia, arrhythmia, infection and electrolyte disturbance, should be identified and reversed. The natural history of moderate heart failure involves increasingly frequent hospital admissions due to symptom exacerbation.

Left heart failure

Causes include:

- ischaemic heart disease (the most common cause)
- systemic hypertension (chronic or 'malignant')
- mitral and aortic valve disease
- cardiomyopathies.

Mitral stenosis causes left atrial hypertension and signs of left heart failure but does not itself cause failure of the left ventricle.

Clinical features

Symptoms are predominantly fatigue, exertional dyspnoea, orthopnoea and paroxysmal nocturnal dyspnoea.

*Physical sig*ns are few and not prominent until a late stage or if ventricular failure is acute. Cardiomegaly is demonstrable with a displaced and often sustained apical impulse. Auscultation reveals a left ventricular third or fourth heart sound that, with tachycardia, is described as a gallop rhythm. Dilatation of the mitral anulus results in functional mitral regurgitation. Crackles are heard at the lung bases. In severe left heart failure the patient has pulmonary oedema (see p. 797).

Right heart failure

This syndrome occurs in association with:

- left heart failure
- chronic lung disease (cor pulmonale)
- pulmonary embolism or pulmonary hypertension
- tricuspid valve disease
- pulmonary valve disease
- left-to-right shunts (e.g. atrial or ventricular septal defects)
- isolated right ventricular cardiomyopathy
- mitral valve disease with pulmonary hypertension.

Clinical features

Symptoms (fatigue, breathlessness, anorexia and nausea) relate to distension and fluid accumulation in areas drained by the systemic veins. *Physical signs* are usually more prominent than the symptoms, with:

- jugular venous distension (± *v* waves of tricuspid regurgitation)
- tender smooth hepatic enlargement
- dependent pitting oedema
- development of free abdominal fluid (ascites)
- pleural transudates (commonly right-sided).

Dilatation of the right ventricle produces cardiomegaly and may give rise to functional tricuspid regurgitation. Tachycardia and a right ventricular third heart sound are usual.

Right heart failure cannot be diagnosed from symptoms and signs alone. Objective evidence of cardiac dysfunction, for example from echocardiography, is needed.

Systolic versus diastolic heart failure

Systolic and diastolic dysfunction usually coexist.

Systolic ventricular dysfunction is most commonly due to coronary artery disease, usually following myocardial infarction. The left ventricle is usually dilated and fails to contract normally.

Diastolic ventricular dysfunction results from impaired myocardial relaxation, with increased stiffness in the ventricular wall and decreased left ventricular compliance leading to impairment of diastolic ventricular filling and hence decreased cardiac output. Coronary artery disease, hypertension and hypertrophic cardiomyopathy are common causes, although infiltrative disease such as amyloid may lead to pure diastolic dysfunction. The incidence remains unclear, although up to 30% of patients with heart failure may have normal systolic contraction. Management is similar to systolic heart failure but there may be an additional place for calcium-channel blockers. Diastolic dysfunction appears to carry a better prognosis.

High-output heart failure

The heart may not be able to meet the demands placed on it in conditions such as anaemia, thyrotoxicosis, beriberi and Gram-negative septicaemia. This form of heart failure presents in much the same manner as low-output states but is associated with tachycardia and a gallop rhythm. Patients are often warm with distended superficial veins. Unlike low-output failure, the oxygen content of systemic venous blood is high owing to the delivery of large amounts of arterial blood to non-metabolizing tissues.

Acute heart failure

The term 'acute heart failure' is often used exclusively to mean acute (cardiogenic) dyspnoea characterized by signs of pulmonary congestion. It is preferable to use the term 'acute pulmonary oedema' or where applicable 'cardiogenic shock'.

Acute failure of the heart most commonly occurs in the setting of acute myocardial infarction when there is extensive loss of ventricular muscle. The condition may also occur with rupture of the interventricular septum producing a ventricular septal defect, or be due to acute valvular regurgitation. Common examples of valvular regurgitation are papillary or chordal rupture producing mitral regurgitation, or sudden aortic valve regurgitation in infective endocarditis. Other causes of acute heart failure include obstruction of the circulation by acute pulmonary embolus and cardiac tamponade. In each case severe cardiac failure can occur with a relatively normal heart size.

Chronic heart failure

Chronic heart failure is often punctuated by acute exacerbations where an abnormality of cardiac function is responsible for the failure of the heart to maintain a physiological circulation. At present no simple objective definition of heart failure is available, since there is no cut-off value or cardiac or ventricular dysfunction or change in flow, pressure, dimension or volume that can be used reliably to identify patients with heart failure.

Cardiac cachexia

The term cardiac cachexia describes the loss of lean (non-oedematous) body mass that occurs in some patients with moderate or severe heart failure. Most patients with cachexia are over 40 years of age, have had heart failure for at least 5 years and are in NYHA (see p. 732) functional class 3/4. Its presence is associated with increased morbidity and mortality.

Several mechanisms are thought to contribute to wasting in heart failure, including malabsorption, anorexia caused by intestinal oedema and drugs, and loss of nutrients through the gastrointestinal and renal tracts. Patients with heart failure also have an increased metabolic rate secondary to increased sympathetic activity in association with reduced anabolic metabolism. Tumour necrosis factor alpha (TNF-α) is increased in patients with cardiac cachexia and contributes to the phenomenon. Possible stimuli to TNF-α release include reduced peripheral blood flow, failing myocardium and prostaglandin release. Natriuretic C-type peptide is also elevated in cachectic patients.

Diagnosis of heart failure

The diagnosis of heart failure should not be based on history and clinical findings; it requires evidence of cardiac dysfunction with appropriate investigation using objective measures of left ventricular structure and function (usually echocardiography). Similarly, the underlying cause of heart failure should be established in all patients (Table 13.21 and Fig. 13.56).

INVESTIGATIONS

Diagnostic

■ **Blood tests** – full blood count, liver biochemistry, urea and electrolytes, cardiac enzymes in acute heart failure to diagnose myocardial infarction, thyroid function.
■ **Chest X-ray** – cardiac size and evidence of pulmonary congestion, initially upper lobe diversion, then fluid in fissures and Kerley B lines (pulmonary venous pressure > 20 mmHg), then frank pulmonary oedema (pulmonary venous pressure > 25 mmHg).
■ **Electrocardiogram** – evidence of ischaemia, hypertension or arrhythmia.
■ **Natriuretic peptide** (B-type NP (BNP) or N terminal (NTproBNP)). A normal plasma level excludes heart failure and is a useful screening test in the investigation of patients with breathlessness.
■ **Echocardiography**. Two-dimensional and Doppler echocardiography establish the presence of systolic and/or diastolic impairment of the left or right ventricle. They may also reveal the aetiology (valve disease, regional wall motion abnormalities in ischaemic heart disease, cardiomyopathy, amyloid), and may detect intracardiac thrombus. An ejection fraction of < 0.45 is generally accepted as evidence for systolic dysfunction.
■ **Stress echocardiography**. Exercise or pharmacological stress echocardiography has no radiation hazard and is a reliable technique for detecting ischaemia as a cause of persistent but reversible cardiac dysfunction and in determining the viability of akinetic myocardium in patients with heart failure. *Dobutamine stress*-induced sustained contractile improvement is observed when flow reserve is appropriate, in the presence of stunning or non-transmural infarction.
■ **Nuclear cardiology**. Radionuclide angiography (RNA) provides accurate measurements of left, and to a lesser extent, right ventricular ejection fractions, cardiac volumes and regional wall motion. Left ventricular filling dynamics (diastolic function) can also be analysed. These measurements are not reliable in the presence of atrial fibrillation. Single-photon-emission computed tomography (SPECT) can be performed at rest or during stress, e.g. dobutamine infusion using different radionuclides, e.g. thallium-201 or technetium-99m, to detect the presence and extent of ischaemia (p. 755).

Table 13.21 Diagnosis of heart failure (European Society of Cardiology guidelines)

Essential features (criteria 1 and 2)
1. Symptoms and signs of heart failure (e.g. breathlessness, fatigue, ankle swelling)
2. Objective evidence of cardiac dysfunction (at rest)

Non-essential features
3. Response to treatment directed towards heart failure (in cases where the diagnosis is in doubt)

Fig. 13.56 Algorithm for the diagnosis of heart failure. Based on the recent European Society of Cardiology and NICE guidelines.

■ **Cardiac MRI**. At present, MRI is only recommended in selected patients with heart failure where other investigations do not provide satisfactory diagnosis. Advanced techniques with high-resolution image quality accurately measure cardiac volumes, wall thicknesses and left ventricular mass. MRI also reliably detects thickened pericardium and quantitates myocardial necrosis, perfusion and function. Quantitative biochemical information and metabolic function can also be obtained.
■ **Positron emission tomography (PET)**. When other tests (e.g. stress echocardiography, SPECT) cannot provide satisfactory results, PET scanning can be used, especially to identify potentially viable muscle that is hibernating. The importance of identifying the pathology is that appropriate treatment (surgical or medical) may restore the function. The technique can determine myocardial blood flow and cellular metabolism very precisely.
■ **Cardiac catheterization** (see p. 757).
■ **Cardiac biopsy** for infiltrative disease, e.g. amyloid.

Functional/prognostic

- **Cardiopulmonary exercise testing.** Peak oxygen consumption (V_{O_2}) is a strong independent predictor of hospital admission and death in patients with heart failure but is not widely available. A 6-minute exercise walk may be used instead.
- **Ambulatory (24–48 hours) ECG monitoring** – if arrhythmia is suspected.
- **Resting and stress radionuclide angiography (MUGA)** – for estimation of ejection fraction, regional wall motion abnormality.

TREATMENT OF HEART FAILURE

Treatment is aimed at relieving symptoms, prevention and control of disease leading to cardiac dysfunction and heart failure, retarding disease progression and improving quality and length of life.

Measures to prevent heart failure include cessation of smoking, alcohol and illicit drugs, effective treatment of hypertension, diabetes and hypercholesterolaemia, and pharmacological therapy following myocardial infarction.

The management of heart failure requires that any factor aggravating the failure should be identified and treated. Similarly the cause of heart failure must be elucidated and where possible corrected. Community nursing programmes to help with drug compliance and to detect early deterioration may prevent acute hospitalization.

General lifestyle advice

Education

Effective counselling of patients and family emphasizing weight monitoring and dose adjustment of diuretics may prevent hospitalization.

Obesity control

Maintain desired weight and body mass index.

Dietary modification

Large meals should be avoided and if necessary weight reduction instituted. Salt restriction is necessary and foods rich in salt or added salt in cooking and at the table should be avoided. A low-sodium diet is unpalatable and of questionable value. In severe heart failure fluid restriction is necessary. Alcohol has a negative inotropic effect and heart failure patients should moderate consumption.

Smoking

Smoking should be stopped, with help from anti-smoking clinics (p. 893) if necessary.

Physical activity, exercise training and rehabilitation

For patients with exacerbations of congestive cardiac failure, bed rest reduces the demands on the heart and is useful for a few days. Migration of fluid from the interstitium promotes a diuresis, reducing heart failure. Prolonged bed rest may lead to development of deep vein thrombosis; this can be avoided by daily leg exercises, low-dose subcutaneous heparin and elastic support stockings. Low-level endurance exercise (e.g. 20–30 minutes walking three or five times per week, or 20 minutes cycling at 70–80% of peak heart rate five times per week) is actively encouraged in patients with compensated heart failure in order to reverse 'deconditioning' of peripheral muscle metabolism. Strenuous isometric activity should be avoided.

Vaccination

While prospective clinical trials are lacking, it is recommended that patients with heart failure be vaccinated against pneumococcal disease and influenza.

Air travel

This is possible for most patients, subject to clinical circumstances. Check with the airline – most have guidelines on who should travel.

Sexual activity

Tell patients on nitrates not to take phosphodiesterase type 5 inhibitors (e.g. sildenafil) as it may induce profound hypotension.

Driving (UK)

DVLA guidance (DVLA Guide to the Current Medical Standards of Fitness to Drive, August 2003) should be followed. Driving motor cars and motorcycles may continue provided there are no symptoms that distract the driver's attention. The DVLA need not be notified. Symptomatic heart failure disqualifies patients from driving large lorries and buses. Re/licensing may be permitted provided that the LV ejection fraction is good (i.e. LVEF is > 0.4), the exercise test requirements can be met and there is no other disqualifying condition.

Monitoring of heart failure patients

The clinical condition of a person with heart failure may fluctuate, and repeated admission to hospital is common. Monitoring of clinical status is necessary and this responsibility should be shared between primary and secondary care health professionals.

Essential monitoring includes assessment of:

- functional capacity (e.g. V_{O_2} max, exercise tolerance test, echocardiography)
- fluid status (body weight, U&Es, clinical)
- cardiac rhythm (ECG, 24-hour tape).

Multidisciplinary team approach

Heart failure care should be delivered by a multidisciplinary team with an integrated approach across the healthcare community. The multidisciplinary team should involve specialist healthcare professionals: heart failure nurse, dietitian, pharmacist, occupational therapist, physiotherapist, palliative care adviser.

Understanding the information needs of patients and carers is vital. Good communication is essential for best clinical management, which should include advice on anxiety, depression and 'end of life' issues.

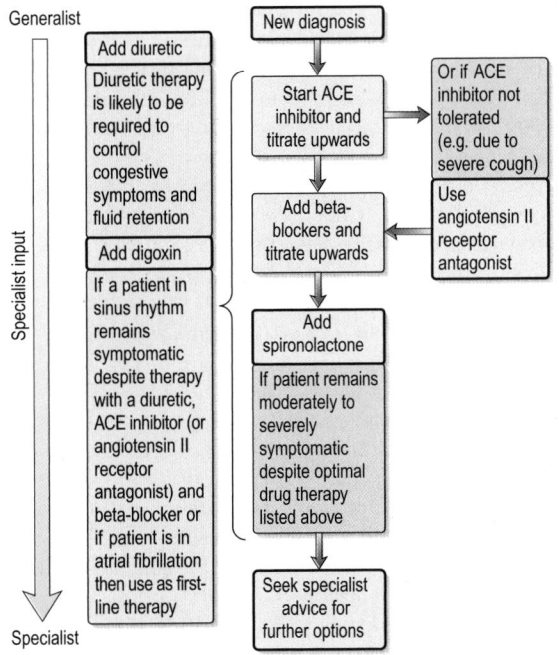

Fig. 13.57 **Heart failure treatment guidelines** (NICE (2003) Chronic heart failure. Clinical Guideline No. 5. Available from www.nice.org.uk)

Drug management (Table 13.23)

The recommendations for pharmacological treatment of heart failure are based on consensus guidelines produced by the European Society of Cardiology and NICE (UK) (Figs 13.57 and 13.58). A summary of treatment is on page 794.

Diuretics

These act by promoting the renal excretion of salt and water by blocking tubular reabsorption of sodium and chloride. The resulting loss of fluid reduces ventricular filling pressures (preload), produces consistent haemodynamic and symptomatic benefits in patients with heart failure, and rapidly improves dyspnoea and peripheral oedema. The intravenous administration of loop diuretics such as furosemide relieves pulmonary oedema rapidly by means of arteriolar vasodilatation reducing afterload, an action that is independent of its diuretic effect.

Diuretics act in various ways.

Loop diuretic (see p. 697)

Loop diuretics such as furosemide and bumetanide have a rapid onset of action (i.v. – 5 min; oral – 1–2 h) and generally short-lived (4–6 h) diuresis as the concentrating power of the kidney is reduced. These agents also produce marked potassium loss and promote hyperuricaemia, and renal function should be monitored.

Thiazide diuretics (see p. 698)

Thiazide diuretics such as bendroflumethiazide have a mild diuretic effect. Potassium excretion is enhanced. Thiazides are less effective in patients with reduced glomerular filtration rates. In some patients with severe congestive heart failure, oedema may persist despite high doses of loop diuretic. Thiazide diuretics in combination with loop diuretics have a synergistic action and greater diuretic effect. Associated metabolic abnormalities are more likely and close supervision is needed. Metolazone is a powerful thiazide, producing profound diuresis acting synergistically with loop diuretics. This combina-

Fig. 13.58 **Stages of heart failure and treatment options for systolic heart failure**. ARA, angiotensin II receptor antagonist; ACE, angiotensin-converting enzyme; VAD, ventricular assisted device. From Jessop M, Brozana S (2003) *New England Journal of Medicine* **348**: 2013, with permission. Copyright © 2003 Massachusetts Medical Society. All rights reserved.

tion is only used for the treatment of severe and resistant heart failure.

Although heart failure symptoms are improved by thiazides and loop diuretic treatment, loop diuretics are not proven to have any survival benefit. In addition, their use may be complicated by overdiuresis and electrolyte depletion (potassium and magnesium), which may predispose to the development of lethal ventricular arrhythmias, hyperkalaemia (potassium-sparing diuretics) and other metabolic disturbances (hyperuricaemia and dyslipidaemia).

Potassium-sparing diuretics (see Table 12.3)

Spironolactone is a specific competitive antagonist to aldosterone, producing a weak diuresis but with a potassium-sparing action. A randomized placebo-controlled study, the Randomized Aldactone Evaluation Study (RALES) showed a 30% reduction in all-cause mortality when spironolactone (up to 25 mg) was added to conventional treatment in patients with moderate to severe heart failure. These results have now been confirmed with another aldosterone antagonist – eplerenone – that has less hormonal side-effects. The risk of hyperkalaemia was low in the trial. Risk factors for developing hyperkalaemia include spironolactone dose > 50 mg/day, high-dose angiotensin-converting enzyme inhibitor (ACEI) and renal impairment. Potassium should be measured 5 days after the initiation of spironolactone until levels are stable and then every 1–3 months, and the dose of spironolactone should not be increased (p. 1000).

Amiloride and *triamterene* act at the distal tubule preventing potassium secretion in exchange for sodium. These drugs are weak diuretics but are useful in combination with more powerful loop diuretics. They should be avoided in the presence of renal failure and in patients taking ACE inhibitors unless there is persistent hypokalaemia. There is no evidence as yet that these two potassium-sparing diuretics have any prognostic effect.

Vasodilator therapy (see Table 13.22)

Diuretics and sodium restriction serve to activate the renin–angiotensin system, promoting formation of angiotensin (a potent vasoconstrictor) and an increase in afterload. A variety of other neural and hormonal reactions also serve to increase preload and afterload. These compensatory mechanisms are initially beneficial in maintaining blood pressure and redistributing blood flow, but in the later stages of heart failure they are deleterious and reduce cardiac output. The high venous pressures found in heart failure are also related to the activation of the sympathetic nervous system and the presence of circulating vasoconstrictors, thus shifting the Starling curve to the right.

Angiotensin-converting enzyme inhibitors ACEI
(Fig. 18.27, p. 1096)

Several large controlled trials (e.g. CONSENSUS and SOLVD), have established the benefit of ACEI in heart failure (Fig. 13.59). The trials have shown that in addition to producing considerable symptomatic improvement in patients with symptomatic heart failure, prognosis is markedly improved and development of heart failure is slowed. The SAVE study confirmed the benefit of ACEI in patients with asymptomatic heart failure following myocardial infarction, in whom the development of overt heart failure was reduced.

ACEI lower systemic vascular resistance and venous pressure, and reduce levels of circulating catecholamines, thus improving myocardial performance. The beneficial haemodynamic effect of these drugs appears to be independent of their inhibition of ACE as they are equally effective when plasma renin activity is normal.

These drugs should be carefully introduced in patients with heart failure because of the risk of first-dose hypotension. This is a particular risk in patients who are receiving large doses of diuretics and who have hyponatraemia (< 130 mmol/L). In such cases a test dose of ACEI should be commenced and the preceding diuretic doses omitted. Some of these agents are pro-drugs (e.g. enalapril) and require conversion to the active metabolite (enalaprilat) by liver enzymes; these drugs have a delayed onset of action and first-dose hypotension may not occur for several hours. Pro-drugs are best avoided if

Table 13.22 Effects of vasodilator drugs used in heart failure

	Reduction in:	
	Preload	Afterload
Nitroprusside	+	+++
Glyceryl trinitrate	+++	+
Isosorbide di/mononitrate	+++	+
β-Adrenoceptor blockers	+	++
ACE inhibitors/antagonists	++	++
Hydralazine	0	+++
Calcium-channel blockers	+	++

ACE, angiotensin-converting enzyme

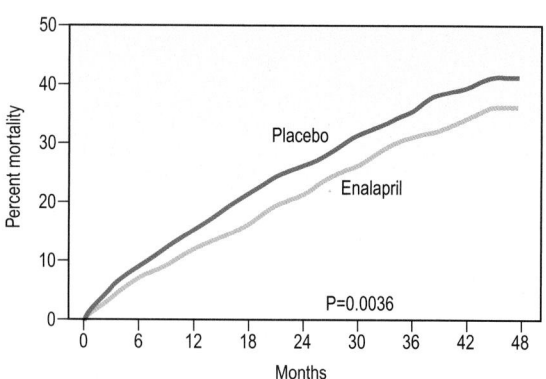

Fig. 13.59 Survival in patients with symptomatic heart failure taking placebo and enalapril (the SOLVD treatment trial). Adapted with permission from *New England Journal of Medicine* (1991) **325**: 293–302. © 1991 Massachusetts Medical Society, all rights reserved.

heart failure results in significantly altered hepatic function. Serious hypotension may result in acute renal failure. Concomitant potassium-sparing diuretics should be discontinued, as ACEI tend to promote potassium retention. Creatinine levels rise by approximately 10–15% during ACE therapy. ACEI are contraindicated in patients with bilateral renal artery stenosis. Between 10% and 15% of patients develop a cough, owing to the inhibition of bradykinin metabolism. A prospective trial looking at dose and survival (ATLAS study) showed no significant mortality difference, although high-dose treatment was associated with a significant reduction in all-cause mortality and hospitalization.

Angiotensin receptor antagonists

Angiotensin II receptor antagonists (ARA) (e.g. losartan, ibersartan, candesartan and valsartan) have similar haemodynamic effects to ACEI, but as they do not affect bradykinin metabolism, they do not produce a cough. A trial comparing losartan with the ACEI enalapril in patients with heart failure (ELITE 2) showed no difference between the AII receptor antagonist and the ACEI.

The combination of ACEI and AII receptor antagonists may confer additional benefit compared to ACEI therapy alone. The Val HeFT study of valsartan and captopril in combination showed that the use of valsartan resulted in a significant reduction in hospitalization but no difference in mortality. However, in a small number of patients (7%) valsartan alone resulted in significant reduction in mortality. The CHARM study showed the value of candesartan in heart failure with an overall 12% reduction in death and hospital admission.

Arteriolar vasodilators (Fig. 13.60)

Drugs such as α-adrenergic blockers (e.g. prazosin) and direct smooth-muscle relaxants (e.g. hydralazine) are potent arteriolar vasodilators but are not very effective in heart failure. Calcium-channel blockers also reduce after-load, but first-generation calcium antagonists (diltiazem, nifedipine) may have a detrimental effect on left ventricular function in patients with heart failure. The PRAISE 2 trial showed that the second-generation calcium antagonist amlodipine showed no prognostic benefit in patients with heart failure.

Venodilators (Fig. 13.60)

Short- and long-acting nitrates (e.g. glyceryl trinitrate and isosorbide mononitrate) act by reducing preload and lowering venous pressure, with resulting reduction in pulmonary and dependent oedema. Reduction of filling pressure does not significantly enhance cardiac output because the heart is operating on the flat portion of the ventricular filling curve. With chronic use, tolerance develops with loss of efficacy and consequent worsening of heart failure. Only combination therapy of nitrate with hydralazine (Veterans Heart Failure Trials, VHeFT) has been shown to improve mortality and exercise performance, and may be useful when ACEI are contraindicated. The benefit of vasodilators is not as great as with ACEI (VHeFT 2).

β-Adrenoceptor blocking agents

There is considerable evidence to support the use of beta-blockers in patients with chronic stable heart failure. The studies MERIT and CIBIS 2 using the beta-blockers metoprolol and bisoprolol respectively have shown improved symptomatic class, exercise tolerance, left ventricular function and mortality in patients with heart failure of any cause. The US Carvedilol Studies using carvedilol, a non-selective vasodilator beta-blocker with additional vasodilator and antioxidant properties, has also demonstrated a significant improvement in mortality. The current guidelines recommend that beta-blockers licensed for use (bisoprolol and carvedilol) in heart failure should be initiated in patients with confirmed heart failure due to left ventricular systolic dysfunction after diuretics and ACE inhibitor therapy, regardless of whether or not symptoms persist. Following the administration of beta-blockers, the ejection fraction may decline, but usually returns to baseline within a month and then increases after 3 months. Thus, initial doses should be low, e.g. carvedilol 3.125 mg twice daily and should be titrated slowly over a period of months rather than days.

Patients who are in heart failure and already on treatment with a beta-blocker for a coexisting condition, such as coronary artery disease or hypertension, should continue with their current beta-blocker initially.

Inotropic agents

Intravenous inotropes are frequently used to support myocardial function in patients with acute left ventricular failure and following cardiac surgery.

Epinephrine (adrenaline), dobutamine, dopexamine and dopamine are intravenous adrenergic agonists. *Dobutamine* predominantly acts on the β₁-adrenoceptor, increasing intracellular cyclic AMP, which in turn increases calcium availability for myocardial contraction. Dobutamine also causes peripheral vasodilatation by an

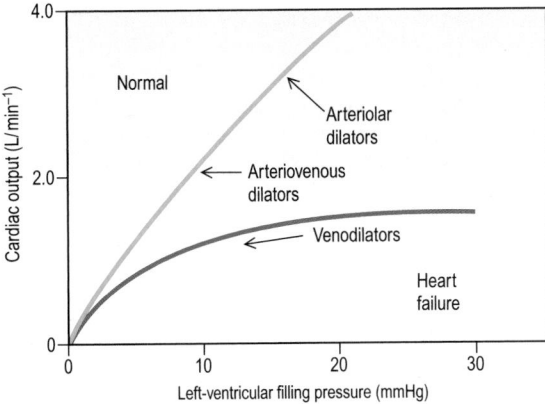

Fig. 13.60 Effect of vasodilators on cardiac output and left ventricular filling pressure in heart failure. Agents with arteriolar and arteriovenous dilating properties reduce the afterload and increase cardiac output. Venodilators reduce the left-ventricular filling pressure (and pulmonary oedema) but do not increase cardiac output.

anti-α-adrenergic effect. *Dopexamine* is a selective β$_2$ agonist with an additional action on peripheral dopamine receptors that theoretically results in improved renal perfusion. *Dopamine* is a less selective inotrope that is often used in a low dose to improve renal perfusion (via dopaminergic receptors) although this renal effect has been questioned (see p. 976).

β-Adrenergic agonists are used in patients with acute left ventricular failure and in patients with end-stage heart failure as a bridge to transplantation. Intermittent intravenous infusions of dobutamine may produce long-lasting improvements in symptoms and exercise performance at the cost of increased mortality.

Several orally active agents have been tested in patients with chronic congestive cardiac failure, but all apart from digoxin have been associated with increased mortality and are not generally used.

Digitalis glycosides

Digitalis glycosides have been used for many years in patients with heart failure and atrial fibrillation. A large prospective trial (Digoxin Investigation Group (DIG) trial) showed that digoxin combined with ACE inhibitors and diuretics, reduced death and hospitalization resulting from progressive heart failure in patients in sinus rhythm. A small significant increase in deaths presumed to be secondary to myocardial infarction and/or arrhythmia meant that the effect on overall mortality was neutral. Therefore patients who are hospitalized or present with severe heart failure in spite of therapy with vasodilators, beta-blockers, diuretics (and also patients with rapid AF), should have digoxin added to their therapeutic regimen.

The half-life of digoxin is approximately 36 hours. It is partly protein-bound, making it liable to drug interaction. As 90% is excreted unchanged in urine, accumulation can occur in renal failure. Digoxin acts as a positive inotrope by competitive inhibition of Na$^+$/K$^+$-ATPase, producing high levels of intracellular sodium. This is then exchanged for extracellular calcium. High levels of intracellular calcium result in enhanced actin–myosin interaction and increased contractility (Fig. 13.3). Digoxin also improves baroreceptor responsiveness, and reduces sympathetic activity and circulating renin.

Digoxin is administered orally (1 mg loading and 0.125–0.25 mg daily according to body mass and renal function). Trough serum levels should be monitored (1.3–2.6 nmol/L) and hypokalaemia should be avoided. The elderly and patients with hyperthyroidism are more prone to digoxin toxicity. In patients with fluctuating renal function, digitoxin, which is metabolized by the liver, is preferable.

With improvement in formulation, digoxin toxicity has become less problematic. The most common features of digoxin toxicity are:

- anorexia, nausea, altered vision
- arrhythmia (e.g. ventricular premature beats especially bigeminy, ventricular tachycardia and AV block)
- digoxin levels > 2.5 nmol/L.

Digoxin toxicity is treated by stopping the drug, restoration of serum potassium and management of arrhythmias. Digoxin antibody (FAB fragments) is a specific antidote that is useful for life-threatening toxicity (p. 1012).

β-Adrenergic agonists

Based on the demonstration that the inotropic state of the failing myocardium is impaired and that the myocardial response to adrenergic stimulation is reduced, several adrenergic agonists have been tested in heart failure. All of these agents consistently increase mortality in the longer term and are therefore restricted in use.

Anticoagulants

Heart failure is associated with a fourfold increase in the risk of a stroke. Oral anticoagulants are recommended in patients with atrial fibrillation and in sinus rhythm with a history of thromboembolism, endocardial thrombus or LV aneurysm. Large-scale prospective randomized controlled trials of antithrombotic treatment in heart failure are in progress.

Antiarrhythmic agents

Precipitating factors should be treated, in particular electrolyte disturbance. Atrial fibrillation is common in heart failure and leads to a deterioration in symptoms. Restoration of sinus rhythm, either by electrical cardioversion or drugs, is desirable but less successful in the presence of structural heart disease and decompensated heart failure. Rate control with digoxin is often preferred.

Arrhythmias are frequent in heart failure and are implicated in sudden death. Although treatment of complex ventricular arrhythmias might be expected to improve survival, there is conflicting evidence that this is so. This may be related to the diverse mechanisms of death in patients with heart failure, death commonly being associated with bradyarrhythmias, particularly in patients with non-ischaemic heart failure. Patients with sustained episodes of ventricular tachycardia should receive empirical treatment, usually with an implantable cardioverter–defibrillator (ICD).

The ICD is likely to improve the survival prospects of patients who have not yet developed serious ventricular arrhythmias and is being evaluated in the SCD-HeFT and MADIT II trials. However, it is already clear that when a life-threatening arrhythmia has already been suffered, an ICD is the best therapy to prevent mortality due to ventricular arrhythmias.

Beta-blockers, ACEI, some statins and spironolactone may reduce sudden cardiac death in patients with coronary heart disease and heart failure. It should be noted that ACEI probably exert an indirect antiarrhythmic effect by reducing high circulating levels of norepinephrine (noradrenaline) and improving cardiac function.

Summary of treatment (see Table 13.23)

All patients with clinical heart failure should receive treatment with diuretics and an ACEI followed by beta-blocker therapy. Spironolactone should be added for severe heart failure. Patients in atrial fibrillation should

Table 13.23 Summary of drug treatment for heart failure				
Medication	Symptoms	Mortality	SCD	Hospitalization
ACEI	↓↓	↓↓	?(↓)	↓↓
AIIRA	↓↓	↔	↔	?(↓)
Beta-blocker	↓↓	↓↓↓	↓↓↓	↓↓
Glycosides	↓	↔	↔	↓
Diuretics	↓↓↓	↔	↔	?
Spironolactone	↓	↓↓↓	↓↓↓	↓↓

ACEI, angiotensin-converting enzyme inhibitor; AIIRA, angiotensin-II receptor antagonists; SCD, sudden cardiac death; ↓, reduce; ↔, no change

be digitalized but patients in sinus rhythm may also be improved by the addition of digoxin or a beta-blocker. Patients with asymptomatic left ventricular dysfunction are at risk of progressive deterioration and should be treated with prophylactic ACEI therapy. Patients with ischaemic heart failure and ongoing ischaemia, and patients intolerant of ACEI or in whom they are contraindicated (hypotension, renal insufficiency or hyperkalaemia) may benefit from nitrate/hydralazine therapy.

The results of the CHARM study show benefits of candesartan (angiotensin II receptor antagonist), which may be used for heart failure treatment as an alternative to ACEI, when ACE inhibitors are ineffective or not tolerated, in patients with systolic or diastolic dysfunction. Heart failure medication must be up-titrated to the maximum dose, particularly of ACEI and beta-blocker, to obtain maximum benefit. Patients with diastolic heart failure have similar prognostic implications to those with systolic heart failure and should be treated in a similar way.

Non-pharmacological treatment of heart failure

Revascularization

While coronary artery disease is the most common cause of heart failure, the role of revascularization in patients with heart failure is unclear. Patients with angina and left ventricular dysfunction have a higher mortality from surgery (10–20%), but have the most to gain in terms of improved symptoms and prognosis. Factors that must be considered before recommending surgery include age, symptoms and evidence for reversible myocardial ischaemia.

Hibernating myocardium and myocardial stunning

'Hibernating' myocardium can be defined as reversible left ventricular dysfunction due to chronic coronary artery disease that responds positively to inotropic stress and indicates the presence of viable heart muscle that may recover after revascularization. It is due to reduced myocardial perfusion, which is just sufficient to maintain viability of the heart muscle. Myocardial hibernation results from repetitive episodes of cardiac stunning that occur, for example, with repeated exercise in a patient with coronary artery disease.

Myocardial stunning is reversible ventricular dysfunction that persists following an episode of ischaemia when the blood flow has returned to normal, i.e. there is a mismatch between flow and function.

The prevalence of hibernating myocardium in patients with coronary artery disease can be estimated from the frequency of improvement in regional abnormalities in wall motion after revascularization and is estimated to be 33% of such patients. Techniques to try to identify hibernating myocardium include stress echocardiography, nuclear imaging techniques and positron emission tomography.

The clinical relevance of the hibernating and stunned myocardium is that ventricular dysfunction due to these mechanisms may be wrongly ascribed to myocardial necrosis and scarring which seems untreatable, whereas reversible hibernating and stunning respond to coronary revascularization.

Biventricular pacemaker or implantable cardioverter-defibrillator (p. 783) (Fig. 13.61)

Pacemakers are indicated in patients with sinoatrial disease and atrioventricular conduction block. Pacemakers are also valuable in patients without AV block but with prolonged PR intervals, left bundle branch block and severe mitral regurgitation. In patients with heart failure and left bundle branch block and NYHA 3 heart failure (MUSTIC study) biventricular pacing is more beneficial than conventional right ventricular pacing. The

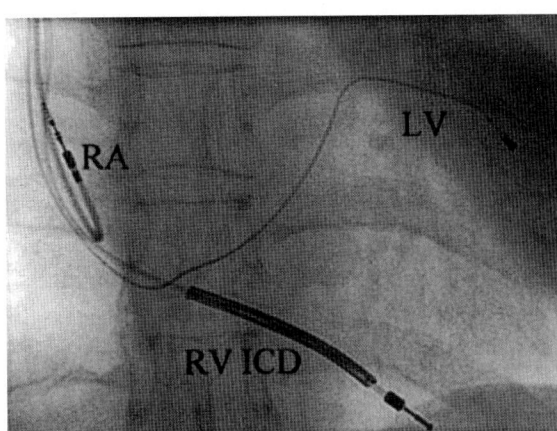

Fig. 13.61 Implanted biventricular pacing with ICD device.

results showed an improvement in symptoms and exercise tolerance. The effect on prognosis is being addressed by an ongoing trial (CARE HF).

Biventricular pacing should also be considered in patients not responding to therapy in the following situations:

- systolic heart failure
- non-reversible cause
- highly symptomatic (New York Heart Association grade 3/4)
- optimal medical therapy
- ventricular dys-synchrony: left bundle branch block QRS > 120 ms
- sinus rhythm, and possibly atrial fibrillation
- significant mitral regurgitation.

New guidelines recommend advanced pacing technologies should be used for cardiac resynchronization therapy (CRT) in selected patients with heart failure. Atrio-biventricular pacing has been shown to improve symptoms and reduce admission to hospital in patients with left bundle branch block and heart failure with poor LV function. The use of combined implantable defibrillators and atrio-biventricular pacemakers for patients with heart failure is likely to increase. One large trial (COMPANION) shows 21% reduction in all-cause mortality and all-cause admissions to hospital in the groups receiving biventricular pacing. ICD therapy in patients with NYHA (Grade 1 and 2, see Table 13.2) has shown a reduction in mortality compared with placebo and amiodarone.

Cardiac transplantation

Cardiac transplantation has become the treatment of choice for younger patients with severe intractable heart failure, whose life expectancy is less than 6 months. With careful recipient selection, the expected 1-year survival for patients following transplantation is over 90%, and is 75% at 5 years. Irrespective of survival, quality of life is dramatically improved for the majority of patients. The availability of heart transplantation is limited.

Heart allografts do not function normally. Cardiac denervation results in a high resting heart rate, loss of diurnal blood pressure variation and impaired renin–angiotensin–aldosterone regulation. Some patients develop 'stiff heart' syndrome, caused by rejection, denervation and ischaemic injury during organ harvest and implantation. Transplantation of an inappropriately small donor heart can also result in elevated right and left heart pressure.

The complications of heart transplantation are summarized in Table 13.24. Many (infection, malignancy, hypertension and hyperlipidaemia) are related to immunosuppression. Allograft coronary atherosclerosis is the major cause of long-term graft failure and is present in 30–50% of patients at 5 years. It is due to a 'vascular' rejection process in conjunction with hypertension and hyperlipidaemia.

There are specific contraindications to cardiac transplantation (Table 13.25); notably, high pulmonary

Table 13.24 Complications of cardiac transplantation

Allograft rejection	**Allograft vascular disease**
'Humoral'	
'Vascular'	**Hypertension**
'Cell-mediated'	
	Hypercholesterolaemia
Infections	
Early: nosocomial	**Malignancy**
organisms – staphylococci,	
Gram-negatives	
Late (2–6 months):	
opportunistic	
(toxoplasmosis,	
cytomegalovirus,	
fungi, *Pneumocystis*)	

Table 13.25 Contraindications for cardiac transplantation

Age > 60 years (some variations between centres)
Alcohol/drug abuse
Uncontrolled psychiatric illness
Uncontrolled infection
Severe renal/liver failure
High pulmonary vascular resistance
Systemic disease with multiorgan involvement
Treated cancer in remission but with < 5 years' follow-up
Recent thromboembolism
Other disease with a poor prognosis

vascular resistance is an absolute contraindication. Several alternatives to transplantation are available: cardiomyoplasty (augmentation of left ventricular contraction by wrapping a latissimus dorsi muscle flap around the ventricle), and the Batista procedure (surgical ventricular size reduction and remodelling the geometry of the left ventricle). Both procedures have a high mortality and limited evidence of substantial benefit in the medium term.

LVAD (left ventricular assist device) and artificial heart

Artificial hearts and left ventricular assist devices are used as bridges to transplantation or corrective surgery. Mechanical devices are also indicated if there is a possibility of spontaneous recovery; for example, acute myocarditis.

The available ventricular assist devices include extracorporeal membrane oxygenation, univentricular and biventricular extracorporeal non-pulsatile devices, extracorporeal and implantable pulsatile devices, and the total artificial heart. A recent study using a total artificial heart improved the rate of survival to cardiac transplantation and survival after transplantation in patients with irreversible biventricular failure. Although most of these devices require the patient to be connected to cumbersome extracorporeal drive systems, miniaturization of control and power-supply components has resulted in the development of wearable left ventricular assist devices.

PULMONARY OEDEMA

This is a very frightening, life-threatening emergency characterized by extreme breathlessness. The dyspnoea may first occur at night in the form of paroxysmal dyspnoea due to pulmonary congestion. This occurs because of reabsorption of dependent oedema when lying flat, and the relative insensitivity of the respiratory centre at night allows pulmonary congestion to develop.

Pathophysiology

A pressure above 20 mmHg causes increased filtration of fluid out of the capillaries into the interstitial space (interstitial oedema). Further accumulation of fluid disrupts intercellular membranes, leading to the collection of fluid in the alveolar spaces (alveolar oedema). Alveolar oedema occurs when the capillary pressure exceeds the total oncotic pressures (approximately 25 mmHg).

Clinical features

Patients with alveolar oedema are acutely breathless, wheezing, anxious and perspiring profusely. In addition, they have a cough productive of frothy, blood-tinged (pink) sputum, which can be copious. The patient is tachypnoeic with peripheral circulatory shutdown. There is a tachycardia, a raised venous pressure and a gallop rhythm. Crackles and wheezes are heard throughout the chest. The arterial Po_2 falls and initially the P_aco_2 also falls, owing to overbreathing. Later, however, the P_aco_2 increases because of impaired gas exchange. The chest X-ray shows diffuse haziness, owing to alveolar fluid, and the Kerley B lines of interstitial oedema (Fig. 13.18). The abnormality can be unilateral, giving the appearance of a tumour that disappears on treatment (a pseudotumour).

Treatment

The patient must be placed in a sitting position. High-concentration oxygen (60% via a variable performance mask) is given. In severe cases it may be necessary to ventilate (non-invasively initially) the patient (see p. 985).

Intravenous diuretic treatment with furosemide or bumetanide is given. These diuretics induce an acute venodilatory response with a reduction in preload that helps to relieve pulmonary congestion in addition to the more delayed diuretic response.

Morphine (10–20 mg i.v. depending on the size of the patient) together with an antiemetic such as metoclopramide (10 mg i.v.) is given. Morphine sedates the patient and causes systemic vasodilatation; it must be avoided if the systolic arterial pressure is less than 90 mmHg. Respiratory depression occurs with large doses of morphine.

Venous vasodilators, such as glyceryl trinitrate, may produce prompt relief by reducing the preload. Cardiac output may be increased by using arterial vasodilatation, such as occurs with hydralazine (Table 13.22 and Fig. 13.60).

Aminophylline (250–500 mg or 5 mg/kg i.v.) is infused over 10 minutes. Aminophylline is a phosphodiesterase inhibitor that causes bronchodilatation, vasodilatation and increased cardiac contractility. It must be given slowly because of the risk of precipitating ventricular arrhythmias. It is usually used when bronchospasm is present.

Venesection and mechanical methods of reducing venous return (e.g. sphygmomanometer cuffs inflated to 10 mmHg below diastolic blood pressure and placed around the thighs) are inefficient and rarely used.

In a severe case, after the acute emergency is controlled, a pulmonary artery balloon catheter may be inserted to monitor progress and treatment. Any factor that precipitated the heart failure, such as cardiac arrhythmias or chest infection, should be corrected. The underlying cardiac problem should be diagnosed and treated.

CARDIOGENIC SHOCK

Shock is a severe failure of tissue perfusion, characterized by hypotension, a low cardiac output and signs of poor tissue perfusion such as oliguria, cold extremities and poor cerebral function. Cardiogenic shock (pump failure) is commonly due to myocardial infarction (10% of MIs). Other causes are acute massive pulmonary embolus, pericardial tamponade and sudden-onset valvular regurgitation.

Diagnosis

Cardiogenic shock is diagnosed when critical impairment of tissue perfusion occurs despite an adequate or elevated pulmonary capillary wedge pressure and in the absence of mechanical circulatory obstruction. An essential element in this diagnosis is the measurement of the pulmonary capillary wedge pressure (see p. 971). In situations where the vascular capacity has expanded or the circulatory fluid volume has decreased, the wedge pressure will be low. In cardiogenic shock the wedge pressure is normal or elevated.

The mortality rate in cardiogenic shock is high, estimated at 90%, because of the vicious downward spiral that occurs: hypotension due to pump failure results in a reduction of coronary flow, which results in further impairment of pump function, and so on.

Treatment

Patients require intensive care, as described in Chapter 15. General measures such as complete rest, continuous 60% oxygen administration and pain and anxiety relief are essential.

The infusion of fluid is necessary if the pulmonary capillary wedge pressure is below 18 mmHg, which is probably the optimal 'filling pressure' with which to prime a failing heart.

Short-acting venous dilators such as glyceryl trinitrate or sodium nitroprusside should be administered intravenously if the wedge pressure is 25 mmHg or more.

Cardiac inotropes such as epinephrine (adrenaline), dobutamine and dopamine may be used to increase aortic diastolic pressure (coronary perfusion pressure). Emergency revascularization of occluded arteries for cardiogenic shock adds benefit compared with medical therapy (including intra-aortic balloon counterpulsation and thrombolytic therapy).

These lead to a temporary improvement; long-term prognosis is not improved unless there is a surgically correctable cause, such as a ruptured interventricular septum or acute mitral regurgitation.

FURTHER READING

Aurigemma SP, Gaasch WH (2004) Diastolic heart failure. *New England Journal of Medicine* **351**: 1097–1105.

Hunt SA, Baker DW, Chin MH et al. (2001) ACC/AHA guidelines for the evaluation and management of chronic heart failure in the adult: executive summary. A report of the American College of Cardiology/American Heart Association Task Force on Practice Guidelines. *Circulation* **104**: 2996–3007.

Jessup M, Brozena S (2003) Heart failure. *New England Journal of Medicine* **348**: 2007–2018.

McMurray JJV, Pfeffer MA (2005) Heart failure. *Lancet:* **365**: 1877–1889.

National Institute for Clinical Excellence (2003) *Chronic Heart Failure – Management of Chronic Sensitivity Failure in Adults in Primary and Secondary Care.* Clinical Guidelines 5. London: NICE.

Task Force for the Diagnosis and Treatment of Chronic Heart Failure, European Society of Cardiology (2001) Guidelines for the diagnosis and treatment of chronic heart failure. *European Heart Journal* **22**: 1527–1560.

ISCHAEMIC HEART DISEASE

Myocardial ischaemia occurs when there is an imbalance between the supply of oxygen (and other essential myocardial nutrients) and the myocardial demand for these substances. The causes are as follows:

Coronary blood flow to a region of the myocardium may be reduced by a mechanical obstruction that is due to:

- atheroma
- thrombosis
- spasm
- embolus
- coronary ostial stenosis
- coronary arteritis (e.g. in SLE).

There can be a decrease in the flow of oxygenated blood to the myocardium that is due to:

- anaemia
- carboxyhaemoglobulinaemia
- hypotension causing decreased coronary perfusion pressure.

An increased demand for oxygen may occur owing to an increase in cardiac output (e.g. thyrotoxicosis) or myocardial hypertrophy (e.g. from aortic stenosis or hypertension).

Myocardial ischaemia most commonly occurs as a result of obstructive coronary artery disease (CAD) in the form of coronary atherosclerosis. In addition to this fixed obstruction, variations in the tone of smooth muscle in the wall of a coronary artery may add another element of dynamic or variable obstruction.

CAD is the largest single cause of death in the UK and many parts of the world. However, over the last decade, the mortality rate in the UK has fallen considerably. Each year there are approximately 60 deaths per 100 000 (giving a standardized mortality rate of about 200 per 100 000). Sudden cardiac death is a prominent feature of CAD. One in every six coronary attacks was found to present with sudden death as the first, last, and only symptom.

The process of coronary atherosclerosis

Coronary atherosclerosis is a complex inflammatory process characterized by the accumulation of lipid, macrophages and smooth muscle cells in intimal plaques in the large and medium-sized epicardial coronary arteries. The vascular endothelium plays a critical role in maintaining vascular integrity and homeostasis. Mechanical shear stresses (e.g. from morbid hypertension), biochemical abnormalities (e.g. elevated and modified LDL, diabetes mellitus, elevated plasma homocysteine), immunological factors (e.g. free radicals from smoking), inflammation (e.g. infection such as *Chlamydia pneumoniae* and *Helicobactor pylori*) and genetic alteration may contribute to the initial endothelial 'injury' or dysfunction, which is believed to trigger atherogenesis. The development of atherosclerosis follows the endothelial dysfunction, with increased permeability to and accumulation of oxidized lipoproteins, which are taken up by macrophages at focal sites within the endothelium to produce lipid-laden foam cells. Macroscopically, these lesions are seen as flat yellow dots or lines on the endothelium of the artery and are known as '*fatty streaks*'. The 'fatty streak' progresses with the appearance of extracellular lipid within the endothelium ('*transitional plaque*'). Release of cytokines such as platelet-derived growth factor and transforming growth factor-β (TGF-β) by monocytes, macrophages or the damaged endothelium promotes further accumulation of macrophages as well as smooth muscle cell migration and proliferation. The proliferation of smooth muscle with the formation of a layer of cells covering the extracellular lipid separates it from the adaptive smooth muscle thickening in the endothelium. Collagen is produced in larger and larger quantities by the smooth muscle and the whole sequence of events cumulates as an '*advanced* or *raised fibrolipid plaque*'. The 'advanced plaque' may grow slowly and encroach on the lumen or become unstable, undergo thrombosis and produce an obstruction ('*complicated plaque*').

Two different mechanisms are responsible for thrombosis on the plaques (Fig. 13.62). The *first process* is superficial endothelial injury, which involves denudation of the endothelial covering over the plaque. Subendocardial connective tissue matrix is then exposed and platelet adhesion occurs because of reaction with

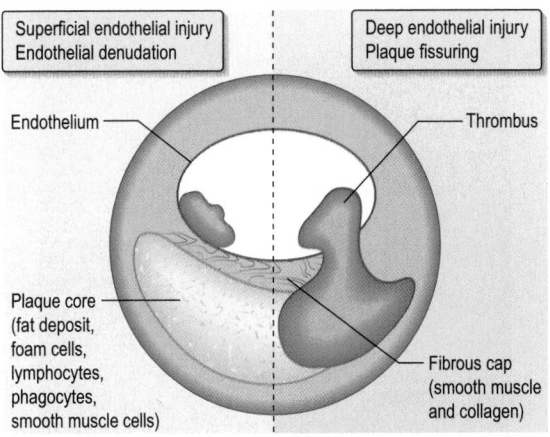

Fig. 13.62 **The mechanisms for the development of thrombosis on plaques.**

Fig. 13.64 **Acute coronary thrombus.** Cross-section (×30) of the epicardial coronary artery, demonstrating a rupture of the shoulder region of the plaque with a luminal thrombus.

collagen. The thrombus is adherent to the surface of the plaque. The *second process* is deep endothelial fissuring, which involves an advanced plaque with a lipid core. The plaque cap tears (ulcerates, fissures or ruptures), allowing blood from the lumen to enter the inside of the plaque itself. The core with lamellar lipid surfaces, tissue factor (which triggers platelet adhesion and activation) produced by macrophages and exposed collagen, is highly thrombogenic. Thrombus forms within the plaque, expanding its volume and distorting its shape. Thrombosis may then extend into the lumen.

A 50% reduction in luminal diameter (producing a reduction in luminal cross-sectional area of approximately 70%) causes a haemodynamically significant stenosis. At this point the smaller distal intramyocardial arteries and arterioles are maximally dilated (coronary flow reserve is near zero), and any increase in myocardial oxygen demand provokes ischaemia.

CAD gives rise to a wide variety of clinical presentations, ranging from relatively stable angina through to the acute coronary syndromes of unstable angina and myocardial infarction (Fig. 13.63). Figure 13.64 shows an actual plaque rupture.

Risk factors for coronary artery disease – primary and secondary prevention

CAD is an atherosclerotic disease that is multifactorial in origin, giving rise to the risk-factor concept. Certain living habits promote atherogenic traits in genetically susceptible persons. A number of 'risk' factors are known to predispose to the condition (Table 13.26). Some of these, such

Fig. 13.63 **The mechanisms for the development of thrombosis on plaques. Relationship between the state of coronary artery vessel wall and clinical syndrome.**
(a) Stable angina pectoris. **(b)** and **(c)** Acute coronary syndromes.

Table 13.26   Risk factors for coronary disease
Fixed
Age
Male sex
Positive family history
Deletion polymorphism in the ACE gene (DD)
Potentially changeable with treatment
Hyperlipidaemia
Cigarette smoking
Hypertension
Diabetes mellitus
Lack of exercise
Blood coagulation factors – high fibrinogen, factor VII
C-reactive protein
Homocysteinaemia
Personality
Obesity
Gout
Soft water
Contraceptive pill
Heavy alcohol consumption
ACE, angiotensin-converting enzyme

as age, gender, race and family history, cannot be changed, whereas other major risk factors, such as serum cholesterol, smoking habits, diabetes and hypertension, can be modified. However, not all patients with myocardial infarction are identified by these risk factors.

Atherosclerotic disease manifest in one vascular bed is often advanced in other territories. Patients with intermittent claudication have a two- to fourfold increased risk of CAD, stroke, or heart failure. Following initial myocardial infarction (MI), there is a three- to sixfold increase in the risk of heart failure and stroke. After stroke, the risk of heart failure and MI is increased twofold.

The disease can be asymptomatic in its most severe form, with one in three myocardial infarctions going unrecognized. Thirty to forty per cent of individuals who present with an acute coronary syndrome have had no prior warning symptom to suggest the presence of underlying disease.

Prevention is now feasible because epidemiological research has identified a number of modifiable predisposing lifestyles and personal attributes that, when corrected, have been shown to reduce the likelihood of the development of clinical atherosclerotic cardiovascular disease (CVD). Atherosclerotic disease begins early in life but those at high risk of CAD cannot be identified at an early age, and therefore prevention must be aimed at the whole population.

Primary prevention can be defined as the prevention of the atherosclerotic disease process and *secondary prevention* as the treatment of the atherosclerotic disease process (i.e. treatment of the disease or its complications). The objective of prevention is to reduce the incidence of first or recurrent clinical events due to CAD, ischaemic stroke and peripheral artery disease.

Traditional risk factors
Age
CAD rates increase with age. Atherosclerosis is rare in childhood, except in familial hyperlipidaemia, but is often detectable in young men between 20 and 30 years of age. It is almost universal in the elderly in the West. Atheromatous lesions in the elderly are often complicated by calcification (Fig. 13.65).

Gender
Men have a higher incidence of coronary artery disease than premenopausal women. However, after the menopause, the incidence of atheroma in women approaches that in men. The reasons for this gender difference are not clearly understood, but probably relate to the loss of the protective effect of oestrogen.

Family history
CAD is often found in several members of the same family. Because the disease is so prevalent and because other risk factors are familial, it is uncertain whether family history, per se, is an independent risk factor. A positive family history is generally accepted to refer to those in whom a first-degree relative has developed ischaemic heart disease before the age of 50 years.

Fig. 13.65 **Electron beam CT scan showing extensive calcification in left anterior descending artery and diagonal branch**. Courtesy of Dr M Rubens, Royal Brompton Hospital, London.

Smoking (see p. 893)
In men, the risk of developing CAD is directly related to the number of cigarettes smoked. It is estimated that about 20% of deaths from CAD in men and 17% of deaths from CAD in women are due to smoking. Evidence suggests that each person stopping smoking will reduce his/her own risk by 25%. The risk from smoking declines to almost normal after 10 years of abstention.

Diet and obesity (see p. 252)
Diets high in fats are associated with ischaemic heart disease, as are those with low intakes of antioxidants (i.e. fruit and vegetables). Supplementation with antioxidants has been shown to be unhelpful in RCTs (p. 247).

It is estimated that up to 30% of deaths from CAD are due to unhealthy diets. The dietary changes which would help to reduce rates of CAD include a reduction in fat, particularly saturated fat intake, a reduction in salt intake and an increase in carbohydrate intake. The consumption of fruit and vegetables should be increased by 50% to about 400 g per day, which is equivalent to at least five daily portions (see Box 5.2).

There is overwhelming evidence from clinical trials that modification of the diet has a significant impact on the risk of CVD in both the primary and secondary prevention settings.

Patients who are overweight and those who are obese have an increased risk of CAD. It is estimated that about 5% of deaths from CAD in men and that 6% of such deaths in women are due to obesity (a body mass index (BMI) of greater than 30 kg/m^2).

The adverse effect of excess weight is more pronounced when the fat is concentrated mainly in the abdomen. This is known as central obesity (visceral fat) and can be identified by a high waist to hip ratio.

Reduction in weight by diet and exercise not only lowers the incidence of CVD but also diabetes/insulin resistance. It is estimated that about 36% of deaths from CAD in men and 38% of deaths from CAD in women are due to lack of physical activity. To produce the maximum benefit the activity needs to be regular and aerobic. Aerobic activity involves using the large muscle groups in the arms, legs and back steadily and rhythmically so that breathing and heart rate are significantly increased.

It is recommended that adults should participate in a minimum of 30 minutes of at least moderate intensity activity (such as brisk walking, cycling or climbing the stairs) on 5 or more days of the week.

Hypertension

Both systolic and diastolic hypertension are associated with an increased risk of CAD. Both drug treatment and lifestyle changes – particularly weight loss, an increase in physical activity, and a reduction in salt and alcohol intake – can effectively lower blood pressure.

It is estimated that 14% of deaths from CAD in men and 12% of deaths from CAD in women are due to a raised blood pressure (defined as a systolic blood pressure of 140 mmHg or over, or a diastolic blood pressure of 90 mmHg or over) and that 6% of deaths from CAD in the UK could be avoided if the numbers of people who have high blood pressure were to be reduced by 50%.

Hyperlipidaemia (see p. 1137)

High serum cholesterol, especially when associated with a low value of high-density lipoproteins (HDL), is strongly associated with coronary atheroma. There is increasing evidence that high serum triglyceride (TG) is also independently linked with coronary atheroma.

Familial hypercholesterolaemia combined with hypertriglyceridaemia and remnant hyperlipidaemia are also associated with increased risk of coronary atherosclerosis.

Measurement of the fasting lipid profile (total cholesterol, low- and high-density lipoproteins and triglycerides) should be performed on all patients.

The risk of CAD is directly related to serum cholesterol levels. Serum cholesterol levels can be reduced by drugs, physical activity and by dietary changes, in particular a reduction in the consumption of saturated fat. It is estimated that 45% of deaths from CAD in men and 47% of deaths from CAD in women are due to a raised serum cholesterol level (in this case greater than 5.2 mmol/L) and that 10% of deaths from CAD in the UK could be avoided if everyone in the population had a serum cholesterol level of less than 6.5 mmol/L.

Different guidelines give slightly different advice for managing high levels of serum cholesterol (hyperlipidaemia). The National Service Framework for coronary heart disease in England includes guidelines on the prevention of CAD in clinical practice and suggests a cholesterol target of less than 5.0 mmol/L for both primary and secondary prevention.

High-density lipoprotein cholesterol (HDL-cholesterol) is the fraction of cholesterol that removes cholesterol (via the liver) from the blood. Low levels of HDL-cholesterol are associated with an increased risk of CAD and a worse prognosis after a heart attack. Guidelines on HDL-cholesterol generally recommend treatment for those with concentrations below 1.0 mmol/L. HDL increases with exercise, alcohol in moderation, not smoking and when TG is lowered.

A 1% reduction in cholesterol levels reduces risks of CAD by 2–3%. Hyperlipidaemia can be treated as follows:

- Statins: 24–30% reduction in mortality in primary and secondary prevention will be achieved if a flat dose of statin (pravastatin or simvastatin) is given. Up to 50% reduction is achieved if the dose of statin (atorvastatin) is titrated to achieve a target LDL of < 2.6 mmol/L.
- Fibrates result in a significant reduction in CAD events in diabetics and patients with high TG and low HDL.
- Diet: the so-called Mediterranean diet (p. 233) has resulted in a 75% reduction in CAD events in post-myocardial infarction patients.

Angiographic studies have shown that lowering the serum cholesterol can slow the progression of coronary atherosclerosis, and can cause regression of disease. Large clinical trials have shown that lipid lowering, usually with a statin, can decrease total mortality and new coronary events, and reduce the need for revascularization. Management of hypercholesterolaemia is described in detail on page 1141.

Diabetes mellitus

Diabetes, an abnormal glucose tolerance or raised fasting glucose is strongly associated with vascular disease.

Diabetes substantially increases the risk of CAD. Men with type 2 diabetes have a two- to fourfold greater annual risk of CAD, with an even higher (three- to fivefold) risk in women with type 2 diabetes.

Diabetes not only increases the risk of CAD but also magnifies the effect of other risk factors for CAD such as raised cholesterol levels, raised blood pressure, smoking and obesity.

Newer risk factors

Although there is general agreement on established cardiovascular risk factors, epidemiological research continues to identify or evaluate additional risk factors that contribute to the occurrence of atherosclerotic CVD and warrant further clarification.

Sedentary lifestyle

Lack of exercise is an independent risk factor for CAD equal to hypertension, hyperlipidaemia and smoking. Regular exercise probably protects against its development (see above).

Psychosocial well-being

Four different types of psychosocial factor have been found to be most consistently associated with an increased risk of CAD: work stress, lack of social support, depression (including anxiety) and personality (particularly hostility).

Alcohol

Moderate alcohol consumption (one or two drinks per day) is associated with a reduced risk of CAD. At high levels of intake – particularly in 'binges' – the risk of CAD is increased. It is currently advised that 'regular consumption of between three and four units a day by men' and 'between two and three units a day by women of all ages will not lead to any significant health risk'.

Genetic factors

A number of genetic factors have been linked with coronary artery disease. The angiotensin-converting enzyme (ACE) gene contains an insertion/deletion (I/D) polymorphism, the DD genotype of which has been associated with a predisposition to coronary artery disease and myocardial infarction.

Lipoprotein (a)

High plasma Lp(a) concentrations are associated with CAD and, although probably not an independent risk factor, elevated plasma Lp(a) increases the CAD risk associated with more traditional risk factors.

Coagulation factors

Serum fibrinogen is strongly, consistently, and independently related to CAD risk. The pathophysiological mechanism by which fibrinogen levels mediate coronary disease risk is related to its effect on the coagulation cascade, platelet aggregation, endothelial function and smooth muscle cell proliferation and migration.

High levels of *coagulation factor VII* are also a risk factor. Polymorphisms of the factor VII gene may increase the risk of myocardial infarction.

Homocysteine, an amino acid regulated by vitamins B_{12}, B_6 and folate, is another factor that has been associated with CAD and atherosclerosis (see p. 248). Homocysteinaemia is a major risk factor in the pathogenesis of CAD and a strong predictor of mortality in this group. Plasma levels of homocysteine are influenced by a variety of genetic and non-genetic factors. The mechanism associating hyperhomocysteinaemia with atherosclerosis is its adverse effect on vascular endothelium. Folic acid in low doses may ameliorate this process.

C-reactive protein (CRP)

CRP is linked with future risk of coronary events independently of the traditional risk factors but its use as a marker for subclinical atherosclerosis and cardiovascular risk has recently been questioned.

Non-steroidal anti-inflammatory drugs (NSAIDs)

NSAIDs that are specific inhibitors against cyclo-oxygenase-2 (COX-2) have been shown to increase cardiovascular risk and mortality. Rofecoxib has already been withdrawn.

Prevention policy

The priorities for CVD prevention in clinical practice are:

- Patients with established CAD, PVD and cerebrovascular atherosclerotic disease.
- Asymptomatic individuals who are at high risk of developing atherosclerotic disease because of multiple risk factors resulting in a 10-year risk of > 5% now (or if extrapolated to age 60) for developing a fatal event, i.e. those with markedly raised levels of single risk factors:
  - cholesterol > 8 mmol/L
  - LDL cholesterol > 6 mmol/L
  - BP > 180/110 mmHg.
- All patients with diabetes.
- Close relatives of:
  - patients with early-onset atherosclerotic cardiovascular disease
  - asymptomatic individuals at a particular high risk.
- Other individuals encountered in routine clinical practice.

How to estimate total cardiovascular risk in asymptomatic people as a guide to prevention strategies

Patients with established CVD have declared themselves to be at high total risk of further vascular events. Therefore they require the most intense lifestyle intervention, and where appropriate drug therapies.

However, in the majority of asymptomatic, apparently healthy people, preventative actions should be guided in accordance with the total CVD risk level. Indeed, risk factor management decisions should usually not be based on considerations of a single modestly raised factor.

To evaluate candidates for the major cardiovascular events cost-effectively, multivariate risk profiles have been formulated; these facilitate targeting those at high risk for preventative measures.

The Joint British Societies, the European Society of Cardiology and the American Heart Association recently emphasized the importance of these risk profiles for motivating as well as reassuring patients and in assisting in selecting therapy. They concluded that these scores direct healthcare professionals to look at the whole patient and to recognize the cumulative nature of risk factors (Fig. 13.66). However, not all practitioners agree with this approach (see pp. 803 and 804).

National Service Framework (NSF)

Plans to reduce CAD-related death in the under-75-year age group by 40% by the year 2010 by the implementation of set standards have been published in the UK by the Department of Health. The NSF includes a nurse-led audited approach to reduce CAD by lowering saturated fat intake, increasing exercise and, most relevant, decreasing/stopping smoking. The hypertension treatment targets are 140/85 mmHg in patients at risk of or with established coronary artery disease and 130/80 mmHg in diabetics. The cholesterol target is either total cholesterol of < 5.0 mmol/L (LDL-cholesterol < 3 mmol/L) or a reduction of 30% (whichever is greater).

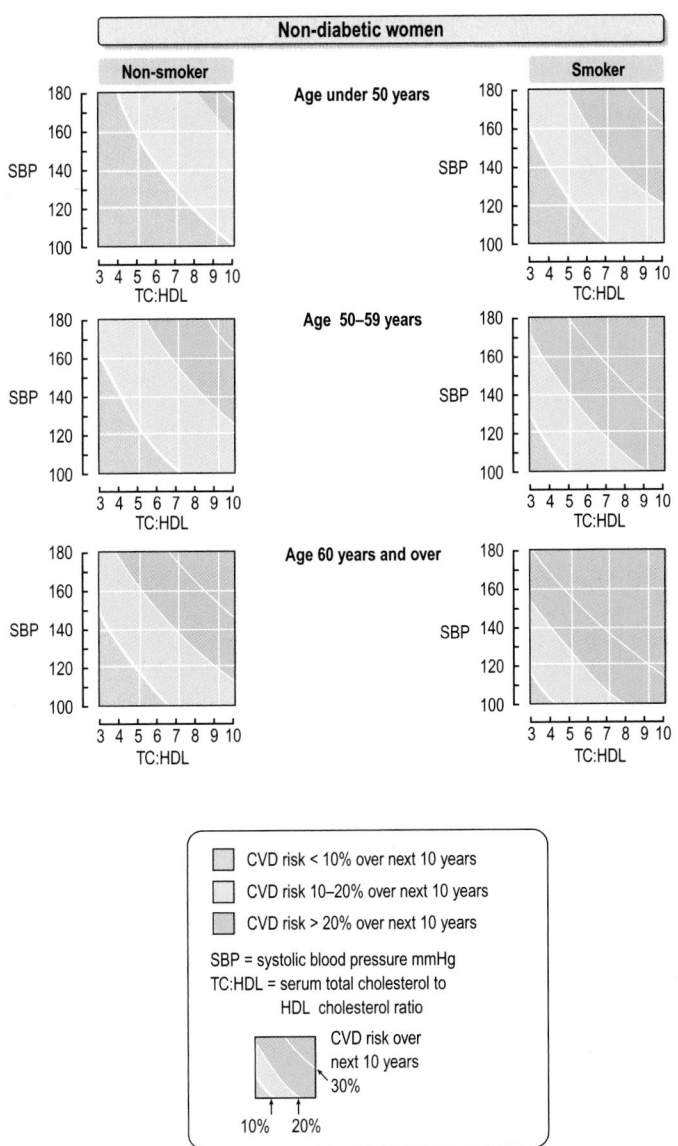

Fig. 13.66 (a) Cardiovascular risk prediction charts for women. Reproduced with permission from The University of Manchester.

Coronary artery disease in women

Until the age of 65, the prevalence of CAD is much less in women than in men and the incidence of MI in women aged 60–70 increases dramatically, corresponding to that in men. Women have a generally poorer survival post-MI than men and have 2–3% higher in-hospital mortality independent of age and other risk factors.

ANGINA (see also p. 732)

The diagnosis of angina is largely based on the clinical history. The chest pain is generally described as 'heavy', 'tight' or 'gripping'. Typically, the pain is central/ retrosternal and may radiate to the jaw and/or arms. *Angina* can range from a mild ache to a most severe pain that provokes sweating and fear. There may be associated breathlessness. CAD is common, fatal and largely preventable. More than 1.4 million people in the UK suffer from angina. CAD accounts for about 3% of all hospital admissions in England. The prevalence of angina is approximately 2% with an incidence of new cases each year approximately 1 per 1000.

Classical or exertional angina pectoris is provoked by physical exertion, especially after meals and in cold,

Fig. 13.66 **(b) Cardiovascular risk prediction charts for men.** Reproduced with permission from The University of Manchester.

windy weather, and is commonly aggravated by anger or excitement. The pain fades quickly (usually within minutes) with rest. Occasionally it disappears with continued exertion ('walking through the pain'). Whilst in some patients the pain occurs predictably at a certain level of exertion, in most patients the threshold for developing pain is variable.

Decubitus angina is that occurring on lying down. It usually occurs in association with impaired left ventricular function, as a result of severe coronary artery disease.

Nocturnal angina occurs at night and may wake the patient from sleep. It can be provoked by vivid dreams. It tends to occur in patients with critical coronary artery disease and may be the result of vasospasm.

Variant (Prinzmetal's) angina refers to an angina that occurs without provocation, usually at rest, as a result of coronary artery spasm. It occurs more frequently in women. Characteristically, there is ST segment elevation on the ECG during the pain. Specialist investigation using provocation tests (e.g. hyperventilation, cold-pressor testing or ergometrine challenge) may be required to establish the diagnosis. Arrhythmias, both ventricular tachyarrhythmias and heart block, can occur during the ischaemic episode.

Cardiac syndrome X refers to those patients with a good history of angina, a positive exercise test and angiographically normal coronary arteries. They form a heterogeneous group, and the syndrome is much more common in women than in men. Whilst they have a good prognosis, they are often highly symptomatic and can be difficult to treat. In women with this syndrome the myocardium shows an abnormal metabolic response to stress, consistent with the suggestion that the myocardial ischaemia results from abnormal dilator responses of the coronary microvasculature to stress. The prognostic and therapeutic implications are not known.

Unstable angina refers to angina of recent onset (less than 1 month), worsening angina or angina at rest, and will be described in more detail as Acute coronary syndrome on page 808.

Examination and diagnosis

There are usually no abnormal findings in angina, although occasionally a fourth heart sound may be heard. Signs to suggest anaemia, thyrotoxicosis or hyperlipidaemia (e.g. lipid arcus, xanthelasma, tendon xanthoma) should be sought. It is essential to exclude aortic stenosis (i.e. slow-rising carotid impulse and ejection systolic murmur radiating to the neck) as a possible cause for the angina. The blood pressure should be taken to identify coexistent hypertension.

Investigations for angina

Resting ECG

This is usually normal between attacks. Evidence of old myocardial infarction (e.g. pathological Q waves), left ventricular hypertrophy or left bundle branch block may be present. During an attack, transient ST depression, T-wave inversion or other changes of the shape of the T wave may appear.

Exercise ECG

Exercise testing can be very useful both in confirming the diagnosis of angina and in giving some indication as to the severity of the CAD. ST segment depression of ≥ 1 mm suggests myocardial ischaemia, particularly if typical chest pain occurs at the same time (Fig. 13.23).

The test has a specificity of 80% and a sensitivity of about 70% for CAD. A strongly positive test (within 6 minutes of starting the Bruce protocol) suggests 'prognostic' disease (see Surgical management below) and helps to identify patients who should be offered coronary angiography. Exercise testing, however, can be misleading:

- A normal test does not exclude CAD (so-called false-negative test) although these patients, as a group, have a good prognosis.
- Up to 20% of patients with positive exercise tests are subsequently found to have no evidence of coronary artery disease (so-called false-positive test).

Cardiac scintigraphy

Myocardial perfusion scans (see p. 755), both at rest and after stress (i.e. exercise or dobutamine), are helpful. Redistribution of the contrast agent is a sensitive indicator of ischaemia and can be particularly useful in deciding if a stenosis seen at angiography is giving rise to ischaemia. A normal perfusion scan makes significant CAD unlikely.

Echocardiography

This can be used to assess ventricular wall involvement and ventricular function. Regional wall motion abnormalities at rest reflect previous ventricular damage. Stress echocardiography, although technically difficult, is useful especially in women with coronary artery disease.

Coronary angiography

This is occasionally useful in patients with chest pain where the diagnosis is unclear. More often, the test is performed to delineate the exact coronary anatomy (Fig. 13.67) in patients being considered for revascularization (i.e. coronary artery bypass grafting or coronary angioplasty). Coronary angiography should be performed only when the benefit in terms of diagnosis and potential treatment outweighs the small risk of the procedure (a mortality rate of less than 1 in 1000 cases). The indications for coronary angiography are outlined in Table 13.27.

Lesions with complex morphology (irregular borders, overhanging edges, thrombus or ulceration) appear to identify a subgroup of stenoses associated with disease progression and adverse clinical outcomes.

Fig. 13.67 Left coronary angiogram. X-ray contrast material is injected into the ostium of the left main coronary artery. In this example, the left main artery divides into three vessels: left anterior descending (top), diagonal and circumflex (bottom) vessels. In the proximal part of the left anterior descending artery is a severe narrowing due to an atherosclerotic plaque (arrow).

Table 13.27 Indications for coronary angiography

Angina refractory to medical therapy
Strongly positive exercise test
Unstable angina
Angina occurring after myocardial infarction
Patients under 50 years with angina or myocardial
  infarction
Where the diagnosis of angina is uncertain
Severe left ventricular dysfunction after myocardial
  infarction
Non-Q-wave myocardial infarction

Treatment of angina

General management

Patients should be informed as to the nature of their condition and reassured that the prognosis is good (annual mortality less than 2%). Underlying problems, such as anaemia or hyperthyroidism, should be treated. Management of coexistent conditions, such as diabetes and hypertension, should be optimized. Risk factors should be evaluated and steps made to correct them where possible; for example, smoking must be stopped, hypercholesterolaemia should be identified and treated (see below), weight loss, where appropriate, and regular exercise should be encouraged.

Choosing between medical therapy and revascularization (coronary artery bypass grafting and angioplasty) can be difficult and will depend on a number of factors including symptoms, angiographic anatomy and patient/physician preference. The various treatment options are not mutually exclusive and should be considered as complementary.

Medical treatment

Prognostic therapies

Aspirin reduces the risk of coronary events in patients with coronary artery disease. All patients with angina, therefore, should take aspirin (75 mg daily is probably adequate) unless contraindicated.

Lipid-lowering therapy (see p. 1141) should be used in patients with total cholesterol above 4.8 mmol/L (particularly if the LDL is > 3.3 mmol/L and the HDL is < 1.0 mmol/L), despite a low fat diet. If the triglycerides (TGs) are under 3.5 mmol/L, then one of the statins (HMG-CoA reductase inhibitors) should be used. If the TGs are above 3.5 mmol/L, a fibrate is indicated. If simple therapy fails to reduce the LDL adequately, then the patient should be referred to a lipidologist. Lipid-lowering therapy can be expected to prevent 20–30 deaths or myocardial infarcts per 1000 patient-years.

Hormone replacement therapy (HRT) is of no value in prevention of CAD.

Symptomatic treatment

Glyceryl trinitrate (GTN) used sublingually, either as a tablet or as a spray, gives prompt relief (peak action 4–8 minutes and lasts 20–30 minutes). It can be used prior to performing activities that the patient knows will provoke angina. Transdermal GTN preparations last up to 24 hours.

All but the most mildly affected patients will probably require regular prophylactic therapy. The choice of drugs is between beta-blockers, nitrates and calcium-channel blockers. There is no commonly accepted algorithm and treatment needs to be tailored to the individual patient. Some patients will require combination therapy, but there is little evidence that adding a third drug is of benefit. Patients not controlled adequately on medical therapy should be considered for revascularization (see below).

Beta-blockers reduce the heart rate (negative chronotropic effect) and the force of ventricular contraction (negative inotropic effect), both of which reduce myocardial oxygen demand, especially on exertion. They are the drugs of choice in patients with previous myocardial infarction because of their proven benefit in secondary prevention. Atenolol, 50–100 mg daily, is the most commonly prescribed. Metoprolol, 25–50 mg twice daily, is often used if renal function is impaired. Beta-blockers may aggravate coronary artery spasm.

Long-acting nitrates (e.g. isosorbide mononitrate) are particularly useful in patients who gain relief from sublingual GTN. They reduce venous return and hence intracardiac diastolic pressures, reduce the impedance to the emptying of the left ventricle and relax the tone of the coronary arteries. Once-daily preparations are available which have a smooth pharmacokinetic profile and avoid the problem of tolerance. Nitrates should be given with care to patients on other hypotensive agents. Sildenafil (or other PDE_5 inhibitors) should not be given to patients taking nitrates.

Calcium-channel blockers block calcium flux into the cell and the utilization of calcium within the cell (Table 13.28). They relax coronary arteries, cause peripheral vasodilatation and reduce the force of left ventricular contraction, thereby reducing the oxygen demand of the myocardium. The non-dihydropyridine calcium antagonists (e.g. diltiazem and verapamil) also reduce the heart rate and are particularly useful anti-anginal agents, but should be used with caution in combination with beta-blockers. Short-acting dihydropyridines (e.g. nifedipine) can cause reflex tachycardia when used alone. Case-control studies have suggested that high-dose nifedipine is associated with adverse outcome. Slow-release formulations and the third-generation agents (e.g. amlodipine) can be used once daily and have a smooth profile of action with no significant effect on the heart rate and no significant negative inotropic effect.

Nicorandil is a potassium-channel activator with a nitrate component; it has both arterial and venous vasodilating properties. Whilst not used as a first-line drug, it is used when there are contraindications to the above agents and in refractory unstable angina.

Coronary angioplasty

Percutaneous transluminal coronary angioplasty (PTCA) refers to the technique of dilating coronary atheromatous obstructions by inflating a balloon within the obstruction (Fig. 13.68). The balloon, which is mounted on the tip of a very thin catheter, is inserted through the obstruction

(a)   (b)   (c)

Fig. 13.68 **Percutaneous transluminal coronary angioplasty (PTCA)**.
(a) Coronary angiography demonstrates a severe stenosis in the proximal left anterior descending artery (arrow).
(b) During PTCA a soft guidewire is passed across the stenosis and then a balloon is expanded that dilates the stenosis.
(c) Post-PTCA.

Table 13.28 **Calcium-channel blockers**		
	Class 1 (non-dihydropyridine) (e.g. verapamil, diltiazem)	**Class 2 (dihydropyridine) (e.g. nifedipine, nicardipine, amlodipine, felodipine, risoldipine)**
Effects		
Sinus node suppression	+++	+
AV node suppression	+++	+
Myocardial depression	++	++
Arteriolar vasodilatation	+	+++
Side-effects		
Flushing, ankle oedema, palpitations	+	++
Bradycardia, impaired AV conduction	++	+
Aggravation of heart failure	++	+
Combination with beta-blockers	No	Yes
AV, atrioventricular		

using X-ray fluoroscopy and is then inflated with dilute contrast material. Multiple inflations of the balloon using a pressure of several atmospheres usually relieve the obstruction. A number of different mechanisms have been postulated, including fracturing and compression of the plaque, and stretching of the artery. Endothelial denudation, local dissection and distal embolization also occur and may account for some of the complications of the procedure. Whilst PTCA is ideally suited to single, discrete stenoses, multiple lesions may be treated and repeat procedures can be undertaken.

Acute coronary occlusion occurs in a small proportion of cases (2–4%), and local dissection of the coronary artery is frequently observed. PTCA improves symptoms of angina, but confers no significant prognostic benefit. The risks associated with PTCA are often understated and comprise mortality (1%), acute myocardial infarction (2%), and the need for urgent coronary artery bypass grafting (CABG) (2%).

A number of trials have compared PTCA with medical therapy for stable angina. PTCA may provide more complete relief from angina, but is associated with higher rates of myocardial infarction or bypass surgery (as a result of this procedure).

Intra-coronary stents

An increasing number of intracoronary stents (Fig. 13.69) are being used both to 'bale out' in cases of dissection and for the primary treatment of stenoses in large vessels (> 3 mm; for example, proximal lesions in big left anterior descending arteries and dominant right coronary arteries), in coronary vein grafts, and in restenotic lesions following PTCA.

Fig. 13.69 **An intracoronary stent.**

Primary stenting or PTCA plus stent implantation is superior to PTCA alone for reducing cardiovascular events and the need for repeat intervention (BENESTENT). Stents have a lower incidence of restenosis, which still complicates up to 30% of PTCA (usually within the first 6 months post-procedure), but are more expensive.

Aspirin plus clopidogrel or ticlopidine are routinely prescribed following stent insertion. The use of monoclonal antibodies to the glycoprotein IIb/IIIa platelet receptor (the final common pathway of platelet aggregation) in selected high-risk cases may reduce peri-procedural complications and reduce the need for re-intervention.

Ongoing studies of new drug-eluting stents (that are coated with agents, e.g. sirolimus, paclitaxel, that reduce in-stent restenosis) and optimal antithrombotic therapies are being carried out. Intracoronary radiation therapy (on the stent) has been used to prevent and treat coronary restenosis.

Surgical management (Fig. 13.70)

There are two principal indications for coronary artery bypass grafting (CABG):

- *Symptom control* in patients who remain symptomatic despite optimal medical therapy and whose disease is not suitable for PTCA. Surgery provides dramatic relief from angina in about 90% of cases.
- *Improved survival* in patients with severe three-vessel CAD (significant proximal stenoses in all three main coronary vessels), particularly those with impaired left ventricular function, and in those with left main stem artery disease. These patients obtain prognostic benefit from CABG, irrespective of symptoms.

Where possible, the left internal mammary artery (LIMA) is used to bypass proximal stenoses in the left anterior descending artery. Similarly, the right internal mammary artery is increasingly being used to bypass stenoses in the right coronary artery. Reverse saphenous vein grafts are still commonly used in addition to arterial grafts, although the long-term patency is less good, with atheromatous occlusion occurring in up to 10% of cases per year. Operative mortality is well below 1% in patients with normal left ventricular function. Perioperative strokes occur in up to 2% of cases, and more subtle neurological deficits are common.

Off-pump coronary surgery is now performed; results show that it is as safe as on-pump surgery and causes less myocardial damage, but the graft patency rate is lower.

Minimally invasive operative procedures for bypass grafting ('MIDCAB') are being developed, including laparoscopic approaches, and may be of use in certain subgroups of patients (e.g. previous CABG and those with coexistent medical conditions which would increase the operative risks of 'full' CABG).

Aggressive lowering of LDL (to less than 2.5 mmol/L) has been shown to be beneficial in patients who have had coronary artery bypass surgery.

PTCA versus bypass surgery

Several studies have compared PTCA with bypass surgery. Both techniques provide excellent symptomatic relief with a similar incidence of major ischaemic complications. The major short-term advantage of PTCA is the avoidance of major open-heart surgery (and a shorter hospital stay). However, up to 50% of patients will require a repeat revascularization procedure within the next 2 years. There is some evidence that diabetic patients have a better 5-year survival after treatment with bypass surgery than with PTCA.

Patients with intractable angina

Some patients remain symptomatic despite medication and are not suitable for (further) revascularization. Transmyocardial laser revascularization (TMR), whereby a laser is used to form channels in the myocardium to allow direct perfusion of the myocardium from blood within the ventricular cavity has been used in some centres but in controlled trials it has not been beneficial.

Spinal cord stimulation (SCS) is accomplished using a flexible electrode in the epidural space at the midthoracic level. Stimulation via a pacemaker-like generator reduces angina and has been shown to reduce indices of ischaemia. Similarly, transcutaneous electrical nerve stimulation has been shown to reduce angina and increase exercise capacity in selected patients.

ACUTE CORONARY SYNDROMES

Acute coronary syndromes (ACS) include ST-elevation myocardial infarction (STEMI), non-ST-elevation myocardial infarction (NSTEMI), and unstable angina. Myocardial infarction occurs when cardiac myocytes die due to myocardial ischaemia, and can be diagnosed on the basis of appropriate clinical history, 12-lead ECG and elevated biochemical markers – troponin I and T, creatinine-kinase-MB (CK-MB). STEMI will be covered in the next section (p. 812).

Fig. 13.70 **Relief of coronary obstruction by surgical techniques**: coronary artery vein bypass grafting (CAVBG) or internal mammary arterial implantation (IMA). In both of these examples, the graft bypasses a coronary obstruction in the left coronary artery (LCA).

Pathophysiology

The common mechanism to all ACS is rupture or erosion of the fibrous cap of a coronary artery plaque. This leads to platelet aggregation and adhesion, localized thrombosis, vasoconstriction, and distal thrombus embolization. The presence of a rich lipid pool within the plaque and a thin fibrous cap, are associated with an increased risk of rupture. Thrombus formation and the vasoconstriction produced by platelet release of serotonin and thromboxane A_2, results in myocardial ischaemia due to reduction of coronary blood flow.

Diagnosis

Clinical presentation

Patients with an ACS may complain of a new onset of *chest pain*, chest pain *at rest*, or a deterioration of pre-existing angina. However, some patients present with *atypical features* including indigestion, pleuritic chest pain or dyspnoea. Physical examination will help to detect alternative diagnoses such as aortic dissection, pulmonary embolism or peptic ulceration and adverse clinical signs such as hypotension, basal crackles, fourth heart sound and cardiac murmurs.

Electrocardiogram

Although the 12-lead ECG may be normal in patients with an ACS, ST depression and T-wave inversion are highly suggestive of an ACS, particularly if associated with anginal chest pain. The ECG should be repeated when the patient is in pain, and continuous ST-segment monitoring is recommended. With STEMI, complete occlusion of a coronary vessel will result in persistent ST-elevation or LBBB pattern, although transient ST elevation is seen with coronary vasospasm (Prinzmetal's angina).

Biochemical markers

The measurement of the *creatinine-kinase-MB* level was until recently the standard marker for myocyte death used in ACS. However. the presence of low levels of CK-MB in the serum of normal individuals and in patients with significant skeletal muscle damage, has limited its accuracy. It can be used to determine re-infarction as levels drop back to normal after 36–72 hours.

The cardiac *troponin* complex is made up of three distinct proteins (I, T and C) that are situated with tropomyosin on the thin actin filament that forms the skeleton of the cardiac myofilament. *Troponin T* attaches the complex to tropomyosin, troponin C binds calcium during excitation–contraction coupling, and troponin I inhibits the myosin binding site on the actin.

The cardiac troponins are not detectable in normal people and so monoclonal antibody tests for cardiac-specific troponin I and cardiac-specific troponin T are highly sensitive markers of myocyte necrosis. If the initial troponin assay is negative, then it should be repeated 9–12 hours after admission. The troponin assay has prognostic information that can determine mortality risk in ACS and define which patients may benefit from aggressive medical therapy and early coronary revascularization (Fig. 13.71).

Myoglobin may be useful for a rapid diagnosis of ACS, as the levels become elevated very early in the time course of an MI, but because of the presence of myoglobin in skeletal muscle the test has poor specificity for ACS. New markers are becoming available, e.g. myeloperoxidase or glutathione peroxidase 1.

Risk stratification

Initial risk in ACS is determined by complications of the acute thrombosis. This may produce recurrent myocardial ischaemia, marked ST depression, dynamic ST changes, a raised troponin level, and be demonstrated with coronary angiography. Long-term risk is defined by clinical risk factors: age, prior myocardial infarction or bypass surgery, diabetes or heart failure. Biological markers such as C-reactive protein, fibrinogen, brain-natriuretic peptide, modified albumin and serum

Fig. 13.71 Relationship between cardiac troponin I levels and risk of death in patients with the acute coronary syndrome (ACS). From Antman EM (1996) *New England Journal of Medicine* **335**: 1342–1349.

Cardiac troponin I (ng/mL)	0 to <0.4	0.4 to <1.0	1.0 to <2.0	2.0 to <5.0	5.0 to <9.0	>9.0
(n)	831	174	148	134	50	67
Mortality (%)	1.0	1.7	3.4	3.7	6.0	7.5
Risk ratio	1.0	1.8	3.5	3.9	6.2	7.8
95% confidence interval	–	0.5–6.7	1.2–10.6	1.3–11.7	1.7–22.3	2.6–23.0

Table 13.29 The TIMI risk score in ACS

Risk factor	Score
Age > 65	1
More than three coronary artery disease risk factors – hypertension, hyperlipidaemia, family history, diabetes, smoking	1
Known coronary artery disease (coronary angiography stenosis > 50%)	1
Aspirin use in the last 7 days	1
Severe angina (more than two episodes of rest pain in 24 hours)	1
ST deviation on ECG (horizontal ST depression or transient ST elevation > 1 mm)	1
Elevated cardiac markers (CK-MB or troponin)	1

Total score	Rate of death/MI in 14 days	Rate of death/MI/urgent revascularization
0–1	3%	4.75
2	3%	8.3%
3	5%	13.2%
4	7%	19.9%
5	12%	26.2%
6–7	19%	40.9%

creatinine, can be used to further stratify patient risk. Left ventricular dysfunction and the presence of left main or triple vessel disease, significantly increase the future cardiovascular risk. The TIMI score can be used in patients with ACS to define risk (Table 13.29).

Investigation and treatment (Table 13.30)

Urgent coronary angiography is indicated for diagnosis and treatment in patients at high risk for progression to myocardial infarction or death.

Low-risk patients (no recurrence of chest pain during observation, normal ECG or minor T wave changes only, normal troponin on the initial assay and at 6–12 hours post-admission) can be managed with oral aspirin and/or clopidogrel, beta-blockers, and nitrates. An exercise test should be performed – a negative result has good prognosis, and an early positive test should direct the patient to an invasive strategy. If the patient is unable to exercise satisfactorily, or if the baseline ECG is abnormal (e.g. LVH or LBBB), then dobutamine stress echocardiography or myocardial perfusion scintigraphy is recommended.

Antiplatelet agents

The platelet is a key part of the thrombosis cascade involved in ACS. Rupture of the atheromatous plaque exposes the circulating platelets to ADP (adenosine diphosphate), thromboxane A$_2$ (TXA$_2$), epinephrine (adrenaline), thrombin, and collagen tissue factor (Fig. 13.72). This causes platelet activation, with thrombin as an especially potent stimulant of such activity. Platelet activation produces the expression of glycoprotein (GP) IIb/IIIa receptors on the platelet surface. These receptors bridge fibrinogen between adjacent platelets, causing platelet aggregates.

Aspirin blocks the formation of thromboxane A$_2$ and so prevents platelet aggregation. In ACS patients 75–150 mg aspirin reduces the relative risk of death or myocardial infarction by about 35–50% and should be given to all patients unless contra-indicated.

Ticlopidine and *clopidogrel* are thienopyridines that inhibit ADP-dependent activation of the GP IIb/IIIa

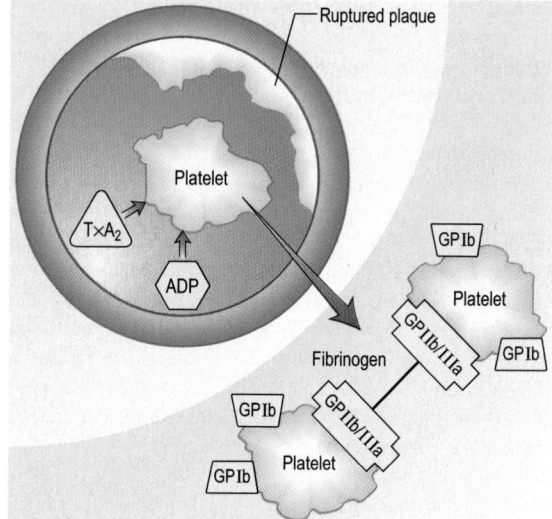

Fig. 13.72 **Platelet aggregation.** Rupture of the atheromatous plaque releases adenosine diphosphate (ADP) and thromboxane A$_2$ (TXA$_2$), which activate platelets causing expression of glycoprotein (GP) IIb/IIIa receptors on their surface. These receptors link with fibrinogen causing platelet aggregation.

complex that allows platelet aggregates to form. Although both ticlopidine and clopidogrel can be used in patients allergic to aspirin, ticlopidine does cause more systemic side-effects, including neutropenia and thrombocytopenia. In ACS patients the addition of 75 mg clopidogrel significantly reduces the risk of cardiovascular death, myocardial infarction, and stroke but increases the risk of bleeding and the evidence of benefit is not compelling.

Activated GP IIb/IIIa receptors on platelets bind to fibrinogen, initiating platelet aggregation (Fig. 13.72). Receptor antagonists have been developed that are powerful inhibitors of platelet aggregation. *Abciximab* is a monoclonal antibody that binds tightly and has a long half-life. *Eptifibatide* is a cyclic peptide that selectively inhibits GP IIb/IIIa receptors, but has a short half-life and wears off in 2–4 hours. *Tirofiban* is a small non-peptide

Table 13.30 Pharmacological therapy in acute coronary syndromes

Drug	Dose	Notes
General myocardial oxygenation		
Oxygen	35–50%	Check ABG in severe COPD
Antiplatelet		
Aspirin	150–300 mg chewable or soluble aspirin, then 75–100 mg p.o. daily	Give PPI with dyspepsia history
Clopidogrel	300 mg p.o. loading dose, then 75 mg p.o. daily	Caution – increased risk of bleeding, avoid if CABG planned
Analgesia		
Diamorphine	2.5–5.0 mg i.v.	Prescribe with antiemetic, metoclopramide 10 mg i.v.
Myocardial energy consumption		
β blockers	e.g. Atenolol 5 mg i.v. repeated after 15 min, then 25–50 mg p.o. daily	Avoid in asthma, heart failure, hypotension, bradyarrhythmias
	or Metoprolol 5 mg i.v. repeated to a maximum of 15 mg, then 25–50 mg p.o. twice daily	Avoid in asthma, heart failure, hypotension, bradyarrhythmias
Coronary vasodilatation		
Glyceryl trinitrate	2–10 mg/h i.v./buccal/or sublingual	Maintain systolic BP above 90 mmHg
Plaque stabilization/ventricular remodelling		
HMG-CoA reductase inhibitors (statins)	e.g. Simvastatin 20–40 mg p.o. daily Pravastatin 20–40 mg p.o. daily Atorvastatin 80 mg p.o. daily	Combine with dietary advice and modification
ACE inhibitors	e.g. Ramipril 2.5–10 mg p.o. daily Lisinopril 5–10 mg p.o. daily	Monitor renal function
Plus for non-ST-elevation myocardial infarction (NSTEMI)		
Antithrombin		
Low-molecular-weight heparins	Enoxaparin 1 mg/kg s.c. twice daily	
Glycoprotein IIB/IIIA inhibitors		
Abciximab	0.25 mg/kg i.v. bolus, then 0.125 mg/kg/min up to 10 mg/min i.v. for 12 h	If coronary intervention likely within 24 h
Eptifibatide	180 mg/kg i.v. bolus, then 2 mg/kg/min i.v. for 72 h	Indicated in high-risk patients managed without coronary intervention or during PCI
Tirofiban	0.4 mg/kg/min i.v. for 30 min, then 0.1 mg/kg/min for 48–108 h	Indicated in high-risk patients managed without coronary intervention or during PCI
Plus for ST-elevation myocardial infarction (STEMI)		
Thrombolysis		
Streptokinase or	1 500 000 units i.v. over 60 min	Antibodies appear after 4 days, which reduces effectiveness
Alteplase (rt-PA) or	15 mg i.v. bolus, then 50 mg over 30 min and 35 mg over 60 min	Dose modification if < 65 kg or 6–12 h post-MI Prescribe LMW heparin i.v. for 48 h
Tenecteplase (TNKase) or	30–50 mg i.v. bolus according to weight	Prescribe LMW heparin i.v. for 48 h or enoxaparin 1 mg/kg twice daily
Reteplase	10 units i.v. bolus repeated after 30 min	Prescribe LMW heparin i.v. for 48 h

ABG, arterial blood gases; CABG, coronary artery bypass grafting; COPD, chronic obstructive pulmonary disease; PCI, percutaneous coronary intervention; PPI, proton pump inhibitor

that rapidly blocks the GP IIb/IIIa receptors, and is reversible in 4–6 hours.

In ACS patients tirofiban reduces the 30-day death or myocardial infarction rate from 7.1% (placebo) to 5.8%.

Troponin-positive patients with diabetes scheduled to have coronary intervention benefit most from GP IIb/IIIa receptor antagonists.

Antithrombins

In ACS patients off aspirin, *low-molecular-weight heparins* (and in particular enoxaparin) can be given subcutaneously twice daily and have replaced unfractionated heparin. They produce a lower rate of refractory angina/myocardial infarction and death than placebo, and when used with aspirin reduce death from myocardial infarction from 10.3% to 7.9%.

Anti-ischaemia agents

In patients with no contraindications (asthma, AV-block, acute pulmonary oedema), beta-blockers are administered intravenously or orally, to reduce myocardial ischaemia by blocking circulating catecholamines. This will reduce the heart rate and blood-pressure, reducing myocardial oxygen consumption. The dose can be titrated to produce a resting heart rate of 50–60 b.p.m.

In patients with ongoing angina, nitrates should be given by either the sublingual, buccal, or intravenous route. They effectively reduce preload and produce coronary vasodilatation. However, tolerance can become a problem, and intravenous administration should be gradually stopped if the patient's symptoms resolve.

Plaque stabilization/remodelling

HMG-CoA reductase inhibitor drugs (statins) and ACE-inhibitors are routinely administered to patients with ACS. These agents may produce plaque stabilization, improve vascular and myocardial remodelling, and reduce future cardiovascular events. Starting the drugs whilst the patient is still in hospital increases the likelihood of patients receiving secondary drug therapy.

Coronary intervention

Coronary revascularization is recommended in high-risk patients with ACS. Coronary stenting may stabilize the disrupted coronary plaque and reduces angiographic restenosis rates compared to PTCA alone.

Pre-procedure clopidogrel and the peri-procedure GP IIb/IIIa inhibitors significantly reduce the complication rate of coronary intervention.

The current rate of CABG in ACS is low (5.4%). The mortality rates with CABG are greater in the high-risk group patients, particularly with a recent myocardial infarction.

Single vessel lesions are usually treated with percutaneous coronary intervention (PCI), unless the anatomy is unfavourable. Conversely, patients with left main stem or triple vessel disease with impaired left ventricular function are best managed with surgery.

Comparing a conservative strategy (coronary intervention only for severe and recurrent angina) versus an interventional strategy (early coronary angiography and intervention) in patients with ACS, the interventional approach significantly reduces the mortality rate, as well as reducing the rate of myocardial infarction, recurrent angina, and hospital readmission. Patients with an increased level of troponin obtain most benefit.

Post-ACS

After the initial management of the ACS (diagnosis, treatment, investigation, revascularization), risk factor modification is necessary to reduce future cardiovascular events.

- Patients should be encouraged to stop cigarette smoking and should be referred to a smoking cessation clinic.
- The patient should maintain optimal weight, exercise daily for 30 minutes, and have a healthy diet.
- Hypertension should be treated to a level < 130/85.
- In patients with diabetes, glycaemic control should be very tight (HbA_{1c} < 7%, p. 1117).
- Low-fat diets should be combined with HMG-CoA reductase inhibitors to reduce LDL cholesterol.

Medication on discharge should include aspirin (clopidogrel), statin, beta-blocker, and an ACE-inhibitor, with a GTN spray for symptomatic relief of angina.

ST ELEVATION MYOCARDIAL INFARCTION (STEMI)

Myocardial infarction occurs when cardiac myocytes die due to prolonged myocardial ischaemia. The diagnosis can be made in patients with an appropriate clinical history together with findings from repeated 12-lead ECGs and elevated biochemical markers – troponin I and T, CK-MB.

Pathophysiology

Rupture or erosion of a vulnerable coronary artery plaque can produce prolonged occlusion of a coronary artery leading to myocardial necrosis within 15–30 minutes. The subendocardial myocardium is initially affected but with continued ischaemia the infarct zone extends through to the subepicardial myocardium, producing a transmural Q-wave myocardial infarction. Early reperfusion may salvage regions of the myocardium, reducing future mortality and morbidity.

The 1-month mortality in patients with a myocardial infarction may be as high as 50% in the community, with 50% of deaths occurring in the first 2 hours of the event. In the pre-thrombolytic era the in-hospital mortality rate was nearly 20% but with modern therapy may be as low as 6–7% at 1 month. Several risk factors can be identified that predict death rate at 30 days (TIMI STEMI score – Table 13.31).

Diagnosis

Symptoms and signs

Any patient presenting with *severe chest pain* lasting more than 20 minutes may be suffering from a myocardial infarction. The pain may not respond to sublingual GTN, and opiate analgesia may be required. The pain may radiate to the left arm, neck or jaw. However, in some patients, particularly with elderly or diabetic patients, the symptoms may be atypical and include *dyspnoea, fatigue,* pre-syncope or *syncope.* Autonomic symptoms are common and on examination the patient may be pale and clammy, with marked sweating. In addition, the pulse may be thready with significant hypotension, bradycardia or tachycardia.

Electrocardiography

An ECG in patients with chest pain should be performed on admission to A&E. The baseline ECG is rarely normal, but if so should be repeated every 15 minutes while the

Table 13.31 TIMI risk score in ST elevation myocardial infarction (STEMI)

Risk factor	Score
Age > 65	2
Age > 75	3
History of angina	1
History of hypertension	1
History of diabetes	1
Systolic BP < 100	3
Heart rate > 100	2
Killip II–IV	2
Weight > 67 kg	1
Anterior MI or LBBB	1
Delay to treatment > 4 hours	1

Total score	Risk of death at 30 days
0	0.8%
1	1.6%
2	2.2%
3	4.4%
4	7.3%
5	12.4%
6	16.1%
7	23.4%
8	26.8%
9–16	35.9%

patient remains in pain. Continuous cardiac monitoring is required because of the high likelihood of significant cardiac arrhythmias. ECG changes (Table 13.32) are usually confined to the ECG leads that 'face' the infarction. The presence of new ST elevation ≥ 0.2 mV at the J-point in leads V_1–V_3, and ≥ 0.1 mV in other leads, suggests anterior MI (Fig. 13.73). An inferior wall MI is diagnosed when ST elevation is seen in leads II, III and AVF (Fig. 13.74). Lateral MI produces changes in leads I, AVL and V_5/V_6. In patients with a posterior MI, there may be ST depression in leads V_1–V_3 with a dominant R wave, and ST elevation in lead V_5/V_6. New LBBB or presumed new LBBB is compatible with coronary artery occlusion requiring urgent reperfusion therapy. The evolution of the ECG during the course of STEMI is illustrated in Figure 13.75.

Investigations

Blood samples should be taken for cardiac troponin I or T levels or CK-MB level according to local hospital

Table 13.32 Typical ECG changes in myocardial infarction (STEMI)

Infarct site	Leads showing ST elements
Anterior:	
Small	V_3–V_4
Extensive	V_2–V_5
Anteroseptal	V_1–V_3
Anterolateral	V_4–V_6, I, AVL
Lateral	I, AVL
Inferior	II, III, AVF
Posterior	V_1, V_2 (reciprocal)
Subendocardial	Any lead
Right ventricle	VR_4

protocol, although treatment should not be deferred until the results are available. Full blood count, serum electrolytes, glucose, and lipid profile should be obtained. Transthoracic echocardiography (TTE) may be helpful to confirm a myocardial infarction, as wall-motion abnormalities are detectable early in STEMI. TTE may detect alternative diagnoses such as aortic dissection, pericarditis, or pulmonary embolism.

Early medical management (Table 13.30)
Accident and emergency
Rapid triage for chest pain (N.B. Time is muscle)

- aspirin 150–300 mg chewed
- sublingual glyceryl trinitrate 0.3–1 mg. Repeat
- oxygen – nasal cannula 2–4 L/min (Fig. 15.22)
- brief history/risk factors. Examination
- intravenous access + blood for markers (plus FBC, biochemistry, lipids, glucose)
- 12 lead ECG
- intravenous opiate, e.g. diamorphine 2.5–5 mg + anti-emetic, e.g. metoclopramide 10 mg
- beta-blocker (if no contra-indication) for ongoing chest pain, hypertension, tachycardia
- if primary PCI available (see p. 815) give GP IIb/IIIa inhibitor. Alternatively give thrombolysis (see below).

Pre-hospital treatment, including thrombolysis, can be given by trained healthcare professions under strict guidelines.

Fibrinolysis
Fibrinolytic agents enhance the breakdown of occlusive thromboses by the activation of plasminogen to form plasmin. The initial thrombolytic agent used in clinical trials was streptokinase. This agent is derived from bacteria, which can lead to the development of neutralizing antibodies that limit its repeated use. In the ISIS 2 study of acute myocardial infarction, patients were randomized to receive a 1-hour intravenous infusion of 1.5 million units of streptokinase, or 1 month of 160 mg/day enteric-coated aspirin, both active treatments, or neither. Both streptokinase and aspirin were significantly better than placebo in reducing vascular mortality at 5 weeks (9.2% versus 12.0%, and 9.4% versus 11.8% respectively). The combination of streptokinase and aspirin was significantly better than either agent alone.

The GISSI 2 and ISIS 3 studies showed no significant difference in the effectiveness of streptokinase and tissue plasminogen activator (t-PA) or anistreplase. In addition there was no mortality benefit from subcutaneous unfractionated heparin versus no heparin.

In the GUSTO trial, accelerated t-PA over 90 minutes with intravenous heparin reduced death by 10/1000 patients versus streptokinase, although there were three more strokes in the t-PA group versus streptokinase and subcutaneous heparin.

In the meta-analysis of fibrinolytics (FTT), fibrinolysis within 6-hours of STEMI or LBBB MI, prevented 30 deaths/1000 patients treated. Between 7 and 12 hours 20/1000 deaths were prevented. After 12 hours the benefits are limited, and there is evidence to suggest less

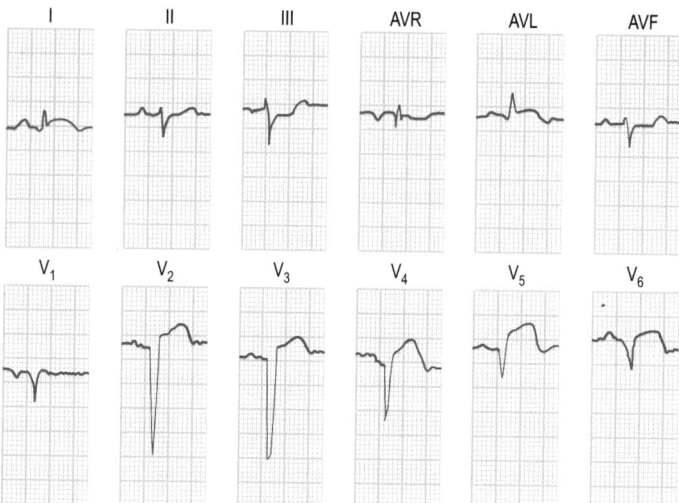

Fig. 13.73 **An acute anterolateral myocardial infarction** shown by a 12-lead ECG. Note the ST segment elevation in leads I, AVL, and V_2–V_6. The T wave is inverted in leads I, AVL and V_3–V_6. Pathological Q waves are seen in leads V_2–V_6.

Fig. 13.74 **An acute inferior wall myocardial infarction** shown by a 12-lead ECG. Note the raised ST segment and Q waves in the inferior leads (II, III and AVF). The additional T wave inversion in V_4 and V_5 probably represents anterior wall ischaemia.

benefit for older patients, possibly because of the increased risk of strokes.

Prompt reperfusion therapy (door to needle time < 30 min) will reduce the death rate following myocardial infarction. Double bolus r-PA (reteplase) and single bolus TNK-t-PA (tenecteplase) facilitate rapid administration of fibrinolytic therapy and can be used for pre-hospital thrombolysis. In patients that fail to reperfuse by 60–90 minutes as demonstrated by 50% resolution of the ST segment elevation, re-thrombolysis or referral for rescue coronary angioplasty is recommended.

Aspirin therapy should be prescribed with fibrinolysis, but there is little additional benefit in combining clopidogrel or abciximab therapy in patients with STEMI/new LBBB. Heparin is recommended with t-PA or tenecteplase, but not with streptokinase. Enoxaparin (low molecular weight heparin) appears to be superior to unfractionated i.v. heparin in patients receiving TNK-t-PA, with less reocclusion and better late patency (ASSENT 3).

The contraindications to thrombolysis are provided in Table 13.33.

Percutaneous coronary intervention (PCI)

PCI performed within 90 minutes is the preferred reperfusion therapy in interventional cardiology centres

Table 13.33	Contraindications to thrombolysis
Absolute contraindications	**Relative contraindications**
Haemorrhagic stroke or stroke of unknown origin at any time	Transient ischaemic attack in preceding 6 months
Ischaemic stroke in preceding 6 months	Oral anticoagulant therapy
Central nervous system damage or neoplasms	Pregnancy or within 1 week postpartum
Recent major trauma/surgery/head injury (within preceding 3 weeks)	Non-compressible punctures
Gastrointestinal bleeding within the last month	Traumatic resuscitation
Known bleeding disorder	Refractory hypertension (systolic blood pressure > 180 mmHg)
Aortic dissection	Advanced liver disease
	Infective endocarditis

Coronary stenting in primary PCI reduces the need for repeat target vessel revascularization but does not appear to reduce mortality rates.

The use of abciximab in STEMI patients undergoing primary angioplasty reduces immediate outcome (death, myocardial infarction, urgent revascularization), but this benefit is minimal by 6-months.

PCI following thrombolysis was discouraged but a recent trial suggests it is safe and improves the 1-year clinical outcome.

Coronary artery bypass surgery

Cardiac surgery is usually reserved for the complications of myocardial infarction such as ventricular septal defect or mitral regurgitation.

Complications of myocardial infarction

Heart failure

Cardiac failure post-STEMI is a poor prognostic feature that necessitates medical and invasive therapy to reduce the death rate. The Killip classification is used to assess patients with heart failure post-MI:

- Killip I – no crackles and no third heart sound
- Killip II – crackles in < 50% of the lung fields or a third heart sound
- Killip III – crackles in > 50% of the lung fields
- Killip IV – cardiogenic shock.

Mild heart failure may respond to intravenous furosemide 40–80 mg i.v., with GTN administration if the blood pressure is satisfactory. Oxygen is required, with regular oxygen monitoring. ACE-inhibitors can be given in < 24–48 hours if the blood pressure is satisfactory. Patients with severe heart failure may require Swan–Ganz catheterization to determine the pulmonary wedge pressure. Intravenous inotropes such as dopamine or dobutamine are used in patients with severe heart failure. If the patient is in cardiogenic shock, then revascularization ± intra-aortic balloon pump insertion, may be required.

Myocardial rupture and aneurysmal dilatation

Rupture of the free wall of the left ventricle is usually an early, catastrophic and fatal event. The patient will have a haemodynamic collapse, then an electromechanical cardiac arrest. A subacute rupture may allow for pericardiocentesis followed by the surgical repair of the rupture. Aneurysmal dilatation of the infarcted myocardium (Figs 13.76 and 13.17) is a late complication that may require surgical repair.

Ventricular septal defect (VSD)

A VSD may occur in 1–2.0% of patients with STEMI, and may be associated with delayed or failed fibrinolysis. However, mortality is very high with a 12-month unoperative mortality of 92%. An intra-aortic balloon pump (IABP) and coronary angiography may allow for patient optimization prior to surgery.

Mitral regurgitation

Severe mitral regurgitation can occur early in the course

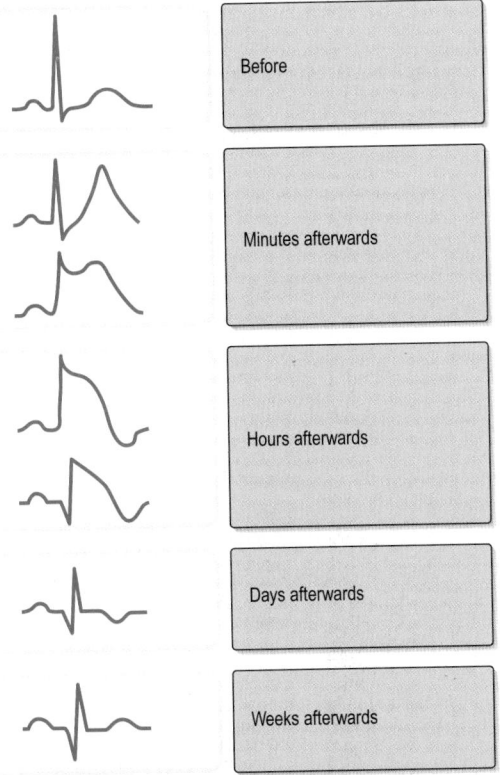

Fig. 13.75 Electrocardiographic evolution of myocardial infarction (STEMI). After the first few minutes the T waves become tall, pointed and upright and there is ST segment elevation. After the first few hours the T waves invert, the R wave voltage is decreased and Q waves develop. After a few days the ST segment returns to normal. After weeks or months the T wave may return to upright but the Q wave remains.

that have the expertise available. In the PAMI (Primary Angioplasty in Myocardial Infarction) trial, patients with a myocardial infarction who presented within 12 hours of the onset of STEMI were randomized to primary PTCA or tissue-type plasminogen activator (t-PA) followed by conservative care. At 2-year follow-up the primary PTCA group had less recurrent ischaemia, lower re-intervention rates and reduced hospital readmission rates. Primary PTCA produced a combined end-point of death or re-infarction of 14.9% compared to 23% for t-PA.

The DANAMI 2 study investigated if rapid transfer of patients with STEMI for primary angioplasty in an interventional centre was superior to thrombolysis. Patients within 12 hours of a high-risk STEMI (> 4 mm elevation) received front-loaded t-PA, primary angioplasty at a local centre, or primary angioplasty at an interventional centre after transfer. Primary PCI significantly reduced the death rate in both local and transferred patients as compared to thrombolytic therapy (8.0% versus 13.7%). The majority of the benefits with primary PCI are obtained by a reduction in recurrent myocardial infarction.

Fig. 13.76 **Two-dimensional echocardiogram (apical four-chamber view) showing a very large apical left ventricular aneurysm** (arrowed).The relatively static blood in the aneurysm produces a swirling 'smoke' effect. This aneurysm was successfully resected surgically. LV, left ventricle; LA, left atrium; RV, right ventricle; RA, right atrium.

of STEMI. Three mechanisms may be responsible for the mitral regurgitation, and a transoesophageal echo-cardiogram (TOE) may be necessary to confirm the aetiology:

- severe left ventricular dysfunction and dilatation, causing annular dilatation of the valve and subsequent regurgitation
- myocardial infarction of the inferior wall, producing dysfunction of the papillary muscle that may respond to coronary intervention
- myocardial infarction of the papillary muscles, pro-ducing sudden severe pulmonary oedema and cardiogenic shock (IABP, coronary angiography, and early surgery may improve patient survival).

Cardiac arrhythmias

Ventricular tachycardia and ventricular fibrillation are common in STEMI, particularly with reperfusion. Cardiac arrest requires defibrillation. Ventricular tachycardia should be treated with intravenous beta-blockers (metoprolol 5 mg, esmolol 25–200 μg/kg/min), lidocaine 50–100 mg, or amiodarone 900–1200 mg per 24 hours. If the patient is hypotensive, synchronized cardioversion may be performed. Ensure that the serum potassium is above 4.5 mmol/L. Refractory ventricular tachycardia or fibrillation may respond to magnesium 8 mmol/L over 15 minutes i.v.

Atrial fibrillation occurs frequently and treatment with beta-blockers and digoxin may be required. Cardio-version is possible but relapse is frequent.

Bradyarrhythmias can be treated initially with i.v. atropine 0.5 mg repeated up to six times in 4 hours. Temporary transcutaneous or transvenous pacemaker insertion may be required in patients with symptomatic heart block.

Conduction disturbances

These are common following MI. AV block may occur during acute MI, especially of the inferior wall (the right coronary artery usually supplies the SA and AV nodes). Heart block, when associated with haemodynamic compromise, may need treatment with atropine or a temporary pacemaker. Such blocks may last for only a few minutes, but frequently continue for several days. Permanent pacing may need to be considered if heart block persists for over 2 weeks.

Post-MI pericarditis and Dressler's syndrome

See Pericardial disease, page 854.

Post-MI drug therapy

Extensive clinical trial evidence has been gathered in post-myocardial infarction patients demonstrating that a range of pharmaceuticals are advantageous in reducing mortality over the following years. Therefore, post-MI most patients should be taking the following medications:

- aspirin 75–100 mg/day
- beta-blocker to maintain heart rate < 60 b.p.m., e.g. metoprolol 50 mg twice daily
- oral nitrates if there is angina, e.g. isosorbide mononitrate 20 mg twice daily
- ACE-inhibitors, e.g. ramipril 2.5 mg twice daily
- statins, e.g. simvastatin 20–80 mg twice daily.

Post-STEMI assessment and risk factor modification

Post-MI, most patients need to modify their lifestyle to reduce the likelihood of future cardiac events, with the same recommendations as for ACS.

If primary angioplasty has not been performed, then it is necessary to identify residual ischaemia and viability, to determine the need for coronary angiography. Uncomplicated patients with no angina during the hospital stay should have a low-level exercise test prior to discharge followed by a formal ETT 6 weeks later. A positive test usually suggests diagnostic/therapeutic coronary angiography/stenting. Alternatively, nuclear scintigraphy or dobutamine stress echocardiography can be used at 5 days to determine the amount of viable myocardium and the extent of myocardial ischaemia. Echocardiography should be performed to guide therapy and to determine baseline ejection fraction. In a patient with an ejection fraction < 30%, ventricular tachycardia on a Holter monitor may warrant an ICD.

SUDDEN CARDIAC DEATH
(see also Table 13.7)

Sudden cardiac death is generally defined as death due to cardiac causes which occurs within 6 hours of the onset of symptoms. The causes of sudden cardiac death tend to mirror, in risk factors and prevalence, the predominant cardiac causes of death in a given population. In developed countries, the majority (80%) are estimated to be due to coronary artery disease, a further 10–15% to cardiomyopathies and 5% to valvular heart disease. Post-mortem studies have revealed that coronary atheroma is present in 80–90% of cases. Forty per cent of all deaths due to coronary atherosclerosis occur suddenly in this way, although up to 50% of patients dying suddenly because of coronary atheroma have no preceding history of coronary disease. The majority of cases of sudden death due to atheroma appear to be due to fatal ventricular arrhythmia, sometimes triggered by acute myocardial ischaemia. Other less common causes of sudden cardiac death are listed in Table 13.34. Patients presenting with a cardiac arrest require immediate cardiopulmonary resuscitation as outlined in Figure 13.35. In those patients that survive a cardiac arrest, an implantable cardioverter–defibrillator is often required, to prevent further cardiac arrest. Antiarrhythmic drugs such as amiodarone may be used as an alternative to an implantable cardioverter–defibrillator but are less effective.

Table 13.34 Causes of sudden cardiac death
Coronary artery disease
Acute myocardial infarction – STEMI
Chronic ischaemic heart disease
Following coronary artery bypass surgery
After successful resuscitation for cardiac arrest
Congenital anomaly of coronary arteries
Coronary artery embolism
Coronary arteritis
Non-coronary artery disease
Hypertrophic cardiomyopathy
Dilated cardiomyopathy (ischaemic or idiopathic)
Arrhythmogenic right ventricular cardiomyopathy
Congenital long QT syndrome
Brugada's syndrome
Valvular heart disease (aortic stenosis, mitral valve prolapse) ± infective endocarditis
Cyanotic heart disease (tetralogy of Fallot, transposition)
Acyanotic heart disease (ventricular septal defect, patent ductus arteriosus)

FURTHER READING
Backer GD et al. (2003) Third Joint Task Force of European and other Societies on CVD Prevention in Clinical Practice. *European Heart Journal* **24**: 1601–1610.

Bertrand ME et al. (2002) Task Force on the Management of Acute Coronary Syndromes of the European Society of Cardiology. Management of acute coronary syndromes in patients presenting without persistent ST-segment elevation. *European Heart Journal* **23**(23): 1809–1840.

Braunwald E et al. (2002) ACC/AHA 2002 guideline update for the management of patients with unstable angina and non–ST-segment elevation myocardial infarction: a report of the American College of Cardiology/American Heart Association Task Force on Practice Guidelines (Committee on the Management of Patients With Unstable Angina). *Journal of the American College of Cardiology* **40**(7): 1366–1374.

Gibbons RJ et al. (2003) ACC/AHA 2002 guideline update for the management of patients with chronic stable angina – summary article: a report of the American College of Cardiology/American Heart Association Task Force on Practice Guidelines (Committee on the Management of Patients With Chronic Stable Angina). *Circulation* **107**(1): 149–158.

Hansson SK (2005) Inflammation, atherosclerosis and coronary artery disease. *New England Journal of Medicine* **352**: 1685–1695.

National Service Framework for Coronary Heart Disease (2000) Department of Health. Online. Available: http://www.doh.gov.uk/nsf/CAD.htm.

VALVULAR HEART DISEASE

MITRAL STENOSIS

Almost all mitral stenosis is due to rheumatic heart disease.

At least 50% of sufferers have a history of rheumatic fever or chorea. The single most common valve lesion due to rheumatic fever is pure mitral stenosis (50%) (Table 13.35). The mitral valve is affected in over 90% of those with rheumatic valvular heart disease. Rheumatic mitral stenosis is much more common in women. The pathological process results after some years in valve thickening, cusp fusion, calcium deposition, a narrowed (stenotic) valve orifice and progressive immobility of the valve cusps.

Other causes include:

- Lutembacher's syndrome, which is the combination of acquired mitral stenosis and an atrial septal defect
- a rare form of congenital mitral stenosis
- in the elderly, a syndrome similar to mitral stenosis, which develops because of calcification and fibrosis of the valve, valve ring and subvalvular apparatus (chordae tendineae)
- carcinoid tumours metastasizing to the lung, or primary bronchial carcinoid.

Pathophysiology

When the normal valve orifice area of 5 cm^2 is reduced to approximately 1 cm^2, severe mitral stenosis is present. In order that sufficient cardiac output will be maintained, the left atrial pressure increases and left atrial hyper-trophy and dilatation occur. Consequently, pulmonary venous, pulmonary arterial and right heart pressures also increase. The increase in pulmonary capillary pressure is

Table 13.35 Rheumatic valvular lesions	
Valves involved	**Percentage of cases**
Mitral valve alone	50
Mitral and aortic valves	40
Mitral, aortic and tricuspid	5
Aortic valve alone	2
All other combinations	3

Table 13.36	Complications of mitral stenosis

Atrial fibrillation
Systemic embolization
Pulmonary hypertension
Pulmonary infarction
Chest infections
Infective endocarditis (rare)
Tricuspid regurgitation
Right ventricular failure

followed by the development of pulmonary oedema. This is partially prevented by alveolar and capillary thickening and pulmonary arterial vasoconstriction (reactive pulmonary hypertension). Pulmonary hypertension leads to right ventricular hypertrophy, dilatation and failure. Right ventricular dilatation results in tricuspid regurgitation. Mitral stenosis is frequently associated with complications (Table 13.36).

Symptoms

Usually there are no symptoms until the valve orifice is moderately stenosed (i.e. has an area of 2 cm^2). In Europe this does not usually occur until several decades after the first attack of rheumatic fever, but children of 10–20 years of age in the Middle or Far East may have severe calcific mitral stenosis.

Because of *pulmonary venous hypertension* and recurrent bronchitis, progressively *severe dyspnoea* develops. A cough productive of blood-tinged, frothy sputum is quite common, and occasionally frank haemoptysis may occur. The development of pulmonary hypertension eventually leads to *right heart failure* and its symptoms of weakness, *fatigue* and abdominal or lower limb swelling.

The large left atrium favours *atrial fibrillation*, giving rise to symptoms such as palpitations. Atrial fibrillation may result in *systemic emboli*, most commonly to the cerebral vessels resulting in neurological sequelae, but mesenteric, renal and peripheral emboli are also seen. Clinical pulmonary embolism as a result of mitral stenosis associated with atrial fibrillation is less commonly seen, but it is likely that subclinical pulmonary emboli occur.

Signs (see Clinical memo in Fig. 13.77)

Face

Severe mitral stenosis with pulmonary hypertension is associated with the so-called mitral facies or malar flush. This is a bilateral, cyanotic or dusky pink discoloration over the upper cheeks that is due to arteriovenous anastomoses and vascular stasis.

Pulse

Mitral stenosis may be associated with a small-volume pulse which is usually regular early on in the disease process when most patients are in sinus rhythm. However, as the severity of the disease progresses, many patients develop atrial fibrillation resulting in an irregularly irregular pulse. The development of atrial fibrillation in these patients often causes a dramatic clinical deterioration.

Jugular veins

If right heart failure develops, there is obvious distension of the jugular veins. If pulmonary hypertension or tricuspid stenosis is present, the *a* wave will be prominent provided that atrial fibrillation has not supervened.

Palpation

There is a tapping impulse felt parasternally on the left side. This is the result of a palpable first heart sound combined with left ventricular backward displacement produced by an enlarging right ventricle. A sustained parasternal impulse due to right ventricular hypertrophy may also be felt.

Auscultation

Auscultation (Fig. 13.77) reveals a loud first heart sound if the mitral valve is pliable, but it will not occur in calcific mitral stenosis. As the valve suddenly opens with the force of the increased left atrial pressure, an 'opening snap' will be heard. This is followed by a low-pitched 'rumbling' mid-diastolic murmur best heard with the bell of the stethoscope held lightly at the apex with the patient lying on the left side. If the patient is in sinus rhythm, the murmur becomes louder at the end of diastole as a result of atrial contraction (presystolic accentuation).

The severity of mitral stenosis is judged clinically on the basis of several criteria:

- The presence of pulmonary hypertension implies that mitral stenosis is severe. Pulmonary hypertension is recognized by a right ventricular heave, a loud pulmonary component of the second heart sound, with eventually signs of right-sided heart failure, such as oedema and hepatomegaly. Pulmonary hypertension results in pulmonary valvular regurgitation that causes an early diastolic murmur in the pulmonary area known as a Graham Steell murmur.
- The closeness of the opening snap to the second heart sound is proportional to the severity of mitral stenosis.
- The length of the mid-diastolic murmur is proportional to the severity.
- As the valve cusps become immobile, the loud first heart sound softens and the opening snap disappears. When pulmonary hypertension occurs, the pulmonary component of the second sound is increased in intensity and the mitral diastolic murmur may become quieter because of the reduction of cardiac output.

Investigations

Chest X-ray

The chest X-ray usually shows a generally small heart with an enlarged left atrium (Fig. 13.16, p. 742). Pulmonary venous hypertension is usually also present. Late in the course of the disease a calcified mitral valve may be seen on a penetrated or lateral view. The signs of pulmonary oedema or pulmonary hypertension may also be apparent when the disease is severe.

Electrocardiogram

In sinus rhythm the ECG shows a bifid P wave owing to

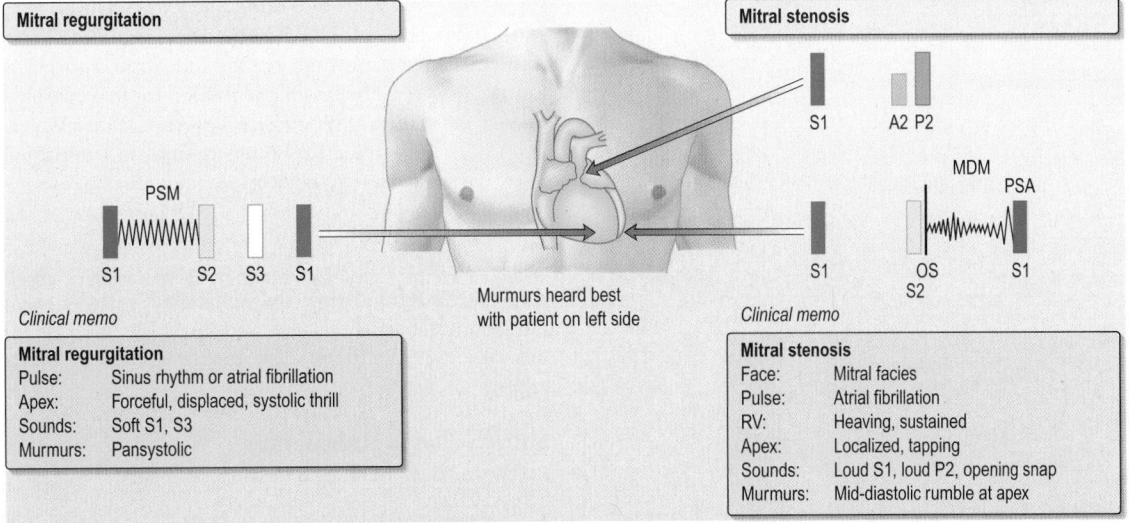

Fig. 13.77 Features associated with mitral regurgitation and mitral stenosis. A2, aortic component of the second heart sound; MDM, mid-diastolic murmur; OS, opening snap; P2, pulmonary component of the second heart sound; PSA, presystolic accentuation; PSM, pansystolic murmur; S1, first heart sound; S2, second heart sound; S3, third heart sound.

delayed left atrial activation (Fig. 13.78). However, atrial fibrillation is frequently present. As the disease progresses, the ECG features of right ventricular hypertrophy (right axis deviation and perhaps tall R waves in lead V_1) may develop (Fig. 13.79).

Echocardiogram (Fig. 13.29)

Two-dimensional echocardiography allows assessment of the mitral valve apparatus and calculation of mitral valve area, thus providing a useful guide in determining whether balloon valvotomy or valve replacement is the treatment of choice in patients symptomatic on medical therapy. Two-dimensional echocardiography also determines left atrial and right ventricular size and function. Continuous wave (CW) Doppler may also be used to measure mitral valve area and provides an estimate of pulmonary artery pressure through measurement of the degree of tricuspid regurgitation. In most cases, echocardiography alone is sufficient to judge the severity of mitral stenosis such that decisions regarding surgery can be made.

Cardiac catheterization

This is required only if an adequate echocardiogram (transthoracic or transoesophageal) is impossible to obtain or if coexisting cardiac problems (e.g. mitral regurgitation or coronary artery disease) are suspected. The typical findings in mitral stenosis are a diastolic pressure that is higher in the left atrium than in the left ventricle (Fig. 13.80). This gradient of pressure is usually proportional to the degree of the stenosis.

Treatment

Mild mitral stenosis may need no treatment other than prompt therapy of attacks of bronchitis. Although

Fig. 13.78 A bifid P wave as seen on the ECG in mitral stenosis (P mitrale). Also shown for comparison are other P wave abnormalities.

Fig. 13.79 Severe mitral stenosis shown by a 12-lead ECG. Note the right axis deviation (frontal plane axis = + 120°), the left atrial conduction abnormality (large terminal negative component of the P wave in V_1) and the right ventricular hypertrophy (R wave in V_1 and right axis deviation).

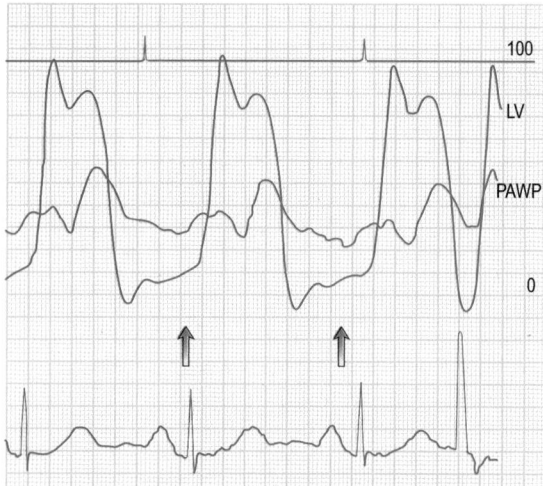

Fig. 13.80 Simultaneous recordings of the ECG, the left ventricular (LV) and the pulmonary arterial wedge pressure (PAWP). The PAWP is almost equivalent to the left atrial pressure. Thus at end-diastole (the onset of the QRS complex) the PAWP is significantly higher than the LV pressure (arrows). The pressure gradient is due to mitral valve stenosis. PAWP is also known as PAOP (occlusion pressure).

infective endocarditis in pure mitral stenosis is uncommon, antibiotic prophylaxis is advised (see p. 31). Early symptoms of mitral stenosis such as mild dyspnoea can usually be treated with low doses of diuretics. The onset of atrial fibrillation requires treatment with digoxin and anticoagulation to prevent atrial thrombus and systemic embolization. If pulmonary hypertension develops or the symptoms of pulmonary congestion persist despite therapy, surgical relief of the mitral stenosis is advised. There are four operative measures.

Trans-septal balloon valvotomy

A catheter is introduced into the right atrium via the femoral vein. The inter-atrial septum is then punctured and the catheter advanced into the left atrium and across the mitral valve. A balloon is passed over the catheter to lie across the valve, and then inflated briefly to split the valve commissures. The procedure is performed under local anaesthesia in the cardiac catheter laboratory. As with other valvotomy techniques, significant regurgitation may result, necessitating valve replacement (see below). This procedure is ideal for patients with pliable valves in whom there is little involvement of the subvalvular apparatus and in whom there is minimal mitral regurgitation. The procedure cannot be performed when there is heavy calcification or more than mild mitral regurgitation. The presence of thrombus in the left atrium is a contraindication to balloon valvotomy; therefore, transoesophageal echocardiography must be performed prior to this technique in order that left atrial thrombus can be excluded.

Closed valvotomy

This operation is advised for patients with mobile, non-calcified and non-regurgitant mitral valves. The fused cusps are forced apart by a dilator introduced through the apex of the left ventricle and guided into position by the surgeon's finger inserted via the left atrial appendage. Cardiopulmonary bypass is not needed for this operation. Closed valvotomy may produce a good result for 10 years or more. The valve cusps often re-fuse and eventually another operation may be necessary.

Open valvotomy

This operation is often preferred to closed valvotomy. The cusps are carefully dissected apart under direct vision. Cardiopulmonary bypass is required. Open dissection reduces the likelihood of causing traumatic mitral regurgitation.

Mitral valve replacement

Replacement of the mitral valve is necessary if:

- mitral regurgitation is also present
- there is a badly diseased or badly calcified stenotic valve that cannot be reopened without producing significant regurgitation
- there is moderate or severe mitral stenosis and thrombus in the left atrium despite anticoagulation.

Artificial valves (see p. 827) may work successfully for more than 20 years. Anticoagulants are generally necessary to prevent the formation of thrombus, which might obstruct the valve or embolize.

MITRAL REGURGITATION

Of the many causes of mitral valve regurgitation, rheumatic heart disease (50%) and a prolapsing mitral valve are the most common. There are many other causes, which include:

- aortic valve disease
- acute rheumatic fever
- myocarditis
- dilated cardiomyopathy
- hypertensive heart disease
- ischaemic heart disease
- infective endocarditis – mitral regurgitation may result from destruction of the mitral valve leaflets
- hypertrophic cardiomyopathy – left ventricular contraction is disorganized and mitral regurgitation often results
- connective tissue disorders – systemic lupus erythematosus (SLE) may cause mitral regurgitation
- collagen abnormalities – Marfan's syndrome and Ehlers–Danlos syndrome cause mitral regurgitation
- degeneration of the valve cusps or mitral annular calcification – results in mitral regurgitation
- rupture of the chordae tendineae (due to myocardial infarction, infective endocarditis or trauma) – results in acute and very severe mitral regurgitation
- drugs, e.g. fenfluramine is associated with mitral regurgitation.

Pathophysiology

Regurgitation into the left atrium produces left atrial

dilatation but little increase in left atrial pressure if the regurgitation is long-standing, as the regurgitant flow is accommodated by the large left atrium. With acute mitral regurgitation the normal compliance of the left atrium does not allow much dilatation and the left atrial pressure rises. Thus, in acute mitral regurgitation the left atrial *v* wave is greatly increased and pulmonary venous pressure rises to produce pulmonary oedema. Since a proportion of the stroke volume is regurgitated, the stroke volume increases to maintain the forward cardiac output and the left ventricle therefore enlarges.

Symptoms

Mitral regurgitation can be present for many years and the cardiac dimensions greatly increased before any symptoms occur. The increased stroke volume is sensed as a 'palpitation'. *Dyspnoea and orthopnoea* develop owing to pulmonary venous hypertension occurring as a direct result of the mitral regurgitation and secondarily to left ventricular failure. *Fatigue and lethargy* develop because of the reduced cardiac output. In the late stages of the disease the *symptoms of right heart failure* also occur and eventually lead to congestive cardiac failure. *Cardiac cachexia* may develop. Thromboembolism is less common than in mitral stenosis, but *subacute infective endocarditis* is much more common.

Signs (see Clinical memo in Fig. 13.77)

The physical signs of uncomplicated mitral regurgitation are:

- laterally displaced (forceful) diffuse apex beat and a systolic thrill (if severe)
- soft first heart sound, owing to the incomplete apposition of the valve cusps and their partial closure by the time ventricular systole begins
- pansystolic murmur, owing to the occurrence of regurgitation throughout the whole of systole, being loudest at the apex but radiating widely over the precordium and into the axilla

- prominent third heart sound, owing to the sudden rush of blood back into the dilated left ventricle in early diastole (sometimes a short mid-diastolic flow murmur may follow the third heart sound).

The signs related to atrial fibrillation, pulmonary hypertension, and left and right heart failure develop later in the disease. The onset of atrial fibrillation has a much less dramatic effect on symptoms than in mitral stenosis.

Investigations

Chest X-ray

The chest X-ray may show left atrial and left ventricular enlargement. There is an increase in the CTR, and valve calcification is seen.

Electrocardiogram

The ECG shows the features of left atrial delay (bifid P waves) and left ventricular hypertrophy (Fig. 13.81) as manifested by tall R waves in the left lateral leads (e.g. leads I and V_6) and deep S waves in the right-sided precordial leads, (e.g. leads V_1 and V_2). (Note that SV_1 plus RV_5 or RV_6 > 35 mm indicates left ventricular hypertrophy.) Left ventricular hypertrophy occurs in about 50% of patients with mitral regurgitation. Atrial fibrillation may be present.

Echocardiogram

The echocardiogram shows a dilated left atrium and left ventricle. There may be specific features of chordal or papillary muscle rupture. CW Doppler can determine the velocity of the regurgitant jet.

The echocardiogram is not as definitive in mitral regurgitation as in mitral stenosis. However, useful information regarding the severity of the condition can be obtained indirectly by observing the dynamics of ventricular function. Transoesophageal echocardiography (TOE) helps to identify structural valve abnormalities before surgery. Intraoperative TOE can also aid assessment of the efficacy of valve repair.

Fig. 13.81 **Left ventricular hypertrophy** shown in a 12-lead ECG. Note the size of the S wave seen in V_1 (21 mm); S in V_1 + R in V_6 = > 35 mm.

Cardiac catheterization

This demonstrates a prominent left atrial systolic pressure wave, and when contrast is injected into the left ventricle it is seen regurgitating into an enlarged left atrium during systole.

Treatment

Mild mitral regurgitation in the absence of symptoms can be managed conservatively by following the patient with serial echocardiograms. Prophylaxis against endocarditis is required (see p. 31). Any evidence of progressive cardiac enlargement generally warrants early surgical intervention by either mitral valve repair or replacement. The advantages of surgical intervention are diminished in more advanced disease. In patients who are not considered appropriate for surgical intervention, or in whom surgery will be considered at a later date, management usually involves treatment with ACE inhibitors, diuretics and possibly anticoagulants. Sudden torrential mitral regurgitation, as seen with chordal or papillary muscle rupture or infective endocarditis, necessitates emergency mitral valve replacement.

Prolapsing (billowing) mitral valve

This is also known as Barlow's syndrome or floppy mitral valve. It is due to excessively large mitral valve leaflets, an enlarged mitral annulus, abnormally long chordae or disordered papillary muscle contraction. Histology may demonstrate myxomatous degeneration of the mitral valve leaflets. It is more commonly seen in young women than in men or older women and it has a familial incidence. Its cause is unknown but it is associated with Marfan's syndrome, thyrotoxicosis, rheumatic or ischaemic heart disease. It also occurs in association with atrial septal defect and as part of hypertrophic cardiomyopathy. Mild mitral valve prolapse is so common that it should be regarded as a normal variant.

Pathophysiology

During ventricular systole, a mitral valve leaflet (most commonly the posterior leaflet) prolapses into the left atrium. This may result in abnormal ventricular contraction, papillary muscle strain and some mitral regurgitation. Usually the syndrome is not haemodynamically serious. Thromboembolism occurs.

Symptoms

Atypical chest pain is the most common symptom. Usually the pain is left submammary and stabbing in quality. Sometimes it is substernal, aching and severe. Rarely it is similar to typical angina pectoris. *Palpitations* may be experienced because of the abnormal ventricular contraction or because of the atrial and ventricular arrhythmias that are commonly associated with mitral valve prolapse. Sudden cardiac death due to fatal *ventricular arrhythmias* is a very rare but recognized complication.

Signs

The most common sign is a mid-systolic click, which is produced by the sudden prolapse of the valve and the tensing of the chordae tendineae that occurs during systole. This may be followed by a late systolic murmur owing to some regurgitation. With more regurgitation, the murmur becomes pansystolic mitral regurgitation.

Investigations

Chest X-ray

The chest X-ray is usually normal unless significant mitral regurgitation is present.

Electrocardiogram

Non-specific ST/T wave changes have been described in 15–30% of cases, but there is no evidence that this is more than in the general population.

Echocardiogram

The diagnosis is confirmed on two-dimensional echocardiography, which typically shows posterior movement of one or both mitral valve cusps into the left atrium during systole.

Cardiac catheterization

Contrast angiograms performed during cardiac catheterization reveal the systolic prolapse of the mitral valve into the left atrium, and mitral regurgitation, if present, is seen. This investigation is not normally required.

Treatment

Usually, beta-blockade is effective for the treatment of the atypical chest pain and palpitations. Sometimes more specific antiarrhythmic drug treatment is necessary. When a prolapsing mitral valve is associated with significant mitral regurgitation and atrial fibrillation, anticoagulation is advised to prevent thromboembolism. Mitral valve prolapse associated with severe mitral regurgitation has a risk of sudden cardiac death. Mitral valve repair is indicated in all such cases. Very occasionally, mitral valve replacement rather than repair may be necessary for severe regurgitation when there is severe prolapse of both leaflets. Prophylaxis against endocarditis (see p. 31) is advised if there is significant mitral valve regurgitation.

AORTIC STENOSIS

Congenital aortic valve stenosis develops progressively because of turbulent blood flow through a congenitally abnormal (usually bicuspid) aortic valve. Most congenitally abnormal aortic valves occur in men and will calcify later in life.

Rheumatic fever results in progressive fusion, thickening and calcification of a previously normal three-cusped aortic valve. In rheumatic heart disease the aortic valve is affected in about 40% of cases and there is usually associated mitral valve disease.

Calcific valvular disease is the commonest cause of aortic stenosis and mainly occurs in the elderly. This is an inflammatory process involving macrophages and T lymphocytes

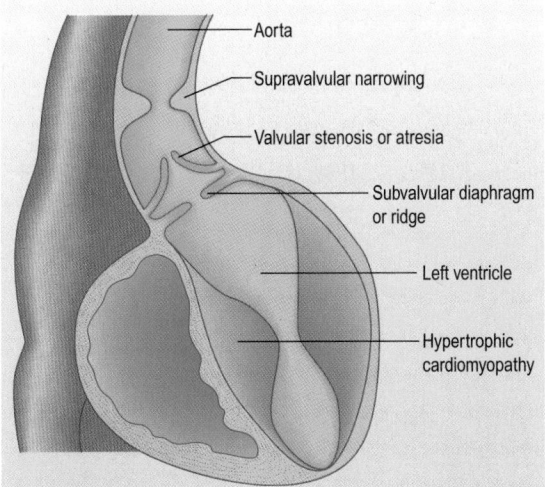

Aorta

Supravalvular narrowing

Valvular stenosis or atresia

Subvalvular diaphragm or ridge

Left ventricle

Hypertrophic cardiomyopathy

Fig. 13.82 **Several forms of left ventricular outflow tract obstruction.**

with initially thickening of the subendothelium with adjacent fibrosis. The lesions contain lipoproteins which calcify, increasing leaflet stiffness and reducing systolic opening.

Valvular aortic stenosis should be distinguished from other causes of obstruction to left ventricular emptying (Fig. 13.82), which include:

- supravalvular obstruction – a congenital fibrous diaphragm above the aortic valve often associated with mental retardation and hypercalcaemia (William's syndrome)
- hypertrophic cardiomyopathy – septal muscle hypertrophy obstructing left ventricular outflow
- subvalvular aortic stenosis – a congenital condition in which a fibrous ridge or diaphragm is situated immediately below the aortic valve.

Pathophysiology

Obstructed left ventricular emptying leads to increased left ventricular pressure and compensatory left ventricular hypertrophy. In turn, this results in relative ischaemia of the left ventricular myocardium, and consequent angina, arrhythmias and left ventricular failure. The obstruction to left ventricular emptying is relatively more severe on exercise. Normally, exercise causes a many-fold increase in cardiac output, but when there is severe narrowing of the aortic valve orifice the cardiac output can hardly increase. Thus, the blood pressure falls, coronary ischaemia worsens, the myocardium fails and cardiac arrhythmias develop. Left ventricular systolic function is typically preserved in patients with aortic stenosis (cf. aortic regurgitation).

Symptoms

There are usually no symptoms until aortic stenosis is moderately severe (when the aortic orifice is reduced to one-third of its normal size). At this stage, *exercise-induced syncope*, *angina* and *dyspnoea* develop. When symptoms

occur, the prognosis is poor – on average, death occurs within 2–3 years if there has been no surgical intervention.

Signs (see Clinical memo in Fig. 13.83)

Pulse

The carotid pulse is of small volume and is slow-rising or plateau in nature (see p. 736).

Precordial palpation

The apex beat is not usually displaced because hypertrophy (as opposed to dilatation) does not produce noticeable cardiomegaly. However, the pulsation is sustained and obvious. A double impulse is sometimes felt because the fourth heart sound or atrial contraction ('kick') may be palpable. A systolic thrill may be felt in the aortic area.

Auscultation

The most obvious auscultatory finding in aortic stenosis is an ejection systolic murmur that is usually 'diamond-shaped' (crescendo–decrescendo). The murmur is usually longer when the disease is more severe, as a longer ejection time is needed. The murmur is usually rough in quality and best heard in the aortic area. It radiates into the carotid arteries and also the precordium. The intensity of the murmur is not a good guide to the severity of the condition because it is lessened by a reduced cardiac output. In severe cases, the murmur may be inaudible.

Other findings include:

- systolic ejection click (see p. 739), unless the valve has become immobile and calcified
- soft or inaudible aortic second heart sound when the aortic valve becomes immobile
- reversed splitting of the second heart sound (splitting on expiration) (see p. 740)
- prominent fourth heart sound (see p. 739), unless coexisting mitral stenosis prevents this.

Investigations
Chest X-ray

The chest X-ray usually reveals a relatively small heart with a prominent, dilated, ascending aorta. This occurs because turbulent blood flow above the stenosed aortic valve produces so-called 'post-stenotic dilatation'. The aortic valve may be calcified. The CTR increases when heart failure occurs.

Electrocardiogram

The ECG shows left ventricular hypertrophy and left atrial delay. A left ventricular 'strain' pattern due to 'pressure overload' (depressed ST segments and T wave inversion in leads orientated towards the left ventricle, i.e. leads I, AVL, V_5 and V_6) is common when the disease is severe. Usually, sinus rhythm is present, but ventricular arrhythmias may be recorded.

Echocardiogram

The echocardiogram readily demonstrates the thickened, calcified and immobile aortic valve cusps. Left ventricular

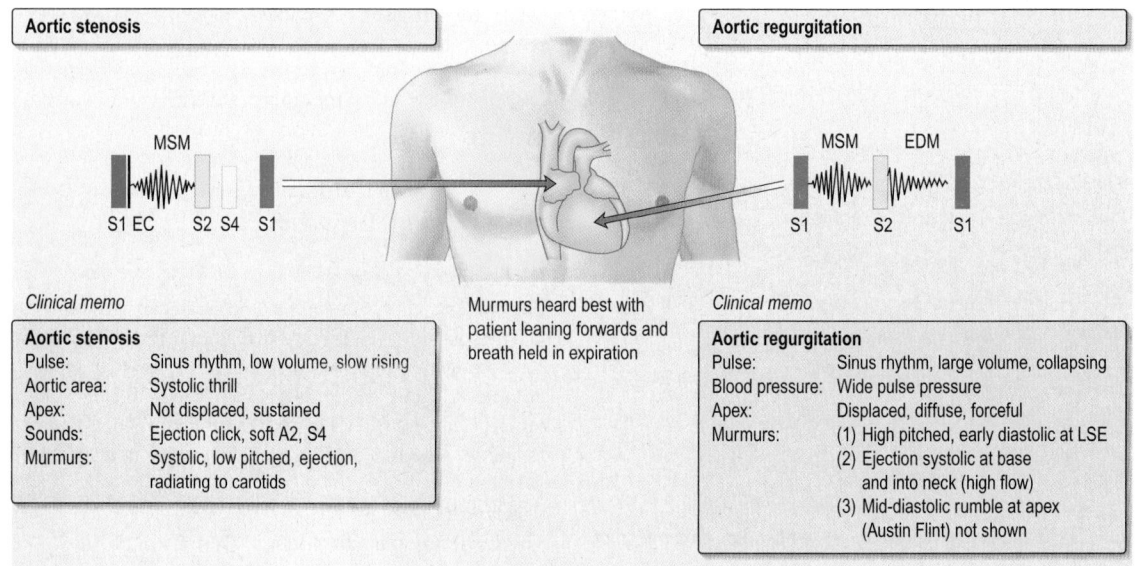

Aortic stenosis

MSM

S1 EC   S2 S4   S1

Aortic regurgitation

MSM   EDM

S1   S2   S1

Murmurs heard best with patient leaning forwards and breath held in expiration

Clinical memo

Aortic stenosis
Pulse:	Sinus rhythm, low volume, slow rising
Aortic area:	Systolic thrill
Apex:	Not displaced, sustained
Sounds:	Ejection click, soft A2, S4
Murmurs:	Systolic, low pitched, ejection, radiating to carotids

Clinical memo

Aortic regurgitation
Pulse:	Sinus rhythm, large volume, collapsing
Blood pressure:	Wide pulse pressure
Apex:	Displaced, diffuse, forceful
Murmurs:	(1) High pitched, early diastolic at LSE
	(2) Ejection systolic at base and into neck (high flow)
	(3) Mid-diastolic rumble at apex (Austin Flint) not shown

Fig. 13.83 **Features of aortic stenosis and aortic regurgitation**. EC, ejection click; EDM, early diastolic murmur; MSM, mid-systolic murmur; S1, first heart sound.

hypertrophy may also be seen. The gradient across the valve can be estimated by CW Doppler, provided the left ventricular function is reasonable (Fig. 13.28, p. 752).

Cardiac catheterization

Cardiac catheterization can be used to document the systolic pressure difference (gradient) between the aorta and the left ventricle (Fig. 13.84) and assess left ventricular function. This is rarely necessary since all of this information can be gained non-invasively with echocardiography. Coronary angiography is necessary before recommending surgery.

Treatment

In patients with aortic stenosis, symptoms are a good index of severity and all symptomatic patients should have aortic valve replacement. Asymptomatic patients should be under regular review for assessment of symptoms and echocardiography. Antibiotic prophylaxis against infective endocarditis is essential (see p. 31).

Provided that the valve is not severely deformed or heavily calcified, critical aortic stenosis in childhood or adolescence can be treated by valvotomy (performed under direct vision by the surgeon or by balloon dilatation using X-ray visualization). This produces temporary relief from the obstruction. Aortic valve replacement will usually be needed a few years later. Balloon dilatation (valvuloplasty) has been tried in adults, especially in the elderly, as an alternative to surgery. Generally results are poor and such treatment is reserved for patients unfit for surgery or as a 'bridge' to surgery (as systolic function will often improve).

AORTIC REGURGITATION

The most common causes of aortic regurgitation are rheumatic fever and infective endocarditis complicating a previously damaged valve. This can be a congenitally abnormal valve (e.g. a bicuspid valve) or one damaged by rheumatic fever. There are numerous other causes and associations (Table 13.37). The majority of patients with

Fig. 13.84 **ECG and pressure trace as a cardiac catheter is withdrawn** from the left ventricle (LV) to the aorta (AO). Note that the peak systolic pressure changes from 250 to 130 mmHg (arrow). The 120 mmHg peak-to-peak systolic gradient indicates severe aortic valvular stenosis.

Table 13.37 Causes and associations of aortic regurgitation

Acute aortic regurgitation	Chronic aortic regurgitation
Acute rheumatic fever	Rheumatic heart disease
Infective endocarditis	Syphilis
Dissection of the aorta	Arthritides:
Ruptured sinus of Valsalva	Reiter's syndrome
aneurysm	Ankylosing spondylitis
Failure of prosthetic	Rheumatoid arthritis
heart valve	Hypertension (severe)
	Bicuspid aortic valve
	Aortic endocarditis
	Marfan's syndrome
	Osteogenesis imperfecta

aortic regurgitation are men (75%), but rheumatic aortic regurgitation occurs more commonly in women.

Pathophysiology

Aortic regurgitation is reflux of blood from the aorta through the aortic valve into the left ventricle during diastole. If net cardiac output is to be maintained, the total volume of blood pumped into the aorta must increase, and consequently the left ventricular size must enlarge. Because of the aortic run-off during diastole, diastolic blood pressure falls and coronary perfusion is decreased. In addition, the larger left ventricular size is mechanically less efficient so that the demand for oxygen is greater and cardiac ischaemia develops.

Symptoms

In aortic regurgitation, significant symptoms occur late and do not develop until *left ventricular failure* occurs. As with mitral regurgitation, a common symptom is '*pounding of the heart*' because of the increased left ventricular size and its vigorous pulsation. *Angina pectoris* is a frequent complaint. Varying grades of *dyspnoea* occur depending on the extent of left ventricular dilatation and dysfunction. *Arrhythmias* are relatively uncommon.

Signs (see Clinical memo in Fig. 13.83)

The signs of aortic regurgitation are many and are due to the hyperdynamic circulation, reflux of blood into the left ventricle and the increased left ventricular size.

The pulse is bounding or collapsing (see p. 736). The following signs, which are rare, also indicate a hyperdynamic circulation:

- Quincke's sign – capillary pulsation in the nail beds
- De Musset's sign – head nodding with each heartbeat
- Duroziez's sign – a to-and-fro murmur heard when the femoral artery is auscultated with pressure applied distally (if found, it is a sign of severe aortic regurgitation)
- pistol shot femorals – a sharp bang heard on auscultation over the femoral arteries in time with each heartbeat.

The apex beat is displaced laterally and downwards and is forceful in quality. On auscultation, there is a high-pitched early diastolic murmur best heard at the left sternal edge in the fourth intercostal space with the patient leaning forward and the breath held in expiration.

Because of the volume overload there is commonly an ejection systolic flow murmur. The regurgitant jet can impinge on the anterior mitral valve cusp, causing a mid-diastolic murmur (Austin Flint).

Investigations
Chest X-ray
The chest X-ray features are those of left ventricular enlargement and possibly of dilatation of the ascending aorta. The ascending aortic wall may be calcified in syphilis, and the aortic valve may be calcified if valvular disease is responsible for the regurgitation.

Electrocardiogram
The ECG appearances are those of left ventricular hypertrophy due to 'volume overload' – tall R waves and deeply inverted T waves in the left-sided chest leads, and deep S waves in the right-sided leads. Normally, sinus rhythm is present.

Echocardiogram
The echocardiogram demonstrates vigorous cardiac contraction and a dilated left ventricle. The aortic root may also be enlarged. Diastolic fluttering of the mitral leaflets or septum occurs in severe aortic regurgitation (producing the Austin Flint murmur, see p. 741). The regurgitant jet can be detected by CW Doppler.

Cardiac catheterization
During cardiac catheterization, injection of contrast medium into the aorta (aortography) will outline aortic valvular abnormalities and allow assessment of the degree of regurgitation.

Treatment
The underlying cause of aortic regurgitation (e.g. syphilitic aortitis or infective endocarditis) may require specific treatment. The treatment of aortic regurgitation usually requires aortic valve replacement but the timing of surgery is critical.

Because symptoms do not develop until the myocardium fails and because the myocardium does not recover fully after surgery, operation is performed before significant symptoms occur. The timing of the operation is best determined according to haemodynamic, echocardiographic or angiographic criteria.

Both mechanical prostheses and tissue valves are used. Tissue valves are preferred in the elderly and when anticoagulants must be avoided, but are contraindicated in children and young adults because of the rapid calcification and degeneration of the valves.

Antibiotic prophylaxis against infective endocarditis (see p. 31) is necessary even if a prosthetic valve replacement has been performed.

TRICUSPID STENOSIS

This uncommon valve lesion, which is seen much more often in women than in men, is usually due to rheumatic heart disease and is frequently associated with mitral and/or aortic valve disease. Tricuspid stenosis is also seen in the carcinoid syndrome.

Pathophysiology

Tricuspid valve stenosis results in a reduced cardiac output, which is restored towards normal when the right atrial pressure increases. The resulting systemic venous congestion produces hepatomegaly, ascites and dependent oedema.

Symptoms

Usually, patients with tricuspid stenosis complain of symptoms due to associated left-sided rheumatic valve lesions. The *abdominal pain* (due to hepatomegaly) and swelling (due to ascites) and *peripheral oedema* that occur are relatively severe when compared with the degree of *dyspnoea*.

Signs

If the patient remains in sinus rhythm, which is unusual, there is a prominent jugular venous *a* wave. This pre-systolic pulsation may also be felt over the liver. There is usually a rumbling mid-diastolic murmur, which is heard best at the lower left sternal edge and is louder on inspiration. It may be missed because of the murmur of co-existing mitral stenosis. A tricuspid opening snap may occasionally be heard.

Hepatomegaly, abdominal ascites and dependent oedema may be present.

Investigations
Chest X-ray
On the chest X-ray there may be a prominent right atrial bulge.

Electrocardiogram
The enlarged right atrium may be manifested on the ECG by peaked, tall P waves (> 3 mm) in lead II.

Echocardiogram
The echocardiogram may show a thickened and immobile tricuspid valve, but this is not so clearly seen as an abnormal mitral valve.

Cardiac catheterization
This demonstrates a diastolic pressure gradient between the right atrium and the right ventricle. Contrast injection will demonstrate a large right atrium.

Treatment

Medical management consists of diuretic therapy and salt restriction. Tricuspid valvotomy is occasionally possible, but tricuspid valve replacement is often necessary. Other valves usually also need replacement because tricuspid valve stenosis is rarely an isolated lesion.

TRICUSPID REGURGITATION

Functional tricuspid regurgitation may occur whenever the right ventricle dilates, e.g. in cor pulmonale, myocardial infarction or pulmonary hypertension.

Organic tricuspid regurgitation may occur with rheumatic heart disease, infective endocarditis, carcinoid syndrome, Ebstein's anomaly (a congenitally mal-positioned tricuspid valve) and other congenital abnormalities of the atrioventricular valves.

Symptoms and signs

The valvular regurgitation gives rise to high right atrial and systemic venous pressure. Patients may complain of the symptoms of *right heart failure* (see p. 788).

Physical signs include a large jugular venous *cv* wave and a palpable liver that pulsates in systole. Usually a right ventricular impulse may be felt at the left sternal edge, and there is a blowing pansystolic murmur, best heard on inspiration at the lower left sternal edge. Atrial fibrillation is common.

Treatment

Functional tricuspid regurgitation usually disappears with medical management. Severe organic tricuspid regurgitation may require operative repair of the tricuspid valve (annuloplasty or plication). Very occasionally, tricuspid valve replacement may be necessary. In drug addicts with infective endocarditis of the tricuspid valve, surgical removal of the valve is recommended to eradicate the infection. This is usually well tolerated in the short term. The insertion of a prosthetic valve for this condition is considered on page 827.

PULMONARY STENOSIS

This is usually a congenital lesion, but it may rarely result from rheumatic fever or from the carcinoid syndrome. Congenital pulmonary stenosis may be associated with an intact ventricular septum or with a ventricular septal defect (Fallot's tetralogy).

Pulmonary stenosis may be valvular, subvalvular or supravalvular. Multiple congenital pulmonary arterial stenoses are usually due to infection with rubella during pregnancy.

Symptoms and signs

The obstruction to right ventricular emptying results in *right ventricular hypertrophy* which in turn leads to right atrial hypertrophy. Severe *pulmonary obstruction* may be incompatible with life, but lesser degrees of obstruction give rise to fatigue, syncope and the symptoms of *right heart failure*. Mild pulmonary stenosis may be asymptomatic.

The physical signs are characterized by a harsh mid-systolic ejection murmur, best heard on inspiration, to the left of the sternum in the second intercostal space. This murmur is often associated with a thrill. The pulmonary closure sound is usually delayed and soft. There may be a pulmonary ejection sound if the obstruction is valvular.

A right ventricular fourth sound and a prominent jugular venous *a* wave are present when the stenosis is moderately severe. A right ventricular heave (sustained impulse) may be felt.

Investigations

Chest X-ray

The chest X-ray usually shows a prominent pulmonary artery owing to post-stenotic dilatation.

Electrocardiogram

The ECG demonstrates both right atrial and right ventricular hypertrophy, although it may sometimes be normal even in severe pulmonary stenosis.

Echocardiogram

Doppler is the investigation of choice.

Cardiac catheterization

The passage of a catheter through the right heart allows the level and degree of the stenosis to be established by measuring the systolic pressure gradient.

Treatment

Treatment of severe pulmonary stenosis requires pulmonary valvotomy (balloon valvotomy or direct surgery).

PULMONARY REGURGITATION

This is the most common acquired lesion of the pulmonary valve. It results from dilatation of the pulmonary valve ring, which occurs with pulmonary hypertension. It is characterized by a decrescendo diastolic murmur, beginning with the pulmonary component of the second sound, that is difficult to distinguish from the murmur of aortic regurgitation. Pulmonary regurgitation usually causes no symptoms and treatment is rarely necessary.

PROSTHETIC VALVES

There is no ideal replacement for our own normally functioning, native heart valves. There are two alternatives for valve prostheses: mechanical or tissue (bioprosthetic) (Fig. 13.85). The valves consist of two basic components: an opening to allow blood to flow through and an occluding mechanism to regulate the flow. Mechanical prostheses rely on artificial concluders: a ball and cage (Starr–Edwards), tilting disc (Bjork–Shiley) or double tilting disc (St Jude). Tissue prostheses are derived from human (homograft), or from porcine or bovine (xenograft) origin. A valve replacement from within the same patient (i.e. pulmonary to aortic valve position) is termed an autograft.

Mechanical vs tissue valves

Mechanical valves, being artificial structures, are more durable than their tissue counterparts, which tend to degenerate after 10 years. However, artificial structures are more thrombogenic. Mechanical valves require formal

(a)

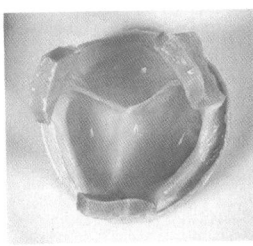

(b)   (c)

Fig. 13.85 **Prosthetic valves.** (a) Bjork–Shiley mechanical prosthetic valve.
(b) St Jude double tilting disc.
(c) Aortic valve tissue prosthesis (aortic view).

anticoagulation for the lifetime of the prosthesis. Tissue valves only require anticoagulation for a limited postoperative period whilst the suture lines endothelialize; it can then be discontinued unless another risk factor for thromboembolism (e.g. atrial fibrillation) persists. The potential lifetime of the prosthetic valve and the patient's tolerance of long-term anticoagulation can inform the choice of valve to be implanted. On auscultation, tissue valve heart sounds are comparable to those of a native valve. Mechanical valve heart sounds are generally louder and both opening and closing sounds can be heard.

Complications

All prostheses carry a risk of infection. Prosthetic valve endocarditis is associated with significant morbidity and mortality; prevention is the cornerstone of management. Patient education about antibiotic prophylaxis is vital and this should be reinforced at clinic visits. Any procedure which results in a breach of the body's innate defences (i.e. dental treatment, catheter insertion) increases the risk of exposing the prosthesis to a bacteraemia. This must be borne in mind when managing a patient with a prosthetic heart valve and steps taken to minimize the risk involved. The prosthetic valve occluding mechanism can be interrupted by vegetations, but also by thrombosis and calcification, resulting in either stenosis or regurgitation. The prosthesis can become detached from the valve ring resulting in a para-prosthetic leak. Evidence of structural failure can be detected by simple auscultation, with echocardiography as the initial investigation of choice. Transthoracic echocardiography is non-invasive, but scattering of echoes by mechanical valves makes their assessment difficult. Transoesophageal echocardiography provides alternative views and higher image resolution, making it the investigation of choice when prosthetic valve endocarditis is suspected.

FURTHER READING

Enrique-Sarano M, Tajik AJ (2004) Aortic regurgitation. *New England Journal of Medicine* **351**: 1539–1546.

Goldsmith I, Turpie AGG, Lip GYH (2002) Valvar heart disease and prosthetic heart valves. *British Medical Journal* **325**: 1228–1231.

Hayek E, Gring KN, Griffin BP (2005) Mitral valve prolapse. *Lancet* **365**: 507–518.

Piper C, Korfer R, Horstkotte D (2001) Prosthetic valve endocarditis. *Heart* **85**: 590–593.

Reimold SC, Rutherford JD (2003) Valvular heart disease in pregnancy. *New England Journal of Medicine* **349**(1): 52–59.

INFECTIVE ENDOCARDITIS

Infective endocarditis is an infection of the endocardial surface of the heart. The disease may occur as an acute, fulminating infection, but more commonly runs an insidious course and is known as subacute bacterial endocarditis (SBE.) The term 'infective endocarditis' is preferred because not all the infecting organisms are bacteria, and fungi can be responsible. The annual incidence in the UK is 6–7 per 100 000, but it is more common in developing countries. Without treatment the mortality approaches 100% and even with treatment there is a significant morbidity and mortality.

Aetiology

Endocarditis is usually the consequence of two factors: the presence of organisms in the bloodstream and abnormal cardiac endothelium facilitating their adherence and growth.

Factors causing a bacteraemia

Anything that results in a breach of the body's innate defences can potentially cause a bacteraemia. In some cases the cause of the bacteraemia is unknown; more often; there is an obvious factor that facilitated the entry of organisms into the bloodstream. This may be patient orientated: poor dental hygiene, intravenous drug use, soft tissue infections; or iatrogenic: dental treatment, intravascular cannulae (especially central), cardiac surgery, or permanent pacemakers.

Local cardiac factors

Damaged vascular endothelium will promote platelet and fibrin deposition. It is these small thrombi that allow organisms to adhere and grow. As they grow, more fibrin and platelets are deposited, forming the characteristic infected vegetation. Abnormal vascular endothelium can be the result of valvular lesions, which create areas of non-laminar blood flow, or jet lesions resulting from ventricular septal defects or a patent ductus arteriosus. Infective endocarditis is less likely to develop where the

haemodynamic disturbance is minimal (i.e. low-pressure systems). Hence it is more common in ventricular septal defects than atrial septal defects, and rare in mitral valve prolapse without significant regurgitation. Aortic and mitral valves are the commonest valves to be affected. Right-sided endocarditis is typically related to intravenous drug use, although the exact pathological mechanisms that underlie this association are not fully known. It may be that damage to right-sided valves results from the injected particulate matter used to cut the drugs. Instrumentation of the right heart (central venous catheter and temporary pacemaker insertion) is also a common cause of right-sided endocarditis.

Virulent pathogens such as *Staphylococcus aureus* and *Streptococcus pneumoniae* may adhere and multiply on previously normal valves.

Organisms responsible

Common organisms and the sources of infections are shown in Figure 13.86.

Rare causes

These include the HACEK group of organisms (*Haemophilus* species (*H. parainfluenzae*, *H. aphrophilus*, and *H. paraphrophilus*, though not *H. influenzae*), *Actinobacillus actinomycetemcomitans*, *Cardiobacterium hominis*, *Eikenella corrodens*, and *Kingella kingae*) and tend towards a more insidious course.

Culture-negative endocarditis

This accounts for 5–10% of endocarditis cases. The usual cause is prior antibiotic therapy (good history taking is vital) but some cases are due to a variety of fastidious organisms that fail to grow in normal blood cultures. These include *Coxiella burnetii* (the cause of Q fever), *Chlamydia* spp., *Bartonella* spp. (organisms that cause trench fever and cat scratch disease) and *Legionella*.

Clinical presentation

Patients can present with an acute illness and the classic features of a new or changing heart murmur and a fever. However, they may present with a subacute insidious illness. A high index of suspicion for the possibility of endocarditis is therefore required; otherwise the diagnosis can easily be delayed with potentially catastrophic consequences.

Clinical signs tend to arise from the following pathological processes: systemic features of infection; cardiac lesions; embolization, and immune complex deposition (Table 13.38).

Distal embolization may result in infarction of the distal organ, and/or spread of infection. The signs and symptoms will depend on the organ involved. For example, cerebral abscess can present with seizures, loss of consciousness or focal neurological signs. Clubbing occurs in 10% (p. 884).

Diagnostic criteria

Criteria for the diagnosis of infective endocarditis have been established. They have subsequently been refined

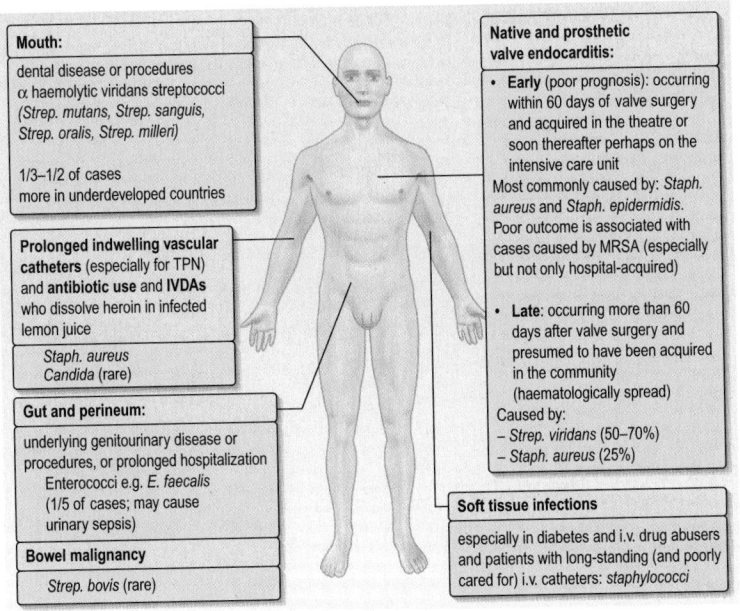

Mouth:

dental disease or procedures
α haemolytic viridans streptococci
(*Strep. mutans, Strep. sanguis,
Strep. oralis, Strep. milleri*)

1/3–1/2 of cases
more in underdeveloped countries

Prolonged indwelling vascular
catheters (especially for TPN)
and antibiotic use and IVDAs
who dissolve heroin in infected
lemon juice

  *Staph. aureus
  Candida* (rare)

Gut and perineum:

underlying genitourinary disease or
procedures, or prolonged hospitalization
  Enterococci e.g. *E. faecalis*
  (1/5 of cases; may cause
  urinary sepsis)

Bowel malignancy

  Strep. bovis (rare)

Native and prosthetic
valve endocarditis

• **Early** (poor prognosis): occurring
  within 60 days of valve surgery
  and acquired in the theatre or
  soon thereafter perhaps on the
  intensive care unit
  Most commonly caused by: *Staph.
  aureus* and *Staph. epidermidis.*
  Poor outcome is associated with
  cases caused by MRSA (especially
  but not only hospital-acquired)

• **Late**: occurring more than 60
  days after valve surgery and
  presumed to have been acquired
  in the community
  (haematologically spread)
  Caused by:
  – *Strep. viridans* (50–70%)
  – *Staph. aureus* (25%)

Soft tissue infections

especially in diabetes and i.v. drug abusers
and patients with long-standing (and poorly
cared for) i.v. catheters: *staphylococci*

Fig. 13.86 **Aetiology and sources of infection in infective endocarditis.**

and are now commonly known as the Duke criteria (Box 13.1).

Investigations

The purpose of these investigations is threefold: *first* to confirm the diagnosis of infective endocarditis; *second*, to identify the causative organism to ensure appropriate therapy; *third*, to monitor the patient's response to therapy.

Microbiology

Blood cultures are the *key diagnostic investigation* in infective endocarditis. At least three sets of samples (i.e.

six bottles) should be taken and there should be liaison with the microbiology department. The yield of any test is increased by the amount of information about the subject given. Serological tests can be sent when the diagnosis is suspected and the blood cultures are negative. They aid diagnosis in cases where the organisms will not grow in standard blood cultures (i.e. *Coxiella, Bartonella, Legionella* and *Chlamydia*).

Other laboratory tests

These are useful to confirm sepsis and monitor response to therapy, though they are non-specific.

- **Full blood count**. A normochromic normocytic anaemia and polymorphonuclear leucocytosis are common. Thrombocytopenia or thrombocytosis can occur.
- **Urea and electrolytes**. Renal dysfunction is a complication of sepsis. Electrolyte disturbance should be identified and corrected primarily in any patient prone to arrhythmias.
- **Liver biochemistry** is often mildly deranged with, in particular, an increased serum alkaline phosphatase.
- **Inflammatory markers**. C-reactive protein and erythrocyte sedimentation rate are non-specific markers of inflammation and are increased in any infection. CRP tends to respond more acutely than ESR.
- **Immunoglobulins and complement**. Serum immunoglobulins are increased, but total complement and C3 complement are decreased owing to immune complex formation. Circulating immune complexes are present in more than 70% of cases, but are not routinely measured.
- **Urine**. Proteinuria may occur and microscopic haematuria is nearly always present.
- **Polymerase chain reaction (PCR)** is used to recover specific DNA or RNA from blood, urine, or surgically excised tissue. It has specific application when the

Table 13.38	Clinical features of infective endocarditis
	Approximate %
General	
Malaise	95
Clubbing	10
Cardiac	
Murmurs	90
Cardiac failure	50
Arthralgia	25
Pyrexia	90
Skin lesions	
Osler's nodes	15
Splinter haemorrhages	10
Janeway lesions	5
Petechiae	50
Eyes	
Roth spots	5
Conjunctival splinter haemorrhages	Rare
Splenomegaly	40
Neurological	
Cerebral emboli	20
Mycotic aneurysm	10
Renal	
Haematuria	70

Box 13.1 Duke criteria for the diagnosis of infective endocarditis (IE)

A diagnosis of IE can be made if two major criteria, one major and three minor, or five minor criteria are present.

Major criteria

Positive blood culture for infective endocarditis

- Expected microorganisms for infective endocarditis from two separate blood cultures – viridans streptococci,* HACEK[†] groups, Streptococcus bovis, or community-acquired Staphylococcus aureus or enterococci, without known primary focus, or
- Persistently positive blood culture, defined as growth and identification of a microorganism consistent with IE originating from:
  - blood cultures that are obtained more than 12 hours apart, or
  - 3/3 or 3/4 or more separate blood cultures, with the first and last blood cultures obtained at least 60 minutes apart

Evidence of endocardial involvement supporting the diagnosis of IE

- Echocardiogram findings
  - (a) Oscillating intracardiac mass present:
    - on valve or supporting structures, or
    - in the path of regurgitant bloodstream flow, or
    - on implanted material, in the absence of an alternative anatomical explanation, or
  - (b) Abscess, or
  - (c) Newly identified partial dehiscence of prosthetic valve, or
- New valvular regurgitation (increase or change in pre-existing murmur does not count as a criterion)

Minor criteria

- Fever: = or > 38°C (100.4°F)
- Predisposition to IE: heart condition predisposing to IE, or intravenous drug abuse (IVDA)
- Echocardiogram: findings may be consistent with IE, but major criteria as stated above are not met
- Immunological phenomena present: Roth spots, Osler's nodes, glomerulonephritis, rheumatoid factor via laboratory analysis
- Microbiological evidence of IE: blood cultures are positive but major criteria are not met as previously described,[‡] or serological studies support an infection that is consistent with the diagnosis of IE
- Vascular phenomena present: major arterial emboli, mycotic aneurysm, septic pulmonary infarcts, conjunctival haemorrhages, intracranial haemorrhage, Janeway lesions

---

* Including nutritional variant strains

[†] HACEK, *Haemophilus aphrophilus, Haemophilus paraphrophilus, Haemophilus parainfluenzae, Actinobacillus actinomycetemcomitans, Cardiobacterium hominis, Eikenella corrodens, Kingella*

[‡] Excluding single positive cultures for coagulase-negative staphylococci and organisms that do not cause endocarditis

---

potential pathogen is slow growing or non-culturable by conventional methods and when phenotypic characterization is essential after two or more organisms are isolated in separate cultures. The latter happens most commonly after contamination with skin commensals during sampling or in case of polymicrobial infection in injecting drug users.

PCR and other novel diagnostic techniques, such as specific fluorescent labelled antibody staining and electron microscopy, should be considered in all cases where cultures have tested negative for infective endocarditis.

Electrocardiogram

This may show evidence of myocardial infarction (emboli) or conduction defects. New atrioventricular block is suggestive of abscess formation. Patients with suspected infective endocarditis therefore should have an ECG on presentation and repeated regularly during their admission depending on their clinical course.

Chest X-ray

This may show evidence of heart failure or, in right-sided endocarditis, multiple pulmonary emboli and/or abscesses. The combination of sepsis and pulmonary infiltrates on chest X-ray should alert the clinician to the possibility of right-sided endocarditis.

Echocardiography

Transthoracic echocardiography (TTE) is rapid, non-invasive and has high specificity for visualizing vegetations (Fig. 13.87) although sensitivity is 60–75%. It is also useful in documenting valvular dysfunction and other local complications, such as aortic root abscesses.

Transoesophageal echocardiography (TOE) has a higher sensitivity and specificity for abscess formation because of the close physical proximity of the transducer to the aortic root. TOE also enhances the visualization of prosthetic valves and is recommended for all cases of suspected prosthetic valve endocarditis.

Echocardiography is an extremely useful tool if used appropriately. A negative echocardiogram does not exclude a diagnosis of endocarditis and it is not an appropriate screening test for patients with a fever or an isolated positive blood culture, where there is a low pre-test probability of endocarditis. However, echocardio-

(a)

(b)

Fig. 13.87 **(a) Two-dimensional echocardiogram (long-axis view) showing vegetations** (arrowed) attached to both the anterior and posterior leaflets of the mitral valve in a patient with infective endocarditis. **(b) M-mode echocardiogram of the left ventricle** demonstrating hyperdynamic contraction associated with volume overloading from severe mitral regurgitation in a patient with endocarditis. IVS, interventricular septum; LV(d) and LV(s), diastolic and systolic left ventricular dimensions; PVW, posterior ventricular wall.

graphy is indicated for all patients suspected of having infective endocarditis.

Principles of therapy

Therapy of endocarditis is difficult because organisms reside within a protected site within the vegetation. High concentrations of intravenous antibiotic are required for prolonged periods to achieve successful treatment. Where possible, synergistic combinations of antibiotics are used, in order to maximize the microbiocidal effect. Given that infective endocarditis carries a substantial morbidity and mortality, a rapid diagnosis and initiation of appropriate antimicrobial therapy is essential. This is best achieved by a multidisciplinary approach consisting of clinicians, cardiologists, cardiothoracic surgeons and microbiologists.

Drug therapy

Empirical antibiotic treatment is started only after cultures are taken. The regimen is then adjusted accord-

ing to culture results. The only exception to this is in those patients who have recently received antibiotics. A delay of 48–72 hours to await culture results prevents further antibiotics confounding the picture and increases the likelihood of identifying the causative organism. This delay is only possible in haemodynamically stable patients. The treatment should continue for 4–6 weeks, although studies of 2-week, short-course therapy have shown that it is highly effective in uncomplicated penicillin-sensitive *Strep. viridans* endocarditis. Typical therapeutic regimens are shown in Table 13.39. The UK guidelines devised by the working party on endocarditis are available from the British Society for Antimicrobial Chemotherapy (BSAC).

Serum levels of gentamicin and vancomycin need to be monitored. In patients with penicillin allergy one of the glycopeptide antibiotics, vancomycin or teicoplanin, can be used. Penicillins, however, are fundamental to the therapy of bacterial endocarditis; allergies therefore seriously compromise the choice of antibiotics. It is essential to confirm the nature of a patient's allergy to ensure that the appropriate treatment is not withheld needlessly. Anaphylaxis would be much more influential in antibiotic choice than a simple gastrointestinal disturbance.

Persistent fever

Most patients with infective endocarditis should respond within 48 hours of initiation of appropriate antibiotic therapy. This is evidenced by a resolution of fever, reduction in serum markers of infection (CRP tends to be the most sensitive) and relief of systemic symptoms of infection. Failure of this to occur needs to be taken very seriously. The following should be considered:

- perivalvular extension of infection and possible abscess formation
- drug reaction (the fever should promptly resolve after drug withdrawal)
- nosocomial infection (i.e. venous access site, UTI)
- pulmonary embolism (as a consequence of right-sided endocarditis or prolonged hospitalization).

In such cases, samples for culture should be taken from all possible sites and evidence sought for the above causes. Changing antibiotic dosage or regimen should be avoided unless there are positive cultures or a drug reaction is suspected. Emergence of bacterial resistance is uncommon. Close liaison with microbiology is recommended and a cardiothoracic surgical opinion should be sought.

Surgery

Surgical intervention should be considered in the following cases:

- extensive damage to a valve
- prosthetic valve endocarditis (valve replacement is usually required)
- persistent infection despite therapy
- large vegetations
- serious embolization

Table 13.39 Antibiotics in endocarditis (adapted from BSAC guidelines)

Clinical situation	Suggested antibiotic regimen to start (all given i.v.)
Clinical endocarditis, culture results awaited, no suspicion of staphylococci	Penicillin 1.2 g 4-hourly, gentamicin 80 mg 12-hourly
Suspected staphylococcal endocarditis (IVDA, recent intravascular devices or cardiac surgery, acute infection)	Vancomycin 1 g 12-hourly, gentamicin 80–120 mg 8-hourly
Streptococcal endocarditis (penicillin sensitive)	Penicillin 1.2 g 4-hourly, gentamicin 80 mg 12-hourly
Enterococcal endocarditis (no high-level gentamicin resistance)	Ampicillin/amoxicillin 2 g 4-hourly, gentamicin 80 mg 12-hourly
Staphylococcal endocarditis	Vancomycin 1 g 12-hourly, OR Flucloxacillin 2 g 4-hourly, OR Benzylpenicillin 1.2 g 4-hourly, PLUS gentamicin 80–120 mg 8-hourly

Note:
1. Monitor vancomycin and gentamicin levels, and adjust if necessary
2. Choice of antibiotic for staphylococci depends on sensitivities
3. Optimum choice of therapy needs close liaison with Microbiology/Infectious Diseases

All antibiotics given i.v.
IVDA, intravenous drug abuse; BSAC, British Society for Antimicrobial Chemotherapy

- myocardial abscess
- fungal endocarditis (this is usually refractory to antimicrobial therapy)
- progressive cardiac failure.

Early liaison with a cardiothoracic surgeon is essential. It is desirable to eradicate active infection before any surgical intervention, but if antibiotic therapy is failing, with progressive cardiac failure, uncontrolled sepsis or severe emboli, it will not be possible to wait. In general, early surgery is preferable.

Antibiotic prophylaxis (see Table 2.9)

Where rheumatic fever is still common, control and prevention will prevent rheumatic heart disease and thus associated endocarditis. In developed countries the focus is on antibiotic prophylaxis. People with valvular lesions who are at moderate to high risk of developing endocarditis are recommended to receive antibiotic therapy before undergoing a procedure likely to result in a bacteraemia, such as dental treatment, endoscopy or surgical instrumentation. There are no randomized placebo-controlled trials to assess the efficacy of such antibiotic prophylaxis, and hence its value has been questioned. It is argued that with uncertain benefits, there is a greater risk of an anaphylactic reaction from widespread penicillin use. Meticulous oral and skin hygiene is probably also significant in preventing endocarditis. Many cases of hospital-acquired endocarditis can be prevented by better care during insertion and handling of intravascular catheters, and prompt removal if they become infected. However, there is enough evidence to recommend the selected use of antibiotic prophylaxis, e.g. with prosthetic valves in those patients who are at a significantly increased risk of developing endocarditis whilst undergoing certain procedures known to cause a bacteraemia.

FURTHER READING
Moreillon P, Que Y-A (2004) Infective endocarditis. *Lancet* **363**: 139–149.
Ramsdale DR, Turner-Stokes L (2004) Prophylaxis and treatment of infective endocarditis in adults. *Clinical Medicine* **4**: 545–550.

CONGENITAL HEART DISEASE

A congenital cardiac malformation occurs in about 1% of live births. There is an overall male predominance, although some individual lesions (e.g. atrial septal defect and persistent ductus arteriosus) occur more commonly in females. As a result of improved medical and surgical management, more children with congenital cardiac disease are surviving into adolescence and adulthood. Thus there is a need for an increased awareness amongst general physicians and cardiologists of the problems posed by these individuals.

Aetiology

The aetiology of congenital cardiac disease is often unknown, but recognized associations include:

- maternal prenatal rubella infection (persistent ductus arteriosus, and pulmonary valvular and arterial stenosis)
- maternal alcohol abuse (septal defects)
- maternal drug treatment and radiation
- genetic abnormalities (e.g. the familial form of atrial septal defect and congenital heart block)
- chromosomal abnormalities (e.g. septal defects and mitral and tricuspid valve defects are associated with Down's syndrome (trisomy 21) or coarctation of the aorta in Turner's syndrome (45, XO)).

Table 13.40 Classification of congenital heart disease

Acyanotic	Cyanotic
With shunts	**With shunts**
Atrial septal defect	Fallot's tetralogy
Ventricular septal defect	Transposition of the great
Patent ductus arteriosus	vessels
Partial anomalous venous	Severe Epstein's anomaly
drainage	
	Without shunts
Without shunts	Severe pulmonary stenosis
Coarctation of the aorta	Tricuspid atresia
Congenital aortic stenosis	Pulmonary atresia
	Hypoplastic left heart

Classification (see Table 13.40)
Symptoms and signs

Congenital heart disease should be recognized as early as possible, as the response is usually better the earlier treatment is initiated. Some symptoms, signs and clinical problems are common in congenital heart disease:

- *Central cyanosis* occurs because of right-to-left shunting of blood or because of complete mixing of systemic and pulmonary blood flow. In the latter case, e.g. Fallot's tetralogy, the abnormality is described as cyanotic congenital heart disease.
- *Pulmonary hypertension* results from large left-to-right shunts. The persistently raised pulmonary flow leads to the development of increased pulmonary artery vascular resistance and consequent pulmonary hypertension. This is known as the Eisenmenger reaction (or the Eisenmenger complex when due specifically to a ventricular septal defect). The development of pulmonary hypertension significantly worsens the prognosis.
- *Clubbing of the fingers* occurs in congenital cardiac conditions associated with prolonged cyanosis.
- *Paradoxical embolism* of thrombus from the systemic veins to the systemic arterial system may occur when a communication exists between the right and left heart. There is therefore an increased risk of cerebrovascular accidents and also abscesses (as with endocarditis).
- *Polycythaemia* can develop secondary to chronic hypoxaemia, leading to a hyperviscosity syndrome and an increased thrombotic risk, e.g. strokes.
- *Growth retardation* is common in children with cyanotic heart disease.
- *Syncope* is common when severe right or left ventricular outflow tract obstruction is present. Exertional syncope, associated with deepening central cyanosis, may occur in Fallot's tetralogy. Exercise increases resistance to pulmonary blood flow but reduces systemic vascular resistance. Thus, the right-to-left shunt increases and cerebral oxygenation falls.
- *Squatting* is the posture adopted by children with Fallot's tetralogy. It results in obstruction of venous return of desaturated blood and an increase in the peripheral systemic vascular resistance. This leads to a reduced right-to-left shunt and improved cerebral oxygenation.

Presentation

Adolescents and adults with congenital heart disease present with specific common problems related to the long-standing structural nature of these conditions and any surgical treatment:

- endocarditis (particularly in association with otherwise innocuous lesions such as small VSDs or bicuspid aortic valve that can give up to 10% lifetime risk)
- progression of valvular lesions (calcification and stenosis of congenitally deformed valves, e.g. bicuspid aortic valve)
- atrial and ventricular arrhythmias (often quite resistant to treatment)
- sudden cardiac death
- right heart failure (especially when surgical palliation results in the right ventricle providing the systemic supply)
- end-stage heart failure (rarely managed by heart or heart–lung transplantation).

Genetic counselling

These conditions necessitate active follow-up of adult patients. Pregnancy is normally safe except if pulmonary hypertension or vascular disease is present when the prognosis for both mother and fetus is poor.

Table 13.41 lists the most common congenital lesions and their occurrence in first-degree relatives.

Genetic factors should be considered in all patients presenting with congenital heart disease. For example, parents with a child suffering from Fallot's tetralogy stand a 4% chance of conceiving another child with the disease, and so fetal ultrasound screening of the mother during pregnancy is essential. Parents with congenital heart disease are also more likely to have affected offspring. Fathers have a 2% risk while mothers have a higher risk (around 5%). Individual families can exhibit even higher risks of recurrence.

Table 13.41 Common congenital lesions

	Percentage of congenital lesions	Occurrence in first-degree relatives (%)
Ventricular septal	39	4
Atrial septal defect	10	2
Persistent ductus arteriosus	10	4
Pulmonary stenosis	7	
Coarctation of the aorta	7	2
Aortic stenosis	6	4
Fallot's tetralogy	6	4
Others	15	

Ventricular septal defect (VSD)

VSD is the most common congenital cardiac malformation (1 in 500 live births). It may occur as an isolated abnormality or in association with other anomalies. Left ventricular pressure is higher than right ventricular pressure; blood therefore moves from left to right and pulmonary blood flow increases. When pulmonary blood flow is very large, progressive obliteration of the pulmonary vasculature eventually causes the pulmonary arterial pressure to equal the systemic pressure (Eisenmenger complex). Consequently, the shunt is reduced or reversed (becoming right-to-left) and central cyanosis may develop.

Clinical features (Fig. 13.88)

Small VSDs ('maladie de Roger') are asymptomatic and usually close spontaneously, with 90% no longer patent by 10 years of age. Unfortunately there is a future risk of the development of aortic regurgitation or endocarditis even after spontaneous closure. A *moderate VSD* produces fatigue and dyspnoea with cardiac enlargement and a prominent apex beat. There is often a palpable systolic thrill at the lower left sternal edge. A loud 'tearing' pansystolic murmur is heard at the same position. A *large VSD* eventually causes pulmonary hypertension.

Investigations

A small VSD produces no abnormal X-ray or ECG findings.

Chest X-ray shows a prominent pulmonary artery owing to increased pulmonary blood flow in larger defects. In Eisenmenger's complex the radiological signs of pulmonary hypertension (i.e. 'pruned' pulmonary arteries) can be seen. Cardiomegaly occurs when a moderate or a large VSD is present. ECG shows features of both left and right ventricular hypertrophy.

2-D echocardiography and CW Doppler (Fig. 13.89) can assess the size and location of the VSD, and its haemodynamic consequences

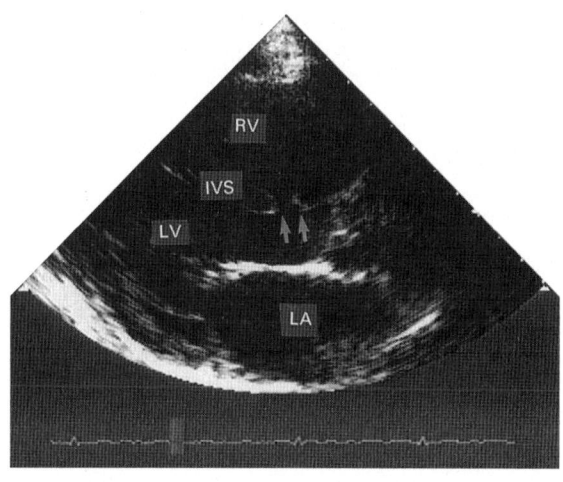

Fig. 13.89 **Two-dimensional echocardiogram (long-axis view) showing a ventricular septal defect** (arrowed). Colour Doppler would provide graphic demonstration of the left-to-right shunt. RV, right ventricle; IVS, interventricular septum; LV, left ventricle; LA, left atrium.

Treatment

Moderate and large VSDs should be surgically repaired before the development of severe pulmonary hypertension. Infective endocarditis prophylaxis (p. 31) should be advised in all cases.

Atrial septal defect (ASD)

Clinical features

This condition is often first diagnosed in adults and represents one-third of all adult congenital heart disease. It is two to three times more common in women than in men. There are two main types of ASD, *ostium secundum* and *ostium primum*. The common form is the ostium secundum defect, which involves the fossa ovalis in the atrial mid-septum. This should not be confused with the

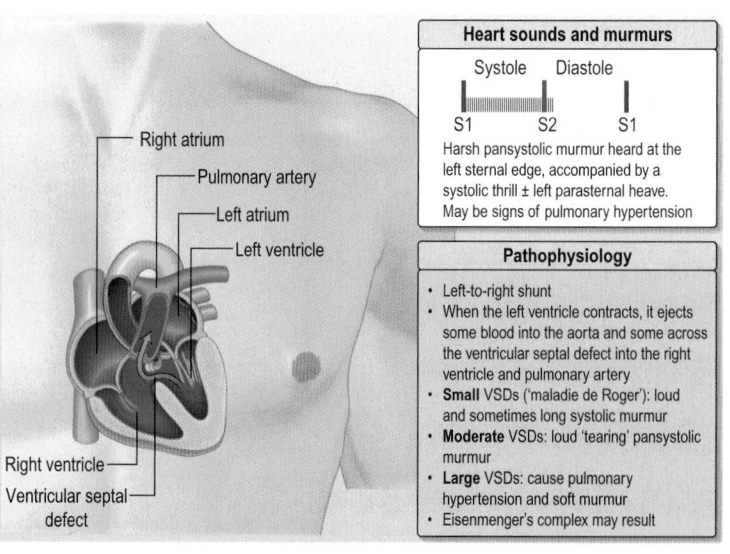

Fig. 13.88 **Ventricular septal defect**: Pathophysiology and auscultatory findings.

Heart sounds and murmurs

Systole   Diastole

S1   S2   S1

Harsh pansystolic murmur heard at the left sternal edge, accompanied by a systolic thrill ± left parasternal heave. May be signs of pulmonary hypertension

Pathophysiology

- Left-to-right shunt
- When the left ventricle contracts, it ejects some blood into the aorta and some across the ventricular septal defect into the right ventricle and pulmonary artery
- **Small** VSDs ('maladie de Roger'): loud and sometimes long systolic murmur
- **Moderate** VSDs: loud 'tearing' pansystolic murmur
- **Large** VSDs: cause pulmonary hypertension and soft murmur
- **Eisenmenger's complex may result

Right atrium
Pulmonary artery
Left atrium
Left ventricle
Right ventricle
Ventricular septal defect

Fig. 13.90 **Atrial septal defect**: Pathophysiology and auscultatory findings.

Heart sounds and murmurs

	Systole	Diastole
Expiration		
Inspiration		
	S1	A2 P2	S1
	Mid-systolic ejection in pulmonary area	Loud P2 Wide fixed splitting of S2	Sometimes diastolic tricuspid flow murmur

Pathophysiology

- Left-to-right shunt through the defect in the interatrial septum
- Dilatation of the pulmonary artery resulting from the shunt
- The murmur is produced by increased flow across pulmonary valve and an increased stroke volume

patent foramen ovale (PFO) which is a normal variant and not a true septal defect. PFO is usually asymptomatic but is associated with paradoxical emboli and an increased incidence of embolic stroke. Communication at the level of the atria allows left-to-right shunting of blood. Because the pulmonary vascular resistance is low and the right ventricle is easily distended (i.e. it is compliant), there is a considerable increase in right heart output. Above the age of 30 years there may be an increase in pulmonary vascular resistance, which gives rise to *pulmonary hypertension*. Atrial arrhythmias, particularly *atrial fibrillation*, are common at this stage.

Most children with ASD are asymptomatic, although they are prone to *pulmonary infection*. Some complain of *dyspnoea* and *weakness*. Palpitations due to atrial arrhythmias are not uncommon. Right heart failure and atrial fibrillation may develop to become the initial presentation in adult life.

The physical signs of ASD reflect the volume over-loading of the right ventricle (Fig. 13.90). A right ventricular heave can usually be felt.

Investigations

- **Chest X-ray** reveals a prominent pulmonary artery and pulmonary plethora. There may be noticeable right ventricular enlargement.
- **ECG** usually shows some degree of right bundle branch block (because of dilatation of the right ventricle) and right axis deviation. Sometimes the ASD is part of a major developmental abnormality involving the ventricular septum and the mitral and tricuspid valves. In this case there is left axis deviation on the ECG.
- **Echocardiogram** is usually abnormal if a significant defect is present. Indirect evidence includes right ventricular hypertrophy and pulmonary arterial dila-tation, and abnormal motion of the interventricular septum. Subcostal views may demonstrate the ASD

(Fig. 13.91). Flow disturbance can be assessed by colour Doppler.

Treatment

A significant ASD (i.e. a pulmonary flow that is more than 50% increased when compared with systemic flow) should be repaired before the age of 10 years or as soon as possible if first diagnosed in adulthood. There is a dilemma with regard to whether less severe shunts should be closed when diagnosed in adulthood. Anecdotal evidence suggests that the shunt might be progressive and that low-risk closure would be appropriate.

There is a good result from surgery unless pulmonary hypertension has developed. Angiographic closure is

Fig. 13.91 **Ostium secundum atrial septal defect** (arrowed) in a young girl, shown by a two-dimensional echocardiogram subcostal four-chamber view (similar to Fig. 13.89, but rotated clockwise). Colour Doppler can demonstrate the left-to-right shunt. LA, left atrium; RA, right atrium; LV, left ventricle; RV, right ventricle.

Fig. 13.92 **The angiographic appearance of a fully deployed ASD closure device.** The device bridges the ASD and wedges against the surfaces of the right and left atrial septa, occluding flow. The metal object in frame is the distal end of a transoesophageal echocardiography probe. Courtesy of Dr D Ward.

now possible with significantly lower risk using a transcatheter clamshell device (Fig. 13.92). A PFO discovered in a patient with an otherwise unexplained thrombotic stroke is now closed in this way to prevent paradoxical thromboembolism. In high-risk groups, for example deep-sea divers, such closures may be undertaken even though the patients are asymptomatic. Uncorrected ASDs do not usually require antibiotic prophylaxis for endocarditis. If there is an accompanying valvular lesion, however, prophylaxis is indicated.

Patent ductus arteriosus (PDA)

The ductus arteriosus connects the pulmonary artery at its bifurcation to the descending aorta immediately distal to the subclavian artery. In fetal life the ductus diverts blood away from the unexpanded, and hence high-resistance, pulmonary circulation into the systemic circulation, where the blood is reoxygenated as it passes through the placenta. At birth, the high oxygen in the lungs and the reduced pulmonary vascular resistance trigger closure of the duct. If the duct is malformed (i.e. it does not contain sufficient elastic tissue) it will not close. This is more common in females and is sometimes associated with maternal rubella. Premature babies are often born with persistent ducts that are anatomically normal but are immature in that they lack the mechanism to close. Other associations include continual prenatal hypoxaemia and high-altitude environments.

Because aortic pressure exceeds pulmonary artery pressure throughout the cardiac cycle, a persistent duct produces continuous aorta-to-pulmonary artery shunting. This leads to an increased pulmonary venous return to the left heart and an increased left ventricular volume load. If the shunt is large, this results in severe left heart failure and pulmonary hypertension. One-third of individuals with an unrepaired ductus die from heart failure, pulmonary hypertension or endocarditis by the age of 40; two-thirds by the age of 60.

Clinical features

There are often no symptoms until later in life when heart failure or infective endocarditis develops.

The characteristic physical sign is a continuous 'machinery' murmur (Fig. 13.93). The peripheral pulse is large in volume ('bounding') because of the increased left heart blood flow and the decompression of the aorta into the pulmonary artery.

Investigations

The aorta and pulmonary arterial system are usually prominent on X-ray, although a small ductus shows no abnormality. There is both a left atrial abnormality and left ventricular hypertrophy on the ECG. With the

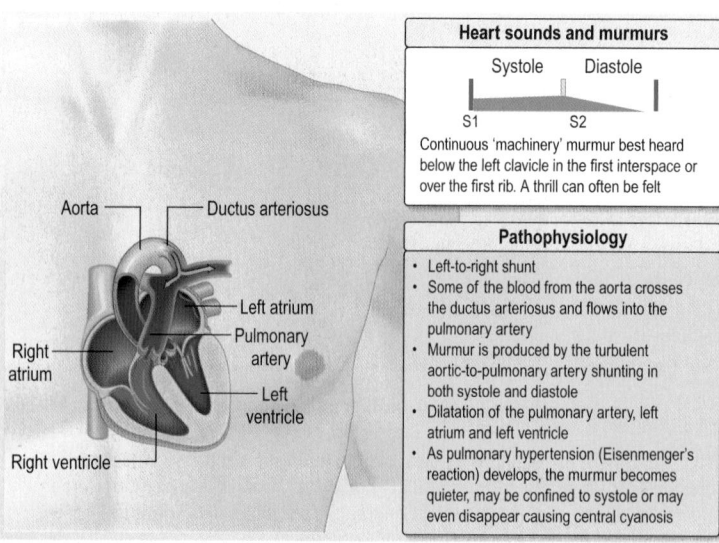

Heart sounds and murmurs

Systole   Diastole

S1   S2

Continuous 'machinery' murmur best heard below the left clavicle in the first interspace or over the first rib. A thrill can often be felt

Pathophysiology

- Left-to-right shunt
- Some of the blood from the aorta crosses the ductus arteriosus and flows into the pulmonary artery
- Murmur is produced by the turbulent aortic-to-pulmonary artery shunting in both systole and diastole
- Dilatation of the pulmonary artery, left atrium and left ventricle
- As pulmonary hypertension (Eisenmenger's reaction) develops, the murmur becomes quieter, may be confined to systole or may even disappear causing central cyanosis

Aorta — Ductus arteriosus
Right atrium
Left atrium
Pulmonary artery
Left ventricle
Right ventricle

Fig. 13.93 **Patent ductus arteriosus**: Pathophysiology and auscultatory findings.

Fig. 13.94 **Coarctation of the aorta**: Pathophysiology and auscultatory findings.

Heart sounds and murmurs

Systole | Diastole

S1 | S2

Mid–late systolic murmur may be heard over the upper precordium or the back. Vascular bruits from the collateral circulation may also be heard

Pathophysiology

Coarctation causes severe obstruction of blood flow in the descending thoracic aorta. The descending aorta and its branches are perfused by collateral channels from the axillary and internal thoracic arteries through the intercostal arteries

development of Eisenmenger's reaction, right ventricular hypertrophy may be seen. The echocardiogram shows a dilated left atrium and left ventricle. Right heart changes are apparent in late disease.

Treatment

Premature infants with a persistent duct are treated medically with indometacin, which inhibits prostaglandin production and stimulates duct closure. In other cases the duct can be ligated surgically or angiographically with very little risk. Surgery should be performed as soon as possible and not later than the age of 5 years. Closure is inappropriate if pulmonary hypertension is severe.

Coarctation of aorta

A coarctation of the aorta is a narrowing of the aorta at, or just distal to, the insertion of the ductus arteriosus, i.e. distal to the left subclavian artery (Fig. 13.94). Rarely it can occur proximal to the left subclavian. It occurs twice as commonly in men as in women. It is also associated with Turner's syndrome (p. 1064). In 80% of cases the aortic valve is bicuspid (and potentially stenotic or endocarditic). Other associations include patent ductus arteriosus, ventricular septal defect, mitral stenosis or regurgitation and circle of Willis aneurysms.

Severe narrowing of the aorta encourages the formation of a collateral arterial circulation involving the periscapular and intercostal arteries. Decreased renal perfusion can lead to the development of systemic hypertension that persists even after surgical correction.

Clinical features

Coarctation of the aorta is often asymptomatic for many years. *Headaches* and *nosebleeds* (due to hypertension) and *claudication* and cold legs (due to poor blood flow in the lower limbs) may be present.

Physical examination reveals hypertension in the upper limbs, and weak, delayed (radiofemoral delay) pulses in the legs.

For heart sounds and murmurs in coarctation of aorta, see Figure 13.94.

Investigations

Chest X-ray may reveal a dilated aorta indented at the site of the coarctation. This is manifested by an aorta (seen in the upper right mediastinum) shaped like a 'figure 3'. In adults, tortuous and dilated collateral intercostal arteries may erode the undersurfaces of the ribs ('rib notching') (Fig. 13.95).

ECG demonstrates left ventricular hypertrophy. Echocardiography sometimes shows the coarctation and other associated anomalies. Aortography will show the defect, and digital vascular imaging allows the coarctation

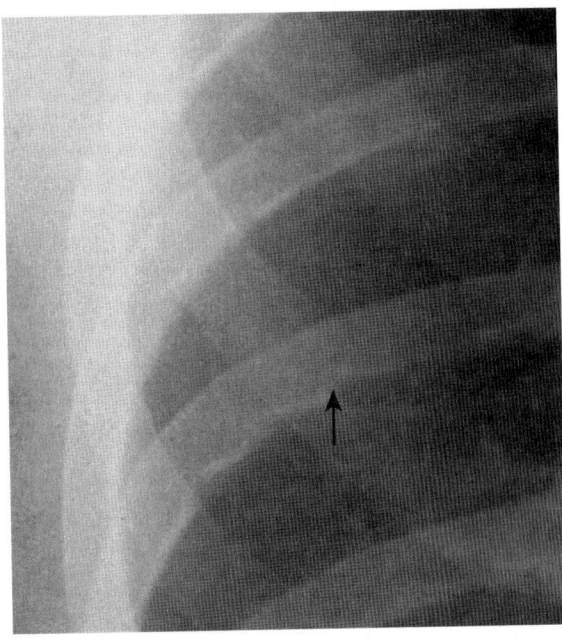

Fig. 13.95 **Chest X-ray close-up of right posterior ribs showing rib-notching** (arrow).

Fig. 13.96 Magnetic resonance angiography image of severe aortic coarctation in an adult.

operation is performed on adolescents or adults the hypertension persists in 70% because of previous renal damage. There is also an increased risk of accelerated atherosclerosis and strokes in these individuals. Balloon dilatation is used in some centres for either primary disease or post-surgical recurrence, although there is a higher incidence of aneurysm formation and post-dilatation recurrence.

Surgical correction in childhood gives a good 25-year survival rate of 83%. If this is delayed until adulthood (20–40), the 25-year survival rate drops to 75%. If coarctation is left uncorrected, however, only 25% of patients are alive at 50, while cardiac failure ensues in two-thirds of surviving patients over 40.

Cyanotic congenital heart disease: Fallot's tetralogy

Most children with cyanotic congenital heart disease do not survive the neonatal period. Fallot's is the most common cyanotic anomaly in those who do survive and is commonest amongst adults. Transposition of the great vessels is more common in the neonatal period but more likely to be fatal. Other cyanotic congenital heart diseases are shown in Table 13.40.

Fallot's tetralogy consists of the four features shown in Figure 13.97.

The level of the right ventricular outflow obstruction may be subvalvular, valvular or supravalvular. The most common obstruction is subvalvular, either alone (50%) or in combination with valvular stenosis (25%).

This combination of lesions leads to a high right ventricular pressure and right-to-left shunting of blood through the VSD. Thus the patient is centrally cyanosed.

to be visualized after the intravenous injection of contrast. CT and MRI (Fig. 13.96) scanning can accurately demonstrate the coarctation and quantify flow.

Treatment

Treatment is usually indicated if the pressure gradient across the coarctation is greater than 30 mmHg. This involves surgical excision of the coarctation and end-to-end anastomosis of the aorta. If the coarctation is extensive, prosthetic vascular grafts may be needed. When surgery is performed in early childhood, hypertension usually resolves completely. However, when the

Clinical features

Children with this condition may present with *dyspnoea* or *fatigue*, or with hypoxic episodes on exertion (Fallot's spells) – *deep cyanosis* and possible *syncope*. These can

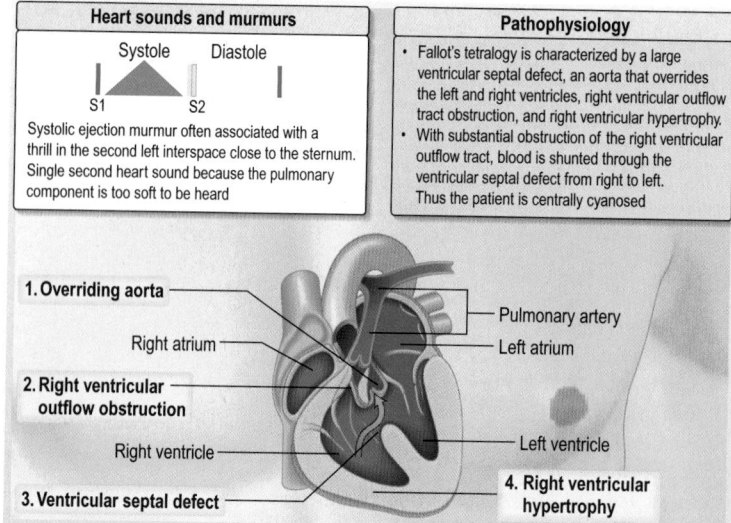

Heart sounds and murmurs	Pathophysiology
Systole Diastole S1 S2 Systolic ejection murmur often associated with a thrill in the second left interspace close to the sternum. Single second heart sound because the pulmonary component is too soft to be heard	• Fallot's tetralogy is characterized by a large ventricular septal defect, an aorta that overrides the left and right ventricles, right ventricular outflow tract obstruction, and right ventricular hypertrophy. • With substantial obstruction of the right ventricular outflow tract, blood is shunted through the ventricular septal defect from right to left. Thus the patient is centrally cyanosed

1. Overriding aorta
Right atrium
Pulmonary artery
Left atrium
2. Right ventricular outflow obstruction
Right ventricle
Left ventricle
3. Ventricular septal defect
4. Right ventricular hypertrophy

Fig. 13.97 Fallot's tetralogy: Pathophysiology and auscultatory findings.

even result in seizures, cerebrovascular events or sudden death. *Squatting* is common.

Adults tend not to suffer 'spells' but fatigue easily with dyspnoea on exertion. *Erythrocytosis* (polycythaemia) secondary to chronic hypoxaemia commonly results in *thrombotic strokes*. *Endocarditis* is common.

A parasternal sustained heave is evident. Central cyanosis is commonly present from birth, and *finger clubbing* and *polycythaemia* are obvious after about 12 months. Growth is usually retarded.

Investigations

- **Chest X-ray** shows a large right ventricle and a small pulmonary artery (classically described as 'boot-shaped').
- **ECG** reveals right ventricular hypertrophy, and the echocardiogram demonstrates discontinuity between the aorta and the anterior wall of the ventricular septum.
- **Cardiac catheterization** is performed to evaluate the size and degree of the right ventricular outflow obstruction.

Treatment

Complete surgical correction of this combination of lesions is possible even in infancy. As adults, however, these individuals are at increased risk of right ventricular failure and ventricular arrhythmias due to the trauma from past corrective surgery. Less-damaging procedures are used presently, the long-term results of which are unknown as yet.

Occasionally a palliative procedure – an anastomosis between a subclavian artery and a pulmonary artery (Blalock shunt) – is performed on very young infants or the premature, in order to increase blood supply to the lungs. Without intervention, 66% survive to 1 year, while only 11% survive to 20 years.

Fallot's spells may need treatment with beta-blockade or, when severe, with diamorphine to relax the right ventricular outflow obstruction. Antibiotic prophylaxis for endocarditis is indicated.

FURTHER READING

Deanfield J et al. (2003) Management of grown up congenital heart disease. Task Force on the Management of Grown Up Congenital Heart Disease, European Society of Cardiology; ESC Committee for Practice Guidelines. *European Heart Journal* **24**(11): 1035–1084.

Hunter S (2000) Congenital heart disease in adolescence. *Journal of the Royal College of Physicians of London* **34**(2): 150–152.

Nevil Thomas Adult Congenital Heart Library: http://www.achd-library.com/

Proceedings of the 32nd Bethesda Conference (2001) Care of the adult with congenital heart disease, October 2–3, 2000. *Journal of the American College of Cardiology*; **37**(5): 1161–1198.

Therrien J, Webb G (2003) Clinical update on adults with congenital heart disease. *Lancet* **362**: 1305–1313.

MARFAN'S SYNDROME (see also p. 1356)

Clinical features

Marfan's syndrome (MFS) is one of the most common autosomal dominant inherited disorders of connective tissue, affecting the heart (aortic aneurysm and dissection, mitral valve prolapse) eye (dislocated lenses, retinal detachment) and skeleton (tall, thin body build with long arms, legs and fingers; scoliosis and pectus deformity) (Fig. 13.98a).

Clinically, two out of three major systems must be affected, to avoid overdiagnosing the condition. Diagnosis may be confirmed by studying family linkage to the causative gene, or by demonstrating a mutation in the Marfan's syndrome gene (*MFS1*) for fibrillin (FBN-1) on chromosome 15q21.

MFS affects approximately 1 in 5000 population worldwide and 25% of patients are affected as a result of a new mutation. This group includes many of the more severely affected patients, with high cardiovascular risk. Other known associations with early death due to aortic aneurysm and dissection are: family history of early cardiac involvement; family history of dissection with an aortic root diameter of < 5 cm; male sex; and extreme physical characteristics, including markedly excessive stature and widespread striae. Histological examination of aortas often shows widespread medial degeneration, described as 'cystic medial necrosis'.

Cardiac investigations

- **Chest X-ray** is often normal but may show signs of aortic aneurysm and unfolding, or of widened mediastinum. Pneumothorax affects 11% and scoliosis is present in 70% of patients.
- **ECG** may be misleadingly normal with an acute dissection. Usually, in conjunction with mitral valve prolapse 40% of patients have arrhythmia, with premature ventricular and atrial arrhythmias.
- **Echocardiography** shows mitral valve prolapse, and mitral regurgitation are seen in the majority of patients. High-quality serial echocardiogram measurements of aortic root diameter in the sinuses of Valsalva, at 90° to the direction of flow are the basis for medical and surgical management (Fig. 13.99b).

Management

Beta-blocker therapy slows the rate of dilatation of the aortic root. Lifestyle alterations, involving sports and career choice, may be indicated, because of ocular, cardiac or skeletal involvement. Sports that necessitate prolonged exertion at maximum cardiac output, such as cross-country running, are to be avoided. Sedentary occupations are usually best, as patients tend to suffer from easy fatiguability and hypermobile painful joints.

The patient should be monitored with yearly echocardiograms up to aortic root diameter 4.5 cm, 6-monthly from 4.5 to 5 cm, and then referred directly to a surgeon who is experienced in aortic root replacement in Marfan's syndrome for elective surgery.

(a)

(b)

Fig. 13.98 **Marfan's syndrome. (a) Photograph of 63-year-old man. (b) Two-dimensional transoesophageal echocardiograms** from a patient with Marfan's syndrome resulting in dissection of the aorta. From its position in the oesophagus, the transducer can be aimed forward to visualize the greatly enlarged ascending aorta (left), or backwards to show the descending thoracic aorta (right). In both views the dissected intima is seen within the aortic lumen. The main entry point to the false lumen is seen in the ascending aorta (arrowed), just above the aortic valve. T, true lumen; F, false lumen.

Pregnancy is generally well tolerated if no serious cardiac problems are present, but is preferably avoided if the aortic root diameter is over 4 cm, with aortic regurgitation. Echocardiography should be performed every 6–8 weeks throughout pregnancy and during the initial 6 months postpartum. Blood pressure should be regularly monitored and hypertension treated actively. Delivery should be by the least stressful method; ideally a vaginal delivery. Caesarean section should not be routinely performed. However, if the aortic root is over 4.5 cm, delivery at 39 weeks by induction or caesarean section should be considered. Beta-blocker therapy may be safely instituted or continued throughout pregnancy, to help prevent aortic dissection.

Careful medical and surgical management have increased the overall survival rate. On average, 13 years of life is added, when surgical survival is compared to that reported in the natural history of MFS.

Genetic counselling

The condition is inherited in an autosomal dominant mode, with each child of one affected parent having a 50:50 chance of inheriting the condition. Males and females are equally often affected. In 25% of all cases, the condition arises as the result of a spontaneous mutation in the sperm or ovum of one of the parents. Fibrillin-1 gene mutations can be identified in 80% of those affected, confirming diagnosis and aiding prognosis. The mutation can also be used to screen at-risk family members, including postnatal or prenatal offspring.

> **FURTHER READING**
>
> Gott VL, Cameron DE, Alejo DE et al. (2002) Aortic root replacement in 271 Marfan patients: a 24-year experience. *Annals of Thoracic Surgery* **73**: 438–443.
>
> Pyeritz RE, Dietz HC (2002) Marfan syndrome and other microfibrillar disorders. In: Royce PM, Steinmann B (eds) *Connective Tissue and its Heritable Disorders: Molecular, Genetic and Medical Aspects*, pp. 585–626. New York: Wiley-Liss.

PULMONARY HEART DISEASE

Introduction

The normal values for mean pulmonary artery pressure (mPAP), mean capillary wedge pressure (mPCWP) and cardiac output (CO) are 12 ± 2 mmHg, 6 ± 2 mmHg and 5 L/min respectively. The fall in pressure across the lung circulation is known as the transpulmonary gradient and reflects the difference between mPAP and mPCWP. The normal transpulmonary gradient is 6 ± 2 mmHg.

The *pulmonary vascular resistance* (PVR) is calculated by the formula:

$$\frac{mPAP - mPCWP}{CO}$$

It is normally about 1.5 mmHg/L/min (1.5 Wood units). Approximately 60% of the body's endothelial surface is in the lungs and the lungs normally offer a low resistance to blood flow. This is because the media of the precapillary pulmonary arterioles is thin as compared with their more muscular systemic counterparts that have to respond constantly to postural changes under the influence of gravity. The fact that the lung circulation normally offers a low resistance to flow explains the preferential passage of blood through the lungs in specific forms of congenital heart disease which may eventually lead to remodelling of the lung circulation and pulmonary hypertension.

Pulmonary hypertension

Definition

Pulmonary hypertension is defined as an mPAP of greater than 25 mmHg at rest or of greater than 30 mmHg during exercise. It may present spontaneously with no apparent underlying disease association (and is then known as primary pulmonary hypertension, PPH) or it can occur in association with other disease processes as listed in Table 13.42.

Causes of pulmonary hypertension

The most common cause of pulmonary hypertension is chronic obstructive pulmonary disease (COPD). In general, the causes of pulmonary hypertension (Table 13.42) can be subdivided depending on whether their effects on the lung circulation are precapillary, capillary or postcapillary.

Precapillary (i.e. in the pulmonary arteries and arterioles). The most severe elevations in PAP and in PVR occur with these disorders. Examples include *PPH, congenital heart disease with Eisenmenger's reaction* and *multiple pulmonary embolism.* In PPH the PCWP is usually normal.

Capillary disorders causing damage to the alveolar capillary mechanisms also cause pulmonary hypertension and these usually fall under the umbrella of parenchymal lung diseases, e.g. emphysema and pulmonary fibrosis. Pulmonary arterial hypoxaemia is a potent cause of vasoconstriction and hence of pulmonary hypertension. Any diseases which lead to low pulmonary artery oxygen levels will give rise to pulmonary hypertension.

Postcapillary (passive) processes involve disease in structures distal to the pulmonary capillary bed. They

Table 13.42 Causes of pulmonary hypertension	
Pulmonary vascular disorders	**Disturbance of respiratory control**
Acute pulmonary thromboembolism (rarely tumour emboli)	Obstructive sleep apnoea
	Morbid obesity (Pickwickian syndrome)
Primary pulmonary hypertension	Cerebrovascular disease
Multiple pulmonary artery stenoses	**Cardiac disorders**
Pulmonary veno-occlusive disease	Mitral stenosis
Chronic pulmonary thromboembolism	Left ventricular failure
	Left atrial myxoma
Parasitic infection, e.g. schistosomiasis	Congenital heart disease with Eisenmenger's reaction
	Miscellaneous
Diseases of the lung and parenchyma	Appetite-suppressant drugs, e.g. dexfenfluramine
COPD	Type 1 glycogen storage diseases
Other chronic lung disorders (Ch. 14)	Lipid storage diseases, e.g. Gaucher's disease
	Connective tissue diseases, e.g. SLE
Musculoskeletal disorders (causing chronic underventilation)	Hepatic cirrhosis
Kyphoscoliosis	Sickle cell disease
Poliomyelitis	
Myasthenia gravis	

cause pulmonary hypertension through elevated venous pressures. Examples include pulmonary veno-occlusive disease, chronic left ventricular failure and mitral valve disease.

A variety of *miscellaneous conditions* can also cause pulmonary hypertension, and these include a history of appetite suppressant drug ingestion and glycogen and lipid storage diseases.

Progressive elevation in PVR ultimately leads to right ventricular dilatation, right ventricular failure and death. When pulmonary hypertension occurs in association with other conditions such as lung disorders or chronic left ventricular failure the primary underlying cause may have the major influence on mortality and the secondary effects of pulmonary hypertension are additive.

Mechanisms of pulmonary hypertension

These depend on the cause and involve hypoxic vasoconstriction, e.g. COPD, decreased surface area of the pulmonary vascular bed, e.g. lung fibrosis, and increased right ventricular volume/pressure, e.g. congenital heart disease.

Following the rise in pulmonary arterial pressure, damage to the pulmonary endothelium leads to excessive release of endothelium-derived vasoconstrictors such as endothelin (ET, see p. 731) which contribute to an increase in PVR. Increased platelet and leukocyte adhesion, elevated serotonin, plasminogen activator inhibitor-1 (PAI-1) and fibrinopeptide A can produce inappropriate intravascular thrombus. ET, angiotensin II and thromboxane A$_2$ can act as growth factors, giving rise ultimately to vasoconstriction, cell proliferation, fibrosis and smooth muscle hypertrophy. Such vascular remodelling increases the PVR.

The symptoms, signs and investigations of pulmonary hypertension are discussed on page 842.

Management

Since pulmonary hypertension is a condition caused by a heterogeneous group of diseases, treatment is directed at the primary cause, e.g. chest physiotherapy, good nutrition and early antibiotics to treat infection in patients with cystic fibrosis and bronchiectasis.

Surgical or medical therapies to optimize cardiac and respiratory function, supplemental oxygen and anticoagulation are necessary together with newer specific therapies designed at modulating pulmonary vasomotor tone.

Patients who have symptoms resulting in marked limitation of physical activity or those who are symptomatic at rest have a poor median survival (32 and 6 months respectively). Adverse factors include right ventricular dysfunction and reduced 6-minute walk distance.

Primary pulmonary hypertension

Primary pulmonary hypertension is a condition of unknown cause characterized by clinical, radiological

and electrocardiographic evidence of pulmonary hypertension and increased PAP and PVR with normal PCWP. It is estimated that one to two individuals per million per year are diagnosed with PPH compared to five to six individuals per million per year with pulmonary hypertension secondary to connective tissue diseases. There is an unexplained predominance of females (approximately a 3 to 1 ratio) with women mainly presenting in the third decade and men in the fourth. Approximately 6–12% of cases are believed to have a familial origin with inheritance in an autosomal dominant fashion.

Some patients with familial PPH have mutations in the gene encoding bone morphogenic protein receptor 2 (BMPR 2) on chromosome 2q33. This gene encodes TGF-β, which acts as a growth suppressor and opposes cellular proliferation. Other gene mutations exist.

PPH has also been linked to certain *drugs*: aminorex fumarate, an amfetamine-like appetite suppressant, talc which is often inhaled with cocaine, fenfluramine and phenteramine in combination (a prescription weight-loss drug).

Plexogenic pulmonary arteriopathy, identical to that seen in PPH, has also been described in patients with connective tissue diseases (limited cutaneous scleroderma, p. 577). These may have a rapidly progressive and fatal disease associated with pulmonary hypertension.

Patients with *systemic lupus erythematosus* can also develop pulmonary hypertension secondary to vascular remodelling, with identical histopathological features to patients with PPH. Patients with *hepatic cirrhosis* and *Eisenmenger reaction* also have identical pathology to patients with PPH.

Clinical presentation

Patients with pulmonary hypertension have an insidious onset and indeed often their condition comes to the attention of the physician late in the course of their illness or when symptoms of right ventricular failure develop. Physical examination may reveal findings consistent with pulmonary hypertension and right ventricular overload (Table 13.43). Clinical signs of right ventricular dysfunction may be present.

Chest X-ray may demonstrate enlargement of the pulmonary arteries and the major branches, with marked tapering (pruning) of peripheral arteries. The lung fields are usually lucent and there may be right atrial and right ventricular enlargement. *ECG* may show right ventricular

Table 13.43 Clinical signs of pulmonary hypertension

Large 'a' wave in jugular venous waveform
Right ventricular (parasternal) heave
Pulmonary ejection sound and flow murmur
Loud pulmonary component to second heart sound
Right ventricular fourth heart sound
Right ventricular failure (hepatomegaly, ascites, peripheral oedema)
Prominent 'v' wave in jugular venous waveform
Right ventricular third heart sound
Tricuspid and pulmonary regurgitation murmurs

hypertrophy and right atrial enlargement (P pulmonale). *Echocardiography* demonstrates enlarged right ventricular dimensions. *Pulmonary function tests* are usually normal.

The *diagnosis* can be confirmed by CT pulmonary angiography.

The differential diagnoses for PPH are an exclusion of secondary causes as shown in Table 13.42. In particular, mitral stenosis, congenital heart disease with Eisenmenger's reaction, connective tissue disease and sickle cell disease should be excluded.

Treatment

Conventional therapy initially consists of warfarin and oxygen followed by oral calcium-channel blockers. A sustained response to this treatment is unlikely (occurring in less than 10% of patients) and advanced treatments include oral endothelin receptor antagonists (bosentan), prostanoid analogues (inhaled illoprost, treprostinil, beraprost) or intravenous epoprostenol.

Prognosis

Several studies have reported a mean survival of 2–3 years from the time of diagnosis. The cause of death is usually right ventricular failure or sudden death. Increased right atrial pressure above 15 mmHg and cardiac index below 2 L/min/m^2 are haemodynamic predictors of poor prognosis. Heart and lung transplantation is used (p. 796).

Chronic cor pulmonale

Cor pulmonale is enlargement of the right ventricle because of increase in afterload that is due to diseases of the thorax, lung and pulmonary circulation; the presence of right ventricular failure is not necessary for the diagnosis of cor pulmonale.

Pathophysiology

The precise mechanism varies according to the cause of cor pulmonale, but chronic obstructive pulmonary disease (COPD), which is discussed here, is illustrative. Pulmonary vascular resistance is increased because of loss of pulmonary vascular tissue and because of pulmonary vasoconstriction caused by hypoxia and acidosis. The increased pulmonary vascular resistance leads to pulmonary hypertension, which initially occurs only during an acute respiratory infection. Eventually, the pulmonary hypertension becomes persistent and progressively more severe. The pulmonary vascular bed is gradually obliterated by muscular hypertrophy of the arterioles and thrombus formation. Right ventricular function is progressively compromised because of the increased pressure load. Hypoxia further impairs right ventricular function and, as it develops, left ventricular function is also depressed.

Clinical features

Chest pain, exertional dyspnoea, syncope and *fatigue* are common symptoms, and *sudden death* occurs. Other symptoms are due to the cause of the pulmonary hypertension.

On *physical examination* (see Table 13.43), there is a prominent 'a' wave in the jugular venous pulse, a right ventricular (parasternal) heave, and a loud pulmonary component to the second heart sound. Other findings include a right ventricular fourth heart sound, a systolic pulmonary ejection click, a mid-systolic ejection murmur, and an early diastolic murmur due to pulmonary regurgitation (Graham Steell murmur). If tricuspid regurgitation develops, there is a pansystolic murmur and a large jugular *cv* venous wave (see p. 741).

Investigations

- **Chest X-ray** may show right ventricular enlargement and right atrial dilatation. The pulmonary artery is usually prominent and the enlarged proximal pulmonary arteries taper rapidly. Peripheral lung fields are oligaemic.
- **ECG** demonstrates right ventricular hypertrophy (right axis deviation, possibly a dominant R wave in lead V$_1$, and inverted T waves in right precordial leads) and a right atrial abnormality (tall peaked P waves in lead II) (Fig. 13.99).
- **Echocardiography** will usually demonstrate right ventricular dilatation and/or hypertrophy. It is often possible to measure the peak pulmonary artery pressure indirectly with Doppler echocardiography. The echocardiogram may also reveal the cause of pulmonary hypertension, such as an intracardiac shunt.

Other investigations may also be required to evaluate the cause of pulmonary hypertension and to look for treatable conditions, such as left-to-right shunts, mitral stenosis or left atrial tumours. With direct measurement of pulmonary artery pressure and pulmonary wedge pressure, *cardiac catheterization* is necessary in some

Fig. 13.99 **Pulmonary hypertension** shown by a 12-lead ECG. There is right axis deviation (+ 120°), right ventricular hypertrophy (dominant secondary R wave [R'] in V$_1$) and a combination of left and right atrial conduction abnormalities.

patients with severe pulmonary hypertension of unknown cause. *Pulmonary angiography* may be indicated if multiple pulmonary emboli are suspected, but is dangerous.

If no other cause is found, then a diagnosis of primary pulmonary hypertension is made (see p. 842).

Treatment

Treatment is determined by the condition underlying pulmonary hypertension. Diuretic treatment is used for right ventricular failure, but care should be taken to avoid excessive fluid depletion as this will result in reduced output from the impaired right ventricle. Hypoxia is avoided by the use of oxygen therapy when safe and necessary. In those with COPD and some others, long-term oxygen therapy improves symptoms and prognosis (p. 905). In contrast to their enormous value in those with left ventricular impairment, angiotensin-converting enzyme inhibitors are seldom useful and may make matters worse.

Pulmonary embolism

Thrombus, usually formed in the systemic veins or rarely in the right heart (less than 10% of cases), may dislodge and embolize into the pulmonary arterial system. Post-mortem studies indicate that this is a very common condition (microemboli are found in up to 60% of autopsies) but it is not usually diagnosed this frequently in life. Ten per cent of clinical pulmonary emboli are fatal.

Most clots which cause clinically relevant pulmonary emboli actually come from the pelvic and abdominal veins, but femoral deep venous thrombosis, and even occasionally axillary thrombosis, can be the origin of the clot. Clot forms as a result of a combination of sluggish blood flow, local injury or compression of the vein and a hypercoagulable state. Emboli can also occur from tumour, fat (long bone fractures), amniotic fluid and foreign material during i.v. drug abuse. Risk factors are shown in Table 8.27 and discussed on page 477.

After pulmonary embolism, lung tissue is ventilated but not perfused – producing an intrapulmonary dead space and resulting in impaired gas exchange. After some hours the non-perfused lung no longer produces surfactant. Alveolar collapse occurs and exacerbates hypoxaemia. The primary haemodynamic consequence of pulmonary embolism is a reduction in the cross-sectional area of the pulmonary arterial bed which results in an elevation of pulmonary arterial pressure and a reduction in cardiac output. The zone of lung that is no longer perfused by the pulmonary artery may infarct, but often does not do so because oxygen continues to be supplied by the bronchial circulation and the airways.

Clinical features

Sudden onset of *unexplained dyspnoea* is the most common, and often the only symptom of pulmonary embolism. *Pleuritic chest pain* and *haemoptysis* are present only when infarction has occurred. Many pulmonary emboli occur silently, but there are three typical clinical presentations. A clinical deep venous thrombosis is not commonly observed, although detailed investigation of the lower limb and pelvic veins will reveal thrombosis in more than half of the cases.

Small/medium pulmonary embolism

In this situation an embolus has impacted in a terminal pulmonary vessel. Symptoms are pleuritic chest pain and breathlessness. Haemoptysis occurs in 30%, often 3 or more days after the initial event. On examination, the patient may be tachypnoeic with a localized pleural rub and often coarse crackles over the area involved. An exudative pleural effusion (occasionally blood-stained) can develop. The patient may have a fever, and cardio-vascular examination is normal.

Massive pulmonary embolism

This is a much more rare condition where sudden collapse occurs because of an acute obstruction of the right ventricular outflow tract. The patient has severe central chest pain (cardiac ischaemia due to lack of coronary blood flow) and becomes shocked, pale and sweaty. Syncope may result if the cardiac output is transiently but dramatically reduced, and death may occur. On examination, the patient is tachypnoeic, has a tachycardia with hypotension and peripheral shutdown. The jugular venous pressure (JVP) is raised with a prominent '*a*' wave. There is a right ventricular heave, a gallop rhythm and a widely split second heart sound. There are usually no abnormal chest signs.

Multiple recurrent pulmonary emboli

This leads to increased breathlessness, often over weeks or months. It is accompanied by weakness, syncope on exertion and occasionally angina. The physical signs are due to the pulmonary hypertension that has developed from multiple occlusions of the pulmonary vasculature. On examination, there are signs of right ventricular over-load with a right ventricular heave and loud pulmonary second sound.

Diagnosis

The symptoms and signs of small and medium-sized pulmonary emboli are often subtle and non-specific, so the diagnosis is often delayed or even completely missed. Pulmonary embolism should be considered if patients present with symptoms of unexplained cough, chest pain, haemoptysis, new-onset atrial fibrillation (or other tachycardia), or signs of pulmonary hypertension if no other cause can be found.

Investigations

Small/medium pulmonary emboli

- **Chest X-ray** is often normal, but linear atelectasis or blunting of a costophrenic angle (due to a small effusion) is not uncommon. These features develop only after some time. A raised hemidiaphragm is present in some patients. More rarely, a wedge-shaped pulmonary infarct, the abrupt cut-off of a pulmonary artery or a translucency of an underperfused distal zone is seen. Previous infarcts may be seen as opaque linear scars.

- **ECG** is usually normal, except for sinus tachycardia, but sometimes atrial fibrillation or another tachyarrhythmia occurs. There may be evidence of right ventricular strain.
- **Blood tests**. Pulmonary infarction results in a polymorphonuclear leucocytosis, an elevated ESR and increased lactate dehydrogenase levels in the serum. Immediately prior to commencing anticoagulants a thrombophilia screen should be checked.
- **Plasma D-dimer** (see p. 468) – if this is undetectable, it excludes a diagnosis of pulmonary embolism.
- **Radionuclide ventilation/perfusion scanning** ($\dot{V}/\dot{Q}$ scan) is a good and widely available diagnostic investigation.

Pulmonary ^{99m}Tc scintigraphy demonstrates underperfused areas (Fig. 13.100a) which, if not accompanied by a ventilation defect on a ventilation scintigram performed after inhalation of radioactive xenon gas (see p. 888), is highly suggestive of a pulmonary embolus. There are limitations to the test, however. For example, a matched defect may arise with a pulmonary embolus which causes an infarct or from emphysematous bullae. This test is therefore conventionally reported as a probability (low, medium or high) of pulmonary embolus and should be interpreted in the context of the history, examination and other investigations.

- **Ultrasound scanning** can be performed for the detection of clots in pelvic or iliofemoral veins (see p. 870).
- **Spiral CT scans** with intravenous contrast (CT pulmonary angiography) show good sensitivity and specificity for medium-sized pulmonary emboli (Fig. 13.100b). They do not exclude pulmonary emboli in small arteries. New multislice CT machines have high sensitivities for even very small thrombi.
- **MR imaging** gives similar results and is used if CT angiography is contraindicated.

Massive pulmonary emboli

- **Chest X-ray** may show pulmonary oligaemia, sometimes with dilatation of the pulmonary artery in the hila. Often there are no changes.
- **ECG** shows right atrial dilatation with tall peaked P waves in lead II. Right ventricular strain and dilatation give rise to right axis deviation, some degree of right bundle branch block, and T wave inversion in the right precordial leads (Fig. 13.101). The 'classic' ECG pattern with an S wave in lead I, and a Q wave and inverted T waves in lead III (S1, Q3, T3), is rare.
- **Blood gases** show arterial hypoxaemia with a low arterial CO_2 level, i.e. type I respiratory failure pattern.
- **Echocardiography** shows a vigorously contracting left ventricle and occasionally a dilated right ventricle and a clot in the right ventricular outflow tract.
- **Pulmonary angiography** is sometimes undertaken if surgery is considered in acute massive embolism. The test is performed by injecting contrast material through a catheter inserted into the main pulmonary artery. Filling defects or obstructed vessels can be delineated

(a)

(b)

Fig. 13.100 **(a) Ventilation** (top) **and perfusion** (bottom) **lung scans** which demonstrate absence of perfusion but normal ventilation in the right upper lobe, i.e. probably pulmonary embolism. **(b) Spiral CT pulmonary angiographic image** at level of the main right and left pulmonary arteries showing a large thrombus in the right pulmonary artery.

(Fig. 13.102). Angiography is hazardous but the risk may be reduced if contrast is injected into each pulmonary artery separately. Although surgical removal of clot may be an option for selected patients it has no proven additional benefit above thrombolysis, and is therefore rarely preformed.

Multiple recurrent pulmonary emboli

- **Chest X-ray** may be normal. Enlarged pulmonary arterioles with oligaemic lung fields indicate advanced disease.
- **ECG** can be normal or show signs of pulmonary hypertension (Fig. 13.99).
- **Leg imaging** with ultrasound and venography may show thrombi.
- $\dot{V}/\dot{Q}$ scan may show evidence of pulmonary infarcts.

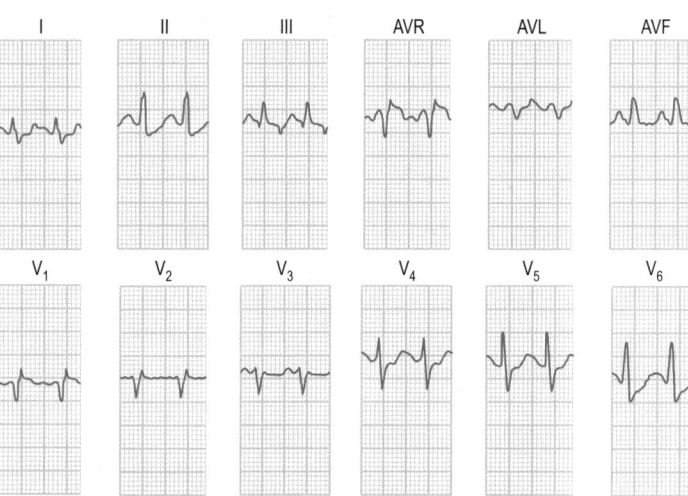

Fig. 13.101 Acute pulmonary embolism shown by a 12-lead ECG. There is an S wave in lead I, a Q wave in lead III and an inverted T wave in lead III (the S1, Q3, T3 pattern). There is sinus tachycardia (160 b.p.m.) and an incomplete right bundle branch block pattern (an R wave in AVR and V_1 and an S wave in V_6).

Fig. 13.102 Pulmonary angiogram (contrast injected directly into the main pulmonary artery) showing a large filling defect in the interlobar segment of the right pulmonary artery and extensive occlusion in the proximal left pulmonary artery.

Further tests looking for exercise-induced hypoxaemia and catheter studies to estimate pulmonary artery pressures are often required.

Treatment

Acute management

All patients should receive high-flow oxygen (60–100%) unless they have significant chronic lung disease. Patients with pulmonary infarcts require bed rest and analgesia. In severe cases, intravenous fluids and even inotropic agents to improve the pumping of the right heart are sometimes required, and very ill patients will require care on the intensive therapy unit (see p. 972).

Prevention of further emboli

A comparison of *low-molecular-weight heparin* (LMWH) with unfractionated heparin has shown no difference. As LMWHs simplify treatment (see p. 480) they are used exclusively if available, although they are more expensive. *Oral anticoagulants* are usually begun immediately and the heparin is tapered off as the oral anticoagulant becomes effective. Oral anticoagulants are continued for 6 weeks to 6 months, depending on the likelihood of recurrence of venous thrombosis or embolism. In some situations, such as after recurrent embolism, lifelong treatment is indicated.

Occasionally, physical methods are required to prevent further emboli. This is usually because recurrent emboli occur despite adequate anticoagulation, but is also indicated in high-risk patients in whom anticoagulation is absolutely contraindicated. The most common method by which pulmonary embolism is treated in this situation is by insertion of a *filter in the inferior vena cava* via the femoral vein to above the level of the renal veins.

Dissolution of the thrombus

Fibrinolytic therapy such as streptokinase (250 000 units by i.v. infusion over 30 minutes, followed by streptokinase 100 000 units i.v. hourly for up to 12–72 hours according to manufacturer's instructions) has been shown in control trials, to clear pulmonary emboli more rapidly and to confer a survival benefit in massive PE. It should be used more often.

Surgery

Surgical *embolectomy* is rarely necessary, but there may be no alternative when the haemodynamic circumstances are very severe.

FURTHER READING

Fedullo PF et al. (2001) Chronic thromboembolic pulmonary hypertension. *New England Journal of Medicine* **345**: 1465–1472.

Loscalzo J (2001) Genetic clues to the cause of primary pulmonary hypertension. *New England Journal of Medicine* **345**: 367–371.

MYOCARDIAL AND ENDOCARDIAL DISEASE

ATRIAL MYXOMA

This is the most common primary cardiac tumour. It occurs at all ages and shows no sex preference. Although most myxomas are sporadic, some are familial or are part of a multiple system syndrome. Histologically they are benign. The majority of myxomas are solitary, usually develop in the left atrium and are polypoid, gelatinous structures attached by a pedicle to the atrial septum. The tumour may obstruct the mitral valve or may be a site of thrombi that then embolize. It is also associated with constitutional symptoms: the patient may present with dyspnoea, syncope or a mild fever. The physical signs are a loud first heart sound, a tumour 'plop' (a loud third heart sound produced as the pedunculated tumour comes to an abrupt halt), a mid-diastolic murmur, and signs due to embolization. A raised ESR is usually present.

The diagnosis is easily made by echocardiography because the tumour is demonstrated as a dense space-occupying lesion (Fig. 13.103). Surgical removal usually results in a complete cure.

Myxomas may also occur in the right atrium or in the ventricles. Other primary cardiac tumours include rhabdomyomas and sarcomas.

MYOCARDIAL DISEASE

Myocardial disease that is not due to ischaemic, valvular or hypertensive heart disease or a known infiltrative, metabolic/toxic or neuromuscular disorder may be caused by:

- an acute or chronic inflammatory pathology (myocarditis)
- idiopathic myocardial disease (cardiomyopathy).

Fig. 13.103 **Atrial myxoma shown by a two-dimensional echocardiogram** (long-axis view). The myxoma is an echo-dense mass obstructing the mitral valve orifice. It was removed surgically. LV, left ventricle; LA, left atrium; M, mass.

Table 13.44   Causes of myocarditis
Idiopathic
Infective
Viral: Coxsackievirus, adenovirus, CMV, echovirus, influenza, polio, hepatitis, HIV
Parasitic: *Trypanosoma cruzi*, *Toxoplasma gondii* (a cause of myocarditis in the newborn or immunocompromised)
Bacterial: Streptococcus (most commonly rheumatic carditis), diphtheria (toxin-mediated heart block common)
Spirochaetal: Lyme disease (heart block common), leptospirosis
Fungal
Rickettsial
Toxic
Drugs Causing hypersensitivity reactions, e.g. methyldopa, penicillin, sulphonamides, antituberculous
Radiation May cause myocarditis but pericarditis more common
Autoimmune An autoimmune form with autoactivated T cells and organ-specific antibodies may occur

Myocarditis

Acute inflammation of the myocardium has many causes (Table 13.44). Establishment of a definitive aetiology with isolation of viruses or bacteria is difficult in routine clinical practice.

In western societies, the commonest causes of infective myocarditis are Coxsackie or adenoviral infection. Myocarditis in association with HIV infection is seen at post-mortem in up to 20% of cases but causes clinical problems in < 10% of cases. Chagas' disease, due to *Trypanosoma cruzi*, which is endemic in South America, is one of the commonest causes of myocarditis world-wide. Additionally toxins (including prescribed drugs), physical agents, hypersensitivity reactions and autoimmune conditions may also cause myocardial inflammation.

Pathology

In the acute phase myocarditic hearts are flabby with focal haemorrhages; in chronic cases they are enlarged and hypertrophied. Histologically an inflammatory infiltrate is present – lymphocytes predominating in viral causes; polymorphonuclear cells in bacterial causes; eosinophils in allergic and hypersensitivity causes (Fig. 13.104).

(a)   (b)

Fig. 13.104 **Biopsies showing (a) normal myocardium and (b) myocarditis, with increased interstitial inflammatory cells.**

Clinical features

Myocarditis may be an acute or chronic process; its clinical presentations range from an asymptomatic state associated with limited and focal inflammation to *fatigue, palpitations, chest pain, dyspnoea* and *fulminant congestive cardiac failure* due to diffuse myocardial involvement. An episode of viral myocarditis, perhaps unrecognized and forgotten, may be the initial event that eventually culminates in an 'idiopathic' dilated cardiomyopathy. Physical examination includes soft heart sounds, a prominent third sound and often a tachycardia. A pericardial friction rub may be heard.

Investigations

- **Chest X-ray** may show some cardiac enlargement, depending on the stage and virulence of the disease.
- **ECG** demonstrates ST and T wave abnormalities and arrhythmias. Heart block may be seen with diphtheritic myocarditis, Lyme disease and Chagas' disease (see below).
- **Cardiac enzymes** are elevated.
- **Viral antibody titres** may be increased. However, since enteroviral infection is common in the general population, the diagnosis depends on the demonstration of acutely rising titres.
- **Endomyocardial biopsy** may show acute inflammation but false negatives are common by conventional criteria. Biopsy is of limited value outside specialized units.
- **Viral RNA** can be measured from biopsy material using polymerase chain reaction (PCR). Specific diagnosis requires demonstration of active viral replication within myocardial tissue.

Treatment

The underlying cause must be identified, treated, eliminated or avoided. Bed rest is recommended in the acute phase of the illness and athletic activities should be avoided for 6 months. Heart failure should be treated conventionally with the use of diuretics, ACE inhibitors/AII receptor antagonists, beta-blockers, spironolactone ± digoxin. *Antibiotics* should be administered immediately where appropriate. *NSAIDs* are contraindicated in the acute phase of the illness but may be used in the late phase. The use of *corticosteroids* is controversial and no studies have demonstrated an improvement in left ventricular ejection fraction or survival following their use. The administration of high-dose intravenous *immunoglobulin* on the other hand appears to be associated with a more rapid resolution of the left ventricular dysfunction and improved survival. Novel and effective antiviral, immunosuppressive (e.g. gamma-interferon) and *immunomodulating* (e.g. IL-10) agents are currently undergoing animal trials and may become available in the future to treat viral myocarditis.

Giant cell myocarditis

This is a severe form of myocarditis characterized by the presence of multinucleated giant cells within the myocardium. The cause is unknown but it may be associated with sarcoidosis, thymomas and autoimmune disease. It has a rapidly progressive course and a poor prognosis. Immunosuppression is recommended.

Chagas' disease

Chagas' disease is caused by the protozoan *Trypanosoma cruzi* and is endemic in South America where upwards of 20 million people are infected. Acutely, features of myocarditis are present with fever and congestive heart failure. Chronically, there is progression to a dilated cardiomyopathy with a propensity towards heart block and ventricular arrhythmias. Treatment is discussed on page 780. Amiodarone is helpful for the control of ventricular arrhythmias; heart failure is treated in the usual way (p. 790).

CARDIOMYOPATHY

Cardiomyopathy is a general term indicating disease of the cardiac muscle. Diseases are classified on predominant clinical presentations:

- dilated cardiomyopathy – ventricular dilatation
- hypertrophic cardiomyopathy – myocardial hypertrophy
- restrictive cardiomyopathy – impaired ventricular filling
- arrhythmogenic right ventricular cardiomyopathy – prominent right ventricular involvement with a high frequency of ventricular arrhythmias
- other rare cardiomyopathies.

Dilated cardiomyopathy (DCM)

DCM is characterized by dilatation and impaired systolic function of the left and/or right ventricle, in the absence of abnormal loading conditions (e.g. hypertension, valve disease) and coronary disease. The aetiology in the majority of cases is unknown and in most patients no cause is found ('idiopathic').

A large number of cardiac and systemic diseases can cause cardiac dilatation and systolic impairment (Table 13.45). Other potential causes of DCM include persistent viral infection and autoimmune disease. Evidence for the latter includes associations with specific HLA subtypes and the frequent finding of circulating cardiac-specific autoantibodies.

At least 25% of the 'idiopathic' cases are known to be familial (Fig. 13.105). In the majority of familial cases inheritance is autosomal dominant, but X-linked and recessive cases occur. In a limited number of cases the responsible genes have been identified. Many of these are genes encoding cytoskeletal or associated myocyte proteins (dystrophin in X-linked cardiomyopathy; actin, desmin, troponin T, beta myosin heavy chain, sarcoglycans, vinculin and lamin a/c in autosomal dominant DCM) (Fig. 13.106). Many of these have prominent associated features such as skeletal myopathy or conduction system disease and therefore differ from the majority of cases of DCM. The aetiology in the majority of cases remains unknown.

Table 13.45	Causes of dilated cardiomyopathy (DCM)
Genetic	e.g. autosomal dominant DCM, X-linked cardiomyopathy
Inflammatory	Post-infective, autoimmune, connective tissue diseases (systemic lupus erythematosus, systemic sclerosis)
Metabolic	e.g. glycogen storage diseases
Nutritional	Thiamin, selenium deficiency
Endocrine	Acromegaly, thyrotoxicosis, myxoedema, diabetes mellitus
Infiltrative	Hereditary haemochromatosis
Neuromuscular	e.g. muscular dystrophy, Friedreich's ataxia, mitochondrial myopathies
Toxic	Alcohol, cocaine, doxorubicin, cyclophosphamide, cobalt
Haematological	Sickle cell anaemia, thrombotic thrombocytopenic purpura

Fig. 13.105 **Pedigree of a family with dilated cardiomyopathy**. Blue symbols are affected family members. The arrow indicates the index case.

Fig. 13.106 **Schematic representation of myocyte proteins implicated in dilated cardiomyopathy (DCM).** See also Fig. 13.4.

Clinical features

Presentation is generally with congestive heart failure and therefore symptoms and signs are those of left and/or right *heart failure*. Additionally, patients may present with *syncope* due to ventricular arrhythmia or conduction disease or with pulmonary or systemic *embolism*. Occasionally, initial presentation is with *sudden cardiac death*. Increasingly, evaluation of relatives of DCM patients is allowing identification of early asymptomatic disease, prior to the onset of these complications. Clinical evaluation should include careful family history and construction of a pedigree where appropriate.

Investigations

- **Chest X-ray** demonstrates generalized cardiac enlargement.
- **ECG** shows diffuse non-specific ST segment and T wave changes. Sinus tachycardia, conduction abnormalities and arrhythmias (i.e. atrial fibrillation, ventricular premature contractions or ventricular tachycardia) are also seen.
- **Echocardiogram** reveals dilatation of the left and/or right ventricle with poor global contraction function (Fig. 13.107).
- **Angiography** should be performed to exclude coronary artery disease in all individuals at risk (generally patients > 40 years or younger if symptoms or risk factors are present).
- **Biopsy** is generally not indicated outside specialist care.

Treatment

The goals of management are to relieve symptoms, retard disease progression and prevent complications. Treatment involves conventional management of heart failure (see p. 790). Diuretics are highly effective for the relief of congestive symptoms but should not be used in isolation since they exacerbate activation of neurohormones that may contribute to disease progression. Disease progression is retarded by the use of ACE-inhibitors, angiotensin II receptor antagonists and spironolactone to antagonize activation of the renin–angiotensin–aldosterone system (RAAS), while beta-blockers act similarly on the sympathetic nervous system. These are indicated in most cases. Beta-blockers may also help prevent arrhythmias. In specific cases, permanent pacing, anti-arrhythmic therapy or implantable cardioverter–defibrillators may be indicated. Severe ventricular dilatation and dysfunction, documented atrial fibrillation or a history of embolization are indications for anti-coagulant treatment. Cardiac transplantation remains the principal option for advanced disease refractory to medical therapy. Potential alternatives to transplantation are discussed in the section on heart failure (see p. 796). There is currently no specific treatment for idiopathic DCM although preliminary studies have investigated the role of growth hormone, immunoadsorption and anti-cytokine therapy.

(b)

Fig. 13.107 **Dilated cardiomyopathy** shown in two-dimensional (apical four-chamber view) and M-mode echocardiograms. The heart has a 'globular' appearance with all four chambers dilated. The extremely impaired left ventricular function can be appreciated from the M-mode recording. Compare the systolic shortening fraction with that of Figures 13.26 and 13.29. LA, left atrium; RA, right atrium; LV, left ventricle; LV(d) and LV(s), diastolic and systolic left ventricular dimensions; IVS, interventricular septum; PVW, posterior ventricular wall.

Hypertrophic cardiomyopathy (HCM)

Hypertrophic cardiomyopathy is characterized by variable myocardial hypertrophy, most commonly involving the interventricular septum, and disorganization ('disarray') of cardiac myocytes and myofibrils (Fig. 13.108). Twenty-five per cent of patients have dynamic left ventricular outflow tract obstruction due to the combined effects of hypertrophy, systolic anterior motion (SAM) of the anterior mitral valve leaflet and rapid ventricular ejection.

The majority of cases are familial, autosomal dominant, and due to mutations in the genes encoding sarcomeric proteins.

The salient clinical and morphological features of the disease vary according to the underlying genetic mutation. For example, marked hypertrophy is common with beta-myosin heavy chain mutations whereas mutations in troponin T may be associated with mild hyper-

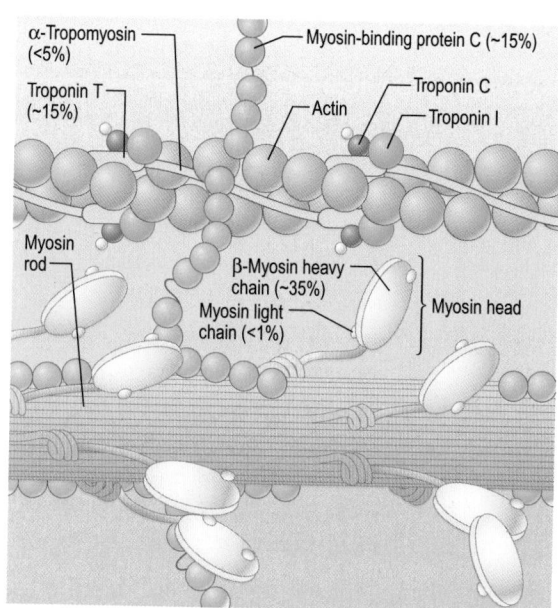

Fig. 13.108 **Sarcomeric proteins implicated in hypertrophic cardiomyopathy**. Reproduced with permission from Spirito P et al. (1997) The management of hypertrophic cardiomyopathy. *New England Journal of Medicine* **336**: 775–785. © Massachusetts Medical Society, all rights reserved.

trophy but a high risk of sudden death. Modifying genetic factors may also influence the phenotype in HCM. These include polymorphisms of components of the renin–angiotensin–aldosterone system which influence myocyte growth.

The hypertrophy may not manifest before completion of the adolescent growth spurt, making the diagnosis in children difficult. HCM due to myosin-binding protein C may not manifest until the sixth decade of life or later. Sporadic cases of HCM occur, but the aetiology is unknown. HCM may also be associated with Noonan's syndrome, Friedreich's ataxia, glycogen storage disease, and mitochondrial myopathies.

Clinical features

Patients with HCM present with *chest pain, dyspnoea, syncope* or *presyncope* (typically with exertion), *cardiac arrhythmias* and *sudden death*. Sudden death may occur at any age but the highest rates (up to 6% per annum) occur in adolescents or young adults. Risk factors for sudden death are discussed below. Dyspnoea is common and is due to impaired relaxation of the heart muscle. Left ventricular filling – and therefore left ventricular emptying – is impaired, compounded by outflow obstruction in about one-third of cases. Systolic ventricular function remains good until the very late stages of disease when progressive dilatation may occur. Atrial fibrillation occurs (the prevalence increasing with increasing duration of disease) and is associated with worsening symptoms due to reduction in ventricular filling and an increased risk of stroke.

The classic physical findings are:

- double apical pulsation (forceful atrial contraction producing a fourth heart sound)
- jerky carotid pulse because of rapid ejection and sudden obstruction to left ventricular outflow during systole
- ejection systolic murmur due to left ventricular outflow obstruction late in systole – it can be increased by manoeuvres that decrease afterload, e.g. standing or Valsalva, and decreased by manoeuvres that increase afterload and venous return, e.g. squatting
- pansystolic murmur due to mitral regurgitation (secondary to SAM)
- fourth heart sound (if not in AF).

Investigations

- **Chest X-ray** is usually unremarkable.
- **ECG** demonstrates left ventricular hypertrophy (Fig. 13.81) and ST and T wave changes. Abnormal Q waves, most commonly in the inferolateral leads occur in 25–50% of patients.
- **Echocardiogram** is usually diagnostic and in the most typical cases shows asymmetric left ventricular hypertrophy (involving septum more than posterior wall), systolic anterior motion of the mitral valve, and a vigorously contracting ventricle (Fig. 13.109). However, any pattern of hypertrophy may be seen, including concentric and apical hypertrophy. Certain mutations, e.g. involving the troponin gene, are associated with minimal or even no hypertrophy.
- **Pedigree analysis** generally reveals autosomal dominant inheritance and may provide prognostic information (e.g. history of sudden death). Genetic analysis where available confirms the diagnosis, may provide prognostic information and facilitates evaluation of relatives.
- **Exercise testing** and ambulatory ECG recording also provide prognostic information.

(a)

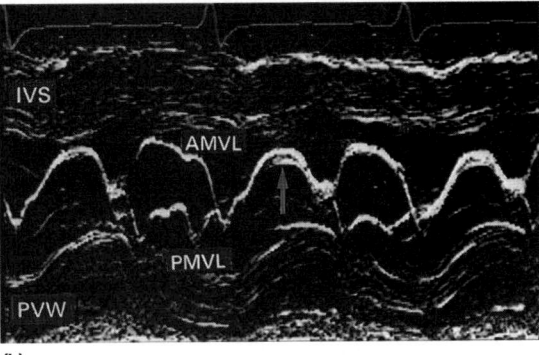

(b)

Fig. 13.109 **Hypertrophic cardiomyopathy** shown by **(a)** a two-dimensional echocardiogram (short-axis view) and **(b)** M-mode recording. The grossly thickened interventricular septum is shown, resulting in a small left ventricular cavity. This condition is associated with an abnormal anterior motion of the mitral valve during systole (arrowed). IVS, interventricular septum; LV, left ventricle; PVW, posterior ventricular wall; AMVL, PMVL, anterior and posterior mitral valve leaflets.

Treatment

The overriding concern in the management of HCM is the prevention of sudden death. Several risk factors for sudden death have been identified. Massive left ventricular hypertrophy (> 30 mm) is a recognized risk factor but the majority of sudden deaths do not occur in individuals with massive hypertrophy, and other risk factors must be considered. These include genotype, family history of sudden cardiac death, abnormal blood pressure response during exercise, non-sustained ventricular tachycardia on Holter monitoring and recurrent syncope. The presence of two or more of these risk factors is associated with a substantial risk of sudden death. Implantable defibrillators effectively prevent sudden death in high-risk cases. In patients in whom the risk is less high, amiodarone is an appropriate alternative. Recent research has suggested that microvascular dysfunction as assessed by PET scanning may be an independent risk factor for sudden death but this requires further validation.

Chest pain and dyspnoea are treated with beta-blockers and verapamil, either alone or in combination. If these are ineffective, disopyramide is a useful second-line therapy for patients with obstruction. In selected cases only (e.g. elderly patients) with significant left outflow obstruction and recalcitrant symptoms, dual-chamber pacing may be of use. Alcohol (non-surgical) ablation of the septum has been investigated and appears to give good results in reduction of outflow tract obstruction and subsequent improvement in exercise capacity. There are, however, significant risks, including the development of complete heart block and massive myocardial infarction. Occasionally, surgical resection of septal myocardium may be indicated. Vasodilators should be avoided because they may aggravate left ventricular outflow obstruction or cause refractory hypotension.

Restrictive cardiomyopathy

Some cardiomyopathies do not present with muscular hypertrophy or ventricular dilatation. Instead, the ventricular filling is restricted (as with constrictive pericarditis), resulting in symptoms and signs of heart failure. Dilatation of the atria and thrombus formation commonly occur.

Conditions associated with this form of cardiomyopathy include amyloidosis (commonest), sarcoidosis, Loeffler's endocarditis and endomyocardial fibrosis; in the latter two conditions there is myocardial and endocardial fibrosis associated with eosinophilia.

The idiopathic form of restrictive cardiomyopathy may be familial and has been associated with mutations in the sarcomeric protein troponin I, suggesting that this form may be part of the spectrum of hypertrophic cardiomyopathy.

Clinical features

Dyspnoea, fatigue and embolic symptoms are the presenting features. Restriction to ventricular filling (especially right) results in persistently elevated venous pressures, consequent hepatic enlargement, ascites, and dependent oedema.

Physical signs are similar to those of constrictive pericarditis – a high jugular venous pressure with diastolic collapse (Friedreich's sign) and elevation of venous pressure with inspiration (Kussmaul's sign). A fourth heart sound is common in early disease and cardiac enlargement, and a third heart sound may be present in advanced disease. In idiopathic restrictive cardiomyopathy, however, cardiac size may remain normal.

Investigations

- **Chest X-ray** may show pulmonary venous congestion. The cardiac silhouette can be normal or show cardiomegaly and/or atrial enlargement.
- **ECG** usually has low-voltage and ST segment and T wave abnormalities.
- **Echocardiogram** shows symmetrical myocardial thickening and often a normal systolic ejection fraction, but impaired ventricular filling.
- **Cardiac catheterization** and haemodynamic studies help distinction from constrictive pericarditis.
- **Endomyocardial biopsy** in contrast with other cardiomyopathies is often useful in this condition and may permit a specific diagnosis such as amyloidosis to be made.

Treatment

There is no specific treatment. Cardiac failure and embolic manifestations should be treated. Cardiac transplantation should be considered in some severe cases, especially the idiopathic variety. In primary amyloidosis, combination therapy with melphalan plus prednisolone with or without colchicine may improve survival. However, patients with cardiac amyloidosis have a worse prognosis than those with other forms of the disease, and the disease often recurs after transplantation. Liver transplantation may be effective in familial amyloidosis (due to production of mutant prealbumin) and may lead to reversal of the cardiac abnormalities.

Fig. 13.110   Gross pathological specimen demonstrating thinning and fibrofatty replacement of RV free wall. From Basso et al. (1996) *Circulation* **94**: 983–991, with permission.

Arrhythmogenic right ventricular cardiomyopathy

Arrhythmogenic right ventricular cardiomyopathy (ARVC) is characterized by progressive fibrofatty replacement of the right ventricular myocardium (Fig. 13.110). This leads to ventricular arrhythmia and risk of sudden death in its early stages and right ventricular or biventricular failure in its later stages. It is familial in at least 50% of cases, most commonly with an autosomal dominant pattern of inheritance. A rare form of ARVC which is associated with dermatological abnormalities (Naxos disease) is caused by a mutation in a gene encoding a myocyte structural protein (plakoglobin) found in desmosomes and gap junctions. There are at least six other loci for ARVC, and mutated genes have been identified in two:

- *human ryanodine receptor 2* (hRyR2), an ion channel protein involved in calcium homeostasis in the sarcoplasmic reticulum of the myocyte (see p. 727)
- *desmoplakin*, a cytoskeletal protein that interacts with plakoglobin.

Clinical features

Presentation is most commonly with severe symptomatic *ventricular arrhythmias* or *syncope*. Occasionally presentation is with right *heart failure*. Heart failure, however, is more commonly associated with a later stage of disease, in which left ventricular dilatation may also occur, and severity of arrhythmia may paradoxically diminish. The condition is often asymptomatic and the first presentation may be with *sudden death* or alternatively it may be diagnosed as a result of routine medical evaluation or family screening.

Fig. 13.111 **Electrocardiogram from an adult with arrhythmogenic right ventricular cardiomyopathy** (ARVC) demonstrating RBBB and precordial T wave insertion with epsilon waves visible at the terminal of the QRS complex (arrow).

Investigations

- **Chest X-ray** is usually unremarkable except in advanced disease.
- **ECG** most commonly demonstrates T wave inversion in precordial leads related to the right ventricle (V_1–V_3). Small-amplitude potentials occurring at the end of the QRS complex (epsilon waves) may be present (Fig. 13.111). Incomplete or complete RBBB is seen.
- **Signal averaged ECG** may indicate the presence of late potentials, the delayed depolarization of individual muscle cells.
- **Echocardiogram**. In early cases this is often normal and in more advanced cases may demonstrate right ventricular dilatation and aneurysm formation, associated in some cases with concomitant left ventricular dilatation.
- **MRI** demonstrates morphological abnormalities of the RV and is capable of demonstrating fatty infiltration.
- **RV angiography** demonstrates enlargement and abnormal motion of right ventricular myocardium.
- **RV biopsy** may demonstrate fibrofatty replacement but is often falsely negative.
- **Holter monitoring** often demonstrates frequent extrasystoles of right ventricular origin and runs of non-sustained or sustained ventricular tachycardia.
- **Genetic testing**, although currently in its infancy, may be a vital diagnostic tool, particularly in variably penetrant disease.

Treatment

Beta-blockers are first-line treatment for patients with non-life-threatening arrhythmias. Amiodarone or sotalol may be used for symptomatic arrhythmias, and for refractory or life-threatening arrhythmias an ICD may be required. Occasionally cardiac transplantation is indicated, either for intractable arrhythmia or cardiac failure.

Other cardiomyopathies

Anderson–Fabry disease (AFD) (p. 1147)

The heart is frequently involved in patients with classical disease. Some male patients with residual enzyme activity present in middle age with few if any of the other typical features of the disease. Cardiac abnormalities that occur in AFD include left ventricular hypertrophy, valvular dysfunction, short PR interval, atrioventricular conduction abnormalities and atrial fibrillation. Patients may also develop systolic impairment and regional wall motion abnormalities.

Left ventricular non-compaction

This cardiomyopathy is inherited as an autosomal dominant and has a poor prognosis. It is characterized by chamber dilatation and prominent sacculation of the ventricle, best seen with echocardiography or magnetic resonance imaging. It presents with dyspnoea, cardiac arrhythmia or sudden death. The responsible gene has not yet been identified.

Inflammatory cardiomyopathy

The association of myocarditis or a prominent history of chronic myocarditis, with left ventricular dysfunction (chamber dilatation and hypokinesis) is termed inflammatory cardiomyopathy. The prognosis depends on the rapidity of its development and the status of left ventricular function.

Cancer chemotherapy with anthracyclines can cause cardiomyopathy that may manifest years later, particularly in individuals treated for childhood cancer.

FURTHER READING

Corrado D, Basso C, Thiene G (2000) Arrhythmogenic right ventricular cardiomyopathy: diagnosis, prognosis and treatment. *Heart* **83**: 588–585.

Maron BJ, et al. (2003) Consensus document on hypertrophic cardiomyopathy. A report of the American College of Cardiology Foundation Task Force on Clinical Expert Consensus Documents and the European Society of Cardiology Committee for Practice Guidelines. *European Heart Journal* **24**(21): 1965–1991.

PERICARDIAL DISEASE

The pericardium acts as a protective covering for the heart. It consists of two separate layers, the inner visceral pericardium and the outer parietal pericardium. The visceral pericardium reflects back upon itself at the level of the great vessels to join the parietal pericardium, thus forming a sac. The pericardial sac contains up to 50 mL of pericardial fluid in the normal heart, although this is a potential space for fluid to collect. The pericardium serves to lubricate the surface of the heart, prevents deformation and dislocation of the heart and acts as a barrier to the spread of infection.

Presentations of pericardial disease include:

- acute pericarditis
- pericardial effusion and cardiac tamponade
- constrictive pericarditis.

Acute pericarditis

This refers to inflammation of the pericardium. Classically, fibrinous material is deposited into the pericardial space and pericardial effusion often occurs. Acute pericarditis has numerous aetiologies (Table 13.46). Most commonly in the UK, it is due to viral infection and myocardial infarction, although in many cases the cause is unknown.

Viral pericarditis. The most common viral causes are Coxsackie B virus and echovirus. Viral pericarditis is usually painful but has a short time course and rarely long-term effects. Increasingly, HIV is implicated in the aetiology of pericarditis, both directly and via immuno-suppression, which predisposes the subject to infective causes.

Post-myocardial infarction pericarditis occurs in about 20% of patients in the first few days following MI. It occurs more commonly with anterior MIs and ST elevation MIs with high serum cardiac enzymes, but its incidence is reduced to 5–6% with thrombolysis. It may be difficult to differentiate this pain from recurrent angina when it occurs early (day 1–2 post-infarct) but a good history of the pain and serial ECG monitoring is helpful. Pericarditis may also occur later on in the recovery phase after infarction. This usually occurs as a feature of

Dressler's syndrome, an autoimmune response to cardiac damage occurring 2–10 weeks post-infarct. Autoimmune reaction to myocardial damage is the main aetiology, and antimyocardial antibodies can often be found. Recurrences are common. Differential diagnosis includes a new myocardial infarction or unstable angina.

Uraemic pericarditis is due to irritation of the pericardium by accumulating toxins. It can occur in 6–10% of patients with advanced renal failure if dialysis is delayed. It is an indication for urgent dialysis as it continues to be associated with significant morbidity and mortality.

Bacterial pericarditis may rarely occur with septicaemia or pneumonia or it may stem from an early postoperative infection after thoracic surgery or trauma or may complicate endocarditis.

Staphylococcus aureus is a frequent cause of purulent pericarditis in HIV patients. This form of pericarditis, especially staphylococcal, is fulminant and often fatal.

Other *endemic infectious pericarditis* includes mycoplasmosis and Lyme pericarditis which are often effusive and require pericardial drainage. The diagnosis is based on serological tests of pericardial fluid and identification of organisms in pericardial or myocardial biopsies.

Tuberculous pericarditis usually presents with chronic low-grade fever, particularly in the evening, associated with features of acute pericarditis, dyspnoea, malaise, night sweats and weight loss. Pericardial aspiration is often required to make the diagnosis. Constrictive pericarditis is a frequent outcome.

Fungal pericarditis is a common complication of endemic fungal infections, such as histoplasmosis and coccidioidomycosis but may be also caused by *Candida albicans,* especially in immunocompromised patients, drug addicts or after cardiac surgery.

Malignant pericarditis. *Carcinoma of the bronchus, carcinoma of the breast* and *Hodgkin's lymphoma* are the most common causes of malignant pericarditis. Leukaemia and malignant melanoma are also associated with pericarditis. A substantial pericardial effusion is very typical and is due to the obstruction of the lymphatic drainage from the heart. The effusion is often haemorrhagic. Radiation and therapy for thoracic tumours may cause radiation injury to the pericardium resulting in serous or haemorrhagic pericardial effusion and pericardial fibrosis. Absence of neoplastic cells in the pericardial fluid in these conditions often helps diagnosis.

Clinical features

Pericardial inflammation produces sharp central *chest pain* exacerbated by movement, respiration and lying down. It is typically relieved by sitting forward. It may be referred to the neck or shoulders. The main differential diagnoses are angina and pleurisy.

Table 13.46   Aetiology of pericarditis

I.   Infectious pericarditis
Viral (Coxsackievirus, echovirus, mumps, herpes, HIV)
Bacterial (staphylococcus, streptococcus, pneumococcus, meningococcus, *Haemophilus influenzae*, mycoplasmosis, borreliosis, *Chlamydia*)
Tuberculous
Fungal (histoplasmosis, coccidioidomycosis, *Candida*)

II.   Post-myocardial infarction pericarditis
Acute myocardial infarction (early)
Dressler's syndrome (late)

III.   Malignant pericarditis
Primary tumours of the heart (mesothelioma)
Metastatic pericarditis (breast and lung carcinoma, lymphoma, leukaemia, melanoma)

IV.   Uraemic pericarditis

V.   Myxoedematous pericarditis

VI.   Chylopericardium

VII.   Autoimmune pericarditis
Collagen–vascular (rheumatoid arthritis, rheumatic fever, systemic lupus erythematosus, scleroderma)
Drug-induced (procainamide, hydralazine, isoniazid, doxorubicin, cyclophosphamides)

VIII.   Post-radiation pericarditis

IX.   Post-surgical pericarditis
Postpericardiotomy syndrome

X.   Post-traumatic pericarditis

XI.   Familial and idiopathic pericarditis

The classical clinical sign is a pericardial *friction rub* occurring in three phases corresponding to atrial systole, ventricular systole and ventricular diastole. It may also be heard as a biphasic 'to and fro' rub. The rub is heard best with the diaphragm of the stethoscope at the lower left sternal edge at the end of expiration with the patient leaning forward. There is usually a *fever, leucocytosis* or *lymphocytosis* when pericarditis is due to viral or bacterial infection, rheumatic fever or myocardial infarction. Features of a *pericardial effusion* may also be present (p. 856). Large pericardial effusion can compress adjacent bronchi and lung tissue and may cause *dyspnoea*.

Investigations

ECG is diagnostic. There is concave-upwards (saddle-shaped) ST elevation (Fig. 13.112). These changes evolve over time, with resolution of the ST elevation, T wave flattening/inversion and finally T wave normalization. The early ECG changes must be differentiated from ST elevation found in myocardial infarction.

Sinus tachycardia may result from fever or haemodynamic embarrassment, and rhythm and conduction abnormalities may be present if myocardium is involved. *Cardiac enzymes* should be assayed as they may be elevated if there is associated myocarditis (see p. 848).

Chest X ray, echocardiograms and radionucleotide scans are of little value in uncomplicated acute pericarditis.

Treatment

If a cause is found, this should be treated. Bed rest and oral NSAIDs (high-dose aspirin, indometacin or ibuprofen) are effective in most patients. In the few days following a myocardial infarction, NSAID use is associated with a higher rate of myocardial rupture and these drugs should not be used. Corticosteroids have been used when the disease does not subside rapidly, but they are associated with side-effects. About 20% of cases of acute pericarditis go on to develop idiopathic relapsing pericarditis. The first-line treatment is again oral NSAIDs. In resistant cases, oral corticosteroids are again used to provide symptomatic relief. However, symptoms commonly recur on dose reduction or withdrawal, and prolonged steroid use is associated with its own side-effects. Numerous other treatments have been studied including azathioprine, colchicine, intravenous corticosteroids and pericardiectomy. Current data tend to favour the use of colchicine to prevent recurrent attacks of pericarditis.

If pericarditis persists for 6–12 months following the acute episode, it is considered chronic. If the pericardium thickens and restricts ventricular filling, constrictive pericarditis is said to have developed.

Pericardial effusion and cardiac tamponade

A pericardial effusion is a collection of fluid within the potential space of the serous pericardial sac (Fig. 13.113), commonly accompanying an episode of acute pericarditis. When a large volume collects in this space, ventricular filling is compromised leading to embarrassment of the circulation. This is known as cardiac tamponade.

Fig. 13.112 **ECGs associated with pericarditis.**
(a) Acute pericarditis. Note the raised ST segment, concave upwards (arrow). **(b) Chronic phase of pericarditis** associated with a pericardial effusion. Note the T wave flattening and inversion and the alternation of the QRS amplitude (QRS alternans). **(c)** The same patient after evacuation of the pericardial fluid. Note that the QRS voltage has increased and the T waves have returned to normal.

Fig. 13.113 **Chest X-ray showing a pericardial effusion;** the heart appears globular.

Clinical features

Symptoms of a pericardial effusion commonly reflect the underlying pericarditis. On examination:

- Heart sounds are soft and distant.
- Apex beat is commonly obscured.
- A friction rub may be evident due to pericarditis in the early stages, but this becomes quieter as fluid accumulates and pushes the layers of the pericardium apart.
- Rarely, the effusion may compress the base of the left lung, producing an area of dullness to percussion below the angle of the left scapula (Ewart's sign).
- As the effusion worsens, signs of cardiac tamponade may become evident:
  - raised jugular venous pressure with sharp rise and *y* descent (Friedreich's sign)
  - Kussmaul's sign (rise in JVP/increased neck vein distension during inspiration)
  - pulsus paradoxus
  - reduced cardiac output.

Investigations

- **ECG** reveals low-voltage QRS complexes.
- **Chest X-ray** (Fig. 13.113) shows large globular or pear-shaped heart with sharp outlines. Typically, the pulmonary veins are not distended.
- **Echocardiography** (Fig. 13.30, p. 755) is the most useful technique for demonstrating the effusion and looking for evidence of tamponade.
- **MRI** should be considered if haemopericardium (blood in the pericardial space) or loculated pericardial effusions are suspected.
- **Pericardiocentesis** is the removal of pericardial fluid with aseptic technique under echocardiographic guidance. It is indicated when a tuberculous, malignant or purulent effusion is suspected.
- **Pericardial biopsy** may be needed if tuberculosis is suspected and pericardiocentesis not diagnostic.

Other tests include looking for underlying causes, e.g. blood cultures, autoantibody screen.

Treatment

An underlying cause should be sought and treated if possible. Most pericardial effusions resolve spontaneously. However, when the effusion collects rapidly, tamponade may result. Pericardiocentesis is then indicated to relieve the pressure – a drain may be left in temporarily to allow sufficient release of fluid.

Pericardial effusions may reaccumulate, most commonly due to malignancy (in the UK). This may require pericardial fenestration, i.e. creation of a window in the pericardium to allow the slow release of fluid into the surrounding tissues. This procedure may either be performed transcutaneously under local anaesthetic or using a conventional surgical approach.

Constrictive pericarditis

Certain causes of pericarditis such as tuberculosis, haemopericardium, bacterial infection and rheumatic heart disease result in the pericardium becoming thick, fibrous and calcified. This may also develop late after open-heart surgery. In many cases these pericardial changes do not cause any symptoms. If, however, the pericardium becomes so inelastic as to interfere with diastolic filling of the heart, constrictive pericarditis is said to have developed. As these changes are chronic, allowing the body time to compensate, this condition is not as immediately life-threatening as cardiac tamponade, in which the circulation is more acutely embarrassed.

Constrictive pericarditis should be distinguished from restrictive cardiomyopathy (see p. 851). The two conditions are very similar in their presentation, but the former is fully treatable, whereas most cases of the latter are not. In the later stages of constrictive pericarditis the subepicardial layers of myocardium may undergo fibrosis, atrophy and calcification.

Clinical features

The symptoms and signs of constrictive pericarditis occur due to:

- reduced ventricular filling (similar to cardiac tamponade, i.e. Kussmaul's sign, Friedreich's sign, pulsus paradoxus)
- systemic venous congestion (ascites, dependent oedema, hepatomegaly and raised JVP)
- pulmonary venous congestion (dyspnoea, cough, orthopnoea, PND) less commonly
- reduced cardiac output (fatigue, hypotension, reflex tachycardia)
- rapid ventricular filling ('pericardial knock' heard in early diastole at the lower left sternal border)
- atrial dilatation (30% of cases have atrial fibrillation).

Investigations

- **Chest X-ray** (Fig. 13.114): shows a relatively small heart in view of the symptoms of heart failure. Pericardial calcification is present in up to 50%. A

Fig. 13.114 **Chest X-ray showing a pericardial calcification** (arrow).

lateral chest film may be useful in detecting calcification that is missed on an AP film. However, a calcified pericardium is not necessarily a constricted one.

- **ECG** reveals low-voltage QRS complexes with generalized T wave flattening or inversion.
- **Echocardiography** shows thickened calcified pericardium, and small ventricular cavities with normal wall thickness. Doppler studies may be useful.
- **CT and MRI** are used to assess pericardial anatomy and thickness (3 mm or greater).
- **Endomyocardial biopsy** may be helpful in distinguishing constrictive pericarditis from restrictive cardiomyopathy in difficult cases.
- **Cardiac catheterization**. End-diastolic pressures in the left and right ventricles measured during this procedure are usually equal, owing to pericardial constriction.

Restrictive cardiomyopathy is a close mimic of constrictive pericarditis and all the above tests may not help to distinguish the two conditions.

Treatment

The treatment for chronic constrictive pericarditis is complete resection of the pericardium. This is a risky procedure with a high complication rate due to the presence of myocardial atrophy in many cases at the time of surgery. Thus early pericardiectomy is suggested in non-tuberculous cases, before severe constriction and myocardial atrophy have developed.

In cases of tuberculous constriction, the presence of pericardial calcification implies chronic disease. Current evidence tends to favour early pericardiectomy with antituberculous drug cover in these cases. If there is no calcification, a course of antituberculous therapy should be attempted first. If the patient's haemodynamic state remains static or deteriorates after 4–6 weeks of therapy, pericardiectomy is recommended.

FURTHER READING

Cairns JA, Camm AJ, Fallen EL, Gersh BJ (2003) Pericardial disease. *Evidence-Based Cardiology* **III**: 407–422.

SYSTEMIC HYPERTENSION

Definitions of hypertension

Elevated arterial blood pressure is a major cause of premature vascular disease leading to cerebrovascular events, ischaemic heart disease and peripheral vascular disease. Blood pressure is a characteristic of each individual, like height and weight, with marked inter-individual variation, and has a continuous (bell-shaped) distribution. The levels of blood pressure observed depend on the characteristics of the population studied – in particular, the age and ethnic background. Blood pressure in industrialized countries rises with age, certainly up to the seventh decade. This rise is more marked for systolic pressure and is more pronounced in men. Hypertension is very common in the developed world. Depending on the diagnostic criteria, hypertension is present in 20–30% of the adult population. Hypertension rates are much higher in black Africans (40–45% of adults).

The definition of an abnormal blood pressure is resolved as indicated in Table 13.47.

The risk of mortality or morbidity rises progressively with increasing systolic and diastolic pressures, with each measure having independent prognostic value; for example, isolated systolic hypertension is associated with a two- to threefold increase in cardiac mortality.

All adults should have blood pressure measured routinely at least every 5 years until the age of 80 years. Seated blood pressure when measured after 5 minutes' resting is usually sufficient, but standing blood pressure

Table 13.47 Classification of blood pressure levels of the British Hypertension Society		
Category	**Systolic blood pressure (mmHg)**	**Diastolic blood pressure (mmHg)**
Blood pressure		
Optimal	< 120	< 80
Normal	< 130	< 85
High normal	130–139	85–89
Hypertension		
Grade I (mild)	140–149	90–99
Grade 2 (moderate)	160–179	100–109
Grade 3 (severe)	≥ 180	≥ 10
Isolated systolic hypertension		
Grade 1	140–149	< 90
Grade 2	≥ 160	< 90

This classification equates with those of the European Society of Hypertension and the World Health Organization–International Society of Hypertension and is based on clinical blood pressure and not values for ambulatory blood pressure measurement. Threshold blood pressure levels for the diagnosis of hypertension using self/home monitoring are greater than 135/85 mmHg. For ambulatory monitoring, 24-hour values are greater than 125/80 mmHg. If systolic blood pressure and diastolic blood pressure fall into different categories, the higher value should be taken for classification should be measured in diabetic and elderly subjects to exclude orthostatic hypotension. The cuff should be deflated at 2 mm/s and the blood pressure measured to the nearest 2 mmHg. Two consistent blood pressure measurements are needed to estimate blood pressure, and more are recommended if there is variation in the pressure. When assessing the cardiovascular risk, the average blood pressure at separate visits is more accurate than measurements taken at a single visit.

Causes

The majority (80–90%) of patients with hypertension have primary elevation of blood pressure (i.e. cause not known – essential hypertension), which can be ameliorated only by life-long pharmacological therapy.

Essential hypertension

Essential hypertension has a multifactorial aetiology.

Genetic factors

Blood pressure tends to run in families and children of hypertensive parents tend to have higher blood pressure than age-matched children of people with normal blood pressure. This familial concordance of blood pressure may be explained, at least in part by shared environmental influences. However, there still remains a large, still largely unidentified genetic component.

Fetal factors

Low birthweight is associated with subsequent high blood pressure. This relationship may be due to fetal adaptation to intrauterine undernutrition with long-term changes in blood vessel structure or in the function of crucial hormonal systems.

Environmental factors

Amongst the several environmental factors that have been proposed, the following seem to be the most significant:

Obesity. Fat people have higher blood pressures than thin people. There is a risk, however, of overestimation if the blood pressure is measured with a small cuff. Adjust the bladder size to the arm circumference. Sleep disordered breathing (see p. 906) often seen with obesity may be an additional risk factor.

Alcohol intake. Most studies have shown a close relationship between the consumption of alcohol and blood pressure level. However, subjects who consume small amounts of alcohol seem to have lower blood pressure level than those who consume no alcohol.

Sodium intake. A high sodium intake has been suggested to be a major determinant of blood pressure differences between and within populations around the world. Populations with higher sodium intake have higher average blood pressures than those with lower sodium intake. Migration from a rural to an urban environment is associated with an increase in blood pressure that is in part related to the amount of salt in the diet. Studies of the restriction of salt intake have shown a beneficial effect on blood pressure in hypertensives. There is some evidence that a high-potassium diet can protect against the effects of a high sodium intake.

Stress. Whilst acute pain or stress can raise blood pressure, the relationship between chronic stress and blood pressure is uncertain.

Humoral mechanisms

The autonomic nervous system, as well as the renin–angiotensin, natriuretic peptide and kallikrein–kinin system, plays a role in the physiological regulation of short-term changes in blood pressure and have been implicated in the pathogenesis of essential hypertension. A low renin, salt-sensitive, essential hypertension in which patients have renal sodium and water retention has been described. However, there is no convincing evidence that the above systems are directly involved in the maintenance of hypertension.

Insulin resistance

An association between diabetes and hypertension has long been recognized and a syndrome has been described of hyperinsulinaemia, glucose intolerance, reduced levels of HDL cholesterol, hypertriglyceridaemia and central obesity (all of which are related to insulin resistance) in association with hypertension. This association (also called the 'metabolic syndrome') is a major risk factor for cardiovascular disease.

Secondary hypertension

Secondary hypertension is where blood pressure elevation is the result of a specific and potentially treatable cause. Secondary forms of hypertension include the following:

Renal diseases

These account for over 80% of the cases of secondary hypertension. The common causes are diabetic nephropathy, chronic glomerulonephritis, adult polycystic disease, chronic tubulointerstitial nephritis, and renovascular disease. Hypertension can itself cause or worsen renal disease. The mechanism of this blood pressure elevation is primarily due to sodium and water retention, although there can be inappropriate elevation of plasma renin levels.

Endocrine causes

These include:

- Conn's syndrome
- adrenal hyperplasia
- phaeochromocytoma
- Cushing's syndrome
- acromegaly.

Congenital cardiovascular causes

The major cause is coarctation of the aorta.

Drugs

There are many drugs that have been shown to cause or aggravate hypertension, or interfere with the response to some antihypertensive agents: NSAIDs, oral contraceptive, steroids, carbenoxolone, liquorice, sympathomimetics and vasopressin.

Patients taking monoamine oxidase inhibitors, who consume tyramine-containing foods, may develop paroxysms of severe hypertension.

Pregnancy

Cardiac output rises in pregnancy but, owing to a relatively greater fall in peripheral resistance, blood pressure in pregnant women is usually lower than in those not pregnant. Hypertension is noted in 8–10% of pregnancies; when detected in the first half of pregnancy or persisting after delivery it is usually due to pre-existing essential hypertension. Hypertension presenting in the second half of pregnancy – or 'pregnancy-induced hypertension' – usually resolves after delivery. When the blood pressure increases to > 160/110 mmHg treatment is warranted for the protection of the mother. Pre-eclampsia is a syndrome consisting of pregnancy-induced hypertension with proteinuria. The primary pathology is unknown, but is likely to involve a disturbance of the uteroplacental circulation and result in intrauterine growth restriction. Hypertension in pregnancy, together with pulmonary embolus, are the most common causes of maternal death, with a rate of 10 per million pregnancies. Furthermore, the critical condition of eclampsia, which is associated with severe hypertension, may ultimately lead to convulsions, cerebral and pulmonary oedema, jaundice, clotting abnormalities and fetal death.

Pathophysiology

The pathogenesis of essential hypertension remains unclear. In some young hypertensive patients, there is an early increase in cardiac output, in association with increased pulse rate and circulating catecholamines. This could result in changes in baroreceptor sensitivity, which would then operate at a higher blood pressure level.

In *chronic hypertension*, the cardiac output is normal and it is an increased peripheral resistance that maintains the elevated blood pressure. The resistance vessels (the small arteries and arterioles) show structural changes in hypertension. These are an increase in wall thickness with a reduction in the vessel lumen diameter. There is also some evidence for rarefaction (decreased density) of these vessels. These mechanisms would result in an increased overall peripheral vascular resistance.

Hypertension also causes changes in the large arteries. There is thickening of the media, an increase in collagen and the secondary deposition of calcium. These changes result in a loss of arterial compliance, which in turn leads to a more pronounced arterial pressure wave. Atheroma develops in the large arteries owing to the interaction of these mechanical stresses and low growth factors (see p. 798). Endothelial dysfunction with alternations in agents such as nitric oxide and endothelins appear to be involved.

Left ventricular hypertrophy, which results from increased peripheral vascular resistance, and increased left ventricular load, is a significant prognostic indicator of future cardiovascular events.

Changes in the *renal vasculature* eventually lead to a reduced renal perfusion, reduced glomerular filtration rate and, finally, a reduction in sodium and water excretion. The decreased renal perfusion may lead to activation of the renin–angiotensin system (renin converts angiotensinogen to angiotensin I, which is in turn converted to angiotensin II by angiotensin-converting enzyme) with increased secretion of aldosterone and further sodium and water retention.

Complications

Cerebrovascular disease and coronary artery disease are the most common causes of death, although hypertensive patients are also prone to renal failure and peripheral vascular disease.

Hypertensives have a sixfold increase in stroke (both haemorrhagic and atherothrombotic). There is a threefold increase in cardiac death (due either to coronary events or to cardiac failure). Furthermore, peripheral arterial disease is twice as common.

Malignant hypertension

Malignant or accelerated hypertension occurs when blood pressure rises rapidly and is considered with severe hypertension (diastolic blood pressure > 120 mmHg) (see p. 864). The characteristic histological change is fibrinoid necrosis of the vessel wall and, unless treated, it may lead to death from progressive renal failure, heart failure, aortic dissection or stroke. The changes in the renal circulation result in rapidly progressive renal failure, proteinuria and haematuria. There is also a high risk of cerebral oedema and haemorrhage with resultant encephalopathy, and in the retina there may be flame-shaped haemorrhages, cotton wool spots, hard exudates and papilloedema (Fig. 13.115). Without effective treatment there is a 1-year survival of less than 20%.

Assessment

Management should be considered in three stages: assessment, non-pharmacological treatment, and drug treatment. During the assessment period, secondary causes of hypertension should be excluded, target-organ damage from the blood pressure should be evaluated, and any concomitant conditions (e.g. dyslipidaemia or diabetes) that may add to the cardiovascular burden should be identified.

History

The patient with mild hypertension is usually asymptomatic. Attacks of sweating, headaches and palpitations may point towards the diagnosis of phaeochromocytoma. Higher levels of blood pressure may be associated with headaches, epistaxis or nocturia. Breathlessness may be present owing to left ventricular hypertrophy or cardiac failure, whilst angina or symptoms of peripheral arterial vascular disease suggest the diagnosis of atheromatous

Fig. 13.115 **Fundus showing hypertensive changes**: Grade 4 retinopathy with papilloedema, haemorrhages and exudates.

Fig. 13.116 **Digital subtraction angiography, showing typical unilateral atheromatous renal artery stenosis with post-stenotic dilatation.**

renal artery stenosis. This is usually a local manifestation of more generalized atherosclerosis, and patients are often elderly with coexistent vascular disease (Fig. 13.116). Fibromuscular disease of the renal arteries encompasses a group of conditions in which fibrous or muscular proliferation results in morphologically simple or complex stenoses and tends to occur in younger patients. Malignant hypertension may present with severe headaches, visual disturbances, fits, transient loss of consciousness or symptoms of heart failure.

Examination

Elevated blood pressure is usually the only abnormal sign. Signs of an underlying cause should be sought, such as renal artery bruits in renovascular hypertension, or

radiofemoral delay in coarctation of the aorta. The cardiac examination may also reveal features of left ventricular hypertrophy and a loud aortic second sound. If cardiac failure develops, there may be a sinus tachycardia and a third heart sound.

Fundoscopy is an essential part of the examination of any hypertensive patient (Fig. 13.115). The abnormalities are graded according to the Keith–Wagener classification:

Grade 1 – tortuosity of the retinal arteries with increased reflectiveness (silver wiring)

Grade 2 – grade 1 plus the appearance of arteriovenous nipping produced when thickened retinal arteries pass over the retinal veins

Grade 3 – grade 2 plus flame-shaped haemorrhages and soft ('cotton wool') exudates actually due to small infarcts

Grade 4 – grade 3 plus papilloedema (blurring of the margins of the optic disc).

Grades 3 and 4 are diagnostic of malignant hypertension.

Ambulatory blood pressure monitoring

Indirect automatic blood pressure measurements can be made over a 24-hour period using a measuring device worn by the patient. The clinical role of such devices remains uncertain, although they are used to confirm the diagnosis in those patients with 'white-coat' hypertension, i.e. in those subjects whose blood pressure is completely normal at all stages except during a clinical consultation (Fig. 13.117a). These patients do not have any evidence of target-organ damage, and unnecessary treatment can be avoided. These devices may also be used to monitor the response of patients to drug treatment and, in particular, can be used to determine the adequacy of 24-hour control with once-daily medication (Fig. 13.117b, c).

Ambulatory blood pressure recordings seem to be better predictors of cardiovascular risk than clinic measurements. Analysis of the diurnal variation in blood pressure suggests that those hypertensives with loss of the usual nocturnal fall in blood pressure ('non-dippers') have a worse prognosis than those who retain this pattern.

Investigations

Routine investigation of the hypertensive patient should include:

- ECG
- urine stix test for protein and blood
- fasting blood for lipids (total and high-density lipoprotein cholesterol) and glucose
- serum urea, creatinine and electrolytes.

If the urea or creatinine is elevated, more specific renal investigations are indicated – creatinine clearance, renal ultrasound (in case of polycystic kidney disease, or parenchymal renal artery disease) and a renal isotope scan or renal angiography if renovascular disease (either atheromatous or fibromuscular dysplasia) is suspected. A low serum potassium may indicate an endocrine disorder (either primary hyperaldosteronism or glucocorticoid

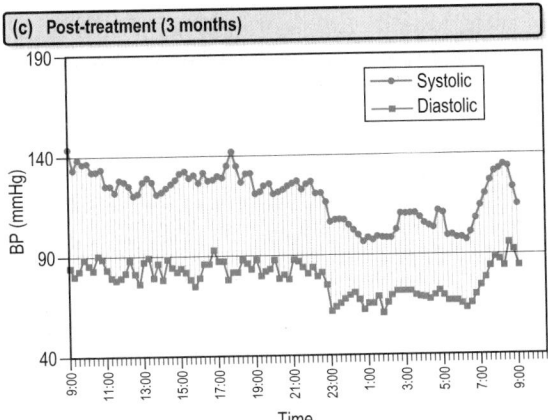

Fig. 13.117 **24-hour ambulatory blood pressure monitoring, showing**:
(a) white-coat hypertension;
(b) pre-treatment;
(c) after 3 months' treatment.

excess), and aldosterone, cortisol and renin measurements must then be made, preferably prior to initiating pharmacological therapy. Clinical suspicion of phaeochromocytoma should be investigated further with measurement of urinary metanephrines and plasma or urinary catecholamines.

If the ECG shows evidence of coronary artery disease the coronary vascular status should be assessed. If left ventricular hypertrophy is suspected *echocardiography* (or

MRI) should be undertaken. A *chest X-ray* is indicated if cardiac involvement or aortic coarctation is likely.

Treatment

Unless the patient has severe or malignant hypertension, there should be a period of assessment with repeated blood pressure measurements, combined with advice and non-pharmacological measures prior to the initiation of drug therapy. The guidelines of the British Hypertension Society (BHS) suggest the following:

Use of non-pharmacological therapy in all hypertensive and borderline hypertensive people:

- weight reduction – BMI should be < 25 kg/m²
- low-fat and saturated fat diet
- low-sodium diet – < 6 g sodium chloride per day
- limited alcohol consumption – ≤ 21 units/week for men and ≤ 14 units/week for women
- dynamic exercise – at least 30 minutes' brisk walk per day
- increased fruit and vegetable consumption
- reduce cardiovascular risk by stopping smoking and increasing oily fish consumption.

Pharmacological therapy should be based on the following:

- The initiation of antihypertensive therapy in subjects with sustained systolic blood pressure (BP) ≥ 160 mmHg, or sustained diastolic BP ≥ 100 mmHg.
- Decide on treatment in subjects with sustained systolic blood pressure between 140 and 159 mmHg, or sustained diastolic BP between 90 and 99 mmHg, according to the presence or absence of target organ damage or a 10-year cardiovascular disease risk > 20%.
- In patients with diabetes mellitus, the initiation of antihypertensive drug therapy if systolic BP is sustained ≥ 140 mmHg, or diastolic BP is sustained ≥ 90 mmHg.
- In non-diabetic hypertensive subjects, treatment goals: BP < 140/85 mmHg. In some hypertensive subjects these levels may be difficult to achieve.
- The main determinant of outcome following treatment is the level of blood pressure reduction that is achieved rather than the specific drug used to lower blood pressure.
- Most hypertensive patients will require a combination of antihypertensive drugs to achieve the recommended targets.
- In most hypertensive patients therapy with statins and aspirin to reduce the overall cardiovascular risk burden. Glycaemic control should be optimized in diabetics (HbA₁c < 7%).

Drug treatment (Table 13.48)
When to initiate treatment

The decision to commence specific drug therapy should usually be made only after a careful period of assessment, of up to 6 months, with repeated measurements of blood pressure. The aim of drug treatment to reduce the risk of complications of hypertension should be carefully

Table 13.48 Advantages and disadvantages of drugs used in hypertension with respect to associated conditions

	Diuretic	Beta-blocker	ACE inhibitor/angiotensin II receptor antagonist	Calcium-channel blockers	Alpha-blocker
Diabetes	Care*	Care*	Yes	Yes	Yes
Gout	No	Yes	Yes	Yes	Yes
Dyslipidaemia	Care†	Care†	Yes	Yes	Yes
Ischaemic heart disease	Yes	Yes	Yes	Yes	Yes
Heart failure	Yes	Yes	Yes	Care‡	Yes
Asthma	Yes	No	Yes	Yes	Yes
Peripheral vascular disease	Yes	Care	Care§	Yes	Yes
Renal artery stenosis	Yes	Care	No	Yes	Yes
Pregnancy	Caution	Not in late pregnancy	No	No	Caution

* Diuretics may aggravate diabetes: beta-blockers worsen glucose intolerance and mask symptoms of hypoglycaemia
† Both diuretics and beta-blockers disturb the lipid profile
‡ Verapamil and diltiazem may exacerbate heart failure, although amlodipine appears to be safe
§ Patients with peripheral vascular disease may also have renal artery stenosis; therefore ACE inhibitors should be used cautiously

explained to the patient and a plan for the patient's treatment (drug dose titration, change of drug, combination of drugs) should be agreed with the patient. All of the drugs used to treat hypertension have side-effects and, since the benefits of drug treatment are not immediate, compliance may be a major problem.

Several classes of drugs are available to treat hypertension. The usual are: (a) ACE inhibitors or angiotensin receptor antagonists; (b) beta-blockers; (c) calcium-channel blockers; or (d) diuretics. It is recommended that drugs are chosen according to the scheme laid out in Figure 13.118.

- The rationale for *step 1* is that young Caucasians are more likely to have high renin hypertension, and older patients and blacks usually have low renin hypertension. If a drug within each pair is not tolerated, the alternative drug type can be used (e.g. if an ACE inhibitor is not tolerated, an angiotensin receptor antagonist or beta-blocker may be used). If a drug is not effective, a drug from the other group should be selected. Thus if a calcium-channel blocker is not helpful, an ACE inhibitor, angiotensin receptor antagonist or beta-blocker should be tried. Almost all patients will need more than one drug to effectively lower blood pressure.
- *Step 2* involves combining one drug from each group. It is not advised to combine a diuretic with a beta-blocker since both aggravate diabetes.
- In *step 3* an ACE inhibitor (or angiotensin receptor antagonist) is combined with a calcium-channel blocker and diuretic. If triple therapy is not sufficient to achieve target blood pressure readings, an alpha-blocker, spironolactone or another agent may be used.

Diuretics
Thiazide diuretics such as bendroflumethiazide (2.5–5 mg daily) and cyclopenthiazide (0.25–0.5 mg daily) are well-established agents which have been shown to reduce the

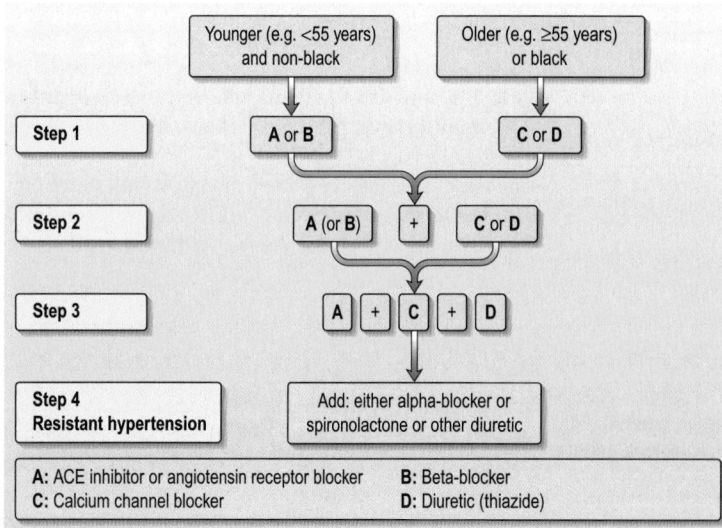

Fig. 13.118 **The British Hypertension Society recommendations for combining blood pressure-lowering drugs.** Adapted from Better blood pressure control: how to combine drugs. *Journal of Human Hypertension* (2003) **17**: 81–86.

risk of stroke in patients with hypertension. The lower doses seems to be equally effective as higher doses in the reduction of blood pressure and most have a duration of up to 24 hours. The major concern with these agents is their adverse metabolic effects, particularly increased serum cholesterol, impaired glucose tolerance, hyperuricaemia (which may precipitate gout) and hypokalaemia. These tend to occur with higher doses of thiazide diuretics.

Loop diuretics such as furosemide (40 mg daily) do have a hypotensive effect, but are not routinely used in the treatment of essential hypertension. Potassium-sparing diuretics such as amiloride (5–10 mg daily) or spironolactone (50–200 mg daily) are not effective agents when used alone, with the exception of spironolactone in the treatment of hypertension and hypokalaemia associated with primary hyperaldosteronism.

Beta-adrenoceptor blockers
The beta-blockers have also been shown to improve the prognosis of hypertensives. They have been suggested to exert their effects by attenuating the effects of the sympathetic nervous and the renin–angiotensin systems. They reduce the force of cardiac contraction, as well as resting and exercise-induced increase in heart rate. But, there are differences between these antihypertensive drugs (Table 13.49):

- *Cardioselectivity.* Some have less effect on the β₂ (non-cardiac) receptors and are therefore said to be relatively cardioselective. These include atenolol and bisoprolol.
- *Intrinsic sympathomimetic activity.* Some agents have partial agonist activity and cause less bradycardia. These include oxprenolol and pindolol.
- *Lipid solubility.* The agents that are less lipid-soluble are less likely to cause central nervous system side-effects. These include atenolol.

The major side-effects of this class of agents are bradycardia, bronchospasm, cold extremities, fatigue, bad dreams and hallucinations. These agents are especially useful in the treatment of patients with both hypertension and angina.

Angiotensin-converting enzyme (ACE) inhibitors
These drugs block the conversion of angiotensin I to angiotensin II, which is a potent vasoconstrictor. They also block the degradation of bradykinin, a potent vasodilator. There is evidence that black African patients respond less well to ACE inhibitors unless combined with diuretics. They are particularly useful in diabetics with nephropathy, where they have been shown to slow disease progression, and in those patients with symptomatic or asymptomatic left ventricular dysfunction, where they have been shown to improve survival.

The major potential side-effects are profound hypotension following the first dose, which is usually seen in sodium-depleted patients or in those on treatment with large doses of diuretics, and deterioration of renal function in those with severe bilateral renovascular disease (in whom the production of angiotensin II is playing a major role in maintaining renal perfusion by causing efferent arteriolar constriction at the glomerulus). They also cause mild dry cough in a number of patients, especially if prescribed at high doses, due to their effect on bradykinin.

These are several ACE inhibitors available and there are no significant differences between them in terms of blood pressure effect other than the half-life and therefore the frequency at which they have to be prescribed for 24-hour blood pressure control; those with the longest duration of action may be taken once-daily, which is clearly a benefit in terms of compliance. The drugs include captopril (50–150 mg daily in divided doses), ramipril (2.5–10 mg daily), enalapril or lisinopril (10–20 mg daily), and trandolapril (1–4 mg daily).

Angiotensin II receptor antagonists
This group of agents selectively block the receptors for angiotensin II. They share many of the actions of ACE inhibitors but, since they do not have any effect on bradykinin, do not cause a cough. They are currently used for patients who cannot tolerate ACE inhibitors because of persistent cough. Angioneurotic oedema and renal dysfunction are encountered less with these drugs than with ACE inhibitors. The agents include losartan (50–100 mg daily), candesartan (16 mg daily) valsartan (80–160 mg daily), irbesartan (75–300 mg daily) and telmisartan (20–80 mg/daily).

Calcium-channel blockers
These agents effectively reduce blood pressure by causing arteriolar dilatation, and some also reduce the force of cardiac contraction. Like the beta-blockers, they are especially useful in patients with concomitant ischaemic

Table 13.49	Main properties of the beta-blockers commonly used for hypertension				
	Cardiac selectivity	Intrinsic sympathomimetic activity	Lipid solubility	Plasma half-life (hours)	Usual dosage
Acebutalol	+	+	0	5	400 mg once or twice daily
Atenolol	+	0	0	6	50 mg once daily
Bisoprolol	++	0	0	10–12	10–20 mg once daily
Celiprolol	0	+	0	5	200 mg once daily
Oxprenolol	0	++	+	1.5	20–80 mg three times daily
Metoprolol	+	0	+	3–10	100–200 mg daily
Propranolol	0	0	+++	5	80–160 mg twice daily
Timolol	0	0	+	5	5–20 mg twice daily

heart disease. The major side-effects are particularly seen with the short-acting agents and include headache, sweating, swelling of the ankles, palpitations and flushing. Many of these side-effects can be lessened by the co-administration of a beta-blocker. The short-acting agents, such as nifedipine (10–20 mg three times daily) are being replaced by once-daily agents that are very well tolerated and include amlodipine (5–10 mg daily) felodipine (5–20 mg daily) and long-acting nifedipine (20–90 mg daily).

Alpha-blockers

These agents cause postsynaptic α_1-receptor blockade with resulting vasodilatation and blood pressure reduction. Earlier short-acting agents caused serious first-dose hypotension, but the newer longer-acting agents are far better tolerated. These include doxazosin (1–4 mg daily). Labetalol is an agent that has combined alpha- and beta-blocking properties, but is not commonly used, except in pregnancy-induced hypertension.

Other vasodilators

These include hydralazine (up to 100 mg daily) and minoxidil (up to 50 mg daily). Both are extremely potent vasodilators that are reserved for patients resistant to other forms of treatment. Hydralazine can be associated with tachycardia, fluid retention and a systemic lupus erythematosus-like syndrome. Minoxidil can cause severe oedema and excessive hair growth and coarse facial features. If these agents are used, it is usually in combination with a beta-blocker.

Centrally acting drugs

Reserpine is used in a low dose of 0.05 mg per day, which provides almost all its antihypertensive action with fewer side-effects than higher doses. It has a slow onset of action (measured in weeks). Methyldopa is still widely used despite central and potentially serious hepatic and blood side-effects. It acts on central α_2-receptors, usually without slowing the heart. Clonidine and moxonidine provide all the benefits of methyldopa with none of the rare (but serious) autoimmune reactions.

Management of severe or malignant hypertension

Patients with severe hypertension (diastolic pressure > 140 mmHg), malignant hypertension (grades 3 or 4 retinopathy), hypertensive encephalopathy or with severe hypertensive complications, such as cardiac failure, should be admitted to hospital for immediate initiation of treatment. However, it is unwise to reduce the blood pressure too rapidly since this may lead to cerebral, renal, retinal or myocardial infarction, and the blood pressure response to therapy must be carefully monitored, preferably in a high-dependency unit. In most cases, the aim is to reduce the diastolic blood pressure to 100–110 mmHg over 24–48 hours. This is usually achieved with oral medication, e.g. atenolol or amlodipine. The blood pressure can then be normalized over the next 2–3 days.

When rapid control of blood pressure is required (e.g. in an aortic dissection), the agent of choice is intravenous sodium nitroprusside. Alternatively, an infusion of labetalol can be used. The infusion dosage must be titrated against the blood pressure response. Fenoldopam, a selective peripheral dopamine receptor agonist, is as effective as nitroprusside.

Management of hypertension in pregnancy

Many antihypertensive agents are contraindicated in pregnancy. Mild hypertension can be treated with methyldopa, which has been established as being safe in pregnancy, or labetalol. Pre-eclamptic hypertension can be treated with the same agents, or nifedipine, although the only method for reversal of overt pre-eclampsia is delivery. More severe hypertension or eclampsia requires treatment with intravenous hydralazine and may even require termination of the pregnancy.

Prognosis

The prognosis from hypertension depends on a number of features:

- level of blood pressure
- presence of target-organ changes (retinal, renal, cardiac or vascular)
- coexisting risk factors for cardiovascular disease, such as hyperlipidaemia, diabetes, smoking, obesity, male sex
- age at presentation.

Several studies have confirmed that the treatment of hypertension, even mild hypertension, will reduce the risk not only of stroke but of coronary artery disease as well.

FURTHER READING

Brown MJ et al. (2003) Better blood pressure control: how to combine drugs. Review. *Journal of Human Hypertension* **17**(2): 81–86.
Caulfield M et al. (2003) Genome-wide mapping of human loci for essential hypertension. *Lancet* **361**(9375): 2118–2123.
Vasan RS et al. (2001) Impact of high-normal blood pressure on the risk of cardiovascular disease. *New England Journal of Medicine* **345**: 1291–1297.
Williams B et al.; British Hypertension Society (2004) Guidelines for management of hypertension: report of the fourth working party of the British Hypertension Society, 2004-BHS IV. *Journal of Human Hypertension* **18**(3): 139–185.

HEART DISEASE IN THE ELDERLY

As the average age of the population increases, and as patients with cardiac disease survive for longer periods of time, the number of elderly patients with heart disease has increased markedly and is likely to continue to escalate in years to come. The elderly are vulnerable to hypertension, coronary artery disease, heart failure, arrhythmias and degenerative pathologies.

Normal findings

Diagnosis of mild forms of heart disease may be difficult in the elderly. The wear and tear of age results in some features that would be regarded as abnormal in the young. For example, a fourth heart sound and a systolic aortic ejection murmur are common findings on examining normal elderly adults. Basal crackles in the elderly are common and may not necessarily imply left-sided heart failure. The ECG often shows slight PR interval prolongation (up to 0.22 s), left axis deviation and T wave flattening. On the chest X-ray there is frequently a degree of tissue calcification. This is seen in the valvular annuli, the aortic arch, and the coronary and pulmonary vasculature, but the cardiac silhouette is usually normal, although changes in the shape of the chest wall may distort normal anatomy. The echocardiogram may show mild myocardial hypertrophy and buckling of the ventricular septum mimicking hypertrophic cardiomyopathy.

It is sometimes difficult to diagnose and define hypertension in the elderly. Cuff blood pressure usually overestimates intravascular pressure since the arterial wall is stiff (pseudohypertension). Normally, blood pressure steadily increases with age, at least up to the age of 70 years; furthermore blood pressure is particularly labile in the elderly.

Disease presentation

Cardiac disease often presents in unexpected ways in an old person. It is not unusual for significant bradycardia to present as a fractured hip owing to a fall resulting from transient asystole. Left heart failure may present as an acute confusional state due to poor cerebral perfusion, rather than with the classical symptom of breathlessness, and frequently accompanies pneumonia. Myocardial infarction may not cause any chest pain ('silent' myocardial infarction) in up to 20% of patients but presents as weakness, abdominal pain, confusion, or a more general deterioration in well-being. Infective endocarditis can cause much diagnostic confusion, particularly in the elderly who may not display fever, and present with symptoms from almost any organ system. Elderly patients may present with heart failure despite a normal-sized heart on X-ray and normal systolic myocardial function on echocardiogram (diastolic heart failure).

Treatment

Age is no bar to effective treatment of heart disease and the principles of treatment of heart disease in the elderly are usually no different from those governing treatment in the young. Drug pharmacokinetics are changed in the elderly: absorption is reduced, renal and hepatic clearance are delayed, body fat increases and lean body mass decreases. Elderly patients frequently have coexistent disease and are taking other medication which interacts with both their cardiac medication and

their heart disease. For example, non-steroidal anti-inflammatory drugs for arthritis may cause fluid retention and worsen heart failure. Old people may forget to take their medication or be confused about the correct dose and timing.

In general, therapy in elderly patients (who have a limited life span) is more likely to be focused on effective relief of symptoms rather than substantial prolongation of life. However, systolic hypertension results in a marked increase in cardiac and cerebrovascular complications, and this risk can be effectively reduced with adequate blood pressure control. Coronary angioplasty, mitral and, less commonly, aortic valvuloplasty can be undertaken in patients too frail for cardiac surgery, which carries a much greater (approximately two to five times) risk in the elderly. As with younger patients, the absolute risk of cardiac surgery is dependent upon the state of the myocardium, the extent of cardiac disease and the condition of other organ systems.

Specific heart problems in the elderly

There are a few cardiac conditions that are largely confined to the elderly.

Aortic sclerosis

Aortic sclerosis results from fibrosis and calcification on the aortic side of an otherwise normal tri-leaflet aortic valve. The resultant obstruction to left ventricular outflow is often trivial; however, true aortic stenosis requiring aortic valve replacement may be necessary if the obstruction is severe.

Mitral annulus calcification

Mitral annulus calcification occurs predominantly in elderly women. It is diagnosed from the chest X-ray and it is not usually responsible for any symptoms.

Endocarditis

A non-bacterial thrombotic form of endocarditis (marantic endocarditis) may occur in the elderly. It is sometimes associated with malignancy and presents with cachexia, thrombosis and embolization. Anticoagulation may be needed.

Lev's disease

Disruption of His–Purkinje conduction by fibrosis and calcification is most common in the old, when it is known as Lev's disease. It presents with Stokes–Adams attacks and must be treated by pacemaker insertion. Age is not a contraindication to pacing, even when the most sophisticated physiological devices are used. Pacemakers should be prescribed on similar criteria in the young and the old.

Carotid sinus hypersensitivity

This is a common cause of syncope in the elderly and is responsible for many admissions for falls, fractures, and dizzy spells. The syndrome is frequently not diagnosed. It is thought to be due to abnormal sensitivity of the carotid baroreceptors resulting in a fall in heart rate, a drop in blood pressure, or both. Diagnosis is made by carotid sinus massage (after excluding carotid stenosis by auscultation). Treatment with a pacemaker may significantly help some patients with the syndrome (see p. 762).

Atrial fibrillation

Atrial fibrillation is much more common in the elderly and is a common cause of stroke in this group of patients. It is often well tolerated and may not need any active treatment for control of heart rate. Anticoagulation is usually advised (see p. 774), except in the very elderly, those prone to falls and those who cannot be relied upon to take their medication regularly.

FURTHER READING

Martin A, Camm AJ (1994) *Heart Disease in the Elderly.* Chichester: John Wiley.

PERIPHERAL VASCULAR DISEASE

PERIPHERAL ARTERIAL DISEASE

Peripheral vascular disease (PVD) is commonly caused by atherosclerosis and usually affects the aorto-iliac or infra-inguinal arteries. It is present in 7% of middle-aged men and 4.5% of middle-aged women but these patients are more likely to die of myocardial infarction or stroke than lose their leg.

Limb ischaemia may be classified as chronic or acute.

Chronic lower limb ischaemia

Symptoms

On exercise, patients complain of a *severe cramp*, usually in the calf, which resolves when they stop walking. They may be unable to continue walking with the *pain* and often the symptoms are worse walking uphill but never occur at rest. This is called intermittent claudication. Patients may experience similar pain in buttocks and thighs associated with male impotence, the 'Leriche syndrome'. *Claudication* can occur in both legs but is often worse in one leg.

Rest pain is defined as a severe unremitting pain in the foot, which stops a patient from sleeping. It is partially relieved by dangling the foot over the edge of the bed or standing on a cold floor. Patients with severe PVD or critical lower limb ischaemia may have *ulceration* or *necrosis* of the tissue (gangrene).

Signs

The lower limbs are cold with dry skin and lack of hair. Pulses may be diminished or absent. Ulceration may occur in association with dark discoloration of the toes or gangrene.

Risk factors

Common risk factors are:

- smoking
- diabetes
- hypercholesterolaemia
- hypertension.

Premature atherosclerosis in patients aged < 45 years may be associated with thrombophilia and hyper-homocysteinaemia.

Differential diagnosis

Symptoms may be confused with those of:

- spinal canal claudication (but all pulses are present)
- osteoarthritis hip/knee (knee pain often at rest)
- peripheral neuropathy (associated with numbness and tingling)
- popliteal artery entrapment (young patients who may have normal pulses)
- venous claudication (bursting pain on walking with a previous history of a DVT)
- fibromuscular dysplasia
- 'Buerger's' disease (young males, heavy smokers).

Investigations

An estimation of the anatomical level of disease may be possible with the examination of pulses. The severity of disease is indicated by *ankle/brachial pressure index* (ABPI). This is a measurement of the cuff pressure at which blood flow is detectable by Doppler in the posterior tibial or anterior tibial arteries compared to the brachial artery (ankle/brachial pressure). Intermittent claudication is associated with an ABPI of 0.4–0.9. Values of < 0.4 are associated with critical limb ischaemia. The sensitivity of the test may be improved by a fall in ABPI after exercise. If the arteries are heavily calcified and incompressible, i.e. in renal or diabetic disease, the ABPI will be falsely elevated. In these patients toe pressure values are more sensitive.

Diagnostic angiograms are now performed less commonly as *Doppler* and *duplex imaging* give an accurate anatomical assessment of the level and degree of disease. Angiograms are performed via a percutaneous arterial catheter and allow therapeutic interventions to be performed (Fig. 13.119).

Magnetic resonance and *CT angiography* are not routinely performed.

Management

Medical

All patients with peripheral vascular disease need aggressive *risk factor management*. Patients are encouraged to stop smoking and need smoking cessation advice. Patients with diabetes mellitus need regular chiropody care and diabetic management. Hypercholesterolaemia should be treated as this reduces disease progression. It has now been shown by the Heart Protection Study that even the reduction of a normal cholesterol level reduces mortality from cardiovascular disease. Low-dose aspirin reduces the risk of myocardial infarction and stroke in patients with peripheral vascular disease. There are as yet no proven oral medications that are of benefit in patients

Fig. 13.119 Angiogram showing occlusion of the right external iliac artery. CI, common iliac; II, internal iliac; EI, external iliac.

with claudication. Supervised exercise programmes significantly improve walking distance and quality of life.

Surgical/radiological

These are only considered in patients who have had their risk factors addressed and who feel that their lifestyle is disabled by their symptoms. For instance a person who can only walk 50 yards before claudicating but who also has severe breathing problems may never need lower limb intervention.

Percutaneous transluminal angioplasty is the first option and is carried out via a catheter inserted into the femoral artery. The long-term patency rates decrease as the angioplasty becomes more distal. The long-term results of angioplasty appear to be similar to those of a continued exercise program. Arterial stents may be deployed in recurrent iliac disease, and drug-eluting stents allowing long-term patency are being investigated.

Bypass procedures may be performed using Dacron, polytetrafluroethylene (PTFE) or autologous veins. Bypasses to distal vessels have poorer long-term patencies. Prosthetic grafts have equal patencies in above-knee bypasses but are inferior to veins below the knee.

In severe ischaemia with unreconstructable arterial disease an *amputation* may be necessary. An amputation may lead to loss of independence, with only 70% of below-knee and 30% of above-knee amputees achieving full mobility.

Acute lower limb ischaemia

Symptoms

Patients complain of the *five P's*. They complain of **p**ain, that the leg looks white (**p**allor), **p**araesthesia, **p**aralysis

and that it feels **p**erishingly cold. The pain is unbearable and normally requires opioids for relief.

Signs

The limb is cold with mottling or marbling of the skin. Pulses are diminished or absent. The sensation and movement of the leg are reduced in severe ischaemia. Patients may develop a compartment syndrome with pain in the calf on compression.

Causes

Acute limb ischaemia (ALI) may occur because of *embolic* or *thrombotic* disease. Embolic disease is commonly due to cardiac thrombus and cardiac arrhythmias. Rheumatic fever is now an uncommon cause and the frequency of cardiac embolic ALI is also on the decline. Emboli may also occur secondary to aneurysm thrombus or thrombus on atherosclerotic plaques. Emboli from atrial myxomas are rare.

Acute limb ischaemia is now often due to thrombotic disease. Acute thrombus may form on a chronic atherosclerotic stenosis in a patient who has previously reported symptoms of claudication. Thrombus may also form in normal vessels in patients, who are hyper-coagulable because of malignancy or thrombophilia defects. Prosthetic or venous grafts may also thrombose either de novo or secondary to a developing stenosis either in the graft or in the native vessels. Popliteal aneurysms may thrombose or embolize distally. Acute upper limb ischaemia may be caused by similar processes or occur secondary to external compression with a cervical rib/band.

Investigation and management

Investigations are similar to those described for chronic lower limb disease.

Medical

Management is dependent on the degree of ischaemia. Patients showing improvement may be treatable with heparin and appropriate treatment of the underlying cause. Patients with emboli following myocardial infarction or atrial fibrillation need long-term warfarin.

Surgical/radiological

Patients with mild to moderate ischaemic symptoms who have occluded a graft may need graft thrombolysis. Intra-arterial thrombolysis may reveal an underlying stenosis within a graft or native vessel that could be treated with angioplasty. Patients with an embolus may benefit from its surgical removal (embolectomy). A bypass graft may be required after occlusion of a popliteal aneurysm or acute-on-chronic lower limb arterial disease. When an ischaemic limb is revascularized, the sudden improvement in blood flow can cause reperfusion injury with release of toxic metabolites into the circulation. In muscle compartments the consequent oedema may lead to a 'compartment syndrome', which requires fasciotomies (release of the fascia to prevent muscle damage). An amputation may be warranted in unreconstructable or severe ischaemia. In patients dying from other causes, acute limb ischaemia may occur and intervention may then be inappropriate.

Aneurysmal disease

Aneurysms are classified as true and false. An aneurysm is defined if there is a permanent dilatation of the artery to twice the normal diameter. In true aneurysms the arterial wall forms the wall of the aneurysm. The arteries most frequently involved are the abdominal aorta, iliac, popliteal, femoral artery and thoracic aorta (in decreasing frequency).

In false aneurysms (pseudoaneurysms) the surrounding tissues form the wall of the aneurysm. False aneurysms can occur following femoral artery puncture. A haematoma is formed because of inadequate compression of the entry site and continued bleeding into the surrounding compressed soft tissue forms the wall of this aneurysm.

Abdominal aortic aneurysm

Abdominal aortic aneurysms (AAA) occur most commonly below the renal arteries (infrarenal). The incidence increases with age, being present in 5% of the population > 60 years. They occur five times more frequently in men and in one in four male children of an affected individual. Aneurysms may occur secondary to atherosclerosis, infection (syphilis, *Escherichia coli*, *Salmonella*) and trauma, or may be genetic (Marfan's syndrome, Ehlers–Danlos syndrome).

Symptoms

Most aneurysms are asymptomatic and are found on routine abdominal examination, plain X-ray or during urological investigations. Rapid expansion or rupture of an AAA may cause *severe pain* (epigastric pain radiating to the back). A ruptured AAA causes *hypotension, tachycardia, profound anaemia* and *sudden death*. The symptoms of rupture may mimic renal colic, diverticulitis and severe lower abdominal or testicular pain. Gradual erosion of the vertebral bodies may cause non-specific back pain. The aneurysm may embolize distally. Inflammatory aneurysms can obstruct adjacent structures, e.g. ureter, duodenum and vena cava. Rarely patients with aneurysms can present with severe haematemesis secondary to an aortoduodenal fistula.

Signs

The aorta is retroperitoneal and in overweight patients there may be no overt signs. An aneurysm is suspected if a pulsatile, expansile abdominal mass is felt. The presence of an AAA should alert a clinician to the possibility of popliteal aneurysms. Patients may present with 'trash feet', dusky discoloration of the digits secondary to emboli from the aortic thrombus.

Investigations

An AAA is first assessed by *ultrasound*.

CT scan is more accurate and relates the anatomical relationship to the renal and visceral vessels.

Management

Like any operation the management of an asymptomatic aneurysm depends on the balance of operative risk and conservative management. The UK Small Aneurysm Trial showed that patients with infrarenal AAA did best with an operation if the aneurysm was:

- ≥ 5.5 cm diameter
- expanding > 1 cm/year
- symptomatic.

Medical

Patients with aneurysmal disease need careful control of hypertension, to stop smoking and to have lipid-lowering medication. Patients with AAA < 5.5 cm are followed up by regular ultrasound surveillance.

Surgical/radiological

Open AAA repair is justified by long-term outcome data but endovascular aneurysm repair (EVAR) is still undergoing assessment within trials. When an aneurysm ruptures, emergency surgery is necessary but the mortality rate is ~ 50%. Elective AAA repair is much less risky (mortality rate ~ 5%) but these patients often have cardiorespiratory and renal disease and need careful preoperative assessment of risk.

Prognosis

After repair, patients with an AAA should return to normal activity within a few months.

Thoraco-abdominal aneurysm (TAA)

The ascending, arch or descending thoracic aorta may become aneurysmal. Ascending TAAs occur most commonly in patients with Marfan's syndrome or hypertension. Descending or arch TAAs occur secondary to atherosclerosis and are now rarely due to syphilis.

Symptoms

Most aneurysms are asymptomatic and are found on routine chest X-ray or cardiological investigation (Fig. 13.120). Rapid expansion may cause severe pain (chest pain radiating to the upper back) and rupture is associated with hypotension, tachycardia and death. Chest symptoms from expansion may include stridor (compressed bronchial tree), haemoptysis (aortobronchial fistula) and hoarseness (compression of the recurrent laryngeal nerve). Aorto-oesophageal fistula uncommonly causes haematemesis.

Investigations

- **CT scan** is used for assessment of a TAA.
- **Aortography** may be used to assess the position of the key branches in relation to the aneurysm
- **Transoesophageal echocardiography** can be helpful by identifying an aortic dissection.

Management

If the aneurysm is > 6 cm then operative repair or stenting may be appropriate but these can be technically difficult

Fig. 13.120 **Plain PA chest X-ray demonstrating a markedly enlarged mediastinum due to an aneurysm of the arch of the aorta (arrows).**

and carry a high risk of mortality and paraplegia. EVAR is at present the procedure of choice for isolated descending thoracic aneurysms but no long-term results are available at present.

Aortic dissection

Aortic dissection usually begins with a tear in the intima. Blood penetrates the diseased medial layer and then cleaves the intimal laminal plain leading to dissection. Thoracic aortic dissection may be classified into:

- *Type A:* involving the aortic arch and aortic valve proximal to the left subclavian artery origin
- *Type B:* involving the descending thoracic aorta distal to the left subclavian artery origin.

Symptoms

Severe and central *chest pain* often radiates to the back and down the arms mimicking myocardial infarction.

Signs

Patients may be shocked and may have neurological symptoms secondary to loss of blood supply to the spinal cord. They may develop renal failure, acute lower limb ischaemia or visceral ischaemia. Peripheral pulses may be absent.

Investigations

The mediastinum may be widened on *chest X-ray*, and *CT scan* or *transoesophageal echocardiography* will confirm the diagnosis (Fig. 13.98b).

Management

At least 50% of patients are hypertensive and they may require urgent antihypertensive medication. Type A dissections should undergo surgery (arch replacement) if fit enough, as medical management carries a high mortality. Type B dissections should be managed medically unless they develop complications.

Raynaud's phenomenon or Raynaud's disease

Raynaud's phenomenon consists of spasm of the digital arteries usually precipitated by cold and relieved by heat. If there is no underlying cause, it is known as Raynaud's disease. This affects 5% of the population, mostly women. The disorder is usually bilateral with fingers affected more commonly than toes.

Symptoms

Vasoconstriction causes *skin pallor* followed by *cyanosis* due to sluggish blood flow, then redness secondary to hyperaemia. The duration of the attacks is variable but they can sometimes last for hours. Numbness, a burning sensation and *severe pain* occur as the fingers warm up. In chronic, severe disease tissue *infarction* and *digital loss* can occur.

Diagnosis

Primary Raynaud's disease needs to be differentiated from secondary treatable causes leading to Raynaud's phenomenon. These are the connective tissue disorders such as systemic sclerosis (see p. 577). It can be associated with atherosclerosis or occupations that involve the use of vibrating tools. Ergot-containing drugs and beta-blockers and smoking can aggravate symptoms.

Management

Patients should avoid cold provocation by wearing gloves and warm clothes and stop smoking. Vasodilators can be prescribed but are often unacceptable as cerebral vasodilatation causes severe headaches. Sympathectomy or prostacyclin infusion can be helpful in severe disease.

Takayasu's disease

This is rare, except in Japan. It is known as the pulseless disease or aortic arch syndrome. It is of unknown aetiology and occurs in females. There is a vasculitis involving the aortic arch as well as other major arteries. There is also a systemic illness, with pain and tenderness over the affected arteries. Absent peripheral pulses and hypertension are common. Corticosteroids help the constitutional symptoms. Eventually heart failure and strokes may occur but most patients survive for at least 5 years. Treatment may require a surgical bypass to improve perfusion of the affected areas.

Thromboangiitis obliterans (Buerger's disease)

This disease, involving the small vessels of the lower limbs, occurs in young men who smoke. It is thought by some workers to be indistinguishable from atheromatous disease. However, pathologically there is inflammation of the arteries and sometimes veins that may indicate a separate disease entity. Clinically it presents with severe claudication and rest pain leading to gangrene. A thrombophlebitis is sometimes present. Treatment is as for all peripheral vascular disease, but patients must stop smoking.

Cardiovascular syphilis

This gives rise to:

- uncomplicated aortitis
- aortic aneurysms, usually in the ascending part
- aortic valvulitis with regurgitation
- stenosis of the coronary ostia.

The diagnosis is confirmed by serology. Treatment is with penicillin. Aneurysms and valvular disease are treated as necessary by the usual methods.

PERIPHERAL VENOUS DISEASE

Varicose veins

Varicose veins are a common problem, sometimes giving rise to pain. They are treated by injection or surgery.

Venous thrombosis

Thrombosis can occur in any vein, but the veins of the leg and the pelvis are the most common sites.

Superficial thrombophlebitis

This commonly involves the saphenous veins and is often associated with varicosities. Occasionally the axillary vein is involved, usually as a result of trauma. There is local superficial inflammation of the vein wall, with secondary thrombosis.

The clinical picture is of a painful, tender, cord-like structure with associated redness and swelling.

The condition usually responds to symptomatic treatment with rest, elevation of the limb and analgesics (e.g. non-steroidal anti-inflammatory drugs). Anticoagulants are not necessary, as embolism does not occur from superficial thrombophlebitis.

Deep-vein thrombosis

A thrombus forms in the vein, and any inflammation of the vein wall is secondary to this.

Thrombosis commonly occurs after periods of immobilization, but it can occur in normal individuals for no obvious reasons. The precipitating factors are discussed on page 477.

A deep-vein thrombosis in the legs occurs in 50% of patients after prostatectomy (without prophylactic heparin) or following a cerebral vascular event. In addition, 10% of patients with a myocardial infarct have a clinically detected deep-vein thrombosis.

Thrombosis can occur in any vein of the leg, but is particularly found in veins of the calf. It is often undetected; autopsy figures give an incidence of over 60% in hospitalized patients. Axillary vein thrombosis occasionally occurs, sometimes related to trauma, but usually for no obvious reason.

Clinical features

The individual may be asymptomatic, presenting with clinical features of pulmonary embolism (see p. 844).

A major presenting feature is *pain* in the calf, often with swelling, redness and *engorged superficial veins*. The affected calf is often warmer and there may be ankle oedema. *Homan's sign* (pain in the calf on dorsiflexion of the foot) is often present, but is not diagnostic and occurs with all lesions of the calf.

Thrombosis in the iliofemoral region can present with severe pain, but there are often few physical signs apart from occasional swelling of the thigh and/or ankle *oedema*.

Complete occlusion, particularly of a large vein, can lead to a *cyanotic discoloration* of the limb and severe oedema, which can very rarely lead to venous gangrene.

Pulmonary embolism can occur with any deep-vein thrombosis but is more frequent from an iliofemoral thrombosis and is rare with thrombosis confined to veins below the knee. In 20–30% of patients, spread of thrombosis can occur proximally without clinical evidence, so careful monitoring of the leg, usually by ultrasound, is required.

Investigations

Clinical diagnosis is unreliable but combined with D-dimer level it has a sensitivity of 80%. Confirmation of an iliofemoral thrombosis can usually be made with *B mode venous compression*, *ultrasonography* or *Doppler ultrasound* with a sensitivity and specificity over 90%.

Below-knee thromboses can be detected reliably only by *venography* with non-invasive techniques, ultrasound, fibrinogen scanning and impedance plethysmography, having a sensitivity of only 70%. A venogram is performed by injecting a vein in the foot with contrast, which will detect virtually all thrombi that are present.

Treatment

The main aim of therapy is to prevent pulmonary embolism, and all patients with thrombi above the knee must be anticoagulated. Anticoagulation of below-knee thrombi is now recommended for 6 weeks as 30% of patients will have an extension of the clot proximally. Bed rest is advised until the patient is fully anticoagulated. The patient should then be mobilized, with an elastic stocking giving graduated pressure over the leg.

Low-molecular-weight heparins (LMWH) (see p. 480) have replaced unfractionated heparin as they are more effective, they do not require monitoring and there is less risk of bleeding. DVTs are being treated at home with low-molecular-weight heparin. Warfarin is started immediately and the heparin stopped when the INR is in the target range. The duration of *warfarin* treatment is debatable – 3 months is the period usually recommended, but 4 weeks is long enough if a definite risk factor (e.g. bed rest) has been present. Recurrent DVTs need permanent anticoagulants. The target INR should be 2.5. Anticoagulants do not lyse the thrombus that is already present. Unfractionated heparin should only be used if LMWH is unavailable.

Thrombolytic therapy (see p. 813) is occasionally used for patients with a large iliofemoral thrombosis.

Prognosis

Destruction of the deep-vein valves produces a clinically painful, swollen limb that is made worse by standing and is accompanied by oedema and sometimes venous eczema. It occurs in approximately half of the patients with clinically symptomatic deep-vein thrombosis, and it means that elastic support stockings are then required for life.

Prevention

Subcutaneous low-molecular-weight heparin (see p. 480) should be given to patients with cardiac failure, a myocardial infarct or surgery to the leg or pelvis.

Early ambulation is indicated, as most thromboses occur within the first 72 hours following surgery. Leg exercises should be encouraged and patients should not sit in a chair with their legs immobilized on a stool. An elastic support stocking should be given to patients at high risk (e.g. those with a history of thrombosis or with obesity).

FURTHER READING

Anderson FA Jr, Spencer FA (2003) Risk factors for venous thromboembolism. *Circulation* **107**: 1–9.

Bates SM, Ginsberg JS (2004) Treatment of deep vein thrombosis. *New England Journal of Medicine* **351**: 268–277.

Block JA, Sequeira W (2001) Raynaud's phenomenon. *Lancet* **357**: 2042–2048.

Burns P, Lima E, Bradbury AW (2002) What constitutes best medical therapy for peripheral arterial disease? *European Journal of Vascular Surgery* **24**: 6–12.

Hiatt WR (2001) Medical management of peripheral arterial disease and claudication. *New England Journal of Medicine* **344**: 1608–1621.

Johnston SL, Lock RJ, Gompels MM (2002) Takayasu arteritis: a review. *Journal of Clinical Pathology* **55**: 481–486.

Kyrle PA, Eichinger S (2005) Deep venous thrombosis. *Lancet* **365**: 1163–1174.

Sakalihasan N et al. (2005) Abdominal aortic aneurysm. *Lancet* **365**: 1577–1589.

SIGNIFICANT WEBSITES

http://www.doh.gov.uk/nsf/coronarych4.htm
UK National Service Framework for Coronary Heart Disease (2000)

http://www.americanheart.org/
American Heart Association

http://www.erc.edu/
European Resuscitation Council

http://www.resus.org.uk
UK Resuscitation Council

http://homepages.enterprise.net/djenkins/ecghome.html
ECG tracings library

Respiratory disease 14

The main role of the respiratory system is to extract oxygen from the external environment and dispose of waste gases, principally carbon dioxide. This requires the lungs to function as an efficient bellows, expelling used air, bringing fresh air in and mixing it efficiently with the air remaining in the lungs. The lungs have to provide a large surface area for gas exchange and the alveoli walls have to present minimal resistance to gas diffusion. For maximum efficiency, ventilation must be matched accurately to blood flow through the pulmonary capillary bed. Altogether, this means the lungs have to present a large area to the environment and this can be damaged by dusts, gases and infective agents. Host defence is therefore a key priority for the lung and is achieved by a combination of structural and immunological defences.

STRUCTURE OF THE RESPIRATORY SYSTEM

The nose, pharynx and larynx

See Chapter 20 (pp. 1156 and 1159).

The trachea, bronchi and bronchioles

The trachea is 10–12 cm in length. It lies slightly to the right of the midline and divides at the carina into right and left main bronchi. The carina lies under the junction of the manubrium sternum and the second right costal cartilage. The right main bronchus is more vertical than the left and, hence, inhaled material is more likely to end up in the right lung.

The right main bronchus divides into the upper lobe bronchus and the intermediate bronchus, which further subdivides into the middle and lower lobe bronchi. On the left the main bronchus divides into upper and lower lobe bronchi only. Each lobar bronchus further divides into segmental and subsegmental bronchi. There are about 25 divisions in all between the trachea and the alveoli.

The first seven divisions are bronchi that have:

- walls consisting of cartilage and smooth muscle
- epithelial lining with cilia and goblet cells
- submucosal mucus-secreting glands
- endocrine cells – Kulchitsky or APUD (amine precursor and uptake decarboxylation) containing 5-hydroxytryptamine.

The next 16–18 divisions are bronchioles that have:

- no cartilage and a muscular layer that progressively becomes thinner
- a single layer of ciliated cells but very few goblet cells
- granulated Clara cells that produce a surfactant-like substance.

The ciliated epithelium is a key defence mechanism. Each cell bears approximately 200 cilia beating at 1000 beats per minute in organized waves of contraction. Each cilium consists of nine peripheral parts and two inner longitudinal fibrils in a cytoplasmic matrix (Fig. 14.1). Nexin links join the peripheral pairs. Dynein arms consisting of ATPase protein project towards the adjacent pairs. Bending of the cilia results from a sliding movement between adjacent fibrils powered by an ATP-dependent shearing force developed by the dynein arms. Absence of dynein arms leads to immotile cilia. Mucus, which contains macrophages, cell debris, inhaled particles and bacteria, is moved by the cilia towards the larynx at about 1.5 cm/min (the 'mucociliary escalator', see below).

The bronchioles finally divide within the acinus into smaller respiratory bronchioles that have alveoli arising from the surface (Fig. 14.2). Each respiratory bronchiole supplies approximately 200 alveoli via alveolar ducts. The term 'small airways' refers to bronchioles of less than 2 mm; there are 30 000 of these in the average lung.

The alveoli

There are approximately 300 million alveoli in each lung. Their total surface area is 40–80 m². The epithelial lining

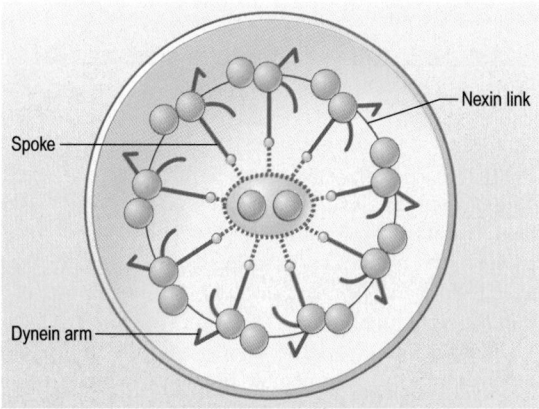

Fig. 14.1 **Cross-section of a cilium.** Nine outer microtubular doublets and two central single microtubules are linked by spokes, nexin links and dynein arms.

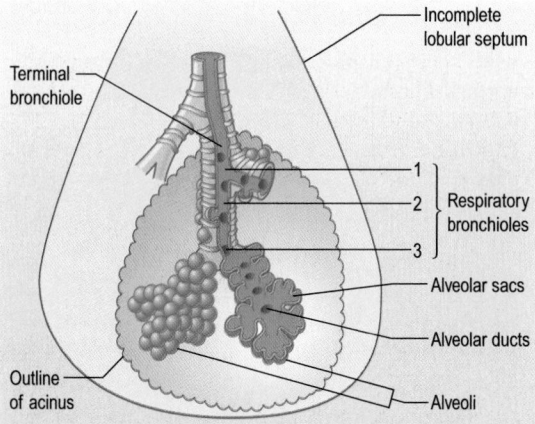

Fig. 14.2 **Branches of a terminal bronchiole ending in the alveolar sacs.**

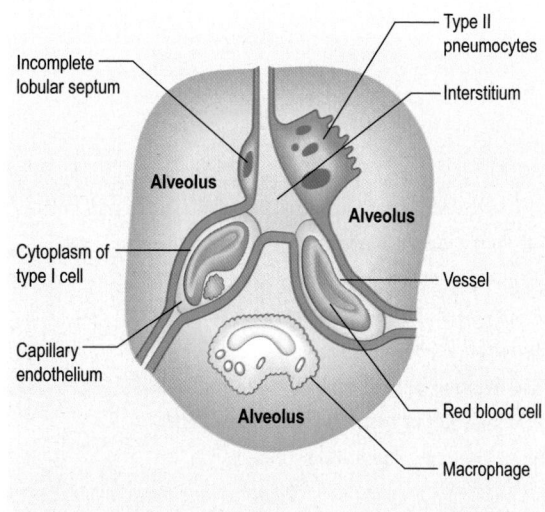

Fig. 14.3 **The structure of alveoli, showing the pneumocytes and capillaries.**

consists largely of *type I pneumocytes* (Fig. 14.3). These cells have an extremely attenuated cytoplasm, and thus provide only a thin barrier to gas exchange. They are derived from type II pneumocytes. *Type I cells* are connected to each other by tight junctions that limit the fluid movements in and out of the alveoli. *Type II pneumocytes* are slightly more numerous than type I cells but cover less of the epithelial lining. They are found generally in the borders of the alveolus and contain distinctive lamellar vacuoles, which are the source of surfactant. Macrophages are also present in the alveoli and are involved in the defence mechanisms of the lung.

The pores of Kohn are holes in the alveolar wall allowing communication between alveoli of adjoining lobules.

The lungs

The lungs are separated into lobes by invaginations of the pleura, which are often incomplete. The right lung has three lobes, whereas the left lung has two. The positions of the oblique fissures and the right horizontal fissure are shown in Figure 14.4. The upper lobe lies mainly in front of the lower lobe and therefore physical signs on the right side in the front of the chest are due to lesions of the upper lobe or the middle lobe. Because of the contrast in density between healthy and diseased lung, plain radiography enables accurate localization of disease processes, especially if postero-anterior (PA) and lateral views are taken (Fig. 14.5).

Each lobe is further subdivided into bronchopulmonary segments by fibrous septa that extend inwards from the pleural surface. Each segment receives its own segmental bronchus.

The bronchopulmonary segment is further divided into individual lobules approximately 1 cm in diameter and generally pyramidal in shape, the apex lying towards the bronchioles supplying them. Within each lobule a terminal bronchus supplies an acinus, and within this

(a) PA

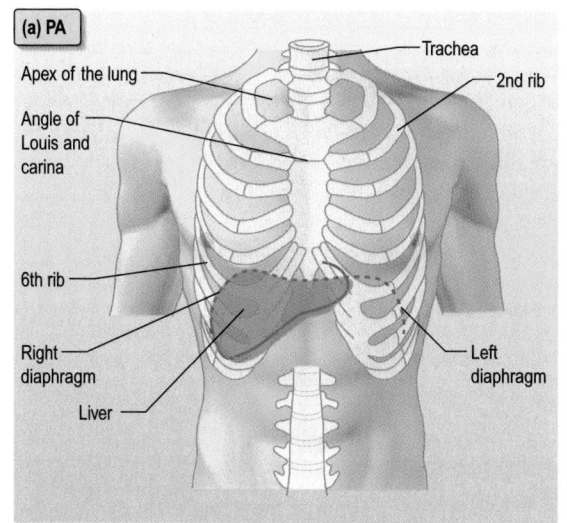

Trachea

Apex of the lung

2nd rib

Angle of
Louis and
carina

6th rib

Right
diaphragm

Left
diaphragm

Liver

(b) Lateral

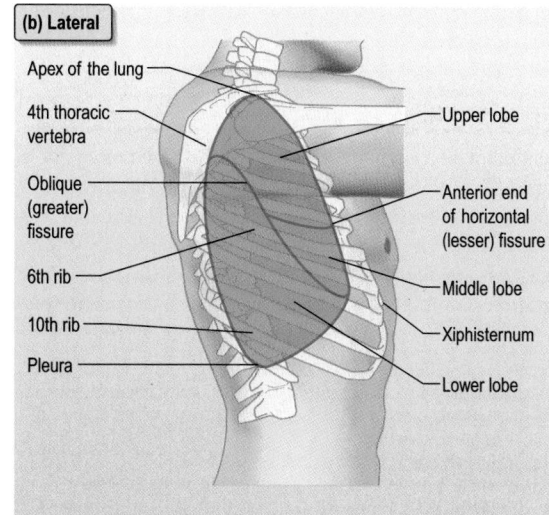

Apex of the lung

4th thoracic
vertebra

Upper lobe

Oblique
(greater)
fissure

Anterior end
of horizontal
(lesser) fissure

6th rib

Middle lobe

10th rib

Xiphisternum

Pleura

Lower lobe

Fig. 14.4 **Surface anatomy of the chest. (a)** PA. **(b)** Lateral.

(a)

(b)

(a) PA

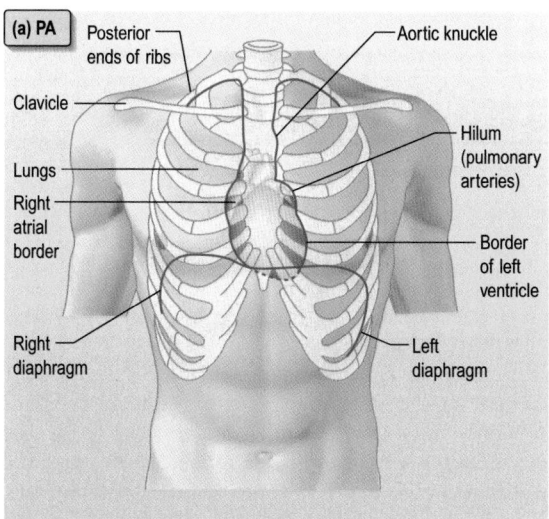

Posterior
ends of ribs

Aortic knuckle

Clavicle

Lungs

Hilum
(pulmonary
arteries)

Right
atrial
border

Border
of left
ventricle

Right
diaphragm

Left
diaphragm

(b) Lateral

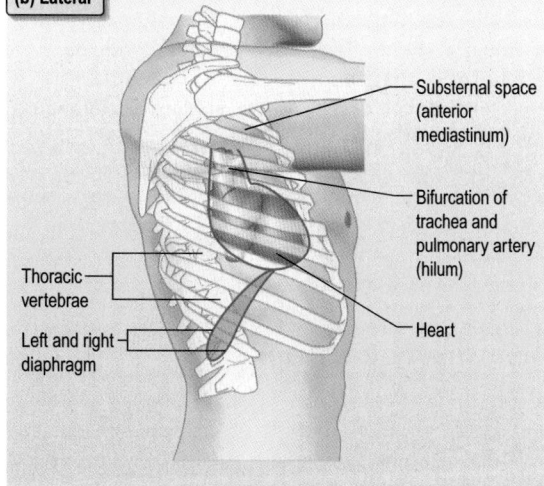

Substernal space
(anterior
mediastinum)

Bifurcation of
trachea and
pulmonary artery
(hilum)

Thoracic
vertebrae

Heart

Left and right
diaphragm

Fig. 14.5 **Chest X-rays. (a)** PA. **(b)** Lateral.

structure further divisions of the bronchioles eventually give rise to the alveoli.

The pleura

The pleura is a layer of connective tissue covered by a simple squamous epithelium. The visceral pleura covers the surface of the lung, lines the interlobar fissures, and is continuous at the hilum with the parietal pleura, which lines the inside of the hemithorax. At the hilum the visceral pleura continues alongside the branching bronchial tree for some distance before reflecting back to join the parietal pleura. In health, the pleurae are in apposition apart from a small quantity of lubricating fluid.

The diaphragm

The diaphragm is covered by parietal pleura above and peritoneum below. Its muscle fibres arise from the lower ribs and insert into the central tendon. Motor and sensory nerve fibres go separately to each half of the diaphragm via the phrenic nerves. Fifty per cent of the muscle fibres are of the slow-twitch type with a low glycolytic capacity; they are relatively resistant to fatigue.

Pulmonary vasculature and lymphatics

The lung is unusual in having a dual blood supply. It receives deoxygenated blood from the right ventricle via the pulmonary artery and also has a systemic supply via the bronchial circulation.

The pulmonary artery divides to accompany the bronchi. The arterioles accompanying the respiratory bronchioles are thin-walled and contain little smooth muscle. The pulmonary venules drain laterally to the periphery of the lobules, pass centrally in the interlobular and intersegmental septa, and eventually join to form the four main pulmonary veins.

The bronchial circulation arises from the descending aorta. These bronchial arteries supply tissues down to the level of the respiratory bronchiole. The bronchial veins drain into the pulmonary vein, forming part of the physiological shunt observed in normal individuals.

Lymphatic channels lie in the interstitial space between the alveolar cells and the capillary endothelium of the pulmonary arterioles.

The tracheobronchial lymph nodes are arranged in five main groups: pulmonary, bronchopulmonary, subcarinal, superior tracheobronchial and paratracheal. In practical terms these form a continuous network of nodes from the lung substance up to the trachea.

Nerve supply to the lung

The innervation of the lung remains incompletely understood. Parasympathetic (from the vagus) and sympathetic (from the adjacent sympathetic chain) nerve supplies entwine in a plexus at the nerve root and branches accompany the pulmonary arteries and the airways. Airway smooth muscle is innervated by vagal afferents,

postganglionic muscarinic vagal efferents and vagally derived non-adrenergic non-cholinergic (NANC) fibres. Neurotransmitters (peptides and purines) may be involved. Three muscarinic receptor subtypes have been identified: M_1 receptors on parasympathetic ganglia, a smaller number of M_2 receptors on muscarinic nerve terminals, and M_3 receptors on airway smooth muscle. The parietal pleura is innervated from intercostal and phrenic nerves but the visceral pleura has no innervation.

> **FURTHER READING**
> Gibson J, Geddes D, Costabel U et al. (2002) *Respiratory Medicine*, 3rd edn, Vols 1 and 2. London: WB Saunders.

PHYSIOLOGY OF THE RESPIRATORY SYSTEM

The nose

The major functions of nasal breathing are:

- to heat and moisten the air
- to remove particulate matter.

About 10 000 L of air are inhaled daily. The relatively low flow rates and turbulence of inspired air are ideal for particle deposition, and few particles greater than 10 microns pass through the nose. Deposited particles are removed from the nasal mucosa within 15 minutes, compared with 60–120 days from the alveolus. Nasal secretion contains many protective proteins in the form of IgA antibodies, lysozyme and interferon. In addition, the cilia of the nasal epithelium move the mucous gel layer rapidly back to the oropharynx where it is swallowed. Bacteria have little chance of settling in the nose. Mucociliary protection against viral infections is more difficult because viruses bind to receptors on epithelial cells. The majority of rhinoviruses bind to an adhesion molecule, intercellular adhesion molecule 1 (ICAM-1), shared by neutrophils and eosinophils. Many noxious gases, such as SO_2, are almost completely removed by nasal breathing.

Breathing

Lung ventilation can be considered in two parts:

- the mechanical process of inspiration and expiration
- the control of respiration to a level appropriate for the metabolic needs.

Mechanical process

Inspiration is an active process and results from the descent of the diaphragm and movement of the ribs upwards and outwards under the influence of the intercostal muscles. In healthy individuals at rest, inspiration is almost entirely due to contraction of the diaphragm. Respiratory muscles are similar to other skeletal muscles but are less prone to fatigue. However, muscle fatigue contributes to respiratory failure in patients with severe

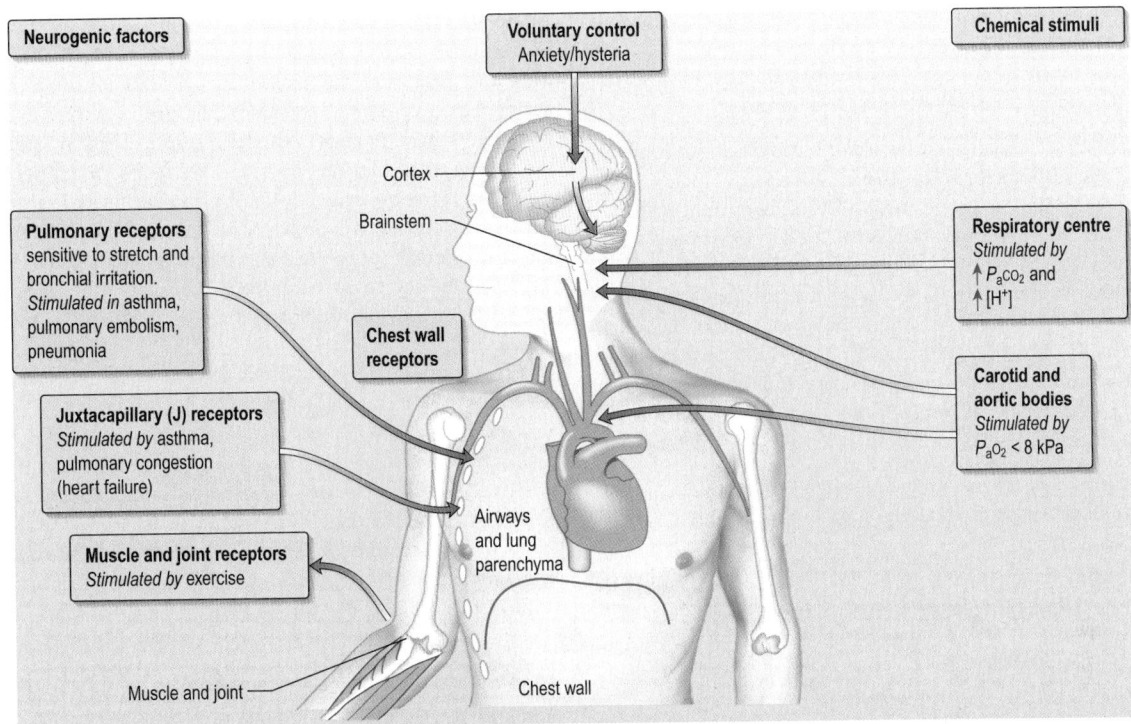

Fig. 14.6 **Chemical and neurogenic factors in the control of ventilation**. The strongest stimulant to ventilation is a rise in $P_a\text{co}_2$ which increases [H$^+$] in CSF. Sensitivity to this may be lost in COPD. In these patients hypoxaemia is the chief stimulus to respiratory drive; oxygen treatment may therefore reduce respiratory drive and lead to a further rise in $P_a\text{co}_2$. An increase in [H$^+$] due to metabolic acidosis as in diabetic ketoacidosis will increase ventilation with a fall in $P_a\text{co}_2$ causing deep sighing (Kussmaul) respiration. The respiratory centre is depressed by severe hypoxaemia and sedatives (e.g. opiates) and stimulated by doxapram, large doses of aspirin and pyrexia. COPD, chronic obstructive pulmonary disease. Derived from Manning HL, Schwartzstein RM (1995) *New England Journal of Medicine* **333**: 1547–1553.

chronic airflow limitation. Muscle weakness can also result from primary neurological and muscle disorders.

Expiration follows passively as a result of gradual relaxation of the intercostal muscles, allowing the lungs to collapse under the influence of their own elastic forces.

Inspiration against increased resistance may require the use of the accessory muscles of ventilation, such as the sternomastoid and scalene muscles. Forced expiration is also accomplished with the aid of accessory muscles, chiefly those of the abdominal wall, which help to push up the diaphragm.

The lungs have an inherent elastic property that causes them to tend to collapse away from the thoracic wall, generating a negative pressure within the pleural space. The strength of this retractive force relates to the volume of the lung; thus, at higher lung volumes the lung is stretched more, and a greater negative intrapleural pressure is generated.

Lung compliance is a measure of the relationship between this retractive force and lung volume. It is defined as the change in lung volume brought about by unit change in transpulmonary (intrapleural) pressure and is measured in litres per kilopascal (L/kPa). At the end of a quiet expiration, the retractive force exerted by the lungs is balanced by the tendency of the thoracic wall to spring outwards. At this point, respiratory muscles are resting and the volume of air in the lung is known as the *functional residual capacity* (FRC).

Diseases that affect the movement of the thoracic cage and diaphragm can have a profound effect on ventilation. These include diseases of the thoracic spine such as ankylosing spondylitis and kyphoscoliosis, neuropathies (e.g. the Guillain–Barré syndrome), injury to the phrenic nerves, and myasthenia gravis.

The control of respiration

Coordinated respiratory movements result from rhythmical discharges arising in an anatomically ill-defined group of interconnected neurones in the reticular substance of the brainstem, known as the respiratory centre. Motor discharges from the respiratory centre travel via the phrenic and intercostal nerves to the respiratory musculature.

The pressures of oxygen and carbon dioxide in arterial blood are closely controlled. In a typical normal adult at rest:

- The pulmonary blood flow of 5 L/min carries 11 mmol/min (250 mL/min) of oxygen from the lungs to the tissues.
- Ventilation at about 6 L/min carries 9 mmol/min (200 mL/min) of carbon dioxide out of the body.

- The normal pressure of oxygen in arterial blood (P_aO_2) is between 11 and 13 kPa (83 and 98 mmHg).
- The normal pressure of carbon dioxide in arterial blood (P_aCO_2) is 4.8–6.0 kPa (36–45 mmHg).

Ventilation is controlled by a combination of neurogenic and chemical factors (Fig. 14.6).

Breathlessness on physical exertion is normal and not considered a symptom unless the level of exertion is very light, such as when walking slowly. Recent surveys of healthy western populations reveal that over 20% of the general population report themselves as breathless on relatively minor exertion. Although breathlessness is a very common symptom, the sensory and neural mechanisms underlying it remain obscure. The sensation of breathlessness is derived from at least three sources:

- *Changes in lung volume.* These are sensed by receptors in thoracic wall muscles signalling changes in their length.
- *Tension developed by contracting muscles.* This is sensed by Golgi tendon organs.
- *Central perception of the sense of effort.*

The airways of the lungs

From the trachea to the periphery, the airways become smaller in size (although greater in number). The cross-sectional area available for airflow increases as the total number of airways increases. The flow of air is greatest in the trachea and slows progressively towards the periphery (as the velocity of airflow depends on the ratio of flow to cross-sectional area). In the terminal airways, gas flow occurs solely by diffusion. The resistance to airflow is very low (0.1–0.2 kPa/L in a normal tracheobronchial tree), steadily increasing from the small to the large airways.

Airways expand as lung volume is increased, and at full inspiration (*total lung capacity*, TLC) they are 30–40% larger in calibre than at full expiration (*residual volume*, RV). In chronic obstructive pulmonary disease (COPD) the small airways are narrowed and this can be partially compensated by breathing at a larger lung volume.

Control of airway tone

Bronchomotor tone is maintained by vagal efferent nerves and, even in a normal subject, is reduced by atropine or β-adrenoceptor agonists. Adrenoceptors on the surface of bronchial muscles respond to circulating catecholamines; there is no direct sympathetic innervation. Airway tone shows a *circadian rhythm*, which is greatest at 04.00 and lowest in the mid-afternoon. Tone can be increased transiently by inhaled stimuli acting on epithelial nerve endings, which trigger reflex broncho-constriction via the vagus. These stimuli include cigarette smoke, solvents, inert dust and cold air; airway responsiveness to these increases following respiratory tract infections even in healthy subjects. In asthma, the airways are very irritable and as the circadian rhythm remains the same, asthmatic symptoms are usually worse in the early morning.

Airflow

Movement of air through the airways results from a difference between the pressure in the alveoli and the atmospheric pressure; alveolar pressure is positive in expiration and negative in inspiration. During quiet breathing the pleural pressure is sub-atmospheric throughout the breathing cycle. With vigorous expiratory efforts (e.g. cough), the central airways are compressed by positive pleural pressures exceeding 10 kPa, but the airways do not close completely because the driving pressure for expiratory flow (alveolar pressure) is also increased.

Alveolar pressure (P_{ALV}) is equal to the pleural pressure (P_{PL}) plus the elastic recoil pressure (P_{EL}) of the lung.

When there is no airflow (i.e. during a pause in breathing) the tendency of the lungs to collapse (the positive recoil pressure) is exactly balanced by an equivalent negative pleural pressure.

As air flows from the alveoli towards the mouth there is a gradual loss of pressure owing to flow resistance (Fig. 14.7a).

Fig. 14.7 **Diagrams showing ventilatory forces.**
(a) During resting at functional residual capacity. **(b)** During forced expiration in normal subjects. **(c)** During forced expiration in a patient with COPD. The respiratory system is represented as a piston with a single alveolus and the collapsible part of the airways within the piston (see text). C, collapse point; P_{ALV}, alveolar pressure; P_{EL}, elastic recoil pressure; P_{PL}, pleural pressure.

In forced expiration, as mentioned above, the driving pressure raises both the alveolar pressure and the intrapleural pressure. Between the alveolus and the mouth, there is a point (C in Fig. 14.7b) where the airway pressure equals the intrapleural pressure, and the airway collapses. However, this collapse is temporary, as the transient occlusion of the airway results in an increase in pressure behind it (i.e. upstream) and this raises the intra-airway pressure so that the airways open and flow is restored. The airways thus tend to vibrate at this point of 'dynamic collapse'.

The elastic recoil pressure of the lungs decreases with decreasing lung volume and the 'collapse point' moves upstream (i.e. towards the smaller airways – see Fig. 14.7c). Where there is pathological loss of recoil pressure (as in chronic obstructive pulmonary disease, COPD), the 'collapse point' starts even further upstream and causes expiratory flow limitation. The measurement of the forced expiratory volume in 1 second (FEV_1) is a useful clinical index of this phenomenon. To compensate, these patients often 'purse their lips' in order to increase airway pressure so that their peripheral airways do not collapse. On inspiration, the intrapleural pressure is always less than the intraluminal pressure within the intrathoracic airways, so there is no limitation to airflow with increasing effort. Inspiratory flow is limited only by the power of the inspiratory muscles.

Flow–volume loops

The relationship between maximal flow rates on expiration and inspiration is demonstrated by the maximal flow–volume (MFV) loops. Figure 14.8a shows this in a normal subject.

In subjects with healthy lungs, effects of flow limitation will not be apparent, since maximal flow rates are rarely achieved even during vigorous exercise. However, in patients with severe COPD, limitation of expiratory flow occurs even during tidal breathing at rest (see Fig. 14.8b). To increase ventilation these patients have to breathe at higher lung volumes and allow more time for expiration which both reduce the tendency for airway collapse. To compensate they increase flow rates during inspiration, where there is relatively less flow limitation.

The measure of the volume that can be forced in from the residual volume in 1 second (FIV_1) will always be greater than that which can be forced out from TLC in 1 second (FEV_1). Thus, the ratio of FEV_1 to FIV_1 is below 1. The only exception to this occurs when there is significant obstruction to the airways outside the thorax, such as with a tumour mass in the upper part of the trachea. Under these circumstances expiratory airway narrowing is prevented by the tracheal resistance (a situation similar to pursing the lips) and expiratory airflow becomes more effort-dependent. During forced inspiration this same resistance causes such negative intraluminal pressure that the trachea is compressed by the surrounding atmospheric pressure. Inspiratory flow thus becomes less effort-dependent, and the ratio of FEV_1 to FIV_1 becomes greater than 1. This phenomenon, and the characteristic flow–volume loop, is used to diagnose extrathoracic airways obstruction (Fig. 14.8c).

Fig. 14.8 **(a and b) Maximal flow–volume loops, showing the relationship between maximal flow rates on expiration and inspiration.** **(a)** In a normal subject. **(b)** In a patient with severe airflow limitation. Flow–volume loops during tidal breathing at rest (starting from the functional residual capacity (FRC)) and during exercise are also shown. The highest flow rates are achieved when forced expiration begins at total lung capacity (TLC) and represent the peak expiratory flow rate (PEFR). As air is blown out of the lung, so the flow rate decreases until no more air can be forced out, a point known as the residual volume (RV). Because inspiratory airflow is only dependent on effort, the shape of the maximal inspiratory flow–volume loop is quite different, and inspiratory flow remains at a high rate throughout the manoeuvre. **(c and d) Flow–volume loops of patients with large airway (tracheal) obstruction, showing plateauing of maximal expiratory flow.** **(c)** Extrathoracic tracheal obstruction with a proportionally greater reduction of maximal inspiratory (as opposed to expiratory) flow rate. **(d)** Intrathoracic large airway obstruction; the expiratory plateau is more pronounced and inspiratory flow rate is less reduced than in (c). In severe airflow limitation the ventilatory demands of exercise cannot be met (cf. a and b), greatly reducing effort tolerance.

When obstruction occurs in large airways within the thorax (lower end of trachea and main bronchi), expiratory flow is impaired more than inspiratory flow but a characteristic plateau to expiratory flow is seen (Fig. 14.8d).

Ventilation and perfusion relationships

For efficient gas exchange there must be a match between ventilation of the alveoli ($\dot{V}_A$) and their perfusion ($\dot{Q}$). There is a wide variation in the $\dot{V}_A/\dot{Q}$ ratio throughout both normal and diseased lung. In the normal lung the extreme relationships between alveolar ventilation and perfusion are:

- ventilation with reduced perfusion (physiological deadspace)
- perfusion with reduced ventilation (physiological shunting).

These and the 'ideal' match are illustrated in Figure 14.9. In normal lungs there is a tendency for ventilation to exceed perfusion towards the apices, with the reverse occurring at the bases.

An increased physiological shunt results in arterial hypoxaemia. The effects of an increased physiological deadspace can usually be overcome by a compensatory increase in the ventilation of normally perfused alveoli. In advanced disease this compensation cannot occur, leading to increased alveolar and arterial $P\text{CO}_2$, together with hypoxaemia which cannot be compensated by increasing ventilation.

Hypoxaemia occurs more readily than hypercapnia because of the different ways in which oxygen and carbon dioxide are carried in the blood. Carbon dioxide can be considered to be in simple solution in the plasma, the volume carried being proportional to the partial pressure. Oxygen is carried in chemical combination with haemoglobin in the red blood cells, and the relationship between the volume carried and the partial pressure is not linear (see Fig. 15.5, p. 960). Alveolar hyperventilation reduces the alveolar $P\text{CO}_2$ and diffusion leads to a proportional fall in the carbon dioxide content of the blood. However, as the haemoglobin is already saturated with oxygen, there is no significant increase in the blood oxygen content as a result of increasing the alveolar $P\text{O}_2$ through hyper-

ventilation. The hypoxaemia of even a small amount of physiological shunting cannot therefore be compensated for by hyperventilation.

In individuals who have mild disease of the lung causing slight $\dot{V}_A/\dot{Q}$ mismatch, the $P_a\text{O}_2$ and $P_a\text{CO}_2$ may still be normal. Increasing the requirements for gas exchange by exercise will widen the $\dot{V}_A/\dot{Q}$ mismatch and the $P_A\text{O}_2$ will fall. $\dot{V}_A/\dot{Q}$ mismatch is by far the most common cause of arterial hypoxaemia.

Alveolar stability

The alveoli of the lung are essentially hollow spheres. Surface tension acting at the curved internal surface tends to cause the sphere to decrease in size. The surface tension within the alveoli would make the lungs extremely difficult to distend were it not for the presence of surfactant. The type II cells within the alveolus secrete an insoluble lipoprotein largely consisting of dipalmitoyl lecithin, which forms a thin monomolecular layer at the air–fluid interface. Surfactant reduces surface tension so that alveoli remain stable.

Fluid surfaces covered with surfactant exhibit a phenomenon known as hysteresis; that is, the surface-tension-lowering effect of the surfactant can be improved by a transient increase in the size of the surface area of the alveoli. During quiet breathing, small areas of the lung undergo collapse, but it is possible to re-expand these rapidly by a deep breath; hence the importance of sighs or deep breaths as a feature of normal breathing. Failure of such a mechanism – which can occur, for example, in patients with fractured ribs – gives rise to patchy basal lung collapse. Surfactant levels may be reduced in a number of diseases that cause damage to the lung (e.g. pneumonia). Lack of surfactant plays a central role in the respiratory distress syndrome of the newborn. Severe reduction in perfusion of the lung causes impairment of surfactant activity and may well account for the characteristic areas of collapse associated with pulmonary embolism.

FURTHER READING

Manning HL, Schwartzstein RM (1995) Pathology of dyspnoea. *New England Journal of Medicine* **333**: 1547–1553.

DEFENCE MECHANISMS OF THE RESPIRATORY TRACT

Pulmonary disease often results from a failure of the many defence mechanisms that usually protect the lung in a healthy individual (Fig. 14.10). These can be divided into physical and physiological mechanisms and humoral and cellular mechanisms.

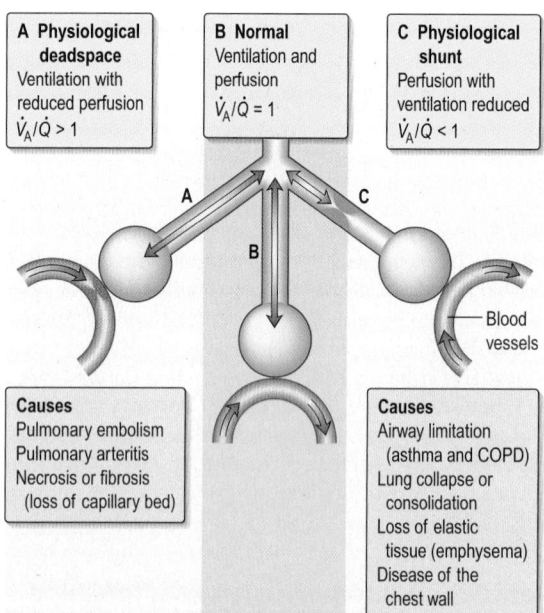

A Physiological deadspace	B Normal	C Physiological shunt
Ventilation with reduced perfusion $\dot{V}_A/\dot{Q} > 1$	Ventilation and perfusion $\dot{V}_A/\dot{Q} = 1$	Perfusion with ventilation reduced $\dot{V}_A/\dot{Q} < 1$

Blood vessels

Causes
Pulmonary embolism
Pulmonary arteritis
Necrosis or fibrosis (loss of capillary bed)

Causes
Airway limitation (asthma and COPD)
Lung collapse or consolidation
Loss of elastic tissue (emphysema)
Disease of the chest wall

Fig. 14.9 **Relationships between ventilation and perfusion: a schematic diagram showing the alveolar–capillary interface.** The centre (B) shows normal ventilation and perfusion. On the left (A) there is a block in perfusion (physiological deadspace), while on the right (C) there is reduced ventilation (physiological shunting).

Physical and physiological mechanisms

Humidification
This prevents dehydration of the epithelium.

Congenital defects in mucociliary transport occur. In the 'immotile cilia' syndrome there is an absence of the dynein arms in the cilia themselves, and in *cystic fibrosis* an abnormal mucus is associated with ciliary dyskinesia. Both diseases are characterized by recurrent infections and eventually with the development of bronchiectasis.

Humoral and cellular mechanisms

Non-specific soluble factors

- α_1-*Antitrypsin* (α_1-antiprotease, see p. 902) is present in lung secretions derived from plasma. It inhibits chymotrypsin and trypsin and neutralizes proteases and elastase.
- *Antioxidant defences* include enzymes such as superoxide dismutase and low-molecular-weight antioxidant molecules (ascorbate, urate) in the epithelial lining fluid. In addition, lung cells are protected by an extensive range of intracellular defences, especially members of the glutathione S-transferase (GST) superfamily.
- *Lysozyme* is an enzyme found in granulocytes that has bactericidal properties.
- *Lactoferrin* is synthesized from epithelial cells and neutrophil granulocytes and has bactericidal properties.
- *Interferon* (see p. 202) is produced by most cells in response to viral infection. It is a potent modulator of lymphocyte function. It renders other cells resistant to infection by any other virus.
- *Complement* is present in secretions and is derived by diffusion from plasma. In association with antibodies, it plays a major cytotoxic role.
- *Surfactant protein* A (SP$_A$) is one of four species of surfactant proteins which opsonizes bacteria/particles, enhancing phagocytosis by macrophages.
- *Defensins* are bactericidal peptides present in the azurophil granules of neutrophils.

Pulmonary alveolar macrophages

These are derived from precursors in the bone marrow and migrate to the lungs via the bloodstream. They phagocytose particles, including bacteria, and are removed by the mucociliary escalator, lymphatics and bloodstream. They are the dominant cell in the airways at the level of the alveoli and comprise 90% of all cells obtained by bronchoalveolar lavage.

Alveolar macrophages work principally as scavengers and are not particularly good at presenting antigens to the immune system. The key antigen-presenting cells in the airways are dendritic cells which form a network throughout the airways.

Lymphoid tissue (see also p. 205)

The lung contains large numbers of lymphocytes which are scattered throughout the airways. In animals, aggregates of bronchus-associated lymphoid tissue (BALT) can be identified but these are not normally found in humans. Sensitized lymphocytes contribute to local immunity through differentiation into IgA-secreting plasma cells. IgG and IgE are found in low concentrations in airway secretions from a combination of local and systemic production.

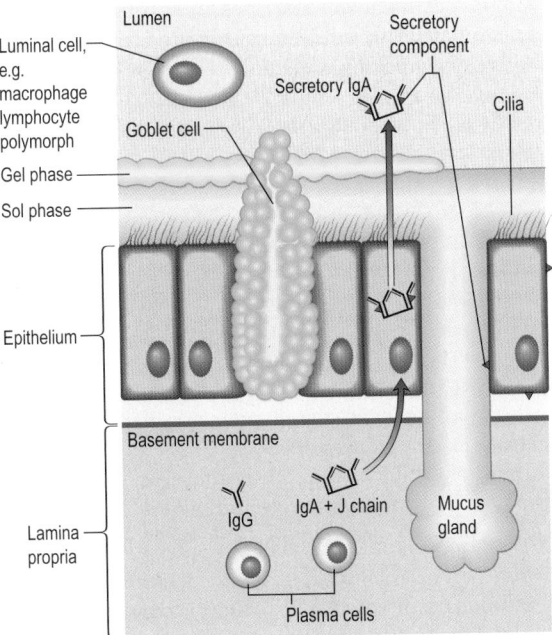

Fig. 14.10 Defence mechanisms present at the epithelial

Particle removal

Over 90% of particles greater than 10 μm diameter are removed in the nostril or nasopharynx. This includes most pollen grains which are typically > 20 microns in diameter. Particles between 5–10 microns become impacted in the carina. Particles smaller than 1 micron tend to remain airborne, thus the particles capable of reaching the deep lung are confined to the 1–5 micron range.

Particle expulsion

This is effected by coughing, sneezing or gagging.

Respiratory tract secretions

The mucus of the respiratory tract is a gelatinous substance consisting chiefly of acid and neutral polysaccharides. The mucus consists of a thick gel that is relatively impermeable to water. This floats on a liquid or sol layer that is present around the cilia of the epithelial cells. The gel layer is secreted from goblet cells and mucous glands as distinct globules that coalesce increasingly in the central airways to form a more or less continuous mucus blanket. Under normal conditions the tips of the cilia are in contact with the under surface of the gel phase and coordinate their movement to push the mucus blanket upwards. Whilst it may only take 30–60 minutes for mucus to be cleared from the large bronchi, there may be a delay of several days before clearance is achieved from respiratory bronchioles. One of the major long-term effects of cigarette smoking is a reduction in mucociliary transport. This contributes to recurrent infection and in the larger airways it prolongs contact with carcinogens. Air pollutants, local and general anaesthetics and bacterial and viral infections also reduce mucociliary clearance.

In addition to these resident cells, the lung has the usual range of acute inflammatory responses and can mobilize neutrophils promptly in response to injury or infection and play a major part in inflammatory conditions such as asthma (p. 916).

FURTHER READING
Kelly FJ (2003) Oxidative stress: its role in air pollution and adverse health effects. *Occupational and Environmental Medicine* **60**: 612–616.

SYMPTOMS (see also p. 911)

Runny, blocked nose and sneezing

Nasal symptoms are extremely common. It can be difficult to distinguish between the common cold or allergic rhinitis as a cause of 'runny nose' (rhinorrhoea), nasal blockage and attacks of sneezing. In allergic rhinitis, symptoms may be seasonal, following contact with grass pollen, or perennial, when the house-dust mite is the allergen. Colds are frequent during the winter but if the symptoms persist for weeks the patient is probably suffering from perennial rhinitis rather than from persistent infection due to a virus.

Nasal secretions are usually thin and runny in rhinitis but thicker and yellowish green in the common cold. Nose bleeds and blood-stained nasal discharge are common occurrences and are not as serious as haemoptysis. However, a blood-stained nasal discharge associated with nasal obstruction and pain may be the presenting feature of a nasal tumour (p. 1158). Total nasal blockage with loss of smell is often a feature of nasal polyps.

Cough (see also p. 911)

Cough is the most common symptom of lower respiratory tract disease. It is caused by the mechanical or chemical stimulation of the cough receptors in the epithelium of the pharynx, larynx, trachea and bronchi. Afferent receptors go to the cough centre in the medulla where efferent signals are generated to the expiratory musculature. Smokers often have a morning cough with little sputum. A productive cough is the cardinal feature of chronic bronchitis, while dry coughing, particularly at night, can be a symptom of asthma. Cough also occurs in asthmatics after mild exertion or following a forced expiration. A cough can also occur for psychological reasons.

A worsening cough is the most common presenting symptom of a bronchial carcinoma. The explosive character of a normal cough is lost when a vocal chord is paralysed – a bovine cough – usually as a result of a carcinoma of the bronchus infiltrating the left recurrent laryngeal nerve. Cough can be accompanied by stridor in whooping cough and in the presence of laryngeal or tracheal obstruction.

Sputum

Approximately 100 mL of mucus is produced daily in a healthy, non-smoking individual. This flows at a regular pace up the airways, through the larynx, and is then swallowed. Excess mucus is expectorated as sputum. The most common cause of excess mucus production is cigarette smoking.

Mucoid sputum is clear and white but can contain black specks resulting from the inhalation of carbon. Yellow or green sputum is due to the presence of cellular material, including bronchial epithelial cells, or neutrophil or eosinophil granulocytes. Yellow sputum is not necessarily due to infection, as eosinophils in the sputum, as seen in asthma, can give the same appearance. The production of large quantities of yellow or green sputum is characteristic of bronchiectasis.

Haemoptysis (blood-stained sputum) varies from small streaks of blood to massive bleeding.

- The most common cause of haemoptysis is acute infection, particularly in exacerbations of chronic obstructive pulmonary disease (COPD) but it should not be attributed to this without investigation.
- Other common causes are pulmonary infarction, bronchial carcinoma and tuberculosis.
- In lobar pneumonia, the sputum is rusty in appearance when blood is present.
- Pink, frothy sputum is seen in pulmonary oedema.
- In bronchiectasis, the blood is often mixed with purulent sputum.
- Massive haemoptyses (> 200 mL of blood in 24 hours) are usually due to bronchiectasis or tuberculosis.
- Uncommon causes of haemoptyses are idiopathic pulmonary haemosiderosis, Goodpasture's syndrome, microscopic polyangiitis, trauma, blood disorders and benign tumours.

Haemoptysis should always be investigated. Often, the diagnosis can be made from a chest X-ray, but a normal chest X-ray does not exclude disease.

Firm plugs of sputum may be coughed up by patients suffering from an exacerbation of allergic bronchopulmonary aspergillosis. Sometimes such sputum may appear as firm threads representing casts from inflamed bronchi.

Breathlessness

Breathlessness should be assessed in relation to the patient's lifestyle. For example, a moderate degree of breathlessness may be totally disabling if the patient has to climb many flights of stairs to reach home.

Dyspnoea is a sense of awareness of increased respiratory effort that is unpleasant and that is recognized by the patient as being inappropriate. It is highly unlikely that this term will be used by the patient. Patients may complain of tightness in the chest; this must be differentiated from angina.

Orthopnoea (see p. 733) is breathlessness on lying down and is partly due to the weight of the abdominal contents pushing the diaphragm up into the thorax. Such patients may also become breathless on bending over.

Tachypnoea and hyperpnoea refer, respectively, to an increased rate of breathing and an increased level of ventilation, which may be appropriate to the situation (e.g. during exercise).

Hyperventilation is inappropriate overbreathing. This may occur at rest or on exertion and results in a lowering of the alveolar and arterial P_{CO_2} (see p. 1298).

Paroxysmal nocturnal dyspnoea is described on page 733.

Wheezing

Wheezing is a common complaint and is the result of airflow limitation due to any cause. The symptom of wheezing is not diagnostic of asthma; it may be absent in the early stages of this disease, and may also occur in patients with bronchiolitis or chronic obstructive pulmonary disease.

Chest pain

The most common type of chest pain encountered in respiratory disease is a localized sharp pain, often referred to as pleuritic. It is made worse by deep breathing or coughing and can be precisely localized by the patient. Localized anterior chest pain may be accompanied by tenderness of a costochondral junction as a symptom of costochondritis. Pain in the shoulder tip suggests irritation of the diaphragmatic pleura, whereas central chest pain radiating to the neck and arms is typically of cardiac origin. Retrosternal soreness may occur in patients with tracheitis, and a constant, severe, dull pain may be the result of invasion of the thoracic wall by carcinoma.

FURTHER READING

Irwin RS, Madison JM (2000) The diagnosis and treatment of cough. *New England Journal of Medicine* **343**: 1715–1721.

Pasterkamp H, Kraman SS, Wodicka GR (1997) Respiratory sounds. Advances beyond the stethoscope. *American Journal of Respiratory and Critical Care Medicine* **156**: 974–987.

EXAMINATION OF THE RESPIRATORY SYSTEM

The nose (p. 1157)

Table 14.1 **Physical signs of respiratory disease**

Pathological process	Chest wall movement (reduced)	Mediastinal displacement	Percussion note	Breath sounds	Vocal resonance	Added sounds
Consolidation (i.e. lobar pneumonia)	Affected side	None	Dull	Bronchial	Increased	Fine crackles
Collapse						
Major bronchus	Affected side	Towards lesion	Dull	Diminished or absent	Reduced or absent	None
Peripheral bronchus	Affected side	Towards lesion	Dull	Bronchial	Increased	Fine crackles
Fibrosis						
Localized	Affected side	Towards lesion	Dull	Bronchial	Increased	Coarse crackles
Generalized (e.g. cryptogenic fibrosing alveolitis)	Both sides	None	Normal	Vesicular	Increased	Fine crackles
Pleural effusion (> 500 mL)	Affected side	Away from lesion (in massive effusion)	Stony dull	Vesicular reduced or absent	Reduced or absent	None
Large pneumothorax	Affected side	Away from lesion	Normal or hyperresonant	Reduced or absent	Reduced or absent	None
Asthma	Both sides	None	Normal	Vesicular Prolonged expiration	Normal	Expiratory polyphonic wheeze
Chronic obstructive pulmonary disease	Both sides	None	Normal	Vesicular Prolonged expiration	Normal	Expiratory polyphonic wheeze and coarse crackles

The chest (Table 14.1)

Examination of the chest

Inspection

Look for mental alertness, cyanosis, breathlessness at rest, use of accessory muscles, any deformity or scars on the chest and movement on both sides. A coarse tremor or flap of the outstretched hands indicates CO_2 intoxication. Prominent veins on the chest may imply obstruction of the superior vena cava.

Cyanosis (see p. 735) is a dusky colour of the skin and mucous membranes, due to the presence of more than 5 g/dL of desaturated haemoglobin. When due to central causes, cyanosis is visible on the tongue (especially the underside) and lips, and indicates a P_aO_2 below 6 kPa. Patients with central cyanosis will also be cyanosed peripherally. Peripheral cyanosis without central cyanosis is caused by a reduced peripheral circulation and is noted on the fingernails and skin of the extremities with associated coolness of the skin.

Finger clubbing is present when the normal angle between the base of the nail and the nail fold is lost. The base of the nail is fluctuant owing to increased vascularity, and there is an increased curvature of the nail in all directions, with expansion of the end of the digit. Some causes of clubbing are given in Table 14.2. Clubbing is not a feature of uncomplicated COPD.

Palpation and percussion

Check the position of the trachea and apex beat. Examine the supraclavicular fossa for enlarged lymph nodes. The distance between the sternal notch and the cricoid cartilage (three to four finger breadths in full expiration) is reduced in patients with severe airflow limitation. Check chest expansion. A tape measure may be used if precise measurements are needed, e.g. in ankylosing spondylitis. Local discomfort over the sternochondral joints may suggest costochondritis. Compression of the chest laterally and anteroposteriorly may produce localized pain suggestive of a rib fracture. On *percussion* liver dullness is usually detected anteriorly at the level of the sixth rib. Liver and cardiac dullness are lost with over-inflated lungs. Other changes are shown in Table 14.1.

Auscultation

The patient is asked to take deep breaths through the mouth. Inspiration sounds more prolonged than expiration. Healthy lungs filter off most of the high-frequency component, which is mainly due to turbulent flow in the larynx. Normal breath sounds are harsher anteriorly over the upper lobes (particularly on the right) and described as vesicular.

Bronchial breathing is heard best over consolidated or collapsed lung and sometimes over areas of localized fibrosis or bronchiectasis. Such areas conduct the high-frequency hissing component of breath sounds well. Characteristically, the noise heard during inspiration and expiration is equally long but separated by a short silent phase. Whispering pectoriloquy (whispered, higher-pitched, sounds heard distinctly through a stethoscope) invariably accompanies bronchial breathing.

Added sounds

Wheeze. Wheeze is usually heard during expiration and results from vibrations in the collapsible part of the airways when apposition occurs as a result of the flow-limiting mechanisms. Wheezes are heard in asthma and in chronic obstructive pulmonary disease, but are not invariably present. In the most severe cases of asthma a wheeze may not be heard, as airflow may be insufficient to generate the sound. Wheezes may be monophonic (single large airway obstruction) or polyphonic (narrowing of many small airways). An end-inspiratory (as opposed to expiratory) 'squeak' may be heard in obliterative bronchiolitis.

Crackles. These brief crackling sounds are probably produced by opening of previously closed bronchioles, and their timing during breathing is of significance – early inspiratory crackles are associated with diffuse airflow limitation, whereas late inspiratory crackles are characteristically heard in pulmonary oedema, fibrosis of the lung and bronchiectasis.

Pleural rub. This is a creaking or groaning sound that is usually well localized. It is indicative of inflammation and roughening of the pleural surfaces, which normally glide silently over one another.

Vocal resonance. Healthy lung attenuates high-frequency notes, leaving the booming low-pitched components of speech. Consolidated lung has the reverse effect, transmitting the high frequencies; the spoken word then takes on a bleating quality. Whispered (and therefore high-pitched) speech can barely be heard over healthy lung, whereas consolidation allows its clear transmission. Sonorous sounds such as 'ninety-nine' are well transmitted across healthy lung to produce vibration that can be felt over the chest wall. Consolidated lung transmits these low-frequency noises less well, and pleural fluid

Table 14.2 Some causes of finger clubbing

Respiratory	Cardiovascular
Bronchial carcinoma, especially epidermoid (squamous cell) type (major cause)	Cyanotic heart disease Subacute infective endocarditis Atrial myxoma
Chronic suppurative lung disease:	**Miscellaneous**
Bronchiectasis Lung abscess Empyema	Congenital – no disease Cirrhosis Inflammatory bowel disease
Pulmonary fibrosis (e.g. cryptogenic fibrosing alveolitis)	
Pleural and mediastinal tumours (e.g. mesothelioma)	
Cryptogenic organizing pneumonia	

severely dampens or obliterates the vibrations altogether. Tactile vocal fremitus is the palpation of this vibration, usually by placing the edge of the hand on the chest wall. For all practical purposes this duplicates the assessment of vocal resonance and is no longer considered a routine part of the chest examination.

Cardiovascular system examination (p. 735) gives additional information about the lungs.

Additional tests

Since so many patients with respiratory disease have airflow limitation, airflow should be routinely measured using a peak flow meter or spirometer. This will provide a much more accurate assessment of airflow limitation than any physical sign.

INVESTIGATION OF RESPIRATORY DISEASE

Haematological and biochemical tests

It is useful to measure:

- haemoglobin, to detect the presence of anaemia or polycythaemia
- packed cell volume (secondary polycythaemia occurs with chronic hypoxia)
- routine biochemistry (often disturbed in carcinoma and infection).
- B-type natriuretic peptide may be a useful test to distinguish cardiac from non-cardiac breathlessness. A rapid bedside test is available but is not yet in routine clinical use.
- D-dimer can be measured to detect intravascular coagulation. A negative test makes pulmonary embolism very unlikely.

Other blood investigations sometimes required include α_1-antitrypsin levels, *Aspergillus* antibodies, viral and mycoplasma serology, autoantibody profiles and specific IgE measurements.

Sputum

Sputum should be inspected for colour:

- yellowish green indicates inflammation (infection or allergy)
- the presence of blood suggests neoplasm or pulmonary infarct (see haemoptysis, p. 882).

Microbiological studies (Gram stain and culture) are not helpful in upper respiratory tract infections or in acute or chronic bronchitis. They are of value in:

- pneumonia
- the diagnosis of tuberculosis (Ziehl–Neelsen or auramine-phenol stains)
- unusual clinical problems
- *Aspergillus* lung disease.

Sputum cytology

This is extremely useful in the diagnosis of bronchial carcinoma. Advantages are:

- a quick result
- cheapness
- it is non-invasive.

However, its value depends on the production of sputum and the presence of a reliable cytologist. Sputum can be induced following the inhalation of nebulized hypertonic saline (5%). This is unpleasant and it is better to proceed to bronchoscopy and bronchial washings (see p. 891), or occasionally, transtracheal aspiration.

Transtracheal aspiration

This technique involves pushing a needle through the cricothyroid membrane, through which a catheter is threaded to a position just above the carina. This procedure induces coughing, and specimens are collected by aspiration or by the introduction and subsequent aspiration of sterile saline. Although not often required, it is an excellent technique for assessing infection in the lower respiratory tract because it avoids contamination of the specimen with bacteria from the pharynx and mouth.

Imaging

Radiology is an essential adjunct to examination of the chest. Diseases such as tuberculosis or lung cancer may not be detectable on clinical examination but are obvious on the chest X-ray. Conversely, the abnormal physical signs in asthma or chronic bronchitis may be associated with a normal chest X-ray. Always try to get previous films for comparison.

Chest X-ray

The following must be taken into account when viewing films:

- *Centring of the film.* The distance between each clavicular head and the spinal processes should be equal.
- *Penetration* (check film is not too dark).
- *The view.* Routine films are taken PA, i.e. the film is placed in front of the patient with the X-ray source behind. Anteroposterior (AP) films are taken only in very ill patients who are unable to stand up or be taken to the radiology department; the cardiac outline appears bigger and the scapulae cannot be moved out of the way. A lateral chest X-ray helps in localization of pathology.

Look at:

- the shape and bony structure of the chest wall
- whether the trachea is central
- whether the diaphragm is elevated or flat
- the shape, size and position of the heart
- the shape and size of the hilar shadows
- the size and shape of any lung abnormalities and vascular shadowing.

X-ray abnormalities

Collapse and consolidation

A chest X-ray showing collapse of a whole lung is shown in Figure 14.11 and causes are shown in Table 14.3. Loss of volume in the relevant hemithorax should raise the possibility of lobar collapse. The lung lobes collapse in characteristic directions. The lower lobes collapse downward and towards the mediastinum, the left upper lobe collapses forwards against the anterior chest wall, while the right upper lobe collapses upwards and outwards, forming the appearance of an arch over the remaining lung. The right middle lobe collapses anteriorly and inward, obscuring the right heart border. If a whole lung collapses, the mediastinum will shift towards the side of the collapse. Consolidated lobes remain the same size; uncomplicated consolidation does not cause mediastinal shift or loss of lung volume.

Pleural effusion (see Fig. 14.45)

Pleural effusions need to be more than 500 mL to cause much more than blunting of the costophrenic angle. On an erect film they produce a characteristic shadow with a curved upper edge rising into the axilla. If very large, the whole of one side of the thorax may be opaque, with shift of the mediastinum to the opposite side.

Table 14.3 Causes of collapse of the lung

Enlarged tracheobronchial lymph nodes due to malignant disease, tuberculosis	Bronchial casts or plugs (e.g. allergic bronchopulmonary aspergillosis)
Inhaled foreign bodies (e.g. peanuts) in children, usually in the right main bronchus	Retained secretions – postoperatively and in debilitated patients

Fig. 14.11 Collapse of the left lung. Chest X-ray showing hazy shadowing in the left upper zone with a raised left diaphragm. There is compensatory emphysema of the right lung.

Labels on figure: Trachea deviated to the left; Heart and apex beat deviated to the left

Table 14.4 Causes of round shadows (> 3 cm) in the lung

Carcinoma	Aspergilloma
Metastatic tumours (usually multiple shadows)	Rheumatoid nodules
	Tuberculoma (may be calcification within the lesion)
Lung abscess (usually with fluid level)	
Encysted interlobar effusion (usually in horizontal fissure)	*Rare causes:* Bronchial carcinoid Cylindroma Chondroma Lipoma
Hydatid cysts (rare and often with a fluid level)	
Arteriovenous malformations (usually adjacent to a vascular shadow)	Other shadows related to mediastinum: Pericardium / Oesophagus / Spinal cord — Seen on lateral chest X-ray

Fibrosis

Localized fibrosis causes streaky shadowing, and the accompanying loss of lung volume causes mediastinal structures to move to the same side. More generalized fibrosis in the lung can lead to a honeycomb appearance (see p. 943), seen as diffuse shadows containing multiple circular translucencies a few millimetres in diameter.

Round shadows

Lung cancer is the commonest cause of large round shadows but many other causes are recognized (Table 14.4).

Miliary mottling

This term describes numerous minute opacities, 1–3 mm in size, which are caused by many pathological processes. The most common causes are miliary tuberculosis, pneumoconiosis, sarcoidosis, fibrosing alveolitis (idiopathic pulmonary fibrosis) and pulmonary oedema (see Fig. 13.18), though the latter is usually perihilar and accompanied by larger, fluffy shadows. A rare but striking cause of miliary mottling is pulmonary microlithiasis.

Computed tomography

Modern CT scanners provide excellent images of the lungs and mediastinal structures. Different settings are required to show the parenchymal tissue and the central structures (Fig. 14.12). Mediastinal structures may be shown more clearly by injecting intravenous contrast medium to enhance the vascular structures.

The advent of rapid *volumetric* or '*spiral*' *scanning* means that scans can be obtained rapidly (within seconds) during contrast injection. This is a useful technique for directly demonstrating pulmonary emboli within pulmonary vessels. *Conventional CT* is valuable in bronchial carcinoma staging to demonstrate mediastinal, pleural or chest wall invasion and to determine operability. CT-guided needle biopsy is the preferred means of obtaining samples from peripheral masses.

Enlarged mediastinal nodes (>1 cm) may be either malignant or reactive and may require biopsy. Scanning should include assessment of liver, adrenals and brain, which are likely sites for metastatic disease.

High-resolution CT scanning (sampling lung parenchyma with 1–2 mm thickness scans at 10–20 mm intervals) allows assessment of diffuse lung parenchymal processes, particularly interstitial disease. It is valuable in the following situations:

- Detection of diffuse interstitial pulmonary involvement in any type of interstitial lung disease, including sarcoidosis, cryptogenic and extrinsic allergic alveolitis, occupational lung disease, and any other form of interstitial pulmonary fibrosis.
- Diagnosis of bronchiectasis. High-resolution CT has a sensitivity and specificity of greater than 90%. Inspiratory and expiratory scans may allow demonstration of air trapping in small airway disease. This technique has replaced bronchography.
- Distinguishing emphysema from interstitial lung disease or pulmonary vascular disease as a cause of a low gas transfer factor with otherwise normal lung function
- Diagnosis of lymphangitis carcinomatosa.

Magnetic resonance imaging

Problems with motion artefact, both respiratory and cardiac, make magnetic resonance imaging (MRI) less valuable than CT in assessment of lung parenchyma. In the mediastinum, MRI with ECG-gating allows accurate images of the heart and aortic aneurysms to be obtained, and MRI retains a place in staging lung cancer, for assessing tumour invasion in the mediastinum, chest wall and at the lung apex, because it produces good images in the sagittal and coronal planes. Vascular structures can be clearly differentiated as flowing blood produces a signal void on MRI.

Positron emission tomography (PET)

Tumours take up a tracer, e.g. fluorodeoxyglucose (FDG), which emits positrons that can be imaged and this helps differentiate benign from malignant tumours. PET scanning is now the investigation of choice for assessing lymph nodes and metastatic disease in bronchial carcinoma.

Scintigraphic imaging

This technique is used widely for the detection of pulmonary emboli although it is now performed less often owing to widespread use of D-dimer measurements to screen for thromboembolism.

Perfusion scan

Macro-aggregated human albumin labelled with technetium-99m is injected intravenously. The particles are of such a size that they impact in pulmonary

Fig. 14.12 **CT scan of the lung.**
(a) Lung setting – showing normal lung markings. 1, right hilum; 2, mediastinum; 3, left hilum; 4, lung vessels; 5, L. main bronchus; 6, R. main bronchus; 7, position of oblique fissure; 8, peripheral lung vessels.
(b) Mediastinal (soft tissue) setting – showing normal mediastinal structures following intravenous contrast enhancement. 1, rib; 2, descending L. pulmonary artery; 3, scapula; 4, subcutaneous fat; 5, L. main bronchus; 6, descending aorta; 7, spinal canal; 8, vertebral body; 9, oesophagus; 10, R. main bronchus; 11, R. pulmonary artery; 12, muscle; 13, R. superior pulmonary vein; 14, superior vena cava; 15, costal cartilage; 16, ascending aorta; 17, sternum; 18, thymic remnant; 19, pulmonary trunk; 20, breast tissue; 21, L. superior pulmonary vein.
(c) Post-contrast scan showing large right upper zone carcinoma (*arrow*) with enlarged lymph nodes in the mediastinum surrounding the trachea.

capillaries, where they remain for a few hours. A gamma camera is then used to detect the position of the macro-aggregated human albumin. The resultant pattern indicates the distribution of pulmonary blood flow; cold areas occur where there is defective blood flow (e.g. in pulmonary emboli).

Ventilation–perfusion scan (see p. 845)

Xenon-133 gas is inhaled into the lung and its distribution is detected at the same time as the perfusion scan. Using the two scans, a pulmonary embolus can be seen to cause a striking diminution of perfusion relative to ventilation. Other lung diseases (e.g. asthma or pneumonia) impair both ventilation and perfusion. Unfortunately, however, a pulmonary embolus often produces substantial changes in the lung substance (e.g. atelectasis) so that such a clear distinction is not always obvious. Nevertheless, this is a better technique than perfusion scan alone.

Respiratory function tests (Table 14.5)

In clinical practice, airflow limitation can be assessed by relatively simple tests that have good intra-subject repeatability. Normal values are required for their interpretation since these tests vary considerably, not only with sex, age and height, but also within individuals of the same age, sex and height. The standard deviation about the mean for a group of individuals is therefore very high; for example, the standard deviation for the peak expiratory flow rate is approximately 50 L/min, and for the FEV_1 it is approximately 0.4 L. Repeated measurements of lung function are useful for assessing the progression of disease in an individual patient.

Tests of ventilatory function

These tests are used mainly to assess the degree of airflow limitation present during expiration.

Peak expiratory flow rate (PEFR)

This is an extremely simple and cheap test. Subjects are asked to take a full inspiration to total lung capacity and then blow out forcefully into the peak flow meter (Fig. 14.13), which is held horizontally. The lips must be placed tightly around the mouthpiece. The best of three tests is recorded.

Table 14.5	Respiratory function tests and exercise tests		
Test	**Use**	**Advantages**	**Disadvantages**
PEFR	Monitoring changes in airflow limitation in asthma	Portable Can be used at the bedside	Effort-dependent Poor measure of chronic airflow limitation
FEV, FVC, FEV₁/FVC	Assessment of airflow limitation The best single test	Reproducible Relatively effort-independent	Bulky equipment but smaller portable machines available
Flow–volume curves	Assessment of flow at lower lung volumes Detection of large airway obstruction both intra- and extrathoracic (e.g. tracheal stenosis, tumour)	Recognition of patterns of flow–volume curves for different diseases	Sophisticated equipment needed for full test but expiratory loop now possible with compact spirometry
Airways resistance	Assessment of airflow limitation	Sensitive	Technique difficult to perform
Lung volumes	Differentiation between restrictive and obstructive lung disease	Effort-independent, complements FEV_1	Sophisticated equipment needed
Gas transfer	Assessment and monitoring of extent of interstitial lung disease and emphysema	Non-invasive (compared with lung biopsy or radiation from repeated chest X-rays and CT)	Sophisticated equipment needed
Blood gases	Assessment of respiratory failure	Can detect early lung disease when measured during exercise	Invasive
Pulse oximetry	Postoperative, sleep studies and respiratory failure	Continuous monitoring Non-invasive	Measures saturation only
Exercise tests (6-min walk)	Practical assessment for disability and effects of therapy	No equipment required	Time-consuming Learning effect At least two walks required
Cardiorespiratory assessment	Early detection of lung/heart disease Fitness assessment	Differentiates breathlessness due to lung or heart disease	Expensive and complicated equipment required

(a) Peak flow meter

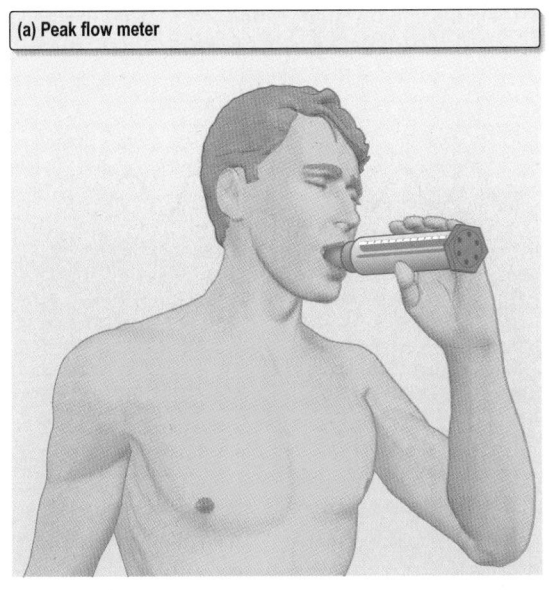

(b) Graph of normal readings

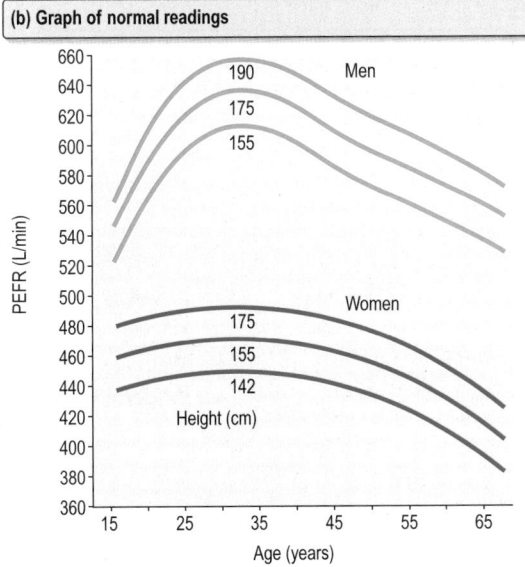

Fig. 14.13 **Peak flow measurements. (a)** Peak flow meter: the lips should be tight around the mouthpiece. **(b)** Graph of normal readings for men and women.

Although reproducible, PEFR is not a good measure of airflow limitation since it measures the expiratory flow rate only in the first 2 ms of expiration and overestimates lung function in patients with moderate airflow limitation. PEFR is best used to monitor progression of disease and its treatment. Regular measurements of peak flow rates on waking, during the afternoon, and before bed demonstrate the wide diurnal variations in airflow limitation that characterize asthma and allow an objective assessment of treatment to be made (Fig. 14.14).

Spirometry

The spirometer measures the FEV_1 and the forced vital capacity (FVC). Both the FEV_1 and FVC are related to height, age and sex. The technique involves a maximum inspiration followed by a forced expiration (for as long as possible) into the spirometer. The act of expiration triggers the moving record chart, which measures volume against time. The record chart moves for a total of 5 s, but expiration should continue until all the air has been expelled from the lungs, as patients with severe airflow limitation may have a very prolonged forced expiratory time. This is demonstrated on the record chart in Figure 14.15.

The FEV_1 expressed as a percentage of the FVC is an excellent measure of airflow limitation. In normal subjects it is around 75%. With *increasing airflow limitation* the FEV_1 falls proportionately more than the FVC, so that the FEV_1/FVC ratio is reduced. With *restrictive lung disease* the FEV_1 and the FVC are reduced in the same proportion and the FEV_1/FVC ratio remains normal or may even increase because of the enhanced elastic recoil.

In chronic airflow limitation (particularly in emphysema and asthma) the total lung capacity (TLC) is usually increased, yet there is nearly always some reduction in the FVC. This is the result of disease in the small airways causing obstruction to airflow before the normal RV is reached. This trapping of air within the lung (giving an increased RV) is a characteristic feature of these diseases.

Other tests

Measurement of airways resistance in a body plethysmograph is more sensitive but the equipment is expensive and the necessary manoeuvres are too exhausting for many patients with chronic airflow limitation.

Flow–volume loops

The ability to measure flow rates against volume (flow–volume loops, see Fig. 14.8) enables a more sophisticated analysis to be made of the site of airflow limitation within the lung. At the start of expiration from TLC, the site of maximum resistance is the large airways, and this

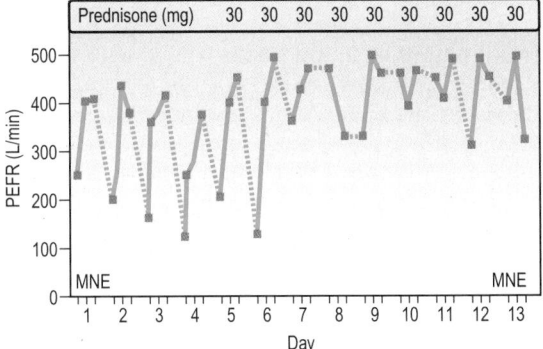

Fig. 14.14 **Diurnal variability in PEFR in asthma, showing the effect of steroids.** M, morning; N, noon; E, evening.

1. Total lung capacity
2. Inspiratory reserve volume
3. Tidal volume
4. Functional residual capacity
5. Vital capacity
6. Residual volume

Fig. 14.16 **The subdivisions of the lung volume.**

Fig. 14.15 **Spirometry.** Volume–time curves showing **(a)** normal patterns for age and sex, **(b)** restrictive pattern (FEV$_1$ and FVC reduced), **(c)** airflow limitation (FEV$_1$ only reduced).

accounts for the flow reduction in the first 25% of the curve. As the lung volume reduces further, so the elastic pressures within the lung holding open the smaller airways reduce, and disease of the lung parenchyma or the small airways themselves becomes apparent. For example, in diseases such as chronic obstructive pulmonary disease (COPD), where the brunt of the disease falls upon the smaller airways, expiratory flow rates at 50% or 25% of the vital capacity may be disproportionately reduced when compared with flow rates at larger lung volumes.

Lung volume

The subdivisions of the lung volume are shown in Figure 14.16. Tidal volume and vital capacity can be measured using a simple spirometer, but the TLC and RV need to be measured by an alternative technique. TLC is measured by connecting the lungs to a reservoir containing a known amount of non-absorbable gas (helium) that can readily be measured. If the concentration of the gas in the reservoir is known at the start of the test and is measured after equilibration of the gas has occurred (when the patient has breathed in and out of the reservoir), the dilution of the gas will reflect the TLC. This technique is known as *helium dilution*. RV can be calculated by subtracting the vital capacity from the TLC.

The TLC measured using this technique is inaccurate if large cystic spaces are present in the lung, because the helium cannot diffuse into them. Under these circumstances the thoracic gas volume can be measured more accurately using a body plethysmograph. The difference between the two measurements can be used to define the extent of non-communicating air space within the lungs.

Transfer factor

This measures the transfer of gas across the alveolar–capillary membrane and reflects the uptake of oxygen from the alveoli into the red cells. A low concentration of carbon monoxide is inhaled and is avidly taken up in a linear fashion by circulating haemoglobin, the amount of which must be known when the test is performed. In normal lungs the transfer factor is a true measure of the diffusing capacity of the lungs for oxygen and depends on the thickness of the alveolar–capillary membrane. In lung disease the diffusing capacity (D_{CO}) also depends on the $\dot{V}_A/\dot{Q}$ relationship as well as on the area and thickness of the alveolar membrane. To control for differences in lung volume, the uptake of carbon monoxide is related to the lung volume; this is known as the transfer coefficient (K_{CO}).

Gas transfer is usually reduced in patients with severe degrees of emphysema and fibrosis. Overall gas transfer can be thought of as a relatively non-specific test of lung function but one that can be particularly used in the early detection and assessment of progress of diseases affecting the lung parenchyma (e.g. cryptogenic pulmonary fibrosis, sarcoidosis, asbestosis).

Measurement of blood gases

This technique is described on page 980.

Measurement of the partial pressures of oxygen and carbon dioxide within arterial blood is essential in the management of cases of respiratory failure and severe asthma, when repeated measurements are often the best guide to therapy.

Arterial oxygen saturation (S_aO_2) can be continuously measured using an oximeter with either ear or finger probes. The oximeter measures the differential absorption of light by oxy- and deoxyhaemoglobin and measures saturation to within 5% of that obtained by blood gas analysis.

Exercise tests

The predominant symptom in respiratory medicine is that of breathlessness. The degree of disability produced by breathlessness can be assessed before and after treatment by asking the patient to walk for 6 minutes along a measured track. This has been shown to be a reproducible and useful test once the patient has undergone an initial training walk to overcome the learning effect.

Exercise tests incorporating assessment of both lung and heart function are of particular value in the investigation of breathlessness. Such tests involve the use of sophisticated equipment enabling measurement of uptake of oxygen ($\dot{V}O_2$), work performed, heart rate and blood pressure together with serial ECGs. Correlation of these variables allows:

- the early detection of lung disease
- the detection of myocardial ischaemia
- the distinction between lung and heart disease
- assessment of fitness.

Pleural aspiration

Diagnostic aspiration is necessary for all but very small effusions. A needle attached to a 20 mL syringe is inserted through an intercostal space over an area of dullness. Fluid is withdrawn and the presence of any blood is noted. Samples are sent for protein estimation, cytology and bacteriological examination, including culture and Ziehl–Neelsen stain for tuberculosis. Large amounts of fluid can be aspirated through a large needle to help relieve extreme breathlessness. Because of the risk of introducing infection into the pleural space, with the subsequent development of an empyema, this technique must be performed using full aseptic precautions.

Pleural aspiration and drainage are now often performed using ultrasound to localize the fluid.

Pleural biopsy

Blind pleural biopsy (Fig. 14.17) is a useful technique if performed by an experienced operator, and will yield positive results in up to 80% of cases of tuberculosis and in 60% of cases of malignancy provided multiple biopsies are taken (Practical box 14.1). Better yields can be obtained by biopsy under direct vision using thoracoscopy.

Intercostal drainage

This is carried out when large effusions are present producing severe breathlessness or for drainage of an empyema (see Practical box 14.2). Pleurodesis is performed for recurrent/malignant effusion.

Mediastinoscopy and scalene node biopsy

This technique can be used in the management of carcinoma of the bronchus. It involves inspection of the mediastinal structures using a mediastinoscope inserted

Fig. 14.17 Technique of pleural biopsy. The biopsy needle is shown penetrating the chest wall. A, lung parenchyma; B, pleural space; C, muscle; D, skin and subcutaneous tissue.

 Practical Box 14.1
Pleural biopsy

- Explain to the patient the nature of the procedure.
- Get written consent.

1. Pleural biopsy is best performed after the aspiration of diagnostic fluid samples but before draining large volumes of fluid.
2. A small skin incision is made, as the end of the Abrams' pleural biopsy needle is blunt.
3. Once in place through the pleura, the back part of the needle is rotated to open the notch; this is kept pointing forward.
4. With lateral pressure the needle is withdrawn so that the notch will snag against the pleura.
5. The needle is held firmly and the hexagonal grip is twisted clockwise to cut the biopsy. To avoid damage to the intercostal vessel or nerve, the notch should never be directed upwards when the biopsy is taken.
6. Several biopsies should be taken at different angles by repeated insertion of the needle.
7. Specimens should be put in sterile saline for culture for tuberculosis and into 10% formol saline for histological examination.

---

by blunt dissection downwards from behind the proximal end of the clavicle. Subsequent biopsy of tissue will reveal the presence or absence of malignant cells in enlarged lymph nodes previously detected by CT, allowing accurate staging of the disease.

Fibreoptic bronchoscopy (Practical box 14.3)

Central bronchial lesions can be biopsied readily.

Washings can be taken from lobes containing more peripheral lesions for cytological examination for malig-

Practical Box 14.2
Intercostal drainage

■ Explain to the patient the nature of the procedure.
■ Get written consent.

1. Carefully sterilize the skin over the aspiration site. Sterile gloves, cap, gown and mask must be worn.
2. Anaesthetize the skin, muscle and pleura with 2% lidocaine.
3. Make a small incision, then push a 28 French gauge Argyle catheter into the pleural space.
4. Attach to a three-way tap and 50 mL syringe.
5. Aspirate up to 1000 mL. Stop aspiration if patient becomes uncomfortable – shock may ensue if too much fluid is withdrawn too quickly.
6. A Silastic pigtail catheter can be inserted under X-ray/ultrasound control and attached to tubing and bag for slower aspiration. For drainage and effusions, an 8–12 French gauge pigtail is inserted using the Seldinger technique in which the needle used to enter the pleural space is withdrawn over a control wire along which the catheter is then passed. A 14–16 French gauge pigtail catheter is used for drainage of empyema.

For pleurodesis
Sterile talc (2–5 g), tetracycline 500 mg or bleomycin 15 units in 30–50 mL sodium chloride 0.9% solution is instilled into the pleural cavity to achieve pleurodesis in recurrent/malignant effusion.

nant cells, and appropriate staining and culture for, for example, *Pneumocystis carinii*, *Mycobacterium*.

Diffuse parenchymal lung disease can be investigated using transbronchial biopsy. The biopsy forceps are pushed as far as possible to the periphery of the lung, the patient is asked to breathe in and the forceps are opened. The patient then breathes out and the jaws of the forceps are closed, removing a small piece of peripheral airway and surrounding lung parenchyma.

Video-assisted thoracoscopic lung biopsy

This technique reduces the need for open thoracotomy when a lung biopsy is required (p. 942).

Bronchoalveolar lavage

This technique can be used both in patients who have disease confined to one lobe and in those with more diffuse lung disease. The tip of the fibreoptic bronchoscope is lodged in the segmental orifice and 20 mL of 0.9% sterile saline is squirted down the suction port of the bronchoscope and immediately aspirated. This is repeated five times; about 40–60% of the total volume is recovered. Fluid is strained through two layers of surgical gauze and the volume is noted. The cells are then spun down and resuspended at a concentration of 1×10^7 cells/mL for differential counting. Since there is a considerable

Practical Box 14.3
Fibreoptic bronchoscopy

This enables the direct visualization of the bronchial tree as far as the subsegmental bronchi under a local anaesthetic. Informed consent should be obtained after explaining the nature of the procedure.

Indications
■ Lesions requiring biopsy seen on chest X-ray.
■ Haemoptysis.
■ Stridor.
■ Positive sputum cytology for malignant cells with no chest X-ray abnormality.
■ Collection of bronchial secretions for bacteriology, especially tuberculosis.
■ Recurrent laryngeal nerve paralysis of unknown aetiology.
■ Infiltrative lung disease (to obtain a transbronchial biopsy).
■ Investigation of collapsed lobes or segments and aspiration of mucus plugs.

Procedure
■ The patient is starved overnight.
■ Atropine 0.6 mg i.m. is given 30 min before the procedure.
■ Topical anaesthesia (lidocaine 2% gel) is applied to the nose, nasopharynx and pharynx.
■ Intravenous sedation (e.g. diazepam 10 mg or midazolam 2.5–10 mg) is given.

■ The bronchoscope is passed through the nose, nasopharynx and pharynx under direct vision to minimize trauma.
■ Lidocaine (2 mL of 4%) is dropped through the instrument on to the vocal cords.
■ The bronchoscope is passed through the cords into the trachea.
■ All segmental and subsegmental orifices should be identified.
■ Biopsies and brushings should be taken of macroscopic abnormalities or occasionally from peripheral lesions under radiographic control.

Disadvantages
■ All patients require sedation to tolerate the procedure.
■ Minor and transient cardiac dysrhythmias occur in up to 40% of patients on passage of the bronchoscope through the larynx.
■ Oxygen supplementation is required in patients with $P_{a}O_{2}$ below 8 kPa.
■ Fibreoptic bronchoscopy should be performed with care in the very sick, and transbronchial biopsies avoided in ventilated patients owing to the increased risk of pneumothorax.
■ Massive bleeding may occur on accidental biopsy of vascular lesions or carcinoid tumours. Rigid bronchoscopy may be required to allow adequate access to the bleeding point for haemostasis.

overlap in the distribution of cells seen in broncho-alveolar wash specimens in different diseases, this technique has no value in diagnosis. However, it can be used to monitor progression of disease, since improvement is characterized by a reduction in the number of cells and a return towards the normal proportions of different cell types.

Skin-prick tests

Allergen solutions are placed on the skin (usually the volar surface of the forearm) and the epidermis is broken using a 1 mm tipped lancet. A separate lancet should be used for each allergen. If the patient is sensitive to the allergen a weal develops and the diameter of the induration should be measured after 10 minutes. A weal of at least 3 mm diameter is regarded as positive provided that the negative control test is truly negative. The results should be interpreted in the light of the history. Skin tests are not affected by bronchodilators or corticosteroids but antihistamines should be discontinued at least 48 hours before testing.

FURTHER READING

Armstrong P, Wilson AG, Dee P et al. (2000) *Imaging of Diseases of the Chest*, 3rd edn. Chicago: Mosby Year Book.

Mueller C, Scholer A, Laule-Kilian K et al. (2004) Use of B-type natriuretic peptide in the evaluation and management of acute dyspnoea. *New England Journal of Medicine* **350**: 647–654.

Murray SJ, Barrett A, Magee JG, Freeman R (2003) Optimisation of acid fast smears for the direct detection of mycobacteria in clinical samples. *Journal of Clinical Pathology* **56**: 613–615.

Ost D et al. (2003) Clinical practice. The solitary pulmonary nodule. *New England Journal of Medicine* **348**: 2535–2542.

SMOKING AND AIR POLLUTION

SMOKING

Prevalence

General household surveys in the UK showed a decline in the prevalence of cigarette smoking in the early nineties. More recent data show that this decline has halted and smoking in the UK is on the increase. At present, 28% of men and women aged 16 years and over smoke. Cigarette smoking is most common between the ages of 16 and 34 years (40% in both sexes) and it is in this age group that the increase has occurred. At the age of 15 more girls (33%) than boys (13%) smoke cigarettes. A greater proportion of manual workers than professional workers smoke. In the USA only 26% of men smoke and 22% of women. However, cigarette consumption is rising in Central and Eastern Europe and many developing countries including China.

Toxic effects

Cigarette smoke contains polycyclic aromatic hydro-carbons and nitrosamines, which are potent carcinogens and mutagens in animals. It causes release of enzymes from neutrophil granulocytes and macrophages that are capable of destroying elastin and leading to lung damage. Pulmonary epithelial permeability increases even in symptomless cigarette smokers, and correlates with the concentration of carboxyhaemoglobin in blood. This altered permeability possibly allows easier access to carcinogens.

The dangers

Cigarette smoking is addictive. People usually start smoking in adolescence for psychosocial reasons and, once it is a regular habit, the pharmacological properties of nicotine play a major part in persistence, conferring some advantage to the smoker's mood. Very few cigarette smokers (less than 2%) can limit themselves to occasional or intermittent smoking. The dangers are listed in Table 14.6.

There is a significant dose–response relationship between the smoking of 0–40 cigarettes daily and lung cancer mortality (Table 14.7). Sputum production and

Table 14.6	The dangers of cigarette smoking
General	**Passive smoking**
Lung cancer	Risk of asthma, pneumonia
COPD	and bronchitis in infants
Carcinoma of the	of smoking parents
oesophagus	An increase in cough and
Ischaemic heart disease	breathlessness in
Peripheral vascular disease	smokers and non-
Bladder cancer	smokers with COPD and
An increase in abnormal	asthma
spermatozoa	Increased cancer risk
Memory problems	
Maternal smoking	
A decrease in birthweight of	
the infant	
An increase in fetal and	
neonatal mortality	
An increase in asthma	

Table 14.7	Effects of smoking on the lung
Large airways	**Small airways**
Increase in submucosal	Increase in number and
gland volume	distribution of goblet cells
Increase in number of	Airway inflammation and
goblet cells	fibrosis
Chronic inflammation	Epithelial
Metaplasia and dysplasia	metaplasia/dysplasia
of the surface epithelium	Carcinoma
	Parenchyma
	Proximal acinar scarring
	Increase in alveolar
	macrophage numbers
	Emphysema (centri-acinar,
	pan-acinar)

airflow limitation increase with daily cigarette consumption, and effort tolerance decreases, partly owing to high levels of carboxyhaemoglobin in bronchitis patients. Smoking and asbestos exposure are synergistic in producing bronchial carcinoma, increasing the risk in asbestos workers by up to five to eight times that of non-smokers exposed to asbestos.

Cigarette smokers who change to other forms of tobacco can reduce the risk, even if they continue to inhale, and are better off changing to cigars or pipes. However, all pipe and cigar smokers also have a greater risk of lung cancer than lifelong non-smokers or former smokers.

Environmental tobacco smoke ('passive smoking') has been shown to cause more frequent and more severe attacks of asthma in children and possibly increases the number of cases of asthma. It is also associated with a small but definite increase in lung cancer.

Stopping smoking

If the entire population could be persuaded to stop smoking, the effect on healthcare use would be enormous. National campaigns, bans on advertising and a substantial increase in the cost of cigarettes are the best ways of achieving this at the population level. Meanwhile, active encouragement to stop smoking remains a useful approach for individuals. Smokers who want to stop should have access to smoking cessation clinics to provide behavioural support. Nicotine replacement therapy (NRT) and buproprion are effective aids to smoking cessation in those smoking more than 10 cigarettes per day. Both should only be used in smokers who commit to a target stop date, and the initial prescription should be for 2 weeks beyond the target stop date. NRT is the preferred choice; there is no evidence that combined therapy offers any advantage. Therapy should be changed after 3 months if abstinence is not achieved.

AIR POLLUTION

Atmospheric air pollution, due to the burning of coal for energy and heat, has been a characteristic of urban living in developed countries for at least two centuries. It consists of black smoke and sulphur dioxide (SO_2). Air pollution of this type peaked in the 1950s in the UK, until legislation led to restrictions on coal burning. Such pollution continues to increase in newly industrialized countries (India, China) and continues in Eastern Europe and Russia. The combustion of petroleum and diesel oil in motor vehicles has led to new air pollution, consisting of primary pollutants such as the oxides of nitrogen (NO and NO_2), diesel particulates, polyaromatic hydrocarbons and the secondary pollutant ozone (O_3) generated by photochemical reactions in the atmosphere. Levels of NO_2 can be higher in poorly ventilated kitchens and living rooms where gas is used for cooking and in fires. In Europe 70% of the particulates present in urban

air result from the combustion of diesel fuel. Very small particles (<2.5 μm, particulate matter $PM_{2.5}$) remain airborne for long periods and are carried into rural areas. In the UK, ozone concentrations are highest in sunny rural areas.

Epidemiology

Classical studies in the 1950s showed that winter-time episodes of severe air pollution (smog) were associated with substantial numbers of deaths from respiratory disease, particularly when temperature inversion trapped black smoke and SO_2 over urban areas. Air pollution of this type continues to cause excess deaths from respiratory and cardiovascular disease in older populations, and symptoms of bronchitis in children. Pollution resulting primarily from motor vehicles has been shown to cause:

- Increased deaths from respiratory and cardiovascular causes in the elderly – particulates less than 10 μm in diameter (PM_{10}).
- Increased respiratory symptoms, hospital admissions and reduced lung function in children and younger adults – SO_2, NO_2, O_3, PM_{10}. Frequently there is a lag of 1–2 days between peaks in air pollution and disease effects.
- Increase in lung cancer – polyaromatic hydrocarbons.

It has been proposed at various times that air pollution is one of the causes of the dramatic increase in asthma and other allergic diseases (Table 14.8). There is no current evidence that this is true, but both NO_2 and ozone have been shown to enhance the nasal and lung airway responses to inhaled allergen, in those with established allergic disease. Air pollution has, however, been shown to have an adverse effect on lung development in teenage children.

Management

Asthmatics are advised to avoid exercising outdoors when air quality is poor and to increase their anti-inflammatory medication (i.e. inhaled corticosteroids).

Short- and long-term measures are required to reduce air pollution, particularly diesel particulates (which are predicted to increase as more diesel engines are used). Such measures include increased motor engine efficiency, catalytic converters, diesel particulate traps, and decreased reliance on cars and trucks.

FURTHER READING

Brunekreef B, Holgate ST (2002) Air pollution and health. *Lancet* **360**: 1233–1242.

Koenig JQ (1999) Air pollution and asthma. *Journal of Allergy and Clinical Immunology* **104**: 717–722.

Kunzil N et al. (2000) Public health impact of outdoor and traffic-related air pollution: a European assessment. *Lancet* **356**: 795–801.

Ware JH (2000) Particulate air pollution and mortality. *New England Journal of Medicine* **343**: 1798–1799.

Table 14.8 Air pollutants and their health effects				
	Average concentration	Poor air quality	Susceptible individuals	Mechanisms of health effects
Sulphur dioxide (SO_2)	5–15 ppb	> 125 ppb	Asthmatics	Bronchoconstriction through neurogenic mechanism
Ozone (O_3)	10–30 ppb	> 90 ppb	All affected, particularly during exercise	Restrictive lung defect Airway inflammation Enhanced response to allergen
Nitrogen dioxide (NO_2)	25–40 ppb	> 100 ppb	Allergic individuals	Airway inflammation Enhanced response to allergen
Particulate matter (PM_{10})	25–30 $\mu g/m^3$	> 70 $\mu g/m^3$	Elderly Allergic individuals	Airway and alveolar inflammation Enhanced production selectively of the allergy antibody (IgE)

ppb, parts per billion

DISEASES OF THE UPPER RESPIRATORY TRACT

The common cold (acute coryza)

This highly infectious illness causes a mild systemic upset and prominent nasal symptoms. It is due to infection by rhinoviruses, the majority of which belong to the picornavirus group and exist in at least 100 different antigenic strains. Infectivity from close personal contact (nasal mucus on hands) or droplets is high in the early stages of the infection, and spread is facilitated by overcrowding and poor ventilation. On average, individuals suffer two to three colds per year; but the incidence lessens with age, presumably as a result of accumulating immunity to the causative virus strains. The incubation is from 12 hours to an upper limit of 5 days.

The clinical features are tiredness, slight pyrexia, malaise and a sore nose and pharynx. Profuse, watery nasal discharge, eventually becoming thick and mucopurulent, persists for up to a week. Sneezing is present in the early stage. Secondary bacterial infection occurs only in a minority.

Sinusitis (see p. 1158)

Rhinitis

Rhinitis is present if sneezing attacks, nasal discharge or blockage occur for more than an hour on most days for:

- a limited period of the year (seasonal rhinitis)
- throughout the whole year (perennial rhinitis).

Seasonal rhinitis

This is often called 'hayfever' and is the most common of all allergic diseases. It is better described as seasonal allergic rhinitis. World-wide prevalence rates vary from 2% to 20%. Prevalence is maximum in the second decade,

and up to 30% of young British people suffer symptoms in June and July.

Nasal irritation, sneezing and watery rhinorrhoea are the most troublesome symptoms, but many also suffer from itching of the eyes and soft palate and occasionally even itching of the ears because of the common innervation of the pharyngeal mucosa and the ear. In addition, approximately 20% suffer from seasonal attacks of asthma. The common seasonal allergens are shown in Figure 14.18. Since pollination of plants that give rise to high pollen counts varies from country to country, seasonal

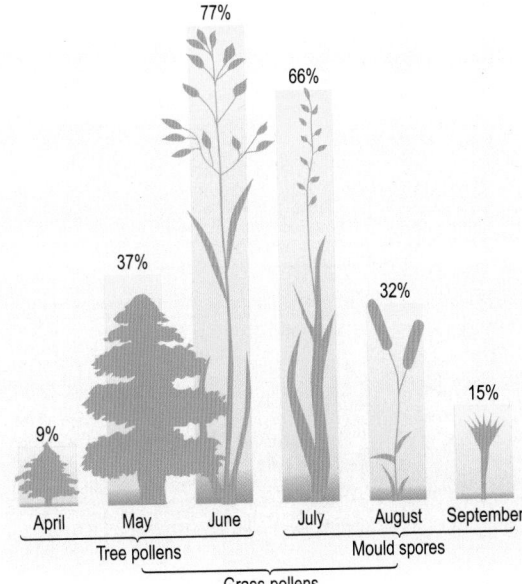

Fig. 14.18 Seasonal allergic rhinitis. Bar graph showing the proportion of patients whose symptoms are worst in the month or months indicated. The causative agents are also shown.

rhinitis and accompanying conjunctivitis and asthma may occur at different times of the year.

Perennial rhinitis

Patients with perennial rhinitis rarely have symptoms that affect the eyes or throat. Half have symptoms predominantly of sneezing and watery rhinorrhoea, whilst the other half complain mostly of nasal blockage. The patient may lose the sense of smell and taste. A swollen mucosa can obstruct drainage from the sinuses, causing sinusitis in half of the patients. Perennial rhinitis is most frequent in the second and third decades, decreasing with age, and can be divided into four main types.

Perennial allergic rhinitis

The major cause of this is allergy to the faecal particles of the house-dust mite *Dermatophagoides pteronyssinus* or *D. farinae*; these particles are approximately 20 μm in diameter (Fig. 14.19), not dissimilar in size to pollen grains. The house-dust mite itself is under 0.5 mm in size, invisible to the naked eye (Fig. 14.19), and is found in dust throughout the house, particularly in older, damp dwellings. It depends for nourishment on desquamated human skin scales and is found in abundance (4000 mites per gram of surface dust) in human bedding.

The next most common allergens come from domestic pets (especially cats) and are proteins derived from urine or saliva spread over the surface of the animal as well as skin protein. Allergy to urinary protein from small mammals is a major cause of morbidity amongst laboratory workers.

Industrial dust, vapours and fumes cause occupationally related perennial rhinitis more often than asthma.

The presence of perennial rhinitis makes the nose more reactive to non-specific stimuli such as cigarette smoke, washing powders, household detergents, strong perfumes and traffic fumes. Although patients often think they are allergic to these stimuli, these are irritant responses and do not involve allergic immune reactions.

Perennial non-allergic rhinitis with eosinophilia

No extrinsic allergic cause can be identified in these patients, either from the history or on skin testing; but, as in patients with perennial allergic rhinitis, eosinophilic granulocytes are present in nasal secretions. Aspirin and NSAID intolerance is found in this group.

Vasomotor rhinitis

These patients with perennial rhinitis have no demonstrable allergy or eosinophilia in nasal secretions. Watery secretions and nasal congestion are triggered by, for example, cold air, smoke, perfume, possibly because of an imbalance of the autonomic nervous system innervating the erectile tissue (sinusoids) in the nasal mucosa.

Nasal polyps

These are round, smooth, soft, semi-translucent, pale or yellow, glistening structures attached to the sinus mucosa by a relatively narrow stalk or pedicle, occurring in patients with both allergic and vasomotor rhinitis. They contain mast cells, eosinophils and mononuclear cells in large numbers and cause nasal obstruction, loss of smell and taste, and mouth breathing, but rarely sneezing, since the mucosa of the polyp is largely denervated. The mechanism(s) of their formation is not known.

Pathogenesis

Sneezing, increased secretion and changes in mucosal blood flow are mediated both by efferent nerve fibres and by released mediators (see p. 916). Mucus production results largely from parasympathetic stimulation, whilst blood vessels are under both sympathetic and parasympathetic control. Sympathetic fibres maintain tonic contraction of blood vessels, keeping the sinusoids of the nose partially constricted with good nasal patency. Stimulation of the parasympathetic system dilates these blood vessels. This stimulation varies spontaneously in a cyclical fashion so that air intake alternates slowly over several hours from one nostril to the other. The erectile cavernous nasal sinusoids can be influenced by emotion, which, in turn, can affect nasal patency.

Allergic rhinitis develops as a result of interaction between the inhaled allergen and adjacent molecules of IgE antibody present on the surface of mast cells found in increased numbers in nasal secretions and within the nasal epithelium. Release of preformed mediators, in particular histamine, causes an increase in permeability of the epithelium, allowing allergen to reach IgE-primed mast cells in the lamina propria. Sneezing, largely caused by histamine, results from stimulation of afferent nerve endings and begins within minutes of the allergen entering the nose. This is followed by nasal exudation and secretion and eventually nasal blockage at a maxi-

Fig. 14.19 Common allergens causing allergic rhinitis and asthma. The house-dust mite, faeces of house-dust mites, pollen grains, domestic pets and moulds. Percentages are those of positive skin-prick tests to these allergens in patients with allergic rhinitis.

Labels within figure:
House-dust mite and faeces (80%) — 500 μm — 20 μm
Pollen grains (70%) — 20 μm
Domestic pets (40%)
Moulds (20%) — 5 μm

mum of 15–20 minutes after contact with the allergen. The cysteinyl leukotrienes and vasodilator prostaglandins (PGD$_2$, PGE$_2$ and PGI$_2$) released from mast cells, eosinophils and macrophages are especially potent in causing nasal blockage.

Although the mast cell contains or can generate many other potent vasomotor and chemotactic factors (see Fig. 14.34), the exact role for each of these is unclear. It is likely that histamine plays a more significant role in the development of allergic rhinitis than of asthma, since the antihistamines are effective treatment for allergic rhinitis but are of little value in the everyday management of asthma. The increase in nasal response observed as the pollen season progresses is in part explained by a progressive increase in mast cells colonizing the mucosa. The mechanisms for recruitment of mast cells under these circumstances probably involve the release of stem cell factor (c-kit) and interleukin-3 from epithelial cells and interleukins -3, -4 and -9 from T cells.

Investigations and diagnosis

The allergic factors causing rhinitis are usually obtained from the history.

Skin-prick testing indicates that the mechanisms leading to allergic rhinitis (or asthma) are present in human skin. A positive test does not necessarily mean that the particular allergen producing the weal causes the respiratory disease. However, if there is a positive clinical history for that allergen, a causative role is likely. Specific serum IgE antibody against the particular allergen (RAST test) provides the same information as the skin-prick test. Blood tests are much more expensive and should be reserved for use in patients who cannot be skin tested for some reason (e.g. dermatographism, active eczema or using antihistamines and unable to stop for 3 days before skin tests).

Treatment

Allergen avoidance

Removal of a household pet or total enclosure of industrial processes releasing sensitizing agents can lead to cure of rhinitis and, indeed, asthma.

Pollen avoidance is impossible. Contact may be diminished by wearing sunglasses, driving with the car windows shut, avoiding walks in the countryside (particularly in the late afternoon when the number of pollen grains is highest at ground level), and keeping the bedroom window shut at night. These measures are rarely sufficient in themselves to control symptoms. Exposure to pollen is generally lower at the seaside, where sea breezes keep pollen grains inland.

The house-dust mite infests most areas of the house, but particularly the bedroom. Mite counts are extremely low in hospitals where carpets are absent, floors are cleaned frequently and mattresses and pillows are covered in plastic sheeting that can be wiped down. Mite allergen exposure can be reduced by enclosing bedding in fabric specifically designed to prevent the passage of mite allergen, while allowing water vapour through. This is both comfortable and reduces symptoms. Acaricides are less effective and cannot be recommended. Increased room ventilation and reduced soft furnishings including carpets, curtains and soft toys are all helpful in reducing the mite load.

Antihistamines

Antihistamines remain the most common therapy for rhinitis, and many can be purchased directly over the counter in the UK. They are particularly effective against sneezing, but are less effective against rhinorrhoea and have little influence on nasal blockage. The first-generation antihistamines cause sedation. Second-generation drugs such as cetirizine (10 mg once daily), loratadine (10 mg once daily), desloratadine (5 mg daily) and fexofenadine (120 mg daily) are highly specific for H$_1$ receptors; they do not cross the blood–brain barrier and are therefore not associated with sedation. Fatal cardiac arrhythmias (torsades de pointes) have been described with terfenadine and astemizole and these drugs should be replaced with those that do not influence the ECG QT interval. Antihistamines also control itching in the eyes and palate.

Decongestants

Drugs with sympathomimetic activity (α-adrenergic agents) are widely used for the treatment of nasal obstruction. They may be taken orally or more commonly as nasal drops or sprays (e.g. ephedrine nasal drops). Xylometazoline and oxymetazoline are widely used because they have a prolonged action and tachyphylaxis does not develop. Secondary nasal hyperaemia can occur some hours later as a rebound effect and rhinitis medicamentosa can develop if patients go on taking increasing quantities of the local decongestant to overcome this phenomenon. Although local decongestants are an effective treatment for vasomotor rhinitis, patients must be warned about rebound nasal obstruction and must use the drug carefully. Usually, such preparations should be prescribed for only a limited period to open the nasal airways for administration of other therapy, particularly topical corticosteroids.

Anti-inflammatory drugs

Sodium cromoglicate and nedocromil sodium influence a number of aspects of inflammation, including mast cell and eosinophil activation and nerve function. They act by blocking an intracellular chloride channel and preventing cell activation. Sodium cromoglicate applied topically in spray or powder form is of limited value in the treatment of allergic rhinitis, though along with nedocromil sodium, it is very effective in the management of allergic conjunctivitis.

Corticosteroids

The most effective treatment for rhinitis is to use small doses of topically administered corticosteroid preparations (e.g. beclometasone spray twice daily or fluticasone propionate spray once daily). The amount used is insufficient to cause systemic effects and the effect is primarily anti-inflammatory. Preparations should be started prior to the beginning of seasonal symptoms. The combination of a topical corticosteroid with a non-sedative antihistamine taken regularly is particularly effective. Special attention needs to be given to teaching patients how to use the aqueous dispensers or metered-dose inhalers to produce optimal drug deposition. It may be necessary to use an α-adrenergic agonist to decongest the nose prior to taking the topical corticosteroid.

If other therapy has failed, seasonal and perennial rhinitis respond readily to a short course (2 weeks) of treatment with oral prednisolone 5–10 mg daily. Nasal polyps respond well to such oral doses of corticosteroids and their recurrence may be prevented by continuous application of topical corticosteroids.

Pharyngitis

The most common viruses causing pharyngitis belong to the adenovirus group, which consists of about 32 serotypes. Endemic adenovirus infection causes the common sore throat, in which the oropharynx and soft palate are reddened and the tonsils are inflamed and swollen. Within 1–2 days the tonsillar lymph nodes enlarge. Occasionally, localized epidemics occur, particularly in schools in the summer-time, with episodes of fever, conjunctivitis, pharyngitis and lymphadenitis of the neck glands; these are due to adenovirus serotype 8. These diseases are self-limiting, and symptomatic treatment is all that is required.

In the past about one-third of sore throats were due to bacterial infections, e.g. haemolytic streptococcus, but this proportion appears to be falling. Persistent and severe tonsillitis requires antibiotic therapy. Phenoxymethylpenicillin (500 mg four times a day) or cefaclor (250 mg three times daily) can be used. Avoid amoxicillin and ampicillin if there is a possibility of infectious mononucleosis (p. 47).

Acute laryngotracheobronchitis

Acute laryngitis is an occasional but striking complication of upper respiratory tract infections, particularly those caused by viruses of the parainfluenza group and the measles virus. Inflammatory oedema extends to the vocal cords and the epiglottis, causing considerable narrowing of the airway; in addition, there may be associated tracheitis or tracheobronchitis. Children under the age of 3 years are most severely affected. The voice becomes hoarse, the cough assumes a barking quality (croup) and there is audible laryngeal stridor. Progressive airways obstruction may occur, with recession of the soft tissue of the neck and abdomen during inspiration, and in severe cases central cyanosis may occur. Inhalation of steam may be helpful; in severe cases endotracheal intubation may be necessary. Oxygen and adequate fluids should be given. Rarely, a tracheostomy may be required.

Acute epiglottitis

H. influenzae type b (Hib) can cause life-threatening infection of the epiglottis, a condition that is rare over the age of 5 years. The young child becomes extremely ill with a high fever, and severe airflow obstruction may rapidly occur. This is a life-threatening emergency and requires urgent endotracheal intubation and intravenous ceftazidime (25–150 mg/kg in children). Chloramphenicol (50–100 mg/kg in children) can also be used. The epiglottis, which is red and swollen, should not be inspected until facilities to maintain the airways are available.

Other manifestations of Hib infection are meningitis, septic arthritis and osteomyelitis. Immunization is achieved with a purified polyribosylribitol phosphate from the capsule of Hib linked to a non-toxic diphtheria toxin PRP-T to increase immunogenicity. It is highly effective when given to infants at 2, 3 and 4 months with primary immunization against diphtheria, tetanus and pertussis (DTP), reducing death rates from Hib infections virtually to zero.

After the advent of the Hib immunization there was an 88% reduction in notification in England and Wales but more recently the rate of infection has increased, for reasons that remain unclear.

Influenza (see also p. 55)

The influenza virus belongs to the orthomyxovirus group and exists in two main forms, A and B. Influenza B is associated with localized outbreaks of milder nature, whereas influenza A is the cause of world-wide pandemics. Influenza A has a capacity to develop new antigenic variants at irregular intervals. Human immunity develops against the haemagglutinin (H) antigen and the neuraminidase (N) antigen on the viral surface. Major shifts in the antigenic make-up of influenza A viruses provide the necessary conditions for major pandemics, whereas minor antigenic drifts give rise to less severe epidemics because immunity in the population is less blunted.

The most serious pandemic of influenza occurred in 1918, and was associated with more than 20 million deaths world-wide. In 1957, a major shift in the antigenic make-up of the virus led to the appearance of influenza A2 type H2N2, which caused a world-wide pandemic. A further pandemic occurred in 1968 owing to the emergence of Hong Kong influenza type H3N2, and minor antigenic drifts have caused outbreaks around the world ever since. In 1997, avian H5N1 strain of influenza A was found in humans and represented a major change in viral surface antigens. In South East Asia it has recently been transmited from poultry to man (avian influenza).

Clinical features

The incubation period of influenza is usually 1–3 days. The illness starts abruptly with a fever, shivering and generalized aching in the limbs. This is associated with severe headache, soreness of the throat and a persistent dry cough that can last for several weeks. Influenza viruses can cause a prolonged period of debility and depression that may take weeks or months to clear; this is known as the postviral syndrome.

Complications

Secondary bacterial infection, particularly with *Strep. pneumoniae* and *H. influenzae*, is common following influenza virus infection. Rarer, but more serious, is the development of pneumonia caused by *Staph. aureus*, which has a mortality of up to 20%. Postinfectious encephalo-myelitis rarely occurs after infection with influenza virus.

Diagnosis and treatment

Laboratory diagnosis is not usually necessary, but a definitive diagnosis can be established by demonstrating a fourfold increase in the complement-fixing antibody or the haemagglutinin antibody when measured before and after an interval of 1–2 weeks or demonstration of the virus in throat or nasal secretion.

Treatment is by bed rest and paracetamol, together with antibiotics for individuals who have chronic bronchitis, heart or renal disease.

The recent introduction of neuraminidase inhibitors may prove helpful in shortening the duration of symptoms in patients with influenza. The cost–benefit of zanamivir and oseltamivir remains unproven but these are currently recommended in the UK for patients with suspected influenza over the age of 65 and 'at-risk' adults, as part of a strategy to reduce admissions to hospital when influenza is circulating in the community.

Prophylaxis

Protection by influenza vaccines is only effective in up to 70% of people and is of short duration, usually lasting for only a year. Influenza vaccine should not be given to individuals who are allergic to egg protein as some are manufactured in chick embryos. New vaccines have to be prepared to cover each change in viral antigenicity and are therefore in limited supply at the start of an epidemic. Nevertheless, routine vaccination is recommended for all individuals over 65 years of age and also for younger people with chronic heart disease, chronic lung disease (including asthma), chronic renal failure, diabetes mellitus and those who are immunosuppressed. During pandemics key hospital and health service personnel should also be vaccinated.

Inhalation of foreign bodies

Children inhale foreign bodies, e.g. peanuts, more commonly than do adults. In the adult, inhalation often occurs after an excess of alcohol or under general anaesthesia (loose teeth or dentures).

When the foreign body is large it may impact in the trachea. The person chokes and then becomes silent; death occurs unless the material is quickly removed (see Emergency box 14.1).

Impaction usually occurs in the right main bronchus and produces:

- choking
- persistent monophonic wheeze
- later, persistent suppurative pneumonia
- lung abscess (common).

Emergency Box 14.1
Treatment of inhaled foreign bodies (Heimlich manoeuvre)

Emergency
The Heimlich manoeuvre is used to expel the obstructing object:

1. Stand behind the patient.
2. Encircle your arms around the upper part of the abdomen just below the patient's rib cage.
3. Give a sharp, forceful squeeze, forcing the diaphragm sharply into the thorax. This should expel sufficient air from the lungs to force the foreign body out of the trachea.

Non-emergency
Rigid bronchoscopy should be performed.

FURTHER READING

Couch RB (2000) Drug therapy: prevention and treatment of influenza. *New England Journal of Medicine* **343**: 1778–1787.

Gubareva LV, Hayden FG (2000) Influenza neuraminidase inhibitors. *Lancet* **355**: 827–835.

Heikkinen T, Jarvinen A (2003) The common cold. *Lancet* **361**: 51–59.

Nichol KL et al. (2003) Influenza vaccination and reduction in hospitalisation rates for cardiac disease and stroke among the elderly. *New England Journal of Medicine* **348**: 1322–1332.

Rijkers GT et al. (2003) Return of *Haemophilus influenzae* type b infection. *Lancet* **361**: 1563–1564.

DISEASES OF THE LOWER RESPIRATORY TRACT

Lower respiratory tract infection accounts for approximately 10% of the world-wide burden of morbidity and mortality. Seventy-five per cent of all antibiotic usage is for these diseases, despite the fact that they are mainly due to viruses.

Acute bronchitis

Acute bronchitis in previously healthy subjects is often viral. Bacterial infection with organisms such as *Strep. pneumoniae* and *H. influenzae* is a common sequel to viral infections, and is more likely to occur in individuals who are cigarette smokers and in those with chronic obstructive pulmonary disease (COPD).

The illness begins with an irritating, unproductive cough, together with discomfort behind the sternum. This may be associated with tightness in the chest, wheezing and shortness of breath. The cough becomes productive, the sputum being yellow or green. There is a mild fever and a neutrophil leucocytosis; wheeze with occasional crackles can be heard on auscultation. In otherwise healthy adults the disease improves spontaneously in 4–8 days without the patient becoming seriously ill.

Treatment with antibiotics is usually given (e.g. amoxicillin 250 mg three times daily), though it is not known whether this hastens recovery in otherwise healthy individuals.

Chronic obstructive pulmonary disease (COPD)

The global Initiative in Obstructive Lung Disease (GOLD) predicts that COPD will become the third most common cause of death and fifth most common cause of disability world-wide by 2020.

The term 'chronic obstructive pulmonary disease' (COPD) was introduced to bring together a variety of clinical syndromes associated with destruction of the lung and airflow obstruction. The terms 'chronic obstructive airways disease' (COAD) and 'chronic obstructive lung disease' (COLD) are used as synonyms in different parts of the world. Prior to 1979, patients with these conditions were often classified by symptoms (chronic bronchitis, chronic asthma), by pathological changes (emphysema) or by physiological correlates (pink puffers, blue bloaters). It was the recognition that these entities overlapped and often coexisted which led to the need for the new term COPD.

Definition of COPD

'COPD is a disease state characterized by airflow limitation that is not fully reversible. The airflow limitation is usually both progressive and associated with an abnormal inflammatory response of the lungs to noxious particles or gases' (GOLD).

Epidemiology and aetiology

COPD is caused by long-term exposure to toxic particles and gases. In developed countries, cigarette smoking accounts for over 90% of cases. In developing countries cigarette smoking, as well as the inhalation of smoke from biomass fuels used in heating and cooking in poorly ventilated areas, are causal factors. However, only 10–20% of heavy smokers develop COPD, indicating individual susceptibility. The development of COPD is also related to the number of cigarettes smoked per day; the risk of death from COPD in patients smoking 30 cigarettes daily is 20 times that of a non-smoker. The bronchitis mortality amongst male doctors in relation to the number of cigarettes smoked is shown in Figure 14.20. Autopsy studies have also shown that substantial numbers of centri-acinar emphysematous spaces are found in the lungs of 50% of British smokers over the age of 60 years and are unrelated to the diagnosis of significant respiratory disease before death.

Climate and air pollution are of less importance, but there is a great increase in mortality from COPD during periods of heavy atmospheric pollution (p. 894). The effect of urbanization, social class and occupation may also play a part in aetiology, but these effects are difficult to separate from that of smoking. Some animal studies suggest that diet could be a risk factor for COPD; but this has not been proven in humans.

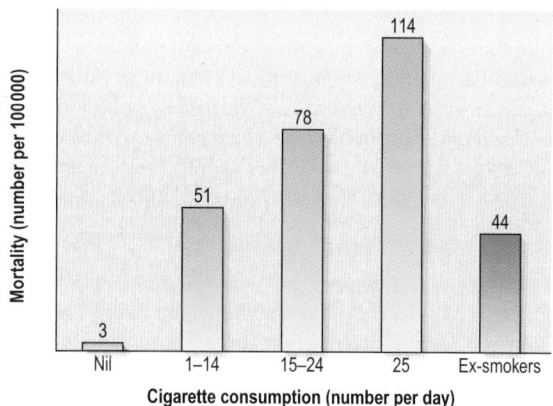

Fig. 14.20 Bronchitis death rates per 100 000 British male doctors according to their smoking habits. From Doll R, Peto R (1976) *British Medical Journal* **2**: 1525.

The socio-economic burden of COPD is considerable. In the UK, COPD causes approximately 18 million lost working days for men and 2.1 million lost working days for women per year, accounting for some 7% of all days of absence from work due to sickness. Nevertheless, the number of patients discharged from hospitals in the UK with this diagnosis has been falling steadily; the death rate has also fallen in the last 25 years from 200 to 70 per 100 000.

Pathophysiology

The most consistent pathological finding is hypertrophy and increase in number of the mucus-secreting goblet cells of the bronchial tree, evenly distributed throughout the lung but mainly seen in the larger bronchi (Fig. 14.21). In more advanced cases, the bronchi themselves are obviously inflamed and pus is seen in the lumen. Microscopically there is infiltration of the walls of the bronchi

Fig. 14.21 COPD. Section of bronchial mucosa stained for mucus glands by PAS showing increase in mucus-secreting goblet cells (courtesy of Dr J Wilson and Dr S Wilson, University of Southampton).

and bronchioles with acute and chronic inflammatory cells and lymphoid follicles in severe disease. In contrast to asthma, the lymphocytic infiltrate is predominantly $CD8^+$. The epithelial layer may become ulcerated and, when the ulcers heal, squamous epithelium may replace the columnar cells. The inflammation is followed by scarring and a remodelling process that thickens the walls and leads to widespread narrowing in the small airways (Fig. 14.22).

The small airways are particularly affected early in the disease, initially without the development of any significant breathlessness. This initial inflammation of the small airways is reversible and accounts for the improvement in airway function if smoking is stopped early. In later stages the inflammation continues, even if smoking is stopped.

Further progression of the disease leads to progressive squamous cell metaplasia, and fibrosis of the bronchial walls. The physiological consequence of these changes is the development of airflow limitation. If the airway narrowing is combined with emphysema (causing loss of the elastic recoil of the lung with collapse of small airways during aspiration) the resulting airflow limitation is even more severe.

Emphysema is defined pathologically as dilatation and destruction of the lung tissue distal to the terminal bronchiole. It is classified according to the site of damage:

- *Centri-acinar emphysema.* Distension and damage of lung tissue is concentrated around the respiratory bronchioles, whilst the more distal alveolar ducts and alveoli tend to be well preserved. This form of emphysema is extremely common; when of modest extent, it is not necessarily associated with disability. Severe centri-acinar emphysema is associated with substantial airflow limitation.
- *Pan-acinar emphysema.* This is less common. Distension and destruction appear to involve the whole of the

acinus, and in the extreme form the lung becomes a mass of bullae. Severe airflow limitation and $\dot{V}_A/\dot{Q}$ mismatch occur. This type of emphysema occurs in α_1-antitrypsin deficiency (see p. 902).
- *Irregular emphysema.* There is scarring and damage affecting the lung parenchyma patchily without particular regard for acinar structure.

Emphysema leads to expiratory airflow limitation and air trapping. The loss of lung elastic recoil results in an increase in TLC while the loss of alveoli with emphysema results in decreased gas transfer.

$\dot{V}_A/\dot{Q}$ mismatch occurs partly because of damage and mucus plugging of smaller airways from chronic inflammation, and partly because of the rapid expiratory closure of the smaller airways owing to loss of elastic recoil from emphysema. This leads to a fall in P_aO_2 and an increase in the work of respiration.

CO_2 excretion is not impaired to the same extent and indeed many patients will show low normal P_aCO_2 values. These patients are the 'pink puffers' who seek to maintain normal blood gases by increasing their respiratory effort. Other patients fail to maintain their respiratory effort and as a consequence their carbon dioxide levels increase. In the short term, the rise in CO_2 leads to stimulation of respiration but in the long term, these patients often become insensitive to CO_2 and come to depend on hypoxaemia to drive their ventilation. These patients appear less breathless and because they run low P_aO_2 values, they start to retain fluid and stimulate the production of erythrocytes (polycythaemia). In consequence they become bloated, plethoric and cyanosed, the typical appearance of the 'blue bloater'. Attempts to abolish hypoxaemia by administering oxygen can make the situation much worse by decreasing respiratory drive in these patients who rely on hypoxia to drive their ventilation.

Carbon dioxide is normally the major stimulant of the respiratory centre. In the face of a prolonged high P_aCO_2 this sensitivity is diminished and hypoxaemia becomes the chief drive to respiration. In this situation an attempt to abolish hypoxaemia by administration of oxygen can result in an increase in P_aCO_2 by decreasing the respiratory drive, worsening respiratory failure.

The classic Fletcher and Peto studies (Fig. 14.23) show that there is a loss of 50 mL per year in FEV_1 in COPD compared to 20 mL per year in healthy people.

In summary, three mechanisms have been suggested for this limitation of airflow in small airways (< 2 mm in diameter).

- Loss of elasticity and alveolar attachments of airways due to emphysema. This reduces the elastic recoil and the airways collapse during expiration.
- Inflammation and scarring cause the small airways to narrow.
- Mucus secretion which blocks the airways.

These all cause narrowing of the small airways and trapping of air leading to hyperinflation of the lungs and breathlessness.

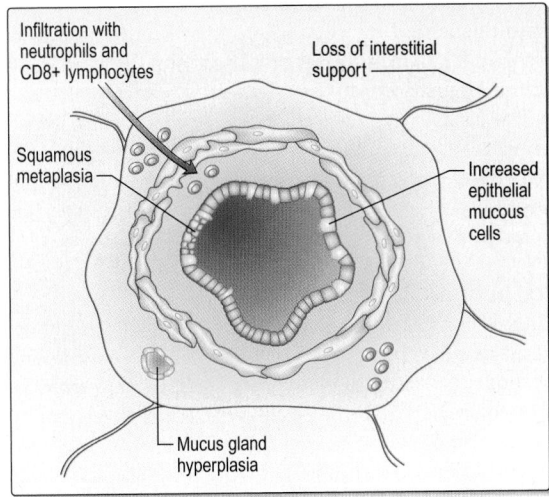

Fig. 14.22 **Pathological changes in the airways in chronic bronchitis and emphysema.**

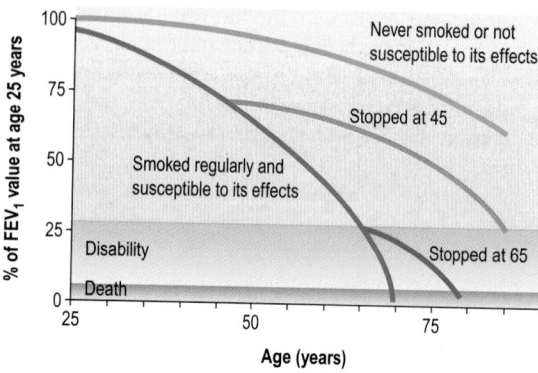

Fig. 14.23 **Influence of smoking on airflow limitation.** From Fletcher CM, Peto R (1977) *British Medical Journal* **1**: 1645.

Pathogenesis

Cigarette smoking

Bronchoalveolar washes have shown that smokers have neutrophil granulocytes present within the lumen of the bronchial tree that are absent in non-smokers. Additionally, the small airways of smokers are infiltrated by granulocytes. These granulocytes are capable of releasing elastases and proteases, which possibly help to produce emphysema. It is suggested that an imbalance between protease and antiprotease activity may produce the damage. α_1-Antitrypsin is a major serum antiprotease which can be inactivated by cigarette smoke (see below).

The hypertrophy of mucous glands in the larger airways is thought to be a direct response to persistent irritation resulting from the inhalation of cigarette smoke. The smoke has an adverse effect on surfactant, favouring overdistension of the lungs.

Infections

Patients with COPD cope badly with respiratory infections, which are often the precipitating cause of acute exacerbations of the disease. However, the role of infection in the development of the progressive airflow limitation that characterizes disabling COPD is far less clear. Prompt use of antibiotics and routine influenza vaccinations are appropriate.

α_1-Antitrypsin deficiency (see also p. 388)

α_1-Antitrypsin inhibitor is an antiproteinase inhibitor produced in the liver, secreted into the blood and which diffuses into the lung. Here it functions as an antiprotease that inhibits neutrophil elastase, a proteolytic enzyme capable of destroying alveolar wall connective tissue.

More than 75 alleles of the α_1-antitrypsin inhibitor gene have been described. The three main phenotypes are MM (normal), MZ (heterozygous deficiency) and ZZ (homozygous deficiency). About 1 child in 5000 in Britain is born with the homozygous deficiency, but not all develop chest disease. Those who do develop breathlessness under the age of 40 years have radiographic evidence of basal emphysema and are usually, but not always, cigarette smokers. Hereditary deficiency of α_1-

antitrypsin inhibitor accounts for about 2% of emphysema cases. A small minority develop liver disease (see p. 388).

Clinical features

Symptoms

The characteristic symptoms of COPD are cough with the production of sputum, wheeze and breathlessness following many years of a smoker's cough. Colds seem to 'go down to the chest' and frequent infective exacerbations occur, giving purulent sputum. Symptoms can be worsened by factors such as cold, foggy weather and atmospheric pollution. With advanced disease, breathlessness becomes severe even after mild exercise such as dressing.

Signs

In mild disease there are no signs apart from 'wheeze' throughout the chest. In severe disease, the patient is tachypnoeic, with prolonged expiration. The accessory muscles of respiration are used and there may be intercostal indrawing on inspiration and pursing of the lips on expiration (see p. 878). Chest expansion is poor, the lungs are hyperinflated, and there is loss of the normal cardiac and liver dullness.

Patients who remain responsive to CO_2 are usually breathless and rarely cyanosed. Heart failure and oedema are rare features except as terminal events. Patients who become insensitive to CO_2 are often oedematous and cyanosed but not particularly breathless. Those with hypercapnia may have peripheral vasodilatation, a bounding pulse, and when the P_aCO_2 is above about 10 kPa, a coarse flapping tremor of the outstretched hands. Severe hypercapnia will lead to confusion and progressive drowsiness. At this stage papilloedema may be present but is neither specific nor sensitive as a diagnostic feature.

Complications

Respiratory failure

The later stages of COPD are characterized by the development of respiratory failure. For practical purposes this is said to occur when there is either a P_aO_2 of less than 8 kPa (60 mmHg) or a P_aCO_2 of more than 7 kPa (55 mmHg) (see Ch. 15).

The persistence of chronic alveolar hypoxia and hypercapnia leads to constriction of the pulmonary arterioles and subsequent pulmonary arterial hypertension. Cardiac output is normal or increased but salt and fluid retention occurs as a result of renal hypoxia.

Cor pulmonale

Patients with advanced COPD may develop cor pulmonale (see p. 843), which is defined as heart disease secondary to disease of the lung. It is characterized by pulmonary hypertension, right ventricular hypertrophy, and eventually right heart failure. On examination, the patient is centrally cyanosed (owing to the lung disease) and, when heart failure develops, the patient becomes more breathless and ankle oedema occurs. Initially a prominent parasternal heave may be felt that is due to

Table 14.9 COPD – Global Initiative in Obstructive Lung Disease (GOLD) criteria

Stage of COPD		FEV$_1$ (%)	Symptoms
0	At risk	≥ 80	None
I	Mild	≥ 80	± Variable
II	Moderate	50–79	+ Mild to moderate
III	Severe	30–49	++ Limit exertion
IV	Very severe	< 30	+++ Limit daily activities

After Fabbri LM, Hurd SS (2003 update) Global strategy for the diagnosis, management and prevention of COPD. *European Respiratory Journal* **22**: 1–2

right ventricular hypertrophy and a loud pulmonary second sound may be heard. In very severe pulmonary hypertension there is incompetence of the pulmonary valve. With right heart failure, tricuspid incompetence may develop with a greatly elevated jugular venous pressure (JVP), ascites and upper abdominal discomfort owing to swelling of the liver.

Diagnosis

This is usually clinical (GOLD criteria, Table 14.9). There is a history of breathlessness and sputum production in a lifetime smoker. In the absence of a history of cigarette smoking a working diagnosis of asthma is usual unless there is a family history of lung disease suggestive of a deficiency of α$_1$-antitrypsin inhibitor.

The patient may have signs of hyperinflation and typical pursed lip respiration. No individual clinical feature is diagnostic. Emphysema is often incorrectly diagnosed on signs of overinflation of the lungs (e.g. loss of liver dullness on percussion), but this may occur with other diseases such as asthma. Furthermore, centri-acinar emphysema may be present without signs of over-inflation. Some elderly men (without emphysema) develop a barrel-shaped chest as a result of osteoporosis of the spine, and a consequent decrease in height.

Investigations

- **Lung function tests** show evidence of airflow limitation (see Figs 14.8 and 14.15). The ratio of the FEV$_1$ to the FVC is reduced and the PEFR is low. In many patients the airflow limitation is reversible to some extent (usually a change in FEV$_1$ of < 15%), and the distinction between asthma and COPD can be difficult. Lung volumes may be normal or increased, and the gas transfer coefficient of carbon monoxide is low when significant emphysema is present.
- **Chest X-ray** is often normal, even when the disease is advanced. The classic features are the presence of bullae, severe overinflation of the lungs with low, flattened diaphragms, and a large retrosternal air space on the lateral film. There may also be a deficiency of blood vessels in the periphery of the lung fields compared with relatively easily visible proximal vessels.
- **Haemoglobin level and PCV** can be elevated as a result of persistent hypoxaemia (secondary polycythaemia, see p. 454).

- **Blood gases** are often normal. In the advanced case there is evidence of hypoxaemia and hypercapnia.
- **Sputum examination** is unnecessary in the ordinary case as *Strep. pneumoniae* or *H. influenzae* are the only common organisms to produce acute exacerbations. Occasionally *Moraxella catarrhalis* may cause infective exacerbations.
- **Electrocardiogram**. In advanced cor pulmonale the P wave is taller (P pulmonale) and there may be right bundle branch block (RSR' complex) and the changes of right ventricular hypertrophy (see p. 845).
- **Echocardiogram** – performed to assess cardiac function.
- **α$_1$-Antitrypsin levels**. The normal range is 2–4 g/L.

Management (Fig. 14.24)

Smoking cessation

Persuading the patient to stop smoking is vital. Even at a late stage of the disease this may slow down the rate of deterioration and prolong the time before disability and death occur (see Fig. 14.23).

Drug therapy

This is used both for the short-term management of exacerbations and for the long-term relief of symptoms. In many cases the drugs used are similar to those used in asthma (see p. 919).

Bronchodilators

Many patients feel less breathless following the inhalation of a β-adrenergic agonist such as salbutamol (200 μg every 4–6 hours). More prolonged and greater bronchodilatation is achieved with antimuscarinic agents: tiotropium (18 μg daily), ipratropium (40 μg four times daily) or oxitropium (200 μg twice daily). Patients find inhalers difficult to use and spacer devices improve delivery. Objective evidence of improvement in the peak flow or FEV$_1$ may be small and decisions to continue or stop therapy should be based on the patient's reported symptoms. Long-acting preparations of theophylline are of little benefit.

Corticosteroids

In symptomatic patients with COPD, a trial of corticosteroids is always indicated, since a proportion of patients have a large, unsuspected, reversible element to their disease and airway function may improve considerably. Prednisolone 30 mg daily should be given for 2 weeks, with measurements of lung function before and after the treatment period. If there is objective evidence of a substantial degree of improvement in airflow limitation (FEV$_1$ increase > 15%), prednisolone should be discontinued and replaced by inhaled corticosteroids (beclometasone 400 μg twice daily in the first instance, adjusted according to response). The long-term value of regular inhaled corticosteroids in all patients with COPD has not been proven.

Antibiotics

Prompt antibiotic treatment shortens exacerbations and should always be given in acute episodes as it may

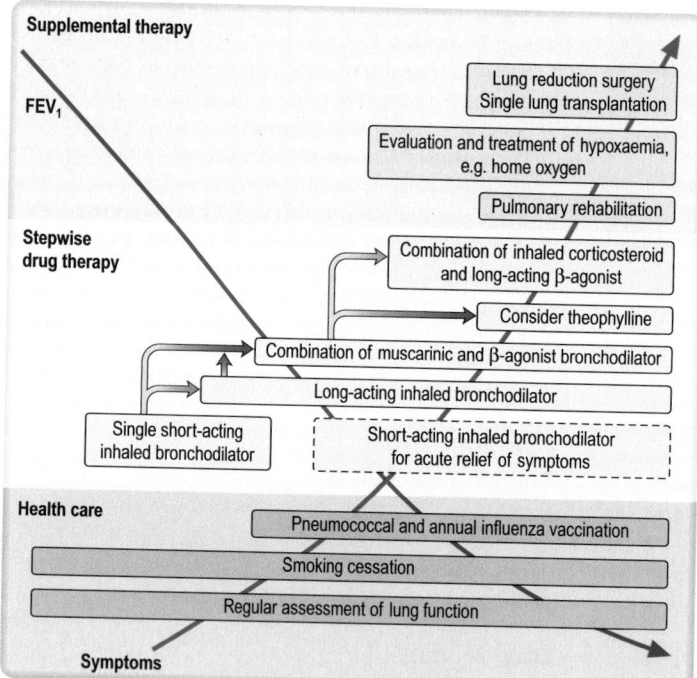

prevent hospital admission and further lung damage. Patients can be given a supply of antibiotics to keep at home to start as soon as their sputum turns yellow or green. Although amoxicillin-resistant *H. influenzae* is increasing (occurring in 10–20% of isolates from sputum) it is not a serious clinical problem. Resistance to cefaclor 500 mg 8-hourly or cefixime 400 mg once daily is significantly less frequent; co-amoxiclav is a useful alternative.

Long-term treatment with antibiotics remains controversial. They were once thought to be of no value, but eradication of infection and keeping the lower respiratory tract free of bacteria may help to prevent deterioration in lung function.

Diuretic therapy (see p. 697)
This is necessary for all oedematous patients. Daily weights should be recorded during acute inpatient episodes.

α_1-Antitrypsin replacement
Weekly or monthly infusions of α_1-antitrypsin have been recommended for patients with serum levels of this compound below 310 mg/L and abnormal lung function. Whether this modifies the long-term progression of the disease has still to be determined.

Vaccines
Patients with COPD should receive yearly influenza vaccine. These patients should also receive one dose of the polyvalent pneumococcal polysaccharide vaccine (a single dose usually provides lifelong immunity).

Other measures
- *Heart failure* should be treated (p. 790).

- *Secondary polycythaemia* – venesection is recommended if the PCV is > 55%.
- *Air travel.* Commercial cabin pressures are equivalent to an altitude of 2750 m. At this level the P_aO_2 will fall from 13.5 to 10 kPa with a fall of 3% in oxygen saturation. This has no effect on healthy travellers but in patients with moderate COPD, a fall in P_aO_2 to below 6.5 kPa can occur and oxygen is necessary. Intended travellers with moderate or severe COPD (Table 14.9) should get medical advice and contact the airline.

Treatment of respiratory failure
There are many causes of respiratory failure (Fig. 14.25) but COPD is by far the most common. The primary aim of the management of respiratory failure is to improve the P_aO_2 by continuous oxygen therapy. In type I respiratory failure (low P_aO_2, normal P_aCO_2) it is safe to administer as much oxygen as is required to return the P_aO_2 to normal. In type II respiratory failure the P_aCO_2 is elevated and giving additional oxygen will nearly always lead to a rise in the P_aCO_2 (see p. 981). Small increases in P_aCO_2 can be tolerated but not if the pH falls dramatically. The pH should not be allowed to fall below 7.25; under such circumstances, increased ventilation must be achieved either by the use of a respiratory stimulant or by artificial ventilation.

Figure 14.26 shows a fixed-performance mask (Venturi mask) for the administration of oxygen. This style of mask is used to deliver low concentrations of oxygen. It should be compared with the variable-performance face mask (see Fig. 15.22).

Initially, 24% oxygen is given, which is only slightly greater than the concentration of oxygen in air. However, because of the shape of the oxygen–haemoglobin dis-

Common	Rare
Chronic obstructive pulmonary disease	Severe asthma Postoperative Diminished chest wall movements Neuromuscular diseases Primary alveolar hypoventilation Obesity

Fig. 14.25 **Algorithm for the treatment of respiratory failure.** LVF, left ventricular failure; CPAP, continuous positive airway pressure; BiPAP, bilevel positive airway pressure.

Fig. 14.26 **'Fixed-performance' device for administration of oxygen to spontaneously breathing patients (Venturi mask).** Oxygen is delivered through the injector of the Venturi mask at a given flow rate. A fixed amount of air is entrapped and the inspired oxygen can be predicted accurately. Masks are available to deliver 24%, 28% and 35% oxygen.

sociation curve (see Fig. 15.5), this small increase in oxygen is valuable. The concentration of inspired oxygen can be gradually increased if the P_aCO_2 does not rise unacceptably.

Additional measures

- *Removal of retained secretions.* The patient should be encouraged to cough to remove secretions. Physiotherapy is helpful. If this fails, bronchoscopy and/or aspiration via an endotracheal tube may be necessary. A tracheostomy is only rarely required.
- *Respiratory support* (see p. 981). Non-invasive ventilatory techniques can be very helpful in avoiding the need for endotracheal intubation. The best current technique uses tight-fitting facial masks to deliver bilevel positive airway pressure ventilatory support (BiPAP). Assisted ventilation with an endotracheal tube is occasionally used for patients with COPD with severe respiratory failure when there is a definite precipitating factor and the overall prognosis is reasonable. Assessing the relative reversibility in an acute setting can present a difficult ethical problem.
- *Respiratory stimulants.* The use of respiratory stimulants has declined in recent years, largely because of the increasing availability of respiratory support services. Doxapram, 1.5–4.0 mg/min by slow i.v. infusion, may help in the short term to arouse the patient and to stimulate coughing, with clearance of some secretions.
- *Corticosteroids, antibiotics and bronchodilators* should be administered in the acute phase and then reassessed once the patient has recovered (see above).

Further management at home
Oxygen

Two controlled trials (chiefly in males) have indicated that life can be prolonged by the continuous administration of oxygen at 2 L/min via nasal prongs to achieve an oxygen saturation of greater than 90% for large proportions of the day and night. Survival curves from these two studies are shown in Figure 14.27.

Only 30% of those not receiving long-term oxygen therapy survived for more than 5 years. A fall in pulmonary artery pressure was achieved if oxygen was given for 15 hours daily, but substantial improvement in mortality was only achieved by the administration of oxygen for 19 hours daily. These results suggest that long-term continuous domiciliary oxygen therapy will benefit patients who have:

- A P_aO_2 of < 7.3 kPa (55 mmHg) when breathing air. Measurements should be taken on two occasions at least 3 weeks apart after appropriate bronchodilator therapy (Box 14.1).
- A P_aO_2 7.3–8 kPa with secondary polycythaemia, nocturnal hypoxaemia, peripheral oedema or evidence of pulmonary hypertension.
- Carboxyhaemoglobin of less than 3% (i.e. patients who have stopped smoking).

The provision of 19 hours of oxygen daily at a flow rate of 1–3 L/min using a 28% oxygen mask is best achieved using an oxygen concentrator. To achieve this with

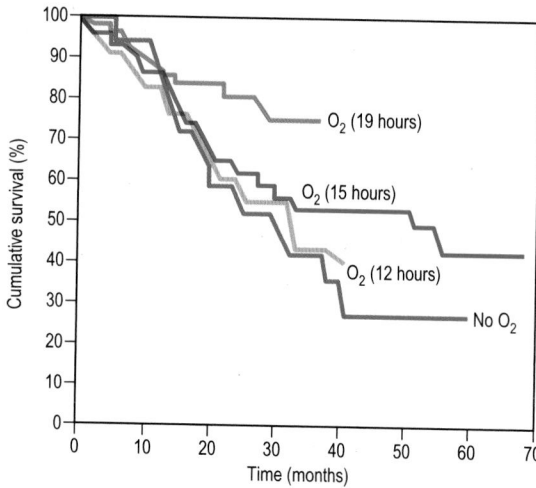

Fig. 14.27 **Cumulative survival curves for patients receiving oxygen.** Oxygen doses are in hours per day.

> **Box 14.1 Guidelines for domiciliary oxygen (Royal College of Physicians, 1999)**
>
> - Chronic obstructive pulmonary disease with P_aO_2 < 7.3 kPa when breathing air during a period of clinical stability.
> - Chronic obstructive pulmonary disease with P_aO_2 7.3–8 kPa in the presence of secondary polycythaemia, nocturnal hypoxaemia, peripheral oedema or evidence of pulmonary hypertension.
> - Diffuse lung disease with P_aO_2 < 8 kPa and in patients with P_aO_2 > 8 kPa with disabling dyspnoea.
> - Cystic fibrosis when P_aO_2 < 7.3 kPa or if P_aO_2 7.3–8 kPa in the presence of secondary polycythaemia, nocturnal hypoxaemia, pulmonary hypertension or peripheral oedema.
> - Pulmonary hypertension without parenchymal lung involvement when P_aO_2 < 8 kPa.
> - Neuromuscular or skeletal disorders, after specialist assessment.
> - Obstructive sleep apnoea despite continuous positive airways pressure therapy, after specialist assessment.
> - Pulmonary malignancy or other terminal disease with disabling dyspnoea.
> - Heart failure with daytime P_aO_2 < 7.3 kPa (on air) or with nocturnal hypoxaemia.

oxygen cylinders would require 20 standard cylinders per week, which is unacceptably expensive. Oxygen concentrators are available through the UK National Health Service for patients who fulfil the above criteria.

Drugs

Pulmonary hypertension can be partially relieved by the use of oral β-adrenergic stimulants such as salbutamol (4 mg three times daily), but whether this is useful in the long term is unknown.

The sensation of breathlessness can be reduced by the use of either promethazine 125 mg daily or dihydrocodeine 1 mg/kg by mouth. Reduced breathlessness and increased exercise tolerance also result from the combined administration of dihydrocodeine and oxygen

delivered from a portable cylinder. Although opiates are the most effective treatment for intractable breathlessness they depress ventilation and carry risk of increasing respiratory failure.

Surgery

Some patients with large emphysematous bullae (which reduce lung capacity) can benefit from bullectomy, enabling adjacent areas of collapsed lung to re-expand and function again. In addition, carefully selected patients with severe COPD (FEV_1 < 1 L), have been offered *lung volume reduction surgery*. This surgery increases elastic recoil, which reduces the expiratory collapse of the airway and decreases expiratory airflow limitation. It also enables the diaphragm to work at a better advantage. Initial studies suggested that ventilation was improved and patients felt less breathless, but mortality was unchanged. A recent controlled trial in severe emphysema, however, showed an increased mortality and no improvement in patients' condition.

Single lung transplantation (see p. 911) is used for end-stage emphysema, with 3-year survival rates of 75%. The principal benefit is to improve quality of life but it does not statistically improve survival.

Pulmonary rehabilitation

A modest increase in exercise capacity with diminution in the sense of breathlessness and improved general well-being can result from exercise training. Regular training periods can be instituted at home; climbing stairs or walking fixed distances can be combined with regular clinic visits for encouragement. Breathing exercises are probably of less value. Quality of life can be improved by a multidisciplinary approach involving physiotherapy, exercise and education, although this does not alter life expectancy or the rate of decline in lung function.

Prognosis

In general, 50% of patients with severe breathlessness die within 5 years (Fig. 14.27), but even in the severe group, stopping smoking will improve the prognosis.

Nocturnal hypoxia

COPD patients with severe arterial hypoxaemia also suffer from profound nocturnal hypoxaemia which may drop the P_aO_2 as low as 2.5 kPa (19 mmHg), particularly during the rapid eye movement (REM) phase of sleep.

Because patients with COPD are already hypoxic, the fall in P_aO_2 produces a much larger fall in oxygen saturation (owing to the steepness of the oxygen– haemoglobin dissociation curve) and desaturation of up to 50% occurs. The mechanism is alveolar hypoventilation due to:

- inhibition of intercostal and accessory muscles in REM sleep
- shallow breathing in REM sleep, which reduces ventilation, particularly in severe COPD
- an increase in upper airway resistance because of a reduction in muscle tone.

These nocturnal hypoxaemic episodes are associated with a further rise in pulmonary arterial pressure owing to vasoconstriction, and the majority of deaths in patients with COPD occur during the night, possibly from cardiac arrhythmias. These patients additionally show severe secondary polycythaemia, partly as a result of the severe nocturnal hypoxaemia.

Each episode of desaturation is usually terminated by arousal from sleep, so that normal sleep is reduced and the patient suffers from daytime sleepiness.

Treatment

Patients with arterial hypoxaemia should not be given sleeping tablets, which will further depress respiratory drive. Treatment is with nocturnal administration of oxygen and ventilatory support.

Positive-pressure ventilation can be administered non-invasively through a tightly fitting nasal mask with bilevel positive airway pressure – inspiratory to provide inspiratory assistance and expiratory to prevent alveolar closure, each adjusted independently. Although these devices to maintain adequate ventilation during sleep and to allow respiratory muscles to rest at night are effective in chronic chest wall disease (e.g. kyphoscoliosis) or neuromuscular disease (e.g. previous poliomyelitis), they do not improve respiratory function, respiratory muscle strength, exercise tolerance or breathlessness in patients with COPD.

Obstructive sleep apnoea

This condition occurs most often in overweight middle-aged men and affects 1–2% of the population. It can occur in children, particularly those with enlarged tonsils. The major symptoms and their frequency are listed in Table 14.10. During sleep, activity of the respiratory muscles is reduced, especially during REM sleep when the diaphragm is virtually the only active muscle. Apnoeas occur when the airway at the back of the throat is sucked closed when breathing in during sleep. When awake this tendency is overcome by the action of opening muscles of the upper airway, the genioglossus and palatal muscles, which become hypotonic during sleep (Fig. 14.28). Partial narrowing results in snoring, occlusion in apnoea and critical narrowing in hypopnoeas. Apnoea leads to hypoxia and increasingly strenuous respiratory efforts until the patient overcomes the resistance. The combination of the effort and the central hypoxic stimulation wakes the patient from sleep. These awakenings are so brief that the patient remains unaware of them but may be woken hundreds of times per night leading to sleep deprivation, especially a reduction in REM sleep,

Fig. 14.28 **Section through head, showing pressure changes (in kPa) in (a) the normal situation and (b) obstructive sleep apnoea.** There is a pressure drop during inspiration as air is sucked through the turbinates. In patients with obstructive sleep apnoea this is sufficient to collapse the pharynx, obstructing inspiration.

with consequent daytime sleepiness and impaired intellectual performance. Contributory factors are obesity, a small pharyngeal opening and coexistent COPD.

Correctable factors occur in about one-third of cases and include:

- encroachment on pharynx – obesity, acromegaly, enlarged tonsils
- nasal obstruction – nasal deformities, rhinitis, polyps, adenoids
- respiratory depressant drugs – alcohol, sedatives, strong analgesics.

Diagnosis

In many cases this can be made on the combination of a good history of the snore–silence–snore cycle reported by the patient's relatives. The Epworth Sleepiness Scale (Table 20.5) helps discriminate apnoea from simple snoring. This can be supported by non-invasive ear or finger oximetry performed at home. Characteristically, arterial oxygen saturation will fall significantly in a cyclical manner. If the oximetry is negative or equivocal, inpatient assessment is indicated, preferably in a room specifically adapted for sleep studies rather than a normal ward side-room. Oximetry is supplemented by video recording. Full polysomnographic studies are rarely necessary for clinical diagnosis but are useful in research labs. These involve oximetry, direct measurements of thoracic and abdominal movement to assess breathing, and electroencephalography to record patterns of sleep and arousal. Some centres also measure oronasal airflow.

The diagnosis of sleep apnoea/hypopnoea is confirmed if there are more than 15 apnoeas or hypopnoeas in any 1 hour of sleep. There is, however, overlap with central sleep apnoea (see p. 1227).

Management

Management consists of correction of treatable factors (see above) with, if necessary, nasal continuous positive

Table 14.10 Symptoms of obstructive sleep apnoea	
Loud snoring (95%)	Nocturnal choking (30%)
Daytime sleepiness (90%)	Reduced libido (20%)
Unrefreshed sleep (40%)	Morning drunkenness (5%)
Restless sleep (40%)	Ankle swelling (5%)
Morning headache (30%)	

airway pressure (CPAP) delivered by a nasal mask during sleep. Such systems raise the pressure in the pharynx by about 1 kPa, keeping the walls apart. CPAP results in improvement of symptoms, quality of life, daytime alertness and survival. Up to 50%, however, cannot tolerate CPAP. Modafinil (a CNS stimulant) is useful in the short term.

Bronchiectasis

The term 'bronchiectasis' is used to describe abnormal and permanently dilated airways. Bronchial walls become inflamed, thickened and irreversibly damaged. The mucociliary transport mechanism is impaired and frequent bacterial infections ensue. Clinically, the disease is characterized by cough production of large amounts of sputum and dilated and thickened bronchi, detected on CT scanning of the thorax.

Aetiology

The causes are shown in Table 14.11. Cystic fibrosis is the most common cause in developed countries.

Clinical features

Patients with mild bronchiectasis only produce yellow or green sputum after an infection. Localized areas of the lung may be particularly affected, when sputum production will depend on position. As the condition worsens, the patient suffers from persistent halitosis, recurrent febrile episodes with malaise, and episodes of pneumonia. Clubbing occurs, and coarse crackles can be heard over the infected areas, usually the bases of the lungs. When the condition is severe there is continuous

Fig. 14.29 CT scan showing bronchiectasis in the right middle lobe. Note dilated bronchi with thickened wall and adjacent artery giving a signet ring appearance.

production of foul-smelling, thick, khaki-coloured sputum. Haemoptysis can occur either as blood-stained sputum or as a massive haemorrhage. Breathlessness may result from airflow limitation.

Investigations

- **Chest X-ray** may be normal or may show dilated bronchi with thickened bronchial walls and sometimes multiple cysts containing fluid.
- **High-resolution CT scanning** (see p. 887) shows bronchial dilatation and wall thickening (Fig. 14.29) with a sensitivity of 97%.
- **Sputum** examination with culture and sensitivity of the organisms is essential for adequate treatment. The major pathogens are *Staph. aureus*, *Pseudomonas aeruginosa*, *H. influenzae* and anaerobes. Other pathogens include *Strep. pneumoniae* and *Klebsiella pneumoniae*. *Aspergillus fumigatus* can be isolated from 10% of sputum specimens in cystic fibrosis, but the role of this organism is uncertain.
- **Sinus X-rays**. Thirty per cent have concomitant purulent rhinosinusitis.
- **Serum immunoglobulins**. Ten per cent of adults have immune deficiency.
- **Sweat electrolytes** – if appropriate (see p. 910).
- **Mucociliary clearance** (nasal clearance of saccharin). A 1 mm cube of saccharin is placed on the inferior turbinate and the time to taste measured (normally less than 30 minutes).

Treatment

Postural drainage

Postural drainage is essential and patients must be trained by physiotherapists to tip themselves into a position in which the lobe to be drained is uppermost at least three times daily for 10–20 minutes. Most patients find that lying over the side of the bed with head and thorax down is the most effective position.

Antibiotics

Experience from the treatment of cystic fibrosis suggests that bronchopulmonary infections need to be eradicated

Table 14.11	Causes of bronchiectasis

Congenital
Deficiency of bronchial
  wall elements
Pulmonary sequestration
	Immunological over-
	response
	Allergic bronchopulmonary
	  aspergillosis
	Post-lung transplant

Mechanical bronchial
obstruction
Intrinsic
Foreign body
Inspissated mucus
Post-tuberculous stenosis
Tumour
	Immune deficiency
	Primary
	Panhypogamma-
	  globulinaemia
	Selective immunoglobulin
	  deficiencies (IgA and IgG$_2$)

Extrinsic Lymph node Tumour	*Secondary* HIV and malignancy

Postinfective bronchial
damage
Bacterial and viral
  pneumonia, including
  pertussis, measles and
  aspiration pneumonia
	Mucociliary clearance
	defects
	Genetic
	Primary ciliary dyskinesia
	  (Kartagener's syndrome
	  with dextrocardia and
	  situs inversus)
	Cystic fibrosis

Granuloma and fibrosis
Tuberculosis, sarcoidosis
  and fibrosing alveolitis
	Acquired
	Young's syndrome –
	  azoospermia, sinusitis

if progression of the disease is to be halted. In mild cases, intermittent chemotherapy with cefaclor 500 mg three times daily or ciprofloxacin 500 mg twice daily may be the only therapy needed. Flucloxacillin 500 mg 6-hourly is the best treatment if *Staph. aureus* is isolated.

If the sputum remains yellow or green despite regular physiotherapy and intermittent chemotherapy, or if lung function deteriorates despite treatment with broncho-dilators, it is likely that there is infection with *P. aeruginosa*. Treatment requires parenteral or aerosol chemotherapy at regular 3-month intervals. Ceftazidime 2 g intravenously 8-hourly or by inhalation (1 g twice daily) has been shown to be effective. Ciprofloxacin 750 mg twice daily orally may be equally effective in the short term, but rapid development of resistance is a problem. High sputum levels of some antibiotics, e.g. tobramycin, can be achieved by inhalation.

Bronchodilators
Bronchodilators are useful in patients with demonstrable airflow limitation.

Anti-inflammatory agents
Inhaled or oral steroids can decrease the rate of progression.

Surgery
Unfortunately, it is rare for bronchiectasis to be suffi-ciently localized for a resection to be performed. Lung or heart–lung transplantation is sometimes required.

Complications
The incidence of complications has fallen with antibiotic therapy. Pneumonia, pneumothorax, empyema and metastatic cerebral abscess can occur. Severe, life-threatening haemoptysis can also occur, particularly in patients with cystic fibrosis.

Massive haemoptysis originates from the high-pressure systemic bronchial arteries and has a mortality of 25%. Other causes of massive haemoptysis are pul-monary tuberculosis (most common), aspergilloma, lung abscess and primary and secondary malignant tumours.

Treatment of the haemoptysis consists of bed rest and antibiotics, when most stop bleeding. Blood transfusion is given if required. Urgent fibreoptic bronchoscopy is occasionally necessary to detect the source of bleeding. If the haemoptysis does not settle rapidly the treatment of choice is bronchial artery embolization. Surgical resection may be required if embolization fails.

Prognosis
The advent of effective antibiotic therapy has greatly improved the prognosis. Ultimately, most patients with severe bronchiectasis will develop respiratory failure because of chronic deterioration of the lung tissue. Cor pulmonale is also a well-recognized complication.

Cystic fibrosis

In cystic fibrosis (CF) there is an alteration in the viscosity and tenacity of mucus produced at epithelial surfaces. The classical form of the syndrome includes broncho-pulmonary infection and pancreatic insufficiency, with a high sweat sodium and chloride concentration. It is an autosomal recessive inherited disorder with a carrier frequency in Caucasians of 1 in 22 (see p. 190). There is a gene mutation on the long arm of chromosome 7 (7q21.3 → 7q22.1). The commonest abnormality is a specific deletion at position 508 in the amino acid sequence [ΔF_{508}] – which results in a defect in a transmembrane regulator protein (see p. 192). This is the cystic fibrosis trans-membrane conductance regulator (CFTR), which is a critical chloride channel (Fig. 14.30). The mutation alters the secondary and tertiary structure of the protein,

Fig. 14.30 **Cystic fibrosis.** Abnormalities and therapeutic advances (see text). CFTR, cystic fibrosis transmembrane conductance regulator.

leading to a failure of opening of the chloride channel in response to elevated cyclic AMP in epithelial cells. This results in decreased excretion of chloride into the airway lumen and an increased reabsorption of sodium into the epithelial cells. With less excretion of salt there is less excretion of water and increased viscosity and tenacity of airway secretions. A possible reason for the high salt content of sweat is that there is a CFTR-independent mechanism of chloride secretion in the sweat gland with an impaired reabsorption of sodium chloride in the distal end of the duct. Many genetic variants are known. The frequency of ΔF_{508} mutation in CF is 70% in the USA and UK, under 50% in southern Europe and 30% in Ashkenazi families.

Clinical features

Respiratory effects

Although the lungs of babies born with CF are structurally normal at birth, frequent respiratory infections soon develop and are often the presenting feature. CF is now the commonest cause of recurrent bronchopulmonary infection in childhood, and is a major cause in early adult life. Sinusitis is almost universal and nasal polyps are common. Breathlessness and haemoptysis occur in the later stages as airflow limitation and bronchiectasis develop. Spontaneous pneumothorax may occur. Respiratory failure and cor pulmonale eventually develop.

Gastrointestinal effects

About 85% of patients have symptomatic steatorrhoea owing to pancreatic dysfunction (see p. 413). Children may be born with meconium ileus owing to the viscid consistency of meconium in CF, and later in life develop the meconium ileus equivalent syndrome, a form of small intestinal obstruction unique to CF. Cholesterol gallstones appear to occur with increased frequency. Cirrhosis develops in about 5% of older patients and there are increased incidences of peptic ulceration and gastrointestinal malignancy.

Nutritional effects

Many patients suffer from malnutrition due to a combination of malabsorption and maldigestion. Poor nutrition is associated with increased pulmonary sepsis.

Other features

Puberty and skeletal maturity are delayed in most CF patients. Males are almost always infertile owing to failure of development of the vas deferens and epididymis. Females are able to conceive, but often develop secondary amenorrhoea as the disease progresses. Arthropathy and diabetes mellitus (in 11% of adults with CF) also occur.

Diagnosis

The diagnosis of CF in older children and adults is based on the clinical history and:

- a family history of the disease
- a high sweat sodium concentration over 60 mmol/L (meticulous technique by laboratories performing

regular sweat analysis is essential, but the test is still difficult to interpret in adults)
- blood DNA analysis of gene defect
- radiology showing features seen in bronchiectasis (see p. 908)
- absent vas deferens and epididymis
- blood immunoreactive trypsin levels – these are not useful diagnostically but may be useful in screening.

Treatment

Oxygen should be given as necessary (Box 14.1). Antibiotic treatment for respiratory infections is as described under bronchiectasis on page 909; treatment of pancreatic insufficiency and malnutrition is described on page 413. Seventy per cent of adults with CF have pseudomonas infection in their sputum. A meta-analysis has demonstrated that nebulized anti-pseudomonal antibiotic therapy improves lung function and decreases the risk of infective exacerbations and hospitalization in these patients. The effects on long-term benefits are still awaited.

Better understanding of the basic abnormality in CF has led to dramatic changes in treatment. Potential treatments to improve hydration of secretions include blocking of sodium reabsorption with amiloride or stimulating chloride secretion with adenosine or uridine triphosphates (ATP or UTP) which stimulate nucleotide receptors by a pathway independent of cAMP. DNA from dead inflammatory cells is a major contributor to the viscosity of sputum. Inhalation of recombinant human DNase (using a jet nebulizer) has been shown to improve FEV_1 by 20% in some patients. Inhaled antibiotics and corticosteroids can also reduce inflammation and improve lung function. Human experimental studies have been conducted on the delivery to the epithelium of the normal CFTR gene using, as a vector, a replication-deficient adenovirus containing normal human CFTR complementary DNA which is trophic for epithelial cells. Gentamicin can suppress premature termination codons, and nasal administration has been shown to correct the physiological abnormality. These studies are in their early stages. The recent difficulties have been in establishing an effective vector. Lung or heart–lung transplantation may be necessary in the later stages of the disease (p. 911).

Prognosis and screening

Almost all CF patients develop progressive respiratory failure but the prognosis has consistently improved. Ninety per cent of children now survive into their teens and the median survival for those born after 1990 is estimated at 40 years. A major problem is sputum infection with *Burkholderia cepacia* (formerly classified as *Pseudomonas*), a plant pathogen, previously considered a harmless commensal. Its acquisition can be associated with accelerated disease and rapid death. Multiple antibiotic resistance is common and spread occurs from person to person. Strategies to limit transmission include rigid segregation of both inpatients and outpatients and advice to CF sufferers not to socialize together. Sadly, groups formed for mutual support and education have been disrupted, leading to considerable distress.

Genetic screening is available for the four most common mutations and this identifies 85–95% of carriers. Screening for the carrier state should be offered to persons or couples with a family history of CF, together with counselling (see p. 191).

Chronic cough (see p. 882)

Pathological coughing results from two mechanisms:

- stimulation of sensory nerves in the epithelium by secretions, foreign bodies, cigarette smoke and tumours
- sensitization of the cough reflex in which there is an abnormal increase in the sensitivity of the cough receptors demonstrable by inhalation of capsaicin or hypotonic chloride solutions.

Sensitization of the cough reflex presents clinically as a persistent tickling sensation in the throat with paroxysms of coughing induced by changes in air temperature, aerosol sprays, perfumes and cigarette smoke. It is found in association with viral infections, oesophageal reflux, postnasal drip, cough-variant asthma, idiopathic cough, and in 15% of patients taking angiotensin-converting enzyme (ACE) inhibitors. The association with ACE inhibitors implicates neuropeptides, prostaglandins E_2 and $F_{2\alpha}$ and bradykinin as a cause of the cough. In the absence of chest X-ray abnormalities, possible investigations include:

- ENT examination (p. 1157) and sinus CT for postnasal drip
- lung function tests and histamine bronchial provocation testing (p. 918) for cough-variant asthma
- ambulatory oesophageal pH monitoring for oesophageal reflux
- CT scan of thorax for interstitial lung disease
- $\dot{V}_A/\dot{Q}$ scans for recurrent pulmonary embolism
- fibreoptic bronchoscopy for inhaled foreign body or tumour
- ECG, echocardiography and exercise testing for cardiac causes
- hyperventilation testing and psychiatric appraisal.

The absence of any pathology makes the management of unexplained cough difficult. Morphine will depress the sensitized cough reflex but its unwanted effects limit its use in the long term. Dihydrocodeine linctus may be of value in some patients. Demulcent preparations and cough sweets provide temporary relief only. Patients taking ACE inhibitors should be changed to an angiotensin-II receptor antagonist, e.g. losartan (see p. 793), which does not block bradykinin.

Lung and heart–lung transplantation

Indications and donor selection

The main diseases treated by transplantation are:

- pulmonary fibrosis
- primary pulmonary hypertension
- cystic fibrosis
- bronchiectasis
- emphysema – particularly α_1-antitrypsin inhibitor deficiency
- Eisenmenger's syndrome.

Indications for this treatment are patients under 60 years with a life expectancy of less than 18 months, no underlying cancer and no serious systemic disease.

Donor selection includes age under 40 years, good cardiac and lung function, and chest measurements slightly smaller than those of the recipient. Matching for ABO blood group is essential, but rhesus blood group compatibility is not essential. Since donor material is limited, single lung transplantation is preferred to double lung or heart–lung transplantation and can be successfully undertaken in pulmonary fibrosis, pulmonary hypertension and emphysema. Bilateral lung transplantation is required in infective conditions to prevent spillover of bacteria from the diseased lung to a single lung transplant. Eisenmenger's syndrome requires heart–lung transplant.

Complications and their treatment

- *Early* – post-transplant pulmonary oedema requires diuretics and respiratory support by ventilation.
- *Infections*, particularly within first 3 months:
  Bacterial pneumonia – antibiotics
  Cytomegalovirus – ganciclovir
  Herpes simplex – aciclovir
- *P. carinii* – prophylactic co-trimoxazole.
- *Immunosuppression* is with ciclosporin or tacrolimus, azathioprine or mycophenolate mofetil and prednisolone.
- *Rejection*:
  Early (first few weeks) – high-dose i.v. corticosteroids
  Late (after 3 months) – in obliterative bronchiolitis, high-dose i.v. corticosteroids are sometimes effective. Post-transplant lymphoproliferative disease may respond to rituximab, a monoclonal antibody which causes lysis of B lymphocytes.

Prognosis. There is a 2-year survival of 75% and 5-year survival of almost 50%.

FURTHER READING

Barnes PJ (2004) Small airways in COPD. *New England Journal of Medicine* **350**: 2635–2637.

British Thoracic Society (1998) Smoking cessation guidelines and their cost-effectiveness. *Thorax* **53** (Suppl 5): S1–S38.

Calverley PMA, Walker P (2003) Chronic obstructive pulmonary disease. *Lancet* **362**: 1053–1061.

Drazen JM, Epstein AM (2003) Guidance concerning surgery for emphysema. *New England Journal of Medicine* **348**: 2134–2136.

Flemons WW (2002) Obstructive sleep apnoea. *New England Journal of Medicine* **347**: 498–505.

Plant PK et al. (2000) Early use of non-invasive ventilation for acute exacerbations of COPD. *Lancet* **355**: 1931–1935.

Ratjen F, Doring G (2003) Cystic fibrosis. *Lancet* **361**: 681–689.

Rowe SM et al. (2005) Cystic fibrosis. *New England Journal of Medicine* **252**: 1992–2001.

Ryan G et al. (2000) Nebulised anti-pseudomonal antibiotics for CF (Cochrane Review). Cochrane Library, Issue 4. Oxford: Update Software.

[Various authors] (2004) Chronic obstructive pulmonary disease. *Lancet* **364**: 613, 709, 883, 896, 985.

ASTHMA

Asthma is a common chronic inflammatory condition of the lung airways whose cause is incompletely understood. Symptoms are cough, wheeze, chest tightness and shortness of breath, often worse at night. It has three characteristics:

- *airflow limitation* which is usually reversible spontaneously or with treatment
- *airway hyperresponsiveness* to a wide range of stimuli (see below)
- *inflammation of the bronchi* with eosinophils, T lymphocytes and mast cells with associated plasma exudation, oedema, marked smooth muscle hypertrophy, mucus plugging and epithelial damage.

In chronic asthma, inflammation may be accompanied by irreversible airflow limitation.

The underlying pathology in pre-school children may be different, in that they may not exhibit appreciable bronchial hyperreactivity. There is no evidence that chronic inflammation is the basis for the episodic wheezing associated with viral infections.

Prevalence

In many countries the prevalence of asthma is increasing, particularly in the second decade of life where this disease affects 10–15% of the population. There is also a geographical variation, with asthma being common in more developed countries, some of the highest rates being in New Zealand, Australia and the UK, but being much rarer in Far Eastern countries such as China and Malaysia, and in Africa and Central and Eastern Europe. Long-term follow-up in developing countries suggests that the disease may become more frequent as individuals become more 'westernized'. Studies of occupational asthma suggest that a high percentage of the workforce, perhaps up to 20%, may become asthmatic if exposed to potent sensitizers.

Classification

Asthma can be divided into:

- *extrinsic* – implying a definite external cause
- *intrinsic* or *cryptogenic* – when no causative agent can be identified.

Extrinsic asthma occurs most frequently in atopic individuals who show positive skin-prick reactions to common inhalant allergens. Positive skin-prick tests to inhalant allergens are shown in 90% of children and 50% of adults with persistent asthma. Childhood asthma is often accompanied by eczema (see p. 1327). An overlooked cause of late-onset asthma in adults is sensitization to chemicals or biological products in the workplace.

Intrinsic asthma often starts in middle age ('late onset'). Nevertheless, many patients with adult-onset asthma show positive skin tests and on close questioning give a history of respiratory symptoms compatible with childhood asthma.

Non-atopic individuals may develop asthma in middle age from extrinsic causes such as sensitization to occupational agents or aspirin intolerance, or because they were given β-adrenoceptor-blocking agents for concurrent hypertension or angina. Extrinsic causes must be considered in all cases of asthma and, where possible, avoided.

Aetiology and pathogenesis

There are two major factors involved in the development of asthma and many other stimuli that can precipitate attacks (Fig. 14.31).

Atopy and allergy

The term 'atopy' was used by clinicians at the beginning of the century to describe a group of disorders, including asthma and hayfever, that appeared:

- to run in families
- to have characteristic wealing skin reactions to common allergens in the environment

Fig. 14.31 **Causes and triggers of asthma.** RSV, respiratory syncytial virus; NSAIDs, non-steroidal anti-inflammatory drugs.

- to have circulating antibody in their serum that could be transferred to the skin of non-sensitized individuals.

The term is best used to describe those individuals who readily develop antibodies of IgE class against common materials present in the environment. Such antibodies are present in 30–40% of the UK population, and there is a link between serum IgE levels and both the prevalence of asthma and airway hyperresponsiveness. Genetic and environmental factors affect serum IgE levels. The use of DNA microsatellite markers to scan the entire genome has uncovered 22 chromosomal regions of interest containing candidate genes. Some of these, in combination with environmental factors, may turn out to play a key role in the development of asthma. The genes controlling the production of the cytokines IL-3, IL-4, IL-5, IL-9, IL-13 and GM-CSF – which in turn affect mast and eosinophil cell development and longevity as well as IgE production – are present in a cluster on chromosome 5q31–33 (the IL-4 gene cluster). A gene on chromosome 2, *PHF11*, which controls IgE synthesis is strongly associated with atopy whereas *ADAM33* on chromosome 20 is more strongly associated with airway hyperresponsiveness and the tissue changes of remodelling.

Early childhood exposure to allergens and maternal smoking have a major influence on IgE production. Much current interest focuses on the role of intestinal bacteria and childhood infections in shaping the immune system in early life. It has been suggested that growing up in a relatively 'clean' environment may predispose towards an IgE response to allergens (the hygiene hypothesis). Conversely, growing up in a 'dirtier' environment may allow the immune system to avoid developing allergic responses. Components of bacteria (e.g. lipopolysaccharide endotoxin; immunostimulatory CpG DNA sequences), viruses (e.g. DS RNA) and fungi (e.g. chiton, a cell wall component) are able to stimulate toll receptors expressed on immune cells to direct the immune and inflammatory response away from the allergic pathways. Thus early life exposure to inhaled and ingested products of microorganisms may be critical in helping shape the subsequent risk of a child becoming allergic and/or developing asthma.

The allergens involved in asthma are similar to those in rhinitis. Allergens from the faecal particles of the house-dust mite are the most significant extrinsic cause of asthma world-wide. Cockroach allergy has been implicated in asthma in US inner-city children, while allergens from furry pets are also becoming increasingly common causes of asthma, rhinitis and urticaria. The fungal spores from *Aspergillus fumigatus* give rise to a complex series of lung disorders, including asthma (see p. 939). Many allergens including those from *Aspergillus* have intrinsic biological properties, e.g. proteolytic enzymes that facilitate their passage through the airway epithelium to increase their sensitizing capacity.

Increased responsiveness of the airways of the lung (airway hyperresponsiveness)

Bronchial hyperresponsiveness can be demonstrated by asking the patient to inhale gradually increasing concentrations of either histamine or methacholine (*bronchial provocation tests*). This induces transient airflow limitation in susceptible individuals (approximately 20% of the population); the dose of the agonist (provocation dose) necessary to produce a 20% fall in FEV_1 is known as the PD_{20} FEV_1 (or PC_{20} FEV_1). Patients with clinical symptoms of asthma respond to very low doses of methacholine; i.e. they have a low PD_{20} FEV_1 (< 11 µmol). In general, the greater the degree of hyperreactivity, the more persistent the symptoms and the greater the need for treatment.

Some patients also react to methacholine but at *higher doses* and include those with:

- attacks of asthma only on extreme exertion
- wheezing or prolonged periods of coughing following a viral infection
- cough variant asthma
- seasonal wheeze in pollen season
- allergic rhinitis, but not complaining of any lower respiratory symptoms until specifically questioned
- some subjects with no respiratory symptoms.

Although the degree of hyperresponsiveness can itself be influenced by allergic mechanisms (see p. 914 and Fig. 14.34), its pathogenesis and mode of inheritance involve a combination of airway inflammation and tissue remodelling.

Precipitating factors
Occupational sensitizers

Over 200 materials encountered at the workplace give rise to occupational asthma. The causes are recognized occupational diseases in the UK, and patients in insurable employment are therefore eligible for statutory compensation provided they apply within 10 years of leaving the occupation in which the asthma developed (Table 14.12).

Table 14.12 Occupational asthma in the UK	
Cause	**Source**
Non-IgE related	
Isocyanates	Polyurethane varnishes
	Industrial coatings
	Spray painting
Colophony fumes	Soldering/welders
	Electronics industry
IgE related	
Allergens from animals, insects and antibiotics	Laboratories
Allergens from flour and grain	Farmers
	Millers/bakers
	Grain handlers
Latex	Health workers
Proteolytic enzymes	Manufacture (but not use) of 'biological' washing powders
Complex salts of platinum	Metal refining
Acid anhydrides and polyamine hardening agents	Industrial coatings

Asthma due to flour, organic dusts and other large protein molecules involves specific IgE antibodies. In contrast, reactive chemicals such as isocyanates and acid anhydrides bond chemically to epithelial cells to activate them as well as provide haptens recognized by T cells. The risk of developing some forms of occupational asthma increases in smokers.

The proportion of employees developing occupational asthma depends primarily upon the level of exposure. Proper enclosure of industrial processes or appropriate ventilation greatly reduces the risk. Atopic individuals develop occupational asthma more rapidly when exposed to agents causing the development of specific IgE antibody. Non-atopic individuals can also develop asthma when exposed to such agents, but after a longer period of exposure.

Non-specific factors

The characteristic feature of bronchial hyperresponsiveness in asthma means that, as well as reacting to specific antigens, the airways will also respond to a wide variety of non-specific direct and indirect stimuli.

Cold air and exercise

Most asthmatics wheeze after prolonged exercise. Typically, the attack does not occur while exercising but afterwards. The inhalation of cold, dry air will also precipitate an attack. Exercise-induced wheeze is driven by histamine and leukotrienes which are released from mast cells when the epithelial lining fluid of the bronchi becomes hyperosmolar owing to drying and cooling during exercise. The phenomenon can be shown by exercise, cold air and hypertonic (e.g. saline or mannitol) provocation tests.

Atmospheric pollution and irritant dusts, vapours and fumes

Many patients with asthma experience worsening of symptoms on contact with cigarette smoke, car exhaust fumes, strong perfumes or high concentrations of dust in the atmosphere. Major epidemics have been recorded when large amounts of allergens are released into the air, e.g. soy bean epidemic in Barcelona. Asthma exacerbations increase in both summer and winter air pollution episodes associated with climatic temperature inversions. Epidemics of the disease have occurred in the presence of high concentrations of ozone, particulates and NO_2 in the summer and particulates, NO_2 and SO_2 in the winter.

Diet

Increased intakes of fresh fruit and vegetables have been shown to be protective, possibly owing to the increased intake of antioxidants. Genetic variation in antioxidant enzymes is associated with more severe asthma.

Emotion

It is well known that emotional factors may influence asthma, but there is no evidence that patients with the disease are any more psychologically disturbed than their non-asthmatic peers.

Drugs

Non-steroid anti-inflammatory drugs (NSAIDs). NSAIDs, particularly aspirin and propionic acid derivatives, e.g. indometacin, have a major role in the development and precipitation of attacks in approximately 5% of patients with asthma. This effect is especially prevalent in those individuals who have both nasal polyps and asthma. It is thought that treatment with these drugs leads to an imbalance in the metabolism of arachidonic acid. NSAIDs inhibit arachidonic acid metabolism via the cyclo-oxygenase (COX) pathway, preventing the synthesis of prostaglandins. It is suggested that under these circumstances there is a reduced production of prostaglandin E_2 which, in a sub-proportion of genetically susceptible subjects, induces the overproduction of cysteinyl leukotrienes by eosinophils, mast cells and macrophages. In such patients there is evidence for polymorphisms involving the promoter region of the LTC_4 synthase gene that controls the level of activity of this terminal enzyme of the leukotriene-generating pathway (Fig. 14.32). Interestingly, asthma in intolerant patients is not precipitated by COX-2 inhibitors, indicating that it is blockade of COX-1 that is linked to impaired PGE_2 production.

Beta-blockers. The airways have a direct parasympathetic innervation that tends to produce bronchoconstriction. There is no direct sympathetic innervation of the smooth muscle of the bronchi, and antagonism of parasympathetically induced bronchoconstriction is critically dependent upon circulating epinephrine (adrenaline) acting through β_2-receptors on the surface of smooth muscle cells. Inhibition of this effect by β-adrenoceptor-blocking drugs such as propranolol leads to bronchoconstriction and airflow limitation, but only in asthmatic subjects. The so-called selective β_1-adrenergic-blocking drugs such as atenolol may still induce attacks of asthma; their use to treat hypertension or angina in asthmatic patients is best avoided.

Allergen-induced asthma

The experimental inhalation of allergen by atopic asthmatic individuals leads to the development of different types of reaction, as illustrated in Figure 14.33.

Immediate asthma (early reaction)

Airflow limitation begins within minutes of contact with the allergen, reaches its maximum in 15–20 minutes and subsides by 1 hour.

Dual and late-phase reactions

Following an immediate reaction many asthmatics develop a more prolonged and sustained attack of airflow limitation that responds less well to inhalation of bronchodilator drugs such as salbutamol. Isolated late-phase reactions with no preceding immediate response can occur after the inhalation of some occupational sensitizers such as isocyanates.

Fig. 14.32 **Arachidonic acid metabolism and the effect of drugs.** The enzyme cyclo-oxygenase occurs in three isoforms, COX-1 (constitutive), COX-2 (inducible) and COX-3 (in brain). PG, prostaglandin.

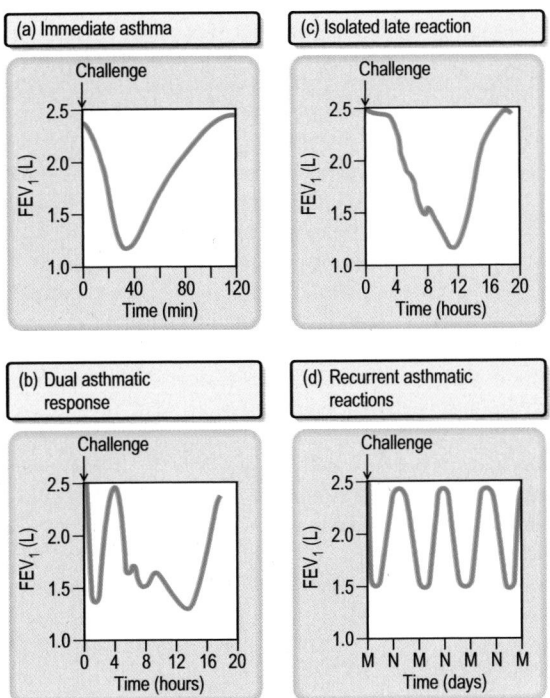

Fig. 14.33 **Different types of asthmatic reactions following challenge with allergen. (a)** Immediate asthma. **(b)** Dual asthmatic response. **(c)** Isolated late reaction. **(d)** Recurrent asthmatic reactions. M, midnight; N, noon.

Recurrent asthmatic reactions

The development of the late-phase reaction is associated with an increase in the underlying level of airway hyperresponsiveness such that individuals may show continuing episodes of asthma on subsequent days.

Pathogenesis

The pathogenesis of asthma is complex and not fully understood. It involves a number of cells, mediators, nerves and vascular leakage that can be activated by several different mechanisms, of which exposure to allergens is among the most significant (Fig. 14.34). The varying clinical severity and chronicity of asthma is dependent on an interplay between airway inflammation and airway wall remodelling. The inflammatory component is driven by Th2-type T lymphocytes which facilitate IgE synthesis through production of IL-4 and eosinophilic inflammation through IL-5 (Fig. 14.34).

Inflammation

Several key cells are involved in the inflammatory response that characterizes all types of asthma.

Mast cells (see also p. 200). These are increased in both the epithelium and surface secretions of asthmatics and can generate and release powerful mediators acting on smooth muscle and small blood vessels, such as histamine, tryptase, prostaglandin D_2 (PGD$_2$) and leukotriene C_4 (LTC$_4$), which cause the immediate asthmatic reaction. Since potent β_2-adrenoceptor agonists such as salbutamol

Fig. 14.34 **Pathogenesis of asthma.** Antigen-presenting cells (dendritic cells) activate Th2 T cells causing them to release cytokines which attract mast cells and eosinophils. IL-9 and IL-4 activate mast cells to release LTC_4, PGD_2 and histamine which act on smooth muscle and blood vessels. IL-3, IL-5 and GM-CSF attract eosinophils; these are also attracted by chemokines which act on type 3 C-C chemokine receptors (CCR-3, e.g. eotaxin, RANTES, MCP-1, –3 and –4). Activated eosinophils release LTC_4, MBP, ECP and peroxidase (EPX) which are toxic to epithelial cells.

IL-4 and IL-13 produced by activated T cells maintain the allergic reaction and cause mucus secretion and smooth muscle contraction. IL, interleukin; GM-CSF, granulocyte–macrophage colony-stimulating factor; RANTES, regulated upon activation, normal T cell expressed and secreted; MBP, major basic protein; ECP, eosinophilic cationic protein; LTC_4, leukotriene C_4; MCP, monocytic chemoattractant protein; PDGF, platelet-derived growth factor; PGD_2, prostaglandin D_2; TGF-β, transforming growth factor-β; VEGF; vascular endothelial growth factor; ET-1, endothelin-1.

have little effect on airway inflammation or hyper-responsiveness but inhibit mast cell mediator release, many other factors are involved in the pathogenesis of late and recurrent asthmatic reactions leading to more severe disease.

Eosinophils. These cells are found in large numbers in the bronchial wall and secretions of asthmatics. They are attracted to the airways by the eosinophilopoietic cytokines IL-3, IL-5 and GM-CSF as well as by chemokines which act on type 3 C-C chemokine receptors (CCR-3) (i.e. eotaxin, RANTES, MCP-1, MCP-3 and MCP-4). These mediators also prime eosinophils for enhanced mediator secretion. When activated, they release LTC_4, and basic proteins such as major basic protein (MBP), eosinophil cationic protein (ECP) and peroxidase (EPX) that are toxic to epithelial cells. Both the number and activation of eosinophils is rapidly decreased by corticosteroids.

Macrophages (dendritic cells) and lymphocytes. These cells are abundant in the mucous membranes of the airways and the alveoli. Dendritic cells have a role in the initial uptake and presentation of allergens to lymphocytes. They can release prostaglandins, thromboxane,

LTC_4 and LTB_4 and platelet-activating factor (PAF). T helper lymphocytes (CD4) show evidence of activation (Fig. 14.34) and the release of their cytokines play a key part in the migration and activation of mast cells (IL-3, IL-4, IL-9) and eosinophils (IL-3, IL-5, GM-CSF). In addition, production of IL-4 leads to the maintenance of the allergic (Th2) T cell phenotype, favouring switching of antibody production by B lymphocytes to IgE. In asthma there occurs a selective upregulation of Th2 T cells with reduced evidence of the Th1 phenotype (producing gamma-interferon and IL-2). This polarization is mediated by dendritic cells and involves a combination of antigen presentation, costimulation and exposure to polarizing cytokines. The activity of both macrophages and lymphocytes is influenced by corticosteroids but not $β_2$-adrenoceptor agonists.

Remodelling

A characteristic feature of chronic asthma is an alteration of structure and functions of the formed elements of the airways. Together, these structural changes interact with inflammatory cells and mediators to cause the characteristic features of the disease. Deposition of matrix proteins, swelling and cellular infiltration cause an expansion of the submucosa beneath the epithelium so that for a given degree of smooth muscle shortening there is excess airway narrowing. Swelling outside the smooth muscle layer spreads the retractile forces exerted by the surrounding alveoli over a greater surface area so that the airways close more easily. Several factors contribute to these changes.

The epithelium. In asthma the epithelium of the conducting airways is stressed and damaged with loss of ciliated columnar cells onto the lumen. Metaplasia occurs with a resultant increase in the number and activity of mucus-secreting goblet cells. The epithelium is a major source of mediators, cytokines and growth factors that serve to enhance inflammation and promote tissue remodelling. Damage and activation of the epithelium make it more vulnerable to infection by common respiratory viruses, e.g. rhinovirus, coronavirus, and to the effects of air pollutants.

Epithelial basement membrane. A pathognomonic feature of asthma is the deposition of repair collagens (types I, III and V) in the *lamina reticularis* beneath the basement membrane. This, along with the deposition of other matrix proteins such as laminin, tenascin and fibronectin, causes the appearance of a thickened basement membrane observed by light microscopy in asthma. This collagen deposition reflects activation of an underlying sheath of fibroblasts that transform into contractile myofibroblasts which also have an increased capacity to secrete matrix. Aberrant signalling between the epithelium and underlying myofibroblasts is thought to be the principal cause of airway wall remodelling, since the cells are prolific producers of a range of tissue growth factors such as epidermal growth factors (EGF), transforming growth factor-β (TGF-β), connective tissue-derived growth factor, platelet-derived growth factor (PDGF), endothelin (ET), insulin-like growth factors (IGF), nerve growth factors and vascular endothelial growth factors (Fig. 14.34). The same interaction between epithelium and mesenchymal tissues is central to branching morphogenesis in the developing fetal lung. It has been suggested that these mechanisms are reactivated in asthma, but instead of causing airway growth and branching, they lead to thickening of the airway wall (remodelling). Increased deposition of collagens, proteoglycans and matrix proteins creates a microenvironment conducive to ongoing inflammation since these complex molecules also possess cell-signalling functions which prolong inflammatory cell survival and prime them for mediator secretion.

Smooth muscle. A prominent feature of asthma is hyperplasia of the helical bands of airways smooth muscle. In addition to increasing in amount, the smooth muscle alters in function to contract more easily and stay contracted because of a change in actin–myosin cross-link cycling. These changes allow the asthmatic airways to contract too much and too easily at the least provocation. Asthmatic smooth muscle also secretes a wide range of cytokines and growth factors that help sustain the chronic inflammatory response. *ADAM33*, the newly described asthma gene, may be involved in driving increased airway smooth muscle and other features of remodelling through increased generation of growth factors.

Nerves. Neural reflexes, both central and peripheral, contribute to the irritability of asthmatic airways. Central reflexes involve stimulation of nerve endings in the epithelium and submucosa with transmission of impulses via the spinal cord and brain back down to the airways where release of acetylcholine from nerve endings stimulates M_2 receptors on smooth muscle causing contraction. Local neural reflexes involve antidromic neurotransmission and the release of a variety of neuropeptides. Some of these are smooth muscle contractants (substance P, neurokinin A), some are vasoconstrictors (e.g. calcitonin gene-related peptide, CGRP) and some vasodilators (e.g. neuropeptide Y, vasoactive intestinal polypeptide). Bradykinin generated by tissue and serum proteolytic enzymes (including mast cell tryptase) is also a potent stimulus of local neural reflexes involving (non-myelinated) nerve fibres.

Clinical features

The principal symptoms of asthma are wheezing attacks and episodic shortness of breath. Symptoms are usually worst during the night. Cough is a frequent symptom that sometimes predominates and is often misdiagnosed as bronchitis. Nocturnal cough can be a presenting feature.

There is a tremendous variation in the frequency and duration of the attacks. Some patients have only one or two attacks a year that last for a few hours, whilst others have attacks lasting for weeks. Some patients have chronic symptoms. Attacks may be precipitated by a wide range of triggers (Fig. 14.31). Asthma is a major cause of impaired quality of life with impact on work, recreational, as well as physical activities and emotions.

Investigations

There is no single satisfactory diagnostic test for all asthmatic patients.

Respiratory function tests

Measurements of peak expiratory flow (PEF) on waking, prior to taking a bronchodilator and before bed after a bronchodilator, are particularly useful in demonstrating the variable airflow limitation that characterizes the disease. An example is shown in Figure 14.14 (p. 889). The diurnal variation in PEF is a good measure of asthma activity and is of help in the longer-term assessment of the patient's disease and its response to treatment. To assess possible occupational asthma, peak flows need to be measured for at least 2 weeks at work and 2 weeks off work.

Spirometry is useful, especially in assessing reversibility. Asthma can be diagnosed by demonstrating a greater than 15% improvement in FEV_1 or PEF following the inhalation of a bronchodilator. However, this degree of response may not be present if the asthma is in remission or in severe chronic asthma when little reversibility can be demonstrated or if the patient is already being treated with long-acting bronchodilators.

The carbon monoxide transfer test is normal in asthma.

Exercise tests

These have been widely used in the diagnosis of asthma in children. Ideally, the child should run for 6 minutes on a treadmill at a workload sufficient to increase the heart rate above 160 beats per minute. Alternative methods use cold air challenge, isocapnoeic hyperventilation (forced overbreathing with artificially maintained P_aCO_2) or aerosol challenge with hypertonic solutions. A negative test does not automatically rule out asthma.

Histamine or methacholine bronchial provocation test (see p. 913)

This test indicates the presence of airway hyper-responsiveness, a feature found in most asthmatics, and can be particularly useful in investigating those patients whose main symptom is cough. The test should not be performed on individuals who have poor lung function ($FEV_1 < 1.5$ L) or a history of 'brittle' asthma.

Trial of corticosteroids

All patients who present with severe airflow limitation should undergo a formal trial of corticosteroids. Prednisolone 30 mg orally should be given daily for 2 weeks with lung function measured before and immediately after the course. A substantial improvement in FEV_1 (> 15%) confirms the presence of a reversible element and indicates that the administration of inhaled steroids will prove beneficial to the patient. If the trial is for 2 weeks or less, the oral steroids can be withdrawn without tailing off the dose, and should be replaced by inhaled corticosteroids in those who have responded and are thought will benefit.

Blood and sputum tests

Patients with asthma may have an increase in the number of eosinophils in peripheral blood (> 0.4×10^9/L). The presence of large numbers of eosinophils in the sputum is a more useful diagnostic tool.

Chest X-ray

There are no diagnostic features of asthma on the chest X-ray, although overinflation is characteristic during an acute episode or in chronic severe disease. A chest X-ray may be helpful in excluding a pneumothorax, which can occur as a complication, or in detecting the pulmonary shadows associated with allergic bronchopulmonary aspergillosis.

Skin tests

Skin-prick tests should be performed in all cases of asthma to help identify allergic causes.

Allergen provocation tests

Allergen challenge is not required in the clinical investigation of patients, except in cases of suspected occupational asthma. Another controversial exception is the investigation of food allergy causing asthma. This diagnosis is difficult, although many patients are concerned about the possibility. If the patient has asthma without any other systemic features, then food allergy is most unlikely to be the cause. Open food challenges are unreliable and if the diagnosis is seriously entertained, blind oral challenges with the food disguised in opaque gelatine capsules are necessary to confirm or refute a causative link (see p. 261).

Management

Asthma is extremely common and causes considerable morbidity. The aims of treatment are to:

- abolish symptoms
- restore normal or best possible lung function
- reduce the risk of severe attacks
- enable normal growth to occur in children
- minimize absence from school or employment.

This involves:

- patient and family education about asthma
- patient and family participation in treatment
- avoidance of identified causes where possible
- use of the lowest effective doses of convenient medications to minimize short-term and long-term side-effects.

Many asthmatics belong to self-help groups whose aim is to further their understanding of the disease and to foster self-confidence and fitness.

Control of extrinsic factors

Measures must be taken to avoid causative allergens such as the house-dust mite, pets, moulds and certain foodstuffs (see allergic rhinitis), particularly in childhood.

Avoidance of the house-dust mite is possible with effective and comfortable covers for bedding and changes to living accommodation. Active and passive smoking should be avoided, as should beta-blockers in either tablet or eyedrop form.

Individuals intolerant to aspirin may benefit by avoiding dietary salicylates and should avoid NSAIDs. Other agents (e.g. preservatives and colouring materials such as tartrazine) should be avoided if shown to be a causative factor. Fifty per cent of individuals sensitized to occupational agents may be cured if they are kept permanently away from exposure. The remaining 50% continue to have symptoms that may be as severe as when exposed to materials at work, especially if they were symptomatic for a long time before the diagnosis was made.

This emphasises:

- the importance of the rapid identification of extrinsic causes of asthma and their removal wherever possible (e.g. occupational agents, family pets)
- once extrinsic asthma is initiated, it may become self-perpetuating possibly by non-immune mechanisms.

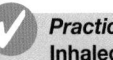

Drug treatment

The mainstay of asthma therapy is the use of therapeutic agents delivered as aerosols or powders directly into the lungs (Practical box 14.4). The advantages of this method of administration are that drugs are delivered direct to the lung and the first-pass metabolism in the liver is avoided; thus lower doses are necessary and systemic unwanted effects are minimized.

Both national and international guidelines have been published on the stepwise treatment of asthma (Box 14.2) based on three principles:

- Asthma self-management with regular asthma monitoring using peak flow meters and individual treatment plans discussed with each patient and written down.
- The appreciation that asthma is an inflammatory disease and that anti-inflammatory (controller) therapy should be started even in mild cases.
- Use of short-acting inhaled bronchodilators (e.g. salbutamol and terbutaline) only to relieve break-through symptoms. Increased use of bronchodilator treatment to relieve increasing symptoms is an indication of deteriorating disease.

A list of drugs used in asthma is shown in Box 14.3.

β_2-adrenergic agonists

The most widely used bronchodilator preparations contain β_2-adrenergic agonists that are selective for the respiratory tract and do not stimulate the β_1-adrenoceptors of the myocardium. These drugs are potent bronchodilators because they cause relaxation of bronchial smooth muscle. Such treatment is very effective in relieving symptoms but does little for the underlying inflammatory nature of the disease. Only the mildest asthmatics with intermittent attacks should rely on bronchodilator treatment alone. Inhalants such as salbutamol (100 µg) or terbutaline (250 µg) should be prescribed as 'two puffs as required'. Some patients use nebulizers at home for self-administration of salbutamol or terbutaline. Such treatment is effective, but patients must not rely on repeated home administration of nebulized β_2-adrenoceptor

agonists for worsening asthma, and must be encouraged to seek medical advice urgently if their condition does not improve. The excessive use of β_2 agonists has been linked to the two epidemics of asthma mortality in the 1960s and 1980s.

Salmeterol and formoterol are highly selective and potent long-acting β_2-adrenoceptor agonists effective by inhalation for up to 12 hours, thereby reducing the need for administration to once or twice daily. Long-acting β_2-adrenoceptor agonists improve symptoms, lung function and reduce exacerbations in patients who are poorly controlled on standard doses of inhaled steroids. They should never be used alone but always in combination with an inhaled corticosteroid.

Practical Box 14.4
Inhaled therapy

Use of a metered-dose inhaler

1. The canister is shaken.
2. The patient exhales to functional residual capacity (not residual volume), i.e. normal expiration.
3. The aerosol nozzle is placed to the open mouth.
4. The patient simultaneously inhales rapidly and activates the aerosol.
5. Inhalation is completed.
6. The breath is held for 10 seconds if possible.
   Even with good technique only 15% of the contents is inhaled and 85% is deposited on the wall of the pharynx and ultimately swallowed.
   NB: Chlorofluorocarbon (CFC) propellants are being replaced by hydrofluoralkane (HFA) propellants. The new aerosols may feel and taste differently and patients will need reassurance of their efficacy.

Spacers

These are plastic conical spheres inserted between the patient's mouth and the inhaler. They are designed to reduce particle velocity so that less drug is deposited in the mouth. Spacers also diminish the need for coordination between aerosol activation and inhalation. They are useful in children and in the elderly and they reduce the risk of candidiasis.

Box 14.2 The stepwise management of asthma

Step		PEFR	Treatment
1	Occasional symptoms, less frequent than daily	100% predicted	As-required bronchodilators If used more than once daily, move to step 2
2	Daily symptoms	≤ 80% predicted	Anti-inflammatory drugs Sodium cromoglicate or low-dose inhaled corticosteroids up to 800 µg If not controlled, move to step 3
3	Severe symptoms	50–80% predicted	High-dose inhaled corticosteroids up to 2000 µg daily
4	Severe symptoms uncontrolled with high-dose inhaled corticosteroids	50–80% predicted	Add regular long-acting β_2 agonists (e.g. salmeterol)
5	Severe symptoms deteriorating	≤ 50% predicted	Add prednisolone 40 mg daily
6	Severe symptoms deteriorating in spite of prednisolone	≤ 30% predicted	Hospital admission

Short-acting bronchodilator treatment taken at any step on as-required basis

Box 14.3 **Drugs used in asthma**

Inhaled oral steroids

Short-acting relievers (salbutamol, terbutaline)

Long-acting relief/disease controllers
Long-acting β_2 agonists – salmeterol, formoterol
Sodium cromoglicate
Leukotriene modifiers – montelukast, zafirlukast,
  pranlukast, zileuton

Other agents with bronchodilator activity

Antimuscarinic agents (ipratropium, oxitropium)
Theophylline preparations

Steroid-sparing agents

Methotrexate
Ciclosporin
Gold
Intravenous immunoglobulin
Anti-IgE monoclonal antibody – omalizumab

β_2-adrenoceptor agonists are less effective when given by mouth than when the drug is inhaled, and to help those who cannot coordinate activation of the aerosol and inhalation, several breath-activated or dry powder devices have been developed.

Antimuscarinic bronchodilators
Muscarinic receptors are found in the respiratory tract; large airways contain mainly M_3 receptors whereas the peripheral lung tissue contains M_3 and M_1 receptors (see p. 876). Non-selective muscarinic antagonists – ipratropium bromide (20–40 µg three or four times daily) or oxitropium bromide (200 µg twice daily) – by aerosol inhalation may be additive to β_2-adrenoceptor stimulants, especially during asthma exacerbations.

Anti-inflammatory drugs
Sodium cromoglicate and nedocromil sodium prevent activation of many inflammatory cells, particularly mast cells, eosinophils and epithelial cells, but not lymphocytes, by blocking a specific chloride channel which in turn prevents calcium influx. These drugs are effective in patients with milder asthma. Sodium cromoglicate is taken regularly either in the form of a Spincap containing 20 mg or in aerosol form from a metered-dose inhaler delivering 5 mg per puff. The dose should be two puffs four times daily from an inhaler, or one Spincap three or four times daily. Nedocromil sodium is taken as an aerosol at a dose of 4 mg (two puffs) two to four times daily. Recent asthma guidelines advise that inhaled corticosteroids are more efficacious than the cromones, but the latter are free of side-effects and, therefore, may offer some advantages in children.

Inhaled corticosteroids
All patients who have regular persisting symptoms need regular treatment with inhaled corticosteroids delivered in a stepwise fashion or as a high dose followed by a reduction to maintenance levels. Beclometasone dipropionate is the most widely used inhaled steroid and is available in doses of 50, 100, 200 and 250 µg per puff. Other inhaled steroids include budesonide, fluticasone, mometasone and triamcinolone.

Much of the inhaled dose does not reach the lung but is either swallowed or exhaled. Deposition in the lung varies between 10% and 25% depending on inhaler technique and the technical characteristics of the aerosol device. Drug which is deposited in the airways reaches the systemic circulation directly, through the bronchial circulation, while any drug that is swallowed has to pass through the liver before it can reach the systemic circulation. Gram for gram, fluticasone and mometasone are more potent than beclometasone with considerably less systemic bioavailability, owing to their greater sensitivity to hepatic metabolism. The newer hydrofluoroalkane (HFA) aerosols of beclometasone deliver a higher proportion of useable drug than the old CFC-based aerosols, and the effective dosage of HFA-beclometasone is equivalent to the same dose of HFA-fluticasone, whereas previously the effective dose ratio was 2 : 1. Absorption of beclometasone and budesonide does not seem to present a risk at doses up to 800 µg/day, but when using high-dose inhaled steroids in patients who have not responded to standard doses, fluticasone or mometasone may be preferred because of their lower bioavailability. The dose–response curve for inhaled corticosteroids is flat beyond 800 µg beclometasone or equivalent, and in patients with moderate asthma who are taking this daily, addition of salmeterol or formoterol is more effective than doubling the dose of inhaled corticosteroid.

The unwanted effects of inhaled corticosteroids are oral candidiasis (5% of patients), and hoarseness due to the effect of corticosteroids on the laryngeal muscles. Subcapsular cataract formation is rare but can occur in the elderly. Abnormalities of bone metabolism can be detected when inhaled corticosteroids are taken in high doses (beclometasone or budesonide > 800 µg daily). In children, inhaled corticosteroids at doses greater than 400 µg daily have been shown to retard short-term growth. Inhaled corticosteroid use should be stepped down once asthma comes under control. Candidiasis and GI absorption can be reduced by using spacers, mouthwashing and teeth cleaning after use.

Oral corticosteroids
Oral corticosteroids may be necessary for those individuals not controlled on inhaled corticosteroids. The dose should be kept as low as possible to minimize side-effects. The effect of short-term treatment with prednisolone 30 mg daily is shown in Figure 14.14 (p. 889). Some patients require continuing treatment with oral corticosteroids. Several studies suggest that treatment with low doses of methotrexate (15 mg weekly) can significantly reduce the dose of prednisolone needed to control the disease in some patients, and ciclosporin also improves lung function in some steroid-dependent asthmatics. Several other steroid-sparing strategies

including methotrexate and immunoglobulin have also been tried but with varying success.

Cysteinyl leukotriene receptor antagonists (LTRAs)

This class of anti-asthma therapy targets one of the principal asthma mediators by inhibiting the cysteinyl LT_1 receptor. A second receptor (cyst LT_2) has recently been identified on inflammatory cells. Montelukast, pranlukast (only available in SE Asia) and zafirlukast are given orally and are effective in a subpopulation of patients. However, it is not possible to predict which individuals will benefit: a 4-week trial of LTRA therapy is recommended before a decision is made to continue or stop. LTRAs should be considered in any patient who is not controlled on low to medium doses of inhaled steroids. Their action is additive to that of long-acting β_2 agonists. LTRAs are particularly useful in patients with aspirin-intolerant asthma and in those patients requiring high-dose inhaled or oral corticosteroids.

Monoclonal antibodies

Newer agents that modulate IgE-associated inflammation are being developed. The most promising of these is a recombinant humanized monoclonal antibody that complexes with free IgE – omalizumab – blocking its interaction with mast cells and basophils. Clinical trials in children and adults with severe asthma despite corticosteroids show good efficacy when omalizumab is given subcutaneously two to four times weekly.

Antibiotics

Although wheezing frequently occurs in infective exacerbations of COPD, there is no evidence that antibiotics are helpful in the management of patients with asthma. Yellow or green sputum containing eosinophils and bronchial epithelial cells may be coughed up in |acute exacerbations of asthma. This is normally due to viral, not bacterial, infection and antibiotics are not required. Occasionally, mycoplasma and chlamydia infections can cause chronic relapsing asthma. The use of appropriate antimicrobials is worthwhile only if a bacterial diagnosis has been established by culture or serology.

Management of asthma exacerbations
(Emergency box 14.2)

The term 'status asthmaticus' was defined as asthma that had failed to resolve with therapy in 24 hours. Although this term is still used occasionally, it has now been discarded and replaced by 'acute severe asthma', i.e. severe asthma that has not been controlled by the patient's use of medication.

Asthma attack

If the PEF is greater than 150 L/min, patients may improve dramatically on nebulized therapy and may not require hospital admission. Their regular treatment should be increased, to include treatment for 2 weeks with 30 mg of prednisolone followed by a gradual reduction in the

> **Emergency Box 14.2**
> **Treatment of severe asthma**
>
> **At home**
> 1. The patient is assessed. Tachycardia, a high respiratory rate and inability to speak in sentences indicate a severe attack.
> 2. If the PEFR is less than 150 L/min (in adults), an ambulance should be called. (All doctors should carry peak flow meters.)
> 3. Nebulized salbutamol 5 mg or terbutaline 10 mg is administered.
> 4. Hydrocortisone sodium succinate 200 mg i.v. is given.
> 5. Oxygen 40–60% is given if available.
> 6. Prednisolone 60 mg is given orally.
>
> **At hospital**
> 1. The patient is reassessed.
> 2. Oxygen 40–60% is given.
> 3. The PEFR is measured using a low-reading peak flow meter, as an ordinary meter measures only from 60 L/min upwards. Measure O_2 saturation with a pulse oximeter.
> 4. Nebulized salbutamol 5 mg or terbutaline 10 mg is repeated and administered 4-hourly.
> 5. Add nebulized ipratropium bromide 0.5 mg to nebulized salbutamol/terbutaline.
> 6. Hydrocortisone 200 mg i.v. is given 4-hourly for 24 hours.
> 7. Prednisolone is continued at 60 mg orally daily for 2 weeks.
> 8. Arterial blood gases are measured; if the $P_a co_2$ is greater than 7 kPa, ventilation should be considered.
> 9. A chest X-ray is performed to exclude pneumothorax.
> 10. One of the following intravenous infusions is given if no improvement is seen:
>   salbutamol 3–20 µg/min, or
>   terbutaline 1.5–5.0 µg/min, or
>   magnesium sulphate 1.2–2 g over 20 min.

oral dose and substitution by an inhaled corticosteroid preparation.

Patients with *acute severe asthma* typically have:

- inability to complete a sentence in one breath
- respiratory rate ≥ 25 breaths per minute
- tachycardia ≥ 110 beats/min (pulsus paradoxus, p. 736, is not useful as it is only present in 45% of cases)
- PEF < 50% of predicted normal or best.

Features of life-threatening attacks are:

- a silent chest, cyanosis or feeble respiratory effort
- exhaustion, confusion or coma
- bradycardia or hypotension
- PEF < 30% of predicted normal or best (approximately 150 L/min in adults).

Arterial blood gases should always be measured in asthmatic patients requiring admission to hospital. Pulse oximetry is useful in monitoring oxygen saturation during the admission and reduces the need for repeated arterial puncture. Features suggesting very severe life-threatening attacks are:

■ a high $P_aCO_2 > 6$ kPa

■ severe hypoxaemia $P_aO_2 < 8$ kPa despite treatment with oxygen

■ a low and falling arterial pH.

Treatment is commenced with 5 mg of nebulized salbutamol or 10 mg terbutaline with oxygen as the driving gas. Nebulized antimuscarinics (e.g. ipratropium bromide) are also helpful. A chest X-ray is taken to exclude a pneumothorax. If no improvement occurs with nebulized therapy, intravenous infusions of β-agonist (salbutamol or terbutaline 250 μg over 10 min) and/or magnesium sulphate (1.2–2 g over 20 min) should be used. Intravenous aminophylline is not now given as trials show no benefit. Hydrocortisone 200 mg i.v. should be administered 4-hourly for 24 hours, and 60 mg of prednisolone should be given orally daily. In patients who do not respond to this regimen, ventilation is often required.

Ideally, patients should be kept in hospital for at least 5 days, since the majority of sudden deaths occur 2–5 days after admission. During this time oxygen saturation should be monitored by oximetry. Oral prednisolone can be reduced from 60 mg to 30 mg once improvement occurs. Further reduction should be gradual on an outpatient basis until an appropriate maintenance dose or substitution by inhaled corticosteroid aerosols can be achieved.

Management of catastrophic sudden severe (brittle) asthma

This is an unusual variant of asthma in which patients are at risk from sudden death in spite of the fact that their asthma may be well controlled between attacks. Severe life-threatening attacks may occur within hours or even minutes. Such patients require a carefully worked out management plan agreed by respiratory physician, primary care physician and patient, and require:

■ emergency supplies of medications at home, in the car and at work

■ oxygen and resuscitation equipment at home and at work

■ nebulized β2 agonists at home and at work

■ self-injectable epinephrine (adrenaline): two Epipens of 0.3 mg epinephrine at home, at work and to be carried by the patient at all times

■ prednisolone 60 mg

■ Medic Alert bracelet.

On developing wheeze, the patient should attend the nearest hospital immediately. Direct admission to intensive care may be required.

Prognosis of asthma

Although asthma often improves in children as they reach their teens, it is now realized that the disease frequently returns in the second, third and fourth decades. In the past the data indicating a natural decrease in asthma through teenage years have led to childhood asthma being treated as an episodic disorder. However, airway inflammation is present continuously from an early age

and usually persists even if the symptoms resolve. Moreover, airways remodelling accelerates the process of decline in lung function over time. This has led to a reappraisal of the treatment strategy for asthma, mandating the early use of controller drugs and environmental measures from the time asthma is first diagnosed.

FURTHER READING

Barnes PJ (2000) New directions in allergic diseases: mechanism-based anti-inflammatory therapies. *Journal of Allergy and Clinical Immunology* **106**: 5–16.

Bousquet J et al. (2000) Asthma: from bronchoconstriction to airways inflammation and remodelling. *American Journal of Respiratory and Critical Care Medicine* **161**: 1720–1745.

British Thoracic Society (2000) Aspirin intolerance and related syndromes. *Thorax* **55** (Suppl 2): S1–S90.

British Thoracic Society (2003) British guideline on the management of asthma. *Thorax* **58** (Suppl 1): i1–i94.

Christiansen SC (2000) Day care siblings and asthma – please sneeze on my child. *New England Journal of Medicine* **343**: 574–575.

Chung KF, Godard P (2000) Difficult therapy-resistant asthma. *European Respiratory Reviews* **10**(69).

Holgate ST (2004) Lessons learnt from the epidemic of asthma. *Quarterly Journal of Medicine* **91**: 247.

Tattersfield AE et al. (2002). Asthma. *Lancet* **360**: 1313–1322.

Venables KM, Chan-Yeung M (1997) Occupational asthma. *Lancet* **349**: 1465–1469.

PNEUMONIA

Pneumonia may be defined as an inflammation of the substance of the lungs. It is usually caused by bacteria. Clinically it presents as an acute illness characterized in the majority of cases by the presence of cough, purulent sputum and fever together with physical signs or radiological changes compatible with consolidation of the lung. The advent of antibiotics has decreased dramatically the mortality from pneumonia among young people but it remains a dangerous condition. Pneumonia is a major cause of death in individuals over the age of 70 years. Bacterial pneumonia is more frequent in HIV-infected individuals than in the general population, particularly in HIV-infected intravenous drug users. The causative agents are the same as found in non-HIV community-acquired pneumonia.

Classification

Pneumonia can be classified both anatomically and on the basis of the aetiology.

Classification by site

Pneumonias are either localized, with the whole of one or more lobes affected, or diffuse, when they primarily affect the lobules of the lung, often in association with the bronchi and bronchioles – a condition referred to as 'bronchopneumonia'.

Table 14.13 The aetiology of pneumonia in the UK

Infecting agent	Frequency as a cause of pneumonia (%)	Clinical circumstances
Streptococcus pneumoniae	50	Community pneumonia patients usually previously fit
Mycoplasma pneumoniae	6	As above
Influenza A virus (usually with a bacterial component)	5	As above
Haemophilus influenzae	5	Pre-existing lung disease: COPD
Chlamydia pneumoniae	5	Community-acquired pneumonia
Chlamydia psittaci	3	Contact with birds (though not inevitable)
Staphylococcus aureus	2	Children, intravenous drug abusers, associated with influenza virus infections
Legionella pneumophila	2	Institutional outbreaks (hospitals and hotels), sporadic, endemic
Coxiella burnetii	1	Abattoir and animal-hide workers
Pseudomonas aeruginosa	< 1	Cystic fibrosis
Pneumocystis carinii		
Actinomyces israelii		
Nocardia asteroides	< 1	AIDS, lymphomas, leukaemias, use of cytotoxic drugs and corticosteroids
Cytomegalovirus		
Aspergillus fumigatus		
Anaerobic organisms	< 1	Inhalation pneumonia, alcohol abuse, postoperative
None isolated	20	–

Classification by aetiology

An aetiological factor can be discovered in approximately 75% of patients. The term 'atypical pneumonia' has been used to describe pneumonia caused by agents such as *Mycoplasma*, *Legionella*, *Chlamydia* and *Coxiella burnetii*. While these pneumonias can differ from pneumococcal disease, there is a considerable overlap in clinical presentation and as these agents account for almost one-fifth of the cases of pneumonia (Table 14.13), the term 'atypical' has been dropped. Pneumonias may also result from:

- chemical causes, such as in the aspiration of vomit (see p. 927)
- radiotherapy (see p. 944)
- allergic mechanisms (see p. 939).

Mycobacterium tuberculosis is a cause of pneumonia; it is considered separately (p. 930), since both its mode of presentation and its treatment are very different from the other infective agents.

Precipitating factors

- *Strep. pneumoniae* – often follows viral infection with influenza or parainfluenza.
- Hospitalized 'ill' patients – often infected with Gram-negative organisms.
- Cigarette smoking (the strongest independent risk factor for invasive pneumococcal disease).
- Alcohol excess.
- Bronchiectasis (e.g. in cystic fibrosis).
- Bronchial obstruction (e.g. carcinoma) – occasionally associated with infection with 'non-pathogenic' organisms.
- Immunosuppression (e.g. AIDS or treatment with cytotoxic agents) – organisms include *Pneumocystis*

carinii, *Mycobacterium avium-intracellulare*, cytomegalovirus.
- Intravenous drug abuse – frequently associated with *Staph. aureus* infection.
- Inhalation from oesophageal obstruction – often associated with infection with anaerobes.

Clinical features

The clinical presentation varies according to the immune state of the patient and the infecting agent. In the most common type of pneumonia – caused by *Strep. pneumoniae* – there is often a preceding history of a viral infection.

With *Strep. pneumoniae* infection the patient rapidly becomes more ill with a high temperature (up to 39.5°C), pleuritic pain and a dry cough. A day or two later, rusty-coloured sputum is produced and at about the same time the patient may develop labial herpes simplex. The patient breathes rapidly and shallowly, the affected side of the chest moves less, and signs of consolidation may be present together with a pleural rub. See Box 14.4 for severe community-acquired pneumonia.

Investigations

Chest X-ray confirms the area of consolidation (Fig. 14.35), but radiological changes lag behind the clinical course so that X-ray changes may be minimal at the start of the illness. Conversely, consolidation may remain on the chest X-ray for several weeks after the patient is clinically cured. The chest X-ray usually returns to normal by 6 weeks, except in patients with severe airflow limitation. Persistent changes on the chest X-ray after this time suggest a bronchial abnormality, usually a carcinoma, with persisting secondary pneumonia. Chest X-rays should rarely be repeated more frequently than at

Fig. 14.35 Chest X-ray showing lobar pneumonia.

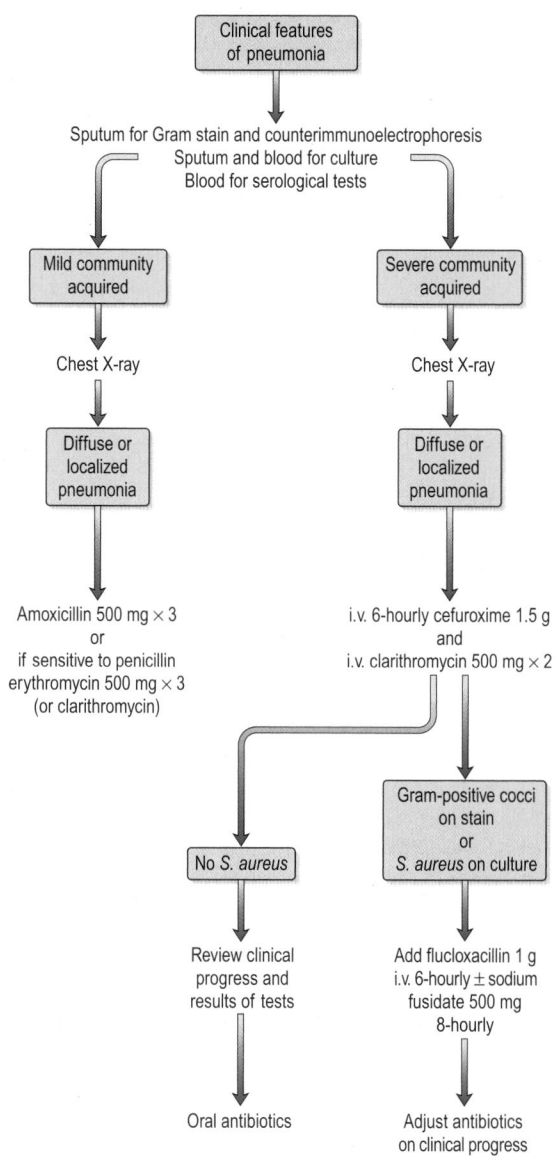

Fig. 14.36 Algorithm for the management of pneumonia (see also p. 928).

weekly intervals during the acute illness and then at 6 weeks after discharge from hospital.

In *Strep. pneumoniae* pneumonia, there is often a white blood cell count that is greater than $15 \times 10^9/L$ (90% polymorphonuclear leucocytosis) and an erythrocyte sedimentation rate (ESR) greater than 100 mm/h.

TYPES OF PNEUMONIA

The individual features of various pneumonias are given below. The overall investigation and management is shown in Figure 14.36 and discussed on page 928.

Mycoplasma pneumonia

Mycoplasma pneumonia is relatively common and occurs in cycles of 3–4 years. It often occurs in patients in their teens and twenties, frequently amongst those living in boarding institutions. Generalized features such as headaches and malaise often precede the chest symptoms by 1–5 days. Cough may not be obvious initially and physical signs in the chest may be scanty.

On chest X-ray, usually only one lobe is involved but sometimes there may be dramatic shadowing in both lungs. There is frequently no correlation between the X-ray appearances and the clinical state of the patient.

The white blood cell count is not raised. Cold agglutinins occur in half of the cases. The diagnosis is confirmed by a rising antibody titre. Treatment is with macrolides, e.g. erythromycin 500 mg four times daily for 7–10 days. Tetracycline is also effective.

Although most patients recover in 10–14 days, the disease can be protracted, with cough and X-ray changes lasting for weeks and relapses occurring. Lung abscesses and pleural effusions are rare.

Extrapulmonary complications can occur at any time during the illness and occasionally dominate the clinical picture. Most are rare but they include:

- myocarditis and pericarditis
- rashes and erythema multiforme
- haemolytic anaemia and thrombocytopenia
- myalgia and arthralgia
- meningoencephalitis and other neurological abnormalities
- gastrointestinal symptoms (e.g. vomiting, diarrhoea).

Viral pneumonia

Primary viral pneumonia is uncommon in adults, influenza A virus or adenovirus infection being the commonest causes. More often, viral infection predisposes patients to bacterial pneumonia by damaging the respiratory epithelium and facilitating bacterial infection.

Influenza A (HSNI) normally does not affect humans but recently has been transmitted from fowls (Avian flu), crossing the species barrier. Patients present with fever, breathlessness, cough (similar to the Hong Kong outbreak in 1997 – H5NI) and diarrhoea. Lymphopenia and thrombocytopenia are present and pulmonary infiltrates are seen on chest X-ray. There is a high mortality. Live poultry markets in Asian countries are the breeding ground, and mass culling of chicken and other poultry was performed in 1997, 1999 and 2004.

Severe acute respiratory syndrome (SARS) is due to a novel coronavirus (see p. 38). The incubation period is approximately 5 days with spread between humans mainly by droplet infection. The outbreak in 2003 affected many healthcare workers. Fever, malaise, headache and rigors were followed in the second week by cough, breathlessness and diarrhoea. Lymphopenia, thrombocytopenia and pulmonary infiltrates (mainly in the lower zones) occur. At the end of the second week 20% of patients deteriorate, developing ARDS, and the mortality is high.

Other pneumonias

Haemophilus influenzae

H. influenzae is a frequent cause of exacerbation of chronic bronchitis and can cause pneumonia in COPD patients. The pneumonia can be diffuse or confined to one lobe. There are no special features to separate it from other bacterial pneumonias. It responds well to treatment with oral amoxicillin 500 mg × 4 daily.

Chlamydia psittaci (see also p. 67)

Typically the individual has been exposed to infected birds, especially parrots, but cases may occur without a history of contact. The incubation period is 1–2 weeks and the disease may pursue a very low-grade course over several months. Symptoms include malaise, high fever, cough and muscular pains. The liver and spleen are occasionally enlarged, and scanty 'rose spots' may be seen on the abdomen. The chest X-ray shows segmental or a diffuse pneumonia. Occasionally the illness presents with a high, swinging fever and dramatic prostration with photophobia and neck stiffness that can be confused with meningitis. The diagnosis is confirmed by the demonstration of a rising titre of complement-fixing antibody. Macrolides or tetracycline are the antibiotics of choice.

Chlamydia pneumoniae

Outbreaks of *C. pneumoniae* have been reported in institutions and within families, suggesting person-to-person spread without any avian or animal reservoir. Serological tests on patients admitted to hospital with community-acquired pneumonia suggest that 5–10% may be the result of *C. pneumoniae* infection. In general, disease is mild with 50% of *C. pneumoniae* infections presenting as pneumonia, 28% as acute bronchitis, 10% with a flu-like illness and 12% with upper respiratory illnesses. Type-specific microimmunofluorescence tests are required to distinguish *C. pneumoniae* from *C. psittaci* and *C. trachomatis*. Treatment is with macrolides or tetracycline.

Staphylococcus aureus

Staph. aureus rarely cause pneumonia except after a preceding influenzal viral illness. The infection starts in the bronchi, leading to patchy areas of consolidation in one or more lobes, which break down to form abscesses. These may appear as cysts on the chest X-ray.

Pneumothorax, effusion and empyemas are frequent. Septicaemia develops with metastatic abscesses in other organs. All patients with staphylococcal pneumonia are very ill; intravenous antibiotics must be administered promptly, but are not always effective. Fulminating staphylococcal pneumonia can lead to death in hours.

Areas of pneumonia (septic infarcts) are also seen in staphylococcal septicaemia. This is frequently seen in intravenous drug abusers, and in patients with central catheters being used for parenteral nutrition. The infected puncture site is the source of the staphylococcus. Pulmonary symptoms are often few but breathlessness and cough occur and the chest X-ray reveals areas of consolidation. Abscess formation is frequent.

Diagnosis and treatment are shown in Figure 14.36.

Coxiella burnetii (Q-fever) (see also p. 78)

The patient develops systemic symptoms of fever, malaise and headache, often associated with multiple lesions on the chest X-ray. The illness may run a chronic course and is occasionally associated with endocarditis. Diagnosis is made by an increase in the titre of complement-fixing antibody. Treatment is usually with macrolides or tetracycline. Severe cases may require rifampicin.

Legionella pneumophila

Three epidemiological patterns of this disease are recognized:

- outbreaks among previously fit individuals staying in hotels, institutions or hospitals where the shower facilities or cooling systems have been contaminated with the organism
- sporadic cases where the source of the infection is unknown; most cases involve middle-aged and elderly men who are smokers, but it is also seen in children
- outbreaks occurring in immunocompromised patients, e.g. on corticosteroid therapy.

Legionella grows well in water up to 40°C in temperature, and the infection is almost certainly spread by the aerosol route. Adequate chlorination and temperature control of the water supply are necessary to prevent the disease.

The incubation period is 2–10 days. Males are affected twice as commonly as females. The infection may be mild, but the characteristic picture is of malaise, myalgia, headache and a fever with rigors and a pyrexia of up to 40°C. Half of the patients have gastrointestinal symptoms, with nausea, vomiting, diarrhoea and abdominal pain. Patients may be acutely ill, with mental confusion and other neurological signs. Haematuria occurs and occasionally renal failure.

The patient is tachypnoeic with an initially dry cough that later may become productive and purulent. The chest X-ray usually shows lobar and then multilobar shadowing, sometimes with a small pleural effusion. Cavitation is rare.

A strong presumptive diagnosis of *L. pneumophila* infection is possible in the majority of patients if they have three of the four following features:

- a prodromal virus-like illness
- a dry cough, confusion or diarrhoea
- lymphopenia without marked leucocytosis
- hyponatraemia.

Hypoalbuminaemia and high serum levels of liver aminotransferases are also common in this disease.

Diagnosis is confirmed by the direct immunofluorescent staining of the organism in the pleural fluid, sputum or bronchial washings. The organism is not seen on Gram staining. Culture on special media is possible but takes up to 3 weeks. A urinary antigen test is commercially available and is highly specific. Retrospective confirmation can be made by demonstrating a four-fold increase in antibody titre in the blood.

Treatment is usually with one of the macrolides, clarithromycin now being the drug of choice. Ciprofloxacin is also effective and rifampicin can be used in addition in ill patients. Mortality can be up to 30% in elderly patients but most patients recover fully.

Gram-negative bacteria

These are the cause of many hospital-acquired pneumonias but they are occasionally responsible for cases in the community.

Klebsiella pneumoniae

Pneumonia due to *Klebsiella* usually occurs in elderly people with a history of heart or lung disease, diabetes, alcohol excess or malignancy. The onset is often sudden, with severe systemic upset. The sputum is purulent, gelatinous or blood-stained. The upper lobes are more commonly affected and the consolidation is often extensive. There is often swelling of the infected lobe so that on the lateral chest X-ray there is bulging of the fissures. The organism can be found in the sputum or in the blood.

Treatment is dependent on the sensitivity of the organism, but a cephalosporin is usually required. The mortality is high, partly owing to the presence of the predisposing condition.

Pseudomonas aeruginosa

Pneumonia due to *Pseudomonas* is of considerable significance in patients with cystic fibrosis, since it correlates with a worsening clinical condition and mortality. It is also seen in patients with neutropenia following cytotoxic chemotherapy. The isolation of *P. aeruginosa* from sputum must be interpreted with care because the organism grows well on bacterial culture medium and may simply represent contamination from the upper airways.

Treatment. *Pseudomonas* and other Gram-negative infections respond well to treatment with the 4-quinolone antibiotic ciprofloxacin (200–400 mg i.v. over 30–60 minutes twice daily) or ceftazidime (2 g bolus i.v. 8-hourly). Ticarcillin (15–20 g daily i.v. infusion) and piperacillin are active against these bacilli. These penicillins are usually given in combination with an aminoglycoside, e.g. gentamicin or netilmicin, for maximum benefit.

Treatment regimens may have to be modified in the light of sensitivity testing. Aminoglycosides are nephrotoxic and ototoxic, so blood levels should be monitored (p. 995).

Moraxella catarrhalis

This organism has been found to be associated with exacerbations of COPD and occasionally with fatal pneumonia. Some strains produce a β-lactamase capable of destroying amoxicillin. The exact role of this organism in bronchopulmonary infection remains to be determined.

Anaerobic bacteria

Infections with these organisms usually occur in patients with an underlying condition, such as diabetes, and are often associated with aspiration. Bacteroides is the most common organism and is sensitive to metronidazole. The prognosis depends largely on the precipitating cause.

Pneumonias due to opportunistic infections

Immunocompromised patients develop pneumonia with all the usual organisms and with a number of organisms which do not normally cause illness in healthy hosts. However, with HAART (p. 143) the incidence of these infections has fallen dramatically in AIDS patients.

Pneumocystis carinii

This is by far the most common opportunistic infection, accounting for 50% of the cases of pneumonia in patients with acquired immunodeficiency syndrome (AIDS) (see p. 136) particularly when the CD4 lymphocyte count is $\leq 200/mm^3$. It is also seen in patients receiving immunosuppressive therapy. In the developing world, however, *Pneumocystis carinii* pneumonia (PCP) is not infrequently found in malnourished children. *P. carinii* is found in the air, and pneumonia arises from reinfection rather than reactivation of persisting organisms acquired in childhood. Clinically the pneumonia is associated with a high fever, breathlessness and dry cough. In patients with

AIDS, the clinical features are described on page 132. The typical radiographic appearance of PCP is of a diffuse bilateral alveolar and interstitial shadowing beginning in the perihilar regions and spreading out in a butterfly pattern. Other chest X-ray appearances include localized infiltration, nodules, cavitation or a pneumothorax. In patients receiving aerosolized pentamidine for prophylaxis, in countries where HAART is not available, infiltrates may be localized to the upper zones. Empirical treatment of PCP is justified in very sick high-risk cases, but wherever possible a firm diagnosis should be obtained by stimulation of sputum with hypertonic saline or fibreoptic bronchoscopy with bronchoalveolar lavage; the diagnosis can be made in 90% of cases by staining sputum using indirect immunofluorescence with monoclonal antibodies.

Other causes of shadowing on the chest X-ray in AIDS patients include:

- cytomegalovirus
- *M. avium-intracellulare*
- *M. tuberculosis*
- *L. pneumophila*
- *Cryptococcus*
- pyogenic bacteria
- Kaposi's sarcoma
- lymphoid interstitial pneumonia
- non-specific interstitial pneumonitis.

Treatment of PCP is with high-dose co-trimoxazole (see p. 136).

Actinomyces israelii (see also p. 90)
The clinical picture is that of severe pneumonia, lung abscess or empyema. Treatment is surgical drainage when appropriate, with high-dose intravenous penicillin for 4–6 weeks.

Nocardia asteroides
This produces a similar picture to *Actinomyces*, though of greater severity. The chest X-ray often shows irregular opacities in one or both lungs, particularly in the mid-zones. Treatment is with sulfadiazine in doses up to 9 g daily.

Cytomegalovirus (see also p. 46)
Bronchitis and pneumonia may occur but these are usually a more minor part of the generalized systemic illness.

Aspergillus fumigatus (see also p. 939)
This fungus gives rise to a widespread invasion of lung tissue in patients who are immunocompromised. It is a serious pneumonia that is usually rapidly fatal. Treatment is with amphotericin and flucytosine.

Mycobacterium avium-intracellulare (MAI)
This bacterium causes lung disease in patients with AIDS primarily as part of disseminated disease when CD4 lymphocyte counts are ≤ 100/mm^3, with the pulmonary complications being of less significance than the extrapulmonary involvement. Therapeutic regimens include combinations of rifabutin or rifampicin, with ethambutol, clofazimine and clarithromycin. Azithromycin and ciprofloxacin with rifabutin and ethambutol is also used.

Cryptococcus
Infection with this fungus is usually disseminated but pulmonary involvement includes intrathoracic lymph node enlargement and effusions.

Kaposi's sarcoma (see also pp. 142 and 1353)
This malignancy affecting HIV-infected homosexual men is seen rarely since the introduction of HAART (see p. 143). Intrathoracic involvement usually follows cutaneous manifestations and includes nodules or infiltrates in the lungs with lymph node enlargement and endobronchial lesions. Symptoms are those of progressive dyspnoea and cough. Chest X-ray appearances are non-specific. Bronchoscopy reveals multiple red or purple flat lesions which are not biopsied because of difficulty with histological diagnosis in crushed fragments and risk of haemorrhage. Treatment is with chemotherapy, vincristine 2 mg and bleomycin 10 mg/m^2 every 3 weeks.

Lymphoid interstitial pneumonia
This condition is more common in children than in adults and is characterized by infiltration with lymphocytes, plasma cells and immunoblasts. It is thought to be a viral pneumonia and causes diffuse reticulonodular infiltrates on the chest X-ray. Corticosteroid therapy appears to be of benefit, as is zidovudine.

Rare causes of pneumonia

Pneumonia may be seen as a minor feature in the course of infection by *Bordetella pertussis*, typhoid and paratyphoid bacillus, brucellosis, leptospirosis and a number of viral infections including measles, chickenpox and glandular fever. Details of these infections are described in Chapter 2.

Aspiration pneumonia

The acute aspiration of gastric contents into the lungs can produce an extremely severe and sometimes fatal illness owing to the intense destructiveness of gastric acid. This has been termed Mendelson's syndrome and can complicate anaesthesia, particularly during pregnancy.

In the absence of a tracheo-oesophageal fistula, aspiration occurs only during periods of impaired consciousness (e.g. during sleep), in reflux oesophagitis with an oesophageal stricture, or in bulbar palsy. Because of the bronchial anatomy, the most usual sites for spillage are the apical and posterior segments of the right lower lobe. The persistent pneumonia is often due to anaerobes and it may progress to lung abscess or even bronchiectasis. It is vital to identify any underlying problem, since appropriate corrective measures can lead to resolution of the pulmonary problems.

Treatment is discussed on page 929.

Cryptogenic organizing pneumonia (COP)

This condition, also called bronchiolitis obliterans organizing pneumonia (BOOP), is an organizing pneumonia of unknown aetiology. No infective agent has been described. Typically, patients present with single or recurrent episodes of malaise associated with cough, breathlessness and fever. Pleuritic chest pain is sometimes present but finger clubbing is very rare. Chest X-rays show confluent bilateral parenchymal shadowing. Lung function tests may show a restrictive defect. The white blood count is normal, but the ESR may be raised. Open lung biopsy will reveal characteristic buds of connective tissue in respiratory bronchioles and in alveolar ducts. These are diagnostic, but the diagnosis is usually made on history and X-ray appearances. The disease responds rapidly to corticosteroid treatment but may recur episodically especially in older women.

Diffuse pneumonia (bronchopneumonia)

Diffuse pneumonia is very common. It is differentiated from severe bronchitis by signs of bronchial breathing or patchy shadows on the chest X-ray. Widespread diffuse pneumonia is a common terminal event, resulting from an inability of patients dying from other conditions (e.g. cancer) to cough up retained secretions, allowing infection to develop throughout the lungs. Decisions on therapy will vary according to the particular clinical circumstances but aggressive antibacterial treatment is rarely appropriate.

GENERAL MANAGEMENT OF PNEUMONIA

Refer to the algorithm given in Figure 14.36. Sputum and blood should always be sent for culture but antibiotic treatment should not be delayed. Severe cases need to be admitted to hospital and a chest X-ray performed. Other investigations, e.g. blood gases, are useful to detect respiratory failure and provide a baseline for comparison if the patient deteriorates.

Further investigations may be necessary for the diagnosis of certain types of pneumonia:

- *Pneumococcal antigen* – counter-immunoelectrophoresis (CIE) of sputum, urine and serum (three to four times more sensitive than sputum or blood cultures)
- *Mycoplasma antibodies* (IgM and IgG) – in acute and convalescent samples – cold agglutinins present in 50%
- *Legionella and Chlamydia antibodies* – immunofluorescent tests
- *Legionella antigen* – in urine.

The choice of antibiotics is inevitably empirical, especially in those patients treated in the community. Empirical therapy is largely directed at *Strep. pneumoniae* infections. Apart from mycoplasma, the other pathogens are responsible for a small minority of infections. Acquired antibiotic resistance of common respiratory bacterial pathogens is recognized as a concern, but is still rare in the UK and

rarely causes clinical failure. There is no convincing evidence that newer antibiotics provide any significant therapeutic advantage over established therapies. For treatment of mild community-acquired pneumonia, oral amoxicillin remains the preferred agent, but should be given at a dose of at least 500 mg 8-hourly. Oral erythromycin (or clarithromycin, which is better tolerated) is an alternative choice for those sensitive to penicillin. For more severe cases treated in hospital, combined therapy with amoxicillin and a macrolide (erythromycin or clarithromycin) is recommended. When oral therapy is contraindicated, parenteral ampicillin or benzylpenicillin should be combined with clarithromycin. If *Staph. aureus* infection is suspected or is proven on culture, intravenous flucloxacillin ± sodium fusidate should be added. Fluoroquinolones are recommended for those intolerant of penicillins or macrolides. For severe cases, parenteral antibiotics should be given with the combination of a broad-spectrum lactamase-stable beta-lactam antibiotic (co-amoxiclav or cefuroxime) and clarithromycin. Parenteral antibiotics should be switched to oral once the temperature has settled for a period of 24 hours and provided there is no contraindication to oral therapy. The choice of antibiotics may be narrowed once microbiological results are available but it should be remembered that up to 10% of pneumonias may have mixed infections.

The overall mortality for patients admitted to hospital with community-acquired pneumonia is currently 5%, except for pneumonia due to *Staph. aureus* where it exceeds 25%. Patients who die from pneumonia usually have not received the appropriate antibiotics in sufficient doses before or during the early stages of hospital admission.

Box 14.4 shows features of *severe community-acquired pneumonia* which indicate a poorer prognosis. In spite of treatment in the intensive care unit, approximately 50% of such patients will die.

General measures

These include care of the mouth and skin. Fluids should be given to avoid dehydration. The patient is normally nursed sitting up or in the most comfortable position.

 Box 14.4 Criteria for the diagnosis of *severe community-acquired pneumonia*

Clinical features
- Respiratory rate ≥ 30/min
- Diastolic blood pressure ≤ 60 mmHg
- Confusion
- High mortality particularly in those > 65 years old
- Co-morbidity

Investigations
- Chest X-ray – more than one lobe involved
- $P_aO_2 < 8$ kPa
- Low albumin (< 35 g/L)
- White cell count (low $< 10^9$/L or high $> 20 \times 10^9$/L)
- Raised serum urea (> 7 mmol/L)
- Blood culture – positive

Cough should normally be encouraged, but if it is unproductive and distressing, suppressants such as codeine linctus can be given. Physiotherapy is needed to help and encourage the patient to cough. Pleuritic pain may require analgesia, but powerful analgesia (e.g. opiates) should be used with care because they cause respiratory depression. In severe hypoxia, oxygen therapy should be given. However, since the hypoxia is often due to a physiological shunt, it makes little difference to the hypoxaemia.

Hospital-acquired (nosocomial) pneumonias

Patients with mild forms of hospital-acquired pneumonias need to be reviewed carefully to make sure that there is nothing else responsible for their deterioration (e.g. heart failure, pulmonary embolism). Although very mild forms of hospital-acquired pneumonia may be treated with co-amoxiclav 500 mg three times daily, most cases will have co-morbidities which will dictate more aggressive anti-biotic therapy. These should be managed in the same way as severe community-acquired pneumonias once appropriate samples for culture and sensitivities have been taken. Gram-negative bacteria are common and treatment should normally include a third-generation cephalosporin (e.g. cefuroxime) and aminoglycosides (e.g. gentamicin). Patients with chronic chest infection and others in whom *Pseudomonas* infection is suspected should receive i.v. ciprofloxacin or ceftazidime. Immunosuppressed patients may require very high-dose broad-spectrum antibiotics as well as antifungal and antiviral agents. Aspiration pneumonia (p. 927) is relatively common in hospital and usually involves infection with multiple bacteria, including anaerobes. The oral route is usually inappropriate in these patients. A combination of metronidazole (intravenous or rectal) and either co-amoxiclav or cefuroxime i.v. is recommended.

COMPLICATIONS OF PNEUMONIA

Lung abscess

This term is used to describe severe localized suppuration in the lung associated with cavity formation on the chest X-ray, often with the presence of a fluid level, and not due to tuberculosis.

There are many causes of lung abscesses, but the most common is aspiration, particularly amongst alcohol abusers following aspiration pneumonia. Lung abscesses also frequently follow the inhalation of a foreign body into a bronchus and occasionally occur when the bronchus is obstructed by a bronchial carcinoma. Chronic or subacute lung abscesses follow an inadequately treated pneumonia.

Abscesses may develop during the course of specific pneumonias, particularly when the infecting agent is *Staph. aureus* or *Klebsiella pneumoniae*. Septic emboli, usually staphylococci, result in multiple lung abscesses. Infarcted areas of lung occasionally cavitate and rarely become infected. Amoebic abscesses may occasionally develop in the right lower lobe following transdiaphragmatic spread from an amoebic liver abscess.

The clinical features are those of persisting and worsening pneumonia associated with the production of large quantities of sputum, which is often foul-smelling owing to the growth of anaerobic organisms. There is usually a swinging fever; malaise and weight loss occur. The chest signs may be few but clubbing often develops if the condition is not rapidly cured. The patient is often anaemic with a high ESR.

Empyema

Empyema means the presence of pus within the pleural cavity. This usually arises from bacterial spread from a severe pneumonia or after the rupture of a lung abscess into the pleural space. Typically an empyema cavity becomes infected with anaerobic organisms and the patient is severely ill with a high fever and a neutrophil granulocytosis.

Investigations

Bacteriological investigation of lung abscess and empyema is best conducted on specimens obtained by transtracheal aspiration, bronchoscopy or percutaneous transthoracic aspiration with ultrasound or CT guidance. Bronchoscopy is helpful to exclude carcinomas and foreign bodies.

Treatment

Although anaerobic organisms are found in up to 70% of lung abscesses and empyemas, there is usually a mixed flora, often with aerobes, particularly *Strep. milleri*. Anaerobic cocci, black-pigmented bacteroids and fusobacteria are the anaerobes found most commonly.

Empyemas should be treated by prompt tube drainage or by rib resection and drainage of the empyema cavity under ultrasound control. Appropriate antibiotic treatment is given for up to 6 weeks. Antibiotics should be given to cover both aerobic and anaerobic organisms. An appropriate initial choice is cefuroxime 1 g i.v. 6-hourly and metronidazole 500 mg i.v. 8-hourly for 5 days, followed by oral cefaclor and metronidazole for a prolonged period depending on bacterial sensitivities. Abscesses occasionally require surgery.

FURTHER READING

British Thoracic Society (2001) BTS guidelines for the management of community acquired pneumonia in adults. *Thorax* **56** (Suppl 4): iv1–iv64.

British Thoracic Society (2002) BTS guidelines for the management of community acquired pneumonia in childhood. *Thorax* **57** (Suppl 1): i1–i24.

File TM (2003) Community acquired pneumonia. *Lancet* **362**: 1991–2001.

Lim WS (2004) Community acquired pneumonia. *Clinical Medicine* **4**(3): 224–228.

Low DE (2003) SARS – one year later. *New England Journal of Medicine* **349**: 2381–2382.

Weinstein RA (2004) Planning for epidemics – the lessons of SARS. *New England Journal of Medicine* **350**: 2332–2334.

Following many decades of decline, tuberculosis is on the increase in developed countries, because of AIDS, the use of immunosuppressive drugs which depress the host defence mechanisms, decreased socio-economic conditions, as well as increased immigration of persons from areas of high endemicity. In developing countries it is 20–50 times more common. There were 9 million new cases in 2000 world-wide. The major reason for this increase was because of the rapid rise in cases from sub-Saharan Africa (due to AIDS) and Russia.

Epidemiology

Tuberculosis is the world's leading cause of death from a single infectious disease, with two million deaths (without HIV infection) in 2000. This is the result of:

- inadequate programmes for disease control with poorly supervised treatment
- multiple drug resistance (MDR)
- co-infection with HIV
- a rapid rise in the world's population of young adults – the age group with the highest mortality from tuberculosis
- overcrowding and poor nutrition.

Tuberculosis is a notifiable disease in the UK; the number of cases is stable, with 6669 notifications in 2001. The incidence of tuberculosis in immigrants from the Asian subcontinent and from the West Indies is respectively forty and four times as common as in the native white population. This has led to great variation in the frequency of the disease in different areas of the UK.

Pathology

The first infection with *M. tuberculosis* is known as primary tuberculosis. It is usually subpleural, often in the mid to upper zones (Ghon focus). Within an hour of reaching the lung, tubercle bacilli reach the draining lymph nodes at the hilum of the lung and a few escape into the bloodstream.

The initial reaction comprises an exudative response and infiltration with neutrophil granulocytes. These are rapidly replaced by macrophages that ingest the bacilli. These interact with T lymphocytes, with the development of cellular immunity that can be demonstrated 3–8 weeks after the initial infection by a positive reaction in the skin to an intradermal injection of protein from tubercle bacilli (tuberculin/PPD). A delayed hypersensitivity-type reaction occurs, resulting in tissue necrosis, and at this stage the classical pathology of tuberculosis can be seen. Granulomatous lesions consist of a central area of necrotic material of a cheesy nature, called caseation, surrounded by epithelioid cells and Langhans' giant cells with multiple nuclei, both cells being derived from the macrophage. Lymphocytes are present and there is a varying degree of fibrosis. Subsequently the caseated areas heal completely and many become calcified. It is known that at least 20% of these calcified primary lesions contain tubercle bacilli, initially lying dormant but capable of being activated by depression of the host defence system. Reactivation leads to typical post-primary pulmonary tuberculosis with cavitation, usually in the apex or upper zone of the lung. 'Post-primary tuberculosis' refers to all forms of tuberculosis that occur after the first few weeks of the primary infection when immunity to the mycobacterium has developed.

Clinical features and investigations

Primary tuberculosis is symptomless in the great majority of individuals. Occasionally there may be a vague illness, sometimes associated with cough and wheeze. A small transient pleural effusion or erythema nodosum may occur, both representing hypersensitivity manifestations of the infective process.

Enlargement of lymph nodes compressing the bronchi can give rise to collapse of segments or lobes of the lung. Apart from cough and a monophonic wheeze, the individual remains remarkably well and the collapse disappears as the primary complex heals. Occasionally, persistent collapse can give rise to subsequent bronchiectasis, often in the middle lobe (Brock's syndrome).

The manifestations of primary and post-primary tuberculosis are shown in Figure 14.37, together with the times when they usually occur. Extrapulmonary manifestations are summarized on page 86. Miliary tuberculosis can occur within a year of the primary infection, or can occasionally occur much later as a manifestation of reactivation or, rarely, reinfection with tubercle bacillus.

Reactivation in the lung, or indeed in any extrapulmonary location, can occur as immunity wanes, usually with age or chronic ill-health. All manifestations are shown in Figure 14.37.

Miliary tuberculosis

This disease is the result of acute diffuse dissemination of tubercle bacilli via the bloodstream. It can be a difficult diagnosis to make, especially in older people, where it is particularly covert. This form of disseminated tuberculosis is universally fatal without treatment.

It may present in an entirely non-specific manner with the gradual onset of vague ill-health, loss of weight and then fever. Occasionally the disease presents as tuberculous meningitis. Usually there are no abnormal physical signs in the early stages, although eventually the spleen and liver become enlarged. Choroidal tubercles are seen in the eyes. These lesions are about one-quarter of the diameter of the optic disc and are yellowish and slightly shiny and raised in nature, later becoming white in the centre. There may be one or many in each eye.

The chest X-ray may be entirely normal in miliary tuberculosis as the tubercles are not visible until uniform miliary shadows 1–2 mm in diameter are seen throughout the lung; they have a hard outline. The lesions can increase in size up to 5–10 mm. Sarcoidosis and staphylococcal or *Mycoplasma* pneumonia can mimic the chest X-ray appearance of miliary tuberculosis. CT scanning may reveal lung parenchymal abnormalities at an earlier stage.

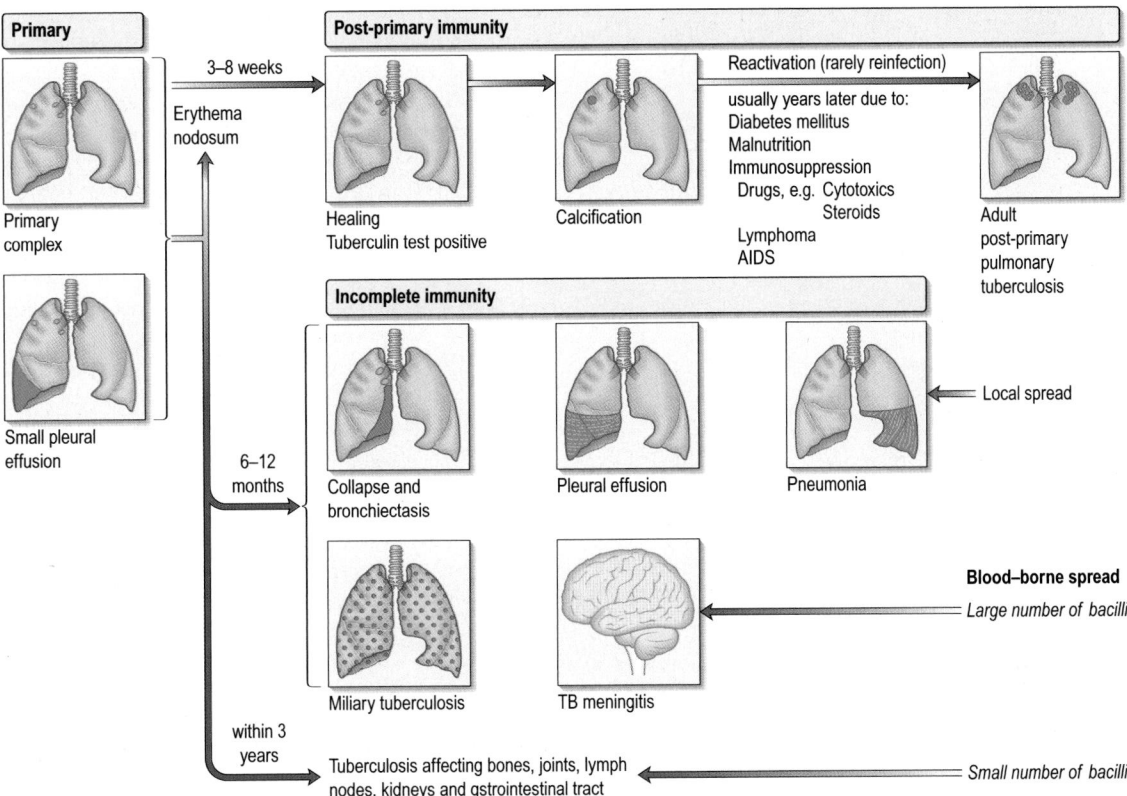

Fig. 14.37 Manifestations of primary and post-primary tuberculosis.

The Mantoux test is usually positive but may be negative in 30–50% of people with very severe disease. Trans-bronchial biopsies are frequently positive before any abnormality is visible on the chest X-ray.

Biopsy and culture of liver and bone marrow may be necessary in patients presenting with a pyrexia of unknown origin (PUO). A trial of antituberculous therapy can be used in individuals with a PUO. The fever should settle within 2 weeks of starting chemotherapy if it is due to tuberculosis. This approach is used in susceptible individuals when a diagnosis cannot be confirmed by other means.

Adult post-primary pulmonary tuberculosis

Typically there is gradual onset of symptoms over weeks or months. Tiredness, malaise, anorexia and loss of weight together with a fever and cough remain the outstanding features of pulmonary tuberculosis. Drenching night sweats are rather uncommon and are more usually due to anxiety. Sputum in tuberculosis may be mucoid, purulent or blood-stained. Many patients suffer a dull ache in the chest and it is not uncommon for patients to complain of recurrent colds. A pleural effusion or pneumonia can be the presenting feature of tuberculosis.

Physical examination reveals little. Finger clubbing is only present if the disease is advanced and associated with considerable production of purulent sputum. There are often no physical signs in the chest even in the presence of extensive radiological changes, though occasionally persistent crackles may be heard. Physical signs of an associated effusion, pneumonia or fibrosis may be present.

Chest X-ray

An abnormal chest X-ray is often found with no symptoms, but the reverse is extremely rare – pulmonary tuberculosis is unlikely in the absence of any radiographic abnormality.

The chest X-ray (Fig. 14.38) typically shows patchy or nodular shadows in the upper zones, loss of volume, and fibrosis with or without cavitation. Calcification may be present. The X-ray appearances alone can strongly suggest tuberculosis, but every effort must be made to obtain microbiological evidence. A single X-ray does not give an indication of the activity of the disease. Very similar chest X-ray appearances occur in histoplasmosis and other fungal infections of the lung, including cryptococcosis, coccidioidomycosis, blastomycosis and aspergillosis, as well as in bronchial carcinoma or cavitating pulmonary infarcts.

Lymph node presentation of tuberculosis

The patient presents with a tender lump or fluctuant mass, usually supraclavicular or in the anterior triangle of the neck.

This form of tuberculosis is discussed on page 87.

Tuberculosis in HIV-infected persons

(see also p. 140)

Tuberculosis in an HIV-infected person is an AIDS-

Fig. 14.38 Chest X-ray showing tuberculosis of left upper lobe with cavitation.

defining illness. Disease may arise from rapid progression of primary infection, by reactivation and by reinfection. The clinical pattern of disease is described on page 141. Treatment is with conventional therapy, but with four rather than three drugs, and it should be supervised (directly observed therapy short course, DOTS). Adverse drug reactions are common and the prognosis may be poor, especially if treatment is not supervised. Multiple drug resistance (MDR) occurs in about 6% of cases of tuberculosis in HIV-positive individuals.

Diagnosis

The diagnosis of tuberculosis is made on the basis of the following investigations:

- **Imaging**. Chest X-ray (see above), and CT scan if necessary.
- **Staining**. The sputum is stained with Ziehl–Neelsen (ZN) stain for acid and alcohol-fast bacilli (AAFB) or an auramine–phenol fluorescent test performed.
- **Culture**. The sputum is cultured on Ogana or Lowenstein–Jensen medium for 4–8 weeks. Liquid culture (Bactec (Becton–Dickinson)) is used in many laboratories and has the advantage of shorter culture times. Cultures to determine the sensitivity of the bacillus to antibiotics take a further 3–4 weeks.
- **Fibreoptic bronchoscopy** with washings from the affected lobes is useful if no sputum is available. This has replaced former techniques such as gastric washings. Transbronchial biopsies can also be obtained for histology and microbiological assessment.
- **Biopsies** of the pleura, lymph nodes and solid lesions within the lung (tuberculomas) may be required to confirm the diagnosis.

The slow growth of *M. tuberculosis* in culture has hindered the ability to make a rapid definitive diagnosis. Radiolabelled DNA and RNA probes specific for various mycobacterial species can identify organisms in culture. The sensitivity of these methods has been enhanced by amplifying target DNA using the polymerase chain reaction. This allows direct testing of sputum and other fluids to provide a laboratory diagnosis within 48 hours and may provide rapid information on the presence or absence of rifampicin resistance. This is still not entirely reliable and should not be accepted as a final diagnosis, particularly in the difficult case when it is most likely to be used. ELISA techniques have been developed which have high specificities, but unfortunately low sensitivity.

Treatment

Bed rest does not affect the outcome of the disease. Some patients will require hospitalization for a brief period; these include ill patients, smear-positive, highly infectious patients (particularly multidrug-resistant TB), those in whom the diagnosis is uncertain and those individuals from whom it is essential to gain cooperation. The most key factor in the successful treatment of tuberculosis is the continuous self-administration of drugs for 6 months; lack of patient compliance is a major reason why 5% of patients do not respond to treatment. In vitro resistance to one or more of the antituberculous drugs used to occur in fewer than 1% of patients in the UK, but the rate of resistance is gradually increasing (isoniazid resistance 4–6%, multidrug resistance 1%).

Directly observed therapy short course (DOTS)

In order to improve compliance, special clinics are used to supervise treatment regimens directly. Incentives to attend (e.g. free meals, cash payments) may be helpful. The effectiveness of DOTS is, however, variable in different countries and compliance is still a problem. Long-stay hospital treatment is required only for persistently uncooperative patients, many of whom are homeless and abuse alcohol.

Six-month regimen

Six-months' treatment with once-daily rifampicin 600 mg and isoniazid 300 mg is standard practice for patients with pulmonary and lymph node disease. (For those whose bodyweight is below 55 kg, rifampicin is reduced to 450 mg daily.) These are given as combination tablets and are taken 30 minutes before breakfast, since the absorption of rifampicin is influenced by food. This is supplemented for the first 2 months by pyrazinamide at a dose of 1.5 g (bodyweight < 50 kg) or 2.0 g daily. Pyrazinamide is of particular value in treating mycobacteria present within macrophages, and for this reason it may have a very valuable effect on preventing subsequent relapse. Pyridoxine 10 mg daily is given to reduce the risk of isoniazid-induced neuropathy. Current recommendations advise the addition of ethambutol (using 1 kg per day) if the risk of drug resistance is increased.

Longer regimens

Treatment of bone tuberculosis should be continued for a total of 9 months, and of tuberculous meningitis for

1 year. The drugs used are the same as for pulmonary tuberculosis, with pyrazinamide prescribed for the first 2 months only and for drug-resistant disease.

Drug-resistant organisms

The development of resistance after initial drug sensitivity (*secondary drug resistance*) occurs in patients who do not comply with the treatment regimens. *Primary drug resistance* is seen in immigrants to the UK and those exposed to others infected with resistant organisms. Multidrug resistance (MDR) is a major therapeutic problem with a high mortality and occurs mainly in HIV-infected patients. Nosocomial transmission of multidrug-resistant tuberculosis to healthcare workers and to other patients is recognized and poses a major public health problem. The drug treatment of suspected drug resistance in HIV-positive and HIV-negative patients is as follows:

- with multiple drug resistance use at least three drugs to which the organism is sensitive
- with resistance to one of the four main drugs, use the other three.

Therapy should be continued for up to 2 years and in HIV-positive patients for at least 12 months after negative cultures. Second-line drugs available for treatment of resistant *M. tuberculosis* are capreomycin, cycloserine, clarithromycin, azithromycin, ciprofloxacin, ofloxacin, ethionamide, kanamycin, amikacin, moxifloxacin and rifabutin.

Unwanted effects of drug treatment

Rifampicin induces liver enzymes, which may be transiently elevated in the serum of many patients. The drug should be stopped only if the serum bilirubin becomes elevated or if transferases are >3× elevated, which is uncommon. Thrombocytopenia has been reported. Rifampicin stains body secretions pink and the patients should be warned of the change in colour of their urine, tears (contact lens) and sweat. Induction of liver enzymes means that concomitant drug treatment may be made less effective (see Ch. 16). Oral contraception will not be effective, so alternative birth-control methods should be used. Rifabutin, a new rifamycin, is similar and is used for prophylaxis against *M. avium-intracellulare* complex infection in HIV patients with CD4 counts < 200 mm^3.

Isoniazid has very few unwanted effects. At high doses it may produce a polyneuropathy but this is extremely rare when the normal dose of 200–300 mg is given daily. Nevertheless, it is customary to prescribe pyridoxine 10 mg daily to prevent this effect. Occasionally, isoniazid gives rise to allergic reactions in the form of a skin rash and fever, with hepatitis occurring in fewer than 1% of cases. The latter, however, may be fatal if the drug is continued.

Pyrazinamide may cause hepatic toxicity, though this is much rarer with present dosage schedules. Pyrazinamide reduces the renal excretion of urate and may precipitate hyperuricaemic gout.

Ethambutol can cause a dose-related optic retrobulbar neuritis that presents with colour blindness for green, reduction in visual acuity and a central scotoma (commoner at doses of 25 mg/kg). This usually reverses provided the drug is stopped when symptoms develop; patients should therefore be warned of its effects. All patients prescribed the drug should be seen by an ophthalmologist prior to treatment and doses of 15 mg/kg should be used.

Streptomycin can cause irreversible damage to the vestibular nerve. It is more likely to occur in the elderly and in those with renal impairment. Allergic reactions to streptomycin are more common than to rifampicin, isoniazid and pyrazinamide. This drug is used only if patients are very ill, have multidrug-resistant TB or are not responding adequately to therapy.

Follow-up

Patients should be seen regularly for the duration of chemotherapy and once more after 3 months, since relapse, though very unlikely, usually occurs within this period of time. Patients with multidrug-resistant TB should be followed up for at least 1 year after treatment is completed.

Chemoprophylaxis

Patients who have any chest X-ray changes compatible with previous tuberculosis and who are about to undergo long-term treatment that has an immunosuppressive effect, such as renal dialysis or treatment with corticosteroids, should receive chemoprophylaxis with isoniazid 300–450 mg daily.

Prevention

BCG vaccination

Vaccination with BCG (bacille Calmette–Guérin) has been given to schoolchildren in the UK since 1954. BCG is live attenuated vaccine derived from *M. bovis* (a bovine strain of *M. tuberculosis*) that lost its virulence after growth in the laboratory for many passages. Early trials showed that it decreases the risk of developing tuberculosis by about 70%. With the continuing decrease in the incidence of tuberculosis in most parts of the UK it is becoming less cost-effective to administer this vaccine, and the procedure is being stopped in many areas of the UK. However, in other areas of the UK with a high immigrant population, the vaccine is being administered at birth rather than at the traditional age of 13 years. This is to prevent the disease from developing in young children, where it can progress extremely rapidly and in whom any delay in diagnosis can be fatal. BCG has been shown to be particularly effective in preventing miliary tuberculosis and tuberculous meningitis. In meta-analysis the protective efficacy is around 50%. However, the efficacy of BCG vaccination varies throughout the world from zero to 94% protection and appears to depend on latitude, being most beneficial in Norway, Sweden and Denmark (80–94%) and least so in the southern states of the USA and in India (0–20%). This lack of efficacy is thought to be related to a number of local factors including the frequency of infection with environmental mycobacteria (e.g. *M. fortuitum, M. kansasii*), which may induce a degree of protection similar to but not enhanced by BCG.

BCG is given only to individuals who are tuberculin-negative; those with positive tests are further screened by a chest X-ray. BCG should be given at a dose of 0.1 mL intradermally to children and adults, but at a dose of 0.05 mL to infants percutaneously.

Contact tracing

Tuberculosis is spread from person to person, and effective tracing of close contacts has helped to limit spread of the disease as well as to identify diseased individuals at an early stage. Screening procedures involve screening all close family members or other individuals who share the same kitchen and bathroom facilities. Close contacts at work or school may also be screened. Contacts who are ill should be thoroughly investigated for tuberculosis. If they are well, a chest X-ray is taken and a tuberculin test is performed (Practical box 14.5).

In adults, even if the tuberculin test is positive, provided the chest X-ray is negative nothing more need be done. Chemoprophylaxis should be considered in patients whose recent tuberculin conversion has been documented and for young adults (16–34 years) who are Heaf Grade 3–4 positive without BCG history and found at new immigrant screening. In patients with HIV infection, who have not had BCG, chemoprophylaxis with isoniazid is given, reducing the relative risk of developing active TB by 40% in highly endemic areas.

In children, a positive tuberculin test is usually taken as evidence of infection, and treatment is instituted. If the tuberculin test is negative in children and young adults (< 35 years), it is repeated at 6 weeks, and if it remains negative then BCG is administered. Children under the age of 1 year who have a family member with tuberculosis are given chemoprophylaxis with a daily dose of isoniazid 5–10 mg/kg for 6 months together with immunization with a strain of BCG that is resistant to isoniazid.

In general, in the UK much greater emphasis is placed on contact tracing and investigation of those under the age of 35 years and in some immigrant groups (African, Asian and Eastern European) in whom the disease is more prevalent.

Other mycobacteria

M. kansasii occurs in water and milk, though not in soil. Disease caused by this mycobacterium has mainly been described in Europe and the USA. It rarely causes a relatively benign type of human pulmonary disease, more common in HIV+ individuals, usually in middle-aged males. Men working in dusty jobs (e.g. miners) appear to be especially at risk, as are those who have underlying COPD. *M. avium-intracellulare* is a cause of pulmonary infection in AIDS patients (see p. 141).

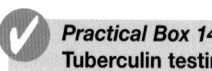

Practical Box 14.5
Tuberculin testing

Mainly used for:
- Contact tracing
- BCG vaccination programmes.

It is rarely of any value in the diagnosis of tuberculosis.

Patients are tested with:
- Purified protein derivative (PPD) of *Mycobacterium tuberculosis*.

The test is based on cell-mediated immunity with the development of induration and inflammation at the site of infection due to infiltration with mainly T lymphocytes. In patients with AIDS the test may be falsely negative owing to impairment of delayed hypersensitivity.

The Mantoux test
This is used for individual patients.

1. 0.1 mL of a 1 : 1000 strength PPD (equivalent to 10 tuberculin units) is injected intradermally.
2. The induration (not the erythema) is measured after 72 hours. The test is positive if the induration is 10 mm or more in diameter.

The Heaf test
This is a simple test used for large-scale screening.

1. A small amount of PPD (100 000 IU/mL) is placed on the flexor surface of the left forearm.
2. The 6-point disposable apparatus is actuated through the solution.
3. The Heaf reaction is graded 0–4 depending on the degree of induration: 0 and 1 (where there is only discrete induration at the puncture site) is a negative result after 3–10 days.

FURTHER READING
British Thoracic Society (2000) Management of opportunist mycobacterial infections. *Thorax* **55**: 210–218.
British Thoracic Society (2000) Control and prevention of tuberculosis in the UK. *Thorax* **55**: 887–901.
Elzinga G et al. (2003) Meeting targets in global tuberculosis control. *Lancet* **363**: 814–819.
Frieden TR et al. (2003) Tuberculosis. *Lancet* **362**: 887–899.
Small PM, Fujiwara PI (2001) Management of tuberculosis in the United States. *New England Journal of Medicine* **345**: 189–200.

DIFFUSE DISEASES OF THE LUNG PARENCHYMA

Diffuse parenchymal lung disorders (DPLD, also referred to as interstitial lung disease) are a heterogeneous group of disorders accounting for about 15% of respiratory clinical practice. Pathological features typically include inflammation of alveolar walls with fluid in alveolar air spaces leading to progressive bilateral destruction of the lung parenchyma.

GRANULOMATOUS LUNG DISEASE

A granuloma is a mass or nodule composed of chronically inflamed tissue formed by the response of the mononuclear phagocyte system (macrophage/histiocyte) to a slowly soluble antigen or irritant. If the foreign substance is inert (e.g. an inhaled dust), the phagocytes turn over slowly; if the substance is toxic or reproducing, the cells turn over faster, producing a granuloma. A granuloma is characterized by epithelioid multinucleate giant cells, as seen in tuberculosis. Granulomas are also seen in other infections, including fungal and helminthic, in sarcoidosis, and in extrinsic allergic alveolitis, and can also be due to foreign bodies (e.g. talc). Granulomatosis with pulmonary vasculitis is discussed on page 938.

Sarcoidosis

Sarcoidosis is a multisystem granulomatous disorder, commonly affecting young adults and usually presenting with bilateral hilar lymphadenopathy, pulmonary infiltration and skin or eye lesions. Beryllium poisoning can produce a clinical and histological picture identical to sarcoidosis, though contact with this element is now strictly controlled.

Epidemiology and aetiology

Sarcoidosis is a common disease of unknown aetiology that is often detected by routine chest X-ray. There is great geographical variation. The prevalence in the UK is approximately 19 in 100 000 of the population. It is common in the USA but is uncommon in Japan. The course of the disease is much more severe in American blacks than in whites. There is no relation with any histocompatibility antigen, but cases of sarcoidosis are seen within families, possibly suggesting an environmental factor. Other aetiological factors suggested are an atypical mycobacterium or fungus, the Epstein–Barr virus, and occupational, genetic, social or other environmental factors (a higher incidence occurs in rural than in urban populations). None of these has been substantiated.

Immunopathology

- Typical sarcoid granulomas consist of focal accumulations of epithelioid cells, macrophages and lymphocytes, mainly T cells.
- There is depressed cell-mediated reactivity to tuberculin and other antigens such as *Candida albicans*.
- There is overall lymphopenia: circulating T lymphocytes are low but B cells are slightly increased.
- Bronchoalveolar lavage shows a great increase in the number of cells; lymphocytes are greatly increased (particularly CD4 helper cells).
- The number of alveolar macrophages is increased but they represent a reduced percentage of the total number of bronchoalveolar lavage cells.
- Transbronchial biopsies show infiltration of the alveolar walls and interstitial spaces with leucocytes, mainly T cells, prior to granuloma formation.

It seems likely that the decrease in circulating T lymphocytes and changes in delayed hypersensitivity responses are the result of sequestration of lymphocytes within the lung. There is no evidence to suggest that patients with sarcoidosis suffer from an overall defect in cellular immunity, since the frequency of fungal, viral and bacterial infections is not increased and there is no substantiated evidence of a greater risk of developing malignant neoplasms.

Clinical features

The peak incidence is in the third and fourth decades, with a female preponderance. Sarcoidosis can affect many different organs of the body. The most common presentation is with respiratory symptoms or abnormalities found on chest X-ray (50%). Fatigue or weight loss occurs in 5%, peripheral lymphadenopathy in 5% and a fever in 4%. A chest X-ray may be negative in up to 20% of non-respiratory cases, though lesions may be detected later.

Bilateral hilar lymphadenopathy

This is a characteristic feature of sarcoidosis. It is often symptomless and simply detected on a routine chest X-ray. Occasionally, the bilateral hilar lymphadenopathy is associated with a dull ache in the chest, malaise and a mild fever.

Although the chest X-ray may not show any evidence of infiltration in the lung fields, evidence from CT scanning (Fig. 14.39), transbronchial biopsies and bronchoalveolar lavage indicates that the lung parenchyma is nearly always involved.

The differential diagnosis of bilateral hilar lymphadenopathy includes:

- lymphoma – though it is rare for this to affect only the hilar lymph nodes
- pulmonary tuberculosis – though it is rare for the hilar lymph nodes to be symmetrically enlarged
- carcinoma of the bronchus with malignant spread to the contralateral hilar lymph nodes – again it is rare for this to give rise to a typical symmetrical picture.

In the early stages it may be difficult to distinguish enlarged lymph nodes on the chest X-ray from the pulmonary arteries, and lymph node enlargement is not always symmetrical. It is for these reasons that, in the

Fig. 14.39 **CT scan in sarcoidosis.** Note enlarged glands at the hilum (black arrow) and nodular shadowing, particularly in right middle lobe (white arrow).

absence of erythema nodosum (see below), further confirmation of the disease process is advisable.

Pulmonary infiltration

This type of sarcoidosis may be progressive and may lead to increasing effort dyspnoea and eventually cor pulmonale and death. The chest X-ray shows a mottling in the mid-zones proceeding to generalized fine nodular shadows. Eventually, widespread pulmonary line shadows develop, reflecting the underlying fibrosis. A honeycomb appearance can occasionally occur. Pulmonary function tests show a typical restrictive lung defect (see below).

The combination of pulmonary infiltration and normal lung function tests is highly suggestive of sarcoidosis. The principal differential diagnoses are tuberculosis, pneumoconiosis, cryptogenic fibrosing alveolitis and alveolar cell carcinoma. However, these other conditions do have their own X-ray appearances and usually cause both symptoms and abnormal lung function tests.

Extrapulmonary manifestations

Skin and ocular sarcoidosis are the most common extrapulmonary presentations.

Skin lesions occur in 10% of cases. Sarcoidosis is the most common cause of erythema nodosum (see p. 1341). The association of bilateral symmetrical hilar lymphadenopathy with erythema nodosum occurs only in sarcoidosis. A chilblain-like lesion known as lupus pernio is also seen, as are skin nodules (see p. 1345).

Ocular and associated effects. Anterior uveitis is common and may present with misting of vision, pain and a red eye, but posterior uveitis may present simply as progressive loss of vision. Although ocular sarcoidosis accounts for about 5% of uveitis presenting to ophthalmologists, evidence of asymptomatic uveitis may be found in up to 25% of patients with sarcoidosis. Conjunctivitis may occur and retinal lesions have also been reported. *Uveoparotid fever* is a syndrome of bilateral uveitis and parotid gland enlargement together with occasional development of facial nerve palsy and is sometimes seen with sarcoidosis.

Keratoconjunctivitis sicca and lacrimal gland enlargement may also occur.

Metabolic manifestations. It is rare for sarcoidosis to present with problems of calcium metabolism, though hypercalcaemia is found in 10% of established cases. Hypercalcaemia and hypercalciuria can lead to the development of renal calculi and nephrocalcinosis. The cause of the hypercalcaemia is due to an increase in circulating 1,25-dihydroxyvitamin D_3, with 1α-hydroxylation occurring in sarcoid macrophages in the lung in addition to that taking place in the kidney.

The central nervous system. Involvement of the central nervous system (CNS) is rare (2%) but can lead to severe neurological disease (see p. 1242).

Bone and joint involvement. Arthralgia without erythema nodosum is seen in 5% of cases. Bone cysts are found, particularly in the digits, with associated swelling. In the absence of swelling, routine X-rays of the hands are unnecessary.

Hepatosplenomegaly Sarcoidosis is a cause of hepatosplenomegaly, though it is rarely of any clinical consequence. A liver biopsy is occasionally performed when the diagnosis is in doubt and shows granulomas.

Cardiac involvement. Cardiac involvement is rare (3%). Ventricular dysrhythmias, conduction defects and cardiomyopathy with congestive cardiac failure are seen.

Investigations

- **Imaging**. Chest X-ray (see above). CT is useful for assessment of diffuse lung involvement.
- **Full blood count**. There is mild normochromic, normocytic anaemia with raised ESR.
- **Serum biochemistry**. Serum calcium is often raised and there is hypergammaglobulinaemia.
- **Transbronchial biopsy** is the most useful investigation. Positive results are seen in 90% of cases of pulmonary sarcoidosis with or without X-ray evidence of lung involvement. Pulmonary non-caseating granulomas are found in approximately one-half of patients with clinically extrapulmonary sarcoidosis in whom the chest X-ray is normal.
- **Serum level of angiotensin-converting enzyme (ACE)** is two standard deviations above the normal mean value in over 75% of patients with untreated sarcoidosis. Raised (but lower) levels are also seen in patients with lymphoma, pulmonary tuberculosis, asbestosis and silicosis, limiting the diagnostic value of the test. However, the test is useful in assessing the activity of the disease and therefore as a guide to treatment with corticosteroids. Reduction of serum ACE during treatment with corticosteroids does not, however, reflect resolution of the disease.
- **Lung function tests** show a restrictive lung defect in patients with pulmonary infiltration. There is a decrease in TLC, a decrease in both FEV_1 and FVC, and a decrease in gas transfer.
- **The tuberculin skin test** is negative in 80% of patients with sarcoidosis; this is of interest but has no diagnostic value.

Treatment

Both the need to treat and the value of corticosteroid therapy are contested in many aspects of this disease. Hilar lymphadenopathy on its own with no evidence on chest X-ray of involvement of the lungs or decrease in lung function tests does not require treatment. Persisting infiltration on the chest X-ray or abnormal lung function tests are unlikely to improve without corticosteroid treatment. If the disease is not improving spontaneously 6 months after diagnosis, treatment should be started with prednisolone 30 mg for 6 weeks, reducing to alternate-day treatment with prednisolone 15 mg for

6–12 months. Although there have been no controlled trials that have proved the efficacy of such treatment, it is difficult to withhold corticosteroids when there is continuing deterioration of lung function. Systemic prednisolone should be given to patients with involvement of the eyes or persistent hypercalcaemia.

If the erythema nodosum of sarcoidosis is severe or persistent it will respond rapidly to a 2-week course of prednisolone 5–15 mg daily, as will patients with uveoparotid fever. Myocardial sarcoidosis and neurological manifestations are also treated with prednisolone.

Prognosis

Sarcoidosis is a much more severe disease in certain racial groups, particularly American blacks, where death rates of up to 10% have been recorded. It is probable that the disease is fatal in fewer than 5% of cases in the UK, most often as a result of respiratory failure and cor pulmonale but, rarely, from myocardial sarcoidosis and renal damage. The chest X-ray provides a guide to prognosis. The disease remits within 2 years in over two-thirds of patients with hilar lymphadenopathy alone, in approximately one-half with hilar lymphadenopathy plus chest X-ray evidence of pulmonary infiltration, but in only one-third of patients with X-ray evidence of infiltration without any demonstrable lymphadenopathy. Lung function tests are the most useful way to monitor progression.

Langerhans' cell histiocytosis (LCH)

This rare disease (a prevalence of 1 per 50 000) is characterized histologically by proliferation of LCH cells identified by the presence of Birbeck granules on electron-microscopy or the CD_{1a} antigen on the surface of the cells. There is a wide variation in clinical presentation, from unifocal bone lesions in older children (which may regress spontaneously), to more disseminated disease in younger children (with a high mortality). Chest X-rays show multiple small cysts (honeycomb lung), fibrosis or widespread nodular shadows. Etoposide treatment is justified for advanced progressive disease.

PULMONARY VASCULITIS AND GRANULOMATOSIS

The classification of pulmonary vasculitis and granulomatous disorders is unsatisfactory. In broad terms it is reasonable to consider two main groups: the respiratory manifestations of systemic connective tissue diseases, and disorders associated with the presence of antineutrophil cytoplasmic antibodies (ANCAs).

Pulmonary vasculitis with connective tissue disease

Rheumatoid disease (see also p. 559)

The features of respiratory involvement in rheumatoid disease are illustrated in Figure 14.40.

Pleural adhesions, thickening and effusion are the most common lesions. The effusion is often unilateral and

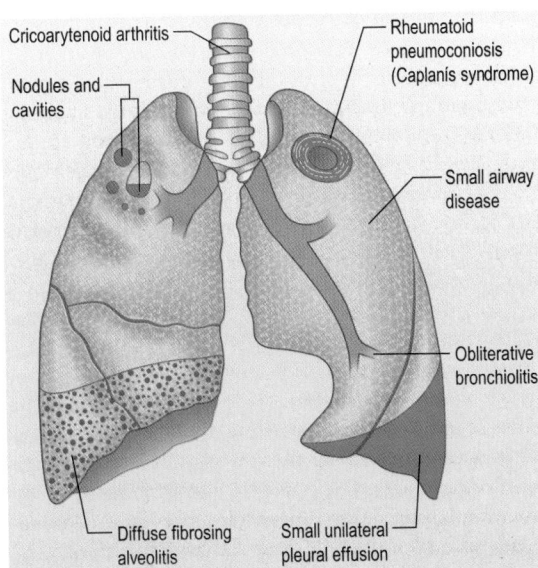

Fig. 14.40 **Respiratory manifestations of rheumatoid disease.**

tends to be chronic. It has a low glucose content but this can occur in any chronic pleural effusion. Several forms of parenchymal disease can occur in patients with rheumatoid arthritis. These include fibrosing alveolitis, rheumatoid nodules, cryptogenic organizing pneumonia, and lymphoid interstitial pneumonia. Moreover, some patients will have modified presentations because they are already on disease-modifying drugs such as prednisolone or methotrexate for their arthritis.

Fibrosing alveolitis occurring in rheumatoid arthritis can be considered as a variant of the cryptogenic form of the disease (see p. 941). The clinical features and gross appearance are the same but the disease is often more chronic. Rheumatoid nodules appear on the chest X-ray as single or multiple nodules ranging in size from a few millimetres to a few centimetres. The nodules frequently cavitate. They usually produce no symptoms but can give rise to a pneumothorax or pleural effusion.

Obliterative disease of the small bronchioles is rare. It is characterized by progressive breathlessness and irreversible airflow limitation. Corticosteroids may prevent progression. Cricoarytenoid joint involvement by rheumatoid arthritis gives rise to dyspnoea, stridor, hoarseness and occasionally severe obstruction necessitating tracheostomy. *Caplan's syndrome* is due to a combination of dust inhalation and the disturbed immunity of rheumatoid arthritis. It occurs particularly in coalworker's pneumoconiosis but it can occur in individuals exposed to other dusts, such as silica and asbestos. Typically the lesions appear as rounded nodules 0.5–5.0 cm in diameter, though sometimes they become incorporated into large areas of fibrosis that are indistinguishable radiologically from progressive massive fibrosis. There may not be much evidence of simple pneumoconiosis prior to the development of the nodule. These lesions may precede the development of the arthritis. Rheumatoid factor is always present in the serum.

Systemic lupus erythematosus (see also p. 575)

Pleurisy is the most common respiratory manifestation of this disease, occurring in up to two-thirds of cases, with or without an effusion. Effusions are usually small and bilateral. Basal pneumonitis is often present, perhaps as a result of poor movement of the diaphragm, or restriction of chest movements because of pleural pain. Pneumonia also occurs, because of either infection or the disease process itself. In contrast to rheumatoid arthritis, diffuse pulmonary fibrosis is rare.

Systemic sclerosis (see pp. 577 and 1343)

Autopsy studies have indicated that there is almost always some diffuse fibrosis of alveolar walls and obliteration of capillaries and the alveolar space. Severe changes result in nodular then streaky shadowing on the chest X-ray, followed by cystic changes, ending up with a honeycomb lung. Lung function tests reveal a restrictive defect and poor gas transfer. Pneumonia may occur owing to aspiration from the dilated oesophagus (see p. 927). Breathlessness may be worsened by restriction of chest wall movement owing to thickening and contraction of the skin and trunk.

Granulomatous vasculitides

Antineutrophil cytoplasmic antibodies
(see also pp. 534 and 633)

Antineutrophil cytoplasmic antibodies (ANCAs) are found in the acute phase of vasculitides, particularly Wegener's granulomatosis, Churg–Strauss syndrome and microscopic polyangiitis (polyarteritis) associated with neutrophil infiltration of the vessel wall.

Two major ANCA reactivities are recognized: proteinase-3 (PR3) ANCA and myeloperoxidase (MPO) ANCA.

About 10% of all vasculitis patients are ANCA-negative: this is more common in Wegener's granulomatosis limited to the upper respiratory tract. Ten to fifteen per cent of cases of progressive glomerulonephritis with anti-glomerular basement membrane (GBM) antibodies are MPO ANCA-positive and these are the most likely to suffer pulmonary haemorrhage.

Wegener's granulomatosis

This granulomatous disease of unknown aetiology is one of the primary systemic vasculitides in which the small arteries are predominantly affected (the other is the Churg–Strauss syndrome, see below). It is characterized by lesions involving the upper respiratory tract, the lungs and the kidneys. Often the disease starts with severe rhinorrhoea with subsequent nasal mucosal ulceration followed by cough, haemoptysis and pleuritic pain. Occasionally there may be involvement of the skin and nervous system. A chest X-ray usually shows single or multiple nodular masses or pneumonic infiltrates with cavitation. The most remarkable radiographic feature is the migratory pattern, with large lesions clearing in one area and new lesions appearing in another. The typical histological changes are usually best

seen in the kidneys, where there is a necrotizing micro-vascular glomerulonephritis. This disease responds well to treatment with cyclophosphamide 150–200 mg daily. A variant of Wegener's granulomatosis called 'midline granuloma' affects the nose and paranasal sinuses and is particularly mutilating; it has a poor prognosis.

The Churg–Strauss syndrome

This condition occurs in patients, usually males in their fourth decade, who have a triad of rhinitis and asthma, eosinophilia and systemic vasculitis. The aetiology is uncertain, with some believing that it represents an unusual progression of allergic disease in a subset of predisposed individuals. Others believe it is a primary vasculitis which presents like asthma because of the involvement of eosinophils.

The pathology of this condition is dominated by an eosinophilic infiltration with a characteristic high blood eosinophil count, vasculitis of small arteries and veins, and extravascular granulomas. Typically it involves the lungs, peripheral nerves and skin but kidney involvement is uncommon. Transient patchy pneumonia-like shadows may occur, but sometimes these can be massive and bilateral. Skin lesions include tender subcutaneous nodules as well as petechial or purpuric lesions. ANCA is usually positive. The disease responds well to corticosteroids. Occasionally Churg–Strauss syndrome may be revealed when oral steroids are withdrawn in patients being treated for asthma. There is no reason to think that other anti-asthma drugs precipitate the condition.

Microscopic vasculitis (polyangiitis)

This involves the kidneys and the lungs where it results in recurrent haemoptysis. ANCA is usually positive. In the early literature there was confusion between this condition, the Churg–Strauss syndrome and polyarteritis nodosa. The latter, however, is ANCA-negative and rarely involves the lungs.

PULMONARY INFILTRATION WITH EOSINOPHILIA

The common types and characteristics of these diseases are shown in Table 14.14. They range from very mild, simple, pulmonary eosinophilias to the often fatal hypereosinophilic syndrome.

Simple and prolonged pulmonary eosinophilia

Simple pulmonary eosinophilia is a relatively mild illness with a slight fever and cough and usually lasting for less than 2 weeks. Occasionally, the disease becomes more prolonged, with a high fever lasting for over a month. There is usually an eosinophilia in the blood and this condition is then called prolonged pulmonary eosinophilia. In both conditions the chest X-ray shows either localized or diffuse opacities. The simple form is probably due to a transient allergic reaction in the alveoli. Many allergens have been implicated, including *Ascaris lumbricoides*,

Table 14.14 Common types and characteristics of pulmonary infiltration with eosinophilia

Disease	Symptoms	Blood eosinophils (%)	Multisystem involvement	Duration	Outcome
Simple pulmonary eosinophilia	Mild	10	None	< 1 month	Good
Prolonged pulmonary eosinophilia	Mild/moderate	> 20	None	> 1 month	Good
Asthmatic bronchopulmonary eosinophilia	Moderate/severe	5–20	None	Years	Fair
Tropical pulmonary eosinophilia	Moderate/severe	> 20	None	Years	Fair
Hypereosinophilic syndrome	Severe	> 20	Always	Months/years	Poor

Ankylostoma, Trichuris, Trichinella, Taenia and *Strongyloides*. Drugs such as aspirin, penicillin, nitrofurantoin and sulphonamides have been implicated. Often, no allergen is identified. The disease is self-limiting and no treatment is required, apart from treating the cause. In the more chronic form all unnecessary treatment should be withdrawn and where appropriate, worms are treated. Corticosteroid therapy is indicated, with resolution of the disease over the ensuing weeks.

Asthmatic bronchopulmonary eosinophilia

This is characterized by the presence of asthma, transient fleeting shadows on the chest X-ray, and blood or sputum eosinophilia. By far the most common cause world-wide is allergy to *A. fumigatus* (see below), although *Candida albicans* and other mycoses may be the allergen in a small number of patients. In many, no allergen can be identified. Whether these cases are intrinsic or driven by an unidentified extrinsic factor is uncertain.

Diseases caused by *Aspergillus fumigatus*

The various types of lung disease caused by *A. fumigatus* are illustrated in Figure 14.41.

The spores of *A. fumigatus* (diameter 5 mm) are readily inhaled and are present in the atmosphere throughout the year, though they are at their highest concentration in the late autumn. They can be grown from the sputum in up to 15% of patients with chronic lung disease in whom they do not produce disease. They are a cause of extrinsic asthma in atopic individuals.

Allergic bronchopulmonary aspergillosis

In this rare disease, *Aspergillus* actually grows in the walls of the bronchi and eventually produces proximal bronchiectasis. There are episodes of eosinophilic pneumonia throughout the year, particularly in late autumn and winter. The episodes present with a wheeze, cough, fever and malaise. They are associated with expectoration of firm sputum plugs containing the fungal mycelium, which results in the clearing of the pulmonary infiltrates on the chest X-ray. Occasionally the large mucus plugs obliterate the bronchial lumen, causing collapse of the lung.

Left untreated, repeated episodes of eosinophilic pneumonia can result in progressive pulmonary fibrosis

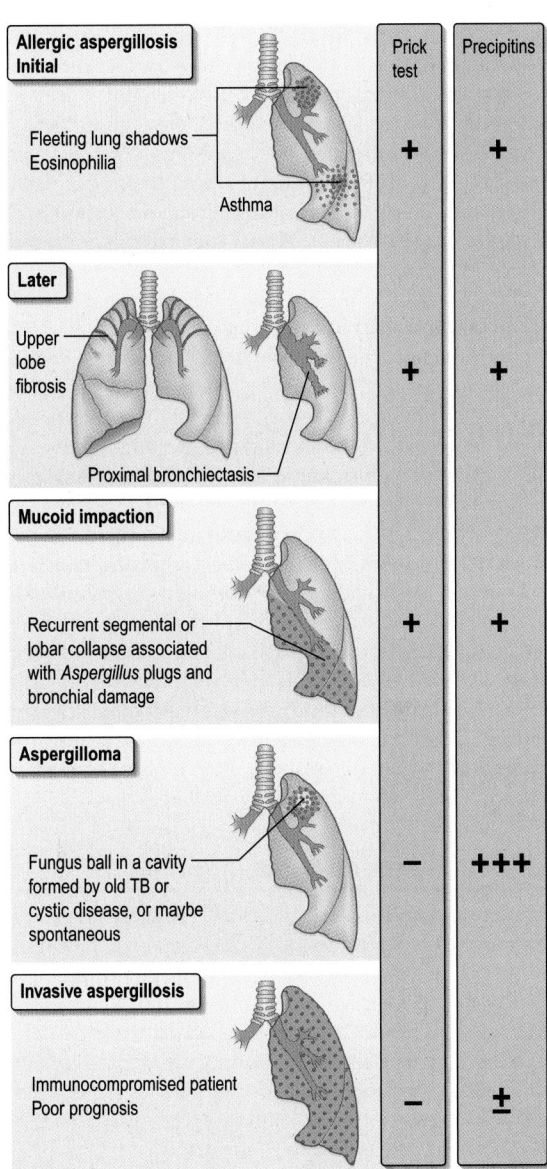

Fig. 14.41 Diseases caused by *Aspergillus fumigatus*.

that usually affects the upper zones and can give rise to a chest X-ray appearance similar to that produced by tuberculosis.

The peripheral blood eosinophil count is usually raised, and total levels of IgE are usually extremely high (both that specific to *Aspergillus* and non-specific). Skin-prick testing to protein allergens from *A. fumigatus* gives rise to positive immediate skin tests. Sputum may show eosinophils and mycelia, and precipitating antibodies are usually, but not always, found in the serum.

Lung function tests show a decrease in lung volumes and gas transfer in more chronic cases, but evidence of reversible airflow limitation can be demonstrated in all cases.

Treatment is with prednisolone 30 mg daily, which causes rapid clearing of the pulmonary infiltrates. Frequent episodes of the disease can be prevented by long-term treatment with prednisolone, but doses of 10–15 mg daily are usually required. Several antifungal agents have been tried in the past without success, but there is now some evidence that treatment with itraconazole helps. The asthma component responds to inhaled corticosteroids, although they do not influence the occurrence of pulmonary infiltrates.

Aspergilloma and invasive aspergillosis

Aspergilloma is the growth of *A. fumigatus* within previously damaged lung tissue where it forms a ball of mycelium within lung cavities. Typically the chest X-ray shows a round lesion with an air 'halo' above it. Continuing antigenic stimulation gives rise to large quantities of precipitating antibody in the serum. The aspergilloma itself causes little trouble, though occasionally massive haemoptysis may occur, requiring resection of the area of damaged lung containing the aspergilloma. Antifungal agents, such as amphotericin, have been tested in aspergilloma, but with little success. Invasive aspergillosis is a well-recognized complication of immunosuppression and requires aggressive antifungal therapy usually with i.v. amphotericin (250 μg/kg daily). Itraconazole or variconazole is used if amphotericin is ineffective, and caspofungin may also work.

Tropical pulmonary eosinophilia

This term is reserved for an allergic reaction to microfilaria from *Wuchereria bancrofti*. The condition is seen in the Asian subcontinent and presents with cough and wheeze together with fever, lassitude and weight loss. The typical appearance of the chest X-ray is of bilateral hazy mottling that is often uniformly distributed in both lung fields. Individual shadows may be as large as 5 mm or may become more confluent, giving the appearance of pneumonia.

The disease is characterized by a very high eosinophil count in peripheral blood. The filarial complement fixation test is positive in almost every case, although the microfilaria are seldom found. The treatment of choice is diethylcarbamazine (see p. 108 for details).

The hypereosinophilic syndrome

This disease is characterized by eosinophilic infiltration in various organs, sometimes associated with an eosinophilic arteritis. The heart muscle is particularly involved, but pulmonary involvement in the form of a pleural effusion or interstitial lung disease occurs in about 40% of cases. Typical features are fever, weight loss, recurrent abdominal pain, persistent non-productive cough and congestive cardiac failure. Corticosteroid treatment may be of value in some cases.

GOODPASTURE'S SYNDROME AND IDIOPATHIC PULMONARY HAEMOSIDEROSIS

Goodpasture's syndrome (see also p. 632)

The disease often starts with symptoms of an upper respiratory tract infection followed by cough and intermittent haemoptysis, tiredness and eventually anaemia, although massive bleeding may occur. The chest X-ray shows transient blotchy shadows that are due to intrapulmonary haemorrhage. These features usually precede the development of an acute glomerulonephritis by several weeks or months. The course of the disease is variable: some patients spontaneously improve while others proceed to renal failure.

The disease usually occurs in individuals over 16 years of age. It is due to a type II cytotoxic reaction driven by antibodies directed against the basement membrane of both kidney and lung. It has been proposed that there may be a shared antigen. ANCA may be positive. An association with influenza A2 virus has been reported.

Treatment is with corticosteroids, but in some cases dramatic improvement has been seen with plasmapheresis to remove the autoantibodies.

Idiopathic pulmonary haemosiderosis

This is clinically similar to Goodpasture's syndrome, but there are no anti-basement-membrane antibodies and the kidneys are less frequently involved. Most cases occur in children under 7 years of age. The child develops a chronic cough and anaemia and the chest X-ray shows diffuse shadows that are due to intrapulmonary bleeding, and eventually miliary nodulation. Characteristically, haemosiderin-containing macrophages are found in the sputum. There is an association with a sensitivity to cow's milk, and an appropriate diet is usually tried.

The prognosis in general is poor and treatment with corticosteroids or azathioprine is usually given.

PULMONARY FIBROSIS AND HONEYCOMB LUNG

Pulmonary fibrosis is the end result of many diseases of the respiratory tract. It may be:

- localized (e.g. following unresolved pneumonia)
- bilateral (e.g. in tuberculosis)

Table 14.15 The main causes of honeycomb lung

Localized	Diffuse
Systemic sclerosis	Cryptogenic fibrosing alveolitis
Sarcoidosis	Rheumatoid lung
Tuberculosis	Langerhans' cell histiocytosis
Asbestosis	Tuberous sclerosis
Berylliosis	Neurofibromatosis

■ widespread (e.g. in cryptogenic fibrosing alveolitis, in industrial lung disease, or due to drugs such as busulfan, bleomycin and cyclophosphamide).

Sometimes a typical radiological appearance is seen that is known as 'honeycomb lung'. This reflects the presence diffusely in both lungs of thick-walled cysts 0.5–2.0 cm diameter. These cystic air spaces probably represent dilated and thickened terminal and respiratory bronchioles. The main causes are shown in Table 14.15.

Cryptogenic fibrosing alveolitis (CFA)

This relatively rare disorder, known in the USA as *idiopathic pulmonary fibrosis*, causes diffuse fibrosis throughout the lung fields, usually in late middle age. The cause is unknown, but in a few cases it may be the

result of occupational exposure to metal or wood dust, while many patients show features of autoimmunity.

Pathogenesis

The pathogenesis of damage and fibrosis is complex and several factors are thought to be involved (Fig. 14.42). Macrophages and alveolar epithelial cells are activated by several mechanisms (see p. 799) and produce growth factors including fibronectin, platelet-derived growth factor, transforming growth factor-β, and insulin-like growth factor-1. These stimulate the deposition of type I and III collagens. Histologically there are two main features:

■ cellular infiltration with T lymphocytes and plasma cells and thickening and fibrosis of the alveolar walls
■ alveolitis – increased cells within the alveolar space (mainly macrophages and type II pneumocytes shed from the alveolar walls).

Clinical features

The main features are progressive breathlessness and cyanosis, which eventually lead to respiratory failure, pulmonary hypertension and cor pulmonale. Gross finger clubbing occurs in two-thirds of cases and fine bilateral end-inspiratory crackles are heard on auscultation. An

Fig. 14.42 **Pathogenesis of pulmonary fibrosis.** Macrophages can be activated by several factors, such as soluble immune complexes and sensitized T lymphocytes, resulting in the release of various cytokines leading to fibrosis.

acute form known as the *Hamman–Rich syndrome* occurs in a small proportion of cases. The chest X-ray is initially of ground-glass appearance, progressing to obvious small nodular shadows with streaky fibrosis and finally a honeycomb lung. A number of autoimmune diseases are seen in association with this condition. For example, autoimmune hepatitis occurs in 5–10% of cases. Similar lung changes are also seen in rheumatoid arthritis, systemic lupus erythematosus, dermatomyositis, systemic sclerosis and Sjögren's syndrome, often associated with Raynaud's phenomenon. CFA has also been reported in association with coeliac disease, ulcerative colitis and renal tubular acidosis.

Investigations

- **Chest X-ray** shows irregular reticulonodular shadowing, often maximal in the lower zones.
- **High-resolution CT scan** shows characteristic changes of peripheral reticular and ground-glass opacification, seen best in the basal regions but extending all over the lungs (Fig. 14.43).
- **Respiratory function tests** show a restrictive ventilatory defect – the lung volumes are reduced, the FEV_1 to FVC ratio is normal to high (with both values being reduced), and carbon monoxide gas transfer is reduced. Peak flow rates may be normal.
- **Blood gases** show an arterial hypoxaemia caused by a combination of alveolar–capillary block and ventilation–perfusion mismatch with normal or low P_aCO_2 owing to hyperventilation.
- **Blood tests**. Antinuclear antibodies and rheumatoid factors are present in one-third of patients. The ESR and immunoglobulins are mildly elevated.
- **Bronchoalveolar lavage** shows increased numbers of cells, particularly neutrophils and macrophages.
- **Histological confirmation** is necessary in some patients. Transbronchial lung biopsy is rarely diagnostic, but can exclude other conditions such as sarcoidosis or lymphangitis carcinomatosa. A video-assisted thoracoscopic lung biopsy is performed to obtain a larger specimen, which is usually needed to make a clear histological diagnosis.

Fig. 14.43 **CT scan showing cryptogenic fibrosing alveolitis.**

Differential diagnosis

The diagnosis of CFA is usually made in a patient presenting with the above signs and characteristic CT changes. The differential diagnosis of the chest X-ray appearance includes extrinsic allergic alveolitis, bronchiectasis, chronic left heart failure, sarcoidosis, industrial lung disease and lymphangitis carcinomatosa.

Prognosis and treatment

The median survival time for patients with CFA is approximately 5 years, although mortality is very high in the acute form. Treatment with prednisolone (30 mg daily) is usually prescribed for disabling disease, though its benefit has still to be proved by appropriate controlled trials. Azathioprine or cyclophosphamide may be added if there is no response. Supportive treatment includes domiciliary oxygen therapy. In severe disease, single lung transplantation can be offered.

Pulmonary alveolar proteinosis

This is a rare disease in which there is accumulation of lipoproteinaceous material within the alveoli. It can be congenital, but most cases are acquired and appear to have an autoimmune basis, with antibodies directed against the cytokine GM-CSF. The disease mostly affects men and presents with progressive exertional dyspnoea and cough. Inspiratory crackles are present in about 50%, and the condition is thus different from fibrosing alveolitis. Diagnosis is made by bronchial lavage, which reveals a milky appearance and many large, foamy macrophages but few other inflammatory cells.

Extrinsic allergic alveolitis

In this disease there is a widespread diffuse inflammatory reaction in both the small airways of the lung and the alveoli. It is due to the inhalation of a number of different antigens, the most common being microbial spores contaminating vegetable matter (e.g. straw, hay, mushroom compost). Some examples are illustrated in Table 14.16. By far the most common of these diseases worldwide is farmer's lung, which affects up to 1 in 10 of the farming community in disadvantaged, wet communities around the world. In the West the incidence is declining as more mechanized farming procedures and better informed animal husbandry are introduced.

Pathogenesis

Histologically there is an initial infiltration of the small airways and alveolar walls with neutrophils followed by T lymphocytes and macrophages, leading to the development of small non-caseating granulomas. These comprise multinucleated giant cells, occasionally containing the inhaled antigenic material. The allergic response to the inhaled antigens involves both cellular immunity and the deposition of immune complexes causing foci of inflammation through the activation of complement via the classical pathway. Some of the inhalant materials may also lead to inflammation by

Table 14.16 Extrinsic allergic (bronchiolar) alveolitis – some causes

Disease	Situation	Antigens
Farmer's lung	Forking mouldy hay or any other mouldy vegetable material	Thermophilic actinomycetes, e.g. *Micropolyspora faeni* Fungi, e.g. *Aspergillus umbrasus*
Bird fancier's lung	Handling pigeons, cleaning lofts or budgerigar cages	Proteins present in the 'bloom' on the feathers and in excreta
Maltworker's lung	Turning germinating barley	*Aspergillus clavatus*
Humidifier fever	Contaminated humidifying systems in air conditioners or humidifiers in factories (especially in printing works)	Possibly a variety of bacteria or amoeba (e.g. *Naegleria gruberi*) Thermoactinomyces
Mushroom workers	Turning mushroom compost	Thermophilic actinomycetes
Cheese washer's lung	Mouldy cheese	*Penicillin casei* *Aspergillus clavatus*
Wine maker's lung	Mould on grapes	Botrytis

directly activating the alternative complement pathway. These mechanisms attract and activate alveolar and interstitial macrophages, so that continued antigenic exposure results in the progressive development of pulmonary fibrosis.

Clinical features

Typically fever, malaise, cough and shortness of breath come on several hours after exposure to the causative antigen. Thus, a farmer forking hay in the morning may notice symptoms during the late afternoon and evening with resolution by the following morning. On examination, the patient may have a fever, tachypnoea, and coarse end-inspiratory crackles and wheezes throughout the chest. Cyanosis caused by ventilation–perfusion mismatch may be severe even at rest. Continued exposure leads to a chronic illness characterized by severe weight loss, effort dyspnoea and cough as well as the features of fibrosing alveolitis (see p. 941).

Investigations

- **Chest X-ray** shows fluffy nodular shadowing with the subsequent development of streaky shadows, particularly in the upper zones. In very advanced cases, honeycomb lung occurs.
- **Lung function tests** show a restrictive ventilatory defect with a decrease in carbon monoxide gas transfer.
- **Polymorphonuclear leucocyte count** is raised in acute cases. Eosinophilia is not a feature.
- **Precipitating antibodies** are present in the serum. One-quarter of pigeon fanciers have precipitating IgG-antibodies against pigeon protein and droppings in their serum, but only a small proportion have lung disease. Precipitating antibodies are evidence of exposure, not disease.
- **Bronchoalveolar lavage** shows increased T lymphocytes and granulocytes.

Differential diagnosis

Although extrinsic allergic alveolitis due to inhalation of the spores of *Micropolyspora faeni* is common among farmers, it is probably more common for these indivi-

duals to suffer from asthma related to inhalation of antigens from a variety of mites that infest stored grain and other vegetable material. These include *Lepidoglyphus domesticus, L. destructor* and *Acarus siro*. Symptoms of asthma resulting from inhalation of these allergens are often mistaken for farmer's lung. Lung function tests will effectively discriminate between the disorders. Pigeon fancier's lung is quite common, but alveolitis from budgerigars, parrots and parakeets is very rare.

Management

Prevention is the aim. This can be achieved by changes in work practice, with the use of silage for animal fodder and the drier storage of hay and grain. Pigeon fancier's lung is more difficult to control since affected individuals remain strongly attached to their hobby. Prednisolone, initially in large doses of 30–60 mg daily, may achieve regression during the early stages of the disease. Established fibrosis will not resolve and in some patients the disease may progress inexorably to respiratory failure in spite of intensive therapy. Farmer's lung is a recognized occupational disease in the UK and sufferers are entitled to compensation, depending upon their degree of disability.

Humidifier fever (Table 14.16)

Humidifier fever, one cause of building-related illnesses (p. 1033), may present with the typical features of extrinsic allergic alveolitis without any radiographic changes. This disease has occurred in outbreaks in factories in the UK, particularly in printing works. In North America it is more commonly found in office blocks with contaminated air-conditioning systems. Humidifier fever may be effectively prevented by sterilization of the re-circulating water used in large humidifying plants.

Drug-induced respiratory reactions
(Table 14.17)

Drugs may produce a wide variety of disorders of the respiratory tract. The mechanisms are varied and include direct toxicity (e.g. bleomycin), immune complex

Table 14.17 Some drug-induced respiratory reactions

Disease	Drugs
Bronchospasm	Penicillins, cephalosporins Sulphonamides Aspirin/NSAIDs Monoclonal antibodies, e.g. infliximab Iodine-containing contrast media β-Adrenoceptor-blocking drugs, (e.g. propranolol) Non-depolarizing muscle relaxants Intravenous thiamine Adenosine
Diffuse parenchymal damage and/or fibrosis	Amiodarone Anakinra (IL-1 receptor antagonist) Nitrofurantoin Paraquat Continuous oxygen Cytotoxic agent (many, particularly busulfan, CCNU, bleomycin, methotrexate)
Pulmonary eosinophilia	Antibiotics: Penicillin Tetracycline Sulphonamides, e.g. sulfasalazine NSAIDs Cytotoxic agents
Acute lung injury	Paraquat
Pulmonary hypertension	Fenfluramine
SLE-like syndrome including pulmonary infiltrates, effusions and fibrosis	Hydralazine Procainamide Isoniazid Phenytoin ACE inhibitors Monoclonal antibodies

CCNU, chloroethyl-cyclohexyl-nitrosourea (lomustine); NSAIDs, non-steroidal anti-inflammatory drugs; SLE, systemic lupus erythematosus

formation with arteritis, hypersensitivity (involving both T cell and IgE mechanisms) and autoimmunity.

Pulmonary infiltrates with fibrosis may result from the use of a number of cytotoxic drugs used in the treatment of cancer. The most common cause of these reactions is bleomycin. The pulmonary damage is dose-related, occurring when the total dosage is greater than 450 mg, but will regress in some cases if the drug is stopped. The most sensitive test is a decrease in carbon monoxide gas transfer, and therefore gas transfer should be measured repeatedly during treatment with the drug. The use of corticosteroids may help resolution. Drugs affecting the respiratory system are shown in Table 14.17, together with the types of reaction they produce. Anaphylaxis with bronchospasm can occur with many drugs. The list

is not exhaustive; for example, over 20 different drugs are known to produce a systemic lupus erythematosus-like syndrome, sometimes complicated by pulmonary infiltrates and fibrosis. Paraquat ingestion (see p. 1018) causes severe pulmonary oedema and death, and pulmonary fibrosis develops in many of those who survive.

Radiation damage

Irradiation of the lung during radiotherapy can cause a radiation pneumonitis. Patients complain of breathlessness and a dry cough. Radiation pneumonitis results in a restrictive lung defect. Corticosteroids should be given in the acute stage.

FURTHER READING

Baughmann RP et al. (2003) Sarcoidosis. *Lancet* **361**: 1111–1118.

British Thoracic Society (1999) The diagnosis, assessment and treatment of diffuse parenchymal lung disease in adults. *Thorax* **54** (Suppl. 1): S1–S30.

Gross TJ, Hunninghake GW (2001) Idiopathic pulmonary fibrosis. *New England Journal of Medicine* **345**: 517–525.

Noth I et al. (2003) Churg–Strauss syndrome. *Lancet* **361**: 587–594.

Porter N et al. (2003) Endocrine and reproductive manifestations of sarcoidosis. *Quarterly Journal of Medicine* **96**: 553–561.

Vassallo R et al. (2000) Pulmonary Langerhans'-cell histiocytosis. *New England Journal of Medicine* **342**: 1969–1978.

OCCUPATIONAL LUNG DISEASE

Exposure to dusts, gases, vapours and fumes at work can cause several different types of lung disease:

- acute bronchitis and even pulmonary oedema from irritants such as sulphur dioxide, chlorine, ammonia or the oxides of nitrogen
- pulmonary fibrosis due to mineral dust
- occupational asthma (see Table 14.12) – this is now the commonest industrial lung disease in the developed world
- extrinsic allergic alveolitis (see Table 14.16)
- bronchial carcinoma due to industrial agents (e.g. asbestos, polycyclic hydrocarbons, radon in mines).

The degree of fibrosis that follows inhalation of mineral dust varies. While iron (siderosis), barium (baritosis) and tin (stannosis) lead to dramatic dense nodular shadowing on the chest X-ray, their effect on lung function and symptoms is minimal. Exposure to silica or asbestos, on the other hand, leads to extensive fibrosis and disability. Coal dust has an intermediate fibrogenic effect and used to account for 90% of all compensated industrial lung diseases in the UK. The term 'pneumoconiosis' means the accumulation of dust in the lungs and the reaction of the tissue to its presence. The term is not wide enough to encompass all occupational lung disease and is now generally used only in relation to coal dust and its effects on the lung.

Coal-worker's pneumoconiosis

Improved conditions and the progressive contraction of the coal industry in the UK have led to a considerable reduction in the number of cases of pneumoconiosis. The disease is caused by dust particles approximately 2–5 μm in diameter that are retained in the small airways and alveoli of the lung. The incidence of the disease is related to total dust exposure, which is highest at the coal face, particularly if ventilation and dust suppression are poor. Two very different syndromes result from the inhalation of coal.

Simple pneumoconiosis
This simply reflects the deposition of coal dust in the lung. It produces fine micronodular shadowing on the chest X-ray and is by far the most common type of pneumoconiosis. It is graded on the chest X-ray appearance according to standard categories set by the International Labour Office (see below). Considerable dispute remains about the effects of simple pneumoconiosis on respiratory function and symptoms. In many cases the symptoms are due to COPD related to cigarette smoking, but this is not always the case. Changes to UK workers' compensation legislation means that coal miners who develop COPD may be compensated for their disability regardless of their chest X-ray appearance.

Categories of simple pneumoconiosis are as follows:

1. small round opacities definitely present but few in number
2. small round opacities numerous but normal lung markings still visible
3. small round opacities very numerous and normal lung markings partly or totally obscured.

Simple pneumoconiosis may lead to the development of progressive massive fibrosis (PMF) (see below). PMF virtually never occurs on a background of category 1 simple pneumoconiosis but occurs in about 7% of those with category 2 and in 30% of those with category 3. Miners with category 1 pneumoconiosis are unlikely to receive compensation unless they also have evidence of COPD. Those with more extensive radiographic changes may be compensated solely on the basis of their X-ray appearances.

Progressive massive fibrosis
In PMF, patients develop round fibrotic masses several centimetres in diameter, almost invariably in the upper lobes and sometimes having necrotic central cavities. The pathogenesis of PMF is still not understood, though it seems clear that some fibrogenic promoting factor is present in individuals developing the disease. At one time this was thought to be *M. tuberculosis*, but it is more probably due to immune complexes, analogous to the development of large fibrotic nodules in coal miners with rheumatoid arthritis (Caplan's syndrome). Rheumatoid factor and antinuclear antibodies are both often present in the serum of patients with PMF, and also in those suffering from asbestosis or silicosis. Pathologically there is apical destruction and disruption of the lung, resulting in emphysema and airway damage. Lung function tests show a mixed restrictive and obstructive ventilatory defect with loss of lung volume, irreversible airflow limitation and reduced gas transfer.

The patient with PMF suffers considerable effort dyspnoea, usually with a cough. The sputum may be black. The disease can progress (or even develop) after exposure to coal dust has ceased and may lead to respiratory failure.

Silicosis

This disease is uncommon though it may still be encountered in stonemasons, sand-blasters, pottery and ceramic workers and foundry workers involved in fettling (removing sand from metal castings made in sand-filled moulds). Silicosis is caused by the inhalation of silica (silicon dioxide). This dust is highly fibrogenic. For example, a coal miner can remain healthy with 30 g of coal dust in his lungs but 3 g of silica is sufficient to kill. Silica seems particularly toxic to alveolar macrophages and readily initiates fibrogenesis (see Fig. 14.42). The chest X-ray appearances and clinical features of silicosis are similar to those of PMF, but distinctive thin streaks of calcification may be seen around the hilar lymph nodes ('eggshell' calcification).

Asbestosis

Asbestos is a mixture of silicates of iron, magnesium, nickel, cadmium and aluminium, and has the unique property of occurring naturally as a fibre. It is remarkably resistant to heat, acid and alkali, and has been widely used for roofing, insulation and fireproofing. Asbestos has been mined in southern Africa, Canada, Australia and eastern Europe. Several different types of asbestos are recognized: about 90% of asbestos is chrysotile, 6% crocidolite and 4% amosite. Chrysotile or white asbestos is the softest asbestos fibre. Each fibre is often as long as 2 cm but only a few microns thick. It is less fibrogenic than crocidolite. Crocidolite (blue asbestos) is particularly resistant to chemical destruction and exists in straight fibres up to 50 mm in length and 1–2 μm in width. Crocidolite is the most likely type of asbestos to produce asbestosis and mesothelioma. This may be due to the fact that it is readily trapped in the lung. Its long, thin shape means that it can be inhaled, but subsequent rotation against the long axis of the smaller airways, particularly in turbulent airflow during expiration, causes the fibres to impact. Crocidolite is also particularly resistant to macrophage and neutrophil enzymatic destruction.

Exposure to asbestos occurred particularly in shipbuilding yards and in power stations, but its ubiquitous use meant that low levels of exposure were common. Up to 50% of urban dwellers have been found to have asbestos bodies (asbestos fibre covered in protein secretions) in their lungs at post-mortem. Regulations in the UK prohibit the use of crocidolite and severely restrict the use of chrysotile. Careful dust control measures are enforced, which should eventually abolish the problem. Workers continue to be exposed to blue asbestos in the course of demolition or in the replacement of insulation, and it should be remembered that there is a considerable time lag between exposure and development of disease, particularly mesothelioma (20–40 years).

A synergistic relationship exists between asbestosis and cigarette smoking and the development of bronchial carcinoma, usually adenocarcinoma; the risk is multiplied fivefold above the risk attributable to smoking. The risk of lung cancer is also increased in non-smokers, especially in those who have parenchymal asbestosis but also in those with pleural plaques without parenchymal fibrosis.

The diseases caused by asbestos are summarized in Table 14.18. Bilateral diffuse pleural thickening, asbestosis, mesothelioma and asbestos-related carcinoma of the bronchus are all eligible for industrial injuries benefit in

the UK, but account for only one-quarter of the number of cases of compensation compared with coal-worker's pneumoconiosis.

Asbestosis is defined as fibrosis of the lungs caused by asbestos dust, which may or may not be associated with fibrosis of the parietal or visceral layers of the pleura. It is a progressive disease characterized by breathlessness and accompanied by finger clubbing and bilateral basal end-inspiratory crackles. Fibrosis, not detectable on chest X-ray, may be revealed on CT scan. No treatment is known to alter the progress of the disease, though corticosteroids are often prescribed.

Mesothelioma

The number of cases of mesothelioma has increased progressively since the mid-1980s and has now reached over 1000 cases per year. Pleural effusions are the most common presentation of mesothelioma, typically with persistent chest wall pain, which should raise the index of suspicion even if the initial pleural fluid or biopsy samples are non-diagnostic. Often a video-assisted thoracoscopic

Table 14.18 The effects of asbestos on the lung

	Exposure	Chest X-ray	Lung function	Symptoms	Outcome
Asbestos bodies	Light	Normal	Normal	None	Evidence of asbestos exposure only
Pleural plaques	Light	Pleural thickening (parietal pleura) and calcification (also in diaphragmatic pleura)	Mild restrictive ventilatory defect	Rare, occasional mild effort dyspnoea	No other sequelae
Effusion	First two decades following exposure	Effusion	Restrictive	Pleuritic pain, dyspnoea	Often recurrent
Bilateral diffuse pleural thickening	Light/moderate	Bilateral diffuse thickening (of both parietal and visceral pleura) more than 5 mm thick and extending over more than one-quarter of the chest wall	Restrictive ventilatory defect	Effort dyspnoea	May progress in absence of further exposure
Mesothelioma	Light (interval of 20–40 years from exposure to disease)	Pleural effusion, usually unilateral	Restrictive ventilatory defect	Pleuritic pain, increasing dyspnoea	Median survival 2 years
Asbestosis	Heavy (interval of 5–10 years from exposure to disease)	Diffuse bilateral streaky shadows, honeycomb lung	Severe restrictive ventilatory defect and reduced gas transfer	Progressive dyspnoea	Poor, progression in some cases after exposure cases
Asbestos-related carcinoma of the bronchus	The features of asbestosis, bilateral diffuse pleural thickening or bilateral pleural plaques plus those of bronchial carcinoma				Fatal

lung biopsy is needed to obtain sufficient tissue for diagnosis. In the event of a positive pleural biopsy diagnosis, local radiotherapy should be given to prevent the seeding of mesothelioma cells down the needle track. No treatment influences the universally fatal outcome.

Byssinosis

This disease occurs world-wide but is declining rapidly in areas where the numbers of people employed in cotton mills are falling. In the UK the disease used to occur in areas of Lancashire and Northern Ireland but is now a historical footnote. The symptoms start on the first day back at work after a break (Monday sickness) with improvement as the week progresses. Tightness in the chest, cough and breathlessness occur within the first hour in dusty areas of the mill, particularly in the blowing and carding rooms where raw cotton is cleaned and the fibres are straightened.

The exact nature of the disease and its aetiology remain disputed. Two important features are that pure cotton does not cause the disease, and that cotton dust has some effect on airflow limitation in all those exposed. Individuals with asthma are particularly badly affected by exposure to cotton dust. The most likely aetiology is endotoxins from bacteria present in the raw cotton causing constriction of the airways of the lung. There are no changes on the chest X-ray and there is considerable dispute as to whether the progressive airflow limitation seen in some patients with the disease is due to the cotton dust or to other factors such as cigarette smoking or co-existent asthma.

Berylliosis

Beryllium–copper alloy has a high tensile strength and is resistant to metal fatigue, high temperature and corrosion. It is used in the aerospace industry, in atomic reactors and in many electrical devices.

When beryllium is inhaled, it can cause a systemic illness with a clinical picture similar to sarcoidosis. The major chronic problem is that of progressive dyspnoea with pulmonary fibrosis. However, strict control of levels in the working atmosphere have made the disease a rarity.

FURTHER READING
Beckett WS (2000) Occupational respiratory disorders. *New England Journal of Medicine* **342**: 406–413.
Parker C, Neville E (2003) Management of malignant mesothelioma. *Thorax* **58**: 809–813.

LUNG CYSTS

These may be congenital, bronchogenic cysts or may result from a sequestrated pulmonary segment. Hydatid disease causes fluid-filled cysts. Thin-walled cysts are due to lung abscesses, which are particularly found in staphylococcal pneumonia, tuberculous cavities, septic

pulmonary infarction, primary bronchogenic carcinoma, cavitating metastatic neoplasm, or paragonimiasis caused by the lung fluke *Paragonimus westermani*.

TUMOURS OF THE RESPIRATORY TRACT

Bronchial carcinoma accounts for 95% of all primary tumours of the lung. Alveolar cell carcinoma accounts for 2% of lung tumours, and other less malignant or benign tumours account for the remaining 3%.

MALIGNANT TUMOURS

Bronchial carcinoma

This is the most common malignant tumour in the West and is the third most common cause of death in the UK after heart disease and pneumonia. Mortality rates world-wide are highest in Scotland, closely followed by England and Wales. In the UK, 32 000 people die each year from bronchial carcinoma, with a male-to-female ratio of 3 : 1. Although the mortality rate from this disease has levelled off in men, it continues to rise in women, and now causes more deaths from malignant disease in women than any other tumour.

The strength of the association between cigarette smoking and bronchial carcinoma overshadows any other aetiological factors (Table 14.19), but there is a higher incidence of bronchial carcinoma in urban compared with rural areas, even when allowance is made for cigarette smoking. Passive smoking (the frequent inhalation of other people's smoke by non-smokers) increases the risk of bronchial carcinoma by a factor of 1.5. Occupational factors include exposure to asbestos, and an association is also claimed for workers in contact with arsenic, chromium, iron oxide, petroleum products and oils, coal tar, products of coal combustion, and radiation. Tumours associated with occupational factors are mostly adenocarcinomas and appear to be less related to cigarette smoking.

Cell types
Based on the characteristics of the disease and its response to treatment bronchial carcinoma maybe divided into small-cell carcinoma and non-small-cell

Table 14.19 Death rates from lung cancer (age standardized) per 100 000 according to smoking habits in male British doctors

Death rate		Number of cigarettes per day	Death rate
Non-smokers	10	1–14	78
Ex-smokers	43	15–24	127
Continuing smokers		25 or more	251
Any tobacco	104		
Pipe/cigar	58		
Cigarettes	140		

carcinoma. Studies of mean doubling times of carcinomas indicate that development from the initial malignant change to presentation takes about 15 years for adeno-carcinoma, 8 years for squamous carcinoma and 3 years for small-cell carcinoma.

Non-small-cell carcinoma

Squamous or *epidermoid carcinoma* is the commonest type, accounting for approximately 40% of all carcinomas. Most present as obstructive lesions of the bronchus leading to infection. It occasionally cavitates (10%) at presentation. The cells are usually well differentiated but occasionally anaplastic. Local spread is common but widespread metastases occur relatively late.

Adenocarcinoma arises from mucous cells in the bronchial epithelium. Invasion of the pleura and the mediastinal lymph nodes is common, as are metastases to the brain and bones. Adenocarcinoma accounts for approximately 10% of all bronchial carcinomas. It is the most common bronchial carcinoma associated with asbestos and is proportionally more common in non-smokers, in women, in the elderly, and in the Far East.

Large cell carcinomas are less-differentiated forms of squamous cell and adenocarcinomas. These account for about 25% of all lung cancers and metastasize early.

Bronchoalveolar cell carcinoma (also termed bronchiolar carcinoma) accounts for only 1–2% of lung tumours and occurs either as a peripheral solitary nodule or as diffuse nodular lesions of multicentric origin. Occasionally this tumour is associated with expectoration of very large volumes of mucoid sputum.

Small-cell carcinoma

This tumour, often called oat-cell carcinoma, accounts for 20–30% of all lung cancers. It arises from endocrine cells (Kulchitsky cells). These cells are members of the APUD system, which explains why many polypeptide hormones are secreted by these tumours. Some of these poly-peptides act in an autocrine fashion: they feed back on the cells and cause cell growth. Small-cell carcinoma spreads early and is almost always inoperable at presentation. The tumour is rapidly growing and highly malignant. It responds to chemotherapy but the prognosis remains poor.

Clinical features

The frequencies of the common symptoms of lung cancer on presentation are shown in Table 14.20. Chest pain and discomfort are often described as fullness and pressure in the chest. Sometimes the pain may be pleuritic owing to invasion of the pleura or ribs.

Often there are no abnormal physical signs. Enlarged supraclavicular lymph nodes may be present. There may be signs of a pleural effusion or of lobar collapse. Signs of an unresolved pneumonia or of associated underlying disease (e.g. diffuse pulmonary fibrosis in asbestosis) may be present.

Direct spread

The tumour may directly involve the pleura and ribs. Carcinoma in the apex of the lung can erode the ribs and

Table 14.20 The frequency of the common presenting symptoms of bronchial carcinoma

Symptom	Frequency (%)
Cough	41
Chest pain	22
Cough and pain	15
Coughing blood	7
Chest infection	< 5
Malaise	< 5
Weight loss	< 5
Shortness of breath	< 5
Hoarseness	< 5
Distant spread	< 5
No symptoms	< 5

involve the lower part of the brachial plexus (C8, T1 and T2), causing severe pain in the shoulder and down the inner surface of the arm (Pancoast's tumour). The sympathetic ganglion can also be involved, producing Horner's syndrome. Hilar tumours may involve the recurrent laryngeal nerve, causing unilateral vocal cord paresis with hoarseness and a bovine cough.

Bronchial carcinoma can also directly invade the phrenic nerve, causing paralysis of the ipsilateral hemi-diaphragm. It can involve the oesophagus, producing progressive dysphagia, and the pericardium, producing pericardial effusion and malignant dysrhythmias. *Superior vena caval obstruction* causes early morning headache, facial congestion and oedema involving the upper limbs; the jugular veins are distended, as are the veins on the chest that form a collateral circulation with veins arising from the abdomen.

Metastatic complications

Bony metastases are common, giving rise to severe pain and pathological fractures. There is frequent involvement of the liver. Secondary deposits in the brain present as a change in personality, epilepsy or as a focal neurological lesion. Spinal cord compression is not uncommon and requires urgent treatment (p. 492). Secondary deposits in the adrenal gland are a very frequent post-mortem finding but are often asymptomatic.

Non-metastatic extrapulmonary manifestations

Although approximately 10% of small-cell tumours produce ectopic hormones at some stage, clinical extrapulmonary manifestations are relatively rare apart from finger clubbing (Table 14.21).

Hypertrophic pulmonary osteoarthropathy (HPOA) (see p. 588) occurs in approximately 3% of all bronchial carcinomas, particularly squamous-cell carcinomas and adenocarcinomas. Symptoms include joint stiffness and severe pain in the wrists and ankles, sometimes associated with gynaecomastia. X-rays show a characteristic proliferative periostitis at the distal ends of long bones, which have an onion-skin appearance. HPOA is invariably associated with clubbing of the fingers. It may regress after resection of the lung tumour or as a result of vagotomy at thoracotomy.

Table 14.21 **Non-metastatic extrapulmonary manifestations of bronchial carcinoma (percentage of all cases)**

Metabolic (universal at some stage) Loss of weight Lassitude Anorexia **Endocrine** (10%) (usually small-cell carcinoma) Ectopic adrenocorticotrophin syndrome Syndrome of inappropriate secretion of antidiuretic hormone (SIADH) Hypercalcaemia (usually squamous cell carcinoma) Rarer: hypoglycaemia, thyrotoxicosis, gynaecomastia **Neurological** (2–16%) Encephalopathies – including subacute cerebellar degeneration Myelopathies – motor neurone disease Neuropathies – peripheral sensorimotor neuropathy Muscular disorders – polymyopathy, myasthenic syndrome (Eaton–Lambert syndrome)	**Vascular and haematological** (rare) Thrombophlebitis migrans Non-bacterial thrombotic endocarditis Microcytic and normocytic anaemia Disseminated intravascular coagulopathy Thrombotic thrombocytopenic purpura Haemolytic anaemia **Skeletal** Clubbing (30%) Hypertrophic osteoarthropathy (± gynaecomastia) (3%) **Cutaneous** (rare) Dermatomyositis Acanthosis nigricans Herpes zoster

Investigations

Chest X-ray

By the time the lung cancer is causing symptoms, it will almost always be visible on chest X-rays. Asymptomatic tumours may be seen on chest X-ray if they are more than 1 cm in diameter. Lateral views are useful to assess the hilum and masses behind the heart. CT scanning will detect smaller masses and is being evaluated for screening. A minority of tumours are confined to the central airways and mediastinum without obvious change on the plain chest X-ray. These will be readily seen at bronchoscopy or on CT scanning. Although investigation of isolated haemoptysis with a normal chest X-ray is often negative, a normal chest X-ray should not deter from further investigation, especially in smokers over the age of 40. About 70% of all primary lung cancers present with a mass, including virtually all small-cell lung cancers and most squamous cell carcinomas. Adenocarcinoma occurs more often in the periphery than the other cell types.

Carcinomas causing partial obstruction of a bronchus interrupt the mucociliary escalator, and bacteria are retained within the affected lobe. This gives rise to the so-called secondary pneumonia that is commonly seen on the chest X-ray.

Bronchial carcinoma can also appear as round shadows on a chest X-ray (see p. 886). Characteristically the edge of the tumour has a fluffy or spiked appearance, though sometimes it may be entirely smooth with cavitation.

The hilar lymph nodes on the side of the tumour are frequently involved. Bronchial carcinoma is also a common cause of large pleural effusions. Carcinoma can spread through the lymphatic channels of the lung to give rise to lymphangitis carcinomatosa; in bronchial carcinoma this is usually unilateral and associated with striking dyspnoea. The chest X-ray shows streaky shadowing throughout the lung. Bilateral lymphangitis carcinomatosa is more often due to metastatic spread, usually from tumours below the diaphragm (the stomach and colon) or from breast cancers.

Computed tomography

CT is useful for identifying disease in the mediastinum, such as enlarged lymph nodes (see Fig. 14.12, p. 887) or local spread of the tumour, and for identifying secondary spread of carcinoma to the opposite lung by detecting masses too small to be seen on the chest X-ray. CT is a poor guide to whether nodes are involved by tumour but a normal CT scan prior to surgery excludes the need for mediastinoscopy and node biopsy. CT scanning should include the liver, adrenal glands and the brain since these are common sites for metastases.

Other imaging modalities

MRI is not useful for the diagnosis of primary lung tumours. PET scanning is now the investigation of choice for assessment of the mediastinum (see p. 887).

Fibreoptic bronchoscopy (see also p. 891, Fig. 14.44)
This technique is used to define the bronchial anatomy

Fig. 14.44 Bronchoscopic view of a bronchial carcinoma obstructing a large bronchus.

and to obtain biopsy and cytological specimens. If the carcinoma involves the first 2 cm of either main bronchus, the tumour is inoperable as there would be insufficient resection margins for pneumonectomy. Widening and loss of the sharp angle of the carina indicates the presence of enlarged mediastinal lymph nodes, either malignant or reactive. These can be biopsied by passage of a needle through the bronchial wall. Vocal cord paresis on the left indicates involvement of the recurrent laryngeal nerve and inoperability.

Percutaneous aspiration and biopsy

Peripheral lung lesions cannot be seen by fibreoptic bronchoscopy and samples may be obtained by direct aspiration or biopsy through the chest wall under appropriate X-ray or CT screening. Fine-needle aspiration samples can be obtained from 75% of peripheral lesions that could not be biopsied transbronchially. Pneumothorax is common (25% of patients), occasionally requiring drainage. Mild haemoptysis occurs in 5%. Implantation metastases do not occur. Although useful if positive, negative FNA is not very helpful. Biopsies obtained with Trucut needles are usually diagnostic.

Other investigations

These include a full blood count for the detection of anaemia, biochemistry for liver involvement, hypercalcaemia and hyponatraemia.

Treatment (see also p. 518)

Treatment of lung cancer involves several different modalities and is best planned by a multidisciplinary team. Treatment decisions need to reflect the poor overall survival rates: only 20% of patients are alive 1 year after diagnosis and only 6–8% after 5 years (cf. 50% for breast or cervix). Patients are staged according to the TNM classification (p. 490) for non-small-cell cancer but small-cell cancer is treated according to whether it is limited or extensive (p. 519).

Surgery

Surgery can be curative in non-small-cell lung cancer (T1, N0, M0) but only 5–10% of all cases are suitable for resection and about 70% of these survive for 5 years. Surgery is rarely appropriate in patients over 65 years as the operative mortality rate exceeds the 5-year survival rate. Trial data suggest that neo-adjuvant chemotherapy may downstage tumours to render them operable and may also improve 5-year survival in patients whose tumours are operable at presentation. Following resection of adenocarcinomas, a recent trial of adjuvant chemotherapy with uracil-tegafir (a pro-drug of fluorouracil) has shown improvements in survival.

Preoperative assessment includes exclusion of metastatic disease by blood tests and imaging as described above. Lung function tests, including walking oximetry, are used to predict postoperative potential. An active life after pneumonectomy is unlikely if the gas transfer is reduced below 50%.

Radiation therapy for cure

In patients who are fit and who have a slowly growing squamous carcinoma, high-dose radiotherapy (65 Gy or 6500 rads) can produce good results. It is the treatment of choice if surgery is declined. Poor lung function is a relative contraindication for radiotherapy. Radiation pneumonitis (defined as an acute infiltrate precisely confined to the radiation area and occurring within 3 months of radiotherapy) develops in 10–15% of cases. Radiation fibrosis, a fibrotic change occurring within a year or so of radiotherapy and not precisely confined to the radiation area, occurs to some degree in all cases. These complications usually cause no problems.

Radiation treatment for symptoms

Bone pain, haemoptysis and superior vena cava obstruction respond favourably to irradiation in the short term.

Chemotherapy is discussed on page 519. Adjuvant chemotherapy with radiotherapy improves response rate and extends median survival in non-small-cell cancer.

Laser therapy, endobronchial irradiation and tracheobronchial stents

These techniques are used in the palliation of inoperable lung cancer in selected patients with tracheobronchial narrowing from intraluminal tumour or extrinsic compression causing disabling breathlessness, intractable cough and complications, including infection, haemoptysis and respiratory failure.

A neodymium-Yag (Nd-Yag) laser passed through a fibreoptic bronchoscope can be used to vaporize inoperable fungating intraluminal carcinoma involving short segments of trachea or main bronchus. Benign tumours, strictures and vascular lesions can also be treated effectively with immediate relief of symptoms.

Endobronchial irradiation (brachytherapy) is useful for the treatment of both intraluminal tumour and malignant extrinsic compression. A radioactive source is afterloaded into a catheter placed adjacent to the carcinoma under fibreoptic bronchoscope control. Radiation dose falls rapidly with distance from the source, minimizing damage to adjacent normal tissue. Reduction in endoscopically assessed tumour size occurs in 70–95% of cases.

Tracheobronchial stents made of silicone or as expandable metal springs are available for insertion into strictures caused by tumour or from external compression or when there is weakening and collapse of the tracheobronchial wall.

Palliative care (see p. 524)

Patients dying of cancer of the lung need attention to their overall well-being. Palliative care must not be ignored simply because the patient cannot be cured. Much can be done to make the patient's remaining life symptom-free and as active as possible. As compared to patients with fatal cancers at other sites, patients with lung cancer tend to remain relatively independent and pain-free, but die more rapidly once they reach the terminal phase.

Daily treatment with prednisolone (up to 15 mg daily) may improve appetite. Morphine or diamorphine are given regularly for pain, either in the form of a sustained-release morphine sulphate tablet twice daily or else as regular elixirs or injections. Many patients benefit from a continuous subcutaneous injection of opiates given by a pump. Candidiasis and other infections in the mouth are common and must be looked for and treated. Patients taking opiates are frequently constipated, so regular laxatives should be prescribed. Short courses of palliative radiotherapy are helpful for bone pain, severe cough or haemoptysis.

Both the patient and the relatives may require counselling, a task that should be shared between the respiratory teams, the primary care team and the nurses, social workers, hospital chaplains and doctors, who make up the palliative care team.

Tracheal carcinoma

Primary tumours of the trachea are rare – their incidence relative to laryngeal and bronchial tumours is 1 : 75 and 1 : 180 respectively. The majority are malignant and cause severe and rapidly progressive dyspnoea and stridor. Flow–volume curves show typical and dramatic reductions in inspiratory flow (extrathoracic tracheal tumours) (see p. 879). Diagnosis is confirmed by bronchoscopy. Rapid and effective destruction of tumour (p. 950) by laser provides temporary relief of symptoms. Radiotherapy is often given and occasionally surgery may be possible but the prognosis is very poor.

Secondary tumours

Metastases in the lung are very common and usually present as round shadows (1.5–3.0 cm diameter). They may be detected on chest X-ray in patients already diagnosed as having carcinoma. *Typical sites for the primary tumour include the kidney, prostate, breast, bone, gastrointestinal tract, cervix or ovary.*

Metastases nearly always develop in the parenchyma and are often relatively asymptomatic even when the chest X-ray shows extensive pulmonary metastases. Rarely metastases may develop in the bronchi, when they may present with haemoptysis.

Carcinoma, particularly of the stomach, pancreas and breast, can involve mediastinal glands and spread along the lymphatics of both lungs (lymphangitis carcinomatosa), leading to progressive and severe breathlessness. On the chest X-ray, bilateral lymphadenopathy is seen together with streaky basal shadowing fanning out over both lung fields.

Occasionally a pulmonary metastasis may be detected as a *solitary round shadow* on chest X-ray in an asymptomatic patient. The most common primary tumour to do this is a renal cell carcinoma.

The differential diagnosis includes:

- primary bronchial carcinoma
- tuberculoma
- benign tumour of the lung
- hydatid cyst.

Single pulmonary metastases can be removed surgically but, as CT scans usually show the presence of small metastases undetected on chest X-ray, surgery is seldom performed.

SCREENING FOR LUNG CANCER

Screening programmes (yearly chest X-ray, 4-monthly sputum cytology) have been tried in high-risk groups but the success rate is minimal, underlining the need for prevention. CT screening is currently being evaluated.

BENIGN TUMOURS

Pulmonary hamartoma
This is the most common benign tumour of the lung and is usually seen on the X-ray as a very well-defined round lesion 1–2 cm in diameter in the periphery of the lung. Growth is extremely slow, but the tumour may reach several centimetres in diameter. Rarely it arises from a major bronchus and causes obstruction.

Bronchial carcinoid
This rare tumour resembles intestinal carcinoid tumour and is locally invasive, eventually spreading to mediastinal lymph nodes and finally to distant organs. It is a highly vascular tumour that projects into the lumen of a major bronchus causing recurrent haemoptysis. It grows slowly and eventually blocks the bronchus, leading to lobar collapse. As foregut derivatives, bronchial carcinoids may produce ACTH but do not usually produce the 5-hydroxytryptamine that is seen in midgut or hindgut carcinoid tumours.

Cylindroma, chondroma and lipoma
These are extremely rare tumours that may grow in the bronchus or trachea, causing obstruction.

Tracheal tumours
Benign tumours include squamous papilloma, leiomyoma, haemangiomas and tumours of neurogenic origin.

FURTHER READING
Hoffman RS (2000) Lung cancer: clinical/pathological features, staging and treatment. *Lancet* **355**: 479–485.
Mulshine JL (2000) Prospects for lung cancer screening. *Lancet* **355**: 592–593.
Seijo LM, Sternman DH (2001) Interventional pulmonology. *New England Journal of Medicine* **344**: 740–749.
Spira A, Ettinger DS (2004) Multidisciplinary management of lung cancer. *New England Journal of Medicine* **350**: 379–392.

DISORDERS OF THE CHEST WALL AND PLEURA

Trauma

Trauma to the thoracic wall can cause penetrating wounds and lead to pneumothorax or haemothorax.

Rib fractures

Rib fractures are caused by trauma or coughing (particularly in the elderly), and can occur in patients with osteoporosis. Pathological rib fractures are due to metastatic spread from carcinoma of the bronchus, breast, kidney, prostate or thyroid. Ribs can also become involved by a mesothelioma. Fractures may not be readily visible on a PA chest X-ray, so lateral X-rays and oblique views may be necessary.

Pain prevents adequate chest expansion and coughing and this can lead to pneumonia.

Treatment is with adequate oral analgesia, by local infiltration or an intercostal nerve block.

Two fractures in one rib can lead to a flail segment with paradoxical movement, i.e. part of the chest wall moves inwards during inspiration. This can produce inefficient ventilation and may require intermittent positive-pressure ventilation, especially if several ribs are similarly affected.

Rupture of the trachea or a major bronchus

Rupture of the trachea or even a major bronchus can occur during deceleration injuries, leading to pneumothorax, surgical emphysema, pneumomediastinum and haemoptysis. Surgical emphysema is caused by air leaking into the subcutaneous connective tissue; this can also occur after the insertion of an intercostal drainage tube. A pneumomediastinum occurs when air leaks from the lung inside the parietal pleura and extends along the bronchial walls.

Rupture of the oesophagus (p. 279)

Rupture of the oesophagus leads to mediastinitis usually with mixed bacterial infections. This is a serious complication of external injury, endoscopic procedures, bougienage or necrotic carcinoma, and requires vigorous antibacterial chemotherapy.

Lung contusion

This causes widespread fluffy shadows on the chest X-ray owing to intrapulmonary haemorrhage. This may give rise to acute respiratory distress syndrome (see p. 986).

Kyphoscoliosis

Kyphoscoliosis may be congenital, owing to disease of the vertebrae such as tuberculosis or osteomalacia, or due to neuromuscular disease such as Friedreich's ataxia or poliomyelitis. The respiratory effects of severe kyphoscoliosis are often more pronounced than might be expected and respiratory failure and death often occur in the fourth or fifth decade. The abnormality should be corrected at an early stage if possible. Positive airway pressure ventilation delivered through a tightly fitting nasal mask is the treatment of choice for respiratory failure (see p. 985).

Ankylosing spondylitis (see also p. 564)

Limitation of chest wall movement is often well compensated by diaphragmatic movement, and so the respiratory effects of this disease are relatively mild. It is occasionally associated with upper lobe fibrosis.

Pectus excavatum and carinatum

Pectus excavatum causes few problems other than embarrassment about the deep vertical furrow in the chest, which can be corrected surgically. The heart is seen to lie well to the left on the chest X-ray. Pectus carinatum (pigeon chest) is often the result of rickets but is rarely seen in the West. No treatment is required.

Pleurisy

This is the term used to describe pain arising from any disease of the pleura. The localized inflammation produces sharp localized pain, made worse on deep inspiration, coughing and occasionally on twisting and bending movements. Pleurisy occurs with pneumonia, pulmonary infarct and carcinoma. Rarer causes include rheumatoid arthritis and systemic lupus erythematosus.

Epidemic myalgia (Bornholm disease) is due to infection by Coxsackie B virus. This illness is common in young adults in the late summer and autumn and is characterized by an upper respiratory tract illness followed by pleuritic pain in the chest and upper abdomen with tender muscles. The chest X-ray remains normal and the illness clears within a week.

Mesothelioma (see p. 946)

Pleural effusion

A pleural effusion is an excessive accumulation of fluid in the pleural space. It can be detected on X-ray when 300 mL or more of fluid is present and clinically when 500 mL or more is present. The chest X-ray appearances (Fig. 14.45) range from the obliteration of the costophrenic angle to dense homogeneous shadows occupying part or all of the hemithorax. Fluid below the lung (a subpulmonary effusion) can simulate a raised hemidiaphragm. Fluid in the fissures may resemble an intrapulmonary mass. The physical signs are shown in Table 14.1 (p. 883).

Diagnosis

This is by pleural aspiration (see p. 892). The fluid that accumulates may be a transudate or an exudate.

Transudates

Effusions that are transudates can be bilateral, but are often larger on the right side. The protein content is less than 30 g/L and the lactic dehydrogenase is less than 200 IU/L. Causes include:

(a)
(b)

Fig. 14.45 Radiographs showing (a) small and (b) large pleural effusions.

- heart failure
- hypoproteinaemia (e.g. nephrotic syndrome)
- constrictive pericarditis
- hypothyroidism
- ovarian tumours producing right-sided pleural effusion
  – Meigs' syndrome.

Exudates

The protein content of exudates is > 30 g/L and the lactic dehydrogenase is > 200 IU/L. Causes include:

- bacterial pneumonia (common)
- carcinoma of the bronchus and pulmonary infarction – fluid may be blood-stained (common)
- tuberculosis
- connective-tissue disease
- post-myocardial infarction syndrome (rare)
- acute pancreatitis (high amylase content) (rare)
- mesothelioma (rare)
- sarcoidosis (very rare)
- yellow-nail syndrome (effusion due to lymphoedema) (very rare)
- familial Mediterranean fever (rare).

Pleural biopsy (see p. 891) may be necessary if the diagnosis has not been established by simple aspiration.

Treatment is of the underlying condition unless the fluid is purulent (empyema) in which case drainage is mandatory.

Management of malignant pleural effusions

Malignant pleural effusions that reaccumulate and are symptomatic can be aspirated to dryness followed by the instillation of a sclerosing agent such as tetracycline or bleomycin. Effusions should be drained slowly since rapid shift of the mediastinum causes severe pain and occasionally shock. This treatment produces only temporary relief.

Chylothorax

This is due to the accumulation of lymph in the pleural space, usually resulting from leakage from the thoracic duct following trauma or infiltration by carcinoma.

Empyema

This is the presence of pus in the pleural space and can be a complication of pneumonia (see p. 929).

Pneumothorax

'Pneumothorax' means air in the pleural space. It may be spontaneous or occur as a result of trauma to the chest. Spontaneous pneumothorax is commonest in young males, the male-to-female ratio being 6 : 1. It is caused by the rupture of a pleural bleb, usually apical, and is thought to be due to congenital defects in the connective tissue of the alveolar walls. Both lungs are affected with equal frequency. Often these patients are tall and thin. In patients over 40 years of age, the usual cause is underlying COPD. Rarer causes include bronchial asthma, carcinoma, a lung abscess breaking down and leading to bronchopleural fistula, and severe pulmonary fibrosis with cyst formation.

Pneumothorax may be localized if the visceral pleura has previously become adherent to the parietal pleura, or generalized if there are no pleural adhesions. Normally the pressure in the pleural space is negative but this is lost once a communication is made with atmospheric pressure; the elastic recoil pressure of the lung then causes it to partially deflate. If the communication between the airways and the pleural space remains open, a bronchopleural fistula is created. Once the communication between the lung and the pleural space is obliterated, air will be reabsorbed at a rate of 1.25% of the total radiographic volume of the hemithorax per day. Thus, a 50% collapse of the lung will take about 40 days to reabsorb completely once the air leak is closed.

It has been postulated that a valvular mechanism may develop through which air can be sucked into the pleural space during inspiration but not expelled during expiration. The intrapleural pressure remains positive throughout breathing, the lung deflates further, the mediastinum shifts, and venous return to the heart decreases, with increasing respiratory and cardiac embarrassment. This is called tension pneumothorax and is very rare unless the patient is on positive ventilation.

The usual presenting features are sudden onset of unilateral pleuritic pain or progressively increasing breathlessness. If the pneumothorax enlarges, the patient becomes more breathless and may develop pallor and tachycardia. There may be few physical signs if the pneumothorax is small.

The characteristic features and management are shown in Figure 14.46. The main aim is to get the patient back to active life as soon as possible.

The procedure for simple aspiration is shown in Practical box 14.6.

FURTHER READING

British Thoracic Society (2003) BTS guidelines for the management of pleural effusions. *Thorax* **58** (Suppl 2): ii8–ii38.

British Thoracic Society (2003) BTS guidelines for the management of pleural disease. *Thorax* **58** (Suppl 2): ii39–ii52.

DISORDERS OF THE DIAPHRAGM

Diaphragmatic fatigue

The diaphragm can become fatigued if the force of contraction during inspiration exceeds 40% of the force it can develop in a maximal static effort. When this occurs acutely in patients with exacerbations of COPD or cystic fibrosis or in quadriplegics, positive-pressure ventilation is required. Further rehabilitation requires exercises to increase the strength and endurance of the diaphragm by breathing against a resistance for 30 minutes a day.

Unilateral diaphragmatic paralysis

This is common and symptomless. The affected diaphragm is usually elevated and moves paradoxically on inspiration. It can be diagnosed when a sniff causes the paralysed diaphragm to rise, the unaffected diaphragm to descend. Causes include:

- surgery
- carcinoma of the bronchus with involvement of the phrenic nerve
- neurological, including poliomyelitis, herpes zoster
- trauma to cervical spine, birth injury, subclavian vein puncture
- infection: tuberculosis, syphilis, pneumonia.

Practical Box 14.6
Simple aspiration

1. Explain the nature of the procedure.
2. Infiltrate 2% lidocaine down to the pleura in the second intercostal space in the mid-clavicular line.
3. Push a 3–4 cm 16 French gauge cannula through the pleura.
4. Connect the cannula to a three-way tap and 50 mL syringe.
5. Aspirate up to 2.5 L of air. Stop if resistance to suction is felt or the patient coughs excessively.
6. Repeat chest X-ray (in expiration) in the X-ray department.

Bilateral diaphragmatic weakness or paralysis

This causes breathlessness in the supine position and is a cause of sleep apnoea leading to daytime headaches and somnolence. Tidal volume is decreased and respiratory rate increased. Vital capacity is substantially reduced when lying down, and sniffing causes a paradoxical inward movement of the abdominal wall best seen in the supine position. Causes include viral infections, multiple sclerosis, motor neurone disease, poliomyelitis, Guillain–Barré syndrome, quadriplegia after trauma, and rare muscle diseases. Treatment is either diaphragmatic pacing or night-time assisted ventilation.

Complete eventration of the diaphragm

This is a congenital condition (invariably left-sided) in which muscle is replaced by fibrous tissue. It presents as marked elevation of the left hemidiaphragm, sometimes associated with gastrointestinal symptoms. Partial eventration, usually on the right, causes a hump (often anteriorly) on the diaphragmatic shadow on X-ray.

Diaphragmatic hernias

These are most commonly through the oesophageal hiatus, but occasionally occur anteriorly, through the foramen of Morgagni, posterolaterally through the foramen of Bochdalek, or at any site following traumatic tears.

Hiccups

Hiccups are due to involuntary diaphragmatic contractions with closure of the glottis and are extremely common. Occasionally patients present with persistent hiccups. This can be as a result of diaphragmatic irritation (e.g. subphrenic abscess) or a metabolic cause (e.g. uraemia). Treatment for persistent hiccups is with chlorpromazine 50 mg three times daily, or diazepam 5 mg three times daily. The cause should be treated, if known.

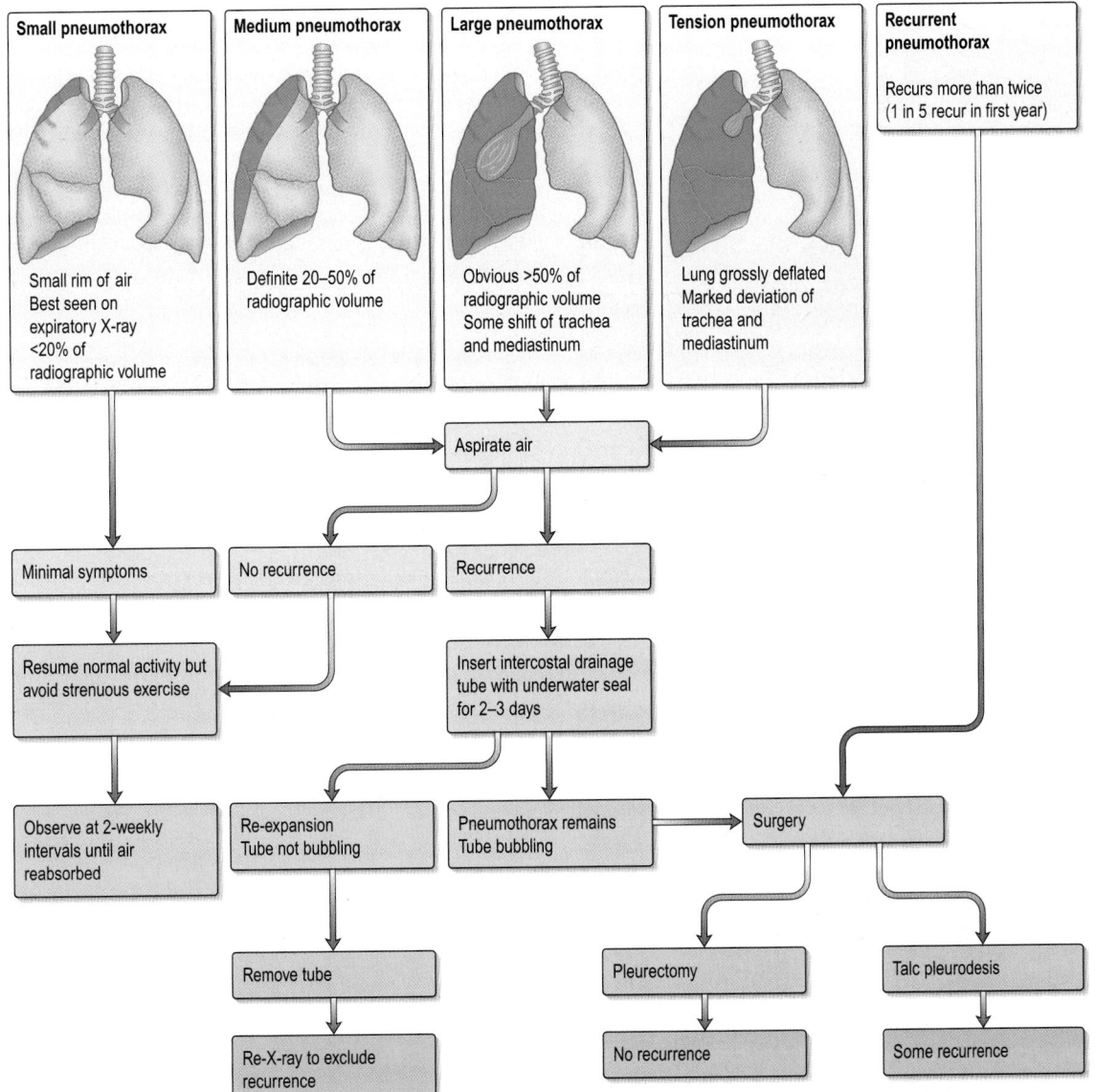

Fig. 14.46 Pneumothorax: an algorithm for management.

MEDIASTINAL LESIONS

The mediastinum is defined as the region between the pleural sacs. It is additionally divided as shown in Figure 14.47. Tumours affecting the mediastinum are rare. Masses are detected very accurately on CT or MR scan (Fig. 14.48).

Retrosternal or intrathoracic thyroid

The most common mediastinal tumour is a retrosternal or intrathoracic thyroid, which is nearly always an extension of the thyroid present in the neck. Enlargement of the thyroid by a colloid goitre, malignant disease or rarely, in thyrotoxicosis, can cause displacement of the trachea and oesophagus to the opposite side. Symptoms of com-

pression develop insidiously before producing the cardinal feature of dyspnoea. Very occasionally an intrathoracic thyroid may be the cause of dysphagia and, rarely, of hoarseness of the voice and vocal cord paralysis from stretching of the recurrent laryngeal nerve. The treatment is surgical removal.

Thymic tumours

The thymus is large in childhood and occupies the superior and anterior mediastinum. It involutes with age but may be enlarged by cysts, which are rarely symptomatic, or by tumours, which may cause myasthenia gravis or lead to compression of the trachea or, rarely, the oesophagus. Surgery is the treatment of choice. Approximately half of the patients presenting with a thymic tumour have myasthenia gravis.

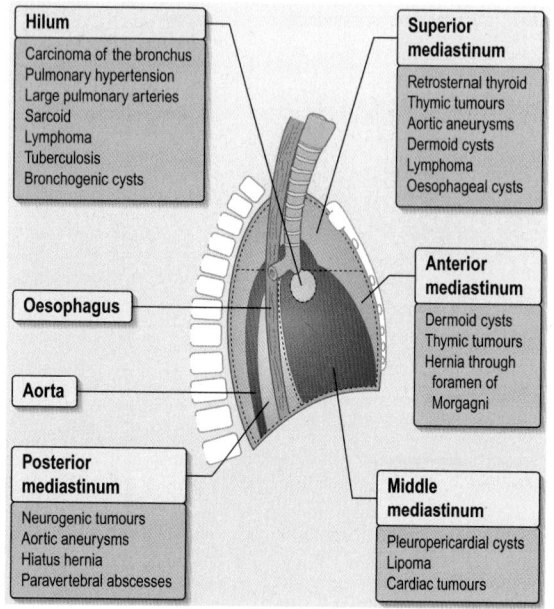

Fig. 14.47 Subdivisions of the mediastinum and mass lesions.

Hilum
Carcinoma of the bronchus
Pulmonary hypertension
Large pulmonary arteries
Sarcoid
Lymphoma
Tuberculosis
Bronchogenic cysts

Superior mediastinum
Retrosternal thyroid
Thymic tumours
Aortic aneurysms
Dermoid cysts
Lymphoma
Oesophageal cysts

Oesophagus

Anterior mediastinum
Dermoid cysts
Thymic tumours
Hernia through foramen of Morgagni

Aorta

Posterior mediastinum
Neurogenic tumours
Aortic aneurysms
Hiatus hernia
Paravertebral abscesses

Middle mediastinum
Pleuropericardial cysts
Lipoma
Cardiac tumours

Pleuropericardial cysts

These cysts, which may be up to 10 cm in diameter, are filled with clear fluid and are usually situated anteriorly in the cardiophrenic angle on the right in 70% of cases. Infection only rarely occurs; malignant change does not occur. The diagnosis is usually made by needle aspiration. No treatment is required, but these patients should be followed up as an increase in cyst size suggests an alternative pathology; surgical excision is then advisable.

SIGNIFICANT WEBSITES

http://www.brit-thoracic.org.uk
British Thoracic Society

http://www.thoracic.org
American Thoracic Society

http://www.asthma.org.uk
UK National Asthma Campaign

http://www.quitsmoking.uk.com
Good site for those waiting to quit or to help patients to quit.

Fig. 14.48 CT scan of a dermoid cyst in the mediastinum.

Intensive care medicine

Intensive care medicine (or 'critical care medicine') is concerned predominantly with the management of patients with acute life-threatening conditions ('the critically ill') in specialized units. As well as emergency cases, such units admit high-risk patients electively after major surgery (Table 15.1). Intensive care medicine also encompasses the resuscitation and transport of those who become acutely ill, or are injured, either elsewhere in the hospital (e.g. in coronary care units, acute admissions wards, postoperative recovery areas, or accident and emergency units) or in the community. Management of

seriously ill patients throughout the hospital, including critically ill patients who have been discharged to the ward ('outreach care') is also undertaken. Teamwork and a multidisciplinary approach are central to the provision of intensive care and are most effective when directed and coordinated by committed specialists. An example of guidelines for involving the critical care team in the management of an acutely ill patient is shown in Box 15.1.

Intensive care units (ICUs) are usually reserved for patients with established or potential organ failure and must therefore provide facilities for the diagnosis, prevention and treatment of multiple organ failure. They are fully equipped with monitoring and technical facilities, including an adjacent laboratory (or 'near patient testing'

Table 15.1   Some common indications for admission to intensive care

Surgical emergencies	Medical emergencies
Acute intra-abdominal catastrophe	*Respiratory failure*
Ruptured/leaking abdominal aortic aneurysm	Exacerbation of chronic obstructive pulmonary disease (COPD)
Perforated viscus, especially with faecal soiling of peritoneum (often complicated by septic shock)	Acute severe asthma
	Severe pneumonia (may be complicated by septic shock)
Trauma (often complicated by hypovolaemic and later septic shock)	Meningococcal infection
Multiple injuries	Status epilepticus
Massive blood loss	Severe diabetic ketoacidosis
Severe head injury	Coma
Obstetric emergencies	**Elective surgical**
Severe pre-eclampsia/ eclampsia	Extensive/prolonged procedure (e.g. oesophagogastrectomy)
Haemorrhage	Cardiothoracic surgery
Amniotic fluid embolism	Major head and neck surgery
	Coexisting cardiovascular or respiratory disease

Box 15.1   Guidance for involving a Medical Emergency or 'Patient at Risk' team

This system should be activated if the following criteria are fulfilled and the patient is being actively treated:

- Heart rate below 40 b.p.m.
- Heart rate above 120 b.p.m.
- Systolic blood pressure above 200 mmHg
- Systolic blood pressure below 80 mmHg
- Urine output less than 0.5 mL/kg/h for 2 consecutive hours
- Respiratory rate above 30 breaths per minute
- Respiratory rate below 8 breaths per minute
- Oxygen saturation less than 90% whilst receiving supplemental oxygen
- Glasgow coma scale less than 8
- Core temperature greater than 39°C
- Core temperature less than 35°C

Modified from Lee A et al. (1995) The medical emergency team. *Anaesthesia and Intensive Care* **23**: 183–186.

devices) for the rapid determination of blood gases and simple biochemical data such as serum potassium, blood glucose and blood lactate levels. Patients can receive continuous expert nursing care and the constant attention of appropriately trained medical staff. High dependency units (HDUs) offer a level of care intermediate between that available on the general ward and that provided in an ICU. They provide monitoring and support for patients with acute (or acute-on-chronic) single organ failure and for those who are at risk of developing organ failure; facilities include short-term ventilatory support and those for immediate resuscitation. They can also provide a 'step-down' facility for patients being discharged from intensive care. These units also provide a more comfortable environment for less severely ill patients who are often conscious and alert. Intermediate care units should not be used for patients requiring multiple organ support or prolonged, sophisticated mechanical ventilation.

The provision of staff and the level of technical support must match the needs of the individual patient and resources are used more efficiently when they are combined in a single critical care facility rather than being divided between physically and managerially separate units.

In the UK only around 2.6% of hospital beds are designated for intensive care, but elsewhere in the developed world the proportion is often much higher.

FURTHER READING
Lyons RA, Wareham K, Hutchings HA et al. (2000) Population requirement for adult critical care beds: a prospective quantitative and qualitative study. *Lancet* **355**: 595–598.
McQuillan P, Pilkington S, Allan A et al. (1998) Confidential inquiry into quality of care before admission to intensive care. *British Journal of Medicine* **316**: 1853–1858.
Vincent JL, Burchardi H (1999) Do we need intermediate care units? *Intensive Care Medicine* **25**: 1345–1349.

GENERAL ASPECTS OF INTENSIVE CARE MANAGEMENT

Critically ill patients require multidisciplinary care with:

- Intensive skilled nursing care (usually 1:1 nurse/patient ratio in the UK).
- Regular physiotherapy.
- Careful management of pain and distress with analgesics and sedation as necessary.
- Constant reassurance and support (critically ill patients easily become disorientated and psychologically disturbed).
- Nutritional support (enteral nutrition should always be used if possible). Studies have shown various nutrients to have positive immunomodulatory effects (immunonutrition) including glutamine, polyun-

saturated fatty acids and nucleotides. Confirmatory randomized studies are awaited. Growth hormone should not be used.
- The use of insulin infusions (if necessary in high doses) to normalize blood sugar appears to improve outcome from critical illness.
- H_2-receptor antagonists in selected cases to prevent stress-induced ulceration.
- TED stockings and subcutaneous heparin to prevent venous thrombosis.
- Care of the mouth, prevention of constipation and of pressure sores.

In many critically ill patients the underlying diagnosis is initially unclear, but in all cases the *immediate objective* is to preserve life and prevent, reverse or minimize damage to vital organs such as the brain, liver and kidneys. This involves a rapid assessment of the physiological derangement followed by prompt institution of measures to support cardiovascular and respiratory function in order to restore perfusion of vital organs, improve delivery of oxygen to the tissues and encourage the removal of carbon dioxide and other waste products of metabolism. The patient's condition and response to treatment should be closely monitored throughout. The underlying diagnosis can then be established as the results of investigations become available, a more detailed history is obtained and a more thorough physical examination is performed.

Discharge of patients from intensive care should normally be planned in advance and should ideally take place during normal working hours. Planned discharge may involve a period in a 'step-down' intermediate care area. Premature or unplanned discharge, especially during the night, has been associated with higher hospital mortality rates. A summary including 'points to review' should be included in the clinical notes and there should be a detailed handover to the receiving team (medical and nursing). The intensive care team should continue to review the patient, who may deteriorate following discharge, on the ward and should be available at all times for advice on further management (e.g. tracheostomy care, nutritional support). In this way deterioration and readmission to intensive care (which is associated with a particularly poor outcome) or even cardiorespiratory arrest may be avoided.

This chapter concentrates on cardiovascular and respiratory problems. Many patients also have failure of other organs such as the kidney and liver; treatment of these is dealt with in more detail in the appropriate chapters.

FURTHER READING
Goldfrad C, Rowan K (2000) Consequences of discharges from intensive care at night. *Lancet* **335**: 1138–1142.
Griffiths RD (2003) Specialized nutrition support in critically ill patients. *Current Opinion in Critical Care* **9**: 249–259.

APPLIED CARDIORESPIRATORY PHYSIOLOGY

OXYGEN DELIVERY AND CONSUMPTION
(Fig. 15.1)

Oxygen delivery (oxygen dispatch) is defined as the total amount of oxygen delivered to the tissues per unit time. It is dependent on the volume of blood flowing through the microcirculation per minute (i.e. the total cardiac output, $\dot{Q}_t$) and the amount of oxygen contained in that blood (i.e. the arterial oxygen content, C_aO_2). Oxygen is transported both in combination with haemoglobin and dissolved in plasma. The amount combined with haemoglobin is determined by the oxygen capacity of the haemoglobin (usually taken as 1.34 mL of oxygen per gram of haemoglobin) and its percentage saturation with oxygen (SO_2), while the volume dissolved in plasma depends on the partial pressure of oxygen (PO_2). Except when hyperbaric oxygen is administered, the amount of dissolved oxygen in plasma is insignificant.

Clinically, however, the utility of this global concept of oxygen dispatch is limited because it fails to account for changes in the relative flow to individual organs and its distribution through the microcirculation (i.e. the efficiency with which oxygen delivery is matched to the metabolic requirements of individual tissues or cells). Furthermore, some organs (such as the heart) have high oxygen requirements relative to their blood flow and may become hypoxic even if the overall oxygen delivery is apparently adequate.

Cardiac output

Cardiac output is the product of heart rate and stroke volume, and is affected by changes in either (Fig. 15.2).

Fig. 15.1 Tissue oxygen delivery and consumption.
Oxygen delivery (DO_2) = cardiac output × (haemoglobin concentration × oxygen saturation (S_aO_2) × 1.34). In normal adults it is roughly 1000 mL/min, of which 250 mL is taken up by tissues. Mixed venous blood is thus 75% saturated with oxygen. $C_{\bar{v}}O_2$, mixed venous oxygen content; $S_{\bar{v}}O_2$, mixed venous oxygen saturation. From Singer M, Grant I (eds) (1999) *ABC of Intensive Care*. London: BMJ Books, with permission.

Fig. 15.2 The determinants of cardiac output.

Heart rate

When heart rate increases, the duration of systole remains essentially unchanged, whereas diastole, and thus the time available for ventricular filling, becomes progressively shorter, and the stroke volume eventually falls. In the normal heart this occurs at rates greater than about 160 beats per minute, but in those with cardiac pathology, especially when this restricts ventricular filling (e.g. mitral stenosis), stroke volume may fall at much lower heart rates. Furthermore, tachycardias cause a marked increase in myocardial oxygen consumption ($\dot{V}_mO_2$) and this may precipitate ischaemia in areas of the myocardium that have reduced coronary perfusion. When the heart rate falls, a point is reached at which the increase in stroke volume is insufficient to compensate for bradycardia and again cardiac output falls.

Alterations in heart rate are often caused by disturbances of rhythm (e.g. atrial fibrillation, complete heart block) in which ventricular filling is not augmented by atrial contraction and stroke volume therefore falls.

Stroke volume

The volume of blood ejected by the ventricle in a single contraction is the difference between the ventricle end-diastolic volume (VEDV) and end-systolic volume (VESV) (i.e. stroke volume = VEDV – VESV). The ejection fraction describes the stroke volume as a percentage of VEDV (i.e. ejection fraction = (VEDV – VESV)/VEDV × 100%) and is an indicator of myocardial performance.

Three interdependent factors determine the stroke volume: preload, myocardial contractility and afterload (see p. 728).

Preload

This is defined as the tension of the myocardial fibres at the end of diastole, just before the onset of ventricular contraction, and is therefore related to the degree of stretch of the fibres. As the end-diastolic volume of the ventricle increases, tension in the myocardial fibres is increased and stroke volume rises (Fig. 15.3). $\dot{V}_mO_2$ increases only slightly with an increase in preload and this is therefore the most efficient way of improving cardiac output.

Myocardial contractility

This refers to the ability of the heart to perform work, independent of changes in preload and afterload. The state of myocardial contractility determines the response of the ventricles to changes in preload and afterload. Contractility is often reduced in intensive care patients, as

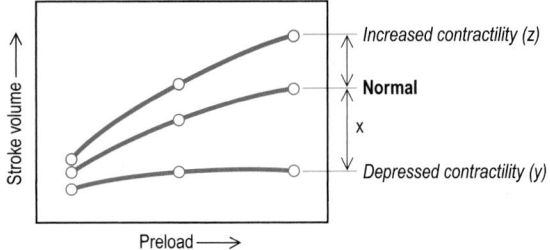

Fig. 15.3 Ventricular function (Starling curve).
As the preload is increased, the stroke volume rises. If the ventricle is overstretched, the stroke volume will fall (x). In myocardial failure, the curve is depressed and flattened (y). Increasing contractility shifts the curve upwards and to the left (z).

a result of either pre-existing myocardial damage (e.g. ischaemic heart disease), or the acute disease process itself (e.g. sepsis). Changes in myocardial contractility alter the slope and position of the Starling curve; the resulting worsening ventricular performance is manifested as a depressed, flattened curve (Fig. 15.3 and Figs 13.0 and 13.0).

Afterload

This is defined as the myocardial wall tension developed during systolic ejection. In the case of the left ventricle, the resistance imposed by the aortic valve, the peripheral vascular resistance and the elasticity of the major blood vessels are the major determinants of afterload. Ventricular wall tension will also be increased by ventricular dilatation, an increase in intraventricular pressure or a reduction in ventricular wall thickness.

Decreasing the afterload can increase the stroke volume achieved at a given preload (Fig. 15.4), whilst reducing $\dot{V}_mO_2$. The reduction in wall tension may also lead to an increase in coronary blood flow, thereby improving the myocardial oxygen supply/demand ratio. Excessive reductions in afterload will cause hypotension.

Increasing the afterload, on the other hand, can cause a fall in stroke volume and is a potent cause of increased $\dot{V}_mO_2$. Right ventricular afterload is normally negligible because the resistance of the pulmonary circulation is very low.

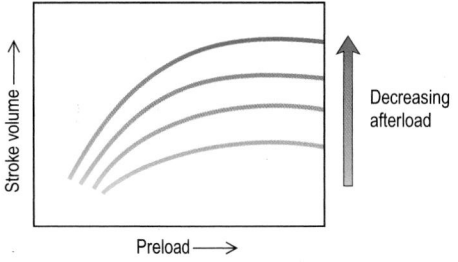

Fig. 15.4 The effect of changes in afterload on the ventricular function curve. At any given preload, decreasing afterload increases the stroke volume.

Oxygenation of the blood

Oxyhaemoglobin dissociation curve

The saturation of haemoglobin with oxygen is determined by the partial pressure of oxygen (PO_2) in the blood, the relationship between the two being described by the oxyhaemoglobin dissociation curve (Fig. 15.5). The sigmoid shape of this curve is significant clinically for a number of reasons:

- Modest falls in the partial pressure of oxygen in the arterial blood (P_aO_2) may be tolerated (since oxygen content is relatively unaffected) provided that the percentage saturation remains above 90%.
- Increasing the P_aO_2 to above normal has only a minimal effect on oxygen content unless hyperbaric oxygen is administered (when the amount of oxygen in solution in plasma becomes significant).
- Once on the steep 'slippery slope' of the curve (percentage saturation below about 90%), a small decrease in P_aO_2 can cause large falls in oxygen content, while increasing P_aO_2 only slightly, e.g. by administering 28% oxygen to a patient with chronic obstructive pulmonary disease (COPD), can lead to a useful increase in oxygen saturation and content.

The P_aO_2 is in turn influenced by the alveolar oxygen tension (P_AO_2), the efficiency of pulmonary gas exchange, and the partial pressure of oxygen in mixed venous blood ($P_{\bar{v}}O_2$).

Fig. 15.5 The oxyhaemoglobin dissociation curve.
a, arterial point; v, venous point; x, arteriovenous oxygen content difference. HbO_2 (%) is the percentage saturation of haemoglobin with oxygen. The curve will move to the right in the presence of acidosis (metabolic or respiratory), pyrexia or an increased red cell 2,3-BPG concentration. For a given arteriovenous oxygen content difference, the mixed venous PO_2 will then be higher. Furthermore, if the mixed venous PO_2 is unchanged, the arteriovenous oxygen content difference increases and more oxygen is offloaded to the tissues (see p. 423). P_{50} (the PO_2 at which haemoglobin is half saturated with O_2) is a useful index of these shifts – the higher the P_{50} (i.e. shift to the right), the lower the affinity of haemoglobin for O_2.

$P_{N_2} = 79$
$P_{O_2} = 21.2$
$P_{H_2O} = 0.8$
$P_{CO_2} = 0.04$

$P_{N_2} = 76$
$P_{O_2} = 13.4$
$P_{H_2O} = 6.3$
$P_{CO_2} = 5.3$

Fig. 15.6 **The partial pressures of inspired and alveolar gas.** Values given in kiloPascals.

Fig. 15.7 **The carbon dioxide dissociation curve.** Note that in the physiological range the curve is essentially linear.

Alveolar oxygen tension (P_AO_2)

The partial pressures of inspired gases are shown in Figure 15.6. By the time the inspired gases reach the alveoli they are fully saturated with water vapour at body temperature (37°C), which has a partial pressure of 6.3 kPa (47 mmHg), and contain CO_2 at a partial pressure of approximately 5.3 kPa (40 mmHg). The P_AO_2 is thereby reduced to approximately 13.4 kPa (100 mmHg).

The clinician can influence P_AO_2 by administering oxygen or by increasing the barometric pressure. Because of the reciprocal relationship between the partial pressures of oxygen and carbon dioxide in the alveoli, a small increase in P_aO_2 can be produced by lowering the P_ACO_2 (e.g. by using mechanical ventilation).

Pulmonary gas exchange

In *normal* subjects there is a small alveolar–arterial oxygen difference ($P_{A-a}O_2$). This is due to:

- a small (0.133 kPa, 1 mmHg) pressure gradient across the alveolar membrane
- a small amount of blood (2% of total cardiac output) bypassing the lungs via the bronchial and thebesian veins
- a small degree of ventilation/perfusion mismatch.

Pathologically there are three possible causes of an increased $P_{A-a}O_2$ difference, as follows:

Diffusion defect

This is not a major cause of hypoxaemia even in conditions such as fibrosing alveolitis, in which the alveolar–capillary membrane is considerably thickened. Carbon dioxide is not affected, as it is more soluble than oxygen.

Right-to-left shunts

In certain congenital cardiac lesions, such as Fallot's tetralogy and when a segment of lung is completely unventilated, a considerable amount of blood bypasses the lungs and causes arterial hypoxaemia. This hypoxaemia cannot be corrected by administering oxygen to increase the P_AO_2, because blood leaving normal alveoli is already fully saturated and further increases in P_O_2 will

not significantly affect its oxygen content. On the other hand, because of the shape of the carbon dioxide dissociation curve (Fig. 15.7), the high P_{CO_2} of the shunted blood can be compensated for by overventilating patent alveoli, thus lowering the CO_2 content of the effluent blood. Indeed, many patients with acute right-to-left shunts hyperventilate in response to the hypoxia or stimulation of mechanoreceptors in the lung, so that the P_aCO_2 is normal or low.

Ventilation/perfusion mismatch (see Ch. 14)

Diseases of the lung parenchyma result in $\dot{V}/\dot{Q}$ mismatch, producing an increase in alveolar deadspace and hypoxaemia. The increased deadspace can be compensated by increasing overall ventilation. In contrast to the hypoxia resulting from a true right-to-left shunt, that due to areas of low $\dot{V}/\dot{Q}$ can be partially corrected by administering oxygen and thereby increasing the P_AO_2 even in poorly ventilated areas of lung.

Mixed venous oxygen tension ($P_{\bar{v}}O_2$) and saturation ($S_{\bar{v}}O_2$)

The $P_{\bar{v}}O_2$ is the partial pressure of oxygen in pulmonary arterial blood that has been thoroughly mixed during its passage through the heart. Assuming P_aO_2 remains constant, $P_{\bar{v}}O_2$ and $S_{\bar{v}}O_2$ will fall if more oxygen has to be extracted from each unit volume of blood arriving at the tissues. A low $P_{\bar{v}}O_2$ therefore indicates either that oxygen delivery has fallen or that tissue oxygen requirements have increased without a compensatory rise in cardiac output. If $P_{\bar{v}}O_2$ falls, the effect of a given degree of pulmonary shunting on arterial oxygenation will be exacerbated. Thus, worsening arterial hypoxaemia does not necessarily indicate a deterioration in pulmonary function but may instead reflect a fall in cardiac output and/or a rise in oxygen consumption.

Conversely, a rise in $P_{\bar{v}}O_2$ and $S_{\bar{v}}O_2$ may reflect impaired tissue oxygen extraction (due to microcirculatory dysfunction) and/or a reduced oxygen uptake utilization (due, for example, to a mitochondrial defect) as may be seen in severe sepsis (see below).

Monitoring the oxygen saturation in central venous, rather than pulmonary artery blood is less invasive and has been shown to be a valuable guide to the resuscitation of critically ill patients (see p. 968).

DISTURBANCES OF ACID–BASE BALANCE

The physiology of acid–base control is discussed on page 716. Acid–base disturbances can be described in relation to the diagram illustrated in Figure 12.14, which shows P_aCO_2 plotted against arterial [H$^+$].

Both acidosis and alkalosis can occur, each of which may be either metabolic (primarily affecting the bicarbonate component of the system) or respiratory (primarily affecting P_aCO_2). Compensatory changes may also be apparent. In clinical practice, arterial [H$^+$] values outside the range 18–126 nmol/L (pH 6.9–7.7) are very rarely encountered.

Blood gas and acid–base values (normal ranges) are shown in Table 15.2. For blood gas analysis, see p. 980.

Respiratory acidosis. This is caused by retention of carbon dioxide. The P_aCO_2 and [H$^+$] rise. A chronically raised P_aCO_2 is compensated by renal retention of bicarbonate, and the [H$^+$] returns towards normal. A constant arterial bicarbonate concentration is then usually established within 2–5 days. This represents a primary respiratory acidosis with a compensatory metabolic alkalosis (see p. 716). Common causes of respiratory acidosis include ventilatory failure and COPD (type II respiratory failure where there is a high P_aCO_2 and a low P_aO_2 – see Ch. 14).

Respiratory alkalosis. In this case the reverse occurs and there is a fall in P_aCO_2 and [H$^+$], often with a small reduction in bicarbonate concentration. If hypocarbia persists, some degree of renal compensation may occur, producing a metabolic acidosis, although in practice this is unusual. A respiratory alkalosis is often produced, intentionally or unintentionally, when patients are mechanically ventilated; it may also be seen with hypoxaemic (type I) respiratory failure (see Ch. 14), spontaneous hyperventilation and in those living at high altitudes.

Metabolic acidosis (p. 716). This may be due to excessive acid production, most commonly lactate and H$^+$ (lactic acidosis) as a consequence of anaerobic metabolism during an episode of shock or following cardiac arrest. A metabolic acidosis may also develop in chronic renal failure or in diabetic ketoacidosis. It can also follow the loss of bicarbonate from the gut, for example, or from the kidney in renal tubular acidosis. Respiratory compensation for a metabolic acidosis is usually slightly delayed because the blood–brain barrier initially prevents the

respiratory centre from sensing the increased blood [H$^+$]. Following this short delay, however, the patient hyperventilates and 'blows off' carbon dioxide to produce a compensatory respiratory alkalosis. There is a limit to this respiratory compensation, since in practice values for P_aCO_2 less than about 1.4 kPa (11 mmHg) are never achieved. It should also be noted that spontaneous respiratory compensation cannot occur if the patient's ventilation is controlled or if the respiratory centre is depressed, for example by drugs or head injury.

Metabolic alkalosis. This can be caused by loss of acid, for example from the stomach with nasogastric suction, or in high intestinal obstruction, or excessive administration of absorbable alkali. Overzealous treatment with intravenous sodium bicarbonate is frequently implicated. Respiratory compensation for a metabolic alkalosis is often slight, and it is rare to encounter a P_aCO_2 above 6.5 kPa (50 mmHg), even with severe alkalosis.

SHOCK AND ACUTE DISTURBANCES OF HAEMODYNAMIC FUNCTION

Shock is difficult to define. The term is used to describe acute circulatory failure with inadequate or inappropriately distributed tissue perfusion resulting in generalized cellular hypoxia.

Causes of shock

Abnormalities of tissue perfusion may result from:

- failure of the heart to act as an effective pump
- mechanical impediments to forward flow
- loss of circulatory volume
- abnormalities of the peripheral circulation.

The causes of shock are shown in Table 15.3. Often shock can result from a combination of these factors (e.g. in sepsis, distributive shock is frequently complicated by hypovolaemia and myocardial depression).

Table 15.2 Arterial blood gas and acid–base values (normal ranges)

H$^+$	35–45 nmol/L	pH 7.35–7.45
P_{O_2}	10–13.3 kPa	(75–100 mmHg)
P_{CO_2}	4.8–6.1 kPa	(36–46 mmHg)
Base deficit	± 2.5	
Plasma HCO$_3^-$	22–26 mmol/L	
O$_2$ saturation	95–100%	

Table 15.3 Causes of shock

Hypovolaemic	**Obstructive**
Exogenous losses (e.g. haemorrhage, burns)	Obstruction to outflow (e.g. pulmonary embolus)
Endogenous losses	Restricted cardiac filling (e.g. cardiac tamponade, tension pneumothorax)
Cardiogenic (e.g. ischaemic cardiac damage)	**Distributive** (e.g. sepsis. anaphylaxis) Vascular dilatation Sequestration Arteriovenous shunting Maldistribution of flow Myocardial depression

PATHOPHYSIOLOGY

The sympatho-adrenal response to shock (Fig. 15.8)

Hypotension stimulates the baroreceptors, and to a lesser extent the chemoreceptors, causing increased sympathetic nervous activity with 'spill-over' of norepinephrine (noradrenaline) into the circulation. Later this is augmented by the release of catecholamines (predominantly epinephrine (adrenaline)) from the adrenal medulla. The resulting vasoconstriction, together with increased myocardial contractility and heart rate, help to restore blood pressure and cardiac output. Reduction in perfusion of the renal cortex stimulates the juxtaglomerular apparatus to release renin. This converts angiotensinogen to angiotensin I, which is in turn converted in the lungs and by the vascular endothelium to the potent vasoconstrictor angiotensin II. Angiotensin II also stimulates secretion of aldosterone by the adrenal cortex, causing sodium and water retention (p. 1096). This helps to restore the circulating volume (see p. 690).

Neuroendocrine response

- There is *release of pituitary hormones* such as adrenocorticotrophic hormone (ACTH), vasopressin (antidiuretic hormone, ADH) and endogenous opioid peptides.
- There is *release of cortisol*, which causes fluid retention and antagonizes insulin.

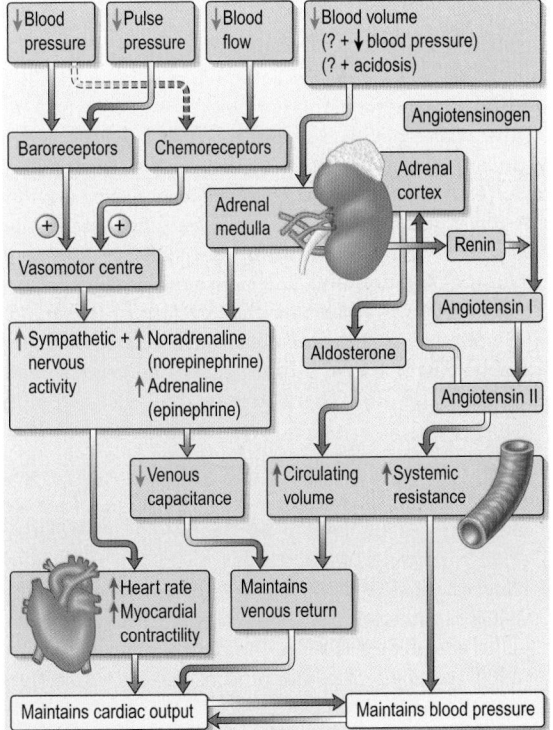

Fig. 15.8 The sympatho-adrenal response to shock.

- There is *release of glucagon*, which raises the blood sugar level.

Although absolute adrenocortical insufficiency (due, for example, to bilateral adrenal haemorrhage or necrosis) is rare, there is evidence that patients with septic shock have blunted response to exogenous ACTH (so-called 'relative' or 'occult' adrenocortical insufficiency) and that this may be associated with an impaired pressor response to norepinephrine (noradrenaline) and a worse prognosis.

Release of pro- and anti-inflammatory mediators (see also Ch. 4)

Severe infection (often with bacteraemia or endotoxaemia), the presence of large areas of damaged tissue (e.g. following trauma or extensive surgery) or prolonged/repeated episodes of hypoperfusion can trigger an exaggerated inflammatory response with systemic activation of leucocytes and release of a variety of potentially damaging 'mediators'. Although beneficial when targeted against local areas of infection or necrotic tissue, dissemination of this 'innate immune' response can produce shock and widespread tissue damage. Characteristically the initial episode of overwhelming inflammation is followed by a period of immune suppression, which in some cases may be profound and during which the patient is at increased risk of developing secondary infections.

Microorganisms and their toxic products

In sepsis/septic shock the inflammatory cascade is triggered by the presence in the bloodstream of microorganisms, their cell wall components (e.g. endotoxin) and/or exotoxins (antigenic proteins produced by bacteria such as staphylococci, streptococci and pseudomonas). Endotoxin is a lipopolysaccharide (LPS) derived from the cell wall of Gram-negative bacteria which is a potent trigger of the inflammatory response. The lipid A portion of LPS can be bound by a protein normally present in human serum known as lipopolysaccharide binding protein (LBP). The LBP/LPS complex attaches to the cell surface marker CD14 and, combined with a secreted protein, this complex then binds to a member of the toll-like receptor family (probably TLR4), which transduces the activation signal into the cell. Another mechanism in this complex area involves TREM-I (triggering receptor expressed in myeloid cells) (see p. 202). Specific kinases then phosphorylate IκB, releasing the nuclear transcription factor NFκB, which passes into the nucleus where it binds to DNA and promotes the synthesis of a wide variety of inflammatory mediators. Cell wall components from Gram-positive bacteria, some of which are similar in structure to LPS (e.g. lipoteichoic acid), can also trigger a systemic inflammatory response, probably through similar, but not identical pathways (see Fig. 15.9).

Activation of complement cascade (see p. 201)

One of the many functions of the complement system is to attract and activate leucocytes, which then marginate

Fig. 15.9 Induction of synthesis of cytokines, free radicals and nitric oxide by bacterial cell wall components. LPS, lipopolysaccharide; LPB, lipopolysaccharide binding protein; LTA, lipoteichoic acid; NFκB, nuclear factor kappa B; IκB inhibitory factor kappa B; PEPG, peptidoglycan-G; TLR, toll-like receptors.

on to endothelium and release inflammatory mediators such as proteases and toxic free radicals of oxygen and other reactive oxygen and nitrogen species (see below).

Cytokines (see also p. 202)

Pro-inflammatory cytokines such as the interleukins (ILs) and tumour necrosis factor (TNF) are also mediators of the systemic inflammatory response. TNF-α release initiates many of the responses to endotoxin, for example, and acts synergistically with IL-1, in part through induction of cyclo-oxygenase, platelet-activating factor (PAF) and nitric oxide synthase (see below). The cytokine network is extremely complex, with many endogenous self-regulating mechanisms. For example, naturally occurring soluble TNF receptors are shed from cell surfaces during the inflammatory response, binding to TNF and thereby reducing its biological activity. An endogenous inhibitory protein that binds competitively to the IL-1 receptor has also been identified.

In addition to pro-inflammatory mediators such as TNF, anti-inflammatory cytokines, e.g. IL-10, are released. The ratio of IL-10 to TNF, and of TNF to TNF receptors, has been shown to be related to mortality in severe sepsis/septic shock. When excessive, this compensatory anti-inflammatory response syndrome (CARS) may be associated with an inappropriate immune hyporesponsiveness.

Platelet-activating factor (PAF)

This vasoactive lipid is released from various cell populations, such as leucocytes and macrophages, in shock. Its effects, which are caused both directly and through the secondary release of other mediators, include hypotension, increased vascular permeability and platelet aggregation.

Products of arachidonic acid metabolism
(see Fig. 14.32)

Arachidonic acid, derived from the breakdown of membrane phospholipid, is metabolized to form prostaglandins and leukotrienes, which are key inflammatory mediators (see p. 198).

Lysosomal enzymes

These can cause myocardial depression and coronary vasoconstriction. Furthermore, lysosomal enzymes can convert inactive kininogens to vasoactive kinins such as bradykinins. These substances cause vasodilatation and increased capillary permeability, as well as myocardial depression. They can also activate clotting mechanisms.

Adhesion molecules (see also p. 198)

Adhesion of activated leucocytes to the vessel wall and their subsequent extravascular migration is a key component of the sequence of events leading to endothelial injury, tissue damage and organ dysfunction. This process is mediated by inducible intercellular adhesion molecules (ICAMs) found on the surface of leucocytes and endothelial cells. Expression of these molecules can be induced by endotoxin and pro-inflammatory cytokines such as IL-1 and TNF-α. Several families of molecules are involved in promoting leucocyte–endothelial interaction. The selectins are 'capture' molecules and initiate the process of leucocyte rolling on vascular endothelium, whilst members of the immunoglobulin superfamily (ICAM-1 and vascular cell adhesion molecule-1) are involved in the formation of a more secure bond which leads to leucocyte migration into the tissues (see Fig. 4.1).

Endothelium-derived vasoactive mediators

Endothelial cells synthesize a number of mediators which contribute to the regulation of blood vessel tone and the fluidity of the blood; these include nitric oxide, prostacyclin and endothelin-1 (a potent vasoconstrictor). Nitric oxide (NO) is synthesized from the terminal guanidino-nitrogen atoms of the amino acid L-arginine under the influence of nitric oxide synthase (NOS). NO inhibits platelet aggregation and adhesion and produces vasodilatation by activating guanylate cyclase in the underlying vascular smooth muscle to form cyclic guanosine monophosphate (cGMP) from guanosine triphosphate (GTP) (Fig. 15.10). There are several distinct NOS enzymes.

- *Constitutive or endothelial NOS* (cNOS or eNOS) present in endothelial cells is responsible for the basal release of NO and is involved in the physiological regulation of vascular tone, blood pressure and tissue perfusion.
- *Neuronal NOS* (nNOS). The role of nerves containing nNOS is uncertain but they probably provide neurogenic vasodilator tone. In the central nervous system nNOS may be a regulator of local cerebral blood flow as well as fulfilling a number of other physiological functions, such as the acute modulation of neuronal firing behaviour.

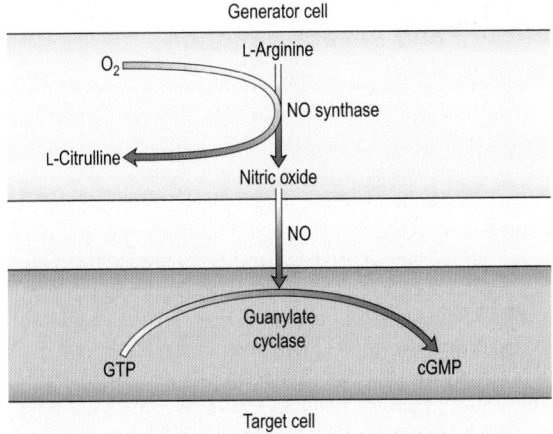

Fig. 15.10 **Synthesis and biochemical action of nitric oxide.**

- *Inducible NOS* (iNOS) is induced in vascular endothelial smooth muscle cells and monocytes within 4–18 hours of stimulation with certain cytokines, such as TNF-α, and endotoxin. The resulting prolonged increase in NO formation is believed to be a cause of the sustained vasodilatation, hypotension and reduced reactivity to adrenergic agonists ('vasoplegia') that characterizes septic shock. This mechanism may also be involved in severe prolonged haemorrhage/traumatic shock. The NO generated by macrophages contributes to their role as highly effective killers of intracellular and extracellular pathogens, in part as a consequence of its ability to bind to cytochrome oxidase and inhibit electron transport, but also via the production of the highly reactive radical peroxynitrite.

Redox imbalance

In health the balance between reducing and oxidizing conditions (redox) is controlled by antioxidants which may either prevent radical formation (e.g. transferrin and lactoferrin which bind iron, a catalyst for radical formation) or remove/inactivate reactive oxygen and nitrogen species (e.g. enzymes such as superoxide dismutases, vitamins C and E, and sulphydryl group donors such as glutathione). There are also mechanisms to remove and repair oxidatively damaged molecules and in particular to preserve DNA integrity. In severe systemic inflammation the uncontrolled production of oxygen-derived free radicals and reactive nitrogen species, e.g. superoxide ($O_2 \bullet^-$), hydroxyl radicals (OH•), hydrogen peroxide (H_2O_2) and peroxynitrite ($ONOO^-$) particularly by activated polymorphonuclear leucocytes can overwhelm these defensive mechanisms and cause:

- lipid and protein peroxidation
- damage to cell membranes
- increased capillary permeability
- impaired mitochondrial respiration
- DNA strand breakage
- apoptosis (p. 162).

Haemodynamic and microcirculatory changes

The dominant haemodynamic feature of septic shock is peripheral vascular failure with:

- vasodilatation
- maldistribution of regional blood flow
- abnormalities in the microcirculation:
  - arteriovenous shunting
  - 'stop-flow' capillaries (flow is intermittent)
  - 'no-flow' capillaries (capillaries are obstructed)
  - failure of capillary recruitment
  - increased capillary permeability with interstitial oedema.

Although these *vascular and microvascular abnormalities* may partly account for the reduced oxygen extraction often seen in septic shock, there is also a *primary defect of cellular oxygen utilization* owing to mitochondrial dysfunction (see above). Initially, before hypovolaemia supervenes, or when therapeutic replacement of circulating volume has been adequate, *cardiac output is usually high and peripheral resistance is low*. These changes may be associated with impaired oxygen consumption, a reduced arteriovenous oxygen content difference, an increased $S_{\bar{v}}O_2$ and a lactic acidosis (so-called 'tissue dysoxia'). Vasodilatation and increased permeability also occur in anaphylactic shock.

In the initial stages of other forms of shock, and sometimes when hypovolaemia and myocardial depression supervene in sepsis and anaphylaxis, cardiac output is low and increased sympathetic activity causes constriction of both precapillary arterioles and, to a lesser extent, the postcapillary venules. This helps to maintain the systemic blood pressure. In addition, the hydrostatic pressure within the capillaries falls and fluid is mobilized from the extravascular space into the intravascular compartment.

Activation of the coagulation system

The production of PGI_2 by the capillary endothelium may be impaired, cell damage (for example to the vascular endothelium) leads to the release of tissue factor (p. 466), which triggers coagulation. In severe cases these changes are compounded by elevated levels of plasminogen activation inhibitor type 1 which impairs fibrinolysis, as well as by deficiencies in physiological inhibitors of coagulation (including antithrombin, proteins C and S and tissue factor-pathway inhibitor). Antithrombin and protein C have a number of anti-inflammatory properties, whereas thrombin is pro-inflammatory.

Ultimately, unregulated activation of the coagulation cascade can progress to disseminated intravascular coagulation (DIC), which is characterized by widespread microvascular thrombosis, inadequate tissue perfusion and organ failure (p. 475).

The inflammatory response to shock, tissue injury and infection is frequently associated with systemic activation of the clotting cascade, leading to platelet aggregation and widespread thrombosis. Plasminogen is converted to plasmin, which breaks down thrombus, liberating fibrin/fibrinogen degradation products (FDPs). Circulating levels of FDPs are therefore increased, the thrombin time, PTT and PT are prolonged and platelet and fibrinogen levels fall. Activation of the coagulation cascade can be confirmed by demonstrating increased plasma levels of 'D' dimers. The development of DIC often heralds the onset of multiple organ failure. Because clotting factors and platelets are consumed in DIC, they are unavailable for haemostasis elsewhere and a coagulation defect results – hence the alternative name for DIC is 'consumption coagulopathy'. In some cases a microangiopathic haemolytic anaemia develops. DIC is particularly associated with septic shock, especially when due to meningococcal infection (see p. 75). Management of the underlying cause is most important. Supportive treatment includes infusions of fresh frozen plasma, platelets and occasionally factor VIII concentrates.

Reperfusion injury

Restoration of flow to previously hypoxic tissues can exacerbate cell damage through the generation of large quantities of reactive oxygen species and activation of polymorphonuclear leucocytes (see above) (Fig. 15.11). The gut mucosa seems to be especially vulnerable to this 'ischaemia–reperfusion injury'.

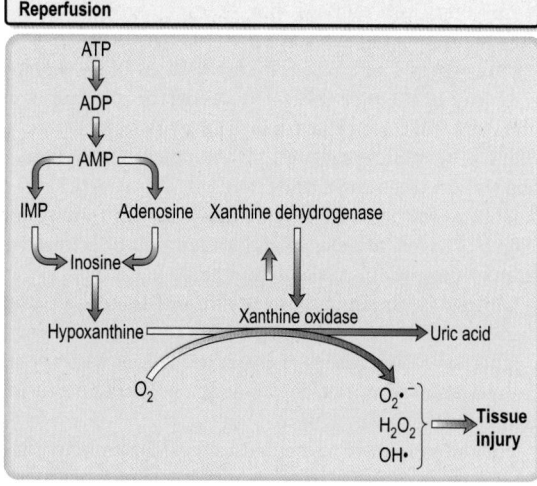

Fig. 15.11 **Generation of reactive oxygen species following ischaemia and reperfusion.**

Metabolic response to trauma, major surgery and severe infection
(see also p. 236)

This is initiated and controlled by the neuroendocrine system and various cytokines (e.g. IL-6) acting in concert, and is characterized by an increase in energy expenditure ('hypermetabolism'). Gluconeogenesis is stimulated by increased glucagon and catecholamine levels, whilst hepatic mobilization of glucose from glycogen is increased. Catecholamines inhibit insulin release and reduce peripheral glucose uptake. Combined with elevated circulating levels of other insulin antagonists such as cortisol, these changes ensure that the majority of patients are hyperglycaemic ('insulin resistance'). Later hypoglycaemia may be precipitated by depletion of hepatic glycogen stores and inhibition of gluconeogenesis. Free fatty acid synthesis is also increased, leading to hypertriglyceridaemia.

Protein breakdown is initiated to provide energy from amino acids, and hepatic protein synthesis is preferentially augmented to produce the 'acute phase reactants' (see p. 200). The amino acid glutamine (which is indispensable in this situation) is mobilized from muscle for use as a metabolic fuel in rapidly dividing cells such as leucocytes and enterocytes. Glutamine is also required for hepatic production of the free radical scavenger glutathione. When severe and prolonged, this catabolic response can lead to considerable weight loss. Protein breakdown is associated with wasting and weakness of skeletal and respiratory muscle, prolonging the need for mechanical ventilation and delaying mobilization. Tissue repair, wound healing and immune function may also be compromised.

CLINICAL FEATURES OF SHOCK

Although many clinical features are common to all types of shock, there are certain aspects in which they differ (Box 15.2).

Hypovolaemic shock

- Inadequate tissue perfusion:
  (a) Skin – cold, pale, blue, slow capillary refill, 'clammy'
  (b) Kidneys – oliguria, anuria
  (c) Brain – drowsiness, confusion and irritability
- Increased sympathetic tone:
  (a) Tachycardia, narrowed pulse pressure, 'weak' or 'thready' pulse
  (b) Sweating
  (c) Blood pressure – may be maintained initially (despite up to a 25% reduction in circulating volume if the patient is young and fit), but later hypotension supervenes
- Metabolic acidosis – compensatory tachypnoea.

Extreme hypovolaemia may be associated with bradycardia.
Additional clinical features may occur in the following types of shock.

Box 15.2 Haemodynamic changes in shock

Hypovolaemic shock
Low central venous pressure (CVP) and pulmonary artery occlusion pressure (PAOP)
Low cardiac output
Increased systemic vascular resistance

Cardiogenic shock
Signs of myocardial failure
Increased systemic vascular resistance
CVP and PAOP high (except when hypovolaemic)

Cardiac tamponade
Parallel increases in CVP and PAOP
Low cardiac output
Increased systemic vascular resistance

Pulmonary embolism
Low cardiac output
High CVP, high pulmonary artery pressure but low PAOP
Increased systemic vascular resistance

Anaphylaxis
Low systemic vascular resistance
Low CVP and PAOP
High cardiac output

Septic shock
Low systemic vascular resistance
Low CVP and PAOP
Cardiac output usually high
Myocardial depression – low ejection fraction
Stroke volume maintained by ventricular dilatation
Cardiac output maintained or increased by tachycardia

Cardiogenic shock (see p. 797)

Signs of myocardial failure, e.g. raised jugular venous pressure (JVP), pulsus alternans, 'gallop' rhythm, basal crackles, pulmonary oedema.

Obstructive shock

- Elevated JVP
- Pulsus paradoxus and muffled heart sounds in cardiac tamponade
- Signs of pulmonary embolism (see p. 844).

Anaphylactic shock (see p. 997)

- Signs of profound vasodilatation:
  (a) Warm peripheries
  (b) Low blood pressure
  (c) Tachycardia
- Erythema, urticaria, angio-oedema, pallor, cyanosis
- Bronchospasm, rhinitis
- Oedema of the face, pharynx and larynx
- Pulmonary oedema
- Hypovolaemia due to capillary leak
- Nausea, vomiting, abdominal cramps, diarrhoea.

Sepsis, severe sepsis and septic shock

- Pyrexia and rigors, or hypothermia (unusual)
- Nausea, vomiting
- Vasodilatation, warm peripheries
- Bounding pulse

- Rapid capillary refill
- Hypotension (septic shock)
- Occasionally signs of cutaneous vasoconstriction
- Other signs:
  (a) Jaundice
  (b) Coma (rare)
  (c) Bleeding due to coagulopathy (e.g. from vascular puncture sites, GI tract and surgical wounds)
  (d) Rash and meningism
  (c) Hyper-, and in more severe cases hypoglycaemia.

The diagnosis of sepsis is easily missed, particularly in the elderly when the classical signs may not be present. Mild confusion, tachycardia and tachypnoea may be the only clues, sometimes associated with unexplained hypotension, a reduction in urine output, a rising plasma creatinine and glucose intolerance.

The clinical signs of sepsis are not always associated with bacteraemia and can occur with non-infectious processes such as pancreatitis or severe trauma. The term 'systemic inflammatory response syndrome' (SIRS) has been suggested to describe the disseminated inflammation that can complicate this diverse range of disorders (Box 15.3). The usefulness of this terminology has, however, been questioned.

MONITORING CRITICALLY ILL PATIENTS

As well as allowing immediate recognition of changes in the patient's condition, monitoring can also be used to establish or confirm a diagnosis, to gauge the severity of the condition, to follow the evolution of the illness and to assess the response to treatment. Invasive monitoring is generally indicated in the more seriously ill patients and in those who fail to respond to initial treatment. These techniques are, however, associated with a small, but significant, risk of complications and should therefore only be used when the potential benefits outweigh the dangers. Likewise, invasive devices should be removed as soon as possible.

Assessment of tissue perfusion

- *Pale, cold skin*, delayed capillary refill and the absence of visible veins in the hands and feet indicate poor perfusion. (Peripheral skin temperature measurements can help clinical evaluation as vasoconstriction is an early compensatory response.)
- *Urinary flow* is a sensitive indicator of renal perfusion and haemodynamic performance.
- *Metabolic acidosis with raised lactate concentration* may suggest that tissue perfusion is sufficiently compromised to cause cellular hypoxia and anaerobic glycolysis. Persistent, severe lactic acidosis is associated with a very poor prognosis. In many critically ill patients, especially those with sepsis, however, lactic acidosis can also be caused by metabolic disorders unrelated to tissue hypoxia and may be exacerbated by reduced clearance owing to hepatic or renal dysfunction.

Box 15.3 Terminology used in systemic inflammation and sepsis

Infection
Invasion of normally sterile host tissue by microorganisms

Bacteraemia
Viable bacteria in blood

Systemic inflammatory response syndrome (SIRS)
The systemic inflammatory response to a variety of severe clinical insults. The response is manifested by two or more of the following:

- Temperature > 38°C or < 36°C
- Heart rate > 90 beats/min
- Respiratory rate > 20 breaths/min or P_aCO_2 < 4.3 kPa
- White cell count > 12×10^9/L, < 4×10^9/L or > 10% immature forms

Compensatory anti-inflammatory response syndrome (CARS)
Release of anti-inflammatory mediators which downregulate the inflammatory response. If excessive, may lead to inappropriate immune hyporesponsiveness

Sepsis
SIRS resulting from documented infection

Severe sepsis
Sepsis associated with organ dysfunction, hypoperfusion or hypotension. Hypoperfusion and perfusion abnormalities may include, but are not limited to, lactic acidosis, oliguria or an acute alteration in mental state

Septic shock
Severe sepsis with hypotension (systolic BP < 90 mmHg or a reduction of > 40 mmHg from baseline) in the absence of other causes for hypotension and despite adequate fluid resuscitation
(Patients receiving inotropic or vasopressor agents may not be hypotensive when perfusion abnormalities are documented)

Refractory shock
Shock unresponsive to conventional therapy (intravenous fluids and inotropic/vasoactive agents) within 1 hour

Fig. 15.12 Gastric tonometry. A Silastic balloon is passed into the stomach. Equilibration of carbon dioxide partial pressure between mucosa and balloon takes up to 30 minutes. Low flow states and tissue ischaemia are associated with a rise in carbon dioxide partial pressure. From Singer M, Grant I (eds) (1999) *ABC of Intensive Care*. London: BMJ Books, with permission.

- *Gastric tonometry* (Fig. 15.12). The earliest compensatory response to hypovolaemia or a low cardiac output, and the last to resolve after resuscitation is splanchnic vasoconstriction. In sepsis, gut mucosal ischaemia may be precipitated by disturbed microcirculatory flow combined with increased oxygen requirements. Mucosal acidosis is therefore an early sign of shock. Changes in intramucosal pH or P_{CO_2} have been suggested as a guide to the adequacy of resuscitation, although the clinical value of this technique is questionable.

Blood pressure

Alterations in blood pressure are often interpreted as reflecting changes in cardiac output. However, if there is vasoconstriction with a high peripheral resistance, the blood pressure may be normal, even when the cardiac output is reduced. Conversely, the vasodilated patient may be hypotensive despite a very high cardiac output.

Hypotension may jeopardize perfusion of vital organs. The adequacy of blood pressure in an individual patient must always be assessed in relation to the premorbid value. Blood pressure is traditionally measured using a sphygmomanometer but if rapid alterations are anticipated, continuous monitoring using an intra-arterial cannula is indicated (Practical box 15.1, Fig. 15.13).

Central venous pressure (CVP)

This provides a fairly simple but appropriate method of assessing the adequacy of a patient's circulating volume and the contractile state of the myocardium. The absolute value of the CVP is not as useful as its response to a fluid challenge (the infusion of 100–200 mL of fluid over a few

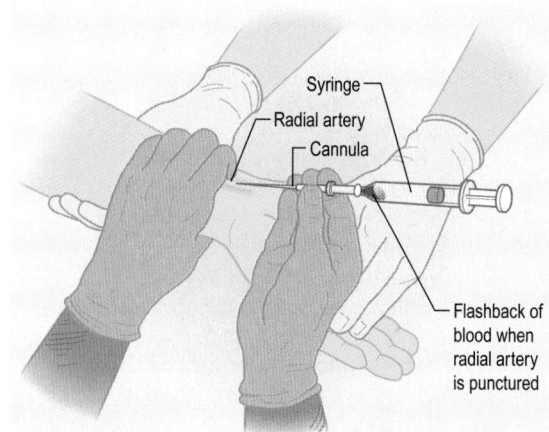

Fig. 15.13 Cannulation of the radial artery.

minutes) (Fig. 15.14). The hypovolaemic patient will initially respond to transfusion with little or no change in CVP, together with some improvement in cardiovascular function (falling heart rate, rising blood pressure and

Fig. 15.14 The effects of rapid administration of a 'fluid challenge' to patients with a central venous pressure within the normal range. From Sykes MK (1963) Venous pressure as a clinical indication of adequacy of transfusion. *Annals of the Royal College of Surgeons of England* 33: 185–197.

 Practical Box 15.1
Radial artery cannulation

Technique
1 The procedure is explained to the patient and if possible consent obtained.
2 The arm is supported, with the wrist extended, by an assistant. (Gloves should be worn.)
3 The skin should be cleaned with chlorhexidine.
4 The radial artery is palpated where it arches over the head of the radius.
5 In conscious patients, local anaesthetic is injected to raise a weal over the artery, taking care not to puncture the vessel or obscure its pulsation.
6 A small skin incision is made over the proposed puncture site.
7 A small parallel-sided cannula (20 gauge for adults, 22 gauge for children) is used in order to allow blood flow to continue past the cannula.
8 The cannula is inserted over the point of maximal pulsation and advanced in line with the direction of the vessel at an angle of approximately 30°.
9 'Flashback' of blood into the cannula indicates that the radial artery has been punctured.
10 To ensure that the shoulder of the cannula enters the vessel the needle and cannula are lowered and advanced a few millimetres into the vessel.
11 The cannula is threaded off the needle into the vessel and the needle withdrawn.
12 The cannula is connected to a non-compliant manometer line filled with heparinized saline. This is then connected via a transducer and continuous flush device to a monitor, which records the arterial pressure.

Complications
■ Thrombosis
■ Loss of arterial pulsation
■ Distal ischaemia, e.g. digital necrosis (rare)
■ Accidental injection of drugs – can produce vascular occlusion
■ Disconnection – rapid blood loss.

increased peripheral temperature). As the normovolaemic state is approached, the CVP usually rises slightly and stabilizes, while other cardiovascular values normalize. At this stage, volume replacement should be slowed, or even stopped, in order to avoid overtransfusion (indicated by an abrupt and sustained rise in CVP, often accompanied by some deterioration in the patient's condition). In cardiac failure the venous pressure is usually high; the patient will not improve in response to volume replacement, which will cause a further, sometimes dramatic, rise in CVP.

The central venous catheter is usually inserted via a percutaneous puncture of a subclavian or internal jugular vein (Practical box 15.2, Fig. 15.15). Techniques using a guidewire are generally safer and more reliable than the catheter over needle devices (Fig. 15.16). They can also be used in conjunction with a vein dilator for inserting introducers of pulmonary artery catheters, multilumen catheters and double lumen cannulae for haemofiltration.

The CVP may be read intermittently using a manometer system (Fig. 15.17) or continuously using a transducer and bedside monitor. It is essential that the pressure recorded always be related to the level of the right atrium. Various landmarks are advocated (e.g. sternal notch with the patient supine, sternal angle or mid-axilla when patient at 45 degrees), but which is chosen is largely immaterial provided it is used consistently in an individual patient. Pressure measurements should be obtained at end-expiration.

The following are common pitfalls in interpreting central venous pressure readings:

Blocked catheter. This results in a sustained high reading, with a damped or absent waveform which often does not correlate with clinical assessment.

Manometer or transducer wrongly positioned. Failure to level the system is a common cause of erroneous readings.

Catheter tip in right ventricle. If the catheter is advanced too far, an unexpectedly high pressure with pronounced oscillations is recorded. This is easily recognized when the waveform is displayed.

Left atrial pressure

In uncomplicated cases, careful interpretation of the CVP provides a reasonable guide to the filling pressures of both sides of the heart. In many critically ill patients, however, this is not the case and there is a disparity in function between the two ventricles. Most commonly, left ventricular performance is worst, so that the left ventricular function curve is displaced downward and to the right (Fig. 15.18). High right ventricular filling pressures, with normal or low left atrial pressures, are less common but may occur with right ventricular dysfunction and in situations where the pulmonary vascular resistance (i.e. right ventricular afterload) is raised, such as in acute respiratory failure and pulmonary embolism.

✓ Practical Box 15.2
Internal jugular vein cannulation

Technique
1 The procedure is explained to the patient and if possible consent obtained.
2 The patient is placed head-down to distend the central veins (this facilitates cannulation and minimizes the risk of air embolism but may exacerbate respiratory distress and is dangerous in those with raised intracranial pressure).
3 The skin is cleaned with an anaesthetic solution such as chlorhexidine. Sterile precautions are taken throughout the procedure.
4 Local anaesthetic (1% plain lidocaine) is injected intradermally to raise a weal at the apex of a triangle formed by the two heads of sternomastoid with the clavicle at its base.
5 A small incision is made through the weal.
6 The cannula or needle is inserted through the incision and directed laterally downwards and backwards in the direction of the nipple until the vein is punctured

just beneath the skin and deep to the lateral head of sternomastoid. *Ultrasound-guided puncture has been recommended, at least for difficult cases, and to reduce the incidence of complications.*
7 Check that venous blood is easily aspirated.
8 The cannula is threaded off the needle into the vein.
9 The CVP manometer line is connected.
10 A chest X-ray should be taken to verify that the tip of the catheter is in the superior vena cava and to exclude pneumothorax.

Possible complications
- Haemorrhage
- Accidental arterial puncture (carotid or subclavian)
- Pneumothorax
- Damage to thoracic duct on left
- Air embolism
- Thrombosis
- Catheter-related sepsis

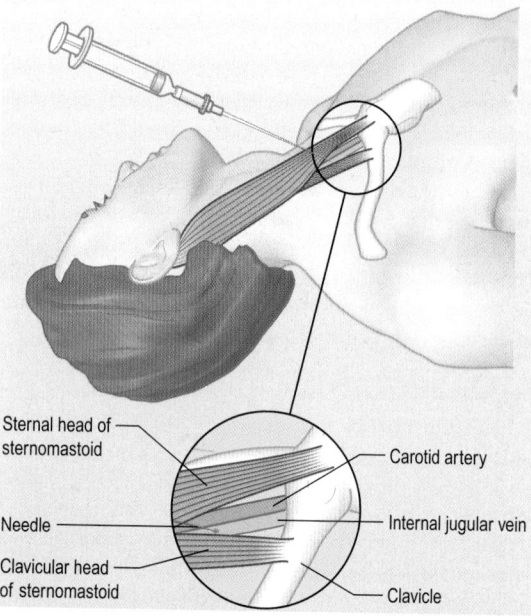

Fig. 15.15 Cannulation of right internal jugular vein with a catheter over the needle device.

Labels: Sternal head of sternomastoid; Needle; Clavicular head of sternomastoid; Carotid artery; Internal jugular vein; Clavicle

Fig. 15.16 **Seldinger technique – insertion of a catheter over guidewire.** (1) Puncture vessel; (2) advance guidewire; (3) remove needle; (4) dilate vessel; (5) advance catheter over guidewire; (6) remove guidewire; (7) catheter in situ. From Hinds CJ, Watson JD (1995) *Intensive Care: A Concise Textbook.* London: Baillière Tindall, with permission.

If there is a disparity in ventricular function after cardiac surgery, then the left atrium can be cannulated directly. If the chest is not open, however, some other means of determining left ventricular filling pressure must be devised.

Pulmonary artery pressure
A 'balloon flotation catheter' enables prompt and reliable catheterization of the pulmonary artery. These 'Swan–Ganz' catheters can be inserted centrally (see Fig. 15.16) or through the femoral vein, or via a vein in the antecubital fossa. Passage of the catheter from the major

veins, through the chambers of the heart, into the pulmonary artery and into the wedged position is monitored and guided by the pressure waveforms recorded from the distal lumen (Fig. 15.19 and Practical box 15.3). A chest X-ray should always be obtained to check the final position of the catheter. In difficult cases screening with an image intensifier may be required.

Once in place, the balloon is deflated and the pulmonary artery mean, systolic and end-diastolic pressures (PAEDP) can be recorded. The pulmonary artery occlusion pressure (PAOP, otherwise known as pulmonary artery wedge pressure – PAWP) is measured by reinflating the

Fig. 15.17 Central venous pressure measurement using a manometer system. The reading must be referred to the level of the right atrium (indicated by the axillary fold or, provided the patient is supine, the sternal notch) using a spirit level.

Fig. 15.18 Left ventricular (LV) and right ventricular (RV) function curves in a patient with left ventricular dysfunction. Since the stroke volume of the two ventricles must be the same (except perhaps for a few beats during a period of circulatory adjustment), left atrial pressure (LAP) must be higher than right atrial pressure (RAP). Moreover, an increase in stroke volume (x) produced by expanding the circulatory volume may be associated with a small rise in RAP (v) but a marked increase in LAP (z).

Practical Box 15.3
Passage of a pulmonary artery balloon flotation catheter through the chambers of the heart into the 'wedged' position

1 A balloon flotation catheter is inserted through the femoral vein or a vein in the ante-cubital fossa.
2 Once in the thorax, marked respiratory oscillations are seen. The catheter should be advanced further towards the lower superior vena cava/right atrium, where oscillations become more pronounced. The balloon should then be inflated and the catheter advanced.
3 When the catheter is in the right ventricle, there is no dicrotic notch and the diastolic pressure is close to zero. The patient should be returned to the horizontal, or slightly head-up, position before advancing the catheter further.

4 When the catheter reaches the pulmonary artery a dicrotic notch appears and there is elevation of the diastolic pressure. The catheter should be advanced further with the balloon inflated.
5 Reappearance of a venous waveform indicates that the catheter is 'wedged'. The balloon is deflated to obtain the pulmonary artery pressure. The balloon is inflated intermittently to obtain the pulmonary capillary artery occlusion (also known as pulmonary artery, or capillary, 'wedge') pressure.

Fig. 15.19 Passage of pulmonary artery balloon flotation catheter through the chambers of the heart into the 'wedged' position to measure the pulmonary artery occlusion pressure. See Practical box 15.3.

Table 15.4 Balloon flotation pulmonary artery catheters: some complications in addition to those associated with central venous cannulation

Complication	Comments
Arrhythmias	Occur during passage of catheter through right ventricle Usually benign Can often be prevented with lidocaine
Sepsis	Occurs at insertion site Bacteraemia or endocarditis may develop
Knotting	Occurs when catheter coils in right ventricle and is then withdrawn
Valve trauma	Occurs if catheter is withdrawn with balloon inflated, also tricuspid and pulmonary valves repeatedly open and close on the catheter
Thrombosis/embolism	
Pulmonary infarction	Occurs if catheter remains in 'wedged' position
Pulmonary artery rupture	Usually fatal May occur if balloon is inflated when catheter already 'wedged'
Balloon rupture/leak/embolism	Rare

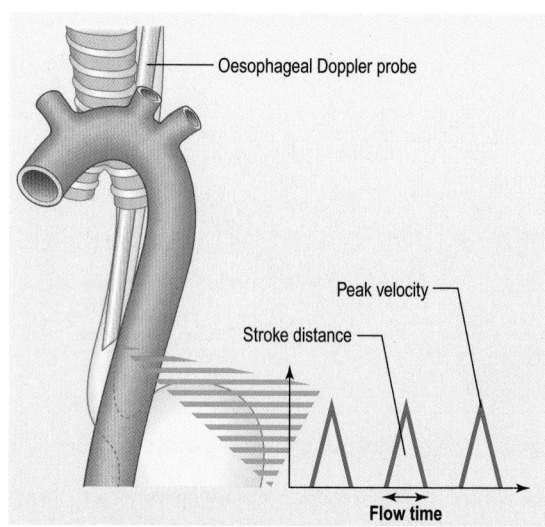

Fig. 15.20 **Doppler ultrasonography.** An oesophageal Doppler probe continuously measures velocity waveforms from the descending thoracic aorta. With a nomogram, stroke distance (area under waveform) provides an estimate of stroke volume. Acceleration and peak velocity indicate myocardial performance, while flow time is related to circulating volume and peripheral resistance. From Singer M, Grant I (eds) (1999) *ABC of Intensive Care.* London: BMJ Books, with permission.

balloon, thereby propelling the catheter distally until it impacts in a medium-sized pulmonary artery. In this position there is a continuous column of fluid between the distal lumen of the catheter and the left atrium, so that PAOP is usually a reflection of left atrial pressure.

The technique is generally safe – the majority of complications are related to user inexperience. Pulmonary artery catheters should preferably be removed within 72 hours, since the incidence of complications, especially infection, then increases progressively (Table 15.4).

Cardiac output

The thermodilution technique is most commonly used clinically. In the past a modified pulmonary artery catheter with a lumen opening in the right atrium and a thermistor located a few centimetres from its tip was used. A known volume (usually 10 mL) of cold 5% dextrose is injected as a bolus into the right atrium. This mixes with, and cools, the blood passing through the heart and the transient fall in temperature is continuously recorded by the thermistor in the pulmonary artery. The cardiac output is computed from the total amount of indicator (i.e. cold) injected, divided by the average concentration, i.e. the amount of cooling, and the time taken to pass the thermistor. It is possible to measure cardiac output continuously using a modified pulmonary artery catheter which transmits low heat energy into the surrounding blood and constructs a 'thermodilution curve'. These catheters also optically measure and continuously display $S_{\bar{v}}O_2$.

In general, pulmonary artery catheters enable the clinician to optimize cardiac output and oxygen delivery,

while minimizing the risk of pulmonary oedema. They can also be used to guide the rational use of inotropes and vasoactive agents. There is increasing evidence however, which suggests that the use of this monitoring device may not lead to improved outcomes and less invasive techniques are increasingly preferred.

Non-invasive techniques for assessing cardiac function

One of the most useful techniques for determining cardiac output and myocardial function non-invasively is Doppler ultrasonography. A probe is passed into the oesophagus to continuously monitor velocity waveforms from the descending aorta (Fig. 15.20). Although reasonable estimates of stroke volume and cardiac output can be obtained, the technique is best used for trend analysis rather than for making absolute measurements. It is particularly valuable for perioperative optimization of the circulating volume and cardiac performance.

If there is disagreement between clinical signs and a monitored variable it should be assumed that the monitor is incorrect until all sources of potential error have been checked and eliminated. Changes and trends in monitored variables are always more informative than a single reading.

MANAGEMENT OF SHOCK (see Fig. 15.21)

Delays in making the diagnosis and in initiating treatment, as well as inadequate resuscitation, contribute to the development of multiple organ failure (MOF) and must be avoided (see p. 978).

Fig. 15.21 **Management of shock.** Patients require intensive nursing care.

A patent airway must be maintained and oxygen must be given. If necessary, an oropharyngeal airway or an endotracheal tube is inserted. The latter has the advantage of preventing aspiration of gastric contents. Very rarely, emergency tracheostomy is indicated (see below). Some patients may require mechanical ventilation.

The underlying cause of shock should be corrected – for example, haemorrhage should be controlled or infection eradicated. In patients with septic shock, every effort must be made to identify the source of infection and isolate the causative organism. As well as a thorough history and clinical examination, X-rays, ultrasonography, CT scanning or a labelled white cell scan may be required to locate the origin of the infection. Appropriate samples (urine, sputum, cerebrospinal fluid, pus drained from abscesses) should be sent to the laboratory for micro-

scopy, culture and sensitivities. Several blood cultures should be performed and 'blind', broad-spectrum antibiotic therapy (p. 30) should be commenced within the first hour of recognition of sepsis. If an organism is isolated later, therapy can be adjusted appropriately. The choice of antibiotic depends on the likely source of infection, previous antibiotic therapy and known local resistance patterns, as well as on whether it was acquired in hospital or in the community. Abscesses must be drained and infected indwelling catheters removed.

Whatever the aetiology of the haemodynamic abnormality, tissue blood flow must be restored by achieving and maintaining an adequate cardiac output, as well as ensuring that arterial blood pressure is sufficient to maintain perfusion of vital organs. Traditionally a mean arterial pressure (MAP) ≥ 60 mmHg, or a systolic blood pressure

≥ 80 mmHg, has been considered adequate but recently published guidelines suggest that initial resuscitation should aim at achieving a MAP ≥ 65 mmHg.

Preload and volume replacement

Optimizing preload is the most efficient way of increasing cardiac output. Volume replacement is obviously essential in hypovolaemic shock but is also required in anaphylactic and septic shock because of vasodilatation, sequestration of blood and loss of circulating volume because of capillary leak.

In obstructive shock, high filling pressures may be required to maintain an adequate stroke volume. Even in cardiogenic shock, careful volume expansion may, on occasions, lead to a useful increase in cardiac output. On the other hand, patients with severe cardiac failure, in whom ventricular filling pressures may be markedly elevated, often benefit from measures to reduce preload (and afterload) – such as the administration of diuretics and vasodilators (see below). Adequate perioperative volume replacement also reduces morbidity and mortality in high-risk surgical patients.

The circulating volume must be replaced quickly (in minutes not hours) to reduce tissue damage and prevent acute renal failure. Fluid is administered via wide-bore intravenous cannulae to allow large volumes to be given quickly, and the effect is continuously monitored.

Care must be taken to prevent volume overload, which leads to cardiac dilatation, a reduction in stroke volume, and a rise in left atrial pressure with a risk of pulmonary oedema. Pulmonary oedema is more likely in very ill patients because of a low colloid osmotic pressure (usually due to a low serum albumin) and disruption of the alveolar–capillary membrane (e.g. in acute lung injury). As a general rule, left ventricular filling pressures should therefore not be allowed to rise to more than 15–18 mmHg in most critically ill patients. Overall, however, many more patients are undertransfused rather than overtransfused.

Choice of fluid for volume replacement
Blood

This is conventionally given for haemorrhagic shock as soon as it is available. In extreme emergencies, crossmatch can be performed in about 30 minutes and is as safe as the standard procedure (see p. 459).

Although red cell transfusion will augment oxygen-carrying capacity, and hence global oxygen delivery, tissue oxygenation is also dependent on microcirculatory flow. This is influenced by the viscosity of the blood and hence the packed cell volume (PCV). Conventionally a PCV of 30–35% has been considered to provide the optimal balance between oxygen-carrying capacity and tissue flow, although it is well recognized that previously fit patients with haemorrhagic shock can tolerate extremely low Hb concentrations provided their circulating volume and cardiac output are maintained. Transfusion of old stored red cells, which are poorly deformable, may be associated with microvascular occlusion and worsening tissue hypoxia.

Complications of blood transfusion are discussed on page 460. Special problems arise when large volumes of stored blood are transfused rapidly. These include:

Temperature changes. Bank blood is stored at 4°C and transfusion may result in hypothermia, peripheral venoconstriction (which slows the rate of the infusion) and arrhythmias. If possible, blood should therefore be warmed during massive transfusion and in those at risk of hypothermia (e.g. during prolonged major surgery with open body cavity).

Coagulopathy. Stored blood has virtually no effective platelets and is deficient in clotting factors. Large transfusions can therefore produce a coagulation defect. This may need to be treated by replacing clotting factors with fresh frozen plasma and administering platelet concentrates. Occasionally cryoprecipitate may be required.

Metabolic acidosis/alkalosis. Stored blood is preserved in citrate/phosphate/dextrose (CPD) solution, and metabolic acidosis attributable solely to blood transfusion is rare and in any case seldom requires correction. A metabolic alkalosis often develops 24–48 hours after a large blood transfusion, probably mainly owing to metabolism of the citrate. This will be exacerbated if any preceding acidosis has been corrected with intravenous sodium bicarbonate.

Hypocalcaemia. Stored blood is anticoagulated with citrate, which binds calcium ions. This can reduce total body ionized calcium levels and cause myocardial depression. This is uncommon in practice, but can be corrected by administering 10 mL of 10% calcium chloride intravenously. Routine treatment with calcium is not recommended.

Increased oxygen affinity. In stored blood, the red cell 2,3-bisphosphoglycerate (2,3-BPG) content is reduced, so that the oxyhaemoglobin dissociation curve is shifted to the left. The oxygen affinity of haemoglobin is therefore increased and oxygen unloading is impaired. This effect is less marked with CPD blood. Red cell levels of 2,3-BPG are substantially restored within 12 hours of transfusion.

Hyperkalaemia. Plasma potassium levels rise progressively as blood is stored. However, hyperkalaemia is rarely a problem as rewarming of the blood increases red cell metabolism – the sodium pump becomes active and potassium levels fall.

Microembolism. Microaggregates in stored blood may be filtered out by the pulmonary capillaries. This process is thought by some to contribute to acute lung injury (ALI) (see p. 460).

Red cell concentrates

Nutrient additive solutions – saline, adenine, glucose and mannitol (SAGM) – are available which allow red cell storage in the absence of plasma (see p. 463).

Concern about the supply, cost and safety of blood, including the risk of disease transmission and immune suppression, has encouraged a conservative approach to transfusion. There is some evidence to suggest that in normovolaemic critically ill patients a restrictive strategy of red cell transfusion (Hb maintained at 7.0–9.0 g/dL) is at least as effective, and may be safer than a liberal transfusion strategy (Hb maintained at 10–12 g/dL). However, in some groups of patient (e.g. the elderly and those with significant cardiac or respiratory disease) it may be preferable to maintain Hb at the higher level.

Blood substitutes
Attempts to develop an effective and safe oxygen-carrying blood substitute have so far been unsuccessful.

Crystalloids and colloids
The choice of intravenous fluid for resuscitation and the relative merits of crystalloids or colloids has long been controversial. Crystalloid solutions such as saline are cheap, convenient to use and free of side-effects, although they are rapidly lost from the circulation into the extravascular spaces. It has been generally accepted that volumes of crystalloid several times that of colloid are required to achieve an equivalent haemodynamic response and that colloidal solutions produce a greater and more sustained increase in circulating volume, with associated improvements in cardiovascular function and oxygen transport.

Nevertheless, a recent large, prospective, randomized, controlled trial has demonstrated that in a heterogeneous group of critically ill patients the use of either physiological saline or 4% albumin for fluid resuscitation resulted in similar outcomes. Moreover the ratio of administered albumin to saline was only 1:4.

Polygelatin solutions (Haemaccel, Gelofusin) have an average molecular weight of 35 000, which is iso-osmotic with plasma. They are cheap and do not interfere with crossmatching. Large volumes can be administered, as clinically significant coagulation defects are unusual and renal function is not impaired. However, because they readily cross the glomerular basement membrane, their half-life in the circulation is only approximately 4 hours and they can promote an osmotic diuresis. Allergic reactions can occur. These solutions are particularly useful during the acute phase of resuscitation, especially when volume losses are continuing; but colloids with a longer half-life are often used later to achieve haemodynamic stability.

Hydroxyethyl starch (HES) has a mean molecular weight of approximately 450 000 and a half-life of about 12 hours. Volume expansion is equivalent to, or slightly greater than, the volume infused. The incidence of allergic reactions is approximately 0.1%. Esterified starch is more expensive than gelatins, but is a useful volume expander.

Dextrans are polymolecular polysaccharides which have a powerful osmotic effect. They interfere with crossmatching and have a small rate of allergic reactions (0.1–1%) which may be life-threatening. Normally a dose of 1.5 g dextran per kilogram of bodyweight (as Dextran 70) should not be exceeded because of the risk of renal damage. In practice, dextrans are rarely used in the UK because of the availability of other agents.

Human albumin solution (HAS) is a natural colloid which has been used for volume replacement in shock and burns, and for the treatment of hypoproteinaemia. HAS is not generally recommended for routine volume replacement, because supplies are limited and other cheaper solutions are equally effective. Controversially a systematic review suggested that the administration of human albumin to patients with hypovolaemia, burns or hypoalbuminaemia might increase mortality. Recent evidence (see above) has, however, demonstrated the safety of 4% albumin when used for fluid resuscitation in such patients.

Myocardial contractility and inotropic agents

Myocardial contractility can be impaired by many factors such as hypoxaemia and hypocalcaemia, as well as by some drugs (e.g. beta-blockers, antiarrhythmics, angiotensin-converting enzyme inhibitors and sedatives).

Severe lactic acidosis can depress myocardial contractility and may limit the response to inotropes. Attempted correction of acidosis with intravenous sodium bicarbonate, however, generates additional carbon dioxide which diffuses across cell membranes, producing or exacerbating intracellular acidosis. Other disadvantages of bicarbonate therapy include sodium overload and a left shift of the oxyhaemoglobin dissociation curve. Ionized calcium levels may be reduced and, combined with the fall in intracellular pH, this may impair myocardial performance. Treatment of lactic acidosis should therefore concentrate on correcting the cause. Bicarbonate should only be administered to correct *extreme persistent metabolic acidosis* (see p. 719).

If the signs of shock persist despite adequate volume replacement, and perfusion of vital organs is jeopardized, pressor agents should be administered to improve cardiac output and blood pressure. Vasopressor therapy may also be required to maintain perfusion in those with life-threatening hypotension, even when volume replacement is incomplete. All inotropes increase myocardial oxygen consumption, particularly if a tachycardia develops, and this can lead to an imbalance between myocardial oxygen supply and demand, with the development or extension of ischaemic areas. For this reason inotropes should be used with caution, particularly in cardiogenic shock following myocardial infarction and in those known to have ischaemic heart disease.

Many of the most seriously ill patients become increasingly resistant to the effects of pressor agents, an observation attributed to 'downregulation' of adrenergic receptors and NO-induced 'vasoplegia' (p. 964).

All inotropic agents should be administered via a large central vein, and their effects monitored. Some of the currently available inotropes are considered here (see also p. 793 and Table 15.5).

Adrenaline (epinephrine)
Epinephrine stimulates both α- and β-adrenergic receptors, but at low doses β effects seem to predominate. This

Table 15.5 Receptor actions of sympathomimetic and dopaminergic agents

	β_1	β_2	α_1	α_2	D_1	D_2	Dose dependence
Adrenaline (epinephrine)							++++
Low dose	++	+	+	±	–	–	
Moderate dose	++	+	++	+	–	–	
High dose	++(+)	+(+)	++++	+++	–	–	
Noradrenaline (norepinephrine)	++	0	+++	+++	–	–	+++
Isoprenaline	+++	+++	0	0	–	–	
Dopamine							+++++
Low dose	±	0	±	+	++	+	
Moderate dose	++	+	++	+	++(+)	+	
High dose	+++	++	+++	+	++(+)	+	
Dopexamine	+	+++	0	0	++	+	++
Dobutamine	++	+	±	?	0	0	++

Receptor	Action
β_1 – postsynaptic	Positive inotropism and chronotropism
	Renin release
β_2 – presynaptic	Stimulates noradrenaline (norepinephrine) release
β_2 – postsynaptic	Positive inotropism and chronotropism
	Vascular dilatation
	Relaxes bronchial smooth muscle
α_1 – postsynaptic	Constriction of peripheral, renal and coronary vascular smooth muscle
	Positive inotropism
	Antidiuresis
α_2 – presynaptic	Inhibition of noradrenaline (norepinephrine) release, vasodilatation
α_2 – postsynaptic	Constriction of coronary arteries
	Promotes salt and water excretion
D_1 – postsynaptic	Dilates renal, mesenteric and coronary vessels
	Renal tubular effect (natriuresis, diuresis)
D_2 – presynaptic	Inhibits adrenaline (epinephrine) release

increases heart rate, cardiac index and reduces peripheral resistance. At higher doses, α-mediated vasoconstriction develops. If this produces a useful increase in perfusion pressure and an increase in urine output, renal failure can be avoided. However, epinephrine can cause excessive vasoconstriction, with worrying reductions in splanchnic flow, particularly at higher doses. Cardiac output may fall, prolonged high-dose administration can cause peripheral gangrene and metabolic acidosis is common. For these reasons the minimum effective dose should be used for as short a time as possible.

Noradrenaline (norepinephrine)

This is predominantly an α-adrenergic agonist. It is particularly useful in those with severe hypotension associated with a low systemic vascular resistance, for example in septic shock. There is a risk of producing excessive vasoconstriction with impaired organ perfusion and increased afterload. Noradrenaline administration should normally therefore be accompanied by comprehensive full haemodynamic monitoring, including invasive or non-invasive determination of cardiac output (see p. 972) and calculation of the peripheral resistance.

Dopamine

Dopamine is a natural precursor of adrenaline (epinephrine) which acts on β receptors and α receptors, as well as dopaminergic D_1 and D_2 receptors.

In low doses (e.g. 1–3 µg/kg/min), dopaminergic vasodilatory receptors in the renal, mesenteric, cerebral and coronary circulations are activated. D_1 receptors are located on postsynaptic membranes and mediate vasodilatation, whilst D_2 receptors are presynaptic and potentiate these vasodilatory effects by preventing the release of adrenaline (epinephrine). Renal and hepatic flow increase and urine output is improved. The value of the renal vasodilator effect of dopamine has, however, been questioned and it has been suggested that the increased urine output is largely attributable to the rise in cardiac output, combined with a decrease in aldosterone concentration and inhibition of tubular sodium reabsorption mediated via D_1 stimulation.

In moderate doses (e.g. 3–10 µg/kg/min), dopamine increases heart rate, myocardial contractility and cardiac output. In some patients the dose of dopamine is limited by β-receptor effects such as tachycardia and arrhythmias.

In higher doses (e.g. >10 µg/kg/min) the increased noradrenaline (norepinephrine) produced is associated with vasoconstriction. This increases afterload and raises ventricular filling pressures.

Dopexamine

Dopexamine is an analogue of dopamine which activates β_2 receptors as well as D_1 and D_2 receptors. Dopexamine is a very weak positive inotrope, but is a powerful splanchnic vasodilator, reducing afterload and improving blood flow to vital organs, including the kidneys. In septic shock, dopexamine can increase cardiac index and heart rate, but causes further reductions in peripheral resistance. It is most useful in those with low cardiac output and peripheral vasoconstriction and has been used as an adjunct to the perioperative management of high-risk patients (see below).

Dobutamine

Dobutamine is closely related to dopamine and has predominantly β_1 activity. Dobutamine has no specific effect on the renal vasculature but urine output often increases as cardiac output and blood pressure improve. It reduces systemic resistance, as well as improving cardiac performance, thereby decreasing afterload and ventricular filling pressures. Dobutamine is therefore useful in patients with cardiogenic shock and cardiac failure. In septic shock, dobutamine increases cardiac output and oxygen delivery.

Phosphodiesterase inhibitors (e.g. milrinone, enoximone)

These agents have both inotropic and vasodilator properties. Because the phosphodiesterase type III inhibitors bypass the β-adrenergic receptor they do not cause tachycardia and are less arrhythmogenic than β agonists. They may be useful in patients with receptor 'downregulation', those receiving beta-blockers, for weaning patients from cardiopulmonary bypass and for patients with cardiac failure. In vasodilated septic patients, however, they may precipitate or worsen hypotension.

Vasopressin

Patients with septic shock have low circulating levels of vasopressin and are hypersensitive to the pressor effects of exogenous vasopressin. Low-dose vasopressin increases blood pressure and systemic vascular resistance in patients with vasodilatory septic shock resistant to catecholamines. A fixed low dose of vasopressin can be used in severe, refractory septic shock, but the results of randomized controlled trials are awaited.

Guidelines for use of inotropic and vasopressor agents

Many still consider dopamine in low to moderate doses to be the first-line agent for restoring blood pressure, although others favour dopexamine as a means of increasing cardiac output and organ blood flow. High-dose dopamine is usually best avoided. Dobutamine is particularly indicated in patients in whom the vasoconstriction caused by dopamine could be dangerous (i.e.

patients with cardiac disease and septic patients with fluid overload or myocardial failure). The combination of dobutamine and norepinephrine (noradrenaline) is popular for the management of patients who are *shocked with a low systemic resistance* (e.g. septic shock). Dobutamine is given to achieve an optimal cardiac output, while noradrenaline (norepinephrine) is used to restore an adequate blood pressure by reducing vasodilatation. In some *vasodilated septic patients* with a high cardiac output, noradrenaline (norepinephrine) is used alone.

Adrenaline (epinephrine), because of its potency, remains a useful agent in patients with *refractory hypotension*, although adverse effects are common. This agent is preferred by some as a cheap, effective agent for the management of septic shock, especially when haemodynamic monitoring is not available.

Targeting 'supranormal' values for oxygen delivery (D_{O_2}) and oxygen consumption (V_{O_2})

Although resuscitation has conventionally aimed at achieving normal haemodynamics, survival of many critically ill patients is associated with raised values for cardiac output, D_{O_2} and V_{O_2}. However, elevation of D_{O_2} and V_{O_2} to these 'supranormal' levels following admission to intensive care produces no benefit and may be harmful. By contrast, *early* goal-directed therapy in the emergency room, aimed at maintaining central venous oxygen saturation at more than 70%, significantly improves outcome in patients with severe sepsis or septic shock.

> **Box 15.4 Patients at risk of developing perioperative multiorgan failure**
>
> - Patients with jeopardized cardiorespiratory function
> - Patients with trauma to two body cavities requiring multiple blood transfusions
> - Patients undergoing surgery involving extensive tissue dissection, e.g. oesophagectomy, pancreatectomy, aortic aneurysm surgery
> - Patients undergoing emergency surgery for intra-abdominal or intrathoracic catastrophic states, e.g. faecal peritonitis, oesophageal perforation
>
> Modified from Shoemaker WC et al. (1988) *Chest* **94**: 1176–1178.

High-risk surgical patients (Box 15.4)

These patients benefit from intensive perioperative monitoring and circulatory support, in particular maintenance of an adequate circulating volume, and postoperative admission to ICU/HDU. In such cases volume replacement and administration of inotropes or vasopressors should be guided by an oesophageal Doppler probe or, in selected cases, pulmonary artery catheterization.

The value of preoperative admission to ICU/HDU for optimization of D_{O_2}, the targeting of survivor values for D_{O_2} and V_{O_2} and the routine use of inodilators such as dopexamine remains unclear.

In conclusion, early resuscitation, aimed especially at achieving an adequate circulating volume, combined with the rational use of inotropes and/or vasoactive agents to maintain blood pressure and cardiac output is essential.

Vasodilator therapy (see p. 792)

In selected cases, afterload reduction may be used to increase stroke volume and decrease myocardial oxygen requirements by reducing the systolic ventricular wall tension. Vasodilatation also decreases heart size and the diastolic ventricular wall tension so that coronary blood flow is improved. The relative magnitude of the falls in preload and afterload depends on the pre-existing haemodynamic disturbance, concurrent volume replacement and the agent selected (see below).

Vasodilator therapy is most beneficial in patients with cardiac failure in whom the ventricular function curve is flat (see Fig. 15.3) and falls in preload have only a limited effect on stroke volume.

This form of treatment, often combined with inotropic support, may therefore be useful in cardiogenic shock and in the management of patients with pulmonary oedema associated with low cardiac output. Vasodilators may also be valuable in shocked patients who remain vasoconstricted and oliguric despite restoration of an adequate blood pressure.

The agents used most commonly to achieve vasodilatation in the critically ill are those which act directly on the vessel wall.

Nitroglycerine (NTG) and *isosorbide dinitrate* (ISDN) are both predominantly venodilators. They are of most value in those with cardiac failure in whom preload reduction may reduce ventricular wall tension and improve coronary perfusion without adversely affecting cardiac performance. Furthermore, these agents may reverse myocardial ischaemia by increasing and redistributing coronary blood flow. They are therefore often used in preference to sodium nitroprusside (see below) in patients with cardiac failure and/or myocardial ischaemia. Both NTG and ISDN reduce pulmonary vascular resistance, an effect that can occasionally be exploited in patients with a low cardiac output secondary to pulmonary hypertension.

Hydralazine predominantly affects arterial resistance vessels. It therefore reduces afterload and blood pressure, while cardiac output and heart rate usually increase. Hydralazine is usually given as an intravenous bolus to control acute increases in blood pressure.

Sodium nitroprusside (SNP) dilates arterioles and venous capacitance vessels, as well as the pulmonary vasculature by donating nitric oxide. SNP therefore reduces the afterload and preload of both ventricles and can improve cardiac output and the myocardial oxygen supply/demand ratio. On the other hand, it has been suggested that SNP can exacerbate myocardial ischaemia by producing a 'steal' phenomenon in the coronary circulation. The effects of SNP are rapid in onset and spontaneously reversible within a few minutes of discontinuing the infusion. A large overdose of SNP can cause cyanide poisoning, with intracellular hypoxia caused by inhibition of cytochrome oxidase, the terminal enzyme of the respiratory chain. This is manifested as a metabolic acidosis and a fall in the arteriovenous oxygen content difference.

Mechanical support of the myocardium

Intra-aortic balloon counterpulsation (IABCP) is the technique used most widely for mechanical support of the failing myocardium. It is discussed on page 763.

Sepsis and multiple organ failure (MOF)
(also known as multiple organ dysfunction syndrome – MODS)

Sepsis is being diagnosed with increasing frequency and is now the commonest cause of death in non-coronary adult intensive care units. The in-hospital incidence of severe sepsis is conservatively in the order of two cases per 100 admissions and length of stay is dramatically longer than for those without sepsis. Mortality rates are high (between 20–70%) and are closely related to the number of organs which fail and the duration of organ dysfunction. Those who die are overwhelmed by persistent or recurrent sepsis, with fever, intractable hypotension and failure of several organs.

Sequential failure of vital organs occurs progressively over weeks, although the pattern of organ dysfunction is variable. In most cases the lungs are the first to be affected (acute lung injury – ALI; acute respiratory distress syndrome – ARDS; see p. 986) in association with cardiovascular instability and deteriorating renal function. Damage to the mucosal lining of the gastrointestinal tract as a result of reduced splanchnic flow followed by reperfusion, allows bacteria within the gut lumen, or their cell wall components, to gain access to the circulation. The liver defences, which are often compromised by poor perfusion, are overwhelmed and the lungs and other organs are exposed to bacterial toxins and inflammatory mediators released by liver macrophages. Some have therefore called the gut the 'motor of multiple organ failure'. Secondary pulmonary infection, complicating ALI/ARDS also frequently acts as a further stimulus to the inflammatory response. Later, renal failure and liver dysfunction develop (see p. 979). Gastrointestinal failure, with an inability to tolerate enteral feeding and paralytic ileus, is common. Ischaemic colitis, acalculous cholecystitis, pancreatitis and gastrointestinal haemorrhage may also occur. Features of central nervous system dysfunction include impaired consciousness and disorientation, progressing to coma. Characteristically, these patients initially have a hyperdynamic circulation with vasodilatation and a high cardiac output, associated with an increased metabolic rate. Eventually, however, cardiovascular collapse supervenes and is the usual terminal event.

Adjunctive treatment

Initial attempts to combat the high mortality associated with sepsis concentrated on cardiovascular and respiratory support in the hope that survival could be prolonged until surgery, antibiotics and the patient's own

Table 15.6 Some of the therapeutic strategies tested in randomized, controlled phase II or III trials in human sepsis

High-dose steroids
Endotoxin antibodies
Bactericidal permeability-increasing protein
TNF antibodies
Soluble TNF receptors
Interleukin-1 receptor antagonists
Platelet-activating factor antagonists
N-acetyl cysteine
Nitric oxide synthase inhibition
Antithrombin
Activated protein C

defences had eradicated the infection and injured tissues were repaired. Despite some success, mortality rates remained unacceptably high. So far, attempts to improve outcome by modulating the inflammatory response (including high-dose steroids) or neutralizing endotoxin (Table 15.6) or inhibiting nitric oxide synthesis (e.g. with *N*-monomethyl-L-arginine) have also proved disappointing and in some cases may even have been harmful.

Recently, however, administration of recombinant human activated protein C (rhAPC), an endogenous anti-coagulant with anti-inflammatory properties, has been shown to improve survival in patients with sepsis-induced organ dysfunction. Also, it seems that the administration of relatively low, 'stress' doses of hydro-cortisone to patients with vasopressor dependent septic shock, may improve outcome. Careful control of the blood sugar level to within the normal range with insulin ('tight glycaemic control') may also reduce mortality rates in critically ill patients.

FURTHER READING
Angus DC, Linde-Zurilke WT, Lidicker J, et al. (2001) Epidemiology of severe sepsis in the United States: analysis of incidence, outcome and associated costs of care. *Critical Care Medicine* **29**: 1303–1310.
Annane D, Bellissant E, Cavaillon J-M (2005) Septic shock. *Lancet* **365**: 63–78.
Dellinger RP et al. for the Surviving Sepsis Campaign Management Guidelines Committee (2004) Surviving sepsis campaign guidelines for management of severe sepsis and septic shock. *Critical Care Medicine* **32**: 858–873.
Hébert PC, Wells G, Blajchman MA et al. (1999) A multicenter, randomised, controlled clinical trial of transfusion requirements in critical care. *New England Journal of Medicine* **340**: 409–417.
Hotchkiss RS, Karl IE (2003) The pathophysiology and treatment of shock. *New England Journal of Medicine* **348**: 138–150.
Landry DW, Oliver JA (2001) The pathogenesis of vasodilatory shock. *New England Journal of Medicine* **345**: 588–595.
SAFE Study Investigators (2004) A comparison of albumin and saline for fluid resuscitation in the intensive care unit. *New England Journal of Medicine* **350**: 2247–2256.

RENAL FAILURE

Acute renal failure is a common and serious complication of critical illness which adversely affects the prognosis. The importance of preventing renal failure by rapid and effective resuscitation, as well as the avoidance of nephrotoxic drugs (especially NSAIDs), and control of infection cannot be overemphasized. Shock and sepsis are the most common causes of acute renal failure in the critically ill, but diagnosis of the cause of renal dysfunction is necessary to exclude reversible pathology, especially obstruction (see Ch. 11).

Oliguria is usually the first indication of renal impairment and immediate attempts should be made to optimize cardiovascular function, particularly by expanding the circulating volume and restoring blood pressure. Restoration of the urine output is a good indicator of successful resuscitation. Evidence now suggests that dopamine is not an effective means of preventing or reversing renal impairment and this agent should not be used for renal protection in sepsis (p. 976). If these measures fail to reverse oliguria, administration of diuretics such as furosemide (frusemide), or less often mannitol, may be indicated. Currently furosemide infusions are most frequently employed (see Ch. 11), but mannitol is specifically indicated in rhabdomyolysis. If oliguria persists, it is necessary to reduce fluid intake and review drug doses.

Intermittent haemodialysis has a number of disadvantages in the critically ill. In particular it is frequently complicated by hypotension and it may be difficult to remove sufficient volumes of fluid. Peritoneal dialysis is also frequently unsatisfactory in these patients and is contraindicated in those who have undergone intra-abdominal surgery. The use of continuous venovenous haemofiltration, usually with dialysis (CVVHD), is therefore preferred (see Ch. 11) and is indicated for fluid overload, electrolyte disturbances (especially hyperkalaemia), severe acidosis and, to a lesser extent, uraemia.

If the underlying problems resolve, renal function almost invariably recovers within a few days to several weeks later.

FURTHER READING
Australian and New Zealand Intensive Care Society (ANZICS) Clinical Trials Group (2000) Low-dose dopamine in patients with early renal dysfunction: a placebo-controlled randomised trial. *Lancet* **356**: 2139–2143.
Schrier RW, Wang W (2004) Acute renal failure and sepsis. *New England Journal of Medicine* **351**: 159–169.

RESPIRATORY FAILURE

Types and causes

The respiratory system consists of a gas-exchanging organ (the lungs) and a ventilatory pump (respiratory muscles/thorax), either or both of which can fail and precipitate respiratory failure. Respiratory failure occurs when pulmonary gas exchange is sufficiently impaired to cause hypoxaemia with or without hypercarbia. In practical terms, respiratory failure is present when the P_aO_2 is < 8 kPa (60 mmHg) or the P_aCO_2 is > 7 kPa (55 mmHg). It can be divided into:

- type I respiratory failure, in which the P_aO_2 is low and the P_aCO_2 is normal or low
- type II respiratory failure, in which the P_aO_2 is low and the P_aCO_2 is high.

Type I or '*acute hypoxaemic*' respiratory failure occurs with diseases that damage lung tissue. Hypoxaemia is due to right-to-left shunts or $\dot{V}/\dot{Q}$ mismatch. Common causes include pulmonary oedema, pneumonia, acute lung injury and, in the chronic situation, fibrosing alveolitis.

Type II or '*ventilatory failure*' occurs when alveolar ventilation is insufficient to excrete the volume of carbon dioxide being produced by tissue metabolism. Inadequate alveolar ventilation is due to reduced ventilatory effort, inability to overcome an increased resistance to ventilation, failure to compensate for an increase in deadspace and/or carbon dioxide production, or a combination of these factors. The most common cause is chronic obstructive pulmonary disease (COPD). Other causes include chest-wall deformities, respiratory muscle weakness (e.g. Guillain–Barré syndrome) and depression of the respiratory centre (e.g. overdose).

Deterioration in the mechanical properties of the lungs and/or chest wall increases the work of breathing and the oxygen consumption/carbon dioxide production of the respiratory muscles. The concept that respiratory muscle fatigue (either acute or chronic) is a major factor in the pathogenesis of respiratory failure is controversial.

MONITORING OF RESPIRATORY FAILURE

A clinical assessment of respiratory distress should be made on the following criteria (those marked with an asterisk may be indicative of respiratory muscle fatigue):

- the use of accessory muscles of respiration
- intercostal recession
- tachypnoea*
- tachycardia
- sweating
- pulsus paradoxus (rarely present)
- inability to speak, unwillingness to lie flat
- agitation, restlessness, diminished conscious level
- asynchronous respiration (a discrepancy in the timing of movement of the abdominal and thoracic compartments)*
- paradoxical respiration (abdominal and thoracic compartments move in opposite directions)*
- respiratory alternans (breath-to-breath alteration in the relative contribution of intercostal/accessory muscles and the diaphragm).*

Blood gas analysis should be performed to guide oxygen therapy and to provide an objective assessment of the severity of the respiratory failure. The *most sensitive clinical* indicator of increasing respiratory difficulty is a rising respiratory rate. *Measurement of tidal volume* is a less sensitive indicator.

Vital capacity is often a better guide to deterioration and is particularly useful in patients with respiratory inadequacy that is due to neuromuscular problems – such as the Guillain–Barré syndrome, in which the vital capacity decreases as weakness increases.

Pulse oximetry

Lightweight oximeters which measure the changing amount of light transmitted through pulsating arterial blood and provide a continuous, non-invasive assessment of S_aO_2 can be applied to an ear lobe or finger. These devices are reliable, easy to use and do not require calibration, although remember that pulse oximetry is not a very sensitive guide to *changes* in oxygenation. An S_aO_2 within normal limits in a patient receiving supplemental oxygen in no way excludes the possibility of hypoventilation. Readings may be inaccurate in those with poor peripheral perfusion.

Blood gas analysis

Errors can result from malfunctioning of the analyser or incorrect sampling of arterial blood.

- The sample should be analysed immediately or the syringe should be immersed in iced water (the end having first been sealed with a cap) to prevent the continuing metabolism of white cells causing a reduction in PO_2 and a rise in PCO_2.
- The sample must be adequately anticoagulated to prevent clot formation within the analyser. However, excessive dilution of the blood with heparin, which is acidic, will significantly reduce its pH. Heparin (1000 i.u./mL) should just fill the deadspace of the syringe, i.e. approximately 0.1 mL. This will adequately anticoagulate a 2 mL sample.
- Air almost inevitably enters the sample. The gas tensions within these air bubbles will equilibrate with those in the blood, thereby lowering the PCO_2 and usually raising the PO_2 of the sample. However, provided the bubbles are ejected immediately by inverting the syringe and expelling the air that rises to the top of the sample, their effect is insignificant.

Disposable pre-heparinized syringes are available for blood gas analysis.

Normal values of blood gas analysis are shown in Table 15.2. Interpretation of the results of blood gas analysis can be considered in two separate parts:

- disturbances of acid–base balance (see pp. 715 and 962)
- alterations in oxygenation.

Correct interpretation requires a knowledge of the history, the age of the patient, the inspired oxygen concentration, any other relevant treatment (e.g. the administration of sodium bicarbonate, and the ventilator settings for those on mechanical ventilation). The oxygen content of the arterial blood is determined by the percentage saturation of haemoglobin with oxygen. The relationship between the latter and the P_aO_2 is determined by the oxyhaemoglobin dissociation curve (Fig. 15.5).

Capnography

Continuous breath-by-breath analysis of expired carbon dioxide concentration can be used to:

- confirm tracheal intubation
- continuously monitor end-tidal P_{CO_2}, which approximates to P_aCO_2 in normal subjects (may be useful when transporting critically ill patients, for example)
- detect apparatus malfunction
- detect alterations in lung function.

MANAGEMENT OF RESPIRATORY FAILURE

Standard management of patients with respiratory failure includes:

- administration of supplemental oxygen
- treatment for airways obstruction
- measures to limit pulmonary oedema
- control of secretions
- treatment of pulmonary infection.

The load on the respiratory muscles should be reduced by improving lung mechanics. Correction of abnormalities which may lead to respiratory muscle weakness, such as hypophosphataemia and malnutrition, is also necessary.

Oxygen therapy

Methods of oxygen administration

Oxygen is initially given via a face mask. In the majority of patients (except patients with COPD and chronically elevated P_aCO_2) the concentration of oxygen given is not vital and oxygen can therefore be given by a 'variable performance' device such as a simple face mask or nasal cannulae (Fig. 15.22).

With these devices the inspired oxygen concentration varies from about 35–55%, with oxygen flow rates of between 6–10 L/min. Nasal cannulae are often preferred because they are less claustrophobic and do not interfere with feeding or speaking, but they can cause ulceration of the nasal or pharyngeal mucosa. Higher concentrations of oxygen can be administered by using a mask with a reservoir bag attached (Fig. 15.22c). Figure 15.22 should be compared with the fixed-performance mask shown in Figure 14.26, with which the oxygen concentration can be controlled. This latter type of mask is used in patients with COPD and chronic type II failure, although the dangers of reducing hypoxic drive have been over-emphasized – hypoxaemia is more dangerous than hypercapnia.

Oxygen toxicity

Experimentally, mammalian lungs have been shown to be damaged by continuous exposure to high concentrations of oxygen, but oxygen toxicity in humans is less well proven. Nevertheless, it is reasonable to assume that high concentrations of oxygen might damage the lungs, and so the lowest inspired oxygen concentration compatible with adequate arterial oxygenation should be used. Dangerous hypoxia should never be tolerated through a fear of pulmonary oxygen toxicity.

Respiratory support

If, despite the above measures, the patient continues to deteriorate or fails to improve, the institution of some form of respiratory support is necessary (Table 15.7). For non-invasive support, see pp 985.

Intermittent positive-pressure ventilation (IPPV) is achieved by intermittently inflating the lungs with a positive pressure delivered by a ventilator via an endotracheal tube or a tracheostomy. A number of refinements and modifications of IPPV have been introduced over the years (Table 15.7). *Controlled mechanical ventilation* (CMV) with the abolition of spontaneous breathing rapidly leads to atrophy of respiratory muscles so that assisted modes that are triggered by the patient's inspiratory efforts (see below) are preferred.

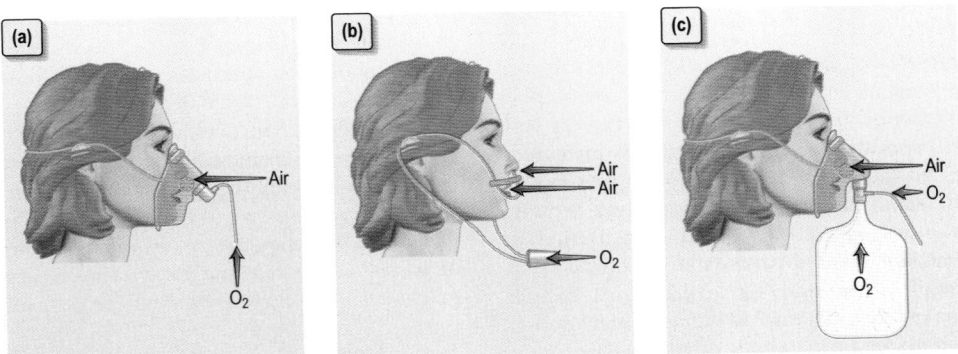

Fig. 15.22 Methods of administering supplemental oxygen to the unintubated patient. (a) Simple face mask. (b) Nasal cannulae. (c) Mask with reservoir bag.

Table 15.7 Techniques for respiratory support

Technique	Comment
Invasive respiratory support	
Intermittent positive-pressure ventilation (IPPV)	May be given with positive end-expiratory pressure (PEEP)
Continuous positive airway pressure (CPAP)	Given via endotracheal tube
Synchronized intermittent mandatory ventilation (SIMV) (volume or pressure controlled)	May be given with pressure support and CPAP
Pressure support ventilation (PSV)	Usually given with CPAP
'Lung-protective' ventilatory strategies to minimize ventilator-associated lung injury	Low tidal volume, reduced airway pressures. Can use with SIMV, PEEP and prolonged inspiratory phase
High-frequency jet ventilation (HFJV)	May be useful in those with lung leak (e.g. bronchopleural fistula)
Extracorporeal techniques	May be useful in severe acute respiratory failure
Non-invasive respiratory support	All given by tight-fitting nasal or facial masks
Continuous positive airway pressure (CPAP)	Inspiratory and expiratory pressures the same
Non-invasive positive support ventilation	± CPAP
Bilevel positive airway pressure (BiPAP)	Inspiratory and expiratory pressures set separately

The rational use of mechanical ventilation depends on a clear understanding of its potential beneficial effects, as well as its dangers.

Beneficial effects of mechanical ventilation

- *Improved carbon dioxide elimination.* By increasing the tidal volume of ventilation, the P_aCO_2 can be controlled.
- *Relief from exhaustion.* Mechanical ventilation reduces the work of breathing, 'rests' the respiratory muscles and relieves the extreme exhaustion that may be present in patients with respiratory failure. In some cases, if ventilation is not instituted, this exhaustion may culminate in respiratory arrest.

Effects on oxygenation. Application of positive pressure can prevent or reverse atelectasis. In those with severe pulmonary parenchymal disease, the lungs may be very stiff and the work of breathing is therefore greatly increased. Under these circumstances the institution of respiratory support may significantly reduce total body oxygen consumption; consequently $P_{\bar{v}}O_2$ and thus P_aO_2 may improve. Because ventilated patients are connected to a leak-free circuit, it is possible to administer high concentrations of oxygen (up to 100%) accurately and to apply a positive end-expiratory pressure (PEEP). In selected cases the latter may reduce shunting and increase P_aO_2 (see below).

Indications for mechanical ventilation

Acute respiratory failure, with signs of severe respiratory distress (e.g. respiratory rate > 40/min, inability to speak, patient exhausted) persisting despite maximal therapy. Confusion, restlessness, agitation, a decreased conscious level, a rising P_aCO_2 (> 8 kPa) and extreme hypoxaemia (< 8 kPa), despite oxygen therapy, are further indications.

Acute ventilatory failure due, for example, to myasthenia gravis or Guillain–Barré syndrome. Mechanical ventilation should usually be instituted when the vital capacity has fallen to 10 mL/kg or less. This will avoid complications such as atelectasis and infection as well as preventing respiratory arrest. The tidal volume and respiratory rate are relatively insensitive indications of respiratory failure in the above conditions and change late in the course of the disease. A high P_aCO_2 (particularly if rising) is an indication for urgent mechanical ventilation.

Other indications include:

- prophylactic postoperative ventilation in high-risk patients
- head injury – to avoid hypoxia and hypercarbia which increase cerebral blood flow and intracranial pressure
- trauma – chest injury and lung contusion
- severe left ventricular failure with pulmonary oedema
- coma with breathing difficulties, e.g. following drug overdose.

Institution of invasive respiratory support

This requires tracheal intubation. If the patient is conscious the procedure must be fully explained before anaesthesia is induced. The complications of tracheal intubation are given in Table 15.8.

Intubating patients in severe respiratory failure is an extremely hazardous undertaking and should only be performed by experienced staff. In extreme emergencies it may be preferable to ventilate the patient by hand using an oropharyngeal airway, a face mask and a self-inflating bag with added oxygen until experienced help arrives.

The patient is usually hypoxic and hypercarbic, with increased sympathetic activity; the stimulus of laryngoscopy and intubation can precipitate dangerous arrhythmias and even cardiac arrest. Except in an extreme emergency, therefore, the ECG and oxygen saturation should be monitored, and the patient preoxygenated with 100% oxygen before intubation. Resuscitation drugs should be immediately available. If time allows, the circulating volume should be optimized and, if necessary, inotropes commenced before attempting intubation. In some cases it may be appropriate to establish intra-arterial and central venous pressure monitoring before instituting mechanical ventilation, although many patients will not tolerate the supine or head-down position. In some deeply comatose patients, no sedation may be required, but in the majority of patients a short-acting intravenous anaesthetic agent followed by muscle relaxation will be necessary.

Tracheostomy

Tracheostomy may be required for the long-term control of excessive bronchial secretions, particularly in those

Table 15.8 Complications of endotracheal intubation

Complication	Comments
Immediate	
Tube in one or other (usually the right) bronchus	Avoid by checking both lungs are being inflated; i.e. both sides of the chest move and air entry is heard on auscultation
	Obtain chest X-ray to check position of tube and to exclude lung collapse
Tube in oesophagus	Gives rise to hypoxia and abdominal distension
	Detected by capnography
Early	
Migration of the tube out of the trachea	
Leaks around the tube	
Obstruction of tube because of kinking or secretions	*A dangerous complication*
	The patient becomes distressed, cyanosed and has poor chest expansion
	The following should be performed immediately:
	■ Manual inflation with 100% oxygen
	■ Endotracheal suction
	■ Check position of tube
	■ Deflate cuff
	■ Check tube for 'kinks'
	If no improvement, remove tube, ventilate with face mask and then insert new endotracheal tube
Late	
Sinusitis	
Mucosal oedema and ulceration	
Laryngeal injury	
Tracheal narrowing and fibrosis	
Tracheomalacia	

with a reduced conscious level, and/or to maintain an airway and protect the lungs in those with impaired pharyngeal and laryngeal reflexes. Tracheostomy is also performed when intubation is likely to be prolonged, for patient comfort and to facilitate weaning from mechanical ventilation.

Tracheostomy can be performed at the bedside in an ICU. A percutaneous dilatational technique, which is quick and economical, is the technique of choice in critically ill patients and can be used in an emergency. Alternatively, the trachea can be opened through the second, third and fourth tracheal rings via a transverse skin incision in theatre.

A life-threatening obstruction of the upper respiratory tract that cannot be bypassed with an endotracheal tube can be relieved by a *cricothyroidotomy*, which is safer, quicker and easier to perform than a formal tracheostomy.

Tracheostomy has a small but significant mortality rate. Complications of tracheostomy are shown in Table 15.9. With any tracheostomy, care should be taken to ensure that the tube is not blocked by secretions.

Minitracheostomy involves inserting a small-diameter uncuffed tube percutaneously into the trachea via the cricothyroid membrane using a guidewire. It can be performed under local anaesthesia. This technique facilitates the clearance of copious secretions in those who are unable to cough effectively, although, because these tubes have no cuff, patients must be able to protect their airway.

Table 15.9 Complications of tracheostomy

As for tracheal intubation (Table 15.8), plus:

Early
Death
Pneumothorax
Haemorrhage
Hypoxia
Hypotension
Cardiac arrhythmias
Tube misplaced in pretracheal subcutaneous tissues
Subcutaneous emphysema

Intermediate
Mucosal ulceration
Erosion of tracheal cartilages (may cause tracheo-oesophageal fistula)
Erosion of innominate artery (may lead to fatal haemorrhage)
Stomal infection
Pneumonia

Late
Failure of stoma to heal
Tracheal granuloma
Tracheal stenosis at level of stoma, cuff or tube tip
Collapse of tracheal rings at level of stoma
Cosmetic

Dangers of mechanical ventilation

Airway complications. There may be complications with tracheal intubation with additional local complications of a tracheostomy (see above) (Tables 15.8 and 15.9).

Disconnection, failure of gas or power supply, mechanical faults. These are unusual but dangerous. A method of manual ventilation, such as a self-inflating bag, and oxygen must always be available by the bedside.

Cardiovascular complications. The application of positive pressure to the lungs and thoracic wall impedes venous return and distends alveoli, thereby 'stretching' the pulmonary capillaries and causing a rise in pulmonary vascular resistance. Both these mechanisms can produce a fall in cardiac output.

Respiratory complications. Mechanical ventilation can be complicated by a deterioration in gas exchange because of $\dot{V}/\dot{Q}$ mismatch and collapse of peripheral alveoli. Traditionally the latter was prevented by using high tidal volumes (10–12 mL/kg) but high inflation pressures, with overdistension of compliant alveoli, perhaps exacerbated by the repeated opening and closure of distal airways, can disrupt the alveolar–capillary membrane. There is an increase in microvascular permeability and release of inflammatory mediators leading to '*ventilator-associated lung injury*'. Extreme overdistension of the lungs during mechanical ventilation with high tidal volumes and PEEP can rupture alveoli and cause air to dissect centrally along the perivascular sheaths. This '*barotrauma*' may be complicated by pneumomediastinum, subcutaneous emphysema, pneumoperitoneum, pneumothorax, and intra-abdominal air. The risk of pneumothorax is increased in those with destructive lung disease (e.g. necrotizing pneumonia, emphysema), asthma or fractured ribs.

A *tension pneumothorax* can be rapidly fatal in ventilated patients. Suggestive signs include the development or worsening of hypoxia, hypercarbia, respiratory distress, an unexplained increase in airway pressure, as well as hypotension and tachycardia, sometimes accompanied by a rising CVP. Examination may reveal unequal chest expansion, mediastinal shift (deviated trachea, displaced apex beat) and a hyperresonant hemithorax. Although, traditionally, breath sounds are diminished over the pneumothorax, this sign can be extremely misleading in ventilated patients. If there is time, the diagnosis can be confirmed by chest X-ray.

Ventilator-associated pneumonia. Nosocomial pneumonia occurs in as many as one-third of patients receiving mechanical ventilation and may be associated with a significant increase in mortality. It can be difficult to diagnose. Leakage of infected oropharyngeal secretions past the tracheal cuff is largely responsible. Bacterial colonization of the oropharynx may be promoted by regurgitation of colonized gastric fluid and the risk of nosocomial pneumonia can be reduced by nursing patients in the semi-recumbent, rather than the supine, position.

Gastrointestinal complications. Initially, many ventilated patients will develop abdominal distension associated with an ileus. The cause is unknown, although the use of opiates may in part be responsible.

Salt and water retention. Mechanical ventilation, particularly with PEEP, causes increased ADH secretion and possibly a reduction in circulating levels of atrial natriuretic peptide. Combined with a fall in cardiac output and a reduction in renal blood flow, these can cause salt and water retention.

Positive end-expiratory pressure (PEEP)

A positive airway pressure can be maintained at a chosen level throughout expiration by attaching a threshold resistor valve to the expiratory limb of the circuit. PEEP re-expands underventilated lung units, and redistributes lung water from the alveoli to the perivascular interstitial space, thereby reducing shunt and increasing the P_aO_2. Unfortunately, however, the inevitable rise in mean intrathoracic pressure that follows the application of PEEP may further impede venous return, increase pulmonary vascular resistance and thus reduce cardiac output. This effect is probably least when the lungs are stiff. The fall in cardiac output can be ameliorated by expanding the circulating volume, although in some cases inotropic support may be required. Thus, although arterial oxygenation is often improved by the application of PEEP, a simultaneous fall in cardiac output can lead to a reduction in total oxygen delivery.

PEEP should be considered if it proves difficult to achieve adequate oxygenation of arterial blood (more than 90% saturation) without raising the inspired oxygen concentration to potentially dangerous levels (conventionally 50%). Many use lower levels of PEEP (5–7 cmH$_2$O) in the majority of mechanically ventilated patients in order to maintain lung volume.

Other techniques for respiratory support

Continuous positive airway pressure (CPAP)

The application of CPAP achieves for the spontaneously breathing patient what PEEP does for the ventilated patient. Oxygen and air are delivered under pressure via an endotracheal tube, a tracheostomy or a tightly fitting face mask (non-invasive ventilation). Not only can this improve oxygenation, but the lungs become less stiff, and the work of breathing is reduced.

Pressure support ventilation (PSV)

Spontaneous breaths are augmented by a pre-set level of positive pressure (usually between 5 and 20 cmH$_2$O) triggered by the patient's spontaneous respiratory effort and applied for a given fraction of inspiratory time or until inspiratory flow falls below a certain level. Tidal volume is determined by the set pressure, the patient's effort and pulmonary mechanics. The level of pressure support can be reduced progressively as the patient improves.

Intermittent mandatory ventilation (IMV)

This technique allows the patient to breathe spontaneously between the 'mandatory' tidal volumes delivered by the ventilator. These mandatory breaths are timed to coincide with the patient's own inspiratory effort (synchronized IMV, or SIMV). SIMV can be used with or without CPAP and spontaneous breaths may be assisted with pressure support.

'Lung-protective' ventilatory strategies

These are designed to avoid exacerbating or perpetuating lung injury by avoiding overdistension of alveoli, minimizing airway pressures and preventing the repeated opening and closure of distal airways. Alveolar volume is maintained with PEEP, and sometimes by prolonging the inspiratory phase, while tidal volumes are limited to 6 mL/kg predicted bodyweight in order to achieve a plateau airway pressure of 30 cmH$_2$O or less. Peak airway pressures should not exceed 35–40 cmH$_2$O. An alternative is to deliver a constant pre-set inspiratory pressure for a prescribed time in order to generate a low tidal volume at reduced airway pressures ('pressure-limited' mechanical ventilation). Respiratory rate can be increased to improve CO$_2$ removal and avoid severe acidosis (pH < 7.2), but hypercarbia is frequent and should be accepted ('permissive hypercarbia'). Both techniques can be used with SIMV. Ventilation with low tidal volumes has been shown to improve outcome in patients with acute lung injury (ALI) or the acute respiratory distress syndrome (ARDS) (see p. 986).

Extracorporeal gas exchange (ECGE)

In patients with severe refractory respiratory failure venovenous bypass through a membrane lung (extracorporeal membrane oxygenation – ECMO, or extracorporeal carbon dioxide removal – ECCO$_2$R) has been used to reduce ventilation requirements, thereby minimizing further ventilation-induced lung damage and encouraging resolution of the lung injury. Although randomized controlled trials have indicated that this technique does not improve outcome in adults, some authorities remain convinced that, when used by experienced teams in specialist centres, extracorporeal gas exchange can significantly reduce the high mortality associated with severe ARDS.

Non-invasive ventilation (NIV)

NIV is used as a therapeutic trial with a view to tracheal intubation if it fails. It is also used as the ceiling of treatment in patients who are not candidates for intubation. It is only suitable for patients who are conscious, cooperative and able to protect their airway; they must also be able to expectorate effectively. Positive pressure is applied to the airways using a tight-fitting full-face or nasal mask so that tracheal intubation is avoided. Techniques include CPAP, and/or bilevel positive airway pressure (BiPAP). With the latter technique, inspiratory and expiratory pressure levels and times are set independently and unrestricted spontaneous respiration is

Box 15.5 Some indications for the use of non-invasive ventilation (NIV)

- Acute exacerbation of COPD (ph <7.35)
- Cardiogenic pulmonary oedema
- Chest wall deformity/neuromuscular disease (hypercapnic respiratory failure)
- Obstructive sleep apnoea
- Severe pneumonia (see Box 14.4)
- Asthma (occasionally)
- Weaning patients from invasive ventilation (p. 985)

Contraindications include facial or upper airway surgery, upper gastrointestinal surgery, inability to protect the airway.

Modified from BTS guidelines after 1997. http://www.british thoracic society.co.uk

possible throughout the respiratory cycle. BiPAP can also be patient triggered. There is a reduced risk of ventilator-associated pneumonia and improved patient comfort, with preservation of airway defence mechanisms, speech and swallowing which allows better nutrition. Spontaneous coughing and expectoration are not hampered, allowing good physiotherapy, and sedation is unnecessary. Institution of non-invasive respiratory support can rest the respiratory muscles, reduce respiratory acidosis and breathlessness, improve clearance of secretions and re-expand collapsed lung segments. The intubation rate, length of ICU and hospital stay and, in some categories of patient, mortality may all be reduced. NIV is particularly useful in acute hypercapnic respiratory failure associated with COPD, provided the patient is not profoundly hypoxic. NIV may also be useful as a means of avoiding tracheal intubation in immunocompromised patients with acute respiratory failure. Box 15.5 shows some indications for the use of NIV when standard medical treatment has failed. Remember NIV should not be used as a substitute for invasion ventilation when the latter is clearly more appropriate.

Weaning

Weakness and wasting of respiratory muscles is an inevitable consequence of the catabolic response to critical illness and may be exacerbated by the reduction in respiratory work during mechanical ventilation. Often abnormalities of gas exchange and lung mechanics persist. Not surprisingly, therefore, many patients experience difficulty in resuming spontaneous ventilation. In a significant proportion of patients who have undergone a prolonged period of respiratory support the situation is further complicated by the development of a neuropathy, a myopathy or both.

Critical illness polyneuropathy and myopathy

Polyneuropathies have most often been described in association with persistent sepsis and multiple organ failure (see below). Polyneuropathy is characterized by a primary axonal neuropathy involving both motor and, to a lesser extent, sensory nerves. Clinically the initial manifestation is often difficulty in weaning the patient from respiratory support. There is muscle wasting, the limbs are weak and flaccid, and deep tendon reflexes are reduced or absent. Cranial nerves are relatively spared. Nerve conduction studies confirm axonal damage. The cerebro-spinal fluid (CSF) protein concentration is normal or minimally elevated. These findings differentiate critical illness neuropathy from Guillain–Barré syndrome, in which nerve conduction studies show evidence of demyelination and CSF protein is usually high.

The cause of critical illness polyneuropathy is not known and there is no specific treatment. Weaning from respiratory support and rehabilitation are likely to be prolonged. With resolution of the underlying critical ill-ness, recovery can be expected after 1–6 months but muscle weakness and fatigue frequently persist.

Myopathies can also occur. A severe quadri-plegic myopathy has been particularly associated with the administration of steroids and muscle relaxants to mechanically ventilated patients with acute, severe asthma.

Often the most severely ill patients will have a combined neuropathy and myopathy.

Criteria for weaning patients from mechanical ventilation

Clinical assessment is the best way of deciding whether a patient can be weaned from the ventilator. The patient's conscious level, psychological state, metabolic function, the effects of drugs and cardiovascular performance must all be taken into account. A subjective evaluation of the patient's response to a short period of spontaneous venti-lation by an experienced clinician (spontaneous breathing trial) is the most reliable predictor of weaning success or failure. Objective criteria are based on an assessment of pulmonary gas exchange (blood gas analysis), lung mechanics and muscular strength.

Techniques for weaning

Patients who have received mechanical ventilation for less than 24 hours – for example, after elective major surgery – can usually resume spontaneous respiration immediately and no weaning process is required. This procedure can also be adopted for those who have been ventilated for longer periods but who tolerate a sponta-neous breathing trial and clearly fulfil objective criteria for weaning. Methods of weaning include:

- The traditional method is to allow the patient to breathe entirely spontaneously for a short time, following which respiratory support is reinstituted. The periods of spontaneous breathing are gradually increased and the periods of respiratory support are reduced. Initially it is usually advisable to ventilate the patient throughout the night. This method can be stressful and tiring for both patients and staff, although this approach is sometimes successful when other methods have failed.
- SIMV has been used as a gradual, controlled method of weaning.

- Gradual reduction of the level of pressure support, with no mandatory breaths is currently considered by many to be the preferred technique.
- CPAP can prevent the alveolar collapse, hypoxaemia and fall in compliance that might otherwise occur when patients start to breathe spontaneously. It is there-fore often used during weaning with SIMV/pressure support and in spontaneously breathing patients prior to extubation.
- Non-invasive ventilation via tightly fitting facial or nasal masks (BiPAP, CPAP).
- Tracheostomy is used frequently in critically ill patients to facilitate weaning from mechanical venti-lation (see above).

Extubation

This should not be considered until patients can cough, swallow, protect their own airway and are sufficiently alert to be cooperative. Patients who fulfil these criteria can be extubated provided their respiratory function has improved sufficiently to sustain spontaneous ventilation indefinitely.

FURTHER READING

Plant PK, Owen JL, Elliott MW (2000) Early use of non-invasive ventilation for acute exacerbations of chronic obstructive pulmonary disease on general respiratory wards: a multicentre randomised controlled trial. *Lancet* **355**: 1931–1935.

Tobin MJ (2001) Advances in mechanical ventilation. *New England Journal of Medicine* **344**: 1968–1996.

Truwit JD, Bernard GR (2004) Noninvasive ventilation. *New England Journal of Medicine* **350**: 2512–2515.

Vincent JL (2003) Nosocomial infections in adult intensive care units. *Lancet* **361**: 2068–2077.

ACUTE LUNG INJURY/ACUTE RESPIRATORY DISTRESS SYNDROME

Definition and causes (see Table 15.10)

Acute lung injury (ALI) and acute respiratory distress syndrome (ARDS) are diagnosed in an appropriate clinical setting with one or more recognized risk factors. ALI/ARDS can be defined as follows:

- Respiratory distress.
- Stiff lungs (reduced pulmonary compliance resulting in high inflation pressures).
- Chest radiograph: new bilateral, diffuse, patchy or homogeneous pulmonary infiltrates.
- Cardiac: no apparent cardiogenic cause of pulmonary oedema (pulmonary artery occlusion pressure < 18 mmHg if measured or no clinical evidence of left atrial hypertension).
- Gas exchange abnormalities: ALI – arterial oxygen tension/fractional inspired oxygen (P_aO_2/F_IO_2) ratio < 40 kPa (< 300 mmHg); ARDS P_aO_2/F_IO_2 (< 26.6 kPa)

Table 15.10 Disorders associated with acute lung injury/acute respiratory distress syndrome

Indirect (non-pulmonary)
Sepsis/septic shock
Systemic inflammatory response (e.g. pancreatitis, cardiopulmonary bypass, severe non-thoracic trauma, severe burns)
Haematological:
    Massive blood transfusion
    Transfusion-associated lung injury
    Disseminated intravascular coagulation
Obstetric:
    Eclampsia
Drug overdose:
    Heroin
    Barbiturates
Miscellaneous:
    High altitude

Direct (pulmonary)
Pneumonia
Pulmonary aspiration:
    Gastric contents
    Near drowning
Inhalation injury:
    Smoke
    Corrosive gases
Lung contusion
Blast injury
Fat embolism
Amniotic fluid embolism

(< 200 mmHg) (in both cases despite normal arterial carbon dioxide tension and regardless of positive end-expiratory pressure). The criterion for arterial oxygen tension/fractional inspired oxygen is arbitrary and the value of differentiating ALI from ARDS has been questioned.

ALI/ARDS can occur as a non-specific reaction of the lungs to a wide variety of direct pulmonary and indirect non-pulmonary insults. By far the commonest predisposing factor is sepsis, and 20–40% of patients with severe sepsis will develop ALI/ARDS (Table 15.10).

PATHOGENESIS AND PATHOPHYSIOLOGY OF ALI/ARDS

Acute lung injury can be considered as the earliest manifestation of a generalized inflammatory response with endothelial dysfunction and is therefore frequently associated with the development of MODS.

Non-cardiogenic pulmonary oedema
This is the cardinal feature of ALI and is the first and clinically most evident sign of a generalized increase in vascular permeability caused by the microcirculatory changes and release of inflammatory mediators described previously (see p. 963), with activated neutrophils playing a particularly key role. The pulmonary epithelium is also damaged in the early stages, reducing surfactant production and lowering the threshold for alveolar flooding.

Pulmonary hypertension
This is a common feature. Initially, mechanical obstruction of the pulmonary circulation may occur as a result of vascular compression by interstitial oedema, whilst local activation of the coagulation cascade leads to thrombosis and obstruction in the pulmonary microvasculature. Later, pulmonary vasoconstriction may develop in response to increased autonomic nervous activity and circulating substances such as catecholamines, serotonin, thromboxane and complement. Those vessels supplying alveoli with low oxygen tensions constrict (the 'hypoxic vasoconstrictor response'), diverting pulmonary blood flow to better oxygenated areas of lung, thus limiting the degree of shunt.

Haemorrhagic intra-alveolar exudate
This exudate is rich in platelets, fibrin, fibrinogen and clotting factors and may inactivate surfactant and stimulate inflammation, as well as promoting hyaline membrane formation and the migration of fibroblasts into the air spaces.

Fibrosis
Within days of the onset of lung injury, formation of a new epithelial lining is underway and activated fibroblasts accumulate in the interstitial spaces. Subsequently, interstitial fibrosis progresses, with loss of elastic tissue and obliteration of the lung vasculature, together with lung destruction and emphysema. In those who recover, the lungs are substantially remodelled.

Physiological changes
Shunt and deadspace increase, compliance falls, and there is evidence of airflow limitation. Although the lungs in ALI and ARDS are diffusely injured, the pulmonary lesions, when identified as densities on a CT scan, are predominantly located in dependent regions. This is partly explained by the effects of gravity on the distribution of extravascular lung water and areas of lung collapse.

CLINICAL PRESENTATION OF ALI/ARDS

The first sign of the development of ALI/ARDS is often an unexplained tachypnoea, followed by increasing hypoxaemia, with central cyanosis, and breathlessness. Fine crackles are heard throughout both lung fields. Later, the chest X-ray shows bilateral diffuse shadowing, interstitial at first, but subsequently with an alveolar pattern and air bronchograms that may then progress to the picture of complete 'white-out' (Fig. 15.23). The differential diagnosis includes cardiac failure and pneumonia.

MANAGEMENT OF ALI/ARDS

This is based on treatment of the underlying condition (e.g. eradication of sepsis), avoidance of complications such as ventilator-associated pneumonia, and supportive measures.

Fig. 15.23 Chest radiograph appearances in acute respiratory distress syndrome. Bilateral diffuse alveolar shadowing with air bronchograms and no cardiac enlargement.

Mechanical ventilation

Strategies designed to minimize ventilator-induced lung injury and encourage lung healing should be used (see p. 985).

Pulmonary oedema limitation. Pulmonary oedema formation should be limited by minimizing left ventricular filling pressure with fluid restriction, the use of diuretics and, if these measures fail, preventing fluid overload by haemofiltration. The aim should be to achieve a consistently negative fluid balance. Some recommend that plasma oncotic pressure should be maintained by using colloidal solutions to expand the intravascular volume. In patients with ALI/ARDS, however, colloids are unlikely to be retained within the vascular compartment; once they enter the interstitial space, the transvascular oncotic gradient is lost and the main determinants of interstitial oedema formation become the microvascular hydrostatic pressure and lymphatic drainage. There is therefore some controversy concerning the relative merits of colloids or crystalloids for volume replacement in patients likely to develop ALI/ARDS, or in whom the condition is established. Cardiovascular support and the reduction of oxygen requirements are also necessary.

Prone position. When the patient is changed from the supine to the prone position lung densities in the dependent region are redistributed and shunt fraction is reduced. A reduced pleural pressure gradient, more uniform alveolar ventilation, caudal movement of the diaphragm, redistribution of perfusion and recruitment of collapsed alveoli may all contribute to the improvement in gas exchange. Body position changes can be achieved with minimal complications despite the presence of multiple indwelling vascular lines. Repeated position changes between prone and supine may allow reductions in airway pressures and the inspired oxygen fraction. The response to prone positioning is, however, variable and it seems that this strategy may not improve overall outcome and, until further trials are performed, should be reserved for those with severe hypoxaemia.

Inhaled nitric oxide. This vasodilator, when inhaled, can improve $\dot{V}/\dot{Q}$ matching by increasing perfusion of ventilated lung units, as well as reducing pulmonary hypertension. It has been shown to improve oxygenation in so-called responders with ALI/ARDS but so far has not been shown to increase survival. Its administration requires specialized monitoring equipment, as products of its combination with oxygen include toxic nitrogen dioxide.

Aerosolized prostacyclin. This appears to have similar effects to inhaled NO and is easier to monitor and deliver. As with inhaled NO, the response to aerosolized prostacyclin is, however, variable and although it has been shown to improve oxygenation its effect on outcome has yet to be established.

Aerosolized surfactant. Surfactant replacement therapy reduces morbidity and mortality in neonatal respiratory distress syndrome and is beneficial in animal models of ALI/ARDS. In adults with ARDS, however, the value of surfactant administration remains uncertain.

High-dose steroids. Administration of high-dose steroids to patients with established ALI/ARDS does not appear to improve outcome, and current evidence suggests that prophylactic administration to those at risk is of no value. There is, however, some anecdotal evidence that the administration of corticosteroids to patients in the fibroproliferative stage of the disease (e.g. 10–14 days after the onset) may reduce mortality, provided there is no evidence of infection.

Prognosis

Mortality from ALI/ARDS has fallen over the last decade, from around 60% to between 30% and 40%, perhaps as a consequence of improved general care, the increasing use of management protocols, and attention to infection control and nutrition, as well as the introduction of novel treatments and lung-protective strategies for respiratory support. Prognosis is, however, still very dependent on aetiology. When ARDS occurs in association with intra-abdominal sepsis, mortality rates remain very high, whereas much lower mortality rates are to be expected in those with 'primary' ARDS (pneumonia, aspiration, lung contusion). Mortality rises with increasing age and failure of other organs. Most of those dying with ARDS do so as a result of MODS and haemodynamic instability rather than impaired gas exchange.

FURTHER READING

Acute Respiratory Distress Syndrome Network (2000) Ventilation with lower tidal volumes as compared with traditional tidal volumes for acute lung injury and the acute respiratory distress syndrome. *New England Journal of Medicine* **342**: 1301–1308.

Ware LB, Matthay MA (2000) The acute respiratory distress syndrome. *New England Journal of Medicine* **342**: 1334–1349.

Wyncoll DLA, Evans TW (1999) Acute respiratory distress syndrome. *Lancet* **354**: 497–501.

PATIENT SELECTION – WITHHOLDING AND WITHDRAWING TREATMENT

For many critically ill patients, intensive care is undoubtedly life-saving and resumption of a normal lifestyle is to be expected. In the most seriously ill patients, however, immediate mortality rates are high, a significant number die soon after discharge from the intensive care unit, and the quality of life for some of those who do survive may be poor. Moreover, intensive care is expensive, particularly for those with the worst prognosis, and resources are limited.

Inappropriate use of intensive care facilities has other implications. The patient may experience unnecessary suffering and loss of dignity, while relatives may also have to endure considerable emotional pressures. In some cases treatment may simply prolong the process of dying, or sustain life of dubious quality, and in others the risk of interventions may outweigh the potential benefits.

Both for a humane approach to the management of critically ill patients and to ensure that limited resources are used appropriately, it is necessary to avoid admitting patients who cannot benefit from intensive care and to limit further aggressive therapy when the prognosis is clearly hopeless. Such decisions can be extremely difficult and every case must be assessed individually, taking into account the patient's previous health and quality of life, the primary diagnosis, the medium- and long-term prognosis of the underlying condition (both in terms of survival and quality of life) and the survivability of the acute illness. Age alone should not be a consideration. When in doubt, active measures should continue but should be reviewed regularly in the light of response to treatment and any further information which may become available. Decisions to limit therapy, not to resuscitate in the event of cardiorespiratory arrest, or to withdraw treatment should be made jointly by the medical staff of the unit, the primary physician or surgeon, the nurses and if possible the patient, normally in consultation with the patient's family. Withdrawal or limitation of active treatment should not be viewed negatively as the cessation of all medical or nursing care. Rather, a positive approach should be adopted to ensuring that the patient dies with dignity, free of pain and distress, and that family and friends receive support and comfort.

Scoring systems

A variety of scoring systems have been developed that can be used to evaluate the severity of a patient's illness. Some have included an assessment of the patient's previous state of health and the severity of the acute disturbance of physiological function (acute physiology, age, chronic health evaluation – APACHE, and simplified acute physiology score – SAPS). Other systems have been designed for particular categories of patient (e.g. the injury severity score for trauma victims).

The APACHE and SAPS scores are widely applicable and have been extensively validated. They can quantify accurately the severity of illness and predict the overall mortality for large groups of critically ill patients, and are therefore useful for defining the 'casemix' of patients when auditing a unit's clinical activity, for comparing results nationally or internationally, and as a means of characterizing groups of patients in clinical studies. Although the APACHE and SAPS methodologies can also be used to estimate risks of mortality, no scoring system has yet been devised that can predict with certainty the outcome in an individual patient. They must not, therefore, be used in isolation as a basis for limiting or discontinuing treatment.

The Therapeutic Intervention Scoring System (TISS) scores interventions and nursing activities for each day of admission. Such information may provide estimates of resource consumption and indices of nursing dependency. This may not only be related to prognosis but can also be used to estimate costs. Current estimates of daily costs of intensive care in the UK vary from £800 to £1600; high dependency and ward care costs are approximately 50% and 20% of intensive care costs respectively.

FURTHER READING

Carlet J, Thys LG, Anteneli M et al. (2004) Challenges in end-of-life care in the ICU. Statement of the 5th International Consensus Conference in Critical Care. *Intensive Care Medicine* **30**: 770–784.

Knaus WA, Wagner DP, Draper EA et al. (1991) The APACHE III prognostic system: risk prediction of hospital mortality for critically ill hospitalized adults. *Chest* **100**: 1619–1636.

BRAIN DEATH

Brain death means 'the irreversible loss of the capacity for consciousness combined with the irreversible loss of the capacity to breathe'. Both these are essentially functions of the brainstem. Death, if thought of in this way, can arise either from causes outside the brain (i.e. respiratory and cardiac arrest) or from causes within the cranial cavity. With the advent of artificial ventilation it became possible to support such a dead patient temporarily, although in all cases cardiovascular failure eventually supervenes and progresses to asystole.

Before considering a diagnosis of brainstem death it is essential that certain preconditions and exclusions be fulfilled.

Preconditions

- The patient must be in apnoeic coma (i.e. unresponsive and on a ventilator, with no spontaneous respiratory efforts).
- Irremediable structural brain damage due to a disorder that can cause brainstem death must have been diagnosed with certainty (e.g. head injury, intracranial haemorrhage).

Exclusions

- The possibility that unresponsive apnoea is the result of poisoning, sedative drugs or neuromuscular blocking agents must be excluded.
- Hypothermia must be excluded as a cause of coma. The central body temperature should be more than 35°C.
- There must be no significant metabolic or endocrine disturbance that could produce or contribute to coma or cause it to persist.
- There should be no profound abnormality of the plasma electrolytes, acid–base balance, or blood glucose levels.

Diagnostic tests for the confirmation of brain death

All brainstem reflexes are absent in brain death.

Tests

The following tests should not be performed in the presence of seizures or abnormal postures.

- Oculocephalic reflexes should be absent: when the head is rotated from side to side, the eyes move with the head and therefore remain stationary relative to the orbit. In a comatose patient whose brainstem is intact, the eyes will rotate relative to the orbit (i.e. doll's eye movements will be present).
- The pupils are fixed and unresponsive to bright light. Both direct and consensual light reflexes are absent. The size of the pupils is irrelevant, although most often they will be dilated.
- Corneal reflexes are absent.
- There are no vestibulo-ocular reflexes on caloric testing (see p. 1189).
- There is no motor response within the cranial nerve territory to painful stimuli applied centrally or peripherally. Spinal reflex movements may be present.
- There is no gag or cough reflex in response to pharyngeal, laryngeal or tracheal stimulation.
- Spontaneous respiration is absent. The patient should be ventilated with 5% CO_2 in 95% O_2 for 10 minutes

and then temporarily disconnected from the ventilator for up to 10 minutes. Oxygenation is maintained by insufflation with 100% oxygen via a catheter placed in the endotracheal tube. The patient is observed for any signs of spontaneous respiratory efforts. A blood gas sample should be obtained during this period to ensure that the P_aCO_2 is sufficiently high to stimulate spontaneous respiration (> 6.7 kPa (50 mmHg)).

The examination should be performed and repeated by two senior doctors.

In the UK it is not considered necessary to perform confirmatory tests such as EEG and carotid angiography.

The primary purpose of establishing a diagnosis of brainstem death is to demonstrate beyond doubt that it is futile to continue mechanical ventilation and other life-supporting measures.

In suitable cases, and provided the assent of relatives has been obtained (easier if the patient was carrying an organ donor card), the organs of those in whom brainstem death has been established may be used for transplantation. In the UK each region has a transplant coordinator who can help with the process, as well as providing information, training and advice about organ donation. They should be informed of all potential donors. In all cases in the UK the coroner's consent must be obtained.

FURTHER READING

Pallis C, Harley DH (1996) *ABC of Brain Stem Death*, 2nd edn. London: BMJ Publishing Group.
Wijdicks EF (2001) The diagnosis of brain death. *New England Journal of Medicine* **344**: 1215–1221.

GENERAL FURTHER READING

Hinds CJ, Watson JD (1996) *Intensive Care: A Concise Textbook*. London: Baillière Tindall.
Society of Critical Care Medicine: www.sccm.org/ professional_resources/guidelines table-of-contents/index.asp.

SIGNIFICANT WEBSITES

http://www.ics.ac.uk
  UK Intensive Care Society

http://www.esicm.org
  European Society of Intensive Care Medicine

http://www.survivingsepsis.org
  Surviving Sepsis Campaign

http://www.sccm.org/professional_resources/ guidelines
  Society of Critical Care Medicine

Drug therapy and poisoning

DRUG THERAPY

Introduction

This chapter provides an introduction to the principles of rational therapeutics whose cardinal features are encompassed within the 1984 'Nairobi Declaration'. This emphasizes the importance of prescribing:

- to the right patient
- the right drug
- at the right dose
- and at an affordable cost.

THE PATIENT

The prerequisite of any form of therapeutic intervention is a reliable diagnosis or, at least, assessment of clinical need. An accurate diagnosis ensures that a patient is not exposed, unnecessarily, to the hazards or costs of a particular intervention. Nevertheless there are some circumstances when treatment is used in the absence of a clear diagnosis. Examples include:

- the symptomatic treatment of severe pain
- the initiation of 'blind' antimicrobial therapy where delay would expose a patient to hazard, or discomfort (e.g. parenteral antimicrobial therapy to a patient in the community with suspected meningococcal meningitis; antimicrobial therapy to a patient with a suspected lower urinary tract infection).

In some instances a particular medicine is only effective in subgroups of patients with a particular disorder. Trastuzumab, for example, is only effective in women with advanced breast cancer whose malignant cells express the HER2 epidermal growth factor receptor. It is likely, in the future, that there will be fragmentation of many diseases we currently consider as single entities, with a more precise definition of sites against which drugs can be targeted.

Medicines are also given to otherwise healthy individuals. In such circumstances there must be a very clear imperative to ensure that the benefits to the individual outweigh the harm. Examples include:

- immunization against serious microbial infections (e.g. influenza vaccination)
- the reduction of individual risk factors for overt disease (e.g. the use of antihypertensive, or lipid-lowering, agents)
- the use of oral contraceptives in sexually active women who wish to avoid pregnancy.

Co-morbidity may also significantly alter the way in which conditions are managed, particular in the elderly. Some examples are shown in Table 16.1.

Prescribing in neonates, infants and children

The use of drugs in the newborn, infants and children poses special problems, as the doses are extrapolated from adult experience (e.g. by adjusting doses solely on the basis of body index). This is rarely wise and may be inappropriate because:

- Dosages are difficult to calculate and precise dosing is often impossible in babies who spit out unpleasant-tasting syrups.
- Percutaneous absorption of topical drugs and disinfecting agents is increased in premature babies (e.g. steroids, iodine or topical aminoglycosides).

Table 16.1 Examples of drugs to be avoided in patients with co-morbidity

Co-morbidity	Avoid	Effect
Parkinson's disease	Neuroleptics	Exacerbates Parkinson's disease
Hypertension	Non-steroidal anti-inflammatory drugs	Sodium retention
Asthma	Beta-blockers, adenosine	Bronchospasm
Respiratory failure	Morphine, diamorphine	Respiratory depression
Atrioventricular block	Digoxin, digitoxin Beta-blockers	Heart block
Renovascular disease	ACE inhibitors/ antagonists	Reduction in glomerular filtration
Epilepsy	Tricyclic antidepressants	Lower convulsive threshold

- Premature babies have approximately 1% of their bodyweight as fat (compared to 20% in adults) causing a marked increase in plasma drug concentrations of fat-soluble drugs when doses are extrapolated from those in adults, even when adjusted for differences in total body mass.
- Hepatic metabolism and renal excretion of drugs are reduced in neonates and infants. Extrapolation from adult dosage regimens, merely adjusted for weight, leads to excessive (and potentially toxic) plasma drug concentrations.

Prescribing for the elderly

The use of drugs in the elderly is often a problem because:

- Compliance with treatment regimens is especially poor if there is cognitive impairment, and is worse with increasing numbers of different prescribed medicines.
- Co-morbidity and the inevitable tendency for poly-pharmacy lead to increased opportunities for drug interactions.
- Changes in drug distribution, associated with a reduction in body mass and changes in body composition, may increase plasma concentrations (especially following intravenous administration).
- Ageing is accompanied by changes in the distribution of cardiac output. In particular, a relatively higher proportion of the stroke volume reaches the brain. This, at least in part, explains why elderly people are so vulnerable to the effects of drugs acting on the central nervous system.

Exaggerated pharmacodynamic effects of drugs acting on cardiovascular and gastrointestinal systems are also common.

Some of the commoner problems that may occur with the use of drugs in the elderly are shown in Table 16.2.

Table 16.2 Common adverse effects of drugs in the elderly

Drug	Effect
Beta-blockers Digoxin	Bradycardia
Nitrates α-Adrenoceptor-blockers Diuretics	Postural hypotension
Diuretics (thiazides)	Glucose intolerance Gout
Anti-muscarinic drugs Tricyclic antidepressants Neuroleptics Minor tranquillizers Anticonvulsants Hypnotics Opioids	Confusion, cognitive dysfunction
Bisphosphonates (mainly alendronic acid)	Oesphageal ulceration and stricture formation
NSAIDs	Gastric erosions Upper gastrointestinal bleeding Perforated peptic ulcer Renal impairment

Drug use in pregnancy

Clinicians should be extremely cautious about prescribing drugs to pregnant women, and only essential treatments should be given. When a known teratogen is needed during pregnancy (e.g. an anticonvulsant drug or lithium) the potential adverse effects should be discussed with the parents preferably before conception. If they decide to go ahead with the pregnancy, they should be offered an appropriate ultrasound scan to assess whether there is any fetal damage. Some known human teratogens are shown in Table 16.3.

Table 16.3 Some human teratogens

Drug	Effect
ACE inhibitors/antagonists	Oligohydramnios
Retinoids, e.g. acitretin	Multiple abnormalities
Amiodarone	Neonatal goitre
Carbimazole	Neonatal hypothyroidism
Warfarin	Dysmorphia Abnormalities of bone growth
Antiepileptics (see p. 1223)	
Carbamazepine Phenytoin	Cleft palate
Valproate	Neural tube defects
NSAIDs	Delayed closure of the ductus arteriosus
Cytotoxic drugs	Most are presumed teratogens
Lithium	Ebstein's anomaly

NB: All drugs should be avoided in pregnancy unless benefit clearly outweighs the risk

Breast-feeding

Although most drugs can be detected in breast milk, the quantity is generally small. This is because, for most drugs, the concentration in milk is in equilibrium with plasma water (i.e. the non-protein-bound fraction). A few drugs (e.g. aspirin, carbimazole) may, however, cause harm to the infant if ingested in breast milk. Relevant drug literature should be consulted when prescribing to a nursing mother.

THE DRUG

Selecting the right drug involves three elements:

- the drug's clinical efficacy for the proposed use
- the balance between the drug's efficacy and safety
- patient preference.

The 'gold standard' approach (see p. 998) to demonstrating the clinical efficacy of a drug is the randomized controlled trial (RCT) although other approaches (p. 999) can be informative. The demonstration of absolute efficacy (against placebo) may, itself, be insufficient. Where there is more than one treatment for the same indication consideration has to be given as to how they compare with one another, taking account the magnitude of their benefits, their individual adverse reaction profiles, and their costs. Comparative randomized controlled trials are particularly useful in this respect.

The preferences of patients themselves should also, wherever possible, be sought. Such discussions should enable them to be equal partners in decision-making about whether and how they wish to undergo treatment. A full understanding of the reasons for considering treatment, the likely benefits, and the possible adverse reactions, has repeatedly been shown to improve 'concordance' with treatment regimens.

THE DOSE

Appropriate drug dosages will have usually been determined from the results of so-called 'dose-ranging' studies during the original development programme. Such studies are generally conducted as RCTs covering a range of potential doses. Drug doses and dosage regimens may be fixed or adjusted.

Fixed dosage regimens

Drugs suitable (in adults) for prescribing at fixed doses for all patients share common features. Efficacy is optimal in virtually all patients; and the risks of dose-related (type A) adverse reactions (see p. 996) are normally low. These drugs have a high 'therapeutic ratio' (i.e. the ratio between the toxic and therapeutic doses). Examples of drugs prescribed at a fixed dose are shown in Table 16.4.

Titrated dosage regimens

For many drugs there are wide interindividual variations in response. As a consequence, whilst a particular dose

Table 16.4 Examples of fixed dose prescribing

Drug	Indication
Aspirin	Secondary prevention of myocardial infarction
Bendroflumethiazide (bendrofluazide)	Hypertension
Amoxicillin	Lower urinary tract infection
	Upper and lower respiratory tract infection
Ferrous sulphate	Iron-deficiency anaemia
Oral contraceptives	Oral contraception

may in one person lack any therapeutic effect, the same dose in another may cause serious toxicity. The reasons for such variability are partly due to pharmacokinetic factors (differences in the rates of drug absorption, distribution or metabolism) and partly due to pharmacodynamic factors (differences in the sensitivity of target organs).

Pharmacokinetics

The intensity of a drug's action, immediately after parenteral administration, is largely a function of its volume of distribution. This, in turn, is predominantly governed by body composition and regional blood flow. Dosage adjustments, for bodyweight or surface area, are therefore common, for example in cancer chemotherapy in order to optimize treatment.

For drugs taken repeatedly, the main determinants of their plasma concentrations (and the intensity of their effects) are the extent of presystemic hepatic metabolism after absorption (Box 16.1), and the rate of systemic clearance (by hepatic metabolism or renal excretion).

Liver drug metabolism occurs in two stages:

- *Phase I* is the modification of a drug, by oxidation, reduction or hydrolysis. Of these, oxidation is the most frequent route and is largely undertaken by a family of isoenzymes known as the cytochrome P450 system (p. 994). Inhibition or induction of cytochrome P450 isoenzymes is a major cause of drug interaction (Table 16.5).
- *Phase II* involves conjugation with glucuronic acid, sulphate, acetate or other substances to render it more soluble and therefore able to be excreted in the urine.

Box 16.1 Some drugs undergoing extensive presystemic (first pass) hepatic metabolism

- Clomethiazole
- Glyceryl trinitrate*
- Isosorbide dinitrate
- Lidocaine*
- Morphine
- Pethidine
- Propanolol
- Verapamil

* For these drugs presystemic metabolism is virtually complete and oral dosing ineffective. Sublingual administration (e.g. glyceryl trinitrate) avoids presystemic metabolism.

Table 16.5 Some inducers and inhibitors of cytochrome P450

Inducers	Barbiturates (esp. phenobarbital)
	Carbamazepine
	Phenytoin
	Rifampicin
	Griseofulvin
	Non-nucleoside reverse transcriptase inhibitors (NNRTI)
	Allopurinol
	Isoniazid
	Protease inhibitors
Inhibitors	Cimetidine
	Quinolones
	Erythromycin
	Imidazoles
	Sulphonamides
	Allopurinol
	Grapefruit juice

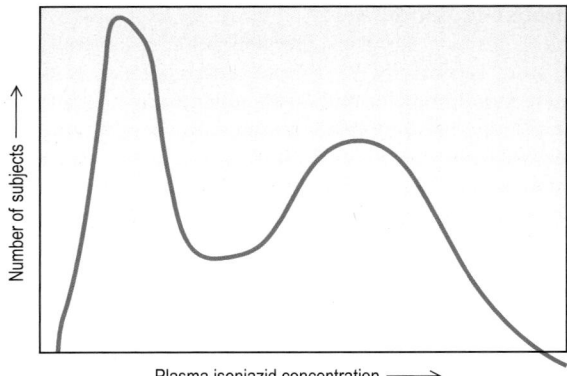

Fig. 16.1 Bimodal distribution of acetylator status.
Plasma isoniazid concentration shows two distinct groups. Modified from Evans DAP et al. (1960) *British Medical Journal* 2: 485.

Genetic causes of altered pharmacokinetics

Both presystemic hepatic metabolism, and the rate of systemic hepatic clearance, may vary markedly between healthy individuals, because of genetic factors governing the expression of drug-metabolizing enzymes (Table 16.6).

The best-known genetic cause of altered drug handling is acetylator phenotype. Certain drugs are metabolized by acetylation in the liver and individuals can be classified as slow acetylators or fast acetylators. Most populations show a distinct bimodal distribution in their acetylator status (see Fig. 16.1), which is likely to be due to a single gene variation. Those who acetylate slowly will have higher plasma concentrations of drug for any given dose and will tend to develop adverse effects more readily. The antituberculous drug isoniazid will cause a polyneuropathy more commonly in patients with slow acetylator status; inhibition of metabolism of the anticonvulsant phenytoin when prescribed concurrently with isoniazid is also more common in slow acetylators. Rapid acetylators may, conversely, be more likely to relapse because of inadequate plasma concentrations of isoniazid. SLE is more likely to develop with procainamide and hydralazine in slow acetylators.

Debrisoquine hydroxylation is also markedly deficient is certain individuals (about 8% of the British population), and such deficiency shows autosomal dominant inheritance. Debrisoquine is rarely used in the treatment of hypertension, not least because almost 1 in 10 patients will have defective metabolism resulting in enhanced adrenergic blockade with the risk of severe hypotension. The same hydroxylase enzyme is involved in metabolism of several beta-blockers and the antidepressant nortriptyline, although it is not clear whether hydroxylation status predicts adverse effects with these drugs.

The rare failure to metabolize suxamethonium resulting in prolonged muscular paralysis is due to a genetic defect in the production of plasma pseudocholinesterase. The condition is autosomal recessive and affects about 1 in 2500 patients.

Table 16.6 Genetic polymorphisms involving drug metabolism

Enzyme	Drug
P450	
Cytochrome CYP1A2	Amitriptyline
	Clozapine
Cytochrome CYP3A4	Quinidine
	Ciclosporin
	Lidocaine
	Verapamil
	Statins
	Protease inhibitors
Cytochrome CYP2C9	Warfarin
	Tolbutamide
	Phenytoin
	Glipizide
	Losartan
Cytochrome CYP2D6	Amitriptyline
	Venlafaxine
	SSRIs
	Codeine
	Beta-blockers
	Flecainide
Cytochrome CYP2C19	Diazepam
	Omeprazole/lansoprazole
Plasma pseudocholinesterase	Succinylcholine
	Mivacurium
Thiopurine methyltransferase	Mercaptopurine
	Azathioprine
UDP-glucuronosyl transferase	Irinotecan
N-acetyl transferase	Procainamide
	Isoniazid
	Hydralazine

Other causes of altered pharmacokinetics

Rates of hepatic drug clearance can also be influenced by environmental factors including diet, alcohol consumption and concomitant therapy with drugs capable of inducing or inhibiting (Table 16.6) drug metabolism. Hepatic drug clearance also decreases with age. By contrast, renal drug clearance does not show substantial

Table 16.7 Some pharmacodynamic genetic polymorphisms

	Drug	Drug effect
ACE	ACE inhibitors, e.g. ranipril	Blood pressure reduction
Bradykinin B_2 receptor	ACE inhibitors	Cough
β_2-Adrenoceptor	Salbutamol	Bronchodilatation
Dopamine receptors (D_2, D_3, D_4)	Haloperidol Clozapine Risperidone	Antipsychotic response Tardive dyskinesia Akathisia
Serotonin transporter	Fluoxetine Paroxetine	Antidepressant response
Oestrogen receptor-α	Oestrogens	Bone mineral density

variation between healthy individuals although it declines with age and in patients with intrinsic renal disease.

Pharmacodynamics

Pharmacodynamic sources of variability in the intensity of drug action are in part due to drug receptor polymorphisms (Table 16.7).

Monitoring the effects of treatment

The combination of pharmacokinetic and pharmacodynamic causes of variability makes careful monitoring of the effects of treatment essential. Three approaches are used.

Pre-treatment dose selection

In patients with known, or suspected, impaired renal function it is usually possible to predict their dose requirements from the serum creatinine concentration. If treatment needs to be started before the serum creatinine concentration is available, or in patients with very advanced renal impairment, or if renal function is fluctuating then start with conventional doses but be prepared to make adjustments within 24 hours. Frequent assessments of renal function, coupled with measurements of plasma drug concentrations, may be necessary.

Measuring plasma drug concentrations

For a few drugs, dosages can be effectively monitored by reference to their plasma concentrations (Table 16.8). This technique is only useful, however, if both the following criteria are fulfilled:

- There is a reliable and available drug assay.
- Plasma concentrations correlate well with therapeutic efficacy and toxicity.

Measuring drug effects

For many drugs, dosage adjustments are made in line with patients' responses. Monitoring can involve dose titration against a therapeutic end-point or a toxic effect. Objective measures (such as monitoring antihypertensive therapy by measuring blood pressure, or cytotoxic therapy with serial white blood cell counts) are most helpful, but subjective ones are necessary in many instances (as with antipsychotic therapy in patients with schizophrenia).

In the future, drug selection and dose requirements may become largely predictable from a knowledge of an individual's pharmacogenetic characteristics (including both drug metabolism and drug receptor polymorphisms) coupled with relevant demographic and clinical data. Currently, only two pharmacogenetic tests are used routinely:

- HER2 expression in patients with advanced breast cancer before treatment with trastuzumab (see p. 520)
- thiopurine methyltransferase activity in children with acute lymphatic leukaemia and patients with Crohn's disease who are to undergo treatment with mercaptopurine and/or azathioprine.

AFFORDABILITY

The money available for healthcare varies widely across the world and there are marked differences even between developed countries (Fig. 16.2). All healthcare systems try to provide their populations with the highest standards of care within the resources they have at their disposal. The expenditure of large sums on a few people may deprive many of cost-effective remedies – a phenomenon known as the 'opportunity cost'.

Table 16.8 Drugs for which therapeutic drug monitoring is used

Drug	Therapeutic plasma concentration range	Toxic level	Optimum post-dose sampling time (hours)
Carbamazepine	20–50 µmol/L	> 50 µmol/L	> 8
Digoxin	1.3–2.6 nmol/L	> 2.6 nmol/L	> 8
Gentamicin	Trough < 2 mg/L	> 14 mg/L	Pre-dose
	Peak 5–10 mg/L	> 12 mg/L	> 1
Lithium	0.6–1.0 mmol/L	> 1.5 mmol/L	> 10
Phenytoin	40–80 µmol/L	> 80 µmol/L	> 10
Theophylline	55–110 µmol/L	> 110 µmol/L	> 4
Ciclosporin	50–200 µg/L	> 200 µg/L	Pre-dose

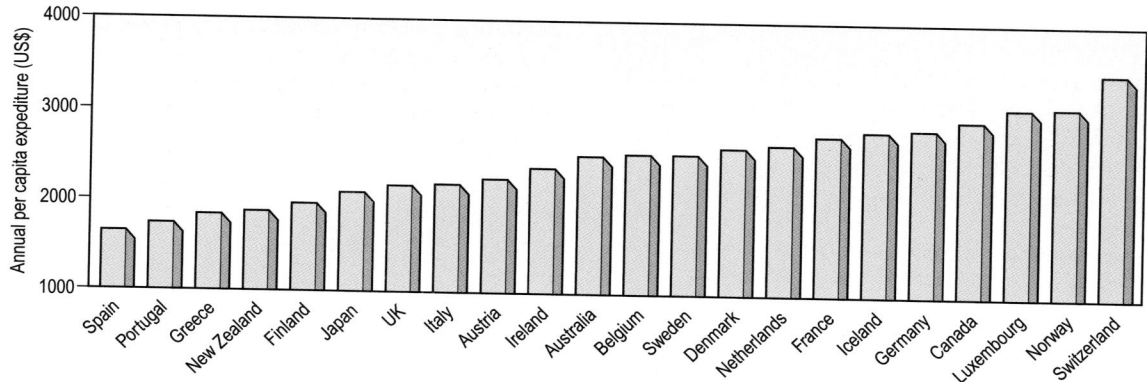

Fig. 16.2 Annual expenditure on healthcare in US $, per head of population, in some developed countries.

In all countries it is therefore inevitable that cost-containment measures will be encouraged (or mandated). For example, to reduce costs all drugs should be prescribed by their generic (approved) names rather than their 'brand' ones because, once their patents have expired, they are cheaper. Despite occasional claims to the contrary, generic products are required to go through the same stringent regulatory processes as their branded counterparts.

ADVERSE DRUG REACTIONS

Adverse drug reactions (ADRs), defined as 'the unwanted effects of drugs occurring under normal conditions of use', are a significant cause of morbidity and mortality. Around 5% of acute medical emergencies are admitted with ADRs; and around 10–20% of hospital inpatients suffer an ADR during their stay. Unwanted effects of drugs are five to six times more likely in the elderly, compared to young adults; and the risk of an ADR rises sharply with the number of drugs administered.

Classification

Two types of ADR are recognized.

Type A (*augmented*) *reactions* (Table 16.9) are:

- qualitatively normal, but quantitatively abnormal, manifestations of a compound's pharmacological or toxicological properties
- predictable from a compound's known pharmacological or toxicological actions
- generally dose-dependent
- usually common
- only occasionally serious.

Whilst some such as hypotension with ACE inhibitors may occur after a single dose, others may develop only after months (pulmonary fibrosis with amiodarone) or years (second cancers with cytotoxic drugs).

Type B (*idiosyncratic*) *reactions* (Table 16.9) have no resemblance to the recognized pharmacological or toxicological effects of the drug. They are:

- qualitatively abnormal responses to the drug
- unpredictable from a compound's known pharmacological or toxicological actions
- generally dose-independent
- usually rare
- often serious.

Table 16.9 Examples of ADRs

Drug	Adverse reaction
Type A	
Anticoagulants	Bleeding
Insulin	Hypoglycaemia
Angiotensin-converting enzyme inhibitors/ antagonists	Hypotension
Antipsychotics	Acute dystonia and dyskinesia
	Parkinson's disease
	Tardive dyskinesia
Tricyclic antidepressants	Dry mouth
Amiodarone	Hyperthyroidism
	Hypothyroidism
	Pulmonary fibrosis
Cytotoxic agents	Bone marrow dyscrasias
	Cancer
Glucocorticoids	Osteoporosis
Type B	
Benzylpenicillin Radiological contrast media	Anaphylaxis
Amoxicillin	Maculopapular rash
Gold salts	Bone marrow dyscrasias
Sulphonamides Lamotrigine	Toxic epidermal necrolysis
Halothane plus suxamethonium	Malignant hyperthermia
Diclofenac Halothane Isoniazid Rifampicin Phenytoin	Hepatotoxicity

Diagnosis

All ADRs mimic some naturally occurring disease, and the distinction between an iatrogenic aetiology and an event unrelated to the drug is often difficult. Although some effects are obviously iatrogenic (e.g. acute anaphylaxis occurring a few minutes after intravenous penicillin), many are less so. There are six characteristics that can help distinguish an adverse reaction from an event due to some other cause:

- *Appropriate time interval.* The time interval between the administration of a drug and the suspected adverse reaction should be appropriate. Acute anaphylaxis usually occurs within a few minutes of administration, whilst aplastic anaemia will only become apparent after a few weeks (because of the life-span of erythrocytes). Drug-induced malignancy, however, will take years to develop.
- *Nature of the reaction.* Some conditions (maculopapular rashes, angio-oedema, fixed drug eruptions, toxic epidermal necrolysis) are so typically iatrogenic that an adverse drug reaction is very likely.
- *Plausibility.* Where an event is a manifestation of the known pharmacological property of the drug, its recognition as a type A adverse drug reaction can be made (e.g. hypotension with an antihypertensive agent, or hypoglycaemia with an antidiabetic drug). Unless there have been previous reports in the literature, the recognition of type B reactions may be very difficult. The first cases of depression with isotretinoin, for example, were difficult to recognize as an adverse drug reaction even though a causal association is now acknowledged.
- *Exclusion of other causes.* In some instances, particularly suspected hepatotoxicity, an iatrogenic diagnosis can only be made after the exclusion of other causes of disease.
- *Results of laboratory tests.* In a few instances, the diagnosis of an adverse reaction can be inferred from the plasma concentration (Table 16.8). Occasionally, an ADR produces diagnostic histopathological features. Examples include putative reactions involving the skin and liver.
- *Results of dechallenge and rechallenge.* Failure of remission when the drug is withdrawn (i.e. 'dechallenge') is unlikely to be an ADR. The diagnostic reliability of dechallenge, however, is not absolute: if the ADR has caused irreversible organ damage (e.g. malignancy) then dechallenge will result in a false negative response. Rechallenge, involving re-institution of the suspected drug to see if the event recurs, is often regarded as an absolute diagnostic test. This is, in many instances, correct but there are two caveats. First, it is rarely ethically justified to subject a patient to further hazard. Second, some adverse drug reactions develop because of particular circumstances which may not necessarily be replicated on rechallenge (e.g. hypoglycaemia with an antidiabetic agent).

Management

As a general rule, type A reactions can usually be managed by a reduction in dosage whilst type B reactions almost invariably require the drug to be withdrawn (and never re-instituted).

Specific therapy is sometimes required for ADRs such as bleeding with warfarin (vitamin K), acute dystonias (benzatropine), or acute anaphylaxis (Emergency box 16.1).

FURTHER READING

Evans WE, McLoed HL (2003) Pharmacogenetics – drug disposition, drug targets and side effects. *New England Journal of Medicine* **348**: 538–549.

Meyer A (2000) Pharmacogenetics and adverse drug reactions. *Lancet* **356**: 1667–1671.

Weinshilourn R (2003) Inheritance and drug response. *New England Journal of Medicine* **348**: 529–537.

Wilkinson GR (2005) Drug metabolism and variability among patients in drug response. *New England Journal of Medicine* **352**: 2211–2221.

Wynne HA (2003) Sensible prescribing for older people. *Clinical Medicine* **3**(5): 409–412.

Emergency Box 16.1
Treatment of acute anaphylaxis

Acute anaphylaxis can occur after insect bites and nut ingestion as well as drugs.

Clinical features
- Bronchospasm
- Facial and laryngeal oedema
- Hypotension
- Nausea, vomiting and diarrhoea

Management
- Position the patient lying flat with feet raised.
- Ensure the airway is free.
- Give oxygen.
- Monitor BP.
- Establish venous access.
- Administer 0.5 mg intramuscular epinephrine (adrenaline) and repeat every 5 min if shock persists.
- Administer intravenous antihistamine (e.g. 10–20 mg chlorphenamine) slowly.
- Administer 100 mg intravenous hydrocortisone.

If hypotension persists, give 1–2 L of intravenous fluid.

If hypoxia is severe, assisted ventilation may be required.

EVIDENCE-BASED MEDICINE

There is now general acceptance that, in so far as is possible, clinical practice should be based on scientific evidence of benefit rather than theoretical speculation, anecdote or pronouncement.

One of the main applications of 'evidence-based medicine' is in therapeutics. From this it is axiomatic that treatments should be introduced into, and used in, routine clinical care only if they have been demonstrated to be effective in formal clinical trials. Three approaches have been used:

- randomized controlled trials
- controlled observational trials
- uncontrolled observational studies.

Randomized controlled trials

Parallel group design.   In this type of study, patients with a particular condition are given, prospectively, one of two (or more) treatments. Treatments are usually allocated randomly (a 'randomized' controlled trial). In order to reduce patient bias, the patients themselves are generally unaware of their treatment allocations (a 'single-blind' trial); and in order to reduce doctor bias the treatment allocation is also withheld from the investigators (a 'double-blind' trial). In order to recruit sufficient numbers of patients, and to examine the effects of treatment in different settings, it is often necessary to conduct the trial at several locations (a 'multicentre' trial). The 'gold standard' for demonstrating the efficacy of a treatment is, thus, the *prospective, randomized, double-blind, multicentre, controlled trial.*

Prospective randomized controlled trials are designed either to show that one treatment is better than another (a 'superiority' trial); or that one treatment is similar to another (an 'equivalence' trial). In a *superiority trial* the study treatment is usually compared to placebo, no treatment, or to current standard practice. With drugs, the comparators may include different doses of the study ('active') drug in order to define the optimum treatment regimen. In an *equivalence trial* the treatment under study is usually compared to another treatment for the same condition.

Although randomized controlled trials were originally introduced to investigate the efficacy of drugs, the methodology can encompass surgical procedures and medical devices.

Cross-over design.   In some circumstances patients can receive both the active and the comparator, in a random sequence, thus acting as their own control. Cross-over trials have the advantage that, since each patient is his/her own control, fewer numbers are required to demonstrate efficacy. Such designs, however, are usually only appropriate in circumstances where the drug is intended to produce improvement in a chronic condition. Examples include hypnotics, bronchodilators and antihypertensive agents.

Assessing randomized controlled trials

In assessing the relevance and reliability of an RCT a number of features need to be taken into account.

- *Was ethical approval obtained?* All clinical trials should have received approval, before the start of the study, from a properly constituted research ethics committee. In particular, patients taking part should have given their full and informed consent to participate.
- *Randomization.* In any randomized controlled trial the method of randomization should be robust. In particular, the investigator should be unaware of which treatment a patient about to enter a trial will receive. This avoids selection bias.
- *Maintaining blindness.* Although, ideally, in RCTs neither the investigator nor the patient is aware of the treatment allocation until the end of the study, this is not always possible. Adverse drug reactions, for example, may make it obvious which treatment a patient has been given. Nevertheless maintaining blindness is necessary where the outcome is subjective (e.g. relief of pain, alleviation of depression) if bias is to be avoided.
- *Were the treated and control groups comparable?* Were the treated and control groups similar in their 'baseline' characteristics? Were they, for example, of similar age, severity and duration of illness? If not, are the differences likely to bias the results? Or has the statistical analysis (using analysis of covariance, or Cox's proportional hazards model) tried to adjust for them? Table 16.10 shows an RCT where the baseline characteristics were comparable.
- *Outcomes.* There are two ways to look at the outcomes of an RCT. One is to include only those who completed the study ('per protocol analysis') and the other is to include all patients from the time of randomization ('intention-to-treat analysis'). Ideally there should be no difference but in reality the results of a per protocol analysis are usually more advantageous to a treatment than an intention-to-treat analysis. The reason is that the intention-to-treat analysis will take account of patients who have withdrawn from the trial because of intolerance of the treatment or adverse drug reactions. It is therefore a much more robust approach. Table 16.10 shows the baseline characteristics and results of an 'intention-to-treat' analysis in an RCT comparing magnesium sulphate and diazepam in the treatment of eclamptic fits. The superiority of magnesium sulphate in this study has resulted in its nearly uniform use.
- *Are the results generalizable?* Were the patients enrolled into the study a reasonable reflection of those likely to be treated in routine clinical practice (a so-called pragmatic trial)? Or were they a selected population that excluded significant patient groups (such as the elderly)? If the latter, view the results with caution.
- *Analysis of a superiority trial.* The aim of a superiority trial is to determine whether one treatment (or dose) is better (or more effective) than another. It is usual to estimate the probability that there is 'no difference' between the treatments; if this is less than 1 in 20 ($p < 0.05$) it is regarded as 'statistically significant'. There are two caveats. First, any difference may still be due to chance and it is better to await the results of two independent studies before adopting a new treatment. Secondly, a trial may show no 'statistically significant' difference when one in fact exists because too few patients have been included. The 'power' of a study (the number of patients needed in each treatment group to detect a predefined difference) should have been defined at the outset. If not, the results of the study should be interpreted with extreme care.

Table 16.10 Randomized comparative trial of parenteral magnesium sulphate and diazepam in the treatment of eclamptic fits

	Baseline characteristics		
	MgSO$_4$ (n = 453)	Diazepam (n = 452)	
Mean age (years)	22.1	22.3	
Primiparous	293	302	
Twins/triplets	14	16	
Previous epileptic history	9	8	
Blood pressure at start of treatment:			
diastolic > 110	238	228	
systolic > 170	161	166	
Gestational age (weeks):			
< 34	119	103	
34–37	110	107	
> 37	168	180	
not known	56	62	
	Results		
	MgSO$_4$ (n = 453)	Diazepam (n = 452)	Relative risk (95% CI)
Further fits	60	126	0.48 (0.36–0.63)
Death	17	23	0.74 (0.40–1.36)
Respiratory depression	35	33	
Pneumonia	9	14	
Renal failure	28	29	
Stroke	13	17	

Collaborative Eclampsia Trialists (1995) Which anticonvulsant for women with eclampsia? Reprinted with permission from Elsevier. *Lancet* **345**: 1455–1462

- *Effect size.* The size of a difference in a superiority trial (the so-called 'effect size') may (or may not) be clinically relevant even if statistically significant. For example, if a trial of a new analgesic for mild pain showed that a new treatment relieved pain in 94% of patients compared to 92% of patients with an older treatment, few clinicians would be impressed even if the effect size (2%) was statistically significant. On the other hand, a reduction in the 30-day mortality after acute myocardial infarction from 8% to 6%, by giving streptokinase, is of real clinical advantage even though the effect size is 2%.

- *Analysis of an equivalence trial.* The aim in this trial is to determine whether two (or possibly more) treatments produce similar benefits. During the design of such trials, it is necessary to decide what difference is unimportant and then to calculate the number of patients needed in order to have an 80% or 90% chance of showing this. In equivalence trials such power calculations show that the number of patients required is invariably greater than those needed for superiority trials. The results of equivalence trials are usually reported as a 'hazard ratio' (the ratio of the response rate to the study treatment to that of the comparator) with its 95% confidence intervals. A hazard ratio of around unity (and with a confidence interval of – say – 0.9–1.1) would indicate that the two treatments were indeed likely to be equivalent. A hazard ratio of 0.5 (confidence interval 0.3–0.7) would suggest inequivalence, and superiority of the study treatment. By contrast, a hazard ratio of 2.0 (confidence interval 1.7–2.3) would suggest that the new treatment was inferior. In equivalence trials, it should be obvious that the comparator itself must have been shown to be effective.

- *Meta-analysis.* An analysis of all controlled trials that have been performed in a particular area can minimize random errors in the assessment of treatment effects because more patients and treatments are included than in any individual trial. Meta-analysis should be performed (and interpreted) carefully because of the heterogeneity of studies.

Controlled observational trials

Three types of observational study have been used to test the clinical effectiveness of therapeutic interventions – historical controlled trials, case-control studies and before and after studies.

Historical controlled trials. Despite the pre-eminence of the prospective randomized controlled trial there are many treatments that have never been subjected to this technique, yet their efficacy is unquestioned. Examples include insulin in the treatment of diabetic ketoacidosis, thyroxine for hypothyroidism, vitamin B$_{12}$ in pernicious anaemia, and defibrillation for ventricular fibrillation.

In a historical controlled trial the outcome in patients treated with the study drug is compared to that of previously untreated patients with the same disease. The circumstances when it is legitimate for a treatment to be accepted into routine use on the basis of favourable comparisons with historical controls are generally limited to the following:

- There should be a biologically plausible reason why the treatment might be effective. From a knowledge of the underlying nature of the condition, and the properties of the treatment, it should be reasonable to infer likely benefit.
- There should be no other effective form of treatment. If there is, then the study treatment should be compared with the alternative in a prospective, randomized controlled trial.
- The disease, if untreated, should result in death or permanent disability.
- The condition should have a known, and predictable, natural history.

New treatments that fulfil these stringent criteria are uncommon. Historical controlled trials are most frequently (though inappropriately) used in the assessment of, for example, new anticancer treatments; in most instances prospective, comparative, randomized, and controlled trials would be more informative.

Case-control studies. This type of study design compares patients with a particular condition (the 'cases') with those without (the 'controls'). The approach has predominantly been used to identify 'risk factors' for specific conditions such as lung cancer (smoking), sudden infant death syndrome (lying prone), or deep venous thrombosis (oral contraceptives). Such a study allows an estimation of the odds ratio:

	Cases	Controls
Risk factor present	*a*	*c*
Risk factor absent	*b*	*d*

The odds ratio (OR) = $a \div b / c \div d$.

An OR that is significantly greater than unity indicates a statistical association that may be causal. The OR for deep venous thrombosis and current use of oral contraceptives equals 2–4 (depending on the preparation): this indicates that the risk of developing a deep venous thrombosis on oral contraceptives is between 2 and 4 times greater than the background rate.

In some studies, the OR for a particular observation has been found to be significantly less than unity, suggesting 'protection' from the condition under study. Some studies of women with myocardial infarction indicated protection in those using hormone-replacement therapies but it has been subsequently shown that the result was due to bias. On the other hand, case-control studies have consistently shown that aspirin and other non-steroidal anti-inflammatory drugs are associated with a reduced risk of colon cancer. This seems to be a causal effect.

Case-control studies claiming to demonstrate the efficacy of a drug need to be interpreted with great care: the possibility of bias and confounding is substantial as was seen in the studies of hormone-replacement therapy

and myocardial infarction. Confirmation from one or more RCTs is usually essential.

Before-and-after studies. It has sometimes been inferred that observed improvements seen in patients before, and after, the application of a particular treatment is evidence of efficacy. Such an approach is fraught with difficulties: the combination of a placebo effect, as well as regression to the mean, is likely to negate most studies using this type of design. Nevertheless there are some circumstances where genuine efficacy can be confidently observed with such designs: the consequences of hip replacement, and cataract surgery, are good examples. Such instances can be regarded as special examples of the use of implicit historical controls.

Uncontrolled observational studies

Uncontrolled case series cannot be considered as providing primary evidence of efficacy unless they are undertaken in circumstances that are virtually those of historical controlled trials. When used in this way to demonstrate clinical effectiveness their validity relies on the use of implicit historical trials. Case series can, however, sometimes be of value in demonstrating the generalizability of the results of RCTs.

Dangers

Drug trials are carried out in specific groups of selected patients under strict supervision. The results, particularly when dramatic, are often used outside these strict criteria. The dramatic effect of spironolactone in heart failure (30% reduction in all-cause mortality) has not been replicated in clinical practice because the wrong patients have been treated, often with higher doses, leading to hyperkalaemia and death.

Evaluation of new drugs

New drugs are subjected to a vigorous programme of preclinical and clinical testing before they are licensed for general use (Table 16.11) and are also monitored for safety following licensing. Doctors are recommended to fill in yellow cards when they suspect an adverse reaction has taken place.

FURTHER READING

Benson K, Hartz AJ (2000) A comparison of observational studies and randomised trials. *New England Journal of Medicine* **342**: 1878–1886.

Collins R, MacMahon S (2001) Reliable assessment of the effects of treatment on mortality and major morbidity. I Clinical trials, II Observational studies. *Lancet* **357**: 373–380, 455–462.

Concato J, Shah N, Horwitz RI (2000) Randomised controlled trials, observational studies and the hierarchy of research designs. *New England Journal of Medicine* **342**: 1887–1892.

Treating individuals (a series of articles starting in January 2005). *Lancet* **365**: 826.

Table 16.11   Evaluation of new drugs

Phase I
Healthy human subjects (usually men)
First use in man
Evaluation of safety and toxicity
Pharmacokinetic assessment
Sometimes pharmacodynamic assessment
Approximately 100 subjects

Phase II
First assessment in patients
Safety and toxicity evaluated
Dose range identified
Pharmacokinetic and pharmacodynamic monitoring
Approximately 500 subjects

Phase III
Use in wider patient population
Efficacy main objective
Safety and toxicity also carefully monitored
Often multicentre trials
Approximately 2000 patients involved

Phase IV
Postmarketing surveillance
All patients prescribed drug monitored
Efficacy, safety and toxicity measured
Quantification of unusual drug adverse effects
Yellow card and Prescription Event Monitoring
Often very large numbers of patients observed

STATISTICAL ANALYSES

The relevance of statistics is not confined to those who undertake research but also to anyone who wants to understand the relevance of research studies to their clinical practice.

The average

Clinical studies may describe, quantitatively, the value of a particular variable (e.g. height, weight, blood pressure, haemoglobin) in a sample of a defined population. The 'average' value (or 'central tendency' in statistical parlance) can be expressed as the mean, median or mode depending on the circumstances:

- The *mean* is the average of a distribution of values that are grouped symmetrically around the central tendency.
- The *median* is the middle value of a sample. It is used, particularly, where the values in a sample are asymmetrically distributed around the central tendency.
- The *mode* is the interval, in a frequency distribution of values, that contains more values than any other.

In a symmetrically distributed population the mean, median and mode are the same.

The average value of a sample, on its own, is of only modest interest. Of equal (and often greater) relevance is the confidence we can place on the sample average as truly reflecting the average value of the population from which it has been drawn. This is most often expressed as a *confidence interval*, which describes the probability of a sample mean being a certain distance from the population mean. If, for example, the mean systolic blood pressure of 100 undergraduates is 124 mmHg, with a 95% confidence interval of ± 15 mmHg, we can be confident that if we replicated the study 100 times the value of the mean would be within the range 109–139 mmHg on 95 occasions. It is intuitively obvious that the larger the sample the less will be the size of the confidence interval.

Correlation

In clinical studies two, or more, variables may be measured in the same individuals in a sample population (e.g. weight and blood pressure). The degree of correlation between the two can be investigated by calculating the *correlation coefficient* (often abbreviated to 'r'). The correlation coefficient measures the degree of association between the two variables and may range from 1 to −1. If $r = 1$, there is complete and direct concordance between the two variables: if $r = -1$, there is complete but inverse concordance; and where $r = 0$ there is no concordance.

Statistical tables are available to inform investigators as to the probability that r is due to chance. As in other areas of statistics, if the probability is less than 1 in 20 ($p < 0.05$) then by custom and practice it is regarded as 'statistically significant'. There are, however, two caveats. First, the 1 in 20 rule is a convention and does not exclude the possibility that a presumed association is due to chance. Second, the fact that there is an association between two variables does not necessarily mean that it is causal. A correlation between blood pressure and weight, with $r = 0.75$ and $p < 0.05$, does not mean that weight has a direct effect on blood pressure (or vice versa).

Correlation analyses can become complicated. The simplest (least squares regression analysis) presumes a straight-line relationship between the two variables. More complicated techniques can be used to estimate r where a non-linear relationship is presumed (or assumed); where the distributions deviate from normal; where the scales of one or both variables are intervals or ranks; or where a correlation between three or more variables is sought.

Hypothesis testing

Much of statistics is concerned with testing hypotheses. The basic assumption – known as the '*null hypothesis*' – is that there is no difference between two variables in one (or more) groups. The reason for this confusing terminology is that statistical techniques are designed to assess the extent to which a zero difference might be due to the play of chance (such as a sampling 'error'). In the analysis of an RCT (p. 998) the null hypothesis asserts that there is no difference between the results in patients treated with placebo and those on active treatment. Statistical tests are used to determine the probability that the observed difference is due to chance. Where this is less than 1 in 20 ($p < 0.05$) it is described as 'statistically significant'. Again, the 1 in 20 rule is arbitrary but is a convention that is widely adopted.

The choice of statistical test to examine the null hypothesis is a complicated one. It is dependent on the type of data collected (whether it is ordinal, cardinal or categorical); and whether it conforms to a normal (parametric) or other (non-parametric) distribution. Those most commonly used include Student's t test (parametric) and χ^2 test, analysis of variance and various tests for non-parametric data. In some circumstances it is possible to use the confidence intervals of the means of two (or more) groups to test the null hypothesis.

When the results of a statistical test indicate that it is reasonable to reject the null hypothesis, and that the probability of the results being due to chance is less than 1 in 20 ($p < 0.05$), it means that 95 times out of a 100 we will be right, but that 5 times out of a 100 we will be wrong. Statisticians call erroneous rejection of the null hypothesis a *type 1 error*. In this situation the null hypothesis is actually true, although we believe it to be false. Erroneous acceptance of the null hypothesis when there is indeed a difference is known as a *type 2 error*. Type 1 errors can be reduced by requiring a higher level of significance (e.g. $p < 0.01$ or $p < 0.005$) but can never be absolutely excluded. Type 2 errors are usually the result of too few participants in the study and can be avoided by estimating the numbers needed to examine specific levels of difference before the trial is started. Such estimates are known as 'power calculations'.

Other statistical techniques

Statisticians have developed a range of sophisticated methods to handle a wide variety of biomedical problems. Unless an investigator is supremely (and usually unwisely) confident it is wise to seek professional advice in analysing numerical data that look complicated. In doing so, it is invariably wiser to do so at the time the study is being designed rather than after the results have been generated!

FURTHER READING

Armitage P, Berry G, Matthews JNS (2002) *Statistical Methods in Medical Research.* Oxford: Blackwell Science.

Bland M (2000) *An Introduction to Medical Statistics,* 3rd edn. Oxford: Oxford University Press.

Daly LE, Bourke GJ (2000) *Interpretation and Use of Medical Statistics.* Oxford: Blackwell Science.

Schulz KF, Grimes DA (2005) Epidemiology I. *Lancet* **365**: 1348–1353.

INFORMATION

Pharmacotherapy moves at a very rapid pace and it is impossible for anyone to keep up with contemporary advances. Details of current prescribing advice can be found in:

- The Summary of Product Characteristics (SmPCs) produced by manufacturers but vetted by the UK drug regulatory authority (the Medicines and Healthcare products Regulatory Agency)
- The British National Formulary (BNF) produced, jointly, by the British Medical Association and the Royal Pharmaceutical Society
- The Technology Appraisals Guidance series from the National Institute for Clinical Excellence (NICE).

Advice on the management of individual conditions, in the form of clinical guidelines (systematically developed statements to assist practitioner and patient decisions about appropriate healthcare for specific clinical circumstances) can be accessed from:

- the National Institute for Clinical Excellence (NICE): http://www.nice-org.uk
- the Scottish Intercollegiate Guidelines Network (SIGN): http://www.sign.ac.uk/
- the National Guidelines Clearing House in the USA: http://www.guideline.gov.

POISONING

The nature of the problem

In many hospitals all over the world, acute poisoning is one of the most common reasons for acute admission to a medical ward. Poisoning is usually by self-administration of prescribed and over-the-counter medicines, or illicit drugs. Poisoning in children aged less than 6 months is most commonly iatrogenic and involves overtreatment with, for example, paracetamol (acetaminophen). Children between 8 months and 5 years of age also ingest poisons accidentally. Drugs may be administered deliberately to cause harm, as in Münchausen's syndrome by proxy, or for financial or sexual gain. Occupational poisoning as a result of dermal or inhalational exposure to chemicals is a common occurrence in the developing world and still occurs in the developed world. Sometimes, inappropriate prescribing by a doctor is responsible for the development of poisoning, for example digoxin intoxication.

In adults, self-poisoning is commonly a 'cry for help'. Those involved are most often females under the age of 35 who are in good physical health. They take an overdose in circumstances where they are likely to be found, or in the presence of others. In those older than 55 years of age, men predominate and the overdose is usually taken in the course of a depressive illness or because of poor physical health.

<table>
<tr><td colspan="2">

> **Box 16.2 Prevention of self-poisoning**
>
> Patients usually take what is readily available at home.
>
> ■ Small amounts only of drugs should be bought.
> ■ Foil-wrapped drugs are less likely to be taken.
> ■ Keep drugs in a safe place.
> ■ Keep drugs and liquids in their original containers.
> ■ Child-resistant drug containers should be used.
> ■ Doctors should be careful in prescribing all drugs.
> ■ Prescriptions for any susceptible patient (e.g. the depressed) must be monitored carefully.
> ■ Household products should be labelled and kept safely, away from children.
>
> **SELF-POISONING CAN KILL**
> All people must be aware of the dangers of drugs and chemicals. Education on safe storage and careful handling of household and workplace chemicals is necessary on a continual basis.

</td></tr>
</table>

> **Box 16.3 Diagnostic process in acute poisoning**
>
> ■ Obtain history if possible from the patient or a relative/friend/paramedic.
> ■ Is there circumstantial evidence of an overdose?
> ■ Are the circumstances in which the patient has been found suggestive of an overdose?
> ■ Was a suicide note left?
> ■ Are the symptoms suggestive of an overdose?
> ■ Do the physical signs suggest an overdose? (Table 16.12)
> ■ Identify the tablets if available with the help of pharmacy and poison information centres. TICTAC is a computer-aided tablet and capsule identification system available in the UK to authorized users. TOX BASE is available over the Internet to registered users (http://www.spib.axl.co.uk).

THE APPROACH TO THE PATIENT

History

Eighty per cent of adults are conscious on arrival at hospital and the diagnosis of self-poisoning can usually be made from the history (Box 16.3). It should be emphasized that in any patient with an altered level of consciousness, drug overdose must always be considered in the differential diagnosis.

Examination

On arrival at hospital the patient must be assessed urgently in the A&E department. Check:

Airways
Breathing
Circulation.

Then:

- *Level of consciousness* – the Glasgow Coma Scale should be used (see p. 1206).
- *Ventilation* – pulse oximetry can be used to measure oxygen saturation. The displayed reading may be inaccurate when the saturation is below 70%, there is poor peripheral perfusion and in the presence of carboxyhaemoglobin and methaemoglobin. Arterial blood gases measure CO_2 as well as oxygenation and is also usually measured.
- *Blood pressure and pulse rate.*
- *Pupil size and reaction to light.*
- Evidence of intravenous drug abuse.
- *A head injury* complicating poisoning.

If the patient is unconscious the following should also be checked:

- *Cough and gag reflex* – present or absent
- *Temperature* – measured with a low-reading rectal thermometer.

Some of the physical signs that may aid identification of the agents responsible for poisoning are shown in Table 16.12.

A third of self-poisoning patients state that they are unaware of the toxic effects of the substance involved; the majority take whatever drug is easily available at their home (Box 16.2). Studies of the agents involved reveal that:

- Acute overdoses usually involve more than one agent.
- Alcohol is the most commonly implicated second agent in mixed self-poisonings – 60% of men and 45% of women consume some alcohol at the same time as the drug.
- There is often a poor correlation between the drug history and the toxicological analytical findings. Therefore, a patient's statement about the type and amount of drug ingested cannot always be relied upon.

In England and Wales there are some 100 000 hospital admissions each year for self-poisoning. The most common agents involved are paracetamol, benzodiazepines, antidepressants and NSAIDs. A similar pattern exists in other developed countries. In contrast, in the developing world, pesticide poisoning is far commoner with some 1 million cases of serious unintentional pesticide poisonings annually and 2 million hospitalized deliberate pesticide ingestions. In addition, ingestion of heating fuels (e.g. petroleum distillates), antimalarials, antituberculous drugs and traditional medicine is reported frequently.

The majority of cases of self-poisoning do not require intensive medical management, but all patients require a sympathetic and caring approach, a psychiatric and social assessment and, sometimes, psychiatric treatment. However, as the majority of patients ingest relatively non-toxic agents, all that is required is good supportive care and, when appropriate, the administration of specific antidotes, such as N-acetylcysteine for paracetamol poisoning. The in-hospital mortality in most developed countries is now ≤ 0.5%. Most deaths from poisoning (80% of some 4500 in the UK) occur outside hospital; the commonest causes are carbon monoxide, tricyclic antidepressants, paracetamol, and analgesic combinations containing paracetamol and an opioid.

Table 16.12 Some physical signs of poisoning	
Features	**Likely poisons**
Constricted pupils	Opioids Organophosphorus insecticides Nerve agents
Dilated pupils	Tricyclic antidepressants Amfetamines Cocaine Antimuscarinic drugs
Convulsions	Tricyclic antidepressants Theophylline Opioids Mefenamic acid Isoniazid Amfetamines
Dystonic reactions	Metoclopramide Phenothiazines
Delirium and hallucinations	Antimuscarinic drugs Amfetamines Cannabis Recovery from tricyclic antidepressant overdose
Loss of vision	Methanol Quinine
Divergent strabismus	Tricyclic antidepressants
Papilloedema	Carbon monoxide Methanol
Nystagmus	Phenytoin Carbamazepine
Hypertonia and hyperreflexia	Tricyclic antidepressants Antimuscarinic drugs
Tinnitus and deafness	Salicylates Quinine
Hyperventilation	Salicylates Phenoxyacetate herbicides Theophylline
Hyperthermia	MDMA (Ecstasy)
Blisters	Usually occur in comatose patients

Box 16.4 Management strategy in acute poisoning

- Provide supportive treatment.
- Reduce poison absorption?
- Take blood for drug levels (Table 16.13).
- Will any other investigations help? (Table 16.14)
- Should urine alkalinization, multiple-dose activated charcoal, or haemodialysis be employed to increase poison elimination?
- Is an antidote helpful? (Table 16.16)

Table 16.13 Agents for which emergency measurement of blood concentrations is appropriate

Aspirin (salicylate)
Digoxin
Ethanol (in monitoring treatment of ethylene glycol and
     methanol poisoning)
Ethylene glycol
Iron
Lithium (NB: Do not use a lithium heparin tube!)
Methanol
Paracetamol
Theophylline

cases. Drug screens on blood and urine are occasionally indicated in severely poisoned patients in whom the cause of coma is unknown. Poison Information Services will advise.

Non-toxicological investigations
(Table 16.14)

Some routine investigations are of value in the differential diagnosis of coma or the detection of poison-induced hypokalaemia, hyperkalaemia, hypoglycaemia, hyperglycaemia and hepatic renal failure or of acid–base disturbances (Table 16.15). Measurement of carboxyhaemoglobin, methaemoglobin and RBC cholinesterase activity are of assistance in the diagnosis and management respectively of cases of poisoning due to carbon monoxide, methaemoglobin-inducing agents such as nitrites, and organophosphorus insecticides and nerve agents.

PRINCIPLES OF MANAGEMENT
(Box 16.4)

Most patients with self-poisoning require only general care and support of the vital systems. However, for a few drugs additional therapy is required.

Toxicological investigations

On admission, or at an appropriate time post-overdose, a timed blood sample should be taken if the agents shown in Table 16.13 have been ingested. The determination of the concentrations of these drugs will be valuable in management and is sometimes useful in medicolegal

CARE OF THE UNCONSCIOUS PATIENT
(see also p. 1206)

In all cases the patient should be nursed in the lateral position with the lower leg straight and the upper leg flexed; in this position the risk of aspiration is reduced. A clear passage for air should be ensured by the removal of any obstructing object, vomit or dentures, and by backward pressure on the mandible. Nursing care of the mouth and pressure areas should be instituted. Immediate catheterization of the bladder in unconscious patients is usually unnecessary as it can be emptied by gentle suprapubic pressure. Insertion of a venous cannula is usual, but administration of intravenous fluids is unnecessary

Table 16.14 Relevant non-toxicological investigations

Serum sodium (e.g. hyponatraemia in MDMA* poisoning) and potassium (e.g. hypokalaemia in theophylline poisoning and hyperkalaemia in digoxin poisoning) concentrations

Serum creatinine concentration (e.g. renal failure in ethylene glycol poisoning)

Acid–base disturbances, including metabolic acidosis (Table 16.15)

Blood glucose concentration (e.g. hypoglycaemia in insulin poisoning or hyperglycaemia in salicylate poisoning)

Serum calcium concentration (e.g. hypocalcaemia in ethylene glycol poisoning)

Liver function (e.g. in paracetamol poisoning)

Serum phosphate (e.g. hypophosphataemia in paracetamol-induced renal tubular damage)

Serum creatine kinase (rhabdomyolysis)

Carboxyhaemoglobin concentration (in carbon monoxide poisoning)

Methaemoglobinaemia (e.g. in nitrite poisoning)

RBC cholinesterase activity (e.g. organophosphorus insecticide and nerve agent poisoning)

ECG (e.g. wide QRS in tricyclic antidepressant poisoning) X-ray for ingestion/injection of radiopaque substances

*MDMA, 3,4-methylenedioxy-methamfetamine (Ecstasy)

Table 16.15 Some poisons inducing metabolic acidosis

Carbon monoxide
Cocaine
Cyanide
Ethanol
Ethylene glycol
Iron
Methanol
Paracetamol
Salicylates
Tricyclic antidepressants

unless the patient has been unconscious for more than 12 hours or is hypotensive.

Respiratory support

If respiratory depression is present, as determined by pulse oximetry or preferably by arterial blood gas analysis, an oropharyngeal airway should be inserted, and supplemental oxygen should be administered. Pulse oximetry alone will not detect hypercapnia. Loss of the cough or gag reflex is the prime indication for intubation. The gag reflex can be assessed by positioning the patient on one side and making him or her gag using a suction tube. In many severely poisoned patients the reflexes are depressed sufficiently to allow intubation without the use of sedatives or relaxants. The complications of endotracheal tubes are discussed on page 983.

If ventilation remains inadequate after intubation, as shown by hypoxaemia and hypercapnia, intermittent positive-pressure ventilation (IPPV) should be instituted.

Cardiovascular support

Although hypotension (systolic blood pressure below 80 mmHg) is a recognized feature of acute poisoning, the classic features of shock – tachycardia and pale cold skin – are observed only rarely. In patients with marked hypotension, volume expansion with saline, gelatins or etherified starches (e.g. hetastarch, hexastarch) should be used, guided by monitoring of central venous pressure (CVP). Urine output (aiming for 35–50 mL/h) is also a useful guide to the adequacy of the circulation.

If a patient fails to respond to the above measures, more intensive therapy is required (see p. 975).

Arrhythmias are observed occasionally in poisoned patients, for example after the ingestion of a tricyclic antidepressant or theophylline. All such patients and those with shock should have ECG monitoring. Known arrhythmogenic factors such as hypoxia, acidosis and hypokalaemia should be corrected.

Other problems

Body temperature

Hypothermia – a rectal temperature below 35°C – is a recognized complication of poisoning, especially in older patients or those who are comatose. The patient should be covered with a 'space blanket' and, if necessary, given intravenous and intragastric fluids at normal body temperature. Inspired gases should also be warmed to 37°C.

Hyperthermia can develop with CNS stimulant ingestion. Removal of clothing and sponging with tepid water will promote evaporation.

Rhabdomyolysis

Rhabdomyolysis can occur from pressure necrosis in drug-induced coma, or it may complicate, for example, MDMA (Ecstasy, p. 1012) abuse in the absence of coma. Patients with rhabdomyolysis are at risk of developing firstly, renal failure from myoglobinaemia, particularly if they are hypovolaemic and have an acidosis, and, secondly, wrist or ankle drop from the development of a compartment syndrome (see p. 547).

Convulsions

These may occur, for example, in poisoning due to tricyclic antidepressants, mefenamic acid or opioids. Usually the fits are short-lived but, if they are prolonged, diazepam 10–20 mg i.v. should be administered. Persistent fits must be controlled rapidly to prevent severe hypoxia, brain damage and laryngeal trauma.

If diazepam in repeated doses is ineffective, the patient should also receive a loading dose of phenytoin (15 mg/kg) administered intravenously at a rate of not more than 50 mg/min, with blood pressure and ECG monitoring.

Stress ulceration and bleeding

Medication to prevent stress ulceration of the stomach should be started on admission in all patients who are unconscious and require intensive care. An H_2-receptor antagonist or a proton pump inhibitor should be administered intravenously.

SPECIFIC MANAGEMENT

Antidotes

Specific antidotes are available for only a small number of poisons (Table 16.16).

Antidotes may exert a beneficial effect by:

- forming an inert complex with the poison (e.g. desferrioxamine, dicobalt edetate, dimercaprol, DMSA,

DMPS, digoxin-specific antibody fragments, hydroxo-cobalamin, pralidoxime, protamine, Berlin (Prussian) blue, sodium calcium edetate)
- accelerating the detoxification of the poison (e.g. N-acetylcysteine, sodium thiosulphate)
- reducing the rate of conversion of the poison to a more toxic compound (e.g. ethanol, fomepizole)
- competing with toxic substances for essential receptor sites (e.g. oxygen, naloxone, vitamin K_1)
- blocking essential receptors through which the toxic effects are mediated (e.g. atropine)
- bypassing the effect of the poison (e.g. oxygen).

Reduction of poison absorption

Inhaled

To reduce poison absorption through the lungs, the casualty should be removed from the toxic atmosphere, without the rescuers themselves being put at risk.

Skin

If clothing is contaminated this should be removed to reduce dermal absorption. In addition, contaminated skin should be washed thoroughly with soap and water.

Gut decontamination

The efficacy of current methods to remove unabsorbed drug from the gastrointestinal tract remains unproven. The two major international societies of clinical toxicology, the American Academy of Clinical Toxicology and the European Association of Poisons Centres and Clinical Toxicologists have produced Position Statements on each method.

Gastric lavage

Gastric lavage involves the insertion of a large-bore orogastric tube into the stomach. Small amounts (200–300 mL in an adult) of warm (38°C) fluid (water or 0.9% saline) are introduced and removed by suction. Lavage is continued until the recovered solution is clear of particulate matter.

Gastric lavage *should not be employed routinely in the management of poisoned patients.* The amount of marker removed by gastric lavage is highly variable and diminishes with time. There is no certain evidence that its use improves clinical outcome and it may cause significant morbidity. Gastric lavage should only be *used*, therefore, if a patient has ingested a potentially life-threatening amount of a poison and the procedure can be undertaken within 1 hour of ingestion. Gastric lavage is contraindicated if airway-protective reflexes are lost (unless the patient is intubated) and also if a hydrocarbon with high aspiration potential or a corrosive substance has been ingested.

Syrup of ipecacuanha

Syrup of ipecacuanha contains two alkaloids, emetine and cephaeline, which induce vomiting by a central action and by a local action (emetine).

Syrup of ipecacuanha *should not be administered to poisoned patients.* The amount of marker removed in

Table 16.16 Antidotes of value in poisoning

Poison	Antidote
Aluminium	Desferrioxamine
Anticoagulants (oral)	Vitamin K_1
Arsenic	Dimercaprol (BAL)
Benzodiazepines	Flumazenil
β-Adrenoceptor blocking drugs	Atropine
	Glucagon
Carbon monoxide	Oxygen
Copper	D-penicillamine
	N-acetylcysteine
	DMPS
Cyanide	Oxygen
	Dicobalt edetate
	Hydroxocobalamin
	Sodium nitrite
	Sodium thiosulphate
Digoxin	Digoxin-specific antibody fragments
Ethylene glycol	Ethanol
	Fomepizole
Iron salts	Desferrioxamine
Lead (inorganic)	Sodium calcium edetate
	DMSA
Methaemoglobinaemia	Methylthioninium chloride (methylene blue)
Methanol	Ethanol
	Fomepizole
Mercury (inorganic)	DMPS
Opioids	Naloxone
Organophosphorus compounds	Atropine
	Pralidoxime
Paracetamol	N-acetylcysteine
Thallium	Berlin (Prussian) blue

DMSA, dimercaptosuccinic acid (succimer); DMPS, dimercaptopropanesulphonate (unithiol).

studies was highly variable and diminished with time. There is no evidence that it improves the clinical outcome and therefore its administration, even in children, should be abandoned.

Single-dose activated charcoal

Activated charcoal has a highly developed internal pore structure which is able to adsorb a wide variety of compounds and drugs, e.g. aspirin, carbamazepine, aminophylline, digoxin, barbiturates, phenytoin, paracetamol. It does not absorb strong acids and alkalis, ethanol, ethylene glycol, iron, lithium, mercury and methanol.

Single-dose activated charcoal *should not be administered routinely in the management of poisoned patients*. Based on volunteer studies, the effectiveness of activated charcoal decreases with time; the greatest benefit is within 1 hour of ingestion. The administration of activated charcoal should only be *used* if a patient (with an intact or protected airway) has ingested a potentially toxic amount of a poison (which is known to be adsorbed to charcoal) up to 1 hour previously. There is no evidence that activated charcoal improves the clinical outcome.

For multiple-dose activated charcoal use, see below.

Cathartics

The administration of a cathartic alone has *no role in the management of the poisoned patient* and is not recommended as a method of gut decontamination. Experimental data are conflicting regarding the use of cathartics in combination with activated charcoal. No clinical studies have been published to investigate the ability of a cathartic, with or without activated charcoal, to reduce the bioavailability of drugs or to improve the outcome of poisoned patients. Based on available data, the routine use of a cathartic in combination with activated charcoal is not recommended.

Whole bowel irrigation

Whole bowel irrigation (WBI) requires the insertion of a nasogastric tube into the stomach and the introduction of polyethylene glycol electrolyte solution 1500–2000 mL/h in an adult. WBI is continued until the rectal effluent is clear.

WBI should not be used routinely in the management of the poisoned patient. Although some volunteer studies have shown substantial decreases in the bioavailability of ingested drugs, no controlled clinical trials have been performed and there is no conclusive evidence that WBI improves the outcome of the poisoned patient. Based on volunteer studies, WBI should be *used* for potentially toxic ingestions of sustained-release or enteric-coated drugs. There are insufficient data to support or exclude the use of WBI for potentially toxic ingestions of iron, lead, zinc, or packets of illicit drugs; WBI remains a theoretical option for these ingestions. WBI is contraindicated in patients with bowel obstruction, perforation, ileus, and in patients with haemodynamic instability or compromised unprotected airways. WBI should be used cautiously in debilitated patients, or in patients with medical conditions that may be further compromised by its use.

FURTHER READING

Bateman N (ed) (2003) Poisons. *Clinical Medicine* **3**(2): 107–130

Bateman DN, Barceloux D, McGuigan M, et al (2004) Position paper: cathartics. *Journal of Toxicology – Clinical Toxicology* **42**: 243–253.

Krenzelok EP, Vale JA, Chyka PA, et al (2005) Position paper: single-dose activated charcoal. *Journal of Toxicology – Clinical Toxicology* **43**: 61–87.

Kulig K, Vale JA (2004) Position paper: gastric lavage. *Journal of Toxicology – Clinical Toxicology* **42**: 933–943.

Lheureux P, Tenenbein M (2004) Position paper: whole bowel irrigation. *Journal of Toxicology – Clinical Toxicology* **42**: 843–854.

Manoguerra AS, Krenzelok EP, McGuigan M, et al (2004) Position paper: Ipecac syrup. *Journal of Toxicology – Clinical Toxicology* **42**: 133–143

Increasing poison elimination

Treatments that speed poison elimination are urine alkalinization, multiple-dose activated charcoal, dialysis and haemoperfusion.

Urine alkalinization

In practice, urine alkalinization is only employed in salicylate and chlorophenoxy herbicide poisoning. (The methodology employed is described under aspirin poisoning p. 1009) There is some controversy regarding the mechanism by which urine alkalinization increases elimination. Most drugs, particularly unionized, lipid-soluble molecules, are largely reabsorbed by the renal tubules. With alkalinization the drug becomes fully ionized and there is a reduction in reabsorption and enhanced elimination. This alkalinization is achieved by increasing urine pH to approximately 7.5 by the administration of intravenous sodium bicarbonate.

Multiple-dose activated charcoal

Multiple doses of activated charcoal aid the elimination of some drugs from the circulation by interrupting their enterohepatic circulation and also by adsorbing the drug that has diffused into the intestinal juices. The adsorptive capacity of charcoal is such that as zero concentrations of free drug are present in luminal fluid, the diffusion gradient still remains as high as possible. The process has been termed 'gut dialysis' since, in effect, the intestinal mucosa is being used as a semipermeable membrane.

Although many studies have demonstrated that multiple-dose activated charcoal increases drug elimination significantly, this therapy has not yet been shown to reduce morbidity and mortality. Multiple-dose activated charcoal should be *used* only if a patient has ingested a life-threatening amount of carbamazepine, dapsone, phenobarbital, quinine or theophylline. In all of these cases there are data to confirm enhanced elimination, though no controlled studies have demonstrated clinical benefit. Adults should receive 50–100 g initially, followed by 50 g 4-hourly or 25 g 2-hourly until charcoal appears in the faeces or recovery occurs.

Haemodialysis

Haemodialysis in acute poisoning is most commonly indicated for the treatment of acute renal failure and only infrequently to increase the elimination of poisons. Haemodialysis is indicated in patients with severe clinical features and high plasma concentrations of ethanol, ethylene glycol, isopropanol, lithium, methanol or salicylate. Haemodialysis is of little value in patients who have ingested poisons with large volumes of distribution, e.g. tricyclic antidepressants, because the plasma contains only a small proportion of the total amount of drug in the body.

Peritoneal dialysis increases the elimination of poisons such as ethylene glycol and methanol but is much less efficient than haemodialysis.

> **FURTHER READING**
>
> Proudfoot AT, Krenzelok EP, Vale JA (2004) Position paper on urine alkalinization. *Journal of Toxicology–Clinical Toxicology* **42**: 1–26.
>
> Vale JA, Krenzelok EP, Barceloux GD (1999) Position Statement and Practice Guidelines on the use of multi-dose activated charcoal in the treatment of acute poisoning. *Journal of Toxicology–Clinical Toxicology* **37**: 731–751.

SPECIFIC POISONS

DRUGS AND CHEMICALS

In this section only specific treatment regimens will be discussed and are in alphabetical order. The general principles of management of self-poisoning will always be required. *All drug doses relate to adults.*

Aluminium and zinc phosphides

Aluminium and zinc phosphides, which are used as rat poison in India and South East Asia, react with moisture in the air and the gastrointestinal tract to produce phosphine, a gas with a garlic-like odour.

Clinical features

Ingestion causes vomiting, epigastric pain, peripheral circulatory failure, severe metabolic acidosis, and renal failure in addition to the features induced by phosphine. Exposure to phosphine causes lacrimation, rhinorrhoea, productive cough, breathlessness, chest tightness, dizziness, headache nausea, and drowsiness. Acute pulmonary oedema, hypertension, cardiac arrhythmias, convulsions and jaundice have been described in severe cases. Ataxia, intention tremor, and diplopia may be found on examination.

Treatment

Treatment is symptomatic and supportive. Gastric lavage should be avoided as it might increase the rate of disintegration of the product ingested and increase toxicity. Activated charcoal is also contraindicated as it will not bind metal phosphides. The value of steroids in preventing pulmonary damage (which may be delayed) has not been established. The mortality is very high despite supportive care.

Amfetamines

Amfetamines are CNS and cardiovascular stimulants. These effects are mediated by increasing synaptic concentrations of epinephrine (adrenaline) and dopamine. Poisoning is usually the result of their use for pleasurable purposes.

Clinical features

These drugs cause euphoria, extrovert behaviour, a lack of desire to eat or sleep, tremor, dilated pupils, tachycardia and hypertension. More severe intoxication is associated with agitation, paranoid delusions, hallucinations and violent behaviour. Convulsions, rhabdomyolysis, hyperthermia and cardiac arrhythmias may develop in severe intoxication. Rarely, intracerebral and subarachnoid haemorrhage occur and can be fatal. There is evidence that long-term neuronal damage is present in abstinent methamfetamine users.

Treatment

Agitation is controlled by diazepam 10–20 mg i.v. or chlorpromazine 50–100 mg i.m. The peripheral sympathomimetic actions of amfetamines may be antagonized by β-adrenoceptor blocking drugs.

> **FURTHER READING**
>
> Ernst T, Chang L, Leonido-Yee M, Speck O (2000) Evidence for long-term neurotoxicity associated with methamphetamine abuse. *Neurology* **54**: 1344–1349.

Antidiabetic agents

In all cases of poisoning with insulin and sulphonylureas, prompt diagnosis and treatment are essential if death or cerebral damage from neuroglycopenia is to be prevented. Metformin overdose rarely causes hypoglycaemia, since its mode of action is to increase glucose utilization, but lactic acidosis is a potentially serious complication.

Clinical features

Features include drowsiness, coma, twitching, convulsions, depressed limb reflexes, extensor plantar responses, hyperpnoea, pulmonary oedema, tachycardia, and circulatory failure. Hypoglycaemia is to be expected, and hypokalaemia, cerebral oedema, and metabolic acidosis might occur. Neurogenic diabetes insipidus and persistent vegetative states are possible long-term complications. Cholestatic jaundice has been described as a late complication of chlorpropamide poisoning.

Treatment

The blood or plasma glucose concentration should be measured urgently and intravenous glucose given.

Glucagon may be ineffective. If the blood sugar is normal, gastric lavage should be considered if the patient has presented within 1 hour of the substantial ingestion of an oral preparation. Recurring hypoglycaemia is highly likely. A continuous infusion of glucose together with carbohydrate-rich meals are required in cases of severe insulin poisoning, though there may be difficulty in maintaining normoglycaemia. In the case of sulphonylurea poisoning, however, further glucose (although its administration may be unavoidable) only serves to increase already high circulating insulin concentrations. Diazoxide 1.25 mg/kg bodyweight intravenously over 1 hour, repeated at 6-hourly intervals if necessary, has therefore been recommended, since it increases blood glucose concentrations and raises circulating catecholamine concentrations while blocking insulin release.

Aspirin

Aspirin is metabolized to salicylic acid (salicylate) by hydrolases present in many tissues, especially the liver, and subsequently to salicyluric acid and salicyl phenolic glucuronide (Fig. 16.3); these two pathways become saturated in overdose, with the following consequences:

- The plasma salicylate concentration increases more than proportionately expected with increasing dose.
- The time needed to eliminate a given fraction of a dose increases with increasing dose.
- Renal excretion of salicylic acid becomes increasingly significant after overdose; this excretion pathway is extremely sensitive to changes in urinary pH, e.g. increasing urinary pH from 7 to 8 (urine alkalinization) increases the renal excretion of salicylates by a factor of 10.

Salicylates stimulate the respiratory centre, increase the depth and rate of respiration, and induce a respiratory alkalosis. Compensatory mechanisms, including renal excretion of bicarbonate and potassium, result in a metabolic acidosis. Salicylates also interfere with carbohydrate, fat and protein metabolism, disrupt oxidative phosphorylation, producing increased concentrations of lactate, pyruvate and ketone bodies, all of which contribute to the acidosis.

Clinical features

After an overdose, symptoms including hyperventilation, sweating, nausea, vomiting, epigastric pain, tinnitus, and deafness can develop. Respiratory alkalosis and metabolic acidosis supervene and a mixed acid–base disturbance is commonly observed. Rarely, in severe cases, non-cardiogenic pulmonary oedema, renal failure, tetany, coma and convulsions ensue.

Management

For all cases (patients must be assessed in hospital):

- Plasma salicylate concentration. The severity of salicylate poisoning can only be assessed accurately by measurement of the salicylate concentration and acid–base status, though the clinical features will also act as a guide. Initial and repeat salicylate levels after 2 hours should be performed.
- Arterial blood gases.
- Serum urea and electrolytes.
- Intravenous fluids and electrolytes to correct any dehydration or electrolyte imbalance.
- Gastric lavage or activated charcoal (50–100 g) is used in patients who have taken a large amount of aspirin less than 1 hour previously, though there is no evidence that lavage and activated charcoal improve the clinical outcome.

Moderate cases – plasma salicylate concentration 500–700 mg/L (3.62–5.07 mmol/L) – should receive *urine alkalinization*: 225 mL of an 8.4% (1 mmol bicarbonate/mL) solution of sodium bicarbonate is infused intravenously over 1 hour to ensure a urine pH (measured by narrow-range indicator paper or pH meter) of more than 7.5; additional boluses are given to maintain alkalinization.

Urine alkalinization is a metabolically invasive procedure requiring frequent biochemical monitoring and medical and nursing expertise. As administration of sodium bicarbonate will exacerbate pre-existing hypokalaemia, this should be corrected before commencing alkalinization.

Severe cases – plasma salicylate concentration > 700 mg/L (5.07 mmol/L) – particularly those with coma and metabolic acidosis, require haemodialysis.

β-Adrenoceptor blocking drugs

Clinical features

In mild poisoning sinus bradycardia is the only feature, but if a substantial amount has been ingested, coma, convulsions and hypotension develop. Less commonly, delirium, hallucinations and cardiac arrest supervene.

Treatment

Atropine 0.6–1.2 mg i.v. may be given but it is usually less effective than glucagon 50–150 μg/kg (typically 5–10 mg

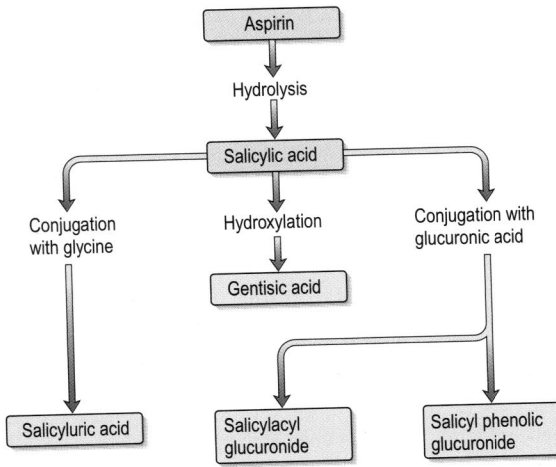

Fig. 16.3 **The metabolism of aspirin.**

in an adult) followed by an infusion of 1–5 mg/h. Glucagon acts by bypassing the blocked β-receptor thus activating adenyl cyclase and promoting formation of cyclic AMP from ATP; cyclic AMP in turn exerts a direct β-stimulant effect on the heart.

FURTHER READING
Lip GYH, Ferner RE (1995) Poisoning with anti-hypertensive drugs: beta-adrenoreceptor blocker drugs. *Journal of Human Hypertension* **9**: 213–221.

Batteries (disc)

Children occasionally ingest disc button batteries, less commonly larger batteries. In the past there was concern that disc batteries might leak and release mercuric oxide but this metal has now been removed in Europe as a result of legislation. Most disc batteries will pass through the gut in 2 or 3 days. If they lodge in the oesophagus, removal by endoscopy is performed.

Benzodiazepines

Benzodiazepines are commonly taken in overdose but rarely produce severe poisoning except in the elderly or those with chronic respiratory disease.

Clinical features

Benzodiazepines produce drowsiness, ataxia and dysarthria. Coma and respiratory depression develop in severe intoxication.

Treatment

If respiratory depression is present, flumazenil 0.5 mg i.v. should be administered in an adult and this dose may be repeated, if necessary.

Cannabis (marijuana)

Cannabis is usually smoked but may be ingested as a 'cake', made into a tea or injected intravenously. It is the drug (other than alcohol) most widely abused in developed countries. The major psychoactive constituent is delta-9-tetrahydrocannabinol (THC). THC possesses activity at the benzodiazepine, opioid and cannabinoid receptors.

Clinical features

Initially there is euphoria followed by drowsiness. A tachycardia is often present. High doses (and chronic use) may lead to psychosis. Intravenous injection leads to watery diarrhoea, tachycardia, hypotension and arthralgia. Whether chronic cannabis abuse causes brain damage remains controversial, though there is increasing evidence that this is the case (p. 1306). Heavy users often become apathetic and suffer impairment of memory and attention. Cannabis use also confers an overall twofold increase in the relative risk for later schizophrenia. Cannabis smoke is carcinogenic.

Treatment

Reassurance is usually the only treatment required, though sedation with intravenous diazepam 10–20 mg i.v. or chlorpromazine 50–100 mg i.m. in adults may be required.

Carbamate insecticides

Carbamate insecticides inhibit acetylcholinesterase but the duration of this effect is comparatively short-lived since the carbamate–enzyme complex tends to dissociate spontaneously.

Clinical features

The features are similar to those of organophosphorus insecticide poisoning (see p. 1016).

Treatment

Occasionally atropine 0.6–2 mg i.v. is required but recovery invariably occurs within 24 hours.

Carbon monoxide

The commonest source of carbon monoxide is an improperly maintained and poorly ventilated heating system. In addition, inhalation of methylene chloride (found in paint strippers) may also lead to carbon monoxide poisoning as methylene chloride is metabolized in vivo to carbon monoxide. The affinity of haemoglobin for carbon monoxide is some 240 times greater than that for oxygen. Carbon monoxide combines with haemoglobin to form carboxyhaemoglobin, thereby reducing the total oxygen-carrying capacity of the blood and increasing the affinity of the remaining haem groups for oxygen. This results in tissue hypoxia. In addition, carbon monoxide also inhibits cytochrome oxidase a_3.

Clinical features

Symptoms of mild to moderate exposure to carbon monoxide may be mistaken for a viral illness. A peak carboxyhaemoglobin (COHb) concentration of less than 10% is not normally associated with symptoms, and peak COHb concentrations of 10–30% may result only in headache and mild exertional dyspnoea. Higher concentrations of COHb are associated with coma, convulsions and cardiorespiratory arrest. Neuropsychiatric features can occur after apparent recovery from carbon monoxide intoxication.

Treatment

In addition to removing the patient from carbon monoxide exposure, high-flow oxygen should be administered using a tightly fitting face mask (p. 985). Endotracheal intubation and mechanical ventilation may be required in those who are unconscious. A recent study using hyperbaric oxygen (HBO) is suggestive of long-term benefit and patients should be referred if they have been unconscious, have a blood carboxyhaemoglobin concentration of > 40% or are pregnant with COHb > 20%.

FURTHER READING
Piantadosi CA (2002) Carbon monoxide poisoning. *New England Journal of Medicine* **347**:1054–1055.
Weaver et al. (2002). Hyperbaric oxygen for acute carbon monoxide poisoning. *New England Journal of Medicine* **347**: 1057–1067.

Chloroquine

Chloroquine poisoning is common in Africa, the Far East and West Pacific.

Clinical features

Hypotension is often the first clinical manifestation of poisoning. It may progress to cardiogenic shock, pulmonary oedema and cardiac arrest. Agitation and acute psychosis, convulsions and coma may ensue. Hypokalaemia is common and is due to chloroquine-induced potassium channel blockade.

Treatment

Severe hypokalaemia (p. 707) should be at least partially corrected (severe hyperkalaemia has been reported in the recovery phase). Adrenaline (epinephrine) is the drug of choice for severe hypotension. The use of high doses of diazepam is controversial but may reduce morbidity and mortality. Multiple-dose activated charcoal may enhance chloroquine elimination.

Cocaine (p. 1306)

Cocaine may be abused by smoking, ingestion, injection or snorting it intranasally. Cocaine blocks the reuptake of biogenic amines. Inhibition of dopamine reuptake is responsible for the psychomotor agitation which commonly accompanies cocaine use. Blockade of norepinephrine (noradrenaline) reuptake produces tachycardia, and inhibition of serotonin reuptake may induce hallucinations. Cocaine also enhances CNS arousal by potentiating the effects of excitatory amino acids.

Clinical features

After initial euphoria, cocaine produces agitation, tachycardia, hypertension, sweating, hallucinations, convulsions, metabolic acidosis, hyperthermia, rhabdomyolysis, and ventricular arrhythmias. Dissection of the aorta, myocarditis, myocardial infarction, dilated cardiomyopathy, subarachnoid haemorrhage, and cerebral haemorrhage also occur.

Treatment

Diazepam 10–20 mg i.v. is used to control agitation and convulsions. Active external cooling should be used for hyperthermia. β-Adrenoceptor blockers are contraindicated for treatment of hypertension and severe tachycardia, as propranolol particularly can cause paradoxical hypertension.

Copper

Copper is used for pipes and roofing material, in alloys and as a pigment. Copper sulphate is used as a fungicide, an algicide and in some fertilizers. Approximately one-third of an ingested copper salt is absorbed and in the blood 80% is bound to caeruloplasmin. Most absorbed copper is deposited in the liver and eliminated mainly in bile.

Clinical features

Acute copper poisoning usually results from the ingestion of contaminated foods or from accidental or deliberate ingestion of copper salts. Copper sulphate is a common cause of poisoning in parts of India. Following substantial ingestion of a copper salt, there is profuse vomiting with abdominal pain, diarrhoea, headache, dizziness, and a metallic taste. Gastrointestinal haemorrhage, haemolysis, and hepatorenal failure may ensue and fatalities have occurred. Body secretions may have a green or blue discoloration.

Occupational exposure to copper fumes (during refining or welding) or to copper-containing dust causes 'metal-fume fever' with upper respiratory tract symptoms, headache, fever and myalgia. Chronic occupational copper exposure causes general malaise, anorexia, nausea, vomiting and hepatomegaly. Contact dermatitis, pulmonary granulomata and pulmonary fibrosis have also been described.

Treatment

Although vomiting occurs invariably following the ingestion of many copper salts, gastric lavage may be of value in reducing copper absorption if presentation is early. Blood copper concentrations correlate well with severity of intoxication, a concentration of < 3 mg/L indicating mild to moderate poisoning and a concentration in excess of 8 mg/L severe intoxication. D-penicillamine, *N*-acetylcysteine and DMPS (unithiol) enhance copper elimination.

FURTHER READING
Barceloux DG (1999) Copper. *Journal of Toxicology–Clinical Toxicology* **37**: 217–230.

Cyanide

Cyanide and its derivatives are used widely in industry. Hydrogen cyanide is also released during the thermal decomposition of polyurethane foams. Cyanide reversibly inhibits cytochrome oxidase a_3 so that cellular respiration ceases.

Clinical features

Inhalation of hydrogen cyanide gas produces symptoms within seconds and death within minutes. In contrast, the ingestion of a cyanide salt may not produce features for 1 hour. After exposure, initial symptoms are non-specific and include a feeling of constriction in the chest and dyspnoea. Coma, convulsions and metabolic acidosis may then supervene.

Treatment

Oxygen should be administered and, if available, dicobalt edetate 300 mg should be given i.v.; the dose may be repeated in severe cases. An alternative antidote is hydroxocobalamin 5 g i.v. (although this is not available in all countries at this dosage and is much more expensive) which may be repeated as necessary. If these two preferred antidotes are not available, sodium nitrite 300 mg i.v. and sodium thiosulphate 12.5 g i.v. should be administered.

Dicobalt edetate (and the free cobalt contained in the preparation) complexes free cyanide. Hydroxocobalamin and sodium thiosulphate enhance endogenous cyanide detoxification mechanisms. Sodium nitrite produces methaemoglobinaemia; methaemoglobin combines with cyanide to form cyanmethaemoglobin.

Digoxin

Toxicity occurring during chronic administration is common, though acute poisoning is infrequent.

Clinical features

These include nausea, vomiting, dizziness, anorexia and drowsiness. Rarely, confusion, visual disturbances and hallucinations occur. Sinus bradycardia is often marked and may be followed by supraventricular arrhythmias with or without heart block, ventricular premature beats and ventricular tachycardia. Hyperkalaemia occurs owing to the inhibition of the sodium/potassium-activated ATPase pump.

Treatment

Sinus bradycardia, atrioventricular block and sinoatrial standstill are often reduced or even abolished by atropine 0.6–2.4 mg i.v. If cardiac output is compromised, however, digoxin-specific antibody fragments 6–8 mg/kg bodyweight should be administered.

Ecstasy (3,4-methylenedioxy-methamfetamine, MDMA) (p. 1305)

Ecstasy is often taken in the setting of a rave where dancing is fast and prolonged. It is likely that the pharmacological effects of the drug (which are similar to those of the closely related amfetamines) are compounded by physical exertion, dehydration or over-hydration.

Clinical features

Mild abuse is characterized by agitation, tachycardia, hypertension, widely dilated pupils, trismus and sweating. In more severe cases, hyperthermia, disseminated intravascular coagulation, rhabdomyolysis, acute renal failure and hyponatraemia (secondary to inappropriate antidiuretic hormone secretion) predominate.

Treatment

Reassurance and rehydration are all that is required. If necessary, diazepam 5–10 mg i.v. should be given for severe agitation or convulsions. If hyperthermia is present, dantrolene 1 mg/kg bodyweight i.v. should be administered. Deaths occur from hyperpyrexia, renal and liver failure. Self-induced water intoxication also occurs.

Ethanol (see p. 262)

Ethanol is commonly ingested in beverages and deliberately with other substances in overdose. It is also present in many cosmetic and antiseptic preparations. Following absorption, ethanol is oxidized to acetaldehyde and then to acetate (Box 5.5, p. 262).

Clinical features

Ethanol is a CNS depressant and the features of ethanol intoxication are generally related to blood concentrations; they are shown in Table 22.15 (p. 1303). In children in particular, severe hypoglycaemia may accompany alcohol intoxication, owing to inhibition of gluconeogenesis. Hypoglycaemia is also observed in adults who are malnourished or who have fasted in the previous 24 hours. In severe cases of intoxication, coma and hypothermia are often present and lactic acidosis, ketoacidosis and acute renal failure have been reported.

Treatment

As ethanol-induced hypoglycaemia is not responsive to glucagon, intravenous glucose 25 g (50 mL of 50% dextrose) should be given. Haemodialysis should be considered if the blood ethanol concentration exceeds 5000 mg/L (32.5 mmol/L) and, particularly, if severe metabolic acidosis is present.

Ethylene glycol

Ethylene glycol is a common constituent of antifreeze fluid used in car radiators. Ethylene glycol itself is non-toxic but is metabolized to toxic products (Fig. 16.4).

Clinical features

Initially the features of ethylene glycol poisoning are similar to ethanol intoxication (though there is no ethanol

Fig. 16.4 **The metabolism of ethylene glycol.** ADH, alcohol dehydrogenase; ALDH, aldehyde dehydrogenase; LDH, lactate dehydrogenase; GLO, glycolic acid oxidase; AO aldehyde oxidase.

on the breath). Coma and convulsions follow and a variety of neurological abnormalities including nystagmus and ophthalmoplegias may be observed. Severe metabolic acidosis, hypocalcaemia and the presence of calcium oxalate crystalluria are well-recognized complications.

Treatment

Supportive measures to combat shock, hypocalcaemia, and metabolic acidosis should be instituted. Inhibitors of alcohol dehydrogenase (either ethanol or fomepizole) should be given to inhibit ethylene glycol metabolism (Fig. 16.4) and, secondly, haemodialysis should be employed to remove ethylene glycol, its aldehyde metabolites and glycolate. A loading dose of ethanol 50 g (conveniently given orally as 125 mL of gin, whisky or vodka) should be administered followed by an intravenous infusion of ethanol 10–12 g/h to produce blood ethanol concentrations of 500–1000 mg/L (11–22 mmol/L). The infusion is continued until ethylene glycol is no longer detectable in the blood. If haemodialysis is employed, the rate of ethanol administration will need to be increased to 17–22 g/h as ethanol is dialysable. Alternatively, fomepizole 15 mg/kg bodyweight can be administered over 30 minutes followed by four 12-hourly doses of 10 mg/kg until ethylene glycol concentrations are less than 200 mg/L. If dialysis is employed the frequency of fomepizole dosing should be increased to 4-hourly during dialysis because fomepizole is dialysable.

FURTHER READING
Barceloux DG, Krenzelok EP, Olson K, Watson W (1999) American Academy of Clinical Toxicology practice guidelines on the treatment of ethylene glycol poisoning. *Journal of Toxicology–Clinical Toxicology* 37: 537–560.

Gamma-hydroxybutyric acid (GHB)

Gamma-hydroxybutyric acid is a short-chain fatty acid that occurs naturally in mammalian brain where it is derived metabolically from gamma-aminobutyric acid (GABA), the primary inhibitory neurotransmitter in the brain. In the last 10 years GHB has emerged as a major recreational drug for body building, weight loss and for producing a 'high'. It has many street names, e.g. cherry meth, liquid X, and is taken as a colourless liquid dissolved in water. Several hundred deaths from GHB poisoning have been reported world-wide in recent years.

Clinical features

Poisoning with GHB is characterized by aggressive behaviour, ataxia, amnesia, vomiting, drowsiness, bradycardia, respiratory depression and apnoea, seizures and coma.

Management

In a patient who is breathing spontaneously, the management of GHB poisoning is primarily supportive with oxygen supplementation and the administration of atropine for persistent bradycardia, as necessary. Those who are severely poisoned will require mechanical ventilation, though recovery is usually complete within 6–8 hours.

Household products

The agents most commonly involved are bleach, cosmetics, toiletries, detergents, disinfectants and petroleum distillates such as paraffin and white spirit. Ingestion of household products is usually accidental and is most common among children less than 5 years of age. If the ingestion is accidental, adverse features very rarely occur except in the case of petroleum distillates where aspiration is a recognized complication because of their low surface tension.

Powder detergents, sterilizing tablets, denture-cleaning tablets and industrial bleaches (which contain high concentrations of sodium hypochlorite) are corrosive to the mouth and pharynx if ingested. Endotracheal intubation or tracheostomy may be required for life-threatening pharyngeal or laryngeal oedema. Gastric aspiration and lavage and dilution or neutralization of the alkali is contraindicated as it causes further damage and a risk of aspiration. Careful upper GI endoscopy is required to estimate the extent of injury. Oesophageal strictures occur.

Nail polish and nail polish remover contain acetone, which may produce coma if ingested in substantial quantities. Inhalation by small children of substantial quantities of talcum powder has occasionally given rise to severe pulmonary oedema and death.

Iron

Unless more than 60 mg of elemental iron per kg bodyweight is ingested (each ferrous sulphate tablet contains 60 mg of iron), adverse features are unlikely to develop. As a result, poisoning is seldom severe but deaths still occur. Iron salts have a direct corrosive effect on the upper gastrointestinal tract.

Clinical features

The initial features are characterized by nausea, vomiting (the vomit may be grey or black in colour), abdominal pain and diarrhoea. Most patients only suffer mild gastrointestinal symptoms. Severely poisoned patients develop haematemesis, hypotension, coma and shock at an early stage. A small minority deteriorate 12–48 hours after ingestion and develop shock, metabolic acidosis, acute renal tubular necrosis and hepatocellular necrosis. Rarely, up to 6 weeks after ingestion, intestinal strictures due to corrosive damage occur.

Treatment

Serum iron should be measured approximately 4 hours after ingestion. Desferrioxamine therapy is not required unless the concentration exceeds the predicted normal iron-binding capacity (> 5 mg/L, 90 μmol/L). If a patient develops coma or shock, desferrioxamine should be given without delay in a dose of 15 mg/kg/h i.v. (total amount of infusion not to exceed 80 mg/kg in 24 hours). If the recommended rate of administration is exceeded, or the therapy is continued for several days, adverse effects including pulmonary oedema have been reported.

FURTHER READING
Tenenbein M (1996) Benefits of parenteral deferoxamine for acute iron poisoning. *Journal of Toxicology–Clinical Toxicology* **34**:485–489.

Lead

Exposure to lead occurs occupationally and the current practice in many countries is to recommend that workers over 18 years of age should cease working with lead when their blood lead concentration is above 600 µg/L (2.9 µmol/L), or 300 µg/L (1.45 µmol/L) for a woman of reproductive capacity, or 500 µg/L (2.4 µmol/L) for all employees aged under 18 years. Children who chew on lead-painted items in their homes (pica) may develop lead poisoning. The use of lead-containing cosmetics or 'drugs' has also resulted in lead poisoning.

Clinical features

Even relatively low blood lead concentrations are of concern in children below the age of 5 years. Each increase of 100 µg/L in lifetime average blood lead concentration is associated with a 4.6 point decrease in IQ. Mild lead intoxication may result in no more than lethargy and occasional abdominal discomfort, though abdominal pain, vomiting, constipation and encephalopathy (seizures, delirium, coma) develop in more severe cases. Encephalopathy is more common in children than in adults but is now rare in the developed world. Renal effects include reversible tubular dysfunction and irreversible renal insufficiency leading to hypertension. Typically, though very rarely, lead poisoning results in foot drop attributable to peripheral motor neuropathy. A bluish discoloration of the gum margins owing to the deposition of lead sulphide is observed occasionally.

The characteristic haematological features include:

- *sideroblastic anaemia,* due to inhibition by lead of several enzymes involved in haem synthesis, including ALA synthetase
- *haemolysis,* which is usually mild, resulting from damage to the red cell membrane
- *punctate basophilia* (or basophilic stippling: the blood film shows red cells with small, round, blue particles), due to aggregates of RNA in red cells owing to inhibition by lead of pyrimidine-5-nucleotidase, which normally disperses residual RNA to produce a diffuse blue staining seen in reticulocytes on blood films (polychromasia).

Treatment

Children and adults, after treatment, must not be returned to their previous environment (and lead exposure).

The decision to use chelation therapy is based not only on the blood lead concentration but on the presence of symptoms. Although sodium calcium edetate 75 mg/kg bodyweight per day for 5 days is probably more efficient in increasing lead excretion than oral dimercaptosuccinic acid (DMSA) 30 mg/kg bodyweight for 5 days, it has to be given intravenously and may result in increased uptake of lead into the brain and zinc depletion. Oral DMSA, if available, is therefore preferred. However, DMSA did not improve scores on tests of cognition, behaviour and neuropsychological function in children with blood lead concentrations of less than 450 µg/L.

FURTHER READING
Canfield RL et al. (2003) Intellectual impairment in children with blood lead concentrations below 10 µg per deciliter. *New England Journal of Medicine* **348**: 1517–1526.

Lithium (see p. 1295)

Lithium toxicity is usually the result of therapeutic over-dose (chronic toxicity) rather than deliberate self-poisoning (acute toxicity).

Chronic toxicity is usually associated with serum concentrations above 1.5 mmol/L (10.4 mg/L). Acute massive overdose may produce concentrations of 5 mmol/L (34.7 mg/L) without causing toxic features (see p. 1296).

Treatment

Forced diuresis with sodium chloride 0.9% is effective in increasing elimination of lithium, though haemodialysis is far superior and should be undertaken particularly if neurological features are present, if renal function is impaired and if chronic toxicity or acute on chronic toxicity are the modes of presentation.

Mercury

Metallic mercury is very volatile and when spilled has a large surface area so that high atmospheric concentrations may be produced in enclosed spaces, particularly when environmental temperatures are high. Thus, great care should be taken in clearing up a spillage of mercury if a thermometer or sphygmomanometer is broken. If ingested, metallic mercury will usually be eliminated per rectum, though small amounts may be found in the appendix. Mercury salts are well absorbed following ingestion as are organometallic compounds where mercury is covalently bound to carbon.

Clinical features

Inhalation of acute mercury vapour causes headache, nausea, vomiting, cough, chest pain, breathlessness and chemical pneumonitis. Proteinuria and nephrotic syndrome are observed rarely. In addition, a fine tremor and neurobehavioural impairment occur and peripheral nerve involvement has also been observed. Ingestion of inorganic and organic mercury compounds causes an irritant gastroenteritis with corrosive ulceration, bloody diarrhoea and abdominal cramps and may lead to circulatory collapse and shock.

Mercurous compounds are less corrosive and toxic than mercuric salts.

Treatment

DMPS (dimercaptopropanesulphonate) is the antidote of choice and is given orally in a dose of 30 mg/kg per day. At least 5 days' treatment is usually required.

FURTHER READING
Clarkson TW, Magos L, Myers GJ (2003) The toxicology of mercury – current exposures and clinical manifestations. *New England Journal of Medicine* **349**: 1731–1737.

Methanol

Methanol is used widely as a solvent and is found in antifreeze solutions. Methanol is metabolized to formaldehyde and formate (Fig. 16.5). The concentration of formate increases greatly and is accompanied by accumulation of hydrogen ions causing metabolic acidosis.

Clinical features

Methanol causes inebriation and drowsiness. After a latent period coma supervenes. Blurred vision and diminished visual acuity occur. The presence of dilated pupils that are unreactive to light suggests that permanent blindness is likely to ensue. A severe metabolic acidosis may develop and be accompanied by hyperglycaemia and a raised serum amylase activity. A blood methanol concentration of 500 mg/L (15.63 mmol/L) confirms serious poisoning. The mortality correlates well with the severity and duration of metabolic acidosis. Survivors may show permanent neurological sequelae including parkinsonian-like signs as well as blindness.

Treatment

Treatment involves the correction of metabolic acidosis, the inhibition of methanol metabolism by the administration of ethanol or fomepizole and the use of haemodialysis to remove methanol and formate and to correct severe metabolic abnormalities. Either of these components is given as described under ethylene glycol poisoning

(p. 1013) until methanol is no longer detectable in the blood.

Folinic acid 30 mg i.v. 6-hourly may protect against ocular toxicity by accelerating formate metabolism.

FURTHER READING
Barceloux DG et al. (2002) American Academy of Clinical Toxicology practice guidelines on the treatment of methanol poisoning. *Journal of Toxicology–Clinical Toxicology* **40**: 415–446.

Monoamine oxidase inhibitors

These are used less frequently in the treatment of depression because of the dangers of dietary and drug interactions. Moclobemide, which acts by reversible inhibition of monoamine oxidase type A (known as a RIMA), is less toxic in overdose.

Clinical features

Features after overdose may be delayed for 12–24 hours. They include excitement, restlessness, hyperpyrexia, hyperreflexia, convulsions, opisthotonos, rhabdomyolysis and coma. Sinus tachycardia and either hypo- or hypertension are also observed.

Treatment

Treatment is supportive with the control of convulsions and the marked excitement; diazepam 10–20 mg i.v. in an adult should be given as necessary and repeated. Dantrolene 1 mg/kg i.v. should be administered if hyperpyrexia develops. Hypotension should be treated with plasma expansion, and hypertension by the administration of a β-adrenoceptor blocker such as chlorpromazine.

Nerve agents

Nerve agents are related chemically to organophosphorus insecticides and have a similar mechanism of toxicity, but a much higher mammalian acute toxicity, particularly via the dermal route. Two classes of nerve agent are recognized: G agents (G allegedly stands for Germany where the early agents were first synthesized) and V agents (V allegedly stands for venomous). G agents include tabun, sarin, soman and cyclosarin. The V agents were introduced later, e.g. VX, and were used by Iraq against that country's own Kurdish population. The nerve agent, sarin, was also employed in two terrorist attacks in Japan in 1994 and 1995. The G agents are both dermal and respiratory hazards, whereas the V agents, unless aerosolized, are contact poisons. Agents used in bioterrorism are described on page 1031.

Clinical features

Systemic poisoning may follow inhalation, ingestion or dermal exposure, though the onset of systemic toxicity is slower by the dermal route.

Systemic features include increased salivation and rhinorrhoea; miosis and eye pain; abdominal pain,

Fig. 16.5 **The metabolism of methanol.** ADH, alcohol dehydrogenase; FDH, formaldehyde dehydrogenase.

nausea, vomiting and diarrhoea; involuntary micturition and defecation; muscle weakness and fasciculation, tremor, restlessness, ataxia and convulsions. Bradycardia, tachycardia and hypotension may occur, dependent on whether muscarinic or nicotinic effects predominate. Death occurs from respiratory failure within minutes but mild or moderately exposed individuals usually recover completely. EEG abnormalities, however, have been reported in those severely exposed to sarin in Japan.

Treatment

The release of a nerve agent among a civilian population requires the deployment of special measures and personnel to ensure the rescue of casualties and the rapid administration of atropine and an oxime, such as pralidoxime. The parenteral administration of atropine to patients presenting with rhinorrhoea and bronchorrhoea may be life-saving. Alternatively, an infusion of pralidoxime can be given. Intravenous diazepam (adult 10–20 mg; child 1–5 mg) is useful in controlling apprehension, agitation, fasciculation and convulsions; the dose may be repeated as required.

Non-steroidal anti-inflammatory agents (NSAIDs)

Self-poisoning with NSAIDs has increased, as several are now widely available.

Clinical features

In most cases minor gastrointestinal disturbance is the only feature but, in more severe cases, coma, convulsions, metabolic acidosis and renal failure have occurred. Poisoning with mefenamic acid commonly results in convulsions, though these are usually short-lived.

Treatment

Treatment is symptomatic and supportive.

Opiates and opioids

Clinical features

Cardinal signs of opiate poisoning are pinpoint pupils, reduced respiratory rate and coma. Hypothermia, hypoglycaemia and convulsions are occasionally observed in severe cases. In severe heroin overdose, non-cardiogenic pulmonary oedema (ARDS) has been reported.

Treatment

Naloxone 0.8–1.2 mg i.v. in an adult (5–10 µg per kg bodyweight in a child) will reverse severe respiratory depression and coma at least partially. In severe poisoning, larger initial doses or repeat doses will be required, as the duration of action of naloxone is often less than that of the drug taken in overdose, e.g. methadone, which has a very long half-life. For this reason an infusion of naloxone may be required. Non-cardiogenic pulmonary oedema should be treated with mechanical ventilation.

Management of the 'body packer'

'Body-packing' is the practice of smuggling drugs in small packets (condoms, foil and cellophane are commonly used) that are swallowed for later retrieval from vomit or faeces, or are inserted into the vagina or rectum. Acute intestinal obstruction may result, and overdose is a hazard if a packet bursts.

Suspected individuals should have abdominal radiography (preferably CT of the abdomen) and a urine screen for drugs. Screens should be repeated daily, or immediately if the patient develops features of intoxication, in case the package is leaking, to confirm the diagnosis.

Packets in the stomach should not be removed by endoscopy or by inducing emesis, as these are potentially dangerous. Packets in the vagina can usually be removed manually. With packets in the small bowel (if there is no clinical, analytical or radiological evidence to support leakage), sorbitol or lactulose to encourage transit through the gut is appropriate. Alternatively, for faster results, whole-bowel irrigation using polyethylene glycol electrolyte solutions can be used. Liquid paraffin should not be used because it can weaken the rubber, leading to bursting of the packets. Activated charcoal is contradicted as it induces constipation when used in substantial doses. Packets in the colon or rectum are probably best managed by giving sorbitol or lactulose and allowing them to pass spontaneously, with least risk of rupture.

Immediate surgery is indicated if acute intestinal obstruction develops, or when packets can be seen radiologically and there is radiological, clinical or analytical evidence to suggest leakage, particularly if the drug involved is a CNS stimulant (e.g. cocaine).

Organophosphorus insecticides

Organophosphorus (OP) insecticides are used widely throughout the world and are a major cause of death in the developing world e.g. rural Bangladesh. Organophosphorus insecticides inhibit acetylcholinesterase, causing accumulation of acetylcholine at central and peripheral cholinergic nerve endings, including neuromuscular junctions.

Clinical features

Poisoning may follow ingestion, inhalation or dermal absorption. As many OP insecticides require biotransformation before becoming active, the features of intoxication are delayed. Poisoning is characterized by anxiety, restlessness, tiredness, headache, and muscarinic features such as nausea, vomiting, abdominal colic, diarrhoea, tenesmus, sweating, rhinorrhoea, bronchorrhoea, and chest tightness. Miosis may be present. Nicotinic effects include muscle fasciculation and flaccid paresis of limb, respiratory, and, occasionally, extraocular muscles. Respiratory failure will ensue in severe cases and is exacerbated by the development of bronchorrhoea and pulmonary oedema. Coma and convulsions occur in severe poisoning. Diagnosis is confirmed by measuring the erythrocyte cholinesterase activity; plasma cholinesterase activity is less specific but may also be depressed.

Treatment

Mild cases require no specific treatment other then the removal of soiled clothing; contaminated skin should be washed with soap and water to prevent further absorption. In patients presenting with systemic features, atropine 0.6–2 mg i.v. should be given to reduce bronchorrhoea and rhinorrhoea, together with an oxime, such as pralidoxime, which reactivates phosphorylated acetylcholinesterase. Pralidoxime may either be administered by slow i.v. injection (30 mg/kg every 4–6 hours) or as an infusion (8–10 mg/kg/h).

Paracetamol (acetaminophen)

Paracetamol is the most common form of poisoning encountered in the UK (48% of all overdoses, cf. USA 7%).

Mechanism of toxicity

In therapeutic dose, paracetamol is conjugated with glucuronide and sulphate. A small amount of paracetamol is metabolized by mixed function oxidase enzymes to form a highly reactive compound (*N*-acetyl-*p*-benzoquinoneimine, NAPQI), which is then immediately conjugated with glutathione and subsequently excreted as cysteine and mercapturic conjugates. In overdose, large amounts of paracetamol are metabolized by oxidation because of saturation of the sulphate conjugation pathway. Liver glutathione stores become depleted so that the liver is unable to deactivate the toxic metabolite (NAPQI). Paracetamol-induced renal damage probably results from a mechanism similar to that which is responsible for hepatotoxicity.

The severity of paracetamol poisoning is dose-related. There is, however, some variation in individual susceptibility to paracetamol-induced hepatotoxicity. Patients with pre-existing liver disease, those with a high alcohol intake and poor nutrition, those receiving enzyme-inducing drugs, those suffering from anorexia nervosa and other eating disorders and HIV infection are at greater risk and are given treatment at lower plasma paracetamol concentrations (Fig. 16.6).

Clinical features

After an overdose of paracetamol, patients usually remain asymptomatic for the first 24 hours or, at the most, develop anorexia, nausea and vomiting. Liver damage is not usually detectable by routine liver function tests until at least 18 hours after ingestion of the drug. Liver damage usually reaches a peak, as assessed by measurement of aminotransferase (ALT/AST) activity and prothrombin time (INR), at 72–96 hours after ingestion. Without treatment, a small percentage of patients will develop fulminant hepatic failure. Renal failure due to acute tubular necrosis occurs in 25% of patients with severe hepatic damage and in a few without evidence of serious disturbance of liver function.

Treatment

N-acetylcysteine (NAC) is an effective protective agent provided it is administered within 8–10 hours of

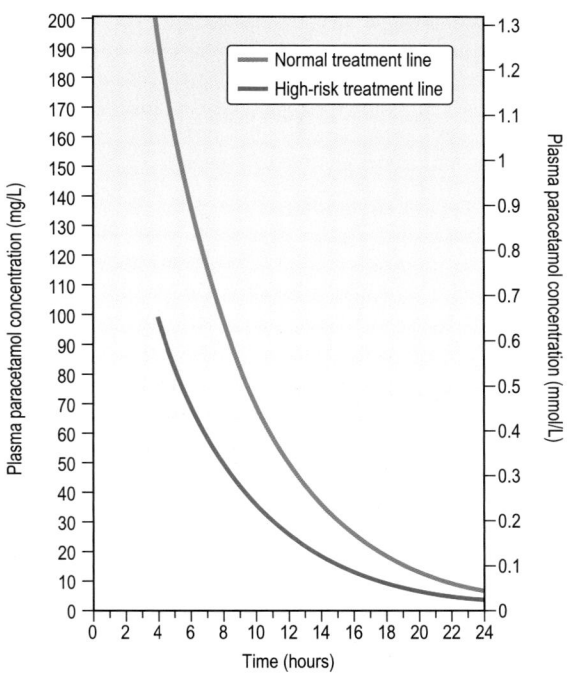

Fig. 16.6 Nomogram of paracetamol. From *British National Formulary* (1998) with permission. For definition of 'High-risk patients', see text.

ingestion of the overdose. It acts by replenishing cellular glutathione stores and may also repair oxidation damage caused by NAPQI. As oral NAC induces vomiting (as does paracetamol ingestion), the intravenous route is preferred. The main treatment regimens used internationally are shown in Box 16.5. Some 5% of patients treated with intravenous NAC develop rash, *angio-*

> ### Box 16.5 Antidote regimens for paracetamol poisoning
>
> **N-acetylcysteine (intravenously in 5% glucose)**
> 150 mg/kg in 200 mL over 15 min, then 50 mg/kg in 500 mL over the next 4 hours and 100 mg/kg in 1000 mL of 5% glucose over the ensuing 16 hours.
>
> Total dose: 300 mg/kg over 20.15 hours
>
> *Note*: A 48-hour regimen is used in some US centres: Patients receive a loading dose of 140 mg/kg, followed by 70 mg/kg every 4 hours for 12 doses, all infused over 1 hour.
>
> **N-acetylcysteine (orally)**
> 140 mg/kg initially, then 60 mg/kg every 4 hours for 17 additional doses.
>
> Total dose: 1330 mg/kg over 72 hours.
>
> **Methionine**
> Oral 2.5 g followed by three similar doses every 4 hours if unable to give *N*-acetylcysteine.

oedema, hypotension and bronchospasm. These adverse effects, which are related to the initial bolus, are seldom serious and discontinuing the infusion is usually all that is required. In more severe cases, chlorphenamine 10–20 mg i.v. in an adult is given.

The overall treatment strategy is to:

- Admit the patient to hospital.
- Take blood for urgent estimation of the plasma paracetamol concentration as soon as 4 hours or more have elapsed since ingestion. Check INR, plasma creatinine and ALT.
- Assess whether the patient is at increased risk of liver damage.
- Give treatment (below) if needed (Fig. 16.6).

The treatment protocol is dependent on the time of presentation.

< 8 hours after ingestion

- If the plasma paracetamol concentration is not available within 8 hours of the overdose and, if 10–15 g or > 150 mg/kg paracetamol has been ingested, treatment should be started at once and stopped if the plasma paracetamol concentration subsequently indicates that treatment is not required.
- Check INR, plasma creatinine and ALT on the completion of treatment and before discharge.

8–15 hours after ingestion

- Urgent action is required because the efficacy of treatment declines progressively from 8 hours after overdose. If > 150 mg/kg paracetamol has been ingested, start treatment immediately.
- In patients already receiving treatment, only discontinue if the plasma paracetamol concentration is below the relevant treatment line (Fig. 16.6) and there is no abnormality of the INR, plasma creatinine or ALT and the patient is asymptomatic. Do not discontinue the infusion if there is any doubt as to the timing of the overdose.
- At the end of treatment, measure INR, plasma creatinine and ALT. If any test is abnormal or the patient is symptomatic, further monitoring is required and expert advice should be sought.
- Patients with normal INR, plasma creatinine and ALT and who are asymptomatic may be discharged.

15–24 hours after ingestion

- Urgent action is required because the efficacy of treatment is limited more than 15 hours after overdose. Start treatment immediately if > 150 mg/kg paracetamol has been ingested.
- The prognostic accuracy of the '200 mg/L line' after 15 hours is uncertain but a plasma paracetamol concentration above the extended treatment line should be regarded as carrying serious risk of severe liver damage.
- At the end of treatment, check INR, plasma creatinine and ALT. If any test is abnormal or the patient is symptomatic, further monitoring is required and expert advice should be sought.

- If liver or renal failure ensues, this should be treated conventionally though there is evidence that a continuing infusion of NAC (continue 16-hour infusion until recovery) will improve the morbidity and mortality. Liver transplantation has been performed successfully in patients with paracetamol-induced fulminant hepatic failure (p. 368).

> **FURTHER READING**
> Vale JA, Proudfoot AT (1995) Paracetamol (acetaminophen) poisoning. *Lancet* **346**: 547–552.

Paraquat

Poisoning with paraquat is very uncommon in the UK but is a common cause of morbidity and mortality in the developing world.

Clinical features

Following ingestion, ulcers in the mouth and oesophagus develop, accompanied by vomiting and diarrhoea, which are induced by paraquat and partly by the co-formulants. In severe cases of poisoning multiple organ failure develops. The prognosis may be determined by measurement of the plasma paraquat concentration.

Treatment

Treatment is supportive.

Phenothiazines

Phenothiazines have varying antimuscarinic, extrapyramidal and sedative effects.

Clinical features

In overdose, impairment of consciousness, hypotension and respiratory depression develop. These effects are less likely to be observed in those who are taking the drug therapeutically.

Treatment

Benzatropine 2 mg i.v. in an adult is occasionally required for the treatment of dyskinesia and oculogyric crisis.

Quinine

Quinine poisoning is relatively common in some countries because of its use for the treatment of leg cramps. It is also ingested in overdose in the developing world where it is employed as an antimalarial.

Clinical features

In addition to the development of tinnitus and deafness, a substantial number of patients develop oculotoxicity including blindness which may be irreversible. Ventricular arrhythmias, convulsions and coma are observed in severe cases.

Treatment

Treatment is supportive. There is evidence that multiple-dose activated charcoal increases quinine elimination (see p. 1007).

Selective serotonin reuptake inhibitors (SSRIs)

Citalopram, fluoxetine, fluvoxamine, paroxetine and sertraline are antidepressants that inhibit serotonin reuptake; venlafaxine additionally inhibits norepinephrine (noradrenaline) reuptake. They lack the antimuscarinic actions of tricyclic antidepressants.

Clinical features

Even large overdoses appear to be relatively safe, unless potentiated by ethanol, though there is some evidence that venlafaxine is more toxic than other SSRIs. Most patients will show no signs of toxicity but drowsiness, nausea, diarrhoea, and sinus tachycardia have been reported. Rarely, junctional bradycardia, seizures, and hypertension have been encountered and influenza-like symptoms may develop.

Treatment

Supportive measures are all that are required.

Theophylline

Poisoning may complicate therapeutic use as well as being the result of deliberate self-poisoning. If a slow-release preparation is involved, peak plasma concentrations may not be attained until 6–12 hours after overdosage and the onset of toxic features is correspondingly delayed.

Clinical features

Nausea, vomiting, hyperventilation, haematemesis, abdominal pain, diarrhoea, sinus tachycardia, supra-ventricular and ventricular arrhythmias, hypotension, restlessness, irritability, headache, hyperreflexia, tremors, and convulsions have been observed. Hypokalaemia probably results from activation of Na^+/K^+-ATPase. A mixed acid–base disturbance is common. Most symptomatic patients have plasma theophylline concentrations in excess of 25 mg/L (430 µmol/L). Convulsions are seen more commonly when concentrations are > 50 mg/L (> 860 µmol/L). Plasma potassium concentrations of < 2.6 mmol/L, acidaemia, hypotension, seizures and arrhythmias are indicators of severe poisoning.

Treatment

There is good evidence that multiple-dose activated charcoal enhances the elimination of theophylline (p. 1007). However, protracted theophylline-induced vomiting may mitigate the benefit of this therapy, unless vomiting is suppressed by ondansetron 8 mg i.v. in an adult. Correction of hypokalaemia to prevent or treat tachyarrhythmias is of great importance. A non-selective β-adrenoceptor blocking drug, such as propranolol, is also useful in the treatment of tachyarrhythmias secondary to hypokalaemia but should only be given to those

without a history of respiratory disease. Convulsions should be treated with diazepam 10–20 mg i.v. in an adult.

FURTHER READING
Shannon M (1999) Life-threatening events after theophylline overdose – a 10-year prospective analysis. *Archives of Internal Medicine* **159**: 989–994.

Tricyclic antidepressants

Tricyclic antidepressants block the reuptake of norepinephrine (noradrenaline) into peripheral and intra-cerebral neurones, thereby increasing the concentration of monoamines in these areas. These drugs also have anti-muscarinic actions and class 1 antiarrhythmic (quinidine-like) activity.

Clinical features

Features of poisoning usually appear within 1 hour after ingestion. Drowsiness, sinus tachycardia, dry mouth, dilated pupils, urinary retention, increased reflexes, and extensor plantar responses are the most common features of mild poisoning. Severe intoxication leads to coma, often with divergent strabismus and convulsions. Plantar, oculocephalic, and oculovestibular reflexes may be temporarily abolished. An ECG will often show a wide QRS interval and there is a reasonable correlation between the width of the QRS complex and the severity of poisoning. Metabolic acidosis and cardiorespiratory depression are observed in severe cases.

Treatment

The majority of patients recover with supportive therapy alone though a small percentage of patients will require mechanical ventilation for 24–48 hours. The onset of supraventricular tachycardia and ventricular tachycardia should be treated with sodium bicarbonate (8.4%) 50 mmol (50 mL) intravenously over 20 minutes, even if there is no acidosis present. In addition, adequate oxygenation, control of convulsions and correction of acidosis should be undertaken. If ventricular tachycardia is compromising cardiac output, lidocaine 50–100 mg i.v. should be administered.

FURTHER READING
Kerr GW, McGuffie AC, Wilkie S (2001) Tricyclic antidepressant overdose: a review. *Emergency Medicine Journal* **18**: 236–241.

Volatile substance abuse (p. 1305)

Volatile substances are either 'bagged' (sprayed into a plastic bag and then inhaled until the subject passes out) or 'huffed' (sprayed on to a cloth held to the mouth). Volatile substances abused in this way include organic solvents, hydrocarbon mixtures such as petrol, and aerosol propellants. Glues (containing toluene) are most often sniffed from a plastic bag, and repeated abuse in this manner leads to the development of erythematous spots around the mouth and nose ('glue-sniffer's rash').

Clinical features

The clinical features are similar to those of alcohol intoxication with initial CNS stimulation followed by depression. Thus, euphoria, blurring of vision, tinnitus, slurring of speech, ataxia, feelings of omnipotence, impaired judgement, irritability and excitement are observed commonly. Convulsions and coma, which is usually short-lived, may occur. Some chronic abusers report psychotic symptoms, listlessness and anorexia. Chronic abuse of toluene-containing glues has also resulted in muscle weakness, gastrointestinal complaints (abdominal pain and haematemesis) and neuropsychiatric disorders (altered mental status, cerebellar abnormalities, polyneuropathy). In addition, hypokalaemia, hypophosphataemia and hyperchloraemia have been reported. Rhabdomyolysis occurs in a substantial minority of these patients.

MARINE ANIMALS

Ciguatera fish poisoning

Over 400 fish species have been reported as ciguatoxic (*Cigua* is Spanish for poisonous snail), though barracuda, red snapper, amberjack and grouper are most commonly implicated. Ciguatera fish contain ciguatoxin, maitotoxin and scaritoxin, which are lipid-soluble, heat-stable compounds that are derived from ingested dinoflagellates such as *Gambierdiscus toxicus*. The mechanisms of toxicity in man appear to involve more than just inhibition of acetylcholinesterase activity, which has been found in vitro.

Clinical features

The onset of symptoms may occur from a few minutes to 30 hours after ingestion of toxic fish. Typically, features appear between 1 and 6 hours and include abdominal cramps, nausea, vomiting and watery diarrhoea. In some cases, numbness and paraesthesiae of the lips, tongue and throat occur. Other features described include malaise, dry mouth, metallic taste, myalgia, arthralgia, blurred vision, photophobia and transient blindness. In more severe cases, hypotension, cranial nerve palsies and respiratory paralysis have been reported. The mortality in severe cases may be as high as 12%. Recovery takes from 48 hours to 1 week in the mild form and from 1 to several weeks in the severe form.

Treatment

Treatment is symptomatic, although atropine has occasionally lessened some of the cardiovascular and gastrointestinal manifestations. Gabapentin may be useful in lessening persistent paraethesiae.

Jelly fish

Most of the jelly fish found in North European coastal waters are non-toxic as their stings cannot penetrate human skin. A notable exception is the 'Portuguese man-o'-war' (*Physalia physalis*), whose sting contains a toxic peptide, phospholipase A, and a histamine-liberating factor.

Clinical features

Local pain occurs followed by myalgia, nausea, griping abdominal pain, dyspnoea and even death.

Treatment

Adhesive tape may be used to remove any tentacles still adherent to the bather. Local analgesia and antihistamine creams provide symptomatic relief.

Paralytic shell fish poisoning

This is uncommon and is caused by bivalve molluscs being contaminated with neurotoxins, including saxitoxin, produced by the toxic dinoflagellates, *Gonyaulax catenella* and *Gonyaulax tamarensis*.

Clinical features

Symptoms develop within 30 minutes of ingestion. The illness is characterized by paraesthesiae of the mouth, lips, face and extremities and is often accompanied by nausea, vomiting and diarrhoea. In more severe cases, dysphonia, dysphagia, muscle weakness, paralysis, ataxia and respiratory depression occur.

Treatment

Treatment is symptomatic and supportive.

Scrombrotoxic fish poisoning

This is due to the action of bacteria such as *Proteus morgani* and *Klebsiella pneumoniae* in decomposing the flesh of fish such as tuna, mackerel, bonito and skipjack if the fish are stored at insufficiently low temperatures. The spoiled fish can contain excessively high concentrations of histamine (muscle histidine is broken down by the bacteria to histamine), though the precise role of histamine in the pathogenesis of the clinical syndrome is uncertain.

Clinical features

The mean incubation period is 30 minutes. The illness is characterized by flushing, headache, sweating, dizziness, burning of the mouth and throat, abdominal cramps, nausea, vomiting and diarrhoea and is usually short-lived; the mean duration is 4 hours.

Treatment

Treatment is symptomatic and supportive. Antihistamines may alleviate the symptoms.

Stings from marine animals

Several species of fish have venomous spines in their fins. These include the weaver fish, short-spine cottus, spiny dogfish and the stingray. Bathers and fishermen may be stung if they tread on or handle these species.

Clinical features

The immediate result of a sting is intense local pain, swelling, bruising, blistering, necrosis and, if the poisoned spine is not removed, chronic sepsis (though this is uncommon). Occasionally, systemic symptoms including vomiting, diarrhoea, hypotension and tachycardia occur.

Treatment

Immersing the affected part in hot water may relieve local symptoms as this denatures the thermolabile toxin.

> **FURTHER READING**
> Currie BJ (2003) Marine antivenoms. *Journal of Toxicology–Clinical Toxicology* **41**: 301–308.
> White J et al. (2003) Clinical toxicology – where are we now? *Journal of Toxicology–Clinical Toxicology* **41**: 263–276.

VENOMOUS ANIMALS

Insect stings and bites

Clinical features

Insect stings from wasps and bees and bites from ants produce pain and swelling at the puncture site. Following the sting or bite, patients should be observed for 2 hours for any signs of evolving urticaria, pruritus, bronchospasm or oropharyngeal oedema.

Treatment

The onset of anaphylaxis requires urgent treatment (see p. 997). Prophylactic immunotherapy has been demonstrated to be of value.

Scorpions

Scorpion stings are a serious problem in North Africa, the Middle East and the Americas. Scorpion venoms stimulate the release of acetylcholine and catecholamines causing both cholinergic and adrenergic symptoms.

Clinical features

Severe pain occurs immediately at the site of puncture, followed by swelling. Signs of systemic involvement, which may be delayed for 24 hours, include vomiting, sweating, piloerection, abdominal colic, diarrhoea. In some cases, depending on the species, shock, respiratory depression and pulmonary oedema may develop.

Treatment

Local infiltration with anaesthetic or a ring block will usually alleviate local pain, though systemic analgesia may be required. Specific antivenom, if available, should be administered as soon possible.

Spiders

The black widow spider (*Latrodectus mactans*) is found in North America and the tropics and occasionally in Mediterranean countries.

Clinical features

The bite quickly becomes painful, and generalized muscle pain, sweating, headache and shock may occur.

Treatment

No systemic treatment is required except in cases of severe systemic toxicity, when specific antivenom should be given, if this is available.

> **FURTHER READING**
> Brown SGA et al. (2003) Ant venom immunotherapy: a double-blind, placebo-controlled, crossover trial. *Lancet* **361**: 1001–1006.

Venomous snakes

Approximately 15% of the 3000 species of snake found worldwide are considered to be dangerous to humans. Snake bite is common in some tropical countries. For example, in Sri Lanka there are some 6 bites per 100 000 population and 900 deaths per year. In Nigeria there are some 500 bites per 100 000 population with a 12% mortality. In Myanmar there are 15 deaths per 100 000 population from snake bites. In the USA (population 250 million) there are some 45 000 bites per year (8000 by venomous species) with some 6 deaths annually. In the UK (population 50 million) approximately 100 people are admitted to hospital annually but no deaths have occurred since 1970. In Australia there are 2–3 deaths annually.

There are three main groups of venomous snakes, representing some 200 species, which have in their upper jaws a pair of enlarged teeth (fangs) that inject venom into the tissues of their victim. These are Viperidae (with two subgroups: Viperinae – European adders and Russell's vipers; and Crotalinae – American rattlesnakes, moccasins, lanceheaded vipers and Asian pit vipers), Elapidae (cobras, kraits, mambas, coral snakes, Australian venomous snakes), and Hydrophiidae (sea snakes). In addition, some members of the family Colubridae are mildly venomous (mongoose snake).

Clinical features

Viperidae

Russell's viper causes most of the snake-bite mortality in India, Pakistan and Burma. There is local swelling at the site of the bite (Fig. 16.7) which may become massive. Local tissue necrosis may occur, particularly with cobra bites. Evidence of systemic involvement occurs within 30 minutes, including vomiting, evidence of shock and hypotension. Haemorrhage due to incoagulable blood can be fatal.

Fig. 16.7 Snake bite showing swelling at site.

Elapidae

There is not usually any swelling at the site of the bite, except with Asian cobras and African spitting cobras – here the bite is painful and is followed by local tissue necrosis. Vomiting occurs first followed by shock and then neurological symptoms and muscle weakness, with paralysis of the respiratory muscles in severe cases. Cardiac muscle can be involved.

Hydrophiidae

Systemic features are muscle involvement, myalgia and myoglobinuria, which can lead to acute renal failure. Cardiac and respiratory paralysis may occur.

Management

As a first aid measure, a firm pressure bandage should be placed over the bite and the limb immobilized. This may delay the spread of the venom. Arterial tourniquets should *not* be used, and incision or excision of the bite area should not be performed. Local wounds often require little treatment. If necrosis is present, antibiotics should be given. Skin grafting may be required later. Antitetanus prophylaxis must be given. The type of snake should be identified if possible.

In about 50% of cases no venom has been injected by the bite. Nevertheless, careful observation for 12–24 hours is necessary in case systemic features (envenomation) develop. General supportive measures should be given, as necessary. These include intravenous fluids with volume expanders for hypotension and diazepam for anxiety. Treatment of acute respiratory, cardiac and renal failure is instituted as necessary.

Antivenoms are not generally indicated unless envenomation is present, as they can cause severe allergic reactions. Antivenoms can rapidly neutralize venom, but only if an amount in excess of the amount of venom is given. Large quantities of antivenom may be required. As antivenoms cannot reverse the effects of the venom, they must be given early to minimize some of the local effects and may prevent necrosis at the site of the bite. Antivenoms should be administered intravenously by slow infusion, the same dose being given to children and adults.

Allergic reactions are frequent, and epinephrine (adrenaline) (1 in 1000 solution) should be available. In severe cases, the antivenom infusion should be continued even if an allergic reaction occurs, with subcutaneous injections of epinephrine being given as necessary.

Some forms of neurotoxicity, such as those induced by the death adder, respond to anticholinesterase therapy with neostigmine and atropine.

FURTHER READING

Gold BS, Dart RC, Barish RA (2002) Bites of venomous snakes. *New England Journal of Medicine* **347**: 347–356.

Theakston RDG, Warrell DA (1991) Antivenoms: a list of hyperimmune sera currently available for the treatment of envenoming by bites and stings. *Toxicon* **29**: 1419–1470.

Warrell DA (ed.) (1999) WHO/SEARO Guidelines for the clinical management of snake bites in the South-East Asian Region. *South East Asian Journal of Tropical Medicine and Public Health* **30** (Suppl. 1): 1–86.

PLANTS

Many plants are known to be poisonous, but it is unusual for severe poisoning to occur in practice. In some regions of the world, however, plant poisonings cause substantial morbidity and mortality. While deaths do occur after unintentional poisoning with plants such as *Atractylis gummifera* (bird-lime or blue thistle) and *Blighia sapida* (ackee tree), the majority of deaths globally occur following intentional self-poisoning with plants such as *Thevetia peruviana* (yellow oleander).

Cicuta species

Cicuta spp. (water hemlock) and the related genus *Oenanthe* contain cicutoxin, a potent central nervous system (CNS) stimulant that produces violent seizure activity. The CNS effects of cicutoxin are similar to those of picrotoxin, a known inhibitor of GABA. Severe gastrointestinal symptoms, diaphoresis, salivation and skeletal muscle stimulation may precede the seizure activity.

Conium maculatum

Conium maculatum (poison hemlock) contains a variety of volatile pyridine alkaloids, including coniine, *N*-methylconiine and gamma-coniceine. Coniceine is significantly more toxic than coniine and is thought to be the precursor to coniine. The toxic activity of the alkaloids is similar to that of nicotine. Large doses produce non-polarizing neuromuscular blockade which may result in respiratory depression and death.

Datura stramonium

Datura stramonium (jimsonweed) and other *Datura* species contain the tropane alkaloids, L-hyoscyamine and scopolamine. These alkaloids are potent antagonists of acetylcholine at muscarinic receptors and produce the anticholinergic syndrome. While morbidity is significant, fatalities are rare and are the consequence of hyperthermia, seizures and/or arrhythmias.

Atropa belladonna

Atropa belladonna (deadly nightshade) contains hyoscyamine and causes antimuscarinic effects – a dry mouth, nausea and vomiting – leading to blurred vision, hallucinations, confusion and hyperpyrexia.

Digitalis purpurea, Nerium oleander, Thevetia peruviana

Ingestion of *Digitalis purpurea,* or the common (*Nerium oleander*) or yellow (*Thevetia peruviana*) oleander can produce a syndrome similar to digoxin poisoning. A randomized controlled trial has shown that digoxin-specific antibody fragments rapidly and safely reverse yellow oleander-induced arrhythmias, restore sinus rhythm, and rapidly reverse bradycardia and hyperkalaemia.

FURTHER READING
Eddleston M et al. (2000) Anti-digoxin Fab fragments in cardiotoxicity induced by ingestion of yellow oleander: a randomised controlled trial. *Lancet* **355**: 967–971.

MUSHROOMS

Most mushrooms and edible fungi are not poisonous, but transient nausea, vomiting and diarrhoea can occur after ingestion of some varieties. There are a few species which are toxic.

Amanita muscaria, Amanita pantherina

Amanita muscaria (fly agaric) and *Amanita pantherina* (false blusher) contain isoxazoles (γ-aminobutyric acid agonists) which cause inebriation, visual disturbances, hallucinations, myoclonic jerks, muscle fasciculation, convulsions and coma.

Amanita phalloides

Amanita phalloides (death cap mushroom) contains amatoxins which inhibit transcription from DNA to mRNA by blockade of nuclear RNA polymerase II, resulting in impaired protein synthesis and cell death. Amatoxins are not inactivated by cooking. Hepatocellular necrosis follows 72 hours after ingestion and some varieties cause renal failure. Treatment is with gastric aspiration and general support; haemodialysis and liver/renal transplantation may be necessary. The value of silibinin and *N*-acetylcysteine is unproven.

Coprinus atramentarius

Coprinus atramentarius (ink cap) contains coprin, an acetaldehyde dehydrogenase inhibitor with a disulfiram-like effect, causing flushing and rash.

Cortinarius orellanus, Cortinarius speciossimus

Cortinarius orellanus and *Cortinarius speciossimus* contain orellanin, a potent nephrotoxin.

'Magic' mushrooms

'Magic' mushrooms, such as *Psilocybe, Panaeolus, Conocybe, Gymnopilus, Stropharia, Pluteus* and *Panaeolina* spp., contain the hallucinogen, psilocybin.

FURTHER READING
Danel VC, Saviuc PF, Garon D (2001) Main features of *Cortinarius* spp. poisoning: a literature review. *Toxicon* **39**: 1053–1060.

Jaeger A et al. (1993) Kinetics of amatoxins in human poisoning: therapeutic implications. *Journal of Toxicology–Clinical Toxicology* **31**: 63–80.

POISONS CENTRE NUMBERS
Australia	(61) 131 126	Malaysia (Penang)	(60) 800 8099
Canada (Vancouver)	(1) 604 682 5050	Republic of Ireland (Dublin)	(353) 1837 9964
Egypt (Cairo)	(20) 26840902	Pakistan (Karachi)	(92) 21 9201 345
France (Paris)	(33) 1 40 054848	UK	0870 600 6266
India (New Delhi)	(91) 11 66 1123	USA	(1) 800 222 1222

SIGNIFICANT WEBSITES
http://www.toxnet.nlm.nih.gov
  National Library of Medicine's Toxnet
http://www.spib.axl.co.uk
  Toxbase – Database of UK National Poisons Information Service

http://www.who/int/ipcs
  Contact details of all poisons centres worldwide

Environmental medicine 17

HEAT

In health, the body core temperature is maintained at 37°C by the hypothalamic thermoregulator centre.

Heat is produced by cellular metabolism, and lost through the skin by both vasodilatation and sweating and through the lungs in expired air. Profuse sweating occurs when the ambient temperature is greater than 32.5°C and during exercise. Evaporation of sweat is the vital mechanism cooling the body.

Heat acclimatization

Acclimatization to hot climates takes several weeks. Sweat volume increases and its salt content falls. Increased evaporation cools down the body.

Heat cramps

Painful muscle (usually leg) cramps often occur in well-acclimatized fit young people when they exercise in hot weather. Cramps are probably the result of low extracellular sodium caused by replenishment of water but not salt during prolonged sweating. They can be prevented by increasing dietary salt and respond to combined salt and water replacement.

Heat illness (heat exhaustion)

In high environmental temperatures, particularly with high humidity, vigorous exercise in clothing which inhibits heat loss can provoke a sudden elevation in core temperature. Weakness/exhaustion, dizziness and syncope, with a core temperature > 37°C define heat *illness* (exertional heat illness after exercise). Temperature elevation is more critical than water and sodium loss. Heat *illness* may progress to heat *injury*, a serious medical emergency.

Management

Remove the patient from any heat source. Cool with cold sponging and fans. Give oxygen by mask. Other causes of hyperpyrexia, e.g. malaria, should be considered.

Oral rehydration with both salt and water (25 g of sodium chloride per 5 L of water) is given in the first 24 hours, with adequate replacement thereafter. In severe heat illness, intravenous fluids are needed. Isotonic saline is usually given, depending on serum sodium. Careful monitoring is required. Secondary potassium loss must be corrected.

Heat injury (heat stroke)

Heat *injury* is an acute life-threatening situation when core temperature rises above 41°C. There is headache, nausea, vomiting and weakness. The skin is hot. Sweating is often absent, but this is not invariable, even in severe heat injury. Brain involvement leads to confusion, delirium and coma.

Heat injury develops in unacclimatized people in hot, humid windless climates, even without exercise. Sweating may be limited by prickly heat. Excessive exercise in inappropriate clothing, e.g. exercising on land in a wetsuit, can lead to heat injury in temperate climates. Old age, diabetes, drugs (e.g. alcohol, antimuscarinics, diuretics and phenothiazines) are all further precipitating factors. The pathogenesis of heat injury is a fall in cardiac output, lactic acidosis and intravascular coagulation. *Diagnosis* is clinical.

Management

- Remove the patient from the hot area immediately.
- Cool with sponging and icepacks.
- Manage in intensive care (monitor biochemistry, clotting and muscle enzymes).
- Give fluids with caution: hypovolaemia is often absent.

Prompt treatment is essential and can lead to rapid and complete recovery. Delay may be fatal. Prevention is by acclimatization, fluids and common sense.

Complications

These are hypovolaemia (shock), intravascular coagulation, cerebral oedema, rhabdomyolysis, and renal and hepatic failure. Their management is described in appropriate chapters.

Malignant hyperpyrexia (see p. 1271)

FURTHER READING
Simon H (1993) Hyperthermia. *New England Journal of Medicine* **329**: 483–487.

COLD

Hypothermia is defined as a core (i.e. rectal) temperature below 35°C. It is frequently lethal when core temperature falls below 32°C.

Frostbite is local cold injury when tissue freezes.

Hypothermia

Hypothermia occurs in many settings.

At home

Hypothermia occurs in cold climates when there is poor heating, inadequate clothing and poor nutrition. Depressant drugs (e.g. hypnotics), alcohol, hypothyroidism or intercurrent illness also contribute. Hypothermia is commonly seen in the poor and elderly, the latter having a diminished ability to sense cold and often loss of insulating fat. Infants and neonates become hypothermic rapidly at room temperature because of their relatively large surface area and lack of subcutaneous fat.

During exposure to extremes of temperature

Hypothermia is a prominent cause of death in climbers, skiers, polar travellers and in wartime. Wet, cold conditions with wind chill, physical exhaustion, injuries and inadequate clothing are contributory.

Following immersion in cold water

Dangerous hypothermia can develop after 1 hour's immersion at water temperatures of 15–20°C. Below 12°C limbs rapidly become numb and paralysed. Recovery takes some hours after rescue.

Clinical features

Mild hypothermia (core 32–35°C) causes shivering and initially quite intense cold. Though alert the subject may not act appropriately to rewarm (e.g. huddling, extra clothing or exercise). As core temperature falls below 32°C, severe hypothermia causes impaired judgement

(including awareness of cold), drowsiness and coma. Death follows, usually from ventricular fibrillation.

Diagnosis

If a thermometer (low-reading) is available, diagnosis is straightforward. If not, a rapid clinical assessment is reliable. A person who *feels* icy to touch – the abdomen, groin and axillae – is hypothermic. If clammy and uncooperative, sleepy or in a coma, core temperature is almost certainly below 32°C – a medical emergency.

Sequelae

Pulse rate and volume fall; respiration becomes shallow and slow. Muscle stiffness develops and tendon reflexes become sluggish. Systemic blood pressure falls. As coma ensues, pupillary and other brainstem reflexes are lost (pupils are fixed and may be dilated in severe hypothermia).

Metabolic changes are variable, either metabolic acidosis or alkalosis developing. Arterial oxygen tension may appear normal since it is measured at room temperature, but the measurement is falsely high as arterial P_{O_2} falls 7% for each degree Celsius (C) fall in temperature.

Ventricular arrhythmias (tachycardia/fibrillation) or asystole is the usual cause of death. 'J' waves – rounded waves above the isoelectric line immediately after the QRS complex – are pathognomonic of hypothermia. Prolongation of PR, QT intervals and QRS complex occurs.

Principles of management

- Rewarm gradually.
- Correct metabolic abnormalities.
- Anticipate and treat dysrhythmias.
- Check for hypothyroidism (see p. 1072).

If the patient is awake, with core temperature above 32°C, place them in a warm room, use a 'space blanket', and give warm fluids orally. Outdoors, add extra dry clothing, huddle together and use a warmed sleeping bag. Rewarming may take several hours. Avoid alcohol: it may add to confusion, boost confidence factitiously, cause peripheral vasodilatation (and further heat loss), or precipitate hypoglycaemia.

Severe hypothermia

In severe hypothermia, people look dead. Always exclude hypothermia before diagnosing brain death (p. 989). Warm gradually, aiming at a 1°C per hour increase in core temperature. Cover with a 'space blanket' and place in a warm room. Direct surface heat from an electric blanket is also helpful. Treat any underlying condition promptly, e.g. sepsis. Monitor all vital functions. Correct dysrhythmias. Drug screening is essential.

Give warm i.v. fluids slowly. Correct metabolic abnormalities. Hypothyroidism, if present, should be treated with triiodothyronine 10 μg i.v. 8-hourly. Various methods of artificial rewarming exist – inhaled humidified air, gastric or peritoneal lavage, and haemodialysis. These are rarely used.

Prevention

Hypothermia prevention is especially necessary in the elderly. Improved home heating and insulation, central heating in bedrooms and electric blankets are helpful. Finance is often needed. Supervision should be given during cold spells; warm food and extra blankets must be provided.

Frostbite

Ice crystals form within skin and superficial tissues when the tissue temperature falls to –3°C: ambient temperatures generally must be below –6°C.

Recognition

Frostbitten tissue is pale, greyish and initially doughy to touch. Later it freezes hard, when it looks and feels like meat taken from a deep freeze. Frostbite can easily occur when working or exercising in low temperatures. Typically it develops without the patient's knowledge. Below –5°C, hands or feet that have lost their feeling are at risk of frostbite.

Management

The frostbitten patient should, if possible, be transported (or walk, even on frostbitten feet) to a place of safety before treatment commences. Warm with a companion's body or by immersion in water at 39–42°C (hand hot). Continue until obvious thawing occurs. This may be painful. Blisters form within several days and, depending on the degree of frostbite, a blackened carapace or shell develops as the blisters regress or burst. Dry, non-adherent dressings and strict aseptic precautions are essential. Frostbitten tissues are anaesthetic and at risk from infection and further trauma. Recovery takes place over many weeks. Surgery may be required, but should be avoided in the early stages.

FURTHER READING
Lazar HL (1997) Editorial: The treatment of hypothermia. *New England Journal of Medicine* **337**: 1545–1547.

HIGH ALTITUDES

The partial pressure of ambient (and hence alveolar and arterial) oxygen falls in a near-linear relationship to altitude (Fig. 17.1).

Below 3000 m there are few clinical effects. Commercial aircraft are pressurized to 2750 m. The resulting hypoxia causes breathlessness only in those with severe cardiorespiratory disease. The incidence of thromboembolism is slightly greater in (sedentary) travellers on long flights than in a similar population at sea level. Above 3000–3500 m hypoxia causes a spectrum of related clinical syndromes that affect visitors to high altitudes, principally climbers, trekkers, skiers and troops (Table 17.1). These occur largely during acclimatization.

Fig. 17.1 The decrease in oxygen and barometric pressure with increasing altitude.

Table 17.1	Conditions caused by sustained hypoxia	
Condition	**Incidence (%)**	**Usual altitude (m)**
Acute mountain sickness	70	3500–4000
Acute pulmonary oedema	2	4000
Acute cerebral oedema	1	4500
Retinal haemorrhage	50	5000
Deterioration	100	6000
Chronic mountain sickness	Rare	4500

Acclimatization takes several weeks and enables humans to live (permanently if necessary) up to about 5600 m. At greater heights, although people can survive for days or weeks, deterioration due to chronic hypoxia is inevitable.

Ascent of the world's highest summits is possible without the use of supplementary oxygen. At the summit of Everest (nearly 9000 m) the barometric pressure is 34 kPa (253 mmHg). An acclimatized mountaineer has an alveolar Po_2 of 4.0–4.7 kPa (30–35 mmHg) – near man's absolute physiological limit.

Acute mountain sickness (AMS)

This describes malaise, nausea, headache and lassitude common for a few days above 3500 m. Following arrival at this altitude there is usually a latent interval of 6–36 hours before symptoms begin. Treatment is rest, with analgesics if necessary. Recovery is usually spontaneous.

Prophylactic treatment with acetazolamide, a carbonic anhydrase inhibitor and a respiratory stimulant is of some value in preventing AMS. Acclimatizing, i.e. ascending gradually, is the best prophylaxis.

In the minority, more serious sequelae of high-altitude pulmonary oedema and high-altitude cerebral oedema develop.

High-altitude pulmonary oedema

Predisposing factors include youth, rapidity of ascent, heavy exertion and severe AMS. Breathlessness, with frothy blood-stained sputum indicates established oedema. Unless treated rapidly this leads to cardiorespiratory failure and death. Milder forms are common, presenting with less severe breathlessness.

High-altitude cerebral oedema

Cerebral oedema is another sequel of hypoxia. It is the result of abrupt increase in cerebral blood flow that occurs even at modest altitudes of 3500–4000 m. Headache is usual, and is accompanied by drowsiness, ataxia, and papilloedema. Coma and death follow if the condition progresses.

Treatment

Any but the milder forms of AMS require urgent treatment. Oxygen should be given if available, and descent to a lower altitude should take place as quickly as possible. Nifedipine reduces pulmonary hypertension and is used in the treatment of pulmonary oedema. Dexamethasone is effective in reducing brain oedema. Portable pressure bags, in which the patient is inserted, are helpful in increasing barometric pressure; these are widely used.

Retinal haemorrhages

Small 'flame' haemorrhages in the retinal nerve fibre layer are common above 5000 m. They are usually symptomless. Rarely they cover the macula, causing painless loss of central vision. Recovery is usual.

Deterioration

Prolonged residence between 6000 and 7000 m leads to weight loss, anorexia and listlessness after several weeks. Above 7500 m, deterioration develops more quickly, although it is possible to survive for a week or more at altitudes over 8000 m.

Chronic mountain sickness

This rare syndrome occurs in long-term residents at high altitudes after several decades. It has been described in the Andes and in central Asia.

Polycythaemia, drowsiness, cyanosis, finger clubbing, congested cheeks and ear lobes, and right ventricular enlargement occur. It is gradually progressive.

By way of contrast, coronary artery disease and hypertension are rare in high-altitude native populations.

FURTHER READING
Clarke C (2001) High altitude and mountaineering expeditions. In: Warrell D, Anderson S (eds) *Expedition Medicine*. London: Royal Geographical Society.
Hackett PH, Roach RC (2001) High-altitude illness. *New England Journal of Medicine* **345**: 107–114.

Information: Wilderness Medical Society, PO Box 2463, Indianapolis, Indiana 462206, USA. Website: http://www.wms.org.
UIAA Mountain Medicine Data Centre leaflets, available from British Mountaineering Council, 177–179 Burton Road, Manchester M20 2BB. Tel: 0161 445 4747; Fax: 0161 445 4500. Website: http://www.thebmc.co.uk.

DIVING

Ambient pressures at various depths are shown in Table 17.2.

Various methods are used to supply air to a diver. With the simplest (e.g. a snorkel), the limiting factor which occurs below 0.5 m, is respiratory effort sucking air into the lungs. At greater depths this 'forced negative-pressure ventilation' causes pulmonary capillary damage and haemorrhagic oedema. Scuba divers – the usual sports diving down to 50 m – carry bottled compressed air.

Divers who work at great depths for commercial purposes or exploration breathe helium–oxygen or nitrogen–oxygen mixtures delivered by hose from the surface.

Complex problems can affect divers at all depths.

Compression problems (descent)

Middle ear barotrauma ('squeeze') is common and caused by inability to equalize pressure in the middle ear – usually the result of Eustachian tube blockage. Deafness occurs and eventual tympanic membrane rupture, with acute vertigo.

Sinus barotrauma ('squeeze') – is due to blockage of the nasal and paranasal sinus ostia, with intense local pain.

Treatment is with decongestants. Avoid diving with any respiratory infection.

Nitrogen narcosis

When compressed air is breathed below 30 m, narcotic effects of nitrogen impair brain function. Changes of mood and performance may be hazardous. These reverse rapidly on ascent.

Nitrogen narcosis is avoided by replacing air with helium–oxygen mixtures, enabling descent to 700 m.

At these great depths direct effect of pressure on neurones can cause tremor, hemiparesis and cognitive impairment.

Table 17.2	Pressure in relation to sea depth	
Sea depth (m)	**Atmospheric pressure (atmospheres)**	**mmHg**
0	1	760
10	2	1520
50	6	4560
90	10	7600

Oxygen narcosis

Pure oxygen is not used for diving because oxygen is toxic. Lung damage (atelectasis, endothelial cell damage and pulmonary oedema) occurs when the alveolar oxygen pressure exceeds 1.5 atmospheres (5 m of water). At around 10 m of water the nervous system is affected. Apprehension, nausea and sweating is followed by muscle twitching and generalized convulsions with possible underwater fatalities.

Decompression problems (i.e. ascent)

Breath-hold (shallow-water) diving

Shallow-water swimmers and free divers deliberately hyperventilate prior to a dive to drive off CO_2 – reducing the stimulus to breathe. The subsequent breath-hold causes a rise in P_aCO_2 and a fall of P_aO_2. However, on surfacing, decompression further lowers P_aO_2. This may cause syncope.

Decompression sickness

Decompression sickness ('the bends') occurs in divers on returning to the surface and is caused by the release of bubbles of inert gases (nitrogen or helium). Bubbles develop only if ascent is too rapid. Decompression tables indicate the time needed for safe return from given depths.

The bends can be mild (type 1 non-neurological bends), with skin irritation, mottling or joint pain only. Type 2 (neurological) bends are more serious – cortical blindness, hemiparesis, sensory disturbances or cord lesions develop. If nitrogen bubbles form in pulmonary vessels, divers experience retrosternal discomfort, dyspnoea and cough ('the chokes'). These develop within minutes or hours of a dive.

Treatment is with oxygen. All but the mildest forms of decompression sickness (i.e. skin mottling alone) require recompression in a pressure chamber.

A long-term problem is aseptic necrosis (e.g. of the hip) due to nitrogen bubbles causing infarction of nutrient arteries of bone. Neurological damage may also persist.

Lung rupture, pneumothorax and surgical emphysema

These emergencies occur principally when divers 'breath-hold' while making emergency ascents after losing their gas supply. There is severe dyspnoea, cough and haemoptysis. Pneumothorax and emphysema usually respond to 100% oxygen. Air embolism may occur and should be treated with recompression and hyperbaric oxygen.

FURTHER READING

Bennett P, Elliot D (2002) *The Physiology and Medicine of Diving*, 5th edn. London: WB Saunders.

Melamed Y, Shupak A, Bitterman H (1992) Medical problems associated with underwater diving. *New England Journal of Medicine* **326**: 30–36.

DIVING INFORMATION

Institute of Naval Medicine, Undersea Medicine Division, Alverstoke, Gosport, Hampshire PO12 2DL. http://www.rnreference. mod.uk/09/inm/undersea.htm

UK Diving emergencies only: Ministry of Defence, Duty Diving Medical Officer. Tel: 07831 151523.

IONIZING RADIATION

Ionizing radiation is either penetrating (X-rays, gamma rays or neutrons) or non-penetrating (alpha or beta particles). Penetrating radiation affects the whole body, while non-penetrating radiation affects only the skin. All radiation effects, however, depend on the type of radiation, the distribution of dose and the dose rate.

Radiation dosage is measured in joules per kilogram (J/kg); 1 J/kg is also known as 1 gray (1 Gy). This is equivalent to 100 rads. Radioactivity is measured in becquerels (Bq); 1 Bq is equal to the amount of radioactive material in which there is one disintegration per second. One curie (Ci) is equal to 3.7×10^{10} Bq.

Radiation differs in the density of ionization it causes. Therefore a dose-equivalent called a sievert (Sv) is used. This is the absorbed dose weighted for the damaging effect of the radiation. The annual background radiation is approximately 2.5 mSv. A chest X-ray gives 0.02 mSv, while a CT scan of the abdomen/pelvis is 10 mSv.

Excessive exposure to ionizing radiation occurs following accidents in hospitals, industry, nuclear power plants and strategic nuclear explosions.

Mild acute radiation sickness

Nausea, vomiting and malaise follow doses of approximately 1 Gy. Lymphopenia occurs within several days, followed 2–3 weeks later by a fall in all white cells and platelets. There is a late risk of leukaemia and solid tumours.

Severe acute radiation sickness

Many systems are affected; the extent of the damage depends on the dose of radiation received. The effects of radiation are summarized in Table 17.3.

Table 17.3 The effects of radiation

Acute effects	Delayed effects
Haemopoietic syndrome	Infertility
Gastrointestinal syndrome	Teratogenesis
CNS syndrome	Cataract
Radiation dermatitis	Neoplasia:
	Acute myeloid leukaemia
	Thyroid
	Salivary glands
	Skin
	Others

Haemopoietic syndrome

Absorption of doses between 2 and 10 Gy is followed by early and transient vomiting in some individuals, followed by a period of relative well-being. Lymphocytes are particularly sensitive to radiation damage, and severe lymphopenia develops over several days. A decrease in granulocytes and platelets occurs 2–3 weeks later as no new cells are being formed by the damaged marrow. Thrombocytopenia with bleeding develops and frequent overwhelming infections occur, with a very high mortality.

Gastrointestinal syndrome

Absorption of doses greater than 6 Gy causes vomiting several hours after exposure. This then stops, only to recur some 4 days later accompanied by severe diarrhoea. Owing to radiation inhibition of cell division, the villous lining of the intestine becomes denuded. Intractable bloody diarrhoea follows, with dehydration, secondary infection and death.

CNS syndrome

Exposures above 30 Gy are followed rapidly by nausea, vomiting, disorientation and coma. Death due to severe cerebral oedema follows within 36 hours.

Radiation dermatitis

Skin erythema, purpura, blistering and secondary infection occur. Total loss of body hair is a bad prognostic sign and usually follows an exposure of at least 5 Gy.

Late effects of radiation exposure

Survivors of the nuclear bombing of Hiroshima and Nagasaki have provided information on the long-term effects of radiation. The risk of developing acute myeloid leukaemia or cancer, particularly of the skin, thyroid and salivary glands, increases. Infertility, teratogenesis and cataract are also late sequelae of radiation exposure.

Treatment

Acute radiation sickness is a medical emergency. Hospitals should be informed immediately of the type and length of exposure so that suitable arrangements can be made to receive the patient. The initial radiation dose absorbed can be reduced by removing clothing contaminated by radioactive materials.

Treatment of radiation sickness is largely supportive and consists of prevention and treatment of infection, haemorrhage and fluid loss. Storage of the patient's white cells and platelets for future use should be considered, if feasible.

Accidental ingestion of, or exposure to, bone-seeking radioisotopes (e.g. strontium-90 and caesium-137) should be treated with chelating agents (e.g. EDTA) and massive doses of oral calcium. Radioiodine contamination should be treated immediately with potassium iodide 133 mg per day. This will block 90% of radioiodine absorption by the thyroid if given immediately before exposure.

ELECTRIC SHOCK

Electric shock may produce clinical effects in several ways:

- *Pain and psychological sequelae.* The common 'electric shock' is usually a painful, but harmless, stimulus but an unpleasant and frightening experience. It produces no lasting neurological damage or skin damage.
- *Cardiac, neurological and muscle damage.* Ventricular fibrillation, muscular contraction and spinal cord damage follow a major shock. These are seen typically following a lightning strike, which is a very high voltage and amperage current.
- *Electrical burns.* These commonly only involve the skin (lightning may cause a fern-shaped burn), but subcutaneous or deep injuries can occur.

SMOKE

Air pollution is discussed on page 894.

Smoke consists of particles of carbon in hot air and gases. These particles are coated with organic acids and aldehydes and synthetic materials. On combustion, other toxins such as carbon monoxide, sulphur dioxide, sulphuric and hydrochloric acids are released. Polyvinyl chloride is no longer used in household goods.

Respiratory symptoms may be immediate or delayed. Patients are dyspnoeic and tachypnoeic. Laryngeal stridor may require intubation. Hypoxia and pulmonary oedema can be fatal.

Patients should breathe through an aspirator or wet towel. Remove the patient from the smoke. Give O_2 and ITU support. Smoke alarms should be used in households.

NOISE

Sound intensity is expressed as the square of sound pressure. The bel is a ratio and is equivalent to a 10-fold increase in sound intensity; a decibel (dB) is one-tenth of a bel. Sound is made up of a number of frequencies ranging from 30 Hz to 20 kHz, with most being between 1 and 4 kHz. When measuring sound, these different frequencies must be taken into account. In practice a scale known as A-weighted sound is used; sound levels are then reported as dB(A). A hazardous sound source is defined as one with an overall sound pressure greater than 90 dB(A).

Repeated prolonged exposure to loud noise, particularly between 2 and 6 kHz, causes first temporary and later permanent hearing loss by physically destroying hair cells in the organ of Corti and, eventually, auditory neurones. This is a common occupational problem, not only in industry and the armed forces, but also in the home (electric drills and sanders), in sport (motor racing), and in entertainment (pop stars, disc jockeys and their audiences).

Serious noise-induced hearing loss is almost wholly preventable by personal protection (ear muffs, ear plugs). Little help can be offered once deafness becomes established.

Other effects of noise

Noise is undoubtedly irritative and increases or produces anxiety. It has been suggested that excess noise affects child development and reading skills.

BIOTERRORISM/BIOWARFARE

Interest in biological warfare and bioterrorism became intense at the time of the 1991 Iraq war especially following the bombing of the Twin Towers in New York when other terrorist attacks were expected. The potential of bacteria as a weapon is illustrated by the fact that a few kilograms of anthrax spores can kill as many people as a Hiroshima size nuclear weapon.

Potential pathogens

The Centers for Disease Control in Atlanta, Georgia, in the United States have developed a classification of potential biological agents which might be used as weapons (Table 17.4). The most likely to be employed are smallpox, anthrax, botulism and plague.

Smallpox

Smallpox is an infectious disease with a mortality of at least 30% for which there is no proven therapy. There is an effective vaccine. However, universal vaccination against smallpox was stopped in the early 1970s and the vast majority of the world's population is unprotected against the virus. The potential therefore exists for a world-wide epidemic of smallpox initiated by a bioterrorist act. One simulated incident outlined an outbreak of smallpox originating in a university function in North America attended by 1000 students. It resulted in

Fig. 17.2 Smallpox rash.

an international outbreak of the infection with exhaustion of the world's supply of smallpox vaccine.

Smallpox has an incubation period of around 12 days, allowing a bioterrorist act to go undetected until a rash (Fig. 17.2), similar to that of chicken pox, develops on the second or third day of the illness. The infection is transmitted by the airborne route and the patient becomes infectious to others 12–24 hours before the rash appears, thus allowing an infected 'volunteer' to pass the infection on to others before being recognized as suffering from the disease. If the vaccine is given within 3 days of contact, the disease may be prevented. The smallpox virus is still stored in two laboratories in the world – one in Russia and the other in the United States of America.

Anthrax

Anthrax is described on page 82. In late 2001, anthrax organisms were sent through the United States mail and infected 22 individuals; 11 had pulmonary anthrax, five of whom died, and 11 suffered from cutaneous anthrax. A major post sorting office became contaminated with anthrax spores.

A simulated anthrax bioterrorist attack postulated the release of anthrax powder from a truck passing a large football stadium containing 74 000 spectators with the infection of 16 000, of whom 4000 died. In an accidental release of anthrax from a bioweapons factory in Russia the death rate in those living in the neighbourhood, especially downwind of the factory, was 75%.

Botulism

Botulism is described on page 73. The toxin produced by the organism *Clostridium botulinum* is the most potent poison known to man. It has been claimed that Iraq at some time had 19 000 L of botulinum toxin, sufficient to kill the entire population of the world three times over.

As a bioweapon, the toxin could be transmitted by food or by the airborne route, e.g. from a crop-spraying plane. It is inactivated by chlorine in domestic water supplies. There is no vaccine available. Following a terrorist event it is possible that many hundreds of intensive care beds with ventilators might be required.

Table 17.4 The critical biological agents (CDC)
Category A pathogens Very infectious and/or readily disseminated organisms which would produce high mortality and have a major impact on public health causing public panic (smallpox, anthrax, botulinism, plague)
Category B pathogens Moderately easy to disseminate organisms causing moderate morbidity and mortality (Q fever, brucellosis, glanders, food/water-borne pathogens, influenza)
Category C pathogens Category includes emerging and possible genetically engineered pathogens (viral haemorrhagic fevers, encephalitis viruses, drug-resistant tuberculosis)
From Khan AS, Morse S, Lillibridge S (2000) Reprinted with permission from Elsevier. *Lancet* **356**: 1179–1182

Plague

Plague (p. 87) could be transmitted as a bioweapon either by airborne dissemination (causing pneumonia) or by infected rats. There is no effective vaccine.

Route of dissemination of biological weapons

Pathogenic microorganisms could be delivered as a weapon by a number of routes, e.g. by aerosol, by crop-spraying aeroplane, via the mail, in food or drink, by a bomb or rocket, or by a human volunteer infected with an organism.

The 'ideal' weapon

An 'ideal' biological weapon could have some, or all, of the following properties:

- Able to produce high morbidity/mortality (e.g. smallpox).
- Capable of being aerosolized or weaponized (e.g. anthrax, plague, smallpox).
- Relatively easy to produce (anthrax).
- Capable of being used against a non-immune target population (smallpox).
- Capable of being made antibiotic-resistant and/or genetically modified to increase pathogenicity (e.g. ? plague; ? smallpox).

Clinical presentations of a bioterrorist attack

Infection associated with a bioterrorist act could present in a number of ways, e.g. with diarrhoea and vomiting (salmonella infection), a respiratory illness (anthrax, plague), a rash (smallpox, viral haemorrhagic fever), a neurological presentation (botulism) or an unexplained febrile illness (Q fever, influenza, tuberculosis). The first indication of an attack could be a cluster of individuals with similar symptoms.

Emergency planning

Most western countries have plans to deal with a bio-terrorist attack. These include the training of healthcare staff, ambulance personnel and police. Such plans stress the importance of awareness of the possibility and preparedness for an attack. Stockpiling of vaccines, antibiotics and protective clothing is essential.

FURTHER READING
Buchler JW, Berkelman RL, Hartley DM (2003) Syndromic surveillance and bioterrorism-related epidemics. *Emerging Infections Diseases* **10**: 1197–1204.
Khan AS, Morse S, Lillibridge S (2000) Public-health preparedness for biological terrorism in the USA. Lancet 356: 1179–1182.

DROWNING AND NEAR-DROWNING

Drowning is the third commonest cause of accidental death in the UK; it caused over 500 000 deaths worldwide in 2000. Approximately 40% of drownings occur in children under five. People also drown after an epileptic seizure or a myocardial infarct whilst in water. Exhaustion, alcohol, drugs and hypothermia all contribute to drowning.

'Dry' drowning

Between 10% and 15% of drownings occur without water aspiration into the lungs. Laryngeal spasm occurs, apnoea, anoxia and cardiac arrest.

'Wet' drowning

Aspiration of fresh water affects pulmonary surfactant, with alveolar collapse and ventilation/perfusion mismatch and hypoxaemia. Aspiration of hypertonic seawater (5% NaCl) pulls additional fluid into the lungs with further ventilation/perfusion mismatch. In practice, however, there is little difference between saltwater and freshwater drowning. In both, severe hypoxaemia develops rapidly after water aspiration. Severe metabolic acidosis develops in the majority of survivors.

Emergency treatment of near-drowning

Patients can survive for up to 30 minutes under water without suffering brain damage – and for longer if the water temperature is near 0°C. This is probably related to the protective role of the diving reflex – submersion causes reflex slowing of the pulse and vasoconstriction. In addition, hypothermia decreases oxygen consumption. CPR should be started immediately (see p. 759).

Resuscitation should always be attempted, even in the absence of a pulse and the presence of fixed dilated pupils. Patients frequently make a dramatic recovery. All patients should be subsequently admitted to hospital for intensive monitoring. Survivors are liable to develop acute lung injury.

Prognosis

This is good if the patient regains consciousness promptly but poor if they remain in coma 30 minutes after resuscitation.

FURTHER READING
Modell JH (1993) Drowning. *New England Journal of Medicine* **328**: 253–256.

TRAVEL

Motion sickness

This common problem, particularly in children, is caused by repetitive stimulation of the labyrinth. It occurs frequently at sea and in cars, but may occur on horseback or on less usual forms of transport such as camels or elephants. It is a major issue in space travel. Nausea, sweating, dizziness, vertigo and profuse vomiting occur, accompanied by an irresistible desire to stop moving.

Prophylactic antihistamines or vestibular sedatives (hyoscine or cinnarizine) are of some value.

Jet-lag

Jet-lag, or circadian dyschronism, is a well-known phenomenon after changing multiple time-zones, particularly from West to East. Fatigue, intense insomnia, headache, irritability, poor concentration and loss of appetite are common. Symptoms last several days.

Mechanisms are poorly understood but relate to the hypothalamic body clock, sited within the suprachiasmatic nuclei. The clock is regulated by various zeitgebers ('time-givers'), e.g. light and melatonin.

Management of jet-lag includes its acceptance as a phenomenon causing poor performance and waiting for 3–5 days to recover. Various hypnotics can help insomnia, but their place is disputed. Oral melatonin is widely used to reduce jet-lag. This increases sleepiness and hastens resetting of the body clock. Melatonin is not available on prescription.

FURTHER READING
Waterhouse J, Reilly T, Atkinson G (1997) Jet-lag. *Lancet* **350**: 1611–1616.

BUILDING-RELATED ILLNESSES

Modern office buildings have a controlled environment with automated heating, ventilation and air-conditioning systems, often without outdoor air. More than half the adult workforce in developed countries work in offices.

Non-specific building-related illness

Headache, fatigue and difficulty in concentrating, sometimes in apparent epidemics, are common complaints of office-workers. Psychological factors may have a role. Temperature, humidity, dust, volatile organic compounds (e.g. paints, solvents) have all been implicated. Maintenance of continuous outdoor air supply is recommended. However, changes in ventilation sometimes fail to improve matters.

Specific building-related illness

Legionnaires' disease (see p. 925) is frequently due to contamination of air-conditioned systems. Humidifier fever (p. 943) is also due to contaminated systems, probably by fungi, bacteria and protozoa. Many common viruses are easily transmitted in the enclosed environment (e.g. the common cold, influenza and rarely pulmonary tuberculosis). Allergic disorders (e.g. rhinitis, asthma and dermatitis) also occur owing to exposure to indoor allergens such as dust mites and plants. Office equipment (e.g. fumes from photocopiers) has also been implicated. Passive smoking (p. 894) is also a problem.

FURTHER READING
Menzies J, Bourbeau T (1997) Building-related illnesses. *New England Journal of Medicine* **337**: 1524–1531.

SIGNIFICANT WEBSITES
http://www.who.int/phe/en/
    WHO guidelines and information on various environmental topics
http://www.hypothermia.org/
    Hypothermia
http://www.high-altitude-medicine.com/
    Altitude sickness

Endocrine disease 18

HORMONAL ACTIVITY

Hormones are chemical messengers produced by a variety of specialized secretory cells. They may be transported in the blood to a distant site of action (the classic 'endocrine' effect) or act directly upon nearby cells ('paracrine' activity). In the hypothalamus, elsewhere in the brain and in the gastrointestinal tract there are many such cells secreting hormones, some of which have true endocrine or paracrine activity, while others behave more like neurotransmitters or neuromodulators. At the molecular level there is little difference in the way cellular activity is regulated between classical neurotransmitters that act across synaptic clefts, intercellular factors acting across gap junctions, classic endocrine and paracrine activity and a variety of other chemical messengers involved in cell regulation – such as cytokines, growth factors and interleukins; progress in basic cell biology has revealed the biochemical similarities in the messengers, receptors and intracellular post-receptor mechanisms underlying all these aspects of cell function.

Synthesis, storage and release of hormones

Hormones may be of several chemical structures: polypeptide, glycoprotein, steroid or amine. Hormone release is the end-product of a long cascade of intracellular events. In the case of polypeptide hormones, neural or endocrine stimulation of the cell leads to increased transcription from DNA to a specific mRNA, which is in turn translated to the peptide product. This is often in the form of a precursor molecule that may itself be biologically inactive. This 'prohormone' may be further processed before being packaged into granules, in the Golgi apparatus. These granules are then transported to the plasma membrane before release, which is itself regulated by a complex combination of intracellular regulators. Hormone release may be in a brief spurt caused by the sudden stimulation of granules, often induced by an intracellular Ca^{2+}-dependent process, or it may be 'constitutive' (immediate and continuous secretion).

Plasma transport

Most classical hormones are secreted into the systemic circulation where they travel to have effects elsewhere in the body. In contrast, hypothalamic releasing hormones are released into the pituitary portal system so that much higher concentrations of the releasing hormones reach the pituitary than occur in the systemic circulation.

Many hormones are bound to proteins within the circulation. In most cases, only the free (unbound) hormone is available to the tissues and thus biologically active. This binding serves to buffer against very rapid changes in plasma levels of the hormone, and some binding protein interactions may also be involved in the active regulation of hormone action. Many tests of

Table 18.1 Plasma hormones with their binding proteins

Hormone	Binding protein(s)
Thyroxine (T₄)	Thyroxine-binding globulin (TBG)
	Thyroxine-binding prealbumin (TBPA)
	Albumin
Triiodothyronine (T₃) (less bound than T₄)	Thyroxine-binding globulin (TBG)
	Albumin
Cortisol	Cortisol-binding globulin (CBG)
Testosterone, estradiol	Sex hormone-binding globulin (SHBG)
Insulin-like growth factor-I (IGF-I)	IGF-binding proteins (mainly IGF–BP3)

endocrine function often measure total rather than free hormone, since binding proteins are frequently altered in disease states. Binding proteins comprise both specific, high-affinity proteins of limited capacity, such as thyroxine-binding globulin (TBG) and other less-specific low-affinity ones, such as prealbumin and albumin. The clinically relevant binding proteins are shown in Table 18.1.

Hormone action and receptors

Hormones act by binding to specific receptors in the target cell, which may be at the cell surface and/or within the cell. Most hormone receptors are proteins with complex tertiary structures, parts of which complement the tertiary structure of the hormone to allow highly specific interactions, while other parts are responsible for the effects of the activated receptor within the cell. Many hormones bind to specific cell-surface receptors where they trigger internal messengers, while others bind to nuclear receptors which interact directly with DNA. Cell-surface receptors usually contain hydrophobic sections which span the lipid-rich plasma membrane, while nuclear receptors contain characteristic amino-acid sequences to bind nuclear DNA (e.g. so-called 'zinc fingers', see p. 167) as in the glucocorticoid receptor.

In order to achieve their intracellular effects, hormone receptors interact with a variety of other regulatory factors within the cell membrane, in the cytosol or within the nucleus of the cell. In each case, binding of the hormone to

its receptor results in a conformational change in the structure of the receptor, which may result in a number of possible outcomes which are illustrated in Figure 3.4 (p. 158):

- activation of, or modified binding to, other regulatory factors within the cell membrane or cytosol (e.g. binding of transmembrane receptors to the cell-membrane G-proteins, thereby activating the stimulatory or inhibitory effects of the latter on other intracellular mediators)
- activation of enzyme activity in the receptor or its regulatory factors (e.g. receptor adenylate cyclase, other protein kinases, phospholipase C) to generate a variety of intracellular 'second messengers' (e.g. cAMP, cGMP, phosphatidylinositol metabolites, calmodulin) which usually form a complex, branching and interacting intracellular cascade of enzyme activation and inhibition and/or mobilization of intracellular stores of ions (primarily calcium)
- altered binding of the receptor to DNA or to nuclear transcription factors in order to stimulate or inhibit transcription of one or more genes
- altered activity of cell-membrane channels or transporters (e.g. for glucose, potassium or for other ions)
- dimerization of the receptor, or internalization of some cell-surface receptors.

These immediate effects of hormone binding may then cause rapid alterations in cell-membrane ion transport or intracellular calcium concentrations, or slower responses such as DNA, RNA and protein synthesis.

In each case, binding of the hormone to its receptor is the first step in a complex cascade of interrelated intracellular events which eventually lead to the overall effects of that hormone on cellular function.

Common 'second messengers' involved in these cascades include *cyclic AMP* (for adrenocorticotrophic hormone (ACTH), luteinizing hormone (LH), follicle-stimulating hormone (FSH) and parathyroid hormone (PTH)), *a calcium–phospholipid system* (for thyrotrophin-releasing hormone (TRH), vasopressin and angiotensin II), *tyrosine kinase* and *other intracellular kinases* (for insulin and insulin-like growth factor-1 (IGF-1)) and *membrane-bound phosphoinositide pathways*.

Some general characteristics of selected hormone systems are shown in Table 18.2.

Table 18.2 Characteristics of some different hormone systems

	Peptides and catecholamines	Steroids and thyroid hormones
Protein binding	Sometimes for growth hormone and insulin-like growth factor	Yes
Changes in plasma concentrations	Rapid changes	Slow fluctuations
Plasma half-life	Short (seconds to minutes)	Long (minutes to days)
Type of receptors	Cell membrane	Intracellular
Mechanism	Activate preformed enzymes	Stimulate protein synthesis
Secretion	Secretory granules	Direct passage rapidly
	Constitutive + bursts	Related to secretion rate
Speed of effect	Rapid (seconds to minutes)	Slow (hours to days)

The sensitivity and/or number of receptors for a hormone are often decreased after prolonged exposure to a high hormone concentration, the receptors thus becoming less sensitive ('downregulation', e.g. angiotensin II receptors, β-adrenoceptors). The reverse is true when stimulation is absent or minimal, the receptors showing increased numbers or sensitivity ('upregulation').

Abnormal receptors are an occasional, though rare, cause of endocrine disease (see p. 1041), but are recognized and characterized more frequently owing to advances in molecular endocrinology.

Control and feedback

Most hormone systems are controlled by some form of feedback; an example is the hypothalamic–pituitary–thyroid axis (Fig. 18.1).

- TRH (thyrotrophin-releasing hormone) is secreted in the hypothalamus and travels via the portal system to the pituitary where it stimulates the thyrotrophs to produce thyroid-stimulating hormone (TSH).
- TSH is secreted into the systemic circulation where it stimulates increased thyroidal iodine uptake and thyroxine (T_4) and triiodothyronine (T_3) synthesis and release.
- Serum levels of T_3 and T_4 are thus increased by TSH; in addition, the conversion of T_4 to T_3 (the more active hormone) in peripheral tissues is stimulated by TSH.
- T_3 and T_4 then enter cells where they bind to nuclear receptors and promote increased metabolic and cellular activity.

- Levels of T_3 (from the blood and from local conversion of T_4) are sensed by receptors in the pituitary and possibly the hypothalamus. If they rise above normal, TRH and TSH production is suppressed, leading to reduced T_3 and T_4 secretion.
- Peripheral T_3 and T_4 levels thus fall to normal.
- If, however, T_3 and T_4 levels are low (e.g. after thyroidectomy), increased amounts of TRH and thus TSH are secreted, stimulating the remaining thyroid to produce more T_3 and T_4; blood levels of T_3 and T_4 may be restored to normal, although at the expense of increased TSH drive, reflected by a high TSH level ('compensated euthyroidism'). Conversely, in thyrotoxicosis when factors other than TSH itself are maintaining high T_3 and T_4 levels, the same mechanisms lead to suppression of TSH secretion.

This is known as a 'negative feedback' system, referring to the effect of T_3 and T_4 on the pituitary and hypothalamus, which represents the most common mechanism for regulation of circulating hormone levels. There are also 'positive feedback' systems, classically seen in the regulation of the normal menstrual cycle (p. 1050).

Patterns of secretion

Hormone secretion is continuous or intermittent. The former is shown by the thyroid hormones, where T_4 has a half-life of 7–10 days and T_3 of about 6–10 hours. Levels over the day, month and year show little variation.

In contrast, secretion of the gonadotrophins, LH and FSH, is normally pulsatile, with major pulses released every 1–2 hours depending on the phase of the menstrual cycle. Continuous infusion of LH to produce a steady equivalent level does not produce the same result (e.g. ovulation in the female) as the intermittent pulsatility, and may indeed produce downregulation. Thus a long-acting superactive gonadotrophin-releasing hormone (GnRH) analogue, such as buserelin, produces downregulation of the GnRH receptors and subsequent very low androgen or oestrogen levels, which are clinically valuable both in carcinoma of the prostate in men and in ovulation-induction regimens in infertile women. In contrast, pulsatile GnRH administration can produce normal menstrual cyclicity, ovulation and fertility in women with hypothalamic amenorrhoea but intact pituitary LH and FSH stores.

Biological rhythms

Circadian means changes over the 24 hours of the day–night cycle and is best shown for the pituitary–adrenal axis. Figure 18.2 shows plasma cortisol levels measured over 24 hours – levels are highest in the early morning and lowest overnight. Additionally, cortisol release is pulsatile, following the pulsatility of pituitary ACTH. Thus 'normal' cortisol levels vary during the day and great variations can be seen in samples taken only 30 minutes apart (Fig. 18.2). The circadian (light–dark) rhythm is seen in reverse with the pineal hormone, melatonin, which shows high levels during dark.

Fig. 18.1 **The hypothalamic–pituitary–thyroid axis.** The green line indicates positive feedback at the hypothalamic and pituitary level.

Fig. 18.2 **Plasma cortisol levels during a 24-hour period.** Note both the pulsatility and the shifting baseline. Normal ranges for 0900h (180–700 nmol/L) and 2400h (less than 100 nmol/L; must be taken when asleep) are shown in the orange boxes. Purple shading shows sleep.

Melatonin may be involved in entraining other hormonal rhythms and systems to the current light–dark cycle, but there is no known clinical syndrome related to abnormalities of this hormone, though a synthetic preparation is widely used for 'jet-lag' (p. 1033).

The *menstrual cycle* is the best example of a longer and more complex (28-day) biological rhythm (see p. 1050).

Other regulatory factors

- *Stress.* Physiological 'stress' and acute illness produce rapid increases in ACTH and cortisol, growth hormone (GH), prolactin, epinephrine (adrenaline) and norepinephrine (noradrenaline). These can occur within seconds or minutes.
- *Sleep.* Secretion of GH and prolactin is increased during sleep, especially the rapid eye movement (REM) phase.
- *Feeding and fasting.* Many hormones regulate the body's control of energy intake and expenditure and are therefore profoundly influenced by feeding and fasting. Thus, secretion of insulin is increased and growth hormone decreased after ingestion of food, and secretion of a number of hormones is altered during prolonged food deprivation.

All these factors must be considered when attempting to measure hormone levels in normal individuals and in patients with disease. For example, cortisol levels will often be high and fail to suppress during standard tests in a patient who is severely stressed by serious illness, and growth hormone will usually be low in postprandial individuals during the daytime.

TESTING ENDOCRINE FUNCTION

Ideally, the *activity* of hormones would be measured at the cellular level, but this is usually impossible. Measurement of hormone *levels* in body fluids is the normal substitute but, although usually an excellent approximation, does not always reflect the current tissue action of the relevant hormone. Most commonly, hormone levels in the blood (or, more technically, levels in plasma or serum) are measured, and all references to hormone levels in this chapter refer to blood/plasma levels unless stated otherwise.

Basal blood levels

Assays for all clinically relevant hormones are available. Obviously the time, day and condition of measurement may make great differences to hormone levels, and the method and timing of samples will depend upon the characteristics of the endocrine system involved. There may also be sex, developmental and age differences.

Basal levels are especially useful for systems with long half-lives (e.g. T_4 and T_3). These vary little over the short term and random samples are therefore satisfactory.

Basal samples for other hormones may also be satisfactory if interpreted with respect to normal ranges for the time of day/month, diet or posture concerned. Examples are FSH, oestrogen and progesterone (varying with time of cycle) and renin/aldosterone (varying with sodium intake, posture and age). For these hormones, all relevant details must be recorded or the results may prove uninterpretable.

Stress-related hormones

Stress-related hormones (e.g. catecholamines, prolactin, GH, ACTH and cortisol) may require samples to be taken via an indwelling needle some time after initial venepuncture; otherwise, high levels may be artefactual.

Urine collections

Collections over 24 hours have the advantage of providing an 'integrated mean' of a day's secretion but in practice are often incomplete or wrongly timed. They also vary with sex and body size or age. Written instructions should be provided for the patient to ensure accurate collection.

Saliva

Saliva is sometimes used for steroid estimations, especially in children.

Stimulation and suppression tests

These tests are used when basal levels give equivocal information. In general, stimulation tests are used to confirm suspected deficiency, and suppression tests to confirm suspected excess of hormone secretion. These tests are valuable in many instances.

For example, where the secretory capacity of a gland is damaged, maximal stimulation by the trophic hormone will give a diminished output. Thus, in the synacthen (SYNthetic-ACTH-en) test for adrenal reserve (Fig. 18.3(a) and Box 18.1), the healthy subject shows a normal response while the subject with primary hypoadrenalism (Addison's disease) demonstrates an impaired cortisol response to ACTH.

A patient with a hormone-producing tumour usually fails to show normal negative feedback. A patient with

Box 18.1 Short tetracosactide (synacthen) test

Indication
Diagnosis of Addison's disease
Screening test for ACTH deficiency

Procedure
Intravenous cannula for sampling
Any time of day, but best at 0900h; non-fasting
Tetracosactide 250 µg, i.v. or i.m. at time 0
Measure serum cortisol at time 0 and time +30 min

Normal response
30 min cortisol > 600nmol/L*
(400–600 nmol/L borderline and may indicate deficiency)

* Precise cortisol normal ranges are variable between laboratories and assays – appropriate local reference ranges must be used

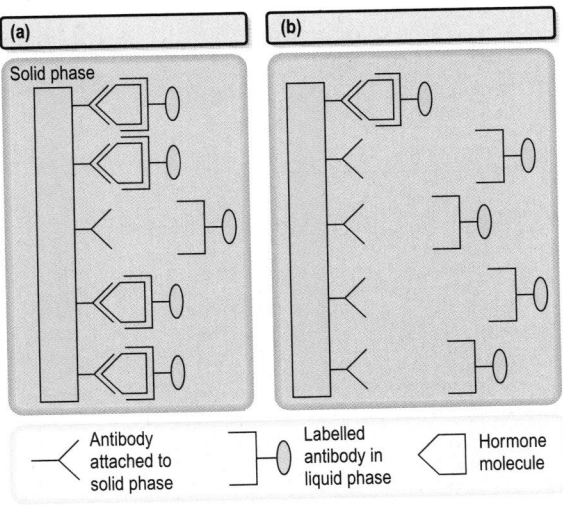

Fig. 18.4 Principles of measurement of hormone levels in plasma by immunoassay (precise details vary with different assays and manufacturers). Immunoassays use two antibodies specific to the hormone being measured – one typically attached to a solid phase and one labelled antibody in the liquid phase.
(a) High hormone levels in plasma: large amount of hormone binds to antibody on solid phase – large amount of labelled antibody linked to solid phase via molecules of the hormone.
(b) Low hormone levels in plasma: less hormone, and therefore less labelled antibody, is linked to the solid phase. Label (radioactive, chemiluminescent, enzymatic or fluorescent) can be measured in either solid or liquid phase after separation of phases; levels of label will be proportional to the amount of hormone in the sample.

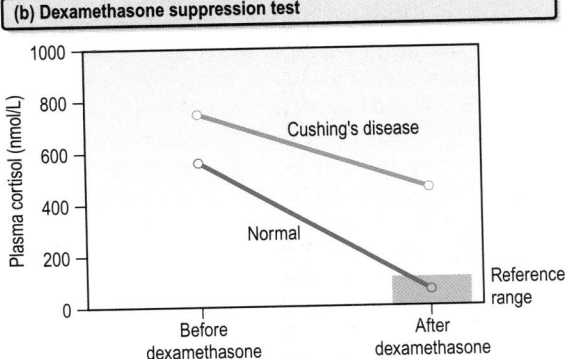

Fig. 18.3 Synacthen and dexamethasone tests.
(a) Short ACTH stimulation test showing a normal response in a healthy subject and a decreased response in a patient with Addison's disease.
(b) Dexamethasone suppression tests in a normal subject and in a patient with Cushing's disease showing inadequate suppression.

Cushing's disease (excess pituitary ACTH) will thus fail to suppress ACTH and cortisol production when given a dose of synthetic steroid, in contrast to normal subjects. Figure 18.3(b) shows the response of a normal subject given dexamethasone 1 mg at midnight; cortisol is suppressed the following morning. The subject with Cushing's disease shows inadequate suppression.

The detailed protocol for each test must be followed exactly, since even slight differences in technique will produce variations in results.

Measurement of hormone concentrations

Circulating levels of most hormones are very low (10^{-9}–10^{-12} mol/L) and cannot be measured by simple chemical techniques. Hormones are therefore usually measured by immunoassays which rely on highly specific antibodies (polyclonal or more usually monoclonal) which bind specifically to the hormone being measured during the assay incubation. This hormone–antibody interaction is measured by use of labelled hormone after separation of bound and free fractions (Fig. 18.4).

Immunoassay is sensitive but has limitations. In particular, the immunological activity of a hormone, as used in developing the antibody, may not necessarily correspond to biological activity. Other measurement techniques include high-pressure liquid chromatography (HPLC).

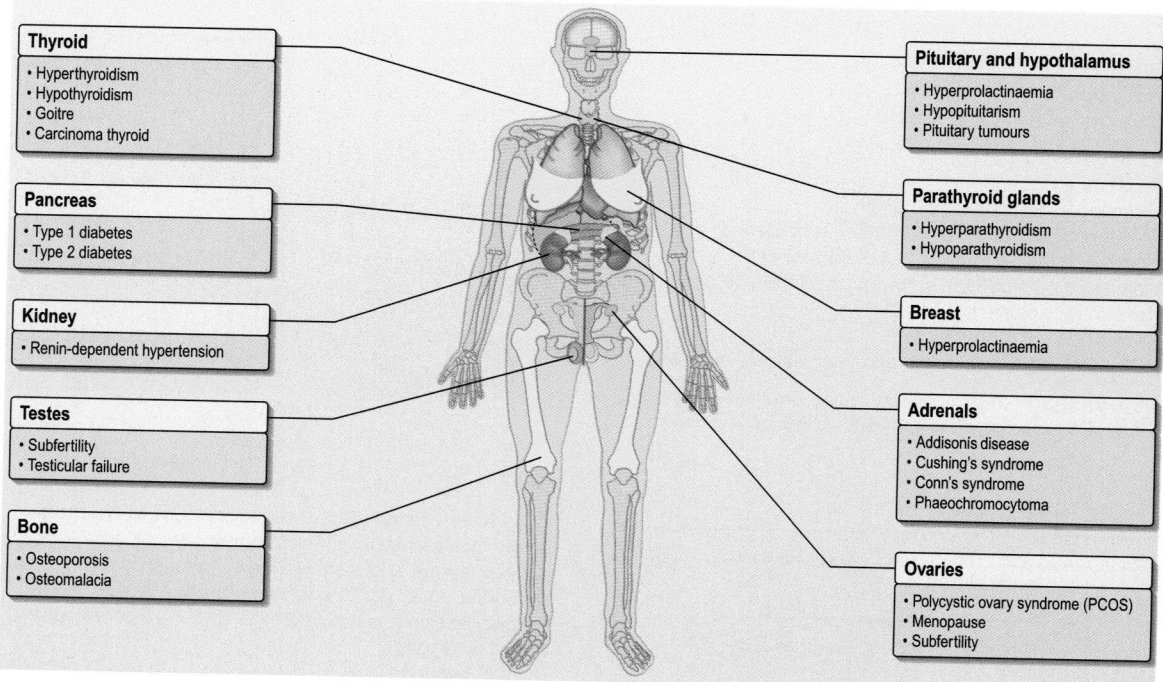

Thyroid • Hyperthyroidism • Hypothyroidism • Goitre • Carcinoma thyroid	**Pituitary and hypothalamus** • Hyperprolactinaemia • Hypopituitarism • Pituitary tumours
Pancreas • Type 1 diabetes • Type 2 diabetes	**Parathyroid glands** • Hyperparathyroidism • Hypoparathyroidism
Kidney • Renin-dependent hypertension	**Breast** • Hyperprolactinaemia
Testes • Subfertility • Testicular failure	**Adrenals** • Addison's disease • Cushing's syndrome • Conn's syndrome • Phaeochromocytoma
Bone • Osteoporosis • Osteomalacia	**Ovaries** • Polycystic ovary syndrome (PCOS) • Menopause • Subfertility

Fig. 18.5 The major endocrine organs and common endocrine problems.

ENDOCRINE DISEASE: AN INTRODUCTION

See Figure 18.5.

Epidemiology

The most common endocrine disorders, excluding diabetes mellitus (Ch. 19), are:

- thyroid disorders, affecting 4–8 new patients per primary care physician each year (the most common problems are thyrotoxicosis, primary hypothyroidism and goitre)
- subfertility, affecting 5–10% of all couples, often with an endocrine component
- menstrual disorders and excessive hair growth in young women, most commonly polycystic ovary syndrome (PCOS)
- osteoporosis, especially in postmenopausal women largely owing to gonadal steroid deficiency
- primary hyperparathyroidism, affecting about 0.1% of the population
- disorders of growth or puberty.

While most other endocrine conditions are uncommon, they often affect young people and are usually curable or completely controllable with appropriate therapy.

Hormones as therapy

Hormones are also widely used therapeutically:

- The oral contraceptive pill is the choice of perhaps 20–30% of women aged 18–35 years using contraception.

- Hormone replacement therapy (HRT; oestrogens ± progestogens) may be used for control of menopausal symptoms in postmenopausal women (see p. 1052).
- Corticosteroid therapy is widely used in non-endocrine disease such as asthma (see p. 918).

Symptoms

Hormones produce widespread effects upon the body, and states of deficiency or excess typically present with symptoms that are generalized rather than focused on the anatomical location of the gland. Many endocrine symptoms are diffuse and vague, and the differential diagnosis is often wide. Symptoms of tiredness, weakness or lack of energy or drive and changes in appetite or thirst are common presentations of endocrine disease, and other typical 'hormonal' symptoms include changes in body size and shape, problems with libido and potency, periods or sexual development, and changes in the skin (dry, greasy, acne, bruising, thinning, thickening) and hair (loss or excess). Endocrine disorders should be always considered when assessing any patient with these common complaints.

History and examination

A detailed history including the past, family and social history is essential for making the diagnosis, planning appropriate management and interpreting results of borderline hormonal blood tests. The past history should include previous surgery or radiation involving endocrine glands, menstrual history, pregnancy and growth in childhood. A full drug history is mandatory as endocrine problems are quite often iatrogenic (Table 18.3). Family history of autoimmune disease, endocrine disease

Table 18.3 Drugs and endocrine disease

Drug*	Effect
Drugs inducing endocrine disease	
Chlorpromazine	
Metoclopramide (and all dopamine antagonists)	Increase prolactin, causing galactorrhoea
Oestrogens	
Iodine	
Amiodarone	Hyperthyroidism
Lithium	
Amiodarone	Hypothyroidism
Chlorpropamide	Inappropriate ADH secretion
Ketoconazole	
Metyrapone, aminoglutethimide	Hypoadrenalism
Chemotherapy	Ovarian and testicular failure
Drugs simulating endocrine disease	
Sympathomimetics	
Amfetamines	Mimic thyrotoxicosis or phaeochromocytoma
Liquorice	Increase mineralocorticoid
Carbenoxolone	activity; mimic aldosteronism
Purgatives	Hypokalaemia
Diuretics	Secondary aldosteronism
ACE inhibitors	Hypoaldosteronism
Drugs affecting hormone-binding proteins	
Anticonvulsants	Bind to TBG – decrease total T_4
Oestrogens	Raise TBG and CBG – increase total T_4/cortisol
Exogenous hormones or stimulating agents	
Use, abuse or misuse, by patient or doctor, of the following:	
Steroids	Cushing's syndrome Diabetes
Thyroxine	Thyrotoxicosis factitia
Vitamin D preparations	
Milk and alkali preparations	Hypercalcaemia
Insulin	
Sulphonylureas	Hypoglycaemia

*Drugs causing gynaecomastia are listed in Table 18.15
Amiodarone may cause both hypo- or hyperthyroidism

including tumours, diabetes and cardiovascular disease is frequently relevant, and knowledge of family members' height, weight, body habitus, hair growth and age of sexual development may aid interpretation of the patient's own symptoms.

Physical signs are listed under the relevant systems.

Aetiology of endocrine disease

Aetiological mechanisms common to many endocrine disorders include:

Autoimmune disease

Organ-specific autoimmune diseases can affect every major endocrine organ (Table 18.4). They are characterized by the presence of specific antibodies in the serum, often present years before clinical symptoms are evident. The conditions are usually more common in women and have a strong genetic component, often with an identical-twin concordance rate of 50% and with HLA associations (see individual diseases). Several of the autoantigens have been identified.

Endocrine tumours

Hormone-secreting tumours occur in all endocrine organs, most commonly pituitary, thyroid and parathyroid. Fortunately, they are more commonly benign than malignant. While often considered to be 'autonomous' – that is, independent of the physiological control mechanisms – many do show evidence of feedback occurring at a higher 'set-point' than normal (e.g. ACTH secretion from a pituitary basophil adenoma).

The molecular basis of some of these tumours is sometimes a very specific mutation of a single gene, such as the mutations of the *Ret*-proto-oncogene in MEN 2 (see p. 1099), but more commonly a wide variety of different lesions in tumour suppressor genes, growth factor receptors and other intracellular mediators have been identified.

Enzymatic defects

The biosynthesis of most hormones involves many stages. Deficient or abnormal enzymes can lead to absent or reduced production of the secreted hormone. In general, severe deficiencies present early in life with obvious signs; partial deficiencies usually present later with mild signs or are only evident under stress. An example of an enzyme deficiency is congenital adrenal hyperplasia (CAH). Again the molecular basis has usually been identified as mutations or deletions of the gene encoding the relevant enzymes.

Receptor abnormalities (see p. 158)

Hormones work by activating cellular receptors. There are rare conditions in which hormone secretion and control are normal but the receptors are defective; thus, if androgen receptors are defective, normal levels of androgen will not produce masculinization (e.g. testicular feminization). There are also a number of rare syndromes of diabetes and insulin resistance from receptor abnormalities (p. 1103); other examples include nephrogenic diabetes insipidus, thyroid hormone resistance and pseudohypoparathyroidism.

CENTRAL CONTROL OF ENDOCRINE FUNCTION

Anatomy

Many peripheral hormone systems are controlled by the hypothalamus and pituitary. The hypothalamus is sited at the base of the brain around the third ventricle and above the pituitary stalk, which leads down to the pituitary

Table 18.4 Types of autoimmune disease affecting endocrine organs

Organ and frequency if known	Antibody	Antigen if known	Clinical syndrome
Stimulating			
Thyroid (1 in 100)	Thyroid-stimulating immunoglobulin (TSI, TSAb)	TSH receptor	Graves' disease, neonatal thyrotoxicosis
Destructive			
Thyroid (1 in 100)	Thyroid microsomal Thyroglobulin	Thyroid peroxidase enzyme (TPO)	Primary hypothyroidism (myxoedema)
Adrenal (1 in 20 000)	Adrenal cortex	21-Hydroxylase enzyme	Primary hypoadrenalism (Addison's disease)
Pancreas (1 in 500)	Islet cell	GAD (see p. 1105)	Type 1 (insulin-dependent) diabetes
Stomach	Gastric parietal cell Intrinsic factor	Gastric parietal cell Intrinsic factor	Pernicious anaemia
Skin	Melanocyte	Melanocyte	Vitiligo
Ovary (1 in 500)	Ovary		Primary ovarian failure
Testis	Testis		Primary testicular failure
Parathyroid	Parathyroid chief cell	Parathyroid chief cell	Primary hypoparathyroidism
Pituitary	Pituitary-specific cells		Selective hypopituitarism (e.g. GH deficiency, diabetes insipidus)

Frequencies are approximate and refer to the population in Northern Europe
GAD, glutamic acid dehydrogenase
NB: Other related diseases include myasthenia gravis and autoimmune liver diseases

itself, carrying the hypophyseal–pituitary portal blood supply.

The anatomical relationships of the hypothalamus and pituitary (Fig. 18.6) include the optic chiasm just above the pituitary fossa; any expanding lesion from the pituitary or hypothalamus can thus produce visual field defects by pressure on the chiasm. Such upward expansion of the gland through the diaphragma sellae is termed 'suprasellar extension'. Lateral extension of pituitary lesions may involve the vascular and nervous structures in the cavernous sinus and may rarely reach the temporal lobe of the brain. The pituitary is itself encased in a bony box; any lateral, anterior or posterior expansion must cause bony erosion.

Embryologically, the anterior pituitary is formed from Rathke's pouch (ectodermal) which meets an out-pouching of the third ventricular floor which becomes the posterior pituitary.

Physiology

Hypothalamus

This contains many vital centres for such functions as appetite, thirst, thermal regulation and sleeping/waking. It acts as an integrator of many neural and endocrine inputs to control the release of pituitary hormone-releasing factors. It plays a role in the circadian rhythm, menstrual cyclicity, and responses to stress, exercise and mood.

Hypothalamic neurones secrete pituitary hormone-releasing and -inhibiting factors and hormones into the portal system which runs down the stalk to the pituitary. As well as the classical hormones described in Table 18.5, the hypothalamus also contains large amounts of other neuropeptides and neurotransmitters such as neuropeptide Y, vasoactive intestinal peptide (VIP) and nitric oxide that can also alter pituitary hormone secretion but whose role is less well defined.

Synthetic hypothalamic hormones and their antagonists are available for the testing of many aspects of endocrine function and for treatment.

Fig. 18.6 MR image of a sagittal section of the brain, showing the pituitary fossa and adjacent structures. (By kind permission of Dr Martin Jeffree.)

Table 18.5 Nomenclature and biochemistry of hypothalamic, pituitary and peripheral hormones

Hypothalamic hormones	Pituitary hormones	Peripheral hormones
Gonadotrophin-releasing hormone (GnRH, LHRH) (*Decapeptide*)	Luteinizing hormone (LH) Follicle-stimulating hormone (FSH) (*Two-chain* α, β *peptides*)	Oestrogens/androgens (*Steroid ring*)
Dopamine (prolactin inhibiting factor, PIF) (*Amine*)	Prolactin (PRL) (*Single chain peptide*)	–
Growth hormone-releasing hormone (GHRH) (*Peptide*) Somatostatin (GHRIH) (*Cyclic peptide*)	Growth hormone (GH) (*Peptide*)	Insulin-like growth factor-1 (IGF-1) (*Peptide*)
Thyrotrophin-releasing hormone (TRH) (*Tripeptide*)	Thyroid-stimulating hormone (TSH) (*Two-chain* α, β *peptide*)	Thyroxine (T_4), triiodothyronine (T_3) (*Thyronines*)
Corticotropin-releasing hormone (CRH) (*Single-chain peptide*)	Adrenocorticotrophic hormone (ACTH) (*Single-chain peptide*)	Cortisol (*Steroid ring*)
Vasopressin (antidiuretic hormone; ADH) (*Nonapeptide*)	–	–
Oxytocin (*Nonapeptide*)	–	–

NB: The α chains of LH, FSH and TSH are identical
GHRIH, growth hormone release inhibitory hormone

Anterior pituitary

Hormone secretion is controlled by hypothalamic releasing or inhibitory hormones (Table 18.5 and Fig. 18.7). Many hormones are under dual control by both stimulatory and inhibitory hypothalamic factors. Examples are:

- Growth hormone release is stimulated by growth hormone-releasing hormone (GHRH) but inhibited by somatostatin (growth hormone release inhibitory hormone, GHRIH).
- TSH release is stimulated by TRH but partially inhibited by somatostatin.

Some hormones have a dual stimulatory control. For example, corticotropin-releasing hormone (CRH) and vasopressin are both endogenous stimulators of ACTH

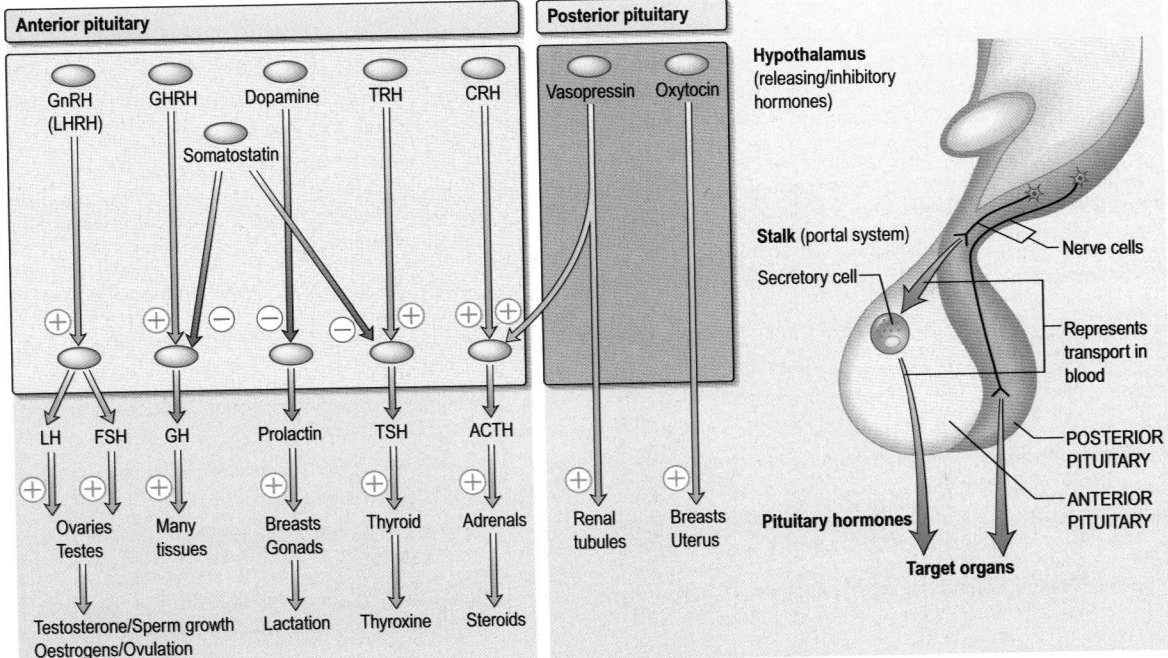

Fig. 18.7 **Hypothalamic releasing hormones and the pituitary trophic hormones.** See the text for abbreviations and an explanation.

release. Uniquely, prolactin is under predominant inhibitory dopaminergic control with some stimulatory TRH control.

Posterior pituitary

This, in contrast, acts merely as a storage organ. Antidiuretic hormone (ADH, vasopressin) and oxytocin, both nonapeptides, are synthesized in the supraoptic and paraventricular nuclei in the anterior hypothalamus. They are then transported along the axon and stored in the posterior pituitary. This means that damage to the stalk or pituitary alone does not prevent synthesis and release of ADH and oxytocin. ADH is discussed on page 1089; oxytocin produces milk ejection and uterine myometrial contraction.

PRESENTATIONS OF HYPOTHALAMIC AND PITUITARY DISEASE

Diseases of the pituitary can cause under- or overactivity of each of the hypothalamo-pituitary–end-organ axes which are under the control of this gland. The clinical features of the syndromes associated with such altered pituitary function can be the presenting symptom of pituitary disease and are discussed later in sections related to the respective hormone axis. First, however, we consider clinical features of pituitary disease which are common to all hormonal axes.

Pituitary space-occupying lesions and tumours

Pituitary tumours (Table 18.6) are the most common cause of pituitary disease, and the great majority of these are benign pituitary adenomas, usually monoclonal in origin. Problems may be caused by excess hormone secretion, by local effects of a tumour, or as the result of inadequate production of hormone by the remaining normal pituitary – hypopituitarism.

Investigations

The investigation of a possible or proven tumour follows three lines.

Is there a tumour?

If there is, how big is it and what local anatomical effects is it exerting? Pituitary and hypothalamic space-occupying lesions, hormonally active or not, can cause symptoms by pressure on, or infiltration of:

- the visual pathways, with field defects and visual loss, and more rarely:
- the cavernous sinus, with III, IV and VI cranial nerve lesions
- bony structures and the meninges surrounding the fossa, causing headache
- hypothalamic centres: altered appetite, obesity, thirst, somnolence/wakefulness or precocious puberty
- the ventricles, causing interruption of cerebrospinal fluid (CSF) flow leading to hydrocephalus
- the sphenoid sinus with invasion causing CSF rhinorrhoea.

Investigations:

- **Lateral skull X-ray.** This may show enlargement of the fossa. Although an X-ray is rarely requested as a definitive investigation, this remains a common incidental finding.
- **Visual fields.** These should be plotted formally by automated computer perimetry or Goldmann perimetry, but clinical assessment by confrontation using a small red pin as target is also sensitive and valuable. Common defects are upper-temporal quadrantanopia and bitemporal hemianopia (see p. 1179). Subtle defects may also be revealed by delay or attenuation of visual evoked potentials (VEPs).

Table 18.6 Characteristics of common pituitary and related tumours

Tumour or condition	Usual size	Most common clinical presentation
Prolactinoma	Most < 10 mm (microprolactinoma)	Galactorrhoea, amenorrhoea, hypogonadism, erectile dysfunction
	Some > 10 mm (macroprolactinoma)	As above plus headaches, visual field defects and hypopituitarism
Acromegaly	Few mm to several cm	Change in appearance, visual field defects and hypopituitarism
Cushing's disease	Most small – few mm (some cases are hyperplasia)	Central obesity, cushingoid appearance (local symptoms rare)
Nelson's syndrome	Often large – > 10 mm	Post-adrenalectomy, pigmentation, sometimes local symptoms
Non-functioning tumours	Usually large – > 10 mm	Visual field defects; hypopituitarism (microadenomas may be incidental finding)
Craniopharyngioma	Often very large and cystic (skull X-ray abnormal in > 50%; calcification common)	Headaches, visual field defects, growth failure (50% occur below age 20; about 15% arise from within sella)

(a)   (b)   (c)

Fig. 18.8 **(a) Coronal MRI of pituitary**, showing a left-sided lucent intrasellar microadenoma (arrowed). The pituitary stalk is deviated slightly to the right. **(b) Coronal MRI of pituitary**, showing macroadenoma with moderate suprasellar extension, and lateral extension compressing left cavernous sinus. The top of the adenoma is compressing the optic chiasm (arrowed). **(c) Sagittal MRI of head**, showing a pituitary macroadenoma with massive suprasellar extension (arrows).

- **MRI of the pituitary.** MRI is superior to CT scanning (Fig. 18.8) and will readily show any significant pituitary mass. However, small lesions within the pituitary fossa on MRI consistent with small pituitary microadenomas are very common, reported in as many as 10% of normal individuals in some studies. Such small lesions are sometimes detected during MRI scanning of the head for other reasons – so-called 'pituitary incidentalomas'.

Is there a hormonal excess?

There are three major conditions usually caused by secretion from pituitary adenomas which will show positive immunostaining for the relevant hormone:

- prolactin excess (prolactinoma or hyperprolactinaemia) – histologically, prolactinomas are 'chromophobe' adenomas (a description of their appearance on classical histological staining)
- GH excess, leading to acromegaly or gigantism – somatotroph adenomas, usually 'acidophil', and sometimes due to specific G-protein mutations (see p. 156)
- Cushing's disease and Nelson's syndrome (excess ACTH secretion) – corticotroph adenomas, usually 'basophil'.

Many tumours are able to synthesize several pituitary hormones, and occasionally more than one hormone is secreted in clinically significant excess (e.g. both GH and prolactin).

The clinical features of acromegaly, Cushing's disease or hyperprolactinaemia are usually (but not always) obvious, and are discussed on pages 1068, 1085, and 1062. Hyperprolactinaemia may be clinically 'silent'. Tumours producing LH, FSH or TSH are well described but very rare.

Some pituitary tumours cause no clinically apparent hormone excess and are referred to as 'non-functioning' tumours, which are common and usually 'chromophobe' adenomas. Laboratory studies such as immunocytochemistry show that these tumours may often produce LH and FSH or the α-subunit of LH, FSH and TSH (see Table 18.5), and occasionally ACTH.

Is there a deficiency of any hormone?

Clinical examination may give clues; thus, short stature in a child with a pituitary tumour is likely to be due to GH deficiency. A slow, lethargic adult with pale skin is likely to be deficient in TSH and/or ACTH. Milder deficiencies may not be obvious, and require specific testing (see Table 18.9).

Treatment

Treatment depends on the type and size of tumour (Table 18.7) and is discussed in more detail in the relevant sections (acromegaly, see p. 1069; prolactinoma, see p. 1063). In general, therapy has three aims:

Removal/control of tumour

Surgery via the trans-sphenoidal route is usually the treatment of choice. Very large tumours are occasionally removed via the open transfrontal route.

Radiotherapy – by an external three-beam technique, stereotactic or rarely via implant of yttrium needles – is usually employed when surgery is impracticable or incomplete, as it controls but rarely abolishes tumour mass. The standard regimen involves a dose of about 45 Gy, given as 20–25 fractions via three fields.

Octreotide or dopamine agonists sometimes cause shrinkage of specific types of tumour (see p. 1069).

Reduction of excess hormone secretion

Reduction is usually obtained by surgical removal but sometimes by medical treatment. Useful control can be achieved with dopamine agonists for prolactinomas or somatostatin analogues for acromegaly, but ACTH secretion usually cannot be controlled by medical means. Growth hormone antagonists are available for acromegaly (p. 1069).

Replacement of hormone deficiencies

Replacement of hormone deficiencies is detailed in Table 18.10.

Small tumours producing no significant symptoms, pressure or endocrine effects may be observed with

Table 18.7 Comparisons of primary treatments for pituitary tumours

Treatment method	Advantages	Disadvantages
Surgical		
Trans-sphenoidal adenomectomy or hypophysectomy	Relatively minor procedure Potentially curative for microadenomas and smaller macroadenomas	Some extrasellar extensions may not be accessible Risk of CSF leakage and meningitis
Transfrontal	Good access to suprasellar region	Major procedure; danger of frontal lobe damage High chance of subsequent hypopituitarism
Radiotherapy		
External (40–50 Gy)	Non-invasive Reduces recurrence rate after surgery	Slow action, often over many years Not always effective Possible late risk of tumour induction
Stereotactic	Precise administration of high dose to lesion	Long-term follow-up data limited
Yttrium implantation	High local dose	Only ever used in a few centres
Medical		
Dopamine agonist therapy (e.g. bromocriptine)	Non-invasive; reversible	Usually not curative Significant side-effects in minority
Somatostatin analogue therapy (octreotide, lanreotide)	Non-invasive; reversible	Usually not curative; expensive; side-effects
Growth hormone receptor antagonist (pegvisomant)	Highly selective	Usually not curative

appropriate clinical, visual field, imaging and endocrine assessments.

Differential diagnosis of pituitary or hypothalamic masses

Although pituitary adenomas are the most common mass lesion of the pituitary, a variety of other conditions may also present as a pituitary or hypothalamic mass and form part of the differential diagnosis.

Other tumours

Craniopharyngioma, a usually cystic hypothalamic tumour, which is often calcified, arising from Rathke's pouch often mimics an intrinsic pituitary lesion. It is the most common pituitary tumour in children but may present at any age.

Uncommon tumours include meningiomas, gliomas, chondromas, germinomas and pinealomas. Secondary deposits occasionally present as apparent pituitary tumours, typically presenting with headache and diabetes insipidus.

Hypophysitis and other inflammatory masses

A variety of inflammatory masses may occur in the pituitary or hypothalamus. These include rare pituitary-specific conditions (e.g. postpartum hypophysitis, lympho-cytic hypophysitis, giant cell hypophysitis), or pituitary manifestations of more generalized disease processes (sarcoidosis, Langerhans' cell histiocytosis, Wegener's granulomatosis).

Other lesions

Carotid artery aneurysms may masquerade as pituitary tumours. Cystic lesions may also present as a pituitary mass, including arachnoid and Rathke cleft cysts.

Hypopituitarism

Pathophysiology

Deficiency of hypothalamic releasing hormones or of pituitary trophic hormones is either selective or multiple. There are, for example, rare isolated deficiencies of LH/FSH and ACTH, some of which may be congenital, autoimmune or idiopathic in nature.

Multiple deficiencies usually result from tumour growth or other destructive lesions. There is generally a progressive loss of anterior pituitary function, usually in the order shown from left to right in Figure 18.7. GH and gonadotrophins are usually first affected. Hyper-prolactinaemia, rather than prolactin deficiency, occurs relatively early because of loss of tonic inhibitory control by dopamine. TSH and ACTH are usually last to be affected. *Panhypopituitarism* refers to deficiency of all anterior pituitary hormones; it is most commonly caused by pituitary tumours, surgery or radiotherapy. Multiple deficiencies can also rarely result from congenital defects, e.g. mutation of the gene for the pituitary-specific transcription factor 'Pit-1' causes deficiency in GH, prolactin and TSH.

Vasopressin and oxytocin secretion will be signi-ficantly affected only if the hypothalamus is involved, either by a hypothalamic tumour or by major supra-sellar extension of a pituitary lesion. Posterior pituitary deficiency is rare in an uncomplicated pituitary adenoma.

Causes

Disorders causing hypopituitarism are listed in Table 18.8. Pituitary and hypothalamic tumours, and surgical or radiotherapy treatment, are the most common.

Table 18.8 Causes of hypopituitarism

Congenital	Traumatic
Isolated deficiency of pituitary hormones (e.g. Kallmann's syndrome)	Skull fracture through base Surgery, especially transfrontal Perinatal trauma
Pit-1 deficiency	**Infiltrations**
Infective	Sarcoidosis
Basal meningitis (e.g. tuberculosis)	Langerhans' cell histiocytosis Hereditary haemochromatosis
Encephalitis	Hypophysitis
Syphilis	Postpartum
Vascular	Lymphocytic
Pituitary apoplexy	Giant cell
Sheehan's syndrome (postpartum necrosis)	**Others**
Carotid artery aneurysms	Radiation damage
Immunological	Fibrosis Chemotherapy
Pituitary antibodies	Empty sella syndrome
Neoplastic	**'Functional'**
Pituitary or hypothalamic tumours	Anorexia nervosa Starvation
Craniopharyngioma	Emotional deprivation
Meningiomas	
Gliomas	
Pinealoma	
Secondary deposits, especially breast	
Lymphoma	

Clinical features

Symptoms and signs depend upon the extent of hypothalamic and/or pituitary deficiencies, and mild deficiencies may not lead to any complaint by the patient. In general, symptoms of deficiency of a pituitary-stimulating hormone are the same as primary deficiency of the peripheral endocrine gland (e.g. TSH deficiency and primary hypothyroidism cause similar symptoms due to lack of thyroid hormone secretion). Thus, secondary hypothyroidism and adrenal failure both lead to tiredness and general malaise; hypothyroidism may cause slowness of thought and action, dry skin and cold intolerance, while hypoadrenalism may cause mild hypotension, hyponatraemia and ultimately cardiovascular collapse during severe intercurrent stressful illness. Loss of libido, loss of secondary sexual hair, amenorrhoea and impotence are symptoms of gonadotrophin and thus gonadal deficiencies, while hyperprolactinaemia may cause galactorrhoea and hypogonadism. GH deficiency may be relatively clinically 'silent' except in children, but may cause markedly impaired well-being in some adults. Weight may increase (due to hypothyroidism) or decrease in severe combined deficiency (pituitary cachexia). Long-standing panhypopituitarism gives the classic picture of pallor with hairlessness ('alabaster skin').

Particular syndromes related to hypopituitarism are:

Kallmann's syndrome

This syndrome is isolated gonadotrophin (GnRH) deficiency (p. 1055).

Sheehan's syndrome

This situation, now rare, is pituitary infarction following postpartum haemorrhage.

Pituitary apoplexy

A pituitary tumour occasionally enlarges rapidly owing to infarction or haemorrhage. This may produce severe headache and sudden severe visual loss sometimes followed by acute life-threatening hypopituitarism.

The 'empty sella' syndrome

An 'empty sella' is sometimes reported on pituitary imaging. This is sometimes due to a defect in the diaphragma and extension of the subarachnoid space (cisternal herniation) or may follow spontaneous infarction of a tumour. All or most of the sella turcica is devoid of apparent pituitary tissue, but, despite this, pituitary function is usually normal, the pituitary being eccentrically placed and flattened against the floor or roof of the fossa.

Investigations

Each axis of the hypothalamic–pituitary system requires separate investigation. However, the presence of normal gonadal function (ovulatory/menstruation or normal libido/erections) suggests that multiple defects of anterior pituitary function are unlikely.

Tests range from the simple basal levels (e.g. free T_4 for the thyroid axis), to stimulatory tests for the pituitary, and tests of feedback for the hypothalamus (Table 18.9). Assessment of the hypothalamo-pituitary–adrenal axis remains critical but controversial: basal 0900h cortisol levels above 400 nmol/L usually indicate an adequate reserve, while levels below 100 nmol/L predict an inadequate stress response. In many cases basal levels are equivocal and a dynamic test is essential: the insulin tolerance test (Box 18.2) is widely regarded as the 'gold standard' but the synacthen test (see Box 18.1), though an indirect measure, is used by many as a routine test of hypothalamic–pituitary–adrenal status. Overall, the assessment of adrenal reserve is best left to an endocrinologist.

Treatment

Steroid and thyroid hormones are essential for life. Both are given as oral replacement drugs, as in primary thyroid and adrenal deficiency, aiming to restore the patient to clinical and biochemical normality (Table 18.10) and levels may be monitored by routine hormone assays. Sex hormone production is replaced with androgens and oestrogens, both for symptomatic control and to prevent long-term problems related to deficiency (e.g. osteoporosis). When fertility is desired, gonadal function may be stimulated directly by human chorionic gonadotrophin (HCG, mainly acting as LH), purified or biosynthetic gonadotrophins, or indirectly by pulsatile gonadotrophin-releasing hormone (GnRH – also known as luteinizing hormone-releasing hormone, LHRH); all are expensive and time-consuming and should be restricted to specialist units.

Table 18.9 Tests for hypothalamic–pituitary (HP) function

- All hormone levels are measured in plasma unless otherwise stated.
- Tests **shown in bold** are those normally measured on a single basal 0900h sample in the initial assessment of pituitary function.

Axis	Basal investigations		Common dynamic tests	Other tests
	Pituitary hormone	End-organ product/function		
Anterior pituitary				
HP-ovarian	**LH** **FSH**	**Estradiol** Progesterone (day 21 of cycle)		Ovarian ultrasound LHRH test*
HP-testicular	**LH** **FSH**	**Testosterone**		Sperm count LHRH test*
Growth	GH	IGF-1 IGF-BP3	Insulin tolerance test	GH response to sleep, exercise or arginine infusion GHRH test*
Prolactin	**Prolactin**	**Prolactin**	–	–
HP-thyroid	**TSH**	**Free T$_4$**, T$_3$		TRH test*
HP-adrenal	ACTH	**Cortisol**	Insulin tolerance test Short synacthen (tetracosactide) test	Glucagon test CRH test* Metyrapone test
Posterior pituitary				
Thirst and osmoregulation		**Plasma/urine osmolality**	Water deprivation test	Hypertonic saline infusion

*Releasing hormone tests were a traditional part of pituitary function testing, but have been largely replaced by the advent of more reliable assays for basal hormones. They test only the 'readily releasable pool' of pituitary hormones and normal responses may be seen in hypopituitarism

Box 18.2 Insulin tolerance test

Indication

Diagnosis or exclusion of ACTH and growth hormone deficiency

Procedure

Should only be performed in experienced, specialist units

Exclude cardiovascular disease (ECG), epilepsy or unexplained blackouts; exclude severe untreated hypopituitarism (basal cortisol must be > 100 nmol/L; normal free T$_4$)

Intravenous hydrocortisone and glucose available for emergency

Overnight fast, begin at 0800–0900h

Soluble insulin, 0.15 Units/kg, i.v. at time 0

Glucose, cortisol and GH at 0, 30, 45, 60, 90, 120 min

Normal response

Cortisol rises above 550 nmol/L*

GH rises above 20 mU/L (severe deficiency = < 9 mU/L (3 ng/L))

Glucose must be < 2.2 mmol/L to achieve adequate stress response

*Precise cortisol normal ranges are variable between laboratories and assays – appropriate local reference ranges must be used

Table 18.10 Replacement therapy for hypopituitarism

Axis	Usual replacement therapies
Adrenal	Hydrocortisone 15–40 mg daily (starting dose 10 mg on rising/5 mg lunchtime/5 mg evening) (Normally no need for mineralocorticoid replacement)
Thyroid	Thyroxine 100–150 µg daily
Gonadal	
Male	Testosterone intramuscularly, orally, transdermally or implant
Female	Cyclical oestrogen/progestogen orally or as patch
Fertility	HCG plus FSH (purified or recombinant) or pulsatile GnRH to produce testicular development, spermatogenesis or ovulation
Growth	Recombinant human GH used routinely to achieve normal growth in children Also advocated for replacement therapy in adults where GH has effects on muscle mass and well-being
Thirst	Desmopressin 10–20 µg one to three times daily by nasal spray or orally 100–200 µg three times daily Carbamazepine and thiazides are rarely used in mild diabetes insipidus
Breast (Prolactin inhibition)	Dopamine agonist (e.g. cabergoline, 500 µg weekly)

GH therapy is given in the growing child, under the care of a paediatric endocrinologist. In adult GH deficiency, GH therapy also produces improvements in body composition, work capacity and psychological well-being, together with reversal of lipid abnormalities associated with a high cardiovascular risk, and this may result in significant symptomatic benefit in some cases. Although symptomatically helpful in many patients and now licensed for such use in most countries, the long-term safety and efficacy of GH therapy in adults is not yet fully established, and its cost is £2500–6000 per annum.

Two points should be noted:

- Thyroid replacement should not commence until normal glucocorticoid function has been demonstrated or replacement steroid therapy initiated, as an adrenal 'crisis' may otherwise be precipitated.
- Glucocorticoid deficiency may mask impaired urine concentrating ability, diabetes insipidus only becoming apparent after steroid replacement.

FURTHER READING

Brook AM, Monson JP (2003) Adult growth hormone deficiency. *Clinical Medicine*, **3**: 15–19.

Lamberts SWJ, de Herder WW, van der Lely AJ (1998) Pituitary insufficiency. *Lancet* **352**: 127–134.

National Institute for Clinical Excellence (2003) Human growth hormone (somatotropin) in adults with growth hormone deficiency: Technology appraisal 64. Online. Available: http://www.nice.org.uk/pdf/TA64_HGHadults_fullguidance.pdf.

REPRODUCTION AND SEX

The normal physiology of the female and male reproductive systems will be considered first, followed by their common disorders. Some relevant terminology is set out in Box 18.3.

Embryology

Up to 8 weeks of gestation the sexes share a common development, with a primitive genital tract including the Wolffian and Müllerian ducts. There are additionally a primitive perineum and primitive gonads.

In the presence of a Y chromosome the potential testis develops while the ovary regresses.

In the absence of a Y chromosome, the potential ovary develops and related ducts form a uterus and the upper vagina.

Production of Müllerian inhibitory factor from the early 'testis' produces atrophy of the Müllerian duct, while, under the influence of testosterone and dihydrotestosterone, the Wolffian duct differentiates into an epididymis, vas

Box 18.3 Definitions in reproductive medicine

Menarche	Age at first period
Primary amenorrhoea	Failure to begin spontaneous menstruation by age 16
Secondary amenorrhoea	Absence of menstruation for 3 months in a woman who has previously had cycles
Oligomenorrhoea	Irregular long cycles; often used for any length of cycle above 32 days
Dyspareunia	Pain or discomfort in the female during intercourse
Libido	Sexual interest or desire; often difficult to assess and is greatly affected by stress, tiredness and psychological factors
Menstruation	Onset of spontaneous (usually regular) uterine bleeding in the female
Impotence (erectile dysfunction)	Inability of the male to achieve or sustain an erection adequate for satisfactory intercourse
Azoospermia	Absence of sperm in the ejaculate
Oligospermia	Reduced numbers of sperm in the ejaculate; normal values are disputed
Virilization	Occurrence of male secondary sexual characteristics in the female

deferens, seminal vesicles and prostate. Androgens induce transformation of the perineum to include a penis, penile urethra and scrotum containing the testes, which descend in response to androgenic stimulation. At birth, testicular volume is 0.5–1 mL.

PHYSIOLOGY

The male

An outline of the hypothalamic–pituitary–testicular axis is shown in Figure 18.9.

1. Pulses of GnRH (LHRH) are released from the hypothalamus and stimulate LH and FSH release from the pituitary.
2. LH stimulates testosterone production from Leydig cells of the testis.
3. Testosterone acts systemically to produce male secondary sexual characteristics, anabolism and the maintenance of libido. It also acts locally within the testis to aid spermatogenesis. Testosterone circulates largely bound to sex hormone-binding globulin (SHBG) (see p. 1036). Testosterone feeds back on the hypothalamus/pituitary to inhibit GnRH secretion.
4. FSH stimulates the Sertoli cells in the seminiferous tubules to produce mature sperm and the inhibins A and B.

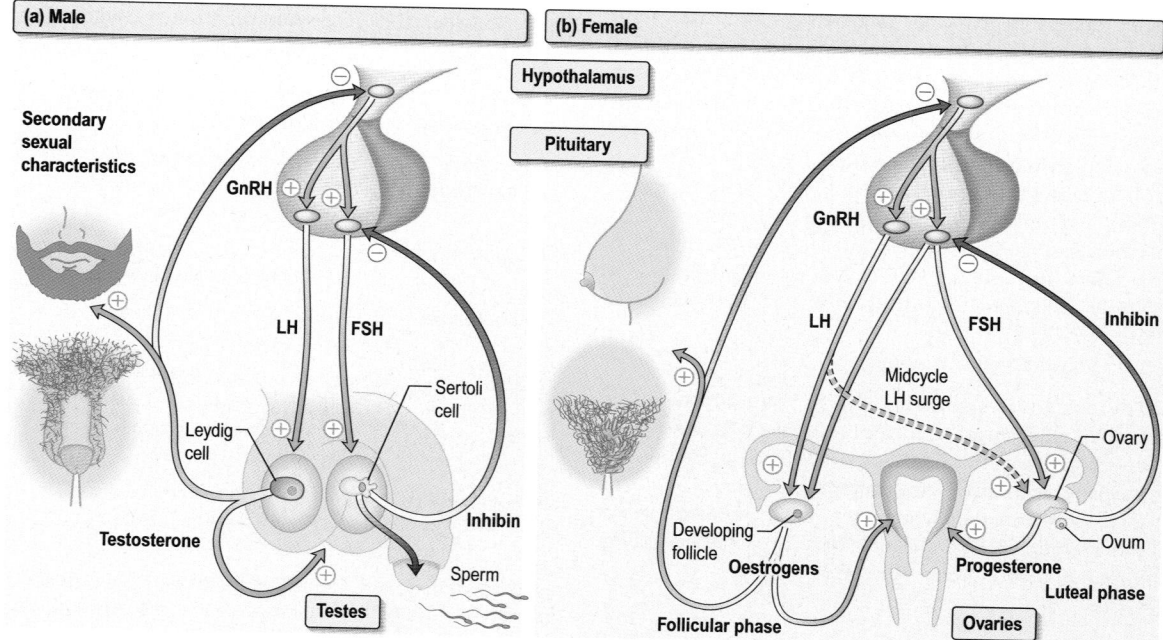

Fig. 18.9 **Male and female hypothalamic–pituitary–gonadal axes.** Note the close parallels. The positive and negative signs indicate feedback.

5. Inhibin causes feedback on the pituitary to decrease FSH secretion.

The secondary sexual characteristics of the male for which testosterone is necessary are the growth of pubic, axillary and facial hair, enlargement of the external genitalia, deepening of the voice, sebum secretion, muscle growth and frontal balding.

The female
The female situation is more complex (Figs 18.9 and 18.10).

1. In the adult female, higher brain centres impose a menstrual cycle of 28 days upon the activity of hypothalamic GnRH.
2. Pulses of GnRH, at about 2-hour intervals, stimulate release of pituitary LH and FSH.
3. LH stimulates ovarian androgen production by the ovarian theca cells.
4. FSH stimulates follicular development and aromatase activity (an enzyme required to convert ovarian androgens to oestrogens) in the ovarian granulosa cells. FSH also stimulates release of inhibin from ovarian stromal cells, which inhibits FSH release.
5. Although many follicles are 'recruited' for development in early folliculogenesis, by day 8–10 a 'leading' (or 'dominant') follicle is selected for development into a mature Graafian follicle.
6. Oestrogens show a double feedback action on the pituitary (Fig. 18.9), initially inhibiting gonadotrophin secretion (negative feedback), but later high-level exposure results in increased GnRH secretion and increased LH sensitivity to GnRH (positive feedback), which leads to the mid-cycle LH surge inducing ovulation from the leading follicle (Fig. 18.10).

7. The follicle then differentiates into a corpus luteum, which secretes both progesterone and estradiol during the second half of the cycle (luteal phase).
8. Oestrogen initially and then progesterone cause uterine endometrial proliferation in preparation for possible implantation; if implantation does not occur, the corpus luteum regresses and progesterone secretion and inhibin levels fall so that the endometrium is shed (menstruation) allowing increased GnRH and FSH secretion.

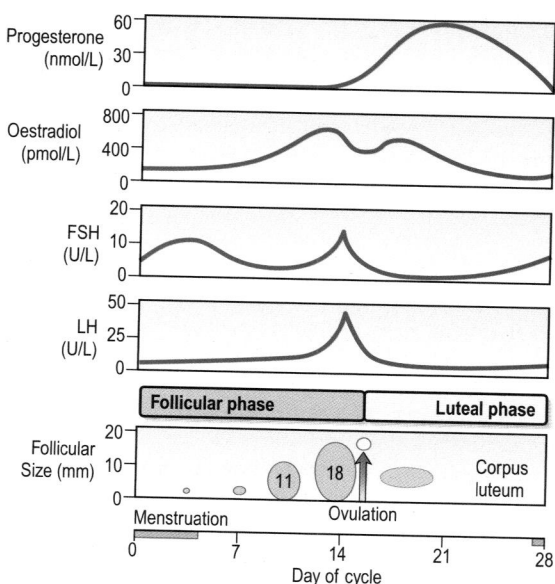

Fig. 18.10 **Hormonal and follicular changes during the normal menstrual cycle.**

9. If implantation and pregnancy follow, human chorionic gonadotrophin (HCG) production from the trophoblast maintains corpus luteum function until 10–12 weeks of gestation, by which time the placenta will be making sufficient oestrogen and progesterone to support itself.

Oestrogens also induce secondary sexual characteristics, especially development of the breast and nipples, vaginal and vulval growth and pubic hair development. They also induce growth and maturation of the uterus and Fallopian tubes. They circulate largely bound to SHBG.

Physiology of prolactin secretion

The hypothalamic–pituitary control of prolactin secretion is illustrated in Figure 18.11.

Prolactin is under tonic dopamine inhibition, while other factors known to increase prolactin secretion (e.g. TRH) are probably of less importance. Prolactin stimulates milk secretion but also reduces gonadal activity. It decreases GnRH pulsatility at the hypothalamic level and, to a lesser extent, blocks the action of LH on the ovary or testis, producing hypogonadism even when the pituitary gonadal axis itself is intact.

Puberty

The mechanisms initiating puberty are poorly understood but are thought to result from withdrawal of central inhibition of GnRH release. Environmental and physical factors are involved in the timing of puberty (including body fat changes, physical exercise) as well as genetic

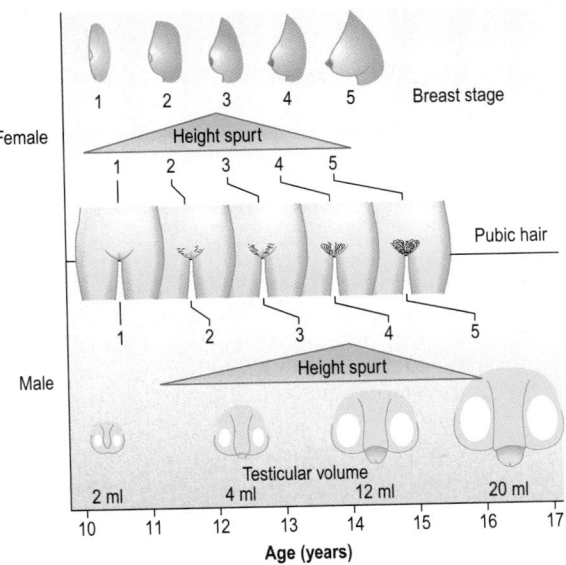

Fig. 18.12 **The age of development of features of puberty.** Stages and testicular size show mean ages, and all vary considerably between individuals. The same is true of height spurt, shown here in relation to other data. Numbers 2 to 5 indicate stages of development (see the text).

factors (e.g. a G protein-coupled receptor gene, *GPR 54*) required for pubertal maturation.

LH and FSH are both low in the prepubertal child. In early puberty, FSH begins to rise first, initially in nocturnal pulses; this is followed by a rise in LH with a subsequent increase in testosterone/oestrogen levels. The milestones of puberty in the two sexes are shown in Figure 18.12.

In boys, pubertal changes begin at between 10 and 14 years and are complete at between 15 and 17 years. The genitalia develop, testes enlarge and the area of pubic hair increases. Peak height velocity is reached between ages 12 and 17 years during stage 4 of testicular development. Full spermatogenesis occurs comparatively late.

In girls, events start a year earlier. Breast bud enlargement begins at ages 9–13 years and continues to 12–18 years. Pubic hair growth commences at ages 9–14 years and is completed at 12–16 years. Menarche occurs relatively late (age 11–15 years) but peak height velocity is reached earlier (at age 10–13 years), and growth is completed much earlier than in boys.

Precocious puberty

Development of secondary sexual characteristics, or menarche in girls, at or before the age of 9 years is premature. All cases require specialist assessment by a paediatric endocrinologist.

Idiopathic (true) precocity is most common in girls and very rare in boys. This is a diagnosis of exclusion. With no apparent cause for premature breast or pubic hair development, and an early growth spurt, it may be normal and may run in families. Treatment with long-acting GnRH analogues (given by nasal spray, by

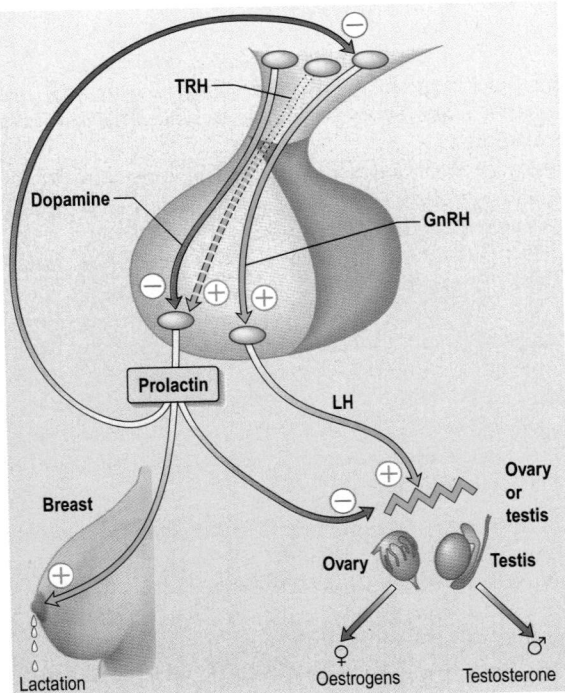

Fig. 18.11 **The control of prolactin secretion.**

subcutaneous injection or by implant) causes suppression of gonadotrophin release via downregulation of the receptor – and therefore reduced sex hormone production – and is moderately effective; cyproterone acetate, an anti-androgen with progestational activity, may also be used.

The following are other forms of precocity:

- *Cerebral precocity.* Many causes of hypothalamic disease, especially tumours, may present in this way. In boys this must be rigorously excluded. MRI scan is almost always indicated to exclude this diagnosis.
- *McCune–Albright syndrome.* This is usually in girls, with precocity, polyostotic fibrous dysplasia and skin pigmentation (café-au-lait). An activating mutation of the *GNAS1* gene encoding the α-subunit of Gs protein has been found.
- *Premature thelarche.* This is early breast development alone, usually transient, at age 2–4 years. It may regress or persist until puberty. There is no evidence of follicular development.
- *Premature adrenarche.* This is early development of pubic hair without significant other changes, usually after age 5 years and more commonly in girls.

Delayed puberty

Over 95% of children show signs of pubertal development by age 14 years. In its absence, investigation should begin by age 15 years. Causes of hypogonadism (see below) are clearly relevant but most cases represent constitutional delay.

In constitutional delay, pubertal development, bone age and stature are in parallel. A family history may confirm that other family members experienced the same delayed development, which is common in boys but very rare in girls.

In boys, a testicular volume > 5 mL indicates the onset of puberty. A rising serum testosterone is an earlier clue.

In girls, the breast bud is the first sign. Ultrasound allows accurate assessment of ovarian and uterine development.

Basal LH/FSH levels may identify the site of a defect, and GnRH (LHRH) tests can indicate the stage of early puberty.

If any progression into puberty is evident clinically, investigations are not required. When delay is great and problems are serious (e.g. severe teasing at school), low-dose short-term sex hormone therapy is used. Specialist assessment is advisable.

The menopause

The menopause, or cessation of periods, naturally occurs about the age of 45–55 years. During the late forties, FSH initially, and then LH concentrations begin to rise, probably as follicle supply diminishes. Oestrogen levels fall and the cycle becomes disrupted. Most women notice irregular scanty periods coming on over a variable period, though in some sudden amenorrhoea or menorrhagia occur. Eventually the menopausal pattern of low estradiol levels with grossly elevated LH and FSH levels (usually > 50 and > 25 U/L, respectively) is established. Menopause may also occur surgically, with radiotherapy to the ovaries and with ovarian disease (e.g. premature menopause).

Clinical features and treatment

Features of oestrogen deficiency are hot flushes (which occur in most women and can be disabling), vaginal dryness and atrophy of the breasts. There may also be vague symptoms of loss of libido, loss of self-esteem, non-specific aches and pains, irritability, depression, loss of concentration and weight gain.

Women show a rapid loss of bone density in the 10 years following the menopause (osteoporosis, see p. 594) and the premenopausal protection from ischaemic heart disease disappears.

Symptomatic patients should usually be treated but the previous widespread use of hormone replacement therapy (HRT) has been thrown into doubt by a number of large prospective studies which have reported in recent years. Although there is no universal agreement, the overall benefits and risks may be summarized as follows (percentages are from the Women's Health Initiative (WHI) study of 16 600 women):

- *Symptomatic improvement in most menopausal symptoms* for the majority of women. Oestrogen-deficient symptoms respond well to oestrogen replacement, the vaguer symptoms generally, but not always, less well. Vaginal symptoms respond to local oestrogen preparations.
- *Protection against fractures of wrist, spine and hip, secondary to osteoporosis (~24–33%)* (see Ch. 10), owing to protection of predominantly trabecular bone (p. 595).
- *A significant reduction in the risk of large bowel cancer (~33%).*
- *A significant increase in the risk of breast cancer (+26%)* – but no change in breast cancer mortality, and some studies suggest breast cancers diagnosed on HRT are easier to treat effectively. This increased risk has been disputed.
- *A significant increase in the risk of endometrial cancer* when unopposed oestrogens are given to women with a uterus.
- *A significant increase in the risk of ischaemic heart disease (+29%) and stroke (+41%).*
- The inconvenience of withdrawal bleeds, unless a hysterectomy has been performed or regimens which include continuous oestrogen and progesterone are used.
- *Other disputed effects* include possible reductions in the incidence of Alzheimer's disease and increase in general well-being.

Absolute risks and benefits for individual women clearly depend on their background risk of that disease, and there is as yet no evidence on the relative risks of different hormone preparations or routes of administration (oral, transdermal or implant). Overall, the WHI study estimated that, over 5 years of treatment, an extra 1 woman in every 100 would develop an illness that would not have occurred had she not been taking HRT. However, the decision about whether or not a woman takes HRT is now very much an individual decision based on the severity of that woman's menopausal symptoms, her personal risk of conditions which may be prevented or made more likely by HRT, and ultimately individual patient choice. For example, the decision is likely to be very different for a non-smoking 50-year-old with severe menopausal symptoms and a family history of osteoporosis, compared to a 60-year-old hypertensive smoker with mild symptoms and a family history of breast cancer. HRT is no longer recommended purely for prevention of postmenopausal osteoporosis in the absence of menopausal symptoms. Where symptomatic treatment is given, use of the lowest effective dose is now advocated, usually for short-term rather than long-term treatment. However, its exact place in therapy is still unclear.

Selective oestrogen receptor modulators, SERMs (e.g. raloxifene), offer a potentially attractive combination of positive oestrogen effects on bone and cardiovascular system with no effects on oestrogen receptors of uterus and breast and possible reduction in breast cancer incidence; long-term outcome studies, however, are still awaited.

Premature menopause

The most common cause of premature menopause in women (before age 40) is ovarian failure, which may be autoimmune or of unknown aetiology. Bilateral oophorectomy causes the same oestrogen-deficiency state. HRT should almost always be given, as the risk of osteoporosis and other conditions related to oestrogen deficiency almost always outweigh the risks at this younger age. HRT may still also be actively recommended when normal menopause occurs relatively early (e.g. before age 50).

The ageing male

In the male there is no sudden 'change of life'. However, there is a progressive loss in sexual function with reduction in morning erections and frequency of intercourse.

The age of onset varies widely, but overall testicular volume diminishes and sex hormone-binding globulin (SHBG) and gonadotrophin levels gradually rise. If premature hypogonadism is present for any reason, replacement testosterone therapy should be given to prevent osteoporosis (see p. 598). More widespread androgen replacement of the ageing male is under evaluation, primarily in the USA, with promising early results, but no long-term follow-up data are available.

Conversely, lowering of androgens forms part of the therapy of prostate hypertrophy and prostate cancer. Finasteride, an inhibitor of 5α-reductase, is used in benign prostatic hypertrophy. It prevents the conversion of testosterone to dihydrotestosterone, which causes prostatic hypertrophy, and is effective, though somewhat delayed in action (see p. 685). GnRH analogues are used to lower testosterone levels and induce disease remission in patients with prostate cancer.

FURTHER READING

Million Women Study Collaborators (2003) Breast cancer and HRT in the Million Women Study. *Lancet* **362**: 419–427.

Riggs BL, Hartmann LC (2003) Selective-estrogen-receptor modulators. *New England Journal of Medicine* **348**: 618–629.

Solomon CG, Dluhy RG (2003) Rethinking post-menopausal hormone therapy. *New England Journal of Medicine* **348**: 579–580.

CLINICAL FEATURES OF DISORDERS OF SEX AND REPRODUCTION

A detailed history and examination of all systems is required (Box 18.4). A man having regular satisfactory intercourse or a woman with regular ovulatory periods is most unlikely to have significant endocrine disease, assuming the history is accurate (check with the partner!).

Tests of gonadal function

Basal measurements of the gonadotrophins, oestrogens/testosterone and prolactin:

- *Low testosterone or estradiol with high gonadotrophins* indicates primary gonadal disease.
- *Low levels of LH/FSH and of testosterone/estradiol* imply hypothalamic–pituitary disease.
- Demonstration of *ovulation* (by measurement of luteal phase serum progesterone and/or by serial ovarian ultrasound in the follicular phase) or a healthy *sperm count* ($20–200 \times 10^6$/mL, > 60% grade I motility and < 20% abnormal forms), provide absolute confirmation of normal female or male reproductive endocrinology, but these tests are not always essential.
- Pregnancy provides complete demonstration of normal male and female function.
- *Hyperprolactinaemia* can be confirmed or excluded by direct measurement. Levels may increase with stress; ideally, a cannula should be inserted and samples taken through it 30 minutes later.

Box 18.4 **Sexual and menstrual disorders**

History
Menstruation – timing of bleeding and cycle
Relationship of symptoms to cycle
Breasts (tenderness/galactorrhoea)
Hirsutism and acne
Libido and potency
Problems with intercourse
Past fertility and future plans

Physical signs
Evidence of systemic disease
Secondary sexual characteristics
Extent/distribution of hair
Genital size (testes, ovaries, uterus)
Clitoromegaly
Breast development, gynaecomastia
Galactorrhoea

Table 18.11 Tests of gonadal function

Test	Uses/comments
Male	
Basal testosterone	Normal levels exclude hypogonadism
Sperm count	Normal count excludes deficiency
	Motility and abnormal sperm forms should be noted
Female	
Basal estradiol	Normal levels exclude hypogonadism
Luteal phase progesterone (days 18–24 of cycle)	If > 30 nmol/L, suggests ovulation
Ultrasound of ovaries	To confirm ovulation
Both sexes	
Basal LH/FSH	Demonstrates state of feedback system for hormone production (LH) and germ cell production (FSH)
HCG test (testosterone or estradiol measured)	Response shows potential of ovary or testis; failure demonstrates primary gonadal problem
Clomifene test (LH and FSH measured)	Tests hypothalamic negative feedback system; clomifene is oestrogen antagonist and causes LH/FSH to rise
LHRH test (rarely used)	Shows adequacy (or otherwise) of LH and FSH stores in pituitary

More detailed tests are indicated in Table 18.11.

DISORDERS IN THE MALE

Hypogonadism

Clinical features

Male hypogonadism may be a presenting complaint or an incidental finding, such as during investigation for subfertility. The testes may be small and soft. Except with subfertility, the symptoms are usually of androgen deficiency, primarily poor libido, impotence and loss of secondary sexual hair (Table 18.12) rather than deficiency of semen production. Sperm makes up only a very small proportion of seminal fluid volume.

Causes of male hypogonadism are shown in Table 18.13.

Investigations

Testicular disease may be immediately apparent but basal levels of testosterone, LH and FSH should be measured. These will allow the distinction between primary gonadal (testicular) failure and hypothalamic–pituitary disease to be made. Depending on the causes, semen analysis, chromosomal analysis (e.g. to exclude Klinefelter's syndrome) and bone age estimation are required.

Table 18.12 Effects of androgens and consequences of androgen deficiency in the male

Physiological effect	Consequences of deficiency
General	
Maintenance of libido	Loss of libido
Deepening of voice	High-pitched voice (if prepubertal)
Frontotemporal balding	No temporal recession
Facial, axillary and limb hair	Decreased hair
Maintenance of erectile and ejaculatory function	Loss of erections/ejaculation
Pubic hair	
Maintenance of male pattern	Thinning and loss of pubic hair
Testes and scrotum	
Maintenance of testicular size/consistency (needs gonadotrophins as well)	Small soft testes
Rugosity of scrotum	Poorly developed penis/scrotum
Stimulation of spermatogenesis	Subfertility
Musculoskeletal	
Epiphyseal fusion	Eunuchoidism (if prepubertal)
Maintenance of muscle bulk and power	Decreased muscle bulk
Maintenance of bone mass	Osteoporosis

Table 18.13 Causes of male hypogonadism

Reduced gonadotrophins (hypothalamic–pituitary disease)
Hypopituitarism
Selective gonadotrophic deficiency (Kallmann's syndrome)
Severe systemic illness
Severe underweight

Hyperprolactinaemia

Primary gonadal disease (congenital)
Anorchia/Leydig cell agenesis
Cryptorchism (testicular maldescent)
Chromosome abnormality (e.g. Klinefelter's syndrome)
Enzyme defects: 5α-reductase deficiency

Primary gonadal disease (acquired)
Testicular torsion
Orchidectomy
Local testicular disease
Chemotherapy/radiation toxicity
Orchitis (e.g. mumps)
Renal failure
Cirrhosis/alcohol
Sickle cell disease

Androgen receptor deficiency/abnormality

In clear-cut gonadotrophin deficiency, pituitary MRI scan, prolactin levels and other pituitary function tests are needed. However, equivocal lowering of serum testosterone (7–10 nmol/L) without elevation of gonadotrophins is a relatively common biochemical finding, and

Table 18.14 Androgen replacement therapy

Preparation	Dose	Route	Remarks
Testosterone mixed esters			Usual first-line maintenance therapy
Testosterone enanthate	250 mg × every 3 weeks	IM	Injection can be painful
Testosterone propionate	50–100 mg 2–3 × weekly	IM	Frequent injections needed as half-life is short
			Good initial therapy
Testosterone undecanoate	80–240 mg daily, in divided doses	Oral	Variable dose, irregular absorption
Testosterone implant	600 mg every 4–5 months	Implant	Requires implant procedure
Testosterone transdermal	2.5–7.5 mg/24 h	Dermal	Patch or gel preparations

is a frequent cause of referral in men with poor libido or erectile dysfunction. Such tests are compatible with mild gonadotrophin deficiency, but may also be seen in acute illness of any cause and often simply represent the lower end of the normal range or the normal circadian rhythm of testosterone when bloods are checked in afternoon or evening surgeries. A therapeutic trial of testosterone replacement is often justified and forms part of the investigation in many patients; full pituitary evaluation may be required in such cases to exclude other pituitary disease. 'Anabolic' steroid (i.e. androgen) abuse causes similar biochemical findings, and an index of suspicion is required if the patient appears well virilized.

Treatment

The cause can rarely be reversed. Replacement therapy should be commenced (Table 18.14). Primary gonadal failure should be treated with androgens. Patients with hypothalamic–pituitary disease are routinely replaced with androgens, but may be given LH and FSH (purified or synthetic) or pulsatile GnRH when fertility is required.

Special instances of hypogonadism

Cryptorchidism

By the age of 5 years both testes should be in the scrotum. After that age the germinal epithelium is increasingly at risk, and lack of descent by puberty is associated with subfertility. Surgical exploration and orchidopexy are usually undertaken but a short trial of HCG occasionally induces descent: an HCG test with a testosterone response 72 hours later excludes anorchia. Intra-abdominal testes have an increased risk of developing malignancy; if presentation is after puberty, orchidectomy is advised.

Klinefelter's syndrome

Klinefelter's syndrome (seminiferous tubule dysgenesis), a chromosomal disorder (47XXY) affecting 1 in 1000 males, involves both loss of Leydig cells and seminiferous tubular dysgenesis. Patients usually present with poor sexual development, small or undescended testes, gynaecomastia or infertility. They are occasionally mentally retarded. Clinical examination shows small pea-sized but firm testes, usually gynaecomastia and often signs of androgen deficiency. Confirmation is by chromosomal analysis. Treatment is androgen replacement therapy unless testosterone levels are normal. No treatment is possible for the abnormal seminiferous tubules and infertility.

Kallmann's syndrome

This is isolated GnRH deficiency. It is often associated with decreased or absent sense of smell (anosmia), and sometimes with other bony (cleft palate), renal and cerebral abnormalities (e.g. colour blindness). It is often familial and is usually X-linked, resulting from a mutation in the *KAL1* gene which encodes anosmin-1 (producing loss of smell); one sex-linked form is due to an abnormality of a cell adhesion molecule. Management is that of secondary hypogonadism (see p. 1056). Fertility is possible.

Oligospermia or azoospermia

These may be secondary to androgen deficiency and can be corrected by androgen replacement. More often they result from primary testicular diseases, in which case they are rarely treatable.

Azoospermia with normal testicular size and low FSH levels suggests a vas deferens block, which is sometimes reversible by surgical intervention.

Lack of libido and erectile dysfunction ('impotence')

Lack of libido is a loss of sexual desire leading to erectile dysfunction. Erectile dysfunction (ED) may be psychological, neurogenic, vascular, endocrine or related to drugs and often includes contributions from several causes. ED is a common symptom in hypogonadism, but most patients with ED have normal hormones and many have no definable organic cause. The *endocrine* causes are those of hypogonadism (see above) and can be excluded by normal testosterone, gonadotrophin and prolactin levels, and the presence of nocturnal emissions and frequent satisfactory morning erections makes endocrine disease unlikely. *Vascular disease* is a common aetiology, especially in smokers, and is often associated with vascular problems elsewhere. *Autonomic neuropathy*, most commonly from diabetes mellitus, is a common partial, if not total, identifiable cause (see p. 1129). Many drugs produce ED (see Table 22.8). A careful history of physical disease, related symptoms, stress and psychological factors, together with drug and alcohol abuse, must be taken.

Psychogenic impotence is frequently a diagnosis of exclusion, though complex tests of penile vasculature and function are available in some centres.

Offending drugs should be stopped. Phosphodiesterase type-5 inhibitors (sildenafil, tadalafil, vardenafil) which increase penile blood flow (see p. 1129) are usually first

Table 18.15	Causes of gynaecomastia
Physiological	**Drugs**
Neonatal	Oestrogenic
Pubertal	oestrogens
Old age	digoxin
	cannabis
Hyperthyroidism	diamorphine
	Anti-androgens
Liver disease	spironolactone
	cimetidine
Oestrogen-producing	cyproterone
tumours (testis, adrenal)	**Others**
HCG-producing tumours	gonadotrophins
(testis, lung)	cytotoxics
Starvation/refeeding	
Carcinoma of breast	

Table 18.16	Effects of oestrogens and consequences of oestrogen deficiency	
Physiological effect		**Consequence of deficiency**
Breast		
Development of connective and duct tissue		Small, atrophic breast
Nipple enlargement and areolar pigmentation		
Pubic hair		
Maintenance of female pattern		Thinning and loss of pubic hair
Vulva and vagina		
Vulval growth		Atrophic vulva
Vaginal glandular and epithelial proliferation		Atrophic vagina
Vaginal lubrication		Dry vagina and dyspareunia
Uterus and tubes		
Myometrial and tubal hypertrophy		Small, atrophic uterus and tubes
Endometrial proliferation		Amenorrhoea
Skeletal		
Epiphyseal fusion		Eunuchoidism (if prepubertal)
Maintenance of bone mass		Osteoporosis

choice for therapy. Other treatments include apomorphine, intracavernosal injections of alprostadil, papaverine or phentolamine, vacuum expanders and penile implants.

If no organic disease is found, or if there is clear evidence of psychological problems, the couple should receive psychosexual counselling.

Gynaecomastia

Gynaecomastia is development of breast tissue in the male. Causes are shown in Table 18.15.

Pubertal gynaecomastia occurs in perhaps 50% of normal boys, often asymmetrically. It usually resolves spontaneously within 6–18 months, but after this duration may require surgical removal, as fibrous tissue will have been laid down. The cause is thought to be relative oestrogen excess, and the oestrogen antagonist tamoxifen is occasionally helpful.

In the older male, gynaecomastia requires a full assessment to exclude potentially serious underlying disease, such as bronchial carcinoma and testicular tumours (e.g. Leydig cell tumour). Drug effects are common (especially digoxin and spironolactone), and once these and significant liver disease are excluded most cases have no definable cause. Surgical removal is occasionally necessary.

DISORDERS IN THE FEMALE

Hypogonadism

Impaired ovarian function, whether primary or secondary, will lead both to oestrogen deficiency and abnormalities of the menstrual cycle. The latter is very sensitive to disruption, cycles becoming anovulatory and irregular before disappearing altogether. Symptoms will depend on the age at which the failure develops. Thus, before puberty, primary amenorrhoea will occur, possibly with delayed puberty; if after puberty, secondary amenorrhoea and hypogonadism will result.

Oestrogen deficiency

The physiological effects of oestrogens and symptoms/ signs of deficiency are shown in Table 18.16.

Amenorrhoea

Absence of periods or markedly irregular infrequent periods (oligomenorrhoea) are the commonest presentation of female gonadal disease. The clinical assessment of such patients is shown in Box 18.5, and common causes listed in Table 18.17.

Polycystic ovary syndrome

Polycystic ovary syndrome is the most common cause of oligomenorrhoea and amenorrhoea in clinical practice

 Box 18.5 Clinical assessment of amenorrhoea

History	**Examination**
? Pregnant	General health
Date of onset	Body shape and skeletal
Age of menarche, if any	abnormalities
Sudden or gradual onset	Weight and height
General health	Hirsutism and acne
Weight, absolute and	Evidence of virilization
changes in recent past	Maturity of secondary
Stress (job, lifestyle,	sexual characteristics
exams, relationships)	Galactorrhoea
Excessive exercise	Normality of vagina, cervix
Drugs	and uterus
Hirsutism, acne, virilization	
Headaches/visual	
symptoms	
Sense of smell	
Past history of	
pregnancies	
Past history of	
gynaecological surgery	

Table 18.17 Amenorrhoea – differential diagnosis and investigation

Diagnosis	LH	FSH	E2	PRL	T	Secondary tests
Polycystic ovary syndrome*	N↑	N	N↓	N↑	N↑	Androstenedione, DHEAS SHBG Ultrasound of ovary Progesterone challenge
Ovarian failure						
Ovarian dysgenesis*	↑↑	↑↑	↓	N	N	Repeat FSH
Premature ovarian failure*	↑↑	↑↑	↓	N	N	Karyotype
Steroid biosynthetic defect*	↑↑	↑↑	↓	N	N	Ultrasound of ovary/uterus
(Oophorectomy)	↑↑	↑↑	↓	N	N	Laparoscopy/biopsy of ovary
(Chemotherapy)	↑↑	↑↑	↓	N	N	HCG stimulation
Resistant ovary syndrome	↑↑	↑↑	↓	N	N	
Gonadotrophin failure (see also hypothalamic causes below)						
Hypothalamic–pituitary disease*	N↓	N↓	↓	N↓	N	Pituitary MRI if diagnosis unclear
Kallmann's syndrome*	N↓	N↓	↓	N	N	Clomifene test
Anorexia*	N↓	N↓	↓	N	N	Possibly LHRH test
Weight loss*	N↓	N↓	↓	N	N	Serum free T$_4$
General illness*	N↓	N↓	↓	N	N	Consider full assessment of pituitary function
Possible hypothalamic causes						
Hypothalamic amenorrhoea*	N↓	N↓	N↓	N	N	Serum free T$_4$
Weight-related amenorrhoea*	N↓	N↓	N↓	N	N	Serum testosterone, SHBG
Exercise-induced amenorrhoea	N↓	N↓	N↓	N	N	
Post-pill amenorrhoea	N↓	N↓	N↓	N	N	Pituitary MRI unless diagnosis clear
Hyperprolactinaemia						
Prolactinoma*	N↓	N↓	N↓	↑/↑↑	N	See p. 1062 (hyperprolactinaemia)
Idiopathic hyperprolactinaemia*	N↓	N↓	N↓	↑	N	
Hypothyroidism*	N↓	N↓	N↓	↑	N	Serum free T$_4$/TSH
Polycystic ovarian disease*	N↑	N↓	N↓	↑	N↑	Pituitary MRI
Other endocrine disease						
Hypothyroidism	N	N	N↓	N↑	N	Serum free T$_4$/TSH
Cushing's syndrome	N↓	N↓	N↓	N↑	N↑	See p. 1085 (Cushing's syndrome)
Androgen excess						
Gonadal or adrenal tumour	N↓	N↓	N↓	N	↑↑	Imaging ovary/adrenal
Congenital adrenal hyperplasia*	N↓	N↓	N↓	N	↑	17α-OH-progesterone
Uterine/vaginal abnormality						
Imperforate hymen*	N	N	N	N	N	Examination under anaesthetic
Absent uterus*	N	N	N	N	N	Ultrasound of pelvis
Lack of endometrium	N	N	N	N	N	Progesterone challenge
Physiological						
Pregnancy	N	N	↑↑	↑	N	Pregnancy test
Lactation	N↓	N↓	N↓	↑	N	

*These conditions may present as primary amenorrhoea
LH, Luteinizing hormone; FSH, follicle-stimulating hormone; E2, Estradiol; PRL, Prolactin; T, Testosterone; DHEAS, dehydroepiandrosterone sulphate; SHBG, sex hormone-binding globulin; HCG, human chorionic gonadotropin; LHRH, luteinizing hormone-releasing hormone
N = Normal; ↓ = Low; ↑ = High; ↑↑ = Very high; N↑ = Normal or high; N↓ = Normal or low

and should always be considered in the context of menstrual dysfunction.

Weight-related amenorrhoea

A minimum body weight is necessary for regular menstruation. While anorexia nervosa is the extreme form (see p. 1310), this condition is common and may be seen at weights with the 'normal' range. The biochemistry is indistinguishable from gonadotrophin deficiency and some patients have additional mild endocrine disease (e.g. polycystic ovarian disease). Restoration of bodyweight to above the 50th centile for height is usually effective in restoring menstruation, but in the many cases where this cannot be achieved then oestrogen replacement is necessary. Similar problems occur with intensive physical training in athletes and dancers.

Hypothalamic amenorrhoea

Amenorrhoea with low oestrogen and gonadotrophins in the absence of organic pituitary disease, weight loss or excessive exercise is described as hypothalamic amenorrhoea. This may be related to 'stress', to previous weight loss or stopping the contraceptive pill, but some patients appear to have defective cycling mechanisms without apparent explanation. Leptin (p. 253) administration for the relative leptin deficiency found in these women has recently been shown to be of benefit.

Hypothyroidism

Oligomenorrhoea and amenorrhoea are frequent findings in severe hypothyroidism in young women.

Other

Pregnancy must always be considered as a possible cause. The possibility of genital tract abnormalities, such as an imperforate hymen, should also be remembered, especially in primary amenorrhoea. Severe illness, even in the absence of weight loss, can lead to amenorrhoea.

Investigations

Basal levels of FSH, LH, oestrogen and prolactin allow initial distinction between primary gonadal and hypothalamic–pituitary causes (Table 18.17). Ovarian biopsy may occasionally be necessary to confirm the diagnosis of primary ovarian failure, although elevation of LH and FSH to menopausal levels is usually adequate. Subsequent investigations are shown in Table 18.17.

Treatment

Treatment is that of the cause wherever possible (e.g. hypothyroidism, low weight, stress, excessive exercise).

Primary ovarian disease is rarely treatable except in the rare condition of 'resistant' ovary, where high-dose gonadotrophin therapy can occasionally lead to folliculogenesis. Hyperprolactinaemia should be corrected (see below). Polycystic ovary syndrome is discussed in detail below. In all other cases oestrogen replacement is usually indicated to prevent the long-term consequences of deficiency.

Hirsutism and polycystic ovary syndrome

Pathophysiology

The extent of normal hair growth varies between individuals, families and races, being more extensive in the Mediterranean and some Asian subcontinent populations. These normal variations in body hair, and the more extensive hair growth seen in patients complaining of hirsutism, represent a continuum from no visible hair to extensive cover with thick dark hair. It is therefore impossible to draw an absolute dividing line between 'normal' and 'abnormal' degrees of facial and body hair in the female. Soft vellous hair is normally present all over the body and this type of hair on the face and elsewhere is 'normal' and is not sex-hormone dependent. Hair in the beard, moustache, breast, chest, axilla, abdominal midline, pubic and thigh areas is sex-hormone dependent. Any excess in the latter regions is thus usually a marker of increased ovarian or adrenal androgen production, most commonly polycystic ovary syndrome (PCOS) but occasionally other rarer causes.

Patients with hirsutism, no elevation of serum androgen levels and no other clinical features are sometimes labelled 'idiopathic hirsutism'. However, studies suggest that most patients with 'idiopathic hirsutism' have some radiological or biochemical evidence of PCOS on more detailed investigation, and indeed several studies have demonstrated evidence of mild PCOS in up to 20% of the normal female population. Therefore, in routine clinical practice, the majority of patients with objective signs of androgen-dependent hirsutism will have PCOS, and investigation is mainly required to exclude rarer and more serious causes of virilization.

PCOS, originally known in its severe form as the *Stein–Leventhal syndrome*, is characterized by multiple small cysts within the ovary and by excess androgen production from the ovaries and to a lesser extent from the adrenals, although whether the basic defect is in the ovary, adrenal, pituitary or a more generalized metabolic defect remains unknown. The precise levels of androgens in blood vary widely from patient to patient. In addition, androgens are normally converted to oestrogens in adipose tissue, but aromatase levels are low (partly due to decreased FSH levels) so that, instead of androgen (mainly androstenedione) being converted to oestrogen, androstenedione is secreted and converted to testosterone in peripheral tissue. Furthermore, SHBG levels are often low (due to high insulin levels), and therefore free androgen levels are high. The response of the hair follicle to circulating androgens also seems to vary between individuals with otherwise identical clinical and biochemical features, and the reason for this variation in end-organ response remains poorly understood.

The ovarian 'cysts' represent arrested follicular development. Studies have shown an association of polycystic ovary syndrome with anovulation, hyperinsulinaemia and insulin resistance, which may also be associated with hypertension, hyperlipidaemia and increased cardiovascular disease (the metabolic syndrome). The precise mechanisms which link the aetiology of polycystic ovaries, hyperandrogenism, anovulation and insulin resistance remain to be elucidated.

Familial or idiopathic hirsutism does occur, but usually involves a distribution of hair growth which is not typically androgenic. Iatrogenic hirsutism also occurs after treatment with androgens, or more weakly androgenic drugs such as progestogens or danazol. Non-androgen-dependent hair growth (hypertrichosis) occurs with drugs such as phenytoin, diazoxide, minoxidil and ciclosporin.

Rarer, and more serious, endocrine causes of hirsutism and virilization include congenital adrenal hyperplasia (CAH, see p. 1087), Cushing's syndrome (p. 1085) and virilizing tumours of the ovary and adrenal. All these conditions should be considered in any patient with hirsutism – as this may be the only presenting complaint.

Clinical features

PCOS usually presents with amenorrhoea/oligomenorrhoea, hirsutism and acne (alone or in combination), usually beginning shortly after menarche. Clinical, biochemical and radiological features of PCOS merge imperceptibly into those of the normal populations. The development of hirsutism commonly provokes severe distress in young women and may lead to avoidance of normal social activities.

The extent and severity of hirsutism

This should be recorded objectively, ideally using a scoring system, to document the problem and to monitor treatment. The method and frequency of physical removal (e.g. shaving, plucking) should also be recorded. Most patients who complain of hirsutism will have an objective excess of hair on examination, but occasionally very little will be found (and appropriate counselling is then indicated).

Age and speed of onset

Hirsutism related to PCOS usually begins around the time of the menarche and increases slowly and steadily in the teens and twenties. Rapid progression and prepubertal or late onset suggest a more serious cause.

Accompanying virilization

Hirsutism due to PCOS may be severe and affect all androgen-dependent areas on the face and body. However, more severe virilization (clitoromegaly, recent-onset frontal balding, male phenotype) implies substantial androgen excess, and usually indicates a rarer cause rather than PCOS. Thinning of head hair in a male pattern – androgenic alopecia – occurs in a proportion of women with uncomplicated PCOS, typically with a familial tendency for premature androgen-related hair loss in both sexes.

Menstruation

Most patients with hirsutism will have some disturbance of menstruation – typically oligo-/amenorrhoea although more frequent erratic bleeding can also occur.

Weight

Many patients with hirsutism are also overweight or obese. This worsens the underlying androgen excess and insulin resistance and inhibits the response to treatment, and is an indication for appropriate advice on diet and exercise. In severe cases the insulin resistance may have a visible manifestation as acanthosis nigricans on the neck and in the axillae (see Fig. 23.24).

Investigations

A variety of investigations may aid the diagnosis of patients with hirsutism:

- **Serum testosterone** may be elevated in PCOS and is invariably substantially raised in virilizing tumours (usually > 5 nmol/L). Patients with hirsutism and normal testosterone level frequently have low levels of sex hormone-binding globulin (SHBG), leading to high free androgen levels.
- **Other androgens.** Androstenedione and dehydroepiandrosterone sulphate are frequently elevated in PCOS, and even more elevated in congenital adrenal hyperplasia and virilizing tumours.
- **17α-Hydroxyprogesterone** is elevated in classical CAH (congenital adrenal hyperplasia), but may be apparent in late-onset CAH only after stimulation tests.
- **Gonadotrophin levels.** LH hypersecretion is a consistent feature of PCOS, but the pulsatile nature of secretion of this hormone means that a 'classic' increased LH/FSH ratio is not always observed on a random sample.
- **Oestrogen levels.** Estradiol is usually normal in PCOS, but estrone levels (which are rarely measured) are elevated because of peripheral conversion. Levels are variable in other causes.
- **Ovarian ultrasound** is a useful investigation (Fig. 18.13), although a skilled observer is necessary. The typical ultrasonic features are those of a thickened capsule, multiple 3–5 mm cysts and a hyperechogenic stroma. It should also be noted that prolonged hyperandrogenization from any cause may lead to polycystic changes in the ovary. Ultrasound may also reveal virilizing ovarian tumours, although these are often small.
- **Serum prolactin.** Mild hyperprolactinaemia is common in PCOS but rarely exceeds 1500 mU/L.

If a virilizing tumour is suspected clinically or after investigation, then more complex tests may include dexamethasone suppression tests, CT or MRI of adrenals, and selective venous sampling.

Differential diagnosis

Most patients presenting with a combination of hirsutism and menstrual disturbance will be shown to have polycystic ovary syndrome, but the rarer alternative diagnoses should be excluded, e.g. late-onset congenital adrenal hyperplasia (early-onset, raised serum 17α-OH-progesterone), Cushing's syndrome (look for other clinical features) and virilizing tumours of the ovary or adrenals (severe virilization, markedly elevated serum testosterone).

Treatments

The underlying cause should be removed in the rare instances where this is possible (e.g. drugs, adrenal or ovarian tumours). Treatment of CAH and Cushing's are discussed on page 1087 and page 1086, respectively. Other therapy depends upon whether the aim is to reduce hirsutism, regularize periods or produce fertility.

Fig. 18.13 **Polycystic ovary syndrome. (a) Longitudinal transvaginal ultrasound of ovary**, revealing multiple cysts with central ovarian stroma showing increased echo texture. **(b) MR image (coronal) of polycystic ovaries**, also showing pelvic anatomy. (Reproduced by kind permission of Barbara Hochstein and Geoffrey Cox, Auckland Radiology Group.)

Local therapy for hirsutism

Cosmetic appearance may be controlled by regular plucking, bleaching, depilatory cream, waxing or shaving. Such removal neither worsens nor improves the underlying severity of hirsutism. More 'permanent' solutions include electrolysis and a variety of 'laser' hair removal systems – all appear effective but have not been evaluated in long-term studies, are expensive, and still often require repeated long-term treatment.

Systemic therapy for hirsutism

This always requires a year or more of treatment for maximal benefit, and long-term treatment is frequently required as the problem tends to recur when treatment is stopped. The patient must therefore always be an active participant in the decision to use systemic therapy and must understand the rare risks as well as the benefits.

- *Oestrogens* (e.g. oral contraceptives) suppress ovarian androgen production and reduce free androgens by increasing SHBG levels. Combined pills, which contain a non-androgenic progestogen (e.g. co-cyprindiol), have an advantage over older combined pills, will result in a slow improvement in hirsutism in a majority of cases and should normally be used first unless there is a contraindication. Long-term follow-up studies of the use of the 'pill' for contraception give firm reassurance about the safety of the long-term treatment which is very often required. After the menopause, HRT preparations which contain medroxyprogesterone (rather than more androgenic progestogens) may be helpful.
- *Cyproterone acetate* (50–100 mg daily) is an antiandrogen but is also a progestogen, teratogenic and a weak glucocorticoid. Given continuously it produces amenorrhoea, and so is normally given for days 1–14

of each cycle. In women of childbearing age, contraception is essential.

- *Spironolactone* (200 mg daily) also has antiandrogen activity and can cause useful improvements in hirsutism in selected cases.
- *Finasteride* (5 mg daily), a 5α-reductase inhibitor which prevents the formation of dihydrotestosterone in the skin, has also been shown to be effective but long-term experience is awaited.

It should be noted that none of these drugs is actually licensed in the UK for the treatment of hirsutism; while spironolactone and cyproterone are widely used, both are subject to Committee of Safety of Medicine (CSM) warnings. Flutamide, another antiandrogen, is not used owing to the high incidence of hepatic side-effects.

Treatment of menstrual disturbance

Cyclical oestrogen/progestogen will regulate the menstrual cycle and remove the symptom of oligo- or amenorrhoea. This is most frequently an additional benefit of the treatment of hirsutism, but may also be used when menstrual disturbance is the only symptom.

Drugs to improve the hyperinsulinaemia associated with PCOS and obesity are increasingly used (and requested by patients). Metformin (500 mg three times daily) improves menstrual cyclicity and ovulation in short-term studies, and some patients also report improvement in hirsutism and ease of weight loss – but gastrointestinal upset may limit use. Glitazones are also effective, but there are few studies of currently-available preparations.

Treatment for fertility

- Metformin alone may improve ovulation and achieve conception.
- Clomifene 50–100 mg can be given daily on days 2–6 of the cycle. This can occasionally cause the *ovarian hyperstimulation syndrome*, an iatrogenic complication of ovulation-induction therapy, causing ovarian enlargement, oedema, hypovolaemia, renal failure, and can lead to shock; specialist supervision is essential. It is recommended that clomifene should not normally be used for longer than six cycles (owing to a possible increased risk of ovarian cancer in patients treated for longer than recommended).
- *Reverse circadian rhythm.* Prednisolone (2.5 mg in the morning, 5 mg on retiring) suppresses pituitary production of ACTH, upon which adrenal androgens partly depend. Regular ovulatory cycles often ensue. A steroid instruction leaflet and a card must be supplied.

More intensive techniques to stimulate ovulation may also be indicated in specialist hands, including low-dose *gonadotrophin therapy*, and ovarian hyperstimulation techniques associated with in vitro fertilization.

Wedge resection of the ovary was a traditional therapy which is rarely required, although laparoscopic ovarian electrodiathermy may be helpful.

Oral contraception

The combined oestrogen–progestogen pill is widely used for contraception and has a low failure rate (< 1 per 100 woman-years). 'Pills' contain 20–40 μg of oestrogen, usually ethinylestradiol, together with a variable amount of one of several progestogens. The mechanism of action is twofold:

- suppression by oestrogen of gonadotrophins, thus preventing follicular development, ovulation and luteinization
- progestogen effects on cervical mucus, making it hostile to sperm, and on tubal motility and the endometrium.

Side-effects of these preparations are shown in Box 18.6. Most of the serious ones are rare and are less common on typical modern 20–30 μg oestrogen pills, although evidence suggests that thromboembolism may be slightly more common on 'third-generation pills' containing desogestrel and gestodene (approx. 30/100 000 woman-years compared with 15/100 000 on older pills and 5/100 000 on no treatment) and on co-cyprindiol. While some problems require immediate cessation of the pill, other milder side-effects must be judged against the hazards of pregnancy occurring with inadequate contraception, especially if other effective methods are not practicable or acceptable.

Box 18.6 Adverse effects and drug interactions of oral contraceptives (mixed oestrogen–progesterone combinations)

General
Weight gain
Loss of libido
Pigmentation (chloasma)
Breast tenderness
Increased growth rate
   of some malignancies

Cardiovascular
Increased blood pressure*
Deep vein thrombosis*
Myocardial infarction
Stroke

Gastrointestinal
Nausea and vomiting
Abnormal liver
   biochemistry*
Gallstones increased
Hepatic tumours

Nervous system
Headache
Migraine*
Depression*

Malignancy
Increase in cancer of the
   breast (but reduced risk
   of ovarian and
   endometrial cancer)

Gynaecological
Amenorrhoea
'Spotting'
Cervical erosion

Haematological
Increased clotting
   tendency

Endocrine/metabolic
Mild impairment of glucose
   tolerance
Worsened lipid profile,
   though variable

Drug interactions
   (reduced contraceptive
   effect owing to enzyme
   induction)
Antibiotics
Barbiturates
Phenytoin
Carbamazepine
Rifampicin
St John's Wort

*Common reasons for stopping oral contraceptives

Hazards of the combined pill are increased in smokers, in obesity, in those with other risk factors for cardiovascular disease (e.g. hypertension, hyperlipidaemia, diabetes) especially in women aged over 35 years (avoid if over 50 years). The 'mini-pill' (progestogen only, usually norethisterone) is less effective but is often suitable where oestrogens are contraindicated (Box 18.6). A progesterone antagonist, mifepristone, in combination with a prostaglandin analogue, induces abortion of pregnancy at up to 9 weeks' gestation. It prevents progesterone-induced inhibition of uterine contraction.

Hyperprolactinaemia

Hyperprolactinaemia has many causes. Common pathological causes include prolactinoma, co-secretion of prolactin in acromegaly, stalk compression due to pituitary adenomas and other pituitary masses, polycystic ovary syndrome, hypothyroidism and 'idiopathic' hyperprolactinaemia; rarer causes are oestrogen therapy (e.g. the 'pill'), renal failure, liver failure, post-ictal and chest wall injury. Dopamine antagonist drugs (metoclopramide, domperidone, phenothiazines) are a common iatrogenic cause, as well as most other antiemetics (except cyclizine) and opiates. Physiological hyperprolactinaemia occurs in pregnancy, lactation and severe stress, as well as during sleep and coitus. The range of serum prolactin seen in common causes of hyperprolactinaemia is illustrated in Figure 18.14. Mildly increased prolactin levels (400–600 mU/L) may be physiological and asymptomatic but higher levels require a diagnosis. Levels above 5000 mU/L always imply a prolactin-secreting pituitary tumour.

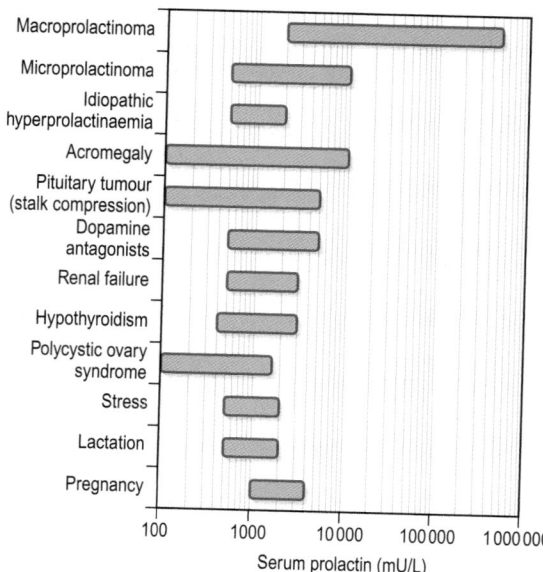

Macroprolactinoma
Microprolactinoma
Idiopathic hyperprolactinaemia
Acromegaly
Pituitary tumour (stalk compression)
Dopamine antagonists
Renal failure
Hypothyroidism
Polycystic ovary syndrome
Stress
Lactation
Pregnancy

100   1000   10 000   100 000   1 000 000
Serum prolactin (mU/L)

Fig. 18.14   **Range of serum prolactin seen in common causes of hyperprolactinaemia.**

Clinical features

Hyperprolactinaemia stimulates milk production in the breast and inhibits GnRH and gonadotrophin secretion per se. It usually presents with:

- galactorrhoea, spontaneous or expressible (60% of cases)
- oligomenorrhoea or amenorrhoea
- decreased libido in both sexes
- decreased potency in men
- subfertility
- symptoms or signs of oestrogen or androgen deficiency – in the long term osteoporosis may result, especially in women
- delayed or arrested puberty in the peripubertal patient.

Additionally, headaches and/or visual field defects may be present if there is a pituitary tumour (more common in men). Not all patients with galactorrhoea have hyperprolactinaemia, but the other causes are poorly understood – 'normoprolactinaemic galactorrhoea' and duct ectasia.

Investigations

Hyperprolactinaemia should be confirmed by repeat measurement. Further tests are appropriate after physiological and drug causes have been excluded:

- **Visual fields** should be checked.
- **Hypothyroidism** must be excluded since this is a cause of hyperprolactinaemia.
- **Anterior pituitary function** should be assessed if there is any clinical evidence of hypopituitarism or radiological evidence of a pituitary tumour (Table 18.9; Box 18.1 and Box 18.2).
- **MRI of the pituitary** is necessary if there are any clinical features suggestive of a pituitary tumour, and desirable in all cases when prolactin is significantly elevated (above 1000 mU/L).

In the presence of a pituitary mass on MRI, the level of prolactin helps determine whether the mass is a prolactinoma or a non-functioning pituitary tumour causing stalk-disconnection hyperprolactinaemia: levels of above 5000 mU/L in the presence of a macroadenoma, or above 2000 mU/L in the presence of a microadenoma (or of no radiological abnormality), strongly suggest a prolactinoma (see p. 1044). Macroprolactinoma refers to tumours above 10 mm diameter, microprolactinoma to smaller ones.

Treatment

Hyperprolactinaemia should usually be treated to avoid the long-term effects of oestrogen deficiency (even if the patient would otherwise welcome the lack of periods!) or testosterone deficiency in the male. Exceptions include minor elevations (400–1000 mU/L) with preservation of normal regular menstruation (or normal male testosterone levels) and postmenopausal patients with microprolactinomas who are not taking oestrogen replacement. Hyperprolactinaemia is controlled with a dopamine agonist. Cabergoline (500 μg once or twice a week judged on clinical response and prolactin levels) is the best tolerated and longest-acting drug. Bromocriptine is the longest-established therapy and therefore preferred if pregnancy is planned: initial doses should be small (e.g. 1 mg), taken with food and gradually increased to 2.5 mg two or three times daily. Side-effects, which prevent effective therapy in a minority of cases, include nausea and vomiting, dizziness and syncope, constipation and cold peripheries. Quinagolide (75–150 µg once daily) is another alternative. These dopamine receptor agonists have been associated with pulmonary, retroperitoneal and pericardial fibrotic reactions and patients need careful monitoring.

Definitive therapy will depend upon the size of the tumour, the patient's wishes, including desire for fertility, and local expertise and facilities. In most cases a dopamine agonist will be the first and only therapy. Prolactinomas usually shrink in size on a dopamine agonist; in macroadenomas any pituitary mass effects commonly resolve and in most cases it is simply sufficient to continue successful dopamine agonist therapy in the long term. Prolactin should therefore always be measured before surgery on any mass in the pituitary region. Microprolactinomas may not recur after several years of dopamine agonist therapy in a substantial minority of cases, but in the majority hyperprolactinaemia will recur if treatment is stopped.

Trans-sphenoidal surgery may restore normoprolactinaemia in patients with microadenoma, but is rarely completely successful with macroadenomas and risks damage to normal pituitary function. Therefore most patients and physicians elect to continue medical therapy rather than proceed to surgery. Some surgeons believe that long-term bromocriptine increases the hardness of the adenoma and makes resection more difficult – but others dissent from this view.

Radiotherapy usually controls adenoma growth and is slowly effective in lowering prolactin but causes progressive hypopituitarism. It may be advocated after medical tumour shrinkage or after surgery in larger tumours, especially where families are complete, but many workers simply advocate continuation of dopamine agonist therapy in responsive cases.

Rarely, tumours enlarge during pregnancy to produce headaches and visual defects. Dopamine agonists, which are traditionally stopped during pregnancy, should be restarted.

SUBFERTILITY

Subfertility, or 'infertility', is defined as the inability of a couple to conceive after 1 year of unprotected intercourse. Investigation requires the combined skills of gynaecologist, endocrinologist and, ideally, andrologist. Both partners must be involved and every aspect of the physiology critically examined.

Causes (Fig. 18.15)
A significant proportion of couples have both male and female contributing factors.

Inadequate intercourse, hostile cervical mucus and vaginal factors are uncommon (5%). Fifteen per cent of cases appear to be idiopathic, and natural fertility decreases with increasing age.

Male factors
About 30–40% of couples have a major identifiable male factor. There is some evidence that male sperm counts are declining in many populations. Untreated male hypogonadism of any cause (see Table 18.13) is likely to be associated with subfertility.

Female factors
Female tubal problems account for perhaps 20%; a similar proportion have ovulatory disorders. Any cause of oligomenorrhoea or amenorrhoea (see Table 18.17) is likely to be associated with suboptimal ovulation or anovulation.

Clinical assessment
Both partners should be seen and the following factors checked:

- *The man.* Look for previous testicular damage (orchitis, trauma), undescended testes, urethral symptoms and venereal problems, local surgery, and use of alcohol and drugs. A semen analysis early in the investigations is essential.
- *The woman.* Look for previous pelvic infection, regularity of periods, previous surgery, alcohol intake and smoking, and adequacy of bodyweight (see p. 1057).
- *Together.* Check the frequency and adequacy of intercourse, and the use of lubricants.

Investigations
Appropriate tests for particular defects are shown in Figure 18.15.

Treatment
Counselling of both partners is essential. Any defect(s) found should be treated if possible. Ovulation can usually be induced by exogenous hormones if simpler measures fail, while in vitro fertilization (IVF) and similar techniques are widely used, especially where there is tubal blockage, oligospermia or 'idiopathic subfertility'. Intracytoplasmic sperm injection (ICSI) appears particularly effective for severe oligospermia and poor sperm function.

DISORDERS OF SEXUAL DIFFERENTIATION

Disorders of sexual differentiation are rare but may affect chromosomal, gonadal, endocrine and phenotypic development (Table 18.18). Such cases always require extensive, multidisciplinary clinical management. An individual's sex can be defined in several ways:

- *Chromosomal sex.* The normal female is 46XX, the normal male 46XY. The Y chromosome confers male sex; if it is not present, development follows female lines.

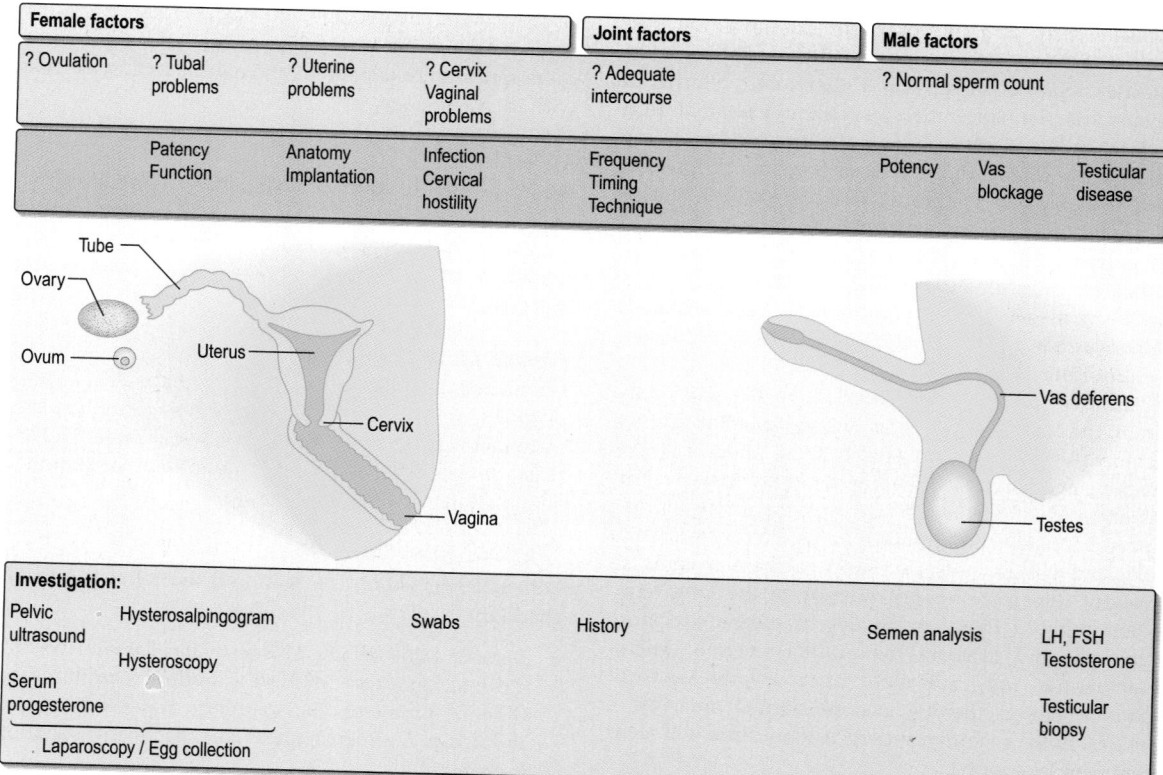

Fig. 18.15 **Major factors involved in subfertility and their investigation.** LH, luteinizing hormone; FSH, follicle-stimulating hormone.

Table 18.18	Disorders of sexual differentiation			
Condition	**Chromosomes**	**Gonads**	**Phenotype**	**Remarks**
Turner's syndrome	45X (50%) 46,X,i (Xq)(5–10%) 45,X, mosaicism (remainder)	Streak	Female	Often morphological features (e.g. short stature, web neck, coarctation of aorta)
Gonadal dysgenesis	46XY	Streak or minimal testes*	Immature female	
Congenital adrenal hyperplasia	46XX	Ovary	Female with variable virilization	Obvious androgen excess
Virilizing tumour	46XX	Ovary	Female with variable virilization	Obvious androgen excess
True hermaphroditism	46XX/XY or mosaic	Testis and ovary	Male or ambiguous	
Klinefelter's syndrome	47XXY	Small testes	Male, often with gynaecomastia	Many are hypogonadal
Testicular feminization	46XY	Testes*	Ambiguous or infantile female	Androgen receptor defective
Testicular synthetic defects	46XY	Testes*	Cryptorchid, ambiguous	
5α-Reductase deficiency	46XY	Testes	Cryptorchid, ambiguous	Impaired conversion of testosterone to dihydrotestosterone
Anorchia	46XY	Absent	Immature female	

*Gonadectomy advised because of high risk of malignancy, i = isochromosome

- *Gonadal sex.* This is obviously determined predominantly by chromosomal sex, but requires normal embryological development.
- *Phenotypic sex.* This describes the normal physical appearance and characteristics of male and female body shape. This in turn is a manifestation of gonadal sex and subsequent sex hormone production.
- *Social sex (gender).* This is heavily dependent on phenotypic sex and normally assigned on appearance of the external genitalia at birth.
- *Sexual orientation* – heterosexual, homosexual or bisexual.

FURTHER READING

Baird DT (1997) Amenorrhoea. *Lancet* **350**: 275–279.
Ehrmann DA (2005) Polycystic ovary syndrome. *New England Journal of Medicine* **352**: 1223–1236.
Greendale GA, Lee NP, Arriola ER (1999) The menopause. *Lancet* **353**: 571–580.
Gruber CJ et al. (2002) Production and actions of estrogens. *New England Journal of Medicine* **346**: 340–352.
Kyel-Mensah AA, Jacobs HS (1995) The investigation of female infertility. *Clinical Endocrinology* **43**: 251–256.
MacLaughlin DT, Donahoe PK (2004) Sex determination and differentiation. *New England Journal of Medicine* **350**: 367–378.
Petitti DB (2003) Combination estrogen–progestin oral contraceptives. *New England Journal of Medicine* **349**: 1443–1450.
Rhoden EL, Morgentaler A (2004) Risks of testosterone replacement therapy. *New England Journal of Medicine* **350**: 482–492.

THE GROWTH AXIS

Physiology and control of growth hormone (GH) (Fig. 18.16)

GH is the pituitary factor responsible for stimulation of body growth in humans. Its secretion is stimulated by GHRH, released into the portal system from the hypothalamus; it is also under inhibitory control by somatostatin. A separate GH stimulating system involves a distinct receptor (GH secretogogue receptor), which interacts with ghrelin (see p. 254). It is not known how these two systems interact. GH acts through a single transmembrane receptor, followed by saturation of Janus kinases (see p. 157). GH acts by binding to a specific (single transmembrane) receptor located mainly in the liver. This induces an intracellular phosphorylation cascade involving the JAK/STAT (signal transducing activators of transcription) pathway (p. 157). This leads to hepatic synthesis and secretion of IGF (insulin-like growth factor-1) which stimulates growth. Plasma levels of IGF-1, however, reflect local growth activity poorly, partly as there are multiple IGF-binding proteins (IGF-

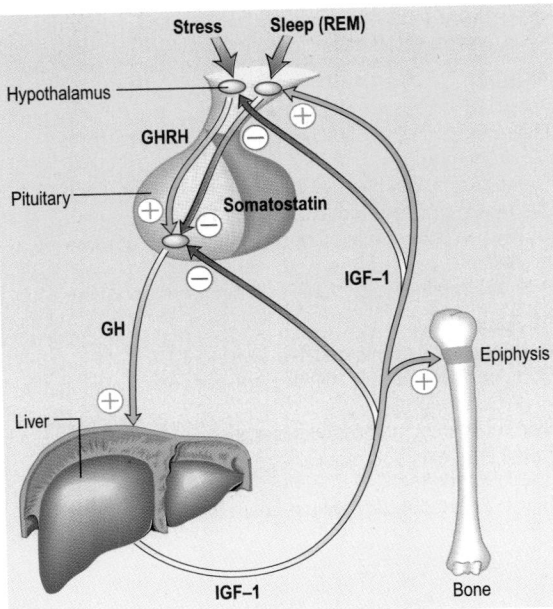

Fig. 18.16   The control of growth hormone (GH) and insulin-like growth factor-1 (IGF-1) secretion and action. Ghrelin is a growth hormone-releasing peptide and is produced in the stomach.

BP) – mainly IGF-BP3. The metabolic actions of the system are:

- increasing collagen and protein synthesis
- promoting retention of calcium, phosphorus and nitrogen, necessary substrates for anabolism
- opposing the action of insulin.

GH release is intermittent and mainly nocturnal, especially during REM sleep. The frequency and size of GH pulses increase during the growth spurt of adolescence and decline thereafter. Acute stress and exercise both stimulate GH release while, in the normal subject, hyperglycaemia suppresses it.

IGF-1 may, in addition, play a major role in maintaining neoplastic growth. A relationship has been shown between circulating IGF-1 concentrations and breast cancer in premenopausal women and prostate cancer in men.

Normal growth

There are factors other than GH involved in linear growth in the human.

- *Genetic factors.* Children of two short parents will probably be short and vice versa.
- *Nutritional factors.* Adequate nutrients must be available. Impaired growth can result from inadequate dietary intake or small-bowel disease (e.g. coeliac disease).
- *General health.* Any serious systemic disease in childhood is likely to reduce growth (e.g. renal failure).
- *Intrauterine growth retardation.* These infants often grow poorly in the long term, while infants with

History
Pregnancy records
Rate of growth (home/school records, e.g. heights on kitchen door)
Comparison with peers at school and siblings
Change in appearance (old photographs)
Change in shoe/glove/hat size or frequency of 'growing out'
Age of appearance of pubic hair, breasts, menarche

Physical signs
Evidence of systemic disease
Body habitus, size, relative weight, proportions (span versus height)
Skin thickness, interdental separation
Facial features
Spade hands/feet
Grading of secondary sexual characteristics

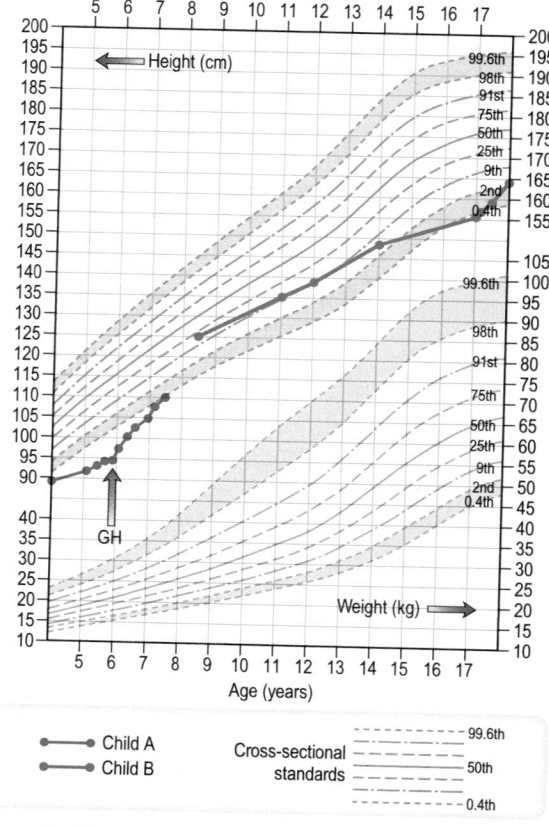

Fig. 18.17 **A height chart for boys. Child A illustrates the course of a child with hypopituitarism**, initially treated with cortisol and thyroxine, but showing growth only after growth hormone treatment. **Child B shows the course of a child with constitutional growth delay without treatment.** (Chart © the Child Growth Foundation.)

simple prematurity usually catch up. There is some evidence that low birthweight may predispose to hypertension, diabetes and other health problems in later adult life (p. 229).

■ *Emotional deprivation and psychological factors*. These can impair growth by complex, poorly understood mechanisms, probably involving temporarily decreased GH secretion.

The relevant aspects of history and examination in the assessment of problems are shown in Box 18.7.

Assessment of growth

Charts showing ranges of height and weight for normal British children are available (Fig. 18.17), and other national data are available. Height must be measured very carefully, ideally at the same time of day on the same instrument by the same observer.

In general, there are three overlapping phases of growth: infantile (0–2 years), which appears largely substrate (food) dependent; childhood (age 2 years to puberty), which is largely GH dependent; and the adolescent 'growth spurt', dependent on GH and sex hormones.

Height velocity is more helpful than current height. It requires at least two measurements some months apart and, ideally, multiple serial measurements. Height velocity is the rate of current growth (cm per year), while already attained height is largely dependent upon previous growth.

Standard deviation scores (SDS) based on the degree of deviation from age–sex norms are widely used by experts – these and growth velocities are far more sensitive than simple charts in assessing growth. Computer programs also allow calculation of many of these indices.

The approximate future height of a child ('mid-parental height') can be simply predicted from the parental heights. For a boy, this is:

[(Maternal height + 14 cm (5.5 inches) + Paternal height)/2]

and for a girl:

[(Paternal height – 14 cm (5.5 inches) + Maternal height)/2].

Thus, with a father of 180 cm and mother of 154 cm, the predicted heights are 174 cm for a son and 160 cm for a daughter.

GROWTH FAILURE: SHORT STATURE

When children or their parents complain of short stature, particular attention should focus on:

■ intrauterine growth retardation, weight and gestation at birth
■ possible systemic disorders – any system, but especially small-bowel disease
■ evidence of skeletal, chromosomal or other congenital abnormalities
■ endocrine status – particularly thyroid
■ dietary intake and use of drugs, especially steroids for asthma
■ emotional, psychological, family and school problems.

Table 18.19 Clinical features of common causes of short stature

Cause	Family history	Growth pattern, clinical features and puberty	Bone age	Remarks
Constitutional delay	Often present	Slow from birth, immature but appropriate with late but spontaneous puberty	Moderate delay	Often difficult to differentiate from GH deficiency Growth velocity measurement vital
Familial short stature	Positive	Slow from birth, clinically normal with normal puberty	Normal	Need heights of family members Growth velocity normal
GH insufficiency	Rare	Slow growth, immature, often overweight, delayed puberty	Moderate delay, increasing with time	Early investigation and treatment vital Increased suspicion if child is plump
Primary hypothyroidism	Rare	Slow growth, immature and delayed puberty	Marked delay	Measure TSH, T_4 in all cases of short stature Clear clinical signs not obvious
Small bowel disease	Sometimes	Slow, immature, usually thin for height, delayed puberty	Delayed	Diarrhoea and/or macrocytosis/anaemia Occasionally no GI symptoms

School, general practitioner, clinic and home records of height and weight should be obtained if possible to allow growth-velocity calculation. If unavailable, such data must be obtained prospectively.

A child with normal growth velocity is unlikely to have significant endocrine disease. However, low growth velocity without apparent systemic cause requires further investigation. Sudden cessation of growth suggests major physical disease; if no gastrointestinal, respiratory, renal or skeletal abnormality is apparent, then a cerebral tumour or hypothyroidism is likeliest.

Consistently slow-growing children require full endocrine assessment. Features of the more common causes of growth failure are given in Table 18.19.

Around the time of puberty, where constitutional delay is clearly shown and symptoms require intervention, then very-low-dose sex steroids in 3- to 6-month courses will usually induce acceleration of growth.

Investigations

Systemic disease having been excluded, the following should be undertaken:

- **Thyroid function tests** – serum TSH and free T_4 to exclude hypothyroidism.
- **GH status.** Basal levels are of little value, though urinary GH measurements may prove to be of some value in screening. Dynamic tests include the GH response to insulin (the 'gold standard'; Box 18.4), arginine, exercise, clonidine and Bovril. Tests should only be performed in centres experienced in their use and interpretation. Normal responses depend on test and GH assay used.
- **Assessment of bone age.** Non-dominant hand and wrist X-rays allow assessment of bone age by comparison with standard charts.

Treatment

Systemic illness should be treated and primary hypothyroidism replaced with thyroxine.

For GH insufficiency, recombinant GH (somatropin) is given as nightly injections in doses of 0.17–0.35 mg/kg per week. Treatment is expensive and should be supervised in expert centres. Human GH (collected from pituitaries) was previously used but was withdrawn as cases of Creutzfeldt–Jakob disease were reported.

GH treatment in so-called 'short normal' children has not been shown to produce any worthwhile increase in final height. In Turner's syndrome (see p. 1064) large doses of GH are effective in increasing final height, especially in combination with appropriate very-low-dose oestrogen replacement. Familial cases of resistance to GH owing to an abnormal GH receptor (Laron-type dwarfism) are well described. They are very rare but may respond to therapy with synthetic IGF-1.

TALL STATURE

The most common causes are hereditary (two tall parents!), idiopathic (constitutional) or early development. It can occasionally be due to hyperthyroidism. Other causes include chromosomal abnormalities (e.g. Klinefelter's syndrome, Marfan's syndrome) or metabolic abnormalities. GH excess is a very rare cause and is usually clinically apparent.

GROWTH HORMONE EXCESS: GIGANTISM AND ACROMEGALY

GH stimulates skeletal and soft-tissue growth. GH excess therefore produces gigantism in children (if acquired before epiphyseal fusion) and acromegaly in adults.

Acromegaly

This is due to a pituitary tumour in almost all cases. Hyperplasia due to GHRH excess is very rare. Overall incidence is approximately 3–4/million per year and prevalence 50–80/million.

Clinical features

Symptoms and signs of acromegaly are shown in Figure 18.18. One-third of patients present with changes in appearance, one-quarter with visual field defects or headaches; in the remainder the diagnosis is made by an alert observer in another clinic, e.g. GP, diabetic, hypertension, dental, dermatology.

Investigations

- **GH levels** may exclude acromegaly if undetectable but a detectable value is non-diagnostic. Normal adult levels are < 1 mU/L for most of the day except during stress or a 'GH pulse'.
- **The glucose tolerance test** is diagnostic. Acromegalics fail to suppress GH below 1 mU/L and some show a paradoxical rise; about 25% of acromegalics have a diabetic glucose tolerance test.
- **IGF-1 levels** are almost always raised in acromegaly – a single plasma level of IGF-1 reflects mean 24-hour GH levels and is useful in diagnosis.
- **Visual field defects** are common.
- **MRI scan of pituitary** – will almost always reveal the pituitary adenoma.
- **Pituitary function** – partial or complete anterior hypopituitarism is common.
- **Prolactin** – mild to moderate hyperprolactinaemia occurs in 30% of patients (Fig. 18.14). In some, the adenoma secretes both GH and prolactin.

Management and treatment

Untreated acromegaly results in markedly reduced survival with most deaths from heart failure, coronary artery disease and hypertension-related causes. In addition, there is an increase in deaths due to neoplasia, particularly large-bowel tumours. Treatment is therefore indicated in all except the elderly or those with minimal abnormalities. There is now consensus agreement that the aim of therapy should be to achieve a mean growth hormone level below 5 mU/L, which has been shown to reduce mortality to normal levels.

Complete cure is often slow, if possible at all. The choice lies between trans-sphenoidal surgery, pituitary radiotherapy, somatostatin analogues, and growth hormone agonists dopamine agonists. Progress can be assessed by monitoring GH and IGF-1 levels. The general pros and cons of surgery, radiotherapy and medical treatment are discussed on page 1045.

When present, hypopituitarism should be corrected (see p. 1048) and concurrent diabetes and/or hypertension should be treated conventionally; both usually improve with treatment of the acromegaly.

Surgery

Trans-sphenoidal surgery is generally agreed as the appropriate first-line therapy. It will result in clinical remission in a majority of cases (60–90%) with pituitary microadenoma, but in only 50% of those with macroadenoma. Surgical success rates are variable and highly dependent upon experience, and a specialist pituitary surgeon is essential. Transfrontal surgery is rarely required except for massive macroadenomas.

Pituitary radiotherapy

External radiotherapy is normally used after pituitary

Symptoms		Signs
Change in appearance		Prominent supraorbital ridge
Increased size of hands/feet		**Prognathism**
Headaches		**Interdental separation**
Excessive sweating		**Large tongue**
Visual deterioration		Hirsutism
Tiredness		Thick greasy skin
Weight gain		**Spade-like hands and feet**
Amenorrhoea		**Tight rings**
oligomenorrhoea		Carpal tunnel syndrome
in women		Visual field defects
Galactorrhoea		Galactorrhoea
Impotence or poor libido		Hypertension
Deep voice		Oedema
Goitre		Heart failure
Breathlessness		Arthropathy
Pain/tingling in hands		Proximal myopathy
Polyuria/polydipsia		Glycosuria
Muscular weakness		(plus possible signs of
Joint pains		hypopituitarism)
Old photographs are		
frequently useful		
Symptoms of		
hypopituitarism may also		
be present		

Fig. 18.18 **Acromegaly – symptoms and signs.** Bold type indicates signs of greater discriminant value.

surgery fails to normalize GH levels rather than as primary therapy. It is often combined with medium-term treatment with a somatostatin analogue or a dopamine agonist because of the slow biochemical response to radiotherapy, which may take 10 years or more. Stereotactic radiotherapy is used in some centres.

Somatostatin analogues

Octreotide and lanreotide are synthetic analogues of somatostatin (p. 1065) which are the treatment of choice in resistant cases, and employed as a short-term treatment while other modalities become effective. They reduce GH and IGF levels in most patients. Both drugs are typically administered as monthly depot injections and are generally well tolerated but are associated with an increased incidence of gallstones and are expensive.

Dopamine agonists

Dopamine agonists were the original medical therapy for acromegaly, and remain useful in some cases. They can be given to shrink tumours prior to definitive therapy or to control symptoms and persisting GH secretion; they are probably most effective in mixed growth-hormone-producing (somatotroph) and prolactin-producing (mammotroph) tumours. The doses are bromocriptine 10–60 mg daily or cabergoline 0.5 mg daily (higher than for prolactinomas) but should be started slowly (see p. 1063). Given alone they reduce GH to 'safe' levels in only a minority of cases – but may be useful for mild residual disease or in combination with somatostatin analogues.

Growth hormone antagonists

Pegvisomant (a genetically modified analogue of GH) is a GH receptor antagonist which has its effect by binding to and preventing dimerization of the GH receptor. It has been shown to normalize IGF-1 levels in 90% of patients. Its main role at the present time is treatment of patients in whom GH and IGF levels cannot be reduced to safe levels with somatostatin analogues alone, surgery or radiotheraphy.

FURTHER READING

Colao A, Lombardi G (1998) Growth-hormone and prolactin excess. *Lancet* **352**: 1455–1461.

Dattani M, Preece M (2004) Growth hormone deficiency and related disorders. *Lancet* **363**: 1977–1987.

Drake WM, Howell SJ, Monson JP, Shalet SM (2001) Optimising GH therapy in adults and children. *Endocrine Reviews* **22**: 425–450.

Orme SM et al. for the UK Acromegaly Study Group (1998) Mortality and cancer incidence in acromegaly: a retrospective cohort study. *Journal of Clinical Endocrinology and Metabolism* **83**: 2730–2734.

Utiger RD (2000) Treatment of acromegaly. *New England Journal of Medicine* **342**: 1210–1211.

THE THYROID AXIS

The metabolic rate of many tissues is controlled by the thyroid hormones, and overactivity and underactivity of the gland are the most common of all endocrine problems.

Anatomy

The thyroid gland consists of two lateral lobes connected by an isthmus. It is closely attached to the thyroid cartilage and to the upper end of the trachea, and thus moves on swallowing. It is often palpable in normal women.

Embryologically it originates from the base of the tongue and descends to the middle of the neck. Remnants of thyroid tissue can sometimes be found at the base of the tongue (lingual thyroid) and along the line of descent. The gland has a rich blood supply from superior and inferior thyroid arteries.

The thyroid consists of follicles lined by cuboidal epithelioid cells. Inside is the colloid, which is an iodinated glycoprotein, thyroglobulin, synthesized by the follicular cells. Each follicle is surrounded by basement membrane, between which are parafollicular cells containing calcitonin-secreting C cells.

Biochemistry

The thyroid hormones, T_4 and T_3, are synthesized within the gland (Fig. 18.19).

More T_4 than T_3 is produced, but T_4 is converted in some peripheral tissues (liver, kidney and muscle) to the more active T_3 by 5′-monodeiodination; an alternative 3′-monodeiodination yields the inactive reverse T_3 (rT_3). The latter step occurs particularly in severe non-thyroidal illness (see below).

In plasma, more than 99% of all T_4 and T_3 is bound to hormone-binding proteins (thyroxine-binding globulin, TBG; thyroid-binding prealbumin, TBPA; and albumin). Only free hormone is available for tissue action, where T_3 binds to specific nuclear receptors within the cell. Factors affecting TBG are shown in Table 18.20; all may result in

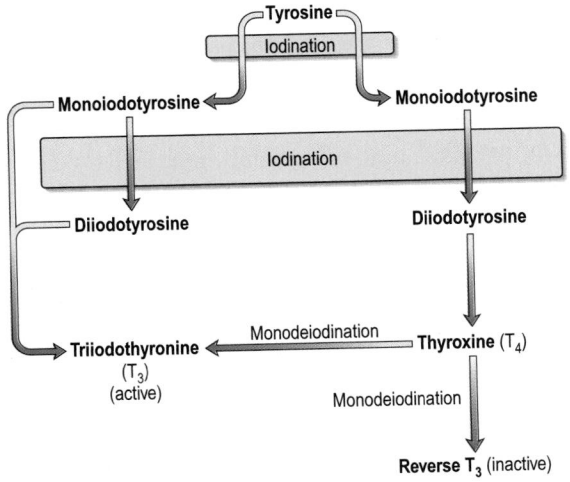

Fig. 18.19 Synthesis and metabolism of the thyroid hormones.

Table 18.20 Factors affecting thyroxine-binding globulin (TBG) levels

Increased TBG
Hereditary
Pregnancy
Oestrogen therapy
Oral contraceptive use
Hypothyroidism
Phenothiazines
Acute viral hepatitis

Decreased TBG
Hereditary
Androgens
Corticosteroid excess
Thyrotoxicosis
Nephrotic syndrome
Major illness
Malnutrition
Chronic liver disease

Drug causing altered binding
Non-steroidal anti-inflammatory drugs
Phenytoin

confusing total T_4 levels in blood, and most laboratories therefore now measure free T_4 levels.

Iodine deficiency

Globally, dietary iodine deficiency is a major cause of thyroid disease, as iodine is an essential requirement for thyroid hormone synthesis. The recommended daily intake of iodine should be at least $140\,\mu g$, and dietary supplementation of salt and bread has reduced the number of areas where 'endemic goitre' still occurs (see below).

Physiology of the hypothalamic–pituitary–thyroid axis (see Fig. 18.1)

1. TRH is released in the hypothalamus and stimulates release of TSH from the pituitary.
2. TSH stimulates the TSH receptor in the thyroid to increase synthesis of both T_4 and T_3 and also to release stored hormone, producing increased plasma levels of T_4 and T_3.
3. T_3 feeds back on the pituitary and perhaps hypothalamus to reduce TRH and TSH secretion.

Thyroid function tests

Immunoassays for free T_4, free T_3 and TSH are widely available. There are only minor circadian rhythms, and measurements may be made at any time. Particular uses of the tests are summarized in Table 18.21, with typical findings in common disorders.

TSH measurement

TSH levels can discriminate between hyperthyroidism, hypothyroidism and euthyroidism. There are pitfalls, however. These are mainly with hypopituitarism, with the 'sick euthyroid' syndrome and with dysthyroid eye disease, all of which may give 'false' (i.e. misleading, not incorrect) low results implying hyperthyroidism. As a single test of thyroid function it is the most sensitive in most circumstances, but accurate diagnosis requires at least two tests – for example, TSH plus free T_4 or free T_3 where hyperthyroidism is suspected, TSH plus serum free T_4 where hypothyroidism is likely.

'Free' T_4 tests

These attempt to measure only the unbound active hormone. Although not perfect, they are in routine clinical use in most laboratories. TBG can also be measured directly.

TRH test

This has been rendered almost obsolete by modern sensitive TSH assays except for investigation of hypothalamic–pituitary dysfunction.

Problems in interpretation of thyroid function tests

There are three major areas of difficulty.

Serious acute or chronic illness

Thyroid function is affected in several ways: (a) reduced concentration and affinity of binding proteins, (b) decreased peripheral conversion of T_4 to T_3 with more rT_3 and (c) reduced hypothalamic–pituitary TSH production. Systemically ill patients can therefore have an apparently low total and free T_4 and T_3 with a normal or low basal TSH (the 'sick euthyroid' syndrome). Levels are usually only mildly below normal and are thought to be mediated by interleukins IL-1 and IL-6; the tests should be repeated after resolution of the underlying illness.

Table 18.21 Characteristics of thyroid function tests in common thyroid disorders (the clinically most informative tests in each situation are shown in bold)

	TSH (0.3–3.5 mU/L)	Free T_4 (10–25 pmol/L)	Free T_3 (3.5–7.5 pmol/L)
Thyrotoxicosis	**Suppressed (< 0.05 mU/L)**	**Increased**	**Increased**
Primary hypothyroidism	**Increased (> 10 mU/L)**	Low/low-normal	Normal or low
TSH deficiency	Low-normal or subnormal	**Low/low-normal**	Normal or low
T_3 toxicosis	Suppressed (< 0.05 mU/L)	Normal	**Increased**
Compensated euthyroidism	**Slightly increased (5–10 mU/L)**	**Normal**	Normal

Pregnancy and oral contraceptives

These lead to greatly increased TBG levels and thus to high or high-normal total T_4. Free T_4 is usually normal. Normal ranges for free T_4 and TSH alter with the normal physiological changes during pregnancy and TSH is often slightly suppressed in the first trimester, but this rarely cause clinical problems.

Drugs

Many drugs affect thyroid function tests by interfering with protein binding. The most common are listed in Table 18.20. Basal TSH should be measured.

Antithyroid antibodies

Serum antibodies to the thyroid are common and may be either destructive or stimulating; both occasionally coexist in the same patient.

Destructive antibodies may be directed against the microsomes or against thyroglobulin; the antigen for thyroid microsomal antibodies is the thyroid peroxidase (TPO) enzyme. TPO antibodies are found in up to 20% of the normal population, especially older women, but only 10–20% of these develop overt hypothyroidism.

TSH receptor IgG antibodies (TRAb) typically stimulate, but occasionally block, the receptor; they can be measured in two ways:

- by the inhibition of binding of TSH to its receptors (TSH-binding inhibitory immunoglobulin, TBII)
- by demonstrating that they stimulate the release of cyclic AMP (thyroid-stimulating immunoglobulin/antibody TSI, TSAb).

HYPOTHYROIDISM

Pathophysiology

Underactivity of the thyroid is usually primary, from disease of the thyroid, but may be secondary to hypothalamic–pituitary disease (reduced TSH drive) (Table 18.22). It is one of the most common endocrine conditions with an overall UK prevalence of over 1% in women, but under 0.1% in men; lifetime prevalence for an individual is higher – perhaps as high as 9% for women and 1% for men with mean age at diagnosis around 60 years.

Causes of primary hypothyroidism
Atrophic (autoimmune) hypothyroidism

This is the most common cause of hypothyroidism and is associated with antithyroid autoantibodies leading to lymphoid infiltration of the gland and eventual atrophy and fibrosis. It is six times more common in females and the incidence increases with age. The condition is associated with other autoimmune disease such as pernicious anaemia, vitiligo and other endocrine deficiencies (p. 1041). In some instances intermittent hypothyroidism occurs with recovery; antibodies which block the TSH receptor may sometimes be involved in the aetiology.

Table 18.22	Causes of hypothyroidism
PRIMARY	**POST-SURGERY**
Congenital	**Post-irradiation**
Agenesis	Radioactive iodine therapy
Ectopic thyroid remnants	External neck irradiation
Defects of hormone synthesis	**Infiltration**
Iodine deficiency	Tumour
Dyshormonogenesis	
Antithyroid drugs	**SECONDARY**
Other drugs (e.g. lithium, amiodarone, interferon)	**Hypopituitarism**
	Isolated TSH deficiency
Autoimmune	
Atrophic thyroiditis	**Peripheral resistance to thyroid hormone**
Hashimoto's thyroiditis	
Postpartum thyroiditis	
Infective	
Post-subacute thyroiditis	

Hashimoto's thyroiditis

This form of autoimmune thyroiditis, again more common in women and most common in late middle age, produces atrophic changes with regeneration, leading to goitre formation. The gland is usually firm and rubbery but may range from soft to hard. TPO antibodies are present, often in very high titres (> 1000 IU/L). Patients may be hypothyroid or euthyroid, though they may go through an initial toxic phase, 'Hashi-toxicity'. Thyroxine therapy may shrink the goitre even when the patient is not hypothyroid.

Postpartum thyroiditis

This is usually a transient phenomenon observed following pregnancy and may involve hyperthyroidism, hypothyroidism or the two sequentially. It is believed to result from the modifications to the immune system necessary in pregnancy, and histologically is a lymphocytic thyroiditis. The process is normally self-limiting, but when conventional antibodies are found there is a high chance of this proceeding to permanent hypothyroidism.

Iodine deficiency

In mountainous areas (the Alps, Himalayas, South America, Central Africa) dietary iodine deficiency still exists, in some areas as 'endemic goitre' where goitre, occasionally massive, is common. The patients may be euthyroid or hypothyroid depending on the severity of iodine deficiency. The mechanism is thought to be borderline hypothyroidism leading to TSH stimulation and thyroid enlargement in the face of continuing iodine deficiency.

Dyshormonogenesis

This rare condition is due to genetic defects in the synthesis of thyroid hormones; patients develop hypothyroidism with a goitre. One particular familial form is associated with sensorineural deafness (Pendred's syndrome).

Symptoms	Signs	
Tiredness/malaise	**Mental slowness**	
Weight gain	Ataxia	
Anorexia	Poverty of movement	Periorbital oedema
Cold intolerance	Deafness	Deep voice
Poor memory	Psychosis/dementia (rare)	Goitre
Change in appearance		
Depression		
Poor libido	'Peaches and	**Dry skin**
Goitre	cream' complexion	Overweight/obesity
Puffy eyes	**Dry thin hair**	
Dry, brittle	Loss of eyebrows	Myotonia
unmanageable hair		Muscular hypertrophy
Dry, coarse skin	Hypertension	Proximal myopathy
Arthralgia	Hypothermia	**Slow-relaxing reflexes**
Myalgia	Heart failure	
Muscle weakness/Stiffness	**Bradycardia**	Anaemia
Constipation	Pericardial effusion	
Menorrhagia or		
oligomenorrhoea	Cold peripheries	
in women	Carpal tunnel syndrome	
Psychosis	Oedema	
Coma		
Deafness		

Fig. 18.20 **Hypothyroidism – symptoms and signs.** Bold type indicates signs of greater discriminant value. A history from a relative is often revealing. Symptoms of other autoimmune disease may be present.

Clinical features (Fig. 18.20)

Hypothyroidism may produce many symptoms. The alternative term 'myxoedema' refers to the accumulation of mucopolysaccharide in subcutaneous tissues. The classic picture of the slow, dry-haired, thick-skinned, deep-voiced patient with weight gain, cold intolerance, bradycardia and constipation makes the diagnosis easy. Milder symptoms are, however, more common and hard to distinguish from other causes of non-specific tiredness. Many cases are detected on biochemical screening.

Special difficulties in diagnosis may arise in certain circumstances:

- *Children with hypothyroidism* may not show classic features but often have a slow growth velocity, poor school performance and sometimes arrest of pubertal development.
- *Young women with hypothyroidism* may not show obvious signs. Hypothyroidism should be excluded in all patients with oligomenorrhoea/amenorrhoea, menorrhagia, infertility or hyperprolactinaemia.
- *The elderly* show many clinical features that are difficult to differentiate from normal ageing.

Investigation of primary hypothyroidism

Serum TSH is the investigation of choice; a high TSH level confirms primary hypothyroidism. A low free T_4 level confirms the hypothyroid state (and is also essential to exclude TSH deficiency if clinical hypothyroidism is strongly suspected and TSH is normal or low).

Thyroid and other organ-specific antibodies may be present. Other abnormalities include the following:

- *anaemia*, which is usually normochromic and normocytic in type but may be macrocytic (sometimes this is due to associated pernicious anaemia) or microcytic (in women, due to menorrhagia)
- *increased serum aspartate transferase levels*, from muscle and/or liver
- *increased serum creatine kinase levels*, with associated myopathy
- *hypercholesterolaemia*
- *hyponatraemia* due to an increase in ADH and impaired free water clearance.

Treatment

Replacement therapy with levothyroxine (thyroxine, i.e. T_4) is given for life. The starting dose will depend upon the severity of the deficiency and on the age and fitness of the patient, especially cardiac performance. In the young and fit, 100 µg daily is suitable, while 50 µg daily (increased to 100 µg after 2–4 weeks) is more appropriate for the small, old or frail. Patients with ischaemic heart disease require even lower initial doses, especially if the hypothyroidism is severe and long-standing. Most physicians would then begin with 25 µg daily and perform serial ECGs, increasing the dose at 3- to 4-week intervals if angina does not occur or worsen and the ECG does not deteriorate.

Adequacy of replacement should be assessed clinically and by thyroid function tests after at least 6 weeks on a steady dose; the aim is to restore T_4 and TSH to well within the normal range. If serum TSH remains high, the dose of T_4 should be increased in increments of 25–50 µg and the tests repeated 6 weeks later. This stepwise progression should be continued until TSH becomes normal, though some physicians believe that complete well-being is only restored in some patients when the T_4 is high-normal and the TSH is slightly suppressed. The usual maintenance dose is 100–150 µg given as a single daily dose; over-replacement may increase the risk of atrial fibrillation in those aged over 60. An annual thyroid function test is recommended – this is usually performed in the primary care setting, often assisted and prompted by district 'thyroid registers'.

Clinical improvement on T_4 may not begin for 2 weeks or more and full resolution of symptoms may take 6 months. The importance of lifelong therapy must be emphasized and the possibility of other autoimmune endocrine disease developing, especially Addison's disease or pernicious anaemia, should be considered. During pregnancy, an increase in T_4 dosage of about 25–50 µg is often needed to maintain normal TSH levels, and the necessity of optimal replacement during pregnancy is emphasized by the finding of reductions in cognitive function in children of mothers with elevated TSH during pregnancy.

Borderline hypothyroidism or 'compensated euthyroidism'

Patients are frequently seen with low-normal serum T_4 levels and slightly raised TSH levels. Sometimes this follows surgery or radioactive iodine therapy when it can reasonably be seen as 'compensatory'. Treatment with thyroxine is normally recommended where the TSH is consistently above 10 mU/L, or when possible symptoms, high-titre thyroid antibodies or lipid abnormalities are present. Where the TSH is only marginally raised, the tests should be repeated 3–6 months later. Conversion to overt hypothyroidism is more common in men or when TPO antibodies are present. In practice, vague symptoms in patients with marginally elevated TSH (below 10 mU/L) rarely respond to treatment, but a 'therapeutic trial' of replacement may be needed to confirm that symptoms are unrelated to the thyroid.

Myxoedema coma

Severe hypothyroidism, especially in the elderly, may present with confusion or even coma. Myxoedema coma is very rare: hypothermia is often present and the patient may have severe cardiac failure, hypoventilation, hypoglycaemia and hyponatraemia. The mortality was previously at least 50% and patients require full intensive care. Optimal treatment is controversial and data lacking; most physicians would advise T_3 orally or intravenously in doses of 2.5–5 µg every 8 hours, then increasing as above. Large intravenous doses should not be used. Additional measures, though unproven, should include:

- oxygen (by ventilation if necessary)
- monitoring of cardiac output and pressures
- gradual rewarming
- hydrocortisone 100 mg i.v. 8-hourly
- glucose infusion to prevent hypoglycaemia.

'Myxoedema madness'

Depression is common in hypothyroidism but rarely with severe hypothyroidism in the elderly the patient may become frankly demented or psychotic, sometimes with striking delusions. This may occur shortly after starting T_4 replacement.

Screening for hypothyroidism

The incidence of congenital hypothyroidism is approximately 1 in 3500 births. Untreated, severe hypothyroidism produces permanent neurological and intellectual damage ('cretinism'). Routine screening of the newborn using a blood-spot, as in the Guthrie test, to detect a high TSH level as an indicator of primary hypothyroidism is efficient and cost-effective; cretinism is prevented if T_4 is started within the first few months of life.

Screening of elderly patients for thyroid dysfunction has a low pick-up rate, is controversial and not currently recommended. However, patients who have undergone thyroid surgery or received radioiodine should have regular thyroid function tests, as should those receiving lithium or amiodarone therapy.

HYPERTHYROIDISM

Hyperthyroidism (thyroid overactivity, thyrotoxicosis) is common, affecting perhaps 2–5% of all females at some time and with a sex ratio of 5 : 1, most often between ages 20 and 40 years. Nearly all cases (> 99%) are caused by intrinsic thyroid disease; a pituitary cause is extremely rare (Table 18.23).

Graves' disease

This is the most common cause of hyperthyroidism and is due to an autoimmune process. Serum IgG antibodies bind to the thyroid TSH receptor stimulating thyroid hormone production, behaving like TSH. These TSH receptor antibodies can be measured in serum. There is an

Table 18.23	Causes of hyperthyroidism

Common
Graves' disease (autoimmune)
Toxic multinodular goitre
Solitary toxic nodule/adenoma

Uncommon
Acute thyroiditis
   viral (e.g. de Quervain's)
   autoimmune
   post-irradiation
   postpartum
Gestational thyrotoxicosis (HCG stimulated)
Neonatal thyrotoxicosis (maternal thyroid antibodies)
Exogenous iodine
Drugs – amiodarone
Thyrotoxicosis factitia (secret T_4 consumption)

Rare
TSH-secreting pituitary tumours
Metastatic differentiated thyroid carcinoma
HCG-producing tumours
Hyperfunctioning ovarian teratoma (struma ovarii)

association with HLA-B8, DR3 and DR2 and 50% concordance is seen amongst monozygotic twins with a 5% concordance rate in dizygotic twins.

Yersinia enterocolitica as well as *Escherichia coli* and other Gram-negative organisms contain TSH binding sites. This raises the possibility that the initiating event in the pathogenesis may be an infection with possible 'molecular mimicry' in a genetically susceptible individual, but the precise initiating mechanisms remain unproven in most cases.

Thyroid eye disease accompanies the hyperthyroidism in many cases (see below) but other components of Graves' disease, e.g. Graves' dermopathy, are very rare. Rarely lymphadenopathy and splenomegaly may occur. Graves' disease is also associated with other autoimmune disorders such as pernicious anaemia, vitiligo and myasthenia gravis.

The natural history is one of fluctuation, many patients showing a pattern of alternating relapse and remission; perhaps only 40% of subjects have a single episode. Many patients eventually become hypothyroid.

Other causes of hyperthyroidism/ thyrotoxicosis

Toxic solitary adenoma/nodule (Plummer's disease)
This is the cause of about 5% of cases of hyperthyroidism. It does not usually remit after a course of antithyroid drugs.

Toxic multinodular goitre
This commonly occurs in older women. Again, antithyroid drugs are rarely successful in inducing a remission – although they can control the hyperthyroidism.

de Quervain's thyroiditis
This is transient hyperthyroidism from an acute inflammatory process, probably viral in origin. Apart from the toxicosis, there is usually fever, malaise and pain in the neck with tachycardia and local thyroid tenderness. Thyroid function tests show initial hyperthyroidism, the erythrocyte sedimentation rate (ESR) and plasma viscosity are raised, and thyroid uptake scans show suppression of uptake in the acute phase. Hypothyroidism, usually transient, may then follow after a few weeks. Treatment of the acute phase is with aspirin, using short-term prednisolone in severely symptomatic cases.

Postpartum thyroiditis
This is described on page 1071.

Clinical features of hyperthyroidism
The symptoms and signs of hyperthyroidism affect many systems (Fig. 18.21).

Symptomatology and signs vary with age and with the underlying aetiology.

- *The eye signs, pretibial myxoedema and thyroid acropachy* occur only in Graves' disease. Pretibial myxoedema is an infiltration on the shin, essentially occurring only with eye disease (see below). Thyroid acropachy is very rare and consists of clubbing, swollen fingers and periosteal new bone formation.
- *In the elderly*, a frequent presentation is with atrial fibrillation, other tachycardias and/or heart failure, often with few other signs. Thyroid function tests are mandatory in any patient with atrial fibrillation.
- *Children* frequently present with excessive height or excessive growth rate, or with behavioural problems

Symptoms	
Weight loss	
Increased appetite	
Irritability/behaviour change	
Restlessness	
Malaise	
Stiffness	
Muscle weakness	
Tremor	
Choreoathetosis	
Breathlessness	
Palpitation	
Heat intolerance	
Itching	
Thirst	
Vomiting	
Diarrhoea	
Eye complaints*	
Goitre	
Oligomenorrhoea	
Loss of libido	
Gynaecomastia	
Onycholysis	
Tall stature (in children)	
Sweating	

*Only in Graves' disease

Signs	
Tremor	Proximal myopathy
Hyperkinesis	Proximal muscle wasting
Irritability	Onycholysis
Psychosis	Palmar erythema
Tachycardia or atrial fibrillation	Graves' dermopathy*
Full pulse	Thyroid acropachy
Warm vasodilated peripheries	Pretibial myxoedema
Systolic hypertension	
Cardiac failure	
Exophthalmos*	
Lid lag and 'stare'	
Conjunctival oedema	
Ophthalmoplegia*	
Periorbital oedema	
Goitre, bruit	
Weight loss	

*Only in Graves' disease

Fig. 18.21 Hyperthyroidism – symptoms and signs. Bold type indicates signs of greater discriminant value.

Table 18.24 Drugs used in the treatment of hyperthyroidism

Drug	Usual starting dose	Side-effects	Remarks
Antithyroid drugs			
Carbimazole	20–40 mg daily, 8-hourly, or in single dose	Rash, nausea, vomiting, arthralgia, agranulocytosis (0.1%), jaundice	Active metabolite is thiamazole (methimazole) Mild immunosuppressive activity
Propylthiouracil	100–200 mg 8-hourly	Rash, nausea, vomiting, agranulocytosis	Additionally blocks conversion of T_4 to T_3
Beta-blocker for symptomatic control			
May need higher doses than normal in hyperthyroidism as metabolism is increased			
Propranolol	40–80 mg every 6–8 hours	Avoid in asthma Use with care in heart failure	Use agents without intrinsic sympathomimetic activity as receptors highly sensitive

such as hyperactivity. They may also show weight gain rather than loss.

- *So-called 'apathetic thyrotoxicosis'* in some elderly patients presents with a clinical picture more like hypothyroidism. There may be very few signs and a high degree of clinical suspicion is essential.

Differential diagnosis

Hyperthyroidism is often clinically obvious but treatment should never be instituted without biochemical confirmation.

Differentiation of the mild case from anxiety states may be difficult; useful positive clinical markers are eye signs, a diffuse goitre, proximal myopathy and wasting. The hyperdynamic circulation with warm peripheries seen with hyperthyroidism can be contrasted with the clammy hands of anxiety.

Investigations

Serum TSH is suppressed in hyperthyroidism (< 0.05 mU/L), except for the very rare instances of TSH hypersecretion. Diagnosis is confirmed with a raised free T_4 or T_3; T_4 is almost always raised but T_3 is more sensitive as there are occasional cases of isolated 'T_3 toxicosis'. TPO and thyroglobulin antibodies are present in most cases of Graves' disease.

TSH receptor antibodies are not measured routinely, but are commonly present: thyroid-stimulating immunoglobin (TSI) 80% positive, TSH-binding inhibitory immunoglobin (TBII) 60–90% in Graves' disease (see p. 1073).

Treatment

Three possibilities are available: antithyroid drugs, radio-iodine and surgery. Practices and beliefs differ widely within and between countries.

Antithyroid drugs

Carbimazole is most often used in the UK, and propylthiouracil is also used. Thiamazole (methimazole), the active metabolite of carbimazole, is used in the USA. These drugs inhibit the formation of thyroid hormones and also have other minor actions; carbimazole/

thiamazole is also an immunosuppressive agent. Initial doses and side-effects are detailed in Table 18.24.

Although thyroid hormone synthesis is reduced very quickly, the long half-life of T_4 (7 days) means that clinical benefit is not apparent for 10–20 days. As many of the manifestations of hyperthyroidism are mediated via the sympathetic system, beta-blockers may be used to provide rapid partial symptomatic control; they also decrease peripheral conversion of T_4 to T_3. Drugs preferred are those without intrinsic sympathomimetic activity, e.g. propranolol (Table 18.24). They should not be used alone for hyperthyroidism except when the condition is self-limiting, as in subacute thyroiditis.

Subsequent management is either by gradual dose titration or a 'block and replace' regimen. Neither regimen has been shown to be unequivocally superior.

Gradual dose titration

1. Review after 4–6 weeks and reduce dose of carbimazole depending on clinical state and T_4/T_3 levels. TSH levels may remain suppressed for several months and are unhelpful at this stage.
2. When clinically and biochemically euthyroid, stop beta-blockers.
3. Review after 2–3 months and, if controlled, reduce carbimazole.
4. Gradually reduce dose to 5 mg daily over 6–24 months if hyperthyroidism remains controlled.
5. When the patient is euthyroid on 5 mg daily carbimazole, discontinue.

Propylthiouracil is used in similar fashion (Table 18.24).

'Block and replace' regimen

With this policy, full doses of antithyroid drugs, usually carbimazole 40 mg daily, are given to suppress the thyroid completely while replacing thyroid activity with 100 µg of thyroxine daily once euthyroidism has been achieved. This is continued usually for 18 months, the claimed advantages being the avoidance of over- or undertreatment and the better use of the immuno-suppressive action of carbimazole. This regimen is contraindicated in pregnancy as T_4 crosses the placenta less well than carbimazole.

Relapse

About 50% of patients will relapse after a course of carbimazole or propylthiouracil, mostly within the following 2 years but occasionally much later. Long-term antithyroid therapy is then used or surgery or radio-therapy is considered (see below). Most patients (90%) with hyperthyroidism have a diffuse goitre but those with large single or multinodular goitres are unlikely to remit after a course of antithyroid drugs. Severe bio-chemical hyperthyroidism is also less likely to remain in remission.

Toxicity

The major side-effect is agranulocytosis that occurs in approximately 1 in 1000 patients usually within 3 months of treatment. All patients must be warned to seek immediate medical attention if they develop unexplained fever or sore throat – written information is essential. Rashes are more frequent and usually require a change of drug. If toxicity occurs on carbimazole, propylthiouracil may be used and vice versa; side-effects are only occasionally repeated on the other drug.

Radioactive iodine

Radioactive iodine (RAI) may be given to patients of all ages, although it is contraindicated in pregnancy and while breast-feeding. RAI is the most common treatment modality in the USA whereas antithyroid drugs tend to be favoured in Europe. Iodine-131 in an empirical dose (usually 200–500 MBq), accumulates in the thyroid and destroys the gland by local radiation – though it takes several months to be fully effective. Strict radiation safety rules apply in the UK and may be inconvenient or dis-concerting for some patients. Patients must be rendered euthyroid before treatment though they have to stop antithyroid drugs at least 4 days before radioiodine, and not recommence until 3 days after radioiodine. (Many patients who are well controlled before RAI do not need to restart at all.)

Early discomfort in the neck and immediate worsening of hyperthyroidism are sometimes seen; if worsening occurs, the patient should receive propranolol (Table 18.24); if necessary carbimazole can be restarted. Euthyroidism normally returns in 2–3 months. Patients with dysthyroid eye disease are more likely to show worsening of eye problems after radioiodine than after antithyroid drugs; this represents a partial contra-indication to RAI, although worsening can usually be prevented by steroid administration.

Apart from the immediate problems above, a major complication is the progressive incidence of subsequent hypothyroidism affecting the majority of subjects over the following 20 years. Though 75% of patients are rendered euthyroid in the short term, a small proportion remain hyperthyroid; increasing the radioiodine dose improves the speed and rate of response but increases the rate of hypothyroidism. Long-term surveillance of thyroid func-

tion is necessary with frequent tests in the first year after therapy, and at least annually thereafter.

Risk of carcinogenesis has been long debated, but it is now clear that overall cancer incidence and mortality are not increased after radioactive iodine (and indeed are significantly reduced in some studies) but the risk of thyroid cancer is significantly increased, although the risk remains very low in absolute terms.

Surgery: subtotal thyroidectomy

Thyroidectomy should be performed only in patients who have previously been rendered euthyroid. Conven-tional practice is to stop the antithyroid drug 10–14 days before operation and to give potassium iodide (60 mg three times daily), which reduces the vascularity of the gland.

The operation should be performed only by experi-enced surgeons to reduce the chance of complications:

- Early postoperative bleeding causing tracheal com-pression and asphyxia is a rare emergency requiring immediate removal of all clips/sutures to allow escape of the blood/haematoma.
- Laryngeal nerve palsy occurs in 1%. Vocal chord movement should be checked preoperatively. Mild hoarseness is more common and thyroidectomy is best avoided in professional singers!
- Transient hypocalcaemia occurs in up to 10% but with permanent hypoparathyroidism in fewer than 1%.
- Recurrent hyperthyroidism occurs in 1–3% within 1 year, then 1% per year.
- Hypothyroidism occurs in about 10% of patients with-in 1 year, and this percentage increases with time. It is likeliest if TPO antibodies are positive. Automated computer thyroid registers with annual TSH screening are used in some regions, and have demonstrated that a high proportion of patients become hypothyroid in the long term.

Choice of therapy

Indications for either surgery or radioiodine are:

- patient choice
- persistent drug side-effects
- poor compliance with drug therapy
- recurrent hyperthyroidism after drugs.

Particular indications for surgery include:

- a large goitre, which is unlikely to remit after anti-thyroid medication.

Special situations in hyperthyroidism

Thyroid crisis or 'thyroid storm'

This rare condition, with a mortality of 10%, is a rapid deterioration of hyperthyroidism with hyperpyrexia, severe tachycardia and extreme restlessness. It is usually precipitated by stress, infection, surgery in an unprepared patient, or radioiodine therapy. With careful management it should no longer occur and most cases referred as 'crisis' are simply severe but uncomplicated thyrotoxicosis.

Treatment is urgent. Propranolol in full doses is started immediately together with potassium iodide, antithyroid drugs, corticosteroids (which suppress many of the manifestations of hyperthyroidism) and full supportive measures.

Hyperthyroidism in pregnancy and neonatal life

Maternal hyperthyroidism during pregnancy is uncommon and usually mild. Diagnosis can be difficult because of misleading thyroid function tests, although TSH is largely reliable. The pathogenesis is almost always Graves' disease. Thyroid-stimulating immunoglobulin (TSI) crosses the placenta to stimulate the fetal thyroid. Carbimazole also crosses the placenta, but T_4 does so poorly so a 'block-and-replace' regimen is contra-indicated. The smallest dose of carbimazole necessary is used and the fetus must be monitored (see below). The paediatrician should be informed and the infant checked immediately after birth – overtreatment with carbimazole can cause fetal goitre. Breast-feeding while on usual doses of carbimazole or propylthiouracil appears to be safe.

If necessary (high doses needed, poor patient compliance or drug side-effects), surgery can be performed, preferably in the second trimester. Radioactive iodine is absolutely contraindicated.

The fetus and maternal Graves' disease

Any mother with a history of Graves' disease may have circulating TSI. Even if she has been treated (e.g. by surgery), the immunoglobulin may still be present to stimulate the fetal thyroid, and the fetus can thus become hyperthyroid, while the mother remains euthyroid.

Any such patient should therefore be monitored during pregnancy. Fetal heart rate provides a direct biological assay of fetal thyroid status, and monitoring should be performed at least monthly. Rates above 160 per minute are strongly suggestive of fetal hyper-thyroidism, and maternal treatment with carbimazole and/or propranolol may be used. To prevent the mother becoming hypothyroid, T_4 may be given as this does not easily cross the placenta. Sympathomimetics, used to prevent premature labour, are contraindicated as they may provoke fatal tachycardia in the fetus.

Hyperthyroidism may also develop in the neonatal period as TSI has a half-life of approximately 3 weeks. Manifestations in the newborn include irritability, failure to thrive and persisting weight loss, diarrhoea and eye signs. Thyroid function tests are difficult to interpret as neonatal normal ranges vary with age.

Untreated neonatal hyperthyroidism is probably associated with hyperactivity in later childhood.

Thyroid hormone resistance

Thyroid hormone resistance is an inherited condition caused by an abnormality of the thyroid hormone receptor. Mutations to the receptor result in the need for higher levels of thyroid hormones to achieve the same intracellular effect. As a result, the normal feedback control mechanisms (see Fig. 18.1, p. 1037) result in high blood levels of thyroxine with a normal TSH in order to maintain a euthyroid state. This has two consequences:

- First, thyroid function tests appear abnormal even when the patient is euthyroid and requires no treatment; this is not a particular problem as free T_4 and TSH levels are measured.
- Second, different tissues contain different thyroid hormone receptors and, in some families, receptors in certain tissues may have normal activity. In this case the level of thyroid hormones to maintain euthyroidism at pituitary and hypothalamic levels (which controls secretion of TSH) may be higher than that required in other tissues such as heart and bone, so that these tissues may exhibit 'thyrotoxic' effects in spite of a normal serum TSH. This 'partial thyroid hormone resistance' can be very difficult to manage effectively.

Long-term consequences of hyperthyroidism

Long-term follow-up studies of hyperthyroidism show a slight increase in overall mortality, which affects all age groups, is not fully explained and tends to occur in the first year after diagnosis. Thereafter, the only long-term risk of adequately treated hyperthyroidism appears to be an increased risk of osteoporosis.

THYROID EYE DISEASE

This is also known as dysthyroid eye disease or ophthalmic Graves' disease.

Pathophysiology

The ophthalmopathy of Graves' disease is due to a specific immune response that causes retro-orbital inflammation. Swelling and oedema of the extraocular muscles lead to limitation of movement and to proptosis which is usually bilateral but can sometimes be unilateral. Ultimately increased pressure on the optic nerve may cause optic atrophy. Histology shows focal oedema and glycosaminoglycan deposition followed by fibrosis. The precise autoantigen which leads to the immune response remains to be identified, but it appears to be an antigen in retro-orbital tissue with similar immunoreactivity to the TSH receptor.

Eye disease is a manifestation of Graves' disease and can occur in patients who may be hyperthyroid, euthyroid or hypothyroid. TSH receptor antibodies are almost invariably found in the serum but their role in the pathogenesis is unclear. Ophthalmopathy is more common in smokers.

Clinical features

The clinical appearances are characteristic (Fig. 18.21) but thyroid eye disease demonstrates a wide range of severity. A high proportion of patients with Graves' disease notice some soreness, painful watering or prominence of the eyes and the 'stare' of lid retraction is relatively common. More severe proptosis occurs in a minority of cases, and limitation and discomfort of eye movement and visual impairment due to optic nerve compression are relatively uncommon. Proptosis and lid retraction may limit the ability to close the eyes completely so that corneal damage may occur. There is periorbital oedema and conjunctival oedema and inflammation.

Eye manifestations do not parallel the degree of biochemical thyrotoxicosis, nor the need for antithyroid therapy, but exacerbation of eye disease is more common after radioiodine treatment (15% vs 3% on antithyroid drugs). Only 5–10% of cases threaten sight, but the discomfort and cosmetic problems cause great patient anxiety.

Investigations

Few investigations are necessary if the appearances are characteristic and bilateral. TSH, T_3 and free T_4 are measured.

There are a variety of grading systems but none is universally accepted. It is essential to clearly document eye movements and the degree of oedema and inflammation. The exophthalmos should be measured to allow progress to be monitored. If appearances or measurements are markedly discrepant in the two eyes, other retro-orbital space-occupying lesions should be considered: MRI of the orbits will exclude other causes and show enlarged muscles and oedema.

Treatment

If the patient is thyrotoxic this should be treated, but this will not directly result in an improvement of the ophthalmopathy, and hypothyroidism must be avoided as this may exacerbate the eye problem. Smokers should be advised to stop. Treatment of the eyes may be either local or systemic, and always requires close liaison between specialist endocrinologist and ophthalmologist:

- *Methylcellulose or hypromellose eyedrops* are given to aid lubrication and improve comfort.
- *Some patients gain relief by sleeping upright.* The eyelids can be taped to ensure closure at night.
- *Systemic steroids* (prednisolone 30–120 mg daily) usually reduce inflammation if more severe symptoms are present. Pulse intravenous methylprednisolone may be more rapidly effective in severe cases.
- *Irradiation of the orbits* (20 Gy in divided doses) is used in severe instances. This improves inflammation and occular motility but has little effect on proptosis.
- *Lid surgery* will protect the cornea if lids cannot be closed.
- *Surgical decompression of the orbit(s)* is occasionally needed.
- *Corrective eye muscle surgery* may improve diplopia due to muscle changes, but should be deferred until the situation has been stable for 6 months. Plastic surgery around the eyes may also be of value.

GOITRE (THYROID ENLARGEMENT)

Goitre is more common in women than in men and may be either physiological or pathological.

Clinical features

Goitres are present on examination in up to 9% of the population. Most commonly a goitre is noticed as a cosmetic defect by the patient or by friends or relatives. The majority are painless, but pain or discomfort can occur in acute varieties. Large goitres can produce dysphagia and difficulty in breathing, implying oesophageal or tracheal compression.

A small goitre may be more easily visible (on swallowing) than palpable. Clinical examination should record the size, shape, consistency and mobility of the gland as well as whether its lower margin can be demarcated (thus implying the absence of retrosternal extension). A bruit may be present. Associated lymph nodes should be sought and the tracheal position determined if possible. Examination should never omit an assessment of the patient's clinical thyroid status.

Specific enquiry should be made about any medication, especially iodine-containing preparations, and possible exposure to radiation.

Particular points of note are:

- Puberty and pregnancy may produce a diffuse increase in size of the thyroid.
- Pain in a goitre may be caused by thyroiditis, bleeding into a cyst or (rarely) a thyroid tumour.
- Excessive doses of carbimazole or propylthiouracil will induce goitre.
- Iodine deficiency and dyshormonogenesis (see above) can also cause goitre.

Assessment

There are two major aspects of any goitre: its pathological nature and the patient's thyroid status.

The nature can often be judged clinically. Goitres (Table 18.25) are usually separable into diffuse and nodular types, the causes of which differ.

Diffuse goitre
Simple goitre
In this instance no clear cause is found for enlargement of the thyroid, which is usually smooth and soft. It may be associated with thyroid growth-stimulating antibodies.

Table 18.25	Goitre – causes and types
Diffuse	**Nodular**
Simple	Multinodular goitre
Physiological (puberty, pregnancy)	Solitary nodular
pregnancy)	Fibrotic (Reidel's thyroiditis)
Autoimmune	Cysts
Graves' disease	
Hashimoto's disease	**Tumours**
Thyroiditis	Adenomas
Acute (de Quervain's thyroiditis)	Carcinoma
thyroiditis)	Lymphomas
Iodine deficiency (endemic goitre)	**Miscellaneous**
goitre)	Sarcoidosis
Dyshormonogenesis	Tuberculosis
Goitrogens (e.g. sulphonylureas)	

Autoimmune thyroid disease

Hashimoto's thyroiditis and thyrotoxicosis are both associated with firm diffuse goitre of variable size. A bruit is often present in thyrotoxicosis.

Thyroiditis

Acute tenderness in a diffuse swelling, sometimes with severe pain, is suggestive of an acute viral thyroiditis (de Quervain's). This is usually associated with a systemic viral illness and may produce transient clinical hyperthyroidism with an increase in serum T_4 (see p. 1074).

Nodular goitres

Multinodular goitre

Most common is the multinodular goitre, especially in older patients. The patient is usually euthyroid but may be hyperthyroid or borderline with suppressed TSH levels but normal T_4 and T_3. Multinodular goitre is the most common cause of tracheal and/or oesophageal compression and can cause laryngeal nerve palsy. It may also extend retrosternally. The classical 'multinodular goitre' is usually readily apparent clinically, but it should be noted that modern, high-resolution ultrasound frequently reports multiple small nodules in glands which are clinically diffusely enlarged and associated with autoimmune thyroid disease. These nodules are also found in up to 40% of the normal population.

Solitary nodular goitre

Such a goitre presents a difficult problem of diagnosis. Malignancy should be considered in any solitary nodule – however, the majority of such nodules are cystic or benign and, indeed, may simply be the largest nodule of a multinodular goitre. The diagnostic challenge is to identify the small minority of malignant nodules, which require surgery, from the majority of benign nodules, which do not. A history of pain, rapid enlargement or associated lymph nodes in such a situation suggests the possibility of thyroid carcinoma, but investigations are paramount. Risk factors for malignancy include previous irradiation, long-standing iodine deficiency and occasional familial cases.

Solitary toxic nodules (Plummer's syndrome) are quite uncommon and may be associated with T_3 toxicosis.

Fibrotic goitre

Fibrotic goitre (Riedel's thyroiditis) is a rare condition, usually producing a 'woody' gland. It is associated with other midline fibrosis and is often difficult to distinguish from carcinoma, being irregular and hard.

Malignancy

In addition to thyroid carcinomas (see below), the thyroid is rarely the site of a metastatic deposit or the site of origin of a lymphoma.

Investigations

Clinical findings will dictate appropriate initial tests:

- **Thyroid function tests** – TSH plus free T_4 or T_3 (see Table 18.21).
- **Ultrasound.** Ultrasound with high resolution is a sensitive method for delineating nodules and can demonstrate whether they are cystic or solid. In addition, a multinodular goitre may be demonstrated when only a single nodule is palpable. Unfortunately, even cystic lesions can be malignant and thyroid tumours may arise within a multinodular goitre; therefore fine-needle aspiration (see below) is often required and performed under ultrasound control at the same time as the scan.
- **Chest and thoracic inlet X-rays** to detect tracheal compression and large retrosternal extensions in patients with very large goitre or clinical symptoms.
- **Fine-needle aspiration (FNA).** In patients with a solitary nodule or a dominant nodule in a multi-nodular goitre, there is a 5% chance of malignancy; in view of this, FNA should be performed. This can be done in the outpatient clinic. Cytology in expert hands can usually differentiate the suspicious or definitely malignant nodule.

  FNA has reduced the need for isotope scans and reduces the necessity for surgery, but there is a 5% false-negative rate which must be borne in mind (and the patient appropriately counselled). Continued observation is required when an isolated thyroid nodule is assumed to be benign without excision.
- **Thyroid scan.** FNA has largely replaced isotope scans in the diagnosis of thyroid nodules. Thyroid scan (^{125}I or ^{131}I) can be useful to distinguish between functioning (hot) or non-functioning (cold) nodules. A hot nodule is rarely malignant; however, a cold nodule is malignant in 10% of cases.

Treatment

Many goitres are small, cause no symptoms and can be observed (including self-monitoring by the patient in the long term). In particular, during puberty and pregnancy a goitre associated with euthyroidism rarely requires intervention and the patient can be reassured that spontaneous resolution is likely. When thyroid function is abnormal the patient should be rendered euthyroid. Indications for surgical intervention are:

- *The possibility of malignancy.* A history of rapid growth, pain, cervical lymphadenopathy, change in voice or previous irradiation to the neck are worrying features. A positive or suspicious FNA makes surgery mandatory and surgery may be necessary if doubt persists even in the presence of a negative FNA (especially if the patient is concerned by the false negative rate).
- *Pressure symptoms on the trachea or, more rarely, oesophagus.* The possibility of retrosternal extension should be excluded.
- *Cosmetic reasons.* A large goitre is often a considerable anxiety to the patient even though functionally and anatomically benign.

Table 18.26 Types of thyroid malignancy

Cell type	Frequency	Behaviour	Spread	Prognosis
Papillary	70%	Occurs in young people	Local, sometimes lung/bone secondaries	Good, especially in young
Follicular	20%	More common in females	Metastases to lung/bone	Good if resectable
Anaplastic	< 5%	Aggressive	Locally invasive	Very poor
Lymphoma	2%	Variable		Sometimes responsive to radiotherapy
Medullary cell	5%	Often familial	Local and metastases	Poor, but indolent course

THYROID CARCINOMA

Types of thyroid carcinoma, their characteristics and treatment are listed in Table 18.26. While not common, these tumours are responsible for 400 deaths annually in the UK. In 90% of cases they present as thyroid nodules (see above), but occasionally with cervical lymphadenopathy (about 5%), or with lung, cerebral, hepatic or bone metastases.

Carcinomas derived from thyroid epithelium may be papillary or follicular (differentiated) or anaplastic (undifferentiated), while medullary carcinomas (about 5% of all thyroid cancers) arise from the calcitonin-producing C cells. Lymphomas also arise within the thyroid. The pathogenesis of thyroid epithelial carcinomas is not understood except for occasional familial papillary carcinoma and those cases related to previous head-and-neck irradiation or ingestion of radioactive iodine (e.g. post-Chernobyl). These tumours are minimally active hormonally and are extremely rarely associated with hyperthyroidism; over 90%, however, secrete thyroglobulin, which can therefore act as a tumour marker.

Papillary and follicular carcinomas

The primary treatment is surgical, normally total or near-total thyroidectomy for local disease. Regional, or more extensive, neck dissection is needed where there is local nodal spread or involvement of local structures.

Most tumours will take up iodine. If initial disease is extensive (or 'high risk') or if thyroglobulin levels rise during follow-up, patients may be given a therapeutic radioiodine dose (high dose: 5.5–7.5 GBq), which will be taken up by remaining thyroid tissue or metastatic lesions. After ablation of normal thyroid in this way, radioiodine scanning may be used to localize residual disease (using low doses) or to treat it (using high doses). Local invasion and lymph node involvement is most common and lungs and bone are the most common sites of distant metastases.

Where surgical excision is histologically complete and/or radioiodine therapy and scanning completed, patients are placed on suppressive doses of thyroxine (sufficient to suppress TSH levels below the normal range). Patient progress is monitored both clinically and biochemically using serum thyroglobulin levels as a tumour marker; levels are low on thyroxine unless there is residual tumour. The measurement of thyroglobulin is either by following the withdrawal of thyroxine therapy (for periods sufficient to significantly raise the TH), or more easily, by using recombinant TSH (thyrotropin alfa, rhTSH).

The prognosis is extremely good when these types of tumour are excised while still confined to the thyroid gland, and the specific therapies available lead to a relatively good prognosis even in the presence of metastases at diagnosis. Age below 40 years and papillary tumours do better than those over 40 and with a follicular histology.

Anaplastic carcinomas and lymphoma

These do not respond to radioactive iodine, and external radiotherapy produces only a brief respite.

Medullary carcinoma

Medullary carcinoma, often associated with multiple endocrine neoplasia (MEN 2, see p. 1099), is usually treated by total thyroidectomy. Local invasion or metastasis is frequent, and the tumour responds poorly to treatment, although progression is often slow. The patient's family should be screened for this and other endocrine neoplastic conditions.

FURTHER READING

Cooper DS (2003) Hyperthyroidism. *Lancet* **362**: 459–468.

Hegedus L (2004) The thyroid nodule. *New England Journal of Medicine* **351**: 1764–1771.

Pearce EN et al. (2003) Thyroiditis. *New England Journal of Medicine* **348**: 2648–2655.

Roberts GGP (2004) Hypothyroidism. *Lancet* **36**: 793–798.

Sherman SI (2003) Thyroid carcinoma. *Lancet* **361**: 501–511.

Weetman AP (2000) Medical progress: Graves' disease. *New England Journal of Medicine* **343**: 1236–1248.

THE GLUCOCORTICOID AXIS

Adrenal anatomy and function

The human adrenals weigh 8–10 g together and comprise an outer cortex with three zones (reticularis, fasciculata and glomerulosa) producing steroids, and an inner medulla that synthesizes, stores and secretes catecholamines (see adrenal medulla, p. 1098).

The adrenal steroids are grouped into three classes based on their predominant physiological effects.

Table 18.27 The major actions of glucocorticoids

Increased or stimulated	Decreased or inhibited
Gluconeogenesis	Protein synthesis
Glycogen deposition	Host response to infection
Protein catabolism	Lymphocyte transformation
Fat deposition	Delayed hypersensitivity
Sodium retention	Circulating lymphocytes
Potassium loss	Circulating eosinophils
Free water clearance	
Uric acid production	
Circulating neutrophils	

Table 18.28 The relative glucocorticoid and mineralocorticoid potency of equal amounts of common natural and synthetic steroids

Steroid	Glucoccorticol effect	Mineralocorticoid effect
Cortisol (hydrocortisone)*	1	1
Prednisolone	4	0.7
Dexamethasone	40	2
Aldosterone	0.1	400
Fludrocortisone	10	400

*Cortisol is arbitrarily defined as 1

Glucocorticoids

These are so named after their effects on carbohydrate metabolism. Major actions are listed in Table 18.27.

The relative potency of common steroids is shown in Table 18.28.

Mineralocorticoids

Their predominant effect is on the extracellular balance of sodium and potassium in the distal tubule of the kidney. Aldosterone, produced solely in the zona glomerulosa, is the predominant mineralocorticoid in humans (about 50%); corticosterone makes a small contribution. The mineralocorticoid activity of cortisol is weak but it is present in considerable excess. However, the mineralocorticoid receptor in the kidney is largely protected from this excess by the intrarenal conversion ('shuttle') of cortisol to the inactive cortisone by the enzyme 11β-hydroxysteroid dehydrogenase.

Androgens

Although secreted in considerable quantities, most have only relatively weak intrinsic androgenic activity until metabolized peripherally to testosterone or dihydrotestosterone.

Biochemistry

All steroids have the same basic skeleton (Fig. 18.22(b)) and the chemical differences between them are slight. The major biosynthetic pathways are shown in Figure 18.22(a).

Physiology

Glucocorticoid production by the adrenal is under hypothalamic–pituitary control (Fig. 18.23).

Corticotropin-releasing hormone (CRH) is secreted in the hypothalamus in response to circadian rhythm, stress and

Fig. 18.22 **(a) The major steroid biosynthetic pathways.** Enzymes catalysing reactions are in red: p450 enzymes are in mitochondria and each catalyses several reaction steps; 3βHSD (hydroxysteroid dehydrogenase) is in cytoplasm, bound to endoplasmic reticulum; 17βHSD and p450$_{aro}$ are found mainly in gonads. **(b) The steroid molecule.**

Fig. 18.23 **Control of the hypothalamic–pituitary–adrenal axis.** CRH, corticotropin-releasing hormone.

other stimuli. CRH travels down the portal system to stimulate ACTH release from the anterior pituitary. ACTH is derived from the prohormone pro-opiomelanocortin, which undergoes complex processing within the pituitary to produce ACTH and a number of other peptides including beta-lipotrophin and beta-endorphin. Many of these peptides, including ACTH, contain melanocyte-stimulating hormone (MSH)-like sequences which cause pigmentation when levels of ACTH are markedly raised.

Circulating ACTH stimulates cortisol production in the adrenal. The cortisol secreted (or any other synthetic corticosteroid administered to the patient) causes negative feedback on the hypothalamus and pituitary to inhibit further CRH/ACTH release. The set-point of this system clearly varies through the day according to the circadian rhythm, and is usually overridden by severe stress.

Following adrenalectomy or other adrenal damage (e.g. Addison's disease), cortisol secretion will be absent or reduced; ACTH levels will therefore rise.

Mineralocorticoid secretion is mainly controlled by the renin–angiotensin system (see p. 1096).

Investigation of glucocorticoid abnormalities

Basal levels

ACTH and cortisol are released episodically and in response to stress. The following precautions are therefore necessary when taking a blood sample:

- Sampling time should be recorded accurately. Conventionally, basal levels are obtained at between 0800h and 0900h near the peak of the circadian variation.
- Stress should be minimized.
- Appropriate reference ranges (for time and assay method) should be used.

Suppression and stimulation tests are used in suspected excess and deficient cortisol production, respectively.

Dexamethasone suppression tests

Administration of a synthetic glucocorticoid to a normal subject produces prompt feedback suppression of CRH and ACTH levels and thus of endogenous cortisol secretion (dexamethasone is not measured by most cortisol assays). Three forms of the test, used in the diagnosis and differential diagnosis of Cushing's syndrome, are available (Table 18.29).

ACTH stimulation tests

Synthetic ACTH (tetracosactide, which consists of the first 24 amino acids of human ACTH) is given to stimulate adrenal cortisol production. Details are given in Table 18.29 and Box 18.1 on page 1039.

Addison's disease: primary hypoadrenalism

Pathophysiology and causes

In this condition there is destruction of the entire adrenal cortex. Glucocorticoid, mineralocorticoid and sex steroid production are therefore all reduced. (This differs from hypothalamic–pituitary disease, in which mineralocorticoid secretion remains largely intact, being predominantly stimulated by angiotensin II. Adrenal sex steroid production is also largely independent of pituitary action.) In Addison's disease reduced cortisol levels lead, through feedback, to increased CRH and ACTH production, the latter being directly responsible for the hyperpigmentation.

Incidence. Addison's disease is rare, with an incidence of 3–4/million/year and prevalence of 40–60/million. Primary hypoadrenalism shows a marked female preponderance and is most often caused by autoimmune disease (> 90% in UK) rather than tuberculosis (< 10%). All other causes are rare (Table 18.30). Autoimmune adrenalitis results from the destruction of the adrenal cortex by organ-specific autoantibodies, with 21-hydroxylase as the common antigen. There are associations with other autoimmune conditions in the polyglandular autoimmune syndromes Types I and II (e.g. type I diabetes mellitus, pernicious anaemia, thyroiditis, hypoparathyroidism, premature ovarian failure).

Clinical features

These are shown in Figure 18.24. The symptomatology of Addison's disease is often vague and non-specific. These symptoms may be the prelude to an Addisonian crisis with severe hypotension and dehydration precipitated by intercurrent illness, accident or operation.

Pigmentation (dull, slaty, grey-brown) is the predominant sign in over 90% of cases.

Table 18.29 Details of dexamethasone suppression and ACTH (synacthen) tests in the diagnosis of Cushing's syndrome and Addison's disease

Test and protocol	Measure	Normal test result or positive suppression	Use and explanation
Dexamethasone (for Cushing's)			
Overnight			
Take 1 mg on going to bed at 2300h	Plasma cortisol at 0900h next morning	Plasma cortisol < 100 nmol/L	Outpatient screening test Some 'false positives'
'Low-dose'			
0.5 mg 6-hourly Eight doses from 0900h on day 0	Plasma cortisol at 0900h on days 0 and +2	Plasma cortisol < 50 nmol/L on second sample	For diagnosis of Cushing's syndrome
'High-dose' used in differential diagnosis			
2 mg 6-hourly Eight doses from 0900h on day 0	Plasma cortisol at 0900h on days 0 and +2	Plasma cortisol on day +2 less than 50% of that on day 0 suggests pituitary-dependent disease	Differential diagnosis of Cushing's syndrome Pituitary-dependent disease suppresses in about 90% of cases
ACTH (synacthen) (for Addison's)			
Short			
Tetracosactide 250 μg i.v. or i.m. at time 0	Plasma cortisol at times 0, +30 min	Cortisol at +30 min > 600 nmol/L	To exclude primary adrenal failure
Long			
Depot tetracosactide 1 mg i.m. at time 0	Plasma cortisol at times 0, +1, +2, +3, +4, +5, +8 and +24 h	Maximum > 1000 nmol/L Rise > 550 nmol/L	To demonstrate or exclude adrenal suppression (rather than primary adrenal failure)

Plasma cortisol values are very dependent upon the assay used – local reference ranges must be consulted

Table 18.30 Causes of primary hypoadrenalism

Autoimmune disease (approx. 90% in UK)	Infiltration Malignant destruction
Tuberculosis (< 10% in UK)	Amyloid
Surgical removal	Schilder's disease
Haemorrhage/infarction) Meningococcal septicaemia Venography	(adrenal leucodystrophy)

Postural systolic hypotension, due to hypovolaemia and sodium loss, is present in 80–90% of cases, even if supine blood pressure is normal. Mineralocorticoid deficiency is the cause of the hypotension.

Investigations

Once Addison's disease is suspected, investigation is urgent. If the patient is seriously ill or hypotensive, hydrocortisone 100 mg should be given intramuscularly together with intravenous saline. Ideally this should be done immediately after a blood sample is taken for later measurement of plasma cortisol. Alternatively, an ACTH stimulation test can be performed immediately. Full investigation should be delayed until emergency treatment (see below) has improved the patient's condition. Otherwise, tests are as follows:

- **Single cortisol measurements** are of little value, although a random cortisol below 100 nmol/L during the day is highly suggestive, and a random cortisol > 550 nmol/L makes the diagnosis unlikely (but not impossible).
- **The short ACTH stimulation test** should be performed (see Table 18.29). An absent or impaired cortisol response is seen, confirmed if necessary by a long ACTH stimulation test to exclude adrenal suppression by steroids or ACTH deficiency.
- **A 0900h plasma ACTH level** – a high level (> 80 ng/L) with low or low-normal cortisol confirms primary hypoadrenalism.
- **Electrolytes and urea** classically show hyponatraemia, hyperkalaemia and a high urea, but they can be normal.
- **Blood glucose** may be low, with symptomatic hypoglycaemia.
- **Adrenal antibodies** are present in many cases of autoimmune adrenalitis.
- **Chest and abdominal X-rays** may show evidence of tuberculosis and/or calcified adrenals.
- **Serum aldosterone** is reduced with high plasma renin activity.
- **Hypercalcaemia and anaemia** (after rehydration) are sometimes seen. They resolve on treatment, but are occasionally the first clue to the diagnosis.

Symptoms
Weight loss
Anorexia
Malaise
Weakness
Fever
Depression
Impotence/amenorrhoea
Nausea/vomiting
Diarrhoea
Confusion
Syncope from postural hypotension
Abdominal pain
Constipation
Myalgia
Joint or back pain

Signs
Pigmentation, especially of new scars and palmar creases
Buccal pigmentation
Postural hypotension
Loss of weight
General wasting
Dehydration
Loss of body hair
(Vitiligo)

Fig. 18.24 **Primary hypoadrenalism (Addison's disease) – symptoms and signs.** Bold type indicates signs of greater discriminant value.

Treatment

Acute hypoadrenalism needs urgent treatment (Emergency box 18.1).

Long-term treatment is with replacement glucocorticoid and mineralocorticoid; tuberculosis must be treated if present or suspected. Replacement dosage details are shown in Table 18.31. Dehydroepiandrosterone (DHEA) replacement has also been advocated, and studies suggest that this may cause symptomatic improvements, although long-term results are awaited.

Adequacy of glucocorticoid dose is judged by:

- clinical well-being and restoration of normal, but not excessive, weight

- normal cortisol levels during the day while on replacement hydrocortisone (cortisol levels cannot be used for synthetic steroids).

Fludrocortisone replacement is assessed by:

- restoration of serum electrolytes to normal
- blood pressure response to posture (it should not fall > 10 mmHg systolic after 2 minutes' standing)
- suppression of plasma renin activity to normal.

Patient advice

All patients requiring replacement steroids should:

- know how to increase steroid replacement dose for intercurrent illness
- carry a 'Steroid Card'
- wear a Medic-Alert bracelet (or similar), which gives details of their condition so that emergency replacement therapy can be given if found unconscious
- keep an (up-to-date) ampoule of hydrocortisone at home in case oral therapy is impossible, for administration by self, family or GP.

> **Emergency Box 18.1**
> **Management of acute hypoadrenalism**
>
> - Clinical context: hypotension, hyponatraemia, hyperkalaemia, hypoglycaemia, dehydration, pigmentation often with precipitating infection, infarction, trauma or operation. The major deficiencies are of salt, steroid and glucose.
> - Assuming normal cardiovascular function, the following are required:
> - One litre of 0.9% saline should be given over 30–60 minutes with 100 mg of intravenous bolus hydrocortisone.
> - Subsequent requirements are several litres of saline within 24 hours (assessing with central venous pressure line if necessary) plus hydrocortisone, 100 mg i.m., 6-hourly, until the patient is clinically stable.
> - Glucose should be infused if there is hypoglycaemia.
> - Oral replacement medication is then started, unless unable to take oral medication, initially hydrocortisone 20 mg, 8-hourly, reducing to 20–30 mg in divided doses over a few days (Table 18.31).
> - Fludrocortisone is unnecessary acutely as the high cortisol doses provide sufficient mineralocorticoid activity – it should be introduced later.

Table 18.31 Average replacement steroid dosages for adults with primary hypoadrenalism	
Drug	**Dose**
Glucocorticoid	
Hydrocortisone	20–30 mg daily e.g. 10 mg on waking, 5 mg at 1200h, 5 mg at 1800h
or	
Prednisolone	7.5 mg daily 5 mg on waking, 2.5 mg at 1800h
rarely	
Dexamethasone	0.75 mg daily 0.5 mg on waking, 0.25 mg at 1800h
Mineralocorticoid	
Fludrocortisone	50–300 µg daily

Secondary hypoadrenalism

This may arise from hypothalamic–pituitary disease (inadequate ACTH production) or from long-term steroid therapy leading to hypothalamic–pituitary–adrenal suppression.

Most patients with the former have panhypopituitarism (see p. 1046) and need T_4 replacement as well as cortisol; in this case hydrocortisone must be started before T_4.

The most common cause of secondary hypoadrenalism is long-term corticosteroid medication for non-endocrine disease. The hypothalamic–pituitary axis and the adrenal may both be suppressed and the patient may have vague symptoms of feeling unwell. The long ACTH stimulation test should demonstrate a delayed cortisol response. Weaning off steroids is often a long and difficult process.

Cushing's syndrome

Cushing's syndrome is the term used to describe the clinical state of increased free circulating glucocorticoid. It occurs most often following the therapeutic administration of synthetic steroids or ACTH (see below). All the spontaneous forms of the syndrome are rare.

Pathophysiology and causes

Spontaneous Cushing's syndrome is rare, with an incidence of < 5/million/year.

Causes of Cushing's syndrome are usually subdivided into two groups (Table 18.32):

- increased circulating ACTH from the pituitary (65% of cases), known as Cushing's disease, or from an 'ectopic',

Table 18.32   Causes of Cushing's syndrome

ACTH-dependent disease
Pituitary-dependent (Cushing's disease)
Ectopic ACTH-producing tumours
ACTH administration

Non-ACTH-dependent causes
Adrenal adenomas
Adrenal carcinomas
Glucocorticoid administration

Others
Alcohol-induced pseudo-Cushing's syndrome

non-pituitary, ACTH-producing tumour elsewhere in the body (10%) with consequential glucocorticoid excess
- a primary excess of endogenous cortisol secretion (25% of spontaneous cases) by an adrenal tumour or nodular hyperplasia, with subsequent (physiological) suppression of ACTH. Rare cases are due to aberrant expression of receptors for other hormones (e.g. glucose-dependant insulinotrophic peptide [GIP], LH or catecholamines) in adrenal cortical cells.

Clinical features

The predominant clinical features of Cushing's syndrome are those of glucocorticoid excess and are illustrated in Figure 18.25.

- *Pigmentation* occurs only with ACTH-dependent causes.

Symptoms	Signs	
Weight gain (central)	Moon face	Oedema
Change of appearance	**Plethora**	**Proximal myopathy**
Depression	Depression/psychosis	Proximal muscle
Insomnia	Acne	wasting
Amenorrhoea/	Hirsutism	Glycosuria
oligomenorrhoea	Frontal balding (female)	
Poor libido	**Thin skin**	
Thin skin/easy bruising	**Bruising**	
Hair growth/acne	Poor wound healing	
Muscular weakness	Pigmentation	
Growth arrest in children	Skin infections	
Back pain	**Hypertension**	
Polyuria/polydipsia	Osteoporosis	
Psychosis	**Pathological fractures**	
	(especially vertebrae and ribs)	
Old photographs may	Kyphosis	
be useful	'Buffalo hump'	
	(dorsal fat pad)	
	Central obesity	
	Striae (purple or red)	
	Rib fractures	

Fig. 18.25   **Cushing's syndrome – symptoms and signs.** Bold type indicates signs of most value in discriminating Cushing's syndrome from simple obesity and hirsutism.

- *A cushingoid appearance* can be caused by excess alcohol consumption (pseudo-Cushing's syndrome) – the pathophysiology is poorly understood.
- *Impaired glucose tolerance* or frank diabetes are common, especially in the ectopic ACTH syndrome.
- *Hypokalaemia* due to the mineralocorticoid activity of cortisol is common with ectopic ACTH secretion.

Diagnosis

There are two phases to the investigation:

1. confirmation of the presence or absence of Cushing's syndrome
2. differential diagnosis of its cause (e.g. pituitary, adrenal or ectopic).

Confirmation

Most obese, hirsute, hypertensive patients do not have Cushing's syndrome, and some cases of genuine Cushing's have relatively subtle clinical signs. Confirmation rests on demonstrating inappropriate cortisol secretion, not suppressed by exogenous glucocorticoids: difficulties occur with obesity and depression where cortisol dynamics are often abnormal. Random cortisol measurements are of no value. Occasional patients are seen with so-called 'cyclical Cushing's' where the abnormalities come and go.

Investigations to confirm the diagnosis include:

- **48-hour low-dose dexamethasone test** (see Table 18.29). Normal individuals suppress plasma cortisol to < 50 nmol/L. Patients with Cushing's syndrome fail to show complete suppression of plasma cortisol levels (although levels may fall substantially in a few cases). This test is highly sensitive (> 97%). The overnight dexamethasone test is slightly simpler, but has a higher false-positive rate.
- **24-hour urinary free cortisol measurements.** This is simple, but less reliable – repeatedly normal values (corrected for body mass) render the diagnosis most unlikely, but some patients with Cushing's have normal values on some collections (approximately 10%).
- **Circadian rhythm.** After 48 hours in hospital, cortisol samples are taken at 0900h and 2400h (without warning the patient). Normal subjects show a pronounced circadian variation (see Fig. 18.2, p. 1038); those with Cushing's syndrome have high midnight cortisol levels (> 100 nmol/L), though the 0900h value may be normal.
- **Other tests.** There are frequent exceptions to the classic responses to diagnostic tests in Cushing's syndrome. If any clinical suspicion of Cushing's remains after preliminary tests then specialist investigations are still indicated, these may include insulin stress test, desmopressin stimulation test and CRH tests.

Differential diagnosis of the cause

This can be extremely difficult since all causes can result in clinically identical Cushing's syndrome. The classical ectopic ACTH syndrome is distinguished by a short history, pigmentation and weight loss, unprovoked hypokalaemia, clinical or chemical diabetes and plasma ACTH levels above 200 ng/L, but many ectopic tumours are benign and mimic pituitary disease closely both clinically and biochemically. Severe hirsutism/virilization suggests an adrenal tumour.

Biochemical and radiological procedures for diagnosis include:

- **Adrenal CT or MRI scan.** Adrenal adenomas and carcinomas causing Cushing's syndrome are relatively large and always detectable by CT scan. Carcinomas are distinguished by large size, irregular outline and signs of infiltration or metastases. Bilateral adrenal hyperplasia may be seen in ACTH-dependent causes or in ACTH-independent nodular hyperplasia.
- **Pituitary MRI.** A pituitary adenoma may be seen but the adenoma is often small and not visible in a significant proportion of cases.
- **Plasma potassium levels.** Hypokalaemia is common with ectopic ACTH secretion. (All diuretics must be stopped.)
- **High-dose dexamethasone test** (Table 18.29). Failure of significant plasma cortisol suppression suggests an ectopic source of ACTH or an adrenal tumour.
- **Plasma ACTH levels.** Low or undetectable ACTH levels (< 10 ng/L) on two or more occasions are a reliable indicator of non-ACTH-dependent disease.
- **CRH test.** An exaggerated ACTH and cortisol response to exogenous CRH suggests pituitary-dependent Cushing's disease, as ectopic sources rarely respond.
- **Chest X-ray** is mandatory to look for a carcinoma of the bronchus or a bronchial carcinoid. Carcinoid lesions may be very small; if ectopic ACTH is suspected, whole-lung and mediastinal CT scanning should be performed.

Further investigations may involve selective catheterization of the inferior petrosal sinus to measure ACTH for pituitary lesions, or blood samples taken throughout the body in a search for ectopic sources. Bronchoscopy, cytology and regional arteriograms are occasionally necessary. Radiolabelled octreotide (^{111}In octreotide) is occasionally helpful in locating ectopic ACTH sites.

Treatment

Untreated Cushing's syndrome has a very bad prognosis, with death from hypertension, myocardial infarction, infection and heart failure. Whatever the underlying cause, cortisol hypersecretion should be controlled prior to surgery or radiotherapy. Considerable morbidity and mortality is otherwise associated with operating on unprepared patients, especially when abdominal surgery is required. The usual drug is metyrapone, an 11β-hydroxylase blocker, which is given in doses of 750 mg to 4 g daily in three to four divided doses. Ketoconazole (200 mg three times daily) is also used and is synergistic with metyrapone. Plasma cortisol should be monitored, aiming to reduce the mean level during the day to 150–300 nmol/L, equivalent to normal production rates.

Aminoglutethimide and trilostane (which reversibly inhibits 3β-hydroxysteroid dehydrogenase/δ-5,4 isomers) are occasionally used.

Choice of further treatment depends upon the cause.

Cushing's disease (pituitary-dependent hyperadrenalism)

- *Trans-sphenoidal removal of the tumour* is the treatment of choice. Selective adenomectomy nearly always leaves the patient ACTH-deficient immediately postoperatively, and this is a good prognostic sign. Overall, pituitary surgery results in remission in 75–80% of cases – but results vary considerably and an experienced surgeon is essential.
- *External pituitary irradiation* alone is slow acting, only effective in 50–60% even after prolonged follow–up and mainly used after failed pituitary surgery. Children, however, respond much better to radiotherapy, 80% being cured.
- *Medical therapy* to reduce ACTH (e.g. bromocriptine, cyproheptadine) is rarely effective.
- *Bilateral adrenalectomy* is an effective last resort if other measures fail to control the disease. This can be performed laparoscopically.

Other causes

Adrenal adenomas should be resected after achievement of clinical remission with metyrapone or ketoconazole. Contralateral adrenal suppression may last for years.

Adrenal carcinomas are highly aggressive and the prognosis is poor. In general, if there are no widespread metastases, tumour bulk should be reduced surgically. The adrenolytic drug op'DDD (Mitotane) may inhibit growth of the tumour and prolong survival, though it can cause nausea and ataxia. Some would also give radiotherapy to the tumour bed after surgery.

Tumours secreting ACTH ectopically should be removed if possible. Otherwise chemotherapy/radiotherapy may be used, depending on the tumour. Control of the Cushing's syndrome with metyrapone or ketoconazole is beneficial for symptoms, and bilateral adrenalectomy may be appropriate to give complete control of the Cushing's syndrome if prognosis from the tumour itself is reasonable.

If the source of ACTH is not clear, cortisol hypersecretion should be controlled with medical therapy until a diagnosis can be made.

Nelson's syndrome

Nelson's syndrome is increased pigmentation (because of high levels of ACTH) associated with an enlarging pituitary tumour, which occurs in about 20% of cases after bilateral adrenalectomy for Cushing's disease. The syndrome is rare now that adrenalectomy is an uncommon primary treatment, and its incidence may be reduced by pituitary radiotherapy soon after adrenalectomy. The Nelson's adenoma may be treated by pituitary surgery and/or radiotherapy (unless given previously).

Incidental adrenal tumours ('incidentalomas')

With the advent of abdominal CT, MRI and high-resolution ultrasound scanning, unsuspected adrenal masses have been discovered in 1% of scans. These obviously include the adrenal tumours described above, but cysts, myelolipomas and metastases are also seen. Functional tests to exclude secretory activity should be performed (adenomas often secrete cortisol at a low level); if none is found then most authorities recommend removal of large (> 4–5 cm) and functional tumours but observation of smaller hormonally inactive lesions.

Congenital adrenal hyperplasia (CAH)

Pathophysiology

This condition results from an autosomal recessive deficiency of an enzyme in the cortisol synthetic pathways. There are six major types, but most common is 21-hydroxylase deficiency which occurs in about 1 in 15 000 births and which has been shown to be due to defects on chromosome 6 near the HLA-region affecting one of the cytochrome p450 enzymes ($p450_{C21}$).

As a result, cortisol secretion is reduced and feedback leads to increased ACTH secretion to maintain adequate cortisol – leading to adrenal hypoplasia. Diversion of the steroid precursors into the androgenic steroid pathways occurs (see Fig. 18.22(a)). Thus, 17-hydroxyprogesterone, androstenedione and testosterone levels are increased, leading to virilization. Aldosterone synthesis may be impaired with resultant salt wasting.

The other forms affect 11β-hydroxylase, 17α-hydroxylase, 3β-hydroxysteroid dehydrogenase and a cholesterol side-chain cleavage enzyme ($p450_{scc}$) (see Fig. 18.22(a)).

Clinical features

If severe, this presents at birth with sexual ambiguity or adrenal failure (collapse, hypotension, hypoglycaemia), sometimes with a salt-losing state (hypotension, hyponatraemia). In the female, clitoral hypertrophy, urogenital abnormalities and labioscrotal fusion are common, but the syndrome may be unrecognized in the male.

Precocious puberty with hirsutism is a later presentation, whereas rare, milder cases only present in adult life, usually accompanied by primary amenorrhoea. Hirsutism developing before puberty is suggestive of CAH.

Investigations

Expert advice is essential in the confirmation and differential diagnosis of 21-hydroxylase deficiency, and with ambiguous genitalia such advice must be sought urgently before any assignment of gender is made.

- 17-Hydroxyprogesterone levels are increased.
- Urinary pregnanetriol excretion is increased.
- Basal ACTH levels are raised.

Treatment

Replacement of glucocorticoid activity, and mineralocorticoid activity if deficient, is as for primary hypoadrenalism (see above). Correct dosage is often difficult to establish in the child but should ensure normal 17-hydroxyprogesterone levels while allowing normal growth; excessive replacement leads to stunting of growth.

Uses and problems of therapeutic steroid therapy

Apart from their use as therapeutic replacement for endocrine deficiency states, synthetic glucocorticoids are widely used for many non-endocrine conditions (Box 18.8). Short-term use (e.g. for acute asthma) carries only small risks of significant side-effects except for the simultaneous suppression of immune responses. The danger lies in their continuance, often through medical oversight or patient default. In general, therapy for 3 weeks or less, or a dose of prednisolone less than 10 mg per day, will not result in significant long-term suppression of the normal adrenal axis.

Long-term therapy with synthetic or natural steroids will, in most respects, mimic endogenous Cushing's syndrome. Exceptions are the relative absence of hirsutism, acne, hypertension and severe sodium retention, as the common synthetic steroids have low androgenic and mineralocorticoid activity.

Excessive doses of steroids may also be absorbed from skin when strong dermatological preparations are used, but inhaled steroids rarely cause Cushing's syndrome, although they commonly cause adrenal suppression.

The major hazards are detailed in Box 18.9. In the long term, many are of such severity that the clinical need for high-dose steroids should be continually and critically assessed. Steroid-sparing agents (e.g. azathioprine) should always be considered and screening and prophylactic therapy for osteoporosis introduced (see p. 596).

Box 18.8 Common therapeutic uses of glucocorticoids

Respiratory disease
Asthma
Chronic obstructive
 pulmonary disease
Sarcoidosis
Hayfever (usually topical)
Prevention/treatment of
 ARDS (see p. 987)

Cardiac disease
Post-myocardial infarction
 syndrome

Renal disease
Some nephrotic syndromes
Some glomerulonephritides

Gastrointestinal disease
Ulcerative colitis
Crohn's disease
Autoimmune hepatitis

Rheumatological disease
Systemic lupus
 erythematosus
Polymyalgia rheumatica
Cranial arteritis
Juvenile idiopathic arthritis
Vasculitides
Rheumatoid arthritis

Neurological disease
Cerebral oedema

Skin disease
Pemphigus, eczema

Tumours
Hodgkin's lymphoma
Other lymphomas

Transplantation
Immunosuppression

Box 18.9 Major adverse effects of corticosteroid therapy

Physiological
Adrenal and/or pituitary
 suppression

Pathological
Cardiovascular
Increased blood pressure

Gastrointestinal
Peptic ulceration
 exacerbation
Pancreatitis

Renal
Polyuria
Nocturia

Central nervous
Depression
Euphoria
Psychosis
Insomnia

Endocrine
Weight gain
Glycosuria/hyperglycaemia/
 diabetes
Impaired growth
Amenorrhoea

Bone and muscle
Osteoporosis
Proximal myopathy and
 wasting
Aseptic necrosis of the hip
Pathological fractures

Skin
Thinning
Easy bruising

Eyes
Cataracts (including inhaled
 drug)

Increased susceptibility to infection
(signs and fever are
 frequently masked)
Septicaemia
Fungal infections
Reactivation of TB
Skin (e.g. fungi)

Supervision of steroid therapy

All patients receiving steroids should carry a 'Steroid Card'. They should be made aware of the following points:

- Long-term steroid therapy must never be stopped suddenly.
- Doses should be reduced very gradually, with most being given in the morning at the time of withdrawal – this minimizes adrenal suppression. Many authorities believe that 'alternate-day therapy' produces less suppression.
- Doses need to be increased in times of serious intercurrent illness (defined as presence of a fever), accident and stress. Double doses should be taken during these times.
- Other physicians, anaesthetists and dentists must be told about steroid therapy.
- Patients should also be informed of potential side-effects and all this information should be documented in the clinical record.
- Regular supervision including, e.g. DXA scan.

Steroids and surgery

Any patient receiving steroids or who has recently received them (within the last 12 months) and may still have adrenal suppression requires careful control of steroid medication around the time of surgery. Details are shown in Table 18.33.

FURTHER READING
Arlt W, Allolio B (2003) Adrenal insufficiency. *Lancet*
361: 1881–1893.
Boscard M et al. (2001) Cushing's syndrome. *Lancet*
357: 783–791.
Howlett TA (1997) An assessment of optimal
hydrocortisone replacement therapy. *Clinical
Endocrinology* 46: 263–268.
Oelkers W (1999) Dehydroepiandrosterone for adrenal
insufficiency. *New England Journal of Medicine* 341:
1073–1074.
Speiser PW and White PC (2003) Congenital adrenal
hyperplasia. *New England Journal of Medicine* 349:
776–788.

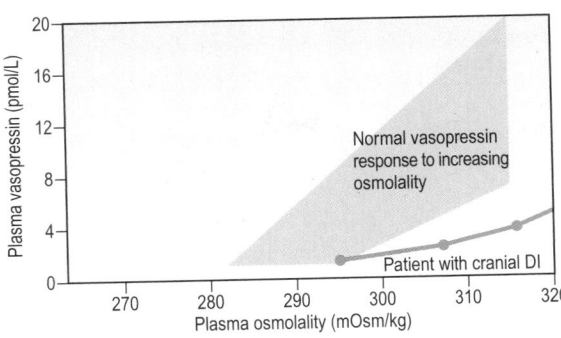

Fig. 18.26 **Plasma vasopressin response to increasing osmolality in normal subjects and in a patient with DI.**

THE THIRST AXIS

Thirst and water regulation are largely controlled by vasopressin, also known as antidiuretic hormone (ADH), which is synthesized in the hypothalamus, and then migrates in neurosecretory granules along axonal pathways to the posterior pituitary. Pituitary disease alone without hypothalamic involvement therefore does not lead to ADH deficiency as the hormone can still 'leak' from the damaged end of the intact axon.

At normal concentrations the kidney is the predominant site of action of vasopressin. Vasopressin stimulation of the V2 receptors allows the collecting tubule to become permeable to water, thus permitting reabsorption of hypotonic luminal fluid (p. 694). Vasopressin therefore reduces diuresis and results in overall retention of water. At high concentrations vasopressin also causes vasoconstriction via the V1 receptors in vascular tissue.

Changes in plasma osmolality are sensed by osmoreceptors in the anterior hypothalamus. Vasopressin

secretion is suppressed at levels below 280 mOsm/kg, thus allowing maximal water diuresis. Above this level, plasma vasopressin increases in direct proportion to plasma osmolality. At the upper limit of normal (295 mOsm/kg) maximum antidiuresis is achieved and thirst is experienced at about 298 mOsm/kg (Fig. 18.26).

Other factors affecting vasopressin release are shown in Table 18.34.

Disorders of vasopressin secretion or activity include:

- deficiency as a result of hypothalamic disease ('cranial' diabetes insipidus)
- inappropriate excess of the hormone
- 'nephrogenic' diabetes insipidus – a rare condition in which the renal tubules are insensitive to vasopressin, an example of a receptor abnormality.

While all these are uncommon, they need to be distinguished from the occasional patient with 'primary polydipsia' and those whose renal tubular function has been impaired by electrolyte abnormalities, such as hypokalaemia or hypercalcaemia.

Table 18.33	Steroid cover for operative procedures		
Procedure	**Premedication**	**Intra- and postoperative**	**Resumption of normal maintenance**
Simple procedures (e.g. gastroscopy, simple dental extractions)	Hydrocortisone 100 mg i.m	–	Immediately if no complications and eating normally
Minor surgery (e.g. laparoscopic surgery, veins, hernias)	Hydrocortisone 100 mg i.m.	Hydrocortisone 20 mg orally 6-hourly or 50 mg i.m. every 6 hours for 24 h if not eating	After 24 h if no complications
Major surgery (e.g. hip replacement, vascular surgery)	Hydrocortisone 100 mg i.m.	Hydrocortisone 50–100 mg i.m every 6 hours for 72 h	After 72 h if normal progress and no complications Perhaps double normal dose for next 2–3 days
GI tract surgery or major thoracic surgery (not eating or ventilated)	Hydrocortisone 100 mg i.m.	Hydrocortisone 100 mg i.m. every 6 hours for 72 h or longer if still unwell	When patient eating normally again Until then, higher doses (to 50 mg 6-hourly) may be needed

Table 18.34 Factors affecting vasopressin release

Increased by:	Decreased by:
Increased osmolality	Decreased osmolality
Hypovolaemia	Hypervolaemia
Hypotension	Hypertension
Nausea	Ethanol
Hypothyroidism	α-Adrenergic stimulation
Angiotensin II	
Epinephrine (adrenaline)	
Cortisol	
Nicotine	
Antidepressants	

Diabetes insipidus (DI)

Clinical features

Deficiency of vasopressin or insensitivity to its action leads to polyuria, nocturia and compensatory polydipsia. Daily urine output may reach as much as 10–15 L, leading to dehydration that may be very severe if the thirst mechanisms or consciousness are impaired or the patient is denied fluid.

Causes of DI are listed in Table 18.35. The most common is hypothalamic–pituitary surgery, following which

Table 18.35 Causes of diabetes insipidus

Cranial diabetes insipidus	Nephrogenic diabetes insipidus
Familial (e.g. DIDMOAD)	
Idiopathic (often autoimmune)	Familial (e.g. vasopressin
Tumours	receptor gene,
Craniopharyngioma	aquaporin-2 gene defect)
Hypothalamic tumour,	Idiopathic
e.g. glioma	Renal disease (e.g. renal
Metastases, especially	tubular acidosis)
breast	Hypokalaemia
Lymphoma/leukaemia	Hypercalcaemia
Pituitary with suprasellar	Drugs (e.g. lithium,
extension (rare)	demeclocycline,
Infections	glibenclamide)
Tuberculosis	Sickle cell disease
Meningitis	
Cerebral abscess	
Infiltrations	
Sarcoidosis	
Langerhans' cell	
histiocytosis	
Post-surgical	
Transfrontal	
Trans-sphenoidal	
Post-radiotherapy (cranial)	
Vascular	
Haemorrhage/thrombosis	
Sheehan's syndrome	
Aneurysm	
Trauma (e.g. head injury)	

Mild temporary nephrogenic DI can occur after prolonged polyuria due to any cause, including cranial DI and primary polydipsia

transient DI is common, frequently remitting after a few days or weeks. Primary overdrinking (polydipsia) is a common differential diagnosis.

DI may be masked by simultaneous cortisol deficiency – cortisol replacement allows a water diuresis and DI then becomes apparent.

DIDMOAD (Wolfram) syndrome is a rare autosomal recessive disorder comprising **D**iabetes **I**nsipidus, **D**iabetes **M**ellitus, **O**ptic **A**trophy and **D**eafness. MR scanning may show an absent or poorly developed posterior pituitary.

Biochemistry

- High or high-normal plasma osmolality with low urine osmolality (in primary polydipsia plasma osmolality tends to be low)
- Resultant high or high-normal plasma sodium
- High 24-h urine volumes (less than 2 L excludes need for further investigation)
- Failure of urinary concentration with fluid deprivation
- Restoration of urinary concentration with vasopressin or an analogue.

The latter two points may be studied with a formal water-deprivation test (Box 18.10). In normal subjects, plasma osmolality remains normal while urine osmolality rises above 600 mOsm/kg. In DI, plasma osmolality rises while the urine remains dilute, only concentrating after exogenous vasopressin is given (in 'cranial' DI) or not concentrating after vasopressin if nephrogenic DI is present. This test can give equivocal results and measurement of vasopressin during the test is helpful.

 Box 18.10 Water deprivation test

Indication
Diagnosis or exclusion of diabetes insipidus

Procedure
Fasting and no fluids from 7.30 a.m. (or overnight if only mild DI is expected and polyuria is only modest)
Monitor serum and urine osmolality, urine volume and weight hourly for up to 8 hours
Abandon fluid deprivation if weight loss > 3% occurs
If serum osmolality > 300 mOsm/kg and/or urine osmolality > 600 mOsm/k give desmopressin, 2 µg i.m. at end of test. Allow free fluid but measure urine osmolality for 2–4 hours

Normal response
Serum osmolality remains within normal range (275–295 mOsm/kg)
Urine osmolality rises to > 600 mOsm/kg

Diabetes insipidus
Serum osmolality rises above normal without adequate concentration of urine osmolality
Response to desmopressin indicates cranial (pituitary) DI rather than nephrogenic DI

Treatment

Alternative agents in mild DI, probably working by sensitizing the renal tubules to endogenous vasopressin, include thiazide diuretics, carbamazepine (200–400 mg daily) or chlorpropamide (200–350 mg daily).

Nephrogenic diabetes insipidus

In this condition, renal tubules are resistant to normal or high levels of plasma vasopressin. It may be inherited as a rare sex-linked recessive, with an abnormality in the vasopressin-2 receptor, or as an autosomal post-receptor defect in an ADH-sensitive water channel, aquaporin-2. More commonly it can be acquired as a result of renal disease, sickle cell disease, drug ingestion (e.g. lithium), hypercalcaemia or hypokalaemia. Wherever possible the cause should be reversed.

Other causes of polyuria and polydipsia

Diabetes mellitus, hypokalaemia and hypercalcaemia should be excluded. In the case of diabetes mellitus the cause is an osmotic diuresis secondary to glycosuria which leads to dehydration and an increased perception of thirst owing to hypertonicity of the extracellular fluid.

Primary or hysterical polydipsia

This is a relatively common cause of thirst and polyuria. It is a psychiatric disturbance characterized by the excessive intake of water. Plasma sodium and osmolality fall as a result and the urine produced is appropriately dilute. Vasopressin levels become virtually undetectable. Prolonged primary polydipsia may lead to the phenomenon of 'renal medullary washout', with a fall in the concentrating ability of the kidney.

Characteristically the diagnosis is made by a water-deprivation test. A low plasma osmolality is usual at the start of the test, and since vasopressin secretion and action can be stimulated, the patient's urine becomes concentrated (albeit 'maximum' concentrating ability may be impaired); the initially low urine osmolality gradually increases with the duration of the water deprivation.

Syndrome of inappropriate antidiuretic hormone (SIADH)

Clinical features

Inappropriate secretion of ADH leads to retention of water and hyponatraemia. The presentation is usually vague, with confusion, nausea, irritability and, later, fits and coma. There is no oedema. Mild symptoms usually occur with plasma sodium levels below 125 mmol/L and serious manifestations are likely below 115 mmol/L. The elderly may show symptoms with milder abnormalities.

The syndrome must be distinguished from those causing similar dilutional hyponatraemia from excess infusion of dextrose/water solutions or diuretic administration (thiazides or amiloride, see p. 698).

Table 18.36   Common causes of the syndrome of inappropriate ADH secretion (SIADH)

Tumours	Metabolic causes
Small-cell carcinoma of lung	Alcohol withdrawal
Prostate	Porphyria
Thymus	
Pancreas	**Drugs**
Lymphomas	Chlorpropamide
	Carbamazepine
Pulmonary lesions	Cyclophosphamide
Pneumonia	Vincristine
Tuberculosis	Phenothiazines
Lung abscess	
CNS causes	
Meningitis	
Tumours	
Head injury	
Subdural haematoma	
Cerebral abscess	
SLE vasculitis	

Diagnosis

The usual features are:

- dilutional hyponatraemia due to excessive water retention
- low plasma osmolality with 'inappropriate' urine osmolality which is higher than plasma osmolality
- continued urinary sodium excretion > 30 mmol/L
- absence of hypokalaemia (or hypotension)
- normal renal and adrenal and thyroid function.

The causes are listed in Table 18.36.

Treatment

The underlying cause should be corrected where possible. Symptomatic relief can be obtained by the following measures:

- Fluid intake should be restricted to 500–1000 mL daily. If tolerated, and complied with, this will correct the biochemical abnormalities in almost every case.
- Plasma osmolality and sodium and bodyweight should be measured frequently.
- If water restriction is poorly tolerated or ineffective, demeclocycline (600–1200 mg daily) may be given; this inhibits the action of vasopressin on the kidney, causing a reversible form of nephrogenic diabetes insipidus. It often, however, causes photosensitive rashes.
- When the syndrome is very severe, rarely hypertonic saline (300 mmol/L slowly i.v.) is given and furosemide may be used. These treatments are potentially dangerous and should only be used with extreme caution.

DISORDERS OF CALCIUM METABOLISM

Serum calcium levels are mainly controlled by parathyroid hormone (PTH) and vitamin D. Hypercalcaemia is much more common than hypocalcaemia and is frequently detected incidentally with multichannel biochemical analysers. Mild asymptomatic hypercalcaemia occurs in about 1 in 1000 of the population, with an incidence of 25–30 per 100 000 population. It occurs mainly in elderly females, and is usually due to primary hyperparathyroidism (primary HPT).

Parathyroid hormone

There are normally four parathyroid glands which are situated posterior to the thyroid, but occasionally additional glands exist or they may be found elsewhere in the neck or mediastinum. PTH, an 84-amino-acid hormone derived from a 115-residue preprohormone, is secreted from the chief cells of the four parathyroid glands. PTH levels rise as serum ionized calcium falls. The latter is detected by specific calcium-sensing receptors on the plasma membrane of the parathyroid cells. PTH has several major actions, all serving to increase plasma calcium by:

- increasing osteoclastic resorption of bone (occurring rapidly)
- increasing intestinal absorption of calcium (a slow response)
- increasing synthesis of 1,25-$(OH)_2D_3$
- increasing renal tubular reabsorption of calcium
- increasing excretion of phosphate.

PTH effects are mediated at specific membrane receptors on the target cells, resulting in an increase of adenyl cyclase messenger activity.

PTH measurements

PTH measurements use two-site immunometric assays that measure only the intact PTH molecule; interpretation requires a simultaneous calcium measurement in order to differentiate most causes of hyper- and hypocalcaemia. Urinary cyclic adenosine monophosphate (cyclic AMP) concentration is an index of the bioactivity of PTH. Vitamin D metabolism is discussed on page 592.

Hypercalcaemia

Pathophysiology and causes

The major causes of hypercalcaemia are listed in Table 18.37; primary hyperparathyroidism and malignancies are by far the most common (> 90% of cases). Hyperparathyroidism itself may be primary, secondary or tertiary. Primary hyperparathyroidism is caused by single (> 80%) parathyroid adenomas or by diffuse hyperplasia of all the glands (15–20%); multiple parathyroid adenomas are rare. Involvement of multiple parathyroid glands may be part of a familial syndrome (e.g. multiple endocrine neoplasia (MEN) syndrome type 1 or 2a). Parathyroid carcinoma is rare (< 1%), though it usually produces severe and intractable hypercalcaemia.

Primary hyperparathyroidism is of unknown cause, though it appears that adenomas are monoclonal. Hyper-

Table 18.37 Causes of hypercalcaemia

Excessive parathormone (PTH) secretion
Primary hyperparathyroidism (commonest by far), adenoma (common), hyperplasia or carcinoma (rare)
Tertiary hyperparathyroidism
Ectopic PTH secretion (very rare indeed)

Malignant disease (second commonest cause)
Myeloma
Secondary deposits in bone
Production of osteoclastic factors by tumours
PTH-related protein secretion

Excess action of vitamin D
Iatrogenic or self-administered excess
Granulomatous diseases, e.g. sarcoidosis, TB
Lymphoma

Excessive calcium intake
'Milk–alkali' syndrome

Other endocrine disease (mild hypercalcaemia only)
Thyrotoxicosis
Addison's disease

Drugs
Thiazide diuretics
Vitamin D analogues
Lithium administration (chronic)
Vitamin A

Miscellaneous
Long-term immobility
Familial hypocalciuric hypercalcaemia

plasia may also be monoclonal. Chromosomal rearrangements in the 5' regulatory region of the parathyroid hormone gene have been identified, and inactivation of some tumour suppressor genes at a variety of sites may also be involved.

Secondary hyperparathyroidism (see p. 668) is physiological compensatory hypertrophy of all parathyroids because of hypocalcaemia, such as occurs in renal failure or vitamin D deficiency. PTH levels are raised but calcium levels are low or normal, and PTH falls to normal after correction of the cause of hypocalcaemia where this is possible.

Tertiary hyperparathyroidism is the development of apparently autonomous parathyroid hyperplasia after long-standing secondary hyperparathyroidism, most often in renal failure. Plasma calcium and phosphate are both raised, the latter often grossly so. Parathyroidectomy is necessary at this stage.

Symptoms and signs

Mild hypercalcaemia (e.g. adjusted calcium < 3 mmol/L) is frequently asymptomatic, but more severe hypercalcaemia can produce a number of symptoms:

- *General features*. There may be tiredness, malaise, dehydration and depression.
- *Renal features*. Renal colic from stones, polyuria or nocturia, haematuria and hypertension occurs. The polyuria results from the effect of hypercalcaemia on renal tubules, reducing their concentrating ability – a

form of mild nephrogenic diabetes insipidus. Primary hyperparathyroidism is present in about 5% of patients who present with renal calculi.

- *Bones.* There may be bone pain. Hyperparathyroidism mainly affects cortical bone, and bone cysts and locally destructive 'brown tumours' occur but only in advanced disease. Only 5–10% of all cases have definite bony lesions even when sought.
- *Abdominal.* There may be abdominal pain.
- *Chondrocalcinosis and ectopic calcification.* These are occasional features.
- *Corneal calcification.* This is a marker of long-standing hypercalcaemia but causes no symptoms.

There may also be symptoms from the underlying cause. Malignant disease is usually advanced by the time hypercalcaemia occurs, typically with bony metastases. The common primary tumours are bronchus, breast, myeloma, oesophagus, thyroid, prostate, lymphoma and renal cell carcinoma. True 'ectopic PTH secretion' by the tumour is very rare, and most cases are associated with raised levels of PTH-related protein. This is a 144-amino-acid polypeptide, the initial sequence of which shows an approximate homology with the biologically active part of PTH, which is necessary in fetal development but does not have a clearly defined role in the adult. Local bone resorbing cytokines and prostaglandins may be involved locally where there are metastatic skeletal lesions, leading to local mobilization of calcium by osteolysis with subsequent hypercalcaemia.

Severe hypercalcaemia (> 3 mmol/L) is usually associated with malignant disease, hyperparathyroidism, renal failure or vitamin D therapy.

Investigations and differential diagnosis

Biochemistry

- *Several* fasting serum calcium and phosphate samples should be performed.
- *Serum PTH.* The hallmark of primary hyperparathyroidism is hypercalcaemia and hypophosphataemia with detectable or elevated intact PTH levels during hypercalcaemia. When this combination is present in an asymptomatic patient then further investigation is usually unnecessary.
- There is often a mild *hyperchloraemic acidosis.*
- *Renal function* is usually normal but should be measured as a baseline.

Where PTH is undetectable or equivocal, a number of other tests may lead to the diagnosis

- *Protein electrophoresis:* to exclude myeloma
- *Serum TSH:* to exclude hyperthyroidism
- *0900h cortisol and/or synacthen test:* to exclude Addison's disease
- *Serum ACE:* helpful in the diagnosis of sarcoidosis
- *Hydrocortisone suppression test:* hydrocortisone 40 mg three times daily for 10 days leads to suppression of plasma calcium in sarcoidosis, vitamin D-mediated hypercalcaemia and some malignancies.

Imaging

Abdominal X-rays may show renal calculi or nephrocalcinosis. High-definition hand X-rays can show subperiosteal erosions in the middle or terminal phalanges. DXA bone density scan is useful to detect bone effects in asymptomatic patients with HPT in whom conservative management is planned.

Parathyroid imaging is generally indicated only for patients who have undergone previous parathyroid surgery, as techniques have an overall sensitivity of just 60–70% and a substantial false-positive rate, which is far less accurate than the expert surgical success rate of at least 90%. Methods include:

- ultrasound which, though insensitive for small tumours, is simple and safe
- high-resolution CT scan or MRI (the most sensitive technique)
- radioisotope subtraction scanning – a picture of the parathyroid tissue derived from the difference in uptake between ^{201}Th (taken up by thyroid and parathyroid) and ^{99m}Tc (by thyroid only).

Treatment of hypercalcaemia

Details of emergency treatment for severe hypercalcaemia are given in Emergency box 18.2. Thereafter, treatment is management of the underlying disease.

Treatment of primary hyperparathyroidism

Medical management

There are no effective medical therapies at present for primary hyperparathyroidism, but a high fluid intake

---

Emergency Box 18.2
Treatment of acute hypercalcaemia

Acute hypercalcaemia often presents with dehydration, nausea and vomiting, nocturia and polyuria, drowsiness and altered consciousness. The serum Ca^{2+} is over 3 mmol/L and sometimes as high as 5 mmol/L. While investigation of the cause is under way, immediate treatment is mandatory if the patient is seriously ill or if the Ca^{2+} is above 3.5 mmol/L. Specialist help is advised.

- Adequate rehydration is essential – usually at least 4–6 L of 0.9% saline on day 1, and 3–4 L for several days thereafter. Central venous pressure (CVP) may need to be monitored to control the hydration rate.
- Intravenous bisphosphonates are the treatment of choice for hypercalcaemia of malignancy or of undiagnosed cause. Pamidronate is preferred (15–60 mg as an intravenous infusion in 0.9% saline or dextrose over 2–8 hours or, if less urgent, over 2–4 days).
- Calcitonin (200 units i.v. 6-hourly) has a short-lived action and is little used.
- Prednisolone (30–60 mg daily) is effective in some instances (e.g. in myeloma, sarcoidosis and vitamin D excess) but in most cases is ineffective.
- Oral phosphate (sodium cellulose phosphate 5 g three times daily) produces diarrhoea. Intravenous phosphate rapidly lowers plasma Ca^{2+} but is dangerous and should not be used.

should be maintained, a high calcium or vitamin D intake avoided, and exercise encouraged. New therapeutic agents that target the calcium-sensing receptors in the kidney may be of value in the future.

Surgery

Indications for surgery in primary hyperparathyroidism remain controversial. There is agreement that surgery is indicated for:

- patients with renal stones or impaired renal function
- bone involvement or marked reduction in cortical bone density
- unequivocal marked hypercalcaemia (> 3.0 mmol/L)
- the uncommon younger patient, below age 50 years
- a previous episode of severe acute hypercalcaemia.

The situation where plasma calcium is mildly raised (2.65–3.00 mmol/L) is more controversial. Most authorities feel that young patients should be operated on, as should those who have reduced cortical bone density or significant hypercalciuria, as this is associated with stone formation.

In older patients without these problems, or in those unfit for or unwilling to have surgery, conservative management is indicated. Regular measurement of serum calcium and of renal function is necessary. Bone density of cortical bone should be estimated every 3–5 years.

Surgical technique and complications

Parathyroid surgery should be performed only by experienced surgeons, as the minute glands may be very difficult to define, and it is difficult to distinguish between an adenoma and normal parathyroid. In expert centres over 90% of operations are successful, involving removal of the adenoma, or removal of all four hyperplastic parathyroids.

Other than postoperative hypocalcaemia (see below), the other rare complications are those of thyroid surgery – bleeding and recurrent laryngeal nerve palsies (< 1%). Vocal cord function should be checked preoperatively.

If initial exploration is unsuccessful, a full work-up including venous catheterization and scanning is essential, remembering that parathyroid tissue can be ectopic.

Postoperative care

The major danger after operation is hypocalcaemia, which is more common in patients with significant bone disease – the 'hungry bone' syndrome. Some authorities pretreat such patients with alfacalcidol 2 µg daily from 2 days preoperatively for 10–14 days. Chvostek's and Trousseau's signs (see p. 1095) should be checked regularly in all these patients. Plasma calcium measurements are performed daily for at least 2–5 days (more often if low) – a mild transient hypoparathyroidism often continues for 1–2 weeks. Depending on its severity, oral or intravenous calcium (for details see p. 1095) should be given temporarily, as only a few patients (< 1%) will develop long-standing surgical hypoparathyroidism.

Familial hypocalciuric hypercalcaemia

This uncommon autosomal dominant, and usually asymptomatic, condition demonstrates increased renal reabsorption of calcium despite hypercalcaemia. PTH levels are normal or slightly raised and urinary calcium is low. It is caused by mutations in the gene on the long arm of chromosome 3 encoding for the calcium-ion-sensing G-protein-coupled receptor in the kidney and parathyroid gland. Family members are often affected, detected by genetic analysis. Parathyroid surgery is not indicated as the course appears benign.

Hypocalcaemia and hypoparathyroidism

Pathophysiology

Hypocalcaemia may be due to deficiencies of calcium homeostatic mechanisms, secondary to high phosphate levels or other causes of hypocalcaemia (Table 18.38). All forms of hypoparathyroidism, except transient surgical effects, are uncommon.

Causes

- *Renal failure* is the most common cause of hypocalcaemia.
- *Hypocalcaemia after thyroid or parathyroid surgery* is common but usually transient – fewer than 1% of thyroidectomies leave permanent damage (see above).
- *Idiopathic hypoparathyroidism* is one of the rarer autoimmune disorders, often accompanied by vitiligo, cutaneous moniliasis and other autoimmune disease.

The *DiGeorge syndrome* (p. 218) is a familial condition where the hypoparathyroidism is associated with intellectual impairment, cataracts and calcified basal ganglia, and occasionally with specific autoimmune disease.

Pseudohypoparathyroidism is a syndrome of end-organ resistance to PTH owing to a mutation in the $G_{s\alpha}$-protein which is coupled to the PTH receptor. It is associated with short stature, short metacarpals, subcutaneous calcifi-

Table 18.38 Causes of hypocalcaemia	
Increased phosphate levels Chronic renal failure (common) Phosphate therapy	**Resistance to PTH** Pseudohypoparathyroidism
Hypoparathyroidism Surgical – after neck exploration (thyroidectomy, parathyroidectomy – common) Congenital deficiency (DiGeorge syndrome) Idiopathic hypoparathyroidism (rare) Severe hypomagnesaemia	**Drugs** Calcitonin Bisphosphonates **Other** Acute pancreatitis (quite common) Citrated blood in massive transfusion (not uncommon) Low plasma albumin, e.g. malnutrition, chronic liver disease Malabsorption, e.g. coeliac disease
Vitamin D deficiency Osteomalacia/rickets Vitamin D resistance	

> **Box 18.11 Causes of tetany**
>
> **In the presence of alkalosis**
> Hyperventilation
> Excess antacid therapy
> Persistent vomiting
> Hypochloraemic alkalosis, e.g. primary
>   hyperaldosteronism
> **In the presence of hypocalcaemia** (see Table 18.38)

FURTHER READING
Bilezikian JP, Silverberg SJ (2004) Asymptomatic primary hyperparathyroidism. *New England Journal of Medicine* **350**: 1746–1751.
Pearce SHS (1998) Calcium homeostasis and disorders of the calcium-sensing receptor. *Journal of the Royal College of Physicians of London* **32**: 10–14.
Strewler GJ (2000) The physiology of parathyroid hormone-related protein. *New England Journal of Medicine* **342**: 177–185.
Thakker RV (2001) Genetic development in hypoparathyroidism. *Lancet* **357**: 974–976.

cation and sometimes by intellectual impairment. Variable degrees of resistance involving other G-protein-linked hormone receptors may also be seen (TSH, LH, FSH).

Pseudo-pseudohypoparathyroidism describes the phenotypic defects but without any abnormalities of calcium metabolism. These individuals may share the same gene defect as pseudohypoparathyroidism and occur in the same families.

Clinical features

Hypoparathyroidism presents as neuromuscular irritability and neuropsychiatric manifestations. Paraesthesiae, circumoral numbness, cramps, anxiety and tetany (Box 18.11) are followed by convulsions, laryngeal stridor, dystonia and psychosis. Two signs of hypocalcaemia are Chvostek's sign (gentle tapping over the facial nerve causes twitching of the ipsilateral facial muscles) and Trousseau's sign, where inflation of the sphygmomanometer cuff above systolic pressure for 3 minutes induces tetanic spasm of the fingers and wrist. Severe hypocalcaemia may cause papilloedema and frequently a prolonged QT interval on the ECG.

Investigations

The clinical history and picture is usually diagnostic and is confirmed by a low serum calcium (after correction for any albumin abnormality). Additional tests include:

- **serum and urine creatinine** for renal disease
- **PTH levels** in the serum: absent or inappropriately low in hypoparathyroidism, high in other causes of hypocalcaemia
- **parathyroid antibodies** (present in idiopathic hypoparathyroidism)
- **25-hydroxy vitamin D serum level** (low in vitamin D deficiency)
- **X-rays** of metacarpals, showing short fourth metacarpals which occur in pseudohypoparathyroidism.

Treatment

Alpha-hydroxylated derivatives of vitamin D are preferred for their shorter half-life, and especially in renal disease as the others require renal hydroxylation. Usual daily maintenance doses are 0.25–2 μg for alfacalcidol (1α-OH-D$_3$). During treatment, plasma calcium must be monitored frequently to detect hypercalcaemia.

ENDOCRINOLOGY OF BLOOD PRESSURE CONTROL

The control of blood pressure (BP) is complex, involving neural, cardiac, hormonal and many other mechanisms.

BP is dependent upon cardiac output and peripheral resistance. Although cardiac output can be increased in endocrine disease (e.g. hyperthyroidism), the main role of hormonal mechanisms is control of peripheral resistance and of circulating blood volume. The oral contraceptive pill is a common endocrine cause of mild hypertension.

When to investigate for secondary hypertension

Endocrine causes account for less than 5% of all hypertension (Table 18.39). It is impracticable and unnecessary to screen all hypertensive patients for secondary causes. The highest chances of detecting such causes are in:

- subjects under 35 years, especially those without a family history of hypertension
- those with accelerated (malignant) hypertension

Table 18.39 Endocrine causes of hypertension	
Excessive renin, and thus angiotensin II, production Renal artery stenosis Other local renal disease Renin-secreting tumours	**Excessive production of other mineralocorticoids** Cushing's syndrome (massive excess of cortisol, a weak mineralocorticoid)
Excessive production of catecholamines Phaeochromocytoma	Congenital adrenal hyperplasia (in some cases)
Excessive GH production Acromegaly	Tumours producing other mineralocorticoids, e.g. corticosterone
Excessive aldosterone production Adrenal adenoma (Conn's syndrome) Idiopathic adrenal hyperplasia Dexamethasone-suppressible hyperaldosteronism	**Exogenous 'mineralocorticoids' or enzyme inhibitors** Liquorice ingestion (inhibits 11β-hydroxylase) Abuse of mineralocorticoid preparations

- those with indications of renal disease (e.g. proteinuria, unequal renal sizes)
- those with hypokalaemia before diuretic therapy
- those resistant to conventional antihypertensive therapy (e.g. more than three drugs)
- those with unusual symptoms (e.g. sweating attacks or weakness).

The renin–angiotensin–aldosterone axis: biochemistry and actions

The renin–angiotensin–aldosterone system is illustrated in Figure 18.27.

Angiotensinogen, an alpha$_2$-globulin of hepatic origin, circulates in plasma. The enzyme, renin, is secreted by the kidney in response to decreased renal perfusion pressure or flow; it cleaves the decapeptide *angiotensin I* from angiotensinogen. Angiotensin I is inactive but is further cleaved by angiotensin-converting enzyme (ACE; present in lung and vascular endothelium) into the active peptide, *angiotensin II*, which has two major actions

(mediated by two types of receptor, AT$_1$ and AT$_2$). The AT$_1$ subtype which is found in the heart, blood vessels, kidney, adrenal cortex, lung and brain mediates the vasoconstrictor effect. AT$_2$ is probably involved in vascular growth. Angiotensin II:

- causes rapid, powerful vasoconstriction
- stimulates the adrenal zona glomerulosa to increase aldosterone production (over hours or days).

As BP increases and sodium is retained, the stimuli to renin secretion are reduced. Dietary sodium excess also suppresses renin secretion, whereas sodium deprivation or urinary sodium loss will increase it.

The renin–angiotensin system can be blocked at several points with renin inhibitors, angiotensin-converting enzyme inhibitors (ACEI) and angiotensin II receptor antagonists (A-IIRA). The latter two are useful agents in treatment of hypertension and heart failure (see pp. 862 and 792) but have differences in action: ACEIs also block kinin production while A-IIRAs are specific for the AT-II receptors.

Atrial and brain natriuretic factors/peptides (ANP and BNP)

Atrial natriuretic peptides, a family of varying length forms, are secreted from atrial granules in response to atrial stretch. They produce marked effects on the kidney, increasing sodium and water excretion and glomerular filtration rate and lowering BP, plasma renin activity and plasma aldosterone (p. 612).

Brain natriuretic peptide is found in the ventricle as well as the brain and has moderate sequence homology with ANP; normally its circulating level is much less than for ANP but may exceed it in congestive cardiac failure.

ANP and BNP appear to play a significant role in cardiovascular and fluid homeostasis, but there is no evidence of primary defects in their secretion causing disease. BNP may accurately reflect the presence and severity of heart failure and appears to be useful in defining prognosis and the need for adjustment of treatment.

Agents that both inhibit the endopeptidases that break down ANP and inhibit ACE (the receptors concerned are similar) are available but long-term clinical studies are awaited.

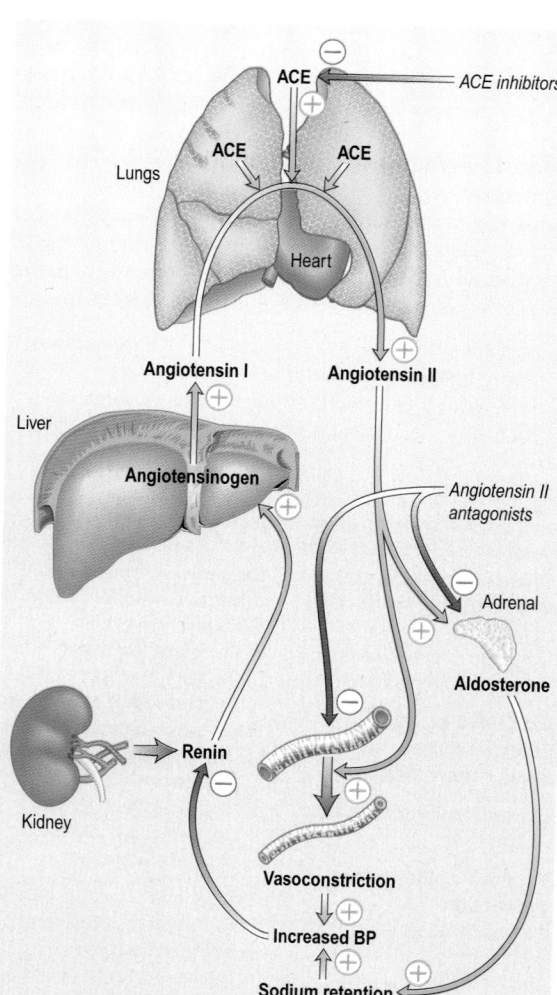

Fig. 18.27 **The renin–angiotensin–aldosterone system.** ACE, angiotensin-converting enzyme.

RENIN (AND ANGIOTENSIN) DEPENDENT HYPERTENSION

Many forms of unilateral and bilateral renal diseases are associated with hypertension. The classic example is renal artery stenosis: the major hypertensive effects of this and other situations such as renin-secreting tumours are directly or indirectly due to angiotensin II.

Angiotensin II receptor antagonists (e.g. losartan, valsartan, candesartan and irbesartan) are effective in hypertension and congestive cardiac failure, similar to angiotensin-converting enzyme inhibitors (ACEI). They produce much the same clinical effects, though with fewer side-effects (e.g. no cough and less hyperkalaemia).

Renal artery stenosis

This is discussed on page 646.

DISORDERS OF ALDOSTERONE SECRETION

Primary hyperaldosteronism

Pathophysiology

This rare condition (< 1% of all hypertension) is caused by excess aldosterone production leading to sodium retention, potassium loss and the combination of hypokalaemia and hypertension.

Causes (see Table 18.39)

Adrenal adenomas (Conn's syndrome) account for 60% of cases; 30% are due to bilateral adrenal hyperplasia of uncertain aetiology.

Clinical features

The usual presentation is with hypertension and hypokalaemia (< 3.5 mmol/L), although 20–40% of patients have initial potassium levels of 3.5–4.2 mmol/L. The few symptoms are non-specific; rarely muscle weakness, nocturia and tetany are seen. The hypertension may be severe and associated with renal, cardiac and retinal damage.

Adenomas, often very small, are more common in young females, while bilateral hyperplasia rarely occurs before age 40 years and is more common in males.

Investigations

The characteristic features are as follows:

- **Hypokalaemia.** A high-salt diet should be given for several days before testing and diuretics must be stopped 3 weeks before investigation; plasma samples must be separated quickly.
- **Urinary potassium loss.** Levels > 30 mmol daily during hypokalaemia are inappropriate.
- **An elevated plasma aldosterone:renin ratio** is a valuable screening test.
- **Elevated plasma aldosterone levels** that are not suppressed with 0.9% saline infusion (300 mmol over 4 hours) or fludrocortisone administration.
- **Suppressed plasma renin activity.** Beta-blockers and other drugs may interfere with renin activity.

Once a diagnosis of hyperaldosteronism is established, differentiation of adenoma from hyperplasia involves adrenal CT or MRI (not infallible as tumours may be very small), complex biochemical testing including diurnal/postural changes in plasma aldosterone levels (which tend to rise with adenomas between 0900h supine and 1300h erect samples; in contrast they fall with hyperplasia), measurement of 18-OH cortisol levels (raised in adenoma), adrenal scintillation scanning, and venous catheterization for aldosterone levels.

A rare cause is glucocorticoid (or dexamethasone)-suppressible hyperaldosteronism caused by a chimeric gene on chromosome 8. A fusion gene resulting from an unusual cross-over at meiosis between the genes encoding aldosterone synthase and adrenal 11β-hydroxylase produces aldosterone which is under ACTH control. Treatment with glucocorticoid resolves the problem.

Treatment

An adenoma should be removed surgically – usually laparoscopically; BP falls in 70% of patients. Those with hyperplasia should be treated with the aldosterone antagonist spironolactone (100–400 mg daily); frequent side-effects include nausea, rashes and gynaecomastia (p. 1056). Spironolactone in long-term use has been linked with tumour development in animals. Amiloride and calcium-channel blockers are moderately effective in controlling the hypertension but do not correct the hyperaldosteronism.

Secondary hyperaldosteronism

This situation arises when there is excess renin (and hence angiotensin II) stimulation of the zona glomerulosa. Common causes are accelerated hypertension and renal artery stenosis, when the patient will be hypertensive. Causes associated with normotension include congestive cardiac failure and cirrhosis, where excess aldosterone production contributes to sodium retention.

Angiotensin-converting enzyme inhibitors (e.g. captopril, enalapril or lisinopril), and angiotensin II antagonists (e.g. losartan, candesartan) are effective in heart failure, both symptomatically and in increasing life expectancy (see p. 792). Spironolactone is of value in both situations, and 25 mg/day has been shown to improve survival in heart failure (see p. 792).

Syndrome of apparent mineralocorticoid excess

This causes the clinical syndrome of primary hyperaldosteronism but with low renin and aldosterone levels. Reduced activity of the enzyme 11β-hydroxysteroid dehydrogenase type 2 (11β-HSD2) prevents the normal conversion in the kidney of cortisol (which is active at the mineralocorticoid receptor) to cortisone (which is not) and therefore 'exposes' the mineralocorticoid receptor in the kidney to the usual molar excess of cortisol over aldosterone in the blood. While the inherited syndrome is rare, the same clinical syndrome can occur with excess ingestion of liquorice – which inhibits the 11β-HSD2 enzyme.

Hypoaldosteronism

Except as part of primary hypoadrenalism (Addison's disease, see p. 1082), this is very uncommon. Causes include hyporeninaemic hypoaldosteronism, aldosterone biosynthetic defects, and drugs (e.g. ACE inhibitors, heparin).

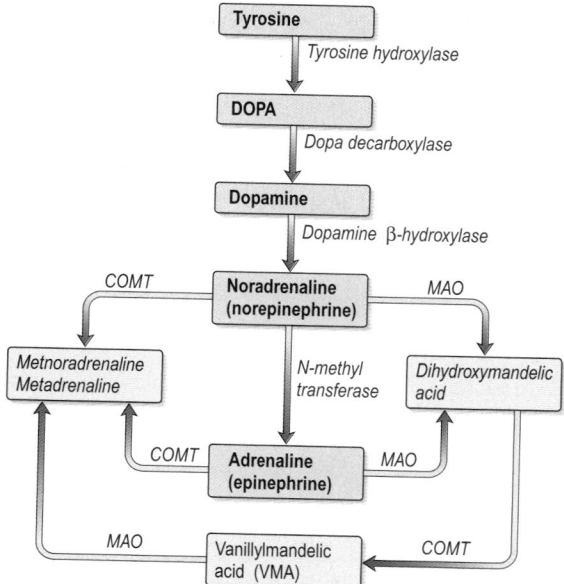

Fig. 18.28 **The synthesis and metabolism of catecholamines.** COMT, catechol-O-methyl transferase; MAO, monoamine oxidase.

Table 18.40 Symptoms and signs of phaeochromocytoma	
Symptoms	**Signs**
Anxiety or panic attacks	Hypertension – intermittent or constant
Palpitations	
Tremor	Tachycardia plus arrhythmias
Sweating	Bradycardia
Headache	Orthostatic hypotension
Flushing	Pallor or flushing
Nausea and/or vomiting	Glycosuria
Weight loss	Fever
Constipation or diarrhoea	(Signs of hypertensive damage)
Raynaud's phenomenon	
Chest pain	
Polyuria/nocturia	

THE ADRENAL MEDULLA

The major catecholamines, noradrenaline (norepinephrine) and adrenaline (epinephrine) are produced in the adrenal medulla (Fig. 18.28), although most noradrenaline is derived from sympathetic neuronal release. While noradrenaline and adrenaline undoubtedly produce hypertension when infused, they probably play little part in BP regulation in normal humans.

Phaeochromocytoma

Phaeochromocytomas, tumours of the sympathetic nervous system, are very rare (less than 1 in 1000 cases of hypertension). Ninety per cent arise in the adrenal, while 10% occur elsewhere in the sympathetic chain. Some are associated with MEN 2 syndromes (see below) and the von Hippel–Lindau syndrome (p. 683). Most tumours release both noradrenaline (norepinephrine) and adrenaline (epinephrine) but large tumours and extra-adrenal tumours produce almost entirely norepinephrine.

Pathology

Oval groups of cells occur in clusters and stain for chromogranin A. Twenty-five percent are multiple and 10% malignant, the latter being more frequent in the extra-adrenal tumours. Malignancy cannot be determined on simple histological examination alone.

Clinical features

The clinical features are those of catecholamine excess and are frequently, but not necessarily, intermittent (Table 18.40). The diagnosis should particularly be considered when cardiovascular instability has been demonstrated, and in severe hypertension in pregnancy.

Diagnosis

Specific tests are:

- **Measurement of urinary catecholamines and metabolites** (preferably metanephrines rather than vanillylmandelic acid (VMA) – Fig. 18.28) is a useful screening test; normal levels on three 24-hour collections of metanephrines virtually exclude the diagnosis. Many drugs and dietary vanilla interfere with these tests.
- **Resting plasma catecholamines** are raised.
- **Plasma chromogranin A** (a storage vesicle protein) is raised.
- **Clonidine suppression and glucagon stimulation** tests may be appropriate, but should only be performed in specialist centres.
- **CT scans**, initially of the abdomen, are helpful to localize the tumours which are often large.
- **MRI** usually shows the lesion clearly.
- **Scanning with [131I]metaiodobenzylguanidine** (mIBG) produces specific uptake in sites of sympathetic activity with about 90% success. It is particularly useful with extra-adrenal tumours.

Treatment

Tumours should be removed if this is possible; 5-year survival is about 95% when not malignant. Medical preoperative and perioperative treatment is vital and includes complete alpha- and beta-blockade with phenoxybenzamine (20–80 mg daily initially in divided doses), then propranolol (120–240 mg daily), plus transfusion of whole blood to re-expand the contracted plasma volume. The alpha-blockade must precede the beta-blockade, as worsened hypertension may otherwise result. Labetolol is not recommended. Surgery in the unprepared patient is fraught with dangers of both hypertension and hypotension; expert anaesthesia and an experienced surgeon are both vital and sodium nitroprusside should be available in case sudden severe hypertension develops.

When operation is not possible, combined alpha- and beta-blockade can be used long term. Radionucleotide treatment with mIBG has been attempted with limited success.

Patients should be kept under clinical and biochemical review after tumour resection as over 10% recur or develop a further tumour. Catecholamine excretion measurements should be performed at least annually.

FURTHER READING
Bouloux PM, Fakeeh M (1995) Investigation of phaeochromocytoma. *Clinical Endocrinology* **43**: 657–664.
Burnie M, Brunner HR (2000) Angiotensin II receptor antagonists. *Lancet* **355**: 637–645.
Stewart PM (1999) Mineralocorticoid hypertension. *Lancet* **353**: 1341–1347.
Taupenot L (2003) The chromogranin-secretogranin family. *New England Journal of Medicine* **348**: 1134–1149.

OTHER ENDOCRINE DISORDERS

DISEASES OF MANY GLANDS

Multiple gland failure (polyglandular autoimmune syndromes)

These are caused by autoimmune disease as detailed in Table 18.4 on page 1042. Most common are the associations of primary hypothyroidism and type 1 diabetes, and either of these with Addison's disease or pernicious anaemia.

Multiple endocrine neoplasia

This is the name given to the simultaneous or metachronous occurrence of tumours involving a number of endocrine glands (Table 18.41). They are inherited in an autosomal dominant manner and arise from the expression of recessive oncogenic mutations, most of which have been isolated. Affected persons may pass on the mutation to their offspring in the germ cell, but for the disease to become evident a somatic mutation must also occur, such as deletion or loss of a normal homologous chromosome. The defect in MEN 1 is in a novel gene (*menin*) on the long arm of chromosome 11 which encodes for a 610-amino-acid protein. MEN 2a and 2b are caused by mutations of the *Ret*-proto-oncogene on chromosome 10. This gene encodes for a transmembrane glycoprotein receptor. For MEN 2a the mutation is in the extracellular domain; for 2b in the intracellular domain.

Management

Treatment is surgical.

For type 1, all four parathyroid glands are removed (as all may be involved), followed by vitamin D (1,25-dihydrocalciferol) replacement therapy. Pancreatic tumours are often multiple and recurrence after partial pancreatectomy is invariable. Other tumours are treated surgically if necessary.

Table 18.41 Multiple endocrine neoplasia (MEN) syndromes

Organ	Frequency	Tumours/manifestations
Type 1		
Parathyroid	95%	Adenomas/hyperplasia
Pituitary	70%	Adenomas – prolactinoma, ACTH or growth hormone secreting (acromegaly)
Pancreas	50%	Islet cell tumours (secreting insulin, glucagon, somatostatin, VIP, pancreatic polypeptide, growth hormone-releasing factor) Zollinger–Ellison syndrome (gastrinoma). Non-functional tumour
Adrenal	40%	Non-functional adenoma
Thyroid	20%	Adenomas – multiple or single
Type 2a		
Adrenal	Most	Phaeochromocytoma (70% bilateral) Cushing's syndrome
Thyroid	Most	Medullary carcinoma (calcitonin producing)
Parathyroid	60%	Hyperplasia
Type 2b		
Type 2a with marfanoid phenotype and intestinal and visceral ganglioneuromas but not hyperparathyroidism Neuromas also present around lips and tongue		

Type 2 tumours may also be recurrent or bilateral and a careful follow-up is necessary.

Screening

A careful family history should first be taken. If the precise gene mutation has been identified in a particular family, then family members at risk can be screened directly for the presence of the mutation. In affected individuals, biochemical screening is then required. If initial biochemical screening is negative, this does not exclude later involvement and needs repeating at regular intervals, typically annually, with more intensive investigation when symptoms arise.

Screening for type 1

Hyperparathyroidism is usually the first manifestation, and serum calcium is the simplest screening test in families with no identified mutation. In an established case (or gene positive family member) other typical screening bloods include prolactin, GH/IGF1 and 'gut hormones'. Repeated imaging is rarely practical.

Screening for type 2

Serum calcium levels will easily detect hyperparathyroidism

- *Medullary carcinoma of thyroid (MCT)* – with the known presence of the gene defect, total thyroidectomy in childhood is recommended. Calcitonin is a useful tumour marker but stimulation (with pentagastrin or calcium infusion test) is needed to pick up 'C' cell hyperplasia which precedes tumour development. Total thyroidectomy is then indicated.
- *Phaeochromocytoma* – metanephrine or catecholamine estimations.

ECTOPIC HORMONE SECRETION

This terminology refers to hormone synthesis, and normally secretion, from a neoplastic non-endocrine cell, most usually seen in tumours that have some degree of embryological resemblance to specialist endocrine cells. The clinical effects are those of the hormone produced, with or without manifestations of systemic malignancy. The most common situations seen are the following:

- *Hypercalcaemia of malignant disease*, often from squamous cell tumours of lung and breast, often with bone metastases. Where metastases are not present, most cases are mediated by secretion of PTH-related protein (PTHrP), which has considerable sequence homology to PTH; a variety of other factors may sometimes be involved, but very rarely PTH itself (see p. 1093). Treatment is also discussed on page 1093.
- *SIADH* (see p. 695). Again, this is most common from a primary lung tumour.
- *Ectopic ACTH syndrome* (see p. 1085). Small-cell carcinoma of the lung, carcinoid tumours and medullary thyroid carcinomas are the most common causes, though many other tumours rarely cause it.
- *Production of insulin-like activity* may result in hypoglycaemia (see p. 1133).

ENDOCRINE TREATMENT OF OTHER MALIGNANCIES

Endocrine forms of treatment for malignancy have been used for many years; for example oophorectomy for breast cancer and orchidectomy for prostatic malignancy. More acceptable therapies include the anti-oestrogen tamoxifen for breast carcinoma and the GnRH analogues, buserelin and goserelin, for prostatic cancer.

FURTHER READING

Mulligan LM, Ponder BA (1995) Genetic basis of endocrine disease: MEN type 2. *Journal of Clinical Endocrinology and Metabolism* **80**: 1989–1995.

Trump D et al. (1996) Clinical studies of MEN type 1. *Quarterly Journal of Medicine* **89**: 653–659.

CHAPTER BIBLIOGRAPHY

Brook CGD, Hindmarsh PC (2001) *Clinical Paediatric Endocrinology*, 4th edn. Oxford: Blackwell Science.
DeGroot L, Jameson JL (2001) *Endocrinology*. Philadelphia: WB Saunders

Wass JAH, Shalet SM (eds) (2002) *Oxford Textbook of Endocrinology and Diabetes*. Oxford: Oxford University Press

SIGNIFICANT WEBSITES

http://www.endocrinology.org
  UK Society of Endocrinology
http://www.endo-society.org
  Endocrine Society
http://www.niddk.nih.gov/health/endo/endo.htm
  US National Institutes of Health, National Institute of Diabetes & Digestive & Kidney Diseases
http://www.endocrineweb.com
  Endocrine web resources

http://www.pituitary.org.uk
  The Pituitary Foundation (UK charity)
http://www.tss.org.uk
  UK Turner Syndrome Support Society
http://www.medicalert.org.uk
  Emergency identification system for people with hidden medical conditions

Diabetes mellitus and other disorders of metabolism

19

HYPERGLYCAEMIA, INSULIN AND INSULIN ACTION

Introduction

Diabetes mellitus (DM) is a syndrome of chronic hyperglycaemia due to relative insulin deficiency, resistance, or both. It affects more than 120 million people world-wide, and it is estimated that it will affect 220 million by the year 2020. Diabetes is usually irreversible and, although patients can have a reasonably normal lifestyle, its late complications result in reduced life expectancy and major health costs. These include macrovascular disease, leading to an increased prevalence of coronary artery disease, peripheral vascular disease and stroke, and microvascular damage causing diabetic retinopathy and nephropathy. Neuropathy is another major complication.

Insulin structure and secretion

Insulin is the key hormone involved in the storage and controlled release within the body of the chemical energy available from food. It is coded for on chromosome 11 and synthesized in the beta-cells of the pancreatic islets. The synthesis, intracellular processing and secretion of insulin by the beta-cell is typical of the way that the body produces and manipulates many peptide hormones. The manufacture and release of insulin from the beta-cell is illustrated in Figure 19.1. Figure 19.2 illustrates the cellular events triggering the release of insulin-containing granules. After secretion, insulin enters the portal circulation and is carried to the liver, its prime target organ. About 50% of secreted insulin is extracted and degraded in the liver; the residue is broken down by the kidneys. C-peptide is only partially extracted by the liver (and hence provides a useful index of the rate of insulin secretion), but is mainly degraded by the kidneys.

An outline of glucose metabolism

Blood glucose levels are closely regulated in health and rarely stray outside the range of 3.5–8.0 mmol/L (63–144 mg/dL), despite the varying demands of food, fasting and exercise. The principal organ of glucose homeostasis is the liver, which absorbs and stores glucose (as glycogen) in the post-absorptive state and releases it into the circulation between meals to match the rate of glucose utilization by peripheral tissues. The liver also combines 3-carbon molecules derived from breakdown of fat (glycerol), muscle glycogen (lactate) and protein (e.g. alanine) into the 6-carbon glucose molecule by the process of gluconeogenesis.

Glucose production

About 200 g of glucose is produced and utilized each day. More than 90% is derived from liver glycogen and hepatic gluconeogenesis, and the remainder from renal gluconeogenesis.

Glucose utilization

The brain is the major consumer of glucose. Its requirement is 1 mg/kg bodyweight per minute, or 100 g daily in

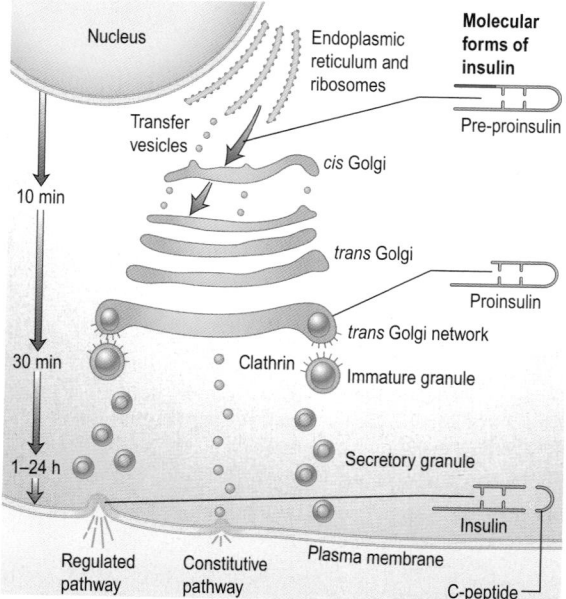

Molecular forms of insulin

Fig. 19.1 Part of a beta-cell. The ribosomes manufacture pre-proinsulin from insulin mRNA. The hydrophobic 'pre' portion of pre-proinsulin allows it to transfer to the Golgi apparatus, and is subsequently enzymatically cleaved off. Proinsulin is parcelled into secretory granules in the Golgi apparatus. These mature and pass towards the cell membrane where they are stored before release. The proinsulin molecule folds back on itself and is stabilized by disulphide bonds. The biochemically inert peptide fragment known as connecting (C) peptide splits off from proinsulin in the secretory process, leaving insulin as a complex of two linked peptide chains. Equimolar quantities of insulin and C-peptide are released into the circulation. A small amount of insulin is secreted by the beta-cell directly via the 'constitutive pathway', which bypasses the secretory granules.

a 70 kg man. Glucose uptake by the brain is obligatory and is not dependent on insulin, and the glucose used is oxidized to carbon dioxide and water. Other tissues, such as muscle and fat, are facultative glucose consumers. The effect of insulin peaks associated with meals is to lower the threshold for glucose entry into cells; at other times, energy requirements are largely met by fatty-acid oxidation. Glucose taken up by muscle is stored as glycogen or broken down to lactate, which re-enters the circulation and becomes a major substrate for hepatic gluconeogenesis. Glucose is used by fat tissue as a source of energy and as a substrate for triglyceride synthesis; lipolysis releases fatty acids from triglyceride together with glycerol, another substrate for hepatic gluconeogenesis.

Hormonal regulation

Insulin is the major regulator of intermediary metabolism, although its actions are modified in many respects by other hormones. Its actions in the fasting and postprandial states differ (Fig. 19.3). In the fasting state its main action is to regulate glucose release by the liver, and in the postprandial state it additionally facilitates glucose uptake by fat and muscle. The effect of counter-regulatory hormones (glucagon, epinephrine (adrenaline), cortisol and growth hormone) is to cause greater production of glucose from the liver and less utilization of glucose in fat and muscle for a given level of insulin.

Glucose transport

Cell membranes are not inherently permeable to glucose. A family of specialized glucose-transporter (GLUT) proteins carry glucose through the membrane into cells.

- GLUT-1 – enables basal non-insulin-stimulated glucose uptake into many cells (see Fig. 6.21).
- GLUT-2 – transports glucose into the beta-cell: a prerequisite for glucose sensing.

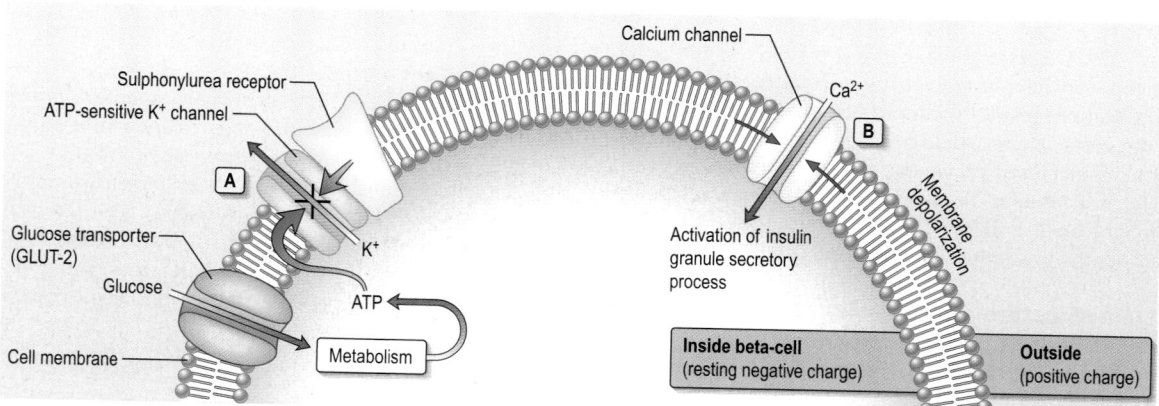

Fig. 19.2 Local forces regulating insulin secretion from beta-cells. Glucose enters the beta-cell via the GLUT-2 transporter protein, which is closely associated with the glycolytic enzyme glucokinase. Metabolism of glucose within the beta-cell generates ATP. ATP closes potassium channels in the cell membrane (A). If a sulphonylurea binds to its receptor, this also closes potassium channels. Closure of potassium channels predisposes to cell membrane depolarization, allowing calcium ions to enter the cell via calcium channels in the cell membrane (B). The rise in intracellular calcium triggers activation of calcium-dependent phospholipid protein kinase which, via intermediary phosphorylation steps, leads to fusion of the insulin-containing granules with the cell membrane and exocytosis of the insulin-rich granule contents. Similar mechanisms produce hormone-granule secretion in many other endocrine cells.

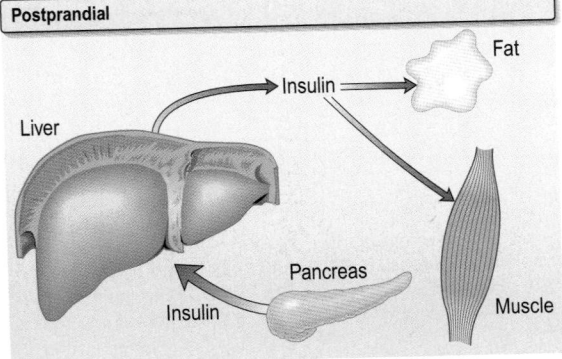

Fig. 19.3 Fasting and postprandial effects of insulin. In the *fasting state* insulin concentrations are low and it acts mainly as a hepatic hormone, modulating glucose production (via glycogenolysis and gluconeogenesis) from the liver. Hepatic glucose production rises as insulin levels fall. In the *postprandial state* insulin concentrations are high and it then suppresses glucose production from the liver and promotes the entry of glucose into peripheral tissues (increased glucose utilization).

- GLUT-3 – enables non-insulin-mediated glucose uptake into brain neurones and placenta.
- GLUT-4 – enables much of the peripheral action of insulin. It is the channel through which glucose is taken up into muscle and adipose tissue cells following stimulation of the insulin receptor (Fig. 19.4).

The insulin receptor

This is a glycoprotein (400 kDa), coded for on the short arm of chromosome 19, which straddles the cell membrane of many cells (Fig. 19.4). It consists of a dimer with two alpha-subunits, which include the binding sites for insulin, and two beta-subunits, which traverse the cell membrane. When insulin binds to the alpha-subunits it induces a conformational change in the beta-subunits, resulting in activation of tyrosine kinase and initiation of a cascade response involving a host of other intracellular substrates. One consequence of this is migration of the GLUT-4 glucose transporter to the cell surface and increased transport of glucose into the cell. The insulin–receptor complex is then internalized by the cell, insulin is degraded, and the receptor is recycled to the cell surface.

FURTHER READING

Shepherd PR, Kahn BB (1999) Glucose transporters and insulin action. *New England Journal of Medicine* **341**: 248–258.

TYPES OF DIABETES

Diabetes may be primary or secondary (Table 19.1). Although secondary diabetes accounts for barely 1–2% of all new cases at presentation, it should not be missed because the cause can often be treated. Type 1 diabetes (insulin-dependent diabetes mellitus) and type 2 diabetes (non-insulin-dependent diabetes mellitus) represent two distinct diseases from the epidemiological point of view, but clinical distinction can sometimes be difficult. The two diseases should, in clinical terms, be seen as a spectrum, distinct at the two ends but overlapping to some extent in the middle (Table 19.2). Varying degrees of insulin secretory failure may be present in both forms of diabetes. For example, some patients with immune-mediated diabetes may not at first require insulin, whereas many with type 2 diabetes will eventually do so.

Type 1 diabetes mellitus

Epidemiology

Type 1 diabetes is a disease resulting in insulin deficiency. In western countries almost all patients have the immune-mediated form of the disease (type 1A). Type 1 diabetes is prominent as a disease of childhood, reaching a peak incidence around the time of puberty, but can present at any age. A 'slow-burning' variant with slower progression to insulin deficiency occurs in later life and is sometimes called latent autoimmune diabetes of adults (LADA). This may be difficult to distinguish from type 2 diabetes. Clinical clues are: considerable weight loss, hyperglycaemia which fails to correct with diet and tablet treatment, the presence of strong or persistent ketonuria at diagnosis, and autoantibody tests indicating autoimmune disease. The highest rates of type 1 diabetes in the world are seen in Finland and other Northern

Table 19.1 Causes of secondary diabetes

Pancreatic disease	**Drug-induced disease**
Cystic fibrosis	Thiazide diuretics
Chronic pancreatitis	Corticosteroid therapy
Malnutrition-related	Atypical antipsychotics
pancreatic disease	Antiretroviral protease
Pancreatectomy	inhibitors
Hereditary haemochromatosis	
Carcinoma of the pancreas	**Insulin-receptor**
	abnormalities
Endocrine disease	Congenital lipodystrophy
Cushing's syndrome	Acanthosis nigricans
Acromegaly	
Thyrotoxicosis	**Genetic syndromes**
Phaeochromocytoma	Friedreich's ataxia
Glucagonoma	Dystrophia myotonica

Fig. 19.4 **Insulin signalling in peripheral cells.** The insulin receptor consists of alpha- and beta-subunits linked by disulphide bridges (top right of figure). The beta-subunits straddle the cell membrane. The transporter protein GLUT-4 is stored in intracellular vesicles. The binding of insulin to its receptor initiates many intracellular actions including translocation of these vesicles to the cell membrane, carrying GLUT-4 with them.

Table 19.2	**The spectrum of diabetes: a comparison of type 1 and type 2 diabetes mellitus**	
	Type 1 (insulin dependent)	**Type 2 (non-insulin dependent)**
Epidemiology	Younger (usually < 30 years of age) Usually lean Increased in those of Northern European ancestry Seasonal incidence	Older (usually > 30 years of age) Often overweight All racial groups. Increased in peoples of Asian, African, Polynesian and American-Indian ancestry
Heredity	HLA-DR3 or DR4 in > 90% 30–50% concordance in identical twins	No HLA links ~ 50% concordance in identical twins
Pathogenesis	Autoimmune disease: Islet cell autoantibodies Insulitis Association with other autoimmune diseases Immunosuppression after diagnosis delays beta-cell destruction	No immune disturbance Insulin resistance
Clinical	Insulin deficiency May develop ketoacidosis Always need insulin	Partial insulin deficiency May develop hyperosmolar state Many come to need insulin when beta-cells fail over time
Biochemical	Eventual disappearance of C-peptide	C-peptide persists

European countries, with the exception of the island of Sardinia, which for unknown reasons has the second highest rate in the world (Fig. 19.5). The incidence of type 1 diabetes appears to be increasing in most populations. In Europe the annual increase is of the order of 3–4%, and is most marked in children under the age of 5 years. A subtype of type 1 diabetes (type 1B) has recently been described in Japanese patients with an abrupt onset, no autoimmune disease and high serum pancreatic enzyme concentrations at diagnosis. This has not been described in other populations. WHO (1995) estimated that there are 19.4 million people with type 1 diabetes and that the number will rise to 57.2 million by 2025.

Causes

Type 1 diabetes belongs to a family of HLA-associated immune-mediated organ-specific diseases. Genetic susceptibility is polygenic, with the greatest contribution

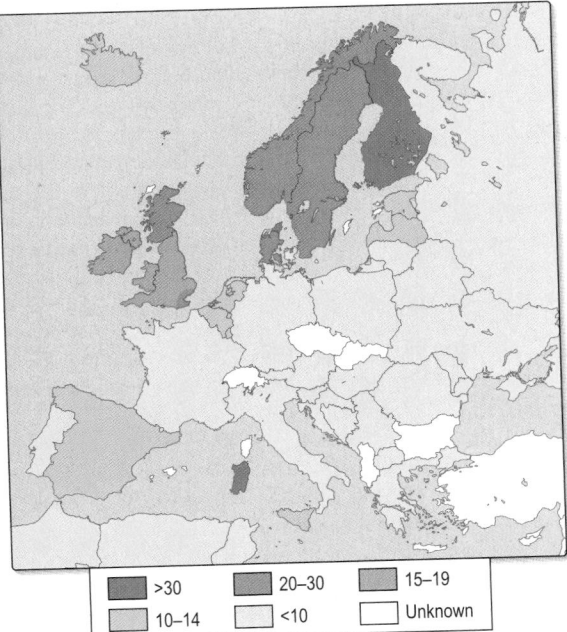

Fig. 19.5 Age-standardized incidence rates of type 1 diabetes (onset 0–14 years) in Europe, per 100 000 per year. From Green A, Gale EAM et al. (1992) *Lancet* **339**: 905–909.

from the HLA region. Autoantibodies directed against pancreatic islet constituents appear in the circulation within the first few years of life, and predate clinical onset by many years. Autoantibodies are also found in older patients with LADA and predict progression to insulin therapy in this group.

Genetic susceptibility

Type 1 diabetes is not genetically predetermined, but increased susceptibility to the disease may be inherited.

Inheritance

The identical twin of a patient with type 1 diabetes has a 30–50% chance of developing the disease. Since twins with identical genes may never develop the disease, non-genetic factors must also be involved. Children of people with type 1 diabetes have an increased chance of developing type 1 diabetes. The risk of developing diabetes by age 20, curiously, is greater with a diabetic father (3–7%) than with a diabetic mother (2–3%). If one child in a family has type 1 diabetes, each sibling has a ~ 6% risk of developing diabetes by age 20. If siblings are HLA-identical (share the same HLA type as the affected child), the risk rises to about 20%. Longer-term follow-up has, however, shown that the lifetime risk of diabetes in first-degree relatives is considerably greater than this.

HLA system. The HLA genes on chromosome 6 are highly polymorphic and modulate the immune defence system of the body. More than 90% of patients with type 1 diabetes carry HLA-DR3-DQ2, HLA-DR4-DQ8, or both, as compared with some 35% of the background popu-

lation. All DQB1 alleles with an aspartic acid at residue 57 confer neutral to protective effects with the strongest effect from DQB1*0602 (DQ6), while DQB1 alleles with an alanine at the same position (i.e. DQ2 and DQ8) confer strong susceptibility. Genotypic combinations have a major influence upon risk of disease. For example HLA DR3-DQ2/HLA DR4-DQ8 heterozygotes have a considerably increased risk of disease. The presence or absence of certain HLA class I alleles substantially modifies the risk conferred by class II susceptibility genes.

Other gene regions. Genome-wide searches for regions conferring susceptibility to, or protection against, type 1 diabetes have been carried out, and 10–20 regions of interest have been identified. These are designated *IDDM1* (HLA locus), *IDDM2* and so on. It is already clear that individually these make a much smaller contribution to genetic susceptibility than the HLA region. An intensive search to identify these genes and their products continues.

A DNA region close to the insulin gene on chromosome 11 is designated *IDDM2*, and short, intermediate and long insertions (see p. 177) have been reported. Homozygosity of the short (class I) allele is found in some 80% of patients with type 1 diabetes as against 40% of controls.

The *CTLA-4* gene has also been implicated in type 1 diabetes and might be a common factor in a variety of HLA-associated autoimmune conditions.

Autoimmunity and insulin-dependent diabetes mellitus

Several pieces of evidence suggest that type 1 diabetes is an immune-mediated disease. These include the HLA associations described above, and associations with other organ-specific autoimmune diseases including auto-immune thyroid disease, Addison's disease and pernicious anaemia. Autopsies of patients who died soon after diagnosis show infiltration of the pancreatic islets by mononuclear cells. This appearance, known as insulitis, resembles that in other autoimmune diseases such as thyroiditis. Autoantibodies directed against islet constituents are also present in some 90% of newly presenting patients. A number of islet antigens have been characterized, and include insulin itself, the enzyme glutamic acid decarboxylase (GAD), and the intracellular portion of two islet peptides from the tyrosine phosphatase family (Fig. 19.6). Confirmation of the autoimmune nature of the disease came from the observation that treatment with immunosuppressive agents such as ciclosporin following diagnosis prolongs beta-cell survival.

Environmental factors

The incidence of childhood type 1 diabetes is rising steadily, suggesting that environmental factor(s) are involved in its pathogenesis. Early exposure to entero-viruses such as Coxsackie B4 has often been suspected, but the role of viruses in the causation of the disease has yet to be confirmed. It has also been suggested that a cleaner environment with less early stimulation of the immune system in childhood may increase susceptibility

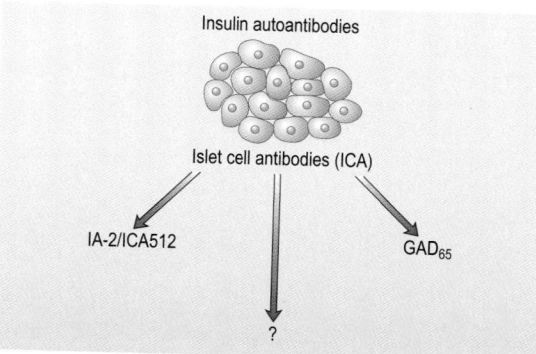

Fig. 19.6 Islet autoantibodies. Islet cell antibodies are detected by a fluorescent antibody technique which detects binding of autoantibodies to islet cells. Much of this staining reaction is due to antibodies specific for glutamic acid decarboxylase (GAD) and protein tyrosine phosphatase – IA-2 (also known as ICA512). Not all the staining seen with ICA is due to these two autoantibodies, so it is assumed that other islet autoantibodies are also involved. Insulin autoantibodies also appear in the circulation but do not contribute to the ICA reaction.

for type 1 diabetes, as for atopic/allergic conditions (the hygiene hypothesis).

Pre-type 1 diabetes and prevention of type 1 diabetes

Prospective studies of first-degree relatives of children with diabetes have shown that islet autoantibodies appear in the circulation in the first few years of life – demonstrating that the process culminating in diabetes is initiated very early – and many years before diagnosis. Further, they can predict development of the disease, especially when present in combination. The ability to predict the disease has opened the way to possible disease prevention, but trials using injected or oral insulin or nicotinamide have all proved unsuccessful.

Type 2 diabetes mellitus

Epidemiology

This is relatively common in all populations enjoying an affluent lifestyle. The four major determinants are increasing age, obesity, ethnicity and family history. Large differences in prevalence exist based on these characteristics. In poor countries diabetes is a disease of the rich, but in rich countries it is a disease of the poor. The disease may be present in a subclinical form for years before diagnosis. The onset may be accelerated by the stress of pregnancy, drug treatment or intercurrent illness. Estimates of prevalence using the WHO criteria (p. 1109) would suggest an overall prevalence of around 2% within the UK. Within the UK, type 2 diabetes is three to four times as prevalent in people of South Asian, African and Caribbean ancestry. High rates have also been found in people of middle Eastern or Hispanic American origin living western lifestyles. Unfortunately, people in westernized countries gain on average nearly 1 gram in weight every day of their adult life between the ages of

25–55 years. This gain, due to a tiny excess in energy intake over expenditure – 90 kcal or one chocolate-coated digestive biscuit per day – is the result of reduced exercise in a population rather than of increased food intake. Further, our sedentary lifestyle means that the proportion of obese young adults is rising rapidly, and epidemic obesity will create a huge public health problem for the future. The increasing numbers of obese adolescents presenting with type 2 diabetes is already a matter for concern in the USA and other parts of the world. Diabetes prevalence increases with age and 10% of people of Northern European stock will develop diabetes by the age of 70. This proportion rises towards 30% in those with a family history of diabetes and in those from some ethnic groups.

The insulin resistant state seen in type 2 diabetes tends to cluster with other conditions which increase cardiovascular risk. These include: hypertension, obesity, hypertriglyceridaemia, a decreased HDL-cholesterol, and the skin condition acanthosis nigricans. High insulin levels are characteristic. This has been called the insulin resistance syndrome, syndrome X or the metabolic syndrome. It seems likely that this is not a distinct entity but one end of a continuum in the relationship between exercise, lifestyle and bodyweight on the one hand, and individuals' genetic make-up on the other – resulting in a state associated with adverse clinical consequences. About a third of the adult population have features of the syndrome, not necessarily associated with diabetes.

Causes of type 2 diabetes
Genetics

Population-based studies show identical twins of patients with type 2 diabetes have a greater than 50% chance of developing diabetes; the risk to non-identical twins or siblings is of the order of 25%. These observations confirm a genetic component to the disease. Type 2 diabetes is a polygenic disorder, but the genes responsible for the great majority of cases have yet to be identified. This situation seems set to change, and as genetic causes are discovered the phenotypic differences between people currently lumped together as having 'type 2 diabetes' will probably be explained.

The genetic causes of some rare forms of type 2 diabetes are shown in Table 19.3.

A rare variant of type 2 diabetes is referred to as 'maturity-onset diabetes of the young' (MODY). This is dominantly inherited. Five variants have been described. The different MODY genotypes are associated with different clinical phenotypes (Table 19.4). MODY should be considered in young people presenting with a typical family history (diabetes affecting a parent and 50% expression of the disease in the family) plus a form of early-onset diabetes which appears easy to control.

Environmental factors: early and late

An association has been noted between low weight at birth and at 12 months of age and glucose intolerance later in life, particularly in those who gain excess weight as adults. The concept is that poor nutrition early in life

Table 19.3 Rare genetic causes of type 2 diabetes

Disorder	Features
Insulin receptor mutations	Obesity, marked insulin resistance, hyperandrogenism in women, acanthosis nigricans (areas of hyperpigmented skin)
Maternally inherited diabetes and deafness (MIDD)	Mutation in mitochondrial DNA. Diabetes onset before age 40. Variable deafness, neuromuscular and cardiac problems, pigmented retinopathy
Wolfram syndrome (DIDMOAD – diabetes insipidus, diabetes mellitus, optic atrophy and deafness)	Recessively inherited. Mutation in the transmembrane gene, *WFS1*. Insulin-requiring diabetes and optic atrophy in the first decade. Diabetes insipidus and sensorineural deafness in the second decade progressing to multiple neurological problems. Few live beyond middle age
Severe obesity and diabetes	Alström, Bardet–Biedl and Prader–Willi syndromes. Retinitis pigmentosa, mental insufficiency and neurological disorders
Disorders of intracellular insulin signalling. All with severe insulin resistance	Leprechaunism Rabson–Mendenhall syndrome Pseudoacromegaly Partial lipodystrophy: lamin A/C gene mutation

impairs beta-cell development and function, predisposing to diabetes in later life. Low birthweight has also been shown to predispose to heart disease and hypertension in later life.

Immunology and inflammation

There is no evidence of immune involvement in the pathogenesis of type 2 diabetes, but as noted earlier, a proportion of late-onset patients carry islet auto-antibodies directed against GAD at diagnosis, and these are more likely to progress to insulin therapy. Such cases are probably type 1 diabetes masquerading as type 2 diabetes.

A recent development is the recognition that subclinical inflammatory changes are characteristic of both type 2 diabetes and obesity. In diabetes, high-sensitivity C-reactive protein (CRP) levels are elevated in association with raised fibrinogen and increased plasminogen activator inhibitor-1 (PAI-1), and contribute to cardiovascular risk. Circulating levels of the proinflammatory cytokines TNF-α and IL-6 are elevated in both diabetes and obesity. Use of anti-inflammatory agents might potentially reduce the vascular risk associated with both conditions.

Abnormalities of insulin secretion and action

There has been considerable controversy as to the relative role of secretory failure versus insulin resistance in the pathogenesis of type 2 diabetes, but both factors are involved. Although insulin can bind normally to its receptor on the surface of cells in type 2 diabetes, unknown abnormalities attenuate insulin signalling within the cell, producing 'insulin resistance'. An excess accumulation of intracellular triglyceride in muscle and liver in type 2 diabetes may contribute to this resistance. Type 2 diabetes develops when a person cannot secrete enough insulin to overcome this burden of insulin resistance. Depleted numbers of beta-cells are thus in a state of high output failure. This leads to increased glucose production from the liver (owing to inadequate suppression by insulin) and inadequate uptake of glucose peripherally.

Patients with type 2 diabetes retain up to 50% of their beta-cell mass at the time of diagnosis. In addition, almost all show islet amyloid deposition at autopsy, derived from a peptide known as amylin or islet amyloid polypeptide (IAPP) which is co-secreted with insulin. It is not known if this is a cause or consequence of beta-cell secretory failure. Abnormalities of insulin secretion manifest early in the course of type 2 diabetes. Normal subjects have a biphasic insulin response to intravenous glucose, but the first-phase insulin response is lost as

Table 19.4 Maturity-onset diabetes of the young (MODY)

	HNF-4a (MODY 1)	Glucokinase (MODY 2)	HNF-1a (MODY 3)	IPF-1 (MODY 4)	HNF-1b (MODY 5)
Chromosomal location	20q	7p	12q	13q	17q
Proportion of all MODY cases	5%	15%	70%	< 1% (MODY)	2%
Onset	Teens to thirties	Present from birth	Teens/twenties	Teens to thirties	Teens/twenties
Progression	Progressive hyperglycaemia	Little deterioration with age	Progressive hyperglycaemia	Progression unclear	Progression unclear
Microvascular complications	Frequent	Rare	Frequent	Few data	Frequent
Other features	None	Reduced birthweight	Sensitivity to sulphonylureas	Pancreatic agenesis in homozygotes	Renal cysts Proteinuria Renal failure

The glucokinase gene is intimately involved in the glucose-sensing mechanism within the pancreatic beta-cell. The hepatic nuclear factor (HNF) genes and the insulin promoter factor-1 (IPF-1) gene control nuclear transcription in the beta-cell where they regulate its development and function. Abnormal nuclear transcription genes may cause pancreatic agenesis or more subtle progressive pancreatic damage hyperglycaemia develops, and insulin secretion in response to oral glucose is delayed and exaggerated. The majority of patients manifest reduced insulin secretion relative to the prevailing glucose concentration, and progressive beta-cell loss occurs in many patients, although not to the extent seen in type 1 diabetes. It is not known whether this is due to 'exhaustion' of surviving beta-cells or to some independent process of damage.

Overview and prevention

Whether an individual develops type 2 diabetes or not is largely due to genetic factors. *When* a person develops diabetes depends on lifestyle and is more relevant. Diabetes diagnosed in a man between the ages of 40–59 can cause a reduction in life expectancy by 5–10 years. In contrast, type 2 diabetes diagnosed after the age of 70 has little appreciable effect on life expectancy in men. Clinical trials have shown that diet, exercise or agents such as metformin have a marked effect in deferring the onset of type 2 diabetes.

FURTHER READING

EURODIAB ACE Study Group (2000) Variation and trends in incidence of childhood diabetes in Europe. *Lancet* **355**: 873–876.

Gale EAM (2002) The rise of childhood type 2 diabetes in the 20th century. *Diabetes* **51**: 3353–3361.

Gerich JE (1998) The genetic basis of type 2 diabetes mellitus: impaired insulin secretion versus impaired insulin sensitivity. *Endocrine Reviews* **19**: 491–503.

Haffner SM (2003) Insulin resistance, inflammation and the prediabetic state. *American Journal of Cardiology* **92** (Suppl); 18J–26J.

Hoppener JWM, Ahren B, Lips CJM (2000) Islet amyloid and type 2 diabetes mellitus. *New England Journal of Medicine* **343**: 411–419.

Taylor R (2004) Causation of type 2 diabetes. *New England Journal of Medicine* **350**: 639–641.

Tooke JE, Pearson ER, Hattersley AT (2000) Unravelling the heterogeneity of non-insulin dependent diabetes. *Journal of the Royal College of Physicians* **34**: 332–335.

CLINICAL PRESENTATION OF DIABETES

Acute and subacute presentations often overlap.

Acute presentation

Young people often present with a 2- to 6-week history and report the classic triad of symptoms:

- polyuria – due to the osmotic diuresis that results when blood glucose levels exceed the renal threshold
- thirst – due to the resulting loss of fluid and electrolytes

- weight loss – due to fluid depletion and the accelerated breakdown of fat and muscle secondary to insulin deficiency.

Ketonuria is often present in young people and may progress to ketoacidosis if these early symptoms are not recognized and treated.

Subacute presentation

The clinical onset may be over several months or years, particularly in older patients. Thirst, polyuria and weight loss are typically present but patients may complain of such symptoms as lack of energy, visual blurring (owing to glucose-induced changes in refraction), or pruritus vulvae or balanitis that is due to *Candida* infection.

Complications as the presenting feature

These include:

- staphylococcal skin infections
- retinopathy noted during a visit to the optician
- a polyneuropathy causing tingling and numbness in the feet
- erectile dysfunction
- arterial disease, resulting in myocardial infarction or peripheral gangrene.

Asymptomatic diabetes

Glycosuria or a raised blood glucose may be detected on routine examination (e.g. for insurance purposes) in individuals who have no symptoms of ill-health. Glycosuria is not diagnostic of diabetes but indicates the need for further investigations. About 1% of the population have renal glycosuria. This is an inherited low renal threshold for glucose, transmitted either as a Mendelian dominant or recessive trait.

Physical examination at diagnosis

Evidence of weight loss and dehydration may be present, and the breath may smell of ketones. Older patients may present with established complications, and the presence of the characteristic retinopathy is diagnostic of diabetes. In occasional patients there will be physical signs of an illness causing secondary diabetes (Table 19.1).

DIAGNOSIS AND INVESTIGATION OF DIABETES

Diabetes is easy to diagnose when overt symptoms are present, and a glucose tolerance test is not necessary for most clinical purposes. The oral glucose tolerance test has, however, allowed more detailed epidemiological characterization based on the existence of separate glucose thresholds for macrovascular and microvascular disease. These correspond with the levels for the diagnosis of impaired glucose tolerance (IGT) and diabetes as specified by the WHO criteria set out in Box 19.1.

Epidemiological studies have shown that for every person with known diabetes, there is another undiagnosed

Box 19.1 WHO diagnostic criteria – 1999

WHO criteria are:

- Fasting plasma glucose > 7.0 mmol/L (126 mg/dL)
- Random plasma glucose > 11.1 mmol/L (200 mg/dL)
- One abnormal laboratory value is diagnostic in symptomatic individuals; two values are needed in asymptomatic people.

The glucose tolerance test is only required for borderline cases and for diagnosis of gestational diabetes.

The glucose tolerance test – WHO criteria

	Normal	Impaired glucose tolerance	Diabetes mellitus
Fasting	Less than 7.0 mmol/L	Less than 7.0 mmol/L	More than 7.0 mmol/L
2 h after glucose	Less than 7.8 mmol/L	Between 7.8 and 11.0 mmol/L	11.1 mmol/L or more

- Adult: 75 g glucose in 300 mL water.
- Child: 1.75 g glucose/kg bodyweight.
- Only a fasting and a 120-min sample are needed.
- Results are for venous plasma – whole blood values are lower.

Note: There is no such thing as mild diabetes. All patients who meet the criteria for diabetes are liable to disabling long-term complications.

in the population. A much larger proportion fall into the intermediate category of impaired glucose tolerance.

Impaired glucose tolerance

This is not a clinical entity but a risk factor for future diabetes and cardiovascular disease. Obesity and lack of regular physical exercise make progression to frank diabetes more likely. The classification is complicated by the poor reproducibility of the oral glucose tolerance test. The group is heterogeneous; some patients are obese, some have liver disease, and others are on medication that impairs glucose tolerance. Individuals with IGT have the same risk of cardiovascular disease as in frank diabetes but do not develop the specific microvascular complications.

Impaired fasting glucose

This diagnostic category (fasting plasma glucose between 6.1 and 6.9 mmol/L) was introduced by the American Diabetes Association, with the practical advantage that it avoids the need for a glucose tolerance test. This is not a clinical entity, but does predict future risk of frank diabetes and cardiovascular disease. This category only overlaps with IGT to a limited extent, and therefore the associated risks of cardiovascular disease and future diabetes are not directly comparable. More recently, the lower cut-off of 5.6 mmol/1 has been recommended by the same association, which will of course greatly increase the number of those affected. This has yet to be considered by the WHO.

Other investigations

No further tests are needed to diagnose diabetes. Other routine investigations include screening the urine for protein, a full blood count, urea and electrolytes, liver biochemistry and random lipids. The latter test is useful to exclude an associated hyperlipidaemia and, if elevated, should be repeated fasting after diabetes has been

brought under control. Diabetes may be secondary to other conditions (see Table 19.1), may be precipitated by underlying illness and be associated with autoimmune disease or hyperlipidaemia. Hypertension is present in 50% of patients with type 2 diabetes and even more in African and Caribbean patients.

TREATMENT OF DIABETES

The role of patient education and community care

The care of diabetes is based on self-management by the patient, who is helped and advised by those with specialized knowledge. The quest for improved glycaemic control has made it clear that whatever the technical expertise applied, the outcome depends on willing cooperation by the patient. This in turn depends on an understanding of the risks of diabetes and the potential benefits of glycaemic control and other measures such as maintaining a lean weight, stopping smoking and taking care of the feet. If accurate information is not supplied, misinformation from friends and other patients will take its place. For this reason the best time to educate the patient is soon after diagnosis. Organized education programmes will involve all health-care workers, including nurse specialists, dietitians and podiatrist.

Diet

The diet for people with diabetes is no different from that considered healthy for everyone. Table 19.5 lists current recommendations on the ideal composition of this diet. To achieve this, food for people with diabetes should be:

- low in sugar (though not sugar free)
- high in starchy carbohydrate (especially foods with a low glycaemic index)

- high in fibre
- low in fat (especially saturated fat).

Table 19.5 Recommended composition of the diet for people with diabetes, with comments on how this may be achieved

Component of diet	Comment
Protein	1 g per kg ideal bodyweight (approx.)
Total fat	< 35% of energy intake. Limit: fat/oil in cooking, fried foods, processed meats (burgers, salami, sausages), high-fat snacks (crisps, cake, nuts, chocolate, biscuits, pastry). Encourage: lower-fat dairy products (skimmed milk, reduced-fat cheese, low-fat yoghurt), lean meat
Saturated and *trans*-unsaturated fat	< 10% of total energy intake
n-6 polyunsaturated fat	< 10% of total energy intake
n-3 polyunsaturated fat	No absolute quantity recommended. Eat fish, especially oily fish, once or twice weekly. Fish oil supplements not recommended
Cis-monounsaturated fat	10–20% of total energy intake (olive oil, avocado)
Total carbohydrate	40–60% of total energy intake. Encourage: artificial (intense) sweeteners instead of sugar (sugar-free fizzy drinks, squashes and cordials). Limit: fruit juices, confectionery, cake, biscuits
Sucrose	Up to 10% of total energy intake, provided this is eaten in the context of a healthy diet (examples: fibre-rich breakfast cereals, baked beans)
Fibre	No absolute quantity recommended. Soluble fibre has beneficial effects on glycaemic and lipid metabolism. Insoluble fibre has no direct effects on glycaemic metabolism, but benefits satiety and gastrointestinal health
Vitamins and antioxidants	Best taken as fruit and vegetables (five portions per day) in a mixed diet. There is no evidence for the use of supplements
Alcohol	Not forbidden. Its energy content should be taken into account, as should its tendency to cause delayed hypoglycaemia in those treated with insulin
Salt	< 6 g per day (lower in hypertension)

The overweight or obese should be encouraged to lose weight by a combination of changes in food intake and physical activity.

Carbohydrates
Slowly absorbed carbohydrates (those with a low glycaemic index) prevent rapid swings in circulating glucose. For example, the glucose peak seen in the blood after eating pasta is much flatter than that seen after eating the same amount of carbohydrate as white potato.

Prescribing a diet
Most people find it extremely difficult to modify their eating habits, and repeated advice and encouragement are needed if this is to be achieved. A diet history is taken, and the diet prescribed should involve the least possible interference with the person's lifestyle. Advice from dietitians is more likely to affect medium-term outcome than is advice from doctors. People taking insulin or oral agents have traditionally been advised to eat roughly the same amount of food (particularly carbohydrate) at roughly the same time each day, so that treatment can be balanced against food intake and exercise. Knowledgeable and motivated patients with type 1 diabetes, who get feedback from regular blood glucose monitoring, can vary the amount of carbohydrate consumed, or meal times, by learning to adjust their exercise pattern and treatment. This is the basis of the DAFNE (Dose Adjustment For Normal Eating) regimen.

Tablet treatment for type 2 diabetes

Diet and lifestyle changes are the key to successful treatment of type 2 diabetes. If satisfactory metabolic control (see 'Measuring control' below) of diabetes is not established by these measures after several weeks, tablets may be needed in addition. Tablets should only be introduced after the patient has witnessed the improvement obtained by changes in diet and lifestyle – this will establish the concept that controlling diabetes is not just a matter of swallowing tablets (but see p. 1123).

Sulphonylureas (Table 19.6)
Their principal action is to promote insulin secretion in response to glucose and other secretagogues.

Sulphonylureas close ATP-sensitive potassium channels on the beta-cell membrane, and the resulting depolarization promotes calcium influx, a signal for insulin release (see Fig. 19.2). Sulphonylureas are ineffective in patients without a functional beta-cell mass and should be avoided in young ketotic patients, who require early insulin therapy, and they are usually avoided in pregnancy (p. 1132).

Sulphonylureas should be used with care in patients with liver disease, and only those primarily excreted by the liver should be given to patients with renal impairment. All encourage weight gain and are therefore not drugs of first choice in obese patients. Tolbutamide is the safest drug in the very elderly because of its short duration of action.

Table 19.6 Properties of the most commonly used sulphonylureas	
Drug	**Features**
Tolbutamide	Lower maximal efficacy than other sulphonylureas
	Short half-life – preferable in elderly
	Largely metabolized by liver – can use in renal impairment
Glibenclamide, glipizide and glimepiride	Long biological half-life
	Active metabolites
	Renal excretion – avoid in renal impairment
Gliclazide	Fairly long biological half-life
	Largely metabolized by liver – can use in renal impairment
	More costly
Chlorpropamide	Very long biological half-life
	Renal excretion – avoid in renal impairment
	1–2% develop inappropriate ADH-like syndrome
	Facial flush with alcohol
	Very inexpensive – major issue for developing countries

Drug interactions and side-effects. All sulphonylureas bind to circulating albumin and may be displaced by other drugs, such as sulphonamides, that compete for their binding sites. They interact with warfarin.

Hypoglycaemia is the most common and dangerous side-effect. Because the action of many sulphonylureas persists for more than 24 hours, recurrent or prolonged hypoglycaemia is likely, and hospital admission is advisable. Skin rashes and other sensitivity reactions do rarely occur.

Meglitinides

Repaglinide and nateglinide are insulin secretagogues known as the meglitinides. Meglitinides are the non-sulphonylurea moiety of glibenclamide. As with the sulphonylureas, they act via closure of the K+-ATP channel in the beta-cells (Fig. 19.2), although their receptor-binding characteristics are different. They are short-acting agents that promote insulin secretion in response to meals, and which might thus reduce between-meal hypoglycaemia. They are more expensive than standard sulphonylureas. Whether they have advantages over established short-acting sulphonylureas such as tolbutamide has not been addressed by clinical trials.

Biguanides

Metformin is currently the best validated primary treatment for type 2 diabetes. Its mechanism of action remains unclear but it reduces gluconeogenesis, thus suppressing hepatic glucose output, and it increases insulin sensitivity. Unlike the sulphonylureas it does not induce hypoglycaemia in normal volunteers. It is particularly helpful in the overweight since it does not promote weight gain.

It may be given in combination with sulphonylureas or thiazolidinediones.

Its side-effects include anorexia, epigastric discomfort and diarrhoea. A colonoscopy should never be ordered without testing the effect of stopping metformin! Lactic acidosis has occurred in patients with severe hepatic or renal disease, and metformin is contraindicated when these are present.

A Cochrane review showed little risk of lactic acidosis with standard clinical use. Most diabetologists withdraw the drug when serum creatinine exceeds 150 μmol/L.

Thiazolidinediones

The thiazolidinediones (more conveniently known as the 'glitazones') reduce insulin resistance by interaction with peroxisome proliferator-activated receptor-gamma (PPAR-gamma), a nuclear receptor which regulates genes involved in lipid metabolism and insulin action. The paradox that glucose metabolism should respond to a drug that binds to nuclear receptors mainly found in fat cells is still not fully understood. One suggestion is that they act indirectly via the glucose–fatty acid cycle, lowering free fatty acid levels and thus promoting glucose consumption by muscle.

The glitazones lower circulating insulin relative to plasma glucose, but do not return glucose levels to normal. They can be used alone or in combination with other agents. The glitazones reduce hepatic glucose production, an effect that is synergistic with that of metformin, and also enhance peripheral glucose uptake. They thus potentiate the effect of endogenous insulin.

Troglitazone, the first agent in this class, was withdrawn because of problems with hepatic toxicity. Rosiglitazone and pioglitazone are currently licensed in the UK and USA. Liver biochemistry should be monitored. They are useful in patients who cannot tolerate metformin or sulphonylureas (NICE guidelines). They cause weight gain and a degree of salt and water retention. Anaemia is an occasional side-effect. The place of this group of agents is not yet clear, whilst the outcome of comparative controlled clinical trials is awaited.

Intestinal enzyme inhibitors

Alpha-glucosidase inhibitors. These offer an alternative approach to the treatment of overweight patients with type 2 diabetes. They inhibit the enzymes involved in carbohydrate digestion in the intestine. Acarbose is a sham sugar that competitively inhibits alpha-glucosidase enzymes situated in the brush border of the intestine. As a result, dietary carbohydrate is poorly absorbed, and the postprandial rise in blood glucose is reduced. Undigested starch may then enter the large intestine where it will be broken down by fermentation. Abdominal discomfort, flatulence and diarrhoea can result, and dosage needs careful adjustment to avoid these side effects. Very little enters the circulation, since it is mainly inactivated in the gut, but liver dysfunction may rarely occur at high doses

Lipase inhibitors. Orlistat causes fat malabsorption by rendering intestinal lipase enzymes less effective, and therefore reducing the absorption of fat from the diet. It can contribute to weight loss in patients who are already under careful dietary supervision possibly because it has the effect of inducing unpleasant steatorrhoea, and patients therefore reduce their fat intake and lose weight. Its place in diabetes management remains unclear.

Insulin treatment

Insulin is found in every creature with a backbone, and the key parts of the molecule show few species differences. Small differences in the amino acid sequence may alter the antigenicity of the molecule. The glucose and insulin profiles in normal subjects are shown in Figure 19.7.

Short-acting insulins

Animal insulins are still used widely in developing countries but have now largely been replaced in most of the West by biosynthetic human insulin. This is produced by adding a DNA sequence coding for insulin or proinsulin into cultured yeast or bacterial cells. The proinsulin is subsequently enzymatically cleaved to insulin.

Short-acting insulins are the standard insulins for use in multiple dose regimens and for continuous intravenous infusion in labour and during medical emergencies. Soluble human or animal insulin formulations have a number of limitations. The short-acting preparations enter the circulation too slowly, reaching a peak 60–90 minutes after injection, and their effect persists too long after meals, predisposing to hypoglycaemia. This delay in absorption is due mainly to the fact that soluble insulin forms hexamers, in which six insulin molecules form

Fig. 19.7 Glucose and insulin profiles in normal subjects.

around a zinc core. These hexamers are too big to be easily absorbed from subcutaneous tissues and dissociate relatively slowly following injection.

Short-acting insulin analogues have the structure of the insulin molecule modified in such a way as to change its pharmacokinetics without altering the biological effect. Insulin analogues such as insulin lispro and insulin aspart have a modification of small numbers of the amino acids on the B chain producing insulins which dissociate much more rapidly from hexamers, and thus enter the circulation more rapidly, and equally disappear from the circulation more rapidly, than soluble insulin (Fig. 19.8).

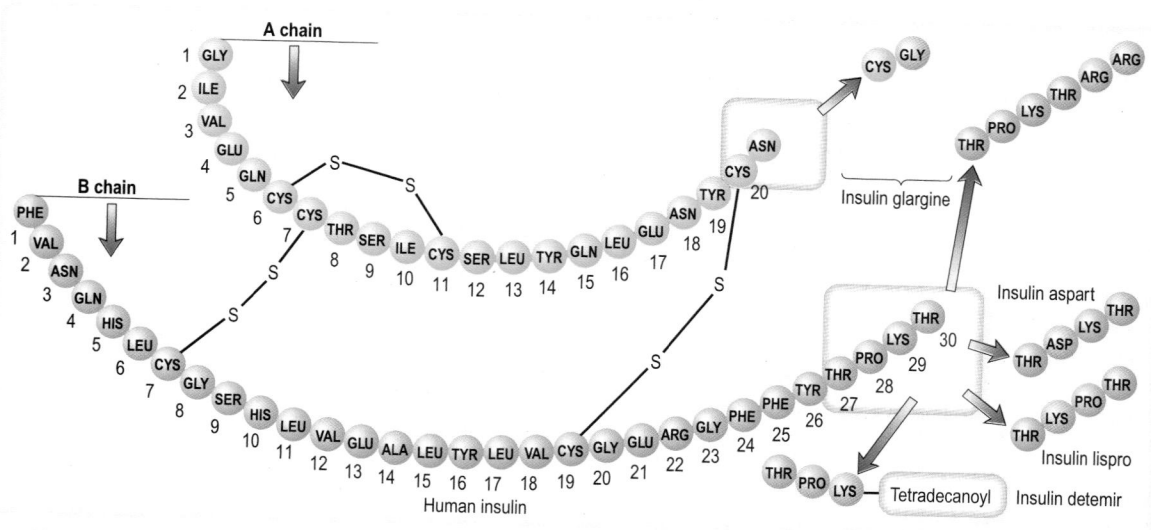

Fig. 19.8 Amino acid structure of human insulin. Lispro is a genetically engineered rapidly acting insulin analogue created by reversing the order of the amino acids proline and lysine in positions 28 and 29 of the B chain. Insulin aspart is a similar analogue created by replacing proline at position 28 of the B chain with an aspartic acid residue. Insulin glargine is a genetically engineered long-acting insulin created by replacing asparagine in position 21 of the A chain with a glycine residue and adding two arginines to the end of the B chain. Insulin detemir discards threonine in position 30 of the B chain and adds a fatty acyl chain to lysine in position B29.

Longer-acting insulins

Protamine or zinc can be added to human and animal insulins to aid the formation of insulin crystals. Crystals dissolve slowly; insulin prepared in this way is cloudy in appearance.

- *Protamine* or NPH (neutral protamine Hagedorn) insulin, also known as isophane insulin, can be premixed with soluble insulin to form stable mixtures. A range of these mixtures is available, but the combination of 30% soluble with 70% NPH is the most widely used.
- *Zinc* insulins are prepared by precipitation of insulin crystals in the presence of excess zinc. The duration of action of the insulin is proportional to the size of the crystals. Since an excess of zinc is present in the vial, these insulins cannot be premixed with soluble insulin, but zinc insulins can be mixed in the syringe with soluble insulin immediately prior to injection.
- *Long-acting analogues* have their structure modified (Fig. 19.8). Insulin glargine has reduced solubility at physiological pH, thus prolonging its duration of action. It is injected as a slightly acidic (pH 4) solution and then precipitates in the tissues. The precipitates then dissolve slowly from the injection site, giving the preparation a longer duration of action and a less peaked concentration profile in the blood than conventional long-acting insulins. Insulin detemir binds to serum albumin, and its slow dissociation from the bound state prolongs its duration of action.

Inhaled insulin will shortly become available, and clinical trials suggest that this may become a feasible means of maintenance therapy. Only short-acting insulin can be administered by this route, so longer-acting insulins still need to be given by injection. The principle is to disperse the insulin into particles sufficiently fine to reach the alveoli. The main limitation is that only about 10% of the inhaled dose reaches the circulation, and this has cost implications. Variability of absorption remains a concern, and it seems unlikely that this form of delivery will ever match the precision of injected insulin.

Practical management of diabetes

All patients with diabetes require diet therapy. Good glycaemic control is unlikely to be achieved with insulin or oral therapy when diet is neglected, especially when the patient is also overweight.

Regular exercise helps to control weight and reduces cardiovascular risk. Walking instead of using transport, gardening regularly, renting an allotment or getting a dog are all to be encouraged. Blood pressure control is vital using an ACE inhibitor or AIIR antagonist (p. 863); virtually all patients require a statin (p. 1123).

Type 2 diabetes

The great majority of patients presenting over the age of 40 will have type 2 diabetes but do not miss the occasional type 1 patient presenting late. An approach to their management is illustrated in Figure 19.9. Diet alone

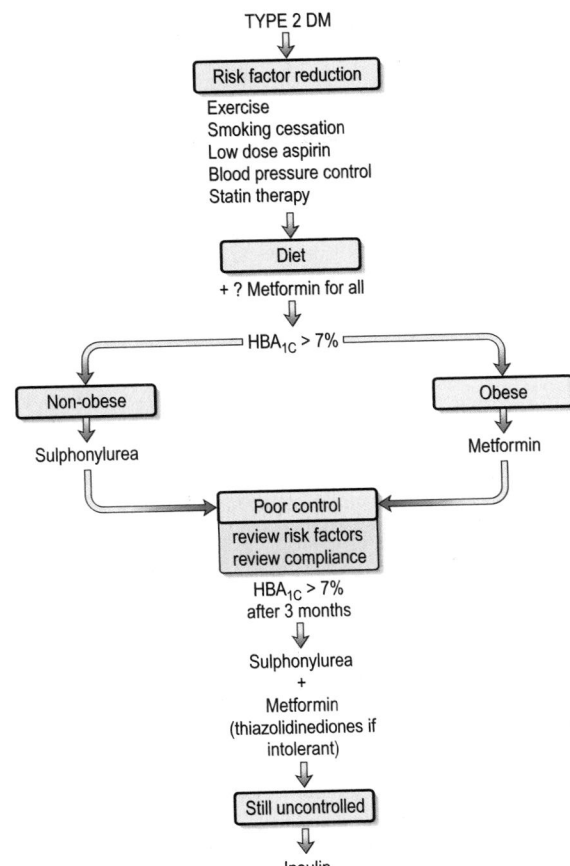

Fig. 19.9 A treatment pathway for type 2 DM.

should be tried in the first instance, and dietary knowledge and compliance should always be reassessed with care before proceeding to the next step. This is of particular importance in the obese patient who fails to lose weight. Metformin is being used in all patients by some diabetologists as it reduces cardiovascular risk. Goals of treatment are described on page 1117.

In type 2 diabetes there is a progressive secretory failure of the beta-cells. The diabetes slowly worsens over years and those patients who are initially adequately controlled with diet, or diet and a tablet, will need gradual increases of their treatment over time, even when adhering well to their diet. An annual review is a convenient way of ensuring that a regular review, and increment, of treatment occurs. For most patients, tablets will eventually fail to achieve adequate metabolic control and a change to insulin treatment will become necessary. The most widespread error in management at this stage is procrastination; the patient whose control is inadequate on oral therapy should start insulin without undue delay. (Consider insulin in all type 2 patients if $HbA_{1c} > 9\%$ and in most cases when $HbA_{1c} > 7.5\%$.)

There is little consensus regarding insulin therapy in type 2 diabetes, but an intermediate insulin given at night with metformin during the day is initially as effective as multidose insulin regimens in controlling glucose levels, and is less likely to promote weight gain. Metformin is a useful adjunct to insulin in those able to tolerate it. A second morning dose of insulin may become necessary to control postprandial hyperglycaemia. Twice-daily injections of premixed soluble and isophane insulins (e.g. Mixtard or Humulin M insulins) are widely used and reasonably effective (Fig. 19.10a). More aggressive treatment, such as with multiple injections or pumps, is increasingly used in younger patients with type 2 diabetes.

Type 1 diabetes

Insulin is always indicated in a patient who has been in ketoacidosis, and is usually indicated in all patients who present under the age of 40 years.

Principles of insulin treatment

Injections

The needles used to inject insulin are very fine and sharp. Even though most injections are virtually painless,

Fig. 19.10 Insulin regimens. Profiles of soluble insulins are shown as dashed lines, intermediate- or long-acting insulin as solid lines (purple) and rapid-acting insulin as dotted lines (blue). The arrows indicate when the injections are given. B, breakfast; L, lunch; S, supper; Sn, snack (bedtime).

patients are understandably apprehensive and treatment begins with a lesson in injection technique. Insulin is usually administered by a pen injection device but can be drawn up from a vial into special plastic insulin syringes marked in units (100 U in 1 mL). Injections are given into the fat below the skin on the abdomen, thighs or upper arm, and the needle is usually inserted to its full length. Slim adults and children usually use a 31 gauge 6 mm needle and fatter adults a 30 gauge 8 mm needle. Both reusable and disposable pen devices are available.

The injection site used should be changed regularly to prevent areas of lipohypertrophy. The rate of insulin absorption depends on local subcutaneous blood flow, and is accelerated by exercise, local massage or a warm environment. Absorption is more rapid from the abdomen than from the arm, and is slowest from the thigh. All these factors can influence the shape of the insulin profile.

Insulin administration

In normal subjects a sharp increase in insulin occurs after meals; this is superimposed on a constant background of secretion (Fig. 19.7). Insulin therapy attempts to reproduce this pattern, but ideal control is usually impossible to achieve for four reasons:

- In normal subjects, insulin is secreted directly into the portal circulation and reaches the liver in high concentration; about 50% of the insulin produced by the pancreas is cleared by the liver. In contrast, insulin injected subcutaneously passes into the systemic circulation before passage to the liver. Insulin-treated patients therefore have lower portal levels of insulin and higher systemic levels relative to the physiological situation.
- Subcutaneous soluble insulin takes 60–90 minutes to achieve peak plasma levels, so the onset and offset of action are too slow.
- The absorption of subcutaneous insulin into the circulation is variable.
- Basal insulin levels are constant in normal people, but injected insulin invariably peaks and declines in people with diabetes, with resulting swings in metabolic control.

A multiple injection regimen with short-acting insulin and a longer-acting insulin at night is appropriate for most younger patients (Fig. 19.10b). The advantages of multiple injection regimens are that the insulin and the food go in at roughly the same time so that meal times and sizes can vary, without greatly disturbing metabolic control. The flexibility of multiple injection regimens is of great value to patients with busy jobs, shift workers and those who travel regularly. Some recovery of endogenous insulin secretion may occur over the first few months (the 'honeymoon period') in type 1 patients and the insulin dose may need to be reduced or even stopped for a period. Requirements rise thereafter. Strict glucose control from diagnosis in type 1 diabetes prolongs beta-cell function, resulting in better glucose levels and less hypoglycaemia. Some type 1 diabetes patients will opt for twice-daily mixed insulin injections (Fig. 19.10a) and put up with the

Table 19.7 Guide to adjusting insulin dosage according to blood glucose test results		
	Blood glucose persistently too high	Blood glucose persistently too low
Before breakfast	Increase evening long-acting insulin	Reduce evening long-acting insulin
Before lunch	Increase morning short-acting insulin	Reduce morning short-acting insulin or increase mid-morning snack
Before evening meal	Increase morning long-acting insulin or lunch short-acting insulin	Reduce morning long-acting insulin or lunch short-acting insulin or increase mid-afternoon snack
Before bed	Increase evening short-acting insulin	Reduce evening short-acting insulin

lifestyle restrictions that this imposes (with twice-daily regimens, the size and timing of meals are fixed more rigidly). Target blood glucose values should normally be 4–7 mmol/L before meals, 4–10 mmol/L after meals.

All patients need careful training for a life with insulin. This is best achieved outside hospital, provided that adequate facilities exist for outpatient diabetes education. A scheme for adjusting insulin regimens is given in Table 19.7.

When to use insulin analogues

Hypoglycaemia between meals and particularly at night is the limiting factor for many patients on multiple injection regimens. The more expensive rapid-acting insulin analogues (Fig. 19.10c) are a useful substitute for soluble insulin in some patients. Curiously, they offer particular benefit in reducing the frequency of nocturnal hypoglycaemia owing to reduced carry-over effect from the day-time. They are often used on grounds of convenience, since patients can inject shortly before meals. This is illogical since standard insulins injected at the same time give equivalent overall control. High or erratic morning blood sugar readings can prove a problem for about a quarter of all patients on conventional multiple injection regimens, because of waning of the bedtime intermediate-acting insulin and variable absorption. The long-acting insulin analogues insulin glargine and insulin detemir help to overcome these problems and reduce the risk of nocturnal hypoglycaemia

Infusion devices

CSII (continuous subcutaneous insulin infusion) is delivered by a small pump strapped around the waist that infuses a constant trickle of insulin via a needle in the subcutaneous tissues. Meal-time doses are delivered when the patient touches a button on the side of the pump.

This approach is particularly useful in the overnight period, since the basal overnight infusion rate can be programmed to fit each patient's needs. Disadvantages include the nuisance of being attached to a gadget, skin infections, and the risk of ketoacidosis if the flow of insulin is broken (since these patients have no protective reservoir of depot insulin) and cost. Infusion pumps should only be used by specialized centres able to offer a round-the-clock service to their patients. This form of treatment has revolutionized the lives of some patients.

Complications of insulin therapy

At the injection site

Shallow injections result in intradermal insulin delivery and painful, reddened lesions or even scarring. Injection site abscesses occur but are extremely rare.

Local allergic responses sometimes occur early in therapy but usually resolve spontaneously. Generalized allergic responses are exceptionally rare. Fatty lumps, known as lipohypertrophy, may occur as the result of overuse of a single injection site with any type of insulin.

Insulin resistance

The most common cause of mild insulin resistance is obesity. Occasional unstable patients require massive insulin doses, often with a fluctuating requirement. There are often associated behavioural problems. Insulin resistance associated with antibodies directed against the insulin receptor has been reported in patients with acanthosis nigricans (see Table 19.3).

Weight gain

Many patients show weight gain on insulin treatment, especially if the insulin dose is increased inappropriately – insulin makes you feel hungry! Sticking to a careful dietary regimen is vital when on insulin. Patients who are in poor control when insulin is started tend to gain most weight.

Whole pancreas and pancreatic islet transplantation

Whole pancreas transplantation has been performed for some 20 years, usually in diabetic patients who require immunosuppression for a kidney transplant. In experienced hands lasting graft function can be achieved, but the procedure adds to the risks of renal transplantation, and long-term prognosis has not improved.

Islet transplantation is performed by harvesting pancreatic islets from cadavers (two or three pancreata are usually needed); these are then injected into the portal vein and seed themselves into the liver. This form of treatment was attempted for many years with poor results, but recent success has been achieved by an improved protocol developed in Edmonton, Canada. It remains an experimental therapy but experience is slowly accumulating. The main disadvantage is the need for powerful immunosuppressive therapy, with associated costs and complications.

Hypoglycaemia during insulin treatment

This is the most common complication of insulin therapy, and limits what can be achieved with insulin treatment. It is a major cause of anxiety for patients and relatives. Symptoms develop when the blood glucose level falls below 3 mmol/L and typically develop over a few minutes, with most patients experiencing 'adrenergic' features of sweating, tremor and a pounding heartbeat. Physical signs include pallor and a cold sweat. Many patients with long-standing diabetes report loss of these warning symptoms and are at a greater risk of progressing to more severe hypoglycaemia. Such patients appear pale, drowsy or detached, signs that their relatives quickly learn to recognize. Behaviour is clumsy or inappropriate, and some become irritable or even aggressive. Others slip rapidly into hypoglycaemic coma. Occasionally, patients develop convulsions during hypoglycaemic coma, especially at night. This must not be confused with idiopathic epilepsy, particularly as patients with frequent hypoglycaemia often have abnormalities on the electroencephalogram. Another presentation is with a hemiparesis that resolves within a few minutes when glucose is administered.

Hypoglycaemia is a common problem. Virtually all patients experience intermittent symptoms and one in three will go into a coma at some stage in their lives. A small minority suffer attacks that are so frequent and severe as to be virtually disabling. Hypoglycaemia results from an imbalance between injected insulin and a patient's normal diet, activity and basal insulin requirement. The times of greatest risk are before meals and during the night. Irregular eating habits, unusual exertion and alcohol excess may precipitate episodes; other cases appear to be due simply to variation in insulin absorption.

Hypoglycaemic unawareness. People with diabetes have an impaired ability to counter-regulate glucose levels after hypoglycaemia. The glucagon response is invariably deficient, even though the alpha-cells are preserved and respond normally to other stimuli. The epinephrine (adrenaline) response may also fail in patients with a long duration of diabetes, and this is associated with loss of warning symptoms. Recurrent hypoglycaemia may itself induce a state of hypoglycaemia unawareness, and the ability to recognize the condition may sometimes be restored by relaxing control for a few weeks.

Nocturnal hypoglycaemia. Basal insulin requirements fall during the night but increase again from about 4 a.m. onwards, at a time when levels of injected insulin are falling. As a result many patients wake with high blood glucose levels, but find that injecting more insulin at night increases the risk of hypoglycaemia in the early hours of the morning. The problem may be helped by the following:

- checking that a bedtime snack is taken regularly
- for patients taking twice-daily mixed insulin to separate their evening dose and take the intermediate insulin at bedtime rather than before supper

- reducing the dose of soluble insulin before supper, since the effects of this persist well into the night
- changing patients on a multiple injection regimen with soluble insulin to a rapid-acting insulin analogue
- changing to a long-lasting insulin analogue at night.

Urgent treatment of hypoglycaemia

Patients and their families quickly learn to recognize and treat the symptoms of hypoglycaemia.

Mild hypoglycaemia

Any form of rapidly absorbed carbohydrate will relieve the early symptoms, and sufferers should always carry glucose or sweets. Drowsy individuals will be able to take carbohydrate in liquid form (e.g. Lucozade). All patients and their close relatives need careful training about the risks of hypoglycaemia. They should be warned not to take more carbohydrate than necessary, since this causes a rebound to hyperglycaemia. The dangers of alcohol excess and hypoglycaemia while driving need to be emphasized.

Severe hypoglycaemia

The diagnosis of severe hypoglycaemia resulting in confusion or coma is simple and can usually be made on clinical grounds, backed by a bedside blood test. If real doubt exists, blood should be taken for glucose estimation before treatment is given. Patients should carry a card or wear a bracelet or necklace identifying themselves as diabetic, and these should be looked for in unconscious patients.

Unconscious patients should be given either intramuscular glucagon (1 mg) or intravenous glucose (25–50 mL of 50% dextrose solution) followed by a flush of normal saline to preserve the vein (since 50% dextrose scleroses veins). Glucagon acts by mobilizing hepatic glycogen, and works almost as rapidly as glucose. It is simple to administer and can be given at home by relatives. It does not work after a prolonged fast. Oral glucose is given to replenish glycogen reserves once the patient revives.

Measuring the metabolic control of diabetes

Urine tests

Some patients will not perform capillary blood glucose monitoring at home. Urine tests give such patients some feedback on whether their diet and treatment are achieving reasonable metabolic control. They are simple to perform using dipsticks, and it can usually be assumed that a patient with consistently negative tests and no symptoms of hypoglycaemia is fairly well controlled. Even so, the correlation between urine tests and simultaneous blood glucose is poor for three reasons:

- Changes in urine glucose lag behind changes in blood glucose.
- The mean renal threshold is around 10 mmol/L but the range is wide (7–13 mmol/L). The threshold also rises with age.

- Urine tests can give no guidance concerning blood glucose levels below the renal threshold.

Home blood glucose testing

The home provides the best place for assessment of day-to-day control. The fasting blood glucose concentration is a useful guide to therapy in tablet-treated type 2 diabetes, but random blood glucose testing (e.g. in the clinic) is of limited value. Patients may easily be taught to provide their own profiles by testing finger-prick blood samples with reagent strips and reading these with the aid of a meter. Most patients are willing and able to provide reasonably accurate results provided they have been properly taught. Blood is taken from the side of a finger tip (not from the tip, which is densely innervated) using a special lancet usually fitted to a spring-loaded device. There is a huge variety of finger-pricking devices and of blood glucose test meters. Patients will normally be able to talk through the use of various devices with a diabetes nurse specialist to select the most appropriate devices for their own purposes. Patients are asked to take regular profiles (e.g. four daily samples on two days each week) and to note these in a diary or record book. Home blood glucose monitoring is an essential aid to good glycaemic control. Patients on insulin are encouraged to adjust their insulin dose as appropriate (Table 19.7) and should ideally be able to obtain advice over the telephone when needed.

Glycosylated haemoglobin (HbA₁ or HbA₁c) and fructosamine

Glycosylation of haemoglobin occurs as a two-step reaction, resulting in the formation of a covalent bond between the glucose molecule and the terminal valine of the β chain of the haemoglobin molecule. The rate at which this reaction occurs is related to the prevailing glucose concentration. Glycosylated haemoglobin is expressed as a percentage of the normal haemoglobin (standardized range 4–6.5%). This test provides an index of the average blood glucose concentration over the life of the haemoglobin molecule (approximately 6 weeks). The figure will be misleading if the life-span of the red cell is reduced or if an abnormal haemoglobin or thalassaemia is present. There is considerable inter-individual variations in HbA₁c levels, even in normal people. Although the glycosylated haemoglobin test provides a rapid assessment of the level of glycaemic control in a given patient, blood glucose testing is needed before the clinician can know what to do about it.

Glycosylated plasma proteins ('fructosamine') may also be measured as an index of control. Glycosylated albumin is the major component, and fructosamine measurement relates to glycaemic control over the preceding 2–3 weeks. It is useful in patients with anaemia or haemoglobinopathy and in pregnancy (when haemoglobin turnover is changeable) and other situations where changes of treatment need a swift means of assessing progress.

Targets

Data from the UK Prospective Diabetic Study (UKPDS) and the Diabetes Control and Complications Trial (DCCT) suggest that under ideal circumstances patients

Table 19.8 Target goals of risk factors for diabetic patients

Parameter	Ideal	Reasonable but not ideal
HbA₁c	< 7%	< 8.5%
Blood pressure (mmHg)	< 130/80	< 140/90
Total cholesterol (mmol/L)	< 4.5	< 6
LDL	< 2.6	
HDL*	> 1.1	
Triglycerides	< 1.7	< 2.0

Standards from American Diabetes Association (2003)
* In women > 1.3 mmol/L.

with both type 1 diabetes and type 2 diabetes would be aiming to run their glycosylated haemoglobin readings in the region of 7.5%, or corrected fructosamine readings of 350 mg/100 g protein, in order to reduce the risk of long-term microvascular complications (Table 19.8). Hypoglycaemia, patterns of eating and lifestyle, weight problems and problems accepting and coping with diabetes limit what can be achieved (see p. 1119). Some will, but most will not, be able to reach these target values, particularly as their duration of diabetes increases. Realistic goals should be set for each patient, taking into account what is likely to be achievable.

Does good metabolic control of diabetes matter?

Blood glucose is just one measure of the diverse metabolic consequence of diabetes which not only affects carbohydrate metabolism but also the metabolism of lipids and proteins. The DCCT in the USA compared standard and intensive insulin therapy in a large prospective controlled trial of young patients with type 1 diabetes. Despite intensive therapy, mean blood glucose levels were still 40% above the non-diabetic range, but even at this level of control, the risk of progression to retinopathy was reduced by 60%, nephropathy by 30% and neuropathy by 20% over the 7 years of the study. Near-normoglycaemia should, therefore, be the goal for all young patients with type 1 diabetes. The unwanted effects of this policy include weight gain and a two- to threefold increase in the risk of severe hypoglycaemia. Control should be less strict in those with a history of recurrent severe hypoglycaemia.

The UKPDS compared standard and intensive treatment in a large prospective controlled trial of type 2 diabetes patients. There was a 25% overall reduction in microvascular disease end-points, a 33% reduction in albuminuria and a 30% reduction in the need for laser treatment for retinopathy in the more intensively treated patients. There appeared to be little difference in outcome between the tools used to achieve good metabolic control (metformin, sulphonylurea or insulin). A proportion of the total patients in the UKPDS were further randomized into standard and intensive blood pressure control groups. Cardiovascular risk was very considerably reduced in the intensive treatment arm.

Can established complications be halted or reversed by intensive insulin therapy? Insulin infusion devices have made near-normal blood glucose control possible for closely supervised groups of patients. Studies in patients with established retinopathy have shown that patients with early retinopathy benefit from intensive therapy, but that patients with more advanced retinal changes generally do not. These observations suggest that microvascular lesions are self-perpetuating once a threshold level of damage has been reached.

Regular checks for patients with diabetes

Box 19.2 is modified from the guidelines set out in *The European Patients' Charter* published by the St Vincent Declaration Steering Committee of the WHO. The charter sets out goals for both the healthcare team and the patient.

> **Box 19.2 Regular checks for patients with diabetes**
>
> **Checked each visit**
> - Review of self-monitoring results and current treatment.
> - Talk about targets and change where necessary.
> - Talk about any general or specific problems.
> - Continued education.
>
> **Checked at least once a year**
> - Biochemical assessment of metabolic control (e.g. glycosylated Hb test).
> - Measure bodyweight.
> - Measure blood pressure.
> - Measure plasma lipids (except in extreme old age).
> - Measure visual acuity.
> - Examine state of retina (ophthalmoscope or retinal photo).
> - Test urine for proteinuria/microalbuminuria.
> - Test blood for renal function (creatinine).
> - Check condition of feet, pulses and neurology.
> - Review cardiovascular risk factors.
> - Review self-monitoring and injection techniques.
> - Review eating habits.

FURTHER READING

Cryer PE (2004) Diverse causes of hypoglycaemia – associated autonomic failure diabetes. *New England Journal of Medicine* 350: 2272–2279.

DCCT/Epidemiology of Diabetes Interventions and Complications Research Group (2000) Retinopathy and nephropathy in patients with type 1 diabetes four years after a trial of intensive insulin therapy. *New England Journal of Medicine* 342: 381–389.

Eckel RH et al. (2005) The metabolic syndrome. *Lancet* 365: 1415–1428.

Hirsch IB (2005) Insulin analogues. *New England Journal of Medicine* 352: 174–183.

Johnston D (2004) NICE guidance on type 1 diabetes in adults. *Clinical Medicine* 4(6): 491–493.

Nutrition Subcommittee (2003) The implementation of nutritional advice for people with diabetes. *Diabetic Medicine* 20: 786–807.

Robertson RP (2004) Islet transplantation as treatment for diabetes. *New England Journal of Medicine* 350: 694–705.

Solomon CG (2003) Reducing cardiovascular risk in type 2 diabetes. *New England Journal of Medicine* 348: 457–459.

Stumuoll M et al. (2005) Type 2 diabetes; pathogenesis and therapy. *Lancet* 365: 1333–1346.

PSYCHOSOCIAL IMPLICATIONS OF DIABETES

Patients starting tablet or insulin treatment should be encouraged to live as normal a life as possible, but this is not easy. Tact, empathy, encouragement and practical support are needed from all members of the clinical team. Diabetes, like any chronic disease, has psychological sequelae. Most patients will experience periods of not coping, of helplessness, of denial and of acceptance often fluctuating over time. Other problems include:

- *It is impossible to take a holiday from diabetes* – yet the human psyche is poorly developed to cope with unremitting adversity.
- *Concessions or sympathy are often denied* to the person with diabetes, since its presence is invisible.
- *The treatment is complex and demanding,* and the person with diabetes is expected to make trade-offs between short-term and long-term well-being.
- *Embarrassing loss of control over personal behaviour* or consciousness can occur in insulin-treated patients after only a slight miscalculation.
- *Risk-taking behaviour* is indulged in by all human beings when emotion is in conflict with logical thought, but its effects can be much greater for the person with diabetes (particularly the risks of unplanned pregnancy, alcohol and tobacco).
- *Poor self-image* is a very common problem.
- *Eating disorders* are more common in people with diabetes – 30–40% of young women with diabetes will exhibit a clinically significant eating disorder.
- *Insulin omission* is common since non-adherence to treatment regimens is universal in all illness. Insulin omission is also very common in young women where the pressure to lose weight overcomes concerns about long-term complications.

Adolescence

Adolescence magnifies the internal conflicts that all human beings cope, or intermittently fail to cope, with during life. A period of poor metabolic control, or dropping out of medical care for a time and re-emerging with complications, is very common. Diabetic Holiday Camps (for example run by Diabetes UK) help prevent a feeling of isolation and not knowing anyone else with the same problem. Separate adolescent clinics allow:

- *Treatment without marginalization* in a larger group of older people
- *Meeting peers with similar problems* in the waiting room
- *Gradual separation from parents* and assumption of personal responsibility for the illness
- *Age-appropriate literature* to be available.

Practical aspects

On a practical level patients need to inform the driving and vehicle licensing authority and their insurance companies after diagnosis. They would also be wise to inform their family, friends and employers in case unexpected hypoglycaemia occurs. Insulin treatment can be undertaken by people in most walks of life; a few jobs are unsuitable. These include driving Heavy Goods or Public Service vehicles, working at heights, piloting aircraft or working close to dangerous machinery in motion. Certain professions such as the police and the armed forces are barred to all diabetic patients. There are few other limitations, although a considerable amount of ill-informed prejudice exists. Doctors can sometimes help support patients in the face of misinformed work practices.

DIABETIC METABOLIC EMERGENCIES

The main terms used are defined in Table 19.9.

Table 19.9 Terms used in uncontrolled diabetes

Ketonuria	Detectable ketone levels in the urine; it should be appreciated that ketonuria occurs in fasted non-diabetics and may be found in relatively well-controlled patients with insulin-dependent diabetes mellitus
Ketosis	Elevated plasma ketone levels in the absence of acidosis
Diabetic ketoacidosis	A metabolic emergency in which hyperglycaemia is associated with a metabolic acidosis due to greatly raised (> 5 mmol/L) ketone levels
Non-ketotic hyperosmolar state	A metabolic emergency in which uncontrolled hyperglycaemia induces a hyperosmolar state in the absence of significant ketosis
Lactic acidosis	A metabolic emergency in which elevated lactic acid levels induce a metabolic acidosis In diabetic patients it is rare and associated with biguanide therapy

Diabetic ketoacidosis

Diabetic ketoacidosis is the hallmark of type 1 diabetes. It is usually seen in the following circumstances:

- previously undiagnosed diabetes
- interruption of insulin therapy
- the stress of intercurrent illness.

The majority of cases reaching hospital could have been prevented by earlier diagnosis, better communication between patient and doctor, and better patient education. The most common error of management is for patients to reduce or omit insulin because they feel unable to eat owing to nausea or vomiting. This is a factor in at least 25% of all hospital admissions. Insulin should never be stopped.

Pathogenesis

Ketoacidosis is a state of uncontrolled catabolism associated with insulin deficiency. Insulin deficiency is a necessary precondition since only a modest elevation in insulin levels is sufficient to inhibit hepatic ketogenesis, and stable patients do not readily develop ketoacidosis when insulin is withdrawn. Other factors include counter-regulatory hormone excess and fluid depletion. The combination of insulin deficiency with excess of its hormonal antagonists leads to the parallel processes shown in Figure 19.11. In the absence of insulin, hepatic glucose production accelerates, and peripheral uptake by

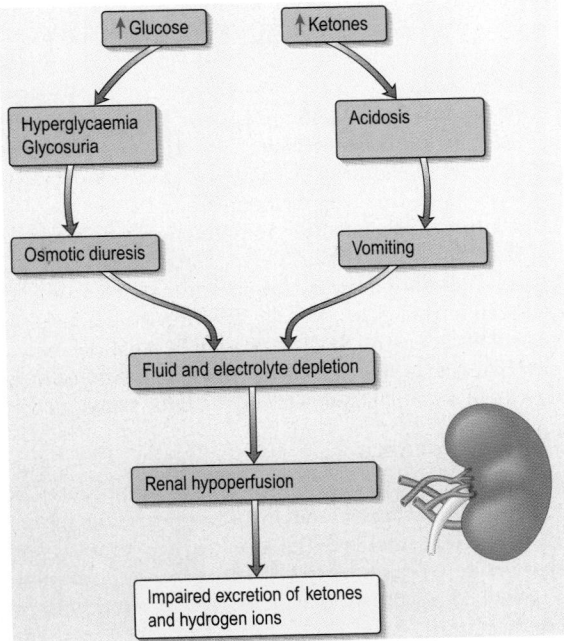

Fig. 19.11 Dehydration occurs during ketoacidosis as a consequence of two parallel processes. Hyperglycaemia results in osmotic diuresis, and hyperketonaemia results in acidosis and vomiting. Renal hypoperfusion then occurs and a vicious circle is established as the kidney becomes less able to compensate for the acidosis.

Fig. 19.12 Ketogenesis. During insulin deficiency, lipolysis accelerates and free fatty acids taken up by liver cells form the substrate for ketone formation (acetoacetate, acetone and β-hydroxybutyrate) within the mitochondrion. These ketones pass into the blood, producing acidosis.

tissues such as muscle is reduced. Rising glucose levels lead to an osmotic diuresis, loss of fluid and electrolytes, and dehydration. Plasma osmolality rises and renal perfusion falls. In parallel, rapid lipolysis occurs, leading to elevated circulating free fatty-acid levels. The free fatty acids are broken down to fatty acyl-CoA within the liver cells, and this in turn is converted to ketone bodies within the mitochondria (Fig. 19.12). Accumulation of ketone bodies produces a metabolic acidosis. Vomiting leads to further loss of fluid and electrolytes. The excess ketones are excreted in the urine but also appear in the breath, producing a distinctive smell similar to that of acetone. Respiratory compensation for the acidosis leads to hyperventilation, graphically described as 'air hunger'. Progressive dehydration impairs renal excretion of hydrogen ions and ketones, aggravating the acidosis. As the pH falls below 7.0 ([H⁺] > 100 nmol/L), pH-dependent enzyme systems in many cells function less effectively. Untreated, severe ketoacidosis is invariably fatal.

Clinical features

The features of ketoacidosis are those of uncontrolled diabetes with acidosis, and include prostration, hyperventilation (Kussmaul respiration), nausea, vomiting and, occasionally, abdominal pain. The latter is sometimes so severe as to cause confusion with a surgical acute abdomen.

Some patients are mentally alert at presentation, but confusion and stupor are common. Up to 5% present in coma. Evidence of marked dehydration is present and the eyeball is lax to pressure in severe cases. Hyperventilation is present but becomes less marked in very severe acidosis owing to respiratory depression. The smell of ketones on

the breath allows an instant diagnosis to be made by those able to detect the odour. The skin is dry and the body temperature is often subnormal, even in the presence of infection; in such cases, pyrexia may develop later.

Diagnosis

This is confirmed by demonstrating hyperglycaemia with ketonaemia or heavy ketonuria, and acidosis. No time should be lost, and treatment is started as soon as the first blood sample has been taken. Hyperglycaemia is demonstrated by dipstick, while a blood sample is sent to the laboratory for confirmation. Ketonaemia is confirmed by centrifuging a blood sample and testing the plasma with a dipstick that measures ketones. Hand-held sensors measuring β-hydroxybutyrate in 30 sec are becoming available. An arterial blood sample is taken for blood gas analysis.

Management

The principles of management are as follows (Emergency box 19.1).

- Replace the *fluid losses* with physiological saline (0.9%).
- Replace the *electrolyte losses*. Potassium levels need to be monitored with great care. Patients have a total body potassium deficit although initial plasma levels may not be low. Insulin therapy leads to uptake of potassium by the cells with a consequent fall in plasma K⁺ levels. Potassium is therefore given as soon as insulin is started.
- *Restore the acid–base balance.* A patient with healthy kidneys will rapidly compensate for the metabolic acidosis once the circulating volume is restored. Bicarbonate is seldom necessary and is only considered if the pH is below 7.0 ([H⁺] > 100 nmol/L), and is best given as an isotonic (1.26%) solution.
- *Replace the deficient insulin.* Modern treatment is with relatively modest doses of insulin, which lower blood glucose by suppressing hepatic glucose output rather than by stimulating peripheral uptake, and are therefore much less likely to produce hypoglycaemia. Soluble insulin is given as an intravenous infusion where facilities for adequate supervision exist, or as hourly intramuscular injections. The subcutaneous route is avoided because subcutaneous blood flow is reduced in shocked patients.
- *Monitor blood glucose closely.* Hourly measurement is needed in the initial phases of treatment.
- *Replace the energy losses.* When plasma glucose falls to near-normal values (12 mmol/L), saline infusion should be replaced with 5% dextrose containing 20 mmol/L of potassium chloride. The insulin infusion rate is reduced and adjusted according to blood glucose.
- *Seek the underlying cause.* Physical examination may reveal a source of infection (e.g. a perianal abscess). Two common markers of infection are misleading: fever is unusual even when infection is present, and polymorpholeucocytosis is present even in the absence

---

Emergency Box 19.1
Guidelines for the diagnosis and management of diabetic ketoacidosis

Diagnosis
- Hyperglycaemia: measure blood glucose.
- Ketonaemia: test plasma with ketostix. Finger prick sample for β-hydroxybutyrate
- Acidosis: measure pH and blood gases.

Investigations
- Blood glucose
- Urea and electrolytes
- Full blood count
- Blood gases
- Blood and urine culture
- Chest X-ray
- ECG
- Cardiac enzymes.

Phase 1 Management
- Admit to HDU
- Insulin: soluble insulin i.v. 6 units/hour by infusion, or 20 units i.m. stat. followed by 6 units i.m. hourly.
- Fluid replacement: 0.9% sodium chloride with 20 mmol KCl per litre. An average regimen would be 1 L in 30 minutes, then 1 L in 1 hour, then 1 L in 2 hours, then 1 L in 4 hours, then 1 L in 6 hours.
- Adjust KCl concentration depending on results of 2 hours' blood K measurement.

IF:
- Blood pressure below 80 mmHg, give plasma expander.
- pH below 7.0 give 500 mL of sodium bicarbonate 1.26% plus 10 mmol KCl. Repeat if necessary to bring pH up to 7.0.

Phase 2 Management
- When blood glucose falls to 10–12 mmol/L change infusion fluid to 1 litre 5% dextrose plus 20 mmol KCl 6-hourly. Continue insulin with dose adjusted according to hourly blood glucose test results.

Phase 3 Management
- Once stable and able to eat and drink normally, transfer patient to four times daily subcutaneous insulin regimen (based on previous 24 hours' insulin consumption, and trend in consumption).

Special measures
- Broad-spectrum antibiotic if infection likely.
- Bladder catheter if no urine passed in 2 hours.
- Nasogastric tube if drowsy.
- Consider CVP pressure monitoring if shocked or if previous cardiac or renal impairment.
- Give s.c. prophylactic LMW heparin in comatose, elderly or obese patients.

Subsequent management
- Monitor glucose hourly for 8 hours.
- Monitor electrolytes 2-hourly for 8 hours.
- Adjust K replacement according to results.

Note: The regimen of fluid replacement set out above is a guide for patients with severe ketoacidosis. Excessive fluid can precipitate pulmonary and cerebral oedema; inadequate replacement may cause renal failure. Fluid replacement must therefore be tailored to the individual and monitored carefully throughout treatment.

---

of infection. Relevant investigations include a chest X-ray, urine and blood cultures, and an ECG (to exclude myocardial infarction). If infection is suspected, broad-spectrum antibiotics are started once the appropriate cultures have been taken.

Problems of management
- *Hypotension.* This may lead to renal shutdown. Plasma expanders (or whole blood) are therefore given if the systolic blood pressure is below 80 mmHg. A central venous pressure line is useful in this situation. A bladder catheter is inserted if no urine is produced within 2 hours, but routine catheterization is not necessary.
- *Coma.* The usual principles apply (see p. 1209). It is essential to pass a nasogastric tube to prevent aspiration, since gastric stasis is common and carries the risk of aspiration pneumonia if a drowsy patient vomits.
- *Cerebral oedema.* This rare, but feared, complication has mostly been reported in children or young adults. Excessive rehydration and use of hypertonic fluids such as 8.4% bicarbonate may sometimes be responsible. The mortality is high.
- *Hypothermia.* Severe hypothermia with a core temperature below 33°C may occur and may be overlooked

unless a rectal temperature is taken with a low-reading thermometer.
- *Late complications.* These include stasis pneumonia and deep-vein thrombosis, and occur especially in the comatose or elderly patient.
- *Complications of therapy.* These include hypoglycaemia and hypokalaemia, due to loss of K⁺ in the urine from osmotic diuresis. Overenthusiastic fluid replacement may precipitate pulmonary oedema in the very young or the very old. Hyperchloraemic acidosis may develop in the course of treatment since patients have lost a large variety of negatively charged electrolytes, which are replaced with chloride. The kidneys usually correct this spontaneously within a few days.

Subsequent management
Intravenous dextrose and insulin are continued until the patient feels able to eat and keep food down. The drip is then taken down and a similar amount of insulin is given as three injections of soluble insulin subcutaneously at meal times and a dose of intermediate-acting insulin at night.

Sliding-scale regimens are unnecessary and may even delay the establishment of stable blood glucose levels. The treatment of diabetic ketoacidosis is incomplete without a careful enquiry into the causes of the episode and advice as to how to avoid its recurrence.

Non-ketotic hyperosmolar state

This condition, in which severe hyperglycaemia develops without significant ketosis, is the metabolic emergency characteristic of uncontrolled type 2 diabetes. Patients present in middle or later life, often with previously undiagnosed diabetes. Common precipitating factors include consumption of glucose-rich fluids (e.g. Lucozade), concurrent medication such as thiazide diuretics or steroids, and intercurrent illness. Non-ketotic coma and ketoacidosis represent two ends of a spectrum rather than two distinct disorders (Box 19.3). The biochemical differences may partly be explained as follows:

- *Age.* The extreme dehydration characteristic of non-ketotic coma may be related to age. Old people experience thirst less acutely, and more readily become dehydrated. In addition, the mild renal impairment associated with age results in increased urinary losses of fluid and electrolytes.
- *The degree of insulin deficiency.* This is less severe in non-ketotic coma. Endogenous insulin levels are sufficient to inhibit hepatic ketogenesis, whereas glucose production is unrestrained.

Clinical features

The characteristic clinical features on presentation are dehydration and stupor or coma. Impairment of consciousness is directly related to the degree of hyperosmolality. Evidence of underlying illness such as pneumonia or pyelonephritis may be present, and the hyperosmolar state may predispose to stroke, myocardial infarction or arterial insufficiency in the lower limbs.

Investigations and treatment

These are, with some exceptions, according to the guidelines for ketoacidosis. The plasma osmolality is usually extremely high. It can be measured directly or calculated as $(2(Na^+ + K^+) + glucose + urea)$ all in mmol/L. Many patients are extremely sensitive to insulin, and the glucose concentration may plummet. The resultant change in osmolality may cause cerebral damage. It is sometimes useful to infuse insulin at a rate of 3 U per hour for the first 2–3 h, increasing to 6 U/h if glucose is falling too slowly. The standard fluid for replacement is 0.9% physiological saline. Avoid 0.45% saline, since rapid dilution of the blood may cause more cerebral damage than a few hours of exposure to hypernatraemia.

Prognosis

The reported mortality ranges as high as 20–30%, mainly because of the advanced age of the patients and the frequency of intercurrent illness. Unlike ketoacidosis, non-ketotic hyperglycaemia is not an absolute indication for subsequent insulin therapy, and survivors may do well on diet and oral agents.

Lactic acidosis

Lactic acidosis may occur in diabetic patients on biguanide therapy. The risk in patients taking metformin is extremely low provided that the therapeutic dose is not exceeded and the drug is withheld in patients with advanced hepatic or renal dysfunction.

 Box 19.3 Electrolyte changes in diabetic ketoacidosis and non-ketotic hyperosmolar state

Examples of blood values

	Severe ketoacidosis	Non-ketotic hyperosmolar state
Na^+ (mmol/L)	140	155
K^+ (mmol/L)	5	5
Cl^- (mmol/L)	100	110
HCO_3^- (mmol/L)	5	30
Urea (mmol/L)	8	15
Glucose (mmol/L)	30	50
Arterial pH	7.0	7.35

The normal range of **osmolality** is 285–300 mOsm/kg. It can be measured directly, or can be calculated approximately from the formula:

Osmolality = $2(Na^+ + K^+)$ + glucose + urea.

For example, in the example of severe ketoacidosis given above:

Osmolality = $2(140 + 5) + 30 + 8 = 328$ mOsm/kg

and in the example of non-ketotic hyperosmolar coma:

Osmolality = $2(155 + 5) + 50 + 15 = 385$ mOsm/kg.

The normal **anion gap** is less than 17. It is calculated as $(Na^+ + K^+) - (Cl^- + HCO_3^-)$. In the example of ketoacidosis the anion gap is 40, and in the example of non-ketotic hyperosmolar coma the anion gap is 20. Mild hyperchloraemic acidosis may develop in the course of therapy. This will be shown by a rising plasma chloride and persistence of a low bicarbonate even though the anion gap has returned to normal.

Patients present in severe metabolic acidosis with a large anion gap normally less than 17 mmol/L), usually without significant hyperglycaemia or ketosis. Treatment is by rehydration and infusion of isotonic 1.26% bicarbonate. The mortality is in excess of 50%.

COMPLICATIONS OF DIABETES

Insulin-treated patients still have a considerably reduced life expectancy. The major cause of death in treated patients is due to cardiovascular problems (70%) followed by renal failure (10%) and infections (6%). There is no doubt that the duration and degree of hyperglycaemia play a major role in the production of complications. Better diabetic control can reduce the rate of progression of both nephropathy and retinopathy and the DCCT showed a 60% reduction in developing complications over 9 years when the HbA_{1c} was kept at around 7% in type 1 diabetes.

Pathophysiology

The mechanisms leading to damage are ill defined. The following are consequences of hyperglycaemia and may play a role:

- *Non-enzymatic glycosylation* of a wide variety of proteins, e.g. haemoglobin, collagen, LDL and tubulin in peripheral nerves. This leads to an accumulation of advanced glycosylated end-products causing injury and inflammation via stimulation of factors, e.g. complement, cytokines.
- *Polyol pathway*. The metabolism of glucose by increased intracellular aldose reductase leads to accumulation of sorbitol and fructose. This causes changes in vascular permeability, cell proliferation and capillary structure via stimulation of protein kinase C and TGF-β.
- *Abnormal microvascular blood flow* impairs supply of nutrients and oxygen. Microvascular occlusion is due to vasoconstrictors, e.g. endothelins and thrombogenesis, and leads to endothelial damage.
- *Other factors* include the formation of reactive oxygen species and growth factors stimulation (TGF-β) and vascular endothelial growth factor (VEGF). These growth factors are released by ischaemic tissues and cause endothelial cells to proliferate. VEGF is currently the favoured angiogenic factor.
- *Haemodynamic changes*, e.g. in kidney (see p. 1126).

It has been proposed that all of the above mechanisms stem from a single hyperglycaemia-induced process of overproduction of superoxide by the mitochondrial electron chain. This exciting new paradigm offers an integrated explanation of how complications of diabetes develop.

Macrovascular complications (Table 19.10)

Diabetes is a risk factor in the development of *atherosclerosis*. This risk is related to that of the background population. For example, Japanese diabetics are much less likely than patients in Europe to develop atherosclerosis, but are

Table 19.10 Diabetic risk factors for macrovascular complications

Duration
Increasing age
Systolic hypertension
Hyperinsulinaemia due to insulin resistance associated with obesity and syndrome X (metabolic syndrome)
Hyperlipidaemia, particularly hypertriglyceridaemia/low HDL
Proteinuria (including microalbuminuria)
Other factors are the same as for the general population

much more likely to develop it than are non-diabetic Japanese. The excess risk to diabetics compared with the general population increases as one moves down the body:

- Stroke is twice as likely.
- Myocardial infarction is three to five times as likely, and women with diabetes lose their premenopausal protection from coronary artery disease.
- Amputation of a foot for gangrene is 50 times as likely.

The UKPDS and DCCT studies have shown that intensive treatment of diabetes has only a small effect upon the cardiovascular risk of type 2 or type 1 diabetes patients. Cardiovascular risk factors occurring together tend to have a multiplicative effect on the overall level of cardiovascular risk. It is vital to tackle all cardiovascular risk factors together in diabetes, and not just to focus on glucose levels.

- *Hypertension*. The UKPDS demonstrated that aggressive treatment of hypertension produces a marked reduction in adverse cardiovascular outcomes, both microvascular and macrovascular. To achieve the target for blood pressure (Table 19.8), the UKPDS found that one-third of patients needed three or more antihypertensive drugs in combination, and two-thirds of treated patients needed two or more.
- *Smoking*: the avoidable risk factor (see p. 893). Never give up efforts to help diabetic patients stop smoking.
- *Lipid abnormalities*. Clinical trials suggest that there is no 'safe' cut-off for serum cholesterol. The lowest achievable level seems best to aim for, and in practice this means that almost all people with type 2 diabetes will be treated with a statin.
- *Low-dose aspirin* can reduce macrovascular risk, but is associated with a morbidity and mortality from bleeding. The benefits of aspirin outweigh the bleeding risk when the risk of a cardiovascular end-point is > 30% in the next 10 years. This risk is reached in patients aged under 45 with three strong additional cardiovascular risk factors, aged 45–54 with three additional risk factors, aged 54–65 with two additional risk factors or aged over 65 with just one additional risk factor.
- *ACE inhibitors/Angiotensin II receptor antagonists*. Treating people with diabetes and at least one other major cardiovascular risk factor with an ACE-inhibitor produces a 25–35% lowering of the risk of heart attack, stroke, overt nephropathy or cardiovascular death. ACE receptor antagonists are sometimes preferred

initially and are also used for those intolerant to ACE inhibitors.

A polypill? From the foregoing, it can be seen that people with diabetes will typically require treatment with several antihypertensives, a statin, an ACE inhibitor and low-dose aspirin.

Microvascular complications

In contrast to macrovascular disease, which is prevalent in the West as a whole, microvascular disease is specific to diabetes. Small blood vessels throughout the body are affected but the disease process is of particular danger in three sites:

- retina
- renal glomerulus
- nerve sheaths.

Diabetic retinopathy, nephropathy and neuropathy tend to manifest 10–20 years after diagnosis in young patients. They present earlier in older patients, probably because these have had unrecognized diabetes for months or even years prior to diagnosis. Genetic factors appear to contribute to the susceptibility to microvascular disease. Diabetic siblings of diabetic patients with renal and eye disease have a three- to fivefold increased risk of the same complication in both type 1 and type 2 patients. There are racial differences in the overall prevalence of nephropathy. In the USA prevalence is thus: Pima American Indians > Hispanic/Mexican > US black > US white patients.

Diabetic eye disease

Diabetes can affect the eyes in a number of ways. The most common and characteristic form of involvement is *diabetic retinopathy*. About one in three young people in this patient population is likely to develop visual problems, and in the UK 5% have in the past become blind after 30 years of diabetes. Indeed, diabetes has been the most common cause of blindness in the population as a whole up to the age of 65 years, but its contribution is falling.

Other forms of eye disease may also occur:

- *The lens* may be affected by reversible osmotic changes in patients with acute hyperglycaemia, causing blurred vision, or by cataracts.
- *New vessel formation* in the iris (rubeosis iridis) may develop as a late complication of diabetic retinopathy and can cause glaucoma.
- *External ocular palsies*, especially of the sixth nerve, can occur (a mononeuritis).

The natural history of retinopathy (Fig. 19.13)

Diabetes causes increased thickness of the capillary basement membrane and increased permeability of the retinal capillaries. Aneurysmal dilatation may occur in some vessels, while others become occluded. These changes are first detectable by fluorescein angiography: a fluorescent dye is injected into an arm vein and photographed in

Fig. 19.13 Features of diabetic eye disease. **(a)** The normal macula (centre) and optic disc. **(b)** Dot and blot haemorrhages (early background retinopathy). **(c)** Hard exudates are present in addition in background retinopathy. **(d)** Multiple cotton-wool spots indicate pre-proliferative retinopathy requiring routine ophthalmic referral. **(e)** Multiple frond-like new vessels, the hallmark of proliferative retinopathy. White fibrous tissue is forming near the new vessels, a feature of advanced retinopathy (this eye also illustrates multiple xenon arc laser burns superiorly). **(f)** Exudates appearing within a disc-width of the macula are a feature of an exudative maculopathy. **(g)** Central and **(h)** cortical cataracts can be seen against the red reflex with the ophthalmoscope.

transit through the retinal vessels. This technique is not necessary to screen effectively for retinal disease. After 20 years of type 1 diabetes, almost all patients have some retinopathy, and 60% progress to sight-threatening proliferative retinopathy (Fig. 19.14). Fifty to eighty per cent of patients with type 2 diabetes will have retinopathy

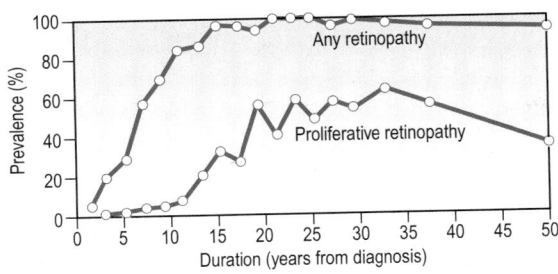

Fig. 19.14 Prevalence of retinopathy in relation to duration of the disease in patients with insulin-dependent diabetes mellitus diagnosed under the age of 33 years. Almost all eventually develop background change and 60% progress to proliferative retinopathy. From *Ophthalmology* (1984) **102**: 520.

after 20 years. Without treatment, 50% of proliferative patients become blind within 5 years.

Non-proliferative/background retinopathy
(Fig. 19.13b,c)
The first abnormality visible through the ophthalmoscope is the appearance of dot 'haemorrhages', which are actually due to capillary microaneurysms. Leakage of blood into the deeper layers of the retina produces the characteristic 'blot' haemorrhage, while exudation of fluid rich in lipids and protein gives rise to hard exudates. These have a bright yellowish white colour and are often irregular in outline with a sharply defined margin. These changes rarely develop in young patients with a duration of diabetes under 10 years, but by 20 years virtually all eyes will manifest at least the occasional microaneurysm on careful ophthalmoscopy. In contrast, retinopathy may be present at diagnosis or shortly thereafter in older patients. Background retinopathy does not in itself constitute a threat to vision but may progress to two other distinct forms of retinopathy: maculopathy or proliferative retinopathy. Both are the consequence of damage to retinal blood vessels and resultant retinal ischaemia.

Diabetic maculopathy
This may lead to blindness in the absence of proliferation and particularly affects the older patient with type 2 diabetes. Macular oedema is the first feature of maculopathy and may in itself result in permanent macular damage if not treated early. The first, and only, sign of this is deteriorating visual acuity and this early condition cannot be diagnosed with standard photography or ophthalmoscopy. This is why it is essential to screen patients with diabetes regularly for changes in visual acuity. In most cases, however, maculopathy does not generate sufficient oedema to cause early loss of acuity. The process may then be detected in its later stages as encroachment of hard exudates on the macular area. These changes are easily visible on standard photography or ophthalmoscopy, through fully dilated pupils.

Pre-proliferative retinopathy
Progressive retinal ischaemia will, in some patients, cause background retinopathy to progress to pre-proliferative, sight-threatening retinopathy. The earliest sign is the appearance of 'cotton-wool spots', representing oedema resulting from retinal infarcts (Fig. 19.13d). They may also occur in severe hypertensive retinopathy. The term 'soft exudate' is often used synonymously but is best avoided. Cotton-wool spots are greyish white, have indistinct margins and a dull matt surface, unlike the glossy appearance of hard exudates. Other features of pre-proliferative retinopathy are described in Table 19.11.

Proliferative retinopathy
Hypoxia is thought to be the signal for formation of new vessels. These lie superficially or grow forward into the vitreous, resembling fronds of seaweed. They branch repeatedly, are fragile, bleed easily (because they lack the normal supportive tissue) and may give rise to a fibrous-tissue reaction (Fig. 19.13e). With advanced retinopathy, haemorrhages can be preretinal or into the vitreous. A vitreous haemorrhage presents as a loss of vision in one eye, sometimes noticed on waking, or as a floating shadow affecting the field of vision. Ophthalmoscopy gives the

Table 19.11	Pathological changes in the retina in diabetic retinopathy: the action needed	
	Fundoscopy/photography findings	**Action needed**
Peripheral retina		
Non proliferative/background	Microaneurysms (dot haemorrhages)	Annual screening only
	Blot haemorrhages	
	Hard exudates	
Pre-proliferative	Multiple cotton wool spots (nerve fibre layer infarcts)	Non-urgent referral to an ophthalmologist
	Venous beading	
	Venous loops	
	Intraretinal microvascular abnormalities	
Proliferative	New blood vessel formation (neovascularization)	Urgent referral to an ophthalmologist
	Preretinal (subhyaloid) haemorrhage	
	Vitreous haemorrhage	
Advanced retinopathy	Retinal fibrosis	Urgent referral to an ophthalmologist – but much vision already lost
	Traction retinal detachment	
Central retina		
Maculopathy	Hard exudates within one disc width of macula	Urgent referral to an ophthalmologist
	Unexplained loss of acuity	

appearance of a featureless, grey haze. Partial recovery of vision is the rule, as the blood is reabsorbed, but repeated bleeds may occur.

Loss of vision may also result from fibrous proliferation associated with new vessel formation. This may give rise to traction bands that contract with the course of time, producing retinal detachment.

Cataracts

Senile cataracts develop some 10–15 years earlier in diabetic patients than in the remainder of the population. The risk of cataracts was lower in the UKPDS intensively controlled group.

Juvenile or 'snowflake' cataracts are much less common. These are diffuse, rapidly progressive cataracts associated with very poorly controlled diabetes. They should be distinguished from temporary lens changes that occasionally appear during hyperosmolar states and resolve when the hyperglycaemia is brought under control.

Examination

Careful systematic examination of the eye is essential. Visual acuity and eye movements are tested, and 15–30 minutes before the eye is examined the pupils are dilated with a mydriatic such as tropicamide 0.5%. Dilating drugs should not be used, however, in patients with a history of glaucoma, except with the advice of an ophthalmologist. The ophthalmologic examination begins at arm's length. At this distance, cataracts are silhouetted against the red reflex of the retina. The ophthalmoscope is advanced until the retina is in focus. The examination begins at the optic disc, moves through each quadrant in turn, and ends with the macula (since this is least comfortable for the patient). The ophthalmoscope is then adjusted to the +10 dioptre lens for examination of the cornea, anterior chamber and lens. The location of abnormalities should always be sketched in the notes for future reference.

Management of diabetic eye disease
(Table 19.11)

The DCCT and UKPDS show that the risk of developing diabetic eye disease can be reduced by striving for aggressive metabolic control of the diabetes. There is no specific medical treatment for background retinopathy. Smoking and hypertension worsen the rate of progression and need treatment. Development or progression of retinopathy may be accelerated by rapid improvement in glycaemic control, pregnancy and in those with nephropathy, and these groups need frequent monitoring. All patients with retinopathy should be examined regularly by a diabetologist or ophthalmologist. Early referral to an ophthalmologist is essential in the following circumstances:

- deteriorating visual acuity
- hard exudates encroaching on the macula
- pre-proliferative changes (cotton-wool spots or venous beading)
- new vessel formation.

The ophthalmologist may perform fluorescein angiography to define the extent of the problem. Maculopathy and proliferative retinopathy are often treatable by retinal laser photocoagulation; in the latter condition early effective therapy reduces the risk of visual loss by about 50%. The value of photocoagulation is particularly marked in those with disc (as against peripheral) new vessels. In one trial, only 15% of treated, as against 50% of untreated, eyes with disc new vessels progressed to legal blindness. Treatment in this case is by panretinal photocoagulation. Surgery can be performed to try to salvage some vision after vitreous haemorrhage and to treat traction retinal detachment in advanced retinopathy.

The diabetic kidney

The kidney may be damaged by diabetes in three main ways:

- glomerular damage
- ischaemia resulting from hypertrophy of afferent and efferent arterioles
- ascending infection.

Diabetic nephropathy
Epidemiology

Clinical nephropathy secondary to glomerular disease usually manifests 15–25 years after diagnosis and affects 25–35% of patients diagnosed under the age of 30 years. It is the leading cause of premature death in young diabetic patients. Older patients also develop nephropathy, but the proportion affected is smaller. Some centres have reported a falling incidence rate of diabetic nephropathy in type 1 diabetes. This may reflect good-quality local care for diabetes rather than a change in the natural history of the disease itself. As people with type 2 diabetes develop diabetes progressively younger, a rising incidence rate of nephropathy is seen.

Pathophysiology

The earliest functional abnormality in the diabetic kidney is renal hypertrophy associated with a raised glomerular filtration rate. This appears soon after diagnosis and is related to poor glycaemic control. As the kidney becomes damaged by diabetes, the afferent arteriole (leading to the glomerulus) becomes vasodilated to a greater extent than the efferent glomerular arteriole. This increases the intraglomerular filtration pressure, further damaging the glomerular capillaries. This increased intraglomerular pressure also leads to increased shearing forces locally which are thought to contribute to mesangial cell hypertrophy and increased secretion of extracellular mesangial matrix material. This process eventually leads to glomerular sclerosis. The initial structural lesion in the glomerulus is thickening of the basement membrane. Associated changes result in disruption of the protein cross-linkages which normally make the membrane an effective filter. In consequence, there is a progressive leak of large molecules (particularly protein) into the urine.

Albuminuria

The earliest evidence of this is 'microalbuminuria' – amounts of urinary albumin so small as to be undetectable by standard dipsticks (see p. 614). Microalbuminuria may be tested for by radioimmunoassay or by using special dipsticks. It is a predictive marker of progression to nephropathy in type 1 diabetes, and of increased cardiovascular risk in type 2 diabetes. Microalbuminuria may, after some years, progress to intermittent albuminuria followed by persistent proteinuria. Light-microscopic changes of glomerulosclerosis become manifest; both diffuse and nodular glomerulosclerosis can occur. The latter is sometimes known as the *Kimmelstiel–Wilson lesion*. At the later stage of glomerulosclerosis, the glomerulus is replaced by hyaline material.

At the stage of persistent proteinuria, the plasma creatinine is normal but the average patient is only some 5–10 years from end-stage renal failure. The proteinuria may become so heavy as to induce a transient nephrotic syndrome, with peripheral oedema and hypoalbuminaemia.

Patients with nephropathy typically show a normochromic normocytic anaemia and a raised erythrocyte sedimentation rate (ESR). Hypertension is a common development and may itself damage the kidney still further. A rise in plasma creatinine is a late feature that progresses inevitably to renal failure, although the rate of progression may vary widely between individuals.

The natural history of this process is shown in Figure 19.15.

Ischaemic lesions

Arteriolar lesions, with hypertrophy and hyalinization of the vessels, can occur in patients with diabetes. The appearances are similar to those of hypertensive disease and lead to ischaemic damage to the kidneys.

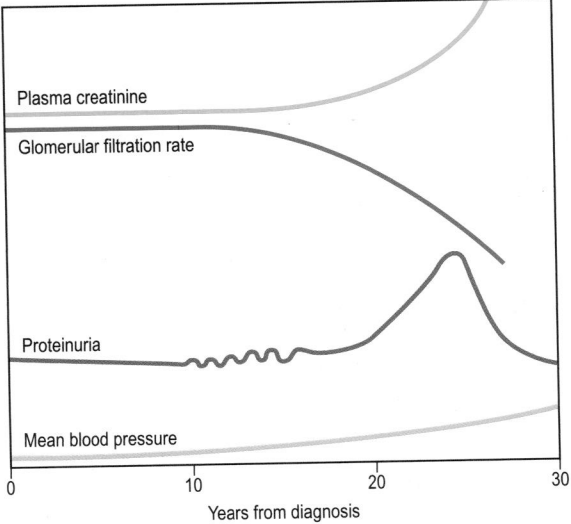

Fig. 19.15 **Schematic representation of the natural history of nephropathy.** The typical onset is 15 years after diagnosis. Intermittent proteinuria leads to persistent proteinuria. In time, the plasma creatinine rises as the glomerular filtration rate falls.

Infective lesions

Urinary tract infections are relatively more common in women with diabetes, but this does not apply to men. Ascending infection may occur because of bladder stasis resulting from autonomic neuropathy, and infections more easily become established in damaged renal tissue. Autopsy material frequently reveals interstitial changes suggestive of infection, but ischaemia may produce similar changes and the true frequency of pyelonephritis in diabetes is uncertain. Untreated infections in diabetics can result in renal papillary necrosis, in which renal papillae are shed in the urine, but this complication is rare.

Diagnosis

The urine of all diabetic patients should be checked regularly for the presence of protein. Many centres also screen younger patients for microalbuminuria since there is evidence that meticulous glycaemic control or early antihypertensive treatment at this stage may delay the onset of frank proteinuria. Once proteinuria is present, other possible causes for this should be considered (see below), but once these are excluded, a presumptive diagnosis of diabetic nephropathy can be made. For practical purposes this implies inevitable progression to end-stage renal failure, although the time course can be markedly slowed by early aggressive antihypertensive therapy. Clinical suspicion of a non-diabetic cause of nephropathy may be provoked by an atypical history, the absence of diabetic retinopathy (usually but not invariably present with diabetic nephropathy) and the presence of red-cell casts in the urine. Renal biopsy should be considered in such cases, but in practice is rarely necessary or helpful. The risk of intravenous urography is increased in diabetes, especially if patients are allowed to become dehydrated prior to the procedure, and a renal ultrasound is preferable but not so informative. A 24-hour urine collection is performed to quantify protein loss and to measure creatinine clearance, and regular measurement is made of the plasma creatinine level.

Investigations to detect other treatable causes of nephropathy include urine microscopy and culture, serum protein electrophoresis, serum calcium, serum urate, ESR and antinuclear factor.

Management

The management of diabetic nephropathy is similar to that of other causes of renal failure, with the following provisos:

- Aggressive treatment of blood pressure with a target below 130/80 mmHg has been shown to slow the rate of deterioration of renal failure considerably. Angiotensin-converting enzyme inhibitors or an angiotensin receptor II antagonist are the drugs of choice (see p. 1096). These drugs should also be used in normotensive patients with persistent microalbuminuria. Reduction in albuminuria occurs with this treatment.
- Oral hypoglycaemic agents partially excreted via the kidney (e.g. glibenclamide) must be avoided.

- Insulin sensitivity increases and drastic reductions in dosage may be needed.
- Associated diabetic retinopathy tends to progress rapidly, and frequent ophthalmic supervision is essential.

Management of end-stage disease is made more difficult by the fact that patients often have other complications of diabetes such as blindness, autonomic neuropathy or peripheral vascular disease. Vascular shunts tend to calcify rapidly and hence chronic ambulatory peritoneal dialysis may be preferable to haemodialysis. The failure rate of renal transplants is somewhat higher than in non-diabetic patients. A segmental pancreatic graft is sometimes performed at the same time as a renal graft. Although pancreatic transplants have a limited viability, owing to progressive fibrosis within the graft, they may give the patient a year or so of freedom from insulin injections.

Diabetic neuropathy

Diabetes can damage peripheral nervous tissue in a number of ways. The vascular hypothesis postulates occlusion of the vasa nervorum as the prime cause. This seems likely in isolated mononeuropathies, but the diffuse symmetrical nature of the common forms of neuropathy implies a metabolic cause. Since hyperglycaemia leads to increased formation of sorbitol and fructose in Schwann cells, accumulation of these sugars may disrupt function and structure.

The earliest functional change in diabetic nerves is delayed nerve conduction velocity; the earliest histological change is segmental demyelination, caused by damage to Schwann cells. In the early stages axons are preserved, implying prospects of recovery, but at a later stage irreversible axonal degeneration develops.

The following varieties of neuropathy occur (Fig. 19.16):

- symmetrical mainly sensory polyneuropathy (distal)
- acute painful neuropathy
- mononeuropathy and mononeuritis multiplex
  (a) cranial nerve lesions
  (b) isolated peripheral nerve lesions
- diabetic amyotrophy
- autonomic neuropathy.

Symmetrical mainly sensory polyneuropathy

This is often unrecognized by the patient in its early stages. Early clinical signs are loss of vibration sense, pain sensation (deep before superficial) and temperature sensation in the feet. At later stages patients may complain of a feeling of 'walking on cotton wool' and can lose their balance when washing the face or walking in the dark owing to impaired proprioception. Involvement of the hands is much less common and results in a 'stocking and glove' sensory loss. Complications include unrecognized trauma, beginning as blistering due to an ill-fitting shoe or a hot-water bottle, and leading to ulceration.

Sequelae of neuropathy. Involvement of motor nerves to the small muscles of the feet gives rise to interosseous wasting. Unbalanced traction by the long flexor muscles leads to a characteristic shape of the foot, with a high arch and clawing of the toes, which in turn leads to abnormal distribution of pressure on walking, resulting in callus formation under the first metatarsal head or on the tips of the toes and perforating neuropathic ulceration. Neuropathic arthropathy (Charcot's joints) may sometimes develop in the ankle. The hands show small-muscle wasting as well as sensory changes, but these signs and symptoms must be differentiated from those of the carpal tunnel syndrome, which occurs with increased frequency in diabetes and may be amenable to surgery.

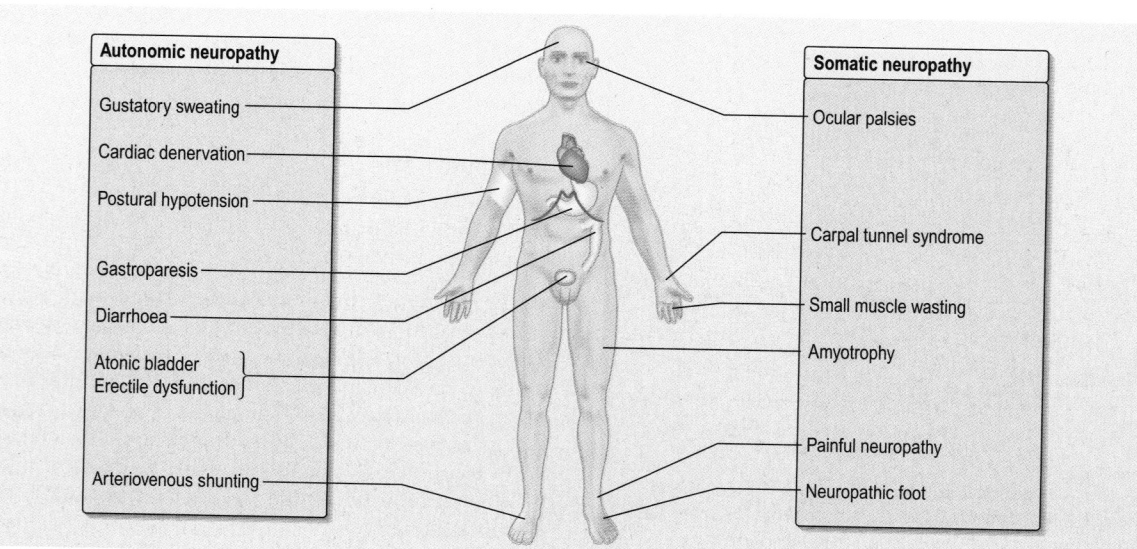

Fig. 19.16 **The neuropathic man.**

Acute painful neuropathy

A diffuse, painful neuropathy is less common. The patient describes burning or crawling pains in the feet, shins and anterior thighs. These symptoms are typically worse at night, and pressure from bedclothes may be intolerable. It may present at diagnosis or develop after sudden improvement in glycaemic control (e.g. when insulin is started). It usually remits spontaneously after 3–12 months if good control is maintained. A more chronic form, developing later in the course of the disease, is sometimes resistant to almost all forms of therapy. Neurological assessment is difficult because of the hyperaesthesia experienced by the patient, but muscle wasting is not a feature and objective signs can be minimal.

Management is firstly to explore for non-diabetic causes (p. 1264). Explanation and reassurance about the high likelihood of remission within months may be all that is needed. Tricyclic antidepressants, gabapentin, mexiletine, valproate and carbamazepine all reduce the perception of neuritic pain somewhat, but usually not as much as patients hope for. Transepidermal nerve stimulation (TENS) benefits some patients. Topical capsaicin-containing creams help occasionally. A few report that acupuncture has helped.

Mononeuritis and mononeuritis multiplex (multiple mononeuropathy)

Any nerve in the body can be involved in diabetic mononeuritis; the onset is typically abrupt and sometimes painful. Radiculopathy (i.e. involvement of a spinal root) may also occur.

Isolated palsies of nerves to the external eye muscles, especially the third and sixth nerves, are more common in diabetes. A characteristic feature of diabetic third nerve lesions is that pupillary reflexes are retained owing to sparing of pupillomotor fibres. Full spontaneous recovery is the rule for most episodes of mononeuritis. Lesions are more likely to occur at common sites for external pressure palsies or nerve entrapment (e.g. the median nerve in the carpal tunnel). The carpal tunnel syndrome (p. 1260) is a common cause for sensory symptoms in the hands in diabetes, but appears to respond less well to decompression.

Diabetic amyotrophy

This condition is usually seen in older men with diabetes. Presentation is with painful wasting, usually asymmetrical, of the quadriceps muscles. The wasting may be very marked and knee reflexes are diminished or absent. The affected area is often extremely tender. Extensor plantar responses sometimes develop and CSF protein content is elevated. Diabetic amyotrophy is usually associated with periods of poor glycaemic control and may be present at diagnosis. It often resolves in time with careful control of the blood glucose.

Autonomic neuropathy

Asymptomatic autonomic disturbances can be demonstrated on laboratory testing in many patients, but symptomatic autonomic neuropathy is rare. It affects both the sympathetic and parasympathetic nervous systems and can be disabling.

The cardiovascular system

Vagal neuropathy results in tachycardia at rest and loss of sinus arrhythmia. At a later stage, the heart may become denervated (resembling a transplanted heart). Cardiovascular reflexes such as the Valsalva manoeuvre are impaired. Postural hypotension occurs owing to loss of sympathetic tone to peripheral arterioles. A warm foot with a bounding pulse is sometimes seen in a polyneuropathy as a result of peripheral vasodilatation.

Gastrointestinal tract

Vagal damage can lead to gastroparesis, often asymptomatic, but sometimes leading to intractable vomiting. Recently implantable devices which stimulate gastric emptying, and injections of botulinum toxin into the pylorus (to partly paralyse the sphincter) have each shown benefit in cases of this previously intractable problem. Autonomic diarrhoea often occurs at night accompanied by urgency and incontinence. Diarrhoea and steatorrhoea may occur owing to small bowel bacterial overgrowth; treatment is with antibiotics such as tetracycline.

Bladder involvement

Loss of tone, incomplete emptying, and stasis (predisposing to infection) can occur, and may ultimately result in an atonic, painless, distended bladder.

Male erectile dysfunction

This is common. The first manifestation is incomplete erection which may in time progress to total failure; retrograde ejaculation also occurs in patients with autonomic neuropathy. Erectile dysfunction in diabetes has many causes including anxiety, depression, alcohol excess, drugs, primary or secondary gonadal failure, hypothyroidism, and inadequate vascular supply owing to atheroma in pudendal arteries. The history and examination should focus on these possible causes. Blood is taken for LH, FSH, testosterone, prolactin and thyroid function. Treatment should ideally include sympathetic counselling of both partners.

Phosphodiesterase type-5 inhibitors (sildenafil, tadalafil, vardenafil), which enhance the effects of nitric oxide on smooth muscle and increase penile blood flow, are used in diabetic patients who do not take nitrates, e.g. for angina. If this therapy succeeds, it is worth trying without it after a few months of success, since sometimes potency will continue unaided after confidence is restored. Sixty per cent of diabetic patients can be expected to benefit from this therapy.

There are alternatives for patients who fail to improve with a phosphodiesterase, who dislike the side-effects (headache and a green tinge to vision the next day) or those in whom it is contraindicated. Apomorphine 2 or 3 mg sublingually 20 minutes before sexual activity is an alternative, but with lower efficacy. Alprostadil (prostaglandin E_1 preparation) may be given after suitable training as a small pellet inserted with a device into the urethra (125 µg initially with a maximum of 1 mg). It has a lower success rate than intracavernosal injection treatment, but is less invasive. If the partner is pregnant, barrier contraception must be used to keep prostaglandin away from the fetus.

Other methods include intracavernosal injection of alprostadil, papaverine and phentolamine. Side-effects include priapism which needs urgent treatment should erection last more than 3 hours. Vacuum devices are also used.

The diabetic foot

Ten to fifteen per cent of diabetic patients develop foot ulcers at some stage in their lives. Diabetic foot problems are responsible for nearly 50% of all diabetes-related hospital admissions. Many diabetic limb amputations could be delayed or prevented by more effective patient education and medical supervision. Ischaemia, infection and neuropathy combine to produce tissue necrosis. Although all these factors may coexist, the ischaemic and the neuropathic foot (Table 19.12) can be distinguished. In rural India foot ulcers are common due to neuropathic and infective causes rather than vascular causes.

Management

Many diabetic foot problems are avoidable, so patients need to learn the principles of foot care (Table 19.13). Older patients should visit a chiropodist regularly and should not cut their own toe-nails. Once tissue damage has occurred in the form of ulceration or gangrene, the aim is preservation of viable tissue. The four main threats to the skin and subcutaneous tissues are:

- *Infection.* This can take hold rapidly in a diabetic foot. Early antibiotic treatment is essential, with antibiotic therapy adjusted in the light of culture results. The organisms grown from the skin surface may not be the organism causing deeper infection. Collections of pus are drained and excision of infected bone is needed if osteomyelitis develops and does not respond to appro-

Table 19.13	Principles of diabetic foot care

Inspect feet daily
Seek early advice for any damage
Check shoes inside and out for sharp bodies/areas before
    wearing
Use lace-up shoes with plenty of room for the toes
Keep feet away from sources of heat (hot sand, hot-water
    bottles, radiators, fires)
Check the bath temperature before stepping in

priate antibiotic therapy. Regular X-rays of the foot are needed to check on progress.
- *Ischaemia.* The blood flow to the feet is assessed clinically and with Doppler ultrasound. Femoral angiography is used to localize areas of occlusion amenable to bypass surgery or angioplasty. Relatively few patients fall into this category, and the risks (deterioration leading to amputation) and benefits of surgical intervention are finely balanced.
- *Abnormal pressure.* An ulcerated site must be kept non-weight-bearing. Resting the affected leg may need to be supplemented with special deep shoes and insoles to move pressure away from critical sites, or by removable or non-removable casts of the leg. After healing, special shoes and insoles are likely to continue to be needed to protect the feet and prevent abnormal pressure repeating damage to a healed area. In neuropathic feet particularly, sharp surgical debridement by a chiropodist is necessary to prevent callus distorting the local wound architecture and causing damage through abnormal pressure on normal skin nearby.
- *Wound environment.* Dressings are used to absorb or remove exudate, maintain moisture, and protect the wound from contaminating agents, and should be easily removable. Expensive new dressings containing growth factors and other biologically active agents may have a role to play in future, but their place is still being assessed.

Foot problems are the major cause of hospital bed occupancy by diabetic patients. Good liaison between physician, chiropodist and surgeon is essential if this period in hospital is to be used efficiently. When irreversible arterial insufficiency is present, it is often quicker and kinder to opt for an early major amputation rather than subject the patient to a debilitating sequence of conservative procedures.

Infections

There is no evidence that diabetic patients with good glycaemic control are more prone to infection than normal subjects. However, poorly controlled diabetes entails increased susceptibility to the following infections:

- *Skin*
  (a) staphylococcal infections (boils, abscesses, carbuncles)
  (b) mucocutaneous candidiasis

Table 19.12	Distinguishing features between ischaemia and neuropathy in the diabetic foot	
	Ischaemia	**Neuropathy**
Symptoms	Claudication	Usually painless
	Rest pain	Sometimes painful neuropathy
Inspection	Dependent rubor	High arch
	Trophic changes	Clawing of toes
		No trophic changes
Palpation	Cold	Warm
	Pulseless	Bounding pulses
Ulceration	Painful	Painless
	Heels and toes	Plantar

- *Gastrointestinal tract*
  - (a) chronic periodontitis
  - (b) rectal and ischiorectal abscess formation (when control very poor)
- *Urinary tract*
  - (a) urinary tract infections (in women)
  - (b) pyelonephritis
  - (c) perinephric abscess
- *Lungs*
  - (a) staphylococcal and pneumococcal pneumonia
  - (b) Gram-negative bacterial pneumonia
  - (c) tuberculosis.

One reason why poor control lends to infection is that chemotaxis and phagocytosis by polymorphonuclear leucocytes are impaired because at high blood glucose concentrations neutrophil superoxide generation is impaired.

Conversely, infections may lead to loss of glycaemic control, and are a common cause of ketoacidosis. Insulin-treated patients need to increase their dose by up to 25% in the face of infection, and non-insulin-treated patients may need insulin cover while the infection lasts. Patients should be told never to omit their insulin dose, even if they are nauseated and unable to eat; instead they should test their blood glucose frequently and seek urgent medical advice. Diabetic patients should receive pneumococcal vaccine (p. 41) and yearly influenza vaccine.

Skin and joints (see also p. 1345)

Joint contractures in the hands are a common consequence of childhood diabetes. The sign may be demonstrated by asking the patient to join the hands as if in prayer; the metacarpophalangeal and interphalangeal joints cannot be apposed. Thickened, waxy skin can be noted on the backs of the fingers. These features may be due to glycosylation of collagen and are not progressive. The condition is sometimes referred to as diabetic cheiroarthropathy.

Osteopenia in the extremities is also described in type 1 diabetes but rarely leads to clinical consequences.

FURTHER READING

Atkinson MA, Eisenbarth GS (2001) Type I diabetes: new perspectives on disease pathogenesis and treatment. *Lancet* **358**: 221–229.

Boulton AJM et al. (2004) Neuropathic diabetic foot ulcers. *New England Journal of Medicine* **351**: 48–55.

Brownlee M (2001) Biochemistry and molecular cell biology of diabetic complications. *Nature* **44**: 813–820.

Colhoun HM et al. (2004) Primary prevention of cardiovascular disease with atorvastatin in type 2 diabetes in the collaborative atorvastatin diabetes study (CARDS). *Lancet* **364**: 685–696.

Diabetes Control and Complications Trial Research Group (1993) The effect of intensive treatment of diabetes on the development and progression of long-term complications in insulin-dependent diabetes mellitus. *New England Journal of Medicine* **329**: 977–986.

Frank RN (2004) Diabetic retinopathy. *New England Journal of Medicine* **350**: 48–58.

Hostetter TH (2001) Prevention of end-stage renal disease in type 2 diabetes. *New England Journal of Medicine* **345**: 910–912.

Mitch WE (2004) Treating diabetic neuropathy. *New England Journal of Medicine* **351**: 1934–1936.

NOTES ON SPECIAL SITUATIONS IN DIABETES

Surgery

Smooth control of diabetes minimizes the risk of infection and balances the catabolic response to anaesthesia and surgery. The procedure for insulin-treated patients is simple:

- Long-acting and/or intermediate insulin should be stopped the day before surgery, with soluble insulin substituted.
- Whenever possible, diabetic patients should be first on the morning theatre list.
- An infusion of glucose, insulin and potassium is given during surgery. The insulin can be mixed into the glucose solution or administered separately by syringe pump. A standard combination is 16 U of soluble insulin with 10 mmol of KCl in 500 mL of 10% glucose, infused at 100 mL/h.
- Postoperatively, the infusion is maintained until the patient is able to eat. Other fluids needed in the perioperative period must be given through a separate intravenous line and must not interrupt the glucose/insulin/potassium infusion. Glucose levels are checked every 2–4 hours and potassium levels are monitored. The amount of insulin and potassium in each infusion bag is adjusted either upwards or downwards according to the results of regular monitoring of the blood glucose and serum potassium concentrations.

The same approach is used in the emergency situation, with the exception that a separate variable-rate insulin infusion may be needed to bring blood glucose under control before surgery.

Non-insulin-treated patients should stop medication 2 days before the operation. Patients with mild hyperglycaemia (fasting blood glucose below 8 mmol/L) can be treated as non-diabetic. Those with higher levels are treated with soluble insulin prior to surgery, and with glucose, insulin and potassium during and after the procedure, as for insulin-treated patients.

Pregnancy and diabetes

Meticulous metabolic control of the diabetes and careful medical and obstetric management is required.

Metabolic control of diabetes in pregnancy

The patient should perform daily home blood glucose profiles, recording blood tests before and 2 hours after meals. The renal threshold falls in pregnancy, and urine tests are therefore of little or no value. Insulin requirements rise progressively, and intensified insulin regimens are generally used. The aim is to maintain blood glucose and fructosamine (or HbA$_{1c}$) levels as close to the normal range as can be tolerated.

General management

The patient is seen at intervals of 2 weeks or less at a clinic managed jointly by physician and obstetrician. Circumstances permitting, the aim should be outpatient management with a spontaneous vaginal delivery at term. Retinopathy and nephropathy may deteriorate during pregnancy. Expert fundoscopy and urine testing for protein should be undertaken at booking, at 28 weeks and before delivery.

Obstetric problems associated with diabetes

Poorly controlled diabetes is associated with stillbirth, mechanical problems in the birth canal owing to fetal macrosomia, hydramnios and pre-eclampsia. Ketoacidosis in pregnancy carries a 50% fetal mortality, but maternal hypoglycaemia is relatively well tolerated.

Neonatal problems

Maternal diabetes, especially when poorly controlled, is associated with fetal macrosomia. The infant of a diabetic mother is more susceptible to hyaline membrane disease than non-diabetic infants of similar maturity. In addition, neonatal hypoglycaemia may occur. The mechanism is as follows: maternal glucose crosses the placenta, but insulin does not; the fetal islets hypersecrete to combat maternal hyperglycaemia, and a rebound to hypoglycaemic levels occurs when the umbilical cord is severed.

These complications are due to hyperglycaemia in the third trimester. Poor glycaemic control around the time of conception carries an increased risk of major congenital malformations. When a pregnancy is planned, optimal metabolic control should be sought before conception.

Gestational diabetes

This term refers to glucose intolerance that develops in the course of pregnancy and usually remits following delivery. The condition is typically asymptomatic. Women who have a previous history of gestational diabetes, older or overweight women, those with a history of large for gestational age babies and women from certain ethnic groups are at particular risk, but many cases occur in women who are not in any of these categories. For this reason some advocate screening of all pregnant women on the basis of random plasma glucose testing in each trimester and by oral glucose tolerance testing if the glucose concentration is, for example, 7 mmol/L or more. There is no consensus concerning the level of blood glucose which is harmful for the baby, and therefore no consensus concerning cut-off levels for screening and intervention.

Treatment is with diet in the first instance, but most patients require insulin cover during the pregnancy. Insulin does not cross the placenta. Many oral agents cross the placenta and are usually avoided because of the potential risk to the fetus.

Gestational diabetes has been associated with all the obstetric and neonatal problems described above for pre-existing diabetes, except that there is no increase in the rate of congenital abnormalities. It is likely to recur in subsequent pregnancies. Gestational diabetes is often the harbinger of type 2 diabetes in later life.

Not all diabetes presenting in pregnancy is gestational. True type 1 diabetes may develop, and swift diagnosis is essential to prevent the development of ketoacidosis. Hospital admission is required if the patient is symptomatic, or has ketonuria or a markedly elevated blood glucose level.

Unstable diabetes

This is used to describe patients with recurrent ketoacidosis and/or recurrent hypoglycaemic coma. Of these, the largest group is made up of those who experience recurrent severe hypoglycaemia.

Recurrent severe hypoglycaemia

This affects 1–3% of insulin-dependent patients. Most are adults who have had diabetes for more than 10 years. By this stage, endogenous insulin secretion is negligible in the great majority of patients. Pancreatic alpha-cells are still present in undiminished numbers, but the glucagon response to hypoglycaemia is virtually absent. Long-term patients are thus subject to fluctuating hyperinsulinaemia owing to erratic absorption of insulin from injection sites, and lack a major component of the hormonal defence against hypoglycaemia. In this situation adrenaline (epinephrine) secretion becomes vital, but this too may become impaired in the course of diabetes. Loss of adrenaline (epinephrine) secretion has been attributed to autonomic neuropathy, but this is unlikely to be the sole cause; central adaptation to recurrent hypoglycaemia may also be a factor.

The following factors may also predispose to recurrent hypoglycaemia:

- *Overtreatment with insulin*. Frequent biochemical hypoglycaemia lowers the glucose level at which symptoms develop. Symptoms often reappear when overall glucose control is relaxed.
- *An unrecognized low renal threshold for glucose*. Attempts to render the urine sugar-free will inevitably produce hypoglycaemia.
- *Excessive insulin doses*. A common error is to increase the dose when a patient needs more frequent injections to overcome a problem of timing.

- *Endocrine causes*. These include pituitary insufficiency, adrenal insufficiency and premenstrual insulin sensitivity.
- *Alimentary causes*. These include exocrine pancreatic failure and diabetic gastroparesis.
- *Renal failure*. Clearance of insulin is diminished.
- *Patient causes*. Patients may be unintelligent, uncooperative or may manipulate their therapy.

Recurrent ketoacidosis

This usually occurs in adolescents or young adults, particularly girls. Metabolic decompensation may develop very rapidly. A combination of chaotic food intake and insulin omission, whether consciously or unconsciously, is now regarded as the primary cause of this problem. It almost always occurs in the context of considerable psychosocial problems, particularly eating disorders. This area needs careful and sympathetic exploration in any patient with recurrent ketoacidosis. It is perhaps not surprising that in an illness where much of one's life is spent thinking of and controlling food intake, 30% of women with diabetes have had some features of an eating disorder at some time. Other causes include:

- *Iatrogenic*. Inappropriate insulin combinations may be a cause of swinging glycaemic control. For example, a once-daily regimen may cause hypoglycaemia during the afternoon or evening and pre-breakfast hyperglycaemia due to insulin deficiency.
- *Intercurrent illness*. Unsuspected infections, including urinary tract infections and tuberculosis, may be present. Thyrotoxicosis can also manifest as unstable glycaemic control.

> **FURTHER READING**
> Kjos SL, Buchanan TA (1999) Gestational diabetes mellitus. *New England Journal of Medicine* **341**: 1749–1756.

HYPOGLYCAEMIA IN THE NON-DIABETIC

Hypoglycaemia develops when hepatic glucose output falls below the rate of glucose uptake by peripheral tissues. Hepatic glucose output may be reduced by:

- the inhibition of hepatic glycogenolysis and gluconeogenesis by insulin
- depletion of hepatic glycogen reserves by malnutrition, fasting, exercise or advanced liver disease
- impaired gluconeogenesis (e.g. following alcohol ingestion).

In the first of these categories, insulin levels are raised, the liver contains adequate glycogen stores, and the hypoglycaemia can be reversed by injection of glucagon. In the other two situations, insulin levels are low and glucagon is ineffective. Peripheral glucose uptake is accelerated by high insulin levels and by exercise, but these conditions are normally balanced by increased glucose output.

The most common symptoms and signs of hypoglycaemia are neurological. The brain consumes about 50% of the total glucose produced by the liver. This high energy requirement is needed to generate ATP used to maintain the potential difference across axonal membranes.

Insulin or sulphonylurea therapy for diabetes accounts for the vast majority of cases of severe hypoglycaemia encountered in an accident and emergency department.

Insulinomas

Insulinomas are pancreatic islet cell tumours that secrete insulin. Most are sporadic but some patients have multiple tumours arising from neural crest tissue (multiple endocrine neoplasia). Some 95% of these tumours are benign. The classic presentation is with fasting hypoglycaemia, but early symptoms may also develop in the late morning or afternoon. Recurrent hypoglycaemia is often present for months or years before the diagnosis is made, and the symptoms may be atypical or even bizarre; the presenting features in one series are given in Table 19.14. Common misdiagnoses include psychiatric disorders, particularly pseudodementia in elderly people, epilepsy and cerebrovascular disease. Whipple's triad remains the basis of clinical diagnosis. This is satisfied when:

- symptoms are associated with fasting or exercise
- hypoglycaemia is confirmed during these episodes
- glucose relieves the symptoms.

A fourth criterion – demonstration of inappropriately high insulin levels during hypoglycaemia – may usefully be added to these.

The diagnosis is confirmed by the demonstration of hypoglycaemia in association with inappropriate and excessive insulin secretion. Hypoglycaemia is demonstrated by:

- Measurement of *overnight fasting* (16 hours) glucose and insulin levels on three occasions. About 90% of patients with insulinomas will have low glucose and non-suppressed (normal or elevated) insulin levels.
- A prolonged 72-hour *supervised fast* if overnight testing is inconclusive and symptoms persist.

Autonomous insulin secretion is demonstrated by lack of the normal feedback suppression during hypoglycaemia. This may be shown by measuring insulin, C-peptide or proinsulin during a spontaneous episode of hypoglycaemia.

Treatment of insulinoma

The most effective therapy is surgical excision of the

Table 19.14 Presenting features of insulinoma
Diplopia
Sweating, palpitations, weakness
Confusion or abnormal behaviour
Loss of consciousness
Grand mal seizures

tumour, but insulinomas are often very small and difficult to localize. Many techniques can be used to attempt to localize insulinomas. Sensitivity and specificity vary between centres and between operators. These include highly selective angiography, contrast-enhanced high-resolution CT scanning, scanning with radio-labelled somatostatin (some insulinomas express somatostatin receptors), and endoscopic and intraoperative ultrasound scanning. Venous sampling for the detection of 'hot spots' of high insulin concentration in the various intra-abdominal veins is still used occasionally.

Medical treatment with diazoxide is useful when the insulinoma is malignant, in patients in whom a tumour cannot be located, and in elderly patients with mild symptoms. Symptoms may also remit on treatment with a somatostatin analogue (octreotide or lanreotide).

Hypoglycaemia with other tumours

Hypoglycaemia may develop in the course of advanced neoplasia and cachexia, and has been described in association with many tumour types. Certain massive tumours, especially sarcomas, may produce hypoglycaemia owing to the secretion of insulin-like growth factor-1. True ectopic insulin secretion is extremely rare.

Postprandial hypoglycaemia

If frequent venous blood glucose samples are taken following a prolonged glucose tolerance test, about one in four subjects will have at least one value below 3 mmol/L. The arteriovenous glucose difference is quite marked during this phase, so that very few are truly hypoglycaemic in terms of arterial (or capillary) blood glucose content. Failure to appreciate this simple fact led some authorities to believe that postprandial (or reactive) hypoglycaemia was a potential 'organic' explanation for a variety of complaints that might otherwise have been considered psychosomatic. An epidemic of false 'hypoglycaemia' followed, particularly in the USA. Later work showed a poor correlation between symptoms and biochemical hypoglycaemia. Even so, a number of otherwise normal people occasionally become pale, weak and sweaty at times when meals are due, and report benefit from advice to take regular snacks between meals.

True postprandial hypoglycaemia may develop in the presence of alcohol, which 'primes' the cells to produce an exaggerated insulin response to carbohydrate. The person who substitutes alcoholic beverages for lunch is particularly at risk. Postprandial hypoglycaemia sometimes occurs after gastric surgery, owing to rapid gastric emptying and mismatching of nutrient absorption and insulin secretion. This is referred to as 'dumping' but it is now rarely encountered (see p. 286).

Hepatic and renal causes of hypoglycaemia

The liver can maintain a normal glucose output despite extensive damage, and hepatic hypoglycaemia is un-

common. It is particularly a problem with fulminant hepatic failure.

The kidney has a subsidiary role in glucose production (via gluconeogenesis in the renal cortex), and hypoglycaemia is sometimes a problem in terminal renal failure.

Hereditary fructose intolerance occurs in 1 in 20 000 live births and can cause hypoglycaemia (see p. 1143).

Endocrine causes of hypoglycaemia

Deficiencies of hormones antagonistic to insulin are rare but well-recognized causes of hypoglycaemia. These include hypopituitarism, isolated adrenocorticotrophic hormone (ACTH) deficiency, and Addison's disease.

Drug-induced hypoglycaemia

Many drugs have been reported to produce isolated cases of hypoglycaemia, but usually only when other predisposing factors are present:

- Sulphonylureas may be used in the treatment of diabetes or may be taken by non-diabetics in suicide attempts.
- Quinine may produce severe hypoglycaemia in the course of treatment for falciparum malaria.
- Salicylates may cause hypoglycaemia; usually accidental ingestion by children.
- Propranolol can induce hypoglycaemia in the presence of strenuous exercise or starvation.
- Pentamidine used in the treatment of resistant pneumocystis pneumonia (p. 136).

Alcohol-induced hypoglycaemia

Alcohol inhibits gluconeogenesis. Alcohol-induced hypoglycaemia occurs in poorly nourished chronic alcoholics, binge drinkers and in children who have taken relatively small amounts of alcohol, since they have a diminished hepatic glycogen reserve. They present with coma and hypothermia.

Factitious hypoglycaemia

This is a relatively common variant of self-induced disease and is much more common than an insulinoma. Hypoglycaemia is produced by surreptitious self-administration of insulin or sulphonylureas. Many patients in this category have been extensively investigated for an insulinoma. Measurement of C-peptide levels during hypoglycaemia should identify patients who are injecting insulin; sulphonylurea abuse can be detected by chromatography of plasma or urine.

FURTHER READING
Markes V, Teale JD (1996) Investigation of hypoglycaemia. *Clinical Endocrinology* **44**: 133–136.

DISORDERS OF LIPID METABOLISM

Lipid physiology

Lipids are insoluble in water, and are transported in the bloodstream as macromolecular complexes. In these complexes, lipids (principally triglyceride, cholesterol and cholesterol esters) are surrounded by a stabilizing coat of phospholipid. Proteins (called apoproteins) embedded into the surface of these 'lipoprotein' particles exert a stabilizing function and allow the particles to be recognized by receptors in the liver and the peripheral tissues. The structure of a chylomicron (one type of lipo-protein particle) is illustrated in Figure 19.17.

Five principal types of lipoprotein particles are found in the blood (Fig. 19.18). They are structurally different and can be separated in the laboratory by their density and electrophoretic mobility. The larger particles give postprandial plasma its cloudy appearance. More than half of all patients aged under 60 with angiographically confirmed coronary artery disease have a lipoprotein disorder.

The genes for all the major apoproteins and that for the low-density lipoprotein (LDL) receptor have been isolated, sequenced and their chromosomal sites mapped. Production of abnormal apoproteins is known to produce, or predispose to, several types of lipid disorder, and it is likely that others will be discovered.

Chylomicrons (Fig. 19.18)

Chylomicrons are synthesized in the small intestine postprandially, passing initially into the intestinal lymphatic drainage, then along the thoracic duct into the bloodstream. They contain triglyceride and a small amount of cholesterol and its ester, and provide the main mechanism for transporting the digestion products of dietary fat to the liver and peripheral tissues. Each newly formed chylomicron contains several different apoproteins (B-48, A-I, A-II), and acquires apoproteins C-II and E by transfer from high-density lipoprotein (HDL) particles in

Fig. 19.18 Schematic representation of the sites of origin, interaction between, and fate of, the major lipoprotein particles.

the bloodstream. Apoprotein C-II binds to specific receptors in adipose tissue and skeletal muscle and the liver and allows the endothelial enzyme, lipoprotein lipase, to remove most of the triglyceride from the particle. The remaining chylomicron remnant particle, which contains the bulk of the original cholesterol, is taken up by the liver by mechanisms which are not fully understood, possibly mediated by apoprotein E.

Very-low-density lipoprotein (VLDL) particles
(Fig. 19.18)

These are synthesized continuously in the liver and contain most of the body's endogenously synthesized triglyceride and a smaller quantity of cholesterol. They are the body's main source of energy during prolonged fasting. Apoprotein B-100 is an essential component of VLDL. Apoproteins C-II and E are incorporated later into VLDL by transfer from HDL particles. As they pass round the circulation, VLDL particles bind through apoprotein C-II allowing triglyceride to be progressively removed by lipoprotein lipase in the capillary endothelium. This leaves a particle, now depleted of triglyceride and apoprotein C-II, called an intermediate-density lipoprotein (IDL) particle.

Fig. 19.17 Schematic diagram of a chylomicron particle (75–1200 nm) showing apoproteins lying in the surface membrane.

Intermediate-density lipoprotein particles
(Fig. 19.18)

These have apoprotein B-100 and apoprotein E molecules on the particle surface. Most IDL particles bind to liver LDL receptors through the apoprotein E molecule and are then catabolized. Some IDL particles have further triglyceride removed (by the enzyme hepatic lipase), producing LDL particles.

Low-density lipoprotein particles (Fig. 19.18)

LDL particles are the main carrier of cholesterol, and deliver it both to the liver and to peripheral cells. The surface of the LDL particle contains a single apoprotein B-100, and also apoprotein E. The apoprotein B-100 is the principal ligand for the LDL clearance receptor. This receptor lies within coated pits on the surface of the hepatocyte. Once bound to the receptor, the coated pit invaginates and fuses with liposomes which destroy the LDL particle (Fig. 19.19). The number of hepatic LDL clearance receptors regulates the circulating LDL concentration, which is also influenced by controlling the activity of the rate-limiting enzyme in the cholesterol synthetic pathway, hydroxymethylglutaryl coenzyme A (HMG-CoA) reductase (Fig. 7.4).

LDL particles can deposit lipid into the walls of the peripheral vasculature. Not all the cholesterol synthesized by the liver is packaged immediately into lipoprotein particles. Some is oxidized into bile salts. Both bile salts and cholesterol are excreted in the bile: both are then reabsorbed through the terminal ileum and recirculated (enterohepatic circulation).

LDL particles become Lp(a) lipoproteins as a result of the linkage of apoprotein (a) to aproprotein B-100 with a single disulphide bond. Raised levels of Lp(a) lipoprotein are a risk factor for cardiovascular disease.

High-density lipoprotein particles (Fig. 19.18)

Nascent HDL particles are produced in both the liver and intestine. They are disc shaped, seemingly inert and contain apoprotein A-I. They are transmuted into mature particles by the acquisition of phospholipids, and the E and C apoproteins from chylomicrons and VLDL particles in the circulation. The more mature HDL particles take up cholesterol from cells in the peripheral tissues aided by cholesterol-efflux regulatory protein – a product of the ATP-binding cassette transporter 1 gene (*ABC1* gene). As it is taken up, the enzyme lecithin-cholesterol acyl-transferase (LCAT), activated by the apoprotein A on the particle's surface, esterifies the sequestered cholesterol. The HDL particle transports cholesterol away from the periphery and may transfer it indirectly to other particles such as VLDL in the circulation or deliver its cholesterol directly to the liver (reverse cholesterol transport) and steroid-synthetic tissues (ovaries, testes, adrenal cortex).

This direct delivery takes place through scavenger-receptor B1. In experimental animals the absence of scavenger-receptor B1 dramatically accelerates the development of atheroma, and genetically programmed overproduction suppresses atheroma formation.

Measurement

When a laboratory measures fasting serum lipids, the majority of the total cholesterol concentration consists of LDL particles with a 20–30% contribution from HDL particles. The triglyceride concentration largely reflects the circulating number of VLDL particles, since chylomicrons are not normally present in the fasted state. If the patient is not fasted, the total triglyceride concentration will be raised owing to the additional presence of triglyceride-rich chylomicrons.

Epidemiology and lipids

LDL and total cholesterol

Population studies have repeatedly demonstrated a strong association between both total and LDL cholesterol concentration and coronary heart risk. There is a strong link between mean fat consumption, mean serum cholesterol concentration and the prevalence of coronary heart disease between countries. The exception is France where the cardiovascular risk is only moderate – perhaps owing to high alcohol consumption. Studies of migrants, particularly of Japanese men migrating to Hawaii, have shown that as diet changes, and cholesterol concentrations rise, so does the cardiovascular risk. Such studies show the role of the environment rather than the genetic make-up of a population.

The Multiple Risk Factor Intervention Trial (MRFIT) screened one-third of a million American men for various cardiovascular risk factors and then followed them for 6 years. Data from this study have shown that although cardiovascular risk rises progressively as total cholesterol

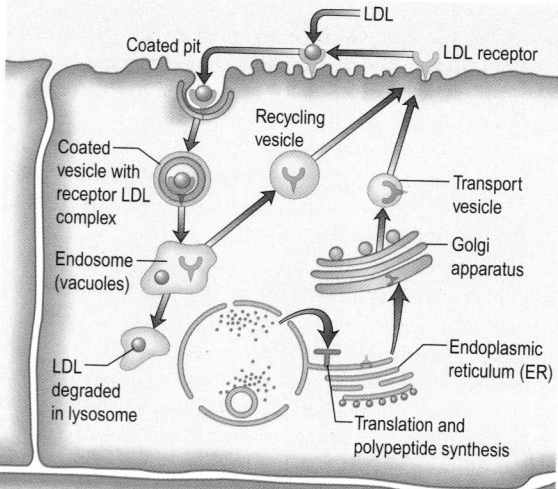

Fig. 19.19 **Receptor-mediated endocytosis.** LDL receptors are formed in the endoplasmic reticulum and transported via the Golgi apparatus to the surface of a hepatocyte. LDLs bind to these receptors, are internalized and taken up by the endosome. The receptor is recycled back to the surface, while the LDL is broken down by the lysosomes, freeing cholesterol needed for membrane synthesis.

Fig. 19.20 The Multiple Risk Factor Intervention Trial. Relationship between levels of serum cholesterol and risks of fatal coronary artery disease in a longitudinal study of more than 361 000 men screened for entry into the trial. From Stamler J, Wentworth D, Neaton JD (1986) *Journal of the American Medical Association* **256**: 2823.

concentration increases (Fig. 19.20), the risk increase is modest for individuals with no other cardiovascular risk factors. With each additional risk factor the effect produced by the same difference in cholesterol concentration becomes greatly magnified. The Framingham Study has reproduced these findings in a separate population.

HDL cholesterol
Epidemiological studies have shown that higher HDL concentrations protect against cardiovascular disease. HDL also has effects on the function of platelets and of the haemostatic cascade. These properties may favourably influence thrombogenesis.

VLDL particles (triglycerides)
There is a relatively weak independent link between raised concentrations of (triglyceride-rich) VLDL particles and cardiovascular risk. Very raised triglyceride concentrations (> 6 mmol/L) cause a greatly increased risk of acute pancreatitis and retinal vein thrombosis. Hypertriglyceridaemia tends to occur in association with a reduced HDL concentration. Much of the cardiovascular risk associated with 'hypertriglyceridaemia' turns out on multivariate analysis to be due to the associated low HDL levels and not to the hypertriglyceridaemia itself.

Chylomicrons
Excess chylomicrons do not confer an excess cardiovascular risk, but raise the total plasma triglyceride concentration.

HYPERLIPIDAEMIA

Hyperlipidaemia results from genetic predisposition interacting with an individual's diet.

Table 19.15 Causes of secondary hyperlipidaemia

Hypothyroidism
Diabetes mellitus (when poorly controlled)
Obesity
Renal impairment
Nephrotic syndrome
Dysglobulinaemia
Hepatic dysfunction
Drugs:
   Oral contraceptives in susceptible individuals
   Retinoids, thiazide diuretics, corticosteroids, op'DDD
      (used in the treatment of Cushing's syndrome),
      sirolimus (and other immunosuppressive agents)

Secondary hyperlipidaemia
If a lipid disorder has been detected it is vital to carry out a clinical history, examination and simple special investigations to detect causes of secondary hyperlipidaemia (Table 19.15), which may need treatment in their own right. Hypothyroidism, diabetes, renal disease and abnormal liver function can all raise plasma lipid levels.

CLASSIFICATION, CLINICAL FEATURES AND INVESTIGATION OF PRIMARY HYPERLIPIDAEMIAS

As the genetic basis of lipid disorders becomes clearer, the genetic classification of Goldstein and colleagues is proving of greater clinical relevance than the Fredrickson (WHO) classification (based on the pattern of lipoproteins found in plasma). The lack of direct correspondence between these two systems of classification can be confusing. For clarity we have used the functional/genetic classification and not the Fredrickson classification. This has the advantage that the genetic disorders may be grouped by the results of simple lipid biochemistry into causes of:

- disorders of VLDL and chylomicrons – hypertriglyceridaemia alone
- disorders of LDL – hypercholesterolaemia alone
- disorders of HDL
- combined hyperlipidaemia.

Disorders of VLDL and chylomicrons – hypertriglyceridaemia alone
The majority of cases appear to be due to multiple genes acting together to produce a modest excess of circulating concentration of VLDL particles, such cases being termed polygenic hypertriglyceridaemia.

In a proportion of cases there will be a family history of a lipid disorder or its effects (e.g. pancreatitis). Such cases are often classified as familial hypertriglyceridaemia. The defect underlying the vast majority of such cases is not understood. The main clinical feature is a history of attacks of pancreatitis or retinal vein thrombosis in some individuals.

Table 19.16 The genetic defects underlying the common lipoprotein disorders

Disorder	Affected gene	Chromosome	Frequency
Common disorders			
Heterozygous familial hypercholesterolaemia	LDL receptor	19	1 : 500
Familial defective apoprotein B	Apo B-100	2	1 : 700
Hypobetalipoproteinaemia	Apo B-100	2	1 : 1000
Familial combined hyperlipidaemia	As yet unknown	As yet unknown	1 : 200
Familial hypertriglyceridaemia	As yet unknown	As yet unknown	1 : 200
Some rarer disorders			
Homozygous familial hypercholesterolaemia	LDL receptor	19	1 : 1 000 000
Lipoprotein lipase deficiency	As yet unknown	As yet unknown	1 : 1 000 000 (homozygous)
Apoprotein C-II deficiency	Apo C-II	19	40 cases

Lipoprotein lipase deficiency and apoprotein C-II deficiency

These are rare diseases which produce greatly elevated triglyceride concentrations owing to the persistence of chylomicrons (and not VLDL particles) in the circulation. The chylomicrons persist because the triglyceride within cannot be metabolized if the enzyme lipoprotein lipase is defective, or because the triglycerides cannot gain access to the normal enzyme owing to deficiency of the apoprotein C-II on their surface. Patients present in childhood with eruptive xanthomas, lipaemia retinalis and retinal vein thrombosis, pancreatitis and hepato-splenomegaly. If not identified in childhood, it can present in adults with gross hypertriglyceridaemia resistant to simple measures. The presence of chylo-microns floating like cream on top of fasting plasma suggests this diagnosis. It is confirmed by plasma electrophoresis or ultracentrifugation. An abnormality of apoprotein C can be deduced if the hyper-triglyceridaemia improves temporarily after infusing fresh frozen plasma, and lipoprotein lipase deficiency is likely if it does not.

Disorders of LDL – hypercholesterolaemia alone

Heterozygous familial hypercholesterolaemia is an autosomal dominant monogenic disorder present in 1 in 500 of the normal population. The average primary care physician would therefore be expected to have four such patients on his or her list, but because of clustering within families the prevalence is lower in some lists and much higher in others. There is an increased prevalence in some racial groups (e.g. French Canadians, Finns, South Africans). Surprisingly, most individuals with this disorder remain undetected. Patients may have no physical signs, in which case the diagnosis is made on the presence of very high plasma cholesterol concentrations which are unresponsive to dietary modification and are associated with a typical family history of early cardio-vascular disease. Diagnosis can more easily be made if typical clinical features are present. These include xanthomatous thickening of the Achilles tendons and xanthomas over the extensor tendons of the fingers. Xanthelasma may be present, but is not diagnostic of familial hypercholesterolaemia.

The genetic defect is the underproduction or malproduction of the LDL cholesterol uptake receptor in the liver (Table 19.16). Over 150 different mutations in the LDL receptor have been described to date. Fifty per cent of men with the disease will die by the age of 60, most from coronary artery disease, if untreated.

Homozygous familial hypercholesterolaemia is very rare indeed. Affected children have no LDL receptors in the liver. They have a hugely elevated LDL cholesterol concentration, and massive deposition of lipid in arterial walls, the aorta and the skin. The natural history is for death from ischaemic heart disease in late childhood or adolescence. Repeated plasmapheresis has been used to remove LDL cholesterol with some success in these patients. Liver transplantation offers the possibility of cure, but the numbers of patients having undergone this procedure is small. The possibility of gene therapy offers a glimmer of hope on the horizon for affected individuals.

Mutations in the apoprotein B-100 gene cause another relatively common single gene disorder. Since LDL particles bind to their clearance receptor in the liver through apoprotein B-100, this defect also results in high LDL concentrations in the blood, and a clinical picture which closely resembles classical heterozygous familial hypercholesterolaemia. The two disorders can be dis-tinguished clearly only by genetic tests. The approach to treatment is the same.

Polygenic hypercholesterolaemia is a term used to lump together patients with raised serum cholesterol concentrations, but without one of the monogenic disorders above. They exist in the right-hand tail of the normal distribution of cholesterol concentration. The precise nature of the polygenic variation in plasma cholesterol concentration remains unknown. Variations in the apoprotein E gene (chromosome 19) appear to contri-bute towards the problem in some individuals in this heterogeneous group.

Disorders of HDL – normal total cholesterol and triglycerides

Tangier disease

Tangier disease is an autosomal recessive disorder characterized by a low HDL cholesterol concentration. Cholesterol accumulates in reticuloendothelial tissue and arteries causing enlarged orange-coloured tonsils and hepatosplenomegaly. Cardiovascular disease, corneal opacities and a polyneuropathy also occur. This has been shown to be due to a mutation in the ATP-binding cassette transporter 1 gene (*ABC1* gene – see HDL physiology above) which normally promotes cholesterol uptake from cells by HDL particles.

Other mutations in this gene have been found in a few families with autosomal dominant HDL deficiency. It is as yet unknown whether abnormalities of this gene contribute to the low HDL cholesterol concentrations commonly seen in cardiovascular disease patients.

Combined hyperlipidaemia (hypercholesterolaemia and hypertriglyceridaemia)

The most common patient group is a polygenic combined hyperlipidaemia. Patients have an increased cardiovascular risk due to both high LDL concentrations and suppression of HDL by the hypertriglyceridaemia.

Familial combined hyperlipidaemia

This is relatively common, affecting 1 in 200 of the general population. The genetic basis for the disorder has not yet been characterized. It is diagnosed by finding raised cholesterol and triglyceride concentrations in association with a typical family history. There are no typical physical signs.

Remnant hyperlipidaemia

This is a rare (1 in 5000) cause of combined hyperlipidaemia. It is due to accumulation of LDL remnant particles and is associated with an extremely high risk of cardiovascular disease. It may be suspected in a patient with raised total cholesterol and triglyceride concentrations by finding xanthomas in the palmar creases (diagnostic) and the presence of tuberous xanthomas, typically over the knees and elbows (Fig. 19.21). Remnant hyperlipidaemia is almost always due to the inheritance of a variant of the apoprotein E allele (apoprotein E2) together with an aggravating factor such as another primary hyperlipidaemia. When suspected clinically the diagnosis can be confirmed using ultracentrifugation of plasma, or phenotyping apoprotein E.

THERAPIES AVAILABLE TO TREAT HYPERLIPIDAEMIA

The lipid-lowering diet

Studies have shown that dietitians helping patients to adjust their own diet to meet the nutritional targets set

Fig. 19.21 Tuberous xanthomata behind the elbow and lipid deposits in the hand creases in a patient with remnant hyperlipidaemia.

out below produce a better lipid-lowering effect than does the issuing of standard diet sheets and advice from a doctor. The main elements of a lipid-lowering diet are set out below.

Reduce the total fat intake

Dairy products and meat are the principal sources of saturated fat in the diet. Intake of these products should therefore be reduced, and fish and poultry should be substituted. Visible fat and skin should be removed before cooking and preparing meat dishes. Meat products including sausages and reconstituted meats (such as 'luncheon meat') should be avoided since the concentration of fat is unknown and often high. Baking and grilling of meats reduces the fat content and is preferred to frying. Low-fat or cottage cheese and skimmed or semi-skimmed milk should be substituted for the standard full-fat varieties. Pastries and cakes contain large quantities of fat and should be avoided. The overall aim should be to decrease fat intake such that it is providing approximately 30% of the total energy intake in the diet. Further reduction in fat intake is unacceptable to many patients.

Substitution with monounsaturates and polyunsaturates

Monounsaturated oils, particularly olive oil, and polyunsaturated oils such as sunflower, safflower, corn and soya oil, should be used in cooking instead of saturated fat-rich alternatives.

Reduce the dietary cholesterol intake

Liver, offal and fish roes should be avoided. Although eggs and prawns are rich in cholesterol their total contribution to the body's cholesterol pool is small and they can still be part of a balanced lipid-lowering diet.

Increase the intake of fibre (non-starch polysaccharides, NSPs)

Foods high in soluble fibre, such as pulses, legumes, root vegetables, leafy vegetables, and unprocessed cereals, help reduce circulating lipid concentrations. These should be substituted in the diet in the place of higher-fat alternatives.

Reduce alcohol consumption

Excess alcohol is a cause of secondary hyperlipidaemia, and may worsen primary lipid disorders.

Achieve an ideal bodyweight

Treatment of obesity is part of the management of hyperlipidaemia, both because it will help the lipid disorder itself, and because obesity is an independent cardiovascular risk factor.

Consider foods containing stanol esters

Plant stanols reduce the absorption of cholesterol from the intestine by competing for space in the micelles that deliver lipid to the mucosal cells of the gut. They are largely unabsorbed and excreted in the stool. Increasing the amount of plant stanol in the diet 10-fold by using a margarine (e.g. Benecol) containing added stanol esters lowers LDL cholesterol by approximately 0.35–0.5 mmol/L. A reduction in the risk of heart disease of about 25% would be expected if this reduction in LDL cholesterol was applied to a population.

Drugs

The classes of drugs used to treat hyperlipidaemia are listed in Table 19.17.

MANAGEMENT OF SPECIFIC HYPERLIPIDAEMIAS

Screening

Most patients with hyperlipidaemia are asymptomatic and have no clinical signs. Many are discovered during the screening of high-risk individuals. Whose lipids should be measured?

There are great doubts as to whether blanket screening of plasma lipids is warranted. Selective screening of people at high risk of cardiovascular disease should be undertaken, to include those with:

- a family history of coronary heart disease (especially below 50 years of age)
- a family history of lipid disorders
- the presence of a xanthoma
- the presence of xanthelasma or corneal arcus before the age of 40 years
- obesity
- diabetes mellitus
- hypertension
- acute pancreatitis
- those undergoing renal replacement therapy.

Where one family member is known to have a monogenic disorder such as familial hypercholesterolaemia (1 in 500

of the population), siblings and children must have their plasma lipid concentrations measured. It is also worth screening the prospective partners of any patients with this heterozygous monogenic lipid disorder because of the small risk of producing children homozygous for the condition.

Acute severe illnesses such as myocardial infarction can derange plasma lipid concentrations for up to 3 months. Plasma lipid concentrations should be measured either within 48 hours of an acute myocardial infarction (before derangement has had time to occur) or 3 months later.

Serum cholesterol concentration does not change significantly after a meal and as a screening test a random blood sample is sufficient. If the total cholesterol concentration is raised, HDL cholesterol, triglyceride, and LDL cholesterol concentrations should be quantitated on a fasting sample. If a test for hypertriglyceridaemia is needed, a fasting blood sample is mandatory.

Hypertriglyceridaemia

A serum triglyceride concentration below 2.0 mmol/L is normal. In the range 2.0–6.0 mmol/L no specific intervention will be needed unless there are coincident cardiovascular risk factors, and in particular a strong family history of early cardiovascular death. In general, patients should be advised that they have a minor lipid problem, offered advice on weight reduction if obese, and advice on correcting other cardiovascular risk factors.

If the triglyceride concentration is above 6.0 mmol/L there is a risk of pancreatitis and retinal vein thrombosis. Patients should be advised to reduce their weight if overweight and start a formal lipid-lowering diet (see below). A proportion of individuals with hypertriglyceridaemia have livers which respond to even moderate degrees of alcohol intake by allowing accumulation or excess production of VLDL particles. If hypertriglyceridaemia persists, lipid measurements should be repeated before and after a 3-week interval of complete abstinence from alcohol. If a considerable improvement results, lifelong abstinence may prove necessary. Other drugs, including thiazides, oestrogens and glucocorticoids, can have a similar effect to alcohol in susceptible patients.

If the triglyceride concentration remains elevated above 6.0 mmol/L, despite the above measures, drug therapy is warranted. A fibric acid derivative is the agent of first choice. Nicotinic acid may be used in addition but its side-effects are often a problem. Fish oil capsules which contain ω-3 long-chain fatty acids are also effective in lowering triglyceride concentrations.

The severe hypertriglyceridaemia associated with the rare disorders of lipoprotein lipase deficiency and apoprotein C-II deficiency may require restriction of dietary fat to 10–20% of total energy intake and the use of special preparations of medium-chain triglycerides in cooking in place of oil or fat. Medium-chain triglycerides are not absorbed via chylomicrons (see p. 296).

Table 19.17 Drugs used in the management of hyperlipidaemia

Drug	Mechanism of action	Contraindications and adverse reactions	Expected therapeutic effect	Long-term safety
Statins e.g. Simvastatin Pravastatin Fluvastatin Atorvastatin	Inhibit the rate-limiting step in cholesterol synthesis (HMG CoA reductase)	*Contraindications:* Active liver disease, pregnancy, lactation *Adverse effects:* Derangement of liver biochemistry, diarrhoea biochemical tests: periodically during treatment. Myositis. Raise ciclosporin level in blood	30–60% reduction in LDL cholesterol Modest triglyceride lowering Tiny effect on HDL cholesterol Atorvastatin and particularly rosuvastatin have the most potent cholesterol-lowering effects	Simvastatin, Atorvastatin and Pravastatin have good long-term safety in large-scale trials and in clinical practice
Cholesterol absorption inhibitors e.g. Ezetimibe	Inhibition of gut absorption of cholesterol from food and also from bile. Mechanism of this inhibition is currently unclear	*Contraindications:* Lactation *Adverse effects:* Occasional diarrhoea, abdominal discomfort	Reduce LDL cholesterol by additional 10–15% if given with a statin Triglyceride concentrations reduced by 10% Increase HDL cholesterol by 5%	Mostly act in gut and little is absorbed. Short term safety good. Not available long enough for medium- or long-term safety to be known
Cholesterol-binding resins e.g. Colestyramine Colestipol	Bind bile acids in the gut preventing enterohepatic circulation. Liver makes more bile acids fromcholesterol, depleting the cholesterol pool	*Adverse effects:* Gastrointestinal side-effects predominate. Palatability is a problem. *Counselling:* Other drugs bind to resins and should be taken 1 h before or 4 h afterwards	8–15% reduction in LDL Little or no effect on HDL cholesterol 5–15% rise in triglyceride concentration	Not systemically absorbed. Safety profile is good and resins are of low risk in women of childbearing age. Fat-soluble vitamin supplements may be required in children, pregnancy and breast-feeding
Fibric acid derivatives e.g. Gemfibrozil Bezafibrate Fenofibrate Ciprofibrate	Complex and not fully understood 1. Limit substrate availability for hepatic triglyceride synthesis 2. Modulate LDL/ligand interaction 3. Promote action of lipoprotein lipase 4. Stimulate reverse transport of cholesterol	*Contraindications:* Severe hepatic or renal impairment, gallbladder disease, pregnancy *Adverse effects:* Reversible myositis, nausea, predispose to gallstones, non-specific malaise, impotence	Reduction of LDL cholesterol by 10–15% and triglycerides by 25–35% HDL cholesterol concentrations increase by 10–50% (newer agents often have greater beneficial effect on HDL)	No knowledge of effect on developing fetus. Avoid in women of child-bearing age. Long-term safety appears good

Cont'd

Hypercholesterolaemia (without hypertriglyceridaemia)

Familial hypercholesterolaemia
Individuals often require treatment with diet and more than one cholesterol-lowering drug. The cholesterol absorption inhibitor ezetimibe is a logical addition to a statin and has a low side-effect profile (Table 19.17). Bile acid sequestrants are an alternative to ezetimibe, but have greater problems with tolerability. Concurrent therapy with statins and fibrates is usually avoided, in view of their overlapping side-effects, but in very severe cases such mixed therapy has been undertaken under close supervision.

Primary prevention for people with risk factors
Lipid-lowering therapy using a statin, or alternatives as above, should be considered in asymptomatic individuals irrespective of the total or LDL cholesterol level in type 2 diabetes alone, or with two or more of: positive family history of cardiovascular disease, albuminuria, hypertension, smoking.

Table 19.17 (Cont'd)   Drugs used in the management of hyperlipidaemia

Drug	Mechanism of action	Contraindications and adverse reactions	Expected therapeutic effect	Long-term safety
Nicotinic acid and derivatives e.g. Nicotinic acid Modified-release nicotinic acid Acipimox	Unclear. Probably inhibit lipid synthesis in the liver by reducing free fatty acid concentrations through an inhibitory effect on lipolysis in fat tissue	*Contraindications:* Pregnancy, breast-feeding. *Adverse effects:* Value limited by frequent side-effects: headache, flushing, dizziness, nausea, malaise, itching, abnormal liver biochemistry. Glucose intolerance, hyperuricaemia, activation of peptic ulcers, hyperpigmentation may occur	Reduce LDL cholesterol by 5–10% Reduce triglycerides by 15–20% HDL cholesterol increased by 10–20%	Medium-term safety but marred by the adverse effects listed. Modified-release preparation reduces side-effect incidence
Omega-3 marine triglycerides	Reduce hepatic VLDL secretion	Occasional nausea and belching	Reduce triglycerides in severe hypertriglyceridaemia No favourable change in other lipids, and may aggravate hypercholesterolaemia in a few patients	Long-term safety is not yet known but seems unlikely to be poor

Primary prevention for people without risk factors

In the absence of risk factors, lipid-lowering therapy should be considered in asymptomatic men with total cholesterol levels persistently above 6.5 mmol/L despite dietary change. Many would use lipid-lowering therapy in an asymptomatic man with this level of total cholesterol if he had a positive family history of cardio-vascular disease and no other risk factors. The situation for women is less clear.

Secondary prevention

As a generality, statin treatment is warranted for any patient with known macrovascular disease (coronary artery disease, TIA or stroke, peripheral vascular disease), irrespective of the total or LDL cholesterol level. If a statin is not tolerated, a fibrate or fibrate/cholesterol absorption inhibitor combination are alternatives.

Risk prevention tables (p. 803)

An array of risk prediction tables (see pp. 803 and 804) are available to allow quantification of the risk of a patient having a cardiovascular event within the next 10 years. Some advocate the use of these risk tables as a guide to treatment – for example if the 10-year risk reaches the 15% or the 30% level. We side with those who have reservations over their use. Such risk analyses are a useful approach in helping to decide whether to use treatments such as aspirin. Aspirin probably has no effect until the day an atherosclerotic plaque ruptures, when it may then prevent thrombosis leading to a heart attack or stroke. Furthermore it has a significant associated morbidity and mortality (from bleeding). At a 10-year cardiovascular risk level of 15% the benefit/risk ratio for

aspirin becomes favourable. At the 30% level the benefits are clear.

In contrast, the use of lipid-lowering agents, if initially tolerated, has a low associated morbidity and mortality. These agents probably reduce the rate of atheroma accumulation over a period of decades. When a patient is young, the chance that atheroma will be bad enough to cause a heart attack or stroke within the next 10 years will be small, even if atheroma is accumulating at a swift rate. The level of cardiovascular risk will only rise to the 15% or 30% level when the patient gets older. Yet it seems bizarre not to treat the gradual accumulation of atheroma when the patient is young with a low 10-year risk, and then to start treatment when age causes the 10-year risk levels to rise to a particular threshold, if all other factors are the same. In choosing whether or not to prescribe, we prefer to consider 'will he/she live long enough to collect some pension and see his/her grandchildren?' rather than 'will he/she have a heart attack or stroke within the next 10 years?'. The answers to these two questions are very different.

Combined hyperlipidaemia (hypercholesterolaemia and hypertriglyceridaemia)

Treatment is the same for all varieties of combined hyperlipidaemia. For any given cholesterol concentration the hypertriglyceridaemia found in the combined hyperlipidaemias increases the cardiovascular risk considerably. Treatment is aimed at reducing serum cholesterol below 6.5 mmol/L and triglycerides below 2.0 mmol/L. Therapy is with diet in the first instance and with drugs if an adequate response has not occurred.

Fibric acid derivatives are the treatment of choice since these reduce both cholesterol and triglyceride concentrations, and also have the benefit of raising cardioprotective HDL concentrations. The combination of a fibric acid derivative and ezetimibe or a bile acid-binding resin is of considerable use when a fibrate alone produces an insufficient reduction in LDL cholesterol. Nicotinic acid can be used in addition, although its unwanted effects render it a third-line agent.

OTHER LIPID DISORDERS

Hypolipidaemia
Low lipid levels can be found in severe protein–energy malnutrition. They are also seen occasionally with severe malabsorption and in intestinal lymphangiectasia.

Hypobetalipoproteinaemia (Table 19.16) is a benign familial condition which is being increasingly recognized. The cholesterol levels are in the range 1–3.5 mmol/L.

Abetalipoproteinaemia
This is described on page 308.

FURTHER READING
Brewer HB (2004) Increasing HDL cholesterol levels. *New England Journal of Medicine* **350**: 1491–1560.
Heart Protection Study Collaborative Group (2004) MRC/BHF Heart Protection Study of cholesterol lowering with simvastatin in 20 536 high risk individuals: a randomized placebo-controlled trial. *Lancet* **363**: 757–767.
Law M (2000) Plant sterol and stanol margarines and health. *British Medical Journal* **320**: 861–864.
Scandinavian Simvastatin Survival Study Group (1994) Randomised trial of cholesterol lowering in 4444 patients with coronary heart disease. *Lancet* **334**: 1383–1389.
Scanu AM (2003) Lp(a) lipoproteins. *New England Journal of Medicine* **349**: 2089–2156.
Smith CR (2004) Lipid lowering therapy – new and established agents reduce risk of cardiovascular events. *Postgraduate Medicine* **115**: 29–30.
Walsh JME, Pignone M (2004) Drug treatment of hyperlipidaemia in women. *Journal of the American Medical Association* **290**: 2243–2252.

INBORN ERRORS OF CARBOHYDRATE METABOLISM

Glycogen storage disease

All mammalian cells can manufacture glycogen, but the main sites of its production are the liver and muscle. Glycogen is a high-molecular-weight glucose polymer. In glycogen storage disease there is either an abnormality in the molecular structure or an increase in glycogen concentration owing to a specific enzyme defect. Almost all these conditions are autosomal recessive in inheritance and present in infancy, except for McArdle's disease, which presents in adults.

Table 19.18 shows the classification and clinical features of some of these diseases.

Galactosaemia

Galactose is normally converted to glucose. However, a deficiency of the enzyme galactose-1-phosphate uridyl-transferase or, less commonly, uridine diphosphate galactase-4-epimerase results in accumulation of galactose-1-phosphate in the blood. The transferase deficiency, inherited as an autosomal recessive, is due in 70% of patients to a glutamine to arginine mis-sense mutation in Q188R. Galactose ingestion (i.e. milk) leads to inanition, failure to thrive, vomiting, hepatomegaly and jaundice, diabetes, cataracts and developmental delay. A lactose-free diet stops the acute toxicity but poor growth and problems with speech and mental development still occur with the transferase deficiency.

Prenatal diagnosis and diagnosis of the carrier state are possible by measurement of the level of galactose-1-phosphate in the blood.

Galactokinase deficiency also results in galactosaemia and early cataract formation.

Defects of fructose metabolism

Absorbed fructose is chiefly metabolized in the liver to lactic acid or glucose. Three defects of metabolism in the liver and intestine occur; all are inherited as autosomal recessive traits:

- *Fructosuria* is due to fructokinase deficiency. It is a benign asymptomatic condition.
- *Hereditary fructose intolerance* is due to fructose-1-phosphate aldolase deficiency. Fructose-1-phosphate accumulates after fructose ingestion, inhibiting both glycogenolysis and gluconeogenesis, resulting in symptoms of severe hypoglycaemia. Hepatomegaly and renal tubular defects occur but are reversible on a fructose- and sucrose-free diet. Intelligence is normal and there is an absence of dental caries.
- *Hereditary fructose-1,6-diphosphatase deficiency* leads to a failure of gluconeogenesis. Infants present with hypoglycaemia, ketosis and lactic acidosis. Dietary control can lead to normal growth.

Pentosuria

Pentosuria is due to reduced activity of NADP-linked sylitol dehydrogenase. It has no clinical significance.

Table 19.18   Some glycogen storage diseases

Type	Affected tissue	Enzyme defect	Clinical features	Tissue needed for diagnosis*	Outcome
Liver glycogenoses					
I (Von Gierke) (25%)	Liver, intestine, kidney	Glucose-6-phosphatase	Hepatomegaly, ketotic hypoglycaemia, stunted growth, obesity, hypotonia	Liver DNA testing	If patients survive initial hypoglycaemia, prognosis is good; hyperuricaemia is a late complication
III (Forbes) (24%)	Liver, muscle (abnormal glycogen structure)	Glycogen debranching enzyme	Like type I	Leucocytes, liver, muscle	Good prognosis but progressive neuropathy and cardiomyopathy
IV (Anderson) (3%)	Liver (abnormal glycogen structure)	Branching enzyme	Failure to thrive, hepatomegaly, cirrhosis and its complications	Leucocytes, liver, muscle	Death in first 5 years Liver transplantation
VI (Hers) (VI and VIII = 30%)	Liver	Liver phosphorylase or phosphorylase kinase	Hepatomegaly with hypoglycaemia in childhood	Liver	Good
VIII	Liver	Phosphorylase 6 kinase deficiency	Hepatomegaly, hypoglycaemic fatiguability	Liver, muscle	No treatment
Muscle glycogenoses					
II (Pompé) (15%)	Liver, muscle, heart	Lysosomal acid α-glucosidase	Heart failure, cardiomyopathy	Fibroblasts, muscles	Death in first 6 months Juvenile and adult variants seen
V (McArdle)	Muscle only	Phosphorylase	Muscle cramps and myoglobinuria after exercise (in adults)	Muscle	Normal life-span; give sucrose prior to exercise
VII (Tarui)	Muscle	Phosphofructokinase	Like type V	Muscle	Like type V

* Tissue obtained is used for the biochemical assay of the enzyme
% = percentage of total number of cases in USA and Europe

INBORN ERRORS OF AMINO ACID METABOLISM

Inborn errors of amino acid metabolism are chiefly inherited as autosomal recessive conditions. The major ones are shown in Table 19.19.

Amino acid transport defects

Amino acids are filtered by the glomerulus, but 95% of the filtered load is reabsorbed in the proximal convoluted tubule by an active transport mechanism. Aminoaciduria results from:

- abnormally high plasma amino acid levels (e.g. phenylketonuria)
- any inherited disorder that damages the tubules secondarily (e.g. galactosaemia)

- tubular reabsorptive defects, either generalized (e.g. Fanconi syndrome) or specific (e.g. cystinuria).

Amino acid transport defects can be congenital or acquired.

GENERALIZED AMINOACIDURIAS

Fanconi syndrome

This occurs in a juvenile form (De Toni–Fanconi–Debré syndrome); in adult life it is often acquired through, for example, heavy metal poisoning, drugs or some renal diseases. There is a generalized defective proximal tubular reabsorption of:

- most amino acids
- glucose
- urate
- phosphate, resulting in hypophosphataemic rickets

Table 19.19 **The major inborn errors of amino acid metabolism**

Disease	Enzyme defect	Incidence	Biochemical and clinical features	Treatment	Prognosis
Albinism	Tyrosinase	1 in 13 000	Amelanosis: whitish hair, pink-white skin, grey-blue eyes Nystagmus, photophobia, strabismus	Symptomatic	Good
Alkaptonuria	Homogentisic acid oxidase	1 in 100 000	Homogentisic acid polymerizes to produce a brown-black product that is deposited in cartilage and other tissues (ochronosis)	None	Good
Homocystinuria Type I	Cystathionine synthase		Homocystine is excreted in urine Learning difficulties Marfan-like syndrome Thrombotic episodes	– – – –	– – – –
Type II	Methylene tetrahydrofolate reductase		Survivors have learning difficulties	–	Many die as neonates
Phenylketonuria	Phenylalanine hydroxylase	1 in 20 000	Brain damage with learning difficulties and epilepsy Phenylpyruvate and its derivatives excreted in urine	Diet low in phenylalanine in first few months of life prevents damage	Good but some intellectual impairment
Histidinaemia	Histidase	Very rare	Learning difficulties	–	–
'Maple syrup' disease	Branched-chain ketoacid dehydrogenase	Very rare	Failure to thrive Fits, neonatal acidosis and severe cerebral degeneration Valine, isoleucine and their derivatives are excreted in urine A milder form is seen	–	Early death
Oxalosis (hyperoxaluria)	Alanine: glyoxylate aminotransferase	Very rare	Nephrocalcinosis, renal stones, renal failure due to deposition of calcium oxalate Prenatal and early diagnosis now possible	–	Liver transplantation ? Gene therapy

There are many other enzyme defects producing, for example, alaninaemia, ammonaemia, argininaemia, citrullinaemia, isovaleric acidaemia, lysinaemia, ornithinaemia or tyrosinaemia

■ bicarbonate, with failure to transport hydrogen ions, causing a renal tubular acidosis that then produces a hyperchloraemic acidosis (p. 717).

Other abnormalities include:

■ potassium depletion, primary or secondary to the acidosis
■ polyuria
■ increased excretion of immunoglobulins and other low-molecular-weight proteins.

Various combinations of the above abnormalities have been described.

The juvenile form begins at the age of 6–9 months, with failure to thrive, vomiting and thirst. The clinical features are as a result of fluid and electrolyte loss and the characteristic vitamin D-resistant rickets.

In the adult, the disease is similar to the juvenile form, but osteomalacia is a major feature.

Treatment of the bone disease is with large doses of vitamin D (e.g. 1–2 mg of 1α-hydroxycholecalciferol with regular blood calcium monitoring). Fluid and electrolyte loss need to be corrected.

Lowe's syndrome (oculocerebrorenal dystrophy)

In this syndrome there is generalized aminoaciduria combined with mental retardation, hypotonia, congenital cataracts and an abnormal skull shape.

SPECIFIC AMINOACIDURIAS

Cystinuria

There is a defective tubular reabsorption and jejunal absorption of cystine and the dibasic amino acids, lysine, ornithine and arginine. Inheritance is either completely or incompletely recessive, so that heterozygotes who have increased excretion of lysine and cystine only can occur. Cystine absorption from the jejunum is impaired but, nevertheless, cystine in peptide form can be absorbed. Cystinuria leads to urinary stones and is responsible for approximately 1–2% of all urinary calculi. The disease often starts in childhood, although most cases present in adult life.

Treatment is with a high fluid intake in order to keep the urinary cystine concentration low. Patients are encouraged to drink up to 3 L over 24 hours and to drink even at night. Penicillamine should be used for patients who cannot keep the cystine concentration of their urine low.

The condition cystinosis must not be confused with cystinuria.

Hartnup's disease

There is defective tubular reabsorption and jejunal absorption of most neutral amino acids but not their peptides. The resulting tryptophan malabsorption produces nicotinamide deficiency (see p. 245). Patients can be asymptomatic, but others develop evidence of pellagra, with cerebellar ataxia, psychiatric disorders and skin lesions. Treatment is with nicotinamide, which often brings about considerable improvement.

Tryptophan malabsorption syndrome (blue diaper syndrome)

This is due to an isolated transport defect for tryptophan: the tryptophan excreted oxidizes to a blue colour on the baby's diaper.

Familial iminoglycinuria

This occurs when there is defective tubular reabsorption of glycine, proline and hydroxyproline. It seems to have few clinical effects.

Methionine malabsorption syndrome

This is due to failure to absorb and excrete methionine, and results in diarrhoea, vomiting and mental retardation. Patients characteristically have an oast-house smell.

LYSOSOMAL STORAGE DISEASES

Lysosomal storage diseases are due to inborn errors of metabolism which are mainly inherited in an autosomal recessive manner.

Glucosylceramide lipidoses: Gaucher's disease

This is the most prevalent lysosomal storage disease and is due to a deficiency in glucocerebrosidase, a specialized lysosomal acid β-glucosidase. This results in accumulation of glucosylceramide in the lysosomes of the reticuloendothelial system, particularly the liver, bone marrow and spleen. Several mutations have been characterized in the glucocerebrosidase gene, the most common being a single base change (N370S) causing the substitution of arginine for serine; this is seen in 70% of Jewish patients. The typical Gaucher cell, a glucocerebroside-containing reticuloendothelial histiocyte, is found in the bone marrow, producing many cytokines such as CD14.

There are three clinical types, the most common presenting in adult life with an insidious onset of hepatosplenomegaly. There is a high incidence in Ashkenazi Jews (1 in 3000 births), and patients have a characteristic pigmentation on exposed parts, particularly the forehead and hands. The clinical spectrum is variable, with patients developing anaemia, evidence of hypersplenism and pathological fractures that are due to bone involvement. Nevertheless, many have a normal life-span.

The diagnosis is made on finding a deficiency of lysosomal B glucocerebrosidase in leucocytes. Plasma chitotriosidase (an enzyme secreted by activated macrophages) is grossly elevated in Gaucher's disease and other lysosomal disorders: it is used to monitor enzyme replacement therapy. Acute Gaucher's disease presents in infancy or childhood with rapid onset of hepatosplenomegaly, with neurological involvement owing to the presence of Gaucher cells in the brain. The outlook is poor.

Some patients with non-neuropathic Gaucher's disease show considerable improvement with infusion of human recombinant glucocerebrosidase (imiglucerase – a human recombinant enzyme). Oral miglustat (an inhibitor of glucosylceramide synthase) is used for mild to moderate Gaucher's disease.

Sphingomyelin cholesterol lipidoses: Niemann–Pick disease

The disease is due to a deficiency of lysosomal sphingomyelinase which results in the accumulation of sphingomyelin cholesterol and glycosphingolipids in the reticuloendothelial macrophages of many organs, particularly the liver, spleen, bone marrow and lymph nodes. The disease usually presents within the first 6 months of life with mental retardation and hepatosplenomegaly; a particular type (11c) presents in adults with dementia. The gene frequency is 1 : 100 in Ashkenazi Jews. Typical foam cells are found in the marrow, lymph nodes, liver and spleen.

The mucopolysaccharidoses (MPSs)

This is a group of disorders caused by the deficiency of lysosomal enzymes (e.g. α-L-iduronidase) required for the catabolism of glycosaminoglycans (mucopolysaccharides).

The catabolism of dermatan sulphate, heparan sulphate, keratin sulphate or chondroitin sulphate may be affected either singularly or together.

Accumulation of glycosaminoglycans in the lysosomes of various tissues results in the disease. Ten forms of MPS have been described; all are chronic but progressive, and a wide spectrum of clinical severity can be seen within a single enzyme defect. The MPS types show many clinical features though in variable amounts, with dysostosis, abnormal facies, poor vision and hearing and joint dysmobility (either stiff or hypermobile) being frequently seen. Mental retardation is present in, for example, Hurler (MPS IH) and San Filippo A (MPS IIIA) types, but normal intelligence and life-span are seen in Scheie (MPS IS). L aronidase infusion reduces lysosomal storage, resulting in clinical improvement.

The GM2 gangliosidoses

In these conditions there is accumulation of GM2 gangliosides in the central nervous system and peripheral nerves. It is particularly common (1 in 2000) in Ashkenazi Jews. *Tay–Sachs disease* is the severest form, where there is a progressive degeneration of all cerebral function, with fits, epilepsy, dementia and blindness, and death usually occurs before 2 years of age. The macula has a characteristic cherry spot appearance.

Fabry's disease

This X-linked recessive condition is due to a deficiency of the lysosomal hydrolase α-galactosidase causing an accumulation of glycosphingolipids with terminal α-galactosyl moieties in the lysosomes of various tissues including the liver, kidney, blood vessels and the ganglion cells of the nervous system. The patients present with peripheral nerve involvement, but eventually most patients develop renal problems in adult life. Treatment is with Agalsidase Beta infusions.

Diagnosis

Many of the sphingolipidoses can be diagnosed by demonstrating the enzyme deficiency, usually in peripheral blood leucocytes.

Prenatal diagnosis is possible in a number of the conditions by obtaining specimens of amniotic cells. Carrier states can also be identified, so that sensible genetic counselling can be given.

FURTHER READING
Cox TM (2001) Gaucher's disease. *Quarterly Journal of Medicine* **94**: 399–402.

AMYLOIDOSIS

Amyloidosis is a disorder of protein metabolism in which there is an extracellular deposition of pathological insoluble fibrillar proteins in organs and tissues. Characteristically, the amyloid protein consists of β-pleated sheets that are responsible for its insolubility and resistance to proteolysis.

Amyloidosis can be acquired or inherited. Classification is based on the nature of the precursor plasma proteins (at least 20) that form the fibrillar deposits. The process for the production of these fibrils appears to be multifactorial and differs amongst the various types of amyloid.

AL amyloidosis (immunoglobulin light chain-associated)

This is a plasma cell dyscrasia, related to multiple myeloma, in which clonal plasma cells in the bone marrow produce immunoglobulins that are amyloidogenic. This may be the outcome of destabilization of light chains owing to substitution of particular amino acids into the light chain variable region. There is a clonal dominance of amyloid light (AL) chains – either the dominant κ or λ isotype – which are excreted in the urine (Bence Jones proteins). This type of amyloid is often associated with lymphoproliferative disorders, such as myeloma, Waldenström's macroglobulinaemia or non-Hodgkin's lymphoma. It rarely occurs before the age of 40 years.

The clinical features are related to the organs involved. These include the kidneys (presenting with proteinuria and the nephrotic syndrome) and the heart (presenting with heart failure). Autonomic and sensory neuropathies are relatively common, and carpal tunnel syndrome with weakness and paraesthesia of the hands may be an early feature. Sensory neuropathy is common. There is an absence of central nervous system involvement.

On examination, hepatomegaly and rarely splenomegaly, cardiomyopathy, polyneuropathy and bruising may be seen. Macroglossia occurs in about 10% of cases and periorbital purpura in 15%.

Familial amyloidoses (transthyretin-associated (ATTR))

These are autosomally dominant transmitted diseases where the mutant protein forms amyloid fibrils, starting usually in middle age. The most common form is due to a mutant – transthyretin – which is a tetrameric protein with four identical subunits. It is a transport protein for thyroxine and retinol-binding protein and mainly synthesized in the liver. Over 80 amino acid substitutions have been described; for example, a common substitution is that of methionine for valine at position 30 (Met 30) in all racial groups, and alanine for threonine (Ala 60) in the English and Irish. These substitutions destabilize the protein, which precipitates following stimulation, and can cause disorders such as familial amyloidotic poly-neuropathy (FAP), cardiomyopathy or the nephrotic syndrome. Major foci of FAP occur in Portugal, Japan and Sweden.

Other less common variants include mutations of apoprotein A-I, gelsolin, fibrinogen Aα and lysozyme.

Clinically, peripheral sensorimotor and autonomic neuropathy are common, with symptoms of autonomic dysfunction, diarrhoea and weight loss. Renal disease is less prevalent than with AL amyloidosis. Macroglossia does not occur. Cardiac problems are usually those of conduction. There may be a family history of unidentified neurological disease.

Other hereditary systemic amyloidoses include other familial amyloid polyneuropathies (e.g. Portuguese, Icelandic, Dutch). There is a familial Creutzfeldt–Jakob disease. In familial Mediterranean fever, renal amyloidosis is a common serious complication.

Reactive systemic (secondary AA) amyloidoses

These are due to amyloid formed from serum amyloid A (SAA), which is an acute phase protein. It is, therefore, related to chronic inflammatory disorders and chronic infection.

Clinical features depend on the nature of the under-lying disorder. Chronic inflammatory disorders include rheumatoid arthritis, inflammatory bowel disease, and untreated familial Mediterranean fever. In developing countries it is still associated with infectious diseases such as tuberculosis, bronchiectasis and osteomyelitis. AA amyloidosis often presents with renal disease, with hepatomegaly and splenomegaly. Macroglossia is not a feature and cardiac involvement is rare.

Other amyloides

Cerebral amyloidosis, Alzheimer's disease and transmissible spongiform encephalopathy

The brain is a common site of amyloid deposition, although it is not directly affected in any form of acquired systemic amyloidosis. Intracerebral and cerebrovascular amyloid deposits are seen in Alzheimer's disease. Most cases are sporadic, but hereditary forms caused by muta-tions have been reported. In hereditary spongiform encephalopathies several amyloid plaques have been seen.

Amyloid deposits are frequently found in the elderly, particularly cerebral deposits of A4 protein. This is also seen in Down's syndrome. Apoprotein E (involved in LDL transport, see p. 1136) interacts directly with β-A4 protein in senile plaques and neurofibrillary tangles in the brain. The gene for apoprotein E is on chromosome 19 and may be susceptibility factor in the aetiology of Alzheimer's disease.

Local amyloidosis

Deposits of amyloid fibrils of various types can be localized to various organs or tissues (e.g. skin, heart and brain).

Dialysis-related amyloidosis

This is due to the β_2-microglobulin producing amyloid fibrils in chronic dialysis patients (p. 678). It frequently presents with the carpal tunnel syndrome.

Diagnosis

This is based on clinical suspicion and, if possible, on tissue histology. Amyloid in tissues appears as an amorphous, homogeneous substance that stains pink with haematoxylin and eosin and stains red with Congo red. It also has a green fluorescence in polarized light. Tissue can be obtained from the rectum or gums. The bone marrow may show plasma cells in amyloidosis or a lymphoproliferative disorder. A paraproteinaemia and proteinuria with light chains in the urine may also be seen in AL amyloidosis. In secondary or reactive amyloidosis there will be an underlying disorder. Scintigraphy using ^{123}I-labelled serum amyloid P component is useful for the assessment of AL, ATTR and AA amyloidosis, but it is not widely available and is expensive.

Treatment

This is symptomatic or the treatment of the associated disorder. The nephrotic syndrome and congestive cardiac failure require the relevant therapies. Treatment of any inflammatory source or infection should be instituted. Colchicine may help familial Mediterranean fever. Chemotherapy (similar to myeloma, p. 578) is showing some efficacy in AL amyloidosis. In ATTR amyloidosis where transthyretin is predominantly synthesized in the liver, liver transplantation (when there would be a disappearance of the mutant protein from the blood) is considered as the definitive therapy.

FURTHER READING

Falk RH, Comenzo RL, Skinner M (1997) The systemic amyloidoses. *New England Journal of Medicine* **337**: 898–909.

Merlini G, Bellotti V (2003) Molecular mechanisms of amyloidosis. *New England Journal of Medicine* **349**: 583–596

THE PORPHYRIAS

This heterogeneous group of rare inborn errors of metabolism is caused by abnormalities of enzymes involved in the biosynthesis of haem, resulting in over-production of the intermediate compounds called 'porphyrins' (Fig. 19.22). The porphyrias show extreme

Fig. 19.22 Porphyrin metabolism showing the various porphyrias. ALA synthase is the rate-limiting enzyme. Deficiencies of the other seven enzymes (crosses) cause the different porphyrias:

1. X-linked sideroblastic anaemia
2. ALA dehydrogenase porphyria (ADP)
3. Acute intermittent porphyria (AIP)
4. Congenital erythropoietic porphyria (CEP)
5. Porphyria cutanea tarda (PCT) and hepatoerythropoietic porphyria (HEP)
6. Hereditary coproporphyria (HCP)
7. Variegate porphyria (VP)
8. Erythropoietic protoporphyria (EPP).

genetic heterogeneity. For example, in acute intermittent porphyria more than 90 mutations have been identified in the porphobilinogen deaminase gene. One mutation has a high prevalence in patients in northern Sweden, suggesting a common ancestor.

Structurally, porphyrins consist of four pyrrole rings. These pyrrole rings are formed from the precursors glycine and succinyl-CoA, which are converted to δ-aminolaevulinic acid (δ-ALA) in a reaction catalysed by the enzyme δ-ALA synthase. Two molecules of δ-ALA condense to form a pyrrole ring.

Porphyrins can be divided into uroporphyrins, coproporphyrins or protoporphyrins depending on the structure of the side-chain. They are termed type I if the structure is symmetrical and type III if it is asymmetrical. Both uroporphyrins and coproporphyrins can be excreted in the urine.

The sequence of enzymatic changes in the production of haem is shown in Figure 19.22. The chief rate-limiting step is the enzyme δ-ALA synthase. This has two isoforms, ALA-N (non-erythroid) and ALA-E (erythroid). ALA-N is under negative feedback by haem but is upregulated by drugs and chemicals; there is no known inherited deficiency and the gene is on 3p21. Conversely ALA-E, encoded by Xp11.21, is unaffected by drugs or haem, and an inherited deficiency causes X-linked sideroblastic anaemia (Fig. 19.22 1).

Consequently:

- Haem (endogenous or exogenous) produces remission of hepatic porphyria.
- Chemicals and drugs can produce disease.
- Erythopoietic porphyria gives constant symptoms and is affected by sunlight.

Clinical features

All of the haem intermediates shown in Figure 19.22 are potentially toxic. Three patterns of symptoms occur in the various types of porphyria.

- neurovisceral (Table 19.20)
- photosensitive
- haemolytic anaemia.

Table 19.20 Porphyria: neurovisceral symptoms	
Neuropsychiatric	**Visceral**

Neuropathy:
    Motor (70%)
    Sensory
Epilepsy (15%)
Psychiatric disorders (50%):
    Depression
    Anxiety
    Psychosis
	Abdominal pain
	Vomiting } up to 90%
	Constipation
	Diarrhoea (occasional)
	Fever (~ 30%)
	Hypertension (up to 50%)
	Tachycardia (up to 80%)
	Muscular pain (~ 50%)

The most common types of porphyria are acute intermittent (AIP), porphyria cutanea tarda (PCT) and erythropoietic porphyria (EPP).

The *diagnosis* of various types is based on urinary excretion levels of aminolaevulinic acid (ALA), porphobilinogen (PBG) and porphyrin in aliquots from a 24-hour collection. Erythrocyte PBG deaminase activity is measured for neurovisceral symptoms. Urinary and plasma porphyrin concentrations are helpful for those with photocutaneous manifestations. Faecal porphyrin analysis is helpful in confirmatory testing.

Neurovisceral

Acute intermittent porphyria (AIP) (Fig. 19.22 ③)

This is an autosomal dominant disorder. Presentation is in early adult life, usually around the age of 30 years, and women are affected more than men. It may be precipitated by alcohol and drugs such as barbiturates and oral contraceptives, but a wide range of lipid-soluble drugs have also been incriminated. Acute attacks present with neurovisceral symptoms (Table 19.20). Symptoms of the rare, autosomal recessive aminolaevulinic acid dehydrogenase porphyria (ADP) ② are similar.

Investigations

The urine turns red-brown or red on standing.

- **Blood count**. This is usually normal, with occasional neutrophil leucocytosis.
- **Liver biochemical tests**. There is elevated bilirubin and aminotransferase.
- **Serum urea** is often raised.
- **ALA and PBG** are raised.
- **Erythrocyte PBG deaminase** is decreased.

Screening

Family members should be screened to detect latent cases. Urinalysis is not adequate but measurement of erythrocyte porphobilinogen deaminase and ALA synthase is extremely sensitive.

Mixed neurovisceral and photocutaneous

Variegate porphyria (VP) (Fig. 19.22 ⑦)

This combines neurovisceral symptoms with those of a cutaneous photosensitive porphyria. A bullous eruption develops on exposure to sunlight owing to the activation of porphyrins deposited in the skin.

Investigation shows an elevated urinary ALA and PBG. Fluorescence emission spectroscopy of plasma differentiates this from other cutaneous porphyrias.

Hereditary coproporphyria (HCP) (Fig. 19.22 ⑥)

This is extremely rare and broadly similar in presentation to variegate porphyria.

Photocutaneous

Porphyria cutanea tarda (cutaneous hepatic porphyria) (PCT) (Fig. 19.22 ⑤)

This condition, which has a genetic predisposition, presents with a bullous eruption on exposure to sunlight; the eruption heals with scarring. Alcohol is the most common aetiological agent but HCV, iron overload or HIV can also precipitate the disease. Evidence of biochemical or clinical liver disease may also be present. Polychlorinated hydrocarbons have been implicated and porphyria cutanea tarda has been seen in association with benign or malignant tumours of the liver.

Hepatoerythropoietic porphyria (HEP, Fig. 19.22 ⑤) is a rare disease clinically very similar to congenital erythropoietic porphyria presenting in childhood; haemolytic anaemia occurs. The defect of HEP is similar to that of PCT.

The diagnosis depends on demonstration of increased levels of urinary uroporphyrin. Histology of the skin shows subepidermal blisters with perivascular deposition of periodic acid–Schiff-staining material. The serum iron and transferrin saturation are often raised. Liver biopsy shows mild iron overload as well as features of alcoholic liver disease.

Congenital erythropoietic porphyria (CEP) (Fig. 19.22 ④)

This is extremely rare and is transmitted as an autosomal recessive trait. Its victims show extreme sensitivity to sunlight and develop disfiguring scars. Dystrophy of the nails, blindness due to lenticular scarring, and brownish discoloration of the teeth also occur.

Erythropoietic protoporphyria (EPP) (Fig. 19.22 ⑧)

This is more common than congenital erythropoietic porphyria and is inherited as an autosomal dominant trait. It presents with irritation and a burning pain in the skin on exposure to sunlight. The liver is usually normal but protoporphyrin deposition can occur. Diagnosis is made by fluorescence of the peripheral red blood cells and by increased protoporphyrin in the red cells and stools.

Management of porphyrias

Neurovisceral

Acute. The management of acute episodes is largely supportive. Precipitating factors, e.g. drugs, should be stopped. Analgesics should be given (avoiding drugs that may aggravate an attack). Intravenous carbohydrates, e.g. glucose, inhibit ALA synthase activity. Intravenous haem arginate (human haemin) infusion reduces ALA and PBG excretion by having a negative effect on ALA synthase-N activity (see Fig. 19.22) and decreases the duration of an attack; this is useful in a severe attack. Calorie and fluid intake should be maintained.

Prevention in remission period. This is by avoidance of possible precipitating factors, e.g. drugs and alcohol.

Stopping smoking, treatment of infections and stress avoidance are helpful. Surgery can precipitate attacks. A high-carbohydrate diet should be maintained and haemin infusions may also help.

Photocutaneous episodes
Acute attacks following exposure to UV light can only be treated symptomatically. However, *venesection*, which reduces urinary porphyria, can be used for PCT in both acute and remission phases. Chloroquine can also aid excretion by forming a water-soluble complex with uroporphyrins.

Liver transplantation is used for severe cases.

Prevention is with avoidance of sunlight, and use of sunscreens and protective clothing.

Oral β-carotene, which quenches free radicals, provides effective protection against solar sensitivity in EPP.

FURTHER READING
American Porphyria Foundation:
    http://www.porphyriafoundation.com.
Kauppinen R (2005) Porphyrias. *Lancet* **365**: 241–252.

Palmieri C et al. (2004) Managing malignant disease in patients with porphyria. *Quarterly Journal of Medicine* **97**: 115–126.

CHAPTER BIBLIOGRAPHY
Scriver CR, Beaudet AL, Sly WS, Valle D (2000) *The Metabolic Basis of Inherited Disease*, 8th edn. New York: McGraw-Hill.
Type I diabetes in adults – national clinical guidelines for diagnosis and management in primary and secondary care. National Collaborating Centre for Chronic Conditions. Royal College of Physicians (2004).
All eyes on the β cell. *Journal of Clinical Investigation* **114**(7): 867–1002.

SIGNIFICANT WEBSITES
http://www.doh.gov.uk/nsf
    UK Government forthcoming National Service Framework draft information
http://www.sign.ac.uk/guidelines/published/index.html
    Scottish Intercollegiate Guidelines Network – guidelines on a range of subjects including diabetes
http://www.dtu.ox.ac.uk
    Diabetes Trials Unit (University of Oxford) – research information, particularly the UK Prospective Diabetes Study results
http://www.eatlas.idf.org
    International Diabetes Federation

http://medweb.bham.ac.uk/easdec/
    Diabetic retinopathy
http://www.diabetes.org.uk
    Diabetes UK charity – information for patients, researchers and health professionals
http://www.diabetes.org
    American Diabetes Association – heavyweight and authoritative, with an American flavour
http://www.diabetes.ca
    Canadian Diabetes Association site – well designed practical site with many links to other diabetes-related sites; a good jumping off point

The special senses 20

DISORDERS OF THE EAR, NOSE AND THROAT

THE EAR

ANATOMY AND PHYSIOLOGY

The ear can be divided into three parts: outer, middle and inner (Fig. 20.1).

The *outer ear* has a skin-lined tube 2.5 cm long leading down to the tympanic membrane (the ear drum). Its outer third is cartilaginous and contains hair, sebaceous and ceruminous glands, but the walls of the inner two-thirds are bony. The outer ear is self-cleaning as the skin is migratory and there are no indications to use cotton wool buds. Wax should only be seen in the outer third.

The *middle ear* is an air-containing cavity derived from the branchial clefts. It communicates with the mastoid air cells superiorly, and the Eustachian tube connects it to the nasopharynx medially. The Eustachian tube ventilates the middle ear and maintains equal air pressure across the tympanic membrane. It is normally closed but opens via the action of the palatal muscles to allow air entry when swallowing or yawning. A defect in this mechanism, such as with a cleft palate, will prevent air entering the middle ear cleft which may then fill with fluid. Lying within the middle ear cavity are the three ossicles (malleus, incus and stapes) that transmit sound from the tympanic membrane to the inner ear. On the medial wall of the cavity is the horizontal segment of the facial nerve, which may be damaged during surgery or by direct extension of infection in the middle ear.

The *inner ear* contains the cochlea for hearing and the vestibule and semicircular canals for balance. There is a semicircular canal arranged in each body plane and these are stimulated by rotatory movement. The facial, cochlear and vestibular nerves emerge from the inner ear and run through the internal acoustic meatus to the brainstem (see Fig. 21.7, p. 1185).

PHYSIOLOGY OF HEARING

The ossicles, in the middle ear, transmit sound waves from the tympanic membrane to the cochlea. They amplify the waves by about 18-fold to compensate for the loss of sound waves moving from the air-filled middle ear to the fluid-filled cochlea. Hair cells in the basilar membrane of the cochlea detect the vibrations and transduce these into nerve impulses which pass to the cochlear nucleus and then eventually to the superior olivary nuclei

Fig. 20.1 The anatomy of the ear.

of both sides; thus lesions central to the cochlear nucleus do not cause unilateral hearing loss.

If the ossicles are diseased, sound can also reach the cochlea by vibration of the temporal bone (bone conduction).

EXAMINATION

The pinna and postauricular region should first be examined for scars or swellings. An auroscope is used to examine the external ear canal whilst the pinna is retracted backwards and upwards to straighten the canal. Look for wax, discharge or foreign bodies. The tympanic membrane should always be seen with a light reflex anteroinferiorly. Previous repeated infections may cause a thickened, whitish drum but fluid in the middle ear may show as dullness of the drum. Perforations are marginal or central.

COMMON DISORDERS

The discharging ear (otorrhoea)

Discharge from the ear is usually due to infection of the outer or middle ear.

Otitis externa is a diffuse inflammation of the skin of the ear canal. The organism may be bacterial, viral or fungal and the patient usually complains of severe pain. Gentle pulling of the pinna is tender and there may be lymphadenopathy of the preauricular nodes.

Examination may reveal debris in the canal which needs to be removed either by gentle mopping or preferably by suction viewed directly under a microscope. In severe cases the canal may be swollen and a view of the tympanic membrane impossible. Any foreign body seen should be removed with great care by trained personnel.

Treatment is with regular cleansing and topical antibiotics combined with corticosteroids; it resolves in 3–4 days.

Otitis media can also present with discharge from the middle ear through a perforation of the tympanic membrane. There are no mucous glands in the external ear canal, however, and if the discharge is serous then middle ear pathology is unlikely.

Treatment is with systemic antibiotics.

Cholesteatoma

Cholesteatoma is defined as keratinizing squamous epithelium within the middle ear cleft and can present with foul smelling otorrhoea. Examination may show a defect in the tympanic membrane full of white cheesy material. Mastoid surgery is required to remove this sac of squamous debris as it can erode local structures such as the facial nerve or even extend intracranially.

Hearing loss

Deafness can be conductive or sensorineural and these

Box 20.1 Hearing loss

Type	Defect	Rinne	Weber
Conductive	Outer or middle ear	Negative	Sound heard louder on the affected side
Sensorineural	Inner ear or more centrally	Positive	Sound heard louder in the normal ear

can be differentiated by the Rinne and the Weber tests (Box 20.1).

Rinne test

Normally a tuning fork, 512 Hz, will be heard as louder if held next to the ear (air conduction) compared to being placed on the mastoid bone (*Rinne positive*). If the tuning fork is perceived louder when placed on the mastoid (bone conduction), then a defect in the conducting mechanism of the external or middle ear is present (*Rinne negative*).

Weber test

A tuning fork placed on the bridge of the nose of a patient with normal hearing (or with symmetrical hearing loss) should be perceived centrally.

Conductive hearing loss may be due to many causes (Table 20.1) but wax is the commonest.

Perforated tympanic membrane

This may arise from trauma or chronic middle ear disease where recurrent infection results in a permanent defect. Surgical repair is only indicated if the patient is symptomatic with hearing loss or recurrent discharge.

Otitis media

This is an acute inflammation of the middle ear, causing severe pain (otalgia) and conductive hearing loss. This occurs because fluid accumulation in the middle ear

---

Table 20.1 Deafness

Conductive	Sensorineural
Congenital – atresia Pendred's syndrome (see p. 1071) Long QT syndrome (see p. 777)	**End organ** Advancing age Occupational acoustic trauma Ménière's disease Drugs (e.g. gentamicin, furosemide (frusemide))

External meatus
Wax
Foreign body
Otitis externa
Chronic suppuration
	Eighth nerve lesions
	Acoustic neuroma
	Cranial trauma
	Inflammatory lesions:
	  Tuberculous meningitis
	  Sarcoidosis
	  Neurosyphilis
	  Carcinomatous meningitis

Drum Perforation/trauma	
Middle ear Otosclerosis Ossicular bone problems Suppuration	**Brainstem lesions (rare)** Multiple sclerosis Infarction

impairs sound conduction to the cochlea. It is often viral in origin, e.g. following a cold, and will settle within 72 hours without antibacterial treatment. In patients with systemic features or after 72 hours, a systemic antibiotic, e.g. amoxicillin, should be given. Topical therapy is of no value. Complications include infection of the mastoid bone.

Acute otitis media may spread to the mastoid area and if there is tenderness and swelling over the mastoid then an urgent ENT opinion should be obtained.

Secretory otitis media with effusion (also called serous otitis media or glue ear) (Fig. 20.2)

This is common in children because of Eustachian tube dysfunction. The effusion resolves naturally in the majority of cases but can persist giving hearing loss, and it predisposes to recurrent attacks of acute otitis media. A grommet is a tube that is inserted into the tympanic membrane and ventilates the middle ear cavity, i.e. it takes over the Eustachian tube's function. Grommets are extruded from the tympanic membrane as it heals (lasting from 6 months to 2 years) but if the Eustachian tube is still not working, fluid will reaccumulate in the middle ear cavity with a return of symptoms. In most children the middle third of the face grows around the age of 7–14 years and Eustachian tube dysfunction is rare after this.

Otosclerosis

This is usually a hereditary disorder where new bony deposits occur within the derivatives of the otic capsule, specifically the stapes footplate and in the cochlea. Characteristically seen in the second and third decades, it is commoner in females and can become worse during pregnancy. The hearing loss may be mixed, and treatment includes a hearing aid or replacement of the fixed stapes with a prosthesis (stapedectomy).

Presbycusis

This is the commonest cause of deafness. It is a degenerative disorder of the cochlea and is seen in old age. The onset is gradual and the higher frequencies are affected most (Fig. 20.3). Speech has two components: low frequencies (vowels) and high frequencies (consonants). When the consonants are lost, speech loses its intelligibility. Increasing the volume merely increases the low frequencies and the characteristic response of 'Don't shout. I'm not deaf!' A high-frequency-specific hearing aid will do much to ease the frustrations of both the patients and their close contacts.

Noise trauma

Cochlear damage can occur, for example, when shooting without ear protectors or from industrial noise (see p. 1030) and characteristically has a loss at 4 kHz.

Acoustic neuroma

This is a slow-growing benign Schwannoma of the vestibular nerve (p. 1245) which can present with progressive sensorineural hearing loss. Any patient with an asymmetric sensorineural hearing loss should be investigated, e.g. with an MRI scan.

Vertigo

Vertigo is usually rotatory when it arises from the ear. The presence of otalgia, otorrhoea, tinnitus or hearing loss suggests an otologic aetiology. Vestibular causes can be classified according to the duration of the vertigo:

- seconds to minutes – benign paroxysmal positional vertigo (BPPV)
- minutes to hours – Ménière's disease
- hours to days – labyrinthine or central pathology.

Fig. 20.3 Audiogram showing presbycusis (high frequency loss).

Fig. 20.2 **Secretory otitis media (glue ear).** Auroscopic view of tympanic membrane which is dull with loss of light reflex.

Benign paroxysmal positional vertigo (BPPV)

BPPV is thought to be due to loose otoliths in the semi-circular canals, commonly the posterior canal. Positional vertigo is precipitated by head movements, usually to a particular position, and may occur when turning in bed or on sitting up. The onset is typically sudden and distressing. The vertigo lasts seconds or minutes and the phenomenon becomes less severe on repeated movements (fatigue). There is no serious underlying cause but it sometimes follows vestibular neuronitis (p. 1190), head injury or ear infection.

Diagnosis

This is made not only on the history but by precipitating an attack by carrying out a positional test in the outpatient clinic. This test, called the *Hallpike manoeuvre*, involves sitting the patient on a couch and then turning the patient's head towards the affected ear. The patient's head is supported by the examiner and the patient then lies down so that the head is just below the horizontal. Nystagmus (following a latent interval of a few seconds) is noted, as is any subjective sensation of vertigo. A positive Hallpike test confirms BPPV, which can be cured in over 90% of cases by the Epley manoeuvre. This involves gentle but specific manipulation and rotation of the patient's head to shift the loose otoliths from the semicircular canals.

A differential diagnosis is a cerebellar mass but here, positional nystagmus (and vertigo) is immediately apparent (no latent interval) and does not fatigue.

Ménière's disease

This condition is characterized by recurring episodic rotatory vertigo lasting 30 minutes to a few hours; attacks are recurrent over months or years. Classically it is associated with a low frequency sensorineural hearing loss, feeling of fullness in the affected ear, loss of balance, tinnitus and vomiting. There is a build-up of endolymphatic fluid in the inner ear, although its precise aetiology is still unclear.

Treatment involves the use of vestibular sedatives, e.g. cinnarizine in the acute phase, low-salt diet, betahistine, and avoidance of caffeine. If the disease cannot be controlled in this way, then a chemical labyrinthectomy, which involves perfusing the round window orifice with ototoxic drugs such as gentamicin is possible. Gentamicin destroys the vestibular epithelium; therefore the patient has severe vertigo for around 2 weeks until the body compensates for the lack of vestibular input on that side. The patient will happily trade occasional mild vertigo when the balance system is challenged to the unpredictable, severe and disabling attacks of vertigo of Ménière's disease.

Labyrinthine or central causes of vertigo

(see Table 21.10)

These are managed with vestibular sedatives in the acute phase. Most patients will settle over a few days but continuous true vertigo with nystagmus suggests a central lesion. A patient with a deficit of vestibular function due to viral labyrinthitis or neuronitis should be able to come off the vestibular sedatives within 2 weeks, as long-term use can give parkinsonian side-effects, delay

central compensation and thus prolong the vertigo. Vestibular rehabilitation by a physiotherapist or audiological scientist can speed up the compensation process, although most patients will be able to do this themselves with time.

Tinnitus

This is a sensation of a sound when there is no auditory stimulus. It can occur without hearing loss. Patients describe a hissing or ringing in their ears and this can cause much distress. It usually does not have a serious cause but vascular malformation, e.g. aneurysms, or vascular tumours may be associated.

Tinnitus associated with deafness is described above.

Treatment

This is difficult. A tinnitus masker (a mechanically produced continuous soft sound) can help. A vestibular sedative, betahistine, is occasionally used.

FURTHER READING

Halmagyi GM (2005) Diagnosis and management of vertigo. *Clinical Medicine* **5**: 159–165.

Hilton M, Pinder D (2003) Benign paroxysmal positional vertigo. *British Medical Journal* **326**: 673.

Lockwood AH (2002) Tinnitus. *New England Journal of Medicine* **348**: 1027–1032.

Luxon LM, Davies RA (eds) (1997) Handbook of vestibular rehabilitation. London: Whurr.

THE NOSE

ANATOMY AND PHYSIOLOGY (Fig. 20.4)

The function of the nose is to facilitate smell and respiration. Smell is a sensation conveyed by the olfactory

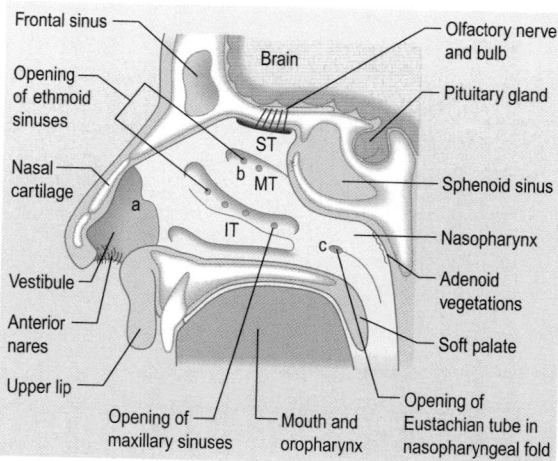

Fig. 20.4 **The anatomy of the nose in longitudinal section**. IT, inferior turbinate; MT, middle turbinate; ST, superior turbinate; a, internal ostium; b, respiratory region; c, choanae.

epithelium in the roof of the nose. The olfactory epithelium is supplied by the first cranial nerve (p. 1179). The nose also filters, moistens and warms inspired air and in doing so assists the normal process of respiration.

The external portion of the nose comprises two nasal bones attached to the rest of the facial skeleton and to the upper and lower lateral cartilages. The internal nose is divided by a midline septum that comprises both cartilage and bone. This separates the internal nose from the external nostril to the posterior choanae. The posterior choanae are in continuity with the nasopharynx posteriorly. The paranasal sinuses open into the lateral wall of the nose and are a system of aerated chambers within the facial skeleton.

The blood supply of the nose is derived from branches of both the internal and external carotid arteries. The internal carotid artery supplies the upper nose via the anterior and posterior ethmoidal arteries. The external carotid artery supplies the posterior and inferior portion of the nose via the superior labial artery, greater palatine artery and sphenopalatine artery. On the anterior nasal septum is an area of confluence of these vessels (Little's area) (Fig. 20.5a).

EXAMINATION

The anterior part of the nose can be examined using a nasal speculum and light source. Endoscopes are required to examine the nasal cavity and postnasal space.

COMMON DISORDERS

Epistaxis

Nose bleeds vary in severity from minor to life-threatening. Little's area (Fig. 20.5a) is a frequent site of nasal haemorrhage. First aid measures should be administered immediately, including compression of the anterior lower portion of the external nose, ice packs and leaning forward. The patient should be asked to avoid

Table 20.2	Aetiology of epistaxis
Local	Idiopathic
	Trauma – foreign bodies, nose-picking and nasal fractures
	Iatrogenic – surgery, intranasal steroids
	Neoplasm – nasal, paranasal sinus and nasopharyngeal tumours
General	Anticoagulants
	Coagulation disorders (p. 469)
	Hypertension
	Osler–Weber–Rendu syndrome (familial haemorrhagic telangiectasia)

swallowing any blood running posteriorly. If the bleeding continues profusely then resuscitation in the form of intravenous access, fluid replacement or blood, and oxygen can be administered. If further intervention is necessary, consideration should be given to intranasal cautery of the bleeding vessel, or intranasal packing may be undertaken using a variety of commercially available nasal packs (Fig. 20.5b). In addition to direct treatment of the epistaxis, a cause and appropriate treatment of a cause should be sought (Table 20.2).

Rhinitis (see p. 895)

Nasal obstruction

Nasal obstruction is a symptom and not a diagnosis. It can significantly affect a patient's quality of life. Causes include:

- *Rhinitis* (p. 895). If an allergen is identified, then allergen avoidance is the mainstay of treatment. Topical steroids and/or antihistamines can be tried. If severe, then oral antihistamines or referral to an allergy clinic for immunotherapy may be warranted.

(a)

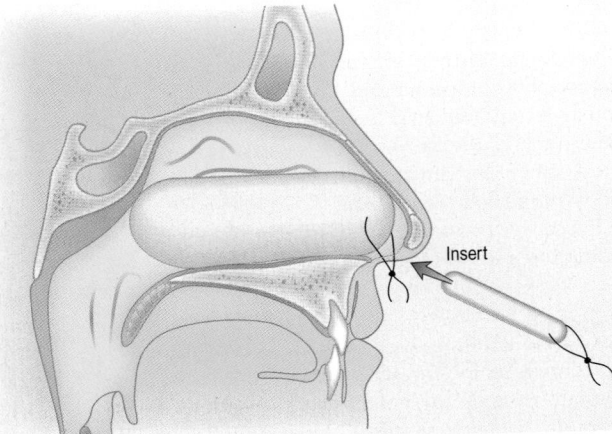

(b)

Fig. 20.5 (a) Blood supply of Little's area on the septum of the nose. (b) Nasal pack.

- *Septal deviation.* Correction of this deviation can be undertaken surgically.
- *Nasal polyps.* This condition occurs with inflammation and oedema of the sinus nasal mucosa. This oedematous mucosa prolapses into the nasal cavity and can cause significant nasal obstruction. In allergic rhinitis (p. 896) the mucosa lining the nasal septum and inferior turbinates are swollen and a dark red or plum colour. Nasal polyps can be identified as glistening swellings which are not tender. Treatment with intranasal steroids may help but if polyps are large or unresponsive to medical treatment then surgery is necessary.
- *Foreign bodies.* These are usually seen in children who present with unilateral nasal discharge. Clinical examination of the nose with a light source often reveals the foreign body, which requires removal either in clinic or in theatre with a general anaesthetic.
- *Sinonasal malignancy.* This is extremely rare. The diagnosis must be considered if unusual unilateral symptoms are seen, including nasal obstruction, epistaxis, pain, epiphoria, cheek swelling, paraesthesia of the cheek and proptosis of the orbit.

Sinusitis

Sinusitis is an infection of the paranasal sinuses that may be bacterial (mainly *Streptococcus pneumoniae* and *Haemophilus influenzae*) or occasionally fungal. It is most commonly associated with an upper respiratory tract infection and can occur with severe asthma. Symptoms include frontal headache, purulent rhinorrhoea, facial pain with tenderness and fever. It can be confused with a variety of other conditions such as migraine, trigeminal neuralgia, and cranial arteritis.

Treatment

Treatment for a bacterial sinusitis includes nasal decongestants, e.g. xylomethazoline, broad-spectrum antibiotics, e.g. co-amoxiclav because *H. influenzae* can be resistant to amoxicillin, anti-inflammatory therapy with topical corticosteroids such as fluticasone propionate nasal spray to reduce mucosal swelling, and steam inhalations.

If the symptoms of sinusitis are recurrent (Box 20.2) or complications such as orbital cellulitis arise, then an ENT opinion is appropriate and a CT scan of the paranasal sinuses is undertaken. Plain sinus X-rays are now rarely used to image the sinuses.

CT scan of the sinuses or an MRI scan can demonstrate soft tissue planes (Fig. 20.6).

Functional endoscopic sinus surgery (FESS) is used for ventilation and drainage of the sinuses.

Anosmia

Olfaction is mainly under the control of cranial nerve I, although irritant, unpleasant nasal sensations are carried by cranial nerves V, IX and X. Anosmia is a complete loss of the sense of smell and *hyposmia* is a decreased sense of smell. If odorant molecules do not reach the olfactory

Box 20.2 Types of sinusitis

Acute sinusitis	Symptoms of sinusitis lasting between 1 week and 1 month
Recurrent acute sinusitis	More than four episodes of acute sinusitis per year
Subacute sinusitis	Symptoms of sinusitis lasting between 1 and 3 months
Chronic sinusitis	Symptoms of sinusitis lasting longer than 3 months

Fig. 20.6 **MRI of sinonasal tumour.** Large soft tissue swelling filling nasal cavity and sinuses on the patient's left side.

epithelium high in the nose, a *conductive deficit* of smell occurs. If the neural transmission of smell is affected then a *sensorineural loss* of smell is incurred. Some conditions may predispose to a mixed (conductive and sensorineural) loss of smell. The main cause of a loss of smell is nasal obstruction due to upper respiratory infection or nasal polyps. Other causes include sinonasal disease, old age, drug therapy and head injury/trauma. It is difficult to predict the speed and extent of recovery in the latter causes.

Idiopathic cases will account for many patients but before this diagnosis is accepted an assessment of the patient for the possibility of an intranasal tumour or intracranial mass should be undertaken.

Fractured nose

Patients with a fractured nose present with epistaxis, bruising of the eyes and nasal bridge swelling. Initially, it is often difficult to assess if the bones are deviated, particularly if there is significant swelling. Reduction of the fracture should be undertaken in the first 2 weeks after injury and can be achieved by manipulation. However, if the fracture sets, a more formal rhinoplasty may have to be undertaken at a later stage. The patient should be examined for a head injury and the nose should also be checked for a septal haematoma. This is painful, can cause nasal obstruction, is fluctuant to touch on the nasal septum and requires immediate drainage.

THE THROAT

ANATOMY AND PHYSIOLOGY

The throat can be considered as the oral cavity, the pharynx and the larynx. The oral cavity extends from the lips to the tonsils. The pharynx can be divided into three areas:

- nasopharynx – extending from the nasal openings to the soft palate
- orpharynx – extending from the soft palate to the tip of the epiglottis
- hypopharynx – extending from the tip of the epiglottis to just below the level of the cricoid cartilage where it is continuous with the oesophagus.

Lying within the hypopharynx is the larynx. This consists of cartilaginous, ligamentous and muscular tissue with the primary function of protecting the distal airway. The pharynx is innervated from the pharyngeal plexus. There are two vocal cords which abduct (open) during inspiration and adduct (close) to protect the airway and for voice production (phonation). The main nerve supply of the vocal cords comes from the recurrent laryngeal nerves (branches of the vagus nerve) which arise in the neck, but on the left side passes down around the aortic arch and then ascends in the tracheo-oesophageal groove to the larynx.

Normal vocal cords vibrate between 90 (male) and 180 (female) times per second, giving the voice its pitch or frequency. A healthy voice requires full closure of the vocal cords with a smooth, regular pattern of vibration, and any pathology that prevents full closure will result in air escaping between the vocal cords during phonation and a 'breathy' voice.

EXAMINATION

Good illumination is essential. Look at teeth, gums, tongue, floor of mouth and oral cavity. Tonsils, soft palate and uvula are easily seen, and a gag reflex (p. 1190) is present. The remainder of the pharynx and larynx can be inspected with a laryngeal mirror or endoscope.

Examination of the neck for lymph nodes and other masses is also performed.

COMMON DISORDERS

Hoarseness (dysphonia)

There are three essential components for voice production: an air source (the lungs); a vibratory source (the vocal cords); and a resonating chamber (the pharynx, the nasal and oral cavities). Although chest and nasal disorders can affect the voice, the majority of hoarseness is due to laryngeal pathology.

Inflammation which increases the 'mass' of the vocal cords will cause the vocal cord frequency to fall, giving a much deeper voice. Thus listening to a patient's voice can often give a diagnosis before the vocal cords are examined.

Nodules

Nodules (always bilateral and commoner in females) and polyps (Fig. 20.7) are found on the free edge of the vocal cord preventing full closure and giving a 'breathy, harsh' voice. They are commonly found in professions that rely on their voice for their livelihood, such as teachers, singers and lawyers. They are usually related to poor technique of voice production and can usually be cured with speech therapy. If surgery is needed, great care must be taken to remain in the superficial layers of the vocal cord in order to prevent deep scarring which may leave the voice permanently hoarse.

Reinke's oedema (Fig. 20.8)

This is due to a collection of tissue fluid in the sub-epithelial layer of the vocal cord. The vocal cord has poor lymphatic drainage, predisposing it to oedema. Reinke's oedema is associated with irritation of the vocal cords: smoking, voice abuse, acid reflux and vary rarely hypothyroidism. Treatment is to remove the irritation in most cases but surgery to thin the cords will also allow the voice to return to its normal pitch.

Acute-onset hoarseness

This, in a smoker is a danger sign. Any patient with a hoarse voice for over 6 weeks should be seen by an ENT surgeon. The voice may be deep, harsh and breathy indicating a mass on the vocal cord or can be weak suggesting a paralysed left vocal cord secondary to mediastinal disease, e.g. bronchial carcinoma.

Early squamous cell carcinoma of the larynx (Fig. 20.9) has a good prognosis. Treatment is with carbon dioxide resection or radiotherapy. Spread of the tumour can lead to referred otalgia which may then require a laryngectomy with possible neck dissection. A patient with a paralysed left vocal cord must have a chest X-ray. Medialization of the paralysed cord to allow contact with the opposite

Fig. 20.7 Vocal cord polyp.

Fig. 20.8 Reinke's oedema of the vocal cords.

Fig. 20.9 Carcinoma of the right cord.

cord can return the voice and give a competent larynx. This can be done under local anaesthesia, giving an immediate result whatever the long-term prognosis of the chest pathology.

Stridor

Stridor or noisy breathing can be divided into inspiratory (source is glottic or above), expiratory (intrathoracic trachea or below) or mixed (subglottis or extrathoracic trachea). All patients with stridor, both paediatric and adult, are potentially at risk of asphyxiation and should be investigated fully. Severe stridor may be an indication for either intubation or a tracheostomy (Table 20.3).

Tracheostomy tubes may be:

- *Cuffed or uncuffed.* A high-volume, low-pressure cuff is used to prevent aspiration and to allow positive-pressure ventilation.
- *Fenestrated or unfenestrated.* This is a small hole on the greater curvature of the tube (both outer and inner) allowing air to escape upwards to the vocal cords and therefore the patient can speak. This tube often has a valve which allows air to enter from the stoma but closes on expiration, directing the air through the fenestration.

Most long-term tracheostomy tubes have an inner and outer tube. The inner tube fits inside the outer tube and projects beyond its lower end. A major problem with a tracheostomy tube is crusting of its distal end with dried secretions and this arrangement allows the inner tube to be removed, cleaned and replaced as frequently as required, without disrupting the outer tube.

When to decannulate a patient is often a difficult issue if laryngeal competence is unclear. Movement of the vocal cords requires an ENT examination but owing to the risk of aspiration, a speech therapist's opinion can also be useful. The tracheostomy tube itself can also give problems due to compression of the oesophagus with a cuffed tube and by preventing the larynx from rising during normal swallowing.

Tonsillitis and pharyngitis

Viral infections of the throat are common and, although many practitioners are under pressure from the patient to give antibiotics, the vast majority are usually self-limiting, settling with bed rest, analgesia and encouraging fluid intake. Fungal infections, usually candidiasis, are uncommon and may indicate an immunocompromised patient or undiagnosed diabetes.

Tonsillitis

Tonsillitis, with a good history of pyrexia, dysphagia, lymphadenopathy and severe malaise is usually bacterial with β-haemolytic streptococcus the commonest organism.

Glandular fever (p. 47)

This can also present with tonsillitis, although clinically the tonsils have a white exudate, there is often a petechial rash on the soft palate and an accompanying lymphadenopathy.

Quinsy

Quinsy is a collection of pus outside the capsule of the tonsil usually located adjacent to its superior pole. The patient often has trismus making examination difficult but the pus pushes the uvula across the midline to the opposite side. The area is usually hyperaemic and smooth but unilateral tonsil ulceration is more likely to be a malignancy. In either case urgent referral to an ENT specialist is essential.

Indications for a tonsillectomy are shown in Table 20.4. This is carried out under a general anaesthetic and current surgical techniques include diathermy dissection, laser excision and coblation (using an ultrasonic dissecting probe). There are strong advocates for each technique and much will depend on the individual surgeon's preference. Some departments now carry out tonsillectomy as a day case procedure as most reactionary bleeding will occur within the first 8 hours postoperatively.

Snoring

Snoring is due to vibration of soft tissue above the level of the larynx. It is a common condition (50% of 50-year-old males will snore to some extent) and can be considered to be related to obstruction of three potential areas; the nose, the palate or/and the hypopharynx (see Fig. 14.28). An Epworth questionnaire (Table 20.5) can also assist in the discrimination of sleep apnoea (p. 907) from simple snoring. Patients with a history of habitual, non-positional, heroic (can be heard through a wall) snoring require a full ENT examination and can be investigated

---

Table 20.3 Indications for tracheostomy

Upper airway obstruction (real or anticipated)
Long-term ventilation
Bronchial lavage
Incompetent larynx with aspiration

Table 20.4 Indications for tonsillectomy

Suspected malignancy
Obstructive sleep apnoea due to tonsillar hypertrophy
Recurrent tonsillitis: five attacks a year for at least 2 years
Quinsy in a patient with a history of recurrent tonsillitis

Table 20.5 Epworth Sleepiness Scale

How likely are you to doze off or fall asleep in the following situations, in contrast to just feeling tired? This refers to your usual way of life in recent time. Even if you have not done some of these things recently, try to work out how they would have affected you. Use the following scale to choose the most appropriate number for each situation.

0 = would never doze
1 = slight chance of dozing
2 = moderate chance of dozing
3 = high chance of dozing

Situation	Chance of dozing
Sitting and reading	
Watching TV	
Sitting and inactive in a public place (theatre or meeting)	
As a passenger in a car for an hour without a break	
Lying down to rest in the afternoon when circumstances permit	
Sitting and talking to someone	
Sitting quietly after lunch (without alcohol)	
In a car, while stopped for a few minutes in the traffic	
TOTAL	

Normal 5 ± 4
Severe obstructive sleep apnoea 16 (±4)
Nacrolepsy 17

by sleep nasendoscopy in which a sedated, snoring patient has a flexible nasendoscope inserted to identify the source of vibration. Nasal pathology such as polyps can be removed surgically with good results and most patients will benefit from lifestyle changes such as weight loss. Stiffening or shortening the soft palate via surgery, often using a laser, can help for palatal snorers but hypopharyngeal snorers require either a dental prosthesis at night to hold the mandible forward or continuous positive airway pressure (CPAP) via a mask (p. 982).

Dysphagia (p. 274)

Difficulty in swallowing is a common symptom but can be the presenting feature of carcinoma of the pharynx and therefore requires investigation.

A pharyngeal pouch is a herniation of mucosa through the fibres of the inferior pharyngeal constrictor muscle (cricopharyngeus) (Fig. 20.10). An area of weakness known as Killian's dehiscence allows a pulsion diverticulum to form. This will collect food which may regurgitate into the mouth or even down to the lungs at night with secondary pneumonia. Diagnosis is made radiologically and treatment is surgical, either via an external approach through the neck where the pouch is excised or more commonly endoscopically with stapling of the party wall (Fig. 20.10c).

Foreign bodies in the pharynx can be divided into three general categories: soft food bolus, coins (smooth), bones (sharp). Soft food bolus can be initially treated conservatively with muscle relaxants for 24 hours. Impacted coins should be removed at the earliest opportunity but sharp objects require emergency removal to avoid perforation of the muscle wall. If the patient perceives the foreign body to be to one side, then it should be above cricopharyngeus and an ENT examination will locate it; common areas are the tonsillar fossae, base of tongue, posterior pharyngeal wall and valleculae. Radiology will identify coins, and it can be a clinical decision to see whether a coin will pass down to the stomach, in which case no further treatment is required as it will exit naturally. Some departments advocate the use of a metal detector to monitor the position of the coin in the patient who is usually a child or has a mental disorder. Fish can be divided into those with a bony skeleton (teleosts) and those with a cartilaginous skeleton (elasmobranchs), and therefore radiology may only be useful in some cases. Radiology can also identify air in the cervical oesophagus indicating a radiolucent foreign body lying distally.

Globus pharyngeus

This is not a true dysphagia. It is a condition with classic

(a) **Normal anatomy of the throat**
Nasopharynx
Mouth (oral cavity)
Soft palate
Oropharynx
Tongue
Hypopharynx
Larynx
Trachea

(b) **Position of pharyngeal pouch**
Constrictor muscles
Larynx
Pharyngeal pouch
Trachea
Oesophagus

(c) **Stapling of the wall between oesophagus and pouch**
Pouch
Oesophagus
Party wall stapled opening pouch into the oesophagus (pouch not removed)

Fig. 20.10 **Pharyngeal pouch**. **(a)** Normal anatomy of the throat. **(b)** Position of pharyngeal pouch. **(c)** Stapling of the party wall between oesophagus and pouch.

symptoms of an intermittent sensation of a lump in the throat. This is perceived to be in the midline at the level of the cricoid cartilage and is worse when swallowing saliva; indeed it often disappears when ingesting food or liquids. ENT examination is usually clear and normal laryngeal mobility can be felt when gently rocking the larynx across the postcricoid tissues. A contrast swallow will show not only the structures below the pharynx but also assess the swallowing dynamically. Any suspicious area will require an endoscopy with biopsy.

FURTHER READING
Burton M (2000) *Diseases of the Ear, Nose and Throat,* 15th edn. Edinburgh: Churchill Livingstone.
Corbridge R (1998) *Essential ENT Practice. A Clinical Text.* London: Arnold.
Roland NJ, McRae RDR, McCombe AW (2000) *Key Topics in Otolaryngology,* 2nd edn. London: Bios Scientific Publishers.

DISORDERS OF THE EYE

A careful and detailed history gives most of the facts needed to make a working diagnosis. The eye has only a few mechanisms by which it can convey a diseased state. Common symptoms include alteration in visual acuity, redness, pain, discharge and photophobia. It is vital that an accurate Snellen visual acuity is recorded in all patients with an eye problem.

Diabetic eye disease (p. 1124) and hypertensive eye disease (p. 860) are discussed elsewhere.

APPLIED ANATOMY AND PHYSIOLOGY

The average diameter of the human eye is 24 mm. The *cornea* occupies the central aspect of the globe and is one of the most richly innervated tissues in the body. This clear, transparent and avascular structure, measuring 12 mm horizontally and 11 mm vertically, provides 78% of the focusing power of the eye. The endothelial cells lining the inner surface of the cornea are responsible for maintaining the clarity of the cornea by continuously pumping fluid out of the tissue. Any factor which alters the function of these cells will result in corneal oedema and cause blurred vision. The anterior surface of the cornea is lined by epithelial cells which, together with the tear film, provide a smooth and regular surface for the refraction of light. The eyelids prevent the cornea from drying and becoming an irregular surface by distributing the tear film over the surface of the globe with each blink. In addition, the lids protect the globe and provide an outflow channel for excess tears via the punctae to the nose (Fig. 20.11).

The cornea and the sclera give mechanical strength and shape to the exposed surface of the globe. The *sclera* is a white opaque structure covering four-fifths of the globe and is continuous with the cornea at the limbus. The six extraocular muscles responsible for eye movements are attached to the sclera and the optic nerve perforates it posteriorly.

The *conjunctiva* covers the anterior surface of the sclera. This richly vascularized and innervated mucous membrane stretches from the limbus over the anterior sclera and is then reflected onto the undersurface of the upper and lower lids. The area of conjunctival reflection under the lids makes up the upper and lower fornix. The conjunctiva over the sclera is referred to as the bulbar conjunctiva whilst that over the lids makes up the tarsal conjunctiva.

The *anterior chamber* is the space between the cornea and the iris, and is filled with aqueous humour (Fig. 20.12). This fluid is produced by the ciliary body (2 μL/min) and provides nutrients and oxygen to the avascular cornea. The outflow of aqueous humour is through the trabecular meshwork and canal of Schlemm adjacent to the limbus. Any factor which impedes its outflow will increase the intraocular pressure. The upper range of normal for intraocular pressure is 21 mmHg.

Sclera covered by conjunctiva
Eyelashes of lower lid

Eyebrow
Pupil
Iris
Limbus
Caruncle
Lower punctum
Lid margin

Fig. 20.11 **Photograph of the right eye.**

Conjunctiva
Pupil
Iris
Cornea
Anterior chamber
Iridocorneal angle
Canal of Schlemm
Ciliary body
Suspensory ligaments (zonule)
Ora serrata
Lens
Posterior chamber
Retina
Choroid
Sclera
Vitreous body
Optic disc
Fovea
Optic nerve
Lamina cribrosa
Central retinal artery

Fig. 20.12 **Section of the eyeball.**

Fig. 20.13 Fundus of the left eye.

Retinal artery
Retinal vein
Optic disc
Macula
Fovea

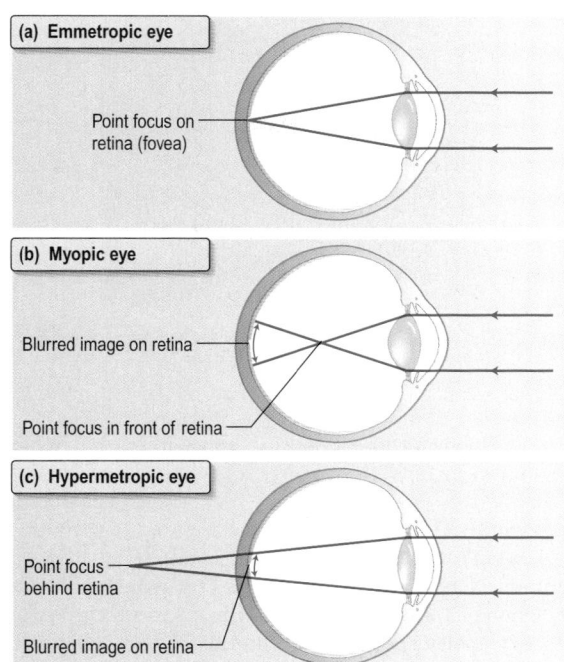

Fig. 20.14 Refraction. **(a)** Emmetropic (normal). **(b)** Myopic (short-sighted). **(c)** Hypermotropic (long-sighted).

(a) **Emmetropic eye**
Point focus on retina (fovea)

(b) **Myopic eye**
Blurred image on retina
Point focus in front of retina

(c) **Hypermetropic eye**
Point focus behind retina
Blurred image on retina

The *iris* is the coloured part of the eye under the transparent cornea. The muscles of the iris diaphragm regulate the size of the pupil, thereby controlling the amount of light entering the eye. Immediately posterior to the pupil and anterior to the vitreous humour lies the lens of the eye. This is a transparent biconvex structure and is responsible for 22% of the refractive power of the eye. By changing its shape it can alter its refractive power and help to focus objects at different distances from the eye. In the fourth decade of life this ability to change shape starts to decline (presbyopia) and the need for reading glasses becomes inevitable. With age the lens starts to become less transparent and cataracts begin to develop.

The inner aspect of the *sclera* is lined by a highly vascular tissue, the choroid, and then the retina. The vitreous humour fills the cavity between the retina and the lens. The retina is the transparent light-sensitive layer, or photographic plate, of the eye. The macula is the area of the retina responsible for detailed fine vision and has the highest density of rods and cones. The axons of the ganglion cells form the optic nerve of the eye (Fig. 20.13).

The *blood supply* to the eye is via the ophthalmic artery and, in particular, the central retinal artery is responsible for supplying the inner retinal layers. Venous return is through the central retinal and ophthalmic veins. Local lymphatic drainage is to the pre-auricular and submental nodes.

The sensory *innervation* of the eye (see p. 1185) is through the trigeminal (V) nerve. Of the six extraocular muscles the abducens (VI) nerve supplies the lateral rectus, the trochlear (IV) nerve supplies the superior oblique, whilst the rest are supplied by the oculomotor (III) nerve. The III nerve also supplies the upper lid and indirectly the pupil (parasympathetic fibres are attached to it). The facial (VI) nerve supplies the obicularis and other muscles of facial expression.

REFRACTIVE ERRORS

The eye projects a sharp and focused image onto the retina. Refractive errors refer to any abnormality in the focusing mechanism of the eye and not to any opacity in the system such as a corneal or retinal scar.

The refraction of light in emmetropic (normal), myopic and hypermetropic eyes is shown in Figure 20.14a, b and c.

Astigmatism occurs when the eye is not of the same radius of curvature for refraction. It may be myopic in one plane and hypermetropic or emmetropic in the other plane. In this situation the front surface of the eye is more rugby ball shaped than football shaped.

Presbyopia is the term used to describe the normal ageing of the lens and leads to a change in the refractive state of the eye. As the lens ages it becomes less able to alter its curvature and this causes difficulty with near vision, especially reading.

Treatment

Errors of refraction can be corrected by using spectacles or contact lenses. The latter result in better quality, but carry the risk of infection. They may be the only option in some refractive states such as keratoconus. There are a number of surgical techniques available with varying degree of accuracy. Currently the most popular method is to use an excimer laser to re-profile the corneal curvature (PRK, LASIK, LASEK). Here the laser either removes corneal tissue centrally to flatten the cornea in myopia or it removes tissue from the peripheral cornea to steepen it in hypermetropia.

DISORDERS OF THE LIDS

The lids afford protection to the eyes and help to distribute the tear film over the front surface of the globe. Excess tears are drained via the punctae and lacrimal system. Malposition of the lids, factors which affect blinking or lacrimal drainage can all cause problems.

Entropion. The lid margin rolls inwards so that the lashes are against the globe (Fig. 20.15). The lashes act as a foreign body and cause irritation, leading to a red eye which can mimic conjunctivitis. Occasionally the constant rubbing of lashes against the cornea causes an abrasion.

Fig. 20.15 **Lid entropion**. The lower lid appears inverted.

Fig. 20.17 **Blepharitis.** Crusty and scaly deposits on the lashes and lash bases.

The commonest cause is ageing and surgery is usually required.

Ectropion. The lid margin is not apposed to the globe. As a result the lacrimal puncta is not in the correct anatomical position to drain tears and patients usually complain of a watery eye. Underlying factors include age, VII nerve palsy and cicatricial skin conditions. Surgery is usually required.

Dacryocystitis. This is inflammation of the lacrimal sac. Patients usually present with a painful lump at the side of the nose adjacent to the lower lid (Fig. 20.16). This should be treated with oral broad-spectrum antibiotics such as cefalexin, and patients should be watched carefully for signs of cellulites. These patients should be referred to the ophthalmologist as some may have an underlying mucocele or dilated sac, and will require surgery.

Blepharitis. This is inflammation of the lid margins. Inflammation may involve the lashes and lash follicles (Fig. 20.17) resulting in styes, or inflammation and blockage of meibomian glands (Fig. 20.18) leading to chalazia (Fig. 20.19). Treatment involves lid toilet and topical antibiotics such as chloramphenicol or fucidic acid. If there is associated cellulites then broad-spectrum oral antibiotics are required. Some patients are left with a lump once the acute inflammatory phase of the chalazion has subsided. Most of these patients find the lump cosmetically unacceptable and require incision and curettage.

Fig. 20.18 **Blepharitis**. Upper lid showing meibomian glands plugged with oily secretions.

Fig. 20.19 **Blepharitis**. Blockage of the meibomian glands leads to swelling of the lid (chalazion).

CONJUNCTIVITIS

This is the commonest cause of a red eye. Inflammation of the conjunctiva leading to a red eye can arise from a number of causes, with viral, bacterial and allergic being the commonest. Common features in all types of conjunctivitis include soreness, redness and discharge, and in general the visual acuity is good. History should include the speed of onset of the inflammation, the colour and consistency of the discharge, whether the eye is itchy and if there has been a recent history of a cold or sore throat. In the neonate it is vital to ensure there has been no associated maternal sexually transmitted disease. The differential diagnosis of conjunctivitis is shown in Table 20.6.

Bacterial conjunctivitis

Bacterial conjunctivitis is uncommon, making up 5% of all cases of conjunctivitis. In the vast majority of patients

Fig. 20.16 **Acute dacryocystitis showing a lump on the side of the nose.**

Table 20.6 Conjunctivitis

	Discharge	Preauricular node	Corneal involvement	Comment
Bacterial	Mucopurulent	-ve except gonococci	+ve Gonococcus	Rapid onset
Viral	Watery	+ve	+ve Adenovirus	Cold and/or sore throat
Chlamydial	Watery	+ve	+ve	GU discharge
Allergic	Stringy	-ve	+ve	Itchy

it causes a sore or gritty eye in the presence of good vision. Bacterial conjunctivitis is invariably bilateral and should be suspected when conjunctival inflammation is associated with a purulent discharge. The rapidity of onset together with the severity of discharge is helpful in determining the underlying organism.

Clinical features

Gonococcal conjunctivitis should be suspected when the onset of symptoms is rapid, the discharge is copious, and ocular inflammation includes chemosis (conjunctival oedema) and lid oedema. Gonococci are a cause of conjunctivitis giving rise to a pre-auricular node.

Less acute or subacute purulent conjunctivitis with moderate discharge can be attributed to organisms such as *Haemophilus influenzae* and *Strep. pneumoniae*. Chronic conjunctivitis is usually associated with mild conjunctival injection and scant purulent discharge. Common organisms include *Staphylococcus aureus* and *Moraxella lacunata*.

Treatment

Prompt treatment with oral and topical penicillin is given in gonococcal conjunctivitis to ensure a reduced rate of corneal perforation. A Gram stain of the conjunctival swab can quickly confirm the presence of diplococci. Gonococcal conjunctivitis is a notifiable disease in the UK.

Empirical treatment for both subacute and chronic conjunctivitis involves a topical broad-spectrum antibiotic such as chloramphenicol. Swabs should be taken if these cases do not respond to this initial treatment.

Chlamydial conjunctivitis

This is a sexually transmitted disease and is most prevalent in sexually active adolescents and young adults. Direct or indirect contact with genital secretions is the usual route of infections but shared eye cosmetics can also be involved. It is caused by *Chlamydia trachomatis* (p. 121). Neonatal chlamydial conjunctivitis is a notifiable disease in the UK and should be suspected in newborns with a red eye. Mothers should be asked about sexually transmitted diseases. Trachoma caused by the same organism is found mainly in the tropics and the Middle East and is a very common cause of blindness in the world (p. 84).

Clinical features

The onset of symptoms is slow, and patients may complain of mild discomfort for weeks. In these cases the red eye is associated with a scanty mucopurulent discharge and a palpable preauricular lymph node. In chronic cases it is not unusual to see superior corneal

vascularization. In neonates the onset of the red eye is typically around 2 weeks after birth, whereas gonococcal conjunctivitis occurs within days of birth. Conjunctival swabs should be taken prior to commencement of treatment.

Treatment

Topical erythromycin twice daily is commenced and patients referred to the genitourinary physicians. Neonates should be started on topical erythromycin and referred to the paediatrician as there may be associated otitis media or pneumonitis.

Viral conjunctivitis

Adenoviral conjunctivitis

This is highly contagious and can cause epidemics in communities. Transmission is through direct or indirect contact with infected individuals. The onset of symptoms may be preceded by a cold or flu-like symptoms. The eye becomes inflamed and this is commonly associated with chemosis, lid oedema and a palpable preauricular lymph node. Some patients may develop a membrane on the tarsal conjunctiva (Fig. 20.20a, b) and haemorrhage on the bulbar conjunctiva. Viral conjunctivitis can cause deterioration in visual acuity owing to corneal involvement (focal areas of inflammation). In 50% of the patients the conjunctivitis is unilateral.

Treatment

The condition is largely self-limiting in the majority of cases. Lubricants together with a cold compress can be soothing for patients. Strict hygiene and keeping towels separate from the rest of the household goes a long way in reducing the spread of the infection. Clinicians also need to ensure good hygiene practice to reduce cross-infection and infecting themselves. In patients with corneal involvement or intense conjunctival inflammation, topical steroids are indicated.

(a)   (b)

Fig. 20.20 (a and b) Viral conjunctivitis; (b) with pseudomembrane on lower lid.

(a)   (b)

Fig. 20.21 **Dendritic ulcers on the cornea.** (a) Stained with fluorescein. (b) Stained with fluorescein and viewed with blue light.

Herpes simplex conjunctivitis

Primary ocular herpes simplex conjunctivitis is typically unilateral. It usually causes a palpable preauricular lymph node and cutaneous vesicles develop on the eyelids and the skin around the eyes in the majority of patients. Over 50% of these patients may develop a dendritic corneal ulcer (Fig. 20.21a, b). The organism responsible for this condition is the herpes simplex virus (HSV), which is usually HSV-1 but HSV-2 can give rise to ocular infection.

Treatment

Primary ocular HSV infection is a self-limiting condition but most clinicians choose to treat it with topical aciclovir in order to limit the risk of corneal epithelial involvement.

Molluscum contagiosum conjunctivitis

This is typically unilateral and produces a red eye that generally goes unrecognized and comes to the forefront because patients fail to improve and the cornea starts to become involved. A closer look at the eyelids and the margin will reveal pearly umbilicated nodules and these are filled with the DNA poxvirus. A high index of suspicion is needed to make an early diagnosis.

Treatment

This includes curetting the central portion of the lesion, freezing the centre or completely excising the lesion. If the corneal involvement is severe or the eye is very inflamed, a short course of topical steroids such as prednisolone 0.5% or dexamethasone 0.1% is helpful.

Allergic conjunctivitis

There are five main types of allergic conjunctivitis: seasonal, perennial, vernal, atopic and giant papillary. The last three are difficult to treat, chronic and can be sight-threatening. They should be referred to an ophthalmologist.

Seasonal/perennial conjunctivitis

Seasonal allergic conjunctivitis and perennial conjunctivitis affect 20% of the general population in the UK. Seasonal allergic conjunctivitis involves an allergic reaction to grass, pollen and fungal spores and occurs mainly in spring and summer. Perennial allergic conjunctivitis occurs all year round but peaks in the autumn and includes allergens such as house-dust mites.

The main symptoms include itching, redness, soreness, watering and a stringy discharge. Occasionally the conjunctiva may become so hyperaemic that chemosis results. This is usually associated with swollen lids.

Treatment

Reducing the allergen load (reducing dust, p. 897) is helpful. Medical treatment includes the use of antihistamine drops such as levocabastine and emedastine together with topical mast cell-stabilizing agents such as sodium cromoglicate and nedocromil. Corticosteroid drops should be avoided. Oral antihistamines help the itching.

CORNEAL DISORDERS

Trauma

Corneal abrasions

Trauma resulting in the removal of a focal area of epithelium on the cornea is very common. Abrasions usually occur when the eye is accidentally poked with a finger, a foreign body (FB) flies into the eye or something brushes against the eye.

Clinical features

Symptoms include severe pain, due to exposure of the corneal nerve endings, lacrimation and inability to open the eye (blepharospasm). Blinking and eye movement can aggravate the pain and foreign body sensation. The visual acuity is usually reduced. Most cases will need topical anaesthetic drops such as oxybuprocaine or amethocaine to be administered before it is possible to examine the eye. The cornea should be inspected with a blue light after instillation of fluorescein drops. The orange dye will stain the area of the abrasion. Under blue light the abrasion lights up as green. Occasionally FBs can lodge on the under surface of the upper lid and give rise to linear vertical abrasions. Eversion of the upper lid is necessary in all cases of abrasions (Fig. 20.22a, b).

Treatment

This involves instillation of a broad-spectrum antibiotic such as chloramphenicol drops or ointment four times a day for 5 days. The role of padding is controversial but common practice is to pad the affected eye for 24 hours once chloramphenicol ointment has been applied to the eye.

(a)   (b)

Fig. 20.22 **Linear corneal abrasion.** (a) Stained with fluorescein. (b) Stained with fluorescein and viewed with blue light.

(a)   (b)

Fig. 20.23 **Foreign bodies. (a)** Corneal. **(b)** Subtarsal.

Corneal foreign body

Occasionally when something flies into the eye it gets stuck on the cornea (Fig. 20.23a). It may be associated with lacrimation and photophobia. Examination is best attempted following instillation of a topical anaesthetic and should include everting the upper lid (Fig. 20.23b). Corneal foreign bodies can usually be seen directly with a white light.

Treatment

The corneal FB should be removed and the patient given a topical antibiotic such as chloramphenicol four times a day for 5 days or fucidic acid twice a day for 5 days.

Trauma

In cases of high-velocity trauma corneal perforation or intraocular FB should be suspected. Examination may show a corneal laceration with or without the FB embedded in the cornea. The FB may be present on the iris or the lens. Other clues of a penetrating injury include a flat anterior chamber or the presence of blood in the anterior chamber (hyphaema) or a large subconjunctival haemorrhage. Urgent referral to the ophthalmologist is mandatory, ensuring that no drops are instilled into the eye and that a plastic shield has been placed over the eye to minimize further risk of trauma.

Blunt trauma usually results in periorbital bruising and gross lid oedema, which can make examination to exclude perforating injury difficult. These patients should be referred to the ophthalmologist for a detailed ocular examination to exclude a perforation retinal detachment or a traumatic hyphaema (Fig. 20.24).

Keratitis

This is a general term to describe corneal inflammation. Common causes include herpes simplex virus, contact lens-associated infection and blepharitis. Symptoms include the sensation of a foreign body or pain (depending on the size and depth of the ulcer), photophobia and lacrimation. Vision is reduced if the ulcer is in the visual axis.

Herpes simplex keratitis

Corneal epithelial cells infected with the virus eventually undergo lysis and form an ulcer which is typically dendritic in shape (see Fig. 20.21). The ulcer stains with fluorescein and can be observed easily with a blue light. Topical immunosuppression, e.g. steroid drops, or systemic immunosuppression, e.g. AIDS, can lead to the centrifugal spread of the virus such that the ulcer increases in area and is referred to as a geographic ulcer. Recurrent attacks of HSV keratitis can be triggered by ultraviolet light, stress and menstruation. All these factors are responsible for activating the virus, which normally lies dormant in the ganglion of the V nerve.

Treatment

Aciclovir ointment five times a day for 2 weeks is usually very effective.

Contact lens-related keratitis

A small number of contact lens wearers develop infective corneal ulcers which are potentially sight-threatening (Fig. 20.25a, b). The organisms usually responsible include Gram-positive and Gram-negative bacteria. Patients should be referred to an ophthalmologist for scraping of the ulcer and commencement of antibiotic treatment.

Blepharitis

This is an extremely common condition where the lid margins are inflamed. Common underlying causes of blepharitis include meibomian gland dysfunction, seborrhoea and *Staphylococcus aureus*. Patients can be asymptomatic or complain of itchy, burning eyes because of tear film instability resulting from meibomian gland dysfunction. *Staphylococcus aureus* is frequently responsible for chronic blepharo-conjunctivitis and some patients may develop keratitis (Fig. 20.26).

Treatment

Lid hygiene is the mainstay of treatment as it helps to reduce the bacterial load and unblock meibomian glands. A short course of topical chloramphenicol is useful in

Fig. 20.24 **Blunt trauma.** Hyphaema and globe rupture with iris prolapse.

Iris prolapse

Hyphaema

(a)   (b)

Ulcer

Fig. 20.25 **Contact lens-related keratitis. (a)** Corneal ulcer. **(b)** Severe keratitis with a corneal abscess and a hypopyon.

Fig. 20.26 **Marginal keratitis.**

Marginal ulcer

Table 20.7 Cataracts: aetiology	
Congenital	Maternal infection
	Familial
Age	Elderly
Metabolic	Diabetes, galactosaemia, hypocalcaemia, Wilson's disease
Drug-induced	Corticosteroids, phenothiazines, miotics, amiodarone
Traumatic	Post-intraocular surgery
Inflammatory	Uveitis
Disease associated	Down's syndrome (p. 175)
	Dystrophia mytonica (p. 1270)
	Lowe's syndrome (p. 1146)

chronic cases but in severe cases or cases where acne rosacea is suspected, oral doxycycline may be required. Patients with keratitis should be referred to the ophthalmologist as they will require topical steroids.

CATARACTS

Cataract (Fig. 20.27a, b) is by far the commonest cause of preventable blindness in the world with an effective surgical treatment. In the UK approximately 250 000 cataract operations are performed each year, making it the commonest surgical procedure.

Aetiology

Age-related opacification of the lens (cataract) is the commonest cause of visual impairment with 30% of people over 65 years having visual acuities below that required for driving (Snellen acuity less than 6/12). The common causes of cataracts are summarized in Table 20.7.

In young patients, familial or congenital causes should be excluded. Any history of ocular inflammation is noted. Cataracts diagnosed in infants demand urgent referral to the ophthalmologist in order to minimize the subsequent development of amblyopia.

Clinical features

Gradual painless deterioration of vision is the commonest symptom. Other symptoms are dependent upon the type of cataract, for example a posterior capsular type would lead to glare and problems with night driving. Early changes in the lens are correctable by spectacles but eventually the opacification needs surgical intervention.

Investigations

Blood glucose, serum calcium and liver biochemistry should be measured to diagnose metabolic disorders.

Treatment

Cataract extraction with the insertion of an intraocular lens is treatment of choice (Fig. 20.27c). The aetiology and density of the cataracts usually determines the technique employed. Currently, small incision surgery called phacoemulsification is the most popular technique used for routine cases.

GLAUCOMA

This refers to a group of diseases where the pressure inside the eye is sufficiently elevated to cause optic nerve damage and result in visual field defects (Fig. 20.28a, b). Normal intraocular pressure (IOP) is between 10 and 21 mmHg. Some types of glaucoma can result in an IOP exceeding 70 mmHg. Glaucoma as a disease entity is the second commonest cause of blindness word-wide and the third commonest cause of blind registration in the UK.

Primary open-angle glaucoma (POAG)

This is the commonest form of glaucoma. High intraocular pressures result from reduced outflow of aqueous

(a)

(b)

Intraocular lens

(c)

Fig. 20.27 **Cataracts. (a)** Early cataract. **(b)** White mature cataract. **(c)** Artificial intraocular lens following phacoemulsification.

Fig. 20.28 **(a) Normal optic disc and (b) glaucomatous optic disc.** The central cup is enlarged and deepened.

Table 20.8 Differential diagnosis of the acute red eye

Cause	Conjunctival injection	Unilateral or bilateral	Pain	Photophobia	Vision	Pupil	Intraocular pressure
Conjunctivitis	Diffuse	Bilateral	Gritty	Occasionally with adenovirus	Normal	Normal	Normal
Anterior uveitis	Circum-corneal	Unilateral	Painful	Yes	Reduced	Constricted	Normal or raised
Acute glaucoma	Diffuse	Unilateral	Severe pain	Mild	Reduced	Mid-dilated	Raised

humour through the trabecular meshwork. The cause of this increased resistance to aqueous outflow at the level of the meshwork is not fully understood. Common risk factors include age (0.02% of 40-year-olds vs 10% of 80-year-olds), race (black Africans are at five times greater risk than whites), positive family history and myopia.

POAG causes a gradual, insidious, painless loss of peripheral visual field. The central vision remains good until the end-stage of the disease. Diagnosis is only made if the IOP is measured. The optic disc is inspected and shows an enlarged cup with a thin neuroretinal rim. Visual fields are performed and show a normal blind spot with scotomas. Most patients are identified as having glaucoma whilst undergoing a routine ophthalmic examination.

Treatment

Treatment aims to reduce the IOP and this is achieved either by reducing aqueous production or increasing aqueous drainage. Beta-blockers such as timolol, carteolol, levobunolol, reduce aqueous production and are the commonest prescribed topical agents. These drugs are contraindicated in patients with COPD, asthma or heart block. Prostaglandin analogues such as latanoprost, travoprost, increase aqueous outflow and are fast becoming the treatment of choice for POAG as they can reduce IOP by 30%. Carbonic anhydrase inhibitors such as acetazolamide reduce aqueous production and are available in both topical and oral form. In its oral form acetazolamide is the most potent drug for reducing ocular pressure. It should not be used in patients with sulphonamide allergy.

Acute angle-closure glaucoma (AACG)

This is an ophthalmic emergency. In this type of glaucoma there is a sudden rise in intraocular pressure to levels greater than 50 mmHg. This occurs due to reduced aqueous drainage as a result of the ageing lens pushing the iris forward against the trabecular meshwork. People most at risk of developing AACG are those with shallow anterior chambers such as hypermetropes and women. The attack is more likely to occur under reduced light conditions when the pupil is dilated.

AACG causes sudden onset of a red painful eye and blurred vision. Patients become unwell with nausea and vomiting and complain of headache and severe ocular pain. The eye is injected, tender and feels hard. The cornea is hazy and the pupil is semi-dilated (Fig. 20.29).

Mid-dilated pupil

Hazy cornea

Fig. 20.29 Acute angle-closure glaucoma.

Table 20.8 shows the differential diagnosis of the acute red eye.

Prompt treatment is required to preserve sight and includes i.v. acetazolamide 500 mg (provided there are no contraindications) to reduce IOP, and instillation of pilocarpine 4% drops to constrict the pupil to improve aqueous outflow and prevent iris adhesion to the trabecular meshwork. Other topical drops such as beta-blockers and prostaglandin analogues can also be instilled if available, provided there are no contra-indications. Analgesia and antiemetics are given as required.

These patients must be referred to an ophthalmologist immediately so that reduction in IOP can be monitored and other agents such as oral glycerol or i.v. mannitol can be administered to non-responding patients. Definitive treatment involves making a hole in the periphery of the iris of both eyes either by laser or surgically.

UVEITIS

Uveitis is inflammation of the uveal tract, which includes the iris, ciliary body and choroid. Inflammation confined to the anterior segment of the eye (in front of the iris) is referred to as iritis or anterior uveitis, that involving the ciliary body is referred to as intermediate uveitis whilst inflammation of the choroid is termed posterior uveitis. If all three regions are involved then the term pan-uveitis is used.

The most common symptoms of uveitis are blurred vision, pain, redness, photophobia and floaters. Each symptom is determined by the location of the inflammation such that photophobia and pain are common features of iritis whilst floaters are commonly seen with posterior uveitis.

Uveitis is commonly encountered with ankylosing spondylitis and positive HLA-B27 (p. 565), arthritis, inflammatory bowel disease, sarcoid, tuberculosis, syphilis,

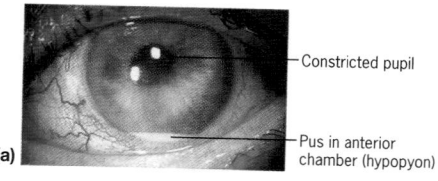

(a) — Constricted pupil — Pus in anterior chamber (hypopyon)

(b)

Fig. 20.30 **Anterior uveitis. (a)** Acute with hypopyon. **(b)** Showing keratic precipitates on the corneal endothelial.

toxoplasmosis, Behçet's syndrome, lymphoma and viruses such as herpes, cytomegalovirus and HIV. In a number of patients no cause is found (idiopathic uveitis).

Anterior uveitis (iritis)

The classic presentation entails a triad of eye symptoms: redness, pain and photophobia. Vision can be normal or blurred depending on the degree of inflammation. The eye can be generally red or the injection can be localized to the limbus. The anterior chamber shows features consistent with inflammation including cells with keratic precipitates (KP) on the corneal endothelium, fibrin or hypopyon (pus), and the pupil may have adhered to the lens (posterior synechiae) (Fig. 20.30a, b). The IOP may be normal or raised either due to cells clogging up the trabecular meshwork or posterior synechiae causing aqueous to build up behind the iris and force the iris against the trabecular meshwork and so reduce aqueous drainage.

Treatment

This consists of reducing inflammation with the use of topical steroids such as dexamethasone 0.1% and dilating the pupil with cyclopentolate 1% to prevent formation of anterior synechiae. Dilatation also allows fundoscopy to exclude posterior segment involvement. If the IOP is raised, this is treated with either topical beta-blockers, prostaglandin analogues, or oral or i.v, acetazolamide. These patients should be referred to the ophthalmologist.

DISORDERS OF THE RETINA

Central retinal vein occlusion (CRVO)

This usually leads to profound sudden painless loss of vision with thrombosis of the central retinal vein at or posterior to the lamina cribrosa where the optic nerve exits the globe. The thrombus causes obstruction to the outflow of blood leading to a rise in intravascular pressure. This results in dilated veins, retinal haemorrhage,

retinal haemorrhage — Disc oedema — Cotton wool spots

Fig. 20.31 **Central retinal vein occlusion.**

cotton wool spots, abnormal leakage of fluid from vessels resulting in retinal oedema (Fig. 20.31). In severe cases an afferent papillary defect is usually present (p. 1182).

Predisposing factors include increasing age, hypertension and cardiovascular disease, diabetes, glaucoma, blood dyscrasias and vasculitis.

Treatment

Treatment of any underlying medical condition is mandatory. Referral to an ophthalmologist is essential to monitor the eye, as some patients can develop retinal ischaemia with resulting neovascularization of the retina and iris. Patients who develop iris neovascularization, rubeosis, are at risk of developing rubeotic glaucoma.

Central retinal artery occlusion (CRAO)

This results in sudden painless severe loss of vision. Retinal arterial occlusion results in infarction of the inner two-thirds of the retina. The arteries become narrow and the retina becomes opaque and oedematous. A cherry red spot is seen at the fovea because the choroid shows up through the thinnest part of the retina (Fig. 20.32). An afferent papillary defect is usually present (p. 1182).

Arteriosclerosis-related thrombosis is the most common cause of CRAO. Emboli from atheromas and diseased heart valves are other causes. Giant cell arteritis (p. 1249) must be excluded.

Treatment

CRAO is an ophthalmic emergency since studies have shown that irreversible retinal damage occurs after 90 minutes of onset. Ocular massage and 500 mg i.v. acetazolamide help to reduce ocular pressure and may help in dislodging the emboli. Breathing into a paper bag allows a build-up of carbon dioxide which acts as a vasodilator and so helps in dislodging the emboli. Other options include making a corneal paracentesis to drain off some aqueous humour, thereby reducing the intraocular pressure.

Cherry red spot — Retinal oedema

Fig. 20.32 **Central retinal artery occlusion.**

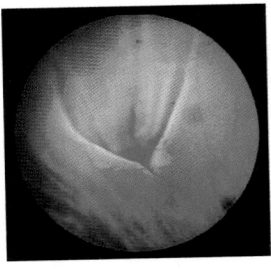

Fig. 20.33 Retinal tear leading to detachment.

Patients with CRAO should have a thorough medical evaluation to determine the aetiology of the emboli or thrombus. Some patients may present with transient loss of vision or amaurosis fugax (p. 1212). All patients with CRAO and amaurosis fugax should be started on oral aspirin if it is not medically contraindicated.

Retinal detachment

This causes a painless progressive visual field loss. The shadow corresponds to the area of detached retina. Following a tear in the retina, fluid collects in the potential space between the sensory retina and the pigment epithelium (Fig. 20.33). Patients usually report a sudden onset of floaters often associated with flashes of light prior to the detachment. These patients should be referred to an ophthalmologist for a detailed fundal examination.

Age-related macular degeneration (AMD)

This is the commonest cause of visual impairment in patients over 50 years in the western world. It is the commonest cause of blind registration in this age group. With age, the macula undergoes degenerative changes which can result in deposition of material (drusen) over the macula or involutional changes at the macula (Fig. 20.34a). Mutations in the fibulin genes (particularly 5) are being described. Not all patients with these changes will be affected visually but a number go on to develop distortion and blurring of their central vision. Some patients develop frank choroidal neovascularization at the macula leading to profound loss of central vision but continuation of good peripheral vision (Fig. 20.34b).

Patients with central distortion or with frank macular pathology should be referred to the ophthalmologist for assessment of treatment. Only a few patients will fulfil the clinical requirement to receive laser treatment or photodynamic therapy (PDT). All patients should be assessed for low-vision aids such as magnifying glasses as this may help to improve their independence. Recently, pegaptanib, an anti-vascular endothelial growth factor (anti-VEGF) has been given by intra-vitreous injection with some benefit and trials continue.

CAUSES OF VISUAL LOSS

Box 20.3 summarizes the causes of visual loss. In developing countries the common causes of blindness are similar to those in the developed world and include trauma, cataract, diabetic retinopathy, glaucoma and macular degeneration. In addition, trachoma due to *Chlamydia trachomatis* (see p. 84) accounts for 10% of global blindness and onchocerciasis (river blindness) due to *Onchocerca volvulus* (p. 108) accounts for blindness in about 1 million people, although this is decreasing with treatment. In leprosy, 70% of patients have ocular involvement, and blindness occurs in 5–10% of these. Ocular involvement is common in cerebral malaria (p. 97), although loss of vision is rare. HIV infection can produce uveitis but the major problem is severe opportunistic infection of the eye when the CD4 count falls (p. 139).

Vitamin A deficiency and xerophthalmia affects millions each year, and the WHO classification of xerophthalmia by ocular signs is shown in Table 5.10 (p. 242).

> ℹ **Box 20.3 Loss of vison: summary**
>
> | Painless loss of vision | Painful loss of vision |
> |---|---|
> | Cataract | Acute angle-closure glaucoma |
> | Open-angle glaucoma | Giant cell arteritis (p. 1249) |
> | Retinal detachment | Optic neuritis (p. 1181) |
> | Central retinal vein occlusion | Uveitis |
> | Central retinal artery occlusion | Scleritis |
> | Diabetic retinopathy (p. 1124) | Keratitis |
> | Vitreous haemorrhage | Shingles |
> | Posterior uveitis | Orbital cellulitis |
> | Age-related macular degeneration | Trauma |
> | Optic nerve compression | |
> | Cerebral vascular disease | |

—Drusen

(a)

—Haemorrhage over macula from choroidal neovascularization of membrane

(b)

Fig. 20.34 Age-related macular degeneration. (a) With deposition of material (drusen) over the macula. **(b)** With choroidal neovascularization.

FURTHER READING

Asbell PA, Dualan I, Mindel J (2005) Age related cataract. *Lancet* **365**: 599–609.

Lynn WA, Lightman S (2004) The eye in systemic infection. *Lancet* **364**: 1439–1450.

Weinreb RN, Khaw PT (2004) Primary open-angle glaucoma. *Lancet* **363**: 1711–1720.

Wilson SE (2004) Lasers for vision correction. *New England Journal of Medicine* **351**: 470–475.

Neurological disease 21

EPIDEMIOLOGY

Clinical neurology is diverse and complex and the epidemiology of these conditions is discussed in individual sections. There s worldwide variation. Conditions seen in UK are summarized in Table 21.1.

HISTORY, SYMPTOMS AND SIGNS

Methods of recording history and basic examination are outside the scope of this chapter. Notes should read chronologically to portray the *story* from the patient or relative. Pattern recognition – interpretation of history, symptoms and examination – is very reliable. Practical experience is vital. There are three critical questions:

- What is/are the site(s) of the lesion(s)?
- What is the likely pathology?
- Does a recognizable disease fit this pattern?

Table 21.1 Incidence rates for commoner neurological conditions/100 000/year in the UK

Headaches (GP consultations)	2200
Cerebrovascular events	205
Shingles (herpes zoster)	140
Diabetic neuropathy	54
Compressive neuropathies	49
Epilepsy	46
Parkinson's disease	19
Post-herpetic neuralgia	11
All CNS tumours	9
Trigeminal neuralgia	8
Meningitis	7
Multiple sclerosis	7
Severe brain injury	7
Subarachnoid haemorrhage	6
Subdural haematoma	6
Presenile dementia (below 65 years)	4
Cerebral palsy	3
Guillain–Barré syndrome	3
Myasthenia gravis	3
Transient global amnesia	3
Motor neurone disease	2

This is the essence of clinical diagnosis. In the text that follows, several common problems are related to core neuroanatomy.

Headaches

Headache is an almost universal experience, and one of the most common symptoms in medical practice. It varies from an infrequent and trivial nuisance to a pointer to serious disease.

Mechanism

Pain receptors are located at the base of the brain in arteries and veins and throughout meninges, extracranial vessels, scalp, neck and facial muscles, paranasal sinuses, eyes and teeth. Curiously, brain substance is almost devoid of pain receptors.

Head pain is mediated by mechanical (e.g. stretching of meninges) and chemical receptors (e.g. 5-hydroxytryptamine and histamine stimulation). Nerve impulses travel centrally via fifth and ninth cranial nerves and via upper cervical sensory roots.

Most headaches are benign, but the diagnostic issue – and usual concern – is the question of serious disease. Here are some useful clinical pointers.

Chronic (benign) and recurrent headaches

Almost all recurring headaches lasting hours/days – band-like, generalized head pains, with a history for several years or months – are vaguely ascribed to muscle tension, and/or migraine (see p. 1247). Depression is a common accompaniment.

In localized pain of short duration (minutes to hours), sinusitis, glaucoma and migrainous neuralgia (p. 1248) should be considered. Malignant hypertension, with arterial damage and brain swelling, occasionally causes headache (see p. 859). Headaches are not caused by high blood pressure alone.

Eyestrain from refractive error does not cause headache, though new prescription lenses sometimes provoke pain.

Pressure headaches

Intracranial mass lesions displace and stretch meninges and basal vessels. Pain is provoked when these structures are shifted either by a mass or by changes in cerebrospinal fluid (CSF) pressure, e.g. coughing. Cerebral oedema around brain tumours causes further shift. These 'pressure headaches' typically become worse on lying down.

Any headache present on waking and made worse by coughing, straining or sneezing may be due to a mass lesion. Vomiting often accompanies pressure headaches. Such headaches are caused early, over days or weeks by posterior fossa masses (see hydrocephalus, p. 1247), but over a longer time scale – months or years – by hemisphere tumours.

A rare cause of prostrating headache with lower limb weakness is an intraventricular tumour causing intermittent hydrocephalus.

Headache of subacute onset

The onset and progression of a headache over days or weeks with or without features of a pressure headache should always raise suspicion of an intracranial mass or serious intracranial disease. Encephalitis (see p. 1239), viral meningitis (p. 1237) and chronic meningitis (p. 1238) should also be considered.

Headaches with scalp tenderness

Patches of exquisite tenderness overlying superficial scalp arteries are caused by giant cell arteritis (see p. 1249), almost exclusively in patients over 50.

Headache following head injury

Subdural haematoma (see p. 1218) must be considered – the majority of post-trauma headaches lasting days, weeks or months are not caused by any serious intracranial pathology.

A single episode of severe headache

This common emergency is caused by one of the following:

- subarachnoid haemorrhage
- migraine, or other benign headaches
- meningitis (occasionally).

Particular attention should be paid to suddenness of onset (suggestive of subarachnoid haemorrhage), neck stiffness and vomiting (meningeal irritation), and to the presence of a rash and/or fever (bacterial meningitis).

Difficulty walking and falls

Change in gait is a common presenting complaint in neurology (see Table 21.2). Arthritis and muscle pain also alter gait, making walking stiff and slow (antalgia). Falls, especially in the elderly, are a common cause of morbidity. The *pattern* of abnormal gait is valuable diagnostically.

Spasticity

Spasticity (see p. 1192), more pronounced in extensor muscles, with or without weakness, causes walking to be stiff and jerky. Toes of shoes become scuffed, catching level ground. Pace shortens but a narrow base is maintained. Clonus – involuntary extensor rhythmic jerking of the legs – may be noticed.

When the problem is predominantly unilateral and weakness is marked (in a hemiparesis), the stiff, weak leg drags and is circumducted.

Table 21.2 Common neurological patterns of difficulty walking
Spasticity/hemiparesis
Parkinson's disease
Cerebellar ataxia
Sensory loss (joint position/loss)
Distal weakness
Proximal weakness
Apraxia of gait

Parkinson's disease (see p. 1227)

There is muscular rigidity throughout extensors and flexors. Power is preserved but walking slows. The pace shortens to a shuffle; its base remains narrow. Falls occur. A stoop and diminished arm swinging become apparent. Gait becomes festinant (hurried) in small rapid steps. There is particular difficulty initiating movement and turning quickly. *Retropulsion* describes small backward steps, taken involuntarily when a patient is halted.

Cerebellar ataxia (see also p. 1195)

In disease of the lateral cerebellar lobes stance becomes broad-based, unstable and tremulous. Ataxia describes this imperfect control. Walking tends to veer towards the more affected cerebellar lobe.

In disease confined to cerebellar midline structures (the vermis) the trunk becomes unsteady without limb ataxia. There is a tendency to fall backwards or sideways – truncal ataxia.

Sensory ataxia

Peripheral sensory lesions (e.g. polyneuropathy, p. 1260) cause ataxia because there is loss of the sense of joint position – *proprioception*. Broad-based, high-stepping, stamping gait develops. This ataxia is made worse by removal of additional sensory input (e.g. vision) and is worse in the dark. First described in sensory ataxia of tabes dorsalis (p. 1240), this is the basis of Romberg's test. Ask the patient to close the eyes while standing: observe whether the patient becomes unstable (and prevent falling).

Lower limb weakness

When weakness is distal, each leg must be lifted over obstacles. When ankle dorsiflexors are weak, such as in a common peroneal nerve palsy (see p. 1260), each foot returns to the ground with a visible and audible *slap*.

Weakness of proximal lower limb muscles (e.g. in polymyositis or muscular dystrophy) leads to difficulty in rising from sitting or squatting. Once upright, the patient walks with a waddling gait, the pelvis being ill-supported by each lower limb as it carries the full weight of the body.

Gait apraxia

With frontal lobe disease (e.g. tumour, hydrocephalus, infarction), the acquired skill of walking becomes disorganized. Leg movement is normal when sitting or lying but initiation and organization of walking fail. This is gait *apraxia* – a failure of the skilled act of walking. Shuffling small steps (*marche à petits pas*), difficulty initiating walking (gait ignition failure) or undue hesitancy may predominate. Urinary incontinence and dementia are often present with frontal lobe disease.

Falls

Falls, especially in the elderly, are a major cause of morbidity and hospital admission, e.g. following hip or upper limb fracture. Often no precise cause can be found. A multidisciplinary approach is essential, e.g. reviewing risk factors such as rugs, stairs, footwear and needs for additional home aids.

Dizziness, vertigo, blackouts, collapse and fatigue

Dizziness covers many complaints, from a vague feeling of unsteadiness to severe, acute vertigo. It is frequently used to describe light-headedness felt in panic and anxiety, during palpitations, and in syncope or chronic ill-health. The real nature of this symptom must be determined.

Vertigo – an illusion of movement – is more definite. It is a sensation of rotation, or tipping. The patient feels that the surroundings are spinning or moving. It is distinctly unpleasant and often accompanied by nausea or vomiting. For causes of vertigo, see page 1188.

Blackout, like dizziness, is a descriptive term implying either altered consciousness, visual disturbance or falling. Epilepsy, syncope, hypoglycaemia, anaemia must be considered. However, commonly no sinister cause is found. A careful history, from an eye-witness, is essential.

Collapse is vague but often used. It is not a diagnosis. Avoid it in medical notes.

Fatigue is another common symptom of neurological disorders.

FURTHER READING

Chaudhuri A, Behan P (2004) Fatigue in neurological disorders. *Lancet* **363**: 978–988.

Davenport R (2004) Diagnosing acute headaches. *Clinical Medicine* **4**(2): 109–112.

Tinetti ME (2003) Preventing falls in the elderly. *New England Journal of Medicine* **348**(1): 42–48.

van Weel C, Vermuelen H, van den Bosch W (1995) Falls: a community perspective. *Lancet* 345: 1549–1551.

NEUROLOGICAL EXAMINATION

A short five-part examination is shown in Practical box 21.1, and a fuller examination in Practical box 21.2.

Formulation

Relevant findings are drawn together in a brief written diagnostic summary. This will form the basis for investigations, transfer of information, and management.

FUNCTIONAL NEUROANATOMY: AN INTRODUCTION

The neurone and synapse (Fig. 21.1)

The neurone is the functional unit of the nervous system. Its cell body and axon terminate in a synapse. The specificity, size and type of each group of neurones vary. A single α-motor neurone within an anterior horn of the

Practical Box 21.1
Five-part short neurological examination

1 **Look at the patient**
   General demeanour
   Speech
   Gait
   Arm swinging

2 **Examine the head**
   Fundi
   Pupils
   Eye movements
   Facial movements
   Tongue

3 **Examine the upper limbs**
   Posture of outstretched arms
   Wasting, fasciculation
   Power, tone
   Coordination
   Reflexes

4 **Examine the lower limbs**
   Power (hip flexion, ankle dorsiflexion)
   Tone
   Reflexes
   Plantar responses

5 **Assess sensation**
   Ask the patient

thoracic spinal cord has an axonal length over 1 metre and innervates between several hundred and 2000 muscle fibres in one leg – a motor unit. By contrast, some spinal or intracerebral internuncial neurones have axons under 100 µm long, terminating solely on one neuronal cell body.

Neurotransmitters

Synaptic transmission is mediated by neurotransmitters released by action potentials passing down an axon.

Neurotransmitters then react with postsynaptic receptors and are removed by transporter proteins. The neurotransmitter–receptor reaction increases ionic permeability and propagates a further action potential. This combination of axonal electrical activity and synaptic chemical release is the basis of all neurological function.

Neurotransmitters include acetylcholine, norepinephrine (noradrenaline), epinephrine (adrenaline), 5-hydroxytryptamine (5-HT), gamma-aminobutyric acid (GABA), opioid peptides, prostaglandins, histamine, dopamine, glutamate, nitric oxide, neuromelanin and vasoactive intestinal peptide (VIP). Of these, glutamate is the principal excitatory neurotransmitter.

The role of neurotransmitters and transporters in pathogenesis continues to be evaluated, but it is thought that a wide variety of acute and chronic neurological disease is mediated by a final common pathway of neuronal injury involving excessive stimulation of glutamate receptors.

Table 21.3 Six grades of muscle power

Grade	Definition
5	Normal power
4	Active movement against gravity and resistance
3	Active movement against gravity
2	Active movement with gravity eliminated
1	Flicker of contraction
0	No contraction

Practical Box 21.2
Ten-part neurological examination

1 **State of consciousness, arousal, appearance** (e.g. coma)

2 **Mental state, attitude, insight** (see Box 22.5, p. 1277)

3 **Cognitive function**
   Orientation in time and place, recall of recent and distant events (memory, level of intellect, language and speech/cerebral dominance, other disorders of skilled function, e.g. apraxia)

4 **Gait and Romberg's test**

5 **Skull shape** – circumference, bruits

6 **Neck** – stiffness, palpation and auscultation of carotid arteries

7 **Cranial nerves** (see Table 21.5)

8 **Motor system**
   Upper limbs:
     Wasting and fasciculation
     Posture of arms: drift, rebound, tremor
     Tone: spasticity or extrapyramidal rigidity
     Power: 0–5 scale (Table 21.3)
     Tendon reflexes: + or ++ normal; +++ increased: 0 absent with reinforcement

   Thorax and abdomen:
     Respiration
     Thoracic and abdominal muscles
     Abdominal reflexes
     Cremasteric reflexes

   Lower limbs:
     Wasting and fasciculation
     Tone, power and tendon reflexes
     Plantar responses

9 **Coordination and fine movements**

10 **Sensory system**
   First, ask whether feeling in the limbs, face and trunk is entirely normal

   Posterior columns:
     Vibration (using a 128 Hz tuning fork)
     Joint position
     Light touch
     2-point discrimination (normal: 0.5 cm finger tips, 2 cm soles)

   Spinothalamic tracts:
     Pain: use a split orange-stick or a sterile pin
     Temperature: hot or cold tubes

   If sensation is abnormal, chart areas involved

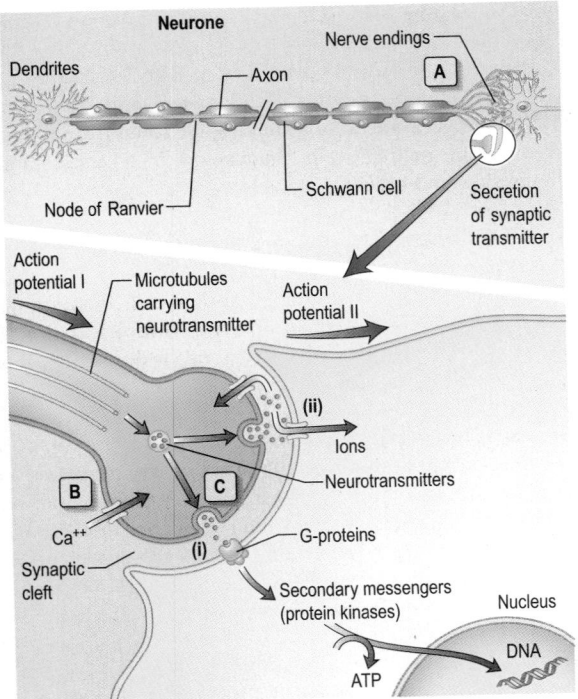

Fig. 21.1 The functional unit: neurone and neurotransmitters. The action potential (i.e. nerve impulse) travels down the axon. Microtubules carry the neurotransmitters to the nerve endings (**A**). Action potential I depolarizes the synaptic membrane, opening the voltage-gated calcium channels (**B**). The influx of calcium causes the vesicles to fuse with the membrane (**C**), allowing the neurotransmitter to (**i**) bind to the receptor and activate the secondary messenger, which then modulates gene transcription (see Ch. 3), and also to (**ii**) open ligand-gated channels. This allows ions to enter, depolarize the membrane and initiate action potential II.

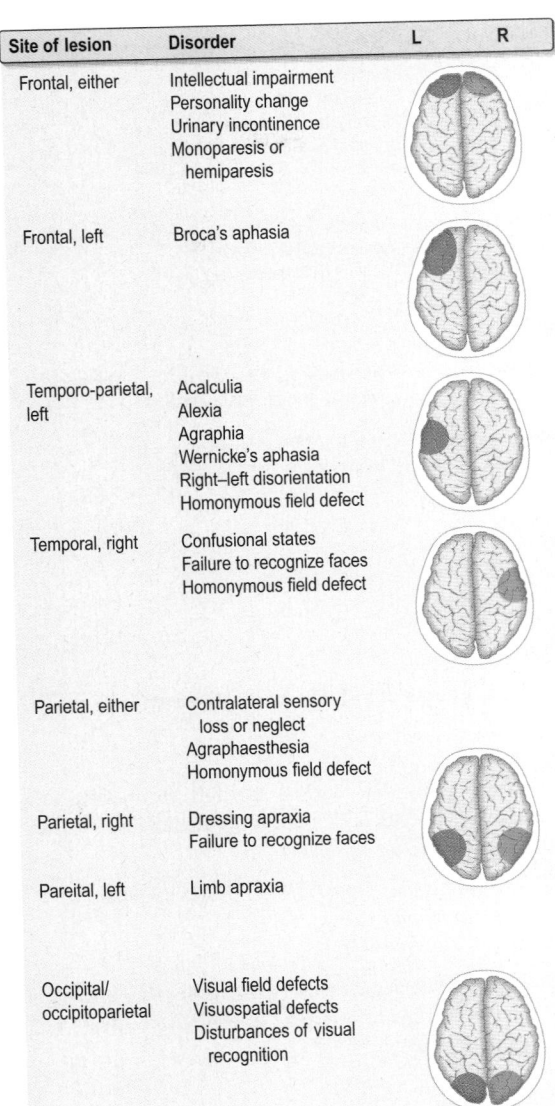

Fig. 21.2 Principal features of destructive cortical lesions (right-handed individual).

Clinical features of focal brain lesions: general mechanisms

Whilst it is unusual to have to recall detailed neuro-anatomy, it is necessary to understand how the nervous system works and how each part is integrated. We can recognize, from symptoms and signs, the part of the nervous system that is malfunctioning – for example, the left frontal lobe, one internal capsule, or a seventh cranial (facial) nerve.

Focal lesions of the cerebral cortex, and throughout the nervous system, cause symptoms and signs by two processes:

- *Suppression or destruction* of neurones and surrounding structures (Fig. 21.2). This is the most common process – part of the system fails to work.
- Synchronous discharge of neurones by *irritative* lesions (Fig. 21.3), e.g. cerebral cortex lesions cause epilepsy, either partial or generalized.

Localization within the cerebral cortex

This subject causes unnecessary difficulty. Work on neuronal networks, functional imaging and plasticity within the brain questions traditional views of highly specific localization of function. However, in practical neurology, it is necessary to understand the main functional roles of the cerebral cortex. The following paragraphs summarize areas of clinical importance.

The dominant hemisphere (usually left)

The concept of cerebral dominance arose with a simple observation. Right-handed stroke patients with acquired language disorders had destructive lesions within the left hemisphere. Almost all right-handed and 70% of left-handed people have language function in the left hemisphere.

Site of lesion	Effects	L	R
Frontal	Partial seizures – focal motor seizures of contralateral limbs Conjugate deviation of head and eyes away from the lesion		
Temporal	Formed visual hallucinations Complex partial seizures Memory disturbances (e.g. déjà vu)		
Parietal	Partial seizures – focal sensory seizures of contralateral limbs		
Parieto-occipital	Crude visual hallucinations (e.g. shapes in one part of the field)		
Occipital	Visual disturbances (e.g. flashes)		

Fig. 21.3 Effects of irritative cortical lesions.

Destructive lesions within the left fronto-temporo-parietal region cause various disorders of human communication:

- spoken language – *aphasia*, also called *dysphasia*
- writing – *agraphia*
- reading – *acquired alexia*.

Developmental dyslexia describes delayed and dis-organized reading and writing ability in children with normal intelligence.

Aphasia

Aphasia is loss of or defective language from damage to the speech centres within the left hemisphere. Numerous varieties have been described.

Broca's aphasia (expressive aphasia, anterior aphasia)

Damage in the left frontal lobe causes reduced speech fluency with comprehension relatively preserved. The patient makes great efforts to initiate language, which becomes reduced to a few disjointed words. There is failure to construct sentences. Patients who recover from this form of aphasia say they knew what they wanted to say, but 'could not get the words out'.

Wernicke's aphasia (receptive aphasia, posterior aphasia)

Left temporo-parietal damage leaves language that is fluent but the words themselves are incorrect. This varies from insertion of a few incorrect or nonexistent words into fluent speech to a profuse outpouring of jargon (that is, rubbish with wholly nonexistent words). Severe jargon aphasia may be bizarre – and confused with psychotic behaviour.

Patients who have recovered from Wernicke's aphasia say that when aphasic they found speech, both their own and others', like a wholly unintelligible foreign language. They could neither stop themselves, nor understand themselves and others.

Nominal aphasia (anomic aphasia or amnestic aphasia)

This means difficulty naming familiar objects. Naming difficulty is an early sign in all types of aphasia. A left posterior temporal/inferior parietal lesion causes a severe, isolated form.

Global aphasia (central aphasia)

This means the combination of the expressive problems of Broca's aphasia and the loss of comprehension of Wernicke's. The patient can neither speak nor understand language. It is due to widespread damage to speech areas and is the commonest aphasia after a severe left hemisphere infarct. Writing and reading are also affected.

Dysarthria

Dysarthria simply means disordered articulation – slurred speech. Language is intact, cf. aphasia. Paralysis, slowing or incoordination of muscles of articulation or local discomfort causes various different patterns of dysarthria. Examples are the 'gravelly' speech of upper motor neurone lesions of lower cranial nerves, the jerky, ataxic speech of cerebellar lesions, the monotone of Parkinson's disease, and speech in myasthenia that fatigues and dies away. Many aphasic patients are also somewhat dysarthric.

The non-dominant hemisphere

Disorders in right-handed patients with right hemisphere lesions are often difficult to recognize. They comprise abnormalities of perception of internal and external space. Examples are losing the way in familiar surroundings, failing to put on clothing correctly (*dressing apraxia*), or failure to draw simple shapes – *constructional apraxia*.

Memory and its disorders (see also p. 1254)

Disorders of memory follow damage to the medial surfaces of both temporal lobes and their brainstem connections – the hippocampi, fornices and mammillary bodies. Bilateral lesions are necessary to cause *amnesia*. It is characteristic of all organic memory disorders that more recent events are recalled poorly, in contrast to the relative preservation of distant memories.

Memory loss (the amnestic syndrome) is part of dementia (p. 1254) but also occurs as an isolated entity (Table 21.4).

Essential elements of neuroanatomy

For clinical purposes, and particularly in general medicine, the extreme complexity of neuroanatomy must be reduced to its core elements. The following sections cover:

Table 21.4   Causes of the amnestic syndrome

Alcohol (Wernicke–Korsakoff syndrome)
Head injury (severe)
Anoxia
Posterior cerebral artery occlusion (bilateral)
Herpes simplex encephalitis
Chronic sedative and solvent abuse
Bilateral invasive tumours
Arsenic poisoning
Following hypoglycaemia

FURTHER READING
Hoffman B, Lefkowitz R, Taylor P (1996)
    Neurotransmission: the autonomic and somatic
    nervous systems. In: *Goodman and Gilman's The
    Pharmacological Basis of Therapeutics*, 9th edn. New
    York: McGraw-Hill.
Masson J, Sagné C, Hamon M, El Mestikawy S (1999)
    Neurotransmitter transporters in the central
    nervous system. *Pharmacological Reviews* **51**: 439–464.

- cranial nerves
- three systems of motor control:
    - corticospinal or pyramidal system
    - extrapyramidal system
    - cerebellum
- motor unit
- reflex arc
- sensory pathways and pain
- control of the bladder and sexual function.

CRANIAL NERVES (see Table 21.5)

I: OLFACTORY NERVE

This sensory nerve arises from olfactory (smell) receptors within nasal mucosa. Branches pierce the cribriform plate and synapse in the olfactory bulb. The olfactory tract then passes to the olfactory cortex in the anteromedial surface of the temporal lobe.

Anosmia (loss of sense of smell) is caused by head injury and tumours of the olfactory groove (e.g. meningioma, frontal glioma). Sense of smell is often lost or diminished, occasionally permanently, after upper respiratory viral infections and when the nostrils are blocked.

II: OPTIC NERVE AND VISUAL SYSTEM

The visual pathway is shown in Figure 21.4. The photic energy of light, its amount regulated by the pupillary

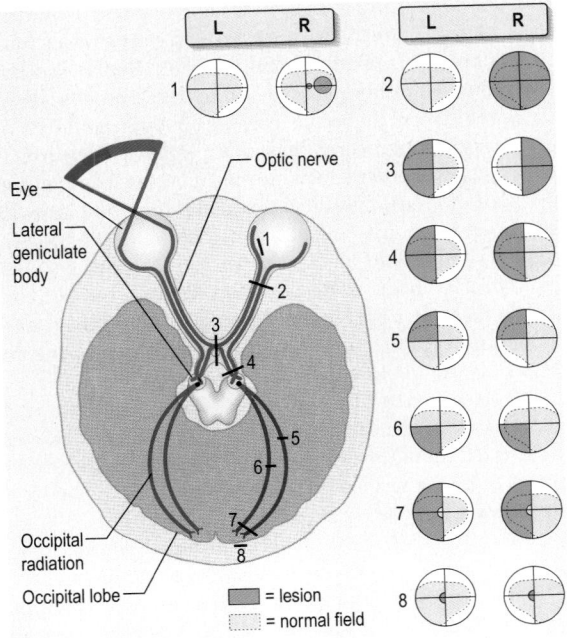

Fig. 21.4 The visual pathway.
1, Paracentral scotoma – retinal lesion.
2, Mononuclear field loss – optic nerve lesion.
3, Bitemporal hemianopia – chiasmal lesion.
4, Homonymous hemianopia – optic tract lesion.
5, Homonymous quadrantanopia – temporal lesion.
6, Homonymous quadrantanopia – parietal lesion.
7, Homonymous hemianopia – occipital cortex or optic radiation.
8, Homonymous hemianopia – occipital pole lesion.

Table 21.5   Cranial nerves

No.	Name	Main clinical action
I	Olfactory	Smell
II	Optic	Vision, fields, afferent light reflex
III	Oculomotor	Eyelid elevation, eye elevation, ADduction, depression in ABduction, efferent (pupil)
IV	Trochlear	Eye intorsion, depression in ADduction
V	Trigeminal	Facial and corneal sensation, muscles of mastication
VI	Abducens	Eye ABduction
VII	Facial	Facial movement, taste fibres
VIII	Vestibular	Balance
	Cochlear	Hearing
IX	Glossopharyngeal	Sensation – soft palate, taste fibres
X	Vagus	Cough, palatal and vocal cord movements
XI	Accessory	Head turning, shoulder shrugging
XII	Hypoglossal	Tongue movement

21 Neurological disease

aperture (see p. 1181), is converted to nerve action potentials by retinal rod, cone and ganglion cells. The lens, under control of the ciliary muscle (see p. 1181), produces the image (inverted) on the retina (1), i.e. an object in the lower part of the visual field is projected to the upper retina, one in a temporal field to the nasal retina. Each optic nerve (2), sheathed in pia–arachnoid meninges, carries axons from retinal ganglion cells to the lateral geniculate bodies.

At the chiasm (3), fibres travelling in the nasal portions of the optic nerves cross, join uncrossed temporal optic nerve fibres and form each optic tract. These fibres synapse at each lateral geniculate body (4). One optic tract thus carries fibres from the temporal ipsilateral retina and the nasal contralateral retina. Some optic tract fibres reaching the lateral geniculate bodies pass to the brainstem (see p. 1181) to control refraction (lens) and pupillary aperture.

From the lateral geniculate body, fibres pass in the optic radiation through the parietal and temporal lobes (5 and 6) to reach the visual, or calcarine, cortex of the occipital lobe (7 and 8). The upper retinae (lower visual fields) project in the optic radiation through the parietal lobes to the upper part of the visual cortex, and the lower retinae (upper fields) through the temporal lobes, beneath the parietal, to the lower visual cortex.

Impulses reach the cortex in strictly maintained vertical topographical order (i.e. upper field to lower retina, tract, radiation and cortex, and vice versa, lower to upper). Within the visual cortex itself there are synaptic connections between groups of cells that detect lines, orientation, shapes, movement, colour, and depth. These are processed by neighbouring visual association areas.

Visual field defects caused by lesions of each optic tract, radiation and cortex are called 'homonymous' to indicate the different (i.e. bilateral) origins of each unilateral pathway. (A homonym is the same word used to denote different things.)

Field defects are hemianopic when half the field is affected by a lesion of the optic tract, radiation or cortex and quadrantanopic when a quadrant is affected. Congruous denotes symmetry and incongruous lack of it. Bitemporal defects (damage to crossing nasal fibres) are caused by lesions of the optic chiasm.

Visual acuity

This is recorded with a Snellen chart and/or Near Vision Reading Types and corrected for refractive errors with lenses or a pinhole. Normal acuity is 6/6 to 6/9; if less, an explanation is necessary.

Visual loss is discussed on page 1171. Causes include:

- Ocular causes, e.g. glaucoma, macular degeneration, cataract, retinal detachment, diabetic vascular disease, trachoma, leprosy, vitamin A deficiency, trauma, onchocerciasis (river blindness). All are of major international health and economic importance.
- Lesions of the visual neural pathway (e.g. optic nerve lesions, chiasmal compression, tract, radiation or cortical lesions).

Visual field defects

These are checked by confrontation with white- and red-headed pins and, if abnormal or in doubt, recorded in detail with a Goldmann (or similar) screen. Examples of field defects are shown in Figure 21.4.

Retinal and local eye lesions (site 1)

Lesions of the retina produce either scotomata (small areas of visual loss) or peripheral visual loss (tunnel vision). Common causes are diabetic retinal vascular disease, glaucoma and retinitis pigmentosa. Local lesions of the eye (e.g. cataract) can also cause visual loss.

Optic nerve lesions (site 2)

Unilateral visual loss, commencing as a central or paracentral (off-centre) scotoma, is the hallmark of an optic nerve lesion. A total optic nerve lesion causes unilateral blindness with loss of pupillary light reflex (direct and consensual) when the blind eye is illuminated (see afferent pupillary defect, p. 1182). For optic nerve lesions, see Table 21.6.

The principal pathological appearances of the visible part of the nerve (optic disc) seen on fundoscopy are:

- disc swelling and hyperaemia (papilloedema)
- pallor (optic atrophy).

Papilloedema and optic neuritis

Papilloedema simply means swelling of the papilla – the optic disc. There are many causes (Table 21.7). In all forms of disc oedema there is axonal swelling within the optic nerve, blockage of axonal transport with capillary and venous congestion. Optic neuritis means swelling of the disc with *inflammation* in the nerve.

The earliest ophthalmoscopic signs of disc swelling are pinkness of the disc followed by fuzziness and heaping up of its margins, the nasal first. There is loss within the disc of the normal, visible, spontaneous pulsation of retinal veins. The physiological cup becomes obliterated, the disc engorged and its vessels dilated. Small haemorrhages often surround the disc.

Various conditions simulate true disc oedema. Marked hypermetropic (long-sighted) refractive errors make the

Table 21.6 Principal causes of an optic nerve lesion
Optic and retrobulbar neuritis
Optic nerve compression (e.g. tumour or aneurysm)
Toxic optic neuropathy (e.g. tobacco, ethambutol, methyl alcohol, quinine)
Syphilis
Ischaemic optic neuropathy (e.g. giant cell arteritis)
Hereditary optic neuropathies
Severe anaemia
Vitamin B_{12} deficiency
Trauma
Infective (spread of paranasal sinus infection or orbital cellulitis)
Papilloedema and its causes (see Table 21.7)
Bone disease affecting optic canal (e.g. Paget's)

Table 21.7 Causes of optic disc swelling (papilloedema)

Raised intracranial pressure	**Venous occlusion**
Brain tumour, abscess, haematoma, intracranial haemorrhage and SAH, idiopathic intracranial hypertension, hydrocephalus, encephalitis	Cavernous sinus thrombosis
	Central retinal vein thrombosis/occlusion
	Orbital mass lesions
	Retinal vascular disease
	Malignant hypertension
	Vasculitis (e.g. SLE)
Optic nerve disease	**Metabolic causes**
Optic neuritis (e.g. multiple sclerosis)	Hypercapnia, chronic hypoxia, hypocalcaemia
Hereditary optic neuropathy	
Ischaemic optic neuropathy (e.g. giant cell arteritis)	**Disc infiltration**
	Leukaemia, sarcoidosis, optic nerve glioma
Toxic optic neuropathy (e.g. methanol ingestion)	
Hypervitaminosis A	

SAH, subarachnoid haemorrhage; SLE, systemic lupus erythematosus

disc appear pink, distant and ill-defined. Opaque (myelinated) nerve fibres at the disc margin and hyaline bodies (drusen) can be mistaken for disc swelling.

Disc infiltration also causes first a prominent, then a swollen disc with raised margins (e.g. in leukaemia).

When there is doubt about disc oedema, fluorescein angiography is diagnostic. Fluorescein is injected intravenously: when there is oedema, retinal leakage is seen and photographed.

Early papilloedema from causes other than optic neuritis (for example a brain tumour) often produces few visual symptoms itself – the underlying disease is the source of the patient's complaints. However, as disc oedema progresses, enlargement of the blind spot and blurring of vision develop. The disc then becomes further engorged, its arterial blood flow falls and, then as papilloedema worsens, infarction of the optic nerve occurs. This causes sudden severe and permanent visual loss.

Optic neuritis

The most common cause of inflammation of the optic nerve is demyelination (e.g. multiple sclerosis). Disc swelling due to optic neuritis is distinguished from other causes of disc oedema by dull ocular pain with early and severe visual loss. Retrobulbar neuritis implies that the inflammatory process is within the optic nerve but behind the bulb (i.e. the eye), so that no abnormality is seen at the disc despite visual impairment.

Leber's hereditary optic neuropathy (LHON)

LHON is a cause of isolated blindness in otherwise healthy young men. Unilateral or bilateral optic nerve neuropathy develops over days or weeks. There is sometimes disc swelling and telangiectasia around the disc in the acute phase, followed by optic atrophy. Severe bilateral visual loss is usual by the age of 40. Maternal inheritance and genetic analysis point to pathogenic mitochondrial DNA mutations, many with a mutation at G11778A. Exceptional cases occur in women.

Optic atrophy

Optic atrophy means disc pallor, from loss of axons, glial proliferation and decreased vascularity that follows many pathological processes, e.g. infarction of the nerve from thromboembolism or following papilloedema, inflammation (demyelinating optic neuritis in MS, syphilis, LHON), optic nerve compression, previous trauma, toxic and metabolic causes (vitamin B_{12} deficiency, quinine and methyl alcohol ingestion). Optic atrophy is described as *consecutive* or *secondary* when it follows papilloedema, of any cause. The degree of visual loss depends upon underlying pathology.

Optic chiasm (site 3)

Bitemporal hemianopic fields are the typical defects seen when a mass compresses the chiasm. Common causes are:

- pituitary neoplasm (p. 1044)
- meningioma
- craniopharyngioma
- secondary neoplasm.

In bilateral visual loss, chiasmal compression must always be considered – and optic nerve compression in unilateral visual failure.

Optic tract and optic radiation (sites 4, 5 and 6)

Optic *tract* lesions (rare) cause field defects that are homonymous, hemianopic and often incomplete and incongruous. Optic *radiation* lesions cause homonymous quadrantanopic defects. Temporal lobe lesions (e.g. tumour or infarction) cause upper quadrantic defects; and parietal lobe, lower.

Occipital cortex (sites 7 and 8)

Homonymous hemianopic defects are produced by unilateral posterior cerebral artery infarction. The macular region (of the cortex, at each occipital pole) is spared because it has a separate blood supply via the middle cerebral artery. Infarction of one occipital pole causes a small, congruous, scotomatous, homonymous hemianopia (8).

Widespread bilateral occipital lobe damage by infarction, trauma or tumour causes cortical blindness (Anton's syndrome). The patient cannot see but characteristically lacks insight into the degree of blindness and may even deny it. The pupillary responses are normal (see also p. 1213).

Pupils

Sympathetic impulses dilate the pupils. Fibres in the nasociliary nerve pass to *dilator pupillae*. These arise from the superior cervical ganglion at C2. Sympathetic *pre*ganglionic fibres to the eye (and face) originate in the hypothalamus, pass uncrossed through the midbrain and lateral medulla, and emerge finally from the spinal cord at T1 (close to the lung apex) and form the superior cervical ganglion at C2. *Post*ganglionic fibres leave the ganglion to form a plexus around the carotid artery bifurcation. Fibres pass to the pupil in the nasociliary nerve from part of this plexus surrounding the *internal* carotid artery. Those fibres to the face (sweating and pilo-erection) arise from the part of the plexus surrounding the *external* carotid artery. This arrangement has some clinical relevance in Horner's syndrome (p. 1183).

Parasympathetic impulses cause pupillary constriction. Fibres in the short ciliary nerves arise from the ciliary ganglion and pass to *sphincter pupillae*, causing constriction. Parasympathetic pathways and the light reflex mechanism are shown in Figure 21.5.

The light reflex

Afferent fibres (1) in each optic nerve (some crossing in the chiasm) pass to both lateral geniculate bodies (2) and relay to the Edinger–Westphal nuclei (4) via the pretectal nucleus (3).

Efferent (parasympathetic) fibres from each Edinger–Westphal nucleus pass via the third nerve to the ciliary ganglion (5) and thence to the pupil (6).

Light constricts the pupil being illuminated (direct reflex) and, by the consensual reflex, the contralateral pupil.

Fig. 21.5 Pupillary light reflex.
Afferent pathway
(1) A retinal image generates action potentials in the optic nerve.
(2) These travel via axons, some of which decussate at the chiasm and pass through the lateral geniculate bodies.
(3) Synapse at each pretectal nucleus.

Efferent pathway
(4) Action potentials then pass to each Edinger–Westphal nucleus of III.
(5) Then, via the ciliary ganglion.
(6) Lead to constriction of pupil.

The convergence reflex

Fixation on a near object requires convergence of the ocular axes and is accompanied by pupillary constriction. Afferent fibres in each optic nerve, which pass through both lateral geniculate bodies, also relay to the convergence centre. This centre receives 1a spindle afferent fibres from the extraocular muscles – principally medial recti – which are innervated by the third nerve.

The efferent route is from the convergence centre to the Edinger–Westphal nucleus, ciliary ganglion and pupils. Voluntary or reflex fixation on a near object is thus accompanied by appropriate convergence and pupillary constriction.

A darkened room makes all pupillary abnormalities easier to see.

Clinical abnormalities of the pupils

Pupillary abnormalities in coma are discussed on page 1208, and in brainstem lesions on page 989.

Physiological changes and old age

A slight difference between the size of each pupil is common (physiological anisocoria) at any age. The pupil tends to become small (3–3.5 mm) and irregular in old age (senile miosis); anisocoria is more pronounced. The convergence reflex becomes sluggish with ageing and a bright light becomes necessary to demonstrate constriction.

Afferent pupillary defect. A blind left eye, for example following complete optic nerve section, has a pupil larger than the right. The features of a left afferent pupillary defect are:

- The left pupil is unreactive to light (i.e. the direct reflex is absent).
- The consensual reflex (constriction of right pupil when the left is illuminated) is absent. Conversely, the left pupil constricts when light is shone in the intact right eye, i.e. the consensual reflex of the right eye remains intact.

Relative afferent pupillary defect (RAPD). When there has been incomplete damage to one afferent pupillary pathway (i.e. of one optic nerve *relative* to the other), the difference between the pupillary reaction, and the relative impairment on one side is called a relative afferent pupillary defect (RAPD). The sign can provide evidence of an optic nerve lesion, when, for example, retrobulbar neuritis occurred many years previously and there has been complete clinical recovery of vision (p. 1235).

After previous left retrobulbar neuritis:

- Light shone in the left eye causes both left and right pupils to constrict.
- When light is shone into the intact right eye, both pupils again constrict (i.e. right direct and consensual reflexes are intact).
- When the light is swung back to the left eye, its pupil dilates slightly, relative to its previous size.

A left RAPD by the *swinging light test*, showing that the consensual reflex is stronger than the direct, indicates

Table 21.8   Causes of Horner's syndrome

Hemisphere and brainstem Massive cerebral infarction Pontine glioma Lateral medullary syndrome 'Coning' of the temporal lobe	**Sympathetic chain in neck** Following thyroid/laryngeal surgery Carotid artery occlusion and dissection Neoplastic infiltration Cervical sympathectomy
Cervical cord Syringomyelia Cord tumours	**Miscellaneous** Congenital Migrainous neuralgia (usually transient) Isolated and of unknown cause
T1 root Bronchial neoplasm (apical) Apical tuberculosis Cervical rib Brachial plexus trauma	

residual damage in the afferent pupillary fibres of the left optic nerve.

Horner's syndrome

This collection of signs – unilateral pupillary constriction with slight ptosis and enophthalmos – indicates a lesion of the sympathetic pathway on the same side. The conjunctival vessels are slightly injected. Causes of Horner's syndrome are given in Table 21.8. There is loss of sweating of the same side of the face or body; the extent depending upon the level of the lesion:

- Central lesions affect sweating over the entire half of the head, arm and upper trunk.
- Neck lesions proximal to the superior cervical ganglion cause diminished facial sweating.
- Lesions distal to the superior cervical ganglion do not affect sweating at all.

Pharmacological tests help to indicate the level of the lesion. For example, a lesion distal to the superior cervical ganglion causes denervation hypersensitivity of the pupil, which dilates when 1 : 1000 epinephrine (adrenaline) is instilled. This dose has little effect on the normal pupil or a Horner's pupil from a proximal lesion. In clinical practice the test is of limited value.

Myotonic pupil (Holmes–Adie pupil)

This common cause of a dilated pupil is more frequent in females. It is usually unilateral, and the pupil is often irregular. There is no reaction (or a very slow reaction) to bright light and also incomplete constriction to convergence. This is due to denervation in the ciliary ganglion, of unknown cause. The myotonic pupil is of no more pathological significance than this, but is sometimes associated with diminished or absent tendon reflexes.

Argyll Robertson pupil

This small, irregular (3 mm or less) pupil is fixed to light but constricts on convergence. The lesion is in the brainstem surrounding the aqueduct of Sylvius.

The Argyll Robertson pupil is (almost) diagnostic of neurosyphilis. Similar changes are occasionally seen in diabetes mellitus.

III, IV, VI: OCULOMOTOR, TROCHLEAR AND ABDUCENS NERVES

Mechanisms controlling eye movement are:

- central upper motor neurone mechanisms driving normal yoked parallel eye movements (conjugate gaze)
- individual movements generated by each oculomotor, abducens and trochlear nerve and muscles they supply.

Conjugate gaze

Fast voluntary and reflex eye movements originate in each frontal lobe. Fibres pass in the anterior limb of the internal capsule and cross in the pons to end in the centre for lateral gaze (paramedian pontine reticular formation – PPRF, Fig. 21.6a), close to each sixth nerve nucleus. The PPRF also receives fibres from:

- the ipsilateral occipital cortex – a pathway concerned with tracking objects
- both vestibular nuclei – pathways linking eye movements with position of the head and neck (doll's head reflexes, p. 990).

Conjugate lateral eye movements are coordinated by the PPRF through the medial longitudinal fasciculus (MLF, Fig. 21.6b). Fibres from the PPRF pass both to the ipsilateral sixth nerve nucleus and, having crossed the midline, the opposite third nerve nucleus via the MLF. Each sixth nerve nucleus (supplying lateral rectus) and the opposite third nerve nucleus (supplying medial rectus and others) are thus linked by the MLF, driving the eyes laterally with parallel axes with the same velocity.

Abnormalities of conjugate lateral gaze

A destructive lesion of one side of the brain allows lateral gaze to be driven by the intact opposite pathway. For example, a destructive left frontal lobe lesion (e.g. an infarct) leads to failure of conjugate lateral gaze to the right. In an acute lesion the eyes are often deviated past the midline to the side of the lesion, here to the left, and therefore look towards the normal limbs, as there is usually a contralateral (i.e. right) hemiparesis.

An irritative left frontal lobe lesion (e.g. an epileptic focus), stimulates the opposite, right, PPRF and drives lateral gaze away from the side of the lesion (i.e. to the right) during an attack.

In the brainstem itself a unilateral destructive lesion involving the PPRF leads to failure of conjugate lateral gaze towards that side. There is usually a contralateral hemiparesis and lateral gaze is deviated towards the side of the paralysed limbs.

Internuclear ophthalmoplegia

Damage to one MLF causes internuclear ophthalmoplegia (INO), one of the more common complex brainstem oculomotor signs and seen frequently in multiple sclerosis. When present bilaterally, INO is almost pathognomonic of this disease.

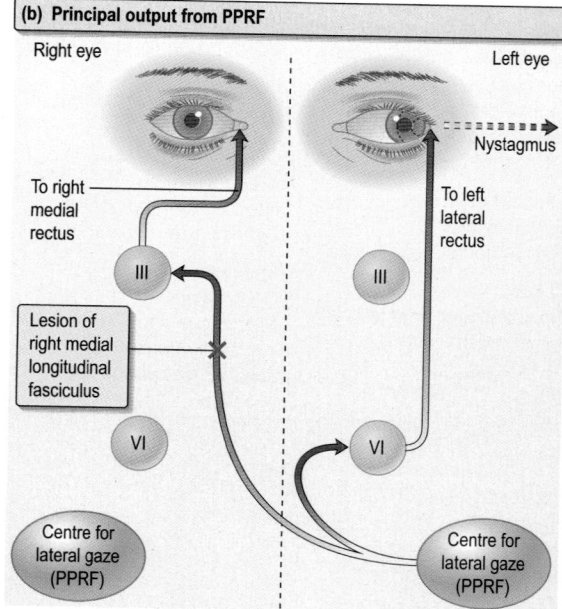

Fig. 21.6 **(a) Principal input to PPRF**. Impulses from the right frontal cortex, the left occipital cortex and both vestibular nuclei (VN) drive the left centre for lateral gaze, or paramedian pontine reticular formation (PPRF).
(b) Principal output from PPRF. Impulses from the PPRF pass via the ipsilateral VIth nerve nucleus to the lateral rectus muscle (ABduction) and via the medial longitudinal fasciculus to the IIIrd nerve nucleus and thus to the opposite medial rectus muscle (ADduction). **X** shows lesion with failure of ADduction of right eye and nystagmus of ABducting left eye.

Unilateral lesions are also caused by small brainstem infarcts. In a right INO there is a lesion of the right MLF (Fig. 21.6b). On attempted left lateral gaze the right eye fails to ADduct. The left eye develops coarse nystagmus in ABduction.

The side of the lesion is on the side of impaired adduction, not on the side of the (obvious, unilateral) nystagmus.

Doll's head reflexes and skew deviation

These are of some diagnostic value in coma (see p. 990).

Abnormalities of vertical gaze

Failure of up-gaze is caused by upper brainstem lesions, such as a supratentorial mass, or a brainstem tumour (e.g. a pinealoma). When the pupillary convergence reflex fails as well, this combination is called Parinaud's syndrome.

Defective up-gaze also occurs in certain degenerative disorders (e.g. progressive supranuclear palsy). Some impairment of up-gaze develops as part of normal ageing.

Weakness of extraocular muscles (diplopia)

Diplopia (double vision) indicates weakness of one or more extraocular muscles. The causes are:

- lesions of the third, fourth and/or sixth cranial nerves or nuclei

- disorders of the neuromuscular junction (e.g. myasthenia gravis)
- disease of, or injury to the ocular muscles
- orbital lesions.

Squint (strabismus)

This describes the appearance of the eyes when the visual axes fail to meet at the fixation point, and is either convergent or divergent.

Paralytic squint. Paralytic or incomitant squint occurs when there is an acquired defect of movement of an eye – the usual situation in neurological disease. There is a squint (and hence diplopia) maximal in the direction of action of the weak muscle.

Non-paralytic squint. Non-paralytic or concomitant squint describes a squint dating from infancy in which the angle between the visual axes does not vary when the eyes are moved – the squint remains the same in all directions of gaze. Diplopia is almost never a symptom. The deviating eye (the one that does not fixate) usually has defective (amblyopic) vision; this is called *amblyopia ex anopsia*.

Non-paralytic squint may be latent (i.e. only visible at certain times), e.g. when tired.

The cover test. The cover test is used principally to assess non-paralytic squint and to recognize latent squint. The patient is asked to fix on a light. When there is no squint a pinpoint reflection is seen in the exact centre of each pupil. One eye that is fixing the light centrally is

Table 21.9 Common causes of an oculomotor nerve lesion

Aneurysm of the posterior communicating artery
'Coning' of the temporal lobe
Infarction of IIIrd nerve:
   in diabetes mellitus
   atheroma
Midbrain infarction
Midbrain tumour

covered quickly. If a squint has been present the other (uncovered) eye moves, to take up central fixation. The test is repeated with the opposite eye. The dominant, fixing eye will not move when the other, squinting, amblyopic eye is covered or uncovered.

III: Oculomotor nerve

The nucleus of the third nerve lies ventral to the aqueduct in the midbrain. Efferent fibres to four external ocular muscles (superior, inferior and medial recti, and inferior oblique), *levator palpebrae superioris* and *sphincter pupillae* (parasympathetic) enter the orbit through the superior orbital fissure.

The common causes of an oculomotor nerve lesion are given in Table 21.9. Signs of a complete third nerve palsy are:

- unilateral complete ptosis
- the eye facing down and out
- a fixed and dilated pupil.

Sparing of the pupil means that parasympathetic fibres that run in a discrete bundle on the superior surface of the nerve remain undamaged, and so the pupil is of normal size and reacts normally. In diabetes, infarction of the third nerve usually spares the pupil.

In a third nerve palsy the eye can still ABduct (sixth nerve) and rotate inwards or intort (fourth nerve). Preservation of intortion (inward rotation) means that the fourth (trochlear) nerve is intact. In a patient with a right third nerve palsy, when the attempt is made to converge and look downwards, the conjunctival vessels of the right eye are seen to twist clockwise, indicating that the eye is intorting and the fourth nerve is intact (see below).

IV: Trochlear nerve

This supplies the superior oblique muscle. The head is tilted away from the side of the lesion and the patient complains of torsional diplopia when attempting to look down and away from the affected side.

VI: Abducens nerve

This supplies the lateral rectus muscle that ABducts the eye. There is an evident convergent squint with diplopia maximal looking to the side of the lesion. The eye cannot be ABducted beyond the midline (see p. 1184 and Fig. 21.6).

The sixth nerve has a long intracranial course The nerve can be damaged in the brainstem (e.g. MS or pontine glioma). In raised intracranial pressure it is compressed against the tip of the petrous temporal bone. The nerve sheath may be infiltrated by tumours, particularly nasopharyngeal carcinoma. An isolated sixth nerve palsy due to infarction occurs in diabetes mellitus and is also a common sequel of head trauma.

Complete external ophthalmoplegia

Complete external ophthalmoplegia describes the immobile eye when III, IV and VI nerves are paralysed by disease at the orbital apex (e.g. a metastasis) or within the cavernous sinus (e.g. sinus thrombosis).

FURTHER READING
Miller NR, Newman NJ (2004) The eye in neurological disease. *Lancet* **364**: 2045–2054.

V: TRIGEMINAL NERVE

This nerve is large, mainly sensory but with some motor fibres.

Sensory fibres (Fig. 21.7; and see Figs 21.11 and 21.12) from the three divisions – ophthalmic (V_1), maxillary (V_2) and mandibular (V_3) – pass to the trigeminal (Gasserian) ganglion within the cavernous sinus at the apex of the petrous temporal bone. From here central fibres enter the brainstem. Ascending fibres transmitting light touch sensation enter the V nucleus in the pons. Descending fibres carrying pain and temperature sensation form the spinal tract of V end in the spinal V nucleus in the medulla. This nucleus extends into the upper cervical cord.

Fig. 21.7 **Sensory input of trigeminal nerve (red) and motor output of facial nerve (blue).** SOF, superior orbital fissure; FO, foramen ovale; FR, foramen rotundum; GG, Gasserian ganglion; SF, stylomastoid foramen.

Motor fibres arise in the upper pons and join the mandibular branch to supply muscles of mastication.

Signs of a V nerve lesion

A complete V nerve lesion causes unilateral sensory loss on the face, tongue and buccal mucosa. When motor fibres are damaged, the jaw deviates to that side as the mouth opens. Diminution of the corneal reflex is an early, and sometimes isolated sign of a fifth nerve lesion.

Central (brainstem) lesions of the lower trigeminal nuclei (e.g. in syringobulbia, p. 1152) produce a characteristic circumoral sensory loss.

When the spinal tract (or spinal nucleus) alone is involved, sensory loss is restricted to pain and temperature sensation, i.e. dissociated (p. 1199).

Causes

Within the *brainstem*, lesions involve fifth nuclei *and* central connections, in, e.g.:

- brainstem glioma
- multiple sclerosis
- infarction
- syringobulbia.

At the *cerebellopontine angle,* the nerve is compressed by:

- acoustic neuroma
- meningioma
- secondary neoplasm.

As these lesions enlarge, the neighbouring seventh and eighth nerves become involved, producing facial weakness and deafness.

At the *apex of the petrous temporal bone,* spreading middle ear infection, or a secondary tumour, damage the nerve. The combination of a painful fifth with a sixth nerve lesion is called Gradenigo's syndrome.

Within the cavernous sinus, the trigeminal (Gasserian) ganglion is compressed by:

- aneurysm of the internal carotid artery
- lateral extension of a pituitary neoplasm
- thrombosis of the cavernous sinus
- secondary neoplasm.

The trigeminal ganglion itself becomes infected in ophthalmic herpes zoster (p. 1240), the most common lesion of the ganglion. Trigeminal postherpetic neuralgia commonly follows, often affecting the first (ophthalmic) division (p. 1240).

Peripheral branches of the trigeminal nerve are affected by neoplastic infiltration of the skull base.

Trigeminal neuralgia

Trigeminal neuralgia (*tic douloureux*) is of unknown cause, seen most commonly in old age. It is almost always unilateral.

Symptoms

Severe paroxysms of knife-like or electric shock-like pain, lasting seconds, occur in the distribution of the fifth nerve. The pain tends to commence in the mandibular division (V_3) and spreads upwards to maxillary (V_2) and ophthalmic divisions (V_1). Spasms occur many times a day.

Each paroxysm is stereotyped, brought on by stimulation of one or more trigger zones in the face. Washing, shaving, a cold wind or eating are examples of trivial stimuli that provoke pain. The face may be screwed up in agony (hence the term *tic*). Pain characteristically does not occur at night. Spontaneous remissions last months or years before recurrence, which is almost inevitable.

Signs

There are no signs of trigeminal nerve dysfunction. The corneal reflex is preserved. The history alone make the diagnosis.

Treatment

The anticonvulsant carbamazepine 600–1200 mg daily reduces severity of attacks in the majority. Phenytoin, gabapentin and clonazepam are used, but are less effective.

If drug therapy fails, surgical procedures (radiofrequency extirpation of the ganglion, neurovascular decompression or sectioning of the sensory root) are useful. Alcohol injection into the trigeminal ganglion or peripheral fifth nerve branches can also be carried out.

Secondary trigeminal neuralgia

Trigeminal neuralgia occurs in MS (p. 1235), with tumours of the fifth nerve (e.g. neuroma) and with cerebellopontine angle lesions (see below). There are usually physical signs – initially a depressed corneal reflex, progressing to trigeminal sensory loss.

Idiopathic trigeminal neuropathy

A chronic isolated fifth nerve lesion sometimes develops without apparent cause. When sensory loss is severe, trophic changes (facial scarring and corneal ulceration) develop.

FURTHER READING

Love S, Coakham HB (2001) Trigeminal neuralgia: pathology and pathogenesis. *Brain* **124**: 2347–2360.

VII: FACIAL NERVE

The facial nerve is largely motor in function, supplying muscles of facial expression. The nerve carries sensory taste fibres from the anterior two-thirds of the tongue via the *chorda tympani*. It also supplies motor fibres to the *stapedius* muscle. The facial nerve (Fig. 21.7) arises from its nucleus in the pons and leaves the skull through the stylomastoid foramen. Part of each facial nucleus supplying the upper face (principally *frontalis* muscle) receives supranuclear fibres from each hemisphere. Therefore in a unilateral upper motor neurone lesion of the facial nerve the upper part of the face is usually spared.

Unilateral facial weakness

Lower motor neurone (LMN) lesions. A unilateral LMN lesion causes weakness of all muscles of facial expression on one side. The angle of the mouth falls, and unilateral dribbling occurs. There is weakness of frowning (*frontalis*) and of eye closure since upper facial muscles are weak. Corneal exposure and ulceration occur if the eye does not close during sleep. The *platysma* muscle is also weak.

Upper motor neurone (UMN) lesions. UMN lesions cause weakness of the lower part only of the face on the side opposite the lesion. *Frontalis* is spared. Thus the normal furrowing of the brow is preserved, and eye closure and blinking are not affected. The earliest sign is simply slowing of one side of the face, for example on baring the teeth. In UMN lesions, too, there is sometimes relative preservation of spontaneous emotional movement (e.g. smiling) compared with voluntary movement.

Causes of facial weakness

A common cause of facial weakness is a supranuclear (UMN) lesion (e.g. cerebral infarction), leading to UMN facial weakness with hemiparesis.

Lesions at four lower levels are recognized by association of LMN facial weakness with other signs.

Pons. Here the sixth (abducens) nerve nucleus is encircled by seventh nerve fibres (Fig. 21.7). The sixth nucleus is thus often involved in pontine lesions of the seventh, causing a convergent squint (lateral rectus palsy) with unilateral facial weakness.

When the neighbouring PPRF and corticospinal tract are involved, there is the triple combination of:

- LMN facial weakness
- failure of conjugate lateral gaze (towards lesion)
- contralateral hemiparesis.

Causes include pontine tumours (e.g. glioma), demyelination and vascular lesions.

The facial nucleus itself is affected unilaterally or bilaterally in poliomyelitis (see p. 49) and in motor neurone disease usually bilaterally (p. 1253) .

Cerebellopontine angle (CPA). The fifth, sixth and eighth nerves are affected with the seventh where they are clustered together in the CPA. Causes are acoustic neuroma, meningioma and secondary neoplasm.

Petrous temporal bone. The geniculate ganglion (sensory for taste) lies at the *genu* (knee) of the facial nerve (Fig. 21.7). Fibres join the facial nerve in the *chorda tympani* and carry taste from the anterior two-thirds of the tongue. The (motor) nerve to *stapedius* leaves the facial nerve distal to the *genu*. Facial nerve lesions within the petrous temporal bone cause the combination of:

- loss of taste on the anterior two-thirds of the tongue
- hyperacusis (unpleasantly loud noise distortion caused by paralysis of *stapedius*).

Causes include:

- Bell's palsy
- trauma
- middle ear infection
- herpes zoster (Ramsay Hunt syndrome, p. 1188)
- tumours (e.g. glomus tumour).

Skull base, parotid gland and in the face itself. Swelling of the facial nerve within the stylomastoid foramen develops in Bell's palsy (see below). The nerve can be compressed by skull base tumours and in Paget's disease of bone. Branches of the nerve that pierce the parotid are damaged by parotid gland tumours, mumps (p. 57), sarcoidosis (p. 935) and trauma. Each facial nerve can also be involved in polyneuritis (e.g. Guillain–Barré syndrome, p. 1260), usually simultaneously.

Weakness of facial muscles is also seen in primary muscle disease and myasthenia. Weakness is usually symmetrical. Causes include:

- dystrophia myotonica (p. 1270)
- facio-scapulo-humeral dystrophy (p. 1270)
- myasthenia gravis (p. 1268).

Bell's palsy

This common, acute, isolated facial palsy is usually due to a viral (often herpes simplex) infection that causes swelling of the nerve within the petrous temporal bone and as it traverses the stylomastoid foramen in the skull base.

The patient notices sudden unilateral facial weakness, sometimes with loss of taste on the anterior two-thirds of the tongue. Pain behind the ear is common at onset. Diagnosis is made on clinical grounds. No other cranial nerves are involved.

Management and course

Weakness progresses over hours or several days. Spontaneous improvement usually begins during the second week. Thereafter, recovery continues but may take 12 months. Occasionally (fewer than 10%) patients are left with an unsightly, residual weakness.

Electrophysiological tests (EMG, p. 1203) are of some help in predicting outcome but seldom used. After the third week, absence of any evoked potential from facial muscles (the nerve is stimulated over the parotid) indicates that full recovery is unlikely.

Steroids (e.g. prednisolone 60 mg daily, reducing to nil over 10 days) with aciclovir have been shown to be more effective than either of these drugs alone.

Suturing the upper to lower lid (tarsorrhaphy) is essential to prevent prolonged corneal exposure if the eye cannot be closed. Adhesive tape to hold the lids closed is an invaluable temporary measure.

Severe late residual paralysis occurs in about 15% and cosmetic surgery is sometimes helpful.

Bell's palsy occasionally recurs and is very rarely bilateral.

Ramsay Hunt syndrome

This is *herpes zoster* (shingles) of the geniculate ganglion. There is a facial palsy (identical in appearance to Bell's) with herpetic vesicles in the external auditory meatus (this receives a sensory twig from the facial nerve) and/or on the soft palate. Deafness, or a fifth nerve lesion may occur. Complete recovery is less likely than in Bell's palsy. Treatment for shingles should be given (famciclovir, p. 1321).

Hemifacial spasm

This is an irregular, painless clonic spasm of the facial muscles, usually occurring after middle age, and more commonly in women. It varies from a mild inconvenience to a severe, disfiguring spasm.

Causes are:

- idiopathic
- following Bell's palsy
- acoustic neuroma
- Paget's disease in the skull base
- pressure from vessels in the cerebellopontine angle (postulated).

There are clonic spasms of facial muscles on one side. Mild LMN facial weakness is common.

Management

Some cases require no treatment. In others, decompression of the facial nerve in the cerebellopontine angle is sometimes helpful. Local injection of botulinum toxin into facial muscles reduces the spasm for some months, and can be repeated. Drugs are of no value.

Myokymia

Facial myokymia describes a rare, continuous, fine, sinuous or wave-like movement of the lower face that is seen in brainstem lesions (e.g. multiple sclerosis, brainstem glioma).

Myokymia is also used to describe innocent twitching around the eye.

FURTHER READING

Gilden DM (2004) Bell's palsy. *New England Journal of Medicine* **315**: 1323–1331.

Johnson RW, Dworkin RH (2003) Treatment of herpes zoster and postherpetic neuralgia. *British Medical Journal* **326**: 748–750.

VIII: VESTIBULOCOCHLEAR NERVE

This nerve has two parts – cochlear and vestibular.

Cochlear nerve

Auditory fibres from the spiral organ of Corti within the cochlea pass to the cochlear nuclei in the pons. Fibres from these nuclei cross the midline and pass upwards through the medial lemnisci to the medial geniculate bodies and thence to the temporal gyri.

Symptoms of a cochlear nerve lesion are deafness and tinnitus (see p. 1156). The deafness is called 'sensorineural' (or perceptive) deafness. Clinical detection is by tuning fork (256 Hz, not 128 Hz) tests, principally Rinne's and Webers tests, which distinguishes conductive from sensorineural deafness (see p. 1154).

Investigations of cochlear lesions

- Pure tone audiometry.
- Auditory evoked potentials. These record from scalp electrodes the response from a repetitive click. The level of the lesion may be detected from the response.

Causes of sensorineural deafness are shown in Table 20.1.

Vestibular nerve

Nerve impulses generated by movement of sensory epithelia of the three semicircular canals, saccule and utricle pass to vestibular nuclei in the pons. The vestibular nuclei are also connected to the cerebellum, nuclei of the ocular muscles, PPRF, extrapyramidal system, reticular formation, temporal lobes and spinal cord.

Balance and posture also depend upon the interaction of proprioceptive (position sense) impulses passing between the neck, spinal muscles and limbs and vestibular system.

The *main symptom* of a vestibular lesion is vertigo and loss of balance. Vomiting frequently accompanies any acute vertigo. Nystagmus is the principal physical sign.

Vertigo

Vertigo, the definite illusion of movement of the subject or surroundings, indicates a disturbance of vestibular, eighth nerve, brainstem or, very rarely cortical function. See Table 21.10.

Deafness and tinnitus accompanying vertigo indicate that its origin is from the ear or eighth cranial nerve (see p. 1154).

Nystagmus

Nystagmus is a rhythmic oscillation of the eyes. It is a sign of disease of either the ocular or vestibular system and its connections. Nystagmus is classified as either *jerk*

Table 21.10	Principal causes of vertigo
Ménière's disease	
Drugs (e.g. gentamicin, anticonvulsant intoxication)	
Toxins (e.g. ethyl alcohol)	
'Vestibular neuronitis'	
Multiple sclerosis	
Migraine	
Acute cerebellar lesions	
Cerebellopontine angle lesions (e.g. acoustic neuroma)	
Partial seizures (temporal lobe focus)	
Brainstem ischaemia or infarction	
Benign paroxysmal positional vertigo	

or *pendular*. For true nystagmus to be present it must be demonstrable and sustained within binocular gaze.

Jerk nystagmus

Jerk nystagmus (the usual nystagmus of neurological disease) has a fast and a slow component. It is seen in vestibular end-organ, eighth nerve, brainstem, cerebellar and (very rarely) cortical lesions. The direction of nystagmus is decided by the fast component, which can be thought of as a reflex attempt to correct the slower, primary movement.

Considerable difficulties exist when attempts are made to use the direction alone of jerk nystagmus as a localizing sign, although nystagmus is both a common and valuable indication of abnormality within the vestibular system as a whole. The following are useful diagnostic starting points:

- **Horizontal jerk or rotary jerk nystagmus** may be either of peripheral origin (middle ear) or central origin (eighth nerve, brainstem, cerebellum and their connections). In peripheral lesions, nystagmus is usually acute and transient (minutes or hours) and associated with severe prostrating vertigo. In central lesions nystagmus is long-lasting (weeks, months or more). Vertigo caused by central lesions tends to wane after days or weeks, the nystagmus outlasting it.
- **Vertical jerk nystagmus.** This is caused only by central lesions.
- **Down-beat jerk nystagmus.** This rarity is caused by lesions around the foramen magnum (e.g. meningioma, cerebellar ectopia).

Pendular nystagmus

Pendular describes movements to and fro similar in both velocity and amplitude. Pendular nystagmus is almost always binocular, horizontal and present in all directions of gaze. Its causes are almost invariably ocular, when there is poor visual fixation (e.g. long-standing, severe visual impairment), or a congenital lesion, when it is sometimes associated with head-nodding. Exceptionally, it occurs in brainstem disease: a fine pendular, jelly-like nystagmus is a sign of a multiple sclerosis (MS) brainstem plaque, or brainstem glioma.

Investigation of vestibular lesions

MRI provides the best structural images of this region.

Caloric tests are used to assess function of the labyrinth. These record the duration of evoked nystagmus when first ice-cold, then warm, water is run into the external meatus. In the normal caloric test:

- ice-cold water in the left ear causes nystagmus with the fast movement to the right
- warm water in the left ear causes nystagmus with the fast movement to the left.

The right ear gives opposite responses. Decreased or absent nystagmus indicates ipsilateral labyrinth, eighth nerve or brainstem involvement. The technique is also used in the diagnosis of brainstem death (p. 989). There are, however, difficulties relating minor abnormalities in caloric tests to clinical symptoms of dizziness.

Vestibular and auditory lesions – central, VIIIth nerve and end organ

Drugs (e.g. anticonvulsant toxicity), alcohol and brainstem vascular disease are common central causes of vertigo. It may also be possible to recognize lesions from clinical features at six distinct levels.

Cerebral cortex. Vertigo is occasionally part of the aura of a partial (temporal lobe) seizure. Vertigo is also a psychological and perceptual sensation when experiencing unaccustomed heights, in panic attacks and agoraphobia. Deafness is very rare in acquired cortical disease; bilateral lesions are necessary.

Pons and brainstem. Vertigo is also common when lesions involve the vestibular nuclei and their connections (MS, vascular, tumour, syrinx). A sixth or seventh nerve lesion, internuclear ophthalmoplegia, lower cranial nerve lesions or contralateral hemiparesis will help localization. Nystagmus is frequently present, while deafness is rare. Transient vertigo occurs in basilar migraine (p. 1248), in syncope, and occasionally in hypoglycaemic attacks; its site of origin is often difficult to ascertain.

Cerebellum. Nystagmus, towards the side of a cerebellar mass (e.g. tumour, haemorrhage or infarct), develops. Limb ataxia is usually present. Bilateral cerebellar, or cerebellar connection disease (e.g. olivo-ponto-cerebellar degeneration) causes bilateral nystagmus. Deafness does not occur.

Cerebellopontine angle. Sensorineural deafness and vertigo occur. Sixth, seventh and fifth nerve lesions develop, followed by cerebellar signs (ipsilateral) and later pyramidal signs (contralateral). Nystagmus is often present. Causes include acoustic neuroma (p. 1245), meningioma and secondary neoplasm, carcinomatous meningitis and inflammatory lesions (Table 21.10).

Petrous temporal bone. Facial weakness (seventh nerve) often accompanies the eighth nerve lesion. Causes include trauma, middle ear infection, secondary neoplasm and Paget's disease of bone (see also Gradenigo's syndrome, p. 1186).

End organs (cochlear and semicircular canals). Causes include:

- Ménière's disease (p. 1156)
- drugs (e.g. gentamicin)
- noise (acoustic trauma, p. 1030)
- middle ear infection (p. 1154)
- mumps
- 'vestibular neuronitis'
- benign paroxysmal positional vertigo (p. 1156)

- advancing age
- intrauterine rubella
- congenital syphilis.

'Vestibular neuronitis'

This common but poorly understood syndrome describes an acute attack of isolated severe vertigo with nystagmus, often with vomiting, but without loss of hearing. It is believed to follow or accompany viral infections that affect the labyrinth or vestibular nerve.

The disturbance lasts for several days or weeks but is self-limiting and rarely recurs. Treatment is with vestibular sedatives; steroids may help. The condition is sometimes followed by benign positional vertigo. Very similar symptoms can be caused by demyelination or vascular lesions within the brainstem, but usually other abnormalities are apparent (see above).

> **FURTHER READING**
> Baloh RW (2003) Vestibular neuritis. *New England Journal of Medicine* **348**: 1027–1032.

LOWER CRANIAL NERVES IX, X, XI, XII

The glossopharyngeal (IX), vagus (X) and accessory (XI) nerves arise in the medulla and leave the skull base together through the jugular foramen. The hypoglossal (XII) also arises in the medulla but leaves through the anterior condylar foramen. All four lower cranial nerves lie close together, just outside the skull, and are related to the carotid artery and ascending sympathetic innervation to the eye.

Glossopharyngeal (IX)

This mixed nerve is largely sensory. Sensory fibres supply all sensation to the tonsillar fossa and pharynx (afferent pathway of gag reflex), and taste to the posterior third of the tongue.

Motor fibres supply the *stylopharyngeus* muscle, autonomic fibres supply the parotid gland, and a sensory branch supplies the carotid sinus.

Vagus (X)

This mixed nerve, largely motor, supplies the striated muscle of the pharynx (efferent pathway of gag reflex), larynx (including vocal cords via the recurrent laryngeal nerves) and upper oesophagus. There are sensory fibres from the larynx. Parasympathetic fibres supply the heart and abdominal viscera.

Accessory (XI)

This motor nerve supplies trapezius and sternomastoid.

Hypoglossal (XII)

This motor nerve supplies the tongue.

Ninth and tenth nerve lesions

Isolated nerve lesions are most unusual, since disease at

> **Table 21.11   Principal causes of ninth, tenth, eleventh and twelfth nerve lesions**
>
> **Within the brainstem**
> Infarction
> Syringobulbia
> Motor neurone disease (motor fibres)
> Poliomyelitis (motor fibres)
>
> **At the skull base (jugular and anterior condylar foramina)**
> Carcinoma of nasopharynx
> Glomus tumour
> Neurofibroma
> Jugular venous thrombosis (XIIth is spared)
> Trauma
>
> **Within the neck and nasopharynx**
> Carcinoma of nasopharynx
> Metastases
> Polyneuropathy
> Trauma

the jugular foramen affects both nerves and sometimes the accessory nerve.

A unilateral ninth nerve lesion causes diminished sensation on the same side of the pharynx. A tenth nerve palsy produces ipsilateral failure of voluntary and reflex elevation of the soft palate, which is drawn over to the opposite side.

Bilateral combined lesions of the ninth and tenth nerves cause visible weakness of elevation of the palate, depression of palatal sensation and loss of the gag reflex. The vagal recurrent laryngeal branches are involved. The cough is depressed and the vocal cords paralysed. The patient complains of difficulty in swallowing, hoarseness, nasal regurgitation and choking (particularly with fluids) – a dangerous situation. Bulbar palsy is a general term describing palatal, pharyngeal and tongue weakness of LMN or muscle origin (p. 1191).

Ninth and tenth nerve lesions often accompany eleventh and twelfth nerve lesions. Causes are given in Table 21.11.

Recurrent laryngeal nerve lesions. Paralysis of this branch of each vagus causes hoarseness (dysphonia) and failure of the forceful, explosive part of voluntary and reflex coughing. There is no visible weakness of the palate but vocal cord paralysis is seen endoscopically. Bilateral acute lesions (e.g. postoperatively) are a serious emergency and cause respiratory obstruction.

The left recurrent laryngeal nerve (which loops beneath the aorta) is more commonly damaged than the right.

Causes of recurrent laryngeal nerve lesions include:

- mediastinal primary tumours (e.g. thymoma)
- secondary spread from carcinoma of the bronchus
- aneurysm of the aorta
- trauma or surgery to the neck
- glossopharyngeal neuralgia (rare).

Glossopharyngeal neuralgia. This describes intensely painful, paroxysmal neuralgic spasms within the pharynx triggered repeatedly by swallowing. There are no physical signs. Treatment of this rare condition is with carbamazepine (see trigeminal neuralgia, p. 1186) or section of the nerve in the pharynx.

Table 21.11 shows the principal causes of lesions.

Eleventh nerve lesions

A lesion of the eleventh nerve causes weakness of sternomastoid (rotation of the head and neck to the opposite side) and trapezius (shoulder shrugging). Table 21.11 shows the principal lesions. Section of the nerve is followed by persistent neuralgic neck pain.

Twelfth nerve lesions

LMN lesions of the twelfth nerve lead to unilateral tongue weakness, wasting and fasciculation. The protruded tongue deviates towards the weaker side. For principal causes, see Table 21.11.

Bilateral supranuclear (UMN) twelfth nerve lesions (see below) produce slow, limited tongue movements; the tongue is stiff and cannot be protruded far. Fasciculation is absent.

BRAINSTEM LESIONS

Bulbar palsy

Bulbar palsy describes weakness of LMN type of muscles whose cranial nerve nuclei lie in the medulla (the 'bulb'). Paralysis of bulbar muscles is caused by disease of lower cranial nerve nuclei (e.g. motor neurone disease), lesions of ninth to twelfth cranial nerves (Table 21.11), malfunction of their neuromuscular junctions (e.g. myasthenia gravis, botulism), or disease of muscles themselves (e.g. muscular dystrophies).

Pseudobulbar palsy

This describes bilateral supranuclear (UMN) lesions of lower cranial nerves producing weakness and poverty of movement of the tongue and pharyngeal muscles. (This resembles, superficially, a bulbar palsy; hence the term *pseudo*bulbar.) The findings in pseudobulbar palsy are a stiff, slow, spastic tongue (that is not wasted), dysarthria with a stiff, slow voice sounding dry and gravelly, and dysphagia. The gag and palatal reflexes are preserved. The jaw jerk is exaggerated. Emotional lability (inappropriate laughing or crying) often accompanies pseudobulbar palsy. Principal causes are:

- motor neurone disease – often both upper UMN and LMN lesions (i.e. elements of both pseudobulbar *and* bulbar palsy)
- multiple sclerosis, mainly as a late event
- cerebrovascular disease, typically in multi-infarct dementia
- following severe head injury.

Great difficulty swallowing, dysarthria and a slow tongue also develop in late stages of Parkinson's disease. This is distinct from both pseudobulbar and bulbar palsy.

MOTOR CONTROL SYSTEMS

There are three systems:

- The *corticospinal* (or pyramidal) system originates in the cerebral cortex and delivers information to spinal cord anterior horn cells. This system enables *purposive*, *skilled*, *intricate*, *strong* and *organized* movement to take place. Defective function is recognized by a distinct pattern of loss of skilled voluntary movement, spasticity and reflex change. This is seen, for example, in a hemiparesis or hemiplegia.
- The *extrapyramidal* system facilitates *fast*, *fluid* movements that the corticospinal system has generated. Defective function is recognized usually by slowness (bradykinesia), stiffness (rigidity) and/or disorders of movement (rest tremor, chorea and other dyskinesias). Frequently, one sign (e.g. stiffness, tremor or chorea) will predominate. Mixtures of these features, and lack of localized pathological anatomy makes classification difficult.
- The *cerebellum* and its connections have a role in coordinating *smooth* movement initiated by the corticospinal system, and in the regulation of balance. Cerebellar disease leads to unsteadiness and jerkiness of movement (ataxia), with characteristic physical signs of past pointing, action tremor and incoordination, with gait ataxia and/or truncal ataxia.

Each of these three motor controllers also relies upon connections with the other two, and with sensory input, from proprioception, reticular formation, vestibular system and special senses.

CORTICOSPINAL OR PYRAMIDAL SYSTEM

The corticospinal tracts originate in neurones of the fifth cortical layer and terminate at motor nuclei of cranial nerves at the lower border of L1 in spinal cord anterior horn cells. The nerve fibre pathways of particular clinical significance (Fig. 21.8) congregate in the internal capsule and cross in the medulla (decussation of the pyramids), passing to the contralateral halves of the spinal cord as the lateral corticospinal tracts. This is the *pyramidal system*, disease of which causes upper motor neurone (UMN) lesions. *Pyramidal* is simply a descriptive term that draws together the anatomy and characteristic physical signs. It is used here interchangeably with the term UMN.

A small proportion of the corticospinal outflow remains uncrossed (the anterior corticospinal tracts) – this is of no relevance in practice.

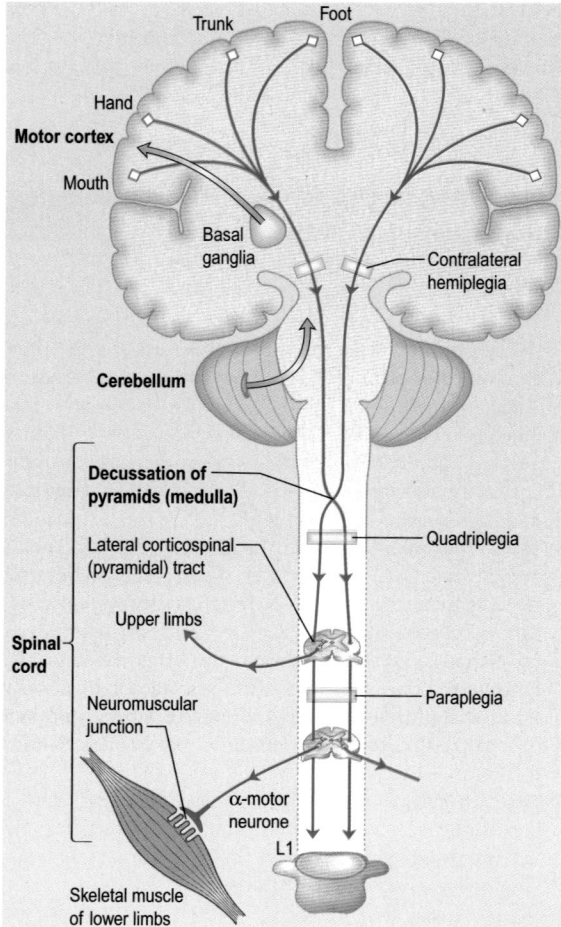

Trunk
Foot
Hand
Motor cortex
Mouth
Basal ganglia
Contralateral hemiplegia
Cerebellum
Decussation of pyramids (medulla)
Lateral corticospinal (pyramidal) tract
Quadriplegia
Upper limbs
Spinal cord
Neuromuscular junction
Paraplegia
α-motor neurone
L1
Skeletal muscle of lower limbs

Fig. 21.8 **The motor system.** Lesions are shown on the right-hand side of the figure.

Characteristics of pyramidal lesions
(see Table 21.12)

Signs of an early pyramidal lesion may be minimal. Weakness, spasticity or changes in superficial reflexes may predominate. Absence of one group of signs does not exclude a UMN lesion.

Pyramidal drift of an upper limb
Normally, the outstretched upper limbs are held symmetrically, even when the eyes are closed. With a

Table 21.12   Evidence of an upper motor neurone lesion
Drift of upper limb
Weakness with a characteristic distribution
Increase in tone of spastic type
Exaggerated tendon reflexes
An extensor plantar response
Loss of fine finger/toe movements
Loss of abdominal reflexes
No muscle wasting
Normal electrical excitability of muscle

pyramidal (UMN) lesion, when both upper limbs are held outstretched, palms uppermost, the affected limb drifts downwards and medially. The forearm tends to pronate and the fingers flex slightly. This sign is often first to occur, sometimes before weakness or reflex changes become obvious.

Weakness and loss of skilled movement
A unilateral pyramidal (UMN) lesion above the decussation in the medulla (e.g. an internal capsule infarct) causes weakness of the opposite limbs, i.e. contralateral hemiparesis. When acute and complete, this weakness will be immediate and dense – e.g. a hemiplegia following an internal capsule infarct. In slowly progressive lesions (e.g. a cortical glioma) a characteristic pattern of increasing weakness emerges in the hemiparetic limbs. In the upper limb flexors remain stronger than extensors, while in the lower limb extensors remain stronger than flexors. In the upper arm the weaker movements are thus shoulder abduction and elbow extension; in the forearm and hand, wrist and finger extensors and abductors are weaker than their antagonists.

In the lower limb weaker movements are hip flexion and abduction, knee flexion, and ankle dorsiflexion and eversion. In addition to weakness, there is loss of skilled movement. For example, fine finger and toe control diminishes. Muscle wasting (except from disuse) is not a feature of pyramidal lesions. Muscles remain normally excitable electrically.

When the UMN lesion is below the decussation of the pyramids, i.e. in the cervical spinal cord, the hemiparesis is on the same side as the lesion. This situation is unusual.

Increase in tone (spasticity)
An acute lesion of one pyramidal tract (e.g. the internal capsule stroke mentioned above) causes initially flaccid paralysis, and loss of tendon reflexes. Increase in tone follows within several days owing to loss of the inhibitory effect of the corticospinal pathways and an increase in spinal reflex activity. This increase in tone affects all muscle groups on the side affected but is detectable most easily in stronger muscles. The pattern is characterized by *changing* resistance to passive movement – the sudden clasp-knife effect. The relevant tendon reflexes become exaggerated and clonus evident.

Changes in superficial reflexes
The normal flexor plantar response becomes extensor (a positive Babinski). In a severe lesion (e.g. the internal capsule infarct) this extensor response can be elicited from a wide area of the affected limb. As recovery progresses, the area that is receptive diminishes until only the posterior third of the lateral aspect of the sole is receptive. The stimulus should be unpleasant (an orange-stick is the correct instrument). An extensor plantar is certain when dorsiflexion of the great toe is accompanied by fanning (abduction) of adjacent toes. Abdominal (and cremasteric reflexes) are abolished on the affected side.

Clinical patterns of UMN disorders

There are two main patterns of UMN (pyramidal) lesions: hemiparesis and paraparesis.

Hemiparesis means a weakness of the limbs of one side; it is usually (but not always, see above) caused by a lesion within the brain. *Paraparesis* means weakness of both lower limbs and is characteristically diagnostic of a spinal cord lesion, though bilateral brain lesions occasionally can also cause a similar picture.

Hemiplegia and *paraplegia* strictly indicate total paralysis, but are often used loosely to describe severe weakness.

Hemiparesis

The level within the corticospinal tract is recognized by various accompanying features.

Motor cortex. Weakness and/or loss of skilled movement confined to one contralateral limb (an arm or a leg – monoplegia) or part of a limb (e.g. a weak hand) is typical of an isolated motor cortex lesion (e.g. a secondary neoplasm). A defect in higher cortical function (e.g. aphasia) and focal epilepsy may occur.

Internal capsule. Since all corticospinal fibres become tightly packed as they reach the internal capsule, occupying about $1\,cm^2$, a small lesion causes a large deficit. For example, an infarct of a small branch of the middle cerebral artery (p. 1212) causes a sudden, dense, contralateral hemiplegia.

Pons. A pontine lesion (e.g. a plaque of multiple sclerosis) is rarely confined only to the corticospinal tract. Since adjacent structures such as the sixth and seventh nuclei, MLF and PPRF (p. 1184), are involved, there are other localizing signs – VI and VII nerve palsies, internuclear ophthalmoplegia (INO) or a lateral gaze palsy, with contralateral hemiparesis.

Spinal cord. An isolated lesion of a single lateral corticospinal tract within the spinal cord (e.g. an injury in the cervical region) causes an ipsilateral UMN lesion, the level indicated by changes in reflexes (e.g. absent biceps C5/6 jerk), presence of a Brown–Séquard syndrome (p. 1199) and muscle wasting at the level of the lesion (p. 1250).

Paraparesis (Table 21.13)

Paraparesis indicates bilateral damage to the corticospinal tracts. Spinal cord compression (p. 1250) or other cord disease is the usual cause, but cerebral lesions occasionally can produce paraparesis. Paraparesis is a feature of many neurological conditions, recognizable by additional features, making this differential diagnosis one of pivotal importance (see page 1250).

EXTRAPYRAMIDAL SYSTEM

The extrapyramidal system is a general term without an absolute definition for motor structures of the basal

Table 21.13 Causes of a spastic paraparesis

Spinal lesions
Spinal cord compression (see Table 21.48)
Multiple sclerosis
Myelitis (e.g. varicella zoster virus)
Motor neurone disease
Subacute combined degeneration of the cord
Syringomyelia
Syphilis
Familial or sporadic paraparesis
Vascular disease of the cord
Non-metastatic manifestation of malignancy
Tropical spastic paraparesis (HTLV-1)
HIV-associated myelopathy

Cerebral lesions*
Parasagittal cortical lesions:
   meningioma
   venous sinus thrombosis
Hydrocephalus
Multiple cerebral infarction

*All are rare causes of a paraparesis
HTLV-1: human T-cell leukaemia virus

ganglia, i.e. corpus striatum (caudate nucleus + globus pallidus + putamen), subthalamic nucleus, substantia nigra and parts of the thalamus. In basal ganglia/extrapyramidal disorders, either or both of two features become apparent in the limbs and axial muscles:

- reduction in speed, known as bradykinesia (slow movement) or akinesia (no movement), with muscle rigidity
- involuntary movements (e.g. tremor, chorea, hemiballismus, athetosis, dystonia).

Extrapyramidal disorders are classified broadly on clinical grounds into akinetic–rigid syndromes (p. 1227) in which poverty of movement predominates, and dyskinesias, in which there are various excessive involuntary movements (p. 1231).

The most common serious extrapyramidal disorder is Parkinson's disease.

Essential anatomy

The corpus striatum lies close to the substantia nigra, thalami and subthalamic nuclei. There are interconnections between these structures, cerebral cortex, cerebellum and reticular formation, cranial nerve nuclei (particularly vestibular) and spinal cord (Fig. 21.9).

Function and dysfunction

The overall function of this complex system is modulation of cortical motor activity by a series of servo loops, between cortex and basal ganglia (Fig. 21.9).

In many involuntary movement disorders there are substantial and specific changes in neurotransmitters (Table 21.14) rather than anatomical lesions discernable on imaging or at autopsy. The main neurotransmitters in

Fig. 21.9 Extrapyramidal system: scheme of connections and neurotransmitters. GLU, glutamate; ENK, enkephalin; GABA, gamma-aminobutyric acid; VA, ventral anterior; VL, ventrolateral; GP*l*, lateral globus pallidus; GP*m*, medial globus pallidus; SN*r*, substantia nigra pars reticulata.

Table 21.14 Changes in the major neurotransmitter profile in Parkinson's and Huntington's diseases

Condition	Site	Neurotransmitter
Parkinson's disease	Putamen	Dopamine ↓ 90% Norepinephrine (noradrenaline) ↓ 60% 5-HT ↓ 60%
	Substantia nigra	Dopamine ↓ 90% GAD + GABA ↓↓
	Cerebral cortex	GAD + GABA ↓↓
Huntington's disease	Corpus striatum	Acetylcholine ↓↓ GABA ↓↓ Dopamine: normal GAD + GABA ↓↓

GABA, γ-amino butyric acid; GAD, glutamic acid decarboxylase, the enzyme responsible for synthesizing GABA; 5-HT, 5-hydroxytryptamine

extrapyramidal pathways are outlined in Figure 21.9; changes in Parkinson's disease, chorea and hemiballismus are discussed below. The complexity of the situation is evident.

A proposed model of principal basal ganglia pathways

1. Direct pathway from striatum to medial globus pallidus (GP*m*) and substantia nigra pars reticulata (SN*r*). Inhibitory **synapse F**, GABA and substance P.
2. Indirect pathway from striatum to globus pallidus; via lateral globus pallidus (GP*l*; inhibitory **synapse C**, GABA, enkephalin) and subthalamic nucleus inhibitory **synapse D**, GABA). Terminates in GP*m*–SN*r* (in excitatory **synapse E**, glutamate).
3. Direct pathways, both inhibitory and excitatory from substantia nigra pars compacta (SN*c*) to striatum. **Synapse A**, dopamine, D_1, excitatory; and **synapse B**, D_2, inhibitory.
4. GP*m* and SN*r* to thalamus. **Synapse G**, GABA.
5. Thalamus to cortex. Excitatory, **synapse H**.
6. Cortex to striatum. Excitatory, glutamate.

The model helps explain how basal ganglia disease can either reduce excitatory thalamo-cortical activity at synapse H, i.e. movement – causing bradykinesia, or increase it, causing hyperkinesia.

Parkinson's disease. This condition is characterized by slowness, stiffness and rest tremor (p. 1227). Degeneration in SN*c* causes loss of dopamine activity in the striatum. Dopamine is excitatory for synapse A and inhibitory for synapse B. Through the direct pathway there is reduced activity at synapse F, leading to increased inhibitory output (G) and decreased cortical activity (H).

Also in Parkinson's disease, in the indirect pathway dopamine deficiency results in disinhibition of neurones synapsing at C. This leads to reduced activity at D, and to increased activity of neurones in the subthalamic nucleus. There is excess stimulation at synapse E, enhancing further inhibitory output of GP*m*–SN*r*.

The net effect via both pathways is to inhibit the ventral anterior (VA) and ventrolateral (VL) nuclei of the thalamus at synapse G. Cortical (motor) activity at H is thus reduced.

Levodopa used in Parkinson's disease (p. 1229) induces its unwanted dyskinesias by increasing dopamine activity at synapses A and B, reversing the sequences in both direct and indirect pathways.

Huntington's disease. This is an inherited dementia (p. 1231) with progressive jerky movements (chorea). Chorea results from damage to neurones (GABA, enkephalin) in the indirect pathway from striatum to GP*l*, reducing activity at synapse C. In turn, there is increased inhibition of subthalamic neurones at D, reduced stimulation at E and decreased inhibition of VA/VL at G. Cortical activity at H increases.

Hemiballismus. This describes wild, flinging limb movements usually caused by a small infarct in the subthalamic nucleus. This reduces excitatory activity at synapse E, causing reduction of inhibition at G with increased activity of thalamo-cortical neurones and increased activity at H.

CEREBELLUM

The third system of motor control modulates coordination, rather than speed. Ataxia, i.e. unsteadiness, is characteristic when it malfunctions.

The cerebellum receives afferent fibres from:

- proprioceptive receptors in joints and muscles
- vestibular nuclei
- basal ganglia
- the corticospinal system
- olivary nuclei.

Efferent fibres pass from the cerebellum to:

- each red nucleus
- vestibular nuclei
- basal ganglia
- corticospinal system.

Each lateral cerebellar lobe coordinates movement of the ipsilateral limbs. The vermis (a midline structure) is concerned with maintenance of axial (midline) posture and balance.

Cerebellar lesions

Expanding mass lesions within the cerebellum obstruct the aqueduct to cause hydrocephalus, with severe pressure headaches, vomiting and papilloedema. Coning of the cerebellar tonsils (p. 1245) through the foramen magnum and respiratory arrest occur, often within hours. Rarely, tonic seizures (sudden attacks of limb stiffness) occur.

Lateral cerebellar lobes

A lesion within one cerebellar lobe (e.g. a tumour or infarction) causes disruption of the normal sequence of movements (dyssynergia) on the same side. Ataxia and other signs develop.

Neurotransmitter changes in cerebellar disease are poorly understood.

Posture and gait. The outstretched arm is held still in the early stages of a cerebellar lesion (cf. the drift of a pyramidal lesion) but there is rebound upward overshoot when the limb is pressed downwards and released. Gait becomes broad and ataxic; the patient falters towards the lesion.

Tremor and ataxia. Movement is imprecise in direction, in force and in distance (dysmetria). Rapid alternating movements (tapping, clapping or rotary hand movements) are clumsy and disorganized (dysdiadochokinesis). Intention tremor (action tremor, with past-pointing) is seen. Speed of movement is preserved, cf. extrapyramidal disease.

Nystagmus. Coarse horizontal nystagmus (p. 1189) develops with lateral cerebellar lobe lesions – the fast component towards the lesion.

Dysarthria. A halting, jerking dysarthria occurs – the scanning speech of cerebellar lesions (usually bilateral).

Other signs. Titubation – rhythmic head tremor in either to and fro ('yes–yes') movements or rotary

Table 21.15 Principal causes of cerebellar syndromes

Tumours	Haemangioblastoma
	Medulloblastoma
	Secondary neoplasm
	Compression by acoustic neuroma
Vascular lesions	Haemorrhage
	Infarction
	Arteriovenous malformation
Infection	Abscess
	HIV
	Kuru
Developmental	Arnold–Chiari malformation
	Basilar invagination
	Cerebral palsy
Toxic and metabolic	Anticonvulsant drugs
	Chronic alcohol abuse
	Following carbon monoxide poisoning
	Lead poisoning
	Solvent abuse
Inherited	Friedreich's ataxia
	Ataxia telangiectasia
	Essential tremor
Miscellaneous	Multiple sclerosis
	Hydrocephalus
	Postinfective cerebellar syndrome of childhood
	Hypothyroidism
	Non-metastatic manifestation of malignancy
	Cerebral oedema of chronic hypoxia

('no–no') movements – also occurs, mainly when cerebellar connections are involved (e.g. in essential tremor and MS, pp. 1231 and 1235). Hypotonia (floppy limbs) and depression of reflexes (and slow, pendular reflexes) are also sometimes seen with cerebellar disease, though of little value as localizing signs.

Midline cerebellar lesions

Midline cerebellar vermis lesions have a dramatic effect on trunk and axial musculature–difficulty standing and sitting unsupported, with a rolling, broad, ataxic gait (truncal ataxia). Lesions of the flocculonodular region of the cerebellum cause vertigo, vomiting and gait ataxia if they extend to the roof of the fourth ventricle.

Table 21.15 summarizes the main causes of cerebellar disease.

TREMOR

Tremor means a regular and sinusoidal oscillation. Different varieties are outlined below. Pathological anatomy and neurotransmitter changes remain largely unknown.

Postural tremor

Everyone has a physiological tremor (often barely perceptible) of the outstretched hands at 8–12 Hz. This is increased with anxiety, caffeine, hyperthyroidism and certain drugs (sympathomimetics, sodium valproate, lithium) or in mercury poisoning. A coarser, postural tremor is seen in benign essential tremor (usually at 5–8 Hz) and in chronic alcohol abuse. Postural tremor does not worsen on movement, though it may become more obvious.

Intention tremor

Tremor exacerbated by action, with past-pointing and accompanying incoordination of rapid alternating movement (dysdiadochokinesis), occurs in cerebellar lobe disease and with lesions of cerebellar connections. Titubation and nystagmus may be present.

Rest tremor

This tremor occurs typically in Parkinson's disease, and is noticeably worst at rest, usually between 4 and 7 Hz – 'pill-rolling' between thumb and index finger.

Other tremors

Coarse tremor is seen following lesions of the red nucleus (e.g. infarction, demyelination) and rarely with frontal lobe lesions.

FURTHER READING
Elble R (2000) Origins of tremor. *Lancet* **355**: 1113–1114.

LOWER MOTOR NEURONE (LMN) LESIONS

The LMN is the motor pathway from anterior horn cell (or cranial nerve nucleus) via peripheral nerve to motor endplate.

The motor unit consists of a single anterior horn cell, the single fast-conducting motor nerve fibre that leaves the spinal cord via the anterior root, and the group of muscle fibres (100–2000) being supplied via the mixed peripheral nerve. Anterior horn cell activity is modulated by impulses from:

- corticospinal tracts
- extrapyramidal system
- cerebellum
- afferent fibres from posterior roots.

Signs of lower motor neurone lesion

These are seen in voluntary muscles, which depend upon an intact nerve supply to produce movement *and* for metabolic integrity. Signs follow rapidly if the LMN is interrupted (Table 21.16). Muscle wasting appears within 3 weeks. Fasciculation (visible twitching) occurs – due to contractions of denervated single motor units. Fibrillation potentials are seen when denervated muscle is sampled electrically (p. 1203).

Causes

Examples of LMN lesions at various levels are:

- cranial nerve nuclei and anterior horn cell – Bell's palsy, motor neurone disease, poliomyelitis

Table 21.16	Signs of a lower motor neurone lesion
Weakness	
Wasting	
Hypotonia	
Reflex loss	
Fasciculation	
Contractures of muscle	} long term effects
'Trophic' changes in skin and nails	

NB: Fibrillation potentials can be detected electromyographically, see page 1203.

- spinal root – cervical and lumbar disc protrusion, neuralgic amyotrophy (see p. 1264)
- peripheral (or cranial) nerve – nerve trauma or entrapment (see p. 1259), mononeuritis multiplex (p. 1260).

SPINAL REFLEX ARC

Components of the spinal reflex arc are illustrated in Figure 21.10. The stretch reflex is the physiological basis for all tendon reflexes. For example, in the knee jerk, a tap on the patellar tendon activates stretch receptors in the quadriceps. Impulses in first-order sensory neurones pass directly to LMNs (L3 and L4) that contract quadriceps.

Loss of a tendon reflex is caused by a lesion anywhere along the spinal reflex path. The reflex lost indicates its level (Table 21.17).

Reinforcement

Distraction of the patient's attention, clenching teeth or pulling interlocked fingers enhances reflex activity. Such

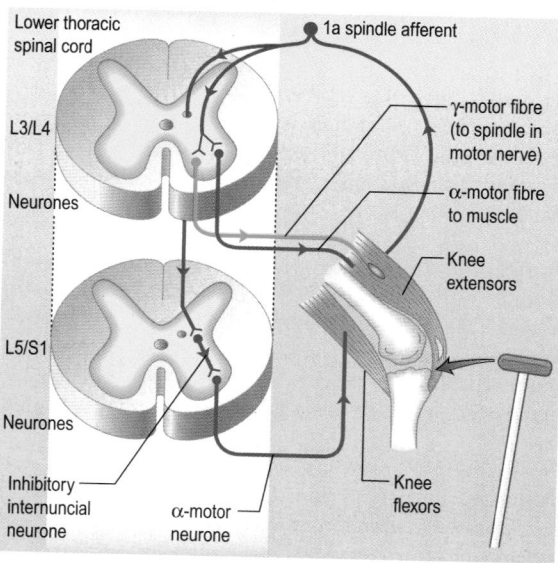

Fig. 21.10 The knee jerk: a spinal reflex arc. Sudden stretching of a tendon generates sensory action potentials in 1a muscle spindle afferents. These synapse with γ motor fibres (to spindles) and α motor fibres. Motor action potentials generated cause muscle contraction. There is also inhibition of knee flexion.

Table 21.17 Spinal levels of tendon reflexes

Spinal level	Reflex
C5–6	Supinator
C5–6	Biceps
C7	Triceps
L3–4	Knee
S1	Ankle

reinforcement manoeuvres should be done before a reflex is recorded 'absent'.

SENSORY PATHWAYS AND PAIN

Peripheral nerves and spinal roots

Peripheral nerves carry all modalities of sensation from either free or specialized nerve endings to dorsal root ganglia and thus to the cord. The sensory distribution of spinal roots (dermatomes) is shown in Figure 21.11.

Spinal cord (Fig. 21.12)

Posterior columns

Axons in the posterior columns whose cell bodies are in

Fig. 21.11 Dermatomes of spinal roots and ophthalmic (V₁), maxillary (V₂) and mandibular (V₃) divisions of the trigeminal nerve.

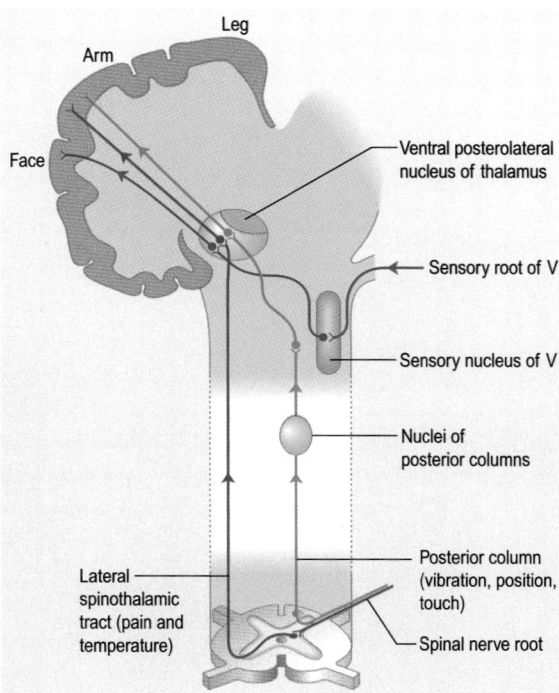

Fig. 21.12 **Principal sensory pathways.** Posterior columns remain uncrossed until the medulla. The spinothalamic tracts cross close to their entry into the spinal cord.

the ipsilateral gracile and cuneate nuclei in the medulla carry the sensory modalities of vibration sense, joint position (proprioception), light touch and two-point discrimination. Axons from second-order neurones then cross the midline in the brainstem to form the medial lemniscus and pass to the thalamus.

Spinothalamic tracts

Axons carrying pain and temperature sensation synapse in the dorsal horn of the cord, cross the cord and pass as the spinothalamic tracts to the thalamus and reticular formation.

Sensory cortex

The projection of fibres from the thalamus to the sensory cortex of the parietal region is shown in Figure 21.12. Connections also exist between the thalamus and the motor cortex.

LESIONS OF THE SENSORY PATHWAYS
(Fig. 21.13)

Altered sensation (paraesthesia), tingling, clumsiness, numbness and pain are the principal symptoms of sensory lesions. The pattern usually suggests the site of pathology.

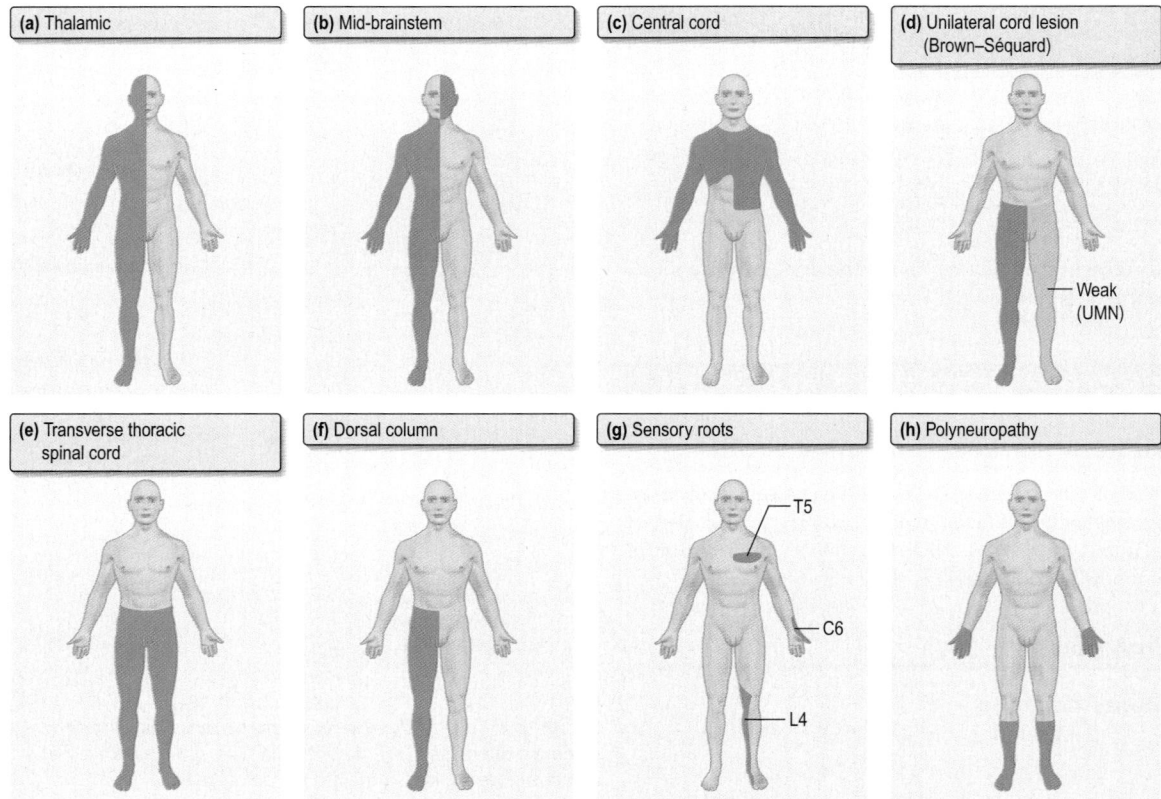

(a) Thalamic **(b)** Mid-brainstem **(c)** Central cord **(d)** Unilateral cord lesion (Brown–Séquard) — Weak (UMN)

(e) Transverse thoracic spinal cord **(f)** Dorsal column **(g)** Sensory roots — T5, C6, L4 **(h)** Polyneuropathy

Fig. 21.13 **Principal patterns of loss of sensation. (a)** Thalamic lesion: sensory loss throughout opposite side (rare). **(b)** Brainstem lesion (rare): contralateral sensory loss below face and ipsilateral loss on face. **(c)** Central cord lesion, e.g. syrinx: 'suspended' areas of loss, often asymmetrical and 'dissociated', i.e. pain and temperature loss but light touch remaining intact. **(d)** 'Hemisection' of cord or unilateral cord lesion = Brown–Séquard syndrome: contralateral spinothalamic (pain and temperature) loss with ipsilateral weakness and dorsal column loss below lesion. **(e)** Transverse cord lesion: loss of all modalities below lesion. **(f)** Isolated dorsal column lesion, e.g. demyelination: loss of proprioception, vibration and light touch. **(g)** Individual sensory root lesions, e.g. C6 (cervical root compression), T5 (shingles), L4 (lumbar root compression). **(h)** Polyneuropathy: distal sensory loss.

Peripheral nerve lesions

Symptoms are felt in the distribution of the affected peripheral nerve (p. 1259).

Section of a sensory nerve is followed by complete sensory loss. Nerve entrapment (p. 1259) causes numbness, pain and tingling. Tapping the site of compression sometimes causes a sharp, electric-shock-like pain in the distribution of the nerve, e.g. Tinel's sign in carpal tunnel syndrome (p. 1260).

Neuralgia

Neuralgia refers to local pain of great severity in the distribution of a damaged nerve. Examples are:

- trigeminal neuralgia (p. 1186)
- postherpetic neuralgia (p. 1240)
- complex regional pain syndrome type II (causalgia) – a chronic burning pain that occasionally follows nerve section (seen after amputation).

Spinal root lesions

Root pain

The pain of root compression is felt in the myotome supplied by that root, and there is also a tingling discomfort in the dermatome. The pain is made worse by manoeuvres that either stretch the nerve root (e.g. limitation of straight leg raising in lumbar disc prolapse) or increase pressure in the spinal subarachnoid space (coughing and straining).

Cervical and lumbar disc protrusions (p. 1265) are common causes of root lesions.

Dorsal spinal root lesions

Section of a dorsal root causes loss of all modalities of sensation in the appropriate dermatome (Fig. 21.11). However, the overlap with adjacent dermatomes may make it difficult to detect anaesthesia if a single root is destroyed.

Lightning pains. Tabes dorsalis (now rare in UK) is a form of neurosyphilis that causes low-grade inflammation of dorsal roots and root entry zones in the spinal cord. Irregular, sharp, momentary stabbing pains (like lightning) involve one or two spots, typically in a calf, thigh or ankle.

Spinal cord lesions

Posterior column lesions

These cause:

- tingling
- electric-shock-like sensations
- clumsiness
- numbness
- band-like sensations.

These symptoms though lateralized are often felt vaguely without a clear sensory level. On examination, position sense, vibration sense, light touch and two-point discrimination are lost below the lesion. Loss of position sense produces the stamping gait of sensory ataxia (p. 1175).

Lhermitte's phenomenon

An electric-shock-like sensation radiates down the trunk and limbs when the neck is flexed. This indicates a cervical cord lesion. Lhermitte's sign is common in acute exacerbations of MS (p. 1253). It also occurs in cervical spondylotic myelopathy (p. 1264), subacute combined degeneration of the cord (p. 1263), radiation myelopathy (p. 1252), and occasionally in cord compression.

Spinothalamic tract lesions

Pure spinothalamic lesions cause isolated contralateral loss of pain and temperature sensation with a clear level below the lesion. This is called *dissociated* sensory loss – pain and temperature are dissociated from light touch, which remains preserved. This is seen typically in syringomyelia where a cavity occupies the central spinal cord (p. 1252).

The spinal level is modified by the lamination of fibres within the spinothalamic tracts. Fibres from the lower spinal roots lie superficially and are therefore damaged first by compressive lesions from outside the cord. As an external compressive lesion (e.g. a midthoracic extradural meningioma; Fig. 21.14) enlarges, the spinal sensory level ascends as deeper fibres become involved. Conversely, a central lesion of the cord (e.g. a syrinx, p. 1252) affects deeper fibres first.

Spinothalamic tract lesions cause loss of pain and temperature perception (e.g. painless burns). Perforating ulcers and neuropathic joints (Charcot joints) develop.

Spinal cord compression (Fig. 21.14)

Cord compression causes a progressive spastic paraparesis (or tetraparesis/quadriparesis) with sensory loss below the level of compression. Sphincter disturbance is common.

Root pain is frequent but not invariable. It is felt characteristically at the level of compression. With thoracic cord compression (e.g. an extradural meningioma), pain radiates around the chest and is made worse by

Fig. 21.14 Clinical features of spinal cord compression.

Labels: Wasted intercostal muscles, sensory loss, root pain; Posterior columns; Spinothalamic tract; Loss of pain and temperature sensation (spinothalamic tract); Lateral corticospinal tract; T4; Compressive lesion, e.g. thoracic meningioma; T5; 'Pyramidal' signs (corticospinal tract); Diminished proprioception and light touch (posterior columns); T6

coughing and straining, as the meningeal root sheaths are stretched.

Involvement of one spinothalamic tract (contralateral loss of pain and temperature) with one corticospinal tract is known as the Brown–Séquard syndrome or hemisection of the cord. The patient complains of numbness on one side and weakness on the other. Paraparesis/spinal cord disease is discussed further on page 1250.

Pontine lesions

Since lesions in the pons (e.g. an MS plaque) lie above the decussation of the posterior columns, and the medial lemniscus and spinothalamic tracts are close together, there is loss of all forms of sensation on the side opposite the lesion. Combinations of III, IV, V, VI and VII cranial nerve nuclei are often also involved (Fig. 21.12) and indicate a level.

Thalamic lesions

Thalamic pain, also called thalamic syndrome, usually follows a small thalamic infarct. A patient has a stroke (hemiparesis and sensory loss). The weakness recovers partially or completely but there develops constant very severe deep-seated burning pain in the paretic limbs. This continues night and day. Extreme anguish is usual and the secondary depression may lead to suicide. Thalamic lesions may also produce loss of sensation on the opposite side of the body; this is a less usual clinical picture.

Parietal cortex lesions

Sensory loss, neglect of one side, apraxia (p. 1175) and subtle disorders of sensation occur. Pain is not a feature of destructive cortical lesions. Irritative phenomena (e.g. partial sensory seizures from a glioma) arising in the parietal cortex cause tingling sensations in a limb, or elsewhere.

FURTHER READING
Donaghy M (1997) *Neurology – Oxford Core Texts.* Oxford: Oxford University Press.

PAIN

Pain is an unpleasant, unique physical and psychological experience. Acute pain serves a biological purpose (e.g. withdrawal) and is typically self-limiting, ceasing when healing is complete. There is sympathetic hypersensitivity. Some forms of chronic pain (e.g. causalgia, p. 1198) last many months, outlasting the time for healing.

Essential physiology of pain

Pain perception is mediated by free nerve endings, terminations of finely myelinated A-delta and of non-myelinated C fibres. Chemicals released following injury either produce pain by direct stimulation or by sensitizing nerve endings. A-delta fibres give rise to perception of sharp, immediate pain, followed by slower-onset, more diffuse and prolonged pain mediated by slower-conducting C fibres.

Sensory impulses enter the cord via dorsal spinal roots. Within it, impulses ascend either in each dorsal (posterior) column or in each spinothalamic tract. The grey matter neurones in the cord are arranged in laminae labelled I to X (dorsal to ventral). A fibres terminate in laminae I and V and excite second-order neurones which send fibres to the contralateral side via the anterior commissure and via the anterolateral column of the direct spinothalamic tract. C fibres mostly terminate in the *substantia gelatinosa* (laminae II and III). A series of short fibres give rise to long axons which pass through the anterior commissure to the contralateral side and up the spino-reticulo-thalamic tract.

The spinothalamic tracts carry impulses that localize pain. Thalamic pathways to and from the cortex mediate emotional components.

Sympathetic activity increases pain, e.g. hyperaemia in a painful limb.

The gate theory of pain

Gate theory, a useful way of thinking about pain, proposes that entry of afferent impulses is monitored first by the substantia gelatinosa. This gate determines whether or not sufficient activity penetrates to fire secondary neurones in the dorsal horn. This, and subsequent gates are influenced by brain and cord 'regulators' that alter how far a gate remains open.

Animal studies show that 'downstream regulatory elements' binding to calcium-regulated transcription factors control CNS endogenous opiate (endorphin) precursors (e.g. pro-dynorphin). These modulate pain.

Endogenous opiates

The endorphin peptides have opioid activity and probably account for placebo effects, the effects of stress, acupuncture and may explain in part why some patients develop 'chronic pain syndromes'. Endorphins are CNS neurotransmitters acting at inhibitory synapses via δ, κ and μ receptors. Dynorphin, from its precursor (above), is believed to modulate nociceptive (pain) impulses entering the spinal cord.

Management of chronic pain (see also p. 524)

Chronic pain is gravely disabling and distressing, and taxing to treat. Multidisciplinary pain-relief clinics are helpful in providing specific and supportive therapy. Pain control should, however, be part of all doctors' skills.

A management plan for intractable pain has seven components:

Diagnostic

Rigorous attention must be paid to the question of diagnosis, reviewing the history (first hand), investigations and radiology. A specific surgical approach may then become apparent (e.g. spinal stenosis, trigeminal neuralgia, glossopharyngeal neuralgia, or syringomyelia).

Psychological

Chronic pain influences quality of life. Depression (p. 1288) is commonly associated with pain when the pathology is benign and antidepressant drugs help. Only a third of patients suffering pain from secondary cancer are clinically depressed, despite the gravity of their disease.

Analgesics (see p. 549)

Perseverance and compliance with therapy is an invariable issue. The WHO analgesic ladder is useful for management of chronic pain.

Co-analgesics

Co-analgesics have a primary use other than for pain but also help either alone or added to analgesics. Examples are tricyclic antidepressants and anticonvulsants (p. 525). Calcium-channel blockers (nifedipine) improve sympathetically mediated pain in, for example, Raynaud's disease. Muscle relaxants (spasticity), antibiotics (infection) and steroids (inflammatory arthropathy) each reduce pain in appropriate situations.

Stimulation

Acupuncture, ice, heat, ultrasound, massage, transcutaneous electrical nerve stimulation (TENS) and spinal cord stimulation all achieve analgesia by a gating effect on large myelinated nerve fibres.

Nerve blocks

Pain pathways can be blocked either temporarily by local anaesthetic or permanently with phenol, or radio-frequency lesions:

somatic blocks:
- **(a)** peripheral nerve and plexus injections
- **(b)** epidural and spinal analgesia
- sympathetic blocks:
- **(a)** sympathetic ganglia and nerve ending injections
- **(b)** central epidural and spinal sympathetic blockade.

Neurosurgery

Highly specialized and sometimes controversial techniques have a place alongside pharmacological remedies. Examples are dorsal rhizotomy, sympathectomy, cordotomy and neurostimulation.

FURTHER READING
Wall PD, Melzack R (1999) *Textbook of Pain*, 4th edn. Edinburgh: Churchill Livingstone.
Lancet (1999) Pain Series. 353: May–June.
Vogt BA (2002) Knocking out the DREAM (downstream regulatory element antagonistic modulator) to study pain. *New England Journal of Medicine* **364**: 362–364.

CONTROL OF THE BLADDER AND SEXUAL FUNCTION

Changes in micturition and failure of normal sexual activity are diagnostic symptoms in sacral, spinal cord and cortical disease.

Essential anatomy and function

The three efferent LMN pathways to the bladder are shown in Table 21.18.

Afferent fibres (T12–S4) record changes in pressure within the bladder and tactile sensation in the genitalia. When the bladder is distended, continence is maintained by reflex suppression of the parasympathetic outflow, and reciprocal activation of the sympathetic, both being subject to cortical (voluntary) control. Voiding takes place by parasympathetic activation of the detrusor muscle, and relaxation of the internal sphincter.

Cortical awareness of bladder fullness is located in the post-central gyrus, parasagittally, while initiation of micturition is in the pre-central gyrus. Voluntary control of micturition is located in the frontal cortex, parasagittally.

Disorders of micturition: incontinence

All three neurological patterns of bladder dysfunction cause urinary incontinence. These may be hard to separate clinically.

Cortical:
- Frontal lesions cause socially inappropriate micturition.
- Pre-central lesions cause difficulty initiating micturition.
- Post-central lesions cause loss of sense of bladder fullness.

Spinal cord. Bilateral UMN lesions (pyramidal tracts) cause frequency of micturition and incontinence. The bladder is small and unusually sensitive to small changes in intravesical pressure (hypertonic bladder). Frontal lobe lesions also sometimes cause a hypertonic bladder.

Lower motor neurone. Sacral lesions (conus medullaris, sacral roots and pelvic nerve lesions – must be bilateral) cause a flaccid, atonic bladder, that overflows unexpectedly.

Male erectile dysfunction

Failure of penile erection often has a mixed aetiology, i.e. an organic and psychological cause. Depression is a common cause and a common effect. Endocrine aspects of sexual dysfunction are discussed on page 1055. Erectile dysfunction is treated with phosphodiesterase type 5 inhibitors, e.g. sildenafil by mouth.

FURTHER READING
Fowler CJ (ed) (1999) *Neurology of Bladder, Bowel and Sexual Dysfunction*. Boston: Butterworth Heinemann.

NEUROLOGICAL INVESTIGATIONS

NEURORADIOLOGY

Skull and spinal X-rays

These show:

- fractures of the skull vault or base
- skull lesions (e.g. metastases, osteomyelitis, Paget's disease, abnormal skull foramina, fibrous dysplasia)
- enlargement or destruction of the pituitary fossa – intrasellar tumour, raised intracranial pressure
- intracranial calcification – tuberculoma, oligodendroglioma, wall of an aneurysm, cysticercosis.

Spinal X-rays show fractures, congenital bone lesions (e.g. cysts), destructive lesions (infection, metastasis) or spondylosis (degenerative change).

Table 21.18 The three efferent pathways to the bladder and genitalia	
Nerve supply	**Function**
Sympathetic T12–L2	Bladder wall relaxation Internal sphincter contraction Orgasm, ejaculation
Parasympathetic S2–4	Bladder wall contraction Internal sphincter relaxation Penis and clitoris erection/engorgement
Pudendal nerves (somatic)	External sphincter (skeletal muscle)

Imaging of the brain and spinal cord

Brain CT is now widely available world-wide and MRI is rapidly becoming a standard test.

Computed tomography: CT

A collimated X-ray beam moves synchronously across a slice of brain between 2 mm and 13 mm thick. Transmitted X-irradiation from a pixel, an element < 1 mm^2, is computer-processed and a Hounsfield number assigned to its density (air = –1000 units; water = 0; bone = +1000 units).

Differences in attenuation (density) between bone, brain and CSF enable recognition of normal and infarcted tissue, tumour, extravasated blood, and oedema.

Enhancement with i.v. contrast media delineates areas of increased blood supply.

Contrast CT imaging of the spinal cord (myelography) and cerebral ventricles (ventriculography) is occasionally performed.

CT is safe apart from occasional systemic reactions to contrast; the irradiation involved is small.

Value of CT

CT scanning demonstrates:

- cerebral tumours
- intracerebral haemorrhage (see p. 1217) and infarction
- subdural and extradural haematoma
- free blood in the subarachnoid space (subarachnoid haemorrhage, see p. 1218)
- lateral shift of midline structures and displacement/enlargement of the ventricular system
- cerebral atrophy
- spinal trauma (with CT myelography)
- skull and scalp lesions.

CT imaging, within its limitations, shows that the brain is anatomically normal, and gives reassurance.

Limitations of CT

- Lesions under 1 cm diameter may be missed.
- Lesions with attenuation close to that of bone may be missed if near the skull.
- Lesions with attenuation similar to that of brain are poorly imaged (e.g. MS plaques, isodense subdural haematoma).
- CT sometimes misses lesions within the posterior fossa.
- The spinal cord is not imaged directly by CT (contrast is necessary).
- Cooperation is required – a general anaesthetic is occasionally needed.

Magnetic resonance imaging: MRI

The hydrogen nucleus is a proton whose electrical charge creates a local electrical field. These protons are aligned by sudden strong magnetic impulses. Protons are then imaged with radiofrequency waves at right angles to their alignment. The protons resonate and spin, then revert to their normal alignment. As they do so, images are made at different phases of relaxation, known as T1, T2, T2 'STIR', diffusion-weighted imaging (DWI) and other sequences. From these sequences, referred to as different weightings, recorded images are compared. Gadolinium is used as an intravenous contrast medium.

Advantages of MRI

- MR distinguishes between brain white and grey matter.
- Spinal cord and nerve roots are imaged directly.
- Pituitary imaging.
- MRI has greater resolution than CT (around 0.5 cm).
- No radiation is involved.
- Magnetic resonance angiography (MRA) images blood vessels without contrast.
- It is useful in muscle disease, e.g. myositis.

Tumours, infarction, haemorrhage, clot, MS plaques, posterior fossa, foramen magnum and spinal cord are demonstrated well on MRI.

Limitations of MRI are principally time and cost. Imaging one region takes about 20 minutes. Patients do need to cooperate. Claustrophobia is an issue but 'open' machines are available. A general anaesthetic may be necessary. Patients with pacemakers or with metallic bodies in the brain cannot be imaged. MR imaging for some days after lumbar puncture (p. 1204) frequently shows diffuse meningeal enhancement with gadolinium.

Doppler studies

B-mode and colour ultrasound are valuable in the detection of stenosis of the carotid arteries.

Digital cerebral and spinal angiography

In many centres where advanced MRI is available, these techniques are little used. Contrast is injected intra-arterially or intravenously. These studies carry a mortality and risk of stroke ($< 1\%$). Sequences of the aorta, carotid and vertebral arteries demonstrate occlusion, stenoses, atheroma and aneurysms. Spinal angiography images cord arteriovenous malformations.

Isotope bone scanning

[^{99m}Tc]-pertechnetate is injected intravenously, it is of value in detection of vertebral and skull lesions (e.g. metastases).

Positron emission tomography (PET) and single proton emission computed tomography (SPECT)

These techniques image function more than anatomy by tracking the uptake and metabolism of radioisotopes.

(a) EEG: 500 µV gain level

Right

Left

Normal activity | Generalized (bilateral) epileptic activity

(b) EEG: 100 µV gain level

Right

Left

E

E

Normal activity | Focal epileptic activity (right)

Fig. 21.15 Examples of EEG traces.
(a) Normal activity followed by generalized epileptic spikes in all leads.
(b) Normal activity followed by focal spikes in right leads. E, eye-movement artefact.

Electroencephalography (EEG)

The EEG (Fig. 21.15) is recorded from scalp electrodes on 16 channels simultaneously. Its main value is in diagnosing epilepsy and diffuse brain diseases. Video-telemetry, which combines EEG with video, is valuable in assessment of 'attacks' that are uncertain clinically.

Epilepsy

Spikes, or spike-and-wave abnormalities, are hallmarks of epilepsy, but it should be emphasized that patients with epilepsy often have a normal EEG between seizures (p. 1222).

Diffuse brain disorders

Recognizable slow-wave EEG abnormalities appear in encephalitis, prion (Creutzfeldt–Jakob) disease and metabolic states (e.g. hypoglycaemia and hepatic coma).

Brainstem death

The EEG is isoelectric (flat), but is no longer necessary to confirm brain death (p. 989).

Electromyography and conduction studies

Electromyography

A concentric needle electrode is inserted into voluntary muscle. The amplified recording is viewed on an oscilloscope and heard through a speaker. Three main features are seen:

- normal interference pattern
- denervation and reinnervation
- myopathic, myotonic or myasthenic changes (p. 1267).

Peripheral nerve conduction (Fig. 21.16)

Four measurements are of principal value in diagnosis of neuropathies and nerve entrapment:

- mean nerve (motor and sensory) conduction velocity
- distal motor latency

- sensory action potentials
- muscle action potentials.

These measurements differentiate between axonal and demyelinating damage and also determine whether the process is focal or diffuse.

Cerebral-evoked potentials

Visual-evoked potentials record the time for a visual stimulus to reach the occipital cortex. Their value is

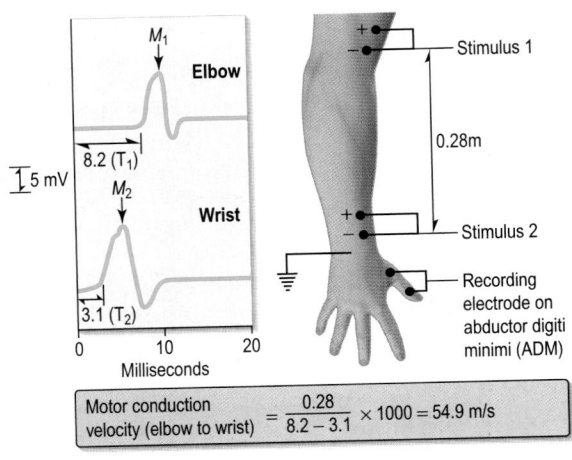

M_1

Elbow

8.2 (T_1)

5 mV

M_2

Wrist

3.1 (T_2)

0   10   20
Milliseconds

Stimulus 1

0.28m

Stimulus 2

Recording electrode on abductor digiti minimi (ADM)

Motor conduction velocity (elbow to wrist)	$= \dfrac{0.28}{8.2 - 3.1} \times 1000 = 54.9$ m/s

Fig. 21.16 Measurement of mean (motor) conduction velocity (MCV) in the ulnar nerve. A recording electrode on the abductor digiti minimi records the muscle action potential (M) from the ulnar nerve at the elbow (Stimulus 1) and at the wrist (Stimulus 2). From these values the motor conduction velocity can be calculated:

M_1 = muscle action potential (MAP) from Stimulus 1
M_2 = MAP from Stimulus 2
T_1 = time from elbow to recording electrode
T_2 = time from wrist to recording electrode

$$MCV = \frac{\text{distance in metres}}{T_1 - T_2} \times 1000 = \text{metres/second.}$$

chiefly to confirm previous retrobulbar neuritis (p. 1181), which leaves a permanently delayed latency despite clinical recovery.

Similar techniques exist for auditory and somatosensory potentials (from a limb) and are also used to monitor brain and cord during neurosurgery.

Examination of the cerebrospinal fluid (CSF) (Table 21.19 and Practical box 21.3)

Indications for lumbar puncture (LP) are:

- diagnosis of meningitis and encephalitis
- diagnosis of subarachnoid haemorrhage (sometimes)
- measurement of CSF pressure, e.g. idiopathic intracranial hypertension (p. 1246)
- removal of CSF therapeutically, e.g. idiopathic intracranial hypertension
- diagnosis of miscellaneous conditions, e.g. MS, neurosyphilis, sarcoidosis, Behçet's disease, neoplastic involvement, polyneuropathies
- intrathecal injection of contrast media and drugs.

Meticulous attention should focus on microbiology in suspected CNS infection. Close liaison between clinician and microbiologist is essential. Specific techniques (e.g. polymerase chain reaction to identify bacteria) can be invaluable. Repeated CSF examination is often necessary

Table 21.19	The normal CSF
Appearance	Crystal clear, colourless
Pressure	60–150 mm of H_2O with patient recumbent
Cell count	< 5/mm^3
	No polymorphs
	Mononuclear cells only
Protein	0.2–0.4 g/L
Glucose	$^2/_3$ to $^1/_2$ of blood glucose
IgG	< 15% of total CSF protein
Oligoclonal bands	Absent

in chronic infections, such as TB. Headache, worse on standing is a common complaint for several days (or more) following LP. Prolonged post-LP headaches can be treated by an autologous intrathecal 'blood patch' – injection of 20 mL of the patient's venous blood.

FURTHER READING

Serpell MG, Rawal N (2000) Headaches after diagnostic dural punctures. *British Medical Journal* **321**: 973–974.

Biopsy

Interpretation of brain, muscle and nerve histology requires a specialist neuropathology service.

Practical Box 21.3
Lumbar puncture

Lumbar puncture should *not* be performed in the presence of raised intracranial pressure or when an intracranial mass lesion is a possibility. The procedure should be explained carefully to the patient, and consent obtained.

Technique

- The patient is placed on the edge of the bed in the left lateral position with the knees and chin as close together as possible.
- The third and fourth lumbar spines are marked. The fourth lumbar spine usually lies on a line joining the iliac crests.
- Using sterile precautions, 2% lidocaine (lignocaine) is injected into the dermis by raising a bleb in either the third or fourth lumbar interspace.
- The special lumbar puncture needle is pushed through the skin in the midline. It is pressed steadily forwards and slightly towards the head, with the head and spine bolstered horizontally with pillows.
- When the needle is felt to penetrate the dura mater, the stylet is withdrawn and a few drops of CSF are allowed to escape.
- The CSF pressure can now be measured by connecting a manometer to the needle. The patient's head must be on the same level as the sacrum. Normal CSF pressure is 60–150 mmH$_2$O. It rises and falls with respiration and the heart beat, and rises on coughing.
- Specimens of CSF are collected in three sterilized test-tubes and sent to the laboratory. An additional sample in which the sugar level can be measured, together

with a simultaneous blood sample for blood sugar measurement, should be taken when relevant (e.g. in meningitis).
- Record the naked-eye appearance of the CSF: clear, cloudy, yellow (xanthochromic), red.
- Patients are usually asked to lie flat after the procedure to avoid a subsequent headache, but this manoeuvre is probably of little value.
- Analgesics may be required for post-LP headaches.

Contraindications for lumbar puncture

- Suspicion of a mass lesion in the brain or spinal cord. Caudal herniation of the cerebellar tonsils ('coning') may occur if an intracranial mass is present and the pressure below is reduced by removal of CSF.
- Any cause of raised intracranial pressure.
- Local infection near the site of puncture.
- Congenital lesions in the lumbosacral region (e.g. meningomyelocele).
- Platelet count below 40×10^9/L and other clotting abnormalities, including anticoagulant drugs.
- Unconscious patients and those with papilloedema must have a CT scan before lumbar puncture.

Notes

- These contraindications are relative. There are circumstances when lumbar puncture is carried out in spite of them.
- The composition of the normal CSF is shown in Table 21.19.

Brain

Brain biopsy (e.g. of a non-dominant frontal lobe) is sometimes used to diagnose inflammatory and degenerative brain diseases. CT- and MR-guided stereotactic biopsy of intracranial mass lesions are now standard procedures.

Muscle

Biopsy, with light microscopy, electron microscopy and biochemical analysis where appropriate, elucidates diagnosis of inflammatory, metabolic and dystrophic disorders of muscle (p. 1267).

Peripheral nerve

Biopsy, usually of one sural nerve (ankle) or superficial branch of a radial nerve aids diagnosis in polyneuropathies (e.g. vasculitis).

Psychometric assessment

Psychometric testing is valuable for measuring cognitive function. Preservation of verbal IQ (a measure of past attainments) in the presence of deterioration of performance IQ (a measure of present abilities) is an indicator of decline of cognitive function, for example following brain injury or in dementia. Low subtest scores (e.g. for block design, various aspects of memory, visual, speech and constructional skills) indicate impaired function of specific brain regions.

The main limitation is that depression and lack of attention also reduce scores. Also, opinions sometimes vary greatly between clinical psychologists about interpretation of agreed numerical values of tests, particularly after brain injury – thus limiting the clinical value of the tests.

Routine tests

See Table 21.20.

Specialized tests in specific diseases

Certain tests are employed in the diagnosis of individual (and often rare) neurological diseases. Examples are:

- anticardiolipin and lupus anticoagulant antibody and detailed clotting studies in stroke (p. 534)
- antibody to acetylcholine receptor protein in myasthenia gravis (p. 1269)
- serum copper and caeruloplasmin in Wilson's disease (p. 387)
- blood lactate studies (failure to rise on exercise) in McArdle's syndrome (p. 1144)
- serum phytanic acid (elevated) in Refsum's disease (p. 1262)
- serum long-chain fatty acid (present) in adrenoleucodystrophy (p. 1235)
- genetic studies – e.g. Huntington's disease, hereditary sensorimotor neuropathies (p. 1263).

Table 21.20 Value of routine investigations in neurology

Test	Yield	Condition
Urinalysis	Glycosuria	Polyneuropathy
	Ketones	Coma
	Bence Jones protein	Cord compression
Blood picture	↑ MCV	B_{12} deficiency
	↑ ESR	Giant cell arteritis
Blood glucose	Hypoglycaemia	Coma
	Hyperglycaemia	Coma
Serum electrolytes	Hyponatraemia	Coma
	Hypokalaemia	Weakness
Serum calcium	Hypocalcaemia	Tetany, spasms
Serum creatine phosphokinase	Raised	Muscle disease
Chest X-ray	Lytic bone or mass lesion	Bronchial cancer, thymoma

FURTHER READING

Blau N et al. (eds) (2003) *Physician's Guide to Laboratory Diagnosis of Metabolic Diseases*. Berlin: Springer.

UNCONSCIOUSNESS AND COMA

The central ascending reticular formation (or reticular activating substance), extending from lower brainstem to thalamus, influences the state of arousal. Our state of consciousness is the product of complex interactions between parts of the reticular formation itself, cortex and brainstem, and all sensory stimuli.

Disturbed consciousness: definitions

Each term simply describes a *recognizable* state, either normal or pathological.

- **Consciousness** means a state of wakefulness with awareness of self and surroundings.
- **Clouding of consciousness** – used more in psychiatry than neurology – means reduced wakefulness and/or self-awareness, sometimes with confusion.
- **Confusion** means altered consciousness – the subject is bewildered and misinterprets his/her surroundings.
- **Delirium** is a state of high arousal (typically *delirium tremens*, p. 1309). There is confusion and often visual hallucination.
- **Sleep** is *normal* mental and physical inactivity from which the subject can be roused.
- **Stupor** is an *abnormal*, sleepy state from which the subject can be aroused by vigorously or repeated stimuli – also used for various psychiatric states, e.g. catatonic and depressive stupor (p. 1307).
- **Coma** means unrousable unresponsiveness. The Glasgow Coma Scale for head injury is shown in Table 21.21.

Table 21.21	Glasgow Coma Scale			
	Score			**Score**
Eye opening (E)		**Verbal response (V)**		
Spontaneous	4	Orientated		5
To speech	3	Confused conversation		4
To pain	2	Inappropriate words		3
No response	1	Incomprehensible sounds		2
		No response		1
Motor response (M)				
Obeys	6			
Localizes	5			
Withdraws	4			
Flexion	3			
Extension	2			
No response	1			

Glasgow Coma Scale = E + M + V
(GCS minimum = 3: maximum = 15)

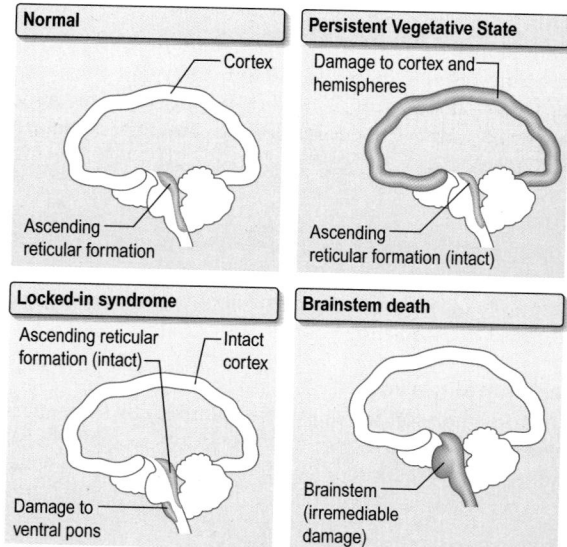

Fig. 21.17 **Basic anatomy of altered consciousness.** Adapted from Bates D Coma and brainstem death *Medicine* 2000; **28:7:** 65–70 with kind permission of the Medicine Publishing Company.

Mechanisms of coma

Altered consciousness is produced by three mechanisms affecting brainstem, reticular formation and cerebral cortex.

- *Diffuse brain dysfunction.* Generalized severe metabolic or toxic disorders (e.g. alcohol abuse, sedative drugs, uraemia and septicaemia) depress/inhibit overall brain function.
- *Direct effect within the brainstem.* A lesion within the brainstem itself damages/inhibits the reticular activating system.
- *Pressure effect on the brainstem.* A mass lesion within the brain compresses the brainstem, inhibiting the ascending reticular activating system.

A single focal hemisphere (or cerebellar) lesion does not produce coma unless it compresses or damages the brainstem. Oedema frequently surrounds masses, contributing to their effects.

Other states of unresponsiveness must be distinguished from coma; this sometimes causes difficulty. The features of these are shown in Table 21.22 and illustrated in Figure 21.17.

Differential diagnosis of the vegetative state

- *Vegetative state* (VS) is a sequel of, for example, widespread cortical damage after head injury. Brainstem function is normal. VS implies loss of sentient behaviour. The patient perceives little or nothing but lies apparently awake, breathing spontaneously.
- *Minimally conscious state* (MCS) describes patients with *some* sentient behaviour, e.g. apparent, vague, pain perception. A patient may emerge from VS into MCS.
- *Locked-in syndrome* is a state of unresponsiveness due to massive brainstem damage below the level of the third nerve nuclei. The patient has a functioning cerebral cortex and is thus unlike a PVS patient, *fully*

aware but cannot move or communicate except by vertical eye movement.
- *Brainstem death* is discussed on page 989.

Distinction between these states is essential before addressing major issues of prognosis, quality of life, and cessation of supportive care.

Unresponsiveness of psychological origin is also a cause of apparent coma.

Causes

Principal causes of coma and stupor are in Table 21.23. A common cause of coma in the UK is self-poisoning. World-wide, cerebral malaria is a frequent cause of coma.

THE UNCONSCIOUS PATIENT

Immediate assessment

Actions that take seconds save lives (Table 21.24).

Get a history from witnesses, paramedics or police. Many people on corticosteroids, with diabetes, epilepsy or hypoadrenalism, carry identification.

Further examination

- Record depth of coma (Table 21.21).
- Full general and neurological examination.

General examination

Many clues point to the cause.

Temperature

Body temperature is raised in infection and hyperpyrexia, and subnormal in hypothermia.

Table 21.22 Differential diagnosis of the vegetative state

Condition	Vegetative state	Minimally conscious state	Locked-in syndrome	Coma	Death confirmed by brainstem tests
Awareness	Absent	Present	Present	Absent	Absent
Sleep–wake cycle	Present	Present	Present	Absent	Absent
Response to noxious stimuli	±	Present	Present (in eyes only)	±	Absent
Glasgow Coma Scale score	E4, M1–4, V1–2	E4, M1–5, V1–4	E4, M1, V1	E1–2, M1–4, V1–2	E1, M1–3, V1
Motor function	No purposeful movement	Some consistent or inconsistent verbal or purposeful motor behaviour	Volitional vertical eye movements or eyeblink preserved	No purposeful movement	None or only reflex spinal movement
Respiratory function	Typically preserved	Typically preserved	Typically preserved	Variable	Absent
EEG activity	Typically slow wave activity	Insufficient data	Typically normal	Typically slow wave activity	Typically absent
Cerebral metabolism (PET)	Severely reduced	Insufficient data	Mildly reduced	Moderately to severely reduced	Severely reduced or absent
Prognosis	Variable: if permanent, continued vegetative state or death	Variable	Depends on cause but full recovery unlikely	Recovery, vegetative state, or death within weeks	Already dead

NB: EEG and measures of cerebral metabolism are not *required* to make these clinical diagnoses
EEG, electroencephalography; PET, positron emission tomography.
From: The vegetative state: guidance on diagnosis and management. *Clinical Medicine* 2003 **3**: 251, with permission from Elsevier.

Table 21.23 Examples of mechanisms of principal causes of coma

Diffuse brain dysfunction
Drug overdose, alcohol abuse
CO poisoning, anaesthetic gases
Hypoglycaemia, hyperglycaemia
Hypoxic/ischaemic brain injury
Hypertensive encephalopathy (p. 859)
Severe uraemia (p. 699)
Hepatocellular failure (p. 368)
Respiratory failure with CO_2 retention (p. 902)
Hypercalcaemia, hypocalcaemia
Hypoadrenalism, hypopituitarism and hypothyroidism (Ch. 18)
Hyponatraemia, hypernatraemia
Metabolic acidosis
Hypothermia, hyperpyrexia
Trauma (following closed head injury)
Epilepsy (following a generalized seizure)
Encephalitis, cerebral malaria, septicaemia
Subarachnoid haemorrhage
Metabolic rarities (e.g. porphyria)
Cerebral oedema from chronic hypoxia (p. 980)
Direct effect within brainstem
Brainstem haemorrhage or infarction
Brainstem neoplasm (e.g. glioma)
Brainstem demyelination
Wernicke–Korsakoff syndrome
Trauma
Pressure effect on brainstem
Hemisphere tumour, infarction, abscess, haematoma, encephalitis or trauma
Cerebellar mass lesions

Table 21.24 The unconscious patient: immediate actions

Examine	Findings	Potential action
Airway	Clear?	Maintain; intubate?
Pulse	Absent?	Cardiopulmonary resuscitation
Pupils	Fixed, dilated?	
Head	Trauma	Observe and investigate
Spinal	Trauma	Immobilize

Skin and skull
Look for cyanosis, jaundice, purpura, rashes, pigmentation, injection marks, trauma. Skin is coarse and dry in hypothyroidism.

Breath
Sniff – for ketones, alcohol, hepatic and uraemic fetor.

Respiration
Depressed but regular respiration occurs in many states of stupor and light coma. As coma deepens, and in normal deep sleep, respiration becomes irregular. *Patterns* of abnormal respiration are of importance:

- *Cheyne–Stokes (periodic) respiration* is alternating hyperpnoea and apnoea. In brain disease this points to bilateral cerebral dysfunction, usually deep in the hemispheres or in the upper brainstem. This pattern, a sign of incipient coning – also occurs slightly in some normal people during sleep, in metabolic comas, with CO_2 retention, and chronic hypoxia at high altitude.

- *Kussmaul* (*acidotic*) *respiration* is deep, sighing hyperventilation seen in diabetic ketoacidosis and uraemia.
- *Central neurogenic* (*pontine*) *hyperventilation* describes sustained, rapid, deep breathing seen with pontine lesions. It may switch abruptly on and off.
- *Ataxic respiration* is shallow, halting, irregular respiration. It frequently precedes death. The medullary respiratory centre is damaged.
- *Vomiting, hiccup and excessive yawning* sometimes indicate a lower brainstem lesion in stupor.

Neurological examination in coma

Head, neck and spine
Note trauma, skull burr-holes and bruits, neck stiffness.

Pupils
Record size and reaction to light.

- *Dilatation of one pupil* that becomes fixed to light, indicates compression of the third nerve as the temporal lobe uncus herniates (coning). This is a neurosurgical emergency (e.g. an extradural haematoma).
- *Horner's syndrome* (ipsilateral pupillary constriction and ptosis, p. 1183) occurs with hypothalamic damage and also, rarely, in coning.
- *Bilateral mid-point reactive pupils* (i.e. normal pupils) are characteristic of metabolic comas and following most CNS-depressant drugs except opiates.
- *Bilateral light-fixed, dilated pupils* are a cardinal sign of brainstem death. They also occur in deep coma of any cause, but particularly in coma due to barbiturate intoxication or hypothermia.
- *Bilateral pinpoint*, light-fixed pupils occur with pontine lesions (e.g. a pontine haemorrhage) that interrupt sympathetic pathways, and with opiate drugs.
- *Bilateral mid-position light-fixed or slightly dilated light-fixed pupils* (4–6 mm), which are sometimes irregular, are seen when brainstem damage interrupts the light reflex.

Mydriatic drugs can confuse diagnosis (see also p. 1004). Previous pupillary surgery can also cause diagnostic difficulty.

Fundi
Look for papilloedema and retinal haemorrhage.

Ocular movements
The ocular axes are usually slightly divergent in coma. In light coma, slow, roving, side-to-side eye movements are seen.

Vestibulo-ocular reflexes. Passive head turning produces conjugate ocular deviation away from the direction of rotation (doll's head reflex). This reflex disappears in very deep coma and is absent in brainstem lesions, and thus in brainstem death. Its real value in coma is somewhat limited.

Calorics. Slow tonic ocular deviation towards the irrigated ear is seen when ice-cold water is run into the external auditory meatus – the caloric or vestibulo-ocular reflex. This indicates an intact brainstem. The test is used in the diagnosis of brainstem death (p. 989).

Abnormalities of conjugate gaze (p. 1183):
- *Sustained conjugate lateral deviation* occurs towards a destructive frontal lesion ('eyes look towards normal limbs'). Rarely, an irritative lesion in one frontal lobe (e.g. an epileptic focus from a glioma) 'drives the eyes away', so conjugate deviation is away from that side. In a pontine, brainstem lesion, when one paramedian pontine reticular formulation (PPRF) itself is damaged (p. 1184), sustained conjugate lateral deviation occurs away from the lesion, towards the paralysed limbs, because the opposite PPRF is active.
- *Skew deviation* (one eye deviated up and the other down) indicates a brainstem or cerebellar lesion.
- *Ocular bobbing* describes sudden, brisk, downward-diving eye movements seen in pontine (or cerebellar) haemorrhage.

Other spontaneous eye movements (other than roving eye movements) are distinctly unusual in true coma.

Lateralizing signs. Coma makes it difficult to recognize focal signs. The following are helpful:

- *Response to visual threat* in a stuporose patient. Asymmetry suggests hemianopia.
- *Facial appearance.* Drooping of one side, unilateral dribbling, or blowing in and out of the paralysed cheek.
- *Tone.* Unilateral flaccidity or spasticity may be the only sign of hemiparesis.
- *Asymmetrical response to painful stimuli.*
- *Asymmetry of plantar responses.* Both are often extensor in deep coma of any cause.
- *Asymmetry of tendon reflexes.*
- *Asymmetry of decerebrate and decorticate posturing.*

Investigations
Often, the cause for coma becomes evident (e.g. head injury, cerebral haemorrhage, self-poisoning). If the explanation remains unclear, further investigations are needed.

Blood and urine
- *Drugs screen* (e.g. salicylates, diazepam, narcotics, amfetamines)
- *Routine biochemistry* (urea, electrolytes, glucose, calcium, liver biochemistry)
- *Metabolic and endocrine studies* (TSH, serum cortisol)
- *Blood cultures*
- *Rarities*, such as cerebral malaria (thick blood film) or porphyria, are often forgotten.

Imaging
CT or MR brain imaging may indicate an otherwise unsuspected mass lesion or intracranial haemorrhage.

CSF examination

Lumbar puncture should be performed in coma only after careful risk assessment. It is usually contraindicated when an intracranial mass lesion is a possibility. CT is necessary to exclude this. CSF examination is likely to alter therapy only if undiagnosed meningoencephalitis or other identifiable infection is present.

Electroencephalography

EEG is of some value in the diagnosis of metabolic coma and encephalitis.

Management

Comatose or stuporose patients – be they at home or outside, on an A&E trolley, in a general ward, or ITU – need immediate careful nursing, meticulous attention to the airway, and frequent monitoring of vital functions.

Longer-term requirements are:

- skin care – turning, removal of jewellery, avoidance of pressure sores and pressure palsies
- oral hygiene – mouth washes, suction
- eye care – taping of lids, prevention of corneal damage, irrigation
- fluids – intragastric or i.v. fluids
- calories – liquid diet through a fine intragastric tube, 1255 kJ (3000 kcal) daily
- sphincters – catheterization only when essential (Paul's tubing if possible); avoid constipation (evacuate rectum).

> **FURTHER READING**
> Royal College of Physician's Working Party Report (2003) The vegetative state: guidance on diagnosis and management. *Clinical Medicine* 3: 249–254.

CEREBROVASCULAR DISEASE AND STROKE

Stroke is the third commonest cause of death in developed countries. The age-adjusted annual death rate from strokes is 116 per 100 000 population in the USA and some 200 per 100 000 in the UK, some 12% of all deaths. It is higher in black African populations than in Caucasian. Stroke is uncommon below the age of 40 and is more common in males. Death rate following stroke is around 25%. Hypertension is the most treatable risk factor. Stroke is decreasing in the 40–60 age range as hypertension is treated. In the elderly, it remains a major cause of morbidity and mortality. Thromboembolic infarction (80%), cerebral and cerebellar haemorrhage (10%) and subarachnoid haemorrhage (about 5%) are the major cerebrovascular problems.

Definitions

These, though valuable clinically, are arbitrary:

- **Stroke**. To the public, stroke means weakness, either permanent or transient on one side, often with loss of

speech. Stroke is *defined* as the clinical syndrome of rapid onset of cerebral deficit (usually focal) lasting more than 24 hours or leading to death, with no apparent cause other than a vascular one. Hemiplegia following middle cerebral arterial thromboembolism is the typical example.

- **Completed stroke** means the deficit has become maximal, usually within 6 hours.
- **Stroke-in-evolution** describes progression during the first 24 hours.
- **Minor stroke**. Patients recover without significant deficit, usually within a week.
- **Transient ischaemic attack (TIA)**. This means a focal deficit, such as a weak limb, aphasia or loss of vision lasting from a few seconds to 24 hours. There is *complete* recovery. The attack is usually sudden. TIAs have a tendency to recur, and may herald thromboembolic stroke.

That vague term 'cerebrovascular accident' should be avoided.

Pathophysiology

Different pathological processes may cause similar clinical events in cerebrovascular disease.

Completed stroke

One of three mechanisms is usual:

- arterial embolism from a distant site (usually the carotid, vertebral or basilar arteries) and subsequent brain infarction
- arterial thrombosis causing occlusion in atheromatous carotid, vertebral or cerebral artery with subsequent brain infarction
- haemorrhage into the brain (intracerebral or subarachnoid).

Less commonly, other processes cause stroke, or look like a common stroke:

- venous infarction
- carotid or vertebral artery dissection
- polycythaemia (hyperviscosity syndromes)
- fat and air embolism (see diving, p. 1028)
- multiple sclerosis – a demyelinating plaque
- mass lesions (e.g. brain tumour, abscess, subdural haematoma)
- rarities: arteritis, neurosyphilis, systemic lupus erythematosus, mitochondrial disease.

Transient ischaemic attack (TIA) (p. 1211)

TIAs are *usually* the result of microemboli, but as in stroke different mechanisms produce similar clinical events. For example, TIAs may be caused by a fall in cerebral perfusion (e.g. a cardiac dysrhythmia, postural hypotension or decreased flow through atheromatous carotid and vertebral arteries). Infarction is usually averted by autoregulation (p. 1211). Small areas of brain infarction following thrombosis or haemorrhage may occasionally cause a clinical TIA. Rarely, brain tumours and subdural

Table 21.25 Reducing stroke risk

Risk factor	Intervention	Reduction in stroke risk		
		Cerebral infarction	Cerebral haemorrhage	Subarachnoid haemorrhage
Hypertension	Treat	++	++	Possible
Smoking	Stop	++	+	Probable
Lifestyle	More active	+	0	0
Alcohol	Moderate intake	+	0	0
Hypercholesterolaemia	Statin therapy	+	0	0
Raised haematocrit	Reduce	+	0	0
Atrial fibrillation	Anticoagulate	+	(Possibly increased risk)	0
Sleep apnoea	Treat	+	0	0
Obesity	Weight reduction	Probable	Probable	0
Diabetes	Good control	Probable	0	0
Carotid artery stenosis	Surgery	++	0	0

++, major correlation with reduced risk; +, moderate correlation with reduced risk

haematomas cause episodes indistinguishable from thromboembolic TIAs. A clinical TIA is thus not an entirely reliable indicator of thromboembolism. Principal sources of emboli to the brain are cardiac thrombi and atheromatous plaques/thrombi within the great vessels, and carotid and vertebral systems. Cardiac thrombi (mural and valvular) follow atrial fibrillation, itself often secondary to valvular disease, or myocardial infarction. A total high red cell volume (e.g. polycythaemia) is also a cause.

Thromboembolism from sources outside the brain generates 70% of all strokes and 80% of TIAs.

Risk factors and prevention

The principal accepted risk factors and effects of altering them are shown in Table 21.25.

The following measures reduce stroke incidence:

- treatment of hypertension (of vital importance)
- cessation of smoking; 50% reduction within 1 year reaching normal risk after 5 years
- active lifestyle (recommend 30–60 min exercise, four to six times per week)
- moderate alcohol consumption
- statin therapy (p. 1141) reduces cerebrovascular disease by up to a third even in people with a low cholesterol level (see Table 19.17)
- anticoagulation in atrial fibrillation
- weight reduction in obesity (see Table 5.14)
- treating polycythaemia.
- surgery for carotid stenosis (see p. 1215).

Low-dose aspirin in symptomless populations and postmenopausal HRT has shown no protective effect.

Cerebral and cerebellar haemorrhage
Hypertension, bleeding disorders, pre-existing cerebral aneurysm, anticoagulant and antiplatelet drug therapy are risk factors.

Rarer risk factors and other causes of stroke
- Thrombocythaemia and thrombophilia (protein C deficiency, factor V Leiden) are weakly associated with arterial stroke but predispose to cerebral venous thrombosis.
- Polycythaemia predisposes to stroke.
- Anticardiolipin and lupus anticoagulant antibodies (i.e. antiphospholipid syndrome p. 577) causes arterial thrombotic stroke in young patients.
- Endocarditis (p. 828) – thromboembolic stroke may be the presenting feature.
- Low-dose oestrogen-containing oral contraceptives do not increase stroke risk significantly in healthy women but probably do so with other risk factors, e.g. uncontrolled hypertension or smoking.
- Migraine is a rare cause of cerebral infarction (p. 1247).
- Vasculitis (SLE, polyarteritis nodosa, giant cell arteritis, granulomatous CNS angiitis) is a rare cause of stroke.
- Amyloidosis can present as recurrent cerebral haemorrhage (p. 1147).
- Hyperhomocysteinaemia predisposes to thrombotic strokes. Folic acid therapy does not reduce the incidence.
- Drugs – illicit drugs, e.g. cocaine and over-the-counter 'cold' remedies containing vasoconstrictors. Chronic use of COX II inhibitors is associated with an increased incidence of stroke (p. 550).

CADASIL (cerebral dominant arteriopathy with subcortical infarcts and leucoencephalopathy) is a rare inherited cause of stroke/vascular dementia. There is a defect in the NOTCH3 gene on chromosome 19. Characteristic damage to small brain arterioles follows with multiple infarcts. Familial migraine and depression in youth occur, progressing to TIA and stroke in the third and fourth decades, and to dementia in the sixth.

Vascular anatomy (Figs 21.18–21.20)

Knowledge of normal arterial anatomy and likely sites of atheromatous plaques and stenoses helps understanding of the main syndromes.

The circle of Willis is supplied by the two internal carotid arteries and by the basilar. The distribution of the

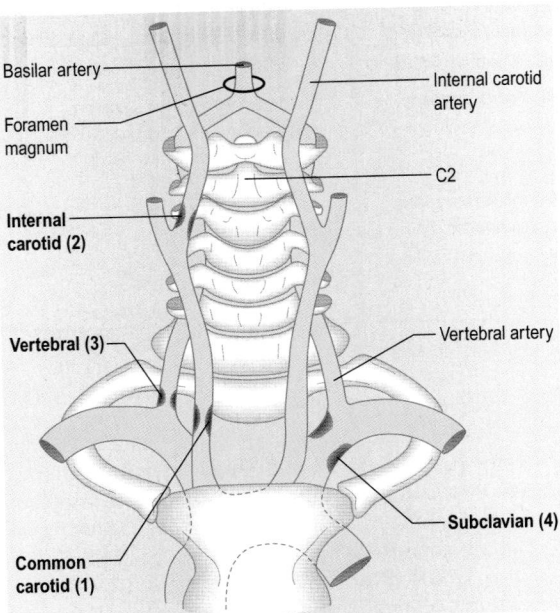

Principal arteries

Anterior cerebral
Middle cerebral
Posterior communicating
Posterior cerebral
Internal carotid
Basilar
Vertebral
Anterior spinal

Circle of Willis

Important smaller arteries

Anterior communicating
Medial striate
Superior cerebellar
Pontine
Labyrinthine
Anterior inferior cerebellar
Posterior inferior cerebellar

Fig. 21.18 Diagram of arteries supplying the brain.

Basilar artery
Foramen magnum
Internal carotid (2)
Vertebral (3)
Common carotid (1)
Internal carotid artery
C2
Vertebral artery
Subclavian (4)

Fig. 21.20 Principal sites of atheromatous stenoses in extracerebral arteries: common carotid (1); internal carotid (2); vertebral (3); subclavian (4).

(a) Medial view of right hemisphere

Anterior cerebral artery
Posterior cerebral artery
Middle cerebral artery branch to macular cortex

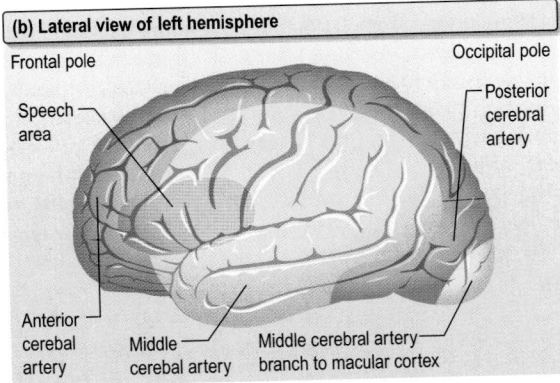

(b) Lateral view of left hemisphere

Frontal pole
Occipital pole
Speech area
Posterior cerebral artery
Anterior cerebral artery
Middle cerebral artery
Middle cerebral artery branch to macular cortex

Fig. 21.19 Distribution of the three major cerebral arteries.

- carotid artery syphon – within the cavernous sinus
- origins of vertebral arteries (3)
- subclavian vessels (4).

Autoregulation

Smooth muscle of small intracerebral arteries responds directly to changes in pressure gradient. In the normal situation, constant cerebral blood flow (CBF) is maintained by mean arterial blood pressures between 60 and 120 mmHg, i.e. CBF is independent of perfusion pressure.

In disease, CBF autoregulation may fail. Contributory causes are:

- severe hypotension with systolic BP < 75 mmHg
- severe hypertension with systolic BP > 180 mmHg
- increase in blood viscosity, e.g. polycythaemia
- raised intracranial pressure
- increase in arterial $P\text{CO}_2$ and/or fall in arterial $P\text{O}_2$.

TRANSIENT ISCHAEMIC ATTACKS

Symptoms

TIAs cause sudden loss of function, usually within seconds, and last for minutes or hours (but by definition < 24 hours). The site is often suggested by the type of attack.

Features

Clinical features of principal forms of TIA are given in Table 21.26. Hemiparesis and aphasia are the commonest but two other events are mentioned briefly here.

anterior, middle and posterior cerebral arteries that supply the cerebrum is shown in Figure 21.19.

Stenoses and plaques proximal to the circle of Willis are common at five sites (positions 1–4 are shown in Fig. 21.20):

- origins of common carotid arteries (1)
- origins of internal carotid arteries (2)

Table 21.26 Features of transient ischaemic attacks

Anterior circulation	Posterior circulation
Carotid system	*Vertebrobasilar system*
Amaurosis fugax	Diplopia, vertigo, vomiting
Aphasia	Choking and dysarthria
Hemiparesis	Ataxia
Hemisensory loss	Hemisensory loss
Hemianopic visual loss	Hemianopic visual loss
	Transient global amnesia
	Tetraparesis
	Loss of consciousness (rare)

Amaurosis fugax

This is a sudden transient loss of vision in one eye. When due to the passage of emboli through the retinal arteries, arterial obstruction is sometimes visible through an ophthalmoscope during an attack. A TIA causing an episode of amaurosis fugax is often the first clinical evidence of internal carotid artery stenosis – and forerunner of a hemiparesis. Amaurosis fugax also occurs as a benign event in migraine.

Transient global amnesia

Episodes of amnesia lasting several hours, occurring principally in people over 65, and followed by complete recovery are presumed to be caused by posterior circulation ischaemia. The exact pathology of this striking but unusual event is unknown. Episodes rarely recur.

Clinical findings in TIA

Diagnosis of TIA is often based solely upon its description. It is unusual to witness an attack. Consciousness is usually preserved in TIA.

There may be clinical evidence of a source of embolus, such as:

- carotid arterial bruit (stenosis)
- atrial fibrillation or other dysrhythmia
- valvular heart disease/endocarditis
- recent myocardial infarction
- difference between right and left brachial BP.

An underlying condition may be evident:

- atheroma
- hypertension
- postural hypotension
- bradycardia or low cardiac output
- diabetes mellitus
- rarely, arteritis, polycythaemia
- antiphospholipid syndrome (p. 577).

Differential diagnosis

TIAs must be distinguished, usually on clinical grounds, from other transient episodes (p. 1226). Occasionally, events identical to TIAs are produced by mass lesions. Focal epilepsy is usually distinguishable by its 'positive' features (e.g. limb jerking) and characteristic progression over minutes. In a TIA, deficit is usually apparent imme-

diately. However, involuntary limb movements do occur occasionally in TIAs.

A focal prodrome in migraine sometimes causes diagnostic confusion. Headache, common but not invariable in migraine, is rare in TIA. Migrainous visual disturbances are not seen in TIA.

Prognosis

Prospective studies show that 5 years after a single thromboembolic TIA:

- 30% have had a stroke, a third in the first year
- 15% have suffered a myocardial infarct.

TIA in the anterior cerebral circulation carries a more serious prognosis than one in the posterior circulation.

TIA: investigations and management

These are discussed with stroke on page 1215.

TYPICAL STROKE SYNDROMES

Cerebral infarction

Major thromboembolic cerebral infarction usually causes an obvious stroke. Some small infarcts may cause TIAs, while others are silent. The clinical picture is thus very variable and depends on the infarct site and extent. Whilst the general site of damage may be deduced from physical signs (e.g. cortex, internal capsule, brainstem), clinical estimation of the precise vascular territory is often inaccurate.

Clinical features

The most common stroke is caused by infarction in the internal capsule following thromboembolism in a middle cerebral artery branch. A similar picture is caused by internal carotid occlusion (Fig. 21.20). Limb weakness on the opposite side to the infarct develops over seconds, minutes or hours (occasionally longer). There is a contralateral hemiplegia or hemiparesis with facial weakness. Aphasia is usual when the dominant hemisphere is affected. Weak limbs are at first flaccid and areflexic. Headache is unusual. Consciousness is usually preserved. Exceptionally, an epileptic seizure occurs at the onset.

After a variable interval, usually several days, reflexes return, becoming exaggerated. An extensor plantar response appears. Weakness is maximal at first; recovery occurs gradually over days, weeks or many months.

Carotid and vertebral artery dissection

Dissection accounts for under one-fifth of strokes below age 40 and is sometimes a sequel of head or neck trauma. Stroke, TIA or migraine-like symptoms occur, often with neck pain at the site of dissection.

Brainstem infarction

This causes complex signs depending on the relationship of the infarct to cranial nerve nuclei, long tracts and brainstem connections (Table 21.27).

Table 21.27 **Features of brainstem infarction**

Clinical feature	Structure involved
Hemiparesis or tetraparesis	Corticospinal tracts
Sensory loss	Medial lemniscus and spinothalamic tracts
Diplopia	Oculomotor system
Facial numbness	Fifth nerve nuclei
Facial weakness (lower motor neurone)	Seventh nerve nucleus
Nystagmus, vertigo	Vestibular connections
Dysphagia, dysarthria	Ninth and tenth nerve nuclei
Dysarthria, ataxia, hiccups, vomiting	Brainstem and cerebellar connections
Horner's syndrome	Sympathetic fibres
Altered consciousness	Reticular formation

- *The lateral medullary syndrome*, also called posterior inferior cerebellar artery (PICA) thrombosis, or Wallenberg's syndrome, is a common example of brainstem infarction presenting as acute vertigo with cerebellar and other signs (Table 21.28 and Fig. 21.21). It follows thrombo-embolism in the PICA or its branches, vertebral artery thrombo-embolism or dissection. The clinical picture depends on the precise structure damaged.
- *Coma* follows damage to the brainstem reticular activating system.
- *The locked-in syndrome* is caused by upper brainstem infarction (p. 1207).
- *Pseudobulbar palsy* (p. 1191) is caused by lower brainstem infarction.

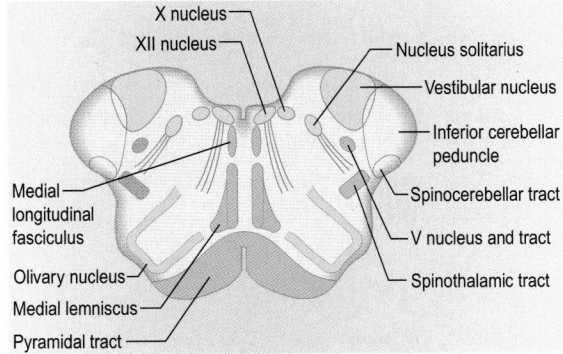

Fig. 21.21 **Cross-section of medulla: structures at risk after brain-stem infarction.**

Table 21.28 **Clinical signs in the lateral medullary syndrome (PICA thrombosis)**

Ipsilateral	Contralateral
Facial numbness (Vth)	Spinothalamic sensory loss
Diplopia (VIth)	Hemiparesis (mild, unusual)
Nystagmus	
Ataxia (cerebellar)	
Horner's syndrome	
IXth and Xth nerve lesions	

Other patterns of infarction

Lacunar infarction

Lacunes are small ($< 1.5 \text{cm}^3$) infarcts seen on MRI or at autopsy. Hypertension is commonly present. Minor strokes (e.g. pure motor stroke, pure sensory stroke, sudden unilateral ataxia and sudden dysarthria with a clumsy hand) are syndromes caused typically by single lacunar infarcts. Lacunar infarction is also often symptomless.

Hypertensive encephalopathy (see also p. 859)

This describes the neurological sequelae of malignant hypertension. Severe headaches, TIA, stroke, and rarely subarachnoid haemorrhage occur. Papilloedema may develop, either as part of an ischaemic optic neuropathy or following brain swelling due to multiple acute infarcts.

Multi-infarct dementia (vascular dementia)

(see also p. 1255)

Multiple lacunes or larger infarcts cause generalized intellectual loss seen with advanced cerebrovascular disease. The condition tends to occur with a stepwise progression over months or years with each subsequent infarct. There is eventually dementia, pseudobulbar palsy and a shuffling gait with small steps – the *marche à petits pas*, sometimes called atherosclerotic parkinsonism. There may be confusion clinically with idiopathic Parkinson's disease. *Binswanger's disease* is an imaging term describing low attenuation in cerebral white matter, with dementia, TIAs and stroke episodes in hypertensive patients.

Infarction in the visual cortex

Posterior cerebral artery infarction or infarction of the middle cerebral artery macular branch causes combinations of hemianopic visual loss and cortical blindness (Anton's syndrome, Fig. 21.19).

Weber's syndrome

This is ipsilateral third nerve paralysis with contralateral hemiplegia due to an infarct in one side of the midbrain. Paralysis of upward gaze is usually present.

Watershed (or borderzone) cerebral infarction

This describes the multiple cortical infarcts that follow prolonged periods of very low perfusion (e.g. from hypotension after massive myocardial infarction or cardiac bypass surgery). Borderzone infarcts occur between areas supplied by the anterior, middle and posterior cerebral arteries. Cortical visual loss, memory loss and intellectual impairment are typical. In severe cases a persistent vegetative state or minimal conscious state develops (p. 1207).

Management of cerebral infarction

The possible sources of embolus should be sought (e.g. carotid bruit, atrial fibrillation, valve lesion, evidence of endocarditis, previous emboli or TIA) and hypertension and postural hypotension assessed. The brachial blood pressure should be measured in each arm; a difference of more than 20 mmHg is suggestive of subclavian artery stenosis. The neurological deficit should be carefully documented.

Stroke: immediate care and thrombolysis
(Box 21.1)

Dedicated units with multidisciplinary, organized team care deliver a higher standard of care than a general ward, reducing stroke mortality and long-term disability. Evidence-based guidelines have contributed to management by establishing clear protocols.

After a stroke, immediate, continued and meticulous attention to the airway and to swallowing is essential. The initial decision to admit a stroke patient to hospital depends upon the clinical state and facilities available. Table 21.29 outlines the current proposals for stroke thrombolysis – unfortunately rarely carried out in the UK. Aspirin 300 mg daily should be given as soon as a diagnosis of ischaemic stroke or thromboembolic TIA is confirmed, reducing to 75 mg after several days.

Management of the unconscious patient is described on page 1209.

Investigations

The purpose of investigations in both stroke and TIA is:

- to confirm clinical diagnosis
- to distinguish between haemorrhage and thrombo-embolic infarction
- to look for underlying causes of disease and to direct therapy, either medical or surgical.

(i) Box 21.1 Stroke: immediate management issues

1. **Admit to multidisciplinary hospital stroke unit if possible.**

2. **General medical measures**
   Care of the unconscious patient (p. 1209)
   Oxygen by mask
   Assessment of swallowing
   Check BP and look for source of emboli.

3. **Is thrombolysis to be considered?**
   If so (see text and Table 21.29) immediate brain imaging is essential.

4. **Brain imaging**
   CT scans will usually be the only emergency imaging available. This will indicate whether there has been brain infarction, haemorrhage or other pathology.

5. **Cerebral infarction**
   If CT shows infarction, give aspirin (300 mg/day initially) antiplatelet therapy if no contraindications, give alteplase thrombolysis, which must be started within 3 hours (aim for 90 min) of stroke; informed consent is essential.

6. **Cerebral haemorrhage**
   If CT shows haemorrhage, do not give any therapy that may interfere with clotting. Neurosurgery may be required.

Table 21.29 Thrombolysis in acute ischaemic stroke

Eligibility
Age ≥ 18 years
Clinical diagnosis of acute ischaemic stroke
Assessed by experienced team
Measurable neurological deficit
Timing of symptom onset well established
CT or MRI and blood test results available
CT or MRI consistent with diagnosis
Treatment could begin within 180 minutes of symptom onset

Exclusion criteria
Symptoms minor or improving rapidly
Haemorrhage on pretreatment CT or MRI
Suspected subarachnoid haemorrhage
Active bleeding from any site
Gastrointestinal or urinary tract haemorrhage in last 21 days
Platelet count $< 100 \times 10^9$/litre
Recent treatment with heparin and activated partial thromboplastin time above normal
Recent treatment with warfarin and INR elevated
Major surgery or trauma in last 14 days
Recent post-myocardial infarction pericarditis
Neurosurgery, serious head trauma or stroke in last 3 months
History of intracranial haemorrhage (any time)
Known arteriovenous malformation or aneurysm
Recent arterial puncture at non-compressible site
Recent lumbar puncture
Blood pressure consistently > 185 systolic or > 110 diastolic
Abnormal blood glucose (< 3 mmol/litre or > 20 mmol/litre)
Suspected or known pregnancy
Active pancreatitis
Epileptic seizure at stroke onset

Dose of intravenous tissue plasminogen activator (alteplase)
Total dose 0.9 mg/kg (maximum 90 mg)
10% of total dose as initial intravenous bolus over 1 minute
Remainder infused intravenously over 60 minutes

Source: National Institute of Neurological Disorders and Stroke protocol; from *Medicine* (2000) **28**(7): 62

Routine investigations in thromboembolic stroke and TIA with their potential yields are listed in Box 21.2.

Imaging TIA and stroke patients
CT and MRI. CT imaging will demonstrate haemorrhage immediately (p. 1217) while a patient with an infarct may have a normal scan. Infarctions are usually detectable at 1 week (Fig. 21.22) although 50% are never detected on CT. CT or MRI should be carried out urgently in the majority of cases.

Diffusion-weighted imaging (DWI) MR can identify infarcted areas within a few minutes of onset. Conventional T2 weighting is no better than CT. Imaging will also show the unexpected, e.g. subdural haematoma, tumour or abscess.

Box 21.2 Stroke: further investigation and management

Further investigation

- Routine bloods (for polycythaemia, infection, vasculitis, thrombophilia, syphilitic serology, clotting studies, autoantibodies, lipids)
- Chest X-ray
- ECG
- Carotid Dopplers
- Angiography

Further management

- Appropriate drugs for hypertension, heart disease, diabetes, other medical conditions
- Other antiplatelet agents, e.g. dipyridamole
- Question of endarterectomy
- Question of anticoagulation – Table 21.30
- Speech therapy, dysphagia care, physiotherapy, occupational therapy
- Specific neurological issues, e.g. epilepsy, pain, incontinence
- Preparations for future care

Fig. 21.22   CT: Massive middle cerebral artery infarct.

Carotid Doppler and duplex scanning.   Ultrasound studies are of value in screening for arterial stenosis and occlusion: in skilled hands they demonstrate accurately the degree of internal carotid artery stenosis.

Vascular imaging.   Magnetic resonance angiography or digital subtraction angiography is valuable in anterior circulation TIAs to confirm surgically accessible arterial stenoses, mainly internal carotid artery stenosis. Most normotensive patients with TIA or stroke in the anterior circulation – who recover well – should have vascular imaging if ultrasound suggests carotid stenosis. The results of endarterectomy are given below.

Lumbar puncture.   This is indicated only in unusual circumstances, such as when blood syphilitic serology is positive.

Long-term management
Medical therapy
All risk factors (Table 21.25) should be identified and, if possible, treated.

Antihypertensive therapy
Recognition and control of high blood pressure in the population is the single most important factor in primary stroke prevention. Transient hypertension often seen after acute stroke usually does not require treatment provided diastolic pressure does not rise higher than 100 mmHg. Sustained severe hypertension needs treatment (p. 864), but the pressure must be lowered slowly to avoid a sudden fall in cerebral perfusion.

Antiplatelet therapy (also p. 478)
Long-term soluble aspirin (75 mg daily) reduces substantially the incidence of further infarction after thromboembolic TIA or stroke. Aspirin inhibits cyclo-oxygenase, which converts arachidonic acid to prostaglandins and thromboxanes. The predominant therapeutic effect is to reduce platelet aggregation. Clopidogrel, dipyridamole and ticlopidine are also used (p. 478). Combined aspirin 75 mg daily and dipyridamole 200 mg twice daily is probably the best prophylaxis against further thromboembolic stroke or TIA.

Anticoagulants
Heparin and warfarin should be given when there is atrial fibrillation, other paroxysmal dysrhythmias or when there are cardiac valve lesions (uninfected) or cardiomyopathies. Brain haemorrhage must be excluded by CT/MRI. All patients on anticoagulants must be aware of the small risk of cerebral (and other) haemorrhage. The drugs are potentially dangerous in the 2 weeks following cerebral infarction because of the risk of provoking cerebral haemorrhage. There are wide differences in clinical practice here. Table 21.30 outlines the issues in secondary stroke prevention.

Other measures
Polycythaemia and clotting abnormalities should be treated if found (p. 453).

Surgical approaches
Internal carotid endarterectomy
Surgery is recommended in TIA or stroke patients shown to have internal carotid artery stenosis greater than 70%. Successful surgery reduces the risk of further TIA/stroke by approximately 75%. Endarterectomy has a mortality around 3%, and a similar risk of stroke. Percutaneous transluminal angioplasty (stenting) is an alternative procedure. Surgery for asymptomatic patients is advocated for some.

Strokes in the elderly
The yield of investigation in stroke falls with age. Age itself is, however, no barrier to recovery, and elderly patients benefit most from high standards of rehabilitation. Consider social isolation in elderly patients, pre-existing cognitive impairment, their nutrition, skin and sphincter care, and reassess swallowing. Carotid endarterectomy over 75 carries little more risk than in younger cases.

Table 21.30 Stroke prevention: indications for considering anticoagulants

Indication	Comment
Valvular heart disease	Heparin/warfarin is of clear benefit in chronic rheumatic heart disease, particularly mitral stenosis
Recent MI Intracardiac thrombus	Heparin/warfarin should be given if there is evidence of intracardiac thrombus
Atrial fibrillation	Anticoagulants long term reduce stroke incidence in atrial fibrillation
Acute internal carotid artery thrombus Acute basilar artery thrombus Internal carotid artery dissection Extracranial vertebral artery dissection	Anticoagulants are reserved for imaging-confirmed cases of arterial thrombosis or dissection. They have not been shown to be beneficial in stroke prevention after thromboembolism from carotid or vertebrobasilar sources
Prothrombic states, e.g. protein C deficiency	Consider anticoagulation in consultation with a haematologist
Recurrent TIAs or stroke on full antiplatelet therapy	If no remediable cause, a trial of anticoagulants may be justified
Cerebral venous thrombosis including sinus thrombosis	Benefits of anticoagulation outweigh risks of haemorrhage

Modified from Brown M (2000) *Medicine* **28**(7): 64

Rehabilitation: physiotherapy and speech therapy

Skilled physiotherapy has particular value in the first few weeks after stroke. It relieves spasticity, prevents contractures and teaches patients to use walking aids. The benefit of physiotherapy for the longer-term outcome is still inadequately researched. Baclofen (a GABA agonist) is sometimes helpful in the management of severe spasticity following stroke.

In aphasia, the speech therapist has a vital understanding of the patient's problems and frustration. It is, however, possible that spontaneous return of speech is hastened as much by normal conversation with a relative as by a therapist. If the patient cannot swallow safely without the risk of aspiration, either nasogastric feeding or percutaneous gastrostomy will be needed. Video-fluoroscopy while attempting to swallow is helpful.

Both physiotherapy and speech therapy have an undoubted psychological role. Stroke is frequently devastating and, particularly when it occurs during working life, radically alters the patient's remaining

years. Many become unemployable, lose independence and are financially embarrassed. Loss of self-esteem makes depression common.

Following early recovery, aids and modifications may be necessary at home. For example: stair rails, portable lavatories, bath rails, hoists, sliding boards, wheelchairs, tripods, altering doorways and sleeping arrangements, stair lifts and kitchen modifications. Liaison between a hospital-based neurology community care team, locally based therapists and primary care physician is valuable.

Prognosis

Twenty-five per cent of patients die within 2 years of a stroke. Around 30% of this group die in the first month. This early mortality is lower for thromboembolic infarction (death in under a quarter) than for intracerebral haemorrhage (death in around three-quarters). A poor outcome is likely when there is coma, a defect in conjugate gaze and severe hemiplegia. Many complications that lead to early death, particularly in the elderly, are preventable – for example, aspiration. Coordinated care reduces risks.

Recurrent strokes are, however, common (10% in the first year) and many patients die subsequently from myocardial infarction. Of initial stroke survivors, some 30–40% remain alive at 3 years.

Gradual improvement usually follows stroke, although the late residual deficit may be severe. Of those who survive, about one-third return to independent mobility and one-third have serious disability requiring permanent institutional care.

The outlook for recovery of language is variable. If, in general, the stroke patient is intelligible at 3 weeks, prognosis for fluent speech is good – but many are left with word-finding difficulties.

Intracranial haemorrhage

This comprises:

- intracerebral and cerebellar haemorrhage
- subarachnoid haemorrhage
- subdural and extradural haemorrhage/haematoma.

Intracerebral haemorrhage

Aetiology

Intracerebral haemorrhage causes around 10% of strokes. Rupture of microaneurysms (Charcot–Bouchard aneurysms, 0.8–1.0 mm diameter) and degeneration of small deep penetrating arteries are the principal pathology. Such haemorrhage is usually massive, often fatal and occurs in chronic hypertension and at well-defined sites – basal ganglia, pons, cerebellum and subcortical white matter.

In normotensive patients, particularly over 60 years, *lobar* intracerebral haemorrhage occurs – in the frontal, temporal, parietal or occipital cortex. Cerebral amyloid angiopathy (rare) is the cause in some of these haemorrhages, and the tendency to rebleed is associated with particular apolipoprotein E genotypes.

Recognition

At the bedside, there is no entirely reliable way of distinguishing between intracerebral haemorrhage and thromboembolic infarction. Both produce stroke. Intracerebral haemorrhage, however, tends to be dramatic with severe headache. It is more likely to lead to coma than thromboembolic stroke.

Brain haemorrhage is seen on CT imaging immediately (cf. infarction, p. 1214) – as intracerebral, intraventricular, or subarachnoid blood. MR imaging may not identify an acute haemorrhage correctly in the first few hours. Thereafter T2 weighted MR is very reliable.

Management: haemorrhagic stroke

The principles are those for cerebral infarction. The immediate prognosis is less good. Antiplatelet drugs and, of course, anticoagulants are contraindicated. Control of hypertension is vital. Urgent neurosurgical clot evacuation is sometimes considered when there is deepening coma and coning (occasionally in lobar haemorrhage but particularly in cerebellar haemorrhage, see below). The outlook is usually poor.

Cerebellar haemorrhage (Fig. 21.23)

There is headache and rapid reduction of consciousness with signs of brainstem origin (e.g. nystagmus, ocular palsies). Gaze deviates towards the haemorrhage. Skew deviation (p. 1183) may develop. There are unilateral or bilateral cerebellar signs, if the patient is awake. Cerebellar haemorrhage sometimes causes acute hydrocephalus. Emergency surgical clot evacuation is often necessary after imaging.

Subarachnoid haemorrhage

Subarachnoid haemorrhage (SAH) means spontaneous arterial bleeding into the subarachnoid space, and is usually clearly recognizable clinically by its dramatic onset. SAH accounts for some 5% of strokes and has an annual incidence of 6 per 100 000.

Causes

The causes of SAH are shown in Table 21.31, though it is unusual to find any contributing disease.

Saccular (berry) aneurysms (Fig. 21.24)

Saccular aneurysms develop on the circle of Willis and

Table 21.31 Underlying causes of subarachnoid haemorrhage	
Saccular ('berry') aneurysms	70%
Arteriovenous malformation (AVM)	10%
No lesion found	20%

Rare associations
Bleeding disorders
Mycotic aneurysms (endocarditis)
Acute bacterial meningitis
Brain tumours (e.g. metastatic melanoma)
Arteritis (e.g. systemic lupus erythematosus)
Spinal AVM (spinal haemorrhage only)
Coarctation of the aorta
Marfan's syndrome, Ehlers–Danlos syndrome
Polycystic kidneys

Fig. 21.24 Digital subtraction angiogram of posterior communicating artery aneurysm.

adjacent arteries. Common sites are at the following arterial junctions:

- between posterior communicating and internal carotid artery – posterior communicating artery aneurysm
- between anterior communicating and anterior cerebral artery – anterior communicating artery aneurysm
- at a bifurcation or at the trifurcation of the middle cerebral artery – middle cerebral artery aneurysm.

Other aneurysm sites are on the basilar, posterior inferior cerebellar, intracavernous internal carotid and ophthalmic arteries. Saccular aneurysms are an incidental finding in 1% of autopsies and can be multiple.

Aneurysms cause symptoms either by spontaneous rupture, when there is usually no preceding history, or by direct pressure on surrounding structures; for example, an enlarging unruptured posterior communicating artery aneurysm is the commonest cause of a painful third nerve palsy (p. 1185).

Arteriovenous malformation (AVM)

This is a collection of arteries and veins of developmental origin, usually within the hemisphere. An AVM may also cause epilepsy, often focal. Once an AVM has ruptured the tendency is to rebleed – 10% will then do so annually.

Cavernous haemangiomas ('cavernomas') are common (< 0.5% of population) and consist of collections of capillary vessels; they are frequently symptomless

Fig. 21.23 CT: Cerebellar haemorrhage.

Fig. 21.25 **MR (T2): Symptomless cavernous haemangioma (arrow).**

(Fig. 21.25). Cavernomas sometimes have a genetic basis, with linkage to two loci on chromosome 7q. Rarely cavernomas cause seizures or bleed; exceptionally they cause sudden death from massive haemorrhage. Surgery is rarely appropriate.

Clinical features of SAH

There is a sudden devastating headache, often occipital. This is usually followed by vomiting and often by coma. The patient remains comatose or drowsy for several hours to several days, or longer. Less severe headaches cause difficulty (p. 1174), but SAH is a *possible* diagnosis in any sudden headache.

After major SAH there is neck stiffness and a positive Kernig's sign. Papilloedema is sometimes present and accompanied by retinal and subhyaloid haemorrhage (tracking beneath the retinal hyaloid membrane). Minor bleeds cause few signs, but almost invariably headache.

Investigations

CT imaging is the initial investigation of choice (Fig. 21.26). Subarachnoid or intraventricular blood is usually seen. Lumbar puncture is not necessary if SAH is confirmed by CT, but should be performed if doubt remains. The CSF becomes yellow (xanthochromic) several hours after SAH. Visual inspection of the supernatant CSF is usually sufficiently reliable for diagnosis, but there is a move to use spectrophotometry to estimate bilirubin released from lysed cells to define

Fig. 21.26 **CT: Subarachnoid haemorrhage showing blood around the brain stem (arrow).**

with certainty SAH in doubtful cases. MR angiography is usually performed in all potentially fit for surgery, i.e. generally below 65 years and not in coma. In some cases, no aneurysm is found despite a definite SAH.

Differential diagnosis

SAH must be differentiated from severe migraine. This is sometimes difficult. *Thunderclap headache* is a term used (confusingly) to describe either SAH or a sudden headache for which no cause is ever found. The onset of acute bacterial meningitis occasionally causes a very abrupt headache, when a meningeal microabscess ruptures. Subarachnoid bleeding also occasionally occurs at the onset of acute bacterial meningitis.

Complications

Blood in the subarachnoid space can lead to obstruction of CSF flow and hydrocephalus. This can be asymptomatic but may cause deteriorating consciousness after SAH. Diagnosis is by CT. Shunting may be required.

Severe arterial spasm (visible on cerebral angiography and a cause of coma or stroke) sometimes complicates SAH. It is a poor prognostic sign.

Management

Immediate treatment of SAH is bed rest and supportive measures. Hypertension should be controlled. Dexamethasone is often prescribed, to reduce cerebral oedema; it also is believed to stabilize the blood–brain barrier. Nimodipine, a calcium-channel blocking agent, reduces mortality.

All surviving SAH cases should be discussed urgently with a specialist neurosurgical centre. Nearly half SAH cases are either dead or moribund before they reach hospital. Of the remainder, a further 10–20% rebleed and die in the next several weeks. Delay or failure to diagnose SAH without coma (e.g. mistaking it for migraine) contributes to this mortality.

Patients who remain comatose or with persistent severe deficits have a poor prognosis. In others, where angiography demonstrates aneurysm, a direct neurosurgical approach to clip the neck of the aneurysm is carried out. In selected cases the results of surgery are excellent. Invasive radiological techniques, such as inserting a fine wire coil into an aneurysm are also used. Direct surgery, microembolism and focal radiotherapy ('gamma knife') are used in AVM.

Subdural and extradural haemorrhage and haematoma

These cause death after head injury unless treated promptly.

Subdural haematoma (SDH) (Fig. 21.27)

SDH means accumulation of blood in the subdural space following rupture of a vein. It usually follows a head injury, which may be trivial. The interval between injury and symptoms may be days, weeks or months. Chronic, unsuspected or spontaneous SDH is common in the elderly and in alcohol abuse.

Fig. 21.27   MR (T1): Bilateral subdural haematomas.

Headache, drowsiness and confusion are common; symptoms are indolent and often fluctuate. Focal deficits such as hemiparesis or sensory loss develop. Epilepsy occasionally occurs. Stupor, coma and coning may follow, but there is a tendency for SDH to resolve spontaneously.

Extradural haemorrhage

This follows a linear skull vault fracture tearing a branch of the middle meningeal artery. Blood accumulates rapidly over minutes/hours in the extradural space. The most characteristic picture is of a head injury with a brief duration of unconsciousness followed by a lucid interval of recovery. The patient then develops a progressive hemiparesis and stupor, and rapid transtentorial coning, with first an ipsilateral dilated pupil, followed by bilateral fixed dilated pupils, tetraplegia and respiratory arrest. An acute *subdural* haemorrhage presents in a similar way.

Management

Suspected extradural or subdural haemorrhage needs immediate imaging.

Extradural bleeding requires urgent neurosurgery. If performed early, the outlook is excellent. When far from specialist neurosurgical help (e.g. in wartime or at sea), surgical drainage through a skull burr-hole has been lifesaving when an extradural has been diagnosed on clinical grounds alone.

Subdural bleeding may allow; more conservative management – even large subdural collections can resolve. Progress is assessed with serial imaging, but close liaison with a neurosurgeon remains essential.

CORTICAL VENOUS THROMBOSIS AND DURAL VENOUS SINUS THROMBOSIS

Intracranial venous thromboses are usually (85%) associated with a pro-thrombotic risk factor e.g. oral contraceptives, pregnancy, genetic and acquired prothrombotic states. Head injury is also a cause but infection e.g. from the paranasal sinus is unusual (6–12%). They may arise apparently de novo.

Cortical venous thrombosis

The venous infarct leads to headache, focal signs (e.g. hemiparesis) and/or epilepsy. There is often a fever.

Dural venous sinus thromboses

Cavernous sinus thrombosis causes ocular pain, fever, proptosis and chemosis. An external and internal ophthalmoplegia with papilloedema develop.

Sagittal and lateral sinus thrombosis cause raised intracranial pressure with headache, fever, papilloedema and often epilepsy.

Management

MRI, MRA and the venous phase of angiography show occluded sinuses and/or veins. Treatment is with heparin initially although its value has been questioned. This is followed by warfarin for six months. Anticonvulsants and anticoagulants are given if necessary.

FURTHER READING

ATLANTIS, ECASS and NINDS rtPA Study Group Investigators (2004) Association of outcome with early stroke treatment. *Lancet* **366**: 768–774.

Dobkin BH (2005) Rehabilitation after stroke. *New England Journal of Medicine* **352**: 1677–84.

Ellegala D, Day A (2005) Ruptured cerebral aneurysms. *New England Journal of medicine* **352**: 121–124.

Levine JS *et al* (2002) The antiphospholipid syndrome. *New England Journal of Medicine* **346**: 752–763.

Miller Fisher C (2002) Transient ischaemic attacks. *New England Journal of Medicine* **347**: 1642–1643.

MRC Asymptomatic Carotid Surgery Trial (ACST) Collaborative Group (2004) Prevention of disabling and fatal strokes by successful carotid endarterectomy in patients without recent neurological symptoms: randomised controlled trial. *Lancet* **363**: 1491–1502.

Outpatient Services Trialists (2004) Rehabilitation therapy services for stroke patients living at home. *Lancet* **363**: 352–356.

Qureshi AI (2004) Endovascular treatment of cerebrovascular disease and intracranial neoplasms. *Lancet* **363**: 804–817.

Rudd AG, Wade D, Irwin P (2000) The national clinical guidelines for stroke. *Journal of the Royal College of Physicians of London* **34**: 131–133

Stam J (2005) Thrombosis of the cerebral veins and sinuses. *New England Journal of Medicine* **352**: 1791–1798.

Warlow C (2003) Seminar: stroke. *Lancet* **362**: 1211–1224.

EPILEPSY AND CAUSES OF LOSS OF CONSCIOUSNESS

EPILEPSY

A seizure is a convulsion or transient abnormal event resulting from a paroxysmal discharge of cerebral neurones. Epilepsy is the continuing tendency to have seizures, even if a long interval separates attacks. A generalized convulsion (i.e. a grand mal fit) is the most common recognized event. Epilepsy is common. Over 2% of the population have two or more seizures during their lives, and in 0.5% epilepsy is an active problem and hence a common one in general practice. In the UK approximately 65 people suffer their first seizure each day. Often no clear cause is found for seizures. Sometimes (though unusually) epilepsy is caused by a brain tumour or follows a stroke. Around 250 000 people take anticonvulsant drugs, the mainstay of treatment. Neurosurgery (temporal lobectomy) is also valuable in carefully selected cases.

Mechanisms

Spread of electrical activity between neurones is normally restricted and *synchronous discharge* of neurones takes place in restricted groups producing the normal EEG rhythms. During a seizure, large groups of neurones are activated repetitively, unrestrictedly and hypersynchronously. Inhibitory synaptic activity between neurones fails. This produces high-voltage spike-and-wave EEG activity, the electrophysiological hallmark of epilepsy.

A partial seizure is epileptic activity confined to one area of cortex with a recognizable clinical pattern (Fig. 21.28). This activity either remains focal or spreads to generate epileptic activity in both hemispheres – and thus a generalized seizure. This spread is called secondary generalization. The focal onset of a seizure may not be apparent. This means that a generalized tonic–clonic seizure may either have started as a focal seizure, or be a primary generalized major convulsion. Brain becomes

epileptogenic either because neurones have a predisposition to be hyperexcitable, for example following abnormal neuronal migration patterns in utero, or because the cells acquire this hyperexcitable tendency. Trauma or brain neoplasms are examples of acquired conditions that alter neuronal seizure threshold.

Seizure threshold

Each individual has a seizure threshold. Experimentally some chemicals (e.g. pentylenetetrazol, a toxic gas) induce seizures in everyone. People who are more likely to have seizures in response to flashing lights, for example, have *low seizure thresholds* – a concept, not a measurement.

Classification

Various classifications of seizures are confusing. Seizures are described here by clinical pattern (Table 21.32).

- *Generalized* implies bilateral abnormal electrical activity, with bilateral motor manifestations and impaired consciousness.
- A *partial (focal) seizure* means a localized seizure:
  (a) simple – without loss of consciousness, e.g. jerking of a limb
  (b) complex – with loss of awareness, e.g. an absence attack.
- *Unclassifiable seizure.*

Generalized seizure types
Tonic–clonic seizures (grand mal seizures, generalized major convulsions)
Following a vague warning, the tonic phase commences. The body becomes rigid, for up to a minute. The patient utters a cry and falls, sometimes suffering serious injury.

Fig. 21.28 Seizure types. (a) Partial (focal) seizure. (b) Primary generalized seizure. (c) Partial seizure with secondary generalization.

Table 21.32   The commoner types of epilepsy
Abridged from International League against Epilepsy

1. **Generalized seizure types**
 A Absence seizures
  (a) Typical absences with 3 Hz spike-and-wave discharge (*petit mal*)
  (b) Atypical absences with other EEG changes
 B Myoclonic seizures
 C Tonic–clonic seizures (*grand mal*, major convulsion)
 D Tonic seizures
 E Akinetic seizures

2. **Partial seizure types** These start by activation of a group of neurones in one part of one hemisphere. They are also called 'focal seizures'   A Simple partial seizures (without impairment of consciousness) (e.g. Jacksonian seizures) B Complex partial seizures (impairment of consciousness) C Partial seizures evolving to tonic–clonic seizures D Apparent generalized tonic–clonic seizures, with EEG but not clinical evidence of focal onset
3. **Unclassifiable seizures** Seizures which do not fit one of the above categories

The tongue is usually bitten. There may be incontinence of urine or faeces.

The clonic phase then begins, a generalized convulsion, with frothing at the mouth and rhythmic jerking of muscles. This lasts from a few seconds to several minutes. Seizures are usually self-limiting, followed by drowsiness, confusion or coma for several hours.

Typical absences (petit mal)

This generalized epilepsy almost invariably begins in childhood. Each attack is accompanied by 3 Hz spike-and-wave EEG activity (Fig. 21.15, p. 1203). Activity ceases, the patient stares and pales slightly for a few seconds. The eyelids twitch; a few muscle jerks may occur. After an attack, normal activity is resumed. Typical absence attacks are never due to acquired lesions such as tumours. They are a developmental abnormality of neuronal control. Children with typical absence attacks tend to develop generalized tonic–clonic seizures in adult life (known as *primary generalized epilepsy*). *Petit mal* describes only these 3 Hz absence seizures. Clinically similar absence attacks are also caused by partial seizures of temporal lobe origin, a source of some confusion.

Other generalized seizure types

Myoclonic seizures describe isolated muscle jerking. *Tonic* seizures describe intense stiffening of the body not followed by convulsive jerking. *Atonic* seizures cause sudden loss of tone, with falling and loss of consciousness.

Partial seizure types
Partial seizures (focal seizures)

A partial or focal seizure (simple or complex, see above) implies that an area of brain (e.g. a temporal lobe) has generated abnormal electrical activity. The seizure frequently has clinical features that provide evidence of its site.

An aura describes the effects of initial focal electrical events, such as an unusual smell, tingling in a limb or a strange inner feeling often recognized as a warning of an impending seizure.

Jacksonian, or focal motor seizures

These simple partial seizures originate in the motor cortex. Jerking movements typically begin at the angle of the mouth or in the hand, spreading to involve the limbs on the side opposite the epileptic focus. Clinical evidence of this spread of activity is called the *march* of the seizure. With a frontal lesion, conjugate gaze (p. 1183) and the head deviate away from the irritative epileptic focus – known as an adversive seizure. Weakness of the convulsing limbs for several hours sometimes follows a seizure – *Todd's paralysis*.

Temporal lobe seizures

These partial seizures, either simple or complex, describe feelings of unreality (*jamais vu*) or undue familiarity (*déjà vu*) with the surroundings. Absence attacks, vertigo, visual hallucinations (i.e. visions or faces) are other examples of temporal lobe seizures.

Table 21.33 Aetiological and precipitating factors in epilepsy
Genetic predisposition
Developmental, e.g. hamartomas, neuronal migration abnormalities
Trauma and surgery
Pyrexia
Intracranial mass lesions, e.g. tumour, neurocysticercosis
Vascular, e.g. cerebral infarction, arteriovenous malformation
Drugs and drug withdrawal
Encephalitis and inflammatory conditions
Metabolic abnormalities, e.g. porphyria, hypocalcaemia
Neural degenerative disorders
Provoked seizures, e.g. photosensitivity, sleep deprivation

Many other types of partial seizure occur, such as autonomic disturbances with piloerection, flushing, and overbreathing, strange smells (frontal cortex), sensory disturbances (parietal cortex), crude visual shapes (occipital cortex), or strange sounds (auditory cortex).

Aetiology and precipitants (Table 21.33)

A definite cause for epilepsy is found in under a third of cases in UK community surveys: cerebrovascular disease accounts for some 15%, cerebral tumours for 6%, alcohol-related seizures for 6% and post-traumatic epilepsy 2%. Rarer causes are hippocampal sclerosis (resection may be possible), malformations of cortical development, vascular malformations, hamartomas, brain abscesses and tuberculomas.

Genetic predisposition and developmental anomalies

Over 200 genetic disorders list epilepsy among their features, giving rise to complex syndromic classifications. These account for < 2% of epilepsy cases. About 30% of epilepsy patients have first-degree relatives with seizures. Usually the mode of inheritance is uncertain. A low seizure threshold appears to run in some families. Generalized typical absence seizures (*petit mal*, 3 Hz spike-and-wave) and primary generalized epilepsy are often inherited as an autosomal dominant trait with variable penetrance. Primary epilepsies are due to complex developmental abnormalities of neuronal control. There are abnormalities in synaptic connections, and anomalies in neurotransmitter distribution and release. Neuronal migration defects in utero, dysplastic areas of cerebral cortex and hamartomas contribute to seizures both in infancy and adult life.

Trauma, hypoxia and surgery

Perinatal trauma (cerebral contusion and haemorrhage) and fetal anoxia are common causes of childhood seizures. Hypoxic damage to the hippocampi (mesial temporal sclerosis) is another childhood cause of epilepsy.

Brain injury is sometimes followed by epilepsy within the first week (early epilepsy) or many months or years later (late epilepsy). To cause epilepsy, the injury must (usually) be sufficient to cause coma. Early epilepsy, a depressed skull fracture, penetrating brain injury, cerebral contusion, dural tear or intracranial haematoma increases the incidence of late post-traumatic epilepsy.

Seizures follow some 10% of neurosurgical operations on the cerebral hemispheres.

Pyrexia

Convulsions sometimes occur when children under 5 years have high fevers (febrile convulsions). In the majority there is no recurrence. Partly for social reasons, febrile convulsions are not usually labelled as epilepsy.

Brain tumours (and abscesses)

Mass lesions in the cortex cause epilepsy – either partial or secondary generalized seizures. If epilepsy develops in adult life, the chance of finding an unsuspected tumour is around 3%.

Hydrocephalus (p. 1247) also lowers seizure threshold.

Vascular

Seizures sometimes follow cerebral infarction, especially in the elderly – there is a peak in incidence late in life. A brain arteriovenous malformation may present with seizures and occasionally a subarachnoid bleed.

Alcohol, drugs and drug withdrawal

Chronic alcohol abuse is a common cause of seizures. These occur either while drinking heavily or during periods of withdrawal. Alcohol-induced hypoglycaemia also provokes attacks (p. 1134).

Phenothiazines, monoamine oxidase inhibitors, tricyclic antidepressants, amfetamines, lidocaine, propofol and nalidixic acid sometimes provoke fits, either in overdose or at therapeutic doses in individuals with a low seizure threshold.

Withdrawal of anticonvulsant drugs (especially phenobarbital) and benzodiazepines may provoke seizures.

Encephalitis and inflammatory conditions

Seizures are frequently presenting features of encephalitis, cerebral abscess, cortical venous thrombosis, and neurosyphilis. They also occur in chronic meningitis (e.g. tuberculosis) and may rarely be the first sign of bacterial meningitis. In countries where the tapeworm is endemic, e.g. India, neurocysticercosis is a frequent cause of seizures.

Metabolic abnormalities

Seizures are seen with:

- hypocalcaemia, hypoglycaemia, hyponatraemia
- acute hypoxia
- uraemia, hepatocellular failure
- mitochondrial disease, porphyria.

Degenerative brain disorders

Seizures can occur in Alzheimer's disease and in many degenerative diseases. Epilepsy is three times commoner in multiple sclerosis patients than in the general population.

Provoked seizures (e.g. photosensitivity)

Seizures are occasionally precipitated by flashing lights or a flickering television screen. Photosensitivity can be recorded on occipital EEG electrodes. Rarely other stimuli (e.g. music) provoke attacks.

Sleep deprivation

A convulsion sometimes follows missing a night's sleep in a susceptible person.

Diagnosis

The history from a witness is crucial, and usually enables one to distinguish other causes of disturbed consciousness (p. 1226). The onset, setting, and stages of attacks are of importance. Neurological examination may be normal or point to a clinical diagnosis (e.g. hemiparesis and papilloedema in a hemisphere tumour). General medical screening, including serum calcium and an ECG should be carried out.

Electroencephalography

The EEG remains a useful test, despite limitations. It should be performed after a first fit.

- *During a seizure* the EEG is almost invariably abnormal, because spikes reach the brain surface.
- *EEG evidence of seizure activity* is shown typically by focal cortical spikes (e.g. over a temporal lobe) or by generalized spike-and-wave activity. Epileptic activity is continuous in *status epilepticus*.
- *3 Hz spike-and-wave activity* occurs specifically in *petit mal* (Fig. 21.15, p. 1203). This is always present during an attack and is frequently seen in between attacks.
- *A normal EEG between attacks* (interictal) does not in any way exclude epilepsy. Many people with epilepsy have normal interictal EEGs.
- *An abnormal interictal EEG* does not prove that one particular attack was epileptic.
- *EEG videotelemetry* is used to study attacks of uncertain nature (e.g. non-epileptic attack disorder, p. 1226).

CT and/or MR imaging

The trend is towards sophisticated imaging of all new cases of epilepsy when resources permit. In practice, CT is a reasonable screening test for tumours in adults but MR is used routinely if available.

Treatment

Emergency measures

When faced with a seizure it is best simply to ensure that the patient comes to as little harm as possible, and that the airway is maintained both during a prolonged seizure and in post-ictal coma. Wooden mouth gags, tongue forceps and physical restraint cause injury.

Most seizures last only minutes and end spontaneously. A prolonged seizure – longer than 3 minutes – or repeated seizures outside hospital are best treated with rectal diazepam (10 mg), or intravenous diazepam. If there is any suspicion of hypoglycaemia, take blood for glucose and give i.v. glucose. Serial epilepsy describes repeated seizures with brief periods of recovery. These may lead to status epilepticus. Sudden death in a seizure is unusual but does occur.

Status epilepticus

This medical emergency means continuous seizures without recovery of consciousness. It should be considered if prolonged serial seizures (two or more) occur with incomplete recovery of consciousness. Status has a mortality of 10–15%. Over 50% of cases occur without a previous history of epilepsy. However, about 25% with apparent refractory status have *pseudostatus* (non-epileptic attack disorder). The iatrogenic morbidity here is significant.

Focal status also occurs. In absence status, for example, status is non-convulsive – the patient is in a continuous, distant, stuporose state. *Epilepsia partialis continua* is continuous seizure activity in one part of the body, such

as a finger or a limb, without loss of consciousness. This is often due to a cortical neoplasm or, in the elderly, a cortical infarct.

Management. See Practical box 21.4.

Anticonvulsant drugs

Drugs are indicated when there is a firm clinical diagnosis of recurrent seizures, or a substantial risk of recurrence. Anticonvulsant use carries the stigma of epilepsy. Concordance is essential, and understanding of potential unwanted effects. For both partial and generalized seizures, prescribe monotherapy with an established anticonvulsant (Table 21.34). The dose is increased until control is achieved or tolerance exceeded. If control is not achieved, a second drug is added. Despite many new anticonvulsants (Table 21.35), there remain different

---

Practical Box 21.4
Management of Status Epilepticus

Several treatment schedules exist. Issues of prime importance are the speed with which convulsive activity is treated, the accuracy of diagnosis and need for continued monitoring and cardiorespiratory support – this must be available. An ITU is essential for optimum management.

- At home, give immediate diazepam 10–20 mg i.v. at 5 mg/min and repeat once. If immediate i.v. access is impossible, give rectally diazepam or paraldehyde.
- Arrange immediate admission to hospital.
- Administer oxygen, monitor ECG, BP, routine bloods (include alcohol, calcium, magnesium, drug screen, anticonvulsant levels). Exclude hypoglycaemia: treat if present.
- Give thiamine i.v. (250 mg) if nutrition poor or alcohol abuse suspected. (In the UK parenteral vitamin B and C, one pair of high-potency i.v. ampoules over 10 minutes.)
- *Anticonvulsants:*
  1. Give lorazepam i.v. 4 mg at 2 mg/min. Respiratory depression, hypotension and cardiac dysrhythmias may occur. (Lorazepam 4 mg vial.)
  2. Reinstate previous anticonvulsant drugs. Establish whether the patient has had adequate phenytoin recently. Measure levels as an emergency if service available.
  3. If seizures continue, consider i.v. phenytoin or fosphenytoin (if patient is not already loaded with these drugs).
     - Phenytoin: give 15 mg/kg i.v. diluted to

10 mg/mL in normal saline into a large vein at less than 50 mg/min. (Phenytoin sodium 250 mg 5 mL ampoule.)
     - Fosphenytoin: this is a pro-drug of phenytoin and can be given faster than phenytoin. Doses are expressed in phenytoin equivalents (PE): fosphenytoin 1.5 mg = 1 mg phenytoin.
     - Give 15 mg/kg (PE) fosphenytoin (15 mg × 1.5 = 22.5 mg) diluted to 10 mg/mL in normal saline at 50–100 mg (PE)/min. (Fosphenytoin sodium 750 mg 10 mL ampoule.)
  4. If status continues, give phenobarbital 10 mg/kg diluted 1 in 10 in water for injection at < 100 mg/min. (Phenobarbital 200 mg/mL 1 mL vial in propylene glycol 90% with water for injection 10%.) Intravenous clonazepam, paraldehyde and clomethiazole are also used.
  5. If, despite these measures, status persists > 90 minutes, use thiopental or propofol anaesthesia with assisted ventilation.
- EEG monitoring is valuable if there is doubt about the nature of status.
- CT scanning may reveal an underlying cause for status.
- Remember: 25% of apparent status turns out to be *pseudostatus.*
- Remember: potential unwanted effects of the drugs (e.g. hypotension, cardiac arrest) and the need for continuous cardiorespiratory monitoring.

Table 21.34	Principal antiepileptic drugs and common seizure types				
Drug	**Partial**	**2° Generalized**	**Tonic–clonic**	**3 Hz absence**	**Myoclonic**
Carbamazepine	+	+	+	−	−
Ethosuximide	0	0	0	+	0
Phenobarbital	+	+	+	0	+ (?)
Phenytoin	+	+	+	−	−
Primidone	+	+	+	0	?
Valproate	+	+	+	+	+

+, efficacy proven/probable; 0, ineffective; − *worsens* seizures; ?, unknown
After Brodie MJ (2000) *Lancet* **356**: 324

Table 21.35 Newer antiepileptic drugs and common seizure types

Drug	Partial	2° Generalized	Tonic–clonic	3 Hz absence	Myoclonic
Gabapentin	+	+	?+	0	?–
Lamotrigine	+	+	+	?	+
Levetiracetam	+	+	+	0	0
Oxcarbazepine	+	+	+	+	+
Tiagabine	+	+	?	?	?
Topiramate	+	+	+	?	+
Vigabatrin	+	+	?+	–	–

+, efficacy proven/probable; 0, ineffective; –, *worsens* seizures; ?, unknown

views about the most appropriate drugs for each seizure type.

Drug levels. Serum levels of most anticonvulsants can be monitored. With phenytoin the therapeutic level is well defined and this should usually be monitored every few months (Table 21.36). Therapeutic serum levels of other anticonvulsants are less useful. Levels are not usually measured routinely unless compliance or toxicity are issues.

Unwanted effects of drugs. Intoxication with all anticonvulsants causes ataxia, nystagmus and dysarthria. Chronic phenytoin causes gum hypertrophy, hypertrichosis, osteomalacia, folate deficiency, polyneuropathy and encephalopathy. A wide range of potential unwanted effects are known. See Table 21.37 for some serious idiosyncratic (i.e. non-dose-related) side-effects. The majority of severe skin reactions (e.g. toxic epidermal necrolysis) following phenytoin, carbamazepine, valproate and phenobarbital occur within the first 8 weeks of treatment.

Three drugs rarely commenced outside a specialist centre are phenobarbital and its derivative primidone (drowsiness, cognitive impairment) – though phenobarbital still has a place in status – and vigabatrin (visual fields defects).

Refractory epilepsy

Despite therapy, seizures persist in some 20–35% of cases of primary generalized epilepsy and partial epilepsy. Rigorous attention to diagnosis, to concordance (compliance), to trials of different drugs and consideration of surgery can help reduce this.

Epilepsy in the elderly

Some 25% of new cases of epilepsy develop over the age of 65. Many patients have cerebrovascular disease, neurodegenerative conditions or brain tumours. The onset of seizures commonly leads to loss of independence and to physical injuries with their complications (e.g. subdural haematomas). With adequate anticonvulsants, control of seizures can be achieved in some 70% of this vulnerable population.

Table 21.36 Doses and therapeutic levels of antiepileptic drugs

	Usual adult daily dose (mg)	Therapeutic range (µmol/L)
Phenytoin	300–500	40–80
Carbamazepine	400–1000	20–50
Valproate	800–2000	200–700

Table 21.37 Some idiosyncratic unwanted effects of anticonvulsant drugs

Drug	Non-dose-related side-effects
Phenytoin	Rashes
	Blood dyscrasias
	Lymphadenopathy
	Systemic lupus erythematosus
	Toxic epidermal necrolysis
Carbamazepine	Rashes
	Blood dyscrasias, particularly severe leucopenia
	Toxic epidermal necrolysis
Sodium valproate	Anorexia
	Hair loss
	Liver damage
Lamotrigine	Toxic epidermal necrolysis
Vigabatrin	Retinal damage (visual field constriction)
	Psychological change

Women, epilepsy and anticonvulsants

Fertility. There is some reduction of fertility in women with epilepsy. This is multifactorial. One-third of women with epilepsy have some ovarian abnormality – irregular menstrual cycles, anovulatory cycles and polycystic ovaries. These are probably more frequent in patients taking sodium valproate.

Birth defects. The overall risk of birth defects in babies of mothers who take one anticonvulsant is around 7%, higher than the 3% in the general population. Counselling before conception is essential. Some women choose to stop anticonvulsants before becoming pregnant. If drugs are continued, monotherapy with a first-line drug is preferable with folic acid (5 mg/day) supplement. Careful ante-natal screening (p. 191) is required. Vitamin K 20 mg orally should also be taken daily during the week before delivery to prevent neonatal haemorrhage (caused by inhibition of vitamin K transplacental transport).

Contraception. Anticonvulsants that induce enzymes (e.g. carbamazepine, phenytoin and phenobarbital) reduce the efficacy of oral contraceptives; valproate does not. A combined contraceptive pill containing either ethinylestradiol 50 µg or mestranol 50 µg provides greater contraceptive security at the risk of side effects. An IUCD or barrier methods of contraception are an alternative.

Breast-feeding. Mothers taking the established drugs (Table 21.34) need not in general be discouraged from breast-feeding – though drug manufacturers are often hesitant in assuring that there is no risk to the baby.

Drug withdrawal

Epilepsy, when controlled, may remain in remission. Drug withdrawal is sometimes possible, and this question often raised. Successful withdrawal is only achieved in less than 50%. Recurrence of seizures can cause considerable difficulty, e.g. when a driving licence has been regained. The UK Driving Licensing Authority (DVLA Swansea) recommend that patients do not drive while anticonvulsants are reduced and for 6 months after stopping them. Careful discussion and full explanation is necessary. Withdrawal should not usually be considered until all fits have been absent for at least 2–3 years.

Neurosurgical treatment

Several surgical approaches are used in epilepsy. Amputation of the non-dominant anterior temporal lobe can be performed in a patient with uncontrolled seizures and hippocampal sclerosis defined by imaging and confirmed by EEG. In these highly selected cases (under 1% of epilepsy patients) in specialist centres this surgical treatment is highly effective – with cure rates (complete seizure cessation) over 50%. Section of the corpus callosum and hemispherectomy are also used.

Social consequences

The majority of patients with epilepsy are managed by a general practitioner or as a hospital outpatient, and suffer infrequent seizures. In a very small minority who have exceedingly frequent seizures, treatment in hospital or even residential care is necessary.

There remains, however, a considerable stigma attached to the word epilepsy and this must be realized when the nature of attacks is uncertain. Employers are reluctant to accept people with epilepsy.

Both adults and children with epilepsy should be encouraged to lead lives as unrestricted as reasonably possible, though with simple, sensible provisos such as avoiding swimming alone and dangerous sports such as rock-climbing or solo canoeing. Domestic issues include leaving the bathroom or lavatory door unlocked. Support groups and information services are valuable.

Driving and epilepsy

It is illegal to drive a motor vehicle if any form of seizure or any episode of unexplained loss of consciousness has occurred during the previous year. There is some variation between different countries. In the UK those who have suffered from epilepsy cannot legally hold a Group 1 driving licence (for a car or motorcycle) unless they satisfy the following legal criteria, whether on or off treatment. The regulations state:

- A person who has suffered an epileptic attack whilst awake must refrain from driving for 1 year from the date of the attack before a driving licence may be issued.
- A person who has suffered a single epileptic attack whilst asleep must also refrain from driving for 1 year from the date of that attack, unless they have had attacks exclusively whilst asleep over a period of 3 years and no awake attacks, i.e. attacks occurring exclusively in sleep must be shown to have occurred over a 3-year period.
- In any event, the driving of a vehicle by such a person should not be likely to cause danger to the public.

For UK Group 2 drivers (vocational and for truck drivers) regulations are stricter. Persons with previous seizures must meet *all* these three criteria:

- They must have been free of attacks for at least 10 years.
- They must not have taken anticonvulsants during this 10 years.
- They do not have any continuing liability to seizures.

Stringent regulations also exist for potential aircraft pilots, sea captains, divers and other similar activities. The correct diagnosis of an attack at any age is therefore of major social and legal importance. It is an essential medical requirement to inform patients of the law. In the UK the patient should then write to the licensing authorities.

FURTHER READING

[Anonymous] (2003) When and how to stop anti-epileptic drugs in adults. *Drug and Therapeutics Bulletin* **41**: 41–43.

Brodie MJ, French JA (2000) Management of epilepsy in adolescents and adults. *Lancet* **356**: 323–329.

Chadwick D, Smith D (2002) The misdiagnosis of epilepsy. *British Medical Journal* **324**: 495–496.

Chang BS (2003) Mechanisms of disease: epilepsy. *New England Journal of Medicine* **349**: 1257–1265.

Driver and Vehicle Licensing Agency (2000) *At a Glance Guide to the Current Medical Standards of Fitness to Drive.* Swansea: Drivers Medical Unit, DVLA.

Elwes R (2002) Surgery for temporal lobe epilepsy. *British Medical Journal* **324**: 496–497.

Kwan P, Brodie MJ (2000) Early identification of refractory epilepsy. *New England Journal of Medicine* **342**: 314–319.

Pedley T et al. (2003) Is refractory epilepsy due to genetically determined resistance to antiepileptic drugs? *New England Journal of Medicine* **348**: 1480–1482.

Reynolds E (2003) Sudden death in the shadows of
epilepsy. *British Medical Journal* **326**: 349–350.
Stephen LJ, Brodie MJ (2000) Epilepsy in elderly
people. *Lancet* **355**: 1441–1446.
Treitman DM et al. (1998) A comparison of four
treatments for generalised convulsive status
epilepticus. *New England Journal of Medicine* **339**:
792–798.

UK PATIENT SUPPORT GROUP
National Society for Epilepsy, Chesham Lane, Chalfont
St Peter, Bucks SL9 0RJ
(http://www.epilepsyuse.org.uk).

OTHER ATTACKS OF DISTURBED CONSCIOUSNESS; FALLS (Table 21.38)

Episodes of transient disturbance of consciousness and
falls are common clinical problems. It is usually possible to
distinguish between a fit (i.e. a seizure), a faint (i.e. syncope),
and other types of attack from the description and an eye-
witness account. Falls must be distinguished from episodes
of disturbed consciousness. The precise cause of falls in the
elderly, with their sequelae such as a femoral fracture, often
remains ill-defined. Falls without loss of awareness are
common in extrapyramidal disease. 'Collapse' is non-
diagnostic and the term should be avoided.

Syncope; vasovagal attacks; drop attacks

The simple faint that over half the population experience at
some time (particularly in childhood, in youth or in
pregnancy) is due to sudden reflex bradycardia with
vasodilatation of both peripheral and splanchnic
vasculature. This simple syncope (also known as neurocardiogenic syncope) is a common response to prolonged
standing, fear, venesection or pain. Syncope almost never
occurs in the recumbent posture. The subject falls to the
ground and is unconscious for less than 2 minutes.
Recovery is rapid. Jerking movements can occur. Incontinence of urine is exceptional.

Syncope occurs with severe anaemia at any age.

Syncope occurs after *micturition in men*, particularly at
night, and in either sex when the venous return to the
heart is obstructed by breath-holding and severe
coughing. *Effort syncope* (on exertion) is of cardiac origin.

Postural hypotension (p. 734) also occurs in autonomic
neuropathy, with phenothiazines, levodopa or tricyclic
antidepressants. Carotid sinus problems (p. 734) and
cardiac arrhythmias (p. 734) cause syncopes.

Transient cerebral (*posterior circulation*) *ischaemia* also
leads to loss of consciousness and patients sometimes
faint during a severe 'basilar' migraine.

Drop attacks are instant unexpected episodes of lower
limb weakness with falling, largely in women over
60 years. They are due to sudden change in lower limb
tone, presumably of brainstem origin, rather than
thromboembolism. Awareness is preserved. Sudden
attacks of leg weakness also occur in hydrocephalus.

Syncope: investigation and management

Syncope and related conditions can usually be
distinguished from epilepsy on clinical grounds. A
witness account is extremely valuable: persistent jerking
movements, incontinence and post-episode confusion
with amnesia are very suggestive of a fit, and unusual in
a faint. Cardiac monitoring is used to detect dysrhythmia.
Tilt testing (p. 749) is sometimes diagnostic in syncope.

The immediate management of syncope, or
impending syncope, is to lay the patient down, to lift the
legs and to record the pulse. In rare circumstances where
cerebral blood flow cannot be restored (e.g. propped
upright in a dentist's chair), cerebral infarction can follow
syncope.

Other conditions

Panic attacks; hyperventilation; non-epileptic attacks.
Panic attacks are usually associated with an autonomic
disturbance, such as tachycardia, sweating and
piloerection. Consciousness is usually preserved and
attacks often easily recognized. Hyperventilation is
common and (see Box 22.11, p. 1298) overbreathing
causes alkalosis. This leads to light-headedness, anxiety
and sometimes circumoral and peripheral tingling and
tetany, e.g. carpopedal spasm (p. 1095). Occasionally
there is loss of consciousness.

Non-epileptic attacks (pseudoseizures) regularly cause
difficulty. Attacks often resemble grand mal fits. Usually
there are bizarre limb movements, but on occasion there
is extreme difficulty in separating these attacks from

Table 21.38 Causes of attacks of disturbed consciousness and falling

Epilepsy
Syncope (situational or vasovagal)
  Simple faints
  Cough
  Effort
  Micturition
  Carotid sinus
  Autonomic failure
  Basilar migraine
Cardiac dysrhythmias
Drop attacks
Hydrocephalus
Transient ischaemic attacks
Panic attacks
Non-epileptic attacks (pseudoseizures)
Hyperventilation
Night terrors ⎤
Breath-holding ⎬ in children
Hypoglycaemia ⎦
Hypocalcaemia
Vertigo
Choking
Drug reactions
Carcinoid syndrome
Phaeochromocytoma

epilepsy. EEG videotelemetry is valuable. Apparent *status epilepticus* can be seen. The serum prolactin level is of some diagnostic value: it rises during a true grand mal seizure but not during a pseudoseizure (or a partial seizure).

Hypoglycaemia (see also p. 1133). Hypoglycaemia causes attacks of loss of consciousness, sometimes with a convulsion. There is often some warning, with hunger, malaise, shaking and sweating. Prompt recovery occurs with i.v. (or oral) glucose. Prolonged hypoglycaemia causes widespread cerebral damage. Hypoglycaemic attacks unrelated to diabetes are rare (but see p. 1133). Feeling faint after fasting or in the early morning does not indicate anything serious.

Hypocalcaemia (see also p. 1094). A grand mal fit may accompany hypocalcaemia – seizure threshold is lowered.

Vertigo. Acute vertigo can be sufficiently severe to cause prostration: a few seconds' unconsciousness sometimes follows.

Choking causes intense coughing and laryngeal spasm when obstruction is partial. However, when a large food bolus completely blocks the larynx, the person becomes blue and silent. Death may follow if the blockage is not relieved promptly, e.g. by the Heimlich manoeuvre (p. 899), or gravity – holding the person upside down.

Drug reactions. Acute dystonic reactions (oculogyric crises, p. 1231) are sometimes mistaken for epilepsy. Consciousness is preserved.

Carcinoid syndrome, phaeochromocytoma and scombroid poisoning (pp. 309 and 1098). Flushing and palpitation is sometimes mistaken for anxiety, allergy or possibly a partial seizure.

Paroxysmal dyskinesias. These are rare causes of attacks of abnormal limb movement.

SLEEP AND ITS DISTURBANCES
(see also p. 1287)

Sleep is required on a regular basis. It preserves recent memory, refreshing cognitive and emotional equilibrium, and avoids neurotransmitter depletion. Poorly understood neurotransmitter pathways – including those involving hypothalamic hypocretin (orexin) neuropeptides – between cortex and reticular formation are involved in the sleep–waking cycle.

In *insomnia*, sleep is fitful (p. 1288). Less time than usual is spent in REM sleep. In old age, sleep requirement falls – sometimes to 4 hours a night. In practice, insomnia is rarely a feature of neurological disease.

Narcolepsy and cataplexy

Narcoleptic attacks are periods of irresistible sleep, i.e. excessive daytime drowsiness, in inappropriate circum-

stances. Episodes occur when there is little distraction, after meals, while travelling in a vehicle, or sometimes without obvious cause (see Table 20.5, p. 1161). Genetically, narcolepsy is strongly associated with HLA-DR2 and HLA-DQBl*0602 antigens. There are suggestions that narcolepsy patients positive for these antigens have subnormal CSF hypocretin 1 (orexin) levels. It is thought to have an autoimmune basis.

Cataplexy is sudden loss of lower limb tone – falling with intact awareness. Attacks are often set off by sudden surprise or emotion.

The two conditions sometimes coexist and are accompanied by vivid hypnagogic hallucinations (on falling asleep), hypnopompic hallucinations (on waking), with sleep paralysis – a frightening inability to move. The EEG remains normal during and between attacks.

Treatment
Methylphenidate, dexamfetamine, modafinil, or small doses of tricyclic antidepressants, particularly clomipramine, are used, rarely with great success. Siberian ginseng (*Elenthrococcus serticosus*) and St John's Wort (*Hypericum perforatum*) are also used.

Central sleep apnoea
This occurs at the onset of sleep and is due to impairment of central ventilatory control due to brainstem pathology. It is seen in the non-obese patient with no history of snoring.

FURTHER READING
Schneerson J (2000) *Handbook of Sleep Medicine*. Oxford: Blackwell.
Zeman A, Reading P (2005) The science of sleep. *Clinical Medicine* **5**: 97–101.

MOVEMENT DISORDERS

Disorders of movement form a substantial part of neurodegenerative diseases. They divide broadly into akinetic–rigid syndromes; slowed movement with increased tone (also called parkinsonism), and dyskinesias – added, uncontrollable movements. Precise anatomical and neurotransmitter profile changes are hard to define. Both parkinsonism and dyskinesia may coexist, leading to confusing classifications. Table 21.39 outlines the principal clinical varieties: idiopathic Parkinson's disease (an akinetic–rigid syndrome) and essential tremor (a dyskinesia) are much the commonest movement disorders.

AKINETIC–RIGID SYNDROMES

Idiopathic Parkinson's disease

In 1817, James Parkinson, a physician in Hoxton, London, published *The Shaking Palsy*, describing this common

Table 21.39　Movement disorders

Akinetic–rigid syndromes
Idiopathic Parkinson's disease
Drug-induced parkinsonism (e.g. phenothiazines)
MPTP-induced parkinsonism
Postencephalitic parkinsonism
Parkinsonism-plus
Childhood akinetic–rigid syndrome

Dyskinesias
Essential tremor
Chorea
Hemiballismus
Myoclonus
Tic or 'habit spasms'
Torsion dystonias
Paroxysmal dyskinesias

world-wide condition, with prevalence of 150/100 000 increasing sharply in those over 70 years. Parkinson's disease is clinically and pathologically distinct from other parkinsonian syndromes.

There are few real clues as to the cause of idiopathic Parkinson's disease (PD). The relatively uniform world-wide prevalence suggests that an environmental agent is not responsible. Some factors possibly involved are:

Nicotine. Several epidemiological studies confirm the curious fact that PD is less prevalent in tobacco smokers than in lifelong abstainers.

MPTP. Minute doses of the pyridine compound, methylphenyltetrahydropyridine (MPTP) cause severe parkinsonism. The link between this and idiopathic PD is tenuous. Suggestions that environmental MPTP-like herbicides are implicated are entirely unsubstantiated.

Encephalitis lethargica. Some survivors of the epidemic, presumed viral encephalitis lethargica, developed severe parkinsonism. However, it is not thought that idiopathic Parkinson's disease is related to an infective agent.

Genetic factors. Whilst not usually familial, there is clustering of early-onset Parkinson's disease in some families. Mutations of the alpha-synuclein gene and ubiquitin carboxyl-terminal hydrolase L1 (UCHL1), on chromosomes 2p13 and 4p14-16.3 respectively, account for occasional cases. Mutations in the parkin gene on chromosome 6 have been found in families with autosomal recessive cases of PD and some young apparently sporadic cases. Parkin mutations probably account for most PD cases with onset below the age of 40. Mutant parkin proteins are unable to interact, and ubiquinate forms of α-synuclein accumulate. The relevance to the common sporadic older PD cases remains doubtful.

Pathology

In the *pars compacta* of the *substantia nigra*, progressive cell

degeneration and neuronal eosinophilic inclusion bodies (Lewy bodies) are seen. These contain protein filaments of ubiquitin and alpha-synuclein. Degeneration also occurs in other basal ganglia nuclei. Biochemically there is loss of dopamine (and melanin) in the striatum. This correlates well with cell loss and with the degree of akinesia.

Clinical symptoms

The combination of tremor, rigidity and akinesia develops slowly, over months or several years, together with changes in posture. The most common initial symptoms are tremor and slowness. Patients complain that limbs and joints feel stiff. They ache. Fine movements become difficult. Slowness causes characteristic difficulty rising from a chair or getting into or out of bed. Writing becomes small (micrographia) and spidery, and tends to tail off. Relatives often notice other features – slowness and an impassive face. Idiopathic PD is almost always initially more prominent on one side.

Clinical signs

Diagnosis is usually evident from the overall appearance.

Tremor

The characteristic 4–7 Hz pill-rolling (movements between thumb and finger) rest tremor usually decreases with action. Tremor is often asymptomatic at first.

Rigidity

Stiffness develops throughout the range of limb movement and is equal in opposing muscle groups – in sharp contrast to the selective increase in tone found in spasticity. This 'lead pipe' increase in tone is usually more marked on one side. It is also present in the neck and axial muscles.

This plastic rigidity is more easily felt when a joint is moved slowly and gently. When one arm is being examined, its tone increases when the opposite arm moves actively. When stiffness occurs with tremor, smooth 'lead-pipe' rigidity is broken up into a jerky resistance to passive movement – known as cogwheeling, or cogging.

Akinesia

Poverty and slowing of movement (bradykinesia) is an additional handicap, distinct from rigidity. There is difficulty initiating movement. Rapid fine finger movements, such as piano-playing, become indistinct, slow and tremulous. Facial immobility gives a mask-like semblance of depression. The frequency of spontaneous blinking is reduced, producing a 'serpentine' stare.

Postural changes

A stoop is characteristic. Gait becomes, hurrying (festinant) and shuffling with poor arm swinging. The posture is sometimes called 'simian' to describe the ape-like forward flexion, immobility and lack of animation. Balance deteriorates, but despite this the gait retains a narrow base. Falls are common in later stages of PD, the sufferer toppling like a falling tree.

Speech

Pronunciation is initially a monotone but progresses to characteristic tremulous slurring dysarthria, the result of combined akinesia, tremor and rigidity. Speech may eventually be lost completely (anarthria).

Gastrointestinal and other symptoms

These include heartburn, dribbling, dysphagia, constipation and weight loss. Urinary difficulties are common, especially in men. Skin is greasy and sweating excessive.

Natural history and other features

Parkinson's disease worsens over some years, beginning as a mild inconvenience but slowly progressing. Remissions are unknown except for rare and remarkable short-lived periods of release. These tend to occur at times of great emotion, fear or excitement, when the sufferer is released for seconds or minutes and able to move quickly.

While bradykinesia and tremor worsen, power remains normal until immobility makes its assessment difficult. Patients often complain bitterly of limb and joint discomfort. There is no sensory loss. The reflexes are brisk; their asymmetry follows the increase in tone. The plantar responses remain flexor. Cognitive function is preserved, at least early on. Dementia often develops in the late stages. Anxiety and depression are common.

The rate of progression is very variable, with a benign form running over several decades. Usually the course is over 10–15 years, with death resulting from bronchopneumonia.

Diagnosis

There is no laboratory test – the diagnosis is made by recognizing physical signs and distinguishing idiopathic PD from other parkinsonian syndromes. Conventional imaging (MR) is normal. Dopamine transporter imaging (available in some specialist centres) discriminates poorly – both between normal and pathological and between PD and other akinetic–rigid syndromes.

Other diffuse and multifocal brain diseases can cause features of parkinsonism, i.e. the slowing, rigidity and tremor seen in idiopathic PD. Examples are Alzheimer's disease, multi-infarct dementia, sequelae of repeated head injury (e.g. in boxers, p. 1250), and the late effects of severe hypoxia or carbon monoxide poisoning. Slowing also occurs in hypothyroidism, and in depression.

Treatment

While no drugs alter the course of Parkinson's disease, levodopa and/or dopaminergic agonists produce striking initial symptomatic improvement. These drugs should be avoided until they are clinically necessary because of delayed unwanted effects (see below). Catechol-*O*-methyl transferase inhibitors are also used as supplementary therapy. Older treatments such as the antimuscarinic trihexyphenidyl (benzhexol) helped little and frequently caused confusion; they are of some value in severe tremor. Selegeline, a monoamine oxidase B inhibitor, may delay the need for levodopa therapy by

Fig. 21.29 **Drugs in Parkinson's disease: a nigrostriatal neurone and striatal dopamine receptors.**
Levodopa crosses the blood–brain barrier, enters a neurone and is converted to dopamine.

A. Carbidopa and benserazide reduce peripheral conversion of levodopa to dopamine by AAAD, thus reducing side-effects of excess circulating dopamine.
B. Dietary amino acids from a high-protein meal may inhibit active transport into brain by competing with levodopa.
C. Levodopa is converted (AAAD) to dopamine in nigrostriatal neurones.
D. At the nerve terminal, amantadine enhances dopamine release.
E. Dopamine agonist drugs react with dopamine receptors.
F. Selegeline, the MAO-B inhibitor, blocks dopamine breakdown.
G. Entacapone, a COMT inhibitor, prolongs dopamine activity by blocking breakdown.

AAAD, aromatic amino acid decarboxylase; COMT, catechol-O-methyl transferase.

some months. Antioxidants are also used with this aim, but their value is unproven. A scheme for the mechanism of action of drugs in Parkinson's disease is shown in Figure 21.29.

Levodopa

Levodopa is combined with an aromatic amino acid decarboxylase inhibitor – benserazide (co-beneldopa, as Madopar) or carbidopa (co-careldopa, as Sinemet). The decarboxylase inhibitor reduces peripheral side-effects, principally nausea, of levodopa and its metabolites. Levodopa treatment is commenced (co-beneldopa 62.5 mg or co-careldopa 110 mg, one tablet three times daily) and gradually increased.

The great majority of patients with idiopathic PD (but not other parkinsonian syndromes) improve initially with levodopa. The response in severe, previously untreated idiopathic PD is sometimes dramatic.

Unwanted effects of levodopa therapy

Nausea and vomiting are the most common immediate symptoms of excess levodopa. Confusion, formed visual pseudo-hallucinations and chorea also occur. There are difficult issues with long-term therapy (e.g. levodopa-induced involuntary movements). After several years levodopa gradually becomes ineffective, even with increasing doses. As treatment continues, episodes of immobility develop (freezing). Falls are common. Fluctuation in response to levodopa also appears, its effect apparently turning on and off, causing freezing alternating with dopa-induced dyskinesias, chorea and dystonic movements. Levodopa's duration of action shrinks, with dyskinesia becoming prominent several hours after a dose (end-of-dose dyskinesia). The patient also begins to suffer from a chronic levodopa-induced movement disorder.

Levodopa therapy does not alter the natural progression of idiopathic PD. After 5 years' treatment, around half of Parkinson's patients suffer from minor or major unwanted effects of therapy. The more distressing problems are often largely insoluble. Approaches to treatment of these complications include:

- Shortening the interval between levodopa doses and increasing each dose.
- Selegiline, a type B monoamine oxidase inhibitor, inhibits catabolism of dopamine in the brain. This sometimes smoothes out the response to levodopa.
- Dopaminergic agonists (see below) are added, or replace levodopa.
- Entacapone (a catechol-O-methyl transferase inhibitor) is used.
- Drug holidays – periods of drug withdrawal – are occasionally helpful. They require close supervision since severe relapse may follow levodopa withdrawal.

Dopamine receptor agonists

Bromocriptine, lisuride, pergolide, cabergoline (ergot derivatives), pramipexole and ropinirole are oral directly acting dopamine receptor agonists, acting principally on D_1 and D_2 receptors, and also on receptors D_{3-5}. These are used as an alternative or an addition to levodopa therapy. The ergot derivatives are associated with pulmonary, retroperitoneal and pericardial fibrotic reactions.

Apomorphine, a potent D_1 and D_2 agonist given by subcutaneous metered infusion is an effective method of smoothing out fluctuations in response to levodopa. Skilled nursing is required to train patients and relatives to set up the infusion pump. Vomiting is common. Haemolytic anaemia is an unusual side-effect.

Dopamine receptor agonists are in general less effective than levodopa in treating symptoms in Parkinson's disease, but cause fewer late unwanted dyskinesias.

There is much variation in clinical practice between different regimens of levodopa and dopamine receptor agonists. There is a trend towards the use of receptor agonists as primary treatment (before levodopa) and to delaying starting any drugs until it is clinically essential. Directly acting agonists are usually used below the age of 70, and levodopa for older cases.

Other agents

Antioxidant compounds such as vitamins C and E (possible neuroprotective agents) are sometimes suggested. Their role is uncertain. Amantadine, originally marketed as an antiviral drug, occasionally has a modest effect. Rivastigmine is helpful for the dementia.

Stereotactic neurosurgery

Stereotactic lesions, usually unilateral in the ventrolateral nucleus of the thalamus (thalamotomy) or in the globus pallidus (pallidotomy), were used widely before levodopa. Surgery still provides effective, if temporary improvement in tremor and dyskinesia with minor relief of bradykinesia. Thalamic stimulation is also used. There has been a revival of interest in surgery in the last decade.

Tissue transplantation

Despite early promise and suggestive laboratory studies in rats with MPTP-induced parkinsonism, tissue transplantation is little used. Experimental transplantation of fetal or autologous dopamine-containing adrenal medulla and glial cell-line neurotrophic releasing factor (GDNF) into the cerebral ventricles or basal ganglia, does not produce any sustained improvement.

Physiotherapy and physical aids

Skilled and determined therapy can improve gait and help overcome particular problems. Practical guidance is of value:

- clothing – avoid zips, fiddly buttons and lace-up shoes
- cutlery – use built-up handles
- chairs – high upright rather than deep, low chairs
- rails – near lavatory and bath
- shoes – should be easy to put on and have smooth soles
- flooring – vinyl is safer than loose carpets.

Walking aids are often a hindrance early on, but later a frame or a tripod may help. All efforts must be made to avoid falls.

Psychiatric aspects

Depression is common as PD progresses. Selective serotonin reuptake inhibitors (SSRIs) are the drugs of choice. Tricyclic antidepressants (e.g. amitriptyline) have extrapyramidal side-effects. Type A monoamine oxidase inhibitors (e.g. phenelzine) are absolutely contraindicated with levodopa.

All antiparkinsonian drugs can cause visual hallucinations, especially at night, and exacerbate cognitive impairment.

OTHER AKINETIC–RIGID SYNDROMES

Drug-induced parkinsonism

Reserpine and methyldopa (drugs once used to treat hypertension), phenothiazines and butyrophenones induce parkinsonism, with slowness and rigidity but usually little tremor. Tricyclic antidepressants also cause some slowing. These unwanted effects tend not to progress and settle when a drug is stopped. They respond negligibly to levodopa.

Neuroleptics and movement disorders

Neuroleptics (i.e. phenothiazines and butyrophenones) also produce movement disorders.

- **Akathisia**. This is a restless, repetitive and irresistible need to move.
- **Acute dystonic reactions**. These occur (dramatically and unpredictably) after single doses of neuroleptics and related drugs widely used as antiemetics and vestibular sedatives (e.g. metoclopramide and prochlorperazine). Spasmodic torticollis, trismus and oculogyric crises (i.e. episodes of sustained upward gaze) occur. These acute dystonias respond promptly to i.v. antimuscarinics, e.g. benzatropine (1–2 mg) or procyclidine 5–10 mg. The offending drug (and all similar) should be avoided forever.
- **Chronic tardive dyskinesias**. These are mouthing and lip-smacking grimaces, disabling disorders that occur several years after commencing neuroleptics. They often become temporarily worse when the neuroleptic dose is reduced. Resolution seldom occurs, even if treatment ceases.

Post-encephalitic parkinsonism and MPTP (see p. 1228)

Parkinsonism-plus

This describes rare disorders in which there is parkinsonism with additional features and pathology. *Progressive supranuclear palsy* (Steele–Richardson–Olzewski syndrome) is the commonest. It consists of parkinsonism, axial rigidity, falls, dementia, and inability to move the eyes vertically or laterally. Other examples are multiple system atrophies, such as olivo-ponto-cerebellar degeneration and primary autonomic failure (Shy–Drager syndrome).

These are progressive, unresponsive to levodopa and usually cause death within a decade.

Akinetic–rigid syndromes in children

Several extremely rare disorders cause akinetic–rigid syndromes with onset under 20 years.

Wilson's disease

This rare but treatable disorder of copper metabolism is inherited as an autosomal recessive. Copper deposition occurs in the brain, particularly in the basal ganglia, in the cornea and liver (p. 387), where it causes cirrhosis. All young patients either with an akinetic–rigid syndrome or with cirrhosis should be screened for Wilson's disease. Neurological damage is reversible with early treatment. This akinetic–rigid syndrome and/or dyskinesias is followed by progressive intellectual impairment. Diagnosis and treatment with the chelating agent penicillamine is discussed on page 388.

Athetoid cerebral palsy

Writhing movements, sometimes with progressive dystonia, occur in cerebral palsy following kernicterus.

This is now rare following prophylactic eradication of rhesus haemolytic disease with anti-D immunoglobulin.

DYSKINESIAS

Benign essential tremor

This common condition, often inherited as an autosomal dominant trait, causes 5–8 Hz tremor, usually worse in the upper limbs. The head is often tremulous (titubation) and also the trunk. Pathologically there is patchy neuronal loss in the cerebellum and its connections. Tremor develops when the hands adopt a posture, such as holding a glass or a spoon. Essential tremor occurs at any age but occurs most frequently in the elderly. It is slowly progressive but rarely produces severe disability. Writing is shaky and untidy: micrographia is absent. Anxiety exacerbates the tremor, sometimes dramatically. In essential tremor, shaking occasionally occurs at rest, as in Parkinson's disease, or on action, as in cerebellar disease.

Treatment is often unnecessary, and unsatisfactory. Many patients are reassured to find they do not have Parkinson's disease, with which essential tremor is often confused.

Small amounts of alcohol, β-adrenergic blockers (propranolol) and the anticonvulsant primidone may help the tremor: sympathomimetics (e.g. salbutamol) make it worse. The antidepressant mirtazapine has some effect. Stereotactic thalamotomy and thalamic stimulation are used in severe cases.

Chorea

Chorea means jerky, quasi-purposive, explosive, fidgety movements, flitting around the body – causes are listed in Table 21.40.

Huntington's disease

Relentlessly progressive chorea and dementia, usually in middle life but sometimes in childhood, are hallmarks of this inherited disease. Prevalence world-wide is about 5 in 100 000. Inheritance is as an autosomal dominant trait with full penetrance: children of an affected parent have a

Table 21.40 Causes of chorea
Huntington's disease
Sydenham's chorea
Benign hereditary chorea
Abetalipoproteinaemia (see p. 308) with chorea
Chorea associated with:
Drugs – phenytoin, levodopa, alcohol
Thyrotoxicosis, pregnancy and oral contraceptive pill
Systemic lupus erythematosus
Polycythaemia vera
Encephalitis lethargica
Stroke (basal ganglia)
Rarities (tumour, trauma, subdural haematoma, following carbon monoxide poisoning, paroxysmal choreoathetosis, Wilson's disease, dentato-rubro-pallido-luysian atrophy)

50% chance of developing Huntington's disease. Previous family history is often concealed, sometimes deliberately. A mutation occurs in the distal short arm of chromosome 4 (4p16.3) with a variable expansion of a CAG-repeat sequence located in exon 1 of a large gene containing 67 exons. This results in translation of an extended glutamine sequence in *huntingtin*, the protein product of the gene. Huntingtin is expressed throughout the body. Its function is unclear. Most adult-onset HD cases have CAG expansions of 40–55 repeats, while greater expansions (> 70 repeats) are seen in childhood-onset HD.

Pathology

Cerebral atrophy progresses, with marked loss of small neurones in the caudate nucleus and putamen.

Changes in neurotransmitters occur:

- *reduced* acetylcholine synthesis (due to reduced choline acetyl transferase) and GABA in the striatum
- *increased* transglutaminase (catalyses aggregates of *huntingtin*) in cortex, cerebellum and corpus striatum
- *depleted* GABA, angiotensin-converting enzyme and met-enkephalin in substantia nigra
- *high* somatostatin levels in the corpus striatum.

These may be secondary to cell damage. In contrast to Parkinson's disease, dopamine and tyrosine hydroxylase remain normal.

Management and course

Other causes of chorea should be investigated. Imaging in Huntington's, if practical with the chorea, shows caudate nucleus atrophy. There is steady progression, of both dementia and chorea. While nothing arrests this, phenothiazines (e.g. sulpiride) and tetrabenazine reduce chorea. Death usually occurs 10–20 years from the onset.

Mutation analysis is used for presymptomatic testing. Test centres have a national protocol for counselling families and addressing the ethical issues.

Sydenham's chorea (St Vitus's dance)

This transient postinfective chorea occurs largely in children and young adults. Streptococcal infection is one cause: under half the cases follow within 3 months of rheumatic fever (p. 76). Sydenham's may recur, or appear, in adult life, during pregnancy as chorea gravidarum and with hormonal contraceptives. There is a diffuse mild encephalitis.

The onset is gradual over a few weeks. Irritability, emotional lability, and inattentiveness herald fidgetiness, sometimes mainly unilateral. A minority of patients become confused. Rheumatic heart disease is sometimes found. Fever is unusual. Antistreptolysin-O (ASO) titre and ESR are typically normal. Sedation may be needed. Recovery occurs spontaneously within weeks or months. Phenoxymethylpenicillin should continue to the age of 20 to prevent rheumatic heart disease.

Hemiballismus (see p. 1194 and Fig. 21.9)

Hemiballismus (also called hemiballism) describes violent swinging movements of one side caused usually by infarction or haemorrhage in the contralateral subthalamic nucleus.

Myoclonus

Myoclonus is sudden, involuntary jerking of a single muscle or a group of muscles. It occurs in a wide range of disorders and is sometimes provoked by sudden stimuli such as loud noise. Piracetam is used for cortical myoclonus.

Benign essential myoclonus

Nocturnal myoclonus – sudden jerking (often with a feeling of falling) on dropping off to sleep – is common and not pathological. Periodic limb movements (repetitive dorsiflexion of the great toe or plantar flexion of the foot during Stage I or II sleep) are brief and occur in restless leg syndrome (p. 666).

Paramyoclonus multiplex describes widespread, random muscle jerking usually occurring in adolescence. Fits do not occur.

Myoclonus in epilepsy

Muscle jerking occurs in many different forms of epilepsy. An antiepileptic drug, e.g. valproate, may be helpful.

Progressive myoclonic epilepsies

These rare conditions include familial and metabolic disorders where myoclonus accompanies progressive encephalopathy. *Lafora body disease* is one example, consisting of myoclonus, epilepsy, dementia, with mucopolysaccharide inclusions in neurones, liver cells and intestinal mucosa.

Static myoclonic encephalopathy

Non-progressive myoclonus sometimes develops following recovery from severe cerebral anoxia.

Non-organic muscle jerking.

This is sometimes volitional, or seen in psychiatric conditions, e.g. somatization, non-epileptic attacks and malingering.

Tics

Some idiosyncratic movement of the face, neck or hand is part of our normal motor gestures. Patients or relatives seek advice when movements become frequent or irritating. Simple transient tics (e.g. sniffing or a particular facial grimace) are common in childhood, but may persist. The borderland between normal and pathological is vague.

Gilles de la Tourette syndrome

This describes multiple tics (motor and speech) with behavioural problems including the attention-deficit-hyperactivity disorder (ADHD) and the obsessive–compulsive disorder (OCD). This develops in childhood or adolescence, more commonly in males, and is lifelong. There is sometimes explosive barking and grunting of obscenities and gestures. The cause is believed to be an

Table 21.41   A classification of dystonias

Generalized dystonia
Primary torsion dystonia (PTD)
Dopamine-responsive dystonia (DRD)
Drug-induced dystonia (e.g. metoclopramide)
Symptomatic dystonia (e.g. after encephalitis lethargica or in Wilson's disease)
Paroxysmal dystonia (very rare, familial, with marked fluctuation)

Focal dystonia
Spasmodic torticollis
Writer's cramp
Oromandibular dystonia
Blepharospasm
Hemiplegic dystonia (e.g. following stroke)
Multiple sclerosis

inherited disorder of synaptic transmission. Haloperidol is sometimes helpful.

Torsion dystonias

Dystonia means movement caused by prolonged muscular contraction – part of the body is thrown into spasm. A brief explanatory classification of these unusual basal ganglia conditions is given in Table 21.41. Their causes are largely unknown.

Primary torsion dystonia (dystonia musculorum deformans)

Dystonia affecting gait and posture in childhood progresses, spreading to all parts of the body over one to four decades. Cognitive function is not impaired. Spontaneous remissions occur occasionally. This rare disease is usually inherited as an autosomal dominant. A PTD gene has been located on chromosome 9 (9q34); this is a deletion of three base pairs encoding an ATP-binding protein torsin A.

Dopamine-responsive dystonia (DRD)

This lower limb dystonia is almost completely abolished by small doses of levodopa. Typically dystonic walking begins in childhood – and may resemble a spastic paraparesis. The usual form is autosomal dominant DRD with a point mutation of the GTP cyclohydrolase 1 gene on chromosome 14q22.3. Patients with other odd dystonic gaits are sometimes given test doses of levodopa.

Spasmodic torticollis

Dystonic spasms gradually develop around the neck, usually in the third to fifth decade. These cause the head to turn (torticollis) or to be drawn backwards (retrocollis) or forwards (antecollis). Minor dystonic movements often also affect the trunk and limbs. A curious feature in some patients is a single trigger area, often on the jaw. A gentle touch with a finger tip at this specific site relieves the spasm temporarily. Torticollis may remit but often persists indefinitely. Similar features are sometimes seen when no organic disease is present.

Writer's cramp

This is a specific inability to perform a previously highly developed repetitive skilled movement, e.g. writing. The movement provokes dystonic posturing. Writer's cramp occurs in those who spend many hours each day *writing*, and is thus seen less frequently than in years past. Other functions of the hand remain normal. There are no other neurological signs. Prolonged rest sometimes helps but the dystonia can cause substantial disability. Similar dystonias occur in other occupations.

Blepharospasm and oromandibular dystonia

These consist of spasms of forced blinking or involuntary movement of the mouth and tongue (e.g. lip-smacking and protrusion of the tongue and jaw). Speech may be affected.

Treatment

All dystonic movement disorders are particularly difficult to help. Butyrophenones (e.g. haloperidol and sulpiride) and antimuscarinics (e.g. trihexyphenidyl (benzhexol)) are sometimes helpful. Botulinum toxin carefully sited by injection can help, temporarily, blepharospasm, torticollis and writer's cramp. Neurosurgical treatment, principally stereotactic thalamotomy for torticollis, or neurostimulation brings some temporary alleviation in selected cases.

FURTHER READING
Bates G (2003) Huntingtin aggregation and toxicity in Huntington's disease. *Lancet* **361**: 1642–1644.
Brooks DJ (2000) Dopamine agonists: their role in the treatment of Parkinson's disease. *Journal of Neurology Neurosurgery and Psychiatry* **68**: 685–690.
Deuschl G (2000) New treatment options for tremor. *New England Journal of Medicine* **342**: 505–507.
Hallett M (1999) One man's poison – clinical applications of botulinum toxin. *New England Journal of Medicine* **341**: 119–120.
Hardy J et al. (2003) Genes and parkinsonism. *Lancet (Neurology)* **2**: 221–228.
Leckman JF (2002) Tourette's syndrome. *Lancet* **360**: 1577–1586.
Lücking C et al. (2000) Association between early-onset PD and mutations in the parkin gene. *New England Journal of Medicine* **342**: 1560–1567.
Nussbaum RL et al. (2003) Genomic medicine: Alzheimer's disease and Parkinson's disease. *New England Journal of Medicine* **348**: 1356–1364.
Samii A, Nutt JG, Ransom BR (2004) Parkinson's disease. *Lancet* **363**: 1783–1793.

MULTIPLE SCLEROSIS (MS)

MS is a chronic inflammatory disorder of the central nervous system. There are multiple plaques of demyelination within the brain and spinal cord. Plaques are 'disseminated in time and place', hence the old name disseminated sclerosis.

Prevalence

MS prevalence varies widely, being directly proportional to distance of residence from the equator. At latitudes of 50–65° N (roughly from southern England to Iceland) prevalence is 60–100 per 100 000; at latitudes less than 30° N prevalence is below 10/100 000. At the equator MS is a rarity. Dietary factors, e.g. high animal fat consumption, had been suggested for this geographical distribution but there is little evidence for this. In the southern hemisphere this trend is similar – increasing prevalence with distance from the equator. Overall, in Europe and N America the annual incidence is 2–10 per 100 000, making it the most common neurological disease in young adults.

Aetiopathogenesis

Although the precise mechanism is unknown, there is an inflammatory process against self molecules in the white matter of the brain and spinal cord mediated by CD4 T cells. In the active lesions (plaques) there is an increase in inflammatory cells, active myelin degradation and phagocytosis. Lymphocytes and monocytes gain access to the brain parenchyma from the circulation by adhering to vascular endothelial cells via the glycoprotein $\alpha_4\beta_1$, integrin expressed on their surface. This integrin (also known as very late antigen VLA_4) is also a regulator of immune-cell activation.

An initial inflammatory demyelinating event may prime autoreactive cellular and humoral immune responses against myelin. Antibody-mediated demyelination, e.g. against myelin basic protein, may present early in MS. Antibodies against myelin oligodendrocyte glycoprotein (MOG) – a protein which is specific to the CNS – have also been found in vitro.

Familial incidence, HLA linkage and migration

First-degree relatives of a patient have an increased chance of developing MS, without a clear-cut pattern of inheritance.

The concordance rate is 31% in monozygotic twins.

In Caucasians in northern Europe and the USA, there is a weak association between MS and antigens HLA-A3, B7, D2 and DR2.

Immigrants from low to high prevalence zones (e.g. from the equator to northern Europe) *acquire* the prevalence of their destination, provided they arrive before the age of 10.

Infection

Efforts to transmit MS experimentally have been uniformly unsuccessful. However, an abnormal immune response in many MS patients produces increased titres of serum and CSF antibodies to many common viruses, particularly measles. Some epidemic transmissible zoonoses, such as scrapie (demyelinating disease in sheep), have some similarities to MS. In man, human T-cell leukaemia virus 1 (HTLV-1) causes tropical spastic paraparesis, but no other features seen in MS. Chlamydia has been questioned as a cause. No known links exist between MS and any infection.

Fig. 21.30 **Multiple sclerosis.** Cross-section of the spinal cord showing demyelination (arrows) in the posterior column and lateral corticospinal tracts. Courtesy of Professor WI Macdonald.

Pathology (Fig. 21.30)

Plaques of demyelination, initially 2–10 mm in size are the cardinal features. Plaques are perivenular with a predilection for distinct CNS sites: optic nerves, the periventricular region, brainstem and its cerebellar connections and the cervical spinal cord (corticospinal tracts and posterior columns).

Acute relapses are caused by focal inflammatory demyelination, which causes a conduction block. Inflammation induces local production of nitric oxide by macrophages, which damages central nerve fibres. *Remission* follows as inflammation subsides. Remyelination occurs and helps recovery. When damage is severe, secondary permanent axonal destruction occurs. In the cord, plaques rarely destroy large groups of anterior horn cells – thus focal muscle wasting (e.g. small hand muscles) is unusual. MS plaques are not seen in myelin sheaths of peripheral nerves.

Clinical features

The commonest age of onset is between 20 and 45 years, a diagnosis before puberty or after 60 years is rare. MS is more common in women. No single group of signs or symptoms is absolutely diagnostic. Despite this, MS is often recognizable clinically by different patterns:

- relapsing and remitting MS (80–90%)
- primary progressive MS (10–20% of cases)
- secondary progressive MS – this follows on from relapsing/remitting disease
- occasionally (<10%) MS runs a fulminating course over some months (fulminant MS).

Three characteristic common presentations of relapsing and remitting MS are described below.

Optic neuropathy (ON)
Symptoms
Blurring of vision in one eye develops over hours or days, varying between a 'looking through frosted glass' sensation to severe unilateral visual loss, but rarely complete blindness. Mild ocular pain is usual. Recovery

occurs, typically within 2 months. Bilateral ON occasionally occurs.

Signs

The optic disc appearance depends upon the site of the plaque within the optic nerve. When the lesion is in the nerve *head* there is disc swelling (optic neuritis, p. 1181). If the lesion is several millimetres *behind the disc* there are often no ophthalmoscopic abnormalities – 'the doctor sees nothing and the patient sees nothing'. This is *retrobulbar neuritis* (p. 1181).

Worsening of vision in ON during a fever, hot weather or after exercise is known as Uthoff's phenomenon – central conduction is slowed by an increase in local body temperature.

Disc swelling from optic neuritis causes early visual acuity loss, thus distinguishing it from disc swelling from raised intracranial pressure – the latter causes little or no visual loss early on, but sudden visual loss in advanced stages.

A relative afferent pupillary defect (p. 1182) in optic neuropathy is often found, and persists after recovery.

Late sequelae of optic neuropathy

There is often no residual loss of vision, but small scotomata and defects in colour vision can be found. Following optic neuropathy, disc pallor appears (optic atrophy), first on the temporal side. Visual evoked responses (VER) remain abnormal (see below and page 1203).

Brainstem demyelination

Acute MS in the brainstem causes combinations of diplopia, vertigo, facial numbness/weakness, dysarthria or dysphagia. Pyramidal signs in the limbs occur when the corticospinal tracts are involved. A typical picture is sudden diplopia, and vertigo with nystagmus, but without tinnitus or deafness. This lasts for some weeks before recovery. Diplopia in MS is produced by many lesions – a sixth nerve lesion and internuclear ophthalmoplegia (INO, p. 1183) are two examples.

Spinal cord lesion

Spastic paraparesis developing over days or weeks (p. 1192) is a typical result of a plaque in the cervical or thoracic cord, causing difficulty in walking and numbness. Lhermitte's sign may be present (p. 1199). Urinary symptoms are common.

Unusual presentations

Epilepsy and trigeminal neuralgia (p. 1186) occur more commonly in MS patients than in the general population. Tonic spasms (brief spasms of one limb) are other unusual presentations. Organic psychosis is occasionally seen in early MS.

End-stage multiple sclerosis

Late MS causes severe disability with spastic tetraparesis, ataxia, optic atrophy, nystagmus, brainstem signs (e.g. bilateral INO), pseudobulbar palsy, and urinary incontinence. Dementia is common. Death follows from uraemia and/or bronchopneumonia.

Differential diagnosis

Few other neurological diseases follow a similar relapsing and remitting course. Thromboembolism causes events with more sudden onset. Other degenerative conditions, such as Friedreich's ataxia, are gradually progressive. Following an isolated neurological event it is often impossible to be sure, even with MR imaging, whether or not MS is the diagnosis. The pattern of subsequent lesions leads to the diagnosis. Remissions may last for several or more years; their length is unpredictable and the mechanism of relapse and remission unclear.

Individual plaques (e.g. in optic nerve, brainstem or cord) must be distinguished from mass, vascular or other inflammatory lesions. Of the latter, CNS sarcoidosis, SLE and Behçet's syndrome may mimic relapsing MS. Adrenoleucodystrophy (an inherited disorder of saturated fatty acid deposition in lipid-containing tissues) can cause a progressive paraparesis identical to chronic progressive MS (p. 1234).

Investigations

- *MRI* of brain and spinal cord is the definitive investigation. Multiple plaques are visible, principally in the periventricular region (Fig. 21.31), brainstem, and cervical cord. Head MRI scans show lesions in 85% of patients with clinical MS. Typical lesions are multifocal with 10 or more lesions seen in a clinical relapse. Plaques are rarely visible on CT.
- *CSF examination* is often unnecessary with diagnostic MR and a compatible clinical picture. CSF analysis shows oligoclonal IgG bands in 80% of cases but these are not specific as they simply indicate immunoglobulin production within the CNS in response to an unknown antigen. The CSF cell count is raised (5–60 mononuclears/mm^3).
- *Electrophysiological tests.* Delay in visual-evoked responses (VER) is seen in optic neuropathy. Some ON attacks are subclinical: a delayed VER provides evidence of a previous optic nerve lesion. This is helpful for diagnosis if there had been, for example, an undiagnosed and apparently solitary spinal cord lesion. Brainstem and somatosensory evoked poten-

Fig. 21.31 **MR (T2): Multiple sclerosis.** The arrows point to the demyelinating lesions.

tials become delayed when these pathways have been damaged. Peripheral nerve studies are normal and EEG unhelpful.

- *Blood/urine* tests are unhelpful.

Management and prognosis

Once diagnosed, practical decisions need to be taken about employment, home and plans for the future in the face of a potentially disabling disease. There is no curative treatment.

The course of MS is unpredictable but a florid MRI lesion load at first presentation is a strong predictor of future disability. There is wide variation in severity. Many patients continue to live self-sufficient, productive lives: others become gravely disabled.

Straightforward advice, tempered with reassurance of the benign course of many cases of MS is necessary. The MS Society, a national UK charity, and others have helpful literature.

MS therapies

Many forms of treatment have been marketed, among them cryotherapy, pyrotherapy, radiotherapy, various vaccines, purified TB protein derivative (PPD), transfer factor, electrical stimulation, gluten-free diets, sunflower seed oil, arsenicals, vitamins and hyperbaric oxygen. None has been shown to improve outcome.

- *Acute relapses.* Short courses of corticosteroids, such as i.v. methylprednisolone 1 g/day for 3 days or high-dose oral steroids, are used widely in relapses and do sometimes reduce severity. They do not influence long-term outcome.
- *Preventing relapse and disability.* Beta-interferon (both INF-β1b and 1a) by self-administered injection is used in relapsing and remitting disease. This is defined as at least two attacks of neurological dysfunction over the previous 2 or 3 years followed by a reasonable recovery. IFN-β1b is also now licensed for secondary progressive MS. Interferon reduces the relapse rate in some patients and prevents an increase in lesions seen on MRI. Long-term outcome seems unaltered. Unwanted effects are flu-like symptoms and irritation at injection sites. Cost–benefit analyses are serious issues: beta-interferons are expensive.
- *Immunosuppressants* (azathioprine, cyclophosphamide) are also used, but controlled trials have shown no benefit
- *Other therapies,* such as glatiramer acetate, reduce relapse frequency. Mitoxantrone is also being evaluated.

The rehabilitative approach in MS

Much can be done for someone with any chronic disabling disease. Practical advice at work, on walking aids, wheelchairs, car conversions, alterations to houses and gardens is needed, from professionals with experience of rehabilitation. Wide-ranging support – for fear, reactive depression and sexual difficulties – is also helpful. Multidisciplinary team liaison between patient, carers, doctors and therapists is essential.

Treat all infections. Urinary infection frequently exacerbates symptoms. Urinary incontinence may be helped by oxybutinin and/or intermittent self-catheterization.

Physiotherapy is of particular value in reducing pain and discomfort of spasticity, particularly lower limb flexor spasms. Muscle relaxants (e.g. baclofen, benzodiazepines, dantrolene and tizanidine) are sometimes helpful. Injected botulinum toxin is used for severe spasticity. Cannabis is used by many patients for painful spasms. Cannabis extracts (e.g. Sativea) are being evaluated. Prevention of pressure sores is vital. Amantadine is sometimes used for general fatigue.

FURTHER READING

Confaureux C et al. (2000) Relapses and progression of disability in multiple sclerosis. *New England Journal of Medicine* **343**: 1430–1438.

Filippi M, Rocca MA, Comi G (2003) The use of quantitative MR-based techniques to monitor the evolution of multiple sclerosis. *Lancet (Neurology)* **2**: 337–346.

Hickman SJ et al. (2002) Management of optic neuritis. *Lancet* **360**: 1953–1962.

Levin LI, Munger KL, Rubertone MV et al. (2003) Multiple sclerosis and Epstein–Barr virus. *Journal of the American Medical Association* **289**: 1533–1536.

Paty DW, Arnold DL (2002) The lesions of multiple sclerosis. *New England Journal of Medicine* **346**: 199–200.

Polman CH, Uitdehaag B (2003) New and emerging treatment options for MS. *Lancet (Neurology)* **2**: 563–566.

UK NATIONAL CHARITY

The MS Society: http://www.mssociety.org.uk

CNS INFECTION AND INFLAMMATION

MENINGITIS

Meningitis means inflammation but usually implies serious infection of the meninges (Table 21.42). Microorganisms reach the meninges either by direct extension from the ears, nasopharynx, cranial injury or congenital meningeal defect, or by bloodstream spread. Immunocompromised patients (e.g. HIV, cytotoxic drugs) are at risk of infection by unusual organisms. Non-infectious causes of inflammation include malignant cells, drugs and blood following subarachnoid haemorrhage.

Pathology

In acute bacterial meningitis, the pia–arachnoid is congested with polymorphs. A layer of pus forms. This may organize to form adhesions, causing cranial nerve palsies and hydrocephalus.

In chronic infection (e.g. TB), the brain is covered in a viscous grey-green exudate with numerous meningeal

Table 21.42   Infective causes of meningitis in the UK

Bacteria
*Neisseria meningitidis**
*Streptococcus pneumoniae**
Staphylococcus aureus
Streptococcus Group B
Listeria monocytogenes
Gram-negative bacilli
Mycobacterium tuberculosis
Treponema pallidum

Viruses
Enteroviruses:
    ECHO
    Coxsackie
Mumps
Herpes simplex
HIV
Epstein–Barr virus

Fungi
Cryptococcus neoformans
Candida
(*Coccidioides immitis, Histoplasma capsulatum,*
Blastomyces dermatitidis in USA)

*These organisms account for 70% of acute bacterial meningitis outside the neonatal period. A wide variety of infective agents are responsible for the remaining 30% of cases. *Haemophilus influenzae* b (Hib) has been eliminated as a cause in many countries by immunization

Table 21.43   Clinical clues in meningitis

Clinical feature	Probable cause
Petechial rash	Meningococcal infection
Skull fracture	Pneumococcal infection
Ear disease	
Congenital CNS lesion	
Immunocompromised patients	HIV opportunistic infection
Rash or pleuritic pain	Enterovirus infection
International travel	Poliomyelitis
	Malaria
	Leptospirosis
Occupational history (working in drains, canals, polluted water, recreational swimming): prostration, myalgia, conjunctivitis, jaundice	

tubercles. Adhesions are invariable. Cerebral oedema occurs in any bacterial meningitis.

In viral meningitis there is a predominantly lymphocytic inflammatory CSF reaction without pus formation, polymorphs or adhesions; there is little or no cerebral oedema unless encephalitis develops.

Clinical features

The meningitic syndrome
This is a simple triad: headache, neck stiffness and fever. Photophobia and vomiting are often present. In acute bacterial infection there is usually intense malaise, fever, rigors, severe headache, photophobia and vomiting. This develops within hours or minutes. The patient is irritable and often prefers to lie still. Neck stiffness and positive Kernig's sign usually appear within hours.

In less severe cases (e.g. many viral meningitides) there are less prominent meningitic signs, but fatal bacterial infection may also be indolent, with a deceptively mild onset. Clinical pictures that are apparently mild are unreliable and lead to fatal misjudgements.

In uncomplicated meningitis, consciousness remains intact, although anyone with high fever may be delirious. Progressive drowsiness, lateralizing signs and cranial nerve lesions indicate complications such as venous sinus thrombosis (p. 1219), severe cerebral oedema, hydrocephalus, or an alternative diagnosis such as cerebral abscess (p. 1243) or encephalitis (p. 1239). Papilloedema may develop.

Specific varieties of meningitis
Clinical clues point to the diagnosis (Table 21.43). If there is access to the subarachnoid space via skull fracture (recent or old) or occult spina bifida, bacterial meningitis can be recurrent – and the infecting organism usually pneumococcus.

Acute bacterial meningitis
Onset is typically sudden, with rigors and high fever. *Meningococcal* meningitis is often heralded by a petechial or other rash, sometimes sparse (see Emergency box 21.1). The meningitis may be part of a generalized meningococcal septicaemia (p. 75). Acute septicaemic shock may develop in any bacterial meningitis.

Viral meningitis
This is almost always a benign, self-limiting condition lasting 4–10 days. Headache may follow for some months. There are no serious sequelae.

Chronic meningitis (see below)

Differential diagnosis
It may be difficult to distinguish between the sudden headache of subarachnoid haemorrhage, migraine and acute meningitis. Meningitis should be considered seriously in anyone with headache and fever and in any sudden headache. Neck stiffness should be assessed carefully – it may not be obvious. Chronic meningitis sometimes resembles an intracranial mass lesion, with headache, epilepsy and focal signs. Cerebral malaria often mimics bacterial meningitis.

Management (Emergency Box 21.1)
Recognition and immediate treatment of acute bacterial meningitis is vital. Minutes save lives. Bacterial meningitis is lethal. Even with optimal care, mortality is around 15%.

When meningococcal meningitis is diagnosed clinically by the petechial rash, immediate i.v antibiotics should be given; lumbar puncture is unnecessary. In other causes of meningitis a lumbar puncture is performed if

> **Emergency Box 21.1**
> **Meningococcal meningitis and**
> **meningococcaemia: emergency treatment**
>
> Suspicion of meningococcal infection is a medical emergency requiring treatment *immediately* medical contact takes place. In meningococcal meningitis, fever, headache and neck stiffness are accompanied or heralded by a petechial, or non-specific blotchy red rash. However, all these features may not be present – and meningococcal infection may sometimes begin like any intercurrent non-serious viral infection.
>
> The ***immediate*** management of suspected meningococcal infection is benzylpenicillin 1200 mg (adult dose) either by slow i.v. injection or intramuscularly, prior to investigations. Cefotaxime 1 g i.v. is an alternative in cases of penicillin allergy. In meningitis, minutes count: delay is unacceptable.
>
> On arrival in hospital, routine tests including blood cultures should be carried out *immediately*, and a close lookout kept for the emergence of septicaemic shock. For further management and prophylaxis, see text.

Table 21.44   Antibiotics and acute bacterial meningitis

Organism	Antibiotic	Alternative (e.g. allergy)
Unknown pyogenic	Cefotaxime	Benzylpenicillin and chloramphenicol
Meningococcus	Benzylpenicillin	Cefotaxime
Pneumococcus	Cefotaxime	Penicillin
Haemophilus	Cefotaxime	Chloramphenicol

there is no clinical suspicion of a mass lesion (p. 1245). If the latter is suspected an immediate CT scan must be performed because coning of the cerebellar tonsils may follow. Typical CSF changes are shown in Table 21.45. CSF pressure is characteristically elevated. If a presumptive diagnosis of the organism can be made (e.g. pneumococcus is likely with skull fracture or sinus infection), targeted treatment should be started immediately. A scheme for immediate antibiotic treatment in acute bacterial meningitis is in Table 21.44.

Blood should be taken for cultures, glucose and routine tests, and chest and skull films if appropriate.

CSF stains demonstrate organisms (e.g. Gram-positive intracellular diplococci – pneumococcus; Gram-negative cocci – meningococcus). Ziehl–Neelsen stain demonstrates acid-fast bacilli (TB), though TB organisms are rarely numerous. Indian ink stains fungi.

It cannot be emphasized enough that meticulous attention should focus on microbiological studies in suspected CNS infection with close liaison between clinician and microbiologist. Specific techniques (e.g. polymerase chain reaction for meningococci and other bacteria) are invaluable. Syphilitic serology should always be carried out.

The clinical picture and CSF examination should thus yield a presumptive cause for acute meningitis within hours. Antibiotics must be started before the actual organism is identified.

If bacterial meningitis is diagnosed, further discussion with the microbiologist should include antibiotics, drug resistance, recent infections in the locality, barrier nursing and prophylaxis.

In bacterial meningitis in children, the use of dexamethasone has declined since the introduction of Hib vaccination. In adults it is recommended for pneumococcal meningitis.

Intrathecal antibiotics are no longer used in meningitis.

Local infection (e.g. paranasal sinus) should be treated surgically if necessary. Repair of depressed skull fracture or meningeal tear may be required.

Prophylaxis

Meningococcal infection should be notified to public health authorities, and advice sought about immunization and prophylaxis of contacts, e.g. with rifampicin or ciprofloxacin. *MenC*, a meningococcal C conjugate vaccine, is part of childhood UK immunization and often given to case contacts. A combined A and C meningococcal vaccine is sometimes used prior to travel to endemic regions, e.g. Africa, Asia; and a quadrivalent ACWY vaccine for specific events, e.g. Hajj and Umrah in Mecca. There is no vaccine for Group B.

A polyvalent pneumococcal vaccine is used after recurrent meningitis, e.g. after a CSF leak following skull fracture.

Hib (*Haemophilus influenzae*) vaccine is given routinely in childhood in the UK, virtually eliminating a common cause of fatal meningitis.

Chronic meningitis

Tuberculous meningitis (TBM) and cryptococcal meningitis commence typically with vague headache, lassitude, anorexia and vomiting. Acute meningitis can occur but is unusual. Meningitic signs usually take some weeks to develop. Drowsiness, focal signs (e.g. diplopia,

Table 21.45   Typical CSF changes in meningitis

	Normal	Viral	Pyogenic	Tuberculosis
Appearance	Crystal-clear	Clear/turbid	Turbid/purulent	Turbid/viscous
Mononuclear cells	< 5 mm³	10–100 mm³	< 50 mm³	100–300 mm³
Polymorph cells	Nil	Nil*	200–300/mm³	0–200/mm³
Protein	0.2–0.4 g/L	0.4–0.8 g/L	0.5–2.0 g/L	0.5–3.0 g/L
Glucose	$\frac{2}{3} > \frac{1}{2}$ blood glucose	$> \frac{1}{2}$ blood glucose	$< \frac{1}{2}$ blood glucose	$< \frac{1}{2}$ blood glucose

*Some polymorph cells may be seen in the early stages of viral meningitis and encephalitis

papilloedema, hemiparesis) and seizures are common. Syphilis, sarcoidosis and Behçet's syndrome also cause chronic meningitis. In some chronic meningitis an organism is never identified.

Management of TBM

TMB is a common and serious disease world-wide. Brain imaging may show meningeal enhancement, hydro-cephalus and tuberculomas (p. 1243), though it may remain normal. See Table 21.45 for CSF changes. In many cases the sparse TB organisms cannot be seen on Ziehl–Neelsen staining. Repeated CSF examination is often necessary and it will be some weeks before cultures are confirmatory. Treatment with anti-TB drugs (p. 932) – rifampicin, isoniazid and pyrazinamide – must commence on a presumptive basis and continue for at least 9 months. Ethambutol should be avoided because of its eye complications. Relapses and complications (e.g. seizures, hydrocephalus) are common in TBM. The mortality remains over 60% even with early treatment.

Malignant meningitis

Malignant cells can cause a subacute or chronic non-infective meningitic process. A meningitic syndrome, cranial nerve palsies, paraparesis and root lesions are seen, often in confusing and fluctuating patterns. The CSF cell count is raised, with high protein and low glucose. Treatment with intrathecal cytotoxic agents is rarely helpful.

Cells in a sterile CSF

Difficulties arise with a raised CSF cell count without evident infecting organism. CSF pleocytosis, a mixture of lymphocytes and polymorphs is the usual situation. See Table 21.46.

Table 21.46 Causes of sterile CSF (pleocytosis)

Partially treated bacterial meningitis	Cerebral venous thrombosis
Viral meningitis	Cerebral infarction
Tuberculosis or fungal infection	Following subarachnoid haemorrhage
Neoplastic meningitis	Encephalitis, including HIV
Parameningeal foci (e.g. paranasal sinus)	Rare causes (e.g. cerebral malaria, sarcoidosis, Behçet's syndrome, Lyme disease, endocarditis, cerebral vasculitis/ angiitis)
Syphilis	
Intracranial abscess	

FURTHER READING

de Gans J et al. (2002) Dexamethasone in adults with bacterial meningitis. *New England Journal of Medicine* **347**: 1549–1556.

Department of Health (1999) *Immunisation Against Infectious Disease*. [PL CMO (99) 4, PL CNO (99) 8, PL CPHO (99) 3].

Hall AJ, Wild CP (2003) Management of bacterial meningitis in adults. *British Medical Journal* **326**: 996–997.

Tunbridge A, Read RC (2004) Management of meningitis. *Clinical Medicine* **4**: 499–505.

INFORMATION FOR PATIENTS
Knowing about meningitis and septicaemia (a leaflet for parents). Department of Health, PO Box 410, Wetherby LS23 7LN.

UK NATIONAL CHARITY
Meningitis Trust: http://www.meningitis-trust.org.uk

ENCEPHALITIS

Encephalitis means inflammation of brain parenchyma, usually viral. Brain inflammation also develops in bacterial and fungal meningitis.

Acute viral encephalitis

The usual organisms cultured from adult UK cases are herpes simplex, ECHO, Coxsackie, mumps and Epstein–Barr viruses. Adenovirus, varicella zoster, influenza, measles and other viruses are rarer. Often, viral aetiology is presumed but never confirmed.

Epidemic and endemic viral encephalitides occur world-wide:

- Japanese encephalitis in South East Asia
- Ross River fever in Australia
- California encephalitis in the USA
- Ömsk haemorrhagic fever in Russia
- Tick-borne flavivirus encephalitis in Sweden and Central Europe
- West Nile encephalitis in Egypt and Sudan.

Epidemic viral encephalitides with unusual organisms are common. For example, encephalitis caused by Nipah-virus, hitherto not known to cause human disease, occurred in 1998 in abattoir workers in Malaysia; in New York in 1999 West Nile virus caused an encephalitis epidemic. In Southern India in 2003 there was an outbreak of encephalitis in children due to the chandipura virus. Rabies (p. 58) is a variety of sporadic viral encephalitis.

Clinical features

Many encephalitides are mild and recovery occurs. In a minority, serious illness develops with high fever, headache, mood change and drowsiness over hours or days. Focal signs, seizures and coma ensue. Death, or brain injury follows. Herpes simplex virus (HSV-1) accounts for many severe cases in Britain. Mortality remains around 20%. In SE Asia, Japanese encephalitis (arbovirus) is more usual, causing a serious illness with higher mortality than HSV-1.

Differential diagnosis

This includes:

- bacterial meningitis with cerebral oedema
- cerebral venous thrombosis
- cerebral abscess
- acute disseminated encephalomyelitis (see below)

- cerebral malaria
- toxic confusional states
- septicaemia, febrile illness, vasculitis
- endocarditis.

Investigations

CT and MR imaging show diffuse areas of oedema, often in the temporal lobes. EEG shows characteristic slow waves, which are useful in some cases; a normal EEG is exceptional. CSF shows a raised cell count. Viral serology (blood + CSF) is helpful. Brain biopsy is occasionally performed.

Treatment

Suspected herpes simplex encephalitis is treated immediately with intravenous aciclovir, the active form of which inhibits DNA synthesis. Phosphorylation of aciclovir is dependent upon viral thymidine kinase; the drug is thus specific for herpesvirus infections. A poor outlook usually follows coma whether or not aciclovir has been given. Supportive measures are required for comatose patients; seizures are treated with anticonvulsants.

Prophylactic immunization against Japanese encephalitis is advised for travellers to endemic areas in Asia.

> **FURTHER READING**
> Editorial (2000) Exotic diseases close to home. *Lancet* **354**: 1221.
> Whitley RJ, Gnann JW (2002) Viral encephalitis. *Lancet* **359**: 507–514.

Acute disseminated encephalomyelitis (ADEM)

ADEM follows many viral infections (e.g. measles, varicella zoster, mumps and rubella) and rarely immunization against rabies, influenza or pertussis. The syndrome is often similar to acute viral encephalitis, with focal brainstem and/or spinal cord lesions due to demyelination (see also MS, p. 1235). Viral particles are not present in these lesions, which are well seen on T2 MR images. Prognosis is variable. Mild cases recover completely. When there is coma, mortality remains c. 25%. Survivors often have permanent brain damage. Treatment is supportive, with steroids and anticonvulsants.

MYELITIS

Myelitis means spinal cord inflammation causing paraparesis or tetraparesis. This occurs with varicella zoster or ADEM. Poliomyelitis is a specific spinal cord anterior horn cell enterovirus infection (p. 49). Transverse myelitis is mentioned on page 1252.

HERPES ZOSTER (SHINGLES)

This is recrudescence of varicella-zoster infection within dorsal root ganglia, the original virus infection having been chickenpox many years previously. Chickenpox and shingles viruses are identical.

Clinical features

For shingles rashes, see page 46.

In the cranial nerves, herpes zoster has a predilection for the fifth and seventh nerves. 'Ophthalmic' herpes is infection of the first division of the fifth nerve. This can lead to corneal scarring and secondary panophthalmitis (p. 1167). Geniculate herpes (geniculate ganglion of VIIth nerve) is also called Ramsay Hunt syndrome (p. 1188). Local complications are secondary bacterial infection, very rarely local purpura with necrosis (*purpura fulminans*), generalized zoster, and postherpetic neuralgia. Myelitis, meningoencephalitis and motor radiculopathy (usually lumbar or brachial) also follow varicella-zoster. Treatment is with aciclovir or its pro-drug valaciclovir.

Postherpetic neuralgia

Postherpetic neuralgia is pain in a previous shingles zone; this occurs in some 10% of patients (often elderly). Burning, continuous pain responds poorly to analgesics. Depression is almost universal. Treatment is unsatisfactory but there is a trend towards gradual recovery over 2 years. Amitryptyline is commonly used. Methylprednisolone intrathecally is sometimes helpful.

> **FURTHER READING**
> Johnson RW, Dworkin RH (2003) Treatment of herpes zoster and postherpetic neuralgia. *British Medical Journal* **326**: 748–750.

NEUROSYPHILIS

Syphilis is described on page 122. A variety of syndromes occur, sometimes mixed.

Asymptomatic neurosyphilis

This describes positive CSF serology without signs.

Meningovascular syphilis

This causes:

- subacute meningitis with cranial nerve palsies and papilloedema
- a gumma – a chronic expanding intracranial mass
- paraparesis caused by a spinal meningovasculitis.

Tabes dorsalis

Demyelination in dorsal roots causes a complex deafferentation syndrome. The elements of tabes are:

- lightning pains (p. 1198)
- ataxia, stamping gait, reflex and sensory loss, muscle wasting
- neuropathic joints (Charcot joints)
- Argyll Robertson pupils (p. 1183)
- ptosis and optic atrophy.

General paralysis of the insane (GPI)

The grandiose title describes madness and weakness. GPI dementia is, however, often similar to Alzheimer's (p. 1254). Progressive cognitive decline, seizures, brisk reflexes, extensor plantars and tremor develop. Death follows within 3 years. Argyll Robertson pupils are usual. GPI and tabes are now rarities.

Other forms of neurosyphilis

In *congenital* neurosyphilis (acquired in utero), features of combined tabes and GPI develop in childhood – taboparesis.

In *secondary* syphilis, a meningeal reaction occurs: this may be symptomless or cause a self-limiting subacute meningitis.

Treatment

Benzylpenicillin 1 g daily by injection for 10 days in primary infection eliminates the risk of neurosyphilis. Established neurological disease can be arrested but not reversed – parenteral penicillin is given for 2–3 weeks. Allergic reactions (Jarisch–Herxheimer reactions) can occur; high-dose steroid cover is usually given with penicillin (p. 124) but there is little evidence of its value.

NEUROCYSTICERCOSIS

The adult pork tapeworm, *Taenia solium*, is endemic in Latin America, India, non-Muslim African countries and rural areas of SE Asia. It is a major global health problem (p. 115).

Epilepsy is a major feature of neurocysticercosis. Other neurological patterns include brainstem dysfunction, cerebellar ataxia, hydrocephalus, and rarely dementia, arachnoiditis, and vasculitis. Most infected people remain symptomless.

Brain CT and MRI are helpful, but not diagnostic. Serological tests indicate infection but not activity. Biopsy of a lesion may be necessary.

Management is primarily the control of seizures with anticonvulsants. The place of anthelminthics (praziquantel and albendazole) is controversial. Neurosurgery is sometimes necessary for giant inflammatory lesions or hydrocephalus.

Prevention (see p. 116)

FURTHER READING
Maguire JH (2004) Tapeworms and seizures. *New England Journal of Medicine* **350**: 215–217.

HIV AND NEUROLOGY (p. 133)

HIV-infected individuals frequently present with or develop neurological conditions. Immunosuppression leads to indolent, atypical clinical patterns. HIV patients also have a high incidence of stroke. These conditions have been dramatically reduced in countries where HAART is available.

Brain and meningeal disease

Meningitis

Acute aseptic meningitis is a primary HIV infection, with spontaneous recovery.

Chronic meningitis occurs with fungal infections (e.g. *Cryptococcus neoformans* or *Aspergillus*), TB, *Listeria*, *E. coli* or other organisms. Aggressive treatment is essential.

Diffuse encephalopathies

AIDS-dementia complex (ADC). This diffuse, progressive, HIV-related dementia, sometimes with cerebellar signs, is still seen where anti-retroviral therapy is unavailable.

Encephalitis and brain abscess. Toxoplasma, cytomegalovirus, herpes simplex, and other organisms cause severe encephalitis, commonly with multiple brain abscesses.

CNS lymphoma. This neoplasm has a poor prognosis (p. 516).

Progressive multifocal leucoencephalopathy. PML is due to papovavirus (JC virus p. 48).

Spinal cord disease

Paraparesis with HIV occurs in several settings:

- acute transverse myelitis – primary HIV myelitis with spontaneous recovery
- myelopathy due to infection, e.g. herpes simplex, zoster, cytomegalovirus or TB
- CNS lymphoma (cord compression or malignant meningitis).

Peripheral nerve disease

Neuropathies (particularly sensory) occur:

- mononeuropathy (e.g. a common peroneal nerve lesion)
- mononeuritis multiplex (p. 1260)
- polyneuropathy (p. 1260).

Autonomic neuropathy also occurs. (p. 1264).

These neuropathies are often a complication of treatment (see Table 2.53).

Management of HIV

See page 143. The incidence of many HIV-related neurological conditions is reduced with HAART.

FURTHER READING
Guiloff R (1999) Infections in the immunocompromised and post transplant patient. I & II. *CPD Bulletin Neurology* **1**: 3–7, 46–50.
Manji H, Miller R (2004) The neurology of HIV infection. *Journal of Neurology, Neurosurgery and Psychiatry* **75**: i29

OTHER INFECTIONS

Many other infections involve the CNS and are discussed in Chapter 2, e.g. rabies, tetanus, botulism, Lyme disease, leprosy and poliomyelitis.

Transmissible spongiform encephalopathy (Creutzfeldt–Jakob disease (CJD)) (p. 60)

This rare, progressive dementia is recognized pathologically by spongiform changes in the brain. CJD, a prion (proteinaceous infectious particle, PrP) disease, occurs world-wide and is transmitted by an agent resistant to many sterilization processes. All PrP diseases are associated with accumulation of a disease-related protein isoform, PrP^{Sc}, derived from a normal cellular precursor, PrP^{C}.

Sporadic, iatrogenic and familial forms. Sporadic CJD cases are usually single. Symptoms develop, usually over the age of 50 years.

Iatrogenic CJD is transmitted from surgical specimens, autopsy, transplant material (e.g. corneal grafts), and human growth hormone. Iatrogenic CJD has a long incubation period, up to 5 years. Death is invariable within 6 months of clinical onset in both sporadic and iatrogenic forms. Quinarine is being used in trials. There is a rare familial form of CJD. CJD pathology is very similar to that of bovine spongiform encephalopathy (BSE, 'mad cow disease'), recognized first in the UK in the early 1980s and in 2003 in the USA.

Incidence. Sporadic CJD occurs world-wide with an annual incidence < 1 per million; some 30–55 cases occur annually in the UK. Numbers have not been rising. Iatrogenic CJD is rarer – 0–6 UK cases annually. Familial CJD cases – 0–4 annually in Britain – are associated with PrP gene mutations. An even rarer form, Gerstmann–Sträussler–Scheinker syndrome, is an inherited autosomal recessive condition, typified by chronic progressive ataxia and terminal dementia, with duration 2–10 years.

Variant CJD (vCJD) was noted in Britain in 1995. Numbers are not increasing. vCJD cases are younger than sporadic cases with a mean age of 29. Early symptoms are neuropsychiatric, followed by ataxia, and dementia with myoclonus or chorea. Diagnosis can be confirmed by tonsillar biopsy and CSF gel electrophoresis. vCJD has a longer course than sporadic CJD – up to several years. vCJD and BSE are caused by the same prion strain, giving rise to speculation that transmission from animal to human food chain occurred, i.e. infection from BSE-infected cattle to humans (p. 60). Transmission via blood transfusion may occur.

Kuru

This dementia and cerebellar ataxia, another prion disease, is described on page 61. Spongiform change occurs, very similar to those in CJD.

OTHER INFLAMMATORY CONDITIONS

Subacute sclerosing panencephalitis (SSPE)

Persistence of measles antigen in the CNS causes this rare late sequel of measles. Progressive mental deterioration, fits, myoclonus and pyramidal signs develop, typically in a child. Diagnosis is made by high measles antibody titre in blood and CSF. Measles immunization protects against SSPE, which is now almost eliminated in the UK.

Progressive rubella encephalitis

Some 10 years after primary rubella infection, this syndrome, which is even rarer than SSPE, causes progressive mental impairment, fits, optic atrophy, cerebellar and pyramidal signs. Antibody to rubella viral antigen is produced locally within the CNS. It has not been seen as a complication of rubella immunization.

Reye's syndrome (see also p. 395)

This severe encephalitic illness of children is accompanied by fatty infiltration of liver with hypoglycaemia.

Mollaret's meningitis

This is recurrent self-limiting episodes of aseptic meningitis (i.e. no bacterial cause found) over many years. Viral (herpes simplex) infection is postulated.

Vogt–Koyanagi–Harada syndrome

This obscure recurrent inflammation of cells of neural crest origin causes uveitis, meningoencephalitis, vitiligo, deafness and alopecia.

Progressive multi-focal leucoencephalopathies (PMFL)

PMFL is usually seen in patients with HIV, is due to the JC virus and is described on page 48. It is also seen in other immunosuppressed patients.

In leucoencephalopathy there is demyelination of the white matter of the cerebral hemispheres. It can also be due to vascular lesions, e.g. CADASIL (p. 1210); toxic and metabolic causes, e.g. drugs (cocaine, Ecstasy), heavy metals, chemotherapy and other immunosuppressive agents (e.g. ciclosporin) when it may be reversible; hereditary factors, e.g. adrenoleucodystrophy; autoimmune and inflammatory causes, e.g. SLE, multiple sclerosis; tumours, e.g. gliomas; and other infections, e.g. Lyme disease, varicella zoster.

Whipple's disease

Whipple's disease is characterized by myoclonus, dementia and supranuclear ophthalmoplegia. It is described on page 305.

Neurosarcoidosis

Neurosarcoid with or without systemic sarcoidosis causes chronic meningoencephalitis, spinal cord lesions, cranial nerve palsies, particularly bilateral seventh nerve lesions, polyneuropathy, and myopathy (p. 935).

Behçet's syndrome (see also p. 584)

Behçet's three principal features are; recurrent oral and/or genital ulceration, inflammatory ocular disease (uveitis, see p. 1169) and neurological syndromes. Brainstem and cord lesions, aseptic meningitis (p. 1239) encephalitis and cerebral venous thrombosis also occur.

Granulomatous (isolated, or primary cerebral) angiitis

In this rare condition there is necrotizing inflammation in the brain and leptomeningeal vessels. Stroke, seizures and confusional states develop. There is some response to steroid and immunosuppressive therapy.

BRAIN AND SPINAL ABSCESSES

Brain abscess (see Fig. 21.32)

Focal bacterial infection behaves as any expanding mass (p. 1245). Typical bacteria are *Streptococcus angiosus*, and *Bacteroides* species (from paranasal sinuses and teeth) and staphylococci (from penetrating trauma). Mixed infections are common. Multiple abscesses develop, particularly in HIV patients. Fungi also cause brain abscesses. A parameningeal infective focus (e.g. ear, nose, paranasal sinus, skull fracture) or a distant source of infection (e.g. lung, heart, abdomen) may be present. Frequently no underlying cause is found. An abscess is 10 times rarer than a brain tumour in the UK.

Clinical features

Headache, focal signs (e.g. hemiparesis, aphasia, hemianopia), epilepsy and raised intracranial pressure develop. Fever, leucocytosis and raised ESR are usual though not invariable. Abscesses may also be indolent, developing over weeks, particularly in the cerebral hemispheres. Cerebellar abscesses tend to develop rapidly over days or hours, producing hydrocephalus.

Management

Urgent imaging is essential. A contrast enhanced T2 weighted MR shows a thin rim of low signalling which is virtually diagnostic of an abscess. The search for a local focus of infection should include a detailed examination of the skull, ears and paranasal sinuses; also include distant foci, such as the heart and abdomen. Lumbar puncture is dangerous and usually unhelpful. Aspiration with stereotactic guidance allows the infective organism to be identified.

Treatment requires liaison between neurosurgeon and microbiologist. Streptococcal and anaerobic infections are treated with cefuroxime 1.5 g IV plus metronidazole 500 mg IV 8 hourly. For staphylococcal infections, flucloxacillin 2–3 g IV 6 hourly with cefuroxime is given. Other bacteria are treated appropriately. Surgical decompression may be necessary if parenteral antibiotics are unsuccessful. Despite treatment, mortality remains high at around 25%. Epilepsy is common in survivors.

Brain tuberculoma

TB bacilli cause chronic caseating intracranial granulomas – tuberculomas. These are the most common intracranial masses in countries where TB is common (e.g. India). Brain tuberculomas either present as mass lesions de novo or develop during tuberculous meningitis. They can be found as symptomless intracranial calcification on imaging. Spinal cord tuberculomas also occur. For treatment, see p. 932.

Subdural empyema and intracranial epidural abscess

Intracranial subdural empyema is a collection of subdural pus, usually secondary to local skull or middle ear infection. Features are similar to those of a cerebral abscess. Imaging is diagnostic.

In intracranial epidural abscess, a thin (1–3 mm) layer of pus tracks along the epidural space causing sequential cranial nerve palsies, typically without evidence of raised intracranial pressure. There is usually evidence of local infection, e.g. in the middle ear. MRI outlines the pus and is the investigation of choice, as CT imaging is sometimes normal. Drainage is required, with appropriate antibiotics.

Spinal epidural abscess

Staphylococcus aureus is the usual organism, reaching the spine via the bloodstream, possibly from a boil. Fever and usually back pain are followed by paraparesis and/or root lesions. Emergency imaging and antibiotics are essential. Surgical decompression is often necessary.

FURTHER READING

Bird S (2004) Recipients of blood or blood products 'at vCJD risk'. *British Medical Journal* **328**: 118–119.

Collins SJ (2004) Transmissible spongiform encephalitis. *Lancet* **363**: 51–61.

Friedlander RM, Gonzalez RG, Afridi NA et al (2003) A 58-year-old woman with left-sided weakness and a right frontal brain mass. *New England Journal of Medicine* **348**: 2125–2132.

Koralnik IJ, Schellingerhout D, Frosch MP (2004) A 66-year-old man with progressive neurologic deficits. *New England Journal of Medicine* **350**: 1882–1893.

BRAIN TUMOURS

Primary intracranial tumours account for some 10% of neoplasms. The most common tumours are outlined in Table 21.47. In the UK, metastases are the commonest

Fig. 21.32 **MR: Pyogenic brain abscess showing the ring enhancing lesion with surrounding oedema.**

Table 21.47 Common brain tumours	
Tumour	**Approximate relative frequency**
Metastases Bronchus Breast Stomach Prostate Thyroid Kidney	50%
Primary malignant tumours of neuroepithelial tissues Astrocytoma Oligodendroglioma Mixed (oligoastrocytomas) gliomas Ependymoma Primary cerebral lymphoma Medulloblastoma	35%
Benign Meningioma Neurofibroma	15%

Oligodendrogliomas

These arise from oligodendrocytes. They grow slowly, usually over several decades. Calcification is common.

Meningiomas (Figs 21.35–21.37)

These benign tumours arise from the arachnoid membrane and may grow to a large size, usually over years. Those close to the skull erode bone. They often occur along the intracranial venous sinuses, which they may invade. They are rare below the tentorium. Common sites are the parasagittal region, sphenoidal ridge, subfrontal region, pituitary fossa and skull base.

Neurofibromas (Schwannomas)

These solid benign tumours arise from Schwann cells and occur principally in the cerebellopontine angle, where they arise from the eighth nerve sheath (acoustic neuroma, p. 1189).

Other neoplasms

Other less common neoplasms include cerebellar haemangioblastoma, ependymoma of the fourth ventricle.

Fig. 21.33 MR (T1): Bilateral cerebellar metastases.

Fig. 21.34 MR (T1): Glioblastoma.

Fig. 21.35 CT: Frontal meningioma.

intracranial tumours (Fig. 21.33). Symptomless meningiomas are also found regularly on imaging or at autopsy.

Gliomas (Fig. 21.34)

These malignant tumours of neuroepithelial origin are usually seen within the hemispheres, but occasionally in the cerebellum, brainstem or cord. Their cause is unknown. Glioma is occasionally associated with neurofibromatosis. They tend to spread by direct extension, virtually never metastasizing outside the CNS.

Astrocytomas

These gliomas arise from astrocytes. They are classified histologically into grades I–IV. Grade I astrocytomas grow slowly over many years, while grade IV tumours (glioblastoma) cause death within several months. *Cystic* astrocytomas of childhood are relatively benign, and usually cerebellar.

Fig. 21.36 MR (T1): Falx (occipital) meningioma.

Fig. 21.37 MR (T1): Suprasellar meningioma.

colloid cyst of the third ventricle, pinealoma, chordoma of the skull base, glomus tumour (of the jugular bulb), medulloblastoma (a cerebellar childhood tumour), craniopharyngioma (p. 1044) and cerebral lymphoma.

Pituitary tumours

These are discussed on page 1044.

Clinical features

Mass lesions within the brain produce symptoms and signs by three mechanisms:

- by direct effect – brain is either destroyed locally or function is impaired
- by secondary effects of raised intracranial pressure and shift of intracranial contents (e.g. papilloedema, vomiting, headache)
- by provoking either generalized or partial seizures.

Although neoplasms, either secondary or primary, are the commonest mass lesions in the UK, cerebral abscess, tuberculoma, subdural and intracranial haematoma can also produce features that are clinically indistinguishable.

Direct effects of mass lesions

The hallmark of a direct effect of a mass is local progressive deterioration of function. Tumours can occur anywhere within the brain. Three examples are given:

- *A left frontal meningioma* caused a frontal lobe syndrome over several years – vague disturbance of personality, apathy and impaired intellect. Expressive aphasia developed, followed by progressive right hemiparesis as the corticospinal pathways became involved. As the mass enlarged further, pressure headaches and papilloedema developed.
- *A right parietal lobe glioma* caused a left homonymous field defect (optic radiation). Cortical sensory loss in the left limbs and left hemiparesis followed over 3 months. Partial seizures (episodes of tingling of the left limbs) developed.
- *A left eighth nerve sheath neurofibroma* (an acoustic neuroma, Schwannoma) in the cerebellopontine angle caused, over 3 years, progressive perceptive deafness (VIII), vertigo (VIII), left facial numbness (V) and weakness (VII), followed by cerebellar ataxia on the same side. Papilloedema was a late sequel.

With a hemisphere tumour, epilepsy and the direct effects commonly draw attention to the problem. The rate of progression varies greatly, from a few days or weeks in a highly malignant glioma, to several years with a slowly enlarging mass such as a meningioma. Cerebral oedema surrounds mass lesions: its effect is difficult to distinguish from that of the tumour itself.

Raised pressure and shift of intracranial contents

Raised intracranial pressure causing headache, vomiting and papilloedema is a relatively unusual presentation of a mass lesion. These symptoms often imply hydrocephalus – obstruction to CSF pathways. Typically this is produced early by posterior fossa masses (that obstruct the aqueduct and fourth ventricle) but later with lesions above the tentorium. Shift of the intracranial contents produces features that coexist with the direct effects of any expanding mass:

- *Distortion of the upper brainstem*, as midline structures are displaced either caudally or laterally by a hemisphere mass (Fig. 21.34). This causes impairment of consciousness.
- *Compression of the medulla*, by herniation of the cerebellar tonsils caudally through the foramen magnum – an example of coning. This causes impaired consciousness, respiratory depression, bradycardia, decerebrate posturing and death.
- *False localizing signs* – false only because they do not point directly to the site of the mass.

Three examples of false localizing signs are:

- *A sixth nerve lesion*, first on the side of a mass and later bilaterally – as the VI nerve is compressed during its long intracranial course.
- *A third nerve lesion* develops as the temporal lobe uncus herniates caudally, compressing the third nerve against the petroclinoid ligament. The first sign is ipsilateral pupil dilatation as parasympathetic fibres are compressed.
- *Hemiparesis on the same side as a hemisphere tumour* (i.e. the side you would not expect) produced by compression of the contralateral cerebral peduncle within the brainstem on the free edge of the tentorium.

These false localizing signs, though unusual, are of importance because they indicate that shift of brain has occurred.

Seizures

Partial seizures, simple or complex, that may evolve into generalized tonic–clonic seizures, are characteristic of many hemisphere masses, whether malignant or benign. The pattern of partial seizure is of localizing value (p. 1221).

Investigations

CT and MR imaging

Imaging is mandatory when a tumour is suspected, though it has limitations. Brain abscess and infarction, benign and malignant tumours have characteristic, but not entirely reliable, appearances.

Technetium brain scan

This is of value in diagnosis of destructive skull vault (e.g. metastases) and skull base lesions.

EEG (p. 1203)

This rarely helps. An exception is cerebral abscess, where characteristic focal slow waves are sometimes seen.

Skull films (p. 1201)

In hemisphere tumours, plain films have no value. With metastases, skull vault lesions may be seen; and with pituitary tumours, enlargement of the pituitary fossa.

Routine tests

Since metastases are common, routine tests, e.g. chest X-ray, should be performed.

More specialized neuroradiology

MR angiography and MR spectroscopy are occasionally used to define changing size or blood supply. Positron emission tomography (PET) is helpful in grading gliomas or locating an occult primary.

Lumbar puncture

Lumbar puncture is initially contraindicated when there is any possibility of a mass, and CSF examination rarely yields useful information in this situation. Withdrawing CSF may provoke immediate herniation of the cerebellar tonsils. LP should be done only after imaging, but is rarely necessary.

Biopsy and tumour removal

Stereotactic biopsy via a skull burr-hole is usually carried out to ascertain the histology of a suspected malignancy. With a symptomatic meningioma, open exploration (craniotomy) is usually performed.

Management

Cerebral oedema surrounding a tumour is rapidly reduced by corticosteroids; i.v. or oral dexamethasone is given. Intravenous mannitol, an osmotic diuretic, is also used to reduce oedema. Epilepsy is treated with anticonvulsants.

Whilst complete surgical removal of a brain tumour is an objective, it is not always possible, nor is surgery always necessary. Follow-up with serial imaging is sometimes preferable. At surgical exploration, some benign tumours can be entirely removed (e.g. acoustic neuromas, some parasagittal meningiomas). With a brain malignancy it is rarely possible to remove an infiltrating mass. Biopsy and debulking are achieved.

Within the posterior fossa, tumour removal is often necessary because of raised pressure and the danger of coning. Overall mortality for posterior fossa exploration remains around 10%.

Radiotherapy is usually given to gliomas and metastases, and improves survival. An isolated posterior fossa metastasis can sometimes be excised successfully. Chemotherapy has little real value in the majority of primary or secondary brain tumours. Vincristine, procarbazine and temozolamide are used. Temozolamide has an active metabolite that interrupts DNA replication by methylation of the 06 position of guanine. Most malignant brain tumours continue to have a poor prognosis despite advances in imaging, surgery, chemotherapy and radiotherapy – less than 50% survival for high-grade gliomas at 2 years. The management involves multidisciplinary care.

Benign (idiopathic) intracranial hypertension (BIH, IIH)

This syndrome, once called *pseudotumor cerebri*, is included with tumours because marked papilloedema develops. There is neither a mass nor an increase in ventricular size. BIH develops mainly in obese young women with vague menstrual irregularities. Headaches and visual blurring (caused by papilloedema) are common. A sixth nerve palsy may develop – a false localizing sign (p. 1185). CSF pressure is elevated with normal constituents. Imaging is normal. Steroid therapy is sometimes thought to be a cause: many other drugs have occasionally been implicated. Other causes of papilloedema should be excluded. Sagittal sinus thrombosis can cause a similar picture.

BIH is benign in the sense that it is not fatal: it is usually self-limiting. However, optic nerve infarction can follow, with consequent blindness when papilloedema is severe and long-standing. Repeated LP, acetazolomide, and thiazide diuretics are used to reduce the intracranial pressure. Weight reduction is helpful. Surgical decompression or shunting is sometimes necessary.

FURTHER READING
Behin A et al. (2003) Primary brain tumours in adults. *Lancet* **361**: 323–331.
Whittle IR et al. (2004) Meningioma. *Lancet* **363**: 1535–1543.

HYDROCEPHALUS

Hydrocephalus means an excessive volume of CSF within the skull. In practice hydrocephalus usually describes different syndromes in which there is, or has been, obstruction to CSF outflow with consequent high pressure and dilatation of the cerebral ventricles. Also, exceptionally an increase in CSF production occurs.

Infantile hydrocephalus

Head enlargement in infancy occurs in 1 in 2000 live births. There are several anatomical causes:

- *Arnold–Chiari malformation*. There is elongation of the medulla. Cerebellar tonsils descend into the cervical canal. Associated spina bifida is common. Syringomyelia may develop (p. 1251).
- *Dandy–Walker syndrome*. There is cerebellar hypoplasia and obstruction to fourth ventricle outflow foramina.
- *Stenosis of the aqueduct of Sylvius* (Fig. 21.38). 'Aqueduct stenosis' is either congenital or acquired following

Fig. 21.38 **MR (T1): Communicating hydrocephalus.**

neonatal meningitis/haemorrhage. Often no evident cause is found.

Hydrocephalus in adult life

Hydrocephalus is often an unsuspected symptomless finding on imaging. However, infantile hydrocephalus can become apparent in adult life (e.g. aqueduct stenosis). Combinations of headache, cognitive impairment, vomiting, papilloedema, ataxia and bilateral pyramidal signs develop. Hydrocephalus may develop in other circumstances:

- *Posterior fossa and brainstem tumours* obstruct the aqueduct or fourth ventricular outflow.
- *Following subarachnoid haemorrhage, head injury or meningitis* (particularly tuberculous).
- *A third ventricle colloid cyst* causes lateral ventricle enlargement, headache and papilloedema. These rare intraventricular tumours also sometimes produce intermittent hydrocephalus – recurrent prostrating headaches with episodes of lower limb weakness.
- *Choroid plexus papilloma* (extremely rare) secretes CSF.

Treatment

Ventriculo-atrial or ventriculo-peritoneal shunting is necessary when progressive hydrocephalus causes symptoms. Neurosurgical removal of tumours is carried out when appropriate, sometimes urgently.

Normal pressure hydrocephalus

This describes enlarged cerebral ventricles, dementia, urinary incontinence and gait apraxia, usually in the elderly. CSF constituents and pressure are normal. There is now doubt about its existence as a true separate entity from dementia. Ventriculo-peritoneal shunting is occasionally carried out.

HEADACHE. MIGRAINE AND FACIAL PAIN

'Tension' headache

The vast majority of chronic and recurrent headaches are believed to be produced by 'neurovascular irritation' and tension within scalp muscles. Despite universal occurrence, precise mechanisms of common headache remain obscure. Tight band sensations, pressure behind the eyes, throbbing and bursting sensations are common. What is clear is that almost all headaches with these features are benign.

There may be obvious precipitating factors such as worry, noise, concentrated visual effort or fumes. Depression is also a frequent underlying feature. Tension headaches are often attributed to cervical spondylosis, refractive errors or high blood pressure. Evidence for such associations is poor. Headaches also follow even minor head injuries. Tenderness/tension in neck and scalp muscles are the only physical signs.

Management

This involves:

- firm reassurance (imaging is often needed)
- avoiding evident causes, e.g. bright lights
- analgesic withdrawal
- physical treatments – massage, icepacks, relaxation
- antidepressants – when indicated
- drugs for recurrent headache/migraine.

Migraine

Migraine is recurrent headache associated with visual and gastrointestinal disturbance. The borderline between migraine and tension headaches is vague. Over 12% of any population world-wide report these symptoms.

Mechanisms

Precise mechanisms of migraine remain unknown. Genetic factors play some part – a rare form of familial migraine is associated with mutation in the alpha-1 subunit of the P/Q-type voltage-gated calcium channel on chromosome 19. The release of the neuropeptide calcitonin-gene-related peptide (CGRP) is thought to play a central role as it is a potent dilator of cerebral and dural vessels.

The headache of migraine, often throbbing, is due to vasodilatation or oedema of blood vessels, with stimulation of nearby nerve endings. Release of vasoactive substances such as nitric oxide has a role. Serum 5-hydroxytryptamine rises with prodromal symptoms and falls during the headache. Magnesium deficiency, neural excitation by glutamate and aspartate, changes in the hypothalamic–pituitary axis and in endogenous opioids have all been suggested.

Cerebral features, such as tingling limbs, aphasia and weakness, are caused by focal depression of cortical function.

Some patients recognize precipitating factors:

- week-end migraine (a time of relaxation)
- chocolate (high in phenylethylamine)
- cheese (high in tyramine)
- noise and irritating lights
- with premenstrual symptoms.

Migraine is common around puberty and at the menopause and sometimes increases in severity or frequency with hormonal contraceptives, in pregnancy and with the onset of hypertension. There is no reason to suppose that the development of migraine is suggestive of any serious intracranial lesion. However, since migraine is so common, an intracranial mass and migraine sometimes occur together by coincidence. Migraine sometimes follows a blow to the head – often minor.

Clinical patterns

Migraine attacks vary from intermittent headaches indistinguishable from tension headaches to discrete episodes that mimic thromboembolic cerebral ischaemia. Distinction between variants is somewhat artificial. Migraine can be separated into phases:

- well-being before an attack (occasional)
- prodromal symptoms
- the main attack (headache, nausea, vomiting)
- sleep and feeling drained afterwards.

Migraine with aura (classical migraine)

Prodromal symptoms are usually visual and related to depression of visual cortical function or retinal function. Unilateral patchy scotomata (retina), hemianopic symptoms (cortex), teichopsia (flashes) and fortification spectra (jagged lines resembling battlements) are common. Transient aphasia sometimes occurs, with tingling, numbness, vague weakness of one side and nausea. The prodrome persists for a few minutes to about an hour. Headache then follows. This is occasionally hemicranial (i.e. splitting the head) but often begins locally and becomes generalized. Nausea increases and vomiting follows. The patient is irritable and prefers a darkened room. Superficial temporal arteries are engorged and pulsating. After several hours the migraine settles, sometimes with a diuresis. Deep sleep often ensues.

Migraine without aura (common migraine)

This is the usual variety. Prodromal visual symptoms are vague. There is recurrent headache accompanied by nausea and malaise.

Basilar migraine

Prodromal symptoms include circumoral and tongue tingling, vertigo, diplopia, transient visual disturbance (even blindness), syncope, dysarthria and ataxia. These occur alone or progress to a typical migraine.

Hemiparetic migraine

This rarity is classical migraine with hemiparetic features, i.e. resembling a stroke but with recovery within 24 hours. Exceptionally, cerebral infarction (stroke) occurs.

Ophthalmoplegic migraine

This rarity is a third nerve, or exceptionally a sixth nerve, palsy with a migraine – and difficult to diagnose without investigation to exclude other conditions.

Facioplegic migraine

This is unilateral facial weakness during a migraine.

Differential diagnosis

The sudden headache may resemble meningitis or SAH.

Hemiplegic, visual and hemisensory symptoms must be distinguished from thromboembolic TIAs (p. 1211). In TIAs maximum deficit is present immediately and headache is unusual.

Unilateral tingling or numbness may resemble sensory epilepsy (partial seizures). In epilepsy, distinct march (progression) of symptoms is usual.

Management

General measures include:

- reassurance and relief of anxiety
- avoidance of dietary factors – rarely helpful.

Patients taking hormonal contraceptives may benefit from a brand change, or trying without. Premenstrual migraine may respond to diuretics. Depot oestrogens are sometimes used. Severe hemiplegic symptoms are an indication for stopping hormonal contraceptives.

During an attack. After ruling out any serious cause for a sudden headache (p. 1174), paracetamol or other simple analgesics should be given, with an antiemetic such as metoclopramide if necessary. Repeated use of analgesics leads to further headaches. Triptans (5-HT$_1$ agonists) are also helpful. In some 30% of cases, where there is recurrent severe migraine, sumatriptan, zolmitriptan, naratriptan and rizatriptan are of value either by prompt self-administered subcutaneous injection, or orally by wafer or inhaler. Triptans should be avoided when there is vascular disease, and not overused. A recent study has shown that an i.v. CGRP antagonist was effective in treating severe attacks.

Prophylaxis. It is difficult to discern placebo effects of prophylactic drugs. The following are used when attacks are frequent:

- pizotifen (antihistamine and 5-HT antagonist) 0.5 mg at night for several days, increasing to 1.5 mg (common side-effects: weight gain and drowsiness)
- propranolol 10 mg three times daily, increasing to 40–80 mg three times daily
- amitriptyline: 10 mg (or more) at night.

Sodium valproate, methysergide, SSRIs, verapamil, topiramate, nifedipine and naproxen are also used.

Facial pain

The face has many pain-sensitive parts – teeth, gums, sinuses, temporomandibular joints, jaw and eyes, all of which can cause pain. Facial pain is also caused by specific neurological conditions.

Trigeminal neuralgia (p. 1186), trigeminal nerve lesions (p. 1186) and postherpetic neuralgia (p. 1240) are described elsewhere.

Cluster headache (migrainous neuralgia)

'Cluster', clinically distinct from migraine despite its name, describes recurrent bouts of excruciating unilateral pain that typically wake the patient. Attacks *cluster* around one eye. 'Cluster' affects adults, mostly males between 30 and 40. Alcohol sometimes provokes an attack, and also experimentally, nitroglycerin. There are changes in grey matter density on functional imaging in the posterior hypothalamus. Intense pain rises to a worse crescendo over half an hour, lasting for several hours. Vomiting occurs. One cheek and nostril feel congested. Transient ipsilateral Horner's syndrome is common.

Despite intense pain there are no serious sequelae. Attacks recur at intervals over several years but tend to disappear after the age of 55. Analgesics are unhelpful. Subcutaneous sumatriptan is the drug of choice. Alternatively oxygen inhalation 7.12 L/min may abort an attack. Most prophylactic migraine drugs are unhelpful. Verapamil, topiramate and lithium carbonate sometimes prevent 'cluster'.

Paroxysmal hemicrania

Episodic paroxysmal hemicrania is a rare condition describing unilateral sudden, brief (< 20 min) pains with some characteristics of cluster headaches. Paroxysms may occur many times each day, and typically respond to indometacin.

Atypical facial pain

Facial pain for which no cause can be found is seen in the elderly, mainly in women. It is believed to be a somatic equivalent of depression. Tricyclic antidepressants are sometimes helpful.

Other causes of facial pain

Facial pain occurs in variants of migraine and in giant cell arteritis (see below).

Giant cell arteritis (GCA) – cranial or temporal arteritis (see also p. 582)

This granulomatous arteritis is described on page 582.

Clinical features

Headache

Headache is almost invariable in GCA. Pain develops over inflamed superficial, temporal or occipital arteries. Touching the skin over an inflamed vessel (e.g. combing hair) causes pain. Arterial pulsation is soon lost; the artery becomes hard, tortuous and thickened. The scalp over inflamed vessels may become red. Rarely, gangrenous patches appear.

Facial pain

Pain in the face, jaw and mouth is caused by inflammation of facial, maxillary and lingual branches of the external carotid artery in GCA. Pain is characteristically worse on eating (jaw claudication). Opening the mouth and protruding the tongue becomes difficult. A painful, ischaemic tongue occurs rarely.

Visual problems

Visual loss from arterial inflammation and occlusion occurs in 25% of untreated GCA cases. Posterior ciliary artery occlusion causes anterior ischaemic optic neuropathy in three-quarters of these. Other mechanisms are central retinal artery occlusion, cilioretinal artery occlusion and posterior ischaemic optic neuropathy. There is sudden monocular visual loss (partial or complete), usually painless. Amaurosis fugax (p. 1212) may precede permanent blindness.

When the posterior ciliary vessels are affected, ischaemic optic neuropathy causes the disc to become swollen and pale; retinal branch vessels usually remain

normal. When the central retinal artery is occluded, there is sudden permanent unilateral blindness, disc pallor and visible retinal ischaemia. Bilateral blindness may develop, with the second eye being affected in 1–2 weeks.

Rare complications

Brainstem ischaemia, cortical blindness, ischaemic microangiopathic neuropathy of peripheral or cranial nerves, and involvement of the aorta, coronary, renal and mesenteric arteries sometimes occur.

Management

The ESR is greatly elevated and the diagnosis should be established immediately by superficial temporal artery biopsy, because of the risk of blindness. Immediate high doses of steroids (prednisolone, initially 60–100 mg daily) should be started in a patient with typical features, even before biopsy (see p. 583). Since the risk of visual loss persists over many years, neurologists and ophthalmologists tend to recommend long-term treatment.

FURTHER READING

Hayreh SS (2000) Steroid therapy for visual loss in patients with GCA. *Lancet* **355**: 1572–1573.
Headache Classification Committee (2004) The International Classification of Headache Disorders, 2nd edition. *Cephalgia* **24** (Suppl 1): 1–160.
Lance J, Goadsby P (1998) *Mechanism and Management of Headache*. Oxford: Butterworth Heinemann.
Silberstein SD (2004) Migraine. *Lancet* **363**: 381–391.

TRAUMATIC BRAIN INJURY

In most western countries head injury accounts for about 250 hospital admissions per 100 000 population annually. Traumatic brain injury (TBI) describes injuries with potentially permanent consequences. For each 100 000 people, 10 die annually following TBI; 10–15 are transferred to a neurosurgical unit – the majority of these require rehabilitation for a prolonged period of 1–9 months. The *prevalence* of survivors with a major persisting handicap is around 100 per 100 000. Road traffic accidents and alcohol abuse are the principal etiological factors in this major cause of morbidity and mortality.

Skull fractures

Linear skull fracture of the vault or base is one indication of the severity of a blow, but is itself not necessarily associated with any brain injury. Healing takes place spontaneously. *Depressed* skull fracture is followed by a high incidence of post-traumatic epilepsy – surgical elevation and debridement are usually necessary.

Principal local complications of skull fracture are:

- *meningeal artery rupture* – causing extradural haematoma (p. 1219)
- *dural vein tears* – causing subdural haematoma (p. 1218) or CSF rhinorrhoea/otorrhoea (risk of meningitis).

Mechanisms of brain damage

Older classifications attempted to separate *concussion* (transient coma for hours followed by apparent complete clinical recovery) from brain *contusion* (prolonged coma, focal signs and lasting brain damage). Pathological support for this division is poor. Mechanisms of TBI are complex and interrelated:

- axonal and neuronal damage – shearing and rotational stresses on decelerating brain, often at sites opposite impact (*contracoup* effect)
- axonal and neuronal damage from direct trauma
- brain oedema and raised intracranial pressure
- brain hypoxia
- brain ischaemia.

Clinical course

In a mild TBI a patient is stunned or dazed for a few seconds or minutes. Following this the patient remains alert with little or no post-traumatic amnesia. Complete recovery is usual. In more serious injuries duration of unconsciousness and particularly of post-traumatic amnesia (PTA) helps grade severity. PTA over 24 hours indicates severe TBI. The Glasgow Coma Scale (GCS, p. 1206) is used to record the degree of coma; this has prognostic value. A GCS below 5/15 at 24 hours implies severe injury; 50% of such patients die or remain in a persistent vegetative or minimal conscious state (p. 1207). However, prolonged coma of up to several weeks is occasionally followed by good recovery.

Recovery after severe TBI takes many weeks/months. During the first few weeks, patients are often intermittently restless or lethargic and have focal deficits, such as hemiparesis or aphasia. Gradually they become more aware, though may remain in post-traumatic amnesia, being unable to lay down any continuous memory despite being awake. This amnesia may last some weeks or more, and may not be obvious clinically. PTA is one predictor of outcome. PTA over 2 weeks implies that persistent organic cognitive deficit is almost inevitable, although return to unsupported paid work may be possible.

Late sequelae

Sequelae of TBI are major causes of morbidity and have important social and medicolegal consequences. They include:

- *Incomplete recovery* – e.g. cognitive impairment, hemiparesis.
- *Post-traumatic epilepsy* (p. 1221).
- *The post-traumatic (post-concussional) syndrome.* This describes the vague complaints of headache, dizziness and malaise that follow even minor head injuries. Litigation is frequently an issue. Depression is prominent. Symptoms may be prolonged.
- *Benign paroxysmal positional vertigo* (BPPV, p. 1156).
- *Chronic subdural haematoma* (p. 1218).
- *Hydrocephalus* (p. 1247).
- *Chronic traumatic encephalopathy* – follows repeated (and often minor) injuries. This 'punch drunk'

syndrome is cognitive impairment, extrapyramidal and pyramidal signs, seen typically in professional boxers.

Immediate management

Attention to the airway is vital. If there is coma, depressed fracture or suspicion of intracranial haematoma, CT imaging and discussion with a neurosurgical unit are essential. Indications for CT imaging vary – from imaging all minor head injuries in some US centres to more considered/stringent criteria elsewhere.

In many severe TBI cases, assisted ventilation will be needed. Intracranial pressure monitoring is valuable. Care of the unconscious patient is described on page 1209. Prophylactic anticonvulsant treatment has been shown to be of no value in prevention of late post-traumatic epilepsy (p. 1221).

Rehabilitation

TBI cases require skilled, prolonged and energetic support. Survivors with severe physical and cognitive deficits require rehabilitation in specialized units. Rehabilitation includes intensive physiotherapy and care from a multidisciplinary team with both physical and psychological skills. Many survivors are left with cognitive problems – amnesia, neglect, disordered attention and motivation, and behavioural/emotional problems – temper dyscontrol, depression and grief reactions. Long-term support for both patients and families is necessary.

FURTHER READING

Bullock MR, Chesnut R, Clipton GL et al. (2000) Guidelines for the management of severe head injury: Brain Trauma Foundation. American Association of Neurological Surgeons. Joint session on Neurotrauma and care. *Neurotrauma* **17**: 449–627.

Haydel MJ et al. (2000) Indications for CT in patients with minor head injury. *New England Journal of Medicine* **343**: 100–105.

Shajar J (2000) Traumatic brain injury. *Lancet* **356**: 923–929.

Wasserberg J (2003). Treating head injuries. *British Medical Journal* **325**: 454–455.

SPINAL CORD DISEASE

The cord extends from C1 (its junction with the medulla) to the vertebral body of L1 where it becomes the conus medullaris. Blood supply is from the anterior spinal artery and a plexus on the posterior cord. This network is supplied by vertebral arteries, thyrocervical trunk and several branches from lumbar and intercostal vessels.

SPINAL CORD COMPRESSION (Table 21.48)

Principal features of chronic and subacute cord compression are spastic paraparesis or tetraparesis, radicular pain at the level of compression, and sensory loss below the compression.

Table 21.48	Causes of spinal cord compression
Spinal cord neoplasms	*Rarities*
Disc and vertebral lesions:	Paget's disease, scoliosis
Chronic degenerative	and vertebral anomalies
Trauma	Epithelial, endothelial and
Inflammatory:	parasitic cysts
Epidural abscess	Aneurysmal bone cyst
Tuberculosis	Vertebral angioma
Granuloma	Haematomyelia, arachnoiditis
Vertebral neoplasms:	Osteoporosis with fracture
Metastases	Arteriovenous malformation
Myeloma	
Epidural haemorrhage	

For example, in compression at T4 (see Fig. 21.14) a band of pain radiates around the thorax, characteristically worse on coughing or straining. Spastic paraparesis develops over months, days or hours, depending upon underlying pathology. Numbness commencing in the feet rises to the level of compression. This is called the *sensory level*. Retention of urine and constipation develop.

Cord compression is a medical emergency. It is sometimes difficult on clinical grounds alone to distinguish chronic progressive cord compression from other (non-surgical) causes of worsening paraparesis and tetraparesis. One reason for this is that pain at the level of compression can be absent.

Spinal cord neoplasms (Table 21.49)

Extramedullary tumours, both extradural and intradural, cause cord compression (Fig. 21.39) gradually over weeks

Table 21.49	Principal spinal cord neoplasms
Extradural	**Extramedullary**
Metastases:	Meningioma
Bronchus	Neurofibroma
Breast	Ependymoma
Prostate	
Lymphoma	**Intramedullary**
Thyroid	Glioma
Melanoma	Ependymoma
	Haemangioblastoma
	Lipoma
	Arteriovenous malformation
	Teratoma

Fig. 21.39 **MR (T2): Thoracic meningioma (cord compression).**

to months, often with root pain and a sensory level (p. 1198).

The rarer intramedullary tumours (e.g. glioma) typically progress slowly over many years. Sensory disturbances similar to syringomyelia may appear (p. 1252).

Tuberculosis

Spinal TB is the commonest cause of cord compression in countries where TB is common. There is destruction of vertebral bodies and disc spaces, with local spread of infection. Cord compression and paraparesis follow, culminating in paralysis – Pott's paraplegia.

Disc and vertebral lesions

Central cervical disc and thoracic disc protrusion causing cord compression are considered on page 1265.

Spinal epidural abscess

This is described on page 1243.

Epidural haemorrhage and haematoma

These are rare sequelae of anticoagulant therapy, bleeding disorders, trauma and after lumbar puncture when clotting is abnormal. A rapidly progressive cord lesion develops.

Management

Early recognition of cord compression is vital. Plain spinal films show degenerative bone disease and destruction of vertebrae by infection or neoplasm. Routine tests (e.g. chest X-ray) may indicate a primary neoplasm or infection. Spinal MR identifies most lesions and has entirely replaced contrast myelography. Surgical exploration is frequently necessary. If decompression is not performed sufficiently promptly, irreversible cord damage may follow. Results are excellent if benign tumours are removed early.

OTHER CAUSES OF PARAPARESIS

Paraparesis (and tetraparesis) occurs in many conditions recognizable by their clinical patterns. The elucidation of the cause of paraparesis has a pivotal place in neurology (see Table 21.13).

Syringomyelia and syringobulbia

The *syrinx*, a fluid-filled cavity within the cervical or thoracic spinal cord, is the essential feature. Syringobulbia means a cavity in the brainstem.

Aetiology and mechanism

Classical syringomyelia is associated with the Arnold–Chiari malformation (see p. 1257). The anatomical abnormality at the foramen magnum probably allows normal pulsatile CSF pressure waves to be transmitted to the fragile tissues of the cervical cord and brainstem, causing secondary cavity formation. The syrinx is in continuity with the central canal of the cord.

Pathological anatomy

The expanding cavity in the cord gradually destroys spinothalamic neurones, anterior horn cells, and lateral corticospinal tracts. In the medulla (syringobulbia), trigeminal nuclei, sympathetic trunk, ninth, tenth, eleventh and twelfth nerve nuclei and the vestibular system are destroyed by the expanding syrinx.

Clinical features

Patients with classical syringomyelia with the Arnold–Chiari malformation usually develop symptoms around the age of 20–30. Upper limb pain exacerbated by exertion or coughing is typical. Spinothalamic sensory loss (pain and temperature) leads to painless upper limb burns, and trophic changes. Difficulty in walking with paraparesis develops. The following are typical signs of a substantial cervical syrinx (Fig. 21.40):

- *Areas of 'dissociated' sensory loss*, i.e. spinothalamic loss without loss of light touch. Bizarre patterns are seen.
- *Loss of upper limb reflexes.*
- *Muscle wasting* in the hand and forearm.
- *Spastic paraparesis* – initially mild and symptomless.
- *Neuropathic joints*, trophic skin changes (scars, nail dystrophy) and ulcers.
- *Brainstem signs* – as the syrinx extends into the brainstem (syringobulbia), there is tongue atrophy and fasciculation, bulbar palsy, nystagmus, Horner's syndrome, hearing loss and impairment of facial sensation.

Course, investigation and management

Syringomyelia is gradually progressive over several decades. Sudden deterioration sometimes follows minor trauma, or spontaneously. MR imaging demonstrates the cavity and herniation of cerebellar tonsils.

There is no curative treatment. Surgical decompression of the foramen magnum sometimes slows deterioration.

Other causes of syrinx formation are bony anomalies at the foramen magnum, spina bifida (p. 1257), arachnoiditis, hydrocephalus (p. 1247), intrinsic cord tumours (e.g. glioma and ependymoma) and trauma.

Fig. 21.40 MR: Cervical syrinx (cavity, arrow).

Metabolic and toxic cord disease

Vitamin B$_{12}$ deficiency (p. 432)

Subacute combined degeneration of the cord resulting from vitamin B$_{12}$ deficiency is the most common example of metabolic disease causing spinal cord damage. Cord lesions probably due to multiple B vitamin deficiencies are also seen in severe malnutrition.

Lathyrism

This curiosity is an endemic spastic paraparesis of central India caused by the toxin beta-(*N*)-oxalylamino-L-alanine. It occurs when excessive quantities of a drought-resistant pulse, *Lathyrus sativa*, are consumed.

Konzo; tropical ataxic neuropathy

In West Africa and the West Indies inadequate preparation of *cassava* root allows ingestion of cyanogenic glycosides. A subacute spastic paraparesis follows – called *konzo*. *Tropical ataxic neuropathy* consists of sensory ataxia, loss of reflexes, deafness and optic atrophy, probably due to chronic low-level exposure to these glycosides.

Acute transverse myelopathy (transverse myelitis)

This term is used to describe a cord lesion and paraparesis (or paraplegia) occurring with viral infections, MS, mixed connective tissue disease and other inflammatory and vascular disorders – e.g. HIV, sarcoid, syphilis, radiation myelopathy, and anterior spinal artery occlusion. MRI is usually required to exclude cord compression.

Anterior spinal artery occlusion

Cord infarction, causing an acute paraplegia or tetraplegia, (or paresis) occurs in many thrombotic or embolic vascular diseases – for example, endocarditis, severe hypotension, atheroma, diabetes mellitus, polycythaemia, syphilis and polyarteritis. Cord infarction sometimes occurs during surgery to the posterior mediastinum, or follows aortic dissection and trauma. It also occurs as an isolated event.

Radiation myelopathy

A mild paraparesis with sensory loss sometimes develops within several weeks to a year after radiotherapy. Care is taken to shield the cord during radiotherapy.

MANAGEMENT OF PARAPLEGIA

General considerations

General health and morale should be reviewed carefully and regularly. Any intercurrent infection is potentially dangerous and should be treated early. Chronic renal failure is a common cause of death. The paraplegic patient needs skilled and prolonged nursing care and training to be aware of problems. Particular issues are discussed below.

Bladder

Catheterization is usually necessary initially. Many patients self-catheterize, or develop reflex bladder emptying, helped by abdominal pressure. Free urinary drainage is essential to avoid stasis, subsequent infection and calculi.

Bowel

Constipation and faecal impaction must be avoided. Manual evacuation is necessary following acute paraplegia, but reflex rectal emptying develops later.

Skin care

The risk of pressure sores and their sequelae is great. Meticulous attention must be paid to cleanliness and to turning the patient every 2 hours. The sacrum, iliac crests, greater trochanters, heels and malleoli should be inspected frequently (see p. 1355). Ripple mattresses and water beds are useful. If pressure sores develop, plastic surgical repair should be considered. Pressure palsies (e.g. of ulnar nerves) must be avoided.

Lower limbs

Passive physiotherapy helps to prevent contractures in paralysed limbs. Severe spasticity, with flexor or extensor spasms, may be helped by baclofen, diazepam, dantrolene, tizanidine or botulinum toxin injections.

Rehabilitation

Many patients with traumatic paraplegia or tetraplegia return to full or partial self-sufficiency despite a wheelchair existence. Specialist advice from a skilled rehabilitation unit is necessary. Lightweight, specially adapted wheelchairs are available. 'Paraplegics' have demanding practical, psychological, sexual and social needs.

> **FURTHER READING**
> Prasad D, Schiff D (2005) Malignant spinal-cord compression. *Lancet Oncology* **6**: 15–24.

DEGENERATIVE NEURONAL DISEASES

Degenerative underlines our incomplete understanding of these progressive nervous system diseases. Their molecular and genetic basis is the subject of intense study.

Motor neurone disease (MND)

In this common disease seen world-wide there is progressive degeneration of lower and upper *motor* neurones in the spinal cord, in cranial nerve motor nuclei and within the cortex. Most MND is sporadic and of unknown cause. It is thought that relentless degeneration of motor nerve cells may be programmed genetically. Abnormal mRNA splicing of the excitatory amino-acid transporter (*EAAT2*) gene, a major glial transporter, was once thought to be specific for MND, but is sometimes found in normal people. Oxidative neuronal damage,

aggregation of abnormal neuronal proteins, glutamate mishandling and abnormalities of neurofilament-mediated axonal transport are also involved. Apoptosis and prolonged neuronal caspase activity (p. 162) are the final mechanisms of cell destruction.

There is a familial form of MND in which there are mutations in the gene (chromosome 21q) encoding the free radical scavenging enzyme copper/zinc superoxide dismutase (SOD-1).

Incidence of the sporadic form is around 2/100 000/ year, with a slight male predominance and onset in middle life.

Clinical features

The sensory system is not involved. In the common, sporadic form of MND, four broad patterns are seen:

- progressive muscular atrophy
- amyotrophic lateral sclerosis (ALS)
- progressive bulbar and pseudobulbar palsy
- primary lateral sclerosis (rare).

Although useful as a means of recognizing MND, these are not distinct aetiological or pathological variants and usually merge as MND progresses. Other classifications are also used.

Progressive muscular atrophy

Wasting beginning in the small muscles of one hand (or both) spreads inexorably. Although it may commence unilaterally, wasting soon follows on the opposite side. Fasciculation is common. It is due to spontaneous firing of abnormally large motor units formed by branching fibres of surviving axons that are striving to innervate muscle fibres that have lost their nerve supply. Cramps may occur. Pain does not.

Physical signs are of wasting and weakness, with fasciculation – often widespread. Tendon reflexes are lost when the reflex arc is interrupted by anterior horn cell loss, but are preserved or exaggerated when there is loss of corticospinal motor neurones.

Amyotrophic lateral sclerosis (ALS)

Lateral sclerosis means disease of the lateral corticospinal tracts (i.e. one cause of spastic paraparesis). Amyotrophy means 'muscle atrophy', i.e. wasting, which is unusual in most other forms of spastic tetraparesis or paraparesis. The course is progressive spastic tetraparesis or paraparesis with added lower motor neurone signs and fasciculation. ALS is the term used for MND in the USA.

Progressive bulbar and pseudobulbar palsy

Here the brunt falls initially upon lower cranial nerve nuclei and their supranuclear connections. Dysarthria, dysphagia, nasal regurgitation of fluids and choking are common symptoms. For reasons unknown, this form of MND is more common in women. Characteristic features are of a bulbar and pseudobulbar palsy, (p. 1191), with mixed UMN and LMN signs in the lower cranial nerves – for example, a wasted fibrillating tongue with a spastic weak palate. Eye movements remain unaffected in all forms of MND. There are neither cerebellar nor extra-pyramidal signs. Awareness is preserved and dementia unusual. Sphincter disturbance occurs late, if at all.

Primary lateral sclerosis

This describes a rare form of MND confined to upper motor neurones. There is progressive tetraparesis with terminal pseudobulbar palsy.

Diagnosis

There are no specific tests. Diagnosis is clinical. Usually MND is easily identifiable and confirmed by EMG and nerve conduction studies. Exclusion of other conditions is necessary in atypical cases. Cervical radiculopathy with myelopathy, syringomyelia, and the rare (almost extinct) syphilitic cervical pachymeningitis can cause diagnostic difficulty. Motor neuropathies and spinal muscular atrophies sometimes resemble the progressive muscular atrophy form of MND – their course is more prolonged. Kennedy's syndrome, an X-linked bulbar and spinal muscular atrophy, sometimes causes confusion: UMN signs are not seen in this condition.

Bulbar myasthenia gravis (p. 1269) may sometimes appear similar in the early stages.

Multifocal motor neuropathy (p. 1260) causes distal weakness with LMN signs; antibodies to GM_1 ganglioside are present and conduction block is seen on electro-physiological studies.

Denervation, a feature of all forms of MND except primary lateral sclerosis, is confirmed by electro-myography. Chronic partial denervation with preserved motor conduction velocity is characteristic. CSF consti-tuents are normal.

Course and management

Remission is unknown. MND progresses, spreading gradually, and causes death, often from broncho-pneumonia. Survival > 3 years is unusual, although there are rare MND cases who survive for a decade or longer.

No treatment has been shown to influence outcome. Riluzole, a sodium-channel blocker that inhibits glutamate release, slows progression slightly, particularly with disease of bulbar onset. Spasticity may be helped by baclofen, and drooling by propantheline or amitriptyline. Ventilatory support and feeding via gastrostomy helps prolong survival. Giving accurate advice to MND patients is particularly difficult. Shared-care protocols between patient, primary care physician, carers and support groups are helpful.

Spinal muscular atrophies

These rare genetic disorders of motor neurones give rise to slowly progressive, usually symmetrical, muscle wasting and weakness. An acute infantile type (Werdnig–Hoffmann disease), a chronic childhood type (Kugelberg–Welander disease) and adult forms are recognized. Clinically these conditions may be confused with muscular dystrophies (p. 1269), hereditary neuropathies or MND.

Table 21.50 Causes of dementia	
Degenerative Alzheimer's disease Dementia with Lewy bodies Frontotemporal dementia Huntington's disease Parkinson's disease Hydrocephalus Primary progressive aphasia	**Traumatic** Punch drunk syndrome (boxers) **Intracranial lesions** Subdural haematoma Tumours
Vascular Cerebrovascular disease Cerebral vasculitis, cranial arteritis	**Infections** Creutzfeldt–Jacob disease HIV infection Neurosyphilis Whipple's disease
Metabolic Uraemia Liver failure Remote effects of cancer	**Endocrine** Hypothyroidism Hypocalcaemia
Toxic Alcohol Occupational exposure (e.g. hydrocarbons) Lead, mercury poisoning	**Psychiatric** Pseudodementia
Vitamin deficiency B_{12} Thiamin	

Dementia

Dementia is used to describe progressive decline of cognitive function, i.e. loss of mind, usually affecting the cerebral cortex as a whole, though sometimes patchily. Memory is especially affected; intellect gradually fails. There is loss of emotional control, a deterioration of social behaviour and loss of motivation. There are many causes of this clinical syndrome, which is common in later life (Table 21.50). Dementia is a very substantial cause of morbidity in any ageing population, with profound social and economic effects. It affects some 10% of any population over 65, and 20% over 80. The commonest causes are Alzheimer's disease, vascular and dementia with Lewy bodies (DLB).

In practice it is difficult to recognize the particular *type* of dementia, and to define landmarks that separate the mild decline in memory and cognitive function often accepted as part of normal ageing.

Differential diagnosis

This includes a depressive disorder with pseudo-dementia, in which many of the features of an early dementia (especially memory impairment, slowed think-ing and lack of spontaneity) are apparent. Patients with pseudodementia often have a previous history of depression or a family history of mood disorder. Success-ful treatment of the mood disorder results in restoration of intellectual function. Delirium and mild or moderate learning difficulties are also differential diagnoses.

Alzheimer's disease

This is the commonest dementia, accounting for over 65% of dementia in any age group. It is a primary degenerative disease of the cerebral cortex. The cardinal clinical features are:

- progressive loss of ability to learn, retain and process new information (memory loss)
- decline in language – difficulty in naming and in understanding what is being said (various aphasias, p. 1178)
- apraxia – impaired ability to carry out skilled motor activities (p. 1175)
- agnosia – failure to recognize objects (e.g. clothing), places or people
- progressive loss of executive function – organizing, planning and sequencing
- behavioural change – agitation, aggression, wandering and persecutory delusions
- loss of insight, relative or complete, into the above
- depression – though severe depression is unusual, because of loss of insight.

The onset is gradual. Alzheimer's disease is rare below the age of 50 but increasingly common thereafter. Disturbance of gait, motor and sensory abnormalities and seizures occur late. The course is progressive over several to 10 or more years, with death in a state of extreme cognitive decline.

Neuropathology and neurochemical changes

Loss of neurones, neurofibrillary tangles, senile plaques and amyloid angiopathy are seen, especially within the frontal, temporal and parietal cortex, hippocampi, substantia innominata and locus ceruleus.

Neurofibrillary tangles in neuronal cell bodies are made up of the microtubular-associated *tau* protein in paired helical filaments. Ubiquitin is also seen in association with tangles. Aggregation of beta-amyloid (Aβ) appears to play a central role, developing progressively in extracellular senile plaques. These plaques contain deposits of amyloid β-protein, produced by enzymes, β and γ secretase. Apoptosis follows, leading to cell death with a marked reduction in choline acetyltransferase, acetylcholine itself, norepinephrine (noradrenaline) and serotonin.

Aetiology

The cause of Alzheimer's disease (AD) is unknown. No environmental toxin has been found. Incidence is increased in Down's syndrome. Increase in free radical formation and failure of antioxidant defences may contribute to neuronal degeneration. Superoxide dismutase (SOD), the free radical defence enzyme is reduced by some 25% in AD frontal cortex and hippocampi.

AD is occasionally familial. Genetic studies have shown linkage between familial (presenile) AD (FAD) and loci on chromosome I (presenilin, PS1 gene), chromosome 14 (presenilin, PS2 gene) and chromosome 21 (amyloid β-protein precursor, APP gene).

Late-onset AD (the great majority) is a heterogeneous disorder. Evidence suggests a link between AD and atherosclerosis, inflammation and cholesterol. A linkage has been found in some cases to a gene locus on chromosome 19q. The gene encoding apolipoprotein E is a possible candidate. This has three alleles, ε2, ε3 and ε4. The ε4 allele is a major risk factor for Alzheimer's disease and the ε2 allele is under-represented. It is possible that beta-amyloid accumulation is more extensive in those with the ε4 allele than in those lacking it.

Dementia with Lewy bodies (DLB)

This accounts for some 25% of all dementias and is characterized by fluctuating cognition with pronounced variation in attention and alertness. Prominent or persistent memory loss may not occur in the early stages. Impairment in attention, frontal, subcortical and visuospatial ability is often prominent. Depression and sleep disorders occur. Recurrent formed visual hallucinations (e.g. strange faces, frightening creatures) are a feature. Parkinsonism (e.g. slowing, rigidity) is common, with repeated falls. Delusions and transient loss of consciousness occur. Cortical Lewy bodies are prominent at autopsy. These inclusions were first described in idiopathic Parkinson's disease, but are a hallmark of DLB. These patients are particularly sensitive to neuroleptic drugs and these should not be used.

Vascular dementia (multi-infarct dementia)

This common cause of dementia is distinguished from Alzheimer's disease by its clinical features and course. There is usually a history of transient ischaemic attacks with brief impairment of consciousness, fleeting pareses or visual loss. The dementia may follow a succession of acute cerebrovascular events or, less commonly, a single major stroke. Vessel occlusion is the most common cause of vascular dementia, and this may produce a variety of cognitive deficits depending on the site of ischaemic damage. Multi-infarct dementia results from involvement of several vessels supplying the cerebral cortex and subcortical structures and is typically associated with signs of cortical dysfunction.

Frontotemporal dementia

Progressive deterioration of social behaviour (disinhibition) and personality develops in middle life, followed by decline in memory, intellect and language. This accounts for some 3% of dementias. Imaging shows selective atrophy of frontal and temporal lobes. There is no excess of either senile plaques or neurofibrillary tangles (both are seen in normal ageing and typically in AD). Cytoplasmic inclusion bodies (silver-staining, Pick's bodies) are seen. These changes separate this condition pathologically from AD.

Other dementias

Subcortical encephalopathies comprise disorders that affect *subcortical* structures such as the basal ganglia. They include dementia occurring in idiopathic Parkinson's disease, Huntington's disease, progressive supranuclear palsy (p. 1231) and dementia occurring in rarities such as cerebral vasculitis. Rare neuropsychiatric conditions such as Creutzfeldt–Jakob disease (p. 1242) and Wilson's disease (p. 387) cause

Table 21.51 Tests in dementia	
Blood tests	**Imaging**
Full blood count	Chest X-ray
ESR, C-reactive protein	CT scan
Urea and electrolytes	MRI
Blood glucose	
Liver biochemistry	**Other**
Serum calcium	EEG
Vitamin B_{12}, folate	CSF
TSH, T_3, T_4	Brain biopsy
Syphilis serology	
HIV antibodies	

progressive dementia. In these conditions, there are usually evident clinical features, e.g. parkinsonism, chorea and/or pseudobulbar palsy. Dementia also occurs commonly in the late stages of multiple sclerosis (p. 1235). Dementia is only a part of the clinical features in these conditions.

Primary progressive aphasia – a language-based dementia – is increasingly recognized; there is a relentless deterioration of language skills with relative preservation of memory.

Investigations

Dementia is diagnosed from the history and basic examination, especially cognitive testing (p. 1277), and confirmed by psychometric testing (e.g. the Wechsler scale). The history should be taken from someone who has known the patient for a long time.

In later life, few cases of dementia are investigated. Defined medical conditions should be excluded (Table 21.51). Investigations in younger cases of dementia include detailed CT, MR and PET imaging, psychometry, EEG, CSF examination and brain biopsy. The latter is usually only carried out in units specializing in the study of dementia.

Management and social consequences

It is rare that a treatable cause for dementia is found, for example hypothyroidism.

Management is supportive, to preserve dignity and to provide care for as long as possible in the familiar home environment. The burden of illness falls frequently on relatives. In an ageing population, medical problems of the carers themselves deserve particular attention.

Recent evidence suggests that participation in cognitively demanding leisure activities in late life can protect against dementia.

Treatment with antioxidants (mainly vitamin E) have shown some slight benefit. Other drugs, principally anticholinesterase inhibitors (donepezil, rivastigmine and galantamine) and memantine, an *N*-methyl D-aspartate (NMDA) receptor antagonist that affects glutamate transmission, have been shown to slow, slightly, the rate of cognitive decline in AD. Whilst there is dispute about the place for these drugs (all are costly), they contribute in some cases to a patient with dementia being able to remain at home for some months. However, the AD2000 randomized controlled trial showed no significant difference between donepezil and placebo. There are thus complex cost–benefit arguments.

FURTHER READING
Casserly I, Topol E (2004) Convergence of atherosclerosis and Alzheimer's disease. *Lancet* **363**: 1139–1146.
Cummings JL (2004) Alzheimer's disease. *New England Journal of Medicine* **351**: 56–57.
Friedlander RM (2003) Apoptosis and caspases in neurodegenerative diseases. *New England Journal of Medicine* **348**: 1365–1374.
Parton MJ, Lyall R, Leigh PN (1999) Motor neurone disease and its management. *Journal of the Royal College of Physicians of London* **33**: 212–218.
Ritchie K, Lovestone S (2002) The dementias. *Lancet* **360**: 1759–1766.
Wilcock GM (2003) Dementia with Lewy bodies. *Lancet* **362**: 1689–1690.

CONGENITAL AND INHERITED DISEASES

CEREBRAL PALSY

This describes disorders apparent at birth or in childhood due to neonatal brain damage. Deficits are non-progressive. Learning problems, mild to severe are frequent, though not exclusive – physical disability is independent of cognitive impairment.

The precise cause of damage in an individual child may be difficult to determine. The following are responsible:

- hypoxia in utero and/or during parturition
- neonatal cerebral haemorrhage and/or infarction
- trauma, neonatal or during parturition
- prolonged seizures – *status epilepticus* or hypoglycaemia
- kernicterus (now rare, with maternal Rh immunization).

Clinical features

Failure to achieve normal milestones is often the earliest feature. More specific motor syndromes become apparent later in childhood or, rarely, in adult life.

Spastic diplegia
This is spasticity (predominantly of lower limbs) with scissoring of gait.

Athetoid cerebral palsy
This is described on page 1231, and now rare.

Infantile hemiparesis
Hemiparesis may be noted at birth or later. One hemisphere is hypotrophic and the contralateral, hemiparetic limbs small (hemiatrophy).

Congenital ataxia
This is incoordination and hypotonia of limbs and trunk.

DYSRAPHISM

Failure of normal fusion of the fetal neural tube leads to a group of congenital anomalies. Folate deficiency during pregnancy is contributory: supplements should always be given (p. 247). Anticonvulsant drugs (e.g. valproate) are also implicated (p. 1224). Bacterial meningitis may follow if there is access to the subarachnoid space.

Anencephaly

This is absence of brain and skull – incompatible with life.

Meningoencephalocele

Brain and meninges extrude through a midline skull defect – protrusion can be minor or massive.

Spina bifida

There is failure of lumbosacral neural tube fusion. Several varieties occur.

Spina bifida occulta

This is isolated failure of vertebral arch fusion (usually lumbar), often seen on X-rays (3% of population). A dimple or a tuft of hair may overlie the anomaly. Clinical abnormalities are rare.

Meningomyelocele with spina bifida

Meningomyelocele consists of elements of spinal cord and lumbosacral roots within a meningeal sac. This herniates through a vertebral defect. In severe cases both lower limbs and sphincters are paralysed. The lumbosacral defect is visible at birth. Meningocele is a meningeal defect alone.

BASILAR IMPRESSION OF SKULL (PLATYBASIA)

This is usually a congenital anomaly. There is invagination of the foramen magnum and skull base upwards. Lower cranial nerves, medulla, upper cervical cord and roots are affected. A syrinx may be present. The *Arnold–Chiari malformation* may coexist, with aberrant cerebellar tonsils extending through the foramen magnum. Basilar invagination also develops in Paget's disease and rarely in osteomalacia (p. 601). Clinical features are spastic tetraparesis, cerebellar and lower brainstem signs.

NEUROECTODERMAL SYNDROMES

Tissue derived from ectoderm forms tumours and hamartomas, with lesions in the skin, eye and nervous system.

Neurofibromatosis (von Recklinghausen's disease)

This is characterized by multiple skin neurofibromas and pigmentation. The neurofibromas arise from the neurilemmal sheath. One new case occurs in every 4000 live births. The mode of inheritance is autosomal dominant with complete penetrance.

Clinical features (see also p. 1345)

Clinically neurofibromatosis is divided into type 1 (peripheral > 70%) and type 2 (central). The abnormal gene for NF1 is on chromosome 17 (q11.2) and for NF2 on chromosome 22 (q12.2) (Table 3.4, p. 179). The main application for these genetic markers is potential antenatal diagnosis and counselling. A wide variety of abnormalities occur.

Peripheral (NF1)

Skin neurofibromas present as subcutaneous, soft, sometimes pedunculated, tumours (p. 1345). They increase in numbers throughout life. Multiple café-au-lait patches are present (p. 1358).

Central (NF2) (see Table 3.4)

The abnormal protein (merlin or schwannomin) is a cytoskeletal protein. Many neural tumours occur:

- meningioma
- acoustic neuroma
- glioma (including optic nerve glioma)
- plexiform neuroma (massive cutaneous overgrowth)
- cutaneous neurofibroma.

Rarely, the benign tumours undergo sarcomatous change.

Associated abnormalities

- Scoliosis
- Orbital haemangioma
- Local gigantism of a limb
- Phaeochromocytoma and ganglioneuroma
- Renal artery stenosis
- Pulmonary fibrosis
- Obstructive cardiomyopathy
- Fibrous dysplasia of bone.

Treatment

Tumours causing pressure symptoms within the nervous system require excision, if feasible.

Tuberous sclerosis (epiloia)

This rare autosomal dominant condition comprises adenoma sebaceum (p. 1345), epilepsy and cognitive impairment (often severe). Retinal phakomas (glial masses), renal tumours, glial overgrowth in brain and gliomas occur.

Sturge–Weber syndrome (encephalofacial angiomatosis)

There is an extensive port-wine naevus on one side of the face (usually in the distribution of a division of the fifth nerve) and a leptomeningeal angioma. Epilepsy is common. Familial occurrence is exceptional.

von Hippel–Lindau syndrome (retinocerebellar angiomatosis)

This is dominantly inherited. Retinal and cerebellar haemangioblastomas develop or, less commonly, haemangioblastomas of the cord and cerebrum. Renal, adrenal and pancreatic tumours (and haemangioblastomas) may also be found. Polycythaemia sometimes develops.

Numerous other disorders can be included here, e.g. ataxia telangiectasia (p. 1258) and Osler–Weber–Rendu syndrome (p. 469).

FURTHER READING
Lonser RR et al. (2003) von Hippel–Lindau disease. *Lancet* **361**: 2059–2066.
Mitchell LE, Adzick NS, Melchionne J, et al (2004) *Spina bifida*. **364**: 1884–1895.

SPINOCEREBELLAR DEGENERATIONS

The classification of this large group of rare inherited disorders is complex. Three conditions will be mentioned here.

Friedreich's ataxia

This is an autosomal recessive progressive degeneration of dorsal root ganglia, spinocerebellar tracts, corticospinal tracts and cerebellar Purkinje cells. Most patients are homozygous for the GAA triplet expansion in the Friedreich's ataxia gene. This gene, mapped to chromosome 9q13, encodes a mitochondrial protein (*fraxatin*) of unknown function. There is abnormal function of mitochondrial ATP. The expression of fraxatin is decreased in Friedreich's patients. Progressive difficulty walking occurs around the age of 12. Death is usual before 40. However, with the identification of the gene, patients mildly affected have been diagnosed in middle age.

Clinical findings are:

- ataxia of gait and trunk
- nystagmus (25%)
- dysarthria
- absent lower limb joint position and vibration sense
- absent lower limb reflexes
- optic atrophy (30%)
- pes cavus
- cardiomyopathy.

Hereditary spastic paraparesis

Isolated progressive paraparesis runs in some families. Inheritance is variable. Additional features including cerebellar signs, pes cavus, wasted hands and optic atrophy are sometimes seen. The paraparesis is usually mild and progresses slowly over many years. Some cases have dystonic features and respond to levodopa.

Ataxia telangiectasia (see also p. 219)

This rare, autosomal recessive condition is a progressive ataxic syndrome in childhood and early adult life. There is striking telangiectasia of the conjunctiva, nose, ears and skin creases. There are also defects in cell-mediated immunity and antibody production. A defect in DNA repair has been demonstrated. Death is usual by the third decade, either from infection or from lymphoreticular malignancy.

FURTHER READING
Wood N, Harding A (2000) Cerebellar and spinocerebellar disorders. In: Bradley W, Daroff RB, Fenichel GM, Marsden CD (eds) *Neurology in Clinical Practice*. Boston: Butterworth Heinemann.

PERIPHERAL NERVE DISEASE

The various nerve fibre types are shown in Table 21.52. All are myelinated except C fibres that carry impulses from pain receptors.

Mechanisms of damage to peripheral nerves

Peripheral nerves consist of two principal cellular structures – the axon and its anterior horn cell, and the myelin sheath, produced by Schwann cells between each node of Ranvier (see Fig. 21.1). Blood supply is via *vasa nervorum*. Six principal mechanisms, some coexisting, cause nerve malfunction.

Demyelination
When the Schwann cell is damaged, the myelin sheath is disrupted. This causes marked slowing of conduction, seen for example in Guillain–Barré syndrome, post-diphtheritic neuropathy and many hereditary sensori-motor neuropathies.

Axonal degeneration
The primary damage is in the axon, which dies back from the periphery. Conduction velocity tends to remain normal (cf. demyelination) because axonal continuity is maintained in surviving fibres. Axonal degeneration occurs typically in toxic neuropathies.

Wallerian degeneration
This describes the changes following nerve section. Both axon and distal myelin sheath degenerate over several weeks.

Table 21.52	A, B and C fibres in peripheral nerves	
Diameter (μ)	**Conduction velocity m/s**	**Function**
Aα (1–20)	70–110	Motor; proprioception
Aβ (5–10)	30–60	Touch
Aγ (3–6)	20–30	Fusimotor, to spindles
Aδ (2–5)	20–30	Sharp pain
B (< 3)	5–15	Autonomic, preganglionic
C (< 1.3)	0.5–2	Slow pain

Compression

Focal demyelination at the point of compression. The myelin sheath is disrupted. This occurs typically in entrapment neuropathies e.g. carpal tunnel syndrome (p. 1260).

Infarction

Microinfarction of *vasa nervorum* occurs in arteritis, e.g. polyarteritis nodosa, Churg–Strauss syndrome (p. 938), and in diabetes mellitus. Wallerian degeneration occurs distal to the ischaemic zone.

Infiltration

Peripheral nerves are infiltrated by inflammatory cells in leprosy, by malignant cells or granulomas in sarcoidosis.

Nerve regeneration

Regeneration occurs either by remyelination, when recovering Schwann cells spin new myelin sheaths around the axon, or by axonal growth down the nerve sheath and sprouting from the axonal stump. Axonal growth takes place at a rate of up to 1 mm daily.

Definitions (Fig. 21.41)

- **Neuropathy** means a pathological process affecting a peripheral nerve or nerves.
- **Mononeuropathy** means a process affecting a single nerve.
- **Mononeuritis multiplex** (multiple mononeuropathy, or multifocal neuropathy) affects several or multiple nerves.
- **Polyneuropathy** describes diffuse, symmetrical disease, usually beginning peripherally. The course is either acute, chronic, static, progressive, relapsing or towards recovery. Polyneuropathies are motor, sensory, sensorimotor (i.e. mixed) and autonomic. They are classified broadly into demyelinating and axonal types, depending upon which principal pathological process predominates. It is often

impossible to separate these clinically. Many different classifications exist. Many systemic diseases cause neuropathies. Widespread loss of tendon reflexes is typical.

- **Radiculopathy** means disease affecting nerve roots.

Diagnosis is made by clinical pattern, electrical tests, nerve biopsy (usually sural or radial) and identification of systemic or genetic disease.

MONONEUROPATHIES

Peripheral nerve compression or entrapment (Table 21.53)

Nerve damage by compression is either acute (e.g. due to a tourniquet or other sustained pressure) or chronic, such as in entrapment neuropathy. In both, focal demyelination predominates at the site of compression, but some distal axonal degeneration also occurs. Acute compression usually affects nerves exposed anatomically, e.g. common peroneal nerve at fibula head, or the ulnar at the elbow. Entrapment develops in relatively tight anatomical passages, e.g. the carpal tunnel.

These neuropathies are recognized largely by clinical features. Diagnosis can be confirmed by nerve conduction

Table 21.53	Nerve compression and entrapment
Nerve	**Site of entrapment or compression**
Median	Carpal tunnel
Ulnar	Cubital tunnel
Radial	Spiral groove of humerus
Posterior interosseous	Supinator muscle
Lateral cutaneous of thigh ('meralgia paraesthetica')	Inguinal ligament
Common peroneal	Neck of fibula
Posterior tibial	Flexor retinaculum (tarsal tunnel)

Fig. 21.41 Peripheral neuropathies – The type of neuropathy (axonal or demyelinating) can be assessed by electrical nerve studies (p. 1203). CIDP, chronic inflammatory demyelinating polyneuropathy; GBS, Guillain–Barré syndrome; DM, diabetes mellitus; HIV, human immunodeficiency virus; OP organophosphate insecticides; FH, family history; HSMN, hereditary sensorimotor neuropathy.

studies. The commonest are mentioned below. All are seen more frequently in people with diabetes. Where leprosy is prevalent (e.g. India) an isolated nerve lesion can occur.

Carpal tunnel syndrome (p. 539)

This is the common condition of median nerve compression at the wrist. Many cases are idiopathic, but this entrapment neuropathy is sometimes seen in:

- hypothyroidism
- diabetes mellitus
- pregnancy (third trimester) and obesity
- rheumatoid arthritis
- acromegaly
- amyloid
- renal dialysis patients
- trauma.

There is nocturnal tingling and pain in the hand (and/or forearm) followed by weakness of thenar muscles. Wasting of abductor pollicis brevis develops, with sensory loss in the palm and radial three-and-a-half fingers. Tinel's sign is often present and Phalen's test positive. Tinel's sign is elicited by tapping the flexor aspect of the wrist: this causes tingling and pain. In a positive Phalen's test, symptoms are reproduced on maximal wrist flexion.

A wrist splint at night or a local steroid injection in the wrist gives relief in mild cases. In pregnancy (fluid retention), it is often self-limiting. Surgical decompression of the carpel tunnel is the definitive treatment.

Ulnar nerve compression

The nerve is compressed in the cubital tunnel (at the elbow). This follows ulnar fractures or prolonged/recurrent pressure.

Clawing of the hand due to wasting of ulnar innervated muscles develops (hypothenar muscles, interossei and medial two lumbricals) with sensory loss in the ulnar one-and-a-half fingers. Decompression and transposition of the nerve at the elbow may be necessary.

The deep branch of the ulnar nerve (solely motor) can be compressed in the palm by recurrent trauma from tools, e.g. a screwdriver handle, crutches or cycle handlebars.

Radial nerve compression

The radial nerve is compressed acutely against the humerus, e.g. when the arm is draped over a hard chair for several hours (Saturday night palsy). Wrist drop and weakness of brachioradialis and finger extension follow. Recovery is usual, though not invariable, within 1–3 months. A rather similar picture occurs with compression of the posterior interosseous nerve in the forearm.

Meralgia paraesthetica (see p. 543)
Common peroneal nerve palsy

When the common peroneal (lateral popliteal) nerve is compressed against the head of the fibula following prolonged squatting, wearing a plaster cast, prolonged bed rest or coma, there is foot drop and weakness of ankle eversion. Frequently no cause is found. A patch of numbness on the anterolateral border of the shin or dorsum of the foot develops. Recovery is usual, though not invariable, within several months.

Multifocal neuropathy (mononeuritis multiplex, multiple mononeuropathy)

This occurs in:

- diabetes mellitus
- leprosy (commonest cause world-wide)
- vasculitis
- sarcoidosis
- amyloidosis
- malignancy
- neurofibromatosis
- HIV infection
- Guillain–Barré syndrome (usually polyneuropathy, p. 1260)
- idiopathic multifocal motor neuropathy.

Diagnosis is largely clinical, supported by electrical studies. Several nerves become affected sequentially or simultaneously, e.g. ulnar, median, radial and lateral popliteal nerves. When multifocal neuropathy is symmetrical, there is difficulty distinguishing it from polyneuropathy.

Idiopathic multifocal motor neuropathy

A distal motor neuropathy (often asymmetrical and predominantly in the hands) of unknown cause develops gradually over months with profuse fasciculation – hence confusion with motor neurone disease (p. 1253). Conduction block and denervation are seen electrically. Antibodies to the ganglioside GM_1 are found in over 50% of cases. This is non-specific – they are sometimes seen in other neuropathies, e.g. Guillain–Barré syndrome.

Treatment with i.v. immunoglobulin, steroids and/or cyclophosphamide slows the condition.

POLYNEUROPATHIES

Many toxins and diseases cause polyneuropathy, though the aetiology sometimes remains obscure. The most common presentation is an acute, chronic or subacute sensorimotor neuropathy. A classification is given in Table 21.54.

Guillain–Barré syndrome (GBS)
Clinical features

This is the most common acute polyneuropathy (3/100 000/year); it is usually demyelinating (occasionally axonal) and probably has an autoallergic basis. GBS is monophasic – it does not recur. GBS is also known as acute inflammatory or postinfective neuropathy, and acute inflammatory demyelinating polyradiculoneuropathy. It has become clear that the clinical spectrum of GBS extends to an acute motor axonal neuropathy, and

Table 21.54 Varieties of polyneuropathy

Guillain–Barré syndrome (acute postinfective
  polyneuropathy)
Chronic inflammatory demyelinating polyneuropathy
Diphtheritic polyneuropathy
Idiopathic sensorimotor neuropathy
Toxic, metabolic and vitamin deficiency neuropathies
  (Table 21.55)
Hereditary sensorimotor neuropathies,
  e.g. Charcot–Marie–Tooth
Other polyneuropathies:
  Neuropathy in cancer
  Neuropathies in systemic diseases
  Autonomic neuropathy
  HIV-associated neuropathy
  Critical illness neuropathy

the Miller–Fisher syndrome – a rare proximal form causing ocular muscle palsies and ataxia.

Paralysis follows 1–3 weeks after an infection that is often trivial, and often unidentified. *Campylobacter jejuni* and cytomegalovirus infections are well-recognized causes of severe GBS. Infecting organisms induce antibody responses against peripheral nerves. 'Molecular mimicry', sharing of homologous epitopes between microorganism liposaccharides and nerve gangliosides (e.g. GM_1), is the potential mechanism.

The patient complains of weakness of distal limb muscles and/or distal numbness. This ascends, progressing over several days to 6 weeks. Loss of tendon reflexes is almost invariable. In mild cases there is little disability before spontaneous recovery begins, but in some 20% respiratory and facial muscles become weak, sometimes progressing to complete paralysis. Autonomic features sometimes develop.

Diagnosis

This is established on clinical grounds and confirmed by nerve conduction studies; these show slowing of conduction in the common demyelinating form, prolonged distal motor latency and/or conduction block. CSF protein is often raised to 1–3 g/L. The cell count and sugar level remain normal.

Differential diagnosis includes other paralytic illnesses, e.g. poliomyelitis, botulism, cord compression or muscle disease.

Course and management

Paralysis may progress rapidly (hours/days) to require ventilatory support. It is essential that ventilation is monitored (vital capacity, blood gases) repeatedly to recognize emerging respiratory muscle weakness. Subcutaneous heparin (p. 480) should be given to reduce the risk of venous thrombosis.

High-dosage intravenous immunoglobulin given within the first 2 weeks reduces the duration and severity of paralysis. There is concern about using this expensive pooled blood product. Patients should be screened for IgA deficiency before immunoglobulin is given – severe allergic reactions due to IgG antibodies may occur when IgA congenital deficiency is present. Angina or myocardial infarction can be precipitated by i.v. immunoglobulin. Plasma exchange is also of proven benefit in shortening disability, though rarely used. Corticosteroids were given for many years but are valueless in GBS. Recovery begins (with or without treatment) between several days and 6 weeks from the outset. Prolonged ventilation may be necessary. Improvement towards independent mobility is gradual over many months but may be incomplete. Fifteen per cent of patients die or are left disabled; fatigue is common.

Chronic inflammatory demyelinating polyneuropathy (CIDP)

This polyneuropathy develops over weeks or months, usually with a persistent but relapsing and remitting course. CSF protein is raised and, usually, segmental demyelination is seen in peripheral nerves. CIDP responds to steroids (long term, low dose) and to i.v. immunoglobulin (for exacerbations). In some cases plaques resembling MS lesions are seen on MRI in brain and spinal cord.

Outlook is variable, but with therapy many CIDP cases run a benign course over many years. Recovery occasionally occurs. There are several CIDP varieties – the usual demyelinating form, an axonal form, and multifocal neuropathy.

Diphtheritic neuropathy (p. 65)

Palatal weakness followed by pupillary paralysis and a sensorimotor neuropathy occur several weeks after the throat infection.

Idiopathic chronic sensorimotor neuropathy

The patient complains of progressive symmetrical numbness and tingling in hands and feet, spreading proximally in glove and stocking distribution. There is distal weakness which also ascends. Rarely cranial nerves are affected. Tendon reflexes become absent. Symptoms may progress over many months, remain static or occasionally remit. Autonomic features are sometimes seen.

Nerve conduction and electromyography show either axonal degeneration or demyelination, or features of both these processes. Peripheral nerve biopsy is helpful in classifying some cases, in particular diagnosing CIDP and unsuspected vasculitis.

Cranial polyneuropathy

This means multiple cranial nerve lesions. This occurs in malignant infiltration, particularly with lymphomas, and with sarcoidosis.

Table 21.55 Toxic, metabolic and vitamin-deficiency neuropathies

Metabolic	Toxic
Diabetes mellitus	Drugs (Table 21.56)
Uraemia	Alcohol
Hepatic disease	Industrial toxins, e.g. lead
Thyroid disease	organophophates
Porphyria	
Amyloid disease	**Vitamin deficiency**
Malignancy	B_1 (thiamin)
Refsum's disease	B_6 (pyridoxine)
Critical illness	Nicotinic acid
	B_{12}

Table 21.56 Drug-related neuropathies

Drug	Neuropathy	Mode/site of action
Phenytoin	M	A
Chloramphenicol	S, M	A
Metronidazole	S, S/M	A
Isoniazid	S, S/M	A
Dapsone	M	A
Anti-retroviral drugs	S > M	A
Nitrofurantoin	S/M	A
Vincristine	S > M	A
Paclitaxel	S > M	A
Disulfiram	S, M	A
Cisplatin	S	A
Amiodarone	S, M	D, A
Chloroquine	S, M	A, D
Suramin	M > S	D, A

A = axonal; D = demyelinating; M = motor

Toxic, metabolic and vitamin-deficiency neuropathies

The most common are shown in Table 21.55. All are due to impaired axonal and/or myelin metabolism.

Metabolic neuropathies
Diabetes mellitus
Several varieties of neuropathy occur in diabetes:

- symmetrical sensory polyneuropathy
- acute painful neuropathy
- mononeuropathy and multiple mononeuropathy:
  - cranial nerve lesions
  - isolated peripheral nerve lesions (e.g. median)
- diabetic amyotrophy
- autonomic neuropathy.

These are discussed in more detail on page 1129.

Uraemia
Progressive sensorimotor neuropathy develops in chronic uraemia. The response to dialysis is variable but the neuropathy usually improves after renal transplantation.

Thyroid disease
A mild chronic sensorimotor neuropathy is sometimes seen in both hyperthyroidism and hypothyroidism (pp. 1074 and 1072). Myopathy also occurs in hyperthyroidism (p. 1074).

Porphyria
In acute intermittent porphyria (p. 1148) there are episodes of a severe, mainly proximal, neuropathy, sometimes associated with abdominal pain, confusion and later coma. Alcohol and barbiturates may precipitate attacks.

Amyloidosis
See page 1147. Polyneuropathy or multifocal neuropathy develops.

Refsum's disease
This is a rare condition inherited as an autosomal recessive. There is a sensorimotor polyneuropathy with ataxia, retinal damage and deafness. It is due to defective phytanic acid metabolism.

Toxic neuropathies
Alcohol
Polyneuropathy, mainly in the lower limbs, occurs with chronic excess alcohol. Calf pain is common. Thiamine is the treatment, but the response is variable, even with complete abstention. Recurrence (and progression) occurs with even small amounts of alcohol.

Drugs and industrial toxins
Many drugs (Table 21.56) and a wide variety of industrial toxins cause polyneuropathy. Toxins include:

- lead poisoning – motor neuropathy
- acrylamide (plastics industry), trichlorethylene, hexane and other fat-soluble hydrocarbons (e.g. glue-sniffing, p. 1305) – progressive sensorimotor polyneuropathy
- arsenic and thallium – polyneuropathy, initially sensory.

Vitamin-deficiency neuropathies
Vitamin deficiencies cause nervous system diseases that are largely preventable and potentially reversible if treated early – and inexorably progressive if not. Deficiencies (often of multiple vitamins) occur in malnutrition.

Thiamin (vitamin B_1)
Dietary deficiency causes *beriberi* (p. 244). Principal features are polyneuropathy and cardiac failure. Thiamin deficiency also leads to an amnestic syndrome (Wernicke–Korsakoff psychosis, p. 245 and below). Alcohol is the commonest cause in western countries and, rarely, anorexia nervosa. For other neurological consequences of alcohol, see Table 21.57.

Wernicke–Korsakoff syndrome. This thiamine-responsive encephalopathy is due to ischaemic damage in the brainstem and its connections. It consists of:

Table 21.57 Neurological effects of ethyl alcohol

Acute intoxication:	Epilepsy (3–10%)
Disturbance of balance, gait and speech	Acute intoxication
	Alcohol withdrawal
Coma	Hypoglycaemia
Head injury and its sequelae	Cerebellar degeneration
	Cerebral infarction
Alcohol withdrawal:	Cerebral atrophy
'Morning shakes'	Dementia
Tremor	Central pontine myelinolysis
Delirium tremens	Marchiafava–Bignami
Thiamin deficiency:	syndrome (a rare
Polyneuropathy	degeneration of corpus
Wernicke–Korsakoff syndrome	callosum)

- *Eye signs* – nystagmus, bilateral lateral rectus palsies, conjugate gaze palsies, fixed pupils and, rarely, papilloedema
- *Ataxia* – broad-based gait, cerebellar signs and vestibular paralysis (absent calorics)
- *Cognitive change* – amnestic syndrome (confabulation), restlessness, stupor, coma
- *Hypothermia and hypotension* – due to hypothalamic involvement (rare).

Wernicke–Korsakoff syndrome is underdiagnosed. Erythrocyte transketolase activity is reduced but of limited practical value – the test is rarely available. Thiamine should be given parenterally if the diagnosis is in question. The vitamin is harmless but should be given slowly as anaphylaxis occurs (p. 245). Untreated Wernicke–Korsakoff syndrome commonly leads to an irreversible amnestic state (Table 21.4, p. 1179).

Pyridoxine (vitamin B₆)
Deficiency causes a mainly sensory neuropathy. In practical terms this is seen as limb numbness developing during anti-TB therapy in slow isoniazid-acetylators (p. 994). Prophylactic pyridoxine 10 mg daily is given with isoniazid.

Vitamin B₁₂ (cobalamin)
Deficiency causes damage to the spinal cord, peripheral nerves and brain.

Subacute combined degeneration of the cord (SACD). Combined spinal cord and peripheral nerve damage is a sequel of Addisonian pernicious anaemia and rarely other causes of vitamin B₁₂ deficiency (p. 432).

The patient complains initially of numbness and tingling of fingers and toes. There is combined distal sensory loss, particularly posterior column, absent ankle jerks (neuropathy), with cord disease – exaggerated knee jerks, extensor plantar responses. Optic atrophy and retinal haemorrhage may occur. In later stages sphincter disturbance, severe generalized weakness and dementia develop. Exceptionally, dementia develops in the early stages. Without treatment, SACD is fatal within 5 years.

Macrocytosis with megaloblastic bone marrow are usual though not invariable in SACD. Parenteral B₁₂

reverses peripheral nerve damage but has little effect on the cord and brain.

Hereditary sensorimotor neuropathies (HSMN)
These are large and complex groups, phenotypically similar but genetically separate.

Charcot–Marie–Tooth disease
(see also pp. 173, 180, 184)
Charcot–Marie–Tooth (CMT) disease is also called peroneal muscular atrophy. CMT describes the common clinical phenotype – distal limb wasting and weakness that slowly progresses over many years, mostly in the legs, with variable loss of sensation and reflexes. In advanced disease, distal wasting is so marked that the legs are said to resemble inverted champagne bottles. Mild cases have pes cavus and clawing of the toes that can pass unnoticed. Multiple genetic variants of the CMT phenotype are now recognized, e.g.:

- HSMN Ia (CMT 1A) – the commonest, autosomal dominant (AD) demyelinating neuropathy caused by duplication (or point mutation) of a 1.5 megabase portion p11.2 of chromosome 17 encompassing the peripheral myelin protein 22 gene (PMP-22, 17p11) (see Table 3.4)
- HSMN Ib (CMT 1B) – the second commonest, an AD demyelinating neuropathy due to mutations in the myelin protein zero gene on chromosome 1 (Po, 1q22)
- HSMN II (CMT 2) – rare axonal neuropathies also caused by Po and other mutations
- distal spinal muscular atrophy – a rare cause of CMT phenotype
- CMT with optic atrophy, deafness, retinitis pigmentosa and spastic paraparesis
- CMT as a sex-linked HSMN form due to abnormality in the connexin gene (p. 184).

HSMN III
This rare demyelinating sensory neuropathy of childhood (Déjérine–Sottas disease) leads to severe incapacity during adolescence. CSF protein is greatly elevated to 10 g/L or more. Nerve roots become greatly hypertrophied. Point mutations either of PMP-22 gene, or of Po, generate this phenotype.

Other polyneuropathies

Neuropathy in cancer
Polyneuropathy is seen as a non-metastatic manifestation of malignancy, sometimes with anti-Hu antibodies. Polyneuropathy occurs in myeloma and other dysproteinaemic states, probably owing to impaired perfusion of nerve trunks or to demyelination associated with allergic reactions affecting peripheral nerves. Individual nerves are sometimes infiltrated with malignant cells.

Neuropathies in systemic diseases

Vasculitic neuropathy occurs in SLE (see p. 575), polyarteritis nodosa (p. 583), Churg–Strauss syndrome (p. 938), rheumatoid disease (p. 560), sarcoidosis and giant cell arteritis (p. 582). Both multifocal neuropathy and symmetrical sensorimotor polyneuropathy develop.

POEMS syndrome. This rare condition consists of chronic inflammatory demyelinating *P*olyneuropathy, *O*rganomegaly (hepatomegaly 50%), *E*ndocrinopathy (gynaecomastia and atrophic testes), an *M* protein band on electrophoresis with less than 5% of plasma cells in bone marrow, and *S*kin hyperpigmentation.

Autonomic neuropathy

Autonomic neuropathy causes postural hypotension, urinary retention, impotence, diarrhoea (or occasionally constipation), diminished sweating, impaired pupillary responses and cardiac arrhythmias. This develops in diabetes mellitus, in amyloidosis and may complicate Guillain–Barré syndrome. Many varieties of neuropathy cause autonomic failure in a mild, and often subclinical, form. Occasionally, when there is damage to small myelinated and non-myelinated B and C fibres, clinical features of the autonomic neuropathy predominate, e.g. in diabetes.

HIV-associated polyneuropathies

Several neuropathies occur. Inflammatory demyelinating neuropathies indistinguishable from Guillain–Barré and CIDP are seen early in HIV infection, particularly during seroconversion. The most common neuropathy is a chronic distal, symmetrical painful neuropathy.

Rarely, a severe lumbosacral polyradiculoneuropathy develops, with profound lower limb flaccid paralysis, areflexia and sphincter dysfunction.

All HIV-associated neuropathies respond poorly to retroviral therapy. These drugs also cause neuropathies (p. 145).

Critical illness polyneuropathy (p. 985)

Some 50% of critically ill ITU patients with multiple organ failure and sepsis develop an axonal poly-neuropathy. The severe inflammatory response following infection or trauma appears to impair the neural microcirculation. Typically distal weakness and absent reflexes are seen during recovery from the critical illness. Resolution is usual.

PLEXUS AND NERVE ROOT LESIONS

The common conditions that cause these are summarized in Table 21.58.

Thoracic outlet syndrome

A fibrous band or cervical rib extending from the tip of the C7 transverse process to the first rib stretches across the lower brachial plexus (roots C8 and T1). There is forearm pain (ulnar border), T1 sensory loss and thenar muscle

---

Table 21.58 **Principal causes of plexus and nerve root lesions**

Plexus
Trauma
Malignant infiltration
Cervical rib (thoracic outlet syndrome)
Neuralgic amyotrophy

Nerve root
Trauma
Herpes zoster
Meningeal inflammation (e.g. syphilis, arachnoiditis)
Tumours (neurofibroma, metastases)
Cervical and lumbar spondylosis

---

wasting, principally abductor pollicis brevis. Horner's syndrome may develop. The rib or band can be excised.

In some patients the rib or band causes subclavian artery or venous occlusion. Neurological and vascular problems rarely occur together. Thoracic outlet syndrome is also used to describe ill-defined upper limb symptoms – usually on poor evidence.

Neuralgic amyotrophy

This is a clinically distinct condition with severe pain in the muscles around one shoulder followed by wasting, usually of infraspinatus, supraspinatus, deltoid and serratus anterior muscles. A demyelinating brachial plexopathy develops over several days. The cause is unknown. Since this sometimes follows viral infection or immunization, an allergic basis is postulated.

Recovery of wasted muscles is usual, over some months.

Malignant infiltration

Metastatic disease of nerve roots of the brachial or lumbo-sacral plexus causes a painful radiculopathy. A common example is an apical bronchial neoplasm (Pancoast's tumour) causing a T1 and sympathetic outflow lesion. There is wasting of small hand muscles, pain, T1 sensory loss with ipsilateral Horner's syndrome. This also occurs in apical TB.

Cervical and lumbar degeneration

Spondylosis (Tables 10.3 and 10.6) describes vertebral degenerative changes that occur during ageing or due to trauma. Several, often related, factors produce neuro-logical signs and symptoms, including:

- osteophytes – local bony overgrowth (spurs or bars)
- congenital narrowing of the spinal canal
- intervertebral disc degeneration with posterior or lateral disc protrusion
- vertebral collapse
- rheumatoid synovitis (p. 557)
- ischaemic changes in the cord and nerve roots.

Narrowing of disc spaces, osteophytes, narrowing of exit foramina, and narrowing of the spinal canal can also be

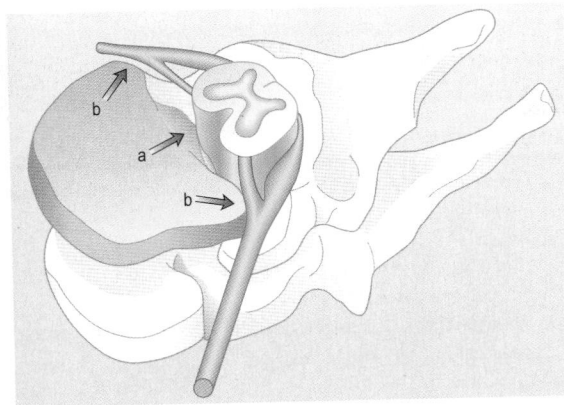

Fig. 21.42 Central and lateral disc protrusions.
(a) Central disc protrusion compressing spinal cord. **(b)** Lateral disc protrusion compressing nerve roots.

seen on X-rays and MR in the symptomless population, commonly in the mid and lower cervical and lower lumbar region.

Lateral cervical disc protrusion (Fig. 21.42)

The patient complains of pain in the arm. A C7 protrusion is the most common problem. There is root pain that radiates to the C7 myotome (triceps, deep to scapula and extensor aspect of forearm), with a sensory disturbance, tingling, and numbness in the C7 dermatome.

In an established C7 root lesion there is:

- weakness/wasting – triceps, wrist and finger extensors
- loss of the triceps jerk (C7 reflex arc)
- C7 dermatome sensory loss.

Although the initial pain is often very severe, most cases recover with rest and analgesics. It is usual to immobilize the neck. Where recovery is delayed, disc protrusion with root compression is seen on MRI. Root decompression is usually helpful.

Lateral lumbar disc protrusion

The L5 and S1 roots are commonly compressed by lateral prolapse of L4–L5 and L5–S1 discs. There is low back pain and sciatica (pain radiating down the buttock and lower limb). The onset is typically acute. It sometimes follows lifting a heavy weight, bending or minor injury. When the pain follows such an event, it is tempting to ascribe the condition entirely to it. However, lateral lumbar disc protrusion is commonly apparently spontaneous, and lifting or injury are usually only precipitating an inevitable event.

Straight-leg raising is limited. There is reflex loss (e.g. ankle jerk in a complete S1 root lesion) and weakness of plantar flexion (S1). Sensory loss is found in the affected dermatome.

Most cases of sciatica resolve with rest and analgesics. In the minority, MRI is necessary. Laminectomy is indicated when a substantial symptomatic disc lesion is shown.

Acute low back pain

Acute low back pain is an extremely common problem. Most cases are of disc origin (discogenic) or pain arises from the facet joints. It is unusual for there to be significant nerve root compression. Bed rest, sleeping on hard boards and lumbar corsets have long been advocated: the evidence base for these measures is poor, and activity and a trial of gentle manipulation is preferred (see also p. 542).

Central disc protrusion (p. 1199)

Central cervical disc protrusion (cervical myelopathy)

Posterior disc protrusion (Fig. 21.43), common at C4–C5, C5–C6 and C6–C7 levels, causes spinal cord compression. Congenital spinal canal narrowing, osteophytic bars and ischaemia are contributory factors. The patient complains of difficulty walking. Frequently there are no neck symptoms. Spastic paraparesis (or tetraparesis) is found, with variable sensory loss. A reflex level in the upper limbs and evidence of lateral disc protrusion may coexist. MRI is necessary to demonstrate the level and extent of cord compression. Neck manipulation should be avoided, and a collar fitted.

Cervical laminectomy or anterior fusion of the vertebral bodies with removal of the disc may be necessary when cord compression is severe or progressive. The results of surgery are variable. Complete recovery of the pyramidal signs is unusual, although progression may be halted.

Central thoracic disc protrusion

Central protrusion of a thoracic disc is a rare cause of paraparesis.

Central lumbosacral disc protrusion

A central disc protrusion causes a *cauda equina* syndrome, i.e. bilateral flaccid (cf. spasticity in higher lesions) lower limb weakness, sacral numbness, retention of urine, impotence and areflexia with back pain. Many nerve roots are involved. Onset is either acute (a cause of an acute flaccid paraparesis) or chronic, when intermittent claudication occurs. A central lumbosacral protrusion should be suspected if a patient with back pain develops

Fig. 21.43 MR (T2): C5/6 disc compressing the cord.

retention of urine or sacral numbness. Urgent imaging and surgical decompression is indicated for this emergency. Neoplasms in the lumbosacral region can cause a similar picture.

Spinal stenosis

A narrow spinal canal is developmental and frequently symptomless. Congenital narrowing of the cervical canal predisposes the cervical cord to damage from minor disc protrusion. In the lumbosacral region, further narrowing of the canal by disc protrusion causes root pain, and/or buttock and lower limb claudication. As the patient walks, nerve roots become hyperaemic and swell, producing buttock and lower limb pain with numbness. Surgical decompression is required.

FURTHER READING

England JD, Ashbury AK (2004) Peripheral neuropathy. *Lancet* **363**: 2151–2161.

Reilly M (2001) Charcot–Marie–Tooth disease: a genetic update. *Current Medical Literature (Neurology)* **17**: 75–78.

Singh A, Crockard HA (1999) Quantitative assessment of cervical spondylotic myelopathy by a simple walking test. *Lancet* **354**: 370–373.

Winer JB (2003) Treatment of Guillain–Barré syndrome. *Quarterly Journal of Medicine* **2002**: 717–721.

NON-METASTATIC MANIFESTATIONS OF MALIGNANCY

Many neurological syndromes may accompany malignancy in the absence of metastases. Clinical pictures include:

- sensorimotor neuropathy (p. 1261)
- mononeuritis multiplex (p. 1260)
- cranial polyneuropathy (p. 1261)
- Lambert–Eaton myasthenic–myopathic syndrome (LEMS, p. 1269)
- motor neurone disease variants (p. 1253)
- spastic paraparesis (p. 1193)
- cerebellar syndrome (p. 1195)
- dementia and encephalopathy (p. 1254)
- progressive multifocal leucoencephalopathy (p. 1242).
- Paraneoplastic stiff-person syndrome. Stiffness of skeletal muscle associated with antibodies to glutamic acid decarboxylase or the synaptic protein amphiphysin. Can be idiopathic as well.

Mechanisms remain obscure. The neurological syndrome sometimes precedes clinical signs of the neoplasm – often a small-cell bronchial carcinoma or lymphoma.

FURTHER READING

Darnell RB, Posner JB (2003) Paraneoplastic syndromes involving the nervous system. *New England Journal of Medicine* **349**: 1543–1554.

DISEASES OF VOLUNTARY MUSCLE

Definitions

- **Myopathy** describes diseases of voluntary muscle generally.
- **Myositis** indicates inflammation.
- **Muscular dystrophy** describes inherited disorders with progressive weakness.
- **Myasthenia** means fatiguable (worse on exercise) weakness.
- **Myotonia** is sustained contraction/slow relaxation seen in myotonias.
- **Channelopathy** describes ion channel disorders in muscle cells.

Weakness without reflex loss is the predominant feature of muscle disease. For classification, see Table 21.59. Only the commoner conditions are mentioned below.

Pathophysiology

Muscle fibres are affected by:

- acute inflammation and fibre necrosis (e.g. polymyositis, infection)
- genetically determined metabolic failure (e.g. Duchenne muscular dystrophy)
- infiltration by inflammatory tissue (e.g. sarcoidosis)

Table 21.59 Classification of muscle disease	
Acquired myopathy	**Genetically determined myopathies**
Inflammatory myopathy Polymyositis: alone with skin lesions (dermatomyositis) with collagen disease with malignancy Viral, bacterial and parasitic infection Sarcoidosis	**Muscular dystrophies** Duchenne muscular dystrophy Facioscapulohumeral dystrophy Limb girdle dystrophy
	Myotonias Dystrophia myotonica Myotonia congenita
Metabolic and endocrine myopathy Corticosteroids/Cushing's syndrome Thyroid disease Calcium metabolism disorders Hypokalaemia Ethanol Drugs	**Channelopathies (periodic paralyses)** Hypokalaemic periodic paralysis Hyperkalaemic periodic paralysis Normokalaemic periodic paralysis
Myasthenic disorders Myasthenia gravis Lambert–Eaton myasthenic– myopathic syndrome (LEMS)	**Specific metabolic myopathies** (e.g.) Myophosphorylase deficiency Other defects of glycogen and fatty acid metabolism Mitochondrial disease (ragged red muscle fibres) Malignant hyperpyrexia

- fibre hypertrophy and regeneration
- immunological, ion channel and mitochondrial disorders.

Examples of the latter are:

- In *myasthenia gravis*, antibodies to the postsynaptic membrane acetylcholine receptor protein block neuromuscular transmission.
- In *Lambert–Eaton myasthenic–myopathic syndrome* (LEMS), antibodies to muscle calcium channel components are found.
- In *myotonias*, defective chloride ion membrane conductance is associated with delayed muscle relaxation.
- In *McArdle's syndrome*, myophosphorylase deficiency produces weakness after exercise.
- In *mitochondrial disease*, various ATP enzyme defects cause weakness.

Investigations

Diagnosis is often made by recognition of the distribution of weakness, wasting or hypertrophy, and muscle consistency (e.g. induration).

Serum muscle enzymes

Serum creatine phosphokinase (and aldolase) is greatly elevated in many dystrophies (e.g. Duchenne dystrophy) and in inflammatory muscle disorders, e.g. polymyositis. These enzymes remain normal in myasthenia gravis and LEMS, and usually remain normal in myotonias and chronic partial denervation.

Neurogenetic tests

Genetic probes in propositus and family members are helpful in the diagnosis of muscular dystrophies.

Electromyography

When a muscle is weak the normal interference pattern is reduced. Changes in interference pattern indicate:

- *Myopathy.* Short-duration spiky polyphasic muscle action potentials are seen. Spontaneous fibrillation is occasionally recorded.
- *Denervation.* Fibrillation potentials (about 1 ms in duration and 50–200 mV in amplitude) are visible.
- *Myotonic discharges.* A characteristic high-frequency whine is heard (on the loudspeaker).
- *Decrement and increment.* In myasthenia gravis, a characteristic decrement in evoked muscle action potential follows repetitive motor nerve stimulation. The reverse occurs (an increment in repetitive response) in the rare LEMS, p. 1269.

Muscle biopsy

Histology of muscle fibre types (type 1, slow; type 2, fast), denervation, inflammation, dystrophic changes and muscle histochemistry are examined. Electron microscopy is sometimes necessary. In chronic partial denervation, fibre type grouping (i.e. groups of atrophic fibres of the same fibre type) is seen. Hypertrophic fibres also occur. In acute denervation, small angulated muscle fibres are seen scattered randomly between normal fibres. In dystrophies and myositis, muscle fibres are diffusely abnormal, nuclei become central, and invasion by inflammatory cells and/or necrosis occurs. Great experience is needed to assess these changes.

Imaging

MRI shows changes within muscles in some cases of myositis.

INFLAMMATORY MYOPATHIES

Polymyositis and dermatomyositis

These conditions are characterized by non-suppurative skeletal muscle inflammation. Muscles are weak and sometimes tender. In many cases there are skin changes (dermatomyositis, p. 1343) or other connective tissue diseases (p. 573). Aetiology is unknown, though HLA-B8/DR3 phenotypes have a predisposition to develop polymyositis – and Cocksackie (and other) viruses are possibly implicated.

Clinical features

Isolated adult polymyositis is a rare disease, seen mainly in the fourth and fifth decades, more commonly in women. Proximal weakness causes difficulty in rising from a chair, climbing stairs or lifting. Weakness typically remains proximal. Weak muscles ache and are sometimes tender and indurated. The course is variable, from a mild condition to a severe progressive disability. If the disease progresses, widespread weakness and wasting develop, with dysphagia, respiratory muscle weakness and cardiac involvement.

Investigations

Serum creatine phosphokinase is usually greatly elevated. EMG shows myopathic changes: occasionally fibrillation potentials cause diagnostic difficulty. Muscle biopsy shows inflammatory changes with mononuclear cell infiltration. ESR is sometimes raised with a mild normochromic normocytic anaemia. ANF may be positive (p. 685).

Differential diagnosis

Muscular dystrophies rarely progress as rapidly as polymyositis and there is no muscle pain. Pseudo-hypertrophy, which occurs in some dystrophies, does not occur in polymyositis. There is no family history. Motor neurone disease is always eventually accompanied by upper motor neurone signs, and prominent fasciculation is common.

Treatment

Corticosteroids with azathioprine or cyclophosphamide reduce symptoms in about 75% of cases. Only rarely does polymyositis cause death.

Table 21.60	Muscle involvement in infections
Myalgia	Influenza viruses
Bornholm disease	Coxsackie B5
Acute polymyositis, with myoglobinuria	Coxsackie B6, ECHO 9
Acute suppurative (tropical) myositis	*Staphylococcus* spp.
Gas gangrene (clostridial myositis)	*Clostridium perfringens*
Necrotizing myositis '	*Streptococcus* spp.
Tuberculous myositis (rare)	*Mycobacterium tuberculosis*
Trichinosis	*Trichinella spiralis*
Cysticercosis	*Taenia solium* (larval form)
Hydatid disease	*Echinococcus granulosus*
Toxoplasma myositis	*Toxoplasma gondii*
Sarcosporidiosis	*Sarcocystis lindemanni*
Chagas' disease	*Trypanosoma cruzi*
Actinomycosis	*Actinomyces* spp.

Viral, bacterial and parasitic myositis

Muscle tissue is involved in many infections; see Table 21.60.

Myopathy in sarcoidosis and rheumatoid disease

In sarcoidosis, a subacute myopathy sometimes develops, either with limb muscle swelling and induration, or with wasting. This is usually during pulmonary sarcoidosis, but occasionally it is isolated. Sarcoid nodules are seen on muscle biopsy. Treatment is with steroids.

In rheumatoid disease, a rare localized nodular myositis causes painful swelling of limb, trunk and facial muscles.

METABOLIC AND ENDOCRINE MYOPATHIES

Corticosteroids and Cushing's syndrome

Proximal weakness occurs with prolonged high-dose steroid therapy, particularly with *9-α*-fluorinated steroids (e.g. dexamethasone and triamcinolone) and in Cushing's syndrome (p. 1085). Selective type-2 fibre atrophy is seen on biopsy.

Thyroid disease (see also p. 1069)

Several myopathies occur. Thyrotoxicosis can be accompanied by severe proximal myopathy. There is also an association between thyrotoxicosis and myasthenia gravis, and between thyrotoxicosis and hypokalaemic periodic paralysis (p. 1271). Both associations are seen more frequently in SE Asia. In ophthalmic Graves' disease, there is swelling and lymphocytic infiltration of extraocular muscles (p. 1077).

Hypothyroidism is sometimes associated with muscle pain and stiffness, resembling myotonia. A proximal myopathy also occurs.

Disorders of calcium metabolism

Proximal myopathy develops in hypocalcaemia, rickets and osteomalacia (p. 1095).

Hypokalaemia

Acute hypokalaemia (e.g. in diuretic therapy) causes a severe flaccid paralysis reversed by potassium, given slowly (p. 707). Chronic hypokalaemia (also commonly caused by diuretics) gives rise to mild, mainly proximal, weakness. See also periodic paralysis (p. 1271).

Alcohol

Severe myopathy with muscle pain, necrosis and myoglobinuria occurs in acute alcoholic excess. A similar syndrome occurs in diamorphine and amfetamine addicts. A subacute proximal myopathy occurs with chronic alcohol abuse.

Drugs

Drug-induced muscle disorders have been described. These include proximal myopathy (steroids), muscle weakness (lithium), painful muscles (fibrates), rhabdomyolysis (fibrate combined with a statin), and malignant hyperpyrexia (p. 1271). All are rare, and most respond to drug withdrawal.

NEUROMUSCULAR JUNCTION

Myasthenia gravis

This acquired condition is characterized by weakness and fatiguability of proximal limb, ocular and bulbar muscles. The heart is not affected. The prevalence is about 4 in 100 000. It is twice as common in women as in men, with a peak age incidence around 30.

The cause is unknown. IgG antibodies to acetylcholine receptor protein are found. Immune complexes (IgG and complement) are deposited at the postsynaptic membranes, causing interference with and later destruction of the acetylcholine receptor.

Thymic hyperplasia is found in 70% of myasthenic patients below the age of 40. In 10% a thymic tumour is found, the incidence increasing with age; antibodies to striated muscle can be demonstrated in these patients. Young patients without a thymoma have an increased association with HLA-B8, and DR3.

There is an association between myasthenia gravis and thyroid disease, rheumatoid disease, pernicious anaemia and SLE. Transient myasthenia gravis is sometimes caused by D-penicillamine treatment.

Clinical features

Fatiguability is seen in many muscles. Proximal limb muscles, extraocular muscles, and muscles of mastication, speech and facial expression are those commonly affected in the early stages. Respiratory difficulties may occur.

Complex extraocular palsies, ptosis and fluctuating proximal weakness are found. The reflexes are initially preserved but may be fatiguable, i.e. disappear. Muscle wasting is sometimes seen after many years.

Investigations

The clinical picture of fluctuating, fatiguable weakness is often diagnostic. Early symptoms of fatigue are frequently dismissed by attending doctors.

Serum acetylcholine receptor antibodies

These disease-specific IgG antibodies are present in 90% of cases of generalized myasthenia gravis. The antibodies are found in no other condition. In pure ocular myasthenia they are detectable in < 50% of cases.

Nerve stimulation

There is a characteristic decrement in the evoked muscle action potential following repetitive motor nerve stimulation.

Tensilon (edrophonium) test

The anticholinesterase edrophonium (10 mg) is injected i.v. as a bolus after a 1–2 mg test dose. Improvement in weakness occurs within seconds and lasts for 2–3 minutes when the test is positive. To be certain, it is wise to have an observer present and to perform a control using saline. Occasionally edrophonium causes bronchial constriction and syncope. The test must not be done without resuscitation facilities.

Other tests

A thymoma on chest X-ray is confirmed by mediastinal MRI. All patients should have a chest CT – even if the chest X-ray is normal. Routine peripheral blood studies are normal – the ESR is not raised, and CPK normal. Autoantibodies to striated muscle (suggests a thymoma), intrinsic factor or thyroid may be found. Rheumatoid factor and antinuclear antibody tests may be positive. Muscle biopsy is usually not performed, though ultrastructural abnormalities can be seen.

Course and management

Myasthenia gravis fluctuates in severity; most cases have a protracted, lifelong course. Respiratory impairment, dysphagia and nasal regurgitation occur; emergency assisted ventilation may be required. Simple monitoring tests, such as the duration the arm can be held outstretched, and the vital capacity, are useful.

Exacerbations (myasthenic crises) are usually unpredictable and unprovoked but may be brought on by infections, by aminoglycosides or other drugs. Enemas (magnesium sulphate) may provoke severe weakness.

Treatment

Oral anticholinesterases

Pyridostigmine (60 mg tablet) is the drug most widely used. Its duration of action is 3–4 hours. The dose (usually 4–16 tablets daily) is determined by the response. Pyridostigmine prolongs acetylcholine action by inhibiting cholinesterase. Overdose of anticholinesterases cause severe weakness (cholinergic crisis). Muscarinic side-effects, e.g. colic and diarrhoea, can be caused by anticholinesterases. Oral atropine (antimuscarinic) 0.5 mg with each dose helps reduce this. Anticholinesterases

help weakness but do not alter the natural history of myasthenia.

Thymectomy

Thymectomy improves prognosis, particularly in women below 40 years with positive receptor antibodies and a history of myasthenia of more than 7 years. Some 60% of non-thymoma cases improve. The precise reason is unclear. If a thymoma is present, surgery is necessary to remove a potentially malignant tumour; it is less usual for myasthenia to improve.

Immunosuppressant drugs

Corticosteroids are often used. There is improvement in 70% of cases, although this may be preceded by an initial relapse. Azathioprine is often used in addition to steroids.

Plasmapheresis and intravenous immunoglobulin therapy

During exacerbations these interventions are of value.

Lambert–Eaton myasthenic–myopathic syndrome (LEMS)

This rare non-metastatic manifestation of small-cell carcinoma of the bronchus is due to defective acetylcholine release at the neuromuscular junction. Proximal muscle weakness, sometimes involving ocular and bulbar muscles is found, with absent tendon reflexes (a cardinal sign). Weakness tends to improve after a few minutes of muscular contraction, and absent reflexes return (cf. myasthenia). Diagnosis is confirmed by EMG and repetitive stimulation of a motor nerve (increment, see above). Antibodies to P/Q-type voltage-gated calcium channels are found in most cases (90%). 3,4-Diaminopyridine (DAP) is a safe and effective therapy.

Other rare myasthenic syndromes exist, for example congenital myasthenia.

FURTHER READING
Chaudhuri A, Behan PE (2004) Fatigue in neurological disorders. *Lancet* **363**: 978–988.

MUSCULAR DYSTROPHIES

These progressive genetically determined disorders of skeletal and sometimes cardiac muscle have a complex clinical and neurogenetic classification.

Duchenne muscular dystrophy (DMD)

This is inherited as an X-linked recessive disorder, though one-third of cases are spontaneous mutants. DMD occurs in 1 in 3000 male infants. The DMD locus has been localized to the Xp21 region of the X chromosome; there is absence of the gene product – the protein *dystrophin*, a rod-shaped cytoskeletal muscle protein. DMD is usually obvious by the fourth year, and often causes death by 20.

Dystrophin is essential for cell membrane stability. Deficiency leads to reduction in three glycoproteins (α-, β- and γ-sarcoglycans) in the dystrophin-associated protein-complex (DAP-complex) that link dystrophin to *laminin* within cell membranes.

Becker's muscular dystrophy (due to an autosomal recessive gene CLC1 on chromosome 7q35) is also disabling, though milder than Duchenne. Weakness becomes apparent in young adults. It is also due to a mutation and abnormalities in dystrophin.

Clinical features

The boy with DMD is noticed to have difficulty running and rising to his feet from the floor – when he has to use his hands to 'climb up his legs' (Gowers' sign). There is initially a proximal limb weakness with calf pseudo-hypertrophy. The myocardium is affected. The boy becomes severely disabled by the age of 10.

Investigations

Diagnosis is often made on clinical grounds alone. Creatine phosphokinase is grossly elevated (100–200 times normal). Muscle biopsy shows characteristic variation in fibre size, fibre necrosis, regeneration and replacement by fat, and on immunochemical staining, absence of dystrophin. EMG shows a myopathic pattern.

Management

There is no curative treatment. Passive physiotherapy helps prevent contractures in the later stages. Portable respiratory support gives a substantially improved life expectancy.

Carrier detection. A female with an affected brother has a 50% chance of carrying the Duchenne gene. In carrier females, 70% have a raised creatine phosphokinase level and usually EMG abnormalities or changes on biopsy. Accurate carrier and prenatal diagnosis (cDNA probes, co-inheritance with DMD locus) are essential.

Genetic advice and counselling should be given to carriers. Many women carriers choose not to have offspring. Determination of fetal sex by amniocentesis and selective abortion of a male fetus is sometimes carried out.

Limb-girdle and facioscapulohumeral dystrophy

These less severe but disabling dystrophies are summarized in Table 21.61. There are many other varieties of muscular dystrophy. Most are associated with a sarcoglycan deficiency. Genes for various limb girdle muscular dystrophies (LGMD) have been located; some of the proteins for which they code, e.g. *calpain*, are known. Type 1 LGMD is a rare autosomal dominant condition. Type 2 LGMD includes all recessive varieties, with complex subdivisions e.g. LGMD2A (calpain III deficiency), LGMD2C (γ-sarcoglycan deficiency).

FURTHER READING
Emery AEH (2002) The muscular dystrophies. *Lancet* **359**: 687–695.

Table 21.61	Limb-girdle and facioscapulohumeral dystrophies	
	Limb-girdle	**Facioscapulohumeral**
Inheritance	Autosomal	Autosomal dominant
Onset	10–20 years	10–40 years
Muscles affected	Shoulder and pelvic girdle	Face, shoulder and pelvis
Progress	Severe disability within 20–25 years	Normal life expectancy slow progression
Pseudo-hypertrophy	Rare	Very rare

MYOTONIAS

Myotonias are characterized by continued, involuntary muscle contraction after cessation of voluntary effort. The EMG is characteristic (p. 1203). Patients with myotonia tolerate general anaesthetics poorly. The two most common myotonias are mentioned below. Since there is defective skeletal muscle cell chloride ion membrane conductance, myotonias are also classified as channelopathies (see below).

Dystrophia myotonica

This autosomal dominant condition is a genetic disorder with triple repeat mutations (p. 184). There is an expanded CTG repeat in the MD protein-kinase gene on chromosome 19q13.3 (*DM1*). There is a correlation between disease severity, age at onset and approximate size of triple repeat mutations. There is progressive distal muscle weakness, with ptosis, weakness and thinning of the face and sternomastoids. Myotonia is typically present. The muscle disease is part of a syndrome comprising:

- cataracts
- frontal baldness
- cognitive impairment (mild)
- oesophageal dysfunction (and aspiration)
- cardiomyopathy and conduction defects
- small pituitary fossa and hypogonadism
- glucose intolerance
- low serum IgG.

This gradually progressive condition usually becomes evident between 20 and 50 years. Phenytoin or procainamide sometimes help the myotonia.

FURTHER READING
Nayanakkara PWB et al. (2003) Case report: a man with fever and a persistent handgrip. *Lancet* **362**: 1038.

CHANNELOPATHIES

Many conditions are now included within this group – see also myotonias (above) and Lambert–Eaton myasthenic–myopathic syndrome (p. 1269).

Myotonia congenita (Thomsen's disease)

An isolated autosomal dominant myotonia, usually mild, becomes evident in childhood. The gene CLC1 is on chromosome 7q35. The myotonia, which persists, is accentuated by rest and by cold. Diffuse muscle hypertrophy occurs – the patient appears to have well-developed muscles.

Hypokalaemic periodic paralysis

This channelopathy is characterized by generalized weakness, including bulbar muscles (speech, swallowing and respiration), that often starts after a heavy carbohydrate meal or after rest following exertion. Attacks last for several hours. It often first comes to light in the teenage years and tends to remit after the age of 35. Serum potassium is usually below 3.0 mmol/L in an attack. The weakness responds to (slow) i.v. potassium chloride. It is usually an autosomal dominant trait caused by mutation in a muscle voltage-gated calcium channel gene (CACLN1A3). Other mutations in the sodium channel (SCNA4 on chromosome 17q13.1–13.3) and potassium channel (KCNE3) also occur. Acetazolimide can prevent attacks. Weakness also occurs in hypokalaemia due to diuretics, and occurs with thyrotoxicosis.

Hyperkalaemic periodic paralysis

This condition, also autosomal dominant, is characterized by attacks of weakness sometimes precipitated by exercise. Attacks start in childhood and tend to remit after the age of 20. Attacks last from 30 minutes to 2 hours. Myotonia may occur. Serum potassium is raised. An attack can be terminated by i.v. calcium gluconate or chloride. There are point mutations in a muscle voltage-gated sodium channel gene (SCN4A) on chromosome 17q13.1–13.3. Acetazolimide or a thiazide diuretic can be helpful.

A very rare normokalaemic, sodium-responsive periodic paralysis also occurs.

FURTHER READING
Benatar MG (1999) Calcium channelopathies. *Quarterly Journal of Medicine* **92**: 133–141.
DiMauro S, Schon, EA (2003) Mitochondrial respiratory chain diseases. *New England Journal of Medicine* **348**: 2656–2666.

METABOLIC MYOPATHIES

This is a large complex group of rare, genetically determined muscle diseases.

Myophosphorylase deficiency (McArdle's syndrome)

This is an autosomal recessive disorder in which lack of skeletal muscle myophosphorylase causes easy fatiguability and severe cramp on exercise, with myoglobinuria. Venous lactate during ischaemic exercise does not increase; this test is specific for the condition. Sucrose ingestion helps (see p. 1144).

Malignant hyperpyrexia

Widespread skeletal muscle rigidity and hyperpyrexia developing as a sequel to general anaesthesia or neuroleptic drugs (e.g. haloperidol) is due to a genetic defect in the sarcoplasmic reticulum calcium-release channel in the skeletal muscle ryanodine receptor (RyR1). Sudden death during or after anaesthesia may occur in this rare condition, sometimes inherited as an autosomal dominant trait. Dantrolene is useful in controlling rigidity.

Mitochondrial diseases (p. 174)

These comprise a complex group of disorders involving muscle, peripheral nerves and CNS. They are characterized by morphological and biochemical abnormalities in mitochondria, with several unusual genetic characteristics, for example the maternal inheritance of mitochondrial DNA. The disease spectrum is wide, ranging from optic atrophy (see Leber's hereditary optic neuropathy, p. 1181) to myopathies, neuropathies and encephalopathy. MELAS (mitochondrial encephalomyopathy, lactic acidosis, stroke-like episodes) is one well-recognized form. Chronic progressive ophthalmoplegia (CPEO) is another, and MERRF describes the occurrence of myoclonic epilepsy and 'ragged red' muscle fibres on biopsy. Further developments in this complex field continue.

INTRODUCTION

Psychiatry is concerned with the study and treatment of disorders of mental function. Psychological medicine, or liaison psychiatry, is the discipline within psychiatry that is concerned with psychiatric and psychological disorders in patients who have physical complaints or conditions. This chapter will primarily concern itself with this particular branch of psychiatry.

The long-held belief that diseases are either physical or psychological has been broken down by the accumulated evidence that the brain is functionally or anatomically abnormal in most if not all psychiatric disorders. Both physical and psychological factors, and their interactions must be considered. This philosophical change of approach rejects the Cartesian dualistic approach of the mind/body *medical model* and replaces it with the more holistic *biopsychosocial model*.

Epidemiology (Box 22.1)

The prevalence of psychiatric disorders in the community in the UK is about 20%, mainly composed of depressive and anxiety disorders and substance misuse (mainly alcohol). The prevalence is about twice as high in patients attending the general hospital, with the highest rates in the accident and emergency department and medical wards. The higher rates in the general hospital are due to several factors, such as admission for deliberate self-harm, a psychiatric disorder or treatment causing physical harm (e.g. alcohol-induced hepatitis or lithium-

Box 22.1 The approximate prevalence of psychiatric disorders in different populations

	% (approx.)
Community	20%
Neuroses	16%
Psychoses	0.5%
Alcohol misuse	5%
Drug misuse	2% (an underestimate)
(total in community 20% due to comorbidity)	
Primary care	25%
General hospital outpatients	30%
General hospital inpatients	40%

related renal failure), and physical presentations of psychiatric disorders (such as weight loss due to anorexia nervosa).

Culture and ethnicity

These can alter either the presentation or the prevalence of psychiatric ill-health. Biological factors in mental illness are usually similar across cultural boundaries, whereas psychological and social factors will vary. For example, the prevalence and presentation of schizophrenia vary little between countries, suggesting that biological/genetic factors are operating independently of cultural factors. In contrast, conditions in which social factors play a greater role vary between cultures, so that anorexia nervosa is found more often in developed cultures. Culture can also influence the presentation of illnesses, such that physical symptoms are more common presentations of depressive illness in Asia than in Europe.

THE PSYCHIATRIC HISTORY

The purpose of the history is to help to make a diagnosis, determine possible aetiology, and estimate prognosis. Data may be taken from several sources, including interviewing the patient, a friend or relative (usually with the patient's permission), or the patient's general practitioner. The patient interview enables a doctor to establish a relationship with the patient and is the primary way to make a psychiatric diagnosis. Box 22.2 gives essential guidance on how to safely conduct such an interview. It is very unlikely that a patient will physically harm a healthcare professional. When interviewing a patient for the first time follow the guidance outlined in Chapter 1 (see p. 14).

The history consists of:

- *Reason for referral* – a brief statement of why and how the patient came to the attention of the doctor.
- *Complaints* – as reported by the patient.
- *Present illness* – a detailed account of the illness from the earliest time at which a change was noted until the patient came to the attention of the doctor.
- *Past psychiatric history* – previous episodes of psychiatric illness and their treatments, including responses and adverse reactions. Always ask after previous episodes of self-harm.
- *Past medical history* – this should include emotional reactions to illness and procedures.
- *Family history* – focusing on the way the parents or carers cared (physically and emotionally) for the patient, and the occurrence of both mental and physical illnesses in first-degree relatives.
- *Personal (biographical) history* – a short biography that covers childhood difficulties including both abuse and neglect, educational problems (e.g. bullying and truanting), qualifications (to judge premorbid intelligence), job problems, sexual relationships, children, present housing, financial situation, bereavements and

life stresses. Ways of asking awkward questions might include:
  - 'Do you feel able to tell me what memory most upsets you/makes you angry?'
  - 'Are you able to say what you have done in the past that you most regret?'
  - 'How well do you get on with your partner? Are you happy in every way? Are there any problems in your sexual life that you think I should know about?'
- A *reproductive history* in women should include menstrual problems, pregnancies, terminations, miscarriages, contraception and the menopause, if relevant.
- *Personality* – this helps to determine prognosis and response to treatment. The doctor should find out how other people would describe the patient. Is the patient generally a worrier, shy, introverted, dependent on others, passive, aggressive, irritable, over-emotional, prone to moodiness, conscientious, or perfectionist? These are all personality traits that predict a poorer outcome in both medical and psychiatric disorders.
- *Drug history* – both prescribed and over-the-counter medication, the use (units per week) and abuse of alcohol, tobacco, caffeine, and illicit drugs.
- *Forensic history* – you should carefully explain that you need to ask about this since ill-health can sometimes lead to problems with the law.
  - 'Have you ever had any legal problems or contact with the police or courts?'
  Particularly note any violent or sexual offences. This is part of a *risk assessment* and is necessary in order to assess potential risks to those close to the patient as well as staff. Ask the patient what is the worst harm they have ever inflicted on someone else, which will give an indication of the potential for violence.
- A *systematic review* of physical symptoms is particularly necessary in patients complaining of physical symptoms.

THE MENTAL STATE EXAMINATION (MSE)

The history will already have assessed several aspects of the MSE, but the interviewer will need to expand several areas as well as test specific areas, such as cognition.

Appearance and general behaviour

State and colour of clothes, facial appearance, eye contact, posture and movement provide information about a patient's affect. Patients with *psychomotor retardation* due to a depressive illness sit with shoulders hunched, immobile, tearful, with a downcast gaze. Depressed individuals tend to wear clothes with dark colours. Agitation (seen with depressive illness) and anxiety cause an easy startle response, sweating, tremor, restlessness, fidgeting, visual scanning (for danger) and even pacing up and down. Patients with mania are often physically

<table>
<tr><td>

ℹ️ **Box 22.2 The essentials of a safe psychiatric interview**

- **Beforehand**: Ask someone senior who knows the patient whether it is safe to interview the patient alone.
- **Access to others**: If in doubt, interview in the view or hearing of others, or accompanied by another member of staff.
- **Setting**: If safe; in a quiet room alone for confidentiality, not by the bed.
- **Seating**: Place yourself between the door and the patient.
- **Alarm**: If available, find out where the alarm is and how to use it.

</td></tr>
</table>

overactive and disinhibited, wearing colourful clothes. Someone who is actively hallucinating will seem distracted and suddenly stop talking or listening and stare intently at a particular place in the room.

Mood and affect

The patient has an *emotion or feeling*, tells the doctor their *mood* and the doctor observes the patient's *affect*. In psychiatric disorders, mood may be altered in three ways:

A persistent change in mood

- *Depression* is a lowering of mood, such as feeling sad, tearful, melancholic or low in spirits. Some patients report *anhedonia*, which is a lack of positive pleasure or loss of interest. Depression is the cardinal feature of depressive illness. Sometimes the word 'depression' is used as shorthand to describe a depressive illness. *Diurnal variation* in mood, feeling worse on waking, suggests a more severe illness, whereas a *reactive mood*, in which the patient can sometimes respond positively, indicates less severity.
- *Anxiety* is a feeling of constant, inappropriate or excessive worry, fear, apprehension, tension or inner restlessness, seen in anxiety and depressive disorders and drug withdrawal.
- *Elation* is a feeling of high spirits, exuberant happiness, vitality and even ecstasy, seen in mania and acute drug intoxication.
- *Irritability* can be either expressed (as in a temper or impatience) or an internal feeling of exasperation or anger, seen in both mania and depressive illness, especially in men.
- *Blunting* of affect is a total absence of emotion, seen most commonly in chronic schizophrenia.

Fluctuating or labile mood

This occurs when different emotions rapidly follow one another, so that a patient is crying one moment and laughing the next. This can occur in mixed affective states (see p. 1288). Alternatively, the patient is easily and excessively emotional over banal events or news, but the emotion is transient. This is seen both in a pseudobulbar palsy, commonly following a cerebrovascular accident (see p. 1191), and with mild depressive illnesses.

Inconsistent or incongruous mood

This occurs when emotional expression fails to match thoughts and actions. For example, a patient may laugh when describing the death of a close relative. This can occur in schizophrenia. Such incongruity needs to be distinguished from the embarrassed laughter that indicates that someone is ill at ease when talking about a distressing subject.

Speech

Disorders of thinking are usually recognized from the patient's speech.

Disorders of the stream of thought

These are abnormalities in the amount and speed of the thoughts experienced.

Pressure of speech occurs in mania and can be recognized by loudness, rapidity, and difficulty in interrupting speech.

Poverty of speech is the opposite experience, when there appears to be an absence of any thought and patients report their minds to be empty. It occurs in depressive illness.

Thought block occurs in schizophrenia. There is an abrupt and complete interruption of the stream of thought, so the mind goes blank. Patients may interpret the experience in an unusual way (e.g. thought withdrawal; see below).

Disorders of the form of thought

Flight of ideas. The patient's thoughts rapidly jump from one topic to another, such that one train of thought is not completed before another appears. It is often produced by clang associations (the use of two or more words with a similar sound: 'sun, son, song'), punning, rhyming, and responding to distracting cues in the immediate surroundings. Flight of ideas is characteristic of mania and often accompanies pressure of speech.

Perseveration is the persistent and inappropriate repetition of the same thoughts or actions. It occurs in frontal lobe disorders.

Loosening of associations is manifested by a loss of the normal structure of thinking. The most striking impression is a lack of clarity so that it is impossible to understand what is being said. There are several forms. Knight's move or derailment denotes an illogical transition from one topic to another, in the absence of flight of ideas. When this abnormality is extreme and disrupts the grammatical structure of speech, it is termed 'word salad'.

Thought broadcast is when the patient experiences their thoughts as being understood by others without talking, as though their thoughts are literally being broadcast to all around them.

Thought insertion occurs when a patient's thought is perceived as being planted in their mind by someone else.

Thought withdrawal occurs when a patient experiences their thoughts being taken away from them, without their control.

The latter three types of thought disorders are all *first rank symptoms*, which Schneider suggested were pathognomonic of schizophrenia (see p. 1307).

Thought content

Thought content refers to the worries and preoccupations manifested by the patient and elicited at interview. Abnormal beliefs and experiences are, of course, part of the thought content, but are regarded as sufficient to be discussed separately (see below).

- An *obsessional rumination* is a recurrent, persistent thought, impulse, image or musical theme that enters the mind despite the individual's effort to resist it. The individual recognizes that the obsessional thought is their own, but it is usually unpleasant and often 'out of character', such as the thought that the patient has accidentally killed someone while driving their car. Common obsessions concern dirt, contamination and orderliness.

- A *compulsion* is a repetitive and seemingly purposeful action performed in a stereotyped way, referred to as a *compulsive ritual*. Compulsions are accompanied by a subjective sense that they must be carried out (or the patient will be overwhelmed by either anxiety or a superstitious belief that something bad will occur) and by an urge to resist. Compulsive rituals are used to counteract ruminations, so patients repetitively wash their hands to diminish the fear of contamination with dirt.

Insight and illness beliefs

Insight is the degree to which a person recognizes that he or she is unwell, and is minimal in patients with a psychosis. Illness beliefs are the patient's own explanations of their ill-health, including diagnosis and causes. These beliefs should be elicited because they can help to determine prognosis and compliance with treatment, with any disease.

Abnormal beliefs

The main form of abnormal belief is the *delusion* (Box 22.3). Delusions can be primary or secondary.

- Primary delusions are rare and appear suddenly and with full conviction but without any preceding mental events. For example, a patient on being offered a glass of wine suddenly believes that this indicates that he is Jesus Christ.
- Secondary delusions are derived from a preceding morbid experience, such as a depressed mood or an auditory hallucination.

Delusions are also classified according to their content, and include persecutory delusions, delusions of reference, guilt, worthlessness, nihilism, religious delusions, and delusions of grandeur, jealousy or control. These are further defined when discussed in relation to specific conditions.

Feelings, thoughts or actions may also be interpreted by the patient as being under the control of some external power. Such *passivity* experiences are first rank symptoms and are regarded as diagnostic of schizophrenia (see p. 1307). Patients may develop secondary delusions that explain this alien control as a result of witchcraft, hypnosis, radio waves or television – so-called delusions of passivity.

Delusions should be distinguished from *overvalued ideas* – deeply held personal convictions that are understandable when the individual's background is known.

Ideas of reference that fall short of delusions are held by people who are particularly self-conscious. Such individuals cannot help feeling that people take particular notice of them in public places, laugh at them or pass comment about them. Such a feeling is not delusional in that individuals who experience it realize that it originates within themselves and that they are no more noticeable than anyone else, but nevertheless cannot dismiss the feeling.

Abnormal perceptions

- *Illusions* are misperceptions of external stimuli and are most likely to occur when the general level of sensory stimulation is reduced.
- *Hallucinations* are defined in Box 22.4. Healthy people occasionally experience hallucinations, such as in normal grief, or during the transition between sleeping and waking (hypnagogic and hypnapompic). Hallucinations can be elementary (e.g. bangs, whistles) or complex (e.g. faces, voices, music), and may affect any of the perceptions: auditory, visual, tactile, gustatory, olfactory or of deep sensation.
- *Pseudohallucinations* are usually auditory, and are either true externally sited hallucinations, but with insight into their imaginary nature, or are sited within internal space (e.g. 'I heard a voice in my head speak to me'). They can occur in mood disorders and do not indicate a psychosis.
- *Depersonalization* is a change in self-awareness such that the person feels unreal or detached from their body. The individual is aware, however, of the subjective nature of this alteration.
- *Derealization* is the unpleasant feeling that the external environment has become unreal and/or remote; patients may describe themselves as though they are in a dream-like state. Both this and depersonalization can occur in healthy people when they are tired, after sensory deprivation and when using hallucinogenic drugs. They also occur in anxiety disorders, schizophrenia and temporal lobe epilepsy.

Box 22.3 Delusion

Delusion is defined as an abnormal belief that is:

- held with absolute conviction
- not amenable to reason or modifiable by experience
- not shared by those of a common cultural or social background
- experienced as a self-evident truth of great personal significance
- usually false.

Box 22.4 Hallucination

An hallucination is defined as a perception in the absence of a stimulus. It is:

- a false perception and not a distortion
- perceived as inhabiting objective space
- perceived as having qualities of normal perception
- perceived alongside normal perceptions
- independent of the individual's will.

- *Déjà vu* is a sudden familiarity with a situation or event as having been encountered before when it is in fact novel.
- *Jamais vu* is the reverse experience when there is failure to recognize a situation or event that has been encountered before. Déjà vu experiences occur in healthy people as well as in extreme anxiety states. Both types of experience can occur in temporal lobe epilepsy (see p. 1221).
- Increased sensitivity of perceptions, such as *photosensitivity* and *phonosensitivity*, occurs in anxiety disorders (e.g. increased sensitivity to the neon striplights and noise in a supermarket in agoraphobia) as well as neurological disorders such as migraine.

Cognitive state

Examination of the cognitive state is necessary to diagnose organic brain disorders, such as delirium and dementia. Poor concentration, confusion and memory problems are the most common subjective complaints. Clinical testing is a screening of cognitive functions, which may suggest the need for more formal psychometry. A premorbid estimate of intelligence can be made from asking the patient the final year level of education and the highest qualifications or skills achieved.

Testing can be divided into tests of diffuse and focal brain functions.

Diffuse functions

Orientation in time, place and person. *Consciousness* can be defined as the awareness of the self and the environment. *Clouding of consciousness* is more accurately a fluctuating level of awareness and is commonly seen in delirium.

Attention is tested by saying the months or days backwards.

Verbal memory. Ask the patient to repeat a name and address with 10 or so items, noting how many times it takes to recall it 100% accurately (normal is 1 or 2) (*immediate recall* or *registration*).

Ask the patient to try to remember it and then ask it of them again after 5 minutes (0 or 1 error is normal) (*short-term memory*).

Long-term memory. Ask the patient to recall the news of that morning or recently. If they are not interested in the news, find out their interests and ask relevant questions (about their football team or favourite soap opera). *Amnesia* is literally an absence of memory and *dysmnesia* indicates a dysfunctioning memory.

Focal functions

Frontal, temporal and parietal function tests are covered on page 1178. *Frontal lobe skills* are difficult to test at the bedside. Note any *disinhibited behaviour* not explained by another psychiatric illness, such as mania. *Sequential tasks* are tested by asking the patient to alternate making a fist with one hand at the same time as a flat hand with the other. Ask the patient to tap a table once if you tap twice and vice versa. Note any *motor perseveration* whereby the patient cannot change the movement once established.

Observe for *verbal perseveration*, in which the patient repeats the same answer as given previously for a different question. *Abstract thinking* is measured by asking the meaning of common proverbs, a literal meaning suggesting frontal lobe dysfunction, assuming reasonable premorbid intelligence.

Mini-mental state examination

Box 22.5 gives the 'mini-mental state' examination of cognitive function. This is a 5-minute bedside test that is useful as a screen and in assessing the degree of cognitive dysfunction in patients with diffuse brain disorders. It correlates well with more time-consuming Intelligence

---

(i) Box 22.5 The mini-mental state examination

Orientation
Score one point for each correct answer:

What is the: time, date, day, month, year?
Maximum: 5 points

What is the name of: this ward, hospital, 5 points
district, town, country?

Registration
Name three objects only once. Score up to 3 points
a maximum of 3 points for each correct repetition.
Repeat the objects until the patient can repeat them accurately (in order to test recall later).

Attention and calculation
Ask the patient to subtract 7 from 100 and 5 points
then 7 from the result four more times.
Score 1 point for each correct subtraction

Recall
Ask the patient to repeat the names of the 3 points
three objects learnt in the registration test.

Language
Score 1 point for each of two simple objects 2 points
named (e.g. pen and a watch)
Score 1 point for an accurate repetition of 1 point
the phrase: 'No ifs, ands or buts'
Give a 3-stage command, scoring 1 point 3 points
for each part correctly carried out; e.g.
'With the index finger of your right hand
touch your nose and then your left ear'
Write 'Close your eyes' on a blank piece 1 point
of paper and ask the patient to follow
the written command. Score 1 point if the
patient closes the eyes.
Ask the patient to write a sentence. 1 point
Score 1 point if the sentence is sensible
and contains a noun and a verb.
Draw a pair of intersecting pentagons 1 point
with each side approximately 1 inch long.
Score 1 point if it is correctly copied

TOTAL MAXIMUM SCORE 30 POINTS

From: Folstein MF, Folstein SE, McHough PR (1975) 'Mini-mental state': a practical method for grading the cognitive state of patients for the clinician. *Journal of Psychiatric Research* **12**: 189–198

Quotient (IQ) tests, but it will not as easily pick up cognitive problems caused by focal brain lesions. A score of 23 or less will pick up about 90% of patients with cognitive impairments, with about 10% false positives.

Defence mechanisms

Although not strictly part of the mental state examination, it is useful to be able to identify psychological defences in ourselves and our patients. Defence mechanisms are mental processes that are usually unconscious. The defence mechanisms described below are among the most commonly used and are useful in understanding many aspects of behaviour.

- *Denial* is similar to repression and occurs when patients behave as though unaware of something that they might be expected to know. One example would be a patient who, despite being told that a close relative has died, continues to behave as though the relative were still alive.
- *Displacement* involves the transferring of emotion from a situation or object with which it is properly associated to another that gives less distress.
- *Identification* refers to the unconscious process of taking on some of the characteristics or behaviours of another person, often to reduce the pain of separation or loss.
- *Projection* involves the attribution to another person of thoughts or feelings that are in fact one's own.
- *Regression* is the adoption of primitive patterns of behaviour appropriate to an earlier stage of development. It can be seen in ill people who become child-like and highly dependent.
- *Repression* is the exclusion from awareness of memories, emotions and/or impulses that would cause anxiety or distress if allowed to enter consciousness.
- *Sublimation* refers to the unconscious diversion of unacceptable behaviours into acceptable ones.

The relevant physical examination

This should be guided by the history and mental state examination. Particular attention should usually be paid to the neurological and endocrinological examinations when organic brain syndromes and affective illnesses are suspected.

Summary or formulation

When the full history and mental state have been assessed, the doctor should make a concise assessment of the case, which is termed a *formulation*. In addition to summarizing the essential features of the history and examination, the formulation includes a differential diagnosis, a discussion of possible causal factors, and an outline of further investigations or interviews needed. It concludes with a concise plan of treatment and a statement of the likely prognosis.

CLASSIFICATION OF PSYCHIATRIC DISORDERS

The classification of psychiatric disorders into categories is mainly based on symptoms, since there are currently few diagnostic tests for psychiatric disorders. The fourth edition text revision (TR) of the *Diagnostic and Statistical Manual of the American Psychiatric Association* (DSM-IV-TR) provides descriptions of diagnostic categories in order to enable clinicians and investigators to diagnose, communicate about, study and treat people with various mental disorders. This scheme has five axes:

I   Psychiatric disorders
II Personality disorders, learning difficulty
III General medical conditions
IV Psychosocial and environmental problems
V   Overall level of functioning

Psychiatric classifications have traditionally divided up disorders into neuroses and psychoses.

Neuroses are illnesses in which symptoms vary only in severity from normal experiences. *Psychoses* are illnesses in which symptoms are qualitatively different from normal experience, with little insight into their nature.

There are several problems with a neurotic–psychotic dichotomy. Firstly, neuroses may be as severe in their effects on the patient and their family as psychoses. Secondly, neuroses may cause symptoms that fulfil the definition of psychotic symptoms. For instance, someone with anorexia nervosa may be convinced that they are fat when they are thin, and this belief would meet all the criteria for a delusional belief. Yet we would traditionally classify the illness as a neurosis.

Another classification system – the *International Classification of Mental and Behavioural Disorders* (ICD-10) – has been published by the World Health Organization. This system has largely abandoned the traditional division between neurosis and psychosis, although the terms are still used. The disorders are now arranged in groups according to major common themes (e.g. mood disorders, schizophrenia and other delusional disorders). A classification of psychiatric disorders derived from ICD-10 is shown in Table 22.1, and this is the classification mainly used in this chapter.

Table 22.1 International classification of psychiatric disorders (ICD-10)

Organic disorders
Mental and behavioural disorders due to psychoactive
   substance use
Schizophrenia and delusional disorders
Mood (affective) disorders
Neurotic, stress-related and somatoform disorders
Behavioural syndromes
Disorders of adult personality and behaviour
Mental retardation

World Health Organization (1992) *The ICD-10 Classification of Mental and Behavioural Disorders.* Geneva: World Health Organization

FURTHER READING
American Psychiatric Association (2000) *Diagnostic and Statistical Manual of Mental Disorders – Fourth Edition Text Revision (DSM–IV-TR)*. Washington, DC: APA.
World Health Organization (1992) *The ICD-10 Classification of Mental and Behavioural Disorders: Clinical Descriptions and Diagnostic Guidelines*. Geneva: World Health Organization.

CAUSES OF A PSYCHIATRIC DISORDER

A psychiatric disorder may result from several causes. It is most helpful to divide causes into the three 'P's: predisposing, precipitating and perpetuating factors.

- *Predisposing factors* often stem from early life and include genetic, pregnancy and delivery, previous traumas and personality factors.
- *Precipitating (triggering) factors* may be physical, psychological or social in nature. Whether they produce a disorder depends on their nature, severity and the presence of predisposing factors. For instance a death of a close, rather than distant, family member is more likely to precipitate a depressive illness or pathological grief reaction in someone who has not come to terms with a previous bereavement.
- *Perpetuating (maintaining) factors* prolong the course of a disorder after it has occurred. Again they may be physical, psychological and/or social, and several are often active and interacting at the same time. For example, high levels of criticism at home combined with taking cannabis, as relief from the criticism, may help to maintain schizophrenia.

PSYCHIATRIC ASPECTS OF PHYSICAL DISEASE

Patients with physical illnesses are more likely to suffer from psychiatric disorders than those who are well. The most common psychiatric disorders in physically ill patients are mood or adjustment disorders and acute organic brain disorders (delirium). The relationship between psychological and physical symptoms may be understood in one of three ways:

- Psychological distress and disorders can precipitate physical diseases (e.g. anorexia nervosa causing cardiac arrhythmias, due to hypokalaemia).
- Physical diseases and their treatments can cause psychological symptoms or ill-health (Table 22.2).
- Physical and psychological symptoms and disorders may be independently co-morbid, particularly in the elderly.

Common psychiatric disorders in the general hospital

Delirium is the commonest psychosis seen in the general hospital, with *dementia* being the commonest chronic organic brain disorder seen. *Mood disorders*, particularly depressive illness, are common in patients with chronic painful conditions (severe arthritis), disabling illnesses (after a stroke), and after being given a life-threatening diagnosis, such as cancer. Other factors also increase the risk of a psychiatric disorder in someone with a physical disease (Table 22.3).

Table 22.2 Psychiatric conditions sometimes caused by physical diseases

Psychiatric disorders/ symptom	Physical disease
Depressive illness	Hypothyroidism Cushing's syndrome Steroid treatment Brain tumour
Anxiety disorder	Thyrotoxicosis Hypoglycaemia (transient) Phaeochromocytoma Complex partial seizures (transient) Alcohol withdrawal
Irritability	Post-concussion syndrome Frontal lobe syndrome Hypoglycaemia (transient)
Memory problem	Brain tumour Hypothyroidism
Altered behaviour	Acute drug intoxication Post-ictal state Acute delirium Dementia Brain tumour

Table 22.3 Factors increasing the risk of psychiatric disorders in the general hospital

Patient factors	Physical conditions
Previous psychiatric history Current social or interpersonal stresses Homeless Recent alcohol misuse	Chronic ill-health Chronic pain Life-threatening illness Recent bad prognostic news Disabling condition Brain disease Recent live birth, stillbirth or miscarriage Functional (psychosomatic) illness
Setting A&E department Neurology, oncology and endocrinology wards Intensive care unit Renal dialysis unit	**Treatment** Certain drugs (e.g. dopamine agonists) Second postoperative day Surgery affecting body image (e.g. emergency stomata)

Differences in treatment

Although the basic principles are the same as in treating psychiatric illnesses in the physically healthy, there are some differences:

- *Uncertainty* regarding the physical diagnosis or prognosis, with its attendant tendency to imagine the worst, is often a triggering or maintaining factor, particularly in an adjustment or mood disorder. Good two-way communication between doctor and patient, with time taken to listen to the patient's concerns, is often the most effective 'antidepressant' available.
- A careful history may reveal the role of a *physical disease* or *treatment* exacerbating the psychiatric condition, which should then be addressed (see Table 22.2). For example, the dopamine agonist bromocriptine can precipitate a psychosis.
- When prescribing psychotropic drugs, the dose should be reduced in disorders affecting *pharmacokinetics*, e.g. fluoxetine in renal or hepatic failure.
- *Drug interactions*, e.g. lithium and non-steroidal anti-inflammatories; lithium and thiazide diuretics. Drug interactions are most likely to occur when a patient taking psychotropic is acutely admitted to hospital and prescribed analgesics.
- Sometimes a physical treatment may be planned that may exacerbate the psychiatric condition. An example would be high-dose steroids as part of the next cycle of chemotherapy in a patient with leukaemia and depressive illness. Careful thought should be given to the particular priority for the patient at that moment. It is often useful to discuss the clinical dilemma with a psychiatrist.
- Always consider the risk of *suicide* in an inpatient with a mood disorder and take steps to reduce that risk; for example, moving the patient to a room on the ground floor and/or having a registered psychiatric nurse attend the patient while at risk.

SEVERE BEHAVIOURAL DISTURBANCE

Patients with aggressive or violent behaviour cause understandable apprehension in all staff, and are most commonly seen in the accident and emergency department. Information from anyone accompanying the patient, including police or carers, can help considerably. Box 22.6 gives the main causes of disturbed behaviour.

Management of the severely disturbed patient

The primary aims of management are control of dangerous behaviour and establishment of a provisional diagnosis.

Box 22.6 Main causes of disturbed behaviour

- Drug intoxication (especially alcohol)
- Delirium (acute confusional state)
- Acute psychosis
- Personality disorder

Three specific strategies may be necessary when dealing with the violent patient:

- reassurance and explanation
- physical restraint
- medication.

The majority of disturbed patients are themselves frightened, as well as frightening, and may feel threatened by those around them, misinterpreting the actions of others. Staff should always explain the situation and their intentions. This simple strategy may calm a patient sufficiently to be interviewed and allow an appropriate examination.

If the behaviour remains severely disturbed, it may be necessary to restrain patients from harming themselves or others. If planned, this should be done with sufficient numbers of trained staff; at least one person per limb and another two in charge or delivering medication. Once brought under physical control, the patient should be held in the prone position, in order to protect the airway and allow access for intramuscular medication. Care must be taken to ensure that neither the airway nor breathing are impeded, by having someone always present at the head of the patient.

It is usually necessary to administer medication while the patient is restrained and they should not be released until they are visibly calmed. Management depends on the provisional diagnosis. 'Rapid tranquillization' should be employed when the patient has a psychosis, so long as the Mental Health Act has been used (see p. 1314) or the situation is so dangerous that the doctor is acting under 'common law'. A deep intramuscular injection of zuclopenthixol acetate in a dose ranging from 50–150 mg together with 0.5–1 mg. lorazepam is now the treatment of choice for rapid effect. Used in combination, they have a synergistic action. Moderate doses of a neuroleptic or benzodiazepine can also be given at regular, comparatively short intervals (30–60 minutes) intramuscularly. Another alternative regimen is intramuscular butyrophenone (haloperidol 5–10 mg) in patients under 60 years old. This dose should be reduced in the elderly and those with known cardiac or hepatic disease. The patient should be observed for up to 1 hour before a further dose is administered. Breathing, pulse rate and blood pressure should be monitored for hypotension, arrhythmias and respiratory difficulty. In the case of continuing disturbance, it may be preferable to administer an adjunctive intramuscular benzodiazepine (lorazepam 2 mg) rather than a further dose of a neuroleptic. Both neuroleptic drugs and benzodiazepines may be used as tranquillizers.

THE SICK ROLE AND ILLNESS BEHAVIOUR

The *sick role* describes behaviour usually adopted by ill people. Such people are not expected to fulfil their normal social obligations. They are treated with sympathy by others and are only obliged to see their doctor and take medical advice or treatments.

Illness behaviour is the way in which given symptoms may be differentially perceived, evaluated and acted (or not acted) upon by different kinds of persons. We all have illness behaviour when we choose what to do about a symptom. Going to see a doctor is generally more likely with more severe and more numerous symptoms and greater distress. It is also more likely in introspective individuals who focus on their health.

Abnormal illness behaviour occurs when there is a discrepancy between the objective somatic pathology present and the patient's response to it, in spite of adequate medical investigation and explanation.

FUNCTIONAL OR PSYCHOSOMATIC DISORDERS: MEDICALLY UNEXPLAINED SYMPTOMS

'*Functional*' disorders are illnesses in which there is no obvious pathology or anatomical change in an organ (thus in contrast to 'organic') and there is a presumed dysfunction in an organ or system. The word *psychosomatic* has had several meanings, including psychogenic, 'all in the mind', imaginary and malingering. The modern meaning is that psychosomatic disorders are syndromes of unknown aetiology in which both physical and psychological factors are likely to be causative. The psychiatric classification of these disorders would be *somatoform disorders*, but they do not fit easily within either medical or psychiatric classification systems, since they occupy the hinterland between them. Medically unexplained symptoms and syndromes are very common in both primary care and the general hospital (over half the outpatients in gastroenterology and neurology clinics have these syndromes). Because orthodox medicine has not been particularly effective in treating or understanding these disorders, many patients perceive their doctors as unsympathetic and seek out complementary treatments of uncertain efficacy. Examples of functional disorders are shown in Table 22.4.

Because epidemiological studies suggest that having one of these syndromes significantly increases the risk of having another, some doctors believe that these syndromes represent different manifestations in time of '*one functional syndrome*', which is indicative of a *somatization* process. Functional disorders also have a significant association with psychiatric disorders, especially depressive and panic disorders as well as phobias. Against this view is the evidence that the majority of primary care patients with most of these disorders do not have either a psychiatric disorder or other functional disorders. It also

seems that it requires a major stress or a psychiatric disorder in order for such sufferers to attend their doctor for help, which might explain why doctors are so impressed with the associations with stress and psychiatric disorders. Doctors have historically tended to diagnose 'stress' or 'psychosomatic disorders' in patients with symptoms that they cannot explain. History is full of such disorders being reclassified as research clarifies the pathology. A recent example is writer's cramp (p. 1233) which most neurologists now agree is a dystonia rather than a neurosis.

Chronic fatigue syndrome (CFS)

There has probably been more controversy over the existence and aetiology of CFS than any other functional syndrome in recent years. This is reflected in its uncertain classification as *neurasthenia* in the psychiatric classification and *myalgic encephalomyelitis* (ME) under neurological disorders. There is good evidence for this syndrome, although the diagnosis is made clinically and by exclusion of other fatiguing disorders. Its prevalence is 0.5% in the UK, although abnormal fatigue as a symptom occurs in 10–20%. It occurs most commonly in women between the ages of 20 and 50 years old. The cardinal symptom is chronic fatigue made worse by minimal exertion. The fatigue is usually both physical and mental, with associated poor concentration, impaired registration of memory, irritability, alteration in sleep pattern (either insomnia or hypersomnia), and muscular pain. The name myalgic encephalomyelitis (ME) is decreasingly used within medicine because it implies a pathology for which there is no evidence.

Aetiology

Functional disorders often have aetiological factors in common with each other (see Table 22.5), as well as more specific aetiologies. For instance, CFS can be triggered by certain infections, such as infectious mononucleosis and viral hepatitis. About 10% of patients with infectious mononucleosis have CFS 6 months after the infectious onset, yet there is no evidence of persistent infection in these patients. Those fatigue states which clearly do follow on a viral infection can be classified as *post-viral fatigue syndromes*. Other aetiological factors include physical inactivity and sleep difficulties. Immune and endocrine abnormalities noted in CFS may be secondary to the inactivity or sleep disturbance commonly seen in patients. Mood disorders are present in a large minority of patients, and can cause problems in diagnosis because of the large overlap in symptoms. These mood disorders may be secondary, independent (co-morbid), or primary with a misdiagnosis of CFS. The role of stress is uncertain, with some indication that the influence of stress is mediated through consequent psychiatric disorders exacerbating fatigue, rather than any direct effect.

Management

The general principles of the management of functional disorders are given in Box 22.7. Specific management of

Table 22.4 Functional or psychosomatic syndromes (medically unexplained symptoms)

'Tension' headaches	Chronic or post-viral fatigue syndrome
Atypical facial pain	Multiple chemical sensitivity
Atypical chest pain	Premenstrual syndrome
Fibromyalgia (chronic widespread pain)	Irritable or functional bowel syndrome
Other chronic pain syndromes	Irritable bladder syndrome

Table 22.5 Aetiological factors commonly seen in functional disorders

Predisposing
Perfectionist, obsessional and introspective personality
  traits
Childhood traumas (physical and sexual abuse)
Similar illnesses in first-degree relatives

Precipitating (triggering)
Infections
Chronic fatigue syndrome (CFS)
Irritable bowel syndrome (IBS)
Psychologically traumatic events (especially accidents)
Physical injuries ('fibromyalgia' and other chronic pain
  syndromes)
Life events that precipitate changed behaviours (e.g. going
  off sick)
Incidents where the patient believes others are responsible

Perpetuating (maintaining)
Inactivity with consequent physiological adaptation (CFS
  and 'fibromyalgia')
Avoidant behaviours – multiple chemical sensitivities
  (MCS), CFS
Maladaptive illness beliefs (that maintain maladaptive
  behaviours) (CFS)
Excessive dietary restrictions ('food allergies')
Stimulant drugs
Sleep disturbance
Mood disorders
Somatization disorder
Unresolved anger or guilt
Unresolved compensation

Box 22.7 Management of functional disorders

The first principle is the identification and treatment of
maintaining factors (e.g. dysfunctional beliefs and
behaviours, mood and sleep disorders).

■ Communication
  Explanation of ill-health, including diagnosis and
    causes
  Education about management (including self-help
    leaflets)
■ Stopping drugs (e.g. caffeine causing insomnia,
    analgesics causing dependence)
■ Rehabilitative therapies
  Cognitive behaviour therapy (to challenge unhelpful
    beliefs and change coping strategies)
  Supervised and graded exercise therapy for
    approximately 3 months (to reduce inactivity and
    improve fitness)
■ Pharmacotherapies
  Specific antidepressants for mood disorders,
    analgesia and sleep disturbance
  Symptomatic medicines (e.g. appropriate analgesia,
    taken only when necessary)

CFS should include a mutually agreed and supervised
programme of gradually increasing activity. However,
few patients regard themselves as cured after treatment.
It is sometimes difficult to persuade a patient to accept

what are inappropriately perceived as 'psychological
therapies' for such a physically manifested condition.
Antidepressants do not work in the absence of a mood
disorder or insomnia.

Prognosis

This is poor without treatment, with less than 10% of
hospital attenders recovered after 1 year. Outcomes are
worse with increasing age, co-morbid mood disorders,
and the conviction that the illness is entirely physical.

Fibromyalgia (chronic widespread pain: CWP)

This controversial condition of unknown aetiology overlaps with chronic fatigue syndrome, with both conditions
causing fatigue and sleep disturbance (see p. 1281).
Diffuse muscle and joint pains are more constant and
severe in CWP, although the 'tender points', previously
considered to be pathognomonic, are now known to be
ubiquitous, associated with psychological distress, and of
no diagnostic importance (p. 547). CWP occurs most
commonly in women aged 40–65 years old, with a
prevalence in the community of between 1 and 11%.
There are associations with depressive and anxiety disorders, other functional disorders, physical deconditioning
and a possibly characteristic sleep disturbance (see
Table 22.5).

Management

Apart from the general principles in Box 22.7, management also consists of symptomatic analgesia, reversing
the sleep disturbance, and a physically orientated rehabilitation programme. A recent meta-analysis suggests
that tricyclic antidepressants that inhibit reuptake of
both serotonin (5-hydroxytryptamine – 5-HT) and
norepinephrine (noradrenaline) (e.g. amitriptyline,
dosulepin (dothiepin)) have the greatest effect on sleep,
fatigue and pain. The doses used were too low for
antidepressant efficacy and the drugs may work through
their hypnotic and analgesic effects.

Other chronic pain syndromes

A chronic pain syndrome is a condition of chronic
disabling pain for which no medical cause can be found.
The psychiatric classification would be a persistent
somatoform pain disorder, but this is unsatisfactory since
the criteria include the stipulation that emotional factors
must be the main cause, and it is clinically difficult to be
that certain. The main sites of chronic pain syndromes are
the head, face, neck, lower back, abdomen, genitalia and
all over (CWP: fibromyalgia). 'Functional' low back pain
is the commonest 'physical' reason for being off sick long-
term in the UK (p. 540). Quite often a minor abnormality
will be found on investigation (such as mild cervical
spondylosis on the neck X-ray), but this will not be severe
enough to explain the severity of the pain and resultant
disability. These pains are often unremitting and respond
poorly to analgesics. Sleep disturbance is almost universal

and co-morbid psychiatric disorders are found in a large minority.

Aetiology

The perception of pain involves sensory (nociceptive), emotional and cognitive processing in the brain. Functional brain scans suggest that the brain may respond abnormally to pain in these conditions, with increased activation in response to chronic pain. This could be related to conditioned behavioural and physiological responses to the initial acute pain. The brain may then adapt to the prolonged stimulus of the pain by changing its central processing. The prefrontal cortex, thalamus and cingulate gyrus seem to be particularly affected and some of these areas are involved in the emotional appreciation of pain in general. Thus it is possible to start to understand how beliefs, emotions and behaviours might influence the perception of chronic pain (see Table 22.5).

Management

Management involves the same principles as used in other functional syndromes (Box 22.7). Since analgesics are rarely effective, and can cause long-term harm, patients should be encouraged to gradually reduce their use. It is often helpful to involve the patient's immediate family or partner, to ensure that the partner is also supported and not unconsciously discouraging progress.

Specific drug treatments are few. Nerve blocks are not usually effective. Anticonvulsants such as carbamazepine and gabapentin may be given a therapeutic trial if the pain is thought to be neuropathic (see p. 1200). The antidepressant *dosulepin* (*dothiepin*) is an effective treatment in half of patients with atypical facial pain, and this effect seems to be independent of dosulepin's effect on mood. Another tricyclic antidepressant, *amitriptyline*, is helpful in tension headaches, which might be related to its independent analgesic effect. Amitriptyline has the added bonus of increasing slow wave sleep, which may be why it is more effective than NSAIDs in chronic widespread pain. Tricyclic antidepressants that affect both serotonin and norepinephrine (noradrenaline) reuptake (e.g. p. 1292) seem to be more effective than more selective norepinephrine reuptake inhibitors, e.g. in neuropathic pain. There is some evidence that tricyclics are generally superior to SSRIs in chronic pain syndromes.

Irritable bowel syndrome

This is one of the commonest functional syndromes, affecting some 10–30% of the population in the UK. The clinical features and management of the syndrome and the related *functional dyspepsia* are described in more detail on page 337. Although the majority of sufferers with the irritable bowel syndrome (IBS) do not have a psychiatric disorder, depressive illness should be excluded in patients with constipation and a poor appetite. Anxiety disorders should be excluded in patients with nausea and diarrhoea. Persistent abdominal pain or a feeling of emptiness may occasionally be the presenting symptom of a severe depressive illness, particularly in the elderly, with a *nihilistic delusion* that the body is empty or dead inside (see p. 1289).

Management

This is dealt with in more detail on page 339 and in Box 22.7. Seeing a physician who provides specific education that particularly addresses individual illness beliefs and concerns can provide lasting benefit. Psychological therapies that help the more severely affected include biofeedback, hypnotherapy, cognitive behaviour therapy and brief interpersonal psychotherapy. If indicated, the choice of antidepressant should be determined by the effects of these drugs on bowel transit times, with tricyclic antidepressants normally slowing and selective serotonin reuptake inhibitors (SSRIs) (p. 1292) normally speeding up transit times.

Multiple chemical sensitivity, candida hypersensitivity, and food allergies

Some complementary health practitioners, doctors, and patients themselves make diagnoses of multiple chemical sensitivities (MCS) (e.g. to foods, smoking, perfumes, petrol), candida hypersensitivity, and allergies (to food, tap-water, and even electricity). Symptoms and syndromes attributed to these putative disorders are numerous and variable and include all the functional disorders, *mood disorders*, and *arthritis*. Scientific support for the existence of these disorders has been hard to acquire, particularly when double-blind methodologies have been used.

Type 1 hypersensitivities to foods such as nuts certainly exist, although they are fortunately uncommon (approximately 3 per 1000) (see p. 220). Direct specific food intolerances also occur (e.g. chocolate with migraine, caffeine with IBS).

Candidiasis can occur in the gastrointestinal tract in immunocompromised individuals, such as those with AIDS. Vaginal candidiasis can occur after antibiotic treatment in otherwise healthy women. A double-blind and controlled study of nystatin in women, diagnosed as having candidiasis hypersensitivity syndrome, showed that vaginal candida was the only symptom relieved more by nystatin than placebo. There is little evidence of candida having a systemic role in other symptoms. In spite of this evidence, the patient is often convinced of the legitimacy and usefulness of these diagnoses and their treatments.

Aetiology

Surveys of patients diagnosed with MCS or food allergies have shown high rates of current and previous psychiatric disorders (especially mood and anxiety disorders) (see Table 22.5). Eating disorders (p. 1310) should be excluded in patients with food intolerances. Some patients, taking very low carbohydrate diets as putative treatments, may develop reactive hypoglycaemia after a high carbohydrate meal, which they then interpret as a food allergy. It has been shown that classical conditioning can produce intolerances to foods and smells in healthy people and this may be a causative mechanism in some patients with intolerance. This study supports the existence of these intolerance conditions, but suggests they may be conditioned responses with attendant physiological consequences. This might explain why double-blinding abolishes the reaction to the stimulus.

Management.

The general principles in Box 22.7 apply. If one assumes a phobic or conditioned response is responsible, graded exposure (systematic desensitization) to the conditioned stimulus may be worthwhile. Preliminary studies do suggest that this approach may successfully treat such intolerances, in the context of cognitive behaviour therapy.

Premenstrual syndrome

The premenstrual syndrome (PMS) consists of both physical and psychological symptoms that regularly occur during the premenstrual phase and substantially diminish or disappear soon after the period starts. Physical symptoms include headache, fatigue, breast tenderness, abdominal distension and fluid retention. Psychological symptoms can include irritability, emotional lability or low mood, and tension. The *premenstrual dysphoric disorder* (PMDD) is a severe form of PMS with marked mood swings, irritability, depression and anxiety accompanying the physical symptoms. Women who generally suffer from mood disorders may be more prone to experience this disorder. The prevalence of PMS does not vary between cultures and is reported by the majority (75%) of women at some time in their lives. Severely disabling PMS (PMDD) occurs in about 3–8% of women. The cause of the premenstrual syndrome remain unclear, although exacerbating factors include some of those outlined in Table 22.5. Research suggests that abnormalities of reproductive hormone receptors may play a role.

Management

The general principles in Box 22.7 apply. Treatments with vitamin B_6 (p. 246), diuretics, progesterone, oral contraceptives, oil of evening primrose and oestrogen implants or patches (balanced by cyclical norethisterone) remain empirical. Psychotherapies aimed at enhancing the patient's coping skills can reduce disability. Two trials suggest that graded exercise therapy improves symptoms. Several studies have demonstrated that SSRIs (p. 1292) are effective treatments for the premenstrual dysphoric syndrome.

The menopause

The clinical features and management of the menopause are described on page 1052. A prospective study has shown that there is no increased incidence of depressive disorders at this time. Such a significant bodily change, sometimes occurring at the same time as children leaving home, is naturally accompanied by an emotional adjustment that does not normally amount to a pathological state.

FURTHER READING

Grady-Weliky TA (2003) Premenstrual dysphoric disorder. *New England Journal of Medicine* **348**: 433–438.

Lishman WA (1998) *Organic Psychiatry: The Psychological Consequences of Cerebral Disorder.* Oxford: Blackwell Science.

Royal College of Physicians and Royal College of Psychiatrists (2003) *The Psychological Care of Medical Patients: A practical guide,* 2nd edn. London: Royal College of Physicians.

White PD, Moorey G (1997) Psychosomatic illnesses are not 'all in the mind'. *Journal of Psychosomatic Research* **42**(4): 329–332.

Whiting G et al. (2001) Interventions for the treatment and management of chronic fatigue syndrome. *Journal of the American Medical Association* **286**: 1360–1368.

SOMATOFORM DISORDERS

As explained in the section on functional disorders (p. 1281), the classification of somatoform disorders is unsatisfactory because of the uncertain nature and aetiology of these disorders. However, there are certain disorders, beyond those described in 'functional disorders', that present frequently and coherently enough to be usefully recognized.

Somatization disorder

One in ten patients presenting with a functional disorder will fulfil the criteria of a chronic somatization disorder, sometimes known as *Briquet's syndrome*. The condition is composed of multiple, recurrent, medically unexplained physical symptoms, usually starting early in adult life. Exhaustion, dizzy spells, headaches, hypersensitivity to light and noise, paraesthesiae, abdominal, neck and back pain, nausea, sexual symptoms, and abnormal skin sensations are among the most common complaints, but symptoms may be referred to almost any part or bodily system. The patient, usually female, has often had multiple medical opinions and repeated negative investigations. Medical reassurance that the symptoms do not have a demonstrable physical cause fails to reassure the patient, who will continue to 'doctor-shop'. The patient is usually reluctant to accept a psychological and/or social explanation for the symptoms even when such a link seems obvious. Abnormal illness behaviour is evident and patients can be attention-seeking and dependent on doctors. Yet they can complain about the medical care and attention they have previously received.

The aetiology is unknown, but both mood and personality disorders are often also present. It is often associated with dependence upon or misuse of prescribed medication, usually sedatives and analgesics. There is often a history of significant childhood traumas, or chronic ill-health in the child or parent, which may play an aetiological role (see Table 22.5). The condition is probably the somatic presentation of psychological distress, although iatrogenic damage (from postoperative and prescribed-drug-related problems) soon complicates the clinical picture. The course of the disorder is chronic and disabling, with long-standing family, marital and/or occupational problems.

Hypochondriasis

The conspicuous feature is a preoccupation with an assumed serious disease and its consequences. Patients commonly believe that they suffer from cancer or AIDS, or some other serious condition. Characteristically, such patients repeatedly request laboratory and other investigations to either prove they are ill or reassure themselves that they are well. Such reassurance rarely lasts long before another cycle of worry and requests begins. The symptom of hypochondriasis may be secondary to or associated with a variety of psychiatric disorders, particularly depressive and anxiety disorders. Occasionally the hypochondriasis is delusional, secondary to schizophrenia or a depressive psychosis. Hypochondriasis may coexist with physical disease but the diagnostic point is that the patient's concern is disproportionate and unjustified.

Management of somatoform disorders

The principles outlined in Box 22.7 also apply to these disorders. Patients very much appreciate a discussion and explanation of their symptoms. Further management consists of ceasing reassurance that no serious disease has been uncovered, since this simply reinforces dependence on the doctor. The doctor should sensitively explore possible psychological and social difficulties, if possible by demonstrating links between symptoms and stresses. Useful questions to ask include:

'When were you last completely well and happy?'

Such a patient may have trouble remembering such a time, which helps to support the diagnosis, and leads to a discussion as to why they have never been well or happy.

'What can't you do now because you are unwell?'
'What changes has your ill-health caused in your close relationships?'

These questions usually give information that can be used to formulate an agreed plan of management. Repeated laboratory investigations should be discouraged. It is vital that all members of staff and close family members adopt the same approach to the patient's problems. Such patients often consciously or unconsciously split both medical staff and family members into 'good' and 'bad' (or caring and uncaring) people, as a way of projecting their distress. Since these disorders have a poor prognosis, the aim is to minimize disability. A contract of mutually agreed care involving the appropriate professionals (general practitioner, and a choice of psycho-therapist, health psychologist, complementary health professional, physician or psychiatrist), with agreed frequency of visits and a review date, can be helpful in managing the condition.

Cognitive behaviour therapy has been shown to provide effective rehabilitation in significant numbers of patients suffering from a somatoform disorder.

FURTHER READING

Boorsky A, Ahern D (2004) Cognitive behaviour therapy for hypochondriasis. *Journal of the American Medical Association* **291**: 1464–1470.

Butler CC et al. (2004) Medically unexplained symptoms. *Journal of the Royal Society of Medicine* **97**: 219–222.

DISSOCIATIVE (CONVERSION) DISORDERS

Until recently these disorders were known as 'hysteria'; but because the word hysteria is sometimes used pejoratively to describe extravagant behaviour, the term is inappropriate.

A *dissociative disorder* is a condition in which there is a profound loss of awareness or cognitive ability without medical explanation. The term dissociative indicates the disintegration of different mental activities, and covers such phenomena as amnesia, fugues, and pseudoseizures (non-epileptic fits).

The term *conversion* was introduced by Freud to explain how an unresolved conflict could be converted into usually symbolic physical symptoms as a defence against it. Such symptoms commonly include paralysis, abnormal movements, sensory loss, aphonia, disorders of gait, and pseudocyesis (false pregnancy). The lifetime prevalence has been estimated at 3–6 per 1000 in women, with a lower prevalence in men. Most cases begin before the age of 35 years. Dissociation is unusual in the elderly.

Table 22.6 Common dissociative/conversion symptoms

Dissociative (mental)	Conversion (physical)
Amnesia	Paralysis
Fugue	Disorders of gait
Pseudodementia	Tremor
Dissociative identity disorder	Aphonia
Psychosis	Mutism
	Sensory symptoms
	Globus hystericus
	Hysterical fits
	Blindness

Clinical features

The various symptoms are usually divided into dissociative and conversion categories (Table 22.6). Dissociative disorders have the following four characteristics that are necessary in order to make the diagnosis:

- They occur in the absence of physical pathology that would explain the symptoms.

- They are produced unconsciously.
- The illness is always triggered by an unresolved conflict or life event.
- Symptoms are not caused by overactivity of the sympathetic nervous system.

Other characteristics include:

- Symptoms and signs often reflect a patient's ideas about illness.
- Patients may take up the symptoms of a relative/ friend who has been ill.
- There is usually abnormal illness behaviour, with obvious exaggeration of disability.
- *Primary gain* is the immediate relief from the emotional conflict.
- *Secondary gain* refers to the social advantage gained by the patient by being ill and disabled (sympathy of family and friends, being off work, disability pension).
- There may be a curious lack of concern about the symptoms or disability ('belle indifference').
- Physical disease is not uncommonly present (e.g. pseudoseizures in someone with epilepsy).

Dissociative *amnesia* commences suddenly. Patients are unable to recall long periods of their lives and may even deny any knowledge of their previous life or personal identity. In a dissociative *fugue,* patients not only lose their memory but wander away from their usual surroundings, and, when found, deny all memory of their whereabouts during this wandering. The differential diagnosis of a fugue state includes post-ictal automatism, depressive illness and alcohol abuse.

Dissociative *pseudodementia* involves memory loss and behaviour that initially suggest severe and generalized dementia. A differential diagnosis is depressive pseudo-dementia (see p. 1289).

Multiple personality disorder is rare, but dramatic, and may be no more than the consequence of suggestion on the part of a psychotherapist. There are rapid alterations between two or more 'personalities' in the same person, each of which is repressed and dissociated from the other 'personalities'. A differential diagnosis is rapid cycling *manic depressive disorder* which would explain sudden apparent changes in personality.

Epidemic or '*mass hysteria*' usually occurs in institutions for girls or young women, in which the combined effects of suggestion and shared anxiety produce outbreaks of sickness or disturbed behaviour, often following sudden illnesses in leaders of the group at a time of threatened or actual social change.

Differential diagnosis

Dissociation is usually a stable and reliable diagnosis over time, although high rates of co-morbid mood and personality disorders are found in chronic sufferers. Particular care should be taken to make the diagnosis on positive grounds, and not simply on the basis of an absence of a medical diagnosis. Care should also be taken to exclude or treat co-morbid psychiatric disorders.

Aetiology

Preliminary research using functional brain scans where healthy controls feigning a motor abnormality were compared with patients with a similar conversion motor symptom suggests that dissociation involves different areas of the brain from stimulation. This supports the theory of unconscious mechanisms first suggested by Charcot (see Fig. 22.1). This research would suggest that there is a disinhibition of voluntary will at an unconscious level, so that the patient can no longer *will* the function to happen.

The psychoanalytical theory of dissociation is that it is the result of emotionally charged memories that are repressed into the unconscious at some point in the past. Symptoms are explained as the combined effects of repression and the symbolic conversion of this emotional energy into physical symptoms. This hypothesis is difficult to test, although there is some evidence that patients with dissociative disorders are more likely to have suffered childhood abuse, particularly when the abuse was both sexual and physical and started early in childhood. Caution should be taken with any such history obtained by therapies that 'recover' childhood memories that were previously completely unknown to the patient.

Patients with dissociative disorders, by definition adopt both the sick role and abnormal illness behaviour, with consequent secondary gains that help to maintain the illness.

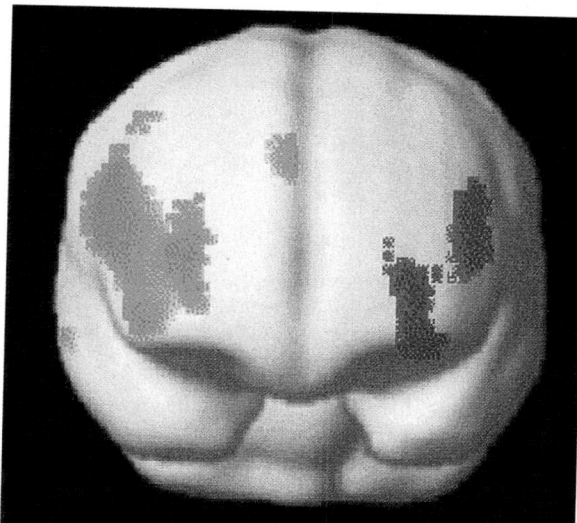

Fig. 22.1 Statistical parametric maps superimposed on an MRI scan of the anterior surface of the brain, orientated as though looking at a person head on. Red region shows hypofunction of patients with conversion motor symptoms. Green region shows hypofunction of healthy controls feigning the same motor abnormality. Reproduced from Spence SA, Crimlisk HL, Cope H, Ron MA, Grasby PM (2000) Discrete neurophysiological correlates in prefrontal cortex during hysterical and feigned disorders of movement. *Lancet* **355**:1243–1244, © The Lancet Ltd. 2000, with permission.

Management

The treatment of dissociation is similar to the treatment of somatoform disorders in general, outlined above and in Box 22.7. The first task is to engage the patient and their family with a model of the illness that makes sense to them, is acceptable, and leads to the appropriate management. An invented example of a suitable explanation is given below:

You told me about the tremendous shock you felt when your mother suddenly died. This was particularly the case since you hadn't spoken to her for so long beforehand, after that big disagreement with her over your wedding to John. You weren't able to say good-bye before she died. Your brain was overloaded with grief, guilt and anger all at once. I wonder whether that is why you aren't able to speak now. I wonder whether it's difficult to think of anything to say that would make things right, particularly since you can't speak with your mother now.

Such an explanation would be modified by mutual discussion until an agreed understanding was achieved, which would serve as a working model for the illness. Provision of a rehabilitation programme that addresses both the physical and psychological needs and problems of the patient would then be planned. A graded and mutually agreed plan of a return to normal function can usually be led by the appropriate therapist (e.g. speech therapist for dysphonia, physiotherapist for paralysis). At the same time, a psychotherapeutic assessment should be made in order to determine the appropriate form of psychotherapy. For instance, couple therapy will address a significant relationship difficulty; individual psychotherapy could ease an unresolved conflict from childhood.

Abreaction brought about by *hypnosis* or by intravenous injections of small amounts of midazolam may produce a dramatic, if short-lived, recovery. In the abreactive state, the patient is encouraged to relive the stressful events that provoked the disorder and to express the accompanying emotions; i.e. to abreact. Such an approach has been useful in the treatment of acute dissociative states in wartime, but appears to be of much less value in civilian life. It should only be contemplated in the presence of an anaesthetist with suitable resuscitation equipment to hand.

Hypnotherapy is psychotherapy while the patient is in a hypnotic trance, the idea being that therapy is more possible because the patient is relaxed and not using repression. This may allow the therapist access to the previously unconscious emotional conflicts or memories. There are no published trials of this technique in dissociation, which Freud gave up as unsuccessful in order to found psychoanalysis, but some hypnotherapists claim good results. Care should be taken to avoid a catastrophic emotional reaction when the patient is suddenly faced with the previously repressed memories.

Prognosis

Most cases of recent onset recover quickly with treatment, which is why a positive diagnosis should be made early, rather than sending the patient on to the next medical specialist. Those cases that last longer than a year are likely to persist, with entrenched abnormal illness behaviour patterns that are hard to shift.

FURTHER READING
Crimlisk HL, Bhatia K, Cope H, David A, Marsden CD, Ron MA (1998) Slater revisited: 6 year follow up study of patients with medically unexplained symptoms. *British Medical Journal* **316**: 582–586.
Mersky H (1995) *The Analysis of Hysteria*, 2nd edn. London: Gaskell.

SLEEP DIFFICULTIES (p. 1227)

Sleep is divided into *rapid eye movement (REM)* and *non-REM* sleep. As drowsiness begins, the alpha rhythm on an EEG disappears and is replaced by deepening slow wave activity (non-REM). After 60–90 minutes, this slow wave pattern is replaced by low amplitude waves on which are superimposed rapid eye movements lasting a few minutes. This cycle is repeated during the duration of sleep, with the REM periods becoming longer. REM sleep is accompanied by dreaming and physiological arousal. Slow wave sleep is associated with release of anabolic hormones and cytokines, with an increased cellular mitotic rate. It helps to maintain host defences, metabolism and repair of cells. For this reason slow wave sleep is increased in those conditions where growth or conservation is required (e.g. adolescence, pregnancy, thyrotoxicosis).

Insomnia is difficulty in sleeping; a third of adults complain of insomnia and in a third of these it can be severe.

Primary sleep disorders include sleep apnoea (p. 1227), narcolepsy (see p. 1227), the *restless legs syndrome (Ekbom's)* (see p. 666) and its related *periodic leg movement disorder*, in which the legs (and sometimes the arms) jerk while asleep.

Delayed sleep phase syndrome occurs when the circadian pattern of sleep is delayed so that the patient sleeps from the early hours until mid-day or later. *Night terrors, sleep-walking* and *sleep-talking* are non-REM phenomena, most commonly found in children, which can recur in adults when under stress or suffering from a mood disorder.

Psychophysiological insomnia commonly occurs with functional, mood and substance misuse disorders, and when under stress (see Box 22.8). It can often be triggered by one of these factors, but then become a habit on its own, driven by anticipation of insomnia and day-time naps. Insomnia causes day-time sleepiness and fatigue, with consequences such as road traffic accidents. Assessment should pay particular attention to mood, life difficulties, and drug intake (especially alcohol, nicotine and caffeine). Initial insomnia (trouble getting off to sleep) is common in mania, anxiety, depressive disorders and substance misuse. Middle insomnia (waking up in the middle of the night) occurs with medical conditions, such as sleep apnoea and prostatism. Late insomnia (early morning waking) is caused by depressive illness and malnutrition (anorexia nervosa).

Habitual alcohol consumption should be carefully estimated since even a small excess can be a potent cause of insomnia, as well as recent withdrawal. *Caffeine* is perhaps the most commonly taken drug in the UK, and its effects are easily underestimated. Six cups (not mugs) of

Box 22.8 Common causes of insomnia

Psychiatric disorders
Mood disorders (mania, depressive and anxiety disorders)
Delirium and dementia

Drug use or misuse
Addictive drug withdrawal (alcohol, benzodiazepines)
Stimulant drugs (caffeine, amfetamines)
Prescribed drugs (steroids, dopamine agonists)

Physical conditions
Pain (classically with carpal tunnel syndrome)
Nocturia (e.g. from prostatism)
Malnutrition

Primary sleep disorders
Sleep apnoea
Restless legs syndrome

real coffee a day are likely to cause insomnia in the average healthy adult. Caffeine is not only found in tea and coffee, but is also found in chocolate, cola drinks and some analgesics. Prescription drugs that can either disturb sleep or cause vivid dreams include most appetite suppressants, glucocorticoids, dopamine agonists, lipid-soluble beta-blockers (e.g. propranolol) and certain psychotropic drugs (especially when first prescribed; e.g. fluoxetine, reboxetine, risperidone).

Hypersomnia is not uncommon in adolescents with depressive illness, occurs in narcolepsy, and may temporarily follow infections such as infectious mononucleosis.

Management of insomnia

This is particularly determined by diagnosis. Where none is immediately apparent, it is worth educating the patient about sleep hygiene. Simple measures such as decreasing alcohol intake, having supper earlier, exercising daily, having a bath prior to going to bed and establishing a routine of going to bed at the same time should be tried. Relaxation techniques and cognitive behaviour therapy have a role in those with intractable insomnia. Short half-life benzodiazepines can be useful for acute insomnia, but should not be used for more than 2 weeks continuously to avoid dependence. Non-benzodiazepine hypnotics (zaleplon, zopiclone, zolpidem) act at the benzodiazepine receptors and occasional dependence has been reported. Certain antihistamines (e.g. promethazine) and anti-depressants (e.g. amitriptyline, trimipramine, trazodone mirtazapine) are not addictive and can be used as hypnotics in low dose, with the added advantage of improving slow wave sleep. The commonest side-effects are morning sedation and weight gain.

FURTHER READING
Sateia MJ, Nowell PD (2004) Insomnia. *Lancet* **364**: 1959–1973.
Wilson S, Nutt D (2005) Assessment and management of insomnia. *Clinical Medicine* **5**: 101–104.

MOOD (AFFECTIVE) DISORDERS

Classification

The central and common feature of these disorders is an abnormality of mood. Mood is best considered in terms of a continuum ranging from severe depression at one extreme to severe mania at the other, with the normal, stable mood at the centre (Fig. 22.2). Mood disorders are divided into bipolar and unipolar affective disorders. In bipolar affective disorder (otherwise known as manic-depressive disorder) patients suffer bouts of both depression and mania. In unipolar affective disorder patients suffer from depressive mood swings alone, although they are commonly recurrent. Although mania can rarely occur by itself without depressive mood swings (thus being classified as unipolar) it is far more commonly found in association with depressive swings, even if sometimes it takes several years for the first depressive illness to appear. Hypomania is mild mania. Dysthymia is a chronic low-grade depressive illness.

DEPRESSIVE DISORDERS

Depressive disorders or 'episodes' are primarily classified as bipolar or unipolar and secondarily as mild, moderate or severe, with or without somatic symptoms. Severe depressive episodes are divided according to the presence or absence of psychotic symptoms. About 10% of patients with depressive illness are eventually found to have bipolar illnesses.

Clinical features of depressive disorder

Whereas everyone will at some time or other feel cheesed off, fed up or down in the dumps, it is when such symptoms become qualitatively different, pervasive, or interfere with normal functioning that a depressive illness has occurred. Depressive disorder, clinical or 'major' depression is characterized by disturbances of mood, speech, energy and ideas (Table 22.7). Patients often describe their symptoms in physical terms. Marked fatigue and headache are the two most common physical symptoms in depressive illness and may be the first

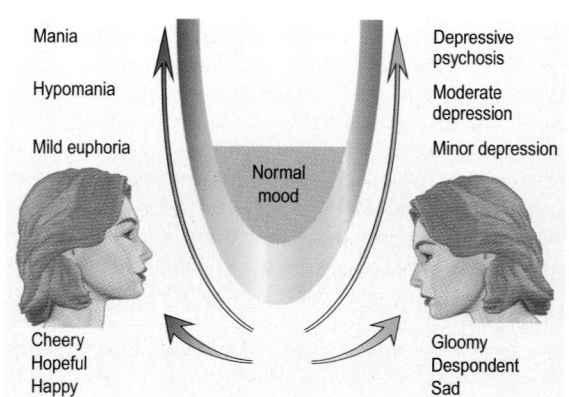

Fig. 22.2 Continuum of normal and abnormal mood.

Table 22.7	Clinical features of depression
Characteristic	**Clinical appearance**
Mood	Depressed, miserable or irritable
Talk	Impoverished, slow, monotonous
Energy	Reduced, lethargic
Ideas	Feelings of futility, guilt, self-reproach, unworthiness, hypochondriacal preoccupations, worrying, suicidal thoughts, delusions of guilt, nihilism and persecution
Cognition	Impaired learning, pseudodementia in elderly patients
Physical	Early waking, poor appetite and weight loss, constipation, loss of libido, erectile dysfunction, fatigue, bodily aches and pains
Behaviour	Retardation or agitation, poverty of movement and expression
Hallucinations	Auditory – often hostile, critical

- physical diseases, particularly if chronic, stigmatizing or painful
- excessive and chronic alcohol use (probably the most depressing drug humans use)
- social stresses, particularly loss events, such as separation, redundancy and bereavement
- interpersonal difficulties with those close to the patient, especially when socially humiliated
- lack of social support, with no confiding relationship.

Depressed patients with another physical disorder view themselves as more sick and visit their doctors almost four times as often as the non-depressed physically ill, stay in hospital longer, comply less with medical advice and medication, and undergo more medical and surgical procedures. Depressive illness may be associated with increased mortality (excluding suicide) in patients with physical illness, such as myocardial infarct.

Dysthymia

Dysthymia is a more mild depressive illness that lasts intermittently for 2 years or more and is characterized by tiredness and low mood, lack of pleasure, low self-esteem, and a feeling of discouragement. The mood relapses and remits, with several weeks of feeling well, soon followed by longer periods of being unwell. It can be punctuated by depressive episodes of more severity; so-called 'double depression'.

Seasonal affective disorder

Seasonal affective disorder is characterized by recurrent episodes of depressive illness occurring during the winter months in the northern hemisphere. Symptoms are similar to those found with *atypical depressive illness*, in that patients complain of hypersomnia, increased appetite (with carbohydrate craving) and weight gain, with profound fatigue. Such patients have a higher prevalence of bipolar affective disorder, and some doctors are uncertain whether the condition is different from normal depressive illness, with the accentuation of mood that naturally occurs by season. However, there is evidence that seasonal depressive illness can be successfully treated with bright light therapy given in the early morning, which causes a phase advance in the circadian rhythm of melatonin. In contrast, the same treatment given in the early evening, with consequent phase delay of melatonin secretion, is less antidepressant. Selective serotonin reuptake inhibitors (SSRIs) are alternative treatments.

Differential diagnosis

The differential diagnoses of depressive illness are shown in Table 22.8. Other psychiatric disorders are the most common misdiagnoses. Ninety per cent of patients presenting with a depressive illness, while misusing alcohol, will no longer be depressed 2 weeks after their last drink.

Pathological (abnormal) and normal grief are described on page 1300. Pathological grief is closely associated with depressive illness.

symptoms to appear. Patients describe the world as looking grey, themselves as lacking a zest for living and devoid of pleasure and interest in life (anhedonia). Anxiety and panic attacks are common; secondary obsessional and phobic symptoms may emerge. Symptoms should last for at least 2 weeks and should cause significant incapacity (e.g. trouble working or relating to others) to be considered an illness.

In the more severe forms, diurnal variation in mood can occur, feeling worse in the morning after waking in the early hours with apprehension. Suicidal ideas are more frequent, intrusive and prolonged. Delusions of guilt, persecution and bodily disease are not uncommon, along with second person auditory hallucinations insulting the patient or suggesting suicide. In severe depressive illness, particular in the elderly, concentration and memory can be so badly affected that the patient appears to have dementia (pseudodementia). Delusions of poverty and non-existence (nihilism) occur particularly in this age group. Suicide is a real risk, with the lifetime risk being approximately 5% in primary care patients, but 15% in those with depressive illness severe enough to warrant admission to hospital.

Epidemiology

About a third of the population will feel unhappy at any one time, but this is not the same as depressive illness. The point prevalence of depressive illness is 5% in the community, with a further 3% having dysthymia (see below). It is more common in women, but there is no increase with age, and no difference by ethnic group or socio-economic class (apart from an inverse relationship only with dysthymia). Married and never married people have similar prevalence rates, with separated and divorced people having two to three times the prevalence. Some studies have suggested that depressive illness is becoming more common.

Depressive illnesses are more common in the presence of:

Table 22.8 Common differential diagnoses of depressive illness

Other psychiatric disorders
Alcohol misuse
Amfetamine (and derivatives) misuse and withdrawal
Borderline personality disorder
Dementia
Delirium
Schizophrenia
Normal and pathological grief

Organic (secondary) affective illness
Physical causes which are both necessary and sufficient as a cause
Cushing's syndrome
Thyroid disease (although sometimes depression persists after treatment)
Hyperparathyroidism
Corticosteroid treatment
Brain tumour (rarely without other neurological signs)

Investigations

A corroborative history can be valuable in helping to exclude differential diagnoses such as alcohol misuse and elucidating maintaining factors such as the relationship with a partner. Physical investigations should be guided by the history and examination. They will often include measurement of free T_4 and TSH (particularly in women), calcium, sodium, potassium, mean corpuscular volume, γ-glutamyl transpeptidase, haemoglobin, white cell count, ESR or plasma viscosity. Less commonly a chest X-ray, antinuclear antibody, morning and evening cortisols, electroencephalogram or a brain scan are indicated.

The aetiology of unipolar depressive disorders

The aetiology of unipolar depressive disorders is multifactorial and a mixture of genetic and environmental factors.

Genetic

Unipolar depression is probably polygenic, but no linkage has been firmly identified. The risk of unipolar depression in a first-degree relative of a patient is approximately three times the risk of the non-affected. The concordance of unipolar depression in monozygotic twins is between 30 and 60%, the concordance increasing with more recurrent illnesses. The issue is complicated by the genetic influence on sleep habits, 'neurotic' personality, and even life events, which are all involved in the genesis of depressive illness.

Biochemical

The monoamine theory of depressive illness is supported by the efficacy of monoamine reuptake inhibitors and the depressive effect of dietary tryptophan depletion. Neuroendocrine tests also suggest that the serotonin neurotransmitter system is downregulated. $5-HT_{1a}$ and $5-HT_2$ receptor subtypes are thought most likely to be involved. Receptor-labelled functional brain scans suggest that

dopamine underactivity is related to psychomotor retardation.

Hormonal

Cushing's syndrome is the most potent cause of 'organic' depressive illness, with 50–80% of patients with Cushing's suffering from a depressive illness. Corticosteroid treatment causes significant mood disturbance. Nearly half of patients with 'functional' depressive illness have raised cortisol levels, and this is associated with adrenal gland enlargement. Hypercortisolaemia can cause hippocampal damage, which has been found in chronic severe depressive illness. All these data suggest that cortisol may play a role in causing depressive illness.

In contrast *atypical depressive illness*, with prominent hypersomnia and weight gain, is associated with a downregulated hypothalamic–pituitary–adrenal axis, supporting the heterogeneity of depressive disorders.

Brain imaging

The use of magnetic resonance imaging (MRI) and positron emission tomography (PET) has revealed a number of abnormalities in the brains of patients with major depression. Increased brain ventricle volume, localized frontal lobe atrophy and reduced blood flow in specific brain areas have been reported, while more recent studies suggest that the hippocampus undergoes selective volume reduction in stress-related neuropsychiatric disorders such as recurrent depression. This may be related to hypercortisolaemia.

Sleep

A reduced time between onset of sleep and REM sleep (shortened REM latency) and reduced slow wave sleep both occur in depressive illness. These abnormalities are persistent in some patients when they are not depressed. Families with several sufferers of depressive illness can share these traits, suggesting that sleep patterns may be inherited and predispose to depression.

Psychological

Poor parenting and physical or sexual abuse in childhood all predispose adults to depressive illness, but the effect is non-specific. Both 'neurotic' (emotional) and perfectionist personality traits are risks for depressive illness, and these may be determined as much by genetic factors as early environment.

Social

Thirty per cent of women will develop a depressive illness after a severe life event or difficulty, such as a divorce, and this is compounded by low self-esteem and a lack of a confiding relationship. Unemployment is a significant risk factor in men.

An integrated model of aetiology

Stress is more likely to trigger depressive illness in a person predisposed by lack of social support and/or certain personality traits. Stress in turn triggers various brain changes in both stress hormones (such as the release of corticotropin-releasing hormone) and neurotransmitters (e.g. serotonin) that are both known to be altered in depressive illness. We can thus start to glimpse the model of an integrated biopsychosocial model of depressive illness. This model challenges dualistic ideas that depressive illnesses are either psychological or physical; depressive illnesses involve both the mind and the body, which are themselves indivisible.

Puerperal affective disorders

Affective illnesses and distress are common in women soon after they have given birth. Such disturbances are usually divided into maternity blues, postpartum (puerperal) psychosis and postnatal depressive illness. *'Maternity blues'* describe the brief episodes of emotional lability, irritability and tearfulness that occur in about 50% of women 2–3 days postpartum and resolve spontaneously in a few days.

Postpartum psychosis occurs once in every 500–1000 births. Over 80% of cases are affective in type and the onset is usually within the first 2 weeks following delivery. In addition to the classical features of an affective psychosis, disorientation and confusion are often noted. Severely depressed patients may have delusional ideas that the child is deformed, evil or otherwise affected in some way, and such false ideas may lead to either attempts to kill the child or suicide. The response to speedy treatment is generally good. The recurrence rate for a psychosis in a subsequent puerperium is 20–30%.

Non-psychotic *postnatal depressive disorders* occur during the first postpartum year in 10% of mothers, especially in the first 3 months. Risk factors are first pregnancy, poor relationship with the partner, ambivalence about the pregnancy, and emotional personality traits. The Edinburgh Postnatal Depression Scale (EPDS) is a 10-item questionnaire and can be used as an effective screening tool. Depressive illness after childbirth is clinically similar to other depressive illnesses, but lack of emotional bonding with the baby is common.

Treatment of depressive illness

The patient needs to know the diagnosis to provide understanding and rationalization of the overwhelming distress inherent in depressive illness. Knowing that self-loathing, guilt and suicidal thoughts are caused by the illness can be 'antidepressant' on its own. The further treatment of depressive disorders involves physical, psychological and social interventions (Box 22.9). Patients who are actively suicidal, severely depressed or with psychotic symptoms should be admitted (necessary for perhaps 1 in 1000 patients with clinical depression in primary care). This provides the patient a break from self-care, and allows support, listening, observation, prevention of suicide, and close monitoring of treatments. Avoid the pitfall of not treating a depressive illness just because it seems an 'understandable' reaction to serious illness or difficult circumstances. This is particularly likely to happen if the patient is elderly, severely or even terminally ill.

Box 22.9 Management of depressive illness

Physical
Stop depressing drugs (alcohol, steroids)
Regular exercise (good for mild to moderate depression)
Antidepressants (choice determined by side-effects, co-morbid illnesses and interactions)
Adjunctive drugs (e.g. lithium; if no response to two different antidepressants)
Electroconvulsive therapy (ECT) (if life-threatening or non-responsive)

Psychological
Education and regular follow-up by same professional
Cognitive behaviour therapy (CBT) (most effective psychotherapy in clinical depression)
Other indicated psychotherapies (couple, family, interpersonal therapies)

Social
Financial: eligible benefits, debt counselling
Employment: acquire or change the job or career
Housing: adequate, secure tenancy, safe, social neighbours
Young children: child-care support

Treatments combined
The most effective treatment is a mixture of CBT and an antidepressant

Drugs used in the treatment of clinical depression

Recreational drugs such as alcohol should be stopped. Prescribed medicines suspected of exacerbating depression, such as corticosteroids, should be gradually stopped or reduced to a safe minimum.

The first course of antidepressant drugs is effective in relieving clinical depression in 60–70% of patients, if given in adequate doses for a sufficient time to the correctly diagnosed patient. Such treatment is more successful when accompanied by sufficient patient education and regular follow-up, particularly in the first 6 weeks of treatment. Dysthymia responds less well to antidepressants than does a depressive episode.

The commonest two pharmacological types of antidepressants are tricyclic antidepressants (TCAs) and selective serotonin reuptake inhibitors (SSRIs). All antidepressants have similar efficacy and speed of onset. Choice depends on their side-effects, which can be used to positive effect (sedating drugs given at night to enhance sleep), and their safety. Patients should be warned about side-effects and that it will take 2 or more weeks before a positive benefit is apparent. Drugs should normally be started at a low dose and increased, depending on side-effects and efficacy. A course of antidepressants should be given until 4 months after recovery to prevent relapse. The two greatest problems with these drugs are persuading the patient to take them and compliance, since 80% of the UK public wrongly believe that they are addictive.

Psychotic depression needs either electroconvulsive therapy or a combination of an antidepressant and an antipsychotic drug.

Selective serotonin reuptake inhibitors (SSRIs)

SSRIs selectively inhibit the reuptake of the monoamine serotonin (5-HT) within the synapse, and are thus termed 'selective serotonin reuptake inhibitors' or SSRIs. Citalopram, and its laevo isomer, escitalopram, fluvoxamine, fluoxetine, paroxetine and sertraline have the advantage of causing less serious or disabling side-effects than tricyclics. For instance, SSRIs do not cause significant weight gain. Because of their long half-lives they can also be given just once a day, normally in the morning after breakfast. For these reasons patients comply more with treatment and therefore SSRIs are now first-line treatments for depressive disorders. Normal doses are between 20 and 60 mg, with sertraline and fluvoxamine needing higher doses. The most common side-effects resemble a 'hangover' and include nausea, vomiting, headache, diarrhoea and dry mouth. Insomnia and paradoxical agitation can occur when first starting the drugs. One in five patients also have sexual side-effects, such as impotence and loss of libido.

A toxic hyperserotonergic state ('serotonin' syndrome) can be caused by the ingestion of two or more drugs that increase serotonin levels, e.g. an SSRI combined with a monoamine oxidase inhibitor (MAOI) or dopaminergic drugs (e.g. selegiline) or a tricyclic antidepressant. Symptoms include agitation, confusion, tremor, diarrhoea, tachycardia and hypertension; hyperthermia is characteristic. Treatment is supportive.

SSRIs have also been associated with a specific withdrawal syndrome (*discontinuity syndrome*). This is characterized by shivering, anxiety, dizziness, headache and nausea. Patients should be warned not to leave out a dose and to gradually reduce SSRIs when stopping them.

Tricyclic antidepressants (TCAs)

Dosulepin (dothiepin), imipramine and amitriptyline are the three most commonly used in the UK, but many related compounds have been introduced, some having fewer autonomic and cardiotoxic effects (e.g. trazodone, lofepramine). These drugs potentiate the action of the monoamines, noradrenaline (norepinephrine) and serotonin, by inhibiting their reuptake into nerve terminals (Fig. 22.3(c)). Other tricyclics in common use include nortriptyline, doxepin and clomipramine. Depending on the particular drug, normal doses are between 75 and 150 mg. Having been available for more than 40 years, there is more evidence of the effectiveness of TCAs in depressive illness than for any other group of antidepressants. They are the drugs most commonly used in severe depressive illness.

TCAs have a number of side-effects (Table 22.9). In long-term treatment or prophylaxis, weight gain is most troublesome. Because of their toxicity in overdose, it is wisest NOT to prescribe them to potentially suicidal outpatients, without careful monitoring or giving the drugs to a reliable family member to look after.

SNaRIs, NaSSAs and NaRIs: antidepressants

The latest generation of antidepressants block a number of different neurotransmitter receptors both at the synapse

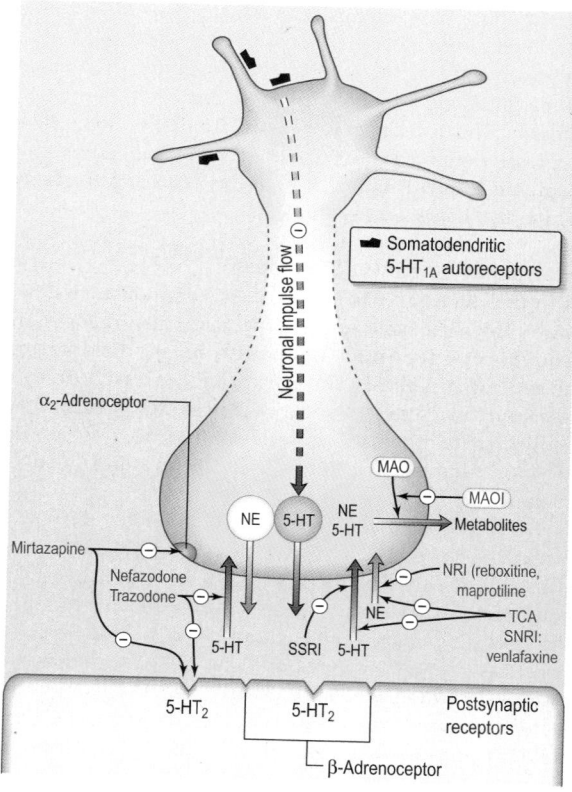

Fig. 22.3 **Sites of action of antidepressants with examples.** In a normal neurone, the stimulation of the somatodendritic 5-HT$_{1A}$ autoreceptors inhibits the neuronal impulse flow down the axon, reducing 5-HT release. In depression, there is a reduction in amine neurotransmissions which results in upregulation of postsynaptic *and* somatodendritic receptors. Using 5-HT, as an example, the depletion of 5-HT results in upregulation of postsynaptic 5-HT$_2$ receptors and presynaptic (somatodendritic) 5-HT$_{1A}$ receptors. The many antidepressants now available have different actions on serotonin and noradrenaline (norepinephrine) neurotransmission. Classical antidepressants (TCA) have less effects on sedation and antimuscarinic and antihistaminergic activities. SSRI, selective serotonin reuptake inhibitors; SNRI, serotonin and noradrenaline (norepinephrine) reuptake inhibitors; NRI, noradrenaline (norepinephrine) reuptake inhibitor (selective); NE, noradrenaline (norepinephrine); MAO, monoamine oxidase; MAOI, monoamine oxidase inhibitor. From Waller DG, Renwick A, Hillier K (eds) (2001) *Medical Pharmacology and Therapeutics*, Edinburgh: Saunders, with permission from Elsevier.

Table 22.9 Side-effects of tricyclic antidepressants

Antimuscarinic effects	Convulsant activity
Dry mouth	Lowered seizure threshold
Constipation	
Tremor	
Blurred vision	**Other effects**
Urinary retention	Weight gain
	Sedation
	Mania (rarely)
Cardiovascular	
QT prolongation	
Arrhythmias	
Postural hypotension	

and elsewhere. Their different receptor profiles cause different side-effects.

Venlafaxine is a potent *blocker* of both *serotonin* and *noradrenaline (norepinephrine) reuptake (SNaRI)*. It has negligible affinity for other neurotransmitter receptor sites and so produces less sedation and fewer antimuscarinic effects. It can be given in slow-release form with the advantage of once-daily dosage. Nausea is the commonest side-effect and high doses can occasionally cause hypertension. It does not cause weight gain.

Mirtazapine is a 5-HT$_2$ and 5-HT$_3$ receptor antagonist and a potent α_2-adrenergic blocker. The consequent effect is to *increase* both *noradrenaline (norepinephrine)* and *selective serotonin transmission*: an *NaSSA*. It can be given at night to aid sleep and rarely causes sexual side-effects. Mirtazapine can be sedating in low dose and can cause weight gain. An uncommon adverse effect is agranulocytosis.

Reboxetine is a *selective noradrenaline (norepinephrine) reuptake inhibitor (NaRI)*. It is not sedating and may help reduced motivation and energy. Weight gain is not reported. Dry mouth, insomnia, constipation, urinary hesitancy and tachycardia are reported side-effects.

Monoamine oxidase inhibitors (MAOIs)

These act by irreversibly inhibiting the intracellular enzymes monoamine oxidase A and B, leading to an increase of norepinephrine (noradrenaline), dopamine and 5-hydroxytryptamine in the brain (see Fig. 22.3(b)). Because of their side-effects and restrictions while taking them, they are rarely used by non-psychiatrists. Psychiatrists use them as a second-line treatment of depressive illnesses, particularly with atypical presentations (p. 1289). The most widely used is phenelzine, which is given in doses of 30–60 mg daily. Side-effects include increased appetite, weight gain, erectile dysfunction and insomnia. MAOIs also produce a severe and dangerous hypertensive reaction with foods containing tyramine or dopamine and therefore a restricted diet is prescribed. Tyramine is present in cheese, pickled herrings, yeast extracts, certain red wines, and any food, such as game, that has undergone partial decomposition. Dopamine is present in broad beans. MAOIs interact with drugs such as pethidine and can also occasionally cause liver damage. MAOIs should not normally be given within 2 weeks of a serotonin reuptake inhibitor, depending on half-lives.

Reversible inhibitors of monoamine A (RIMAs)

An example is moclobemide; usual dose 300 mg daily. These drugs appear to have fewer side-effects (insomnia and headache, but some sexual problems) and constitute a low risk in overdose. Patients prescribed such antidepressants should be told that they can eat a normal diet, but should be careful to avoid excessive amounts of food rich in tyramine (see above).

Antidepressant use in general medicine

In patients with cardiac disease, SSRIs, lofepramine and trazodone are preferred over more quinidine-like compounds. MAOIs and mirtazapine do not affect epileptic thresholds. SSRIs are metabolized by the cytochrome P450 system, unlike venlafaxine, mirtazapine and reboxetine; the latter therefore have fewer drug interactions. Care should be taken not to prescribe antidepressants while a patient is taking the herbal antidepressant St John's wort, which interacts with serotonergic drugs in particular. Doses of antidepressants should initially be halved in the elderly and in patients with renal or hepatic failure.

Antidepressants should be avoided if possible in pregnancy and breast-feeding. If other treatments are ineffective, the risks of drug therapy should be balanced against no treatment, which can affect fetal progress and the future mother–child bonding. Tricyclic antidepressants are generally believed to be safe in pregnancy, with no statistical increase in congenital malformations in fetuses exposed to them. However, occasionally their antimuscarinic side-effects produce jitteriness, sucking problems and hyperexcitability in the new-born. Postpartum plasma levels of babies breast-fed by treated mothers are negligible. SSRIs do not seem to be teratogenic but manufacturers advise against their use in pregnancy until more data are available. MAOIs should be avoided during pregnancy because of the possibility of a hypertensive reaction in the mother.

Electroconvulsive therapy (ECT)

Although the use of ECT is declining in the UK, it is still the treatment of choice in severe life-threatening depressive illness, particularly when psychotic symptoms are present. It is sometimes essential treatment when the patient is dangerously suicidal or refusing to eat and drink. The treatment involves the passage of an electric current across two electrodes applied to the anterior temporal areas of the scalp, in order to induce an epileptic fit. The fit is the essential part of the treatment. Before the treatment is given, the patient is given a general anaesthetic and receives a muscle relaxant to prevent injury during the fit. Treatments are normally given twice a week for 3–6 weeks.

ECT is a controversial treatment, yet it is remarkably safe and free of serious side-effects. Post-ictal confusion and headache are not uncommon, but transient. Short-term retrograde amnesia and a temporary defect in new learning can occur during the weeks of treatment, but these are short-lived effects.

Uncommonly used treatments

Transcranial magnetic stimulation (TMS) is an experimental treatment, with promising early results. *Psychosurgery* is very occasionally considered in patients with severe intractable depressive illness, when all other treatments have failed (see p. 1302). A third improve remarkably, while a further third improve somewhat. *Vagus nerve stimulation* may represent a major advance in the management of chronic and treatment-refractory depressive disorders but definitive clinical trials are awaited.

Psychological treatments
Cognitive behaviour therapy (CBT)

Aaron Beck developed CBT in the 1960s to reverse the negative cognitive triad with which patients regarded themselves, their situation and their futures. It involves the identification of the automatic dysfunctional thinking that maintains the negative perceptions that feed depression. They commonly include catastrophizing (e.g. making a 'mountain out of a mole-hill'), overgeneralizing (e.g. 'I failed an exam; therefore I am a failure as a person.'), categorical ('black or white') thinking (e.g. 'My work is either perfect or abysmal.'). CBT then involves identifying the links between these thoughts, consequent behaviour, and feeling low, and then testing their logic. This is done by considering the evidence either in the therapy sessions (e.g. Q: 'Did you pass the other exams you took?' A: 'Yes; I guess I did.') or by behavioural 'experiments' (e.g. showing the 'abysmal' work to a colleague and asking their opinion).

There is good evidence that CBT is as effective as antidepressant drugs for mild and moderate depressive illness. CBT is also effective in preventing a relapse of clinical depression. CBT is an effective treatment not only for depressive illness, but also for anxiety disorders and functional disorders (see pp. 1297 and 1281). It has even been shown to help reduce the severity of delusions in schizophrenia.

Interpersonal psychotherapy

This psychotherapy is probably as effective as antidepressants in mild and moderate clinical depression. The therapist focuses on a patient's interpersonal relationships involved in or affected by their illness (especially relationship changes or deficiencies), using problem-solving techniques to help the patient to find solutions.

Other psychotherapies

Couple therapy is particularly effective when a patient with clinical depression is in a relationship with problems (practical, emotional or sexual). Both the patient and partner attend therapy. *Family therapy* is effective not only in a family with problems, but also as a way of helping the family to help the patient get better. It may involve understanding one family member's 'depression' as a systemic 'solution' for a wider problem within the family.

Social treatments

Many patients with clinical depression have associated social problems (see Box 22.9). Assistance with social problems can make a significant contribution to clinical recovery. Other social interventions include the provision of group support, social clubs, occupational therapy and referral to a social worker. Educational programmes, self-help groups, and informed and supportive family members can help improve outcome.

Prognosis

The majority of patients have recovered by 6 months in primary care and 12 months in secondary care. About a quarter of patients attending hospital with depressive illnesses will have a recurrence within a year, and three-quarters will have a relapse within 10 years. Patients with recurrent depressive illnesses should be offered prevention. This may involve CBT that concentrates on relapse prevention, other forms of psychotherapy, or antidepressant medication. Full-dose antidepressants are the most effective prophylaxis in recurrent depressive disorders.

FURTHER READING

Alexopoulus GS (2005) Depression in the elderly. *Lancet* **365**: 1961–1970.

Belmaker RH (2004) Bipolar disorders. *New England Journal of Medicine* **351**: 476–486.

Brockington I (2004) Postpartum psychiatric disorders. *Lancet* **363**: 303–310.

Lader M, Cowan P (2001) Depression. *British Medical Bulletin* **57**.

UK ECT Review Group (2003) Efficacy and safety of electroconvulsive therapy in depressive disorders. Review. *Lancet* **361**: 799–808.

Whooley MA, Simon GE (2000) Managing depression in medical outpatients. *New England Journal of Medicine* **343**: 1942–1950.

MANIA AND HYPOMANIA

The clinical features of mania reflect a marked elevation of mood, characterized by euphoria, overactivity and disinhibition (Table 22.10). Hypomania is the mild form of mania. Hypomania lasts a shorter time and is less severe, with no psychotic features and less disability. Hypomania can be distinguished from normal happiness by its persistence, non-reactivity (not provoked by good news and not affected by bad news) and social disability. Mania almost always occurs as part of a bipolar affective disorder. The social disability of mania can be severe, with disinhibited behaviour leading to significant debts (from overspending and over-generosity), lost relationships (from promiscuity), social ostracism and lost employment (from reckless or disinhibited behaviour).

Some patients have a *rapid cycling* illness, with frequent swings from one mood state to another. A *mixed affective state* occurs when features of mania and depressive illness are seen in the same episode. *Cyclothymia* is a personality trait with spontaneous swings in mood not sufficiently severe or persistent to warrant another diagnosis.

Table 22.10	Clinical features of mania
Characteristic	**Clinical appearance**
Mood	Elevated or irritable
Talk	Fast, pressurized, flight of ideas
Energy	Excessive
Ideas	Grandiose, self-confident, delusions of wealth, power, influence or of religious significance, sometimes persecutory
Cognition	Disturbance of registration of memories
Physical	Insomnia, mild to moderate weight loss, increased libido
Behaviour	Disinhibition, increased sexual activity, excessive drinking or spending
Hallucinations	Fleeting auditory or, more rarely, visual

Differential diagnosis

Acute intoxication with recreational drugs, such as amfetamines, amfetamine derivatives (MDMA: Ecstasy), and cocaine can mimic mania. Long-term use of cannabis can also induce an illness with manic features. In one study a quarter of patients with Cushing's syndrome had a secondary manic illness during their illness. Similarly corticosteroids can induce mania less commonly than depressive illness. Dopamine agonists (e.g. bromocriptine) are also known to sometimes induce secondary mania. The excited phase of catatonic schizophrenia can sometimes be mistaken for mania.

Epidemiology

The lifetime prevalence of bipolar affective disorder is 1% across the world. Unlike unipolar depressive illness, it is equally common in men and women, supporting its different aetiology. There is no variation by socio-economic class or race. The mean age of onset is 21; earlier than unipolar depression. The higher prevalence found in divorced people is probably a consequence of the condition.

Aetiology

Genetic

There is strong evidence for a genetic aetiology in this disorder. There is a 60–80% concordance rate in monozygotic twins, compared to 15% in dizygotic twins, suggesting a high rate of heritability. Adoption studies show similar rates, so this high rate is probably genetic and not due to the family environment. Linkage studies have so far proved disappointing, with several suggestive chromosome linkages being found, suggesting there is no single gene with a large effect. Instead it is likely that the condition will prove to be caused by several genes acting together.

Biochemical

It is difficult to carry out research on patients with acute mania, so studies are few. Brain monoamines seem to be increased in mania. Dexamethasone tends not to suppress cortisol levels in patients with mania, suggesting a similar pattern of non-suppression to that seen in severe depressive illness.

Psychological

The effect of life events is much weaker in bipolar compared to unipolar illnesses, with most effect apparent at first onset. Similarly, personality does not seem to be a major influence, in contrast to unipolar depression, although there is some evidence of a link with the creativity and divergent thinking that is an advantage in the right occupation.

Treatment of mania

Acute mania

Acute mania is treated with lithium and/or antipsychotic (neuroleptic) drugs. Lithium is the treatment of choice for acute mania in the absence of severe hyperactivity. The advantage of lithium is the lack of motor side-effects seen with neuroleptics (bipolar patients are particularly prone to tardive dyskinesia). The main disadvantage is slow speed of response (normally 2 weeks). The dose of lithium depends on whether the citrate or carbonate salt is used.

Haloperidol and the more sedating chlorpromazine are commonly used neuroleptics, given orally or intramuscularly. Doses are similar to those used in schizophrenia. The behavioural excitement and over-activity are usually reduced within days, but elation, grandiosity and associated delusions often take longer to respond. Severe mania is best treated with a combination of lithium and a neuroleptic, allowing the neuroleptic to be withdrawn after the first 2 or 3 weeks. First attacks of mania usually require treatment for up to 3 months. The anticonvulsants carbamazepine and sodium valproate are also helpful in hypomania or in rapidly cycling illnesses (see below). Recent work suggests it can be sometimes helpful to add to the regimen a benzodiazepine, such as clonazepam or lorazepam.

Prevention

Since bipolar illnesses tend to be relapsing and remitting, prevention of relapse is the major therapeutic challenge in the management of bipolar affective disorder. A patient who has experienced more than two episodes of affective disorder within a 5-year period is likely to benefit from preventative treatments.

Lithium

Lithium (carbonate or citrate) is the main agent used for prophylaxis in patients with repeated episodes of bipolar illness. It is rapidly absorbed into the gastrointestinal tract and more than 95% is excreted by the kidneys; small amounts are found in the saliva, sweat and breast milk. Renal clearance of lithium correlates with renal creatinine clearance. Lithium is a mood-stabilizing drug that prevents mania more than depression. It reduces the frequency and severity of relapses by half and significantly reduces the likelihood of suicide. Its mode of action is unknown, but lithium is known to act on the serotoninergic system. Poor responses to lithium are associated with a negative family history, an unstable premorbid personality, and a rapid cycling illness.

Patients should be screened for thyroid (free T_4, TSH and thyroid autoantibodies) and renal disease (serum urea and creatinine, 24-hour urinary volume) before starting on lithium. Lithium interferes with thyroid function and can produce frank hypothyroidism. The presence of thyroid autoantibodies increases the risk, so it is worthwhile measuring these before treatment. Long-term treatment with lithium causes two renal problems; nephrogenic diabetes insipidus (DI) and reduced creatinine clearance (see p. 609). The therapeutic range for prophylaxis is 0.5–1.0 mmol/L. Lithium levels should be checked every 3 months, along with regular thyroid (free T_4 and TSH) and renal function tests. The best screen for DI is to ask the patient about polyuria and polydipsia. Tests should include serum urea and creatinine, and 24-hour urinary volume if DI is suspected. A creatinine clearance should be carried out if glomerular disease is suspected. Patients should carry a lithium card with them at all times. Other side-effects of lithium include:

- nausea and diarrhoea
- a fine tremor (15%)
- polyuria and polydipsia (see above)
- weight gain, mainly through increased appetite.

Lithium toxicity begins to occur when the serum concentration exceeds 1.5 mmol/L. Symptoms include drowsiness, nausea, vomiting, blurred vision, a coarse tremor, ataxia and dysarthria. Toxicity is more likely when the patient is dehydrated or with a drug interaction increasing concentrations. Such symptoms progress to delirium and convulsions, and coma and death can occur. As a rule, lithium is not advised during pregnancy, particularly in the first trimester, because of an increased risk of fetal malformation (Ebstein's anomaly). Between 25–30% of women with a history of bipolar disorder relapse within 2 weeks of delivery. Restarting lithium within 24 hours of delivery (if the mother is prepared to forgo breast-feeding) markedly reduces the risk of relapse.

Anticonvulsant, mood-stabilizing drugs

Carbamazepine and *sodium valproate* are used both in prophylaxis and treatment of manic states. Some patients who do not respond to lithium may respond to these anticonvulsants or a combination of both. Patients with rapid cycling illnesses show a better response to anticonvulsants than to lithium. For antimanic treatment, dosage in the initial stage of treatment will be 200 mg twice daily of carbamazepine, increasing to a normal dose of 800–1000 mg. Other drugs which appear to exercise a prophylactic mood-stabilizing effect include sodium valproate, olanzapine and risperidone. Both carbamazepine and valproate can be teratogenic (neural tube defects) and should be avoided in pregnancy. Other side-effects of these drugs are given on page 1224.

Prognosis

The average duration of a manic episode is 2 months, with 95% making a full recovery in time. Recurrence is the rule in bipolar disorders, with up to 90% relapsing within 10 years.

> **FURTHER READING**
> Daly I (1997) Mania. *Lancet* **349**: 1157–1160.

SUICIDE AND ATTEMPTED SUICIDE (DELIBERATE SELF-HARM) (see also p. 1002)

Suicide accounts for 2% of male and 1% of female deaths in England and Wales each year, equivalent to a rate of 8 per 100 000. The rate increases with age, peaking for women in their sixties and for men in their seventies. Suicide is the second most common cause of mortality in 15- to 34-year-olds. Approximately 15% of people who have suffered a severe depressive disorder (requiring admission) will eventually commit suicide, with 6% doing so in the 10 years after their first admission. Suicide rates in schizophrenia sufferers are likewise high, being 20–50 times the rate in the general population; 20–40% of people with schizophrenia make suicide attempts, and 9–13% are successful. A Finnish study suggests that the suicide rate is higher in women who have sustained a miscarriage or undergone an induced abortion, whereas it is significantly reduced in women who are pregnant. The highest rates of suicide have been reported in rural southern India (148 per 100 000 in young women and 58 per 100 000 in young men) and in Hungary (40 per 100 000), while the lowest are those of Spain (3.9 per 100 000) and Greece (2.8 per 100 000), but such variations may reflect differences in reporting, which may be related to religion, as much as genuine differences. Factors that increase the risk of suicide are indicated in Table 22.11.

A distinction must be drawn between those who attempt suicide – deliberate self-harm (DSH) – and those who succeed (suicides):

- The majority of cases of DSH occur in people under 35 years of age.
- The majority of suicides occur in people aged over 60.
- Suicides are more common in men, while DSH is more common in women.
- Suicides are more common in older men, although rates are falling. Rates in young men are rising fast throughout the UK and Western Europe.
- Suicides in women are slowly falling in the UK.
- Approximately 90% of cases of DSH involve self-poisoning.
- A formal psychiatric disorder is common retrospectively in suicide, but unusual in DSH.

There is, however, an overlap between DSH and suicide. Between 1–2% of people who attempt suicide will kill themselves in the year following DSH. The risk of suicide stays elevated in those with DSH, with 0.5% per annum committing suicide in the following 20 years. In the UK, over 100 000 suicide attempts are made each year, and the overwhelming majority of these are seen and treated within accident and emergency departments.

Table 22.11 Factors that increase the risk of suicide
Male sex
Older age
Living alone
Immigrant status
Recent bereavement, separation or divorce
Recent loss of a job or retirement
Living in a socially disorganized area
Family history of affective disorder, suicide or alcohol abuse
Previous history of affective disorder, alcohol or drug abuse
Previous suicide attempt
Addiction to alcohol or drugs
Severe depression or early dementia
Incapacitating painful physical illness

The guidelines (Box 22.10) for the assessment of such patients will help ensure that the risk factors relating to suicide are covered. Indications for referral to a psychiatrist before discharge from hospital are also given.

In general, it is worth trying to interview a family member or close friend and check these points with them. Requests for immediate represcription on discharge should be denied, except in cases of essential medication (e.g. for epilepsy). In such cases, however, only 3 days' supply of medication should be given, and the patient should be requested to report to their general practitioner or to their psychiatric outpatient clinic for further supplies. Occasionally involuntary admission under the Mental Health Act (1983) will be required (p. 1314).

FURTHER READING

Kim WJ, Singh T (2004) Trends and dynamics of youth suicides in developing countries. *Lancet* **363**: 1090–1091.

Maris RW (2002) Suicide. *Lancet* **360**: 319–326.

Box 22.10 Guidelines for the assessment of patients who harm themselves

Questions to ask: be concerned if positive answer
- Was there a clear precipitant/cause for the attempt?
- Was the act premeditated or impulsive?
- Did the patient leave a suicide note?
- Had the patient taken pains not to be discovered?
- Did the patient make the attempt in strange surroundings (i.e. away from home)?
- Would the patient do it again?

Other relevant factors
- Has the precipitant or crisis resolved?
- Is there continuing suicidal intent?
- Does the patient have any psychiatric symptoms?
- What is the patient's social support system?
- Has the patient inflicted self-harm before?
- Has anyone in the family ever taken their life?
- Does the patient have a physical illness?

Indications for referral to a psychiatrist
Absolute indications include:
- Clinical depression
- Psychotic illness of any kind
- Clearly preplanned suicidal attempts which were not intended to be discovered
- Persistent suicidal intent (the more detailed the plans, the more serious the risk)
- A violent method used.

Other common indications include:
- Alcohol and drug abuse
- Patients over 45 years, especially if male, and young adolescents
- Those with a family history of suicide in first-degree relatives
- Those with serious (especially incurable) physical disease
- Those living alone or otherwise unsupported
- Those in whom there is a major unresolved crisis
- Persistent suicide attempts
- Any patients who give you cause for concern.

THE ANXIETY DISORDERS

These are conditions in which anxiety dominates the clinical symptoms. They are classified according to whether the anxiety is persistent (general anxiety) or episodic, with the episodic conditions classified according to whether the episodes are regularly triggered by the same cue (phobia) or not (panic disorder). The differential diagnoses of anxiety disorders are given in Table 22.12.

General anxiety disorder

This occurs in 4% of the population and is more common in women. Symptoms are persistent and often chronic. General anxiety disorder (GAD) and its related panic disorder are differential diagnoses for medically unexplained symptoms, owing to the many physical symptoms that are caused by these conditions.

Clinical features

The physical and psychological symptoms are outlined in Table 22.13. The patient looks worried, has a tense posture, restless behaviour, a pale and sweaty skin. The

Table 22.12 Anxiety disorders – the differential diagnosis

Psychiatric disorder	Physical disorder
Depressive illness	Hyperthyroidism
Obsessive compulsive disorder	Hypoglycaemia
Presenile dementia	Phaeochromocytoma
Alcohol dependence	
Drug dependence	
Benzodiazepine withdrawal	

Table 22.13 Physical and psychological symptoms of anxiety

Physical symptoms	Nervous system
Gastrointestinal	Fatigue
Dry mouth	Blurred vision
Difficulty in swallowing	Dizziness
Epigastric discomfort	Headache
Aerophagy	Sleep disturbance
'Diarrhoea' (usually frequency)	
Respiratory	**Psychological symptoms**
Feeling of chest constriction	Apprehension and fear
Difficulty in inhaling	Irritability
Overbreathing	Difficulty in concentrating
	Distractability
Cardiovascular	Restlessness
Palpitations	Sensitivity to noise
Awareness of missed beats	Depersonalization
Feeling of pain over heart	Derealization
Genitourinary	
Increased frequency	
Failure of erection	
Lack of libido	

Box 22.11 The hyperventilation syndrome

Features

Panic attacks – fear, terror and impending doom – accompanied by some or all of the following:

- dyspnoea (trouble getting a good breath in)
- palpitations
- chest pain or discomfort
- choking sensation
- dizziness
- paraesthesiae
- sweating
- carpopedal spasms.

Cause

Overbreathing leading to a decrease in $P_a\text{co}_2$ and an increase in arterial pH.

Diagnosis

- A provocation test – voluntary overbreathing for 2–3 minutes – provokes similar symptoms; rebreathing from a large paper bag relieves them.
- Blood gases

Management

- Explanation and reassurance is given.
- The patient is trained in relaxation techniques and slow breathing.
- The patient is asked to breathe into a closed paper bag.

patient takes time to go to sleep, and when asleep wakes intermittently with worry dreams. Associated conditions include the hyperventilation syndrome, which is even more common in panic disorder (Box 22.11). The patient will sigh deeply, particularly when talking about the stresses in their life.

Mixed anxiety and depressive disorder

This disorder is probably the commonest mood disorder in primary care, in which there are equal elements of both anxiety and depression, showing how closely associated these two abnormal mood states are.

Panic disorder

Panic disorder is diagnosed when the patient has repeated sudden attacks of overwhelming anxiety, accompanied by severe physical symptoms, usually related to both hyperventilation (Box 22.11) and sympathetic nervous system activity. The prevalence is 1%. Patients with panic disorder often have catastrophic illness beliefs during the panic attack, such as convictions that they are about to die from a stroke or heart attack, or that they suffer from multiple sclerosis (MS). The fear of a stroke is related to dizziness and headache. Fear of a heart attack accompanies chest pain (atypical chest pain), and the fear of MS follows paraesthesiae.

Aetiology

General anxiety and panic disorder occurs four or more times as commonly in first-degree relatives of affected

Box 22.12 Phobias

A phobia is an abnormal fear and avoidance of an everyday object or situation.

Phobias are common (8% prevalence), disabling, and treatable with behaviour therapy.

patients, suggesting a genetic influence. Sympathetic nervous system overactivity, increased muscle tension and hyperventilation are the common pathophysiological mechanisms. Psychodynamic theory suggests that anxiety is the emotional response to the threat of a loss, whereas depression is the response to the loss itself. There is some evidence that being bullied, with the explicit threats involved, leads to anxiety disorders in young people.

Phobic (anxiety) disorders

Phobias are common conditions in which intense fear is triggered by a single stimulus, or set of stimuli, that are predictable and normally cause no particular concern to others (e.g. agoraphobia, claustrophobia, social phobia). This leads to avoidance of the stimulus (see Box 22.12). The patient knows that the fear is irrational, but cannot control it. The prevalence of all phobias is 8%, with many patients having more than one. Many phobias of 'medical' stimuli exist (e.g. of doctors, dentists, hospitals, vomit, blood and injections) which affect the patient's ability to receive adequate healthcare.

Aetiology

Phobias may be caused by classical conditioning, in which a response (fear and avoidance) becomes conditioned to a previously benign stimulus (a lift) often after an initiating shock (being stuck in a lift). In children, phobias can arise through imagined threats (e.g. stories of ghosts told in the playground). Women have twice the prevalence of most phobias than men. Phobias aggregate in families, but genetic factors are probably weak.

Agoraphobia

Translated as 'fear of the market place', this common phobia (4% prevalence) presents as a fear of being away from home, with avoidance of travelling, walking down a road, and shops being common presentations. This can be a very disabling condition, since the patient can be too unwell to ever leave home, particularly by themselves. It is often associated with *claustrophobia*, a fear of enclosed spaces.

Social phobia

This is the fear and avoidance of social situations: crowds, strangers, parties and meetings. Public speaking would be the sufferer's worst nightmare. It is suffered by 2% of the population.

Simple phobias

The commonest is the phobia of spiders (arachnophobia), particularly in women. The prevalence of simple phobias is 7% in the general population. Other common phobias include insects, moths, bats, dogs, snakes, heights, thunderstorms and the dark. Children are particularly phobic about the dark, ghosts and burglars, but the large majority grow out of these fears.

Treatment of anxiety disorders
Psychological treatments

For many people with brief episodes of an anxiety disorder, a discussion with a doctor concerning the nature of anxiety is usually sufficient.

- *Relaxation* techniques can be effective in mild/moderate anxiety. This can be achieved in many ways, including complementary techniques such as meditation and yoga. Conventional relaxation training involves slow breathing, muscle relaxation, and mental imagery.
- *Anxiety management training* involves two stages. In the first stage, verbal cues and mental imagery are used to arouse anxiety. In the second stage, the patient is trained to reduce this anxiety by relaxation, distraction and reassuring self-statements.
- *Biofeedback* is useful for showing patients that they are not relaxed, even when they fail to recognize it, having become so used to anxiety. Biofeedback involves feeding back to the patient a physiological measure that is abnormal in anxiety. These measures may include electrical resistance of the skin of the palm, heart rate, muscle electromyography, or breathing pattern.
- *Behaviour therapies* are treatments derived from experimental psychology that are intended to change behaviour and thus symptoms. The most common and successful behaviour therapy (with 80% success in some phobias) is *graded exposure*, otherwise known as *systematic desensitization*. This is the treatment of choice for a phobia. Firstly, the patient rates the phobia into a hierarchy or 'ladder' of worsening fears (e.g. in agoraphobia: walking to the front door with a coat on; walking out into the garden; walking to the end of the road). Secondly, the patient practises exposure to the least fearful stimulus until no fear is felt. The patient then moves 'up the ladder' of fears until they are cured.
- *Cognitive behaviour therapy* (CBT) (see p. 1293) is the treatment of choice for panic disorder and general anxiety disorder because the therapist and patient need to identify the mental cues (thoughts and memories) that may subtly provoke exacerbations of anxiety or panic attacks. CBT also allows identification and alteration of the patient's 'schema', or way of looking at themselves and their situation, that feeds anxiety.

Drug treatments

Drugs used in the treatment of anxiety can be divided into two groups: those that act primarily on the central nervous system, and those that block peripheral autonomic receptors.

Table 22.14 Withdrawal syndrome with benzodiazepines
Insomnia
Anxiety
Tremulousness
Muscle twitchings
Perceptual distortions
Hypersensitivities (light, sound, touch)
Convulsions

- *Benzodiazepines* are centrally acting anxiolytic drugs. They bind to specific receptors that stimulate release of the inhibitory transmitter γ-aminobutyric acid (GABA). Diazepam (5 mg twice daily, up to 10 mg three times daily in severe cases) and chlordiazepoxide have relatively long half-lives (20–40 hours) and are used as anti-anxiety drugs in the short term. Side-effects include sedation and memory problems, and patients should be advised not to drive while on treatment. They can cause dependence and tolerance within 4–6 weeks, particularly in dependent personalities. The withdrawal syndrome (Table 22.14) can occur after just 3 weeks of continuous use and is particularly severe when high doses have been given for a longer time. Thus, if a benzodiazepine drug is prescribed for anxiety, it should be given in as low a dose as possible and for not more than 2 weeks continuously. A withdrawal programme from chronic use includes changing the drug to the long-acting diazepam, followed by a very gradual reduction in dosage.
- *Buspirone* (5–10 mg three times daily) is a 5-HT_{1A} partial agonist that is anxiolytic after 2 weeks of treatment. It is not yet established as a treatment in the UK. It does not seem to help panic disorder.
- Most SSRIs (e.g. paroxetine, sertraline, citalopram), venlafaxine, MAOIs (phenelzine) and moclobemide (a RIMA) are useful symptomatic treatments for general anxiety and panic disorders, as well as some phobias (social phobia). Imipramine is an established symptomatic treatment for panic disorder, and other tricyclics such as amitriptyline and clomipramine are probably equally effective. Treatment response is often delayed several weeks; a trial of treatment should last 3 months.
- Many of the symptoms of anxiety are due to an increased or sustained release of epinephrine (adrenaline) and norepinephrine (noradrenaline) from the adrenal medulla and sympathetic nerves. Thus, *beta-blockers* such as propranolol (20–40 mg two or three times daily) are effective in reducing peripheral symptoms such as palpitations, tremor and tachycardia, but do not help central symptoms such as anxiety.

Acute stress reactions and adjustment disorders

Acute stress reaction

This occurs in individuals without any other psychiatric disorder, in response to exceptional physical and/or psychological stress. While severe, such a reaction usually subsides within hours or days. The stress may be an overwhelming traumatic experience (e.g. accident, battle, physical assault, rape) or a sudden change in the social circumstances of the individual, such as a bereavement. Individual vulnerability and coping capacity play a role in the occurrence and severity of an acute stress reaction, as evidenced by the fact that not all people exposed to exceptional stress develop symptoms. Symptoms usually include an initial state of feeling 'dazed' or numb, with inability to comprehend the situation. This state may be followed either by further withdrawal from the situation or by anxiety and overactivity. Autonomic signs of arousal, including tachycardia, sweating and hyper-ventilation, are commonly present. The symptoms usually appear within minutes of the stressor and disappear within 2–3 days.

Adjustment disorder

This disorder can follow an acute stress reaction and is common in the general hospital. This is a more prolonged (up to 6 months) emotional reaction to bad news or a significant life event, with low mood joining the initial shock and consequent anxiety, but not of sufficient severity to fulfil a diagnosis of a mood or anxiety disorder. Supportive counselling is usually a successful treatment, allowing facilitation of unexpressed feelings, elucidation of unspoken fears, and education about the likely future.

Pathological (abnormal) grief

This is a particular kind of adjustment disorder. It can be characterized as excessive and/or prolonged grief, or even absent grieving with abnormal denial of the bereavement. Usually the relative will be stuck in grief, with insomnia and repeated dreams of the dead person, anger at doctors or even the patient for dying, consequent guilt in equal measure, and an inability to 'say good-bye' to the loved person by dealing with their effects. *Guided mourning* uses cognitive and behavioural techniques to allow the relative to stop grieving and move on in life.

Normal grief immediately follows bereavement, is expressed openly, and allows a person to go through the social ceremonies and personal processes of bereavement. The three stages are firstly shock and disbelief, secondly the emotional phase (anger, guilt and sadness) and thirdly acceptance and resolution. This normal process of adjustment may take up to a year, with movement between all three stages occurring in a sometimes haphazard fashion.

Post-traumatic stress disorder (PTSD)

This arises as a delayed and/or protracted response to a stressful event or situation of an exceptionally threatening nature, likely to cause pervasive distress in almost anyone. Causes include natural or human disasters, war, serious accidents, witnessing the violent death of others, being the victim of sexual abuse, rape, torture, terrorism or hostage-taking. Predisposing factors such as personality, previously unresolved traumas, or a history of psychiatric illness may prolong the course of the

syndrome. These factors are neither necessary nor sufficient to explain its occurrence, which is most related to the intensity of the trauma, the proximity of the patient to the traumatic event, and how prolonged or repeated it was. Recent functional brain scan research suggests a possible neurophysiological relationship with OCD (p. 1301).

Clinical features

The typical symptoms of PTSD include:

- *'flashbacks'* – repeated vivid reliving of the trauma in the form of intrusive memories, often triggered by a reminder of the trauma
- *insomnia*, usually accompanied by nightmares, the nocturnal equivalent of flashbacks
- *emotional blunting*, emptiness or 'numbness', alternating with …
- *intense anxiety* at exposure to events that resemble an aspect of the traumatic event, including anniversaries of the trauma
- *avoidance* of activities and situations reminiscent of the trauma
- *emotional detachment* from other people
- *hypervigilance* with autonomic hyperarousal and an enhanced startle reaction.

This clinical picture represents the severe end of a spectrum of emotional reactions to trauma, which might alternatively take the form of an adjustment or mood disorder. The course is often fluctuating but recovery can be expected in two-thirds of cases at the end of the first year. Complications include depressive illness and alcohol misuse. In a small proportion of cases the condition may show a chronic course over many years and a transition to an enduring personality change.

Treatment and prevention

Compulsory *psychological debriefing* immediately after a trauma does not prevent PTSD and may be harmful. Behaviourally based therapies should be offered for those with symptoms and CBT is often effective. It can be normalizing to have therapy in groups with other patients who have suffered similar trauma. Randomized controlled trials have now shown that *eye movement desensitization and reprocessing* (EMDR) is an effective treatment for PTSD. SSRIs, venlafaxine and nefazodone have a place in the management of chronic PTSD, but drop-out from pharmacotherapy is common.

The adult consequences of childhood sexual and physical abuse

Estimates of the prevalence of childhood sexual abuse (CSA) vary depending on definition but there is reasonable evidence that 20% of women and 10% of men suffered significant, coercive and inappropriate sexual activity in childhood. The abuser is usually a member of the family or known to the child, and preadolescent girls are at greatest risk. The likelihood of long-term consequences is determined by:

- an earlier age of onset
- the severity of the abuse
- the repeated nature and duration of the period of abuse
- the association with physical abuse.

Consequent adult psychiatric disorders include depressive illness, substance misuse, eating disorders, borderline personality disorder and deliberate self-harm. Other negative outcomes include a decline in socio-economic status, sexual problems, prostitution, and difficulties in trusting those closest to the patient.

Psychodynamic psychotherapy

Psychodynamic psychotherapy is derived from psychoanalysis and is based on a number of key analytical concepts. These include Freud's ideas about psychosexual development, defence mechanisms, free association as the method of recall, and the therapeutic techniques of interpretation, including that of transference, defences and dreams. Such therapy usually involves once-weekly 50-minute sessions, the length of treatment varying between 3 months and 2 years. The long-term aim of such therapy is twofold: symptom relief and personality change. Psychodynamic psychotherapy is classically indicated in the treatment of unresolved conflicts in early life, as might be found in non-psychotic and personality disorders, but to date there is a lack of convincing evidence concerning its superiority over other forms of treatment.

FURTHER READING

Fricchione G (2004) Generalized anxiety disorders. *New England Journal of Medicine* **351**: 675–682.

Sher L (2004) Recognising post-traumatic stress disorder. *Quarterly Journal of Medicine* **97**: 1–5.

OBSESSIVE–COMPULSIVE DISORDER

Obsessive–compulsive disorder (OCD) is characterized by obsessional ruminations and compulsive rituals. It is particularly associated with and/or secondary to both depressive illness and *Gilles de la Tourette syndrome* (p. 1232). The prevalence is up to 2% in the general population, although it is probably undiagnosed. There is an equal distribution by gender, and the mean of onset ranges from 20–40 years.

Clinical features

The obsessions and compulsions are so persistent and intrusive that they greatly impede a patient's functioning and cause considerable distress. There is a constant need to check that things have been done correctly, and no amount of reassurance can remove the small amount of doubt that persists. Some rituals are derived from superstitions, such as actions repeated a fixed number of times, with the need to start again if interrupted. When severe and primary, OCD can last for many years and is resistant to treatment. However, obsessional symptoms commonly occur in other disorders, most notably general anxiety disorder, depressive illness and schizophrenia, and disappear with the resolution of the primary disorder.

Minor degrees of obsessional symptoms and compulsive rituals or superstitions are common in people who are not ill or in need of treatment, particularly in times of stress. The mildest grade is that of obsessional personality traits such as over-conscientiousness, tidiness, punctuality and other attitudes and behaviours indicating a strong tendency towards conformity and inflexibility. Such individuals are *perfectionists* who are intolerant of shortcomings in themselves and others, and take pride in their high standards. When such traits are so marked that they dominate other aspects of the personality, in the absence of clear-cut OCD, the diagnosis is obsessional (anankastic) personality (see p. 1313).

Aetiology

Genetic

OCD is found in 5–7% of the first-degree relatives. Twin studies showed a 80–90% concordance in monozygotic twins and about 50% in dizygotic twins.

Basal ganglia dysfunction

OCD is associated with a number of neurological disorders involving dysfunction of the striatum, including Parkinson's disease, Sydenham's and Huntington's chorea. OCD can follow head trauma. Neuroimaging suggests that abnormalities exist in the frontal lobe and basal ganglia (Fig. 22.4). Hyperactivity of the orbitofrontal cortex has been a consistent finding in brain imaging research on OCD patients. The PET images shown here are from the initial report of this finding by a research group at the University of California at Los Angeles. Other work suggests the caudate nucleus is smaller than in healthy controls.

Serotonin

Serotonin function is probably abnormal in patients with OCD. Serotonin reuptake inhibitors are effective drugs. Postsynaptic serotonin receptor hypersensitivity may follow chronically low levels of synaptic serotonin.

Fig. 22.4 **PET images of (left) a normal patient and (right) an obsessive–compulsive disorder (OCD) patient.** The right image shows the hyperactivity of the orbitofrontal cortex which is a consistent finding in this condition. Baxter R et al. *Archives of General Psychiatry* **44**: 211, with permission.

Conditioning

This suggests that compulsive rituals are classically conditioned avoidance responses, which therefore lend themselves to treatment with graded exposure therapy.

Treatment

Psychological treatments

A behaviour therapy that is particularly effective for rituals is *response prevention*. Patients are instructed not to carry out their rituals. There is an initial rise in distress but with persistence both the rituals and the distress diminish. Patients are encouraged to practise response prevention, while returning to situations that normally make them worse.

Modelling involves the therapist demonstrating to the patient what is required and encouraging the patient to follow this example. In the case of hand-washing rituals, this might involve holding an allegedly contaminated object and carrying out other activities without washing, the patient being encouraged to follow suit.

Thought stopping can reduce obsessional ruminations. The patient is taught to arrest the obsessional thought by arranging a sudden intrusion (e.g. snapping an elastic band, clicking the fingers).

Cognitive behaviour therapy involves exposure to the provocative stimulus plus cognitive therapy.

Physical treatment

Anxiolytic drugs provide short-term symptomatic relief for overwhelming anxiety on a short-term basis.

Selective *serotonin reuptake inhibitors* are the mainstay of drug treatment. Their efficacy is independent of their antidepressant action but the doses required are usually some 50–100% higher than those effective in depression. Three months' treatment with high doses may be necessary for a positive response. Positive correlations between reduced severity of OCD and decreased orbitofrontal and caudate metabolism following behavioural and SSRI treatments have been demonstrated in a number of studies. Clomipramine is the tricyclic most commonly used in the UK.

Psychosurgery

Psychosurgery is very occasionally recommended in cases of chronic and severe OCD that has not responded to other treatments. The development of stereotactic techniques has led to the replacement of the earlier, crude leucotomies with more precise surgical interventions such as subcaudate tractotomy and cingulotomy, with small yttrium radioactive implants, which induce lesions in the cingulate area or the ventromedial quadrant of the frontal lobe. Psychosurgery is performed only in a few specialist centres in the UK, and formal and detailed consent requirements are laid down in the appropriate mental health act.

Prognosis

Two-thirds of cases improve within a year. The remainder run a fluctuating or persistent course. The prognosis is worse when the personality is anankastic and the OCD is primary and severe.

FURTHER READING

Jenike MA (2004) Obsessive–compulsive disorder. *New England Journal of Medicine* **350**: 259–265.

ALCOHOL MISUSE AND DEPENDENCE

A wide range of physical, social and psychiatric problems are associated with excessive drinking. *Alcohol misuse* occurs when a patient is drinking in a way that regularly causes problems to the patient or others.

- The *problem drinker* is one who causes or experiences physical, psychological and/or social harm as a consequence of drinking alcohol. Many problem drinkers, while heavy drinkers, are not physically addicted to alcohol.
- *Heavy drinkers* are those who drink significantly more in terms of quantity and/or frequency than is safe to do so long term.
- *Binge drinkers* are those who drink excessively in short bouts, usually 24–48 hours long, separated by often quite lengthy periods of abstinence. Their overall monthly or weekly alcohol intake may be relatively modest.
- *Alcohol dependence* is defined by a physical dependence on or addiction to alcohol. The term 'alcoholism' is a confusing one with off-putting connotations of vagrancy, 'meths' drinking and social disintegration. It has been replaced by the term '*alcohol dependence syndrome*'.

Epidemiology of alcohol misuse

A survey of drinking in England and Wales found that 15% of men admitted drinking more than 35 units per week and 4% of women drank more than 25 units per week. In the survey, 4% of men and 2% of women reported alcohol withdrawal symptoms.

Approximately one in five male admissions to acute medical wards are directly or indirectly due to alcohol. Between 33–40% of accident and emergency attenders have blood alcohol concentrations above the present UK legal limit for driving. People with serious drinking problems have a two to three times increased risk of dying compared to members of the general population of the same age and sex.

Table 22.15 provides an approximate estimate of what can be expected in an average individual in the way of behavioural impairment resulting from a particular blood alcohol level. The usual drink (1 unit of alcohol: $\frac{1}{2}$ pint of ordinary beer (3.5%), a pub measure of wine) contains about 8 g of absolute alcohol and raises the blood alcohol concentration by about 15–20 mg/dL, the amount that is metabolized in 1 hour.

Detection

Alcohol misuse should be suspected in any patient presenting with one or more physical problems commonly associated with excessive drinking (see p. 263). Alcohol

Table 22.15 Approximate correlation between blood alcohol level and behavioural/motor impairment

Rising blood alcohol (mg/dL)	Expected effect
20–99	Impaired coordination, euphoria
100–199	Ataxia, poor judgement, labile mood
200–299	Marked ataxia and slurred speech; poor judgement, labile mood, nausea and vomiting
300–399	Stage 1 anaesthesia, memory lapse, labile mood
400+	Respiratory failure, coma, death

Table 22.16 Common alcohol-related psychological and social problems

Psychological	Social
Depression	Marital and sexual difficulties
Anxiety and phobias	Family problems
Memory disturbances	Child abuse
Personality disturbances	Employment problems
Delirium tremens	Financial difficulties
Attempted suicide	Accidents at home, on the roads, at work
Pathological jealousy	Delinquency and crime
	Homelessness

misuse may also be associated with a number of psychiatric symptoms/disorders and social problems (Table 22.16).

Guidelines

The patient's frequency of drinking and quantity drunk during a typical week should be established. Alcohol consumption can be assessed on the basis of units of alcohol.

- Drinking up to 21 units of alcohol a week for men and 14 units for women carries no long-term health risk.
- There is unlikely to be any long-term health damage with 21–35 units (men) and 14–25 units (women), provided the drinking is spread throughout the week.
- Beyond 36 units a week in men and 24 units a week in women, damage to health becomes increasingly likely.
- Drinking above 50 units a week in men (35 units in women) is a definitive health hazard.

Diagnostic markers of alcohol misuse

Laboratory parameters indicating alcohol misuse are often called markers of recent alcohol misuse. Elevated γ-glutamyl transpeptidase (γ-GT) and mean corpuscular volume (MCV) may indicate alcohol excess in the last few weeks. Blood or breath alcohol are useful tests in anyone suspected of very recent drinking.

Alcohol dependence syndrome

DSM-IV TR describes dependence as 'a pattern of repeated self-administration that usually results in tolerance,

withdrawal and compulsive drug-taking behaviour', the essential element of which is the continued use of the substance despite significant substance-related problems. Figure 22.5 outlines the main characteristics of the syndrome but these do not necessarily present in any particular order. Symptoms of alcohol dependence in a typical order of occurrence are shown in Table 22.17. Diagnostic criteria for alcohol withdrawal syndrome are shown in Table 22.18.

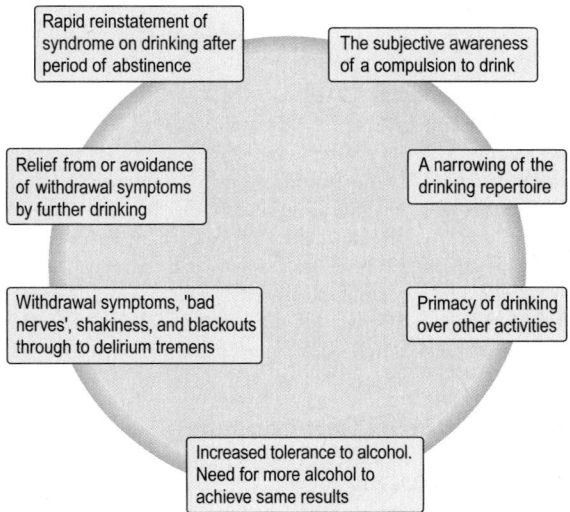

Fig. 22.5 Elements of the alcohol-dependence syndrome.

Table 22.17 Symptoms of alcohol dependence

Unable to keep a drink limit	Trembling after drinking the day before
Difficulty in avoiding getting drunk	Morning retching and vomiting
Spending a considerable time drinking	Sweating excessively at night
Missing meals	Withdrawal fits
Memory lapses, blackouts	Morning drinking
Restless without drink	Increased tolerance
Organizing day around drink	Hallucinations, frank delirium tremens

Table 22.18 Diagnostic criteria for alcohol withdrawal syndrome

Any three of the following:
Tremor of outstretched hands, tongue or eyelids
Sweating
Nausea, retching or vomiting
Tachycardia or hypertension
Anxiety
Psychomotor agitation
Headache
Insomnia
Malaise or weakness
Transient visual, tactile or auditory hallucinations or illusions
Grand mal convulsions

The course of the alcohol dependence syndrome

About 25% of all cases of alcohol misuse will lead to chronic alcohol dependence. This most commonly ends in social incapacity, death or abstinence. Alcohol dependence syndrome usually develops after 10 years of heavy drinking (3–4 years in women). In some individuals who use alcohol to alter consciousness, obliterate conscience and defy social canons, dependence and apparent loss of control may appear in only a few months or years.

Delirium tremens (DTs)

Delirium tremens is the most serious withdrawal state and occurs 1–3 days after alcohol cessation, so is commonly seen a day or two after admission to hospital. Patients are disorientated, agitated, and have a marked tremor and visual hallucinations (e.g. insects or small animals coming menacingly towards them). Signs include sweating, tachycardia, tachypnoea and pyrexia. Complications include dehydration, infection, hepatic disease or the Wernicke–Korsakoff syndrome (p. 245).

Causes of alcohol dependence

Genetic factors. Sons of alcohol-dependent people who are adopted by other families are four times more likely to develop drinking problems than are the adopted sons of non-alcohol misusers. Genetic markers include dopamine-2 receptor allele A1, alcohol dehydrogenase subtypes and monoamine oxidase B activity, but they are not specific.

Environmental factors. A Boston follow-up study showed that one in ten boys who grew up in a household where neither parent misused alcohol subsequently became alcohol dependent, compared with one in four of those reared by alcohol-misusing fathers and one in three of those reared by alcohol-misusing mothers.

Biochemical factors. Several factors have been suggested, including abnormalities in alcohol dehydrogenase, neurotransmitter substances and brain amino acids, such as GABA. There is no conclusive evidence that these or other biochemical factors play a causal role.

Psychiatric illness. This is an uncommon cause of addictive drinking but it is a treatable one. Some depressed patients drink excessively in the hope of raising their mood. Patients with anxiety states or phobias are also at risk.

Excess consumption in society. The prevalence of alcohol dependence and problems correlates with the general level (per capita consumption) of alcohol use in a society. This, in turn, is determined by factors that may control overall consumption – including price, licensing laws, the number and nature of sales outlets, and the customs of society concerning the use and misuse of alcohol.

Treatment
Psychological treatment of problem drinking

Successful identification at an early stage can be a helpful intervention in its own right. It should lead to:

- the provision of information concerning safe drinking levels
- a recommendation to cut down where indicated
- simple support and advice concerning associated problems.

Successful alcohol counselling involves *motivational enhancement* (*motivational therapy*), feedback, education about adverse effects of alcohol, and agreeing drinking goals. A motivational approach is based on five stages of change: precontemplation, contemplation, determination, action and maintenance. The therapist uses motivational interviewing and reflective listening to allow the patient to persuade himself along the five stages to change.

This technique, cognitive behaviour therapy and 12-step facilitation (as used by Alcoholics Anonymous (AA)) have all been shown to reduce harmful drinking. With addictive drinking, self-help group therapy, which involves the long-term support by fellow members of the group (e.g. AA), is helpful in maintaining abstinence. Family and marital therapy involving both the alcohol misuser and spouse may also be helpful.

Drug treatments of problem drinking
Alcohol withdrawal and DTs

Addicted drinkers often experience considerable difficulty when they attempt to reduce or stop their drinking. Withdrawal symptoms are a particular problem and delirium tremens needs urgent treatment (Box 22.13). In the absence of DTs, alcohol withdrawal can be treated on an outpatient basis, using one of the fixed schedules in Box 22.13, so long as the patient attends daily for medication and monitoring, and has good social support. Outpatient schedules are sometimes given over 5 days. Long-term treatment with benzodiazepines should not be prescribed in those patients who continue to misuse alcohol. Many alcohol misusers add dependence on diazepam or clomethiazole to their problems.

Drugs for prevention of alcohol dependence

Naltrexone, the opioid antagonist (50 mg per day), reduces the risk of relapse into heavy drinking and the frequency of drinking. *Acamprosate* (1–2 g per day) acts on several receptors including those for GABA, norepinephrine (noradrenaline) and serotonin. There is good evidence that it reduces drinking frequency. Neither drug seems particularly helpful in maintaining abstinence. Both drug effects are enhanced by combining them with counselling

Drugs such as *disulfiram* react with alcohol to cause unpleasant acetaldehyde intoxication and histamine release. A daily maintenance dose means that the patient must wait until the disulfiram is eliminated from the body before drinking safely. There is mixed evidence of efficacy.

Box 22.13 Management of delirium tremens (DTs)

General measures

Admit the patient to a medical bed.

Correct electrolyte abnormalities and dehydration.

Treat any co-morbid disorder (e.g. infection).

Give oral thiamine (200 mg daily) in the absence of Wernicke–Korsakoff (W–K) syndrome.

Give parenteral thiamine in the presence of a W–K encephalopathy (NB: beware anaphylaxis).

Give prophylactic phenytoin or carbamazepine, if previous history of withdrawal fits.

Specific drug treatment

One of the following orally:

- Diazepam 10–20 mg
- Chlordiazepoxide 30–60 mg
- Lorazepam 2–4 mg.
  Repeat 1 hour after last dose depending on response.

Fixed-schedule regimens

- Diazepam 10 mg every 6 hours for 4 doses, then 5 mg 6-hourly for 8 doses OR
- Chlordiazepoxide 30 mg every 6 hours for 4 doses, then 15 mg 6-hourly for 8 doses OR
- Lorazepam 2 mg every 6 hours for 4 doses, then 1 mg 6-hourly for 8 doses.
  Provide additional benzodiazepine when symptoms and signs are not controlled.

Table 22.19 Commonly used drugs of misuse and dependence

Stimulants	Narcotics
Methylphenidate	Morphine
Phenmetrazine	Heroin
Phencyclidine ('angel dust')	Codeine
Cocaine	Pethidine
Amfetamine derivates	Methadone
Ecstasy (MDMA)	
Hallucinogens	**Tranquillizers**
Cannabis preparations	Barbiturates
Solvents	Benzodiazepines
Lysergic acid diethylamide (LSD)	
Mescaline	

One trial has suggested that fluoxetine is helpful in the treatment of patients who have both a depressive illness and alcohol dependence.

Outcome

Research suggests that 30–50% of alcohol-dependent drinkers are abstinent or drinking very much less up to 2 years following traditional intervention. It is too early to be certain of the long-term outcome of patients treated with the latest psychological and pharmacotherapies.

FURTHER READING

Fiellin DA, Reid MC, O'Connor PG (2000) New therapies for alcohol problems: application to primary care. *American Journal of Medicine* **108**: 227–237.

Kasten TR, O'Connor PG (2003) Management of drug and alcohol withdrawal. *New England Journal of Medicine* **348**: 1786–1795.

Mayo-Smith MF (1997) Pharmacological management of alcohol withdrawal: a meta-analysis and evidence-based practice guideline. *Journal of the American Medical Association* **278**: 144–151.

DRUG MISUSE AND DEPENDENCE

In addition to alcohol and nicotine, there are a number of psychotropic substances that are taken for their effects on mood and other mental functions (Table 22.19).

Causes of drug misuse

There is no single cause of drug misuse and/or dependence. Three factors appear commonly, in a similar way to alcohol problems:

- the availability of drugs
- a vulnerable personality
- social pressures, particularly from peers.

Once regular drug-taking is established, pharmacological factors determine dependence.

Solvents

One per cent of adolescents in the UK sniff solvents for their intoxicating effects. Tolerance develops over weeks or months. Intoxication is characterized by euphoria, excitement, a floating sensation, dizziness, slurred speech and ataxia. Acute intoxication can cause amnesia and visual hallucinations. About 300 teenagers die in the UK each year from asphyxiation or acute poisoning.

Amfetamines and related substances

These have temporary stimulant and euphoriant effects that are followed by fatigue and depression, with the latter sometimes prolonged for weeks. Psychological rather than true physical dependence is the rule with 'Speed'. In addition to a manic-like presentation, amfetamines can produce a paranoid psychosis indistinguishable from acute paranoid schizophrenia.

Ecstasy

'Ecstasy' (E, white burger, white dove) is the street name for 3,4-methylenedioxy-methamfetamine (MDMA), a psychoactive phenylisopropylamine, synthesized as an amfetamine derivative. It is a psychodelic drug which is often used as a 'dance' drug. It has a brief duration of action (4–6 hours). There is evidence that repeated use of MDMA can cause permanent neurotransmitter changes in the brain. Deaths have been reported from malignant hyperpyrexia and dehydration. Acute renal and liver failure can occur.

Cocaine

Cocaine is a central nervous system stimulant (with similar effects to amfetamines) derived from *Erythroxylon coca* trees grown in the Andes. In purified form it may be taken by mouth, sniffed or injected. If cocaine hydrochloride is converted to its base ('crack') it can be smoked. This causes an intense stimulating effect and 'free-basing' is common. Compulsive use and dependence occur more frequently among users who are free-basing. Dependent users take large doses and alternate between the withdrawal phenomena of depression, tremor and muscle pains, and the hyperarousal produced by increasing doses. Prolonged use of high doses produces irritability, restlessness, paranoid ideation and occasionally convulsions. Persistent sniffing of the drug can cause perforation of the nasal septum. Overdoses cause death through myocardial infarction, hyperthermia and arrhythmias (p. 1011).

Hallucinogenic drugs

Hallucinogenic drugs, such as lysergic acid diethylamide (LSD) and mescaline, produce distortions and intensifications of sensory perceptions, as well as frank hallucinations in acute intoxication. Psychosis is a long-term complication.

Cannabis

Cannabis (grass, pot, spliff, reefer) is a drug widely used in some subcultures. It is derived from the dried leaves and flowers of the plant *Cannabis sativa*. It can cause tolerance and dependence. Hashish is the dried resin from the flower tops whilst marijuana refers to any part of the plant. The drug, when smoked, seems to exaggerate the pre-existing mood, be it depression, euphoria or anxiety. It may have specific analgesic properties. An amotivational syndrome has been reported with chronic daily use. Cannabis may of itself sometimes cause psychosis in the right circumstances (see below).

Tranquillizers

Drugs causing dependence include barbiturates and benzodiazepines. Benzodiazepine dependence is common and may be iatrogenic, when the drugs are prescribed and not discontinued. Discontinuing treatment with benzodiazepines may cause withdrawal symptoms (see Table 22.14). For this reason, withdrawal should be supervised and gradual.

Opiates

Physical dependence occurs with morphine, heroin and codeine as well as with synthetic and semisynthetic opiates such as methadone and pethidine. These substances display cross-tolerance – the withdrawal effects of one are reduced by administration of one of the others. The psychological effect of such substances is of a calm, slightly euphoric mood associated with freedom from physical discomfort and a flattening of emotional

Table 22.20 Opiate withdrawal syndrome	
Yawning Rhinorrhoea Lacrimation Pupillary dilatation Sweating Piloerection Restlessness	12–16 hours after last dose of opiate
Muscular twitches Aches and pains Abdominal cramps Vomiting Diarrhoea Hypertension Insomnia Anorexia Agitation Profuse sweating Weight loss	24–72 hours after last dose of opiate

response. This is believed to be due to the attachment of morphine and its analogues to receptor sites in the CNS normally occupied by endorphins. Tolerance to this group of drugs is rapidly developed and marked, but is rapidly lost following abstinence. *The opiate withdrawal syndrome* consists of a constellation of signs and symptoms (Table 22.20) that reaches peak intensity on the second or third day after the last dose of the opiate. These rapidly subside over the next 7 days. Withdrawal is dangerous in patients with heart disease or other chronic debilitating conditions.

Opiate addicts have a relatively high mortality rate, owing to both the ease of accidental overdose and the blood-borne infections associated with shared needles. Heart disease (including infective endocarditis), tuberculosis and AIDS are common causes of death, while tetanus, malaria and the complications of hepatitis B and C are also common.

Treatment of chronic misuse

Blood and urine screening for drugs are required in circumstances where drug misuse is suspected (Table 22.21). When a patient with an opiate addiction is admitted to hospital for another health problem, advice should be sought from a psychiatrist or the patient's drug

Table 22.21 Length of time urine toxicology screens are likely to remain positive after abstinence	
Substance	**Usual time positive**
Amfetamines	48 hours
Barbiturates	
Short-acting	24 hours
Long-acting	7+ days
Benzodiazepines	3+ days
Cannabinols	5+ days
Cocaine	3+ days
Codeine	48 hours
Morphine	48 hours

clinic regarding management of their addiction while an inpatient.

The treatment of chronic dependence is directed towards helping the patient to live without drugs. Patients need help and advice in order to avoid a withdrawal syndrome. Alternatively, patients can be helped to minimize harm to themselves and others. Some patients with opiate addiction who cannot manage such a regimen may be maintained on oral methadone. In the UK, only specially licensed doctors may legally prescribe heroin and cocaine to an addict for maintenance treatment of addiction. An overdose should be treated immediately with the opioid antagonist naloxone.

Drug psychoses

Drug-induced psychoses have been reported with amfetamine and its derivatives, cocaine, and hallucinogens. It can occur acutely after drug use, but is more usually associated with chronic misuse. Psychoses are characterized by vivid hallucinations (usually auditory, but often in more than one sensory modality), misidentifications, delusions and/or ideas of reference (often of a persecutory nature), psychomotor disturbances (excitement or stupor) and an abnormal affect. ICD-10 requires that the condition occurs within 2 weeks and usually within 48 hours of drug use and that it should persist for more than 48 hours but not more than 6 months.

Cannabis use can result in acute anxiety, depression or hallucinations. Manic-like psychoses occurring after long-term cannabis use have been described, but seem more likely to be related to the toxic effects of heavy ingestion. However, there are now five prospective studies which suggest, when taken together, that cannabis doubles the risk of schizophrenia, and that perhaps 8% of schizophrenia in the UK would be prevented if cannabis use ceased. This risk is higher in people taking cannabis early in their lives and heavily.

FURTHER READING

Arsenault L et al. (2004) Causal association between cannabis and psychosis: examination of the evidence. *British Journal of Psychiatry* **184**: 110–117.

Cami J, Farre M (2004) Drug addiction. *New England Journal of Medicine* **349**: 975–986.

SCHIZOPHRENIA

The group of illnesses conventionally referred to as 'schizophrenia' is diverse in nature and covers a broad range of perceptual, cognitive and behavioural disturbances. The point prevalence of the condition is 0.5% throughout the world, with equal gender distribution. A physician primarily needs to know how to recognize schizophrenia, what problems it might present with in the general hospital, and how it is treated.

Table 22.22 Genetic risk for schizophrenia

General population	1%
Second-degree relative	2.5%
Parent	4%
Sibling	8%
Child of one affected parent	12%
Child of two affected parents	30–40%
Dizygotic twin	8–19%
Monozygotic twin	40–60%

Causes

No single cause has been identified. Schizophrenia is likely to be a disease of neural disconnection caused by an interaction of genetic and multiple environmental factors that affect brain development. It is likely that cannabis use is a risk factor. The genetic aetiology is likely to be polygenic and non-mendelian. Schizophrenia has a heritability of about 80%. The genetic risk in the general population and relatives of affected individuals is shown in Table 22.22. Brain scans and histology often show ventricular enlargement and disorganized cytoarchitecture in the hippocampus, supporting the neurodevelopmental theory of aetiology. Dopamine receptors are upregulated in the mesolimbic system, but the serotonin system may also be involved.

Clinical features

The illness can begin at any age but is rare before puberty. The peak age of onset is in the early twenties. The symptoms that have been considered as diagnostic of the condition have been termed *first rank symptoms* and were described by the German psychiatrist Kurt Schneider. They consist of:

- auditory hallucinations in the third person, and/or voices commenting on their behaviour
- thought withdrawal, insertion and broadcast
- primary delusion
- delusional perception
- somatic passivity and feelings – patients believe that thoughts, feelings or acts are controlled by others.

The more of these symptoms a patient has the more likely the diagnosis is schizophrenia. Other symptoms of *acute* schizophrenia include behavioural disturbances, other hallucinations, secondary (usually persecutory) delusions and blunting of mood. Schizophrenia is sometimes divided into 'positive' (type 1) and 'negative' (type 2) types:

Positive schizophrenia is characterized by acute onset, prominent delusions and hallucinations, normal brain structure, a biochemical disorder involving dopaminergic transmission, good response to neuroleptics, and better outcome.

Negative schizophrenia is characterized by a slow, insidious onset, a relative absence of acute symptoms, the presence of apathy, social withdrawal, lack of motivation, underlying brain structure abnormalities, and poor neuroleptic response.

Chronic schizophrenia

This is characterized by long duration and 'negative' symptoms of underactivity, lack of drive, social withdrawal and emotional emptiness.

Differential diagnosis

Schizophrenia should be distinguished from:

- organic mental disorders (e.g. partial complex epilepsy)
- mood (affective) disorders (e.g. mania)
- drug psychoses (e.g. amfetamine psychosis)
- personality disorders (schizotypal).

In older patients, any acute or chronic brain syndrome can present in a schizophrenia-like manner. A helpful diagnostic point is that clouding of consciousness and disturbances of memory do not occur in schizophrenia, and visual hallucinations are unusual.

A *schizoaffective psychosis* describes a clinical presentation in which clear-cut affective and schizophrenic symptoms coexist in the same episode.

Prognosis

The prognosis of schizophrenia is variable. A review of treatment studies suggests that 15–25% of people with schizophrenia recover completely, about 70% will have relapses and may develop mild to moderate negative symptoms, while about 10% will become seriously disabled.

Treatment

The best results are obtained by combining drug and social treatments.

Antipsychotic (neuroleptic) drugs

These act by blocking the D_1 and D_2 groups of dopamine receptors. Such drugs are most effective against acute, positive symptoms and are least effective in the management of chronic, negative symptoms. Complete control of positive symptoms can take up to 3 months, and premature discontinuation of treatment can result in relapse.

As antipsychotic drugs block both D_1 and D_2 dopamine receptors, they usually produce extrapyramidal side-effects. This limits their use in maintenance therapy of many patients. They also block adrenergic and muscarinic receptors and thereby cause a number of unwanted effects (Table 22.23).

An infrequent but potentially dangerous unwanted effect is the *neuroleptic malignant syndrome*. This occurs in 0.2% of patients on neuroleptic drugs, particularly the potent dopaminergic antagonists, e.g. haloperidol. Symptoms occur a few days to a few weeks after starting therapy and consist of hyperthermia, muscle rigidity, autonomic instability (tachycardia, labile BP, pallor) and a fluctuating level of consciousness. Investigations show a raised creatine phosphokinase, raised white cell count and abnormal liver biochemistry. Treatment consists of stopping the drug and general management, e.g. temperature reduction. Bromocriptine enhances dopaminergic activity and dantrolene will reduce muscle tone but no treatment has proven benefit.

Table 22.23	Unwanted effects of neuroleptic drugs	
Common effects	**Rare effects**
Motor	Hypersensitivity
Acute dystonia	Cholestatic jaundice
Parkinsonism	Leucopenia
Akathisia	Skin reactions
Tardive dyskinesia	
	Others
Autonomic	Precipitation of glaucoma
Hypotension	Galactorrhoea
Failure of ejaculation	Amenorrhoea
	Cardiac arrhythmias
Antimuscarinic	Seizures
Dry mouth	
Urinary retention	
Constipation	
Blurred vision	
Metabolic	
Weight gain	

Pregnancy. Data on the potential teratogenicity of antipsychotic (neuroleptic) medications are still limited. The disadvantages of not treating during pregnancy have to be balanced against possible developmental risks to the fetus. The butyrophenones (e.g. haloperidol) are probably safer than the phenothiazines. Subsequent management decisions on dosage will depend primarily on the ability to avoid side-effects, since the antiparkinsonian agents are still believed to be teratogenic and should be avoided.

Phenothiazines

Phenothiazines are the group of neuroleptics used most extensively. Chlorpromazine (100–1000 mg daily) is the drug of choice when a more sedating drug is required. Trifluoperazine is used when sedation is undesirable. Fluphenazine decanoate is used as a long-term prophylactic to prevent relapse, as a depot injection (25–100 mg i.m. every 1–4 weeks).

Butyrophenones

The butyrophenones (e.g. haloperidol 2–30 mg daily) are also powerful antipsychotics, used in the treatment of acute schizophrenia and mania. They are highly likely to cause a dystonia and/or extrapyramidal side-effects, but are much less sedating than the phenothiazines. A third of patients with acute schizophrenia will have a good response to haloperidol and a further third will make a partial response.

Atypical antipsychotics

These drugs are 'atypical' in that they block D_2 receptors less than D_1 and thus cause fewer extrapyramidal side-effects and less tardive dyskinesia. They are now being used as first-line drugs for newly diagnosed schizophrenia.

Clozapine. Clozapine is also used in patients with intractable schizophrenia who have failed to respond to at least two conventional antipsychotic drugs. This drug is a dibenzodiazepine with a relative high affinity for D_1 compared with D_2 dopamine receptors, muscarinic and α-adrenergic receptors. It also blocks 5-HT$_2$ and 5-HT$_1$

receptors. Functional brain scans have shown that clozapine selectively blocks limbic dopamine receptors more than striatal ones, which is probably why it causes considerably fewer extrapyramidal side-effects.

Clozapine has been shown to exercise a dramatic therapeutic effect on both intractable positive and negative symptoms. However, clozapine is expensive and produces severe agranulocytosis in 1–2% of patients. Therefore it can only be prescribed in the UK to registered patients by doctors and pharmacists registered with the Clozaril patient-monitoring service. The starting dose is 25 mg per day with a maintenance dose of 150–300 mg daily. White cell counts should be monitored weekly for 18 weeks and then 2-weekly for the length of treatment. In addition to its antipsychotic actions, clozapine may also help reduce aggressive and hostile behaviour and the risk of suicide. It can cause considerable weight gain and sialorrhoea. There is an increased risk of diabetes mellitus.

Risperidone is a benzisoxazole derivative with combined dopamine D_2 receptor and $5-HT_{2A}$-receptor blocking properties. Dosage ranges from 6–10 mg per day. The drug is not markedly sedative and the overall incidence and severity of extrapyramidal side-effects is lower than with more conventional antipsychotics.

Olanzapine has affinity for $5-HT_2$, D_1, D_2, D_4, and muscarinic receptor sites. Clinical studies indicate it to have a lower incidence of extrapyramidal side-effects. The apparent better compliance with the drug may be related to its lower side-effect profile and its once-daily dosage of 5–10 mg. Weight gain is a problem with long-term treatment and there is an increased risk of diabetes mellitus.

Neither risperidone nor olanzapine seem as specific a treatment for intractable chronic schizophrenia as clozapine.

Other atypical antipsychotics include sulpiride, ziprasidone and quietiapine.

Psychological treatment
This consists of reassurance, support and a good doctor–patient relationship. Psychotherapy of an intensive or exploratory kind is contraindicated. In contrast, recent research shows that cognitive behaviour therapy can help reduce the intensity of delusions.

Social treatment
Social treatment involves attention being paid to the patient's environment and social functioning. Family education can help relatives and partners to provide the optimum amount of emotional and social stimulation, so that not too much emotion is expressed (a risk for relapse). Sheltered employment is usually necessary for the majority of sufferers if they are to work.

Medical presentations related to treatment
The motor side-effects of neuroleptics are the commonest reason for a patient with schizophrenia to present to a physician, followed by deliberate self-harm. *Acute dystonia* normally arises in patients newly started on neuroleptics, causing a *torticollis*. Extrapyramidal side-effects are common and present in the same way as Parkinson's disease. *Akathisia* is a motor restlessness, most commonly affecting the legs. It is similar to the restless legs syndrome (p. 666), but apparent during the day.

Amenorrhoea and galactorrhoea can be caused by dopamine antagonists. Postural hypotension can affect the elderly, and neuroleptics can be the cause of delirium in the elderly, if their antimuscarinic effects are prominent.

FURTHER READING
Freedman R (2003) Schizophrenia. *New England Journal of Medicine* **349**: 1738–1749.
Mueser KT, McGurk SR (2004) Schizophrenia. *Lancet* **363**: 2063–2072.

ORGANIC MENTAL DISORDERS

Organic brain disorders result from structural pathology, as in dementia (see p. 1254), or from disturbed central nervous system (CNS) function, as in fever-induced delirium. They do not include mental and behavioural disorders due to alcohol and misuse of drugs, which are classified separately.

Delirium

Delirium, also termed *toxic confusional state* and *acute organic reaction*, is an acute or subacute brain failure in which impairment of attention is accompanied by abnormalities of perception and mood. It is the most common psychosis seen in the general hospital. Ten to twenty per cent of older surgical and medical inpatients have delirium during their admission. Confusion is usually worse at night, with consequent sleep reversal, so that the patient is asleep in the day and awake all night. During the acute phase, thought and speech are incoherent, memory is impaired and misperceptions occur. Episodic visual hallucinations (or illusions) and persecutory delusions occur. As a consequence, the patient may be frightened, suspicious, restless and uncooperative.

A developing, deteriorating or damaged brain predisposes a patient to develop delirium (Table 22.24).

A large number of diseases may cause delirium, particularly in elderly patients. Some causes of delirium are listed in Table 22.25. Delirium tremens should be considered in the differential diagnosis (p. 1304) as well as Lewy body dementia (p. 1255). Diagnostic criteria are given in Box 22.14.

Management
History should be taken from a witness. Examination may reveal the cause. Investigation and treatment of the underlying physical disease should be undertaken (Table 22.25). The patient should be carefully nursed and rehydrated in a quiet single room with a window that does not allow exits. If a high fever is present, the

Table 22.24   Predisposing factors in delirium

Extremes of age (developing or deteriorating brain)
Damaged brain:
    Any dementia (most common predisposition)
    Previous head injury
    Alcoholic brain damage
    Previous stroke
Dislocation to an unfamiliar environment (e.g. hospital
    admission)
Sleep deprivation
Sensory extremes (overload or deprivation)
Immobilization

Table 22.25   Some common causes of delirium

Systemic infection	Intracranial causes
Any infection, particularly with high fever (e.g. malaria, septicaemia)	Trauma Tumour Abscess Subarachnoid haemorrhage Epilepsy
Metabolic disturbance Hepatic failure Renal failure Disorders of electrolyte balance Hypoxia	**Drug intoxication** Anticonvulsants Antimuscarinics Anxiolytic/hypnotics Tricyclic antidepressants Dopamine agonists Digoxin
Vitamin deficiency Thiamin (Wernicke–Korsakoff syndrome, beriberi) Nicotinic acid (pellagra) Vitamin B$_{12}$	**Drug/alcohol withdrawal** **Postoperative states**
Endocrine disease Hypothyroidism Cushing's syndrome	

Box 22.14 Delirium – diagnostic criteria (derived from DSM-IV-TR)

- Disturbance of consciousness:
  ↓ clarity of awareness of environment
  ↓ ability to focus, sustain or shift attention
- Change in cognition:
  memory deficit, disorientation,
  language disturbance, perceptual disturbance
- Disturbance develops over a short period (hours or days)
- Fluctuation over course of day
- Disturbance is caused by the consequences of a general medical condition or medication

patient's temperature should be reduced. All current drug therapy should be reviewed and, where possible, stopped. Psychoactive drugs should be avoided if possible (because of their own risk of exacerbating delirium). In severe delirium, haloperidol is an effective choice, the daily dose usually ranging between 1.5 mg (in the elderly) to 30 mg per day. If necessary, the first dose can be administered intramuscularly. Olanzapine is an effective alternative, especially if given at night for insomnia.

Prognosis of delirium

Delirium usually clears within a week or two, but brain recovery usually lags behind the recovery of the causative physical illness. The prognosis depends not only on the successful treatment of the causative disease, but also on the underlying state of the brain. Twenty-five per cent of the elderly with delirium will have an underlying dementia; 15% of patients do not survive their underlying illness; 40% are in institutional care at 6 months.

FURTHER READING
Nayeem K, O'Keefe ST (2003) Delirium. *Clinical Medicine* **3**(5): 412–415.

EATING DISORDERS

Obesity

This is the commonest eating disorder (see p. 252), which has become epidemic in some developed countries. It is usually caused by a combination of constitutional and social factors, but a binge eating disorder and psychological determinants of 'comfort eating' should be excluded.

Anorexia nervosa

The main clinical criteria for diagnosis are:

- a bodyweight more than 15% below the standard weight, or a body mass index (BMI) below 17.5 (ICD-10)
- weight loss is self-induced by avoidance of fattening foods, vomiting, purging, exercise, or appetite suppressants
- a distortion of body image so that the patient regards herself as fat when she is thin
- a morbid fear of fatness
- amenorrhoea in women.

Clinical features include:

- onset usually in adolescence
- a previous history of chubbiness or fatness
- the patient generally eats little
- amenorrhoea – an early symptom; in 20% it precedes weight loss
- binge eating
- usually a marked lack of sexual interest
- lanugo hair.

The physical consequences of anorexia include sensitivity to cold, constipation, hypotension and bradycardia. In most cases, amenorrhoea is secondary to the weight loss. Vomiting and abuse of purgatives may lead to hypokalaemia and alkalosis.

Prevalence

Case register data suggest an incidence rate of 19 per 100 000 females aged between 15 and 34 years. Surveys have suggested a prevalence rate of approximately 1% among schoolgirls and university students. However, many more young women have amenorrhoea accompanied by less weight loss than the 15% required for the diagnosis. The condition is much less common among men (ratio of 1 : 10). The onset in women is usually at between 16–17 years of age and it seldom occurs after the age of 30 years.

Aetiology

Biological factors

Genetic. Six to ten per cent of siblings of affected women suffer from anorexia nervosa. There is an increased concordance amongst monozygotic twins, suggesting a genetic predisposition.

Hormonal. The reductions in sex hormones and the hypothalamic–pituitary–adrenal axis are secondary to malnutrition and usually reversed by refeeding.

Psychological factors

Individual. Anorexia nervosa has often been seen as an escape from the emotional problems of adolescence and a regression into childhood. Patients will often have had dietary problems in early life. Perfectionism and low self-esteem are common antecedents. Studies suggest that survivors of childhood sexual abuse are at risk of developing an eating disorder, usually anorexia nervosa, in adolescence.

Family. Families of such patients are allegedly characterized by overprotection, inflexibility and lack of conflict resolution. Anorexia is alleged to prevent dissension in families. However, a case control study suggested that there is no more evidence of these factors in families of patients with anorexia nervosa than in control families with a child with an established physical disease.

Social and cultural factors

There is a higher prevalence in higher social classes, and a high rate in certain occupational groups (e.g. ballet dancers and nurses) and in societies where cultural value is placed on thinness.

Prognosis

The condition runs a fluctuating course, with exacerbations and partial remissions. Long-term follow-up suggests that about two-thirds of patients maintain normal weight and that the remaining one-third are split between those who are moderately underweight and those who are seriously underweight. Indicators of a poor outcome include:

- a long initial illness
- severe weight loss
- older age at onset
- bulimia (see below), vomiting or purging
- personality difficulties
- difficulties in relationships.

Suicide has been reported in 2–5% of patients with chronic anorexia nervosa. The mortality rate per year is 0.5% from all causes. More than one-third have recurrent affective illness, and various family, genetic and endocrine studies have found associations between eating disorders and depression. Fifty per cent of patients make a full recovery, 30% a partial recovery and 20% none.

Treatment

Treatment can be conducted on an outpatient basis unless the weight loss is severe and accompanied by marked physical symptoms, dizziness and weakness and/or electrolyte and vitamin disturbances. Hospital admission may then be unavoidable and may need to be on a medical ward initially. Rarely, the patient's weight loss may be so severe as to be life-threatening. If the patient cannot be persuaded to enter hospital, compulsory admission may have to be used. Inpatient treatment goals include:

- establishing a good relationship with the patient
- restoring the weight to a level between the ideal body-weight and the patient's ideal weight
- the provision of a balanced diet, building up to 12.6 MJ (3000 calories) in three to four meals per day
- the elimination of purgative and/or laxative use and vomiting.

Outpatient treatment can be conducted on cognitive behavioural or dynamic psychotherapeutic lines or on a combination of both. Setting up a therapeutic alliance is vital. Individual psychotherapy is better than family therapy if the patient has left home, and vice versa. Motivational enhancement techniques are being used with some success.

Drug treatment has met with limited success, except to symptomatically treat insomnia and depressive illness.

Bulimia nervosa

This refers to episodes of uncontrolled excessive eating, which are also termed 'binges'. There is a preoccupation with food and a habitual adoption of certain behaviours that can be understood as the patient's attempts to avoid the fattening effects of periodic binges. These behaviours include:

- self-induced vomiting
- laxative abuse
- misuse of drugs – diuretics, thyroid extract or anorectics.

Additional clinical features include:

- physical complications of vomiting:
  (a) cardiac arrhythmias
  (b) renal impairment – consequences of low K+
  (c) muscular paralysis
  (d) tetany – from hypokalaemic alkalosis
  (e) swollen salivary glands – from vomiting
  (f) eroded dental enamel
- associated psychiatric disorders:
  (a) depressive illness
  (b) alcohol misuse
- fluctuations in bodyweight within normal limits
- menstrual function – periods irregular but amenorrhoea rare
- personality – perfectionism and low self-esteem present premorbidly.

The prevalence of bulimia in community studies is high; it affects between 5% and 30% of girls attending high schools, colleges or universities in the USA. Bulimia is sometimes associated with anorexia nervosa. A pre-morbid history of dieting is common. The prognosis for bulimia nervosa is better than for anorexia nervosa.

Treatment

Cognitive behaviour therapy has been shown to be more effective than both interpersonal psychotherapy and drug treatments. SSRIs (e.g. fluoxetine) are also an effective treatment, even in the absence of a depressive illness.

Atypical eating disorders

These include eating disorders that do not conform clinically to the diagnostic criteria for anorexia nervosa or bulimia nervosa. Binge eating disorders consist of bulimia without the vomiting and other weight-reducing strategies.

FURTHER READING

Fairburn CG, Harrison PJ (2003) Eating disorders. *Lancet* **361**: 407–417.

Mehler PS (2003) Bulimia nervosa. *New England Journal of Medicine* **349**: 875–881.

Wilson GT, Shafran R (2005) Eating disorders guidelines from NICE *Lancet* **365**: 79–81.

SEXUAL DISORDERS

Sexual disorders can be divided into sexual dysfunctions, deviations, and gender role disorders (Table 22.26).

Sexual dysfunction

Sexual dysfunction in men refers to repeated inability to achieve normal sexual intercourse, whereas in women it refers to a repeatedly unsatisfactory quality of sexual satisfaction. Problems of sexual dysfunction can usefully be classified into those affecting sexual desire, arousal and orgasm. Among men presenting for treatment of sexual dysfunction, erectile dysfunction is the most frequent complaint. The prevalence of premature ejaculation is low, while ejaculatory failure is rare.

Sexual drive is affected by constitutional factors, ignorance of sexual technique, anxiety about sexual performance, medical and psychiatric conditions and certain drugs (Tables 22.27 and 22.28).

The treatment of sexual dysfunction involves careful assessment, the participation (where appropriate) of the patient's partner, and specific therapeutic techniques, including relaxation, behavioural therapy (Masters and Johnson) and psychotherapy. The introduction of phosphodiesterase type 5 inhibitors (e.g. sildenafil) has introduced an effective therapy for the treatment of erectile dysfunction (see p. 1055).

Sexual deviation

Sexual deviations are regarded as unusual forms of behaviour rather than as an illness. Doctors are only likely to be involved when the behaviour involves break-

Table 22.26 Classification of sexual disorders

Sexual dysfunction	Sexual deviations	Disorders of the gender role
Affecting sexual desire	**Variations of the sexual 'object'**	Transsexualism
Low libido	Fetishism	
	Transvestism	
Impaired sexual arousal	Paedophilia	
	Bestiality	
Erectile dysfunction	Necrophilia	
Failure of arousal in women		
	Variations of the sexual act	
Affecting orgasm		
Premature ejaculation	Exhibitionism	
Retarded ejaculation	Voyeurism	
Orgasmic dysfunction in women	Sadism	
	Masochism	
	Frotteurism	

Table 22.27 Medical conditions affecting sexual performance

Endocrine	**Neurological**
Diabetes mellitus	Neuropathy
Hyperthyroidism	Spinal cord lesions
Hypothyroidism	
	Musculoskeletal
Cardiovascular	Arthritis
Angina pectoris	
Previous myocardial infarction	**Respiratory**
Disorders of peripheral circulation	Asthma
	COPD
Hepatic	
Cirrhosis, particularly alcohol-related	**Psychiatric**
	Depressive illness
Renal	Substance misuse
Renal failure	

Table 22.8 Drugs affecting sexual arousal

Male arousal	Female arousal
Alcohol	Alcohol
Benzodiazepines	CNS depressants
Neuroleptics	Antidepressants (SSRIs)
Cimetidine	Oral combined contraceptives
Opiate analgesics	Methyldopa
Methyldopa	Clonidine
Clonidine	
Spironolactone	
Antihistamines	
Metoclopramide	
Diuretics	
Beta-blockers	
Cannabis	

Alcohol increases the desire but diminishes the performance

ing the law (e.g. paedophilia or bestiality) and when there is a question of an associated mental or physical disorder. Homosexuality was formerly classified as an illness but it is now an accepted alternative sexual lifestyle. Men are more likely than women to have sexual deviations.

Gender role disorders

Transsexualism involves a disturbance in gender identity in which the patient is convinced that their body is the wrong gender. A person's gender identity refers to the individual's sense of masculinity or femininity as distinct from sex. It is thought to arise from a biological component (prenatal endocrine influences), psychological imprinting and social conditioning. Disturbances in these three areas have variously been blamed for the cause of transsexualism.

For males, treatment includes oestrogen administration and, if surgery is to be recommended, a period of living as a woman as a trial beforehand. In the case of female transsexuals, treatment involves surgery and the use of methyltestosterone.

FURTHER READING
Halaris A (ed.) (1997) Sexual dysfunction. In: *Baillière's Clinical Psychiatry: International Practice and Research*, Vol 3. London: Baillière Tindall.
Tomlinson J (1997) *ABC of sexual health*. London: British Medical Books.

PERSONALITY DISORDERS

These disorders comprise deeply ingrained and enduring patterns of behaviour which manifest themselves as inflexible responses to a broad range of personal and social situations. Personality disorders are developmental conditions that appear in childhood or adolescence and continue into adult life. They are not secondary to another psychiatric disorder or brain disease, although they may precede or coexist with other disorders. In contrast, personality change is acquired, usually in adult life, following severe or prolonged stress, extreme environmental deprivation, serious psychiatric disorder or brain injury or disease.

Personality disorders are usually subdivided according to clusters of traits that correspond to the most frequent or obvious behavioural manifestations. The main categories of personality disorder are described below.

Borderline (emotionally unstable). Such people act impulsively and develop intense, but short-lived, emotional attachments to others. They describe chronic internal emptiness with frequent self-harm, self-abuse (eating disorders, substance misuse) and they may develop transient psychotic features of uncertain significance. There is often a strong family history of mood disorders.

Paranoid. A paranoid personality is characterized by extreme sensitiveness, suspiciousness, litigiousness, a tendency to excessive self-importance, and a preoccupation with unsubstantiated conspiratorial explanations of events.

Schizoid. A schizoid personality is characterized by emotional coldness and detachment, a limited capacity to express emotions, indifference to praise or criticism, an almost invariable preference for solitary activities, lack of close friendships, and a marked insensitivity to prevailing social norms and conventions.

Antisocial. An antisocial personality is characterized by a callous unconcern for the feelings of others, an incapacity to maintain enduring relationships, a very low tolerance of frustration, an incapacity to experience guilt and to profit from experience, and a marked proneness to rationalize and blame others.

Histrionic. A histrionic personality is characterized by self-dramatization, theatricality, suggestibility, shallow and labile emotions, a continual seeking for excitement and appreciation by others, and an inappropriate seductiveness in appearance or behaviour.

Anankastic (obsessive–compulsive). Such a personality is characterized by feelings of excessive doubt and caution, preoccupation with details, rules, lists, order, perfectionism, excessive conscientiousness, scrupulousness, excessive pedantry, rigidity and stubbornness, and intrusion of unwelcome thoughts or impulses.

Dependent. People with dependent personality encourage others to make their personal decisions, subordinate their needs to others on whom they are dependent, are unwilling to make demands on others, feel unable to care for themselves, are preoccupied with fears of being abandoned. Such patients have a limited capacity to make everyday decisions without an excessive amount of advice and reassurance from others.

Many individuals with disturbed personalities do not fit neatly into such categories, but manifest a mixture of features.

PSYCHIATRY AND THE LAW

The law in most developed countries provides for the compulsory admission and/or treatment of mentally disordered persons for their own protection and/or the protection of others and for mitigation in the case of mentally disordered individuals who commit a criminal offence (see also p. 6). In England and Wales the Act of Parliament that is crucially involved is the Mental Health Act 1983, although a new Act is about to go through parliament. The Mental Health (Scotland) Act 1984 and the Mental Health (Northern Ireland) Order 1986 contain clauses broadly similar to those in England and Wales.

Apart from one provision of the National Assistance Act 1948, the Mental Health Act 1983 is the only method whereby individuals can legally be deprived of their liberty without having committed a crime or being suspected of committing a crime. It is, therefore, necessary that doctors understand the seriousness of their responsibility and the details of the legislation.

There are three conditions that need to be met before an appropriate compulsory section form is signed. The patient must be:

- suffering from a defined mental disorder
- at risk to his/her and/or other people's health or safety
- unwilling to accept hospitalization voluntarily.

The reasons why there is no alternative approach to the treatment suggested for the patient should be outlined. Sexual deviance or alcohol/drug dependence are not defined mental disorders, but otherwise the definition of mental disorder is broad. Any registered medical practitioner may sign a medical recommendation under the Act, but the added signature of a specialist psychiatrist is needed for compulsory orders lasting for more than 72 hours. Unless the patient is already in hospital, the nearest relative or an approved mental health social worker is also required to sign the application form. Relevant sections of the Act are detailed in Table 22.29.

Physicians are likely to be involved in sections 5(2) and 2. It should be remembered that a section does not give a doctor the right to treat a physical disease, although it could be argued that a section would apply if the physical disease was causing the mental disorder (e.g. delirium). This has never been legally tested.

Although much of the process of detention against one's will is formalized, there is no liability for a doctor who acts in good faith with a patient's best interests at heart. Clearly written medical notes, accepted forms of treatment and common sense remain the basis of good practice.

Table 22.29	**Commonly used sections of the Mental Health Act 1983**		
Section	**Duration**	**Signatures required**	**Purpose**
2	28 days	Two doctors (one approved) plus nearest relative or social worker	Assessment and treatment
3	6 months	Two doctors (one approved) plus nearest relative or social worker	Treatment
4	72 hours	One doctor plus relative or social worker	Emergency admission
5(2)	72 hours	Doctor in charge of patient's care	Emergency detention of a patient already in hospital
5(4)	6 hours	Nurse (RMN)	Emergency detention of a patient already in hospital
136	72 hours	Police officer	Psychiatric assessment of those in public places thought by police to be mentally ill and in need of a place of safety

FURTHER READING

Duggan C (ed.) (1997) Assessing risk in the mentally disordered. *British Journal of Psychiatry* **170** (Suppl 32).

CHAPTER BIBLIOGRAPHY

Davies T, Craig TKJ (1998) *ABC of Mental Health*. London: BMJ Books.
Gelder M, López-Ibor JJ, Andreasen N (2000) *New Oxford Textbook of Psychiatry*, 3rd edn. Oxford: Oxford University Press.
Goldberg D (ed.) (1997) *Maudsley Handbook of Practical Psychiatry*, 3rd edn. Oxford: Oxford University Press.

Johnstone EC, Freeman CPL, Zealley AK (1998) *Companion to Psychiatric Studies*, 6th edn. Edinburgh: Churchill Livingstone.
Shorter E (1998) *A History of Psychiatry*. Chichester: John Wiley.
Stahl SM (2000) *Essential Psychopharmacology*, 2nd edn. Cambridge: Cambridge University Press

SIGNIFICANT WEBSITES

http://www.rcpsych.ac.uk
UK Royal College of Psychiatrists

http://www.connects.org.uk
Website for mental health in general

http://www.cebmh.com
Centre for Evidence-Based Mental Health

http://www.mentalhealth.org.uk
Mental Health Foundation – charity

http://www.sleepfoundation.org
National Sleep Foundation

http://www.edauk.com
Eating Disorders Association

http://psych.org
American Psychiatric Association

Skin disease 23

Introduction

Skin diseases have a high prevalence throughout the world. In developing countries infectious diseases such as tuberculosis, leprosy and onchocerciasis are common, whereas in developed countries inflammatory disorders such as eczema and acne are common. Skin disorders can be inherited, e.g. Ehlers–Danlos syndrome, a part of normal development, e.g. acne vulgaris, or may present as part of a systemic disorder, e.g. systemic lupus erythematosus (SLE).

Approximately 25% of the UK population will develop a skin problem and, although self-medication is common, skin disease still accounts for 10% of the workload of family doctors. The common reasons for this are itching or pain, which can interfere with people's ability to function normally or to sleep; rashes which cause anxiety, depression and lack of self-confidence and can lead to social isolation if obviously visible; and an inability to work, because certain dermatoses (such as allergic hand eczema in a builder or hairdresser) can interfere with or even prevent working.

Rarely skin disease can be fatal. Examples are malignant melanoma, toxic epidermal necrolysis and pemphigus.

STRUCTURE AND FUNCTION OF THE SKIN

The skin consists of four distinct layers: the epidermis, the basement membrane zone, the dermis and the subcutaneous layer (Fig. 23.1). The functions are summarized in Box 23.1.

The epidermis

The epidermis is a stratified epithelium of ectodermal origin that arises from dividing basal keratinocytes. The downward projections of the epidermis into the dermis are called the 'rete ridges'. The lower epidermal cells (basal layer) produce a variety of keratin filaments and desmosomal proteins (e.g. desmoglein and desmoplakin),

(a) Whole skin

Figure labels:
- Hair
- Stratum corneum (cornified layer)
- Granular cell layer
- Spinous layer
- Basal cell layer
- Sweat duct
- Sweat gland
- Hair follicle
- Blood vessels
- Sebaceous gland
- Epidermis
- Collagen and elastin fibres
- Arrector pili muscle
- Dermis
- Subcutaneous fat
- Nerves

(b) Epidermis

Figure labels:
- Intercellular lamellae
- Flattened keratinocytes
- Lamellar bodies
- Keratohyalin granules
- Keratin filaments
- Desmosome
- Melanocyte
- Hemidesmosome
- Stratum corneum
- Granular layer
- Spinous layer
- Basal layer
- Basal lamina
- Basal keratinocytes

Fig. 23.1 **The structure of the skin.**

Box 23.1 Functions of the skin

- Physical barrier against friction and shearing forces
- Protection against infection (immune and innate), chemicals, ultraviolet irradiation
- Prevention of excessive water loss or absorption
- Ultraviolet-induced synthesis of vitamin D
- Temperature regulation
- Sensation (pain, touch and temperature)
- Antigen presentation/immunological reactions/wound healing

which make up the 'cytoskeleton'. This confers strength to the epidermis and prevents it shedding off. Higher up in the granular layer, complex lipids are secreted by the keratinocytes and these form into intercellular lipid bilayers which act as a semipermeable skin barrier. The upper cells (stratum corneum) lose their nuclei and become surrounded by a tough impermeable 'envelope' of various proteins (loricrin, involucrin, filaggrin and keratin). Changes in lipid metabolism and protein expression in the outer layers allow normal shedding of keratinocytes.

Keratinocytes can secrete a variety of cytokines (e.g. interleukins, gamma-interferon, tumour necrosis factor alpha) in response to tissue injury or in certain skin diseases. These play a role in specific immune function, cutaneous inflammation and tissue repair. There is a further layer of protection against microbial invasion, called the innate immune system of the skin. This includes neutrophils and macrophages as well as keratinocyte-produced antimicrobial peptides (called β-defensins and cathelicidins). Expression of these peptides is both constitutive and induced by skin inflammation, and they are active against bacterial, viral and fungal pathogens. There is evidence to suggest a deficiency of these peptides may account for the susceptibility of patients with atopic eczema to skin infection.

Other cells in the epidermis

Melanocytes are found in the basal layer and secrete the pigment melanin. These protect against UV irradiation.

Racial differences are due to variation in melanin production not melanocyte numbers.

Merkel cells are also found in the basal layer and originate from either neural crest or epidermal keratinocytes. They are numerous on finger tips and in the oral cavity and play a role in sensation.

Langerhans' cells are dendritic cells found in the suprabasal layer. They derive from the bone-marrow and as they express the cytokine CCR6, they are guided to normal skin, which contains a CCR6 agonist called macrophage inflammatory protein 3α. Langerhans' cells endocytose extracellular antigens in the skin and then migrate to local lymph nodes for T cell presentation and thus act as antigen-presenting cells.

Basement membrane zone (see Fig. 23.27)

The basement membrane zone is a complex proteinaceous structure consisting of type IV and VII collagen, hemidesmosomal proteins, integrins and laminin. Collectively they hold the skin together keeping the epidermis firmly attached to the dermis. Inherited or autoimmune-induced deficiencies of these proteins can cause skin fragility and a variety of blistering diseases (see p. 1346).

The dermis

The dermis is of mesodermal origin and contains blood and lymphatic vessels, nerves, muscle, appendages (e.g. sweat glands, sebaceous glands and hair follicles) and a variety of immune cells such as mast cells and lymphocytes. It is a matrix of collagen and elastin in a ground substance.

The sweat glands

Eccrine sweat glands are found throughout the skin except the mucosal surfaces.

Apocrine sweat glands are found in the axillae, anogenital area and scalp and do not function until puberty.

The sweat glands and vasculature are involved in temperature control.

The sebaceous glands

These are inactive until puberty. They are responsible for secreting sebum or grease onto the skin surface (via the hair follicle) and are found in high number on the face and scalp.

Nerves

The skin is richly innervated. These fibres allow sensation of touch, pain, itch, vibration and change in temperature.

Hair

Hairs arise from a downgrowth of epidermal keratinocytes into the dermis. The hair shaft has an inner and outer root sheath, a cortex and sometimes a medulla. The lower portion of the hair follicle consists of an expanded bulb (which also contains melanocytes) surrounding a richly innervated and vascularized dermal papilla. The hair regrows from the bulb after shedding.

There are three types of hair:

- *terminal* – medullated coarse hair, e.g. scalp, beard, pubic
- *vellus* – non-medullated fine downy hairs seen on the face of women and in prepubertal children
- *lanugo* – non-medullated soft hair on newborns (most marked in premature babies) and occasionally in people with anorexia nervosa.

All hair follicles follow a growth cycle: anagen (growth phase), catagen (involution phase), telogen (shedding phase). At any one time most hairs (> 90%) will be in the anagen phase, which is typically 3–5 years for scalp hair.

Grey hair is due to decreased tyrosinase activity in the hair bulb melanocytes. White hair is due to total loss of these melanocytes.

Nails

Nails are tough plates of hardened keratin which arise from the nail matrix (just visible as the moon-shaped lunula) under the nail fold. It takes 6 months for a fingernail to grow out fully and 1 year for a toe-nail.

The subcutaneous layer

The subcutaneous layer consists predominantly of adipose tissue as well as blood vessels and nerves. This layer provides insulation and acts as a lipid store.

APPROACH TO THE PATIENT

The *history* should aim to elicit the following points:

- time course of rash
- distribution of lesions
- symptoms (e.g. itch or pain)
- family history (especially of atopy and psoriasis)
- drug/allergy history
- past medical history
- provocating factors (e.g. sunlight or diet)
- previous skin treatments.

Examination entails looking at and feeling a rash (for terminology, see Table 23.1). It should include an assessment of nails, hair, and mucosal surfaces, even if these are recorded as unaffected. The following terms are used to describe distribution: flexural, extensor, acral (hands and feet), symmetrical, localized, widespread, facial, unilateral, linear, centripetal (trunk more than limbs), annular and reticulate (lacy network or mesh like).

Investigation. With regard to investigation, clinical acumen remains the most useful tool in dermatology but a variety of tests are useful in confirming a diagnosis (Table 23.2).

FURTHER READING

Montagna W, Kligman AM, Carlisle KS (1992) *Atlas of normal human skin*. New York: Springer Verlag.

Ong PY, Ohtake T, Brandt C et al. (2002) Endogenous antimicrobial peptides and skin infections in atopic dermatitis. *New England Journal of Medicine* **347**: 1151–1160 (and editorial, pp. 1199–1200).

Paus R, Cotsarelis G (1999) The biology of hair follicles. *New England Journal of Medicine* **341**: 491–497.

Rees J (1999) Understanding barrier function of the skin. *Lancet* **354**: 1491–1492.

Robert C, Kupper TS (1999) Inflammatory skin diseases, T cells, and immune surveillance. *New England Journal of Medicine* **341**: 1817–1828.

Table 23.1   Morphological description of skin lesions

Atrophy	Thinning of the skin
Bulla	A large fluid-filled blister
Crusted	Dried serum or exudate on the skin
Ecchymosis	Large confluent area of purpura ('bruise')
Erosion	Denuded area of skin (partial epidermal loss)
Excoriation	Scratch mark
Fissure	Deep linear crack or crevice (often in thickened skin)
Lichenified	Thickened epidermis with prominent normal skin markings
Macule	Flat, circumscribed non-palpable lesion
Nodule	Large papule (> 0.5 cm)
Papule	Small palpable, circumscribed lesion (< 0.5 cm)
Petechia	Pinpoint-sized macule of blood in the skin
Plaque	Large flat-topped, elevated, palpable lesion
Purpura	Larger macule or papule of blood in the skin which does not blanch on pressure
Pustule	Yellowish white pus-filled lesion
Scaly	Visible flaking and shedding of surface skin
Telangiectasia	Abnormal visible dilatation of blood vessels
Ulcer	Deeper denuded area of skin (full epidermal and dermal loss)
Vesicle	A small fluid-filled blister
Weal	Itchy raised 'nettle rash'-like swelling due to dermal oedema

INFECTIONS

BACTERIAL INFECTIONS (see also p. 62)

The skin's normal bacterial flora prevents colonization by pathogenic organisms. A break in epidermal integrity by trauma, leg ulcers, fungal infections (e.g. athlete's foot) or abnormal scaling of the skin (e.g. in eczema) can allow infection. If reinfection occurs this may be due to asymptomatic nasal carriage of bacteria or the presence of other infected close contacts.

Table 23.2   Investigations used in skin disorders

Test	Use	Clinical example
Skin swabs	Bacterial culture	Impetigo
Blister fluid	Electron microscopy and viral culture	Herpes simplex
Skin scrapes	Fungal culture Microscopy	Tinea pedis Scabies
Nail sampling	Fungal culture	Onychomycosis
Wood's light	Fungal fluorescence	Scalp ringworm Erythrasma
Blood tests	Serology	Streptococcal cellulitis
	Autoantibodies	Discoid lupus erythematosus
	HLA typing	Dermatitis herpetiformis
	DNA analysis	Epidermolysis bullosa
Skin biopsy	Histology	General diagnosis
	Immunohistochemistry	Cutaneous lymphoma
	Immunofluorescence	Immunobullous disease
	Culture	Mycobacteria/fungi
Patch tests	Allergic contact eczema	Hand eczema
Urine	Dipstick (glucose) Cytology (red cells)	Diabetes mellitus Vasculitis
Dermatoscopy (direct microscopy of skin)	Assessment of pigmented lesions	Malignancy

Impetigo

Impetigo is a highly infectious skin disease most common in children (Fig. 23.2). It presents as weeping, exudative areas with a typical honey-coloured crust on the surface. It is spread by direct contact. The term 'scrum pox' is impetigo spread between rugby players. Group A β haemolytic streptococci and staphylococci are the causative agents: skin swabs should be taken. *Bullous impetigo* is caused by bacterial toxins (exfoliation A and B) from *Staphylococcus aureus*.

Treatment

Localized disease is treated with topical fucidic acid and mupirocin is used for MRSA (three times daily). The antiseptic povidone iodine is used to soften crusts and exudates for 1 week. Extensive disease is treated with oral antibiotics for 7–10 days (flucloxacillin 500 mg four times daily for *Staphylococcus*; penicillin V 500 mg four times daily for *Streptococcus*). Other close contacts should be examined, and children should avoid school for 1 week after starting therapy. If impetigo appears resistant to treatment or is

Fig. 23.2 **Impetigo** – crusted blistering lesions on the chin.

(a) (b)

Fig. 23.3 **Erythrasma of the axilla**, showing pink fluorescence under a Wood's lamp.

recurrent, take nasal swabs and check other family members. Nasal mupirocin (three times daily for 1 week) is useful to eradicate nasal carriage in hospitals.

Cellulitis

Cellulitis presents as a hot, sometimes tender area of confluent erythema of the skin owing to infection of the deep subcutaneous layer. It often affects the lower leg, causing an upwards-spreading, hot erythema, and occasionally will blister, especially if oedema is prominent. It may also be seen affecting one side of the face. Patients are often unwell with a high temperature. It is usually caused by a streptococcus or a staphylococcus. In the immunosuppressed or diabetic patient, Gram-negative organisms or anaerobes should be suspected. There may be an obvious portal of entry for infection such as a recent abrasion or a venous leg ulcer. The web spaces of the toes should be examined for evidence of fungal infection. Skin swabs are usually unhelpful. Confirmation of infection is best done serologically by streptococcal titres (antistreptolysin O titre (ASOT) and ADB).

Erysipelas is the term used for a more superficial infection (often on the face) of the dermis and upper subcutaneous layer that clinically presents with a well-defined edge. However, both erysipelas and cellulitis overlap, so it is often impossible to make a meaningful distinction.

Necrotising fasciitis: (see p. 64).

Treatment

Treatment is with penicillin V (or erythromycin) and flucloxacillin (all 500 mg four times daily). If disease is advanced, treatment may need to be given intravenously for 3–5 days followed by 1–2 weeks of oral therapy. Treat any identifiable underlying cause. If cellulitis is recurrent, low-dose antibiotic prophylaxis (e.g. penicillin V 500 mg twice daily) should be given, as each episode will cause further lymphatic damage.

Ecthyma

Ecthyma is also an infection due to *Streptococcus* sp. or *Staphylococcus aureus* or occasionally both. It presents as chronic well-demarcated, deeply ulcerative lesions sometimes with an exudative crust. It is commoner in developing countries, being associated with poor nutrition and hygiene. It is rare in the UK but is seen more commonly in intravenous drug abusers and people with HIV.

Treatment is with penicillin V and flucloxacillin (both 500 mg four times daily) for 10–14 days.

Erythrasma

Erythrasma is caused by *Corynebacterium minutissimum*. It usually presents as an orange-brown flexural rash, and is often seen in the axillae or toe web spaces (Fig. 23.3). It is frequently misdiagnosed as a fungal infection. The rash shows a dramatic coral pink fluorescence under Wood's (ultraviolet) light.

Treatment is with topical fucidin three times daily for 7 days or oral erythromycin 500 mg four times daily for 7–10 days.

Folliculitis

Folliculitis is an inflammation of the hair follicle. It presents as itchy or tender papules and pustules. *Staphylococcus aureus* is frequently implicated. It is commoner in humid climates and when occlusive clothes are worn. A variant occurs in the beard area (called 'sycosis barbae') which is commoner in black Africans. This is probably caused by the ability of shaved hair to grow back into the skin, especially if the hair is naturally curly. Extensive, itchy folliculitis of the upper trunk and limbs should alert one to the possibility of underlying HIV infection. Folliculitis following exposure in hot tubs is due to pseudomonas ovale.

Treatment is with topical antiseptics, topical antibiotics (e.g. fucidin) or oral antibiotics (e.g. flucloxacillin 500 mg or erythromycin 500 mg both four times daily for 2–4 weeks).

Boils (furuncles)

Boils are a rather more deep-seated infection of the skin, often caused by *Staphylococcus*. These can cause painful red swellings. They are commoner in teenagers and often recurrent. Recurrent boils may rarely occur in diabetes mellitus or in immunosuppression. Large boils are sometimes called 'carbuncles'.

Treatment is with oral antibiotics (e.g. erythromycin 500 mg four times daily for 10–14 days) and occasionally by incision and drainage. Antiseptics such as povidone iodine, chlorhexidine (as soap) and a bath oil (e.g. Oilatum plus™) can be useful in prophylaxis.

Hidradenitis suppurativa

This is a rare condition characterized by a painful, discharging, chronic inflammation of the skin at sites rich in apocrine glands (axillae, groins, natal cleft). The cause is unknown but it is commoner in females, and within some families it appears to be inherited in an autosomal dominant fashion. Clinically it presents after puberty with papules, nodules and abscesses which often progress to cysts and sinus formation. With time, scarring may arise. The condition follows a chronic relapsing/remitting course and is often worse in obese individuals.

Treatment is very difficult but weight loss, antibiotics, oral retinoids and co-cyprindiol ('2 mg cyproterone acetate + 35 µg ethinylestradiol' in females only) have been tried. They should be used as for acne vulgaris (p. 1338). Severe recalcitrant cases have been treated occasionally with surgery and skin grafting and more recently intravenous infliximab, a monoclonal antibody (p. 498).

Pitted keratolysis

This is a superficial infection of the horny layer of the skin caused by a *Corynebacterium*. It frequently involves the sole of the forefoot and appears as numerous small punched-out circular lesions of a rather macerated skin (e.g. as seen after prolonged immersion). There may be an associated hyperhidrosis of the feet and a prominent odour.

Treatment. Topical antibiotics (e.g. fucidin or clindamycin, applied three times daily for 2–4 weeks) and topical anti-sweating lotions are effective therapies.

Erysipeloid

This is a very rare infection due to *Erysipelothrix insidiosa*. It is seen in people who handle raw meat (especially pork) and fish. The organism gains entry through breaks in the skin. It presents as a spreading well-demarcated purplish red lesion, usually on the fingers, hands or forearms. There are no systemic symptoms.

Treatment is with penicillin V or oxytetracycline (both 500 mg four times daily for 7–10 days).

MYCOBACTERIAL INFECTIONS

Leprosy (Hansen's disease) (p. 80)

Leprosy usually involves the skin, and the clinical features depend on the body's immune response to the organism *Mycobacterium leprae*.

Indeterminate leprosy is the commonest clinical type, especially in children. This presents as hypopigmented or erythematous circular macules with occasional mild anaesthesia and scaling. This may resolve spontaneously or progress to one of the other types. Biopsy reveals a perineural granulomatous infiltrate and scant acid-fast bacilli.

Tuberculoid leprosy presents with a few hypopigmented or erythematous plaques with an active erythematous, raised rim. Lesions are usually markedly anaesthetic, dry and hairless reflecting the nerve damage. Nerves may be enlarged and palpable. Biopsy shows a granulomatous infiltrate centred on nerves, but no organisms.

Lepromatous leprosy presents with multiple inflammatory papules, plaques and nodules. Loss of the eyebrows ('madarosis') and nasal stuffiness are common. Skin thickening and severe disfigurement may follow. Anaesthesia is much less prominent. Biopsy shows numerous acid-fast bacilli.

Diagnosis and treatment are discussed on page 81.

Skin manifestations of tuberculosis

Tuberculosis can occasionally cause skin manifestations:

- *Lupus vulgaris* usually arises as a post-primary infection. It usually presents on the head or neck with red-brown nodules which look like apple jelly when pressed with a glass slide. They heal with scarring, and new lesions slowly spread out to form a chronic solitary erythematous plaque. Chronic lesions are at high risk of developing squamous cell carcinoma.
- *Tuberculosis verrucosa cutis* arises in people who are partially immune to tuberculosis but who suffer a further direct inoculation in the skin. It presents as warty lesions on a 'cold' erythematous base.
- *Scrofuloderma* arises when an infected lymph node spreads to the skin causing ulceration, scarring and discharge.
- *The tuberculides* are a group of rashes caused by an immune manifestation of tuberculosis rather than direct infection. Erythema nodosum is the commonest and is discussed on page 1341. Erythema induratum ('Bazin's disease') produces similar deep red nodules but these are usually found on the calves rather than the shins and they often ulcerate.

Atypical mycobacteria

Atypical (non-tuberculous) mycobacteria can occasionally infect the skin. *Mycobacterium marinum* is found in fish tanks and occasionally swimming pools. It can gain access via a break in the skin and then causes deep granulomatous nodules, often in a linear fashion.

VIRAL INFECTIONS

Viral exanthem

This, probably the commonest type of virally induced rash, presents clinically as a widespread non-specific erythematous maculopapular rash. It probably arises because of circulating immune complexes of antibody and viral antigen localizing to dermal blood vessels. The rash can be caused by many different viruses (e.g. echo-, parvo-, human herpes virus-6, Epstein–Barr virus; see p. 47) and so is rarely diagnostic. The rash will resolve spontaneously in 7–10 days.

Slapped cheek syndrome (erythema infectiosum, fifth disease)

This affects children and is caused by parvovirus B19 (see p. 48). It is a mild viral illness which is followed by an intense erythema on the cheeks ('slapped cheeks') and a reticulate erythema on the proximal limbs.

Herpes simplex virus (see also p. 43)

Herpes simplex virus (HSV) occurs as two genomic subtypes. HSV type 1 is spread by direct contact and droplet infection. Most people are affected in early childhood but the infection is usually subclinical. Occasionally it can cause a self-limiting pyrexial primary illness with either clusters of painful blisters on the face or a painful gingivostomatitis. Once infected, cell-mediated immunity develops. In some individuals this response is poor and they may get recurrent attacks of HSV, often manifest as cold sores. Immunosuppression can also cause a recrudescence of HSV. HSV can also autoinoculate into sites of trauma and present as painful blisters/pustules. For example they may be seen on the fingers of healthcare workers ('herpetic whitlow').

HSV type 2 infections occur mainly after puberty and usually affect the genital area. Infections are often symptomatic and transmitted sexually. However, HSV type 1 can also be found in the genital area due to orogenital contact.

Other rare complications of HSV infection include corneal ulceration, eczema herpeticum (p. 1327), chronic perianal ulceration in AIDS patients and erythema multiforme (p. 1342).

Treatment

Oral valaciclovir (500 mg twice daily for 5 days) is used for primary HSV and painful genital HSV. Recurrent cold sores are treated with aciclovir cream but this must be used early to be effective in shortening an attack. Attacks of genital herpes become less frequent with time. Intravenous aciclovir must be used in immunosuppressed patients.

Varicella zoster virus

Varicella zoster virus (VZV) causes the common child-

Fig. 23.4 **Herpes zoster in an African** (courtesy of Dr P Matondo, Lusaka, Zambia).

hood infection called chickenpox. It is discussed on page 45. It also causes herpes zoster.

Herpes zoster (shingles)

'Shingles' results from a reactivation of the VZV. It may be preceded by a prodromal phase of tingling or pain, which is then followed by a painful and tender blistering eruption in a dermatomal distribution (Fig. 23.4 and Fig. 2.15, p. 46). The blisters occur in crops, may become pustular and then crust over. The rash lasts 2–4 weeks and is usually more severe in the elderly. Occasionally more than one dermatome is involved.

Complications of shingles include severe, persistent pain (post-herpetic neuralgia), ocular disease (if ophthalmic nerve involved) and rarely motor neuropathy.

Treatment

Herpes zoster requires adequate analgesia and antibiotics (if secondary bacterial infection is present). Valaciclovir 1 g or famciclovir 500 mg three times daily for 7 days is used, or oral aciclovir 800 mg, five times daily for 7 days helps shorten the attack if given early in the illness. High-dose intravenous aciclovir is needed for immunosuppressed patients. It remains unclear how useful aciclovir therapy is in preventing prolonged post-herpetic neuralgia.

Human papilloma virus

Human papilloma virus (HPV) is responsible for the common cutaneous infection of 'viral warts'. There are more than 70 subtypes as detected by DNA hybridization. All can cause overgrowth of differentiated squamous epithelium.

Common warts are papular lesions with a coarse roughened surface, often seen on the hands and feet, but also on other sites. Small black dots (bleeding points) are often seen within the lesion (Fig. 23.5). Children and adolescents are usually affected. Spread is by direct contact and is also associated with trauma.

Plantar warts (verrucae) is the term used for lesions on the soles of the feet. They often appear flat ('inward

Fig. 23.5 **Viral wart.**

growing') although they have the same papillomatous surface change and black dots are often revealed if the skin is pared down (unlike callosities). Warts may be painful or tender if they are over pressure points or around nail folds.

Filiform warts occur on the face, at the nasal vestibule or around the mouth. They are elongated with a horny cap.

Plane warts are much less common and are caused by certain HPV subtypes. They are clinically different and appear as very small, flesh-coloured or pigmented, flat-topped lesions (best seen with side-on lighting) with little in the way of surface change and no black dots within them. They are usually multiple and are frequently found on the face or the backs of the hands.

Anogenital warts are usually seen in adults and are normally transmitted by sexual contact. They are rare in childhood and, whilst child sex abuse should always be considered, it should be remembered they may well have been transmitted through non-sexual contact. HPV subtypes 16 and 18 are potentially oncogenic and are associated with cervical and anal carcinomas.

Treatment

Common warts on the skin are surprisingly difficult to treat effectively but they almost always resolve spontaneously after months to years (with no scarring), presumably because of cell-mediated immune recognition. When they do resolve, they tend to do so rapidly within a few days.

Regular use of a topical keratolytic agent (e.g. 2–10% salicylic acid) over many months with weekly paring of the lesion helps speed up resolution in some patients and remains the mainstay of treatment. A course of cryotherapy (freezing) can also help. Cautery, surgery, carbon dioxide laser, alpha-interferon injection and bleomycin injection have all been used with variable success but are not recommended, as treatments may be very painful and can cause permanent scarring. Experimental usage of a complex of α-lactalbumin and oleic acid (human α-lactalbumin made lethal to tumour cells – HAMLET) is promising.

Genital warts (see p. 126) are usually treated with either cryotherapy, trichloracetic acid, 5% imiquimod cream or topical podophyllin. Patients with genital warts (and their sexual partners) must be screened for other sexually transmitted diseases.

Molluscum contagiosum ('water blisters')

Molluscum contagiosum is a common cutaneous infection of childhood caused by a pox virus. The virus can be seen in the fluid under EM. Clinically, lesions are multiple, small (1–3 mm) translucent papules which often look like fluid-filled vesicles but are in fact solid. Individual lesions may have a central depression called a punctum. They exhibit the Köbner phenomenon (p. 1332). They can occur at any body site including the genitalia. Transmission is by direct contact. Occasionally lesions may be up to 1 cm in diameter ('giant molluscum'). They are said to be more extensive in children with atopic eczema, which may just reflect that scratching aids their spread.

They usually continue to occur in crops over 6–12 months and rarely require treatment as they spontaneously resolve. Any form of localized trauma including scratching, helps speed up resolution and cryotherapy may be considered in an older child. Molluscum in an adult, especially if giant, should raise the underlying possibility of immunosuppression, especially HIV infection.

Orf

Orf is a disease of sheep (and occasionally goats) due to a pox virus infection. It causes a vesicular and pustular rash around the mouths of young lambs. People who come into contact with the affected fluid may develop lesions on the hands. Clinically they appear as 1–2 cm reddish papules with a surrounding erythema which usually become pustular. The lesion(s) resolves spontaneously after 4–6 weeks and immunity lasts lifelong. Occasionally orf is complicated by erythema multiforme (p. 1342).

FUNGAL INFECTIONS

Fungi are primitive, saprophytic organisms found throughout our environment. Fungal skin disease (mycosis) has a high prevalence in humans, with 'thrush' and 'athlete's foot' being two of the commonest examples. In the immunosuppressed, mycoses can be widespread and life-threatening. There are three groups of pathogenic fungi that commonly affect the outer layer of skin or keratinizing epithelium: dermatophytes, *Candida albicans* and pityrosporum.

Dermatophyte infection

By definition, dermatophytes cause a 'ringworm' type of rash. The three main genera responsible are *Trichophyton*, *Microsporum* and *Epidermophyton*. These organisms are identified by microscopy and culture of skin, hair or nail samples. The clinical appearance of mycoses depends in

Fig. 23.6 **Tinea cruris** – ringworm of the groin.

part on the organism involved, the site affected and the host reaction. All are spread by direct contact from other humans or from infected animals. The use of communal showers and swimming baths and the sharing of towels or sportswear aids indirect fomite transmission.

Tinea corporis

Ringworm of the body usually presents with slightly itchy, asymmetrical, scaly patches which show central clearing and an advancing, scaly, raised edge. Occasionally vesicles or pustules may be seen in the edge. Central clearing is not a universal feature and it is recommended that all asymmetrical scaly lesions should be scraped for fungus. Ringworm of the face (tinea faciei) often arises after the use of topical steroids. It tends to be more erythematous and less scaly than trunk lesions and it may become itchy after sun exposure.

Tinea cruris

Ringworm of the groin is extremely common world-wide. Early on, the lesions appear as well-demarcated red plaques with an arc-like border extending down the upper thigh (Fig. 23.6). Central clearing may appear and a few pustules or vesicles may be seen if inflammation is intense. Satellite lesions, suggestive of *Candida*, are not present.

Tinea pedis

Athlete's foot may be confined to the toe clefts, where the skin looks white, macerated and fissured. It may also be more diffuse, usually causing a diffuse scaly erythema of the soles, spreading on to the sides of the foot. Annular lesions are rare and can be misdiagnosed. There may be an associated hyperhidrosis and fungal involvement of one or more toe-nails. In severe infection, a strong inflammatory reaction can occur causing pustules or blistering and this often leads to a misdiagnosis of pompholyx-type eczema.

Tinea manuum

Ringworm of the hands also presents with a diffuse erythematous scaling of the palms with variable skin peeling and skin thickening. Annular lesions are rare at this site.

Tinea capitis

The fungus is either within the hair shaft (endothrix) or spread out over the hair surface (ectothrix). The latter can cause fluorescence under a Wood's lamp (ultraviolet light). Scalp ringworm is spread by close contact (especially in schools and households) and may also be spread indirectly by hairdressers. The number of new cases has risen enormously in the large cities in developed countries. Increase in travel and immigration has allowed the spread of different pathogenic fungi (e.g. *Trichophyton tonsurans* from Central America, *Trichophyton violaceum* from India and Pakistan) into new countries where there is overcrowding and poor social conditions. The majority of UK cases are due to *T. tonsurans* (which does not show fluorescence).

Tinea capitis is much commoner in children, especially those of black African origin, whose scalp and hair seems more susceptible to fungal invasion. The clinical appearance of scalp ringworm is highly variable from a mild diffuse scaling with no hair loss (similar to dandruff) to the more typical appearance of circular scaly patches in the scalp with associated alopecia and broken hairs. As the hosts immune response increases, a few pustules may appear and an exudate may be present. At worst, a full-blown 'kerion' develops; a boggy swollen mass with copious quantities of discharging pus and exudate accompanied by severe alopecia. This is still poorly recognized and inappropriately treated with antibiotics and attempted surgical drainage.

Extensive infection is occasionally accompanied by a widespread papulopustular rash on the trunk. This is a so-called 'Id reaction' and probably relates to the host immune response to the fungus. It seems commoner in black African children. It resolves when the fungal infection is treated.

Tinea unguium

Ringworm of the nails is increasingly common with age and frequently ignored as it is often asymptomatic. Clinically this presents as asymmetrical whitening (or yellowish black discoloration) of one or more nails, which usually starts at the distal or lateral edge before spreading throughout the nail (Fig. 23.7). The nail plate appears

Fig. 23.7 **Dermatophyte infection of the nail showing white crumbling dystrophy.**

thickened. Crumbly white material appears under the nail plate and this is the best specimen to obtain for mycology sampling. The nail plate may become destroyed with advanced disease.

'Tinea incognito'

This is the term used to describe a fungal skin infection that has been modified by therapy with a topical steroid. The clinical appearance is variable but may show a non-specific erythema with little in the way of scaling or a few reddish nodules. The history of the rash improving with steroid treatment (owing to the suppression of inflammation) but worsening and spreading every time it is stopped is typical. Skin scrapings for mycology or even a biopsy should confirm the diagnosis.

Treatment

Localized ringworm of the body or flexures is treated with topical antifungal creams (clotrimazole, miconazole, terbinafine or amorolofine applied three times daily for 1–2 weeks). More widespread infection, including tinea pedis, tinea manuum and tinea capitis, requires oral antifungal therapy. Itraconazole (100 mg daily) and terbinafine (250 mg daily) are the most effective drugs used for periods of 1–2 months, but are not licensed for use in children. High-dose griseofulvin is still used in children for scalp ringworm (15–20 mg/kg per day for 8 weeks).

Tinea unguium of the toe-nails is the most resistant to treatment. Itraconazole (100 mg daily or 200 mg twice daily for 1 week per month 'pulsed therapy') or terbinafine (250 mg daily) given for 3 months will cure up to about 80% of cases.

Candida albicans (see also p. 91)

Candida albicans is a yeast that is sometimes found as part of the body's flora, especially in the gastrointestinal tract. It acts as an opportunist, taking hold in the skin when there is a suitable warm moist environment such as in nappy rash (p. 1362) or intertrigo in obese individuals (Fig. 23.8).

The flexural areas affected are red with a rather ragged peeling edge that may contain a few small pustules. Small circular areas of erythema or small papules and pustules may be seen in front of the advancing edge (satellite lesions). *Candida* may also affect the moist interdigital clefts of the toes and mimic tinea pedis. In people who have their hands immersed frequently in water (e.g. cleaners, nurses) *Candida* may cause infection in the macerated skin of the finger web spaces or the damaged skin around the nail folds ('chronic paronychia'). Nail infection may mimic tinea unguium. It can infect mucosal surfaces of the mouth or genital tract. This tends to occur in patients taking broad-spectrum antibiotics (due to suppression of protective bacterial flora) or in immunosuppressed patients. Clinically superficial white or creamy pseudomembranous plaques appear which can be scraped off leaving raw areas underneath.

Fig. 23.8 Intertrigo with satellite lesions typical of candidiasis.

Treatment

Treatment is aimed at removing any underlying predisposing factor and applying topical antifungal creams, e.g. clotrimazole or miconazole (or the equivalent as mouth lozenges/pessaries). *Candida* nail infections require systemic antifungal therapy with an imidazole such as itraconazole (100 mg daily for 3 months). Recurrent candidiasis is relatively common, especially in women. Diabetes mellitus should always be excluded. Repeated topical treatment or an oral imidazole may be needed.

Pityrosporum

This yeast occurs as part of the normal flora of human skin. Colonization is prominent in the scalp, flexures and upper trunk. There are two morphological variants called *Pityrosporum ovale* and *Pityrosporum orbiculare*, and the mycelial form of this yeast is called *Malassezia furfur*. *Pityrosporum* can overgrow in some individuals and has been implicated in three dermatoses:

- pityriasis versicolor
- seborrhoeic eczema (p. 1329)
- pityrosporum folliculitis.

Pityriasis versicolor

This is a relatively common condition of young adults caused by infection with *Pityrosporum*. In Caucasians it presents most commonly on the trunk with reddish brown scaly macules which are asymptomatic. In black-skinned individuals (or in whites who are sun-tanned) it more commonly presents as macular areas of hypo-pigmentation. Inappropriate use of topical steroids tends to spread the rash.

Diagnosis can be confirmed by skin scrapings or Wood's light examination (yellow fluorescence).

Treatment is with selenium sulphide shampoo (apply to body and remove after 30 minutes and repeat daily for 1 week) or a topical imidazole cream (twice daily for 10 days). Oral itraconazole (100 mg twice daily for 1 week) can be used for resistant cases. The pigmentation takes months to recover even after successful treatment. The condition may recur but can be retreated.

Pityrosporum folliculitis

This is common in young adult males and characterized by small itchy papules and pustules on the upper back which are centred on hair follicles. It is commoner in people with Down's syndrome. It responds well to ketoconazole shampoo or a topical imidazole cream (twice daily for 2 weeks).

INFESTATIONS

Scabies

Scabies is an intensely itchy rash caused by the mite *Sarcoptes scabiei*. It can affect all races and people of any social class. It is most common in children and young adults but can affect any age group. There are 300 million cases of scabies in the world each year. It is commoner in poorer countries with social overcrowding.

Scabies is spread by prolonged close contact such as within households or institutions, and by sexual contact. It presents clinically with itchy red papules (or occasionally vesicles and pustules), which can occur anywhere in the skin but rarely on the face, except in neonates. The distribution of lesions is often suggestive of the diagnosis (Fig. 23.9). Sites of predilection are between the web spaces of the fingers and toes, on the palms and soles, around the wrists and axillae, on the male genitalia, and around the nipples and umbilicus.

Fig. 23.9 **Scabies** – itchy papules and pustules centred on the web spaces of the hand.

The pathognomonic sign is of linear or curved skin burrows but these are not always present. The pruritus is normally worse at night. Excoriations and secondary bacterial infection may complicate the rash. Scabies can be confirmed by taking skin scrapings of a lesion and examining a potassium hydroxide preparation for the mite and/or its eggs by microscopy.

Treatment

This involves application of a topical scabicide (e.g. 5% permethrin or malathion). For the treatment to be successful the following factors should be noted:

- All the skin below the neck should be treated, including the genitalia, palms and soles, and under the nails. Treat the head and neck regions in infants (up to age 2 years).
- All close contacts should be treated at the same time even if asymptomatic.
- Reapply scabicide to the hands if they are washed during the treatment period.
- Patients should be warned that the pruritus may persist for up to 4 weeks after successful treatment. Adjunct treatment with crotamiton cream, an emollient or a mild topical steroid is helpful.
- A patient information leaflet about therapy helps improve compliance.

Benzyl benzoate is still used occasionally but it can be very irritant. Lindane is a cheap therapy which is still used in many countries but there are concerns about resistance to this drug and possible neurotoxic side-effects.

Crusted scabies (Norwegian scabies)

Crusted scabies is a clinical variant that occurs in immunosuppressed individuals where huge numbers of mites are carried in the skin. Patients are not always itchy but they are extremely infectious after relatively minimal contact, which is unfortunate as the diagnosis is often delayed. Clinically this presents as hyperkeratotic crusted lesions, especially on the hands and feet. Lesions may progress such that the patient has a widespread erythema with irregular crusted plaques. It can therefore mimic infected eczema or psoriasis.

Treatment is with careful barrier nursing, repeated applications of a scabicide and, in resistant cases, oral ivermectin (100–200 μg/kg – two doses 1 week apart) may be given but this is an unlicensed use.

Lice infection

Lice are blood-sucking ectoparasites that can affect man in three ways.

Head lice (pediculosis capitis)

Head lice is a common infection world-wide, affecting predominantly children and being commoner in females. Spread is by direct contact and encouraged by overcrowding. It usually presents with itch or scalp excoriations. Occasionally, erythematous papules on the neck may be seen.

Diagnosis can be confirmed by the presence of eggs ('nits') seen tightly bound to the hair shaft. Adult lice may be seen rarely in heavy infection. School nurses and parents are usually adept at this.

Treatment. Eradication is difficult because of non-compliance as well as resistance patterns. Malathion, carbaryl or permethrin applications (two applications 7 days apart) are the most commonly used. Nit combing of wet hair is not as effective as chemical treatment. District policies of rotating insecticides are outmoded. If one treatment fails, a different insecticide is used for the next course in an individual. Treatment is usually repeated after 7 days and metal nit combs may help remove the eggs. Some areas in the UK have given up with specific anti-lice treatments but have a policy of treating schools and family members with regular nit-combing, shampooing and conditioning of the hair. However, a recent study showed that chemical therapies are more effective than physical treatments, but more studies are needed.

Body lice (pediculosis corporis)

Body lice is a disease of poverty and neglect. It is rarely seen in developed countries except in homeless individuals and vagrants. It is spread by direct contact or sharing infested clothing. The lice and eggs are rarely seen on the patient but are commonly found on the clothing. It presents with itch, excoriations and sometimes post-inflammatory hyperpigmentation of the skin.

Treatment consists of malathion or permethrin for the patient and high-temperature washing and drying of clothing.

Pubic lice (crabs, phthiriasis pubis)

Pubic lice are transmitted by direct contact, usually sexual. It presents with itching, especially at night. Lice can be seen near the base of the hair with eggs somewhat further up the shaft. Occasionally eyebrows, eyelashes and the beard area are affected.

Treatment is as for head lice but all sexual contacts should be treated and other sexually transmitted diseases should be screened for. Pubic lice of the eyelashes is treated with white soft paraffin three times daily for 1–2 weeks.

Arthropod-borne diseases ('insect bites' or papular urticaria)

These depend on contact with an animal (e.g. dog, cat, bird) that is infected with fleas ('*Ctenocephalides*') or on bites from flying insects (e.g. midges, mosquitoes). In the case of flea bites the animal itself may be itchy with scaly and thickened skin. These fleas can also live in soft furnishings (e.g. carpets and beds) even after the animal

has been removed. Bites present as itchy urticated lesions which are often grouped in clusters. The legs are most commonly affected. It is not unusual for an individual to react badly to bites when other family members seem unaffected. Anti-flea treatment of the animal and furnishings is required. Insect repellents and appropriate clothing help reduce bites from flying insects.

FURTHER READING

Chosidow O. (2000) Scabies and pediculosis. *Lancet* **355**: 819–826.

Gnann JW, Whitley RJ (2002) Herpes zoster. *New England Journal of Medicine* **347**: 340–346

Ko CJ et al. (2004) Pediculosis. *Journal of the American Academy of Dermatology* **50**: 1–12.

Manders SM (1998) Toxin-mediated streptococcal and staphylococcal disease. *Journal of the American Academy of Dermatology* **39**: 383–398.

Sterling JC et al. (2001) Guidelines for the management of cutaneous warts. *British Journal of Dermatology* **144**: 4–11.

Swartz MN (2004) Cellulitis. *New England Journal of Medicine* **350**: 908–912.

PAPULO-SQUAMOUS/ INFLAMMATORY RASHES

ECZEMA

The term 'eczema' derives from the Greek word for 'boiling', which reflects that the skin can become so acutely inflamed that fluid weeps out or vesicles appear. It is synonymous with the term dermatitis and the two words are interchangeable. In the developed world eczema accounts for a large proportion of skin disease, both in hospital and community-based populations. It is estimated that 10% of people have some form of eczema at any one time, and up to 40% of the population will have an episode of eczema during their lifetime.

All eczemas (see Table 23.3) have some features in common and there is a spectrum of clinical presentation from acute through to chronic. Vesicles or bullae may appear in the acute stage if inflammation is intense. In subacute eczema the skin can be erythematous, dry and flaky, oedematous, and crusted (especially if secondarily infected). Chronic persistent eczema is characterized by thickened or lichenified skin. Eczema is nearly always itchy. Histologically 'eczematous change' refers to a col-

Table 23.3 Classification of eczema	
Endogenous	**Exogenous**
Atopic eczema	Contact eczema – irritant
Discoid eczema	Contact eczema – allergic
Hand eczema	Photosensitive eczema
Seborrhoeic eczema	Lichen simplex/nodular prurigo
Venous ('gravitational') eczema	
Asteatotic eczema	

lection of fluid in the epidermis between the keratinocytes ('spongiosis') and an upper dermal perivascular infiltrate of lymphohistiocytic cells. In more chronic disease there is marked thickening of the epidermis ('acanthosis').

Atopic eczema

This type of eczema (often called 'endogenous eczema') occurs in individuals who are 'atopic' (p. 912). It is common, occurring in up to 5% of the UK population. It is commoner in early life, occurring at some stage during childhood in up to 10–20% of all children.

Aetiology

The exact pathophysiology is not fully understood but there is a selective activation of Th2-type CD4 lymphocytes in the skin which drives the inflammatory process. In at least 90% of cases there is a raised serum total IgE level. Atopic eczema is a genetically complex, familial disease with a strong maternal influence. A positive family history of atopic disease is often present: there is a 90% concordance in monozygotic twins but only 20% in dizygotic twins. If one parent has atopic disease the risk for a child of developing eczema is about 20–30%, and 50% if both parents are affected. Genetic studies in atopy have so far shown linkage to several different loci where pathologically relevant candidate genes exist: e.g. the β-subunit of the high-affinity IgE receptor (11q13); Th2 cytokine genes (5q31-33); the α-subunit of IL-4 (16q12); and RANTES (17q11). Both eczema and psoriasis have been linked to chromosome 1q21 and 17q25, suggesting common candidate genes controlling skin inflammation.

Genetic heterogeneity is likely and it may be that certain genes are more involved in developing eczema rather than asthma, and other genes may be significant in determining severity of the disorder or age of onset. The disease is also significantly influenced by environmental factors.

Exacerbating factors

Infection either in the skin or systemically can lead to an exacerbation, possibly by a superantigen effect. Paradoxically, lack of infection (in infancy) may cause the immune system to follow a Th-2 pathway and allow eczema to develop (the so-called 'hygiene hypothesis'). Strong detergents, chemicals and even woollen clothes can be irritant and exacerbate eczema. Teething is another factor in young children. Severe anxiety or stress appear to exacerbate eczema in some individuals. Cat and dog fur can certainly make eczema worse, possibly by both allergic and irritant mechanisms. The role of house dust mite and diet is less clear cut. There is some evidence that food allergens may play a role in triggering atopic eczema and that dairy products may exacerbate eczema in a few selected infants under 12 months of age.

Clinical features

Atopic eczema can present as a number of distinct morphological variants. The commonest presentation is of itchy erythematous scaly patches, especially in the

Fig. 23.10 **Atopic eczema behind the knees.**

flexures such as in front of the elbows and ankles, behind the knees (Fig. 23.10) and around the neck. In infants eczema often starts on the face before spreading to the body. Very acute lesions may weep or exude and can show small vesicles. Scratching can produce excoriations, and repeated rubbing produces skin thickening (lichenification) with exaggerated skin markings.

In patients with pigmented skin, eczema often shows a reverse pattern of extensor involvement. Also, the eczema may be papular or follicular in nature and lichenification is common. A final problem in pigmented skin is of post-inflammatory hyper- or hypopigmentation which is often very slow to fade after control of the eczema.

Associated features

Involvement of the nail bed may produce pitting and ridging of the nails. In some atopic individuals the skin of the upper arms and thighs may feel roughened because of follicular hyperkeratosis ('keratosis pilaris'). The palms may show very prominent skin creases ('hyperlinear palms'). There may be an associated dry 'fish-like' scaling of the skin which is non-inflammatory and often prominent on the lower legs ('ichthyosis vulgaris').

Complications

Broken skin commonly becomes secondarily infected by bacteria. This is usually due to *Staphylococcus aureus* although streptococci can colonize eczema, especially in macerated flexural areas such as the neck and groin. Clinically this infection may appear as crusted, weeping impetigo-like lesions. Occasionally *Pseudomonas* can be grown from skin swabs but this rarely causes a clinical problem. Cutaneous viral infections (e.g. viral warts and molluscum) are often widespread in atopic eczema and are probably spread by scratching. HSV can cause a widespread eruption called eczema herpeticum (Kaposi's varicelliform eruption). This can occasionally be a very severe infection and rarely can be fatal. This appears as multiple small blisters or punched-out crusted lesions associated with malaise and pyrexia, and needs rapid treatment with oral (or intravenous if severe) aciclovir. Ocular complications of atopic eczema include conjunctival irritation and less commonly keratoconjunctivitis and cataract. Retarded growth may be seen in children with chronic severe eczema; it is due to the disease itself and not the use of topical steroids.

Investigations

The diagnosis of atopic eczema is normally clinical. Atopy is characterized by high serum IgE levels or high specific IgE levels to certain ingested or inhaled antigens. The latter can be tested by radio-immunoabsorbent assay (RAST tests) of blood, or indirectly by skin prick testing (p. 918). A peripheral blood eosinophilia may also be seen.

Prognosis

The majority (90%) of children with early-onset atopic eczema will spontaneously improve and 'clear' before the teenage years, 50% being clear by the age of 6. A few will get a recurrence as adults, even if just as hand eczema. However, if the onset of eczema is late in childhood or in adulthood, the disorder follows a more chronic remitting/relapsing course.

Treatment (Box 23.2)

General measures

These include avoiding known irritants (especially soaps or furry animals), wearing cotton clothes, and not getting too hot. Manipulating the diet (e.g. dairy-free diet) is rarely beneficial except in children under 12 months with a hereditary risk of eczema. Any change in diet should be done under supervision, especially with growing children who may need supplements such as calcium.

Topical therapies

Topical therapies (p. 1364) are sufficient to control atopic eczema in most people. The 'triple' combination of topical steroid, frequent emollients (see Table 23.16) and bath oil and soap substitute (e.g. aqueous cream) helps.

Written information or a practical demonstration of how to apply these treatments improves compliance.

Use of topical steroids. Unjustified fear about the dangers of topical steroids has often led to under-treatment of eczema. Providing appropriate-strength steroid preparations are used for the right body site, these

Box 23.2 Management of atopic eczema

- Education and explanation
- Avoidance of irritants/allergens
- Emollients
- Bath oils/soap substitutes
- Topical therapies:
  - steroids
  - immunomodulators
- Adjunct therapies:
  - oral antibiotics
  - sedating antihistamines
  - bandaging
- Phototherapy/systemic therapy (for severe cases)

Table 23.4 Classification of topical steroids by potency

Potency	Steroid
Very potent	0.05% clobetasol propionate
	0.3% diflucortolone valerate
Potent	0.1% betamethasone valerate
	0.025% fluocinolone acetonide
Diluted potent	0.025% betamethasone valerate
	0.00625% fluocinolone acetonide
Moderately potent	0.05% clobetasone butyrate
	0.05% alclometasone dipropionate
Mild	2.5% hydrocortisone
	1% hydrocortisone

compounds can be used quite safely on a long-term inter-mittent basis. Topical steroids can be divided into five groups depending on their potency (Table 23.4).

The following guidelines should be followed to allow their safe use in common chronic inflammatory skin conditions.

- The face should be treated with mild steroids.
- In adults the body should be treated with either mild, moderately potent or diluted potent steroids.
- In young children the body should be treated with mild and moderately potent steroids.
- Potent steroids may be used for short courses (7–10 days).
- Treatment of the palms and soles (but not the dorsal surfaces) may require potent or very potent steroids as the skin is much thicker.
- Regular use of emollients may lessen the need for steroid use.
- Only use steroids on inflamed skin. Do not use as an emollient.
- 'Apply sparingly' means use sufficient to leave a glistening surface to the skin after application.
- Use weaker steroid preparations in flexures (e.g. the groin, and under breasts) as apposition of the skin at these sites tends to occlude the treatment and increase absorption.

Topical immunomodulators

Tacrolimus ointment (0.1% and 0.03%) and the less potent pimecrolimus (a skin-selective inflammatory cytokine inhibitor) cream have recently been licensed for atopic eczema in patients over 2 years old. They have the advantage over potent steroids of not causing atrophy and are thus very useful for treating sensitive areas such as the face and eyelids. They can be very irritant when first used (although this settles with continued use) and 9% of patients develop flushing after alcohol. The long-term side-effects remain unknown. They do not work so well on lichenified eczema, probably because of poor absorption. Current advice is to avoid vaccinations and sun exposure when using these agents. The milder potency steroid creams should still be considered as first-line therapy but tacrolimus is a useful alternative to excessive use of potent steroids.

Antibiotics

These are needed for bacterial infection and are usually given orally for 7–10 days. Flucloxacillin (500 mg four times daily) is effective against *Staphylococcus*, and penicillin V (500 mg four times daily) acts against *Streptococcus*. Erythromicin (500 mg four times daily) is useful if there is allergy to penicillin. Topical antiseptics may be useful in cases of recurrent infection but they can be irritant. They are usually added to the bath water rather than directly onto the skin. Combination topical steroid/antibiotic creams are used for short periods but there is little evidence that they are better than topical steroids alone.

Sedating antihistamines

These (e.g. oral hydroxyzine 25 mg) are useful at night-time. They help by their sedative properties, not by their antihistamine activity.

Bandaging

Paste bandaging can be useful for resistant or lichenified eczema of the limbs. It helps absorption of treatment and acts as a barrier to prevent scratching. Wet tubular gauze bandages are useful for inpatient therapy but are difficult and time-consuming to use at home.

Second-line agents

These may be considered in severe non-responsive cases, especially if the eczema is significantly interfering with an individual's life (e.g. growth, sleeping, schoolwork or job). Ultraviolet phototherapy (see p. 1339), prednisolone (initial doses up to 30 mg daily), ciclosporin (3–5 mg/kg daily) and azathioprine (1–2 mg/kg daily) (p. 1347) can all be effective treatments. However, they all have side-effects and the risk/benefit ratio must be openly discussed with the patient before they are used.

Use of ciclosporin. Ciclosporin is a selective immuno-suppressant that inhibits interleukin-2 production by T lymphocytes. A large number of other drugs interact with ciclosporin (e.g. erythromycin, NSAIDs) and should be avoided. Renal damage and hypertension are the two most serious side-effects so blood pressure and serum creatinine should be measured every 6–12 weeks. Creatinine clearance should be measured yearly in people on long-term therapy. Renal damage becomes increasingly common with time and tends to be dose-dependent but is mostly reversible. Hypertrichosis, paraesthesia and nausea are less serious side-effects. Pregnancy should be avoided.

Discoid eczema (nummular eczema)

Discoid eczema is a morphological variant of eczema, characterized by well-demarcated scaly patches especially on the limbs, and this can be confused sometimes with psoriasis. It is commoner in adults and can occur in both atopic and non-atopic individuals. It tends to follow an acute/subacute course rather than a chronic pattern. There is often an infective component (*Staphylococcus aureus*).

Fig. 23.11 **Pompholyx eczema** (courtesy of Dr A Bewley, London).

Hand eczema

Eczema may be confined to the hands (and feet). It can present with:

- itchy vesicles or blisters of the palm and along the sides of the fingers (also called 'pompholyx') (Fig. 23.11)
- a diffuse erythematous scaling and hyperkeratosis of the palms
- a scaling and peeling most marked at the finger tips.

Hand eczema is not unusual in atopics but more frequently occurs in non-atopic individuals, and a cause is not always found. A history of contact with irritants (e.g. detergents, chemicals) and an occupational history should be sought, especially in finger-tip eczema. Patch testing for specific allergic or contact eczema should always be considered, as up to 10% of individuals with hand eczema will show a positive test. Finally look for evidence of fungal infection, as this can occasionally induce a secondary pompholyx of the hands or feet (a so-called 'Id reaction').

Seborrhoeic eczema

Aetiology

Overgrowth of *Pityrosporum ovale* (also called *Malassezia furfur* in its hyphal form) together with a strong cutaneous immune response to this yeast produces the characteristic inflammation and scaling of seborrhoeic eczema. The condition is more common in parkinsonism as well as in HIV disease.

Clinical features

Seborrhoeic eczema affects body sites rich in sebaceous glands, although these do not appear to be involved in its cause. Three age groups are affected:

- *In childhood* it is common and presents in the first few months of life as 'cradle cap' in most babies. This may in part be due to the effect of maternal androgens on infant sebaceous glands. Yellowish, greasy, thick crusts are seen on the scalp. A more widespread erythematous, scaly rash can be seen over the trunk,

Fig. 23.12 Seborrhoeic eczema affecting the sides of the nose.

especially affecting the nappy area. Unlike with atopic eczema, the child is normally unbothered as there is little associated pruritus. The rash normally improves spontaneously after a few weeks.

- *In young adults* (especially males) it occurs in 1–3% of the population. The rash is more persistent and presents as an erythematous scaling along the sides of the nose (Fig. 23.12), in the eyebrows, around the eyes and extending into the scalp (which shows marked dandruff). It affects the skin over the sternum, axillae and groins, and the glans penis. A blepharitis may also be present.
- *In elderly people* seborrhoeic eczema can be more severe and progress to involve large areas of the body and even cause erythroderma.

Treatment

This is suppressive rather than curative. A combination of a mild steroid ointment (e.g. 1% hydrocortisone applied twice daily) and a topical antifungal cream (e.g. miconazole cream applied twice daily) will help to control the eruption. Two per cent sulphur or 2% salicylic acid can be added to help control resistant cases. Recent studies have shown 0.1% tacrolimus ointment to be very effective. Ketoconazole shampoo and arachis oil are useful for the scalp. Emollients and a soap substitute are useful adjuncts.

Venous eczema (varicose eczema, gravitational eczema)

This type of eczema occurs on the lower legs because of chronic venous hypertension (usually of more than 2 years' duration) (see p. 1353). The exact cause remains unknown but it has been suggested that venous hypertension causes endothelial hyperplasia and extravasation of red and white blood cells, which in turn causes inflammation, purpura and pigmentation.

Clinical features

Venous eczema tends to occur in older people, especially women. It usually appears on the lower legs around the ankles. There may be a past history of venous thrombosis or previous surgery for varicose veins. Brownish pigmentation (haemosiderin) is seen in the skin and a venous leg ulcer or varicose veins may be present.

Superimposed contact eczema is common in venous eczema patients, especially when there have been chronic venous leg ulcers. This is usually due to an allergic reaction to topical therapies or skin dressings. Patch testing is useful in treatment-resistant cases.

Treatment

This should include emollients and a moderately potent topical steroid. Support stockings or compression bandages, together with leg elevation, help reverse the underlying venous hypertension (p. 1353).

Asteatotic eczema (winter eczema, eczema craquelé, senile eczema)

This is a dry plate-like cracking of the skin with a red, eczematous component which occurs in elderly people. It occurs predominantly on the lower legs and the backs of the hands, especially in winter. The exact cause is unknown but the repeated use of soaps in the elderly may be causal. The loss of the stratum corneum lipids with age may also be of some relevance. Rarely, asteatotic eczema can be the presenting sign of myxoedema or can follow the commencement of diuretic therapy.

Treatment

Avoiding soaps, and the regular use of emollients and bath oils should be encouraged. Humidifying centrally heated rooms may help. If the skin is very inflamed, a mild topical steroid can be used.

Contact and irritant eczema

These types of eczema can be caused by many environmental agents (exogenous eczema); they are often in an unusual or localized distribution (Fig. 23.13). There is no personal or family history of atopic disease. A history of an exacerbation of eczema at the workplace is also

Fig. 23.13 Contact eczema secondary to perfume allergy.

suggestive. This can happen by two mechanisms: direct irritation or an allergic reaction (type IV delayed hypersensitivity, p. 226). A detailed history of occupation, hobbies, cosmetic products, clothing and contact with chemicals is necessary.

Allergic contact eczema occurs after repeated exposure to a chemical substance but only in those people who are susceptible to develop an allergic reaction. It is common, occurring in up to 4% of some populations. Many substances can cause this type of reaction but the commoner culprits are nickel (in costume jewellery and buckles), chromate (in cement), latex (in surgical gloves), perfume (in cosmetics and air fresheners), and plants (such as primula or compositae). A good history is necessary and if suspicious, patch testing should be arranged to prove any allergy.

Irritant contact eczema can occur in any individual. It often occurs on the hands after repeated exposures to irritants such as detergents, soaps or bleach. It is therefore common in housewives, cleaners, hairdressers, mechanics and nurses.

Treatment

Treatment is as for atopic eczema as well as strict avoidance of any causative agent. This may also involve the wearing of protective clothing such as gloves, or in extreme cases (such as with chromate sensitivity in builders) even changing occupation or hobbies.

Photosensitive eczema

This is discussed on page 1340.

Lichen simplex/nodular prurigo (neurodermatitis)

These two terms are applied to a pattern of cutaneous response to scratching or rubbing in the absence of an underlying dermatosis. They are more common in Asians and also in black African and Oriental patients.

Lichen simplex appears as thickened, scaly and hyperpigmented areas of lichenification (Fig. 23.14). It starts with intense itching that becomes tender with increased rubbing or scratching. It is rare before adolescence and is commoner in females. Common sites are the nape of the neck, the lateral calves, the upper thighs, the upper back and the scrotum or vulva but any accessible site can be affected.

Nodular prurigo is a different pattern of cutaneous response to scratching, rubbing or picking. Individual, itchy papules and domed nodules appear especially on the upper trunk and the extensor surfaces of the limbs. They show significant surface damage from scratching. This is a chronic unremitting condition which is often resistant to treatment

These two conditions overlap, with some patients showing mixed features. Atopic individuals seem predisposed to develop these conditions (in the absence of obviously active eczema). However, they can occur in non-atopics. Emotional stress appears to be a contributory factor in many of these patients.

The diagnosis is made by exclusion of other pathologies and may require a skin biopsy. General medical causes of pruritus should be excluded (p. 1344). In the elderly, nodular prurigo may be an early sign of bullous pemphigoid, before the more typical blistering phase has appeared.

Treatment

Treatment is often difficult as symptoms can be intractable. Very potent topical steroids (e.g. 0.05% clobetasol propionate) with occlusive tar bandaging sometimes help. Intralesional steroids can also be useful but there is a risk of atrophy. For resistant cases (especially of prurigo lesions), phototherapy (p. 1339) and even ciclosporin (3–5 mg/kg/day) can be used but the risk/benefit ratio must be discussed with the patient as these therapies are potentially toxic.

PSORIASIS

Psoriasis is a common papulo-squamous disorder affecting 2% of the population and is characterized by well-demarcated, red scaly plaques. The skin becomes inflamed and hyperproliferates to about 10 times the normal rate. It affects males and females equally and can affect all races. The age of onset occurs in two peaks. Early onset (age 16–22) is commoner and is often associated with a positive family history. Late-onset disease peaks at age 55–60 years.

Aetiology

The condition appears to be polygenic but is also dependent on certain environmental triggers. Twin studies show 73% concordance in monozygotic twins compared with 20% of dizygotic pairs. Five genetic regions (on chromosomes 6-21p, 17q, 4q, 1q and 3q) have been linked to psoriasis but as yet no genes have been identified. Infection (group A *Streptococcus*), drugs (e.g. lithium), ultraviolet light, alcohol abuse and possibly stress may trigger or exacerbate disease in certain individuals. The exact aetiology is unknown but it is likely that psoriasis is a T-lymphocyte driven disorder to

Fig. 23.14 **Lichen simplex from chronic rubbing.**

Fig. 23.15 **Psoriasis – pathogenesis.** The figure shows the interaction of T cells with antigen-presenting cells and keratinocytes. Novel T-cell-targeted therapies are shown (red). NFAT, nuclear factor of activated T cells; ICAM, intracellular adhesion molecule; LFA, lymphocyte function-associated antigen; MHC, major histocompatibility complex; TNF, tumour necrosis factor; IL, interleukin; CLA, cutaneous lymphocyte antigen; B7 = CD80.

an unidentified antigen(s) with a possible altered response from the keratinocyte (Fig. 23.15). The initial T cell activation requires a complex interaction between T lymphocyte and antigen-presenting cell and this has provided a number of potential 'targets' for the newly developed biological therapies. This activation results in upregulation of Th1-type T cell cytokines, e.g. gamma-interferon (INF-γ), interleukins (IL-1, -2, -8), growth factors (TGF-α and TNF-α) and adhesion molecules (ICAM-1) and these are all potential therapeutic targets. The cytokine TNF-α is also produced by keratinocytes and this may be involved in both initiation and maintenance of psoriatic lesions. TNF-α blockade seems to be the most promising of the new biological agents (see Fig. 23.15).

Pathology

Skin biopsy shows acanthosis and parakeratosis, reflecting the increase in skin turnover. The granular layer is often absent. Polymorphonuclear abscesses may be seen in the upper epidermis. The epidermal rete ridges appear elongated and clubbed as they fold down into the dermis. Dermal changes include capillary dilatation surrounded by a mixed neutrophilic and lymphohistiocytic perivascular infiltrate.

Clinical features

Psoriasis can present in different clinical patterns but there is an overlap between the different forms. Certain drugs can make psoriasis worse – notably lithium, antimalarials and rarely beta-blockers.

Chronic plaque psoriasis

This is the 'common' type of psoriasis. It is characterized by pinkish red scaly plaques, especially on extensor surfaces such as knees (Fig. 23.16a) and elbows. The lower back, ears and scalp are also commonly involved. New plaques of psoriasis occur at sites of skin trauma – the so-called Köbner phenomenon. The lesions can become itchy or sore.

Flexural psoriasis

This tends to occur in later life. It is characterized by well-demarcated, red glazed plaques confined to flexures such as the groin, natal cleft and sub-mammary area. As these sites are apposed there is rarely any scaling. In the absence of psoriasis elsewhere the rash is often mis-diagnosed as candida intertrigo but the latter will normally show satellite lesions.

Guttate psoriasis

'Raindrop-like' psoriasis is a variant most commonly seen in children and young adults (Fig. 23.16b). An explosive eruption of very small circular or oval plaques appears over the trunk about 2 weeks after a streptococcal sore throat.

Erythrodermic and pustular psoriasis

These are the most severe types of psoriasis reflecting a widespread intense inflammation of the skin. They can occur together ('Von Zumbusch' psoriasis) and may be associated with malaise, pyrexia and circulatory disturb-

(a)

Fig. 23.17 **Psoriasis of the nail** – yellowish brown discoloration and distal nail plate separation (onycholysis).

(b)

Fig. 23.16 **(a) Psoriasis of the knees.**
(b) Guttate psoriasis in an African (courtesy of Dr P Matondo, Lusaka, Zambia).

ance. This form can be life-threatening. The pustules are not infected but are sterile collections of inflammatory cells. There is also a more localized variant of pustular psoriasis that confines itself to the hands and feet (palmo-plantar psoriasis) but is not associated with severe systemic symptoms. This latter type is more common in heavy cigarette smokers.

Associated features
Nails. Up to 50% of individuals with psoriasis develop nail changes (Fig. 23.17) and, rarely, these can precede the onset of skin disease. There are five types of nail change: (a) pitting of the nail plate; (b) distal separation of the nail plate (onycholysis); (c) yellow-brown discoloration; (d) subungual hyperkeratosis; (e) rarely, a damaged nail matrix and lost nail plate. Treatment of nail dystrophy is very difficult.

Arthritis. From 5–10% of individuals develop psoriatic arthritis and most of these will have nail changes.

Treatment
This is concerned with control rather than cure. It should

be tailored to the patient's wishes and not just to the doctor's assessment of disease severity. Treatments include topical agents (dithranol, tar, calcipotriol, tazarotene and corticosteroids), UVB and PUVA therapy (p. 1340) and systemic immunosuppressive/immuno-modulating agents. Severe cases may require inpatient treatment.

Chronic plaque psoriasis: emollients should always be used to hydrate the skin. Mild to moderate topical steroids, synthetic vitamin D_3 analogues (e.g. calcipotriol, calcitriol, tacalcitol), 0.05% tazarotene (a vitamin A antagonist, i.e. a retinoid) and purified coal tar are the most popular specific therapies. Salicylic acid can be a useful adjunct. All should be applied once to twice daily to palpable lesions. Once lesions have flattened, therapy can be discontinued. Dithranol can also be helpful but it causes staining of the skin and clothing and it may prove difficult to use at home on a regular basis. It is normally applied for 20–60 minutes and then washed off. It must be applied carefully to the lesions as it causes irritation to normal skin. Dithranol is more likely to induce remission than other topical therapies. Tazarotene and calcipotriol can be very irritant (calcitriol somewhat less so) so they are often used in combination with steroid creams. Vitamin D analogues should be used with caution in erythrodermic or pustular psoriasis because of hypercalcaemia.

Topical therapies are sometimes used in combination with UVB or PUVA. The 'Goeckerman regimen' consists of tar and UVB; the 'Ingram's regimen' consists of dithranol and UVB. The latter has similar results to oral PUVA in terms of clearance rates and lengths of remission – approximately 75% in 6 weeks.

Flexural psoriasis is usually treated with mild steroid and/or tar topical creams. Calcitriol and 0.1% tacrolimus ointment are also useful for treating flexural (facial and genital) psoriasis where irritation can be a problem.

Guttate psoriasis is usually treated with topical therapies and/or UVB phototherapy.

Palmo-plantar psoriasis is treated with very potent topical steroids, coal tar paste or local hand and foot PUVA.

Systemic therapy (such as methotrexate, acitretin, mycophenolate, ciclosporin or hydroxycarbamide (hydroxyurea)) are used for resistant cases.

Erythrodermic psoriasis also requires systemic therapy (but not phototherapy) as well as general supportive measures (p. 1341).

All systemic treatments must be monitored for toxicity.

Use of methotrexate. Methotrexate is normally given once weekly. Some patients experience severe nausea on the day they take it, which can be lessened by folic acid therapy. Both males and females should avoid conception during and for 3 months after therapy. Some patients are allergic to methotrexate and develop a pyrexia and mouth ulceration. Regular blood tests need to be done to monitor for bone marrow suppression and liver damage. Alcohol must be avoided as this increases the risk of hepatotoxicity. NSAIDs should also be avoided as these inhibit renal excretion. Lower doses should be used in the elderly. Long-term users will need either a liver biopsy every 2–3 years to monitor for hepatic damage or, if available, regular monitoring of their serum procollagen III peptide. Patients with concomitant psoriatic arthritis are more likely to develop pulmonary fibrosis.

Biological agents (see Fig. 23.15)

A large number of specific biological agents are being developed but only one is licensed in the UK for use in cutaneous psoriasis. They show variable efficacy and all need to be given by injection. All are prohibitively expensive.

The *TNF-α blockers* infliximab, adalimumab and etanercept (p. 563) seem to be the most effective with almost 60–80% of patients having at least a 75% improvement within 12 weeks. Many of the other agents show a disappointing lower efficacy with only 30–50% of patients showing such improvement, i.e. less than with phototherapy or methotrexate. Alefacept (a fusion protein of LFA-3 and IgG which binds to CD2) was the first biological agent to be licensed for cutaneous psoriasis, but so far only in the USA. Efalizumab is now licensed in Europe.

Long-term side-effects of these new biological agents are unknown. Infection (especially reactivation of tuberculosis) and increased malignant disease (such as skin cancer and lymphoma) remain real concerns. It seems sensible to restrict these new therapies to those patients who have failed to respond to (or cannot tolerate because of toxicity) all the conventional systemic treatments.

Prognosis

Most individuals who develop chronic plaque psoriasis will have the condition lifelong but 80% will get a remission at times. It fluctuates in severity and there are no available tests to predict outcome. Guttate psoriasis resolves spontaneously over 1–2 months and in up to a third of individuals does not recur. However, two-thirds will go on to get recurrent guttate attacks or will progress to chronic plaque psoriasis.

Fig. 23.18 Urticaria.

URTICARIA

Urticaria (hives, 'nettle rash') is a common skin condition characterized by the acute development of itchy weals or swellings in the skin because of leaky dermal vessels (Fig. 23.18). Urticaria is described as 'acute' if it lasts less than 6 weeks and 'chronic' if it persists beyond this.

Aetiology

The final event in pathogenesis involves degranulation of cutaneous mast cells, which releases a number of inflammatory mediators (including histamine) that in turn make the dermal capillaries leaky. In most cases the underlying cause is unknown. Occasionally urticaria is secondary to viral or parasitic infection, drug reactions (e.g. aspirin or penicillin allergy), food allergy (e.g. to strawberries, food colourings or seafood), or rarely systemic lupus erythematosus. There is evidence for an autoimmune aetiology in some of the 'idiopathic' cases as certain individuals develop autoantibodies against the high-affinity IgE receptor α-subunit of the mast cell. Urticaria is commoner in atopic individuals and usually presents in children and young adults.

Clinical features

The history is of cutaneous swellings or weals developing acutely over a few minutes. They can occur anywhere on the skin and last between minutes and hours before resolving spontaneously. Lesions are intensely itchy and show no surface change or scaling. Lesions are normally erythematous but if very acutely swollen, they may appear flesh-coloured or whitish and people often mistake them for blisters. Severe urticaria with subcutaneous involvement can present as soft tissue swelling (angio-oedema) especially around the eyes, the lips and the hands. This can be very alarming to the patient. It can also be dangerous if mucosal areas such as the mouth and larynx are involved but fortunately this is very rare.

Physical urticarias

Occasionally urticaria can be caused by physical stimuli such as cold (cold urticaria), deep pressure (delayed pressure urticaria), stress or heat (cholinergic urticaria), sunlight (solar urticaria, p. 1340), water (aquagenic urticaria) or chemicals such as latex (contact urticaria).

Cholinergic urticaria is one of the commonest physical urticarias and has rather different clinical lesions from the other forms. Small itchy papules rather than weals appear on the upper trunk and arms after exercise or anxiety.

Pressure can cause two types of urticaria. More superficial pressure can cause *dermographism*, which is relatively common. This presents as urticated weals occurring a few minutes after application of light pressure. Even scratching or rubbing will bring up linear weals in dermographic individuals. *Delayed pressure urticaria* is rare and occurs as deep swellings some hours after pressure is removed (e.g. on the soles of the feet or under a tight belt).

Investigations

The history is often the best guide to determining the cause of urticaria. Investigation is probably not justified unless the history suggests one of the underlying causes listed above. The physical urticarias should be reproducible by applying the relevant stimulus.

Treatment

Any identifiable underlying cause should be treated. Patients should avoid salicylates and opiates as they can degranulate mast cells. Oral antihistamines (H_1 blockers) are the most useful in treating idiopathic cases. Therapy should be started with regular use of a non-sedating antihistamine (e.g. cetirizine 10 mg daily or loratadine 10 mg daily). If control proves difficult, addition of a sedating antihistamine or an H_2 blocker may be helpful. Dietary manipulation (e.g. additive and colouring free diets) helps a small proportion of patients with chronic urticaria but it is generally unrewarding. Angio-oedema of the mouth and throat may require urgent treatment with intramuscular epinephrine (adrenaline) and intravenous steroids (see Emergency box 16.1).

Prognosis

Most cases of 'idiopathic' urticaria last a few weeks to months before disappearing spontaneously. A small percentage of people go on to develop chronic urticaria which can last for several months or years. The physical urticarias (especially cholinergic urticaria) are more persistent, often lasting for years, and they are often resistant to therapy.

Urticarial vasculitis

This is a variant of urticaria and should be suspected if individual urticarial lesions last longer than 24 hours and leave bruising behind after resolution. There is often an associated arthralgia or myalgia and a small proportion may go on to develop a connective tissue disease. The diagnosis is confirmed by skin biopsy. A full vasculitis screen should be carried out for an underlying cause (p. 581).

Treatment is with antihistamines, oral dapsone (50–100 mg daily) or immunosuppressants.

Hereditary angio-oedema.   This is an extremely rare autosomal dominant condition due to an inherited deficiency of C1-esterase inhibitor, a component of the complement system. The defect may be due to either reduced function or reduced absolute levels. Serum C2 and C4 levels are normally low but C1 and C3 are normal. Rarely this condition is acquired and associated with lymphoma or SLE. These types show low C1 esterase inhibitor levels but also low C1 levels.

Clinical features

It presents with attacks of non-itchy cutaneous angio-oedema (but no urticaria) which may last up to 72 hours. It may also present with recurrent abdominal pain (due to intestinal oedema) and there may be a family history of sudden death (due to laryngeal involvement). A non-specific erythematous rash may precede an attack of angio-oedema but urticaria is not a feature.

Treatment

In the acute setting treatment is with C1 esterase inhibitor concentrates and fresh frozen plasma. Epinephrine (adrenaline) and steroids are often ineffective. Maintenance treatment with the anabolic steroid stanozolol (or danazol) stimulates an increase in hepatic synthesis of C1 esterase inhibitor but this should not be used in children. Family members should be screened.

PITYRIASIS ROSEA

Pityriasis rosea is a self-limiting rash seen in adolescents and young adults. The cause is unknown but it is thought to be viral or post-viral. There is an increased incidence in spring and autumn and outbreaks may occur in institutions.

Clinical features

The rash consists of circular or oval pink macules with a collarette of scale and is more prominent on the trunk than on the limbs. The long axis of the oval lesions tends to run along dermatomal lines giving a 'Christmas tree' pattern on the back. The rash may be preceded by a large solitary patch with peripheral scaling ('herald patch') and this is most commonly found on the trunk. The rash is usually asymptomatic and spontaneously resolves over 4–8 weeks.

Treatment

Treatment is not normally required but 1% menthol in aqueous cream helps relieve any itch. In persistent cases UVB may be helpful.

LICHEN PLANUS

Lichen planus is a pruritic inflammatory dermatosis that is commonly associated with mucosal involvement and rarely with nail dystrophy and scarring alopecia.

The cause is unknown but a T-cell driven immune mechanism is postulated, as an almost identical rash can be caused by certain drugs (e.g. gold, levamisole,

Fig. 23.19   **Lichen planus.**

penicillamine or antimalarials) or by graft-versus-host disease.

Pathology

A mixed lymphohistiocytic infiltrate is seen at the dermoepidermal junction, which becomes ragged and saw-toothed. The basal layer shows liquefactive degeneration with the production of colloid bodies in the upper dermis. There may be acanthosis and a hyperkeratosis of the epidermis.

Clinical features

The rash is characterized by small, purple flat-topped, polygonal papules that are intensely pruritic (Fig. 23.19). It is common on the flexors of the wrists and the lower legs but can occur anywhere. There may be a fine lacy white pattern on the surface of lesions (Wickham's striae). Lesions may fuse into plaques, especially on the lower legs and in black Africans. Hyperpigmentation is common after resolution of lesions, especially in patients with pigmented skin. Atrophic, hypertrophic and annular variants can occur. Lichen planus lesions often localize to scratch marks. If lesions occur in the scalp they may cause a scarring alopecia.

Mucosal involvement is common. The mouth is the most commonly affected but the oesophagus and the anogenital region can be involved. It can present as lacy white streaks, white plaques or as ulceration. The prominent mucosal symptom is of severe pain rather than itch. Nails may be dystrophic and can be lost altogether (with scarring and 'wing' formation) in severe disease.

Prognosis

The condition often clears by 18 months but can recur at intervals. The hypertrophic and atrophic variants and mucosal disease are more persistent, lasting years. Ulcerative mucosal disease is premalignant.

Treatment

This requires the use of potent topical steroids (0.05% clobetasol propionate) and occasionally oral prednisolone (30 mg daily for 2–4 weeks). Occlusion of topical treatments can be helpful. Resistant cases may respond to PUVA, oral retinoids (0.5 mg/kg/day) or azathioprine (1–2 mg/kg daily). Topical 0.1% tacrolimus ointment has proved a very useful off-license therapy for painful mucosal disease.

GRANULOMA ANNULARE

Granuloma annulare is a dermatosis predominantly of children and young adults. It is characterized by clusters of small dermal papules (with no surface change) that often form into rings or part of a ring. They are common on the dorsal surface of the hands and feet. They are flesh coloured or slightly erythematous and are usually asymptomatic. As they heal the centre becomes dusky and altered in texture. A deep form, which is tender, exists in children. Diffuse granuloma annulare may be associated with diabetes mellitus. The pathology shows a granulomatous dermal infiltrate with foci of degeneration of collagen (necrobiosis). Spontaneous resolution often occurs but cryotherapy or triamcinolone injection may help localized disease.

LICHEN SCLEROSUS ET ATROPHICUS

Lichen sclerosus et atrophicus is a common inflammatory dermatosis that occurs in all age groups and particularly affects the anogenital region. It is more common in females. It presents with atrophic ivory-white macules with a well-defined edge, on the vulva, glans penis, foreskin or perianal skin. Telangiectasia is seen over the surface. Occasionally lesions involve the shaft of the penis and the urethral meatus. Lesions are often itchy but are sore at times. Long-standing vulval lesions are associated with fissuring and a marked loss of architecture, especially of the clitoral hood and the labium minora, which may become fused. Early lesions in young girls present as haemorrhagic blisters and these are occasionally mistaken as signs of sexual abuse. Involvement of the foreskin can cause phimosis, and urethral disease may interfere with micturition. Perianal lesions can fissure and cause constipation.

Rarely lichen sclerosus can affect non-genital skin. It is most common in females and shows rather more hyperkeratosis and follicular plugging than is seen in the anogenital region.

If the clinical picture is unclear, diagnosis may require biopsy to exclude genital lichen planus and extramammary Paget's disease. Vulval scarring can also occur with cicatricial pemphigoid (p. 1348), so occasionally immunofluorescence studies are needed.

The underlying cause is unknown but HLA associations and recent studies showing antibodies to extracellular matrix protein-1 suggest an autoimmune aetiology.

Treatment with very potent topical steroids helps control the symptoms. Hydroxychloroquine (200 mg twice daily) is used in resistant cases. The condition can burn itself out after many years, especially in children. There is a risk of developing squamous cell carcinoma in long-standing lesions. Male patients may require circumcision if phimosis does not respond to medical therapy.

FURTHER READING

Burden AD (2000) Identifying a gene for psoriasis on chromosome 6. *British Journal of Dermatology* **143**: 237–243.

Grattan C et al. (2001) Management and diagnostic guidelines for urticaria and angio-oedema. *British Journal of Dermatology* **144**: 708–714.

Heydendael VMR et al. (2003) Methotrexate versus ciclosporine in moderate-to-severe psoriasis. *New England Journal of Medicine* **349**: 658–665.

Kupper TS (2003) Immunological targets in psoriasis. *New England Journal of Medicine* **349**: 1987–1990.

Leung DYM, Bieber T (2003) Atopic dermatitis. *Lancet* **361**: 151–160.

Oyama N et al. (2003) Autoantibodies to extracellular matrix protein 1 in lichen sclerosus. *Lancet* **362**: 118–123.

Powell JJ et al. (1999) Lichen sclerosus – seminar. *Lancet* **353**: 1777–1783.

Schön W, Boehncke WH (2005) Psoriasis. *New England Journal of Medicine* **352**: 1899–1912.

FACIAL RASHES

Facial rashes often cause diagnostic confusion but a close examination of the clinical signs should help differentiate the underlying cause (Table 23.5). All facial rashes, by virtue of their visibility, can cause significant distress to the patient and this should never be underestimated.

Acne vulgaris

Acne is a common facial rash occurring in adolescence and rarely in early and mid-adult life. The cause is multifactorial but the blockage of pilosebaceous units with surrounding inflammation is the main pathological process and this can be due to a number of different factors (Fig. 23.20a).

Clinical features

Acne presents in areas rich in sebaceous glands such as the face, back and sternal area. The three cardinal features are:

Table 23.5	Causes of facial rashes
Acne vulgaris	Perioral dermatitis
Rosacea	Photosensitivity
Seborrhoeic eczema	Sarcoidosis
Atopic eczema	Chronic discoid lupus erythematosus
Contact eczema	Systemic lupus erythematosus
Dermatomyositis	Subacute lupus erythematosus

Fig. 23.20 (a) Pathophysiology of acne vulgaris (b) Acne vulgaris.

- open comedones (blackheads) or closed comedones (whiteheads)
- inflammatory papules
- pustules (Fig. 23.20b).

The skin may be very greasy (seborrhoea). Rupture of the inflamed lesions may lead to deep-seated dermal inflammation and nodulocystic lesions, which are more likely to cause facial scarring. A premenstrual exacerbation of acne is sometimes noticed. There is a tendency for spontaneous improvement over a number of years but acne can persist unabated into adult life.

A number of clinical variants exist:

- *Infantile acne.* Facial acne is occasionally seen in infants and is sometimes cystic. It is thought to be due to the influence of maternal androgens and resolves spontaneously.
- *Steroid acne.* Acne may occur secondary to corticosteroid therapy or Cushing's syndrome. Comedones and cysts are rare in this variant but involvement of the back and shoulders (rather than the face) is common. Clinically the rash often appears as a pustular folliculitis.

- *Oil acne.* This is an industrial disease seen in workers who have prolonged contact with oils or other hydrocarbons and is common on the legs and other exposure sites.
- *Acne fulminans.* This is a rare variant seen most commonly in young male adolescents. Severe necrotic and crusted acne lesions appear, associated with malaise, pyrexia, arthralgia and bone pain (due to sterile bone cysts). It requires urgent treatment with oral prednisolone (30–40 mg daily) and analgesics followed by a course of oral isotretinoin (see below).
- *'Follicular occlusion triad'.* This is a rare disorder most commonly seen in black Africans. It is characterized by the presence of severe nodulocystic acne, dissecting cellulitis of the scalp (p. 1361) and hidradenitis suppurativa (p. 1320). It has been suggested that this is caused by a problem of follicular occlusion rather than having an infective aetiology.

Treatment

Treatment is aimed at decreasing sebum production, decreasing bacteria, normalizing duct keratinization or decreasing inflammation.

Regular washing with acne soaps to remove excess grease should be encouraged (normal soaps can be comedogenic). 'Picking' should be discouraged.

First-line therapy

Topical agents are used for mild acne such as antibiotics (tetracycline, clindamycin) and keratolytics (benzoyl peroxide); these are similar in efficacy and the latter have the advantage of not causing antibiotic resistance. Topical retinoids (tretinoin) or retinoid-like agents (adapalene) are also used. If these fail, second-line agents should be added.

Second-line therapy

- *Low-dose oral antibiotic therapy* often helps but must be given for at least 3–4 months. Oxytetracycline 500 mg twice daily is often used first. Minocycline 100 mg daily, erythromycin 500 mg twice daily or trimethoprim 100 mg twice daily is also used.
- An extra treatment 'cyproterone acetate 2 mg/ ethinylestradiol 35 μg' (co-cyprindol) is of value in females if there is no contraindication to oral contraception. This acts as a normal combined contraceptive but has antiandrogen activity. It may take 6–8 months to have its maximum effect.
- *UVB phototherapy* can be helpful but is rarely used now owing to the development of retinoid drugs.

Third-line therapy

Third-line treatment with a retinoid drug (isotretinoin) should be given if:

- the above measures fail
- there is nodulocystic acne with scarring
- there is severe psychological disturbance.

Use of retinoids (isotretinoin or acitretin). Retinoids are synthetic vitamin A analogues that affect cell growth and differentiation. They are very teratogenic.

Isotretinoin is a 'hospital-only drug' in most countries because of its teratogenicity and is restricted to the use of dermatologists. A pregnancy test and contraceptive advice are mandatory prior to its use in fertile women, and new UK regulations demand that this is done monthly during treatment. It is given as a 4-month course at a dose of 0.5–1 mg/kg/day. Over 90% of individuals will respond to this therapy and 65% of people will obtain a long-term 'cure'.

Patients must avoid pregnancy during therapy and for 1 month after stopping isotretinoin (but for 2 years after stopping acitretin as it is very lipophilic). Both drugs cause drying of the skin, especially of the lips and nasal mucosa. Hair thinning and exercise-induced myalgia are not uncommon. Blood count, liver function and fasting lipids need to be monitored during therapy. In a few individuals retinoids may cause depression but it should also be remembered that acne itself has been a cause of suicide.

Potential new treatment

A single study has shown pulsed-dye laser therapy to have some benefit in mild to moderate acne but was not curative. Further work is needed to establish its effectiveness, the optimum 'dosing' schedule and long-term safety.

Rosacea

Rosacea (Fig. 23.21) is a common inflammatory rash predominantly affecting the face. The onset is usually in middle age and it is commoner in women. It often causes significant psychological distress.

The cause is unknown. Theories have suggested an underlying problem in vasomotor stability of blood vessels or a role of the skin mite *Demodex* but there is little evidence to confirm these speculations.

Fig. 23.21 **Rosacea.** Papules and pustules on a background erythema. There are no comedones.

Clinical features

The cardinal features are of facial flushing, inflammatory papules and pustules affecting the nose forehead and cheeks. The flushing may precede the other signs by some years. There are no comedones. Additional features may include dilated blood vessels (telangiectasia), inflammation of the eyelid margins (blepharitis), keratitis and sebaceous gland hypertrophy especially of the nose. The latter is commoner in men and can cause a disfiguring enlargement of the nose called rhinophyma. The flushing may be exacerbated by alcohol, hot drinks, sunlight and changes in ambient temperature. Prolonged use of topical steroids can exacerbate or trigger the condition. As the disease progresses the flushing may be replaced by a permanent erythema.

Treatment

This is suppressive rather than curative. Long-term use of topical 0.075% metronidazole may help. Avoid topical steroids. A 3-month course of oral tetracycline (500 mg twice daily) is also helpful. Oral metronidazole (400 mg twice daily) or oral isotretinoin (0.5–1 mg/kg/day) is occasionally given in resistant cases (p. 1338). The papules and pustules tend to respond best to therapy but repeat courses may be necessary. The flushing and erythema are often resistant to treatment but cosmetic camouflage can be helpful for these features. Intense pulse light or pulsed-dye laser therapy can help the erythema and telangiectasia but often needs to be repeated as they tend to recur. Rhinophyma can be treated with plastic surgery or by carbon dioxide laser.

Perioral dermatitis

Perioral dermatitis is a common rash found around the mouth, especially in young females. The exact cause is unknown but it often has an iatrogenic component as topical steroids often exacerbate the condition in the long term.

Clinical features

It presents with erythema, scaling, papules and occasionally pustules around the mouth. It usually spares a halo of skin immediately adjacent to the lips.

Treatment

Treatment involves stopping topical steroids, although they may have to be withdrawn slowly to prevent too severe a rebound after withdrawal. The mainstay of treatment is with a 3- to 4-month course of low-dose oxytetracycline or erythromycin (both 500 mg twice daily) and topical metronidazole.

FURTHER READING

[Anonymous] (2003) Acne isotretinoin and depression. (Review) *Drugs and Therapeutics Bulletin* **41**: 76–78.

James WD (2005) Acne. *New England Journal of Medicine* **352**: 1463–1472

Seaton ED et al. (2003) Pulsed-dye laser treatment for inflammatory acne vulgaris: randomised controlled trial. *Lancet* **362**: 1347–1352 (and editorial, p. 1342).

PHOTODERMATOLOGY

Sunlight – light in the ultraviolet (UV) part of the spectrum – combines short, medium and long wavelengths (UVC, UVB, and UVA respectively). Both UVB and UVA can penetrate the atmosphere and reach the skin. This light energy is potentially mutagenic and carcinogenic but it can also suppress cutaneous inflammation. Thus UV irradiation can both *cause* skin disease and be used to *treat* it.

Photosensitive rashes usually appear on sites exposed to the sun's rays, such as the face, the anterior 'V' of the chest, the ears and the backs of the hands. Certain 'protected' areas are characteristically spared such as under the chin or the upper eyelid and between the finger webs. Porphyria, drug sensitivity and lupus erythematosus should be excluded in all photosensitive patients.

Photosensitive rashes may be divided into photoexacerbated/provoked rashes and the idiopathic photodermatoses (Table 23.6). The former are discussed on pages 574 (SLE), 245 (pellagra) and 1148 (porphyria).

Phototherapy and photoprotection

Phototherapy

UVB and UVA are both used in the treatment of inflammatory dermatoses. They have a suppressive effect on cutaneous inflammation and there is evidence that they can suppress systemic immunoreactivity to some degree. However, both types can cause skin ageing and predispose to skin malignancy if excessive doses are used. This is more of a problem in white-skinned

Table 23.6   Differential diagnosis of photosensitive rashes

Photoexacerbated/provoked rashes

Systemic disease	SLE, CDLE, SCLE (p. 574)
Metabolic disease	Porphyrias (pp. 1148 and 1346), pellagra (p. 245)
Drugs	Thiazides, phenothiazines, tetracyclines, amiodarone
Plant phototoxins	Phytophotodermatitis (photosensitivity induced by contact of the skin with certain plants, e.g. celery, hogweed, rue)
Skin disease	Rosacea
	Rarely atopic eczema, psoriasis, lichen planus (these normally improve in sunlight)

Idiopathic photodermatoses

Polymorphic light eruption
Chronic actinic dermatitis
Solar urticaria

CDLE, chronic discoid lupus erythematosus
SCLE, subacute cutaneous lupus erythematosus

individuals. Unaffected regions of skin or high-risk areas like the scrotum can be screened during phototherapy.

UVB is less carcinogenic than UVA. *Narrow-band UVB* (311 nanometre) is used more than broad-band UVB because it is much more effective and less likely to burn. It is used in the treatment of eczema and psoriasis (especially in children) and is given three times per week for 6–10 weeks. Eye protection needs to be worn during therapy.

UVA is relatively ineffective on its own so is used in conjunction with a photosensitizer ('psoralen') hence the term 'PUVA'. The psoralen can be given by mouth or applied to the skin in bath water. PUVA is given twice per week and eye protection must been worn *for the whole of the treatment day* as the psoralen sensitizes the retina. It is more effective than narrow-band UVB but is limited by its carcinogenic potential, especially squamous cancer. A maximum dose is given over a lifetime depending on skin type (1000 joules or 200 sessions approximately). It is used for many conditions including psoriasis, eczema, cutaneous T cell lymphoma, some photosensitive dermatoses and vitiligo.

Sunbeds are used for tanning and consist of predominantly UVA light; they are therefore rarely effective in treating skin disease. If used frequently there is an increased risk of skin cancer and premature ageing.

Photoprotection

There are two broad classes of sunblock cream: they either absorb UV light (e.g. aminobenzoic acid or methoxycinnamate) or reflect it (e.g. titanium dioxide). Most modern creams protect against UVA and UVB to varying degrees. UVB protection is graded by the 'sun protection factor' (SPF): an SPF of 15 implies you can spend 15 times as long in the sun before burning providing it is applied correctly. SPFs above 15 confer little extra protection. There is no standardized way of assessing efficiency against UVA. Some sunscreens (especially aminobenzoates) may rarely cause photo-sensitization. This can be proven by photopatch testing.

IDIOPATHIC PHOTODERMATOSES

Polymorphic light eruption (PLE)

This is the most common photosensitive eruption in temperate regions, affecting up to 10–20% of the population. It is most common in young women. In many it is mild and often goes undiagnosed. An itchy rash appears some hours after sun exposure which is strictly confined to the exposed sites. Lesions may be papules, vesicles or plaques. They can last for several hours or several days. The condition starts in spring and often improves during the summer because of skin 'hardening'.

Treatment

Avoidance of sunlight and the use of sunblocks are helpful in mild cases. Topical steroids help treat an attack. In those individuals who only get PLE after very intense sun exposure (e.g. on sunny holidays) a short course of oral prednisolone (30 mg daily for 7–10 days) will often prevent or treat an attack. For resistant cases 'desensitization' with low-dose PUVA (or narrow-band UVB) in the springtime may be required but patients will need to 'top up' their sun exposure from natural sunlight during the summer to keep their skin desensitized.

Chronic actinic dermatitis (photosensitive eczema, actinic reticuloid)

This is a relatively rare type of eczema occurring in a photosensitive distribution over the face, neck and hands. It typically affects middle-aged or elderly males. There may be a pre-existing eczema, so the subsequent development of photosensitivity is often missed. This is further confounded by the fact that the eczema usually will spread to affect skin not exposed to sunlight, and in fact the patient can become erythrodermic. The skin has typical features of eczema but there is often marked skin thickening. Histology is often atypical and can look almost lymphoma-like. The diagnosis can be confirmed by specialist monochromator light-testing. The most severe cases can be exacerbated by even artificial lighting, as these patients can become exquisitely photosensitive.

Treatment

This consists of strict avoidance of sunlight, including high-factor sunblocks and screening of house and car windows. Topical steroids and emollients are useful in milder cases. Oral prednisolone may be needed and azathioprine (1–2 mg/kg daily) should be considered for long-term suppression. Low-dose PUVA under steroid cover may help with 'desensitization'.

Solar urticaria

This is extremely rare. Itchy urticarial lesions occur within minutes of sun exposure and characteristically settle within 1–2 hours. Sun avoidance, sunblocks, H_1 antihistamines and low-dose PUVA are all used in treatment.

FURTHER READING
Hawk JLM (ed) (1999) *Photodermatology*, London: Arnold.
Stern RS (2004) Treatment of photoaging. *New England Journal of Medicine* **350**: 1526–1534.

ERYTHRODERMA

Erythroderma, meaning 'red skin', refers to the clinical state of inflammation or redness of all (or nearly all) of the skin. It is sometimes called *exfoliative dermatitis*, but dermatitis is not always present.

Aetiology

There are a number of underlying causes (Table 23.7); previous skin disease and drugs are the most common.

Table 23.7 Causes of erythroderma

Common
Atopic eczema
Psoriasis
Drugs (e.g. sulphonamides, gold, sulphonylureas, penicillin, allopurinol, captopril)
Seborrhoeic eczema
Idiopathic

Rare
Chronic actinic dermatitis
Cutaneous T-cell lymphoma (Sézary syndrome) (p. 1353)
Malignancy (especially leukaemias)
Pemphigus foliaceus
Pityriasis rubra pilaris (a hereditary disorder of keratinization)
HIV infection
Toxic shock syndrome (p. 64)

Clinical features

It is commoner in males and later in life. Patients often complain of their skin feeling 'tight' as well as itchy. Long-standing erythroderma is often associated with hair loss, ectropion of the eyelids and even nail shedding. Systemic symptoms are common such as malaise, pyrexia, widespread lymphadenopathy and other complications (see below). Erythroderma can occasionally lead to death so it should be regarded as a medical 'emergency'.

Examination should specifically look for pustules and nail changes suggestive of psoriasis.

A skin biopsy may elucidate the cause, especially of cutaneous lymphoma. Techniques such as T-cell receptor gene rearrangement studies (looking for evidence of clonal T cell expansion in the skin and blood) are also useful in the diagnosis of lymphoma.

A number of cases defy an exact diagnosis and a lymph node biopsy is required. If there is no malignancy, lymph nodes normally show non-specific, reactive (dermatopathic) changes.

Complications

The skin is one of the largest organs of the body; perhaps it is no surprise that inflammation of the whole organ can cause metabolic and haemodynamic problems including:

- high-output cardiac failure from increased blood flow
- hypothermia from heat loss
- fluid loss by transpiration
- hypoalbuminaemia
- increased basal metabolic rate
- 'capillary leak syndrome'.

Capillary leak syndrome is the most severe complication and has been responsible for a fatal outcome in some cases of psoriasis, although this is extremely rare. It is thought that the inflamed skin releases large quantities of cytokines that cause a generalized vascular leakage. This can cause cutaneous oedema and leaky vessels in the lungs, resulting in acute lung injury (p. 986).

Treatment

Treatment of erythroderma is best initiated in hospital. Patients must be kept very warm (with space blankets and heaters), with fluid-balance charts. Their vital signs should be monitored regularly. Changes in electrolytes, albumin and circulatory status should be monitored regularly. Swabs should be taken to detect any secondary skin infection.

The skin condition is treated with bed rest and either a bland emollient or a mild topical steroid. All non-essential drugs should be stopped. Where known, the underlying cause should be treated. The blanket use of systemic steroid therapy for erythroderma remains controversial in view of possible side-effects.

Advanced capillary leak syndrome will require specialized haemodynamic management in an intensive care unit.

FURTHER READING
Rothe MJ et al. (2000) Erythroderma. *Dermatologic Clinics* **18**: 405–415.

CUTANEOUS SIGNS OF SYSTEMIC DISEASE

Some dermatoses are associated with a variety of underlying systemic diseases. Furthermore some medical conditions may present with cutaneous features.

Erythema nodosum

Erythema nodosum has a number of underlying causes (Table 23.8). It presents as painful or tender dusky blue-red nodules, commonly over the shins or lower limbs, which fade over 2–3 weeks leaving a bruised appearance (see Fig. 23.39). It is most common in young adults, especially females. It may be associated with arthralgia, malaise and fever. The inflammation involves the dermis and the subcutaneous layer (panniculitis).

Treatment

Symptomatic therapy with non-steroidal anti-inflammatory drugs (avoid in pregnancy), light compression bandaging and bed rest are all that are necessary as the condition resolves spontaneously. The underlying cause

Table 23.8 Causes of erythema nodosum

Streptococcal infection*
Drugs* (e.g. sulphonamides, oral contraceptive)
Sarcoidosis*
Idiopathic*
Yersinia infection
Fungal infection (histoplasmosis, blastomycosis)
Tuberculosis
Leprosy
Inflammatory bowel disease
Chlamydia infection

*Common causes in the UK

should be treated. In very persistent cases dapsone (100 mg daily), colchicine (500 µg twice daily) or prednisolone (up to 30 mg daily) can be useful.

Erythema multiforme

Erythema multiforme (EM) is a hypersensitivity rash of acute onset frequently caused by infection or drugs. A cell-mediated T lymphocytic response is seen in the skin, which causes epidermal cell death.

In 50% of cases, the cause is not found but the following should be considered:

- herpes simplex virus (the most common identifiable cause)
- other viral infections (e.g. EBV, orf disease)
- drugs (e.g. sulphonamide, anticonvulsants)
- mycoplasma infection
- connective tissue disease (e.g. SLE, polyarteritis nodosa)
- HIV infection
- Wegener's granulomatosis
- carcinoma, lymphoma.

Clinically the lesions can be erythematous, polycyclic, annular or show concentric rings called 'target lesions' (Fig. 23.22). Frank blistering is not uncommon. The rash tends to be symmetrical and commonly affects the limbs, especially the hands and feet where palms and soles may be involved. Occasionally there is severe mucosal involvement leading to necrotic ulcers of the mouth and genitalia, and a conjunctivitis ('EM major' – previously called Stevens–Johnson syndrome – see Box 23.3). The term 'EM minor' may be used for cases without mucosal involvement.

Fig. 23.22 **Erythema multiforme major** – target lesions of **(a)** the palm and **(b)** with mucosal involvement around the mouth.

 Box 23.3 **Stevens–Johnson syndrome**

This term is now used for a mild form of toxic epidermal necrolysis (p. 1359) which shares similar mucosal lesions to 'erythema multiforme major' but does not show typical target lesions. Both Stevens–Johnson syndrome and toxic epidermal necrolysis are more likely to be drug induced.

Erythema multiforme usually resolves in 2–4 weeks. Rarely, recurrent erythema multiforme can occur and this is triggered by herpes simplex infection in 80% of cases.

Treatment

This is symptomatic and involves treating the underlying cause. Some advocate the use of oral steroids in severe disease but this remains controversial.

Recurrent erythema multiforme can be treated with prophylactic oral aciclovir (200 mg twice daily) even if no cause has been found, as 80% appear to be driven by herpes simplex virus. In resistant cases, azathioprine (1–2 mg/kg daily) is used.

Pyoderma gangrenosum

Pyoderma gangrenosum is of unknown aetiology and presents with erythematous nodules or pustules which frequently ulcerate (Fig. 23.23). The ulcers can be large and grow at an alarming speed. The ulcer has a typical bluish black ('gangrenous') undermined edge and a purulent surface ('pyoderma'). There may be an associated pyrexia and malaise. Biopsy through the ulcer edge shows an intense neutrophilic infiltrate and occasionally a vasculitis but the diagnosis depends mostly on the clinical appearance. The main causes are:

- inflammatory bowel disease
- rheumatoid arthritis
- myeloma, leukaemia, lymphoma
- liver disease (primary biliary cirrhosis)
- idiopathic (> 20% in some series).

Treatment

This is with very potent topical steroids or 0.1% tacrolimus ointment. High-dose oral steroids may be needed to prevent rapidly progressive ulceration. Oral dapsone and minocycline may help. Other immuno-suppressants, such as ciclosporin, are useful in resistant cases. The underlying cause should be treated.

Fig. 23.23 **Pyoderma gangrenosum.**

Fig. 23.24 Acanthosis nigricans.

Acanthosis nigricans

Acanthosis nigricans presents as thickened, hyper-pigmented skin predominantly of the flexures (Fig. 23.24). It can appear warty or velvety when advanced. In early life it is seen in obese individuals who have very high levels of insulin owing to insulin resistance (and this is sometimes termed 'pseudo-acanthosis nigricans'). In older people it normally reflects an underlying malignancy (especially gastrointestinal tumours). Rarely it is associated with hyperandrogenism in females.

Treatment

Topical or oral retinoids (0.5 mg/kg/day) may help (p. 1338) and weight loss is advised in the obese. Any underlying malignancy should be treated.

Dermatomyositis (see also p. 579)

The rash is distinctive. Facial erythema and a magenta-coloured rash around the eyes with associated oedema are often present. Bluish red nodules or plaques may be present over the knuckles and extensor surfaces. The nail folds are frequently ragged with dilated capillaries. The diagnosis is made from the clinical appearance, muscle biopsy, EMG and a serum creatine phosphokinase. Skin biopsy is not diagnostic.

There is a childhood form which usually occurs before the age of 10 and which eventually resolves. This type is often associated with calcinosis in the skin and can cause significant long-term functional problems with weak muscles and contractures. Life-threatening bowel infarction can also occur in the childhood form. The adult form usually occurs after the age of 40. Some cases are associated with an underlying malignancy, whereas others appear to reflect a 'connective tissue disease'. This latter group may overlap with scleroderma and lupus erythematosus.

Treatment

Skin disease may respond to hydroxychloroquine (200 mg twice daily) as well as immunosuppressants, e.g. azathioprine or ciclosporin.

Scleroderma (see also p. 577)

The term scleroderma refers to a thickening or hardening of the skin owing to abnormal dermal collagen. It is not a diagnostic entity in itself. Systemic sclerosis and morphoea both show sclerodermatous changes but are separate conditions.

Systemic sclerosis (often called scleroderma) has cutaneous and systemic features and is discussed fully on page 577.

Morphoea is confined to the skin and usually presents in children or young adults. It is commoner in females and the cause is unknown. Lesions are usually on the trunk and appear as bluish red plaques which progress to induration and then central white atrophy. A linear variant exists in childhood which is more severe as it can cause atrophy of underlying deep tissues and thus can cause unequal limb growth or scarring alopecia.

Rarely, sclerodermatous skin changes may be seen in chronic Lyme disease (acrodermatitis chronica atrophicans), chronic graft-versus-host disease, polyvinyl chloride disease, eosinophilic myalgia syndrome (due to tryptophan therapy) and bleomycin therapy.

Lupus erythematosus (LE)

There are three clinical variants to this disease but some patients may show features of more than one type.

- chronic discoid lupus erythematosus (CDLE)
- subacute lupus erythematosus (SCLE)
- systemic lupus erythematosus (SLE).

The aetiology is unknown but is due to abnormality in immune function as variable autoantibodies may be found in all types. Very rarely it can be induced by certain drugs such as phenothiazines, hydralazine, methyldopa, isoniazid, tetracycline, mesalazine and penicillin.

Chronic discoid lupus erythematosus (CDLE)

CDLE is the most common type of LE seen by dermatologists and more frequently affects females. Clinically it presents with fixed erythematous, scaly, atrophic plaques with telangiectasia, especially on the face or other sun-exposed sites (Fig. 23.25). Hypo-pigmentation is common and follicular plugging occurs. Scalp involvement leads to a scarring alopecia. Oral involvement (erythematous patches or ulceration) occurs in 25% of cases.

CDLE can be triggered and exacerbated by UV exposure. A few patients also suffer with Raynaud's phenomenon or unusual chilblain-like lesions (chilblain lupus). Only 5% of cases will go on to develop SLE but this is more common in children. Serum antinuclear antibody (ANA) is positive in 30% of cases.

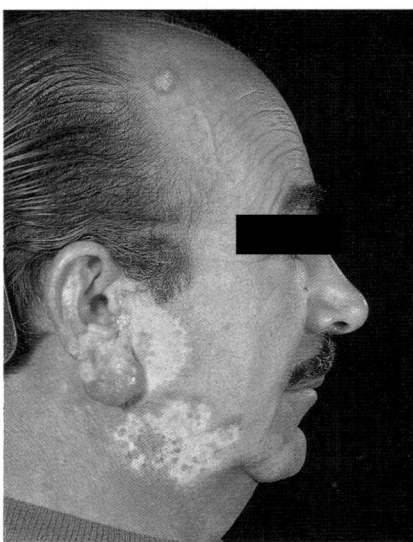

Fig. 23.25 **Chronic discoid lupus erythematosus**, showing scaling, atrophy and hypopigmentation.

Fig. 23.26 **Systemic lupus erythematosus** – showing the structural sites of damage in bullous disorders. LAD, linear IgA disease; EB, epidermolysis bullosa.

Skin biopsy shows a dense patchy, dermal lymphohistiocytic infiltrate which often is centred on appendages. Epidermal basal layer damage, follicular plugging and hyperkeratosis may be present. Direct immunofluorescence studies of lesional skin may show the presence of IgM and C3 at the dermoepidermal junction ('lupus band').

Treatment

First-line therapy is with sunscreens and potent topical steroids. Certain oral antimalarials (hydroxychloroquine 100–200 mg twice daily and mepacrine 100 mg daily) can prove very useful and are generally safe for long-term intermittent use. Oral prednisolone is beneficial but its use is limited by its side-effect profile. Azathioprine, retinoids, ciclosporin and thalidomide can be useful in resistant cases.

Prognosis

The disease is usually chronic, although it may fluctuate in severity. CDLE remains confined to the skin in most patients and it will eventually go into remission in up to 50% of cases (after many years).

Subacute lupus erythematosus (SCLE)

SCLE is a rare cutaneous variant of LE. It presents with widespread indurated, sometimes urticated, erythematous lesions, often on the upper trunk. The lesions can also be annular. Photosensitivity is often a prominent feature. Complications, such as arthralgia and mouth ulceration, are seen but significant organ involvement is rare. ANF and extractable nuclear antibodies (anti-Ro and anti-La) are usually positive (see p. 534).

Treatment is with oral dapsone, antimalarials or systemic immunosuppression (prednisolone and ciclosporin).

Systemic lupus erythematosus (SLE)
(see also p. 574)

The cutaneous involvement of SLE is one of the minor problems of the disease but it may be the presenting feature.

Features include macular erythema over the cheeks, nose and forehead ('butterfly rash', Fig. 23.26). Palmar erythema, dilated nail fold capillaries, splinter haemorrhages and digital infarcts of the finger tips may also be seen but are not always noticed by the patient. Joint swellings, livedo reticularis and purpura are occasionally seen. Rarely SLE can be complicated by an atypical erythema multiforme-like rash ('Rowell's syndrome'). Treatment (p. 576) is usually managed by a rheumatologist.

Pruritus

The pathophysiology of pruritus is poorly understood but is due to peripheral mechanisms (e.g. skin disease), central or neuropathic mechanisms (e.g. multiple sclerosis), neurogenic (e.g. cholestasis/μ-opioid receptor stimulation, p. 386) or psychogenic mechanisms (e.g. parasitophobia). Evidence suggests that low stimulation of unmyelinated C-fibres in the skin is associated with the sensation of itch (high stimulation produces pain). Histamine, tachykinins (e.g. substance P) and cytokines (e.g. interleukin-2) may also play a role peripherally in the skin. The major nerve pathways for itch and the influence of the central nervous system are not well characterized but opioid μ-receptor-dependent processes can regulate the perception and intensity of itch.

Pruritus (see lichen simplex, nodular prurigo/neurodermatitis) in the absence of a demonstrable rash can be caused by a number of different medical problems (Table 23.9).

Table 23.9 Medical conditions associated with pruritus

Iron deficiency anaemia
Internal malignancy (especially lymphoma)
Diabetes mellitus
Chronic renal failure
Chronic liver disease (especially primary biliary cirrhosis)
Thyroid disease
HIV infection
Polycythaemia vera

Asteatotic eczema and cholinergic urticaria are common causes of pruritus where the rash is often missed. The term idiopathic pruritus or 'senile' pruritus probably overlaps with asteatotic eczema and this is common in the elderly.

Treatment involves avoiding soaps and using symptomatic measures (as for asteatotic eczema). Phototherapy may help intractable cases. Oral opiate antagonists, which act centrally, are under assessment. Underlying medical problems should be treated.

Sarcoidosis (see also p. 934)

Sarcoidosis is a multisystem granulomatous disorder of unknown aetiology. It can present as reddish brown dermal papules and nodules, especially around the eyelid margins and the rim of the nostrils. More polymorphic lesions (papules nodules and plaques) may appear on the body. It is most common in black Africans where it is often accompanied by hypo- or hyperpigmentation. Rarely it can present with a bluish red infiltrate or swelling, especially of the nose or ears, called lupus pernio. Both these types of lesion can be seen anywhere on the body but are common on the face. Erythema nodosum (p. 1341) of the shins is sometimes seen in acute-onset sarcoidosis. Erythema nodosum is an immunological reaction and not due to sarcoid tissue infiltration. Swollen fingers from a dactylitis occur. Whilst sarcoidosis may be confined to the skin, all patients should be investigated for evidence of systemic disease (p. 934).

Treatment of cutaneous lesions includes very potent topical steroids (0.05% clobetasol propionate), intralesional steroids, oral steroids and occasionally methotrexate or antimalarials.

Neurofibromatosis type 1 (von Recklinghausen's disease) (see also p. 1257 and Table 3.4)

Type 1 neurofibromatosis is an autosomal dominant condition with complete penetrance. It often presents in childhood with a variety of cutaneous features. Many cases are new mutations in the *NF1* gene. Early signs include *café-au-lait* spots (brown macules, greater than 2.5 cm in diameter and more than five lesions) and axillary freckling. Lisch nodules (hyperpigmented iris hamartomas) may be seen in the eyes by slit lamp examination. Later on, fleshy skin tags and deeper soft tumours (neurofibromas) appear and they may progress to completely cover the skin causing significant cosmetic disability. Learning difficulties and skeletal dysplasias occur. A number of endocrine disorders may be rarely associated including phaeochromocytoma, acromegaly and Addison's disease.

Tuberous sclerosis (epiloia)

Tuberous sclerosis is also an autosomal dominant condition of variable severity which may not present until later childhood. It is characterized by a variety of hamartomatous growths. The three cardinal features are (a) mental retardation, (b) epilepsy, and (c) cutaneous abnormalities – but not all have to be present. The skin signs include:

- adenoma sebaceum (reddish papules/fibromas around the nose)
- periungual fibroma (nodules arising from the nail bed)
- shagreen patches (firm, flesh-coloured plaques on the trunk)
- ash-leaf hypopigmentation (pale macules best seen with UV light)
- forehead plaque (indurated flesh-coloured patch)
- *café-au-lait* patches
- pitting of dental enamel.

Internal hamartomas can arise in the heart, kidney, retina and CNS. Parents of a suspected case should be carefully examined (under UV light) as they may have a forme fruste of the condition which can manifest just as hypopigmented patches. This would have genetic implications for future offspring.

Diabetes mellitus (see also p. 1131)

Diabetes mellitus can have a number of cutaneous features. Complications of diabetes itself include:

- fungal infection (e.g. candidiasis)
- bacterial infections (e.g. recurrent boils)
- xanthomas
- arterial disease (ulcers, gangrene)
- neuropathic ulcers.

Specific dermatoses of diabetes include:

- necrobiosis lipoidica (a patch of spreading erythema over the shin which becomes yellowish and atrophic in the centre and may ulcerate)
- diffuse granuloma annulare (p. 1336)
- diabetic dermopathy (red-brown flat-topped papules)
- blisters (usually on the feet or hands)
- diabetic stiff skin (tight waxy skin over the fingers with limitation of joint movement owing to thickened collagen – also called cheiroarthropathy).

Chronic liver disease (see also p. 357)

Chronic liver disease may present with jaundice, palmar erythema, spider naevi, white nails, hyperpigmentation and pruritus.

Porphyria cutanea tarda (PCT, p. 1149) is a rare genetic disorder associated with liver disease usually due to hepatic damage from excessive alcohol consumption or hepatitis C infection: 75% of cases are sporadic, 25% familial. Overall, 20% of cases have underlying hereditary haemochromatosis (p. 386). It presents clinically on exposed skin with sun-induced blisters, skin fragility, scarring, milia and hypertrichosis. Treatment of the cutaneous features is with repeated venesection and/or very low-dose chloroquine plus an avoidance of alcohol. There is anecdotal evidence that specific treatment of hepatitis C (p. 373) will also help the skin, presumably through improving liver function. All forms of PCT are at risk of hepatic carcinoma.

Chronic renal failure (see also p. 668)

Chronic renal failure is commonly associated with intractable pruritus. Pallor, hyperpigmentation and ecchymoses are commonly seen. Rarely it is associated with non-inflammatory blisters, pseudo-porphyria cutanea tarda and cutaneous calcification. Long-standing renal transplant patients often suffer with recurrent viral warts and squamous cell carcinomas due to the immunosuppression.

Thyroid disease (see also p. 1069)

Hypothyroidism may cause dry firm gelatinous (myxoedematous) skin with diffuse hair thinning and a loss of the outer third of the eyebrows. Hyperthyroidism may be associated with warm sweaty skin and a diffuse alopecia. Graves' disease is rarely associated with thyroid acropachy ('clubbing' with underlying bone changes) and pretibial myxoedema (a red-brown mucinous infiltration of the shins which can become lumpy and tender).

Cushing's syndrome (see also p. 1085)

Cushing's syndrome may cause hirsutism, a moon face, a buffalo hump, stretch marks (striae) and a pustular folliculitis (often called steroid acne) of the skin.

Hyperlipidaemias (see also p. 1138)

Hyperlipidaemias can present with xanthomas, which are abnormal collections of lipid in the skin. All patients with xanthomas should be investigated for hyperlipidaemia although the most common type called xanthelasma (yellow plaques around the eyes) are usually associated with normal lipids. There are a number of other clinical variants of xanthomas such as (i) tuberous xanthoma (firm orange-yellow nodules and plaques on extensor surfaces), (ii) tendon xanthoma (firm subcutaneous swellings attached to tendons), (iii) plane xanthoma (orange-yellow macules often affecting palmar creases), (iv) eruptive xanthoma (numerous small yellowish papules commonly on the buttocks).

Table 23.10 Non-metastatic cutaneous manifestations of underlying malignancy

Dermatosis	Tumour
Dermatomyositis	Lung, GI tract, GU tract
Acanthosis nigricans	GI tract, lung, liver
Paget's disease (localized patch of eczema around the nipple)	Ductal breast carcinoma
Erythroderma	Lymphoma/leukaemia
Tylosis (thickened palms/soles)	Oesophageal carcinoma
Ichthyosis (dry flaking of skin)	Lymphoma
Erythema gyratum repens (concentric rings of erythema which change rapidly)	Lung, breast
Necrolytic migratory erythema (burning, geographic and spreading annular areas of erythema)	Glucagonoma

Cutaneous amyloid

Cutaneous amyloid can be confined to the skin or be part of systemic disease (p. 1148). Macular amyloid is a common, purely cutaneous variant seen in Asians. It is characterized by itchy brown rippled macules on the upper back.

Systemic amyloid may be associated with reddish brown papules, nodules or plaques, especially around the eyes, the flexural areas and mucosal surfaces. Distinctive periorbital bruising and macroglossia may also be present.

Systemic malignant disease

Certain rashes may be a non-metastatic manifestation of an underlying malignancy (Table 23.10). Rarely tumours can metastasize to the skin where they normally present as papules or nodules which may proceed to ulceration.

FURTHER READING
Crawford GH et al. (2002) Skin signs of systemic disease: an update. *Advances in Dermatology* **18**: 1–27.
English JC et al. (2001) Sarcoidosis. *Journal of the American Academy of Dermatology* **44**: 725–743.
Robinson-Boston L (2000) Cutaneous manifestations of end-stage renal disease. *Journal of the American Academy of Dermatology* **43**: 975–986.
Sommer S et al. (2002) Connective tissue disease and the skin. *Clinical Medicine* **2**: 9–14.
Twycross R et al. (2003) Itch: scratching more than the surface. *Quarterly Journal of Medicine* **96**: 7–26.
Yosipovitch G et al. (2003) Itch. *Lancet* **361**: 690–694.

BULLOUS DISEASE

Primary blistering diseases of the skin are rare. A variety of skin proteins hold the skin together. Inherited abnormalities or immune damage of these proteins causes abnormal cell separation, inflammation, fluid accumulation

Fig. 23.27 **Section of the basemet membrane zone**, showing the structural sites of damage in bullous disorders. LAD, linear IgA disease; EB, epidermolysis bullosa.

and blistering (Fig. 23.27). The level of blistering determines the clinical picture as well as the prognosis. Therefore skin biopsy for light and electron microscopy together with immunofluorescence (IMF) studies is paramount in diagnosis. However, remember that the commonest causes of skin blistering are chickenpox, herpes, impetigo, pompholyx eczema and insect bite reactions, although these are often localized.

IMMUNOBULLOUS DISEASE

Pemphigus vulgaris

Pemphigus vulgaris is a potentially fatal blistering disease occurring in all races but commoner in Ashkenazi Jews and possibly in people from the Indian subcontinent. Onset is usually in middle age and both sexes are affected equally. Prior to the development of oral steroids this condition was frequently fatal. The development of autoantibodies against the desmosomal protein, desmoglein 3, is pathogenic in this disease and they can be measured experimentally as markers of disease activity. Rarely the disease can be drug induced (e.g. penicillamine or captopril).

Skin biopsy shows a superficial intraepidermal split just above the basal layer with acantholysis (separation of individual cells). In the rarer variant, pemphigus foliaceous (characterized by anti-desmoglein 1 autoantibodies), the split is higher in the upper epidermis. Both direct IMF of skin (perilesional) and indirect IMF using patients' serum show intercellular staining of IgG within the epidermis.

Clinical features

Mucosal involvement (especially oral ulceration) is common and is the presenting sign in up to 50% of cases.

This is followed by the appearance of flaccid blisters, particularly involving the trunk. They tend to be sore rather than itchy. Blistering usually becomes widespread but they rapidly denude; thus pemphigus often presents with erythematous, weeping erosions. Blisters can be extended with gentle sliding pressure (Nikolsky's sign). Flexural lesions often have a vegetative appearance. In *pemphigus foliaceus* the blisters and erosions often start in a seborrhoeic distribution (scalp, face and upper chest) before becoming more widespread.

Treatment

This is with very high-dose oral prednisolone (60–100 mg daily) or pulsed methylprednisolone, and this may need to be lifelong. Other immunosuppressants such as azathioprine, or mycophenolate mofetil (or occasionally cyclophosphamide or ciclosporin) are used as steroid-sparing agents but they often take many weeks to be effective. Intravenous immunoglobulin infusions may help gain quick control whilst waiting for these other drugs to work. Anti-CD20 monoclonal antibody (rituximab) has recently been reported to help multidrug-resistant cases.

Whilst treatment is normally effective, perhaps up to 10% of patients may die, either because of complications of the disease or more commonly from side-effects of the treatment.

Use of azathioprine. Azathioprine can cause bone marrow suppression and an allergic hepatitis. Therefore blood count and liver function tests should be regularly monitored during therapy (every 6 weeks). Long-term use with other immunosuppressants causes a slightly increased risk of malignancy, especially of the skin.

Fig. 23.28 **Bullous pemphigoid.**

Bullous pemphigoid

Bullous pemphigoid is more common than pemphigus. It presents in later life (usually over 60 years old) and mucosal involvement is rarer. Autoantibodies against a 230 kDa or 180 kDa hemidesmosomal protein ('bullous pemphigoid antigens 1 and 2') play an aetiological role.

Skin biopsy shows a deeper blister (than in pemphigus) owing to a subepidermal split through the basement membrane. Direct and indirect IMF studies show linear staining of IgG along the basement membrane.

Clinical features

Large tense bullae appear anywhere on the skin (Fig. 23.28) but often involve limbs, hands and feet. They may be centred on an erythematous or urticated background and they can be haemorrhagic. Pemphigoid can be very itchy. Mucosal ulceration is uncommon but a variant of pemphigoid exists which predominantly affects mucosal surfaces with scarring (cicatricial pemphigoid).

Treatment

This is with high-dose oral prednisolone (30–60 mg daily) and steroid-sparing agents such as azathioprine or mycophenolate mofetil. Weekly methotrexate is also occasionally used. In general disease control is easier than with pemphigus. Treatment can often be withdrawn after 2–3 years. Pemphigoid treatment frequently causes side-effects, especially as most patients are elderly. Occasionally localized or mild disease can be controlled with superpotent topical steroids, oral dapsone or high-dose oral minocycline.

Dermatitis herpetiformis (see also p. 303)

Dermatitis herpetiformis (DH) is a rare blistering disorder associated with gluten-sensitive enteropathy (coeliac disease). DH and celiac disease are associated with other organ-specific autoimmune disorders.

Skin biopsy shows a subepidermal blister with neutrophil microabscesses in the dermal papillae. Direct IMF studies of uninvolved skin show IgA in the dermal papillae and patchy granular IgA along the basement membrane. The jejunal mucosa usually shows a partial villous atrophy.

Clinical features

Dermatitis herpetiformis is commoner in males and can present at any age but is most likely to appear for the first time in young adult life. It presents with intensely itchy, small blisters of the skin. The lesions have a predilection for the elbows, extensor forearms, scalp and buttocks. The tops of the blisters are usually scratched off; thus crusted erosions are often seen at presentation. Remissions and exacerbations are common.

Treatment

This should always be with a gluten-free diet (GFD). Control of the skin disease can be obtained with oral dapsone (50–200 mg daily) or sulphonamides. If a strict GFD is adhered to, oral medication can often be withdrawn after 2 years. The GFD will need to be lifelong. It protects against the rare complication of small bowel lymphoma.

Use of dapsone. Dapsone frequently causes a mild, dose-related haemolytic anaemia but the haemolysis can be devastating if there is G6PD deficiency. Liver damage, peripheral neuropathy and aplastic anaemia can also rarely occur, so regular monitoring of a blood count and liver function is needed.

Linear IgA disease (chronic bullous dermatosis of childhood)

Linear IgA disease is a subepidermal blistering disorder of adults and children. Pathogenic IgA autoantibodies can bind to a variety of basement membrane proteins including ladinin, BP 180 antigen and laminin 5 (see Fig. 23.27). It is the most common immunobullous disease seen in children. Rarely it is drug induced by vancomycin.

Clinical features

Linear IgA disease can present with circular clusters of large blisters, a pemphigoid type of blistering or a dermatitis herpetiformis picture. Mucosal involvement of the mouth, vulva and eyes is not uncommon and can cause scarring. Direct IMF studies of skin show linear IgA deposition along the basement membrane.

Treatment

This is with oral dapsone (50–200 mg daily) or sulphonamides. Occasionally immunosuppression is needed. Many patients show spontaneous resolution after 3–6 years.

MECHANOBULLOUS DISEASE (EPIDERMOLYSIS BULLOSA, 'EB')

These are due to inherited abnormalities in structural skin proteins which lead to 'skin fragility'. The resultant blistering tends to arise secondary to trauma and often appears at or shortly after birth. These conditions can be a mild inconvenience, severely disabling or fatal but fortunately are very rare. There are three groups of disorders in which the fundamental gene/protein abnormalities have been characterized. This enables prenatal amniocentesis diagnosis.

Epidermolysis bullosa simplex

This is a group of autosomal dominant genodermatoses characterized by 'superficial' blistering owing to mutations of cytoskeleton proteins within the basal layer of the epidermis, e.g. keratin 5 (chromosome 12q) or keratin 14 (chromosome 17q). Most forms of EB simplex show mild disease with intermittent blistering of the hands and feet, especially in hot weather. The teeth and nails are normal and scarring is absent.

Epidermolysis bullosa dystrophica

This group of genodermatoses is characterized by 'deeper' blistering associated with scarring and milia formation. The level of split is deep within the basement membrane and is due to a mutation in the *COL-7A1* gene (locus at chromosome 3p21.1) which causes a loss of collagen VII in the anchoring fibrils. Nails, mucosae and even the larynx are often involved. The autosomal dominant variety is milder but the autosomal recessive type produces severe disease with disabling scarring, fusion of digits, joint contractures and dysphagia. Life expectancy is significantly reduced. Repeated scarring results in the development of multiple squamous cell carcinomas and most die from this complication in early adult life. The average life expectancy after the appearance of the first squamous cell carcinoma is 5 years.

Junctional epidermolysis bullosa

This, the most severe form, is characterized by a split in the lamina lucida of the basement membrane and is due to mutations in various proteins, mainly laminin 5 but also $\alpha_6\beta_4$ integrin or the 180 kDa bullous pemphigoid-2 antigen. It presents at birth with widespread blistering and areas of absent skin. Erosions of the central face and hoarseness from laryngeal involvement are common. Nail and teeth abnormalities are also common. Both a lethal and a rarer non-lethal form of junctional EB exist and they show an autosomal recessive inheritance. The lethal form causes death in infancy or early childhood.

Investigation and treatment

Investigation and treatment of EB should be carried out in a specialist centre. Diagnosis at birth on clinical grounds is difficult and should be avoided. Exact diagnosis depends on ultrastructural analysis of induced blisters in the skin and immunohistochemistry. Only then can prognosis and genetic counselling be given accurately to parents. Prenatal diagnosis is available for the more severe forms of EB.

FURTHER READING

Allen J et al. (2003) Linear IgA disease. *British Journal of Dermatology* **149**: 977–985, 1055–1058.

Cooper et al. (2003) Treatment of resistant pemphigus vulgaris with an anti-CD20 monoclonal antibody (rituximab). *Clinical and Experimental Dermatology* **28**: 366–368.

Diaz LA, Giudice GJ (2000) End of the century overview of skin blisters. *Archives of Dermatology* **136**: 106–112.

Fine J-D et al. (2000) Inherited epidermolysis bullosa comes into the new millennium. *Journal of the American Academy of Dermatology* **43**: 135–137.

Harman KE et al. (2003) Guidelines for the management of pemphigus. *British Journal of Dermatology* **149**: 926–937.

Trent JT et al. (2003) Epidermolysis bullosa: identification and treatment. *Advances in Skin & Wound Care* **16**: 284–290.

Wojnarowska F et al. (2002) Guidelines for the management of bullous pemphigoid. *British Journal of Dermatology* **147**: 214–221.

SKIN TUMOURS

BENIGN CUTANEOUS TUMOURS

Melanocytic naevi (moles)

Moles are a benign overgrowth of melanocytes that are common in white-skinned people. They appear in childhood and increase in number and size during adolescence and early adult life. They often start as flat brown macules with proliferation of melanocytes at the dermoepidermal junction (junctional naevi). The melanocytes continue to proliferate and grow down into the dermis (compound naevi), which causes an elevation of the mole above the skin surface. The pigmentation is usually even and the border regular. They eventually mature into a dermal naevus (cellular naevus) often with a loss of pigment.

Blue naevus is an acquired asymptomatic blue-looking mole. It is due to a proliferation of melanocytes deep in the mid-dermis.

Basal cell papilloma (seborrhoeic wart)

This is a common benign overgrowth of the basal cell layer of the epidermis. The lesion can be flesh coloured, brown or even black and often has a greasy appearance. The surface is irregular and warty and the lesions appear very superficial as though stuck on to the skin (Fig. 23.29).

Fig. 23.29 **Seborrhoeic warts** (basal cell papillomas).

Tiny keratin cysts may be seen on the surface. They can be treated with cryotherapy or curettage.

Dermatofibroma (histiocytoma)

Dermatofibromas appear as firm, elevated pigmented nodules which may feel like a button in the skin. A peripheral ring of pigmentation is sometimes seen. They are often found on the leg and are commoner in females. There may be a preceding history of trauma or insect bite. The lesion consists of histiocytes, blood vessels and varying degrees of fibrosis. If symptomatic, excision is required.

Epidermoid cyst (previously 'sebaceous cyst')

Epidermoid cysts present as cystic swellings of the skin with a central punctum. They contain 'cheesy' keratin rather than sebum; thus the old term 'sebaceous cyst' should be avoided. These cysts occasionally rupture causing significant dermal inflammation which is not infected.

Pilar cyst (trichilemmal cyst)

Pilar cysts are smooth cysts without a punctum, usually found on the scalp. They may be multiple and familial.

Keratoacanthoma

Keratoacanthomas are rapidly growing epidermal tumours which develop central necrosis and ulceration (Fig. 23.30). They occur on sun-exposed skin in later life and can grow up to 2–3 cm across. Whilst they may resolve spontaneously over a few months, they are best excised, both to exclude a squamous cell carcinoma (which they can mimic) and to improve the cosmetic outcome.

Pyogenic granuloma (granuloma telangiectaticum)

Pyogenic granulomas are a benign overgrowth of blood vessels. They present as rapidly growing pinkish red nodules which are friable and readily bleed. They may follow trauma and are often found on the fingers and lips. They are best excised to exclude an amelanotic malignant melanoma.

Cherry angioma (Campbell de Morgan spots)

They are benign angiokeratomas that appear as tiny pinpoint red papules, especially on the trunk, and increase with age. No treatment is required.

POTENTIALLY PRE-MALIGNANT CUTANEOUS TUMOURS

Solar keratoses (actinic keratoses)

These frequently develop later in life in white-skinned people who have had significant sun exposure. They appear on exposed skin as erythematous silver-scaly papules or patches with a conical surface and a red base (Fig. 23.31). The background skin is often inelastic, wrinkled and may show flat brown macules ('liver spots' or solar lentigos) reflecting diffuse solar damage. A small proportion of these keratoses can transform into squamous cell carcinoma but only after many years.

Treatment of lesions is with cryotherapy, topical 5-fluorouracil cream or 5% imiquimod cream.

Bowen's disease

This is a form of intraepidermal carcinoma-in-situ which rarely can become invasive. It presents on exposed skin as an isolated scaly red patch or plaque, looking rather like psoriasis, although it has a rather irregular edge. The lesions do not clear but slowly increase in size with time.

A variant which can show partial or full-thickness dysplasia can involve the epidermis of the mucosa or neighbouring skin – this can affect the vulva, the glans penis and perianal skin. It is termed vulval- (penile-, or anal-) intraepithelial dysplasia. Clinically it can present as non-specific erythema or as a warty thickening. These diseases have a stronger link with HPV and probably have a higher premalignant potential than Bowen's disease. They are commoner in immunosuppressed individuals. The anal form is increasingly reported in HIV-positive patients and extension into the rectum has been reported.

Fig. 23.30 **Keratoacanthoma.**

Fig. 23.31 **Solar keratoses with background actinic damage.**

Treatment is with topical 5-fluorouracil, 5% imiquimod cream, cryotherapy, curettage, photodynamic therapy or a tissue-destructive laser.

Atypical mole syndrome (dysplastic naevus syndrome)

This is often familial. A large number of melanocytic naevi begin to appear in childhood, even on unexposed sites. Individual lesions may be large with irregular pigmentation and border, and histologically they may show cytological and architectural atypia but no frank malignant change. Individuals with this condition have an increased risk of developing malignant melanoma. They should have their moles photographed and be regularly reviewed. Suspicious lesions should be excised.

Giant congenital melanocytic naevi

These are very large moles present at birth. They show an increased risk of developing malignant melanoma. Approximately 10% of lesions larger than 20 cm across will develop a malignant melanoma in childhood. Excision should be undertaken if possible.

Lentigo maligna

This is a slow-growing macular area of pigmentation seen in elderly people, commonly on the face. The border and pigmentation are often irregular. Some people regard this lesion as a melanoma-in-situ. There is an increased risk of developing invasive malignant melanoma. Treatment is by excision if possible but 5% imiquimod cream is currently under assessment in the very large lesions where surgery would be so disfiguring.

MALIGNANT CUTANEOUS TUMOURS

Basal cell carcinoma (rodent ulcer)

Basal cell carcinomas are the most common malignant skin tumour and most relate to excessive sun exposure. They are common later in life on exposed sites although rare on the ear. They present as a slow-growing papule or nodule (or rarely be cystic) which may go on to ulcerate (Fig. 23.32). Telangiectasia over the tumour or a skin-coloured jelly-like 'pearly edge' may be seen. A flat, diffuse superficial form exists and an ill-defined 'morphoeic' variant. Basal cell carcinomas will slowly grow and erode structures if untreated but these tumours almost never metastasize.

Treatment

Treatment is usually with surgical excision with a 3–5 mm border. Radiotherapy, photodynamic therapy, cryotherapy or 5% imiquimod cream can be useful for large superficial forms but follow-up for recurrence is required. Curettage is occasionally used in older patients, although not for central facial lesions as they often recur. Recurrent tumour or morphoeic basal cell carcinoma is best treated with Mohs' micrographic surgery to ensure adequate clearance.

Fig. 23.32 **Ulcerating basal cell carcinoma.**

Squamous cell carcinoma

Squamous cell carcinoma is a more aggressive tumour than basal cell carcinoma as it can metastasize if left untreated. Most relate to sun exposure and daily application of sun cream has been shown to reduce the incidence in Australia. They can arise in pre-existing solar keratoses or Bowen's disease or be due to chronic inflammation such as in lupus vulgaris. Rarely multiple tumours arise because of arsenic ingestion in early life. Multiple tumours occur in people who have had prolonged periods of immunosuppression, such as renal transplant patients where certain human papilloma virus subtypes may be involved in malignant transformation.

Clinically the lesions are often keratotic, rather ill-defined nodules which may ulcerate (Fig. 23.33). They can grow very rapidly. Examination of regional lymph

Fig. 23.33 **Squamous cell carcinoma.**

nodes is essential. They are most common on sun-exposed sites in later life. One should have a high index of suspicion for ulcerated lesions on the lower lip or ear.

Treatment is with excision or occasionally radiotherapy. Curettage should be avoided.

Malignant melanoma

Malignant melanoma is the most serious form of skin cancer as metastases can occur early and it causes a number of deaths even in young people. As with other types of skin cancer the incidence is continuing to increase, probably because of excessive exposure to sunlight. The history of childhood sun exposure and intermittent sun exposure appears to play a role in the development of malignant melanoma. Other risk factors include atypical mole syndrome, giant congenital melanocytic naevi, lentigo maligna and a positive family history of malignant melanoma. Malignant melanoma is commoner in later life; young adults are also affected. The tumour suppressor gene *p16* (on chromosome 9p) is frequently mutated or deleted in melanoma cell lines and its role in atypical mole syndrome/familial melanoma is currently under investigation.

Diagnosis of melanoma is not always easy but the clinical signs listed in Table 23.11 help distinguish malignant from benign moles. Examination with a dermatoscope can further help in detecting malignant lesions.

Four clinical types exist:

- *Lentigo maligna melanoma* is where a patch of lentigo maligna develops a papule or nodule signalling invasive tumour.
- *Superficial spreading malignant melanoma* is a large flat irregularly pigmented lesion which grows laterally before vertical invasion develops.
- *Nodular malignant melanoma* (Fig. 23.34) is the most aggressive type. It presents as a rapidly growing pigmented nodule which bleeds or ulcerates. Rarely they are amelanotic (non-pigmented) and can mimic pyogenic granuloma.

Fig. 23.34 Nodular malignant melanoma.

- *Acral lentiginous malignant melanoma* arises as pigmented lesions on the palm, sole or under the nail and it usually presents late.

Treatment

This consists of urgent wide excision (2 cm margin) of the lesion. Histological analysis will determine the depth of invasion ('Clark's level') and the thickness of the tumour ('Breslow thickness'). These two factors are significant in predicting prognosis and 5-year survival rates: 96% for local lesions, 60% for regional spread and 14% for distant metastases. For localized melanomas the thickness and presence or absence of ulceration are the strongest independent predictors of outcome. Excision and histology interpretation should only be done by experts to ensure optimum treatment and assessment of prognosis. Sentinel node biopsy for patients with thicker lesions is required for predicting prognosis: 15% will be positive without clinical lymphadenopathy. Metastatic disease is best managed by an oncologist with a multidisciplinary team and can involve surgery to lymph nodes, radiotherapy, immunotherapy and chemotherapy. Initial optimism for high-dose alpha-interferon therapy in advanced disease has recently been challenged with a systematic review suggesting no clear benefit.

The role of governments and medical personnel in public health education to discourage sunbathing and to use sunscreens is of the utmost importance in skin cancer prevention.

Cutaneous T-cell lymphoma (mycosis fungoides)

This is a rare type of skin tumour which often follows a relatively benign course. It presents insidiously with scaly patches and plaques which can look eczematous or psoriasiform. Lesions often appear initially on the buttocks. These lesions may come and go or remain persistent over many years. Patients may well die of unrelated causes. Skin biopsy confirms the diagnosis, showing invasion by atypical lymphocytes. T-cell receptor gene rearrangement studies show that the there is often a monoclonal expansion of lymphocytes in the skin.

Table 23.11 Clinical criteria for the diagnosis of malignant melanoma

ABCDE criteria (USA)
Asymmetry of mole
Border irregularity
Colour variegation
Diameter > 6 mm
Elevation

The Glasgow 7-point checklist

Major criteria	Change in size
	Change in shape
	Change in colour
Minor criteria	Diameter more than 6 mm
	Inflammation
	Oozing or bleeding
	Mild itch or altered sensation

Occasionally the disease can progress to a cutaneous nodular or tumour stage which may be accompanied by systemic organ involvement. In elderly males the disease may progress rarely to an erythrodermic variant accompanied by lymphadenopathy and peripheral blood involvement ('Sézary syndrome').

All patients should be staged at the time of diagnosis to assess for any systemic involvement.

Treatment

Early cutaneous disease can be left untreated or treated with topical steroids or PUVA. More advanced disease of the skin, or systemic involvement, may require radiotherapy, chemotherapy, immunotherapy or electron beam therapy. Bexarotene, an agonist at the retinoid X receptor, can cause regression.

Kaposi's sarcoma

This is a tumour of vascular and lymphatic endothelium that presents as purplish nodules and plaques. There are three types:

- *The 'classic' or 'sporadic' form* (as described by Kaposi) occurs in elderly males, especially Jews from Eastern Europe. It presents as slow-growing purple tumours in the foot and lower leg which rarely cause any significant problem.
- *The 'endemic' form* occurs in males from central Africa and shows more widespread cutaneous involvement as well as lymph node (or occasionally systemic) involvement. Oedema is a prominent feature.
- *The immunosuppression-related form* is more severe and is most common in homosexual patients with HIV (p. 142). Lesions are widespread and often affect the skin, bowel, oral cavity and lungs.

All three types have a strong association with herpes virus type 8 but other factors must be involved as herpes type 8 seroprevalence in the general population is up to 10% in the USA and 50% in some African countries. HAART (p. 143) has significantly reduced the incidence of Kaposi's sarcoma in HIV.

Treatment

Treatment of advanced Kaposi's sarcoma is with radiotherapy, immunotherapy or chemotherapy.

FURTHER READING
Antman K, Chang Y (2000) Kaposi's sarcoma. *New England Journal of Medicine* **342**: 1027–1038.
Girardi M, Heald PW, Wilson LD (2004) The pathogenesis of mycosis fungoides. *New England Journal of Medicine* **350**: 1978–1988.
Hill D (1999) Efficacy of sunscreens in protection against skin cancer. *Lancet* **354**: 699–700 (see also pp. 723–729).
Perrott RE et al. (2003) Reassessing the role of lymphatic mapping and sentinel lymphadenectomy in the management of cutaneous malignant melanoma. *Journal of the American Academy of Dermatology* **49**: 567–588.

Ready N et al. (2003) Adjuvant high-dose interferon therapy for high-risk melanoma. *Archives of Dermatology* **139**: 1635–1637.
Thomas JM et al. (2004). Excision margins in high risk malignant melanoma. *New England Journal of Medicine* **350**: 757–766 (and editorial, p. 823).
Thompson JF et al. (2005) Cutaneous melanoma. *Lancet* **365**: 687–701.

DISORDERS OF BLOOD VESSELS/LYMPHATICS

LEG ULCERS

Venous ulcers

Leg ulcers are common in western societies and can have many causes (Table 23.12). Venous ulcers are the most common type in developed countries.

Venous ulcers are the result of sustained venous hypertension in the superficial veins, owing to incompetent valves in the deep or perforating veins or to previous deep vein thrombosis. The increased pressure causes extravasation of fibrinogen through the capillary walls, giving rise to perivascular fibrin deposition, which leads to poor oxygenation of the surrounding skin.

Venous ulcers are common in later life and cause a significant drain on healthcare budgets as they are often chronic and recurrent; they affect 1% of the population over the age of 70 years. They are most commonly found on the lower leg in a triangle above the ankles (Fig. 23.35), and are associated with:

- venous eczema (p. 1330)
- brown pigmentation from haemosiderin
- varicose veins
- lipodermatosclerosis (the combination of induration, reddish brown pigmentation and inflammation)
- scarring white atrophy with telangiectasia (atrophie blanche).

Treatment

High-compression bandaging (e.g. Unna boot or four-layer bandaging) and leg elevation are used to try to

Table 23.12 Causes of leg ulceration

- Venous hypertension
- Arterial disease (e.g. atherosclerosis)
- Neuropathic (e.g. diabetes, leprosy)
- Neoplastic (e.g. squamous or basal cell carcinoma)
- Vasculitis (e.g. rheumatoid arthritis, SLE, pyoderma gangrenosum)
- Infection (e.g. ecthyma, tuberculosis, deep mycoses, tropical ulcer, syphilis, yaws)
- Haematological (e.g. sickle cell disease, spherocytosis)
- Drug (e.g. hydroxycarbamide (hydroxyurea))
- Other (e.g. necrobiosis lipoidica, trauma, artefact)

Fig. 23.35 Venous leg ulcer.

decrease the venous hypertension. Doppler studies should always be done before bandaging to exclude arterial disease. This treatment is best delivered in the community by appropriately trained nurses. 'Four-layer bandaging' is increasingly popular as this provides high levels of graduated compression (with pressures decreasing up the leg). The choice of ulcer dressing is less critical but one should be chosen to keep the ulcer moist and free of slough and exudate. Up to 80% of ulcers can be healed within 26 weeks. Slower healing rates occur in patients with decreased mobility and if the ulcers are very large, present for longer than 6 months or are bilateral. Diuretics are sometimes helpful to reduce the oedema. Antibiotics are necessary only for overt bacterial infection. Unusual fungal infection ('tinea incognito') is increasingly reported under compression bandaging.

Venous leg ulcers can be very painful so adequate analgesia should be given, including opiates if required. Underlying venous disease is best investigated with duplex ultrasound or plethysmography. Split-thickness skin grafting is used in resistant cases. Life-long support stockings (individually fitted) should be worn after healing as this lessens recurrence.

Surgery for purely superficial venous disease can occasionally be useful for ulcer healing but, in general, venous surgery is unhelpful.

Arterial ulcers

Arterial ulcers may present as punched-out, painful ulcers higher up the leg or on the feet. There may be a history of claudication, hypertension, angina or smoking. Clinically the leg may be cold and show pallor. Absent peripheral pulses, arterial bruits and loss of hair may be present. Doppler ultrasound studies will confirm arterial disease (p. 866) and digital subtraction angiography will further delineate the extent and site of the disease.

Treatment depends on keeping the ulcer clean and covered, adequate analgesia and vascular reconstruction if appropriate.

Neuropathic ulcers

Neuropathic ulcers tend to be seen over pressure areas of the feet, such as the metatarsal heads, owing to repeated trauma. These are most commonly seen in diabetics because of peripheral neuropathy. In developing countries leprosy is a common cause.

Treatment depends on keeping the ulcer clean and removing pressure or trauma from the affected area. Diabetics should pay particular attention to foot care and correctly fitting shoes with the help of a specialist podiatrist (p. 1130).

PRESSURE SORES (DECUBITUS ULCERS, BEDSORES)

These occur in the elderly, immobile, unconscious or paralysed patients. They are due to skin ischaemia from sustained pressure over a bony prominence, most commonly the heel and sacrum. Normal individuals feel the pain of continued pressure, and even during sleep, movement takes place to change position continually. Pressure sores may be graded:

- Stage I: non-blanchable erythema of intact skin
- Stage II: partial-thickness skin loss of epidermis/dermis (blister or shallow ulcer)
- Stage III: full-thickness skin loss involving subcutaneous tissue but not fascia
- Stage IV: full-thickness skin loss with involvement of muscle/bone/tendon/joint capsule.

There are numerous risk factors for development of pressure sores (Table 23.13).

The majority of pressure sores occur in hospital. Seventy per cent appear in the first 2 weeks of hospitalization, and 70% are in orthopaedic patients, especially those on traction. Between 20% and 30% of pressure sores occur in the community.

Table 23.13 Risk factors for the development of pressure sores

- Prolonged immobility:
  paraplegia
  arthritis
  severe physical disease
  apathy
  operation and postoperative states
  plaster casts
  intensive care
- Decreased sensation:
  coma, neurological disease, diabetes mellitus
  drug-induced sleep
- Vascular disease:
  atherosclerosis, diabetes mellitus, scleroderma, vasculitis
- Poor nutrition:
  anaemia
  hypoalbuminaemia
  vitamin C or zinc deficiency

Eighty per cent of patients with deep ulcers involving the subcutaneous tissue die in the first 4 months.

The early sign of red/blue discoloration of the skin can lead rapidly to ulcers in 1–2 hours. Leaving patients on hard emergency room trolleys, or sitting them in chairs for prolonged periods, must be avoided.

Management
Prevention
Prevention is better than cure. Specialist 'tissue-viability nurses' help identify at-risk patients and train other medical staff. Several risk-assessment tools have been devised for the immobile patient based on the known risk factors. The 'Norton scale' and Waterlow Pressure Sore Risk Assessment (Box 23.4) are two such validated systems which produce a numerical score, enabling staff to identify those at most risk.

Treatment
- Bed rest with pillows and fleeces to keep pressure off bony areas (e.g. sacrum and heels) and prevent friction.
- Air-filled cushions for patients in wheelchairs.
- Special pressure-relieving mattresses and beds.
- Regular turning but avoid pressure on hips.
- Ensure adequate nutrition.
- Non-irritant occlusive moist dressings (e.g. hydro-colloid).
- Adequate analgesia (may need opiates).

- Plastic surgery (debridement and grafting in selected cases).
- Treatment of underlying condition.

VASCULITIS (see also p. 581)
Vasculitis is the term applied to an inflammatory disorder of blood vessels which causes endothelial damage. Cutaneous vasculitis (confirmed by skin biopsy) may be an isolated problem but occasionally is associated with vasculitis in other organs. The most commonly used classification is based on the size of blood vessel involved (see Tables 10.18 and 10.19).

The cutaneous features are of haemorrhagic papules, pustules, nodules or plaques which may erode and ulcerate. These purpuric lesions do not blanche with pressure. Occasionally a fixed livedo reticularis pattern may appear which does not disappear on warming. Pyrexia and arthralgia are common associations even in the absence of significant systemic involvement. Other clinical features depend on the underlying cause.

The most common cutaneous vasculitis affects small vessels and is called leucocytoclastic vasculitis (LCV) or angiitis. This usually appears on the lower legs as a symmetrical palpable purpura. It is rarely associated with systemic involvement. This can be caused by drugs (15%), infection (15%), inflammatory disease (10%), malignant disease (< 5%) but often no cause is found (55–60%). Extensive investigations are probably best reserved for

---

Box 23.4 Pressure sore risk-assessment tools

Norton Scale for Pressure Sores

Physical		Neurology		Activity		Mobility		Incontinence	
4	Good	4	Alert	4	Ambulant	4	Full	4	None
3	Fair	3	Apathetic	3	Walks with help	3	Slightly	3	Occasionally
2	Poor	2	Confused	2	Not bound	2	Limited*	2	Usually
1	Very poor	1	Stupor	1	Bedfast	1	Very limited Immobile	1	Double

*Norton Scale for Pressure Sores. Low scores carry a high risk

Waterlow Pressure Sore Risk Assessment

Build/weight for height		Visual skin type		Continence		Mobility		Sex Age		Appetite	
Average	0	Healthy	0	Complete	0	Fully mobile	0	Male	1	Average	0
Above average	2	Tissue paper	1	Occasionally incontinent	1	Restricted/ difficult	1	Female	2	Poor	1
Below average	3	Dry	1	Catheter/ incontinent	2	Restless/ fidgety	2	14–18	1	Anorectic	2
		Oedematous	1					50–64	2		
		Clammy	1	of faeces		Apathetic	3	65–75	3		
		Discoloured	2	Doubly	3	Inert/traction	4	75–80	4		
		Broken/spot	3	incontinent				81+	5		

Special risk factors

			Assessment value	
1. Poor nutrition; e.g. terminal cachexia	8		At risk	10
2. Sensory deprivation, e.g. diabetes, paraplegia, cerebrovascular accident	6		High risk	15
3. High-dose anti-inflammatory or steroids in use	3		Very high risk	20
4. Smoking 10+ per day	1			
5. Orthopaedic surgery/fracture below waist	3			

those with persistent lesions or associated signs and symptoms. Whilst LCV often settles spontaneously, treatment with analgesia, support stockings, dapsone or prednisolone may be needed to control the pain and to heal up any ulceration. Urticarial vasculitis is discussed on page 1335.

LYMPHATICS

Lymphoedema

Lymphoedema refers to a chronic non-pitting oedema due to lymphatic insufficiency. It is most commonly seen affecting the legs and tends to progress with age. The legs can become enormous and prevent wearing of normal shoes. Chronic disease may cause a secondary 'cobblestone' thickening of the skin. Lymphoedema can be primary (and present early in life) owing to an inherited deficiency of lymphatic vessels (e.g. Milroy's disease) or can be secondary because of obstruction of lymphatic vessels (e.g. filarial infection or malignant disease).

Treatment is with compression stockings and physical massage. If there is recurrent cellulitis, long-term antibiotics are advisable as each episode of cellulitis will further damage the lymph vessels. Surgery should be avoided.

Lymphangioma circumscriptum

Lymphangioma circumscriptum is a rare hamartoma of lymphatic tissue. It usually presents in childhood with multiple small vesicles in the skin which weep lymphatic fluid and sometimes blood. They reflect deeper vessel involvement so surgery should be avoided. Cryotherapy or CO_2 laser treatment may help the superficial lesions.

FURTHER READING

Cullum N et al. (2003) Pressure sores. *Clinical Evidence* **9**: 2167–2176.

Fiorentino DF (2003) Cutaneous vasculitis. *Journal of the American Academy of Dermatology* **48**: 311–340.

Health Technology Assessment Programme – Systematic Reviews of Wound Care Management (1999) Vol. 3, No. 17 (parts I and II); (2000) Vol. 4, No. 21; (2001) Vol. 5 No. 9. London: Department of Health. Online. Available: http://www.ncchta.org.

Topham EJ et al. (2002) Chronic lower limb oedema. *Clinical Medicine* **2**: 28–31.

Valencia IC et al. Chronic venous insufficiency and venous leg ulceration (2001) *Journal of the American Academy of Dermatology* **44**: 401–421.

DISORDERS OF COLLAGEN AND ELASTIC TISSUE

Ehlers–Danlos syndrome (see also p. 602)

Ehlers–Danlos syndrome can be subdivided into at least 10 variants. They are all inherited disorders causing abnormalities in collagen of the skin, joints and blood vessels. Clinically this causes increased elasticity of the skin, hypermobile joints and fragile blood vessels causing easy bruising or in some cases internal haemorrhage. The skin is hyperextensible but recoils normally after stretching. It is easily injured and heals slowly with scarring like tissue paper. Pseudotumours may occur at the sites of scarring (such as elbows and knees) consisting mainly of fat, but calcification can occur.

Pseudoxanthoma elasticum

Pseudoxanthoma elasticum is a rare group of disorders characterized by abnormalities in collagen and elastic tissue affecting the skin, eye and blood vessels. The skin may be loose, lax and wrinkled. It can look yellowish and papular ('plucked chicken skin') and tends to lose its elastic recoil when stretched. Skin changes are best seen in the flexures especially the sides of the neck. Noncutaneous features are not always present but they include recurrent gastrointestinal bleeding, early myocardial infarction, claudication and angioid streaks on the retina reflecting disruption of vascular elastic tissue.

Marfan's syndrome (see also p. 839)

Marfan's syndrome, an autosomal dominant disorder of connective tissue, is described on page 839. The syndrome is characterized by tall stature and long thin digits (arachnodactyly) (Fig. 13.98). The arm span can exceed the height of the patient and a high arched palate may be present. Lax ligaments result in frequent dislocation of joints. Inguinal and femoral hernias are common. Scoliosis and flat feet may be present. Pulmonary changes include emphysema, diaphragmatic hernia and spontaneous pneumothorax. Dislocation of the ocular lens is common. Skin changes are usually absent but striae may develop. Patients with homocystinuria (see p. 602), type III and VI Ehlers–Danlos syndrome (EDS) and 'marfanoid phenotype' have some similar features but often do not develop the life-threatening complications of Marfan's syndrome, so accurate diagnosis by an expert is essential.

Treatment

Patients should be reviewed by an ophthalmologist, an orthopaedic surgeon and a cardiologist to screen for and deal with the above complications. Genetic counselling should be offered to families.

Striae

Striae are visible linear scars due to dermal collagen damage and stretching. Histologically a thinned epidermis overlies parallel bundles of fine collagen. They occur commonly over the abdomen and breasts in pregnancy but also occur on the thighs and trunk in rapidly growing adolescents as well as in some obese individuals. They are also seen in Cushing's syndrome and corticosteroid therapy. Striae are initially reddish blue but fade

Fig. 23.36   **Keloid scar of the lobe of the ear.**

Fig. 23.37   **Vitiligo of the hands showing areas of depigmentation.**

to white atrophic marks. Puberty-related striae normally disappear completely.

Keloid scars

Keloid scars are characterized by smooth hard nodules (Fig. 23.36) due to excessive collagen production. They may occur spontaneously or follow skin trauma/surgery, and they are often itchy. They tend to affect young adults and are much commoner in black Africans. Sites of predilection include the shoulders, upper back and chest, ear lobes and the chin. Unlike hypertrophic scars (which fade within 12 months) keloids are persistent and may fade with time.

Treatment is with triamcinolone injection, compression with silica gels or surgery but the latter must be followed by steroid injection or superficial radiotherapy or it may make the problem worse.

FURTHER READING
Hu X et al. (2003) ABCC6/MRP6 mutations: further insight into the molecular pathology of pseudoxanthoma elasticum. *European Journal of Human Genetics* **11**: 215–224.
Ohtani T et al. (2002) Pseudoxanthoma elasticum. *Journal of Dermatology* **29**: 615–620.
Wordsworth P et al. (2001) The real connective tissue diseases. *Clinical Medicine* **1**: 21–24.

DISORDERS OF PIGMENTATION

HYPOPIGMENTATION

Vitiligo
Vitiligo is a common disorder of depigmentation which probably has an autoimmune aetiology. Sufferers often have relatives with other organ-specific autoimmune disorders. It presents in childhood or early adult life with well-demarcated macules of complete pigment loss. There is no history of preceding inflammation. Patients are very susceptible to sunburn. Lesions are often symmetrical and frequently involve the face, hands (Fig. 23.37) and genitalia. The hair can also depigment. Trauma may induce new lesions. Spontaneous repigmentation can occur and often starts around hair follicles, giving a speckled appearance. However, repigmentation is rare if a lesion has persisted for more than 1 year or if the hair is depigmented. The psychological consequences of vitiligo can be devastating especially in Asian or black African people.

Treatment is very unsatisfactory and has no impact on the long-term outcome. Sunblocks should be used to prevent burning. Potent topical steroids or phototherapy help some individuals. Treatment with 0.1% tacrolimus ointment is currently under assessment, with conflicting early results. If vitiligo is almost universal and fixed, depigmentation with monobenzone may be considered. Finally, referral to a specialist camouflage clinic is often the most helpful 'treatment'.

Post-inflammatory hypopigmentation
This is one of the most common causes of pale skin. It is much more common in people with pigmented skin. It is seen as a consequence of eczema, acne or psoriasis and may even be the reason for individuals presenting to a doctor. Providing the skin disease is controlled, the pigmentation will recover slowly after many months. Post-inflammatory hyperpigmentation can also occur.

Oculocutaneous albinism
This is a group of rare autosomal recessive disorders affecting the pigmentation of skin, hair and eyes. It can affect all races. Melanocytes are in normal number but have abnormal function. Clinically it presents with universal pale skin, white or yellow hair and a pinkish iris. Photophobia, nystagmus and a squint are also present in most cases.

Treatment involves obsessive protection against sunlight to avoid sunburning and development of skin cancer.

Idiopathic guttate hypomelanosis

This occurs most commonly in black African people and is of unknown aetiology. It presents with small (2–4 mm) asymptomatic porcelain-white macules, often on skin exposed to sunlight. The borders are often sharply defined and angular. There is no effective treatment.

Leprosy (see also p. 80)

Both tuberculoid leprosy and indeterminate leprosy can present with anaesthetic patches of depigmentation and should always be considered in people from endemic regions. Loss of hair and decreased sweating may also be present in the lesions.

HYPERPIGMENTATION

Freckles (ephelides)

These appear in childhood as small brown macules after sun exposure. They fade in the winter months.

Lentigos

These are a more permanent macule of pigmentation similar to freckles but they tend to persist in the winter. Solar lentigos (also called 'liver spots') occur in older people on exposed skin because of actinic damage.

Chloasma

These are brown macules often seen symmetrically over the cheeks and forehead and are most common in women. They can occur spontaneously but are also associated with pregnancy and the oral contraceptive pill.

Metabolic/endocrine effects

A generalized skin darkening can occur with chronic liver disease, especially haemochromatosis. It also is seen sometimes in Cushing's syndrome, Addison's disease (more marked in palmar creases and buccal mucosa) and Nelson's syndrome.

Peutz–Jeghers syndrome (p. 309)

This is an autosomal dominant genetic condition. It presents with brown macules of the lips and perioral region. It is associated with gastrointestinal polyposis which occasionally become malignant.

Urticaria pigmentosa (cutaneous mastocytosis)

This presents most commonly with multiple pigmented macules in children. These lesions tend to become red, itchy and urticated if they are rubbed (Darier's sign). Occasionally lesions may blister and in the rare congenital, diffuse form of the disease the skin can become thickened and leathery.

Occasionally, systemic symptoms are present, such as wheeze, flushing, syncope or diarrhoea, reflecting extensive mast cell degranulation from the skin. Anaphylaxis occurs very rarely and may be precipitated by mast cell degranulators such as aspirin or opiates. The condition spontaneously resolves after some years in children but is persistent in adults.

Skin biopsy shows an excess of mast cells in the skin. Recently a mutation in the proto-oncogene *c-kit* has been demonstrated, resulting in mast cell proliferation and mast cell apoptosis. Monoclonal antibodies against mast cell markers (tryptase and CD117) on immunohisto-chemistry confirm the diagnosis.

Treatment of the skin, if required, is with anti-histamines or PUVA.

Rarely there may be infiltration of internal organs with mast cells (*systemic mastocytosis*), especially in adult disease or neonatal disease. This can involve any organ but especially the bone (where it can cause severe pain), gastrointestinal tract, liver and spleen. There is a small risk of developing leukaemia if the bone marrow is heavily infiltrated.

Other conditions with pigmentation

Café-au-lait macules are seen in neurofibromatosis types 1 and 2. They also occur in a wide variety of disorders including tuberous sclerosis, ataxia, telangiectasia, Fanconi's anaemia, multiple endocrine neoplasia type 1, McCune–Albright syndrome.

Multiple lentigines: apart from in Peutz–Jeghers syndrome these are also seen in xeroderma pigmentosum.

Acquired melanocytic naevi are seen in Turner's syndrome (p. 1064) and familial atypical mole–melanoma syndrome (dysplastic naevi, p. 1351).

FURTHER READING
Tharp MD et al. (2003) Mastocytosis. *Advances in Dermatology* **19**: 207–236.

DRUG-INDUCED RASHES

Drugs can be toxic and teratogenic but they can also cause problems through allergic reactions. This frequently presents in the skin where just about any type of skin rash can arise (Table 23.14) although a widespread symmetrical maculopapular rash is the most common type (Fig. 23.38). 'Fixed drug eruptions' may occur where a rash evolves and resolves at a specific site. The rash is reproduced at exactly the same site after a repeated exposure.

A thorough history is of great value and always think of a drug cause for any skin condition. The use of prick-testing and patch-testing is rarely helpful and not without risk. Drug allergy can only be proven by rechallenging but this is rarely justified as it carries some risks. Rechallenging is occasionally justified for anti-tuberculosis drugs or antiretroviral drugs but this should be carried out as an inpatient as there is a risk of anaphylaxis. Certain individuals (e.g. those with HIV infections) are more susceptible to drug rashes (Fig. 23.39).

Most rashes will settle spontaneously once the offending agent is removed. The commonest culprits in a hospital setting are antibiotics and chemotherapy agents.

Table 23.14 Morphological types of drug rashes and some common causes

Maculopapular	Penicillin/amoxicillin
Urticaria	Penicillin, aspirin
Vasculitis	Gold, hydralazine
Fixed drug rash	Phenolphthalein in laxatives, tetracyclines, paracetamol
Pigmentation	Minocycline (black), amiodarone (slate grey)
Lupus erythematosus	Penicillamine, isoniazid
Photosensitivity	Thiazides, chlorpromazine, sulphonamide, amiodarone
Pustular	Carbamazepine
Erythema nodosum	Sulphonamide, oral contraceptive
Erythema multiforme	Barbiturates
Acneiform	Corticosteroids
Lichenoid	Chloroquine, thiazides, gold, allopurinol
Psoriasiform	Methyldopa, gold, lithium, beta-blockers
Toxic epidermal necrolysis	Penicillin, co-trimoxazole, carbamazepine, NSAIDs
Pemphigus	Penicillamine, ACE inhibitors
Erythroderma	Gold, sulphonylureas, allopurinol

Fig. 23.38 Morbilliform drug rash due to penicillin allergy.

Fig. 23.39 Erythema nodosum in a patient with HIV on co-trimoxazole.

The three most serious types of drug rashes are:

- erythroderma (p. 1340)
- toxic epidermal necrolysis
- anticonvulsant hypersensitivity syndrome.

Toxic epidermal necrolysis is characterized by a widespread subepidermal blistering and sloughing of most of the skin. The skin may be itchy but typically takes on a burning quality. Fever and mucosal involvement are common. The internal epithelial surfaces (lung, bladder, gastrointestinal tract) are also involved. Multiorgan failure and sepsis often occur. Toxic epidermal necrolysis can be fatal even after drug withdrawal and intensive care support. Patients should be managed in intensive care or a specialized burns unit. Occlusive cutaneous dressings significantly reduce the pain. Ophthalmological assessment and oral hygiene are necessary. Specific medical treatment with steroids or ciclosporin is controversial. Intravenous immunoglobulin may be beneficial if given early in the disease.

A variant exists called *Stevens–Johnson syndrome* where the damage is restricted to the mucosal surfaces with milder bullous involvement of the skin.

Anticonvulsant hypersensitivity syndrome is characterized by a generalized mucocutaneous rash, fever and lymphadenopathy with variable arthralgia, pharyngitis, periorbital oedema and hepatosplenomegaly. Rarely pustulation of the skin and conjunctivitis are present. The blood may show a peripheral eosinophilia, lymphocytosis with atypical lymphocytes, and a hepatitic picture. It can progress to multiorgan failure. This reaction occurs typically 3–4 weeks into therapy. It can occur with any of the aromatic anticonvulsants (carbamazepine, phenytoin, phenobarbital, primidone and clonazepam). As they often cross-react, all these drugs must be avoided in the future. Sodium valproate is a suitable alternative. There is also potential for cross-reaction with the newer anticonvulsants vigabatrin and lamotrigine.

FURTHER READING

Baba M et al. (2003) The anticonvulsant hypersensitivity syndrome. *Journal of the European Academy of Dermatology and Venereology* **17**: 399–401.

Breathnach SM (2002) Adverse cutaneous reactions to drugs. *Clinical Medicine* **2**: 15–19.

Campione E et al. (2003) High-dose intravenous immunoglobulin for severe drug reactions: efficacy in toxic epidermal necrolysis. *Acta Dermatovenereologica* **83**: 430–432.

Fiszenson-Albala F et al. (2003) A 6-month prospective survey of cutaneous drug reactions in a hospital setting. *British Journal of Dermatology* **149**: 1018–1022.

Sullivan et al. (2001) The drug hypersensitivity syndrome. *Archives of Dermatology* **137**: 357–364.

DISORDERS OF NAILS

Psoriasis and fungal nail infection are the commonest causes of nail dystrophy and are discussed on pages 1333 and 1323.

- *Nail pitting* can be caused by psoriasis, alopecia areata and atopic eczema. A few pits can be present because of trauma.
- *Onycholysis* (distal nail plate separation) is caused by psoriasis, thyrotoxicosis, following trauma and rarely due to a photosensitive reaction to drugs such as tetracyclines.
- *Koilonychia* (thin spoon-shaped nails) can be caused by iron deficiency anaemia or rarely is congenital.
- *Leuconychia* (white nails) is seen in hypoalbuminaemia. A striate congenital leuconychia exists.
- *Beau's lines* (transverse lines) appear as solitary depressions which grow out slowly over many months. They arise due to a severe illness or shock which causes a temporary arrest in nail growth.
- *Yellow-nail syndrome* is a rare disorder of lymphatic drainage. It presents with thickened, slow-growing, yellow nails with associated pleural effusions, bronchiectasis and lymphoedema of the legs.
- *Onychogryphosis* is a gross thickening of the nail which is seen in later life especially in the big toe-nail. There is often a history of preceding trauma. Both psoriasis and fungal infection can also cause nail thickening.
- *Nail–patella syndrome* is an autosomal dominant condition which presents with triangular rather than half-moon-shaped lunulae, especially of the thumb and forefingers. The nail plates may be small or dystrophic. The patellae are hypoplastic or absent. Other skeletal anomalies can be present and renal impairment (glomerulonephritis) occurs in up to 30% of individuals.
- *Melanonychia* (longitudinal brown streaks) are seen as a normal variant in black-skinned patients. In a white patient it may reflect an underlying subungual melanoma, especially if the pigmentation progresses proximally onto the nail fold ('Hutchinson's sign').
- *Clubbing* is discussed on page 884.

FURTHER READING
Baran R, Dawber RPR (eds.) (2001) *Diseases of the Nails and their Management*, 3rd edn. Oxford: Blackwell Scientific Publications.

DISORDERS OF HAIR

HAIR LOSS

Hair loss can be due to a disorder of the hair follicle in which the scalp skin looks normal (non-scarring alopecia) or due to a disorder within the scalp skin that causes permanent loss of the follicle (scarring or cicatricial alopecia). This latter form causes shiny atrophic bald areas in the scalp which are devoid of follicular openings. There are many causes of alopecia (Table 23.15).

Androgenic alopecia

Androgenic alopecia (male pattern baldness) is the most common type of non-scarring hair loss and depends on

Table 23.15 Causes of alopecia

Scarring alopecia	Non-scarring alopecia
Discoid lupus erythematosus	Androgenic alopecia
Kerion (tinea capitis)	Telogen effluvium
Lichen planus	Alopecia areata
Dissecting cellulitis	Trichotillomania (self-induced hair-pulling)
X-irradiation	Tinea capitis
Idiopathic ('pseudopelade')	Traction alopecia
	Metabolic (iron deficiency, hypothyroidism)
	Drug (e.g. heparin, isotretinoin, chemotherapy)

genetic factors and an abnormal sensitivity to androgens. It presents in young men with frontal receding followed by thinning of the crown and there is often a positive family history. It also occurs in females but tends to occur at a later age, be milder and show little in the way of frontal recession. If acne and menstrual disturbance are also present, polycystic ovary syndrome and other endocrine disorders of androgens can be present.

Treatment. This may not be required. Topical 5% minoxidil lotion or oral finasteride (1 mg daily) can help arrest progression and may cause a small amount of regrowth, providing it is used early in disease but the treatment needs to be continued possibly lifelong. Approximately one-third of patients will not respond to either therapy. Finasteride is a selective inhibitor of 5α-reductase type II and it can cause side-effects in 1% of patients such as loss of libido. It should not be used in females as it can affect the sexual development of a male fetus. However, antiandrogen therapy (e.g. cyproterone acetate or spironolactone) helps some women.

Alopecia areata

Alopecia areata is an immune-mediated type of hair loss. It is associated with other organ-specific autoimmune diseases. It presents in childhood or young adults with patches of baldness. These may regrow to be followed by new patches of hair loss. The presence of broken exclamation mark hairs (narrow at the scalp/wider and more pigmented at the tip) at the edge of a bald area is diagnostic. Regrowth may initially be with white hairs and often occurs slowly over months. Occasionally all of the scalp hair is lost (alopecia totalis) and rarely all body hair is lost (alopecia universalis). The nails may be pitted or roughened.

Treatment has no effect on the long-term progression. Potent topical or injected steroids are of limited use. Topical immunotherapy with diphencyprone, PUVA or topical 5% minoxidil are occasionally tried but often do not help. Wigs can be provided for severe cases and patient support groups are often beneficial.

Traction alopecia

This refers to the 'mechanical damage' type of hair loss that arises from pulling the hair back into a bun or tight plaiting. It is more common in black Africans.

Telogen effluvium

Telogen effluvium refers to the pattern of diffuse hair loss that occurs some 3 months after pregnancy or a severe illness. It occurs because 'stress' puts all the hairs into the telogen phase of hair shedding at the same time. The hair fully recovers and the normal staggered hair growth/hair shedding cycle resumes within a few months.

Dissecting cellulitis

This is a chronic folliculitis affecting predominantly young black males. It presents with papules and pustules over the occipital region of the scalp with hair loss. If severe, the back of the scalp becomes a boggy swelling (discharging pus) with areas of scarring alopecia. It can be complicated by keloid scar formation ('acne keloidalis nuchae').

Treatment is difficult but prolonged courses of low-dose antibiotics are worth trying in early disease. Prolonged courses of isotretinoin can help a few individuals and deep surgical excision can be used in recalcitrant cases.

INCREASED HAIR GROWTH

Hirsutism (p. 1058)

Hirsutism refers to the male pattern of hair growth seen in females. The racial variation in hair growth must be considered. Certain races (e.g. Mediterranean and Asian) have more male pattern hair growth than northern European females. This is not due to excess androgens but may reflect a genetically determined altered sensitivity to them. If virilizing features (deep voice, clitoromegaly, dysmenorrhoea, acne) are present, one should carry out a full endocrine assessment. Hirsutism can cause severe psychological distress to some individuals.

Treatment involves physical methods such as bleaching, waxing, electrolysis and laser therapy. Antiandrogen therapy is occasionally helpful.

Hypertrichosis

Hypertrichosis refers to the state of excessive hair growth at any site and occurs in both sexes. It can be seen in anorexia nervosa, porphyria cutanea tarda, and underlying malignancy and is caused by certain drugs (e.g. ciclosporin, minoxidil).

FURTHER READING

Barth JH (2000) Should men still go bald gracefully? *Lancet* **355**: 161–162.

MacDonald Hull SP et al. (2003) Guidelines for the management of alopecia areata. *British Journal of Dermatology* **149**: 692–699.

Price VH (1999) Treatment of hair loss. *New England Journal of Medicine* **341**: 964–973.

Wendelin DS et al. (2003) Hypertrichosis. *Journal of the American Academy of Dermatology* **48**: 161–179.

BIRTH MARKS/NEONATAL RASHES

Strawberry naevus (cavernous haemangioma)

Strawberry naevus affects up to 1% of infants. It presents at, or shortly after, birth as a single red lumpy nodule (Fig. 23.40) that grows rapidly for the first few months. Multiple lesions can be present. They will spontaneously resolve with good cosmesis but this may take up to 7 years for complete resolution. Occasionally plastic surgery is needed after resolution to remove residual slack skin. Reassurance of parents is usually all that is required.

Treatment is indicated if:

- the lesion interferes with feeding or vision
- the lesion ulcerates or bleeds frequently
- the lesion is associated with high-output cardiac failure from shunting of large volumes of blood
- the lesion consumes platelets and/or clotting factors causing potentially life-threatening haemorrhage ('Kasabach–Merritt syndrome').

The latter two complications are very rare and only tend to occur in large lesions with significant deep vessel involvement.

Treatment modalities include intralesional or oral corticosteroids, surgery (for selected lesions), and tunable

Fig. 23.40 **Strawberry naevus** (cavernous haemangioma).

dye laser (for treating ulceration). Alpha-interferon injections, vincristine or embolization is only used for life-threatening events.

Port-wine stain (naevus flammeus)

Port-wine stain is also called a capillary haemangioma but strictly speaking it is not a haemangioma but is just an abnormal dilatation of dermal capillaries. It presents at birth as a flat red macular area and is commonly found on the face. It does not improve spontaneously and it may become thickened with time. If the lesion is found in the distribution of the first division of the trigeminal nerve it may be associated with ipsilateral meningeal vascular anomalies which can cause epilepsy and even hemiplegia (Sturge–Weber syndrome, p. 1257). If a port-wine stain involves the skin near the eye, glaucoma is a risk and ophthalmic assessment is mandatory.

Treatment of port-wine stains is ideally carried out with the tunable dye laser.

Milia

'Milk spots' are small follicular epidermal cysts. They are small pinhead white papules commonly found on the face of infants. They resolve spontaneously.

Mongolian blue spot

This appears in infants as a deep blue-grey bruise-like area, usually over the sacrum or back, and is occasionally mistaken as a sign of child abuse. It is due to deep dermal melanocytes. It is very common in Oriental children, less common in black Africans and rare in Caucasians. It has usually disappeared by the age of 7 years.

Toxic erythema of the newborn (erythema neonatorum)

Toxic erythema of the newborn is a term used to describe a common transient blotchy maculopapular rash in newborns. The rash is occasionally pustular but the child is not toxic or unwell. It disappears within a few days, spontaneously.

Nappy rash ('diaper dermatitis')

This is an irritant eczema caused by occlusion of faeces and urine against the skin. It is almost universal in babies. The flexures are usually spared, which is a useful differentiating feature from seborrhoeic and atopic eczema. If satellite lesions are present around the edge, it may indicate a superimposed *Candida* infection. This rash can also occur in the elderly incontinent.

Treatment involves frequent changing of the nappy and regular application of a barrier cream.

Acrodermatitis enteropathica (p. 249)

This is due to a rare inherited deficiency of zinc absorption. It presents 4–6 weeks after weaning, or earlier in bottle-fed babies. There is an erythematous, sometimes blistering, rash around the perineum, mouth, hands and feet. It may be associated with photophobia, diarrhoea and alopecia.

Treatment is with lifelong oral zinc, which seems to override the poor absorption. The response is rapid.

> **FURTHER READING**
> Bruckner AL et al. (2003) Hemangiomas of infancy. *Journal of the American Academy of Dermatology* **48:** 477–493.
> Harper J, Oranje A, Prose N (eds) (2000) *Textbook of Pediatric Dermatology.* Oxford: Blackwell Scientific.

HUMAN IMMUNODEFICIENCY VIRUS AND THE SKIN (p. 134)

HIV infection commonly causes significant dermatological problems. A rash may even be the presenting feature of underlying HIV infection. It is estimated that 90% of HIV-positive patients will suffer with a mucocutaneous disorder during the illness. It is also estimated that up to 30% of people with AIDS will suffer from three different dermatoses. These rashes can often be clinically atypical and difficult to diagnose. One must have a low threshold for skin biopsy and skin culture. On top of this many of the skin problems are resistant to standard treatments. Most of these dermatoses have become less prevalent since the advent of HAART (p. 144).

Cutaneous infection and opportunistic infection

Not surprisingly, infections are increased because of the HIV-induced immune deficiency. Molluscum contagiosum are particularly common especially on the face. They are often multiple and of a 'giant' size measuring over 1 cm across. Molluscum are rarely seen in adults and they can be the presenting feature of HIV. Other viral infections such as extensive ulcerative herpes or widespread viral warts may be seen. Bacterial infections (e.g. staphylococcal boils) and fungal infections (e.g. ringworm and *Candida*) are also common. Recalcitrant and recurrent oropharyngeal candidiasis is a particular problem.

Opportunistic infections such as cutaneous cytomegalovirus (pustules or necrotic ulcers), sporotrichosis (linear nodules) or cryptococcus (red papules, psoriasiform or molluscum-like lesions) can pose diagnostic difficulties, stressing the need for skin biopsy and culture.

Inflammatory dermatoses

Inflammatory dermatoses show an increased incidence with HIV infection, probably due to an immune dysfunction or imbalance rather than as a consequence of immune suppression. Severe, extensive seborrhoeic eczema is very common and may be a presenting sign of HIV. Other types of eczema, psoriasis, ichthyosis (dry scaly skin), nodular prurigo and pruritus are all common in HIV infection and can be very severe. Granuloma annulare and lichen planus are probably increased in incidence. The treatment of these conditions is difficult as oral immunosuppressive therapies (e.g. prednisolone, ciclosporin) are best avoided in patients with low CD4 counts. Topical therapies and phototherapy seem relatively safe. Oral retinoids are useful in the management of psoriasis.

'Autoimmune dermatoses'

Bullous pemphigoid, thrombocytopenic purpura, and vitiligo seem to be increased in incidence. The polyclonal stimulation of B lymphocytes by HIV and the resulting abnormal antibody production may be involved in their aetiology. Erythroderma is sometimes seen in HIV disease where skin biopsy suggests a 'graft-versus-host disease' mechanism. This presumably reflects a severe underlying immune dysfunction of T lymphocyte control.

Drug rashes

Adverse drug rashes are much commoner in HIV patients. Reactions to co-trimoxazole, dapsone and antiretroviral drugs appear particularly common. Drug rashes may be severe (especially with nevirapine) resulting in erythroderma or toxic epidermal necrolysis. Other unusual rashes include a striking nail/mucosal pigmentation from zidovudine, paronychia from indinavir and facial lipodystrophy mostly from protease inhibitors.

Cutaneous tumours

Kaposi's sarcoma (p. 142) is much commoner in homosexuals with HIV than in other groups. Basal and squamous cell carcinomas and benign melanocytic naevi are also a little increased in incidence, presumably reflecting a loss of immune surveillance.

'Specific' HIV dermatoses

'Itchy folliculitis' of HIV (also called papular pruritic eruption)

Itchy follicular eruptions are common in HIV as CD4 counts decline. The previously described staphylococcal folliculitis, eosinophilic folliculitis, pityrosporum folliculitis, and demodex mite folliculitis are probably all part of a spectrum and the term itchy folliculitis is useful to encompass these. It presents with intensely itchy papules centred on hair follicles and occurring most commonly over the upper trunk and upper arms. The face is more commonly involved in black patients. Individual lesions frequently have the top scratched off, leaving a crateriform appearance. The aetiology is unknown but may reflect a hypersensitivity reaction as high IgE and eosinophil counts may be present.

Treatment with oral minocycline, potent topical steroids and emollients may help. Phototherapy or oral isotretinoin is useful in resistant cases.

Oral hairy leucoplakia

This is characterized by white plaques with vertical ridging on the sides of the tongue. Unlike with oral *Candida*, the lesions cannot be peeled off to leave raw areas underneath. It was first recognized in HIV disease but can rarely occur in other forms of immunosuppression. It is thought to be due to co-infection with Epstein–Barr virus.

Treatment with aciclovir, ganciclovir or foscarnet may help.

FURTHER READING
Osborne GE et al. (2003) The management of HIV-related skin disease. Part I: infections. *International Journal of STD & AIDS* **14**: 78–86.
Osborne GE et al (2003) The management of HIV-related skin disease. Part II: neoplasms and inflammatory disorders. *International Journal of STD & AIDS* **14**: 235–240.

DERMATOSES OF PREGNANCY

There are a number of minor skin changes during pregnancy. There is an increase in spider naevi, melanocytic naevi, skin tags and chloasma. The abdomen shows midline pigmentation (linea nigra) and striae (stretch marks). There are four less common skin problems associated with pregnancy.

Polymorphic eruption of pregnancy (PEP)

This rash tends to appear in the last trimester of a first pregnancy in 1 in 160 cases. It is of unknown aetiology and recurs only rarely in subsequent pregnancies. It presents with very itchy urticated papules and plaques and occasionally small vesicles. Lesions usually start on the abdomen and striae but may spread to the upper arms and thighs. The umbilicus may be spared. PEP is commoner in twin pregnancies. The rash is not associated with any maternal or fetal risk. PEP has been shown to be associated with low maternal serum cortisol levels.

Treatment is with reassurance, bland emollients and mild topical steroids. The rash disappears after childbirth.

Prurigo of pregnancy

This affects 1 in 300 pregnancies. It usually starts on the abdomen in the third trimester but may persist for some months after delivery. Clustered excoriated papules (prurigo-like lesions) occur on the abdomen and extensor surfaces of the limbs. The cause is unknown but pregnancy-related itch (pruritus gravidarum) may be due to cholestasis (p. 393). Rarely liver function tests are abnormal and urinary HCG levels may be elevated. It can recur in subsequent pregnancies. Some authors believe the condition is associated with an increase in fetal mortality but this remains controversial.

Treatment is with topical steroids and oral antihistamines.

Pruritic folliculitis of pregnancy

This occurs in the second or third trimester of pregnancy and is characterized by an itchy folliculitis which looks similar to steroid-induced 'acne'. It is not associated with any increased maternal or fetal risk.

Treatment with topical benzoyl peroxide and hydrocortisone cream help relieve symptoms.

Pemphigoid gestationis (herpes gestationis)

This is the rarest of the pregnancy-related rashes (1 in 60 000). The immune changes of pregnancy appear to set off bullous pemphigoid. It is characterized by an itchy blistering urticated eruption starting on the abdomen but may become widespread. Large bullae may be present. Unlike PEP it can occur early, starting in the second or even first trimester of pregnancy, and the umbilicus is often involved. It tends to recur in subsequent pregnancies and at an earlier stage. Diagnosis is confirmed by immunofluorescence studies.

A transient bullous eruption occurs in 5% of infants, presumably owing to transplacental passage of the offending antibody. There is no increase in fetal mortality but there is an increased incidence of prematurity and low birth weight, which is probably due to the autoantibody causing placental insufficiency. Therefore, it seems sensible to keep such pregnancies closely monitored and to advise on hospital rather than home delivery.

Treatment of mild cases may be with potent topical steroids but most cases will require oral corticosteroids. The steroid dose may need to be increased after delivery as there is often a postpartum flare-up of the disease. The rash can be set off again by the oral contraceptive pill and this should be avoided.

FURTHER READING
Kroumpouzos G et al. (2001) Dermatoses of pregnancy. *Journal of the American Academy of Dermatology* **45**: 1–19.

PRINCIPLES OF TOPICAL THERAPY

Dermatology is unique in having such direct accessibility

to the affected organ. This allows the use of topical treatments, which can avoid certain systemic side-effects.

A topical therapy consists of an *active ingredient*, an appropriate *vehicle* or *base* to deliver this, and often a *preservative* or *stabilizer* to maintain the product's shelf-life. Cosmetically acceptable products need to be found and patients should be instructed about their correct usage. Without this, compliance tends to be poor. Perfumed or scented products should be avoided.

Bases and their uses

Creams
These are a semisolid mixture of oil and water held together by an emulsifying agent. They need to have added preservatives such as parabens. They are 'lighter' and rub in more easily than ointments. They have a high cosmetic acceptability and are useful for topical treatments of the face and hands. Aqueous cream is particularly useful as a soap substitute.

Ointments
These are semisolid and contain no water, being based usually on oils or greases such as polyethylene glycol (water soluble) or paraffin (fatty). They feel greasy or sticky to the touch. They are the best treatment for dry, flaky skin disorders as they are good at hydrating the stratum corneum and they deliver an active ingredient (e.g. a steroid) more effectively.

If patients dislike the greasy nature of ointments, a cream is better than no treatment at all, but creams are less effective and do have to be used more frequently. A compromise may be to use a cream on the face and an ointment elsewhere (Table 23.16).

Lotions
These are based on a liquid vehicle such as water or alcohol. They are usually volatile and rapid evaporation promotes a cooling effect on the skin. They are useful for weeping skin conditions and are ideal for use on hairy skin (e.g. the scalp). The cooling effect can be a useful antipruritic. Alcohol-based lotions should be avoided on broken skin as they cause stinging.

Gels
These are semisolid preparations of high molecular weight polymers. They are non-greasy and liquefy on contact with the skin. They are useful for treating hairy skin (e.g. the scalp).

Table 23.16 **Emollients commonly used in the UK**

Greasy emollients	Lighter creams
Diprobase ointment*	E45 cream*
Oily cream	Diprobase cream*
Unguentum Merck*	Aveeno cream*
50 : 50 white soft paraffin/liquid paraffin	Aqueous cream

*Trade names

Pastes

Pastes contain a high percentage (> 40%) of powder in an ointment base. They are thick and stiff and difficult to remove from the skin. They are useful when a treatment needs to be applied precisely to a skin lesion without it smearing on to surrounding normal skin. An example would be dithranol in Lassar's paste (used on plaques of psoriasis) as dithranol will burn the surrounding normal skin.

Safety of topical steroids

Providing that preparations of appropriate strength are used for the body site being treated, these compounds can be used safely on a long-term intermittent basis (p. 1328). If potent steroids are misused they will cause skin atrophy manifest as striae, wrinkling, fragility and telangiectasia.

Problems with topical therapies

- *Systemic absorption* may occur but only if very large areas of inflamed skin are treated topically and especially if the treatment is occluded with bandages or polyurethane films. Neonates are particularly susceptible to this owing to the relative increase in body surface area to volume.
- *Contact allergy* to topical preparations is not uncommon and may be suspected by unusually resistant disease or by apparent worsening of a condition after application of a substance. It is more common with creams as it often the result of allergy to the preservative or emulsifying agent. Allergy can also be due to the active ingredient itself (e.g. neomycin or hydrocortisone).
- *Folliculitis* can occur because of blockage of hair follicles. Creams and ointments should be applied to the skin in the same direction as hair growth to try to prevent this blockage. It is a particular problem with the use of ointments in hot weather (especially if under occlusive bandages) and a lighter cream may be more appropriate at this time.

CHAPTER BIBLIOGRAPHY
Champion RH, Burton JL, Ebling FJG (eds) (1998) *Textbook of Dermatology,* 6th edn. Oxford: Blackwell Scientific.
Harper J, Oranje A, Prose N (eds) (2000) *Textbook of Pediatric Dermatology.* Oxford: Blackwell Scientific.

Omary MB, Coulombe PA, Mclean I (2004) Mechanisms of disease: intermediate filament proteins and their associated diseases. *New England Journal of Medicine* **351**: 2087–100.
Weedon D (ed) (2002) *Skin Pathology,* 2nd edn. Edinburgh: Churchill Livingstone.

UK PATIENT SUPPORT GROUPS (for full list see http://www.bad.org.uk/patientsindex.htm)
British Association of Skin Camouflage: c/o Resources for Business, South Park Road, Macclesfield SK11 6SH
DEBRA (Dystrophic Epidermolysis Bullosa Research Association): DEBRA House, 13 Wellington Business Park, Duke's Ride, Crowthorne, Berkshire RG11 6LS

Hairline International: 1668 High Street, Knowle, West Midlands B93 0LY
National Eczema Society: Hill House, Highgate Hill, London N19 5NA
Psoriasis Association: Milton House, 7 Milton Street, Northampton NN2 7JG
Vitiligo Society: 125 Kennington Road, London SE11 6SF

SIGNIFICANT WEBSITES
http://www.bad.org.uk
British Association of Dermatologists
http://www.aad.org/MedWebGuide.html
American Academy of Dermatology web guide
http://tray.dermatology.uiowa.edu/Dermlmag.htm
Dermatologic image database (adult)
http://www.usc.edu/hsc/nml/e-resources/info/dermis.html
Dermatologic image database (paediatric)
http://www.eczema.org
UK National Eczema Society (atopic eczema)
http://www.paalliance.org
Psoriatic Athropathy Alliance (psoriasis)

http://www.skin-camouflage.net
British Association of Skin Camouflage
http://www.debra.org.uk
Dystrophic Epidermolysis Bullosa Association
http://www.hairlineinternational.co.uk
Hairline International
http://tray.dermatology.uiowa.edu/Dermimag.htm
Dermatology images (atlas)
http://www.usc.edu/hsc/nml/index.html
Dermatology images (atlas)
http://www.psoriasis-association.org.uk
Psoriasis Association
http://www.vitiligosociety.org.uk
Vitiligo Society

Index

O

X